Procedures

5TH EDITION

Today's MEDICAL ASSISTANT

Clinical & Administrative Procedures

Kathy Bonewit-West, BS, MEd
Professor Emeritus
Medical Assistant Program
Hocking College
Nelsonville, Ohio
Former Member, Curriculum Review Board of the
American Association of Medical Assistants

Julie Pepper, CMA (AAMA), BS
Professor Emeritus
Medical Assisting Program
Chippewa Valley Technical College
Eau Claire, Wisconsin

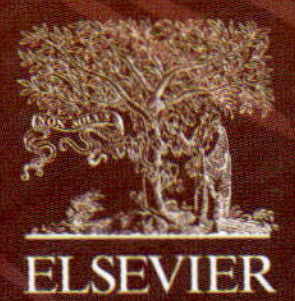

ELSEVIER

Elsevier
3251 Riverport Lane
St. Louis, Missouri 63043

TODAY'S MEDICAL ASSISTANT: CLINICAL & ADMINISTRATIVE PROCEDURES, FIFTH EDITION

ISBN: 978-0-443-12177-7

Notice

Practitioners and researchers must always rely on their own experience and knowledge in evaluating and using any information, methods, compounds or experiments described herein. Because of rapid advances in the medical sciences, in particular, independent verification of diagnoses and drug dosages should be made. To the fullest extent of the law, no responsibility is assumed by Elsevier, authors, editors or contributors for any injury and/or damage to persons or property as a matter of products liability, negligence or otherwise, or from any use or operation of any methods, products, instructions, or ideas contained in the material herein.

Previous editions copyrighted 2021, 2016, 2013, and 2009.

Senior Content Strategist: Yvonne Alexopoulos
Senior Content Development Specialist: Kathleen Nahm
Publishing Services Manager: Julie Eddy
Senior Project Manager: Rachel E. McMullen
Design Direction: Amy Buxton

Printed in India

Last digit is the print number: 9 8 7 6 5 4 3 2 1

For Emersyn
Who dares to dream and has the courage to pursue those dreams.
You turn obstacles into stepping stones!
With love,
KBW

For Jeff, Megan, and Callie
Your support throughout this project has been amazing! Thank you!
JKP

Reviewers

Andrew A. Conte, AAS, CCMA, NREMT, CEHRS
Clinical Medical Assistant Instructor
Northlands Job Corps Center
Vergennes, Vermont

Cheryl DeCoff, BS, CMA (AAMA)
Program Director, Assistant Professor
Quinsigamond Community College
Worcester, Massachusetts

Donielle R. Garrett, MBA-HCM, BS, CCMA, AHI
Instructor
Western Governors University
Salt Lake City, Utah

Belinda Glover, MEd, CMA (AAMA), PBT (ASCP)
Faculty
Herzing University
Milwaukee Falls, Wisconsin

Rudayna Jebara, CMA (AAMA)
Medical Assisting Program Director/Professor
Joliet Junior College
Joliet, Illinois

Rhonda Johns, MS, CMA (AAMA)
Professional Faculty/Medical Assistant Program Director
Washtenaw Community College
Ann Arbor, Michigan

Judith Kimelman Kline, RMA(AMT), NCMA, CCMA, CMAA, AHI, NCET, NCICS, NCPT
Professor
D A Dorsey Technical College
Miami, Florida

Denise Lash, MEd, CMA (AAMA)
Program Director Medical Assisting/Associate Professor
Lakeland Community College
Kirtland, Ohio

Dawn Sexton, MS, MBA, CMA
Allied Health Instructor
Senior Project Consultant
Oracle Health and Charter College
Great Falls, Montana

Preface

Medical assistants, for many years an integral part of most providers' staff, now fulfill an ever-expanding and varied role in the medical office, both clinically and administratively. With increased responsibilities, however, comes a greater need for professional knowledge and skills. This text has been designed to provide the basics of administrative and clinical competency combined with background knowledge of anatomy and physiology.

The underlying principle of this book is to provide a format for the achievement of professional competency in skills performed in the medical office, and the understanding of their application to real-life or on-the-job situations. When professional competency is achieved in the classroom, less of a gap should exist between the academic world and the real world, and thus the transition from student to practicing medical assistant is made more easily.

Although the book's usefulness to students in medical assisting educational programs has been emphasized, the practicing medical assistant will also find this text helpful as a learning and reference source. The organization of the text lends itself well to individualized instruction and convenient reference use.

FEATURES IN THIS TEXTBOOK

This fifth edition provides up-to-date information in both the administrative and clinical areas, and it incorporates current trends in technology.

IMPORTANT UPDATES INCLUDE THE FOLLOWING:

- Information about compliance to all aspects of HIPAA in the medical office
- Current information on the OSHA Bloodborne Pathogens Standard
- Over 200 newly updated photographs
- Current information on gloving and masking in the medical office
- Information on COVID-19 theory and testing procedures
- Updated information on the autoclave
- New procedure for the non-contact forehead thermometer
- New procedure for automated blood pressure measurement
- Updated pediatric immunization schedule
- Information on asthma action plans
- Information and procedure for the Cologuard FIT-DNA test
- New procedure for performing a CLIA-waived glucose test
- Revised and updated information on food labels and the USDA Dietary Guidelines for Americans
- Expanded information on computer storage options
- New information on telehealth
- Fully updated filing rules regarding names of married people
- Up-to-date information on ICD-10 coding
- New information on the changes in CPT coding of evaluation and management codes
- Information on submitting claims electronically
- Completely modernized and updated throughout to comply with general curriculum updates and industry standards
- Maps and corresponds to the updated ABHES competencies and curriculum standards, as well as the most recent CAAHEP core curriculum, content areas, and competencies

STANDARD PEDAGOGICAL FEATURES IN THIS TEXTBOOK

Other very important features include valuable learning aids:

- The organizational format of this textbook facilitates the learning process by providing students and educators with detailed objectives and an in-depth study of the most current and up-to-date administrative and clinical procedures performed in the medical office. Presented at the beginning of each chapter are **Learning Objectives** and related **Procedures,** a **Chapter Outline,** and **Key Terms.** The learning objectives address the cognitive knowledge required to perform the procedures. Procedures coincide with the objectives to delineate the task or skill to be mastered by the student. (In the student Study Guide, most procedures are expanded into detailed performance objectives, including outcomes, and conditions and standards of acceptable performance.) The chapter outline provides a quick reference of the cognitive knowledge included in that chapter. The Key Terms list designates the terms and definitions that should be mastered for each chapter.

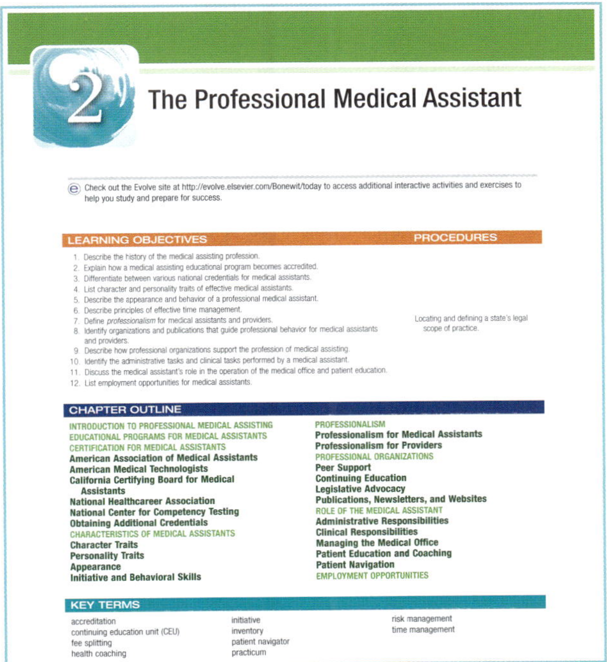

2 The Professional Medical Assistant

Check out the Evolve site at http://evolve.elsevier.com/Bonewit/today to access additional interactive activities and exercises to help you study and prepare for success.

LEARNING OBJECTIVES

1. Describe the history of the medical assisting profession.
2. Explain how a medical assisting educational program becomes accredited.
3. Differentiate between various national credentials for medical assistants.
4. List character and personality traits of effective medical assistants.
5. Describe the appearance and behavior of a professional medical assistant.
6. Describe principles of effective time management.
7. Define *professionalism* for medical assistants and providers.
8. Identify organizations and publications that guide professional behavior for medical assistants and providers.
9. Describe how professional organizations support the profession of medical assisting.
10. Identify the administrative tasks and clinical tasks performed by a medical assistant.
11. Discuss the medical assistant's role in the operation of the medical office and patient education.
12. List employment opportunities for medical assistants.

PROCEDURES

Locating and defining a state's legal scope of practice.

CHAPTER OUTLINE

INTRODUCTION TO PROFESSIONAL MEDICAL ASSISTING
EDUCATIONAL PROGRAMS FOR MEDICAL ASSISTANTS
CERTIFICATION FOR MEDICAL ASSISTANTS
American Association of Medical Assistants
American Medical Technologists
California Certifying Board for Medical Assistants
National Healthcareer Association
National Center for Competency Testing
Obtaining Additional Credentials
CHARACTERISTICS OF MEDICAL ASSISTANTS
Character Traits
Personality Traits
Appearance
Initiative and Behavioral Skills
PROFESSIONALISM
Professionalism for Medical Assistants
Professionalism for Providers
PROFESSIONAL ORGANIZATIONS
Peer Support
Continuing Education
Legislative Advocacy
Publications, Newsletters, and Websites
ROLE OF THE MEDICAL ASSISTANT
Administrative Responsibilities
Clinical Responsibilities
Managing the Medical Office
Patient Education and Coaching
Patient Navigation
EMPLOYMENT OPPORTUNITIES

KEY TERMS

accreditation
continuing education unit (CEU)
fee splitting
health coaching
initiative
inventory
patient navigator
practicum
risk management
time management

- The **knowledge** or **theory** that the student must acquire to perform each skill is presented in a clear and concise manner. **Numerous illustrations** accompany the theory section to aid the student in acquiring the knowledge relating to each skill.

- **Procedures** for each skill follow the theory section and are designed to help the student perform the skill with the level of competency required on the job. Each procedure is presented in an organized step-by-step format, with underlying principles and illustrations accompanying the techniques. A documentation example follows each clinical procedure to provide the student with a guide for documenting their own procedure. Where appropriate, examples of documenting in the electronic health record (EHR) are also included. Students should find it much easier to acquire competency in documenting with these examples.

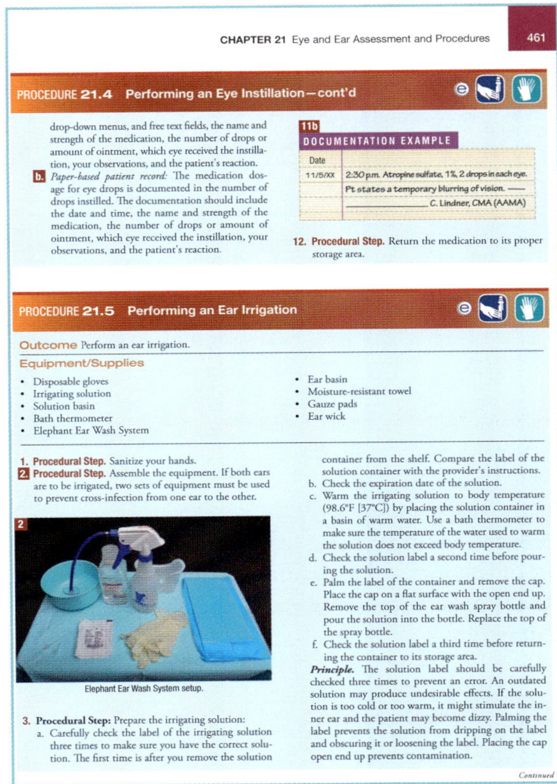

CHAPTER 21 Eye and Ear Assessment and Procedures 461

PROCEDURE 21.4 Performing an Eye Instillation—cont'd

drop-down menus, and free text fields, the name and strength of the medication, the number of drops or amount of ointment, which eye received the instillation, your observations, and the patient's reaction.

b. *Paper-based patient record:* The medication dosage for eye drops is documented in the number of drops instilled. The documentation should include the date and time, the name and strength of the medication, the number of drops or amount of ointment, which eye received the instillation, your observations, and the patient's reaction.

11b DOCUMENTATION EXAMPLE

Date	
11/5/XX	2:30 p.m. Atropine sulfate, 1%, 2 drops in each eye.
	Pt states a temporary blurring of vision. ——
	______________ C. Lindner, CMA (AAMA)

12. **Procedural Step.** Return the medication to its proper storage area.

PROCEDURE 21.5 Performing an Ear Irrigation

Outcome Perform an ear irrigation.

Equipment/Supplies

- Disposable gloves
- Irrigating solution
- Solution basin
- Bath thermometer
- Elephant Ear Wash System
- Ear basin
- Moisture-resistant towel
- Gauze pads
- Ear wick

1. **Procedural Step.** Sanitize your hands.
2. **Procedural Step.** Assemble the equipment. If both ears are to be irrigated, two sets of equipment must be used to prevent cross-infection from one ear to the other.

2 Elephant Ear Wash System setup.

3. **Procedural Step:** Prepare the irrigating solution:
   a. Carefully check the label of the irrigating solution three times to make sure you have the correct solution. The first time is after you remove the solution container from the shelf. Compare the label of the solution container with the provider's instructions.
   b. Check the expiration date of the solution.
   c. Warm the irrigating solution to body temperature (98.6°F [37°C]) by placing the solution container in a basin of warm water. Use a bath thermometer to make sure the temperature of the water used to warm the solution does not exceed body temperature.
   d. Check the solution label a second time before pouring the solution.
   e. Palm the label of the container and remove the cap. Place the cap on a flat surface with the open end up. Remove the top of the ear wash spray bottle and pour the solution into the bottle. Replace the top of the spray bottle.
   f. Check the solution label a third time before returning the container to its storage area.

   Principle. The solution label should be carefully checked three times to prevent an error. An outdated solution may produce undesirable effects. If the solution is too cold or too warm, it might stimulate the inner ear and the patient may become dizzy. Palming the label prevents the solution from dripping on the label and obscuring it or loosening the label. Placing the cap open end up prevents contamination.

Continued

- The unique and memorable medical assistant biographical profiles (**Memories from Practicum** and **Putting It All into Practice**) help students "connect" with their future beyond the classroom. The medical assistants featured are real people sharing their fears, likes, hopes, and aspirations, providing a "real-world" feel to the book and an inspiration for the student.

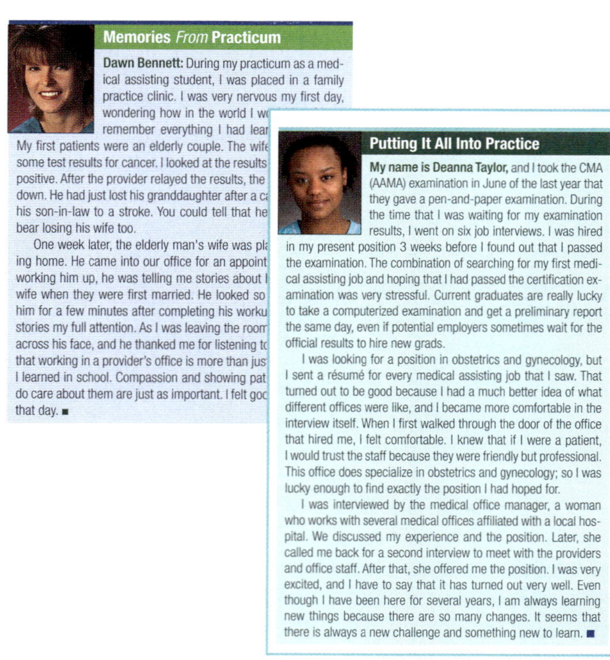

Memories *From* Practicum

Dawn Bennett: During my practicum as a medical assisting student, I was placed in a family practice clinic. I was very nervous my first day, wondering how in the world I w
remember everything I had lear
My first patients were an elderly couple. The wife
some test results for cancer. I looked at the results
positive. After the provider relayed the results, the
down. He had just lost his granddaughter after a c
his son-in-law to a stroke. You could tell that he
bear losing his wife too.
One week later, the elderly man's wife was pl
ing home. He came into our office for an appoint
working him up, he was telling me stories about
wife when they were first married. He looked so
him for a few minutes after completing his work
stories my full attention. As I was leaving the room
across his face, and he thanked me for listening t
that working in a provider's office is more than jus
I learned in school. Compassion and showing pat
do care about them are just as important. I felt go
that day. ■

Putting It All Into Practice

My name is Deanna Taylor, and I took the CMA (AAMA) examination in June of the last year that they gave a pen-and-paper examination. During the time that I was waiting for my examination results, I went on six job interviews. I was hired in my present position 3 weeks before I found out that I passed the examination. The combination of searching for my first medical assisting job and hoping that I had passed the certification examination was very stressful. Current graduates are really lucky to take a computerized examination and get a preliminary report the same day, even if potential employers sometimes wait for the official results to hire new grads.

I was looking for a position in obstetrics and gynecology, but I sent a résumé for every medical assisting job that I saw. That turned out to be good because I had a much better idea of what different offices were like, and I became more comfortable in the interview itself. When I first walked through the door of the office that hired me, I felt comfortable. I knew that if I were a patient, I would trust the staff because they were friendly but professional. This office does specialize in obstetrics and gynecology; so I was lucky enough to find exactly the position I had hoped for.

I was interviewed by the medical office manager, a woman who works with several medical offices affiliated with a local hospital. We discussed my experience and the position. Later, she called me back for a second interview to meet with the providers and office staff. After that, she offered me the position. I was very excited, and I have to say that it has turned out very well. Even though I have been here for several years, I am always learning new things because there are so many changes. It seems that there is always a new challenge and something new to learn. ■

- **Patient Coaching** boxes emphasize this important aspect of the medical assistant's job and present it in context to make it more relevant, thereby making it more memorable.

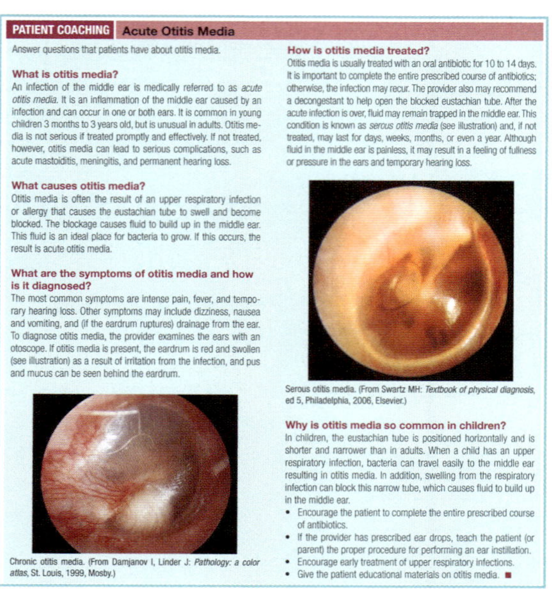

PATIENT COACHING Acute Otitis Media

Answer questions that patients have about otitis media.

What is otitis media?
An infection of the middle ear is medically referred to as *acute otitis media*. It is an inflammation of the middle ear caused by an infection and can occur in one or both ears. It is common in young children 3 months to 3 years old, but is unusual in adults. Otitis media is not serious if treated promptly and effectively. If not treated, however, otitis media can lead to serious complications, such as acute mastoiditis, meningitis, and permanent hearing loss.

What causes otitis media?
Otitis media is often the result of an upper respiratory infection or allergy that causes the eustachian tube to swell and become blocked. The blockage causes fluid to build up in the middle ear. This fluid is an ideal place for bacteria to grow. If this occurs, the result is acute otitis media.

What are the symptoms of otitis media and how is it diagnosed?
The most common symptoms are intense pain, fever, and temporary hearing loss. Other symptoms may include dizziness, nausea and vomiting, and (if the eardrum ruptures) drainage from the ear. To diagnose otitis media, the provider examines the ears with an otoscope. If otitis media is present, the eardrum is red and swollen (see illustration) as a result of irritation from the infection, and pus and mucus can be seen behind the eardrum.

Chronic otitis media. (From Damjanov I, Linder J: *Pathology: a color atlas*, St. Louis, 1999, Mosby.)

How is otitis media treated?
Otitis media is usually treated with an oral antibiotic for 10 to 14 days. It is important to complete the entire prescribed course of antibiotics; otherwise, the infection may recur. The provider also may recommend a decongestant to help open the blocked eustachian tube. After the acute infection is over, fluid may remain trapped in the middle ear. This condition is known as *serous otitis media* (see illustration) and, if not treated, may last for days, weeks, months, or even a year. Although fluid in the middle ear is painless, it may result in a feeling of fullness or pressure in the ears and temporary hearing loss.

Serous otitis media. (From Swartz MH: *Textbook of physical diagnosis*, ed 5, Philadelphia, 2006, Elsevier.)

Why is otitis media so common in children?
In children, the eustachian tube is positioned horizontally and is shorter and narrower than in adults. When a child has an upper respiratory infection, bacteria can travel easily to the middle ear resulting in otitis media. In addition, swelling from the respiratory infection can block this narrow tube, which causes fluid to build up in the middle ear.

- Encourage the patient to complete the entire prescribed course of antibiotics.
- If the provider has prescribed ear drops, teach the patient (or parent) the proper procedure for performing an ear instillation.
- Encourage early treatment of upper respiratory infections.
- Give the patient educational materials on otitis media. ■

- **Case Studies** are designed to assist the student in responding to "real-life" situations that occur in the medical office. A practitioner's response is given for each case study too, as a means of comparison for the student.

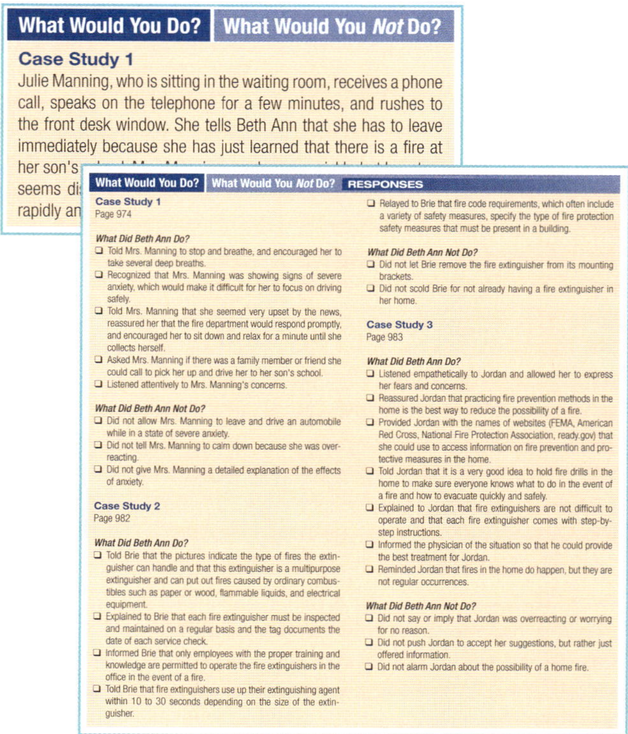

What Would You Do? What Would You *Not* Do?

Case Study 1
Julie Manning, who is sitting in the waiting room, receives a phone call, speaks on the telephone for a few minutes, and rushes to the front desk window. She tells Beth Ann that she has to leave immediately because she has just learned that there is a fire at
her son's
seems di
rapidly an

What Would You Do? What Would You *Not* Do? RESPONSES

Case Study 1
Page 974

What Did Beth Ann Do?
- Told Mrs. Manning to stop and breathe, and encouraged her to take several deep breaths.
- Recognized that Mrs. Manning was showing signs of severe anxiety, which would make it difficult for her to focus on driving safely.
- Told Mrs. Manning that she seemed very upset by the news, reassured her that the fire department would respond promptly, and encouraged her to sit down and relax for a minute until she collects herself.
- Asked Mrs. Manning if there was a family member or friend she could call to pick her up and drive her to her son's school.
- Listened attentively to Mrs. Manning's concerns.

What Did Beth Ann Not Do?
- Did not allow Mrs. Manning to leave and drive an automobile while in a state of severe anxiety.
- Did not tell Mrs. Manning to calm down because she was overreacting.
- Did not give Mrs. Manning a detailed explanation of the effects of anxiety.

Case Study 2
Page 982

What Did Beth Ann Do?
- Told Brie that the pictures indicate the type of fires the extinguisher can handle and that this extinguisher is a multipurpose extinguisher and can put out fires caused by ordinary combustibles such as paper or wood, flammable liquids, and electrical equipment.
- Explained to Brie that each fire extinguisher must be inspected and maintained on a regular basis and the tag documents the date of each service check.
- Informed Brie that only employees with the proper training and knowledge are permitted to operate the fire extinguishers in the office in the event of a fire.
- Told Brie that fire extinguishers use up their extinguishing agent within 10 to 30 seconds depending on the size of the extinguisher.
- Relayed to Brie that fire code requirements, which often include a variety of safety measures, specify the type of fire protection safety measures that must be present in a building.

What Did Beth Ann Not Do?
- Did not let Brie remove the fire extinguisher from its mounting brackets.
- Did not scold Brie for not already having a fire extinguisher in her home.

Case Study 3
Page 983

What Did Beth Ann Do?
- Listened empathetically to Jordan and allowed her to express her fears and concerns.
- Reassured Jordan that practicing fire prevention methods in the home is the best way to reduce the possibility of a fire.
- Provided Jordan with the names of websites (FEMA, American Red Cross, National Fire Protection Association, ready.gov) that she could use to access information on fire prevention and protective measures in the home.
- Told Jordan that it is a very good idea to hold fire drills in the home to make sure everyone knows what to do in the event of a fire and how to evacuate quickly and safely.
- Explained to Jordan that fire extinguishers are not difficult to operate and that each fire extinguisher comes with step-by-step instructions.
- Informed the physician of the situation so that he could provide the best treatment for Jordan.
- Reminded Jordan that fires in the home do happen, but they are not regular occurrences.

What Did Beth Ann Not Do?
- Did not say or imply that Jordan was overreacting or worrying for no reason.
- Did not push Jordan to accept her suggestions, but rather just offered information.
- Did not alarm Jordan about the possibility of a home fire.

- **Key Terms** identified at the beginning of the chapter are defined at the end of the chapter in the **Terminology Review,** providing students with a valuable terminology overview for each chapter. The Terminology Review contains a helpful "Word Parts" column for key terms that are easily broken down into meaningful word portions.

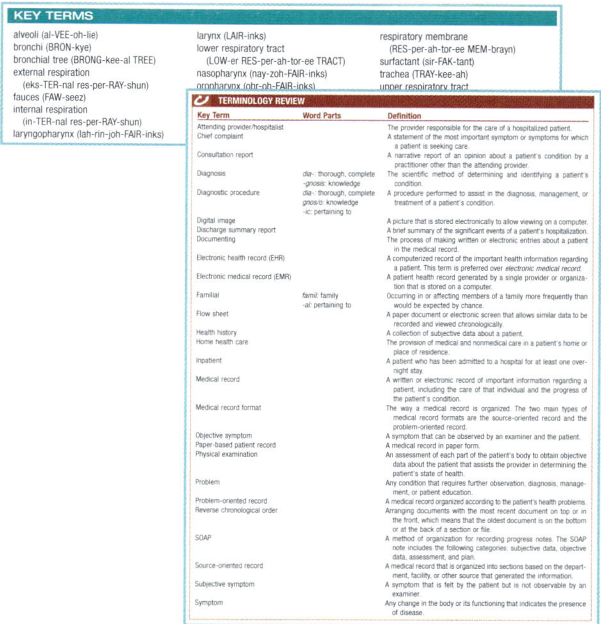

KEY TERMS

alveoli (al-VEE-oh-lie)
bronchi (BRON-kye)
bronchial tree (BRONG-kee-al TREE)
external respiration
(eks-TER-nal res-per-RAY-shun)
fauces (FAW-seez)
internal respiration
(in-TER-nal res-per-RAY-shun)
laryngopharynx (lah-rin-joh-FAIR-inks)
larynx (LAIR-inks)
lower respiratory tract
(LOW-er RES-per-ah-tor-ee TRACT)
nasopharynx (nay-zoh-FAIR-inks)
oropharynx (ohr-oh-FAIR-inks)
respiratory membrane
(RES-per-ah-tor-ee MEM-brayn)
surfactant (sir-FAK-tant)
trachea (TRAY-kee-ah)
upper respiratory tract

TERMINOLOGY REVIEW

Key Term	Word Parts	Definition
Attending provider/hospitalist		The provider responsible for the care of a hospitalized patient.
Chief complaint		A statement of the most important symptom or symptoms for which a patient is seeking care.
Consultation report		A narrative report of an opinion about a patient's condition by a practitioner other than the attending provider.
Diagnosis	*dia-*: thorough, complete *-gnosis*: knowledge	The scientific method of determining and identifying a patient's condition.
Diagnostic procedure	*dia-*: thorough, complete *gnos/o*: knowledge *-ic*: pertaining to	A procedure performed to assist in the diagnosis, management, or treatment of a patient's condition.
Digital image		A picture that is stored electronically to allow viewing on a computer.
Discharge summary report		A brief summary of the significant events of a patient's hospitalization.
Documenting		The process of making written or electronic entries about a patient in the medical record.
Electronic health record (EHR)		A computerized record of the important health information regarding a patient. This term is preferred over *electronic medical record*.
Electronic medical record (EMR)		A patient health record generated by a single provider or organization that is stored on a computer.
Familial	*famil*: family *-al*: pertaining to	Occurring in or affecting members of a family more frequently than would be expected by chance.
Flow sheet		A paper document or electronic screen that allows similar data to be recorded and viewed chronologically.
Health history		A collection of subjective data about a patient.
Home health care		The provision of medical and nonmedical care in a patient's home or place of residence.
Inpatient		A patient who has been admitted to a hospital for at least one overnight stay.
Medical record		A written or electronic record of important information regarding a patient, including the care of that individual and the progress of the patient's condition.
Medical record format		The way a medical record is organized. The two main types of medical record formats are the source-oriented record and the problem-oriented record.
Objective symptom		A symptom that can be observed by an examiner and the patient.
Paper-based patient record		A medical record in paper form.
Physical examination		An assessment of each part of the patient's body to obtain objective data about the patient that assists the provider in determining the patient's state of health.
Problem		Any condition that requires further observation, diagnosis, management, or patient education.
Problem-oriented record		A medical record organized according to the patient's health problems.
Reverse chronological order		Arranging documents with the most recent document on top or in the front, which means that the oldest document is on the bottom or at the back of a section or file.
SOAP		A method of organization for recording progress notes. The SOAP note includes the following categories: subjective data, objective data, assessment, and plan.
Source-oriented record		A medical record that is organized into sections based on the department, facility, or other source that generated the information.
Subjective symptom		A symptom that is felt by the patient but is not observable by an examiner.
Symptom		Any change in the body or its functioning that indicates the presence of disease.

Continuing education is of utmost importance in such a rapidly changing profession. New techniques and developments in the field of medicine have a direct influence on the medical assisting profession. Continuing education helps the medical assistant maintain and improve existing skills and learn new skills.

The authors hope that individuals who use this approach to medical assisting will view this text not as a stopping place but as a means of opening doors to new paths to be explored in the medical assisting profession.

EXTENSIVE SUPPLEMENTAL RESOURCES

PROCEDURAL VIDEOS

The most impressive feature of this textbook is the inclusion of clinical and administrative skills videos on the Evolve site, which present many of the skills outlined in the textbook. An icon (e) is placed within the procedural title bar of the procedures in this text that have accompanying procedural videos. Students will have the invaluable opportunity to watch these procedures at home or at school, using any computer and internet connection. This should greatly enhance the learning of these clinical and administrative skills and provide the medical assistant graduate with competence and confidence to perform clinical and administrative skills in the medical office.

EVOLVE RESOURCES

An Evolve site accompanies the textbook and is designed for students to apply the theory and skills learned throughout the textbook. Organized by chapter, the site includes **Apply Your Knowledge** questions (multiple-choice questions that give students an opportunity to "apply the knowledge" they learned in that particular chapter), **Procedure Videos, Video Evaluations** (true/false questions that quiz students on their knowledge of the procedures shown in the procedure videos which are marked with an (e) icon), **Practicum Activities** for your practicum, and various games and interactive activities (e.g., "Quiz Show" and "Road to Recovery") that provide entertainment while learning important concepts related to selected chapters, matching exercises, labeling exercises, identification exercises, and other helpful activities for the student.

STUDY GUIDE

The student **Study Guide** that accompanies the textbook greatly enhances the learning value of the textbook. Full of practice, critical-thinking questions, and various other ways students can practice their content knowledge, the Study Guide is a valuable supplemental resource for any student who is looking to get the most out of their textbook. In addition, its outcome-based approach meets the criteria required for outcome-based program accreditation as stipulated by the Commission on Accreditation of Allied Health Educational Programs (CAAHEP) and the Curriculum Review Board of the American Association of Medical Assistants (AAMA), as well as meeting all of the most recently updated ABHES and CAAHEP competencies and curriculum standards. Included are extensive exercises for each chapter, as well as performance checklists for all textbook procedures (and even a few extras not included in the textbook). The Study Guide also includes pretests and posttests, which help better prepare students for chapter tests, a student Study Guide assignment sheet for documenting completion of assignments and calculating points earned for each assignment, a laboratory assignment sheet to keep track of student procedure performance, and various ways for students to practice their content knowledge, through multiple-choice questions, true/false questions, critical-thinking exercises, and other stimulating practice activities.

Acknowledgments

The completion of the fifth edition of this text permits the opportunity to relay appreciation to the medical assisting educators who so eagerly and enthusiastically use and enjoy this text. To them, the authors are also indebted for their helpful assistance and suggestions for this new text.

The photographs in the textbook were taken by Brian Blauser and Jack Foley, professional photographers. We are indebted to them for their careful precision and patience in taking and editing the photographs, thus greatly enhancing the learning value of this text.

We would like to gratefully acknowledge the following practicing medical assistants for contributing many hours to be photographed for demonstration of the clinical procedures in the text: Megan Baer, Trudy Browning, Janet Canterbury, Theresa Cline, Marlyne Cooper, Hope Fauber, Dori Glover, Jennifer Hawk, Kevin Hickey, Cammie Lindner, Judy Markins, Korey McGrew, Natalie Morehead, Traci Powell, Linda Proffitt, Latisha Sharpe, Dawn Shingler, Michelle Shockey, Kara Van Dyke, Michelle Villers, and Huang Ying.

We would also like to acknowledge the following individuals who portrayed patients and other individuals in the text: Brian Adevc, Travis Allman, Jessica Bennett, Kim Bingham, Pamela Bitting, Hollie Bonewit-Cron, Caitlin Brennan, Sarah Buckley, Phillip Carr, Chloe Cline, Angie Coffin, Brittany Cogar, Chad Cron, Dawn Decaminada, Elizabeth Feeny, Aja Fox, Markly Georges, Erika Giertz, Ciera Hart, Connie Hazlett, Gary Hazlett, Isabella Ipacs, Joey Ipacs, Susan Ipacs, Charles Larimer, Pam Larimer, Christopher Mace, Leah Moran, Deborah Murray, Delaney Murray, Michael Nkrumah, Heather Pike, Megan Powell, Quincy Sheets, Dawn Shingler, Jan Six, Megan Skidmore, Colton Smith, Janice Smith, Sydney Smith, Melissa Spencer, Clinton Swart, Faye Townsend, Tristen West, Devin White, Lynn Witkowski, and Judith Zappala.

We would like to extend our appreciation to the authors, publishers, and equipment companies who have granted us permission to use their illustrations.

The publication of this text was accomplished through the capable guidance of many talented individuals at Elsevier. First and foremost, this book could not have attained this level of excellence without the exceptional capabilities of Kathleen Nahm. Also, many thanks to Rachel McMullen for her outstanding production work and Ravishankar Raju for his extensive multimedia knowledge and expertise. And, finally, we want to relay a very special thank you to Kristin Wilhelm, Content Director, for her dedication to quality medical assisting education and her encouragement in helping us achieve our very best in this edition.

With warm regard, we would like to recognize those very important individuals—the medical assisting students, graduates, and practicing medical assistants—who continually strive for excellence in meeting the demands and ever-increasing requirements of such a challenging profession. A quote by an unknown author really says it better: “Celebrate your talents, for they are what make you unique.”

Kathy Bonewit-West, BS, MEd
Julie Pepper, CMA AAMA, BS

Clinical Procedure Icons

The OSHA Bloodborne Pathogens Standard must be followed when performing many of the clinical procedures presented in this text. To assist the student in following the OSHA Standard, icons have been incorporated into the procedures. An illustration of each icon along with its description is outlined below.

HAND HYGIENE is an important medical aseptic practice and is crucial in preventing the transmission of pathogens in the medical office. The medical assistant should sanitize the hands frequently, using proper technique. When performing clinical procedures, the hands should always be sanitized before and after patient contact, before applying gloves and after removing gloves, and after contact with blood or other potentially infectious materials.

CLEAN DISPOSABLE GLOVES should be worn when it is reasonably anticipated that you will have hand contact with the following: blood and other potentially infectious materials, mucous membranes, nonintact skin, and contaminated articles or surfaces.

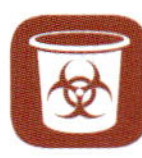

BIOHAZARD CONTAINERS are closable, leakproof, and suitably constructed to contain the contents during handling, storage, transport, or shipping. The containers must be labeled or color coded and closed before removal to prevent the contents from spilling.

APPROPRIATE PROTECTIVE CLOTHING such as gowns, aprons, and laboratory coats should be worn when gross contamination can reasonably be anticipated during performance of a task or procedure.

FACE SHIELDS OR MASKS IN COMBINATION WITH EYE-PROTECTION DEVICES must be worn whenever splashes, spray, spatter, or droplets of blood or other potentially infectious materials may be generated, posing a hazard through contact with your eyes, nose, or mouth.

Contents

The Health Care System

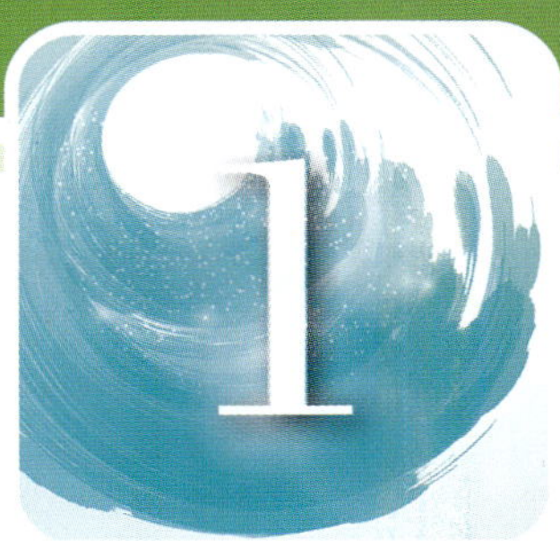

Check out the Evolve site at http://evolve.elsevier.com/Bonewit/today to access additional interactive activities and exercises to help you study and prepare for success.

LEARNING OBJECTIVES

1. Describe the role of medical office care in the health care system.
2. Describe the historical development of managed care.
3. Identify the flow of activity in ambulatory care.
4. Identify the various types of health care professionals and describe the job responsibilities of each professional.
5. State the educational requirements for physicians.
6. List and describe the parts of the medical office.
7. Identify and describe the various types of medical specialties.
8. Describe the philosophy of the patient-centered medical home as a means of delivering primary care.
9. Identify three medical practice types.
10. Compare and contrast various complementary and traditional medical treatments.

CHAPTER OUTLINE

KEY TERMS

ambulatory (AM-byoo-la-toe-ree) care
capitation (cap-ih-TAY-shun)
curative (KYUR-a-tive) treatment
empirical (em-PEER-ih-cle)
fee-for-service
formulary (FORM-you-lay-ree)
health insurance
holistic (hole-IH-stick)
managed care
medicaid
medicare
palliative (PAL-ee-a-tive) treatment
patient-centered medical home (PCMH)
quality assurance
residency (RES-ih-dense-ee)
symptomatic (simp-toe-MA-tick) treatment
tricare
utilization review

INTRODUCTION TO HEALTH AND THE HEALTH CARE SYSTEM

The World Health Organization (WHO) defines *health* as the absence of illness or disease and a state of being in which the individual feels well and is able to carry out the daily functions of life with no difficulties and no pain. In reality, no one reaches this optimum level of health. Everyone has aches and pains, psychological if not physical.

In our health care system, the provider's responsibility is to examine hundreds of people in the course of a week and to try to focus on medical problems that meet the following criteria: the problem is causing or can cause severe difficulties in carrying out the daily functions of life, and the problem can be treated either by reducing the effects of the symptoms or by eradicating the problem altogether.

Each individual the provider sees has a different group of presenting physical symptoms and a different set of social circumstances and emotional issues. The provider listens to the patient's description of their life, performs objective laboratory and diagnostic tests, identifies medical problems, and assesses the nature of each problem.

Providers know that the vast majority of medical problems do not pose a long-term threat to health. Most medical conditions get better over time. Effective treatments are available to cure many conditions **(curative treatment)**. In other cases the provider can reduce the symptoms even if the underlying medical condition is not significantly affected. This type of treatment is called **symptomatic treatment** (responding to symptoms) or **palliative treatment** (seeking to reduce the effects of a disease or condition without curing the underlying disease). For example, a patient with a urinary tract infection who is given a prescription for antibiotics receives curative treatment, whereas a patient who has diabetes mellitus type I receives palliative treatment. The patient is prescribed insulin, which alleviates the symptoms of the diabetes; however, the treatment does not cure the diabetes.

Most treatments are based on scientific study. In Western scientific medicine, as in no other medical tradition, approaches to diagnosis and treatment have been studied and tested over hundreds of years. As long ago as the 4th century BCE, a physician named Hippocrates in Greece believed that disease was not a punishment for transgressions against the gods but rather the result of physiologic and environmental factors that could be studied. Since the time of Hippocrates, the practice of medicine has changed considerably in response to scientific discoveries.

MODERN TRENDS IN HEALTH CARE

Several trends running through modern medicine have a strong influence on the way in which health care is provided in ambulatory settings.

The first trend is the desire of those who pay the bills—employers, the federal and state governments, and insurance companies—to reduce the costs of health care, especially care for chronic diseases, and to make health care providers responsible for effective management of patients who require care over time without duplication of services and without medical errors. Medicare is encouraging several initiatives to encourage doctors and other health care providers to coordinate patient care and to be accountable for value in the care provided; these initiatives include Accountable Care Organizations (ACOs), formed voluntarily by groups of physicians, hospitals, and other health care providers to give coordinated and high-quality care to Medicare patients.

A second trend is to encourage the general public to become more responsible for their own good health and management of chronic conditions. There are several public initiatives to improve dietary practices, especially for children, to prevent obesity. Within the health care system there is an increasing emphasis on coaching patients to manage their health and to initiate changes that will improve their health (including dietary changes, smoking cessation, and adherence to a healthy exercise program.) The current epidemic of addiction to pain medication has led to restrictions in most states on the amount of controlled substances that a provider can prescribe. Many states are also requiring continuing education for practitioners in pain management. There is a strong emphasis on avoiding dependency on controlled substances for treatment of chronic pain by following guidelines issued by the Centers for Disease Control (CDC) in 2016.

The third trend is an increased understanding, through **empirical** evidence (information learned from experimental research), that people *feel better* the less they must be confined to a hospital or go to a hospital for treatment. Being able to be diagnosed and treated in an outpatient setting with follow-up at home allows people to feel more in control of their lives as medical patients. There is increasing development of remote medicine and telemedicine applications so that patients can be monitored and coached to health at any time.

This is especially important for people who have frequent contact with the medical system, such as the parents of infants and children, the elderly, and those with chronic illnesses. Many people who would have been hospitalized for long periods or possibly even institutionalized 50, 25, or even 10 years ago are currently living independently in the community.

Currently the hospital's role is primarily to provide acute care and diagnostic services. For a patient to be hospitalized, their condition must be unstable or necessitate constant regulation of therapy. Patients who do not meet these strict criteria go home to be followed as an outpatient; are transferred to a rehabilitation facility for intense, regular rehabilitative treatment; or are sent to a nursing home for long-term maintenance care.

HEALTH INSURANCE AND PATIENT CARE: COMPETING FORCES FACING THE MEDICAL OFFICE

FEE-FOR-SERVICE INSURANCE PLANS

Traditionally, medical care in the United States was paid for on a **fee-for-service** basis. Each service was billed and paid for as a separate charge: so much for the office visit, so much for the electrocardiogram, so much for the urinalysis, and so on. Fee-for-service payments can be thought of as ordering food at a restaurant à la carte: so much for the main course, so much for a salad, so much for coffee.

During the first part of the 20th century, health insurance (if the patient had any) paid only for hospitalization, and usually the patient completed most of the paperwork. **Health insurance** is a system by which a person or the person's employer pays an insurance company a yearly amount of money, and the insurance company pays some or most of the person's medical expenses for that year. The theory behind insurance is that although a few people will have large medical bills over the course of the year, most people will have small bills. By setting the fee for everyone at a level above the actual cost of care for most people, the insurance company can pay for the care of the well, the occasionally ill, and the often ill and still make a profit.

This system encouraged health care providers to provide a high level of care for everyone with health insurance because the insurance paid for every test and every procedure. Providers' incomes soared between the end of World War II and the early 1980s. With the increasing costs of laboratory and diagnostic testing, hospital services, and office visits, the cost of medical care increased far more rapidly than the cost of other goods and services in the U.S. economy. (In economic terms, health care inflation increased much more rapidly than the general rate of inflation.)

During this time, ever-better health insurance became a standard employee benefit at many companies. The first kind of health insurance offered, in the 1950s and 1960s, was coverage for hospital care. Coverage for office visits became standard in the 1970s.

HIGHLIGHT on the History of Medical Treatment of Infectious Disease

Historians generally place the beginning of Western medicine with Hippocrates, an ancient Greek physician who saw medicine as an independent discipline based on clinical practice rather than prayer and ritual. For several centuries there were few treatment methods other than rest, exercise, diet, and a few medications derived from plants. The intensive study of the human body in the 1500s fostered a better understanding of physiologic processes. For example, the English scientist William Harvey, who rejected the traditional belief that blood was made up of "spirits" and that body fluids were "humors," developed a theory, later proved true, that blood flows from the heart to the lungs, throughout the body via arteries, and back to the heart via veins.

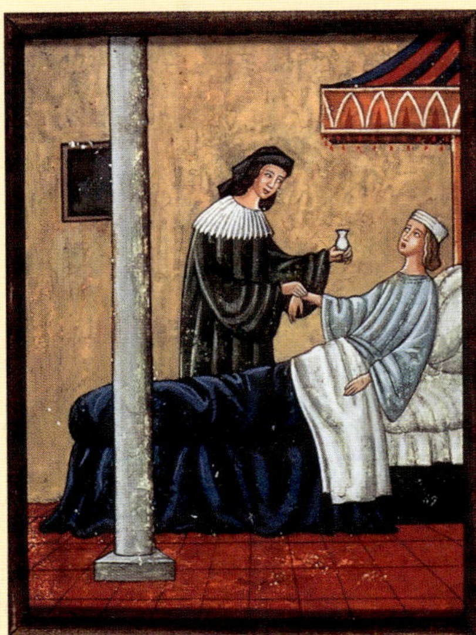

Physician in the Middle Ages taking a patient's pulse and holding a flask of urine. (Courtesy Blocker History of Medicine Collections, Moody Medical Library, University of Texas Medical Branch, Galveston, TX.)

The first microscopic lens was invented in 1677 by Antony van Leeuwenhoek. Through his microscope, van Leeuwenhoek saw yeasts, molds, and algae, adding evidence to the theory that diseases could be caused by particles too small to be seen with the eyes. He also identified red blood cells passing through capillaries.

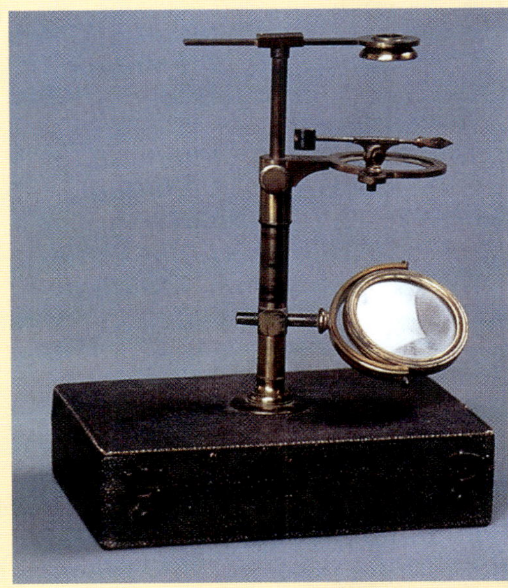

Early microscope, circa 1765. (Courtesy Blocker History of Medicine Collections, Moody Medical Library, University of Texas Medical Branch, Galveston, TX.)

Continued

HIGHLIGHT on the History of Medical Treatment of Infectious Disease—cont'd

Throughout the 19th century, other scientists and physicians advanced the understanding of the cause of disease. Some found ways to combat disease without understanding the mechanism by which the disease acted; others determined the actual cause of a particular disease.

In the 1840s the Viennese obstetric assistant Ignaz Semmelweis discovered that the number of cases of puerperal fever, or so-called "childbed fever," a fatal illness of women who had just given birth, could be reduced if physicians washed their hands.

Semmelweis conducted what currently would be called an *epidemiologic study.* He studied the records of women who had died and determined which physicians and medical students had attended which birth. His study of the records led him to conclude that most of the women who died had been attended to by physicians and medical students who had come into the birthing room directly from the anatomy laboratory, where they had worked with cadavers, without first washing their hands. Most of Semmelweis's colleagues dismissed his notion that simple handwashing could reduce childbirth deaths as nonsense, and during his lifetime Semmelweis was ridiculed. It was not until decades later that physicians regularly began washing their hands.

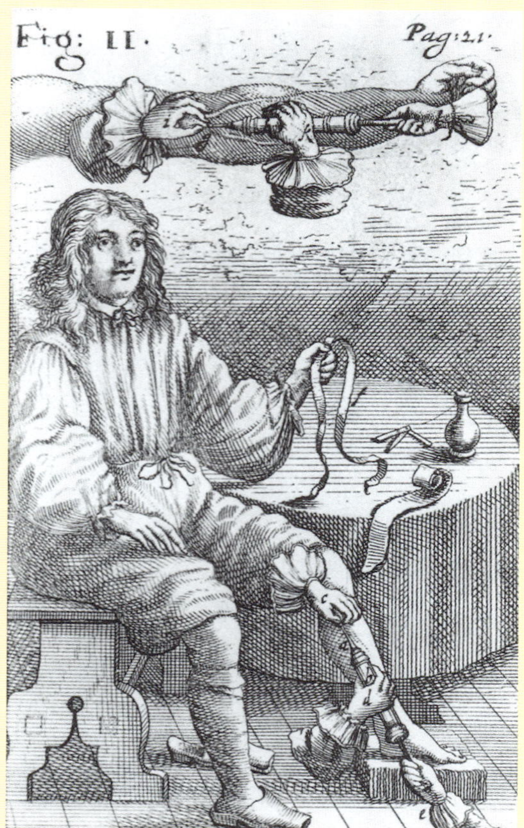

Extracting blood for a transfusion, 18th century. (Courtesy National Library of Medicine.)

The Scottish surgeon Joseph Lister worked on similar ideas to develop the first practice of antisepsis (cleaning areas where germs may be) and later asepsis (creating a germ-free environment). Lister started by pouring carbolic acid on the wounds of those who had just undergone surgery. Over time, he found milder substances. Lister found that far fewer patients who were treated with these substances died from gangrene that developed in the open wounds.

Semmelweis, Lister, and others worked empirically, which means they sought results through experiments that could be repeated with the same results. Although they were able to decrease infection rates, they never completely understood what caused infectious diseases. Other scientists sought to determine that bacteria caused specific diseases.

The German physician Robert Koch is called the "Father of Microbiology" because of his work with specific bacteria. Koch isolated the bacterial agent that causes anthrax. Koch grew the anthrax bacillus in a number of different liquid media in his laboratory, used the microscope to identify it, injected the organism into a healthy animal, waited for the animal to become sick, and then recovered the same organism from the sick animal. This proved that one specific type of bacteria causes one specific disease. We currently know that it is possible to break the chain of illness by keeping those who are contagious away from those who are vulnerable to disease.

The work of Louis Pasteur and Koch, among others, helped set the stage for the understanding of infectious disease and for worldwide vaccination programs to eradicate smallpox and to try to eradicate the "childhood illnesses" of mumps, measles, and rubella (German measles).

The first vaccination actually had been performed a century earlier. Edward Jenner, an English physician in the farming country of Gloucestershire, used the pus from one person's cowpox lesion to vaccinate another individual against smallpox in 1796.

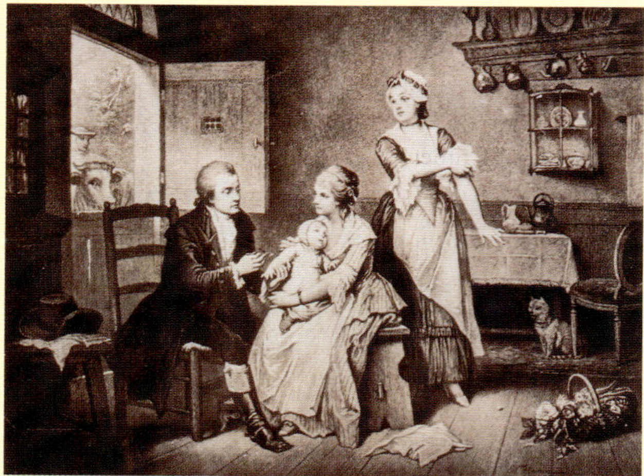

Edward Jenner vaccinating an infant. (Courtesy National Library of Medicine.)

Cowpox is a variant of smallpox. It is lethal to animals but relatively harmless to humans. For centuries, people had realized that people who had been infected with cowpox did not develop smallpox. We currently understand what happened—their immune systems had developed antibodies to cowpox that also prevented smallpox infection by attacking the smallpox virus.

HIGHLIGHT on the History of Medical Treatment of Infectious Disease—cont'd

Jenner used "humanized cowpox" to establish immunity by taking pus from a lesion on a human infected with cowpox and rubbing it into an open wound on another human. A couple of weeks later, he inoculated the second person with smallpox. Not only did the individual not become ill, but he also was not contagious. A century later Pasteur would discover fully the mechanism by which vaccination works. Vaccines were discovered for many diseases. By the beginning of the 20th century, vaccines had been developed for diphtheria and tetanus, and most children received these vaccines as infants by the middle of the 20th century. New immunizations continue to be developed not only for infants but also for adolescents, adults, and the elderly.

Medications to kill bacteria were another important tool in the fight against infectious disease. Paul Ehrlich is credited with the development of the first medication to kill bacteria. In 1909 he developed a drug called *Salvarsan* (arsphenamine), which could be used to effectively treat syphilis. Unfortunately the medication itself was extremely toxic. The first of the sulfanilamide drugs, Prontosil, was developed in 1932 in Germany. It was effective against infections caused by streptococci and some other types of bacteria. The sulfanilamides became popular before and during World War II because they were the only antiinfective agents widely available. Penicillin, a mold that kills bacteria, had been discovered in 1922 by Alexander Fleming in London after it attacked bacteria that he was growing on agar plates. Initially the scientific community did not believe that it would be effective inside the body, and little follow-up research was done. During World War II, two medical researchers, Howard Florey and Ernst Chain, took up the research on penicillin and managed to prove that the medication was effective. The first human was treated in 1941, and within a few years mass production had been established and penicillin was in widespread use.

Discovery of the first virus is credited to Dimitri Ivanowski, a Russian botanist, in 1892. He discovered that a substance could pass through a ceramic filter that trapped all known bacteria and still cause a disease of tobacco called *mosaic tobacco disease.* We now know that the culprit is the tobacco mosaic virus. Yellow fever was the first viral disease of humans to be identified. During construction of the Panama Canal, workers were devastated by this disease. Research done by Walter Reed established that the disease was caused by a virus transmitted by mosquitoes and not direct contact. Controlling mosquitoes facilitated the work on the canal. The development of the electron microscope in 1930 allowed viruses to be seen, but progress to control viral diseases was slow. For most viruses the body has adequate defenses to overcome the infection, but there are some significant exceptions. The retroviruses, such as human immunodeficiency virus (HIV), are notable because they are able to overcome the body's immune system. In the 1970s the first deaths from acquired immunodeficiency syndrome (AIDS) were reported in the United States. Within the next 20 years, a worldwide epidemic occurred. By 1997 more than 6 million deaths worldwide had been caused by the AIDS virus. Treatments have been able to control the progression of the disease for many years, but to date there is no effective immunization or cure for this disease. The ability of viruses to mutate rapidly has resulted in recent viral pandemics from diseases such as severe acute respiratory syndrome (SARS) in 2004, H1N1 influenza in 2009, and SARS-CoV-2 virus (COVID-19) in 2019. ■

GOVERNMENT INSURANCE PLANS

Recognizing that there were large numbers of the population without insurance because they were not employed, the federal government began to provide health insurance to large segments of the population starting in the 1960s. **Medicaid** began to provide health insurance for low-income children without parental support and later expanded to cover all the medically indigent. **Medicare** initiated health insurance for the elderly, the disabled, and those with end-stage kidney disease. The Civilian Health and Medical Program of the Uniformed Services (CHAMPUS; currently called **TRICARE**) provided health insurance for dependents of active-duty military personnel. With these programs, the federal government has become the primary insurer for more than 75 million Americans. These plans, which included payments for office visits for illness, greatly increased the number of Americans who had medical insurance. There was little incentive for the consumer (the patient) to control costs because insurance was covering those costs and care in most cases was "free" to the consumer.

Although most Americans who were insured did not feel that they were "paying" for their medical care, they were, indirectly. The huge increases in health care costs were one of the major sources of the generally high rates of inflation in the 1970s. Employers who paid for the insurance had to pay ever-rising premiums and offset these large premium increases with small increases in cash wages, which did not keep up with inflation. So American workers did, in fact, pay for health insurance and health care costs in lower purchasing power for the cash they received as salary.

MANAGED CARE

Health Maintenance Organizations (HMOs) were originally formed with a belief that consistent, routine care would help to prevent later expensive care. Managed care was based on the belief that increasing prevention and promoting early detection and diagnosis of chronic and life-threatening medical conditions would reduce costs. At that time traditional health insurance covered only office visits for illness or injury and did not cover so-called "routine care" (well-child visits, immunizations, regular checkups, or physical examinations). The HMO movement, which gained acceptance in the 1970s, pushed traditional health insurance companies to begin providing coverage for routine care.

In the late 1970s, insurance companies began to respond to escalating health care costs by reviewing care to find out if it was medically necessary. This process, called **utilization review**, identifies patients who, according to the insurance companies, no longer need to be hospitalized. Originally, utilization review was used by Medicare and Medicaid and only for hospitalized patients. Other insurance companies soon realized that shortening hospital stays was an important way of reducing overall health care costs. The combination of HMO insurance plans and strict utilization review for hospitalized patients is the basis of what we call **managed care**. Utilization review is currently used for both inpatients and outpatients to control health care costs.

The original HMO model had two components: insurance and services including diagnostic tests and pharmacy. HMO plans set up full-service medical clinics. Providers were employees. The HMO established a contractual relationship with a hospital for inpatient services, and patients had to go to the specific hospital with which the HMO had a contract.

In the late 1980s HMO services began to separate from HMO insurance. A second type of HMO model based on networks of providers who agreed to provide care for HMO patients came into being. Some of these networks operated under the old fee-for-service plans but agreed to discounted fees from the HMOs in exchange for access to the rapidly growing patient populations enrolled in HMOs. In an effort to reduce payments, HMOs tried to have providers accept a flat monthly fee for each subscriber in their practice and agree to provide all necessary primary care for that fee. This type of payment is called **capitation**. This reduces the incentive to provide extra services because their cost will not be reimbursed separately.

A quality assurance plan is required by each state for HMO insurance plans. **Quality assurance** ensures that patients receive safe and appropriate services. This is accomplished by planned review of data about the types and effectiveness of services provided to patients of the HMO.

The managed care movement in general, as well as the trend to decrease reimbursement for primary care in particular, put the burden on providers to compete with one another to provide the most care for the least money. As a result, providers often feel pressure to limit diagnostic tests, reduce hospitalizations and the number of days patients stay in the hospital, and use generic instead of brand-name drugs. (Generics are identical in chemical formulation to brand-name drugs and can be manufactured only after the brand-name drug's patent protection has expired.)

Managed care also puts pressure on providers to see more patients, spend less time with each patient, and justify all services including diagnostic tests and referrals. The expense of handling sicker patients is expected to be balanced by those patients who use less than the average amount of medical services.

In addition, insurance plans have tried to reduce their costs for prescription medications by restricting drug coverage to lists of approved drugs. Such a list, called a **formulary**, usually includes one or two of the less expensive drugs for each possible medical condition. Exceptions are made if the provider can show that the less expensive drugs have been ineffective for their patient or cannot be used because the patient is allergic to them and that a more expensive drug is necessary. In some plans the patient can receive a more expensive medication by paying more of the cost.

HEALTH CARE REFORM

Despite these measures, beginning in the late 1990s, both insurance premiums and health care costs began to increase at more than double and even triple the underlying rate of inflation. There has also been an increase in the number of individuals and families who do not qualify for government insurance plans and also do not have health insurance through their employers. This may be because they work part-time or are self-employed. The Patient Protection and Affordable Care Act, which became law in March 2010, expanded insurance coverage to an estimated 32 million Americans who were previously uninsured. Among the provisions that went into effect in September 2010, insurance companies are no longer allowed to exclude children with preexisting health conditions or to drop customers after discovering technical mistakes on applications. As of 2014 this law required all individuals to purchase health insurance or pay an annual fine. Even though this part of the law is no longer in force, a strong belief persists that society has an obligation to make appropriate health care accessible to all citizens.

AMBULATORY CARE

There is no such thing as a "typical" medical office. The style of any particular medical office depends on the personality of the provider or providers who practice there, as well as the general population of patients who come there. Regardless of the provider's personality and the patients' personal backgrounds, the same kinds of activities occur in any provider's office setting.

Currently, the trend in medical care is toward an increasing amount of **ambulatory care**—defined as the patient coming to the care rather than the patient receiving care in a home or hospital setting (Fig. 1.1). To take advantage of ambulatory care, the patient must be able to walk into the provider's office or at least be brought to the office in a wheelchair. In addition to private providers'offices, offices of providers who make up a staff model HMO, community health centers, multispecialty clinics, and hospitals are increasingly making more space available for outpatient care.

FLOW OF ACTIVITY IN AMBULATORY CARE

The flow of activities for each patient in an outpatient setting is similar. The patient will do the following:

- Enter the office.
- Approach the reception desk, identify the provider and time of appointment, provide the office staff with

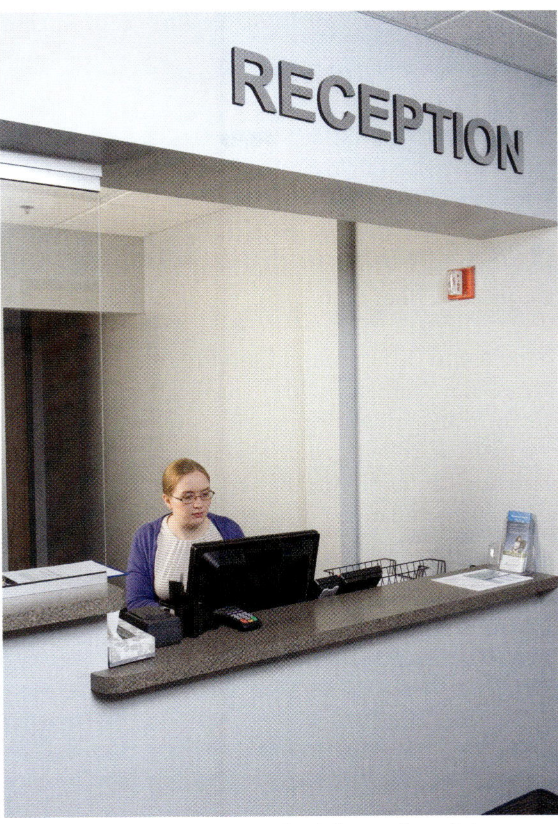

Fig. 1.1 The patient check-in area in a clinic.

personal and payment information, and make a copayment (if necessary).

- Be seen by a physician (or by a nurse practitioner [NP] or physician assistant [PA] if the practice uses such personnel).
- Undergo diagnostic or laboratory tests in the office.
- Receive a diagnosis, treatment, or a referral to another health care provider.
- Receive instruction for follow-up care and any laboratory or diagnostic tests to be done elsewhere before leaving the medical office; if seriously ill, the patient may be admitted to the hospital.

Fig. 1.2 is a flowchart of how a patient moves through the medical office.

Once a patient has been seen in the medical office, the office begins the process of obtaining payment for its services. The medical payment may come from a private insurance plan, a government-funded insurance program, and/or from the patient. The patient may be responsible for a percentage of the charges or the entire bill if they do not have insurance.

After the examination, the patient receives instructions to prepare for a test or procedure to be performed or information about medication that has been prescribed. Patients who are seen regularly because of a chronic illness may spend time with a provider or medical assistant reviewing the patient's individual treatment plan. A follow-up appointment is made if necessary.

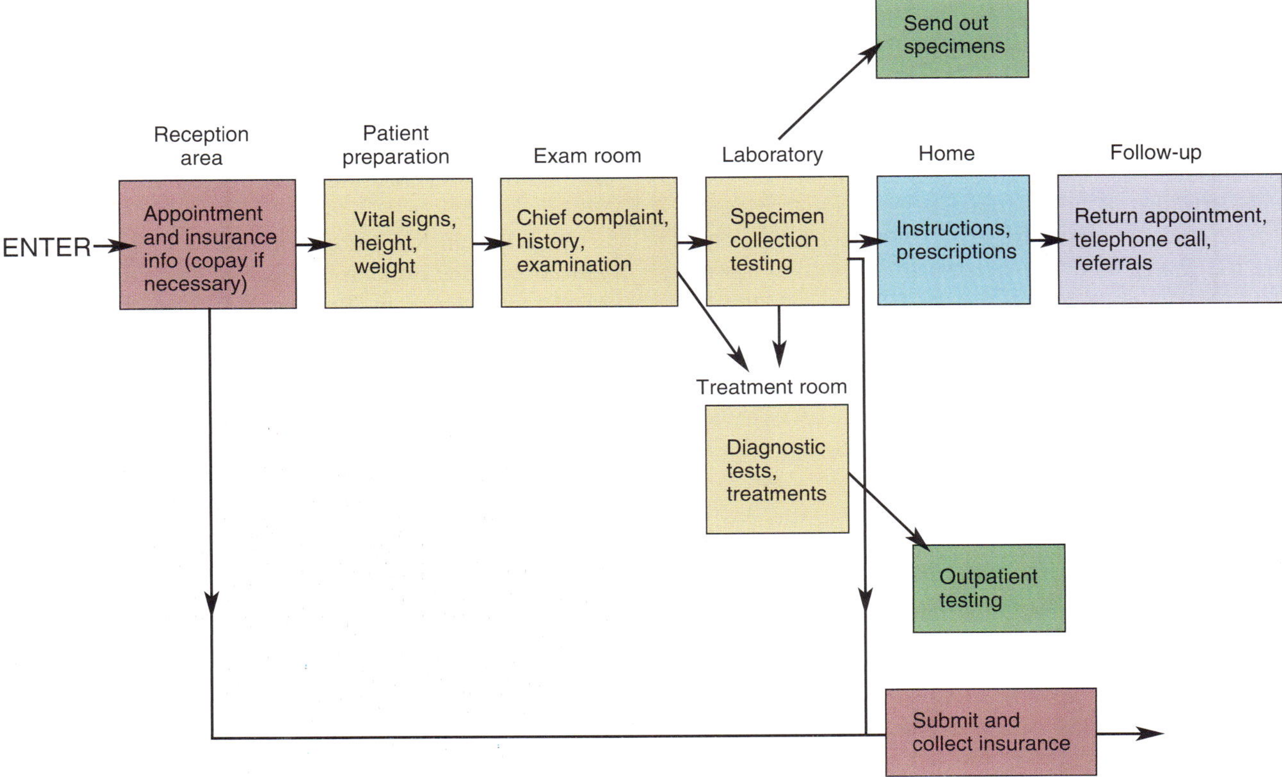

Fig. 1.2 Patient progress through a medical office.

Most medical offices provide health education materials in print or online. These materials may consist of pamphlets, article reprints, health education videos, or health news reports specially prepared for viewing in the medical office.

THE HEALTH CARE TEAM

A medical assistant works as a member of a dedicated health care team. The provider or group of providers expects each medical assistant to fill a slightly different role within the office team. This role will depend on the style of the practice, the region of the country where the practice is located, and what types of medical professionals make up the team.

As the operations of a medical practice become more complex, providers may employ individuals with more specialized medical business and medical management experience to run the business side of the office. In these offices, medical assistants play more of a clinical role. In smaller offices, medical assistants usually perform both clinical and administrative activities.

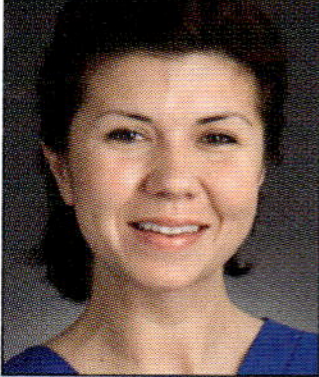

Putting It All Into Practice

My name is Aida Reyes, and I am the Medical Assistant for a primary care provider. I have been working here for 12 years, and in that time it has gotten busier and busier. We used to see about 15 patients in a typical morning or afternoon, and now we are seeing an average of 20–25. When I first took the job, I thought it would be a fairly relaxed environment. How busy could it be with only one provider? Since I first began, our practice has merged with another practice and expanded, so that there are now four physicians and two nurse practitioners. We are now affiliated with a large medical group that does the billing centrally, so that I primarily work with my provider, preparing patients for examination, queuing up medications that need to be refilled for the provider, keeping the examination rooms stocked, taking vital signs and doing other previsit work, then preparing patients for follow-up laboratory testing and making sure that we receive all test results back. I also call patients who have not come in when they are scheduled and help with referrals for my provider's patients (because so many patients have some type of managed care insurance). ■

Members of the Health Care Team

The members of the medical team who typically work in ambulatory care, be it a private practice, a community or public health clinic, or a hospital clinic, include physicians, NPs, PAs, medical assistants, registered nurses (RNs) or licensed practical nurses, a business manager, a receptionist, a medical secretary, file clerks, and one or more insurance specialists. Medical transcription is occasionally done in the medical office, but increasingly it is outsourced or replaced by the electronic health record or voice recognition software. If the office performs moderate- or high-complexity laboratory tests, a certified medical technologist may also be on the staff or serve as a consultant.

Hospital or community-based clinics will possibly also have a staff of social workers, outreach workers, and case managers to provide social services to patients. Practices specializing in women's health (obstetrics and gynecology) may also have certified nurse-midwives.

Table 1.1 lists various nurses and allied health professionals and describes their roles.

Physicians and Other Health Care Providers

Physicians have either an MD (medical doctor) or a DO (doctor of osteopathy) degree, either of which is awarded after 4 years of college, then 4 years of medical or osteopathic school. In addition, they complete a hospital-based, intensive postgraduate training period, traditionally called a **residency**, which lasts from 2 to 7 years, depending on the specialty. To receive a medical license from the state where they will practice, the physician must pass parts I, II, and III of the U.S. Medical Licensing Examination (USMLE). The first two parts of the examination are taken during medical school, but part III cannot be taken until the physician has completed at least 1 year of residency (sometimes called an *internship*).

If a physician wants to be "board certified" in a specialty, they must pass another examination, administered by the certification board of the particular specialty. The physician does not need to be board certified to obtain a state license to practice medicine.

A PA must have at least 2 years of college plus 2 years of PA school, although most PA programs award a master's degree. A PA usually specializes (e.g., in pediatrics, in adult medicine) and manages a group of patients receiving routine care. A PA must practice with a physician. All states have laws regulating PAs, and students must pass the national certification examination to obtain a state license.

An NP is an RN who has completed a program in advanced practice nursing, a program that usually grants a Master of Science in Nursing (MSN) or higher degree. NPs can specialize in pediatrics, family practice, gerontology, or other specialty areas. In primary care, NPs help with all aspects of patient care, including physical examination, diagnosis, treatment, consultations, and patient education. They may serve as a patient's primary care provider. They are licensed as NPs by the state in which they practice.

The educational requirements and scope of an NP's ability to practice independently are determined by each state. In all states, NPs are allowed to carry a caseload and manage routine patient care. All states allow NPs to write prescriptions with varying degrees of supervision. In some states, NPs are also allowed to practice independently, but in most they must practice in an office with supervision by a physician. In a few states, NPs are allowed to admit patients to hospitals.

Table 1.1 Nurses and Allied Health Professionals

Occupation	Credentials	Responsibilities
Certified Professional Coder Certified Coding Associate Certified Coding Specialist	CPC CCA CCS	Assigns codes to patient charges and diagnoses for insurance billing. There are many additional coding certifications depending on knowledge and specialty.
Diagnostic Medical Sonographer	DMS	Performs ultrasound scans in hospitals and ambulatory care facilities. Ultrasound uses high-frequency sound waves to produce images. A sonographer may specialize in ultrasound of the heart (echocardiography).
Emergency Medical Technician Paramedic	EMT, paramedic	Provides emergency services and life support in the community. Several levels of emergency service personnel exist, depending on training and experience.
Health Information Specialist Registered Health Information Administrator Registered Health Information Technician	RHIA; RHIT RHIA RHIT	Works with patient medical records; may provide assistance in planning, managing information, gathering data for medical research, and policy making.
Medical Assistant Certified Medical Assistant (AAMA) Registered Medical Assistant	CMA (AAMA) RMA	Performs administrative and clinical tasks in ambulatory care. There are also other certifications.
Medical (Laboratory) Technologist	MT; MLT	Performs laboratory tests in the clinical laboratory and may supervise laboratory operations or provide consulting services.
Medical Secretary Certified Medical Secretary	CMS	Secretary who specializes in administrative procedures in a health care setting.
Nuclear Medicine Technologist Certified Nuclear Medicine Technologist	CNMT	Operates devices that detect and map absorption of radioactive substances given by injection to create diagnostic images.
Nurse, Practical Licensed Practical Nurse Licensed Vocational Nurse	LPN LVN	Performs direct patient care and clinical procedures. May work in hospitals, nursing homes, and ambulatory care settings.
Nurse Practitioner	NP	Specializes in a specific area such as internal medicine, pediatrics, or women's health, and often manages routine patient care in ambulatory care settings.
Nurse, Registered	RN	Plans and provides nursing care in inpatient settings. Provides supervision for caregivers in both inpatient and outpatient settings.
Occupational Therapist Occupational Therapy Assistant	OT OTA	Plans therapeutic activities for rehabilitation, especially for activities of daily living (ADLs). Implements treatment plans.
Physical Therapist Physical Therapy Assistant	PT PTA	Plans exercises for large muscle groups for rehabilitation and implements treatment plans.
Physician Assistant	PA	Manages routine patient care under the supervision of a physician. Usually works in ambulatory care.
Radiologic Technologist	RT	Takes radiographs and assists with special radiographic examinations. After completing education, may specialize in computed tomography, mammography, or therapeutic radiation.
Registered Dietician	RD	Assists with nutrition of patients in hospitals and ambulatory care. Performs nutrition screening and counseling. Coordinates all aspects of food service in many settings.
Respiratory Therapist	CRT; RRT	Provides respiratory treatments and manages patients on ventilators.
Surgical Technologist	CST	Assists during surgery in hospital and day surgery centers by setting up operating rooms, preparing instruments and equipment, and passing instruments during surgery.

Source: CMS (Centers for Medicare and Medicaid Services).

What Would You Do? What Would You *Not* Do?

Case Study 1

In the examination room, Alicia Darwin, a new patient, tells Aida that she has switched providers because she had often been seen by a nurse practitioner in the medical office where she used to go. "I don't think a nurse practitioner has as much experience as a doctor," she says, "and besides, the nurse practitioner can't give me medication if I need it." She asks Aida to confirm that she will always be seen by the physician in this office. She adds, "I don't have anything against nurses like you; I just want to have a real doctor take care of me." ■

Effective Teamwork

Working as an effective health care team does not just happen. To be effective, team members work together to provide appropriate care for each patient. The more people involved, the more crucial this teamwork is. Each member of the team must be committed to problem solving, communicating, and coordinating effective care.

Teamwork is reinforced at regular staff meetings, which can be directed by either the medical or the business director of the office, depending on the particular topics of the meeting. However, the true test of teamwork occurs on a daily basis as health care is provided.

Each health care team member has certain responsibilities and restrictions on activities and areas about which they are allowed to make decisions. Sometimes this scope is defined by federal or state law. For example, medical assistants are allowed to administer injections in some states, but in others they cannot. The medical assistant must learn what areas fall within the proper scope of practice and decision-making responsibility in their state.

The specific education and role of the medical assistant is discussed in Chapter 2. The medical assistant plays an important role by keeping the work of the office flowing smoothly. They must communicate well with other health team members. Because a patient will not always repeat all information to the provider, the medical assistant must communicate anything related to the patient's health verbally or through the medical record. At the same time, the medical assistant must be careful to avoid giving medical advice to the patient (unless following specific guidelines established by the physician).

Teamwork is enhanced when each team member helps and supports other members and avoids blaming or criticizing others. Because the number of employees in a medical office is often small, it is important for everyone to do their best to get along and deal with conflict. When a problem arises, it is important to try to find solutions to the problem rather than focusing on who caused the problem or whose fault it is. It is also helpful to maintain perspective and accept that things do go wrong and that most problems can be dealt with. In any conflict situation, it is important to listen to the point of view of others and validate their feelings. Effective communication techniques are discussed in more detail in Chapter 4.

PARTS OF THE MEDICAL OFFICE

A physician's office has a number of different physical spaces in it. Each space has a particular purpose. Every provider's office has three basic areas: a reception area and waiting room, examination and treatment rooms, and an area for other activities. This may include medical records storage, if the office uses paper medical records; storage for supplies; and staff offices or cubicles.

In most offices, providers also have their own offices, separate from examination rooms, but some providers have examination tables in their offices, combining the two spaces in one room.

Larger offices may have several additional areas such as an office laboratory; separate treatment rooms or special procedure rooms; a business office, which is separate from the front office (reception, telephones, appointments); and a lunch or break room for the staff.

All providers' offices must meet a number of specifications laid out by regulatory agencies. These include the federal Occupational Safety and Health Administration (OSHA), which regulates workplace health and safety. Providers' offices also must meet the specifications of the Americans with Disabilities Act, which requires that doorways be at least 3 feet wide and hallways at least 5 feet wide. Restroom facilities must be available for both patients and staff. Office laboratories are regulated by the Clinical Laboratory Improvement Amendments of 1988 (CLIA '88). Local boards of health also inspect and regulate hospitals and clinics.

Fig. 1.3 shows the layout of a small medical office.

RECEPTION AREA AND WAITING ROOM

The reception area and waiting room are the first place any new or prospective patient will see. First impressions are important. The waiting room should be clean and well lit. Furniture should be arranged and not haphazardly placed. Up-to-date, general-interest reading material should be available; many providers also have patient education materials available in the waiting room. Waiting rooms in pediatric and family practice offices also have toys available for children. Large pediatric practices may have a separate waiting room for sick children or for adolescents.

The waiting room should have enough chairs for two people per patient visit, multiplied by the number of patients seen in 2 hours. It needs to present a calm atmosphere and look professional. Usually the waiting area is carpeted. It should have comfortable chairs, grouped in blocks, if possible, rather than just lined up around the walls. Colors should be muted, and music should be soft. Red, yellow, and orange are typically avoided; currently, provider's office

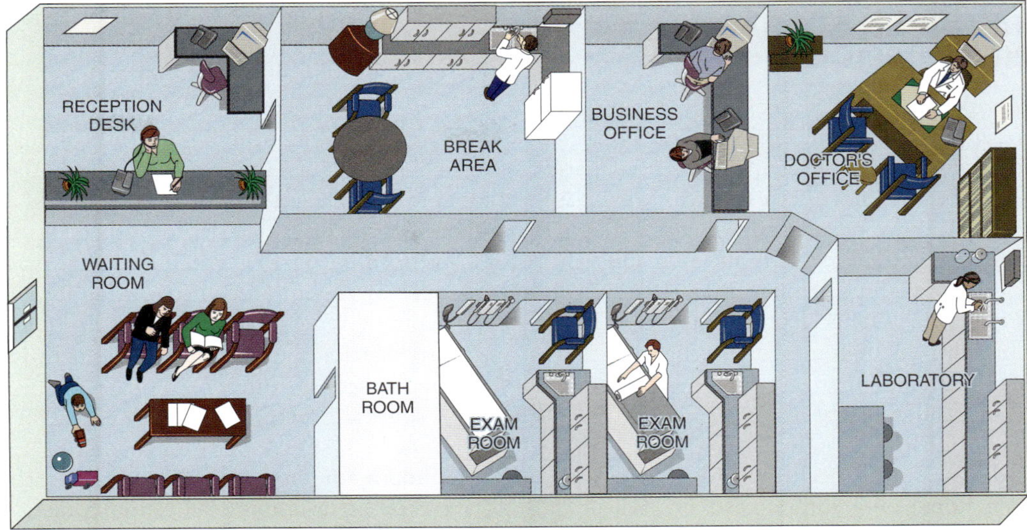

Fig. 1.3 Layout of a small medical office.

decor often uses shades of green, dusty pink, or salmon. Music may be played from a CD or radio station of the "easy listening" variety, or there may be a television in the waiting room.

The reception area adjoins the waiting room. The medical assistant at the reception desk should greet each patient as they enter the waiting room. Most reception areas have a counter so that the patient can fill out or sign forms, and many have a sliding window so that patients cannot hear the conversations occurring behind the receptionist.

Patients check in here when they enter the office. New patient forms are received here, and health insurance cards are copied or scanned. Copayments are taken from patients whose insurance requires them. Appointments may be made by the receptionist or in a separate area of the office.

EXAMINATION ROOMS AND LABORATORY

Examination rooms are designed for the convenience of the provider and assisting personnel who will work there. However, they also need to be as comfortable and calming to the patient as possible. Reading material should be available in each examination room. Although good scheduling will ensure that patients will not wait too long in these rooms for a provider, most providers do see patients in at least two examination rooms. Additional delays may occur if the provider has to respond to urgent telephone calls or office emergencies.

Fig. 1.4 shows a typical examination room.

Many providers perform treatments or diagnostic procedures in examination rooms, but complex procedures (such as suturing a laceration) are often performed in larger rooms with extra equipment and/or supplies. These are called *treatment rooms.*

If laboratory tests are performed in the medical office, there is a special room or area set aside for this. CLIA

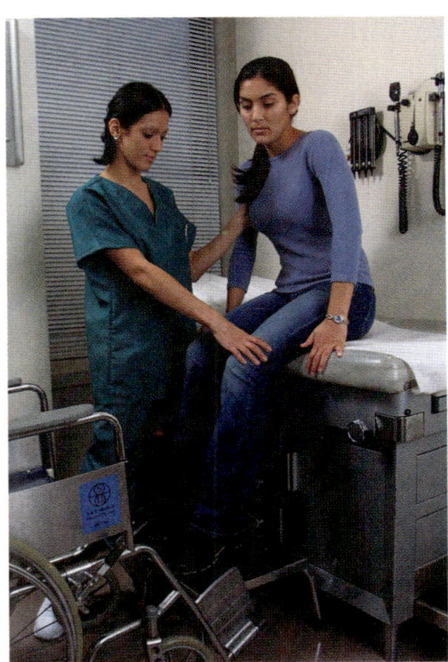

Fig. 1.4 Examination rooms are usually compact, but each should be large enough to accommodate a wheelchair. (From Proctor D, Adams A: *Kinn's The medical assistant*, ed 12, St. Louis, 2014, Saunders.)

regulates laboratory testing. Medical assistants are trained to perform low-complexity tests (CLIA-waived tests) such as dipstick urinalysis, urine pregnancy tests, and rapid strep tests. They may also perform more complex texts with special training.

CLIA specifies who can supervise laboratories and lays out the process for inspection and accreditation. It sets strict guidelines for quality control, quality assurance, handling of hazardous materials, documentation, and proficiency training. Offices that perform only CLIA-waived laboratory tests may perform laboratory testing in the patient preparation area. Ideally the bathroom is adjacent to this area, with an opening in the wall so that urine samples can be passed directly into the laboratory area.

MEDICAL RECORDS STORAGE AND BUSINESS OFFICE

If the office uses paper records, the medical records may be stored near the reception area, in the business areas, adjacent to the patient preparation area, or in a separate room. Charts of active patients—those who have been seen within the past 2 to 3 years—are kept in the records storage area in the office. Inactive charts are removed regularly and stored in a less accessible location such as the basement of the building or off-site in a facility that maintains records in storage. Charts needed for patients who will be coming in during a specified period—morning, afternoon, or an entire day—are removed from the storage area and prepared for use.

The majority of medical practices have moved away from paper records to eletronic health records. In this case, patient records are stored on a computer's hard disk or in the cloud and are simply pulled up as needed. The process of placing old records into the computerized record is lengthy, and some offices that use an electronic health record store the former paper records of established patients in an accessible area for 1 to 2 years after the transition to the electronic health record.

Posting of patient charges, billing, and computer operations may be performed in an area behind the reception desk or in a separate business office. If the practice has one or more satellite locations, the billing and insurance tasks are usually done in the practice's main office for all locations. Some offices contract billing and insurance claim processing to an outside company, which may even be located in another state.

What Would You Do? What Would You *Not* Do?

Case Study 2

The provider complains to Aida that there are always dishes in the sink in the break room and crumbs and used paper coffee cups on the table. Even though the area is not seen by patients, the provider is concerned that an insect or rodent problem could develop. Aida knows that the part-time file clerk and the part-time receptionist have a tendency to leave dirty dishes and trash after their afternoon break. She herself is so busy that she rarely has time to either clean or sit down in the break room. ■

ADDITIONAL AREAS FOUND IN MANY OFFICES

Providers' private offices are often a reflection of their personal tastes. This room is where a provider meets privately with patients, patients' families, and other visitors. The provider usually displays degrees and certificates of membership in professional organizations on the walls of the office. Even if the practice has a small library for the use of all staff, providers will usually have at least a few important references in this office. Art and memorabilia that show the provider's personal taste also help to make the private office a pleasant place for the provider to do quiet work and hold meetings.

Recognizing the needs of staff for a quiet place to take their breaks and eat their lunch, newer offices and large offices often include a staff break or lunchroom. This room may have a refrigerator and microwave for staff to prepare lunches they bring from home. There should be at least one table and chairs. The lunch or break room should not double as a storage area, and staff should avoid using the room for meetings that deprive others of use of the room.

Depending on the type of medical practice, particular rooms may be set aside for specific treatments or diagnostic procedures. Types of special rooms include the following:

- A pediatrics examination or treatment room in a family practice group's office
- A surgical procedure room in a general surgery group's office
- A room for more complex testing such as colposcopy and pelvic ultrasounds in a group practice specializing in obstetrics and gynecology
- A trauma room in a large clinic or community health center

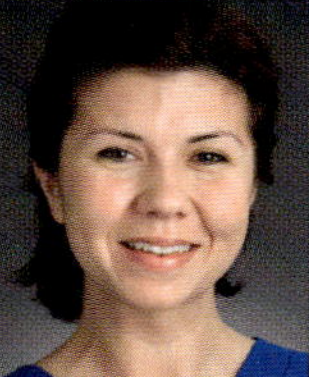

Memories *from* Practicum

Aida Reyes: The clinic where I did my practicum was so large that at first I kept getting lost. Another thing that confused me was the doors that the staff used to get from one part of the clinic to another. It was arranged by department, but the layout of rooms in each department was different. I spent the majority of my time in internal medicine working with one medical assistant and one provider, but my preceptor arranged for me to spend time in other departments such as medical records, billing, and pediatrics and with the referral coordinator. In addition to the full-time providers, there were some specialists who came in once or twice a week, including a neurologist, an orthopedic surgeon, and an ophthalmologist. The clinic also employed a social worker and a dietician. In each department there was a nurse and there were at least two medical assistants in addition to the receptionist. The amazing thing was how quickly I adapted and became comfortable finding my way around. After only a few weeks, it felt like I belonged there. I was so proud when my preceptor said, "Aida, you have become one of the team. I don't know how we ever got along without you." ■

MEDICAL SPECIALTIES

Since the middle of the 20th century, the practice of medicine has been broken down into fields of specialty and subspecialty. In 1950 most Americans received their medical care from a general practitioner, who took care of adults and children, often delivered babies, and performed many general surgical procedures.

Currently, Americans may see two, three, or more providers routinely. Box 1.1 describes the medical specialties in which a providers can be board certified according to the

BOX 1.1 Specialties in Which the American Board of Medical Specialties Offers Certification

Allergy and Immunology (Allergist, Immunologist): Treats adults and/or children with allergies and problems of the immune system. Many individuals experience allergies and/or asthma in the presence of allergens. The immune system can also malfunction either through inherited or acquired diseases. Allergists and immunologists diagnose, manage, and treat allergic diseases, immunodeficiency conditions, and autoimmune diseases.

Anesthesiology (Anesthesiologist): Provides anesthesia during surgery and other procedures, as well as medical care to patients before, during, and after surgery. The anesthesiologist also supervises other anesthesia personnel in the operating room such as nurse anesthetists and anesthesiology residents.

Colon and Rectal Surgery: Performs surgical treatment of the large intestine and rectum. These surgeons specialize in the diagnosis and treatment of diseases of the colon and rectum in addition to full training in general surgery. They perform diagnostic and screening procedures and perform surgery when necessary.

Dermatology (Dermatologist): Specializes in conditions of the skin. Dermatologists diagnose skin diseases and perform surgery on the skin. Laser treatments are commonly used for skin conditions in addition to medication, cryotherapy, and surgery.

Emergency Medicine: Treats patients for emergency conditions, usually in the emergency department of a hospital. Emergency medicine focuses on the treatment of acute illnesses and injuries that require immediate care. The physician is often an employee of a hospital emergency department or other urgent care center.

Family Medicine (Family Practitioner): Treats adults and children for routine care and complaints; often the primary care physician for all family members. The family practitioner is concerned with the total health of the individual and the family.

Internal Medicine (Internist): Provides medical treatment for conditions of various body systems. The internist may be the primary care provider for adults. Within the discipline of internal medicine there are several subspecialties based on patient age groups, body system, or type of disease.

Medical Genetics and Genomics: Provides diagnostic procedures and treatment for individuals with genetically linked diseases. Also provides genetic counseling and prenatal diagnosis.

Neurological Surgery (Neurosurgeon): Performs prevention, diagnosis, surgical and nonsurgical treatment, and rehabilitation for conditions of the brain, spine, and nervous system. Also provides surgical and nonsurgical treatment of pain.

Nuclear Medicine: Specializes in diagnosis using radionuclides, atoms that give off electromagnetic radiation. Nuclear medicine physicians (also called nuclear radiologists) are usually employed by a hospital or university (or both) and have little direct patient care. They are responsible for diagnosis and recommending treatment of abnormalities detected through the various imaging modalities used in the nuclear medicine department.

Obstetrics (Obstetrician) and Gynecology (Gynecologist): Specializes in care during pregnancy and delivery (obstetrician); specializes in other care and surgery of the female reproductive system (gynecologist). The gynecologist is responsible for screening procedures, diagnostic procedures, and both medical and surgical treatments. They also frequently uses hormone-modulating treatments.

Ophthalmology (Ophthalmologist): Specializes in the care of the eye. The ophthalmologist manages diseases and conditions of the eye with both medical and surgical treatment including laser treatments. May also manage errors of refraction and prescribe corrective lenses, although this is often delegated to an optometrist.

Orthopedic Surgery (Orthopedic Surgeon): Specializes in diagnosis and treatment of acute and traumatic injuries of the musculoskeletal system, as well as diseases of the muscular or skeletal system. Both surgical and nonsurgical treatments are used. A subspecialty is sports medicine.

Otolaryngology (Otolaryngologist or ENT): Specializes in the care of the ear, nose, throat, head, and neck. The physician, often called an ENT (for ear, nose, and throat), is responsible for the diagnosis and surgical or nonsurgical treatment of a variety of disorders affecting the specified organs.

Pathology (Pathologist): Examines cells, tissues, and other specimens to determine whether their structure is normal or abnormal; attempts to determine the nature or cause of disease. Pathologists examine tissue biopsies and other specimens to identify abnormal cells. They also perform autopsies. They may be trained within two primary specialty areas: clinical pathology and/or anatomic pathology.

Pediatrics (Pediatrician): Specializes in the care of children from birth through adolescence. In the United States, pediatricians are considered to be primary care practitioners. However, many pediatricians specialize, and almost every specialty for adult medicine is represented as a pediatric subspecialty.

Physical Medicine and Rehabilitation (Physiatrist): Specializes in the treatment and rehabilitation of patients with disabling conditions such as spinal cord injury and stroke. A physiatrist sees patients across several age groups and specialty areas and focuses on restoring maximal function to patients. They may specialize in specific age groups or types of injury, such as spinal cord injury.

Plastic Surgery: Specializes in surgical and nonsurgical treatment of physical defects of various areas of the body. The plastic surgeon performs procedures for cosmetic enhancement or reconstruction of various parts of the body. Cosmetic surgery has become popular in the past two decades. Reconstructive surgery includes craniofacial surgery, hand surgery, and maxillofacial surgery to repair congenital defects and problems that result from injury or disease.

Preventative Medicine: Includes aerospace medicine, occupational medicine, and public health. In this medical specialty, physicians practice in one of the specialty areas or one of the subspecialties (addiction medicine, clinical informatics, medical toxicology, or undersea and hyperbaric medicine).

Psychiatry (Psychiatrist) and Neurology (Neurologist): Specializes in preventing, diagnosing, and treating mental illness and/or diseases of the nervous system. Psychiatrists have completed the same general training as any other physician, and they

Continued

BOX 1.1 Specialties in Which the American Board of Medical Specialties Offers Certification—cont'd

are able to prescribe medication for mental illness and monitor the effects of medication therapy. Like other mental health professionals, they usually also have training in psychotherapy, psychoanalysis, and/or cognitive behavioral therapy. Neurologists have training in diseases of the central and peripheral nervous system. Subspecialties include addiction psychiatry, brain injury medicine, neurodevelopmental disabilities, pain medicine, sleep medicine, and others.

Radiology (Radiologist): Specializes in the use of x-ray and other ionizing radiation for diagnosis (diagnostic radiology), treatment (radiation oncology), or medical physics. A diagnostic radiologist has the training to manage several types of diagnostic imaging including x-ray studies, computed tomography (CT) scans, and magnetic resonance imaging (MRI).

Surgery (General Surgeon): Performs general surgical procedures. A general surgeon performs primarily abdominal or vascular surgery using traditional methods or laparoscopic methods. Hand surgery may be performed by a general surgeon or a plastic surgeon.

Thoracic Surgery (Thoracic Surgeon): Performs surgery of the chest including cardiac surgery, although thoracic surgeons usually specialize in surgery of the chest or cardiac surgery.

Urology (Urologist): Specializes in the care of the urinary system in males and females and the reproductive tract in males; also specializes in surgery of the urinary tract and male reproductive tract. The urologist may provide medical treatment for infections or surgical repair for abnormal growths or correction of congenital malformations.

American Board of Medical Specialties. In many areas, there are several subspecialties. If the provider wants to become certified in a subspecialty, after the residency training they participate in additional training called a *fellowship* for 2 to 3 years. It is not possible to be board certified in any specialty or subspecialty without completing a residency.

PRIMARY CARE AND THE PATIENT-CENTERED MEDICAL HOME

Primary care providers specialize in internal medicine (treatment of the internal organs of adults by other than surgical means), pediatrics (general medical care of children and adolescents), or family medicine (general medical care of children, adolescents, and adults—the current equivalent of general practice).

Over the course of time, the activities of different types of providers have shifted. For instance, currently fewer family practitioners deliver babies than did general practitioners in the 1950s and 1960s, preferring to leave that task to obstetricians, owing in part to the cost of malpractice insurance. Although some women continue to see a gynecologist for an annual pelvic examination and Pap test, the primary care provider is usually also willing to perform these activities.

Primary care has been greatly influenced in the past decade by the movement to establish a **patient-centered medical home (PCMH)** as the provider of a patient's primary care. The PCMH is a model of primary care that emphasizes patient-centered health care based on a personal relationship between a patient, a physician, and the patient's care team. The PCMH movement incorporates several elements:

- It is patient-centered, and health care teams are jointly responsible for patient care and safety.
- It is comprehensive, including prevention, acute care, and chronic care.
- Care is coordinated across the entire health care system including specialty care, hospitals, home care, and community services.
- Patients receive high-quality care; both patients and families are encouraged to make informed decisions about their health.

Most states have adopted an initiative to support the PCMH movement and encourage primary care practices to become recognized PCMHs. There is a strong relationship between PCMH practices and ACOs mandated by the Centers for Medicare and Medicaid Services (CMS), which are intended to increase the quality of care of Medicare patients. Within the PCMH movement, medical assistants play an important role in enhancing access to care. They are often expected to undertake more advanced duties than were formerly assigned to them.

OSTEOPATHY

Osteopathy is a mix of traditional scientific medicine and **holistic** medicine, which focuses more on healing the entire person than a specific disease or condition. This branch of medical practice seeks to balance the structure and function of the body through manipulation of muscles and joints. Osteopathy was started in the late 1800s by Andrew Taylor Still (1828–1917). Osteopaths see disease as the result of dysfunction in the skeletal and muscular systems. Pain, "asymmetry" (the difference in anatomy or joint movement between one side of the body and the other), and tissue tenderness are used to gauge symptoms. Osteopaths, who hold DO degrees, currently are given all the privileges of those with MD degrees. The majority of osteopaths practice as primary care doctors, where they believe their holistic and structural approach can be most effective.

PODIATRY

Podiatrists use traditional medical and surgical techniques but are limited in their practice to treatment of disorders of the feet and ankles. Since the 1970s, podiatry has worked to enlarge its area of practice by focusing on surgery of the foot to alleviate such problems as bone spurs and bunions. Podiatrists work closely with primary care doctors in the management of diabetic patients and the elderly, who often require specialized foot care.

CHIROPRACTIC

Contemporary chiropractic care focuses on the evaluation of neuromuscular and skeletal disorders within the context of overall well-being and health. Begun in 1895 by Daniel David Palmer (1845–1913), chiropractic holds that the body has its own ability to heal and maintain balance. According to chiropractic theory, the nervous system is the center of all disease and healing. Traditionally chiropractors believed that subluxation was often the root cause of disease. Currently chiropractors, who are licensed by the state in which they practice, specialize in the manipulative treatment of the spine and joints, but they also include dietary modification, nutritional supplementation, physical therapies, and exercise in their treatments.

PRACTICE TYPES

Seventy years ago most physicians who were not full-time members of hospital staffs worked by themselves in an office, either in their home or in an office building. They paid their office expenses, taxes, and liability insurance out of their income, and the difference was considered their "net income" from their practice. As their practice got busier, their income increased. Currently many physicians work with other providers. Some of them have an ownership position in the practice or facility in which they work, but others are employees and receive a salary from their employer. The following categories refer to the way the office is structured, not the business arrangement or ownership.

SOLO PRACTICE

It is still possible for a physician to work in a solo practice, but to do so, the physician provider must make a number of trade-offs. Solo practices are limited in their size by the number of patients one physician can manage. When a physician practices alone, the medical assistant is usually responsible for aspects of both administrative and clinical support.

Even if a solo practitioner employs an NP or a PA to see additional patients, the physician still must factor into their workday some time to oversee the work of these nonphysician professionals. In addition, the physician, as the employer, is usually responsible for paying the malpractice insurance premiums for all of the licensed professionals in their office. Physicians in solo practice are also completely responsible for their patients. Usually, they make arrangements with other physicians to share after-hours and weekend call responsibilities and to cover for vacations.

GROUP PRACTICE

Currently many providers participate in a group practice. The most common type of group practice includes three or four providers of the same medical specialty who band together to share resources such as office space and personnel. In these groups, medical assistants usually specialize in either clinical or administrative work, although they expect to help out in other areas.

Depending on the business form used, patients are the responsibility of either one provider or "the group." In either case, if a patient's regular provider is not available, another provider in the office can see the patient. In addition, providers who work in group practices usually share after-hours and weekend call responsibilities. They usually split the cost of malpractice insurance, and the policy is written for the group rather than for each individual. Group practices are commonly owned by hospitals, and the physicians and other providers are employees rather than owners.

Large medical groups with providers who provide primary care, as well as providers with other medical specialties, are becoming increasingly common throughout the country. Their names often include the words "associates" or "medical associates." This organizational form allows a sharing of resources that, in turn, allows each provider in the group to provide a broader range of services. In the past, these groups were more common in particular regions and in rural areas where a single group of providers has the responsibility of being both the providers in town and the staff of a small, rural hospital. HMOs that provide all services in one building, so-called "closed-panel HMOs," also operate as multispecialty groups.

These practices often have separate administrative departments for billing, appointment scheduling, and referrals and separate clinical departments for phlebotomy, electrocardiography, laboratory work, and radiography. In such practices, medical assisting jobs can be limited in scope, and specific responsibilities depend on the department in which the medical assistant works.

CLINIC

Traditionally a clinic was connected to a hospital and provided ambulatory care, often to patients with limited financial resources. Patients were either seen at no charge or billed by the clinic, and providers were paid a salary for their services and/or saw patients as part of their residency program. Currently a *clinic* usually refers to a public or nonprofit facility that provides outpatient public health services, although private solo or group practices may use the word "clinic" in their name. Community health centers, established by the federal government in the late 1960s, operate as clinics and have physicians and NPs, PAs, and nurse-midwives all on salary.

COMPLEMENTARY AND ALTERNATIVE MEDICINE

Numerous other practices are used for the treatment of illness, some of which have a long tradition and some of which have developed more recently. Studies from the early 1990s found that Americans annually spend literally millions of dollars on therapies that are not part of their provider's standard approach. Patients often do not even tell their providers about these other treatments. When practices have been used for extended periods in specific cultures, they may be called *traditional medicine*. The term *complementary medicine* is usually used for medical treatments that patients use in addition to standard medical treatments. The term *alternative medicine* refers to practices that are used instead of standard medical treatment. For many patients, these may overlap. For example, acupuncture has been a definitive method of treatment in traditional Chinese medicine for centuries (Fig. 1.5). In the United States it has become a popular treatment method used in addition to standard treatment. It has become so popular that there are many schools to train practitioners, and the practice of acupuncture requires a license in most states.

Since the early 1990s, scholars of medicine have begun to take an interest in studying complementary and alternative practices scientifically. The federal government has since established the National Center for Complementary and Integrative Health within the National Institutes of Health. This agency coordinates and funds scientific research to study the effectiveness of these health practices. The most well-respected medical journals such as the *New England Journal of Medicine* and *JAMA* have published a number of studies about the effectiveness of various nonstandard therapies, and numerous specialized journals have also been established to publish research about such therapies. When research demonstrates that a practice is effective, physicians trained in the classic Western medical tradition are more accepting and may even incorporate some of these practices or refer patients to practitioners.

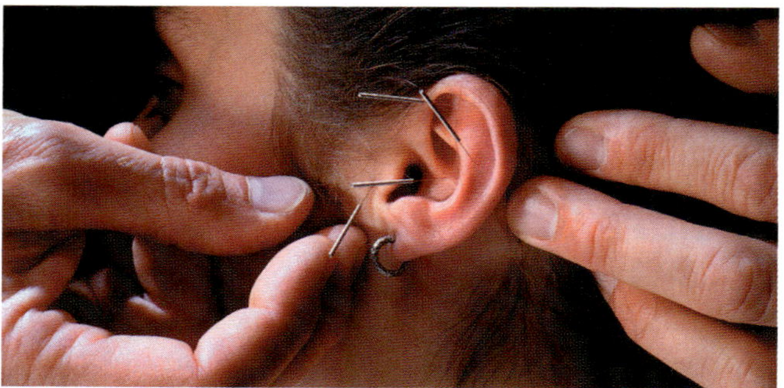

Fig. 1.5 Acupuncture involves the placement of several extremely thin needles in various parts of the body.

What Would You Do? What Would You *Not* Do?

Case Study 3

While Aida is taking John Carter's medical history, he mentions that he has been getting acupuncture and taking several herbal preparations that he buys at a health food store. He also says that he wears shoe insoles with magnets in them because he has had heel pain for several months. He says, "You should try them. They have really helped my heel pain." ■

What Would You Do? What Would You *Not* Do? RESPONSES

Case Study 1

Page 10

What Did Aida Do?

- ❑ Accepted Alicia Darwin's reason for changing medical offices without making a judgment.
- ❑ Stated that she hopes Alicia will feel comfortable as a patient in their practice.
- ❑ Stated that she is a medical assistant, not a nurse, and explained the difference briefly.
- ❑ Clarified the legal position of a nurse practitioner in her state related to prescribing medications.

What Did Aida Not Do?

- ❑ Agreed verbally or by implication that she is a nurse.
- ❑ Asked for additional information about Alicia's previous provider or medical office.
- ❑ Made any critical remarks about nurse practitioners or Alicia's previous provider.
- ❑ Made any statement that could be interpreted as a guarantee that Alicia will like this provider better.

Case Study 2

Page 12

What Did Aida Do?

- ❑ Agreed that the condition of the break room could be improved.
- ❑ Promised to talk to all staff members about keeping the break room clean.
- ❑ Arranged time to speak to staff members either individually or as a group to discuss ways to keep the break room clean and make a plan.
- ❑ Encouraged all staff members to take an active part in developing a plan to keep the break room clean.

What Would You Do? What Would You *Not* Do? RESPONSES—cont'd

- ❑ Followed up to be sure that any plan made was implemented and was effective.

What Did Aida Not Do?

- ❑ Did not focus on identifying who was responsible when talking to either the provider or other staff members.
- ❑ Did not become defensive when talking to the provider or other staff members.
- ❑ Did not single out any staff member(s) as responsible for the problem.
- ❑ Did not complain about one staff member's behavior to any other staff member.

Case Study 3

Page 16

What Did Aida Do?

- ❑ Accepted John Carter's description of his complementary and alternative medical practices.
- ❑ Documented all practices in the medical record.
- ❑ Asked questions to explore the underlying problems such as heel pain or the reason for acupuncture.

What Did Aida Not Do?

- ❑ Did not tell John that he might be endangering his health because of his use of complementary or alternative medical practices.
- ❑ Did not tell John that acupuncture, magnets, or herbs would not help him.
- ❑ Did not ask John where to buy foot insoles with magnets.
- ❑ Did not dismiss John's practices as insignificant and fail to document them.

TERMINOLOGY REVIEW

Key Term	Word Parts	Definition
Ambulatory care	*ambulare:* to walk *-ory:* pertaining to	Medical care that is provided on an outpatient basis. The patient is able to come to the facility providing care and return home after having received services.
Capitation		A set payment provided by managed care insurance per patient per month regardless of the amount of service the patient receives.
Curative treatment		Treatment that cures disease.
Empirical	*empiricus:* experienced *-al:* pertaining to	Learned from observation or experiment.
Fee-for-service		A means of payment for health care in which the cost for each service provided is reimbursed in full or in part.
Formulary		A list of prescription drugs covered or preferred by a managed care insurance company.
Health insurance		Purchase of protection for covered services related to health care.
Holistic	*holos:* whole *-ic:* pertaining to	Considering the whole; in medicine, considering the entire person when providing health care.
Managed care		A system that manages the delivery of health care with the intention of controlling costs.
Medicaid		Health insurance for all medically indigent people.
Medicare		Health insurance for the elderly, the disabled, and those with end-stage kidney disease.
Palliative treatment		Therapy that reduces the effects of a disease or condition but does not remove the disease itself.
Patient-centered medical home (PCMH)		A model of primary care that emphasizes patient-centered health care based on a personal relationship among a patient, a provider, and the patient's care team.
Quality assurance		Measures to ensure that patients receive safe and appropriate services.
Residency		A program to provide training in a medical specialty to a physician who has finished medical school.
Symptomatic treatment		Therapy for symptoms of a disease or condition that does not remove the disease itself.
Tricare		Health insurance for dependents of active-duty miliatry personnel.
Utilization review		Assessment of medical services to determine whether they are appropriate, necessary, and of high quality.

The Professional Medical Assistant

Check out the Evolve site at http://evolve.elsevier.com/Bonewit/today to access additional interactive activities and exercises to help you study and prepare for success.

LEARNING OBJECTIVES

1. Describe the history of the medical assisting profession.
2. Explain how a medical assisting educational program becomes accredited.
3. Differentiate between various national credentials for medical assistants.
4. List character and personality traits of effective medical assistants.
5. Describe the appearance and behavior of a professional medical assistant.
6. Describe principles of effective time management.
7. Define *professionalism* for medical assistants and providers.
8. Identify organizations and publications that guide professional behavior for medical assistants and providers.
9. Describe how professional organizations support the profession of medical assisting.
10. Identify the administrative tasks and clinical tasks performed by a medical assistant.
11. Discuss the medical assistant's role in the operation of the medical office and patient education.
12. List employment opportunities for medical assistants.

PROCEDURES

Locating and defining a state's legal scope of practice.

CHAPTER OUTLINE

KEY TERMS

accreditation
continuing education unit (CEU)
fee splitting
health coaching
initiative
inventory
patient navigator
practicum
risk management
time management

INTRODUCTION TO PROFESSIONAL MEDICAL ASSISTING

Medical assisting came into existence as a career during the second half of the 20th century. Around the middle of the 1900s, most physicians established their own practice when they completed their medical education and hospital training. A physician (almost always a man) usually saw patients and had no assistance, except possibly from his wife who answered the telephone and often did the billing.

The physician spent a large portion of each day making house calls. During a house call the physician would examine a patient with only the equipment he could carry in his medical bag. The physician's office was often located in a room in his house or the first floor of a building, with the physician living in an apartment above. Patients who went to the physician's office may or may not have had an appointment. They expected to wait to be seen.

In the first 20 years after World War II (before the increasing use of technology caused medical costs to skyrocket), a physician usually charged $2 to $5, possibly $10, for an office visit, a sum that currently seems small. However, for some patients, even this small charge was more than a day's pay. For physicians the low fee was enough because the expenses of the practice were also low. In fact, physicians rarely pressed poor patients for full payment. They always had many patients who owed them money, and it was not uncommon for patients to pay small amounts on a weekly basis for many months or even years, especially the parents of young children. Sometimes physicians would even barter by exchanging medical care for goods or services provided by the patient. For example, a patient might pay for his medical care by bringing the physician fresh produce from his farm.

During the past 70 years, the practice of medicine has changed dramatically. This, in turn, has changed the way in which physicians operate their medical practices. With the advent of government insurance programs, not only were office visits covered by insurance, but the medical office was also expected to complete and submit the insurance forms to receive payment. Physicians and other providers soon discovered that the cost of employing a person to complete these forms was offset by improved collections and cash flow. Gradually almost all insurance billing shifted to the health care provider. As practices are consolidated, centralized billing is common.

Advances in medical science made many more diagnostic tests, laboratory tests, and treatments available and even necessary for good medical care. It made sense to have an assistant in the office to perform these tests and allow the providers to concentrate on seeing patients.

Even as laboratory and diagnostic testing has increased in amount and in complexity, so too have the administrative equipment and technology used in a provider's office. Currently there are computers, wireless electronic devices, printers, fax machines, photocopiers, intercoms, and voicemail systems.

Providers send claims to a number of different insurance companies. Many insurance plans require prior approval for certain medical procedures, referrals to specialists, or surgical procedures. Insurance companies and government programs prefer electronic claims filing and often make electronic payments directly into providers' office accounts at banks. This creates a need not only for more staff but also for more highly trained staff.

Providers have also almost completely stopped making house calls. Because of this, providers need more office space. In addition, patients with more complex needs are seen in providers' offices rather than in the hospital emergency department or outpatient department. Sometimes a patient must occupy an examination or treatment room for an extended period of time, such as when an individual with asthma is receiving an inhalation treatment.

Another change that has had an impact on the medical practice involves the increase in medical litigation. Since the 1970s, providers have practiced what has come to be called "defensive medicine." Because of the fear of a malpractice lawsuit and the high cost of malpractice insurance, providers began to perform more laboratory and diagnostic tests to rule out even the most unlikely cause of an illness. Another factor stimulating the expanded use of laboratory tests in outpatient care is the increased number of Clinical Laboratory Improvement Amendments (CLIA)-waived tests that are available.

As services expanded, physicians employed nurses to help them in their offices. This helped ease their burden of performing procedures and caring for patients, but nurses were often unable and unwilling to assist with the administrative aspects of the practice. As a result, many physicians found a willing candidate and trained that person to assist first with administrative duties and then with both patient care and administrative duties. This evolved over time into what is currently the medical assistant profession.

In 1956, medical assistants from 15 states organized to form the American Association of Medical Assistants (AAMA). In 1978 the profession was recognized by the U.S. Department of Education. The AAMA and other organizations, especially the American Medical Technologists (AMT), have worked to define professional training for the medical assistant and to provide certification for medical assistants through national examinations.

EDUCATIONAL PROGRAMS FOR MEDICAL ASSISTANTS

Initially, medical assistants received on-the-job training, but as the profession grew, formal educational programs were established. These programs vary in length from 6 months to 2 years. Medical assisting programs include theoretical and practical preparation in all aspects of the medical assisting profession. To maintain quality, many of these programs seek **accreditation**, credit, or recognition from a regional or national organization for maintaining certain standards. The two recognized accrediting agencies for medical assisting programs are the Commission on Accreditation of Allied Health Education Programs (CAAHEP), in collaboration with the AAMA, and the Accrediting Bureau of Health Education Schools (ABHES). It is important to distinguish program accreditation from institutional accreditation. There are many medical assistant programs in accredited institutions of higher learning that have not obtained specific program accreditation.

A medical assistant program seeking accreditation from one of the aforementioned agencies must prepare a written report showing how the educational standards of that agency are being met. After the report has been submitted, an accreditation visit is made to validate the information presented in the report. Once accreditation has been granted, graduates of the program are eligible to take either the certified medical assistant (CMA) AAMA or registered medical assistant (RMA) certification examination. Accredited programs must include at least 160 hours of practical work experience in a medical office or clinic, known as a **practicum** or practical experience (formerly called an *externship*).

CERTIFICATION FOR MEDICAL ASSISTANTS

Medical assistants usually graduate from an educational program that may vary in length from 6 months to 2 years. If the medical assistant graduates from a program accredited by CAAHEP or ABHES, they are automatically eligible to take a national certification examination. Certification is a process by which an organization, often a national body, validates the credentials of an individual or a program. Certification is important for health care professionals. Professionals such as physicians and nurses require certification (by passing a national examination) as a condition for obtaining a state license to practice their profession. Certification is also important for medical assistants, especially those who live in a state that does not regulate unlicensed health professionals. When an unbiased national organization validates knowledge and skills, the employer can be sure that the medical assistant has excellent qualifications.

Several organizations provide certification for medical assistants. Each has different requirements for eligibility, and some organizations offer more than one certification. In many areas, employers hire only medical assistants who have passed a certification examination. As medical assistants perform more specialized clinical tasks, employers have become increasingly concerned about validating skills and knowledge before hiring them.

AMERICAN ASSOCIATION OF MEDICAL ASSISTANTS

The AAMA administers the CMA (AAMA) examination. To take the examination, an individual must have graduated from a medical assistant program accredited by CAAHEP or ABHES or be a CMA (AAMA) seeking recertification.

The examination is computer-based and is administered online at testing centers. Most states have several testing locations.

Application materials can be obtained from the AAMA Certification Department, 20 North Wacker Dr., Suite 1575, Chicago, IL 60606-2903; from the director of accreditation at the medical assistant program attended; or a medical assistant can apply online at the AAMA website (www.aama-ntl.org).

Passing this examination allows a medical assistant to use the title CMA (AAMA) after their name on all official documents, including patient records and business cards.

AMERICAN MEDICAL TECHNOLOGISTS

The AMT is an organization that offers several certifications. Medical assistants may take an examination to be certified as an RMA, a certified medical administrative specialist (CMAS), and/or a registered phlebotomy technician (RPT). In addition, this organization certifies medical technologists and medical laboratory technicians.

To take the RMA examination, an individual must have (1) graduated from a medical assisting program that includes at least 720 hours of training that includes at least 160 hours of externship (practicum) in an institution that is accredited by an organization approved by the U.S. Department of Education; (2) graduated from a formal medical services program of the U.S. Armed Forces and have graduated within the last 4 years; (3) been employed full-time in the profession of medical assisting for at least 3 of the previous 7 years; (4) completed a medical assisting work-study/training program within the last 4 years; (5) been instructing in an accredited MA program for between 1 and 5 years and have at least 3 years of full-time clinical work experience in a health care profession.

Applications for the RMA examination can be obtained from the Registrar's Office, AMT, 10700 W. Higgins, Suite 150, Rosemont, IL 60018, or the applicant can apply online. Information about the examination can be obtained from the AMT website (www.americanmedtech.org). The RMA examination may be given at a student's school, or an applicant may take the test online at testing centers located throughout the country.

Passing this examination entitles the medical assistant to use the initials RMA after their name on all official documents.

CALIFORNIA CERTIFYING BOARD FOR MEDICAL ASSISTANTS

The California Certifying Board for Medical Assistants (CCBMA) is one of the three organizations recognized by the Medical Board of California for certification of medical assistants (with the AAMA and the AMT). The CCBMA administers the California Certified Medical Assistant examination (CACMA) which is primarily taken by residents of California. Information is available on the CCBMA website at www.ccbma.org.

NATIONAL HEALTHCAREER ASSOCIATION

The National Healthcareer Association (NHA) offers certifications for several allied health professions. Medical assistants may be interested in obtaining certification as a certified clinical medical assistant (CCMA), certified medical administrative assistant (CMAA), certified electrocardiogram (ECG) technician (CET), and/or certified phlebotomy technician (CPT). The NHA also has certifications for certified administrative medical assistants (CMAA), certified billing and coding specialists (CBCS), and other health professions. Information is available on the NHA website at www.nhanow.com.

NATIONAL CENTER FOR COMPETENCY TESTING

The National Center for Competency Testing (NCCT) offers testing for graduates of affiliated programs, as well as medical assistants with experience or training through the military. It is possible to become certified as a medical assistant (NCMA), a medical office assistant (NCMOA), an ECG technician (NCET), and/or a phlebotomy technician (NCPT). The NCCT also certifies insurance and coding specialists and other health professions. Information is available on the NCCT website at www.ncctinc.com.

OBTAINING ADDITIONAL CREDENTIALS

A medical assistant may need to validate other skills as a condition of employment.

Training in cardiopulmonary resuscitation (CPR) is offered directly through the American Red Cross (ARC) and the American Heart Association (AHA) and by hospitals and other health care agencies. Like other health professionals, medical assistants recertify at the health care provider level every 2 years to be sure their skills are current as required by their professional organization and/or employer. Most health care facilities require current CPR credentials.

Medical assistants may also take courses in performing first aid, hearing tests, limited x-ray examinations, or other specialized tests, depending on state law and the needs of the medical practice. In many areas, medical assistant certification or registration is a valid qualification to perform phlebotomy, but some states and/or institutions require separate certification in phlebotomy. This can be obtained through organizations listed earlier, as well as the American Society for Clinical Pathology (ASCP) or the American Society of Phlebotomy Technicians. The websites of these organizations are listed at the end of the chapter.

A medical assistant who obtains experience working for a podiatrist or an ophthalmologist may want to obtain certification as a podiatric medical assistant, certified (PMAC) or a certified ophthalmic assistant (COA) or technician (COT).

If the medical assistant has specialized in the administrative area, additional credentials can be obtained as a medical administrative specialist. It is also possible to obtain one of the various certifications in medical billing and/or coding with additional education, such as a certified professional coder (CPC) from the AAPC, an organization that specializes in coding training and certification. A medical assistant might also obtain certification as a certified coding associate (CCA), a certified coding specialist (CCS), or a certified coding specialist–physician-based (CCS-P) from the American Health Information Management Association (AHIMA).

CHARACTERISTICS OF MEDICAL ASSISTANTS

Medical assistants possess or develop a number of characteristics that make them effective in their work. Although a person's character and personality have been shaped by heredity and environment, a medical assisting student can work to enhance the traits that are important for health care delivery. Appearance and behavior are also an important means of projecting competence in the medical office (Fig. 2.1).

CHARACTER TRAITS

The most important character traits of a competent medical assistant are dependability, honesty, and tolerance. Character is closely related to the moral and ethical values of an individual. It is often regarded as the true self and reveals itself through actions over time. As an integral part of the office practice, for example, medical assistants must arrive at work on time and be ready to get the day started. Medical assistants who come to work promptly every day demonstrate that dependability is part of their character.

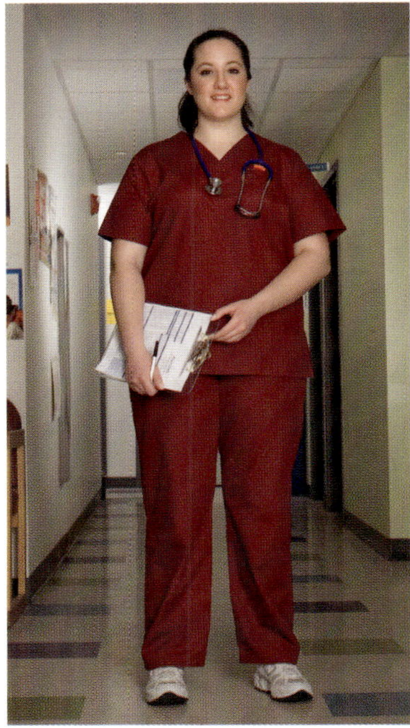

Fig. 2.1 A professional appearance projects competence and increases the patient's confidence in the medical assistant.

A medical assistant projects honesty by working within their "scope of practice"—that is, doing only what they are trained to do and being comfortable in saying "I don't know" or "I don't know how to" when appropriate. State laws regulating the scope of practice for medical assistants vary greatly, so it is important always to be aware of legal restrictions (Procedure 2.1). Medical assistants must always maintain confidentiality and behave ethically. They must recognize that a high level of trust is an important component of high-quality patient care. Tolerance or a willingness to accept the beliefs and practices of others is another important character trait. Tolerance allows medical assistants to work effectively with coworkers and patients from a variety of religious, ethnic, and cultural backgrounds. The patient-centered medical home (PCMH) in primary care emphasizes seeing each patient as a whole person and responding to needs throughout the life span.

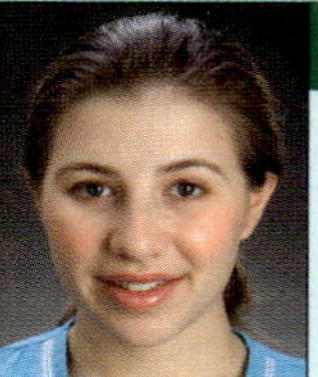

Putting It All Into Practice

My name is Beth Ann Wilson, and I am a certified medical assistant. I attended a medical assistant training program at the community college near my home. I was the first person in my family to go to college, and my family was very proud of me. After the first year (two semesters), I received a certificate in medical assisting, and I found a job in our town at a group practice specializing in obstetrics and gynecology. My instructor encouraged me to take the CMA (AAMA) examination, and I was glad when I found out that I had passed it. I continued to take night classes so that I could get my associate's degree. I also attend the state and local chapter meetings of the AAMA so that I can get the continuing education I need to renew my CMA (AAMA) certification.

When I started working, I spent most of my time at the front desk answering the telephone and checking patients in, but after about 8 months I began to escort patients back to the examination rooms, prepare them for examinations, perform laboratory tests, and assist during examinations. We do some specialized tests in our office, including colposcopy, and I was trained to set up for the test and assist the providers. Janice, our office manager, who is also a CMA (AAMA), has asked me to be responsible for ordering all the supplies for the office and taking inventory. She has also encouraged me to take business courses and attend seminars related to using the electronic health record that we are using. Not too long ago, Janice told me that she is planning to cut back her hours in the spring, and she hopes that I will be able to take over some of her duties in running the practice. That will be a big challenge, but I think I am ready for it. I have a few ideas of my own, and I will be glad for an opportunity to try them out. ■

PERSONALITY TRAITS

Certain personality traits are essential to being a successful medical assistant. Personality is closely related to character, but it refers more to the outward way that a person acts with others. Personality traits include being genuinely interested in helping people; being outgoing, warm, and caring; and having a sense of humor. The ability to remain calm in challenging or difficult situations is also important.

The practice of medicine is one of the "caring professions." Each professional in the medical office needs to have a serious interest in helping people and be able to communicate that when interacting with others. Although the medical assistant must know how to perform the necessary administrative activities effectively and efficiently, the first priority is the care of patients who visit the office.

The concepts of warmth and caring are discussed in more detail in Chapter 4 in the section on communication. For now, it is important to say that being able to interact in a caring manner is a valuable personality trait. Some aspects of caring can be learned and practiced. If an individual does not have a naturally caring personality, they will find it much harder to learn the communication skills needed to express caring.

The ability to put the needs of others first is important. The medical assistant must not allow personal circumstances to interfere with interactions with patients, colleagues, or providers. Remaining objective and concentrating on the situation at hand are important. The patient's needs take precedence over the needs of the medical assistant.

The atmosphere in a medical office may change quickly from calm and orderly to rushed and somewhat disorganized. The medical assistant who can remain calm when things do not go as planned will be more successful than one who is thrown completely off balance by sudden changes in schedule or plans and who becomes emotionally unable to respond effectively.

What Would You Do? What Would You *Not* Do?

Case Study 1

It is a busy Monday and Beth Ann is getting ready to leave the office for her lunch break at 1:30 p.m. when a male provider steps out of an examination room and asks her to assist him with a Pap test and pelvic examination. Beth Ann knows that it is office policy to always have a female staff member in the examination room when a pelvic examination is done. She tells the provider that she is about to go for lunch, but she will find someone to assist him. She goes to the front and finds the receptionist at the desk checking in patients, but neither of the two other medical assistants working that day is in sight. ■

APPEARANCE

Personal appearance influences both the feelings and the behavior of the medical assistant. It also influences the way in which the patients respond to the medical assistant. Psychologists have long recognized the importance of physical appearance. Important judgments are made within seconds of meeting a stranger on the basis of appearance and body language.

When the medical assistant calls a patient to come from the waiting room to the examination or treatment room, the patient immediately forms an impression of the quality of care the medical assistant—and the provider—are going to provide (Fig. 2.2). A medical assistant who is neat, clean, and well groomed projects a sense of professionalism, authority, and competence. When medical assistants are courteous, they project respect for a person's dignity. This is important because many patients feel awkward, especially when dressed in underwear and an examination gown. In the same way, anything that the patient experiences as negative can result in an instant feeling of doubt in the medical assistant's ability. This may be generalized to a general feeling of doubt about all office staff. Patients often react negatively to rumpled clothing, dirty or worn shoes, unpleasant body odor, strong scent from perfume or personal products, piercings, tattoos, or an appearance that seems too "dressed up" because of jewelry, false nails, heavy makeup, and/or elaborate hairstyle.

Most medical offices require that medical assistants wear a uniform when performing clinical tasks. The uniform worn by most medical assistants consists of scrub pants with a scrub top or short-sleeved shirt; clean, white, soft-soled shoes; and a laboratory coat or jacket as needed. The top and/or jacket may be patterned, especially in a pediatric practice. Both top and bottom should fit well without being too tight. Pants should be hemmed neatly so that they do not drag on the ground. In some practices all staff wear coordinated uniforms. When performing administrative tasks, the medical assistant wears scrubs or street clothes. If street clothes are worn, they should project a businesslike appearance (Fig. 2.3). For example, jeans are always unacceptable attire in the medical office.

Neatness and good grooming are also important for health and safety reasons. It can convey professionalism, competency, and confidence and increase the trust of the patient in the medical assistant. Hair carries bacteria, even if regularly washed. Medical assistants who have long hair and perform clinical activities should pull their hair back and tie it, usually in a ponytail. A little bit of makeup can enhance a medical assistant's professional image, but too much is not appropriate for a work environment. Medical assistants should always present a businesslike appearance.

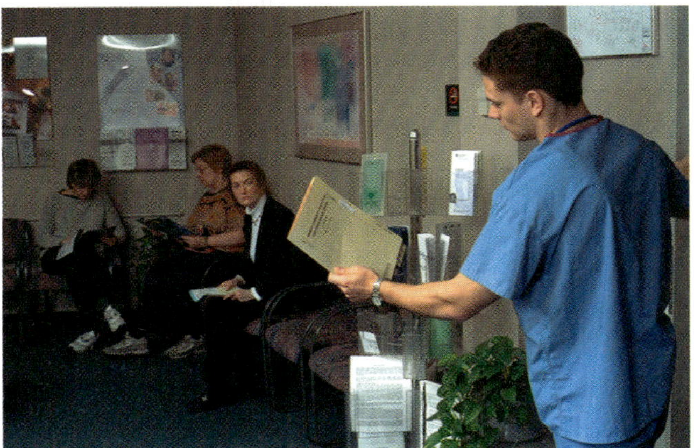

Fig. 2.2 The patient judges the medical assistant's professionalism when called from the waiting room.

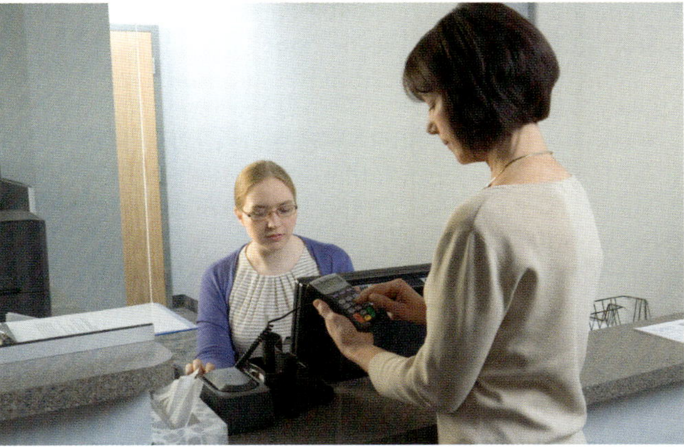

Fig. 2.3 Street clothes may be worn for administrative tasks in some offices.

Medical assistants should maintain scrupulous personal hygiene and avoid perfume or scented personal care products. Many patients have allergies or respiratory problems that can be aggravated by perfumes, colognes, and scented hairspray or deodorants.

Nails should be kept relatively short and should not be polished. Long nails are not functional for keyboard work, patient care, or laboratory procedures. The Centers for Disease Control and Prevention (CDC) recommends that artificial nails not be worn and fingernails be kept ¼ inch or shorter when one is caring for patients at high risk of acquiring infections.

Traditionally, health professionals were allowed to wear only "functional" jewelry—a wristwatch and a plain wedding band—because jewelry is not regularly washed and can become tangled in equipment. Currently, most medical offices allow staff to wear small earrings that do not dangle below the earlobe and necklaces that can be tucked into the shirtfront. Wearing rings other than a plain wedding band is not a good idea. Rings, other than a plain band, can cut through protective gloves or scrape a patient. In addition, they need to be taken off frequently for handwashing. Most medical offices do not allow visible piercings or implants, except for the ears. It may also be a policy of the medical office that visible tattoos and implants (microdermal or subdermal) must be covered. Those on the arms can be covered with a long-sleeved jersey worn under the scrub top or special sleeves designed specifically to cover tattoos or implants. A professional appearance helps to avoid embarrassment during physical examinations and procedures.

INITIATIVE AND BEHAVIORAL SKILLS

Initiative is the ability to begin or follow through on a plan without being supervised. Initiative is an important quality for a medical assistant. The willingness to take initiative and perform tasks that need to be done without being specifically instructed to do so improves the functioning of the office as a whole.

However, initiative does not mean taking over. The office is the provider's place of business, and the provider expects to run it. Initiative does not mean redecorating the waiting room without asking permission. It does mean doing things that need to be done without being asked, keeping up with current issues in practice without being told, and identifying helpful educational opportunities and asking permission to attend. It also means finding useful things to do when the office is slow, such as restocking supplies, ordering supplies, and cleaning out cabinets and cupboards.

Office managers who supervise medical assistant students during practicum relay that some medical assistant students do not take enough initiative. Taking appropriate initiative is an important skill to develop. While in school, students learn to wait for someone to tell them exactly what to do and how to do it. In the workplace the opposite quality is valued. A medical assistant is expected to figure out what needs to be done and how to help out—even during a practicum.

When a medical assistant begins a practicum or a new position, they must learn when to jump in and perform a task without being asked. The task that is most comfortable for the medical assistant to perform may not be the one that shows the most initiative. Medical assistant students can make an independent decision to restock examination rooms or clean the break room if they have no other pressing duties.

Initiative is a quality that employers look for in new medical assistants. An employer may even test a new employee's initiative by showing them how to do something, such as restocking an examination room at the end of the day and then watching to see if the new medical assistant restocks the examination room without being told.

Managing activities, tasks, and schedules efficiently requires attention and effort first as a student and later as a professional medical assistant. This concept of **time management** goes beyond day-to-day use of time to include planning, setting goals, prioritizing, and analyzing the effectiveness of how time has been used.

Getting organized requires a method to keep track of personal, class, and/or work schedules. An effective schedule includes classes, work schedules, meetings, and/or other regular activities, but it can also be helpful to schedule time for specific tasks such as homework (for a student) or preparing an inventory (for a working medical assistant). There is a tendency to put off tasks that seem difficult or unappealing. Scheduling specific times to work on these types of tasks increases the likelihood of completing them so that they are done well and on time.

For class and work activities, it may be helpful to create and update a task list. In its simplest form, this is created daily as a list of tasks to be done; each task is checked off or crossed off when it is completed. Task lists do not have to be limited to a single day, and they can be prioritized, with the tasks placed in order from most important to least important. In analyzing a schedule, some unimportant activities may stand out as items that can be eliminated or reduced in frequency. It may provide a psychological boost to limit the task list to tasks that can really be completed within the allotted time span.

To perform many tasks efficiently, it is important to have easy access to information including names, addresses, and telephone numbers of friends, classmates, or business contacts. Reference materials needed for the job or for schoolwork should also be easily accessible.

There are many tools to facilitate effective use of time, including a personal organizer, or personal planning book, or scheduling and information management software on a smartphone or computer. Address books and reference materials can also be in book or index card format or electronic format.

The willingness to adapt to change is important for medical assistants, as well as all health care workers. The pace of change within ambulatory care is fairly rapid, so it is unwise to become attached to one way of doing things. Changes in equipment, procedures, staff, and setting can occur quite frequently, but patient care needs to remain excellent. When the medical assistant approaches changes with tolerance and even enthusiasm, the office runs more smoothly. The medical assistant needs to adapt to the office setting rather than expecting the office to adapt to their preferences.

Finally, it is important for the medical assistant to work well with others and be a team player. Behavior that enhances patient care includes helping others, maintaining a positive attitude and not complaining, avoiding gossip, working within the established chain of command, and handling stress without losing emotional control or creating emotional scenes. Keeping perspective, accepting corrections or criticism without becoming defensive, and learning from mistakes are important. These behaviors facilitate working with others over the long term with a minimum of discord.

What Would You Do? What Would You *Not* Do?

Case Study 2

Dawn Elliot, a 48-year-old woman, brings her mother, Ruth Mitchell, who is 70 years old, to the office with complaints of vaginal bleeding. The provider asks for blood to be drawn in the office to determine if Mrs. Mitchell has anemia from blood loss. Diane, a medical assistant practicum student who has been working with Mrs. Mitchell, comes to Beth Ann and says, "Can you draw the blood from my patient? She says she doesn't want a student to draw her blood." ■

PROFESSIONALISM

Professionalism is behavior based on a body of knowledge and ethical standards to serve the public. The particular body of knowledge is different for each profession, but ethical standards for professionals are similar.

PROFESSIONALISM FOR MEDICAL ASSISTANTS

The AAMA maintains a Code of Ethics for medical assistants, and the AMT also maintains Standards of Practice that define professional practice. These codes of ethics can be viewed at the websites of each organization.

The medical assistant's ethical responsibilities are to admit mistakes, stay within their training and legal scope of practice, maintain confidentiality, stay current, and uphold the honor of the profession. This may mean having to confront a coworker who is not adhering to such principles.

Dealing with a coworker's inappropriate conduct is difficult, especially for a new employee or if the coworker is higher in the organizational hierarchy. We live in a society that does not like "tattletales." On the other hand, unprofessional behavior in a medical office is disruptive to the concept of teamwork. Even if the unprofessional behavior does not pose an immediate threat to a patient, any behavior that results in people not working well together can lead to an uncomfortable or dangerous situation. The medical assistant should first discuss the situation with the coworker by calmly and objectively describing the actions or behavior that they consider unprofessional. If the person does not correct the situation, it is appropriate to report the behavior to the office manager. If the behavior of a coworker is illegal or threatens the health or safety of others, the medical assistant should report it as soon as possible to the individual's supervisor. Larger institutions often have a safety hotline where both patients and staff can report concerns anonymously. States maintain websites where complaints can be filed if health care professionals are believed to have performed illegal or unethical activities.

What Would You Do? What Would You *Not* Do?

Case Study 3

Before examining Ruth Mitchell, the provider asks Beth Ann to recheck Mrs. Mitchell's blood pressure. It is 190/100 in the right arm and 186/98 in the left arm. Beth Ann notices that the blood pressure had been taken that day by Diane, a medical assistant practicum student, who had recorded it as 130/80. Beth Ann asks Diane if she is confident about the blood pressure reading she obtained from Mrs. Mitchell. Diane says, "It was really faint, and I didn't hear it that well, so I wrote down the same blood pressure as she had the last time she was here. I didn't want to look incompetent. Besides, I was afraid it might affect my grade if you thought I was having trouble hearing the blood pressure." ■

PROFESSIONALISM FOR PHYSICIANS

For physicians, *professionalism* means treating patients based on the body of scientific knowledge the physicians have accumulated, and continue to accumulate, over their working lifetime. In addition, physicians are bound by both ethical standards and legal regulations.

One source of guidance for physicians is the American Medical Association's (AMA's) *Principles of Medical Ethics.* The AMA code of ethics is reviewed and updated periodically by that organization.

Other sources of professional guidance for physicians include the following:

- State and federal regulations
- Regulations of the hospital(s) to which the physicians admit patients
- Any open-panel health maintenance organizations or preferred provider organizations in which the physicians participate
- The national medical board of their specialty or subspecialty

Physicians may have traditionally taken guidance from Hippocrates (c. 460–377 BCE). Hippocrates was an ancient Greek physician who wrote the Hippocratic Oath. The Hippocratic Oath served as a guide to good conduct for ancient physicians, and parts of it are still currently applicable. Its philosophic underpinnings are still taught in medical school and adhered to by physicians, especially the key concept: "First, do no harm."

Each state has its own definition of unprofessional conduct. The state makes the decision on whether to suspend or revoke the physician's license to practice medicine if they have been involved in unprofessional behavior. For more information on unprofessional activities of physicians, and by extension all office staff, see *Highlight on Unprofessional Conduct for a Physician.*

PROFESSIONAL ORGANIZATIONS

The AAMA and the AMT are professional organizations for medical assistants. For an annual membership fee, many benefits are available. Medical assisting students can join either the AAMA or the AMT for a reduced annual rate and receive member services. Membership information is available at the website for each organization.

PEER SUPPORT

Through local and national meetings and workshops, medical assistants are able to enter a network of peers with whom they can share and from whom they can learn. They can also obtain insurance at reasonable cost, professional journals, and access to other sources of information important to the profession.

CONTINUING EDUCATION

With the constant change in the medical field, it is not merely important but necessary to keep skills up to date, attain new skills, and obtain new information about

HIGHLIGHT on Unprofessional Conduct for a Physician

Even if they are not illegal, many activities are considered unprofessional for physicians, and by extension for their employees, including the following:

- Receiving payment for referrals to other physicians, laboratories, treatment centers, or pharmacies. Although physicians often make specific referrals, it is unethical for them to have arrangements to receive payments for those referrals, and especially to refuse to refer a patient unless a payment is made. This practice is sometimes called **fee splitting**. It is also unethical to charge a patient simply for being admitted to a hospital, without any other service being provided.
- Prescribing medication or diagnostic tests for financial gain rather than because of the patient's need for the test.
- Pressuring patients to use pharmacies or laboratories in which the physician has a financial interest. It is also unethical to prescribe medication, tests, or procedures that are not medically necessary. Billing an insurance company for unnecessary procedures is illegal.
- Accepting gifts from pharmaceutical companies or medical equipment manufacturers or suppliers in return for promoting the company's product or prescribing only the company's drug. Physicians may accept inexpensive or educational gifts if allowed by state law with the understanding that they have no obligation to promote the product.
- Allowing another physician or surgeon to perform surgery without informing the patient. The patient has the right to know who is performing a procedure.
- Failing to disclose the source of sperm used for artificial insemination (e.g., husband, sperm bank, paid donor). The physician may not substitute sperm without informing the patient.
- Failing to practice medicine appropriately.
- Practicing medicine under the influence of mind-altering drugs, alcohol, or any prescription medication that may impair mental function, alertness, or physical performance.
- Allowing an unlicensed person to practice medicine.
- Failing to order a consultation regarding any medical problem that is beyond a physician's personal experience and expertise. For example, a gynecologist should not treat a patient for renal failure.
- Withholding information about a patient's medical care from another medical facility just because the patient has an outstanding bill.
- Putting a patient at risk of human immunodeficiency virus (HIV) infection or refusing to treat a patient who is HIV positive.
- Performing a procedure that might transmit HIV to a patient if a physician or any other health care worker is HIV positive.
- Engaging in a sexual relationship with a patient. Something inherent in the relationship between two individuals in which one is perceived to be more influential than the other puts pressure on the "weaker" party to please the more powerful party. Because this makes it difficult to determine if consent is freely given, such a relationship should never be sexual in nature. Sexual relationships between professionals and the people they serve (e.g., physician–patient, attorney–client, teacher–student) are thus considered unethical and unprofessional.

professional practices. Most health professions require a certain amount of continuing education for licensure or certification renewal. These are designed either as contact hours or **continuing education units (CEUs)**. A CEU is a unit of participation in professional continuing education.

Medical assistant contact hours and CEUs can be obtained from educational programs that have been approved by the particular certifying agency. The AAMA validates continuing education programs given through the state and national organization. Attending meetings of professional organizations is the best way to find educational programs specifically for the needs of professional medical assistants. Home study programs are also available to obtain continuing education credit.

An individual must be recertified as a CMA (AAMA) every 5 years. This can be accomplished by retaking the certification examination or by successfully completing the required continuing education programs. Sixty points must be accumulated during the 5-year period: 10 in the administrative area, 10 in the clinical area, and 10 in the general area, with 30 additional hours in any of the three categories. Of these, 30 points must be CEUs (1 contact hour each) from AAMA-approved programs.

RMAs must accumulate 30 points of continuing education every 3 years. (One contact hour is equivalent to one point.) Medical assistants who become certified through other organizations must meet their requirements for recertification.

LEGISLATIVE ADVOCACY

One of the tasks of professional organizations is to monitor legislative initiatives at the state and national levels that may affect the profession. For example, the AAMA petitioned the CMS to designate medical assistants with a national certification as qualified for computerized provider order entry (CPOE) for Stage 2 of Meaningful Use of the electronic health record. This was allowed, and the wording of the CMS Stage 2 Final Rule was updated.

PUBLICATIONS, NEWSLETTERS, AND WEBSITES

Both the national and the state organizations provide a means for communication among professional medical assistants, including *CMA Today*, published by the AAMA, and the *Journal of Continuing Education Topics and Issues*, published by the AMT. The national organizations have state associations, often with several chapters within the state. The state organizations may produce newsletters and maintain websites. Conferences are held annually both nationally and at the state level to enhance communication and contact among members of the profession.

ROLE OF THE MEDICAL ASSISTANT

ADMINISTRATIVE RESPONSIBILITIES

Various administrative responsibilities must be performed on a daily basis in a medical office. We like to think of a provider's office as a place where patients receive medical treatment, but in reality much of the activity in a provider's office involves managing the logistics of scheduling patients, preparing to provide services, and receiving payment for services. The medical assistant may be responsible for a number of these activities, although larger offices may employ specialists to perform these tasks.

1. Scheduling appointments, both over the telephone and in person, is a primary responsibility of the medical assistant. A patient may also need to have appointments made with other medical facilities; examples include a consultation with a specialist, a diagnostic procedure, outpatient surgery, continuing therapy or rehabilitation, and a hospital admission. Some patients may need to schedule multiple appointments with other facilities as the result of a single office visit. The medical assistant must learn the procedure for making and documenting each type of appointment.
2. Maintaining the medical record and filing records and reports have traditionally been some of the medical assistant's roles. With the increasing use of electronic medical records, there is less manual filing in many offices, but it still may be necessary to scan paper reports and keep track of laboratory and diagnostic test results. Each patient encounter with a clinician—physician, nurse practitioner (NP), or physician assistant (PA)—is followed by documentation of the patient's visit. Clinicians may enter information directly into an electronic medical record, or they may create handwritten or dictated patient notes. If the dictation method is used, it may be transcribed using voice recognition software or it may be sent to an outside service electronically. In this case the medical assistant prints the reports after they have been returned and files them after the provider has approved them. The medical assistant may prepare letters and other documents for the provider. Patients often receive printed summaries of their visit before leaving the office.
3. Every patient visit generates activities that are necessary for the provider to be paid for the services provided. The medical assistant must know how to accept and document payments, total and enter charges, code the procedures and/or diagnostic tests performed, and enter payments received. These charges and payments are entered into the office computer to keep track of money owed to and received by the practice. In turn, the charges are used to generate insurance claims and patient bills. In larger offices and clinics, a separate business office usually handles financial matters. Small offices often send billing information to an outside billing service. If billing is performed in the office, the medical assistant must be able to create patient bills and submit insurance claims.
4. On a regular basis, checks and cash need to be deposited into the office's bank account. Preparing bank deposits and recording the deposits in the office's checkbook are activities that medical assistants often perform.
5. Every business has bills to pay. These include rent (or mortgage, if the office is owned), utilities, lease payments on equipment, staff salaries, and a number of other regular payments, such as liability and malpractice insurance. Medical assistants or business office personnel usually pay these bills and maintain records of these and other bills owed by the office. (Some offices have an outside bookkeeping service perform these tasks. Even in offices that pay their own regular bills, salary may be managed by an outside payroll service.)
6. In the patient-centered medical home, the medical assistant may have additional administrative responsibilities to enter health registry data into the medical record and to monitor patient progress by the use of disease-specific registries and tools. Previsit administrative tasks may be more extensive than in other types of medical practices.

CLINICAL RESPONSIBILITIES

Depending on the type of medical office, clinical activities may make up the bulk of the medical assistant's responsibilities. The medical assistant prepares patients for examination, performs diagnostic tests, performs treatments, and assists the provider with examination and treatment.

1. Medical assistants are often asked to collect and process specimens. Some specimens are tested in the office, and others are sent to an outside laboratory.
2. Medical assistants perform several diagnostic tests, such as ECGs and respiratory testing.
3. Medical assistants prepare patients for examination, including taking medical histories, measuring the patient's height, weighing the patient, measuring vital signs, and obtaining information about allergies, current medications, and the chief complaint. Having this done by a medical assistant may allow the provider to see at least one extra patient per hour.
4. After each patient appointment, the medical assistant prepares the examination and/or treatment room for the next patient (Fig. 2.4). This involves making sure that there is fresh paper on the table, the proper instruments and supplies are available for the next examination or procedure, and the necessary equipment is available and in working order.
5. Medical assistants help the provider with examinations and procedures. The medical assistant settles a patient into an examination room and positions and drapes the patient for portions of the examination. Another duty is

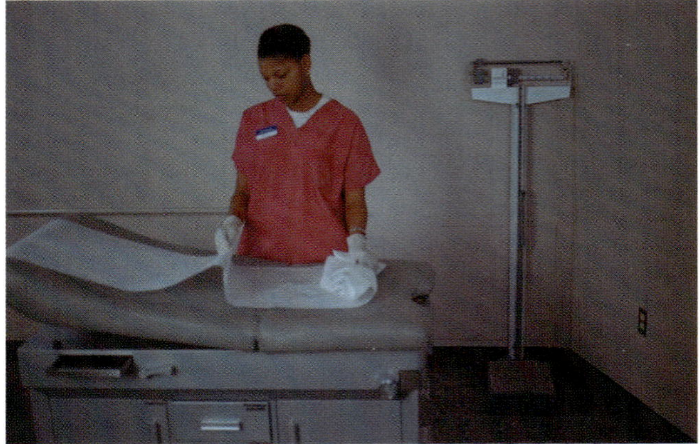
Fig. 2.4 Medical assistant preparing an examination room.

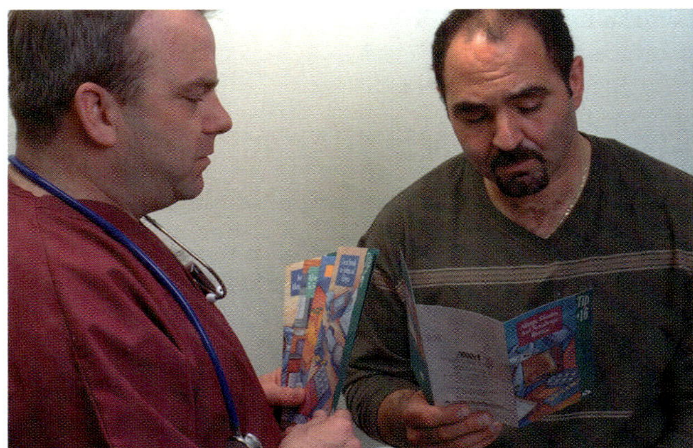
Fig. 2.5 The medical assistant uses brochures to teach a patient.

to pass instruments and supplies to the provider during procedures. The medical assistant may also remove sutures and change sterile dressings. If minor surgery or sterile procedures are performed in the office, the medical assistant sets up the equipment and supplies and then assists the provider as needed.

6. Medical assistants may perform treatments, including nebulizer treatments and application of hot and cold packs or compresses.
7. Medical assistants prepare and administer medications and immunizations depending on state law and office policy. The administration of medication requires concentration and precision. All medications must be documented according to office procedure.
8. Sometimes a medical assistant also has to perform emergency care and administer first aid or assist with an office emergency. This does not happen often, but every medical assistant must be prepared.

MANAGING THE MEDICAL OFFICE

The medical assistant may have many responsibilities to keep the medical office running smoothly.

1. Operational activities involve maintaining the **inventory** of supplies. This can include everything from purchasing tongue blades and gauze to contracting with a uniform service to launder the staff's laboratory coats or patient gowns. It may also involve evaluating and recommending changes in the supplies purchased and evaluating new equipment for potential purchase or lease.
2. A second group of activities involves personnel policy and procedures. Businesses are always reviewing their policies and procedures and updating and revising them as needed. As offices move from one or two providers and a small staff to a larger organization, policies and procedures become more important to standardize the way all employees are dealt with.
3. **Risk management** is the development of policies and procedures that minimize the chances of the practice being sued by a patient or disciplined by a regulatory agency. Every provider's office needs to have one person responsible for risk management, which involves, among other areas, the promotion of health and safety for office personnel and patients, implementation of a quality assurance program, maintenance of proper infection control measures, fire prevention, and the proper disposal of hazardous waste and controlled substances.
4. Record keeping is an important activity for the individual who manages a medical office. In addition to patient records, many other kinds of records must be kept, including office insurance records, quality assurance records, maintenance contracts, personnel records, and financial records.

PATIENT EDUCATION AND COACHING

Instructing and coaching patients are important roles for medical assistants. The medical assistant instructs the patient in several types of situations.

1. The medical assistant is often responsible for educating the patient about office procedures, including giving information to a new patient who is making the first appointment, as well as instructing an established patient whose circumstances have changed.
2. The medical assistant may provide information about maintaining health to patients directly as directed by the provider or by making educational materials available in the office. These are always reviewed by the provider before being given to patients (Fig. 2.5).
3. The medical assistant may teach a patient about ways to manage their disease or condition, especially if the patient is newly diagnosed. For example, a provider might ask a medical assistant to teach a patient how to take their own blood pressure using a sphygmomanometer and a stethoscope and keep a record of the results.

Maintaining the highest possible level of health requires more than knowledge. Patients must be motivated to make healthy choices to maintain their current level of health, as well as to prevent disease and comply with treatment plans prescribed by the provider. **Health coaching** is defined as a process that helps patients to identify their values related to health, set health goals, and take steps to meet their personal goals. Coaching requires listening to patients, validating their concerns, and also encouraging them to make the changes that their own beliefs tell them are important. Medical assistants can work with patients to help them maintain health through proper diet, exercise and rest, and social interaction. They can also assist patients, especially those with risk factors, to take positive steps to prevent disease by identifying a specific target (e.g., a lower cholesterol or low-density lipoprotein [LDL] level), setting goals to meet that target, and following up with the necessary behavior changes. Health coaching can also be an effective way to help a patient stick to a prescribed treatment plan. If the provider has prescribed a regimen of home glucose testing, insulin, and dietary modifications, a medical assistant might coach the patient to improve compliance after initial teaching has been completed. If a patient needs services from the community, the medical assistant may provide brochures from community agencies or locate community resources for a patient—such as an exercise class given without cost at a center for senior citizens—but it might also be necessary to coach the patient to make specific plans to use those services. A patient might also require coaching to adapt to decreased balance or strength by avoiding behaviors that tend to cause falls.

PATIENT NAVIGATION

A **patient navigator** is a person whose role is to remove the obstacles patients face in accessing and receiving treatment. The concept was originally developed in relation to the treatment of cancer, which can involve a maze of doctors' offices, hospitals, outpatient centers, and patient-support organizations, as well as numerous problems with insurance and payment systems. The patient-centered medical home model attempts to coordinate a patient's care through the office of the primary care provider; in this type of office or in any other type of medical office, the medical assistant may function as a patient navigator to help a patient with complex medical needs to access and receive appropriate referrals to community services or additional health care services.

EMPLOYMENT OPPORTUNITIES

According to the U.S. Department of Labor Bureau of Labor Statistics, medical assisting is projected to grow 16% between 2021 and 2031. An increase in the elderly population as baby-boomers age will increase the demand for preventative services. Certification may help to distinguish a medical assistant who meets recognized standards from an entry-level assistant.

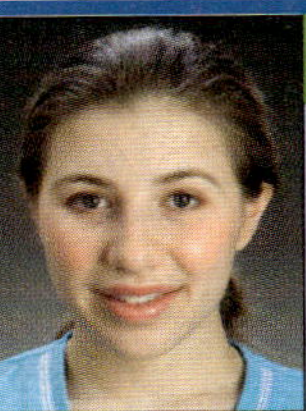

Memories *from* Practicum

Beth Ann Wilson: I couldn't believe how nervous I was before I went to my practicum the first day. I had worked at several jobs and even done filing at a medical office during the summer when I was in high school, but it felt totally different to know that I would be responsible to act like a "real" medical assistant. Fortunately, the staff members at my placement were wonderful. They let me shadow one of the medical assistants until I felt comfortable to work with patients on my own. They were also careful to expose me gradually to each part of the medical office, so it didn't get overwhelming. The person who helped me the most was Cheryl, the office manager. Every day she sought me out and asked how it was going. There was one time when a provider asked me to take out a patient's sutures, and I hadn't even seen someone perform that procedure. I didn't know what to say, but I told him I would find another medical assistant to help him. Then I went to Cheryl. She found someone else to perform the procedure and made sure that I had an opportunity to observe. I never could decide whether I liked checking patients in up front or assisting the providers better, as long as I had a chance to interact with patients. It has always made me feel good to know that I am helping others. ■

The majority of medical assistants work in providers' offices. Other common places of employment include hospitals and offices of other health practitioners, such as chiropractors, podiatrists, and optometrists. Medical assistants also work in outpatient care centers, schools or other educational facilities, medical laboratories, government agencies, insurance companies, employment services, and nursing care facilities.

The median annual income reported by medical assistants in 2021 was $37,190/year $17.88/hour), but salaries vary depending on geographic location, skill level, and type of facility in which the medical assistant is employed.

The most direct route for career advancement is probably to become an office, practice, or department manager. This may require additional education, especially in business administration, but often management skills can be learned mainly on the job. To become a medical assistant instructor, it is necessary to have an Associate in Science degree or a higher degree in a related field and to be a CMA. Clinical advancement usually requires additional training in a formal educational program preparing for a health career, such as dental hygiene, laboratory technology, nursing, radiologic technology, or respiratory therapy.

What Would You Do? What Would You *Not* Do? RESPONSES

Case Study 1
Page 22

What Did Beth Ann Do?
- ❑ Looked for an available staff member.
- ❑ Asked the receptionist if she knew where one of the other medical assistants was.
- ❑ Used the intercom to locate a medical assistant.
- ❑ Checked the examination rooms with open doors to see if a medical assistant might be almost finished checking in a patient.
- ❑ Assisted the provider if she was unable to find another medical assistant to do it.

What Did Beth Ann Not Do?
- ❑ Did not leave for lunch without finding someone to assist the provider.
- ❑ Did not tell the provider that she was sorry she could not assist him at this time.

Case Study 2
Page 24

What Did Beth Ann Do?
- ❑ Agreed to draw the blood without complaining.
- ❑ Tried to make the patient feel comfortable and confident.
- ❑ Explained to Diane later that some patients do not want students to perform certain procedures.
- ❑ Told Diane that she was glad Diane called her to help.
- ❑ Reinforced that even if Diane's pride was slightly hurt, Diane did the correct thing by not showing this to the patient.

What Did Beth Ann Not Do?
- ❑ Did not make the patient feel as if she were asking for special treatment.
- ❑ Did not tell Diane that she looked very young or unprofessional.
- ❑ Did not talk about the incident as a funny story in the break room to other staff.

Case Study 3
Page 25

What Did Beth Ann Do?
- ❑ Told the patient that the provider asked her to recheck the blood pressure because it sometimes changes when patients sit in a quiet examination room.
- ❑ Found a private place to speak to Diane and agreed with her that sometimes it is really hard to hear the blood pressure.
- ❑ Explained to Diane that it is important to take and record the blood pressure correctly even if she has to ask for assistance.
- ❑ Reminded Diane that the staff understands she is a student and will not be able to perform every procedure perfectly.
- ❑ Offered to work with Diane to improve her technique.

What Did Beth Ann Not Do?
- ❑ Did not talk down to Diane or try to make her feel bad.
- ❑ Did not tell others in the office not to rely on Diane's blood pressure measurements.
- ❑ Did not tell the patient that Diane had not been sure of her measurement.

TERMINOLOGY REVIEW

Key Term	Word Parts	Definition
Accreditation		Credit or recognition from a regional or national organization for maintaining certain standards.
Continuing education unit (CEU)		A standard unit of measure of continuing education for professionals defined as 1 contact hour by the AAMA but also commonly 10 contact hours of participation.
Fee splitting		The practice of sharing fees with colleagues, especially for making referrals.
Health coaching		A process that helps patients to identify their values related to health, set health goals, and take steps to meet their personal goals.
Initiative		The ability to begin or carry through a plan of action independently.
Inventory		A complete list and accounting of supplies.
Patient navigator		A person whose role is to remove obstacles that patients face in accessing and receiving treatment.
Practicum		A supervised work experience that is required in an educational program and usually unpaid. Formerly called an *externship.*
Risk management		Processes to protect a health care facility from the risk of legal action.
Time management		Skills and techniques used to manage time to accomplish tasks and meet goals.

PROCEDURE 2.1 Locating and Defining a State's Legal Scope of Practice

Outcome Locate and define the legal scope of practice of one's own state.

Equipment/Supplies:

- Paper
- Pen
- Computer and printer
- Blank index cards

1. **Procedural Step.** Research the legal scope of practice for a medical assistant in your state.
2. **Procedural Step.** Write a brief report summarizing what is included in the scope of practice for the medical assistant and what is not. Include a discussion of the consequences for medical assistants and patients if the medical assistant performs activities that are not included in the legal scope of practice. Describe what procedures can and cannot be delegated to the medical assistant by a physician, by a nurse (nurse practitioner or registered nurse) and by a physician assistant.
   Principle. It is important to know how each state defines (or is vague about) the scope of practice for a medical assistant if one is to practice professionally.
3. **Procedural Step.** Imagine two situations, one in which a medical assistant practices within the legal scope of practice and one in which the medical assistant practices beyond the legal scope of practice. Summarize each on an index card. On the back of the card explain how the situation relates to the scope of practice for a medical assistant.
4. **Procedural Step.** Working in a small group, role-play the situations created by another classmate. When everyone in the group has finished the role play, engage in a group discussion to identify the scenarios that do and do not fall within the legal scope of practice for a medical assistant.
   Principle. Discussion helps a person to clarify and digest new information.
5. **Procedural Step.** Hand in your report and index cards to your instructor.

Ethics and Law for the Medical Office

 Check out the Evolve site at http://evolve.elsevier.com/Bonewit/today to access additional interactive activities and exercises to help you study and prepare for success.

LEARNING OBJECTIVES	PROCEDURES
Ethics and Health Care	
1. Identify key differences between law and ethics.	
2. List reasons for medical assistants to study ethics.	
3. Identify specific rights that patients have in relation to health care.	
4. Correlate the concept of duties to the actions expected of health professionals.	Demonstrating appropriate response to ethical issues.
5. Be a patient advocate.	
6. Report illegal and/or unsafe activities and behaviors affecting patient care to proper authorities.	
7. Describe how certain ethical issues generate ethical conflict in society.	
8. Describe ways to separate and prioritize personal and professional ethics.	Separating personal and professional ethics.
Law and Professional Liability	
9. Identify similarities and differences between public law and private law.	
10. Differentiate between criminal law and civil law.	
11. List and explain the elements of a valid contract.	
12. State the rights and duties of each party in the provider–patient relationship.	
13. Incorporate the Patients' Bill of Rights into personal practice.	Incorporating the Patients' Bill of Rights.
14. Define *standard of care* and describe how this concept affects the behavior of health professionals.	
15. Describe the medical assistant's role in obtaining informed consent.	
16. Explain the principles of negligence and professional negligence as they apply to the behavior of health professionals.	
17. Explain the purpose and need for professional liability insurance.	
Federal and State Laws Affecting the Medical Office	
18. Describe and explain the laws regulating controlled substances and prescription medications.	
19. List and explain several laws that protect employees of medical offices.	
20. Describe how the provisions of the Health Insurance Portability and Accountability Act (HIPAA) affect the medical office.	
21. List and explain the situations where mandatory reporting is required by the medical office.	Reporting illegal activities and comply with public health statutes.
22. Describe how states regulate the practice of medicine and health occupations.	
23. Differentiate between licensing and voluntary accreditation for health care facilities.	

CHAPTER OUTLINE

KEY TERMS

abandonment
advocate (ADD-va-kit)
arbitration
autonomy (ah-TAH-noe-mee)
beneficence (ben-IH-fih-sens)
civil law
cloning (KLOH-ning)
controlled substance
crime
criminal law
defendant
do-not-resuscitate (DNR) orders
Drug Enforcement Administration (DEA)
duty
emancipated minor
ethics
expressed consent
felony
fidelity
fraud
gene therapy
genetic engineering
health care proxy (PROX-ee)
implied consent
informed consent
liability
license
licensure (LI-sen-sur)
litigation (lih-tih-GAY-shun)
living will
locum tenens (LOW-come TEN-ens)
malpractice
mature minor
mediation
medical durable power of attorney
misdemeanor (mis-de-MEAN-or)
morals
negligence (NEG-lih-jhens)
nonmalfeasance (non-mal-FEE-suns)
patient incompetence
plaintiff (PLANE-tiff)
prescription
prudent
reciprocity (re-sip-RAW-city)
res ipsa loquitur (ress-IHP-sah LOW-kwee-tour)

respondeat superior (ray-SPON-day-at sue-PEER-ee-or)
right
risk management
standard of care
statute (STA-chewt) of limitations
stem cells
subpoena (su-PEE-na)
subpoena *duces tecum* (su-PEE-na DEW-chess TAY-come)
tort
veracity (ver-ASS-ih-tee)

INTRODUCTION TO MEDICAL ETHICS

A democratic society tolerates a wide range of beliefs about **morals** (beliefs about what is right and wrong) and creates rules to regulate public behavior using laws created by the democratic process. Change and flexibility are possible because laws are continually reviewed through the judiciary process.

It is important to remember that society's beliefs about right and wrong precede laws and also influence their interpretation. Currently the rapid pace of technologic innovation and changing beliefs places considerable stress on the social structure.

There is also a wide diversity of expectations about normal, acceptable behavior, sometimes called etiquette or manners. Breaches of etiquette pose no true threat to the integrity of an individual or society. However, individuals may have just as strong an emotional reaction to what they see as bad manners as they would have to a true ethical breach.

In the context of the medical office, a patient may feel that being rushed by the provider and treated "as a number, not a name" by the front office staff is being treated without dignity. The patient's emotional response to how they are treated may seem more important than the actual quality of care.

REASONS TO STUDY ETHICS

The branch of knowledge that deals with standards of behavior or beliefs is called **ethics**. Although it is an abstract discipline, medical assistants should study ethics for a number of reasons.

First, it is an important part of an individual's education to develop the intellectual skills needed to analyze complex problems and justify the choices made in particular situations. In the case of ethics, the choice is between alternative courses of action that have moral and social consequences.

Second, as society has become increasingly complex, average citizens are more aware that choices affect not only people living now but also those who will live in the future. People hesitate to see only elected and appointed officials dealing with these choices. Learning about ethics and social issues encourages ordinary people to have input into social beliefs and expectations. There is also a greater sense of interconnectedness involving the whole world, sometimes called *globalism*. Many individuals feel some level of responsibility for all human beings and indeed for all living beings.

Third, in the specific realm of medicine and science, often referred to as bioethics, more sophisticated medical treatment and new technologies are constantly becoming available. However, society does not have unlimited resources to provide everything to everyone, even in the developed world. There is a need to make informed choices about what care will be provided to whom and when rather than simply responding to special interests.

Fourth, every year new biomedical research makes it possible to do more things with which the world has no previous experience. Society must have informed citizens who can analyze issues and guide the future. Within the health care system, health professionals, including medical assistants, must be able to consider ethical questions as they strive to improve health care for individuals as well as society as a whole.

ETHICS AND HEALTH CARE

ETHICAL CONCEPTS

Current thinking about biomedical ethics identifies several rights (very strong claims) for patients and duties (requirements) for the institutions and individuals who provide health care. The sources of these ideas include religious traditions, social belief systems, and political documents such as the Declaration of Independence, the U.S. Constitution, and the Bill of Rights as well as ethical theories developed by individual philosophers.

Rights

A **right** is a claim that is expected to be honored. It is stronger than a wish or a need.

The early leaders of the American government believed in natural rights and the duty of any government to preserve them. Natural rights were considered to exist through the natural order or to be granted by God. Such rights include the following:

1. Right to life
2. Right to privacy
3. Right to autonomy
4. Right to the means to sustain life

Right to Life

One of the rights mentioned in the Declaration of Independence is the right to life.

Since the 1970s, the term *right to life* has come to be associated with the movement against abortion. But in a broader context it reflects the belief that no human being has the right to kill another. A belief in the right to life is found in all major religions and traditions.

The right to life has many implications for medicine. Historically, physicians and other health care workers were prohibited from harming patients because this could threaten patients' lives. They could not assist with suicide; this is expressly stated in the Hippocratic Oath. In the United States today, however, many individuals want some control over their own deaths, including the choice of suicide assisted by a physician.

Two important areas of conflict appeared in the middle of the 20th century. First, advances in medical care made it possible to keep people alive even though they could not recover their health. Sometimes this extension of life came at the cost of prolonged suffering.

Second, the absolute right to life of an unborn fetus conflicts with the right of a woman to control her own reproductive capacity. Birth-control methods, artificial conception methods, and abortion, are measures aimed at controlling the size of a family. Many women and their physicians have come to believe that they have a right to make decisions related to reproduction, including use of available technology, as they see fit.

Right to Privacy

The U.S. Supreme Court has ruled that there is an implicit right to privacy in the Bill of Rights, specifically in the Fourth Amendment. A series of court decisions affirming a woman's right to use mechanical birth control and to have an abortion hinged on justices' perceiving this right to privacy.

Patient confidentiality, which has been upheld by courts, is another manifestation of the right to privacy. Patient confidentiality is discussed in detail later in this chapter.

Right to Autonomy

Currently medical ethics takes the position that individuals have the right to **autonomy**, which means the right to make independent decisions about their health care according to their individual values and concerns without constraint or coercion by others. This right is preserved even when the individual's decisions do not match the values of the medical community or the individual provider. The right of autonomy is the basis for **informed consent**, which is consent based on the understanding of a medical procedure and its possible outcomes. Health care professionals must provide their patients with complete information so that those patients will be able to make informed decisions. The patient must have the mental capacity to reason and consider alternatives. Because of this, the law limits the autonomy of children or individuals with decreased mental capacity, such as the mentally retarded or individuals whose mental capacity has been impaired by illness, those acting under the influence of drugs or alcohol, and those experiencing a mental illness.

Respect for autonomy does not derive from the Hippocratic Oath. Rather, it comes from the thinking of European philosophers such as Immanuel Kant and John Locke.

Right to the Means to Sustain Life

Every society must grapple with the problem of equitable distribution of goods and services to its citizens and how to regulate that distribution over time.

This is not a problem when the supply is adequate or when supply is greater than demand. For instance, in ordinary circumstances the supply of oxygen is more than adequate to meet the needs of the entire population.

It is when the amount of a particular resource is less than the desire for that resource that problems develop. In this case, resources are said to be scarce, and the society's government may take measures to determine who will have access to the scarce resources.

At a minimum, every individual should have access to what is necessary to sustain life and preserve human dignity. Consideration of justice in distribution and access is especially important in social and political movements. Any society must find ways to respond to need while also rewarding contribution and providing for stability within the social system.

Duties

A **duty** is a commitment to act in a certain way on the basis of religious beliefs, moral principles, or a particular professional code of conduct. Traditionally, five main duties of a health care professional have been identified.

Putting It All Into Practice

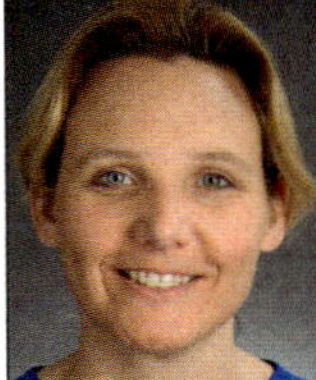

My name is Vicki Edmonds, and I have worked in a family practice for about 6 years. There are two physicians and two nurse practitioners in my practice, and I usually assist one of the physicians. Of course, if it is busy or one of the other medical assistants is ill, we all pitch in and help out. Neither of the physicians in my practice has ever been sued, and we all work together to be sure it stays that way. We do everything we can so that our patients not only receive great care but also are satisfied with their treatment. We also document everything carefully because our physicians are aware that you cannot prove that care was given if it isn't documented. Every once in a while, we have a patient who constantly misses appointments or doesn't take their medication, and if the physician thinks that it is harmful to the patient's health, sometimes he will instruct the patient to find another practitioner to care for them. I remember one time when the patient lived far away and she said that it was difficult for her to make the trip to our office. After she missed three appointments in a row, the physician had me write a letter suggesting that she find another physician nearer her home. He explained that he couldn't be responsible for her if she was unable to keep appointments. In the letter he gave her a month to find another physician, and he offered to help her if she was having difficulty. We sent that letter by certified mail and obtained a return receipt. Then we documented everything in the patient's medical record. The patient sent a letter back saying that she was going to an office much closer to home and she thought that this would work out better for her. ■

Do No Harm

The concept of **nonmalfeasance** means, first of all, doing no harm in any treatment given. This duty is found in the Hippocratic Oath. It is not taken in a literal sense, because many treatments can have adverse effects. Rather, it is taken to mean that medical benefits should outweigh adverse effects.

This concept applies especially to scientific research. Guidelines for ethical research not only require informed consent but also restrict research with possible harmful effects to those patients whose conditions are so serious that doing nothing is likely to be as dangerous as the treatment or procedure being studied.

Do the Best Possible

The concept of **beneficence**, doing the best possible, is seen in some systems of ethics as a separate duty, whereas in others it is considered an extension of doing no harm. It is often difficult to pinpoint exactly what harm and good are; they may vary with a particular individual's viewpoint.

Be Faithful to Reasonable Expectations

The concept of **fidelity**, being faithful, comes from the Latin term *fides,* which means "faith." In the case of medical practice, fidelity is usually interpreted as meaning being faithful to reasonable expectations. Although patients' expectations vary, there is general agreement that a patient can reasonably expect to be treated with dignity by competent providers who honor their agreements. Patients can also expect that they will be cared for by individuals who adhere to the ethical standards of their profession, to statutory law, and to accepted medical and scientific practice.

Be a Patient Advocate

The concept of fidelity includes the expectation that patients' needs come first. An **advocate** is a person who intercedes on behalf of another person. A medical assistant functions as an advocate for patients by suggesting appropriate community referrals to the physician, by making sure that all insurance claims are complete, by following up to help patients receive insurance coverage if additional information will make that possible, and in general by working to protect patients' rights.

To protect patients' safety, it may even be necessary for a medical assistant to report unsafe or illegal behavior to proper authorities, including errors in patient care. The first step is always to follow up within the organization by documenting and reporting to the supervisor any incident or situation that could cause harm. If no action is taken after a reasonable period of time, the situation should be reported to the next person in the chain of command. If a medical assistant has followed up within the organization without resolution of an unsafe or illegal situation, they should report the incident to the appropriate government agency. Information about professionals whose **licenses** have been revoked or suspended is available online in many states.

Tell the Truth

The concept of **veracity** has increased in importance since the 19th century. Veracity is not found in the Hippocratic Oath. It has developed with the evolution of the scientific tradition. Today it is seen as a proactive duty—physicians and other health care professionals must provide truthful information without having to be asked. It is a tenet of modern science that scientific knowledge belongs to all. Results of experiments must be accurate and reviewed by other scientists to see if the results can be replicated; then they should be published for the benefit of all.

Give Each Person a Fair Share

The concept of *justice* requires that each individual be given their due and implies that they deserve a fair share of resources. However, there is often an underlying belief that an individual must contribute or bear a portion of the burden before being allowed to obtain certain resources. Justice in the context of medical practice appears not only in terms of distribution of medical resources but also in a belief in the right to compensation should a mistake be made.

Deciding what is "fair" is difficult because different situations may require different guidelines. In the United States, the tendency is to believe in "first come, first served." But in an emergency department, serious conditions must take precedence.

What Would You Do? What Would You *Not* Do?

Case Study 1

Denise Fitzgerald, a 16-year-old girl, has come to the office with complaints of a sore throat and fever. While Vicki is taking vital signs, she notices a circular wound on Denise's arm that looks like a cigarette burn. It is red and has some crusted areas. When she asks Denise about it, the patient blushes and says in a low voice that her boyfriend burned her a few days ago to teach her a lesson. Then Denise says, "Please don't tell the doctor because he will tell my mother, and I'm afraid she will make me break up with my boyfriend." ■

ETHICAL CONFLICT

Many issues become controversial when there is a disagreement within society about the relative hierarchy of certain rights and duties.

Reproductive Issues

Conflict surrounds the issues of contraception, abortion, and others related to reproduction. With regard to pregnancy, some people feel that the duty to follow divine law or natural measures takes precedence over an individual's right to autonomy. This results in differing beliefs about how appropriate it is to use contraception and artificial measures to become pregnant. There has been controversy about the "morning-after pill." The pill is taken as soon as possible after having had sex, if the woman's method of birth control is unreliable or unused. It could also be used if a woman has been sexually assaulted. It has been found to be relatively safe and was approved as an over-the-counter medication for women older than age 18 by the U.S. Food and Drug Administration (FDA) in 2006.

Another controversial issue is abortion. Some argue that the fetus's right to life outweighs the woman's right to privacy in determining—with her physician—the proper course of her medical care. Since the original U.S. Supreme Court decision in 1973 upholding a woman's right to obtain an abortion in any state *(Roe* v. *Wade),* the Court has been called on to rule many times on various state laws that seek to limit this right. The Partial-Birth Abortion Ban Act of 2003, which prohibits a specific abortion procedure that can be done in the second trimester of pregnancy, is an example of a federal law that restricts a woman's right to abortion in some cases. It was upheld in the Supreme Court case of *Gonzales* v. *Carhart* in 2007. In June of 2022 the U.S. Supreme Court reversed its decision on *Roe* v. *Wade*. This reversal means that there is no longer a constitutional right to abortion. At the time of the writing of this chapter there is much debate going on about this decision.

Stem Cell Research

A promising area of research for medical treatment involves the use of embryonic **stem cells.** These cells, taken from fetal tissue, can mature into different types of tissue. Embryonic cells may be able to reduce or possibly even reverse the symptoms of Parkinson disease and other diseases.

An ethical conflict arises because the cells of live human embryos may be killed in the course of research. In addition, embryonic cell tissue may be harvested from aborted fetuses or fertilized ova not used for in vitro fertilization. Researchers who use fetal tissue stress that they use only tissue from spontaneous abortions (miscarriages). Antiabortion advocates argue that if there is an increased need for fetal tissue, a time may come when a woman might be influenced in her decision regarding whether or not to have an abortion if she could sell her fetus's tissue for research and/or treatment.

Adult stem cells can also be used to treat certain conditions. There is not quite the versatility with adult stem cells as there is with embryonic stem cells. If stem cells are taken from the skin, bone marrow, or brain it will develop into those types of cells, i.e. stem cells from the brain will make more brain cells. This is still an important part of stem cell therapy. There is little ethical controversy about research on adult stem cells.

Genetic Engineering and Cloning

A number of ethical issues surround the practices of **genetic engineering** (making, altering, or repairing genetic material) and **cloning** (reproducing genetically identical cells or individuals).

One is the issue of genetically engineered crops and other food products. This encompasses practices as diverse as injecting milk cows with growth hormones to get them to produce more milk, to incorporating material from bacteria into plant seeds. Opponents argue that we cannot predict all of the possible effects of manipulating genetic material and are likely to see unexpected and unwanted consequences to ourselves or other species.

Gene therapy is a term used for experimental treatments that attempt to treat or cure disease by giving patients new genes or parts of genes that may have been synthesized in the laboratory, taken from human tissue, or engineered from the genetic material of animals or other species. Research efforts are overseen by the Recombinant DNA Advisory Committee of the National Institutes of Health (NIH). One of the problems with advances in gene therapy is that treatment for one individual can be extremely expensive and yet the treatment may not restore complete function.

Human cloning is prohibited by several states, but efforts to pass legislation on the federal level have not succeeded to date. Experiments in animal cloning continue, although critics claim that it results in unhealthy animals and needless suffering.

Refusing or Withholding Treatment and Physician-Assisted Suicide

The right to refuse treatment is well established for adults. The 1990 Patient Self-Determination Act (PSDA) establishes the duty of hospitals, nursing homes, and health maintenance organizations (HMOs) to inform patients or new subscribers of their right to express their wishes related to health care and to refuse treatment. The act also establishes the right of an individual to prepare an advance directive that specifies what treatments they would like to receive, and what ones they would not wish to receive if the individual were to become incapable of making those decisions at a later time. Courts have held an individual's right to refuse treatment in such high regard that they have allowed mentally ill patients to refuse treatment for their mental illness.

When an individual requires resuscitation or life support to stay alive, there may come a point where the treatment seems to be resulting in more suffering (harm) than benefit. This is especially true if it is unlikely that the person could recover their health or normal function. If there is a written document expressing the person's wishes, life support may be removed or discontinued. In the absence of an advance directive, an individual's family may bring to court a petition to remove life support. Such a petition must be supported by witnesses other than those who file the petition, stating that the incompetent individual expressed a desire to avoid being kept alive by artificial means. Life support has been interpreted to include ventilators, antibiotics, and even tube feedings.

Physician-assisted suicide and euthanasia (literally, "good death"), sometimes called *mercy killing,* evokes fears that the power to take life will be abused—that it will be used more for the convenience of others than for the well-being of those who are dying. Advocates for the disabled have argued that allowing physician-assisted suicide or euthanasia could be the first step in society's determining that the severely disabled are too much of a financial and physical burden and therefore having them euthanized.

In 1997, Oregon became the first state to legalize physician-assisted suicide, allowing physicians to write a prescription for a patient of a lethal dose of pain killer or other medication. The physician is not allowed to administer the medication. The U.S. Supreme Court upheld a challenge to the Oregon law in 2006. Discussion regarding physician-assisted suicide occurs in every state, but to date only five other states (Washington, Montana, Vermont, Colorado, California), and the District of Columbia allow physician-assisted suicide. Most other states have specific laws prohibiting assisted suicide, and a few states prohibit it by common law. Patients with a terminal illness and their families are often looking for a trusted advisor with whom they can discuss their fears and concerns. Even when a physician is not morally willing or legally able to provide a means for a patient to end their life, there is increasing recognition of the value of frank discussion and reassurance that patients will not be left to cope alone.

Advance Directives

On the basis of personal beliefs, patients can formalize their decisions about treatment in terminal or end-of-life situations in a number of ways. These include **do-not-resuscitate (DNR) orders**, living wills, health care proxies, and organ donor cards, all of which fall under the heading of "advance directives" (Box 3.1). An advance directive may specify care to be given or avoided and name a person to make medical decisions for the individual should they become incompetent. This is usually a spouse, child older than age 18, member of the clergy, or close friend. Medical advance directives should always name a single individual to make decisions, with an alternative if possible. This is often a difficult choice, especially for an elderly person with several children (Fig. 3.1). In addition, the patient may want to provide for the donation of any useful organs. Organ donation (or donation of one's entire body) and procedures for determining who may give permission if the patient has not left a directive are outlined in the Uniform Anatomical Gift Act. The PSDA of 1990 requires hospitals, nursing homes, HMOs, and other facilities to provide information about advance directives to patients.

Signed originals rather than photocopies of the advance directives should be held by the named surrogate, and the patient should keep copies with their important papers. It should also be noted in the primary care physician's records with a copy, if possible, so that the surrogate can be contacted if necessary.

DNR orders should be in the medical record, and the staff should be informed of the patient's wishes. If the patient is at home, the family must have a copy of the DNR order to show emergency personnel, who otherwise will be legally obliged to resuscitate the patient.

Removal of life support means that no form of support—including mechanical breathing, feeding, or medications to prolong life—should be given. If necessary, pain medication and sedation are continued after the removal of life support.

A **living will** is a document executed by an individual that gives medical professionals instructions about how they wish to be treated in the event of becoming incompetent.

BOX 3.1 Advance Directives

Do-Not-Resuscitate Order

Requested by either a patient or health care agent. A written order from the provider in the patient's medical record that allows medical staff not to resuscitate in the event of cardiac or respiratory arrest.

Living Will

Executed by an individual before or during illness. Identifies the patient's wishes about which life-prolonging actions should or should not be taken. In states that accept it, it provides instructions to health professionals about treatment to be provided and may include instructions to a health care agent as to which treatments they should authorize. Provisions for organ donation, autopsy, or donation of remains to a medical school are also usually included in a living will.

Health Care Proxy

Executed by an individual before or during illness. Names a health care agent who has the ability to make decisions about care, including signing a do-not-resuscitate order. It may also outline the types of care that the individual does or does not wish to receive. It becomes effective only when the individual becomes incapable of making their own decisions.

Durable Power of Attorney

Provides a written authorization to act on the behalf of another that remains in effect even if the grantor becomes incapacitated. An ordinary power of attorney, used in business affairs, expires when a person becomes incapacitated. An authorization limited to health care decisions only is called a *durable power of attorney for health care decisions* or a **medical durable power of attorney**.

Organ Donation Status

Authorization to donate organs after death either by signing up with a website or including in a license application. Many states have done away with a separate organ donor card, preferring to place the organ-donor designation on an individual's driver's license or ID card. If a person has signed up using a state database, a separate card is not usually issued.

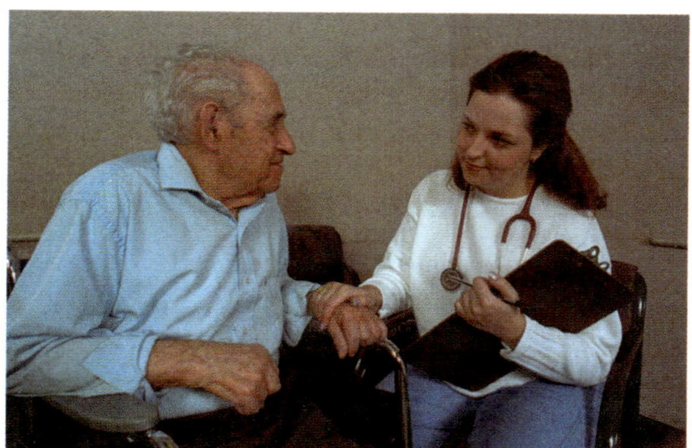

Fig. 3.1 Elderly patients are grateful when office staff respond to their fears and concerns.

A living will may also give instructions regarding organ donation, autopsy, or donation of the remains to a medical school for anatomy dissection. Many states allow an individual's wishes to donate organs to be noted on their driver's license or on an organ donor card that can be carried in one's wallet. In the event of a fatal auto accident, the police—who usually use the license or other documents to make identification—can notify ambulance personnel that the deceased is an organ donor.

A person usually names an agent to carry out their wishes if they are unable to do so. A **health care proxy** names the person who is charged with this responsibility and may also give specific instructions to the designated person concerning medical issues. Laws regulating living wills and health care proxies vary from state to state, and it is important for patients to use forms that will be valid where they live. This may require the assistance of an attorney.

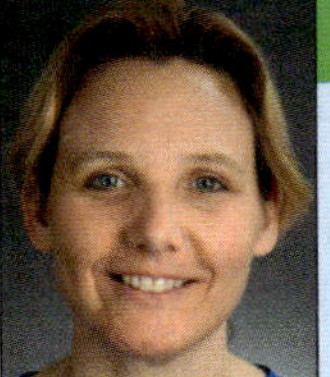

Memories *from* Practicum

Vicki Edmonds: When I was at my practicum at a clinic affiliated with a community hospital, the employees were implementing a plan for the providers to discuss advance directives with all patients. They hoped to have each patient prepare a written health care proxy and provide the office with a copy. As we viewed each patient's medical record for the visit, we checked to see if there was already a completed form. If not, we printed a blank health care proxy form and had it available for the provider to give to the patient. Then, when patients checked out, we would remind them to return the completed form. At first I found this embarrassing because it seemed like such a private thing. Then one of our elderly patients told me that she was so grateful that her husband had signed a health care proxy before he had a stroke, which left him completely paralyzed and unable to speak. She said that the discussions they had had when he was preparing the form had helped her understand exactly what his wishes were. On the basis of those discussions, she had asked the hospital staff not to resuscitate him if he stopped breathing or his heart stopped. She told me that before they talked about it, she would not have been comfortable making that decision. I was impressed by this patient's ability to talk frankly about her family's preparations to face serious illness, and I was grateful because it helped me become more comfortable with the subject. ■

PERSONAL, PROFESSIONAL, AND ORGANIZATIONAL ETHICS

It is important to distinguish between personal and professional ethics. In the work situation, professional ethics usually takes precedence over personal ethics and morals. For example, a medical assistant may believe that a parent who is paying the medical bill should be given the results of laboratory tests done on their child. Legally, however, after age 18, information about a patient can be given only with the patient's consent. In this case, professional ethics requires that the medical assistant follows the law to maintain patient confidentiality no matter what they believe personally.

Acting according to professional ethics means that the medical assistant cannot ethically withhold from the physician information given by the patient related to the medical condition. Even if the medical assistant does not agree with how the physician is managing a patient's care, the medical assistant cannot ethically (or legally) suggest another treatment plan for the patient.

It is important to clarify one's personal set of ethics, moral values, and beliefs and identify areas where there may be potential conflict with professional ethics to avoid having to make a difficult decision on the spot. The medical assisting student should determine their own personal beliefs related to issues of potential ethical conflict. Then they should decide what professional ethics requires in those situations (Procedure 3.1).

An individual or medical practice can look to a professional organization for guidance related to ethical questions. Medical associations publish guidelines related to medical ethics. Professional associations for medical assistants can be a source of information and guidelines. For problems affecting the medical office, a discussion including all office staff may assist in decision making (Fig. 3.2).

Organizational ethics includes the guidelines of an entire organization that influence the policies of the organization and conduct of employees in the workplace. An organization's mission statement is usually the best place to identify the specific principles and guidelines that are most important to it. The policy and procedure manual provides specific guidelines as well. In addition, there are several generally accepted principles for organizations. No organization should depend on unfair means to earn money. Employees should not manipulate or falsify information. Monetary transactions should be fair. Employees should not take or use office property for their own benefit. Employees should be treated fairly, and they should not be exploited. Employees should not be exposed to hazardous conditions without being provided with the means to protect their own safety (Procedure 3.2).

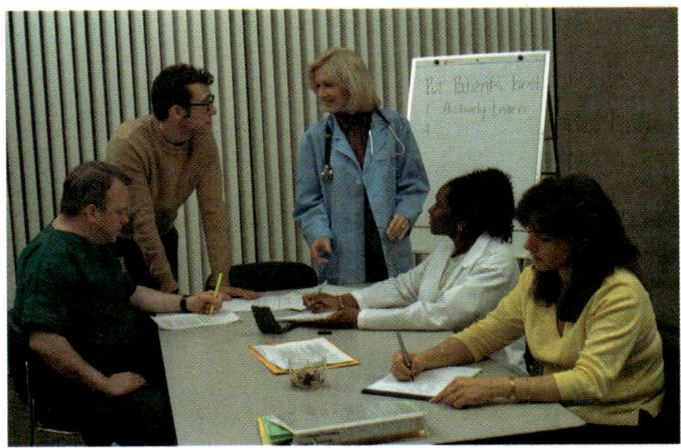

Fig. 3.2 A staff meeting to discuss problems affecting the medical office may be helpful.

INTRODUCTION TO LAW

DIFFERENCE BETWEEN PUBLIC LAW AND PRIVATE LAW

The legal system in the United States is primarily divided into two parts, public law and private law. *Public law* refers to laws that define the relationship between the individual and society as a whole. The term **criminal law** is used to refer to the set of laws that protect society. Examples include laws against robbery, rape, and operating a motor vehicle while under the influence of alcohol or a controlled drug. Private law, also called **civil law**, comprises the laws that deal with relationships and disputes between individuals and/or groups of people. This may involve two individuals or groups of people; individuals and corporations, government, or other organizations; or it may involve one corporate, government, or organizational entity and another such entity. Contracts are considered a part of civil law, and disputes about contracts that go to court are tried as part of the civil court system.

LAWSUITS

Both civil and criminal action disputes can lead to lawsuits that are tried in the court system. In any court proceeding, there is a **plaintiff**, the person or entity that makes the complaint, and a **defendant**, the person or entity against whom a lawsuit is brought. In a criminal lawsuit, the plaintiff is the district's or state's attorney, a representative of the government. In a civil lawsuit, the plaintiff is the injured party.

In criminal law, the criminal activity itself is held to be harmful or potentially harmful to society or individual members of society. The act itself is punishable regardless of whether anyone was actually harmed by the act. In civil law, an injury or damage that results because of someone's wrongful act results in **liability** (legal responsibility). The same misdeed can provoke both a criminal charge and a civil lawsuit. The criminal lawsuit will determine if the person is guilty of committing a crime punishable by an imprisonment or fine paid to the government. The civil lawsuit will determine what liability the person has to the injured party, if any.

A well-known example of this dual legal picture is the O. J. Simpson case. Simpson was found not guilty by a jury of the murder of his ex-wife, Nicole, and her friend, Ronald Goldman. However, her estate filed a civil suit against him on the grounds of "wrongful death." In the civil case, he was found liable for their deaths, and more than 30 million dollars was awarded in damages. In a criminal case the charge must be proven "beyond a reasonable doubt," but in a civil case the burden of proof is only to a level at which the supporting evidence is more convincing than the opposing evidence ("a preponderance of the evidence").

SPECIALIZED AREAS OF LAW

Specialized areas of law include constitutional law, international law, and administrative law. Constitutional law is the study of the law of countries and other political organizations. International law concerns the relationships among countries and includes maritime law and regulations applying to ocean-going vessels. Administrative law arises from the actions of federal government agencies, such as the Social Security Administration and the Internal Revenue Service.

CREATION OF LAWS

Law was created by tradition through accepted social practices and decisions of the courts. Today most laws are created through a vote by a legislative body. Legislators are elected by popular vote to serve in either the state or the federal legislature. One of their important duties is to draft and vote on new legislation, which is called a *bill* while it is under consideration. Once passed by either the House of Representatives or the Senate, a bill that contains several parts becomes an *act*. Once passed by both houses, the act is signed into law by the president (for a federal law) or a state governor (for a law applicable to one state). Cities and towns can also enact laws, called *ordinances*; these usually have to do with local issues, such as smoking in public places, parking, leash laws for pets, and curfews at parks.

All employees of the medical office must be aware of the federal and state laws that regulate the provision of health care and insurance reimbursement as well as those related to the operation of a business.

CRIMINAL LAW

The branch of law that describes offenses against the public welfare is called *criminal law*. A **crime** is an offense in violation of a law that prohibits or requires certain behavior. When a person is convicted of a crime (or pleads guilty to a crime), punishment is imposed. A **felony** is a serious crime punishable by death or imprisonment in a state or federal penal institution for more than 1 year. A **misdemeanor** is a less serious crime punishable by a fine or imprisonment for less than 1 year, often in a local or county penal institution.

Nonviolent Crimes

Occasionally a provider is charged with manslaughter or criminal **negligence** if a patient dies or sustains serious injury as a result of incorrect or negligent treatment. This is usually in addition to a civil lawsuit brought by the patient or family for wrongful death (see the discussion of professional malpractice later in this chapter). Euthanasia and assisted suicide—except for physician-assisted suicide in states that allow it—are usually considered murder whether performed by a health professional or family member.

Two or more people who have joined together to commit an unlawful act may be accused of conspiracy; this may be applied to actions that are illegal in and of themselves or actions to prevent detection of a prior crime.

Stealing another person's property (without violence) is called *larceny*. In the medical office, this may take the form of *embezzlement*—appropriation of funds from a client, customer, or employer.

A growing problem in the health care industry is **fraud**—deliberate deception carried out to secure unfair or unlawful gain. Billing for services not provided, billing for services provided to imaginary patients, performing unneeded services, and even deliberately using codes from a higher level of service than what was provided are all forms of insurance fraud. Every instance of such a billing can be considered a separate act. If the fraud involves the use of mail (mail fraud) or electronic resources (wire fraud), it becomes a federal offense.

In the mind of an office employee, there may be a difference between billing an insurance company using a code for more complex service than was actually provided, "because they pay us so little anyway," and billing for procedures that were never performed. But from a legal perspective, both are considered fraud; if proved, both carry serious penalties.

Insurance companies and agencies of the federal and state governments are victims of billions of dollars in fraudulent claims each year. They have increasing incentives to investigate health care facilities they suspect of fraudulent billing.

CIVIL LAW

The branch of law that regulates interactions among individuals, groups, organizations, and the government is civil law. Disputes arise when one individual or group believes that the actions of another individual or group have caused personal injury or damage to property. In medical offices these usually relate to the actual care received by the patient and/or the relationship between the patient and the provider or office staff. Two types of obligations that may give rise to civil lawsuits are contracts and torts.

Contract law involves agreements between two or more parties and these are discussed in detail later. If a contract exists, failure to meet the terms of the contract by either party is called a *breach of contract.* A **tort** is an injury or wrong against a person or property that does not involve breach of contract. If a person knows or should know the consequences of their action, the wrong is called an *intentional tort.* If the action is a mistake or has unintended consequences, it is called an *unintentional tort.* See Box 3.2 for a list of torts. Keep in mind that intentional torts may also be prosecuted as criminal acts if they are performed with specific intent to cause injury.

BOX 3.2 Intentional and Unintentional Torts

Intentional Torts

Abandonment Failure to continue to provide medical care to a patient without proper notification.

Assault Threat to touch another person or their property without permission in a way that will cause pain, injury, or damage or that is offensive.

Battery Touching of another person or their property without permission in a way that will cause pain, injury, or damage or that is offensive.

Defamation Making a false claim that may harm a person's reputation, business, or group. If the claim is made verbally, it is called *slander.* If the claim is made in writing, it is called *libel.*

False imprisonment Confining a person without legal authority, such as using restraints without a proper physician order.

Invasion of privacy Public disclosure of private information, such as releasing medical information or photographs without the consent of the patient.

Misrepresentation Providing information with knowledge that it is incorrect or with reckless disregard for the truth.

Unintentional Torts

Negligence Failure to act with reasonable prudence in a situation. Negligence by a professional is also called *malpractice.*

Strict liability Responsibility for injury even if there was no negligence. This is often applied when individuals are injured by products or equipment.

LAW AND PROFESSIONAL LIABILITY

PROVIDER–PATIENT RELATIONSHIP

The provider–patient relationship is a contractual relationship. Each party has certain rights and responsibilities under the relationship.

The following elements must be present for there to be a contract:

1. There must be a mutual agreement.
2. There must be intent to do (or not do) something that is legal.
3. The action must occur in exchange for service (called *consideration*) or for payment.
4. The parties must be legally able to enter into a contract.

A contract does not have to be written or sometimes even discussed in detail. When clothes are left for dry cleaning, it is assumed that there will be an obligation to pay for the service. The same is true if a patient makes a visit to a medical office. Written contracts are used when there is a considerable amount of money at stake (such as a car loan or mortgage). In the medical office a patient may be asked to sign a statement confirming that payment will be made for any charges not covered by insurance.

Certain groups of people are not legally able to be a party to contracts, including most medical care contracts. These people are also not able to give informed consent. Such groups include the following:

1. Children younger than the age of 18
2. Mentally ill adults or adults with severe intellectual disabilities
3. Individuals who are temporarily mentally incapacitated (including those who have received narcotic analgesics or other mind-altering medications)
4. Individuals who are under threat or duress (fear of a threat)
5. Individuals who have been found incompetent to handle their affairs (as determined by a physician or court)

When it is a case of **patient incompetence** (legal inability to consent to medical treatment decisions), all consent forms should be signed and all implied contracts made with a competent party acting as a willing health care decision maker for the child or incompetent person. In some circumstances, adult rights, including the right to consent to medical treatment, are given to individuals younger than 18 years of age. Such an individual is called an **emancipated minor.** In most states, an individual between the ages of 14 and 18 years can obtain a court order from a judge to become free of control of a parent or guardian after proving the ability to be financially independent. If a minor is not emancipated, they may still be considered to have the maturity to choose or reject a particular health care treatment with or without parental consent. In this case the individual may be considered to be a **mature minor**, an individual younger than age 18 with the maturity to provide informed consent for certain medical procedures. Depending on the jurisdiction, there may be specific laws or it may be a common law policy.

The Provider

Within the provider–patient relationship, the physician provides skillful care to the patient and continues to treat the patient unless the provider informs the patient that the relationship will be terminated. In this case the provider must give the patient time to make other arrangements for care. The provider arranges for someone else to treat the patient if the provider is unavailable (such as on nights, on weekends, and during vacations). The provider informs the patient about treatments or procedures and carries out only those treatments and procedures to which the patient consents. The provider informs the patient of test results, diagnoses, and medical conditions and gives the patient instructions for follow-up care and procedures to follow at home.

A provider has the following rights:

- To accept or decline to treat a patient
- To choose to limit the medical practice to a particular size or certain specialty
- To decide where to practice

Decisions not to treat particular patients must be based on general principles (such as limiting a practice to urology) rather than arbitrary decisions (based on a whim or subjective judgment).

If a provider is going to be away for a period of time, a substitute may be hired on a temporary basis. This individual is called a *locum tenens*, a Latin term that literally means "place holder." This term may be used for any temporary worker.

Conflict of Interest

Providers are often sought after to endorse certain products or activities and are then compensated for that endorsement. They may have a financial interest in a medical product or organization and then they use or prescribe that particular product. These are examples of conflict of interest. It is important that this is addressed. The medical assistant should let their supervisor know of the possible incident of conflict of interest.

The Patient

The patient agrees to keep appointments, give accurate information about their medical condition, provide an accurate medical history, follow directions, and pay for service.

The patient has the following rights:

- To refuse treatment
- To receive complete information about procedures
- To select a provider
- To expect continuity of care
- To expect confidentiality of verbal and written communication with the provider and the provider's agents
- To be treated with respect and dignity
- To receive complete information about the treatment suggested, alternatives, and possible consequences of alternatives or no treatment

To ensure that every patient receives the care that they need, all health care agencies need to follow the principles of risk management. **Risk management** is a complex set of procedures that are involved in the process of investigating conditions that may cause issues for patients. It involves determining what the issues are that the patient may encounter when they visit our facility and what can our facility do to prevent an issue from occurring.

Patients' rights may be legally defined by the state or an institution. The *Patients' Bill of Rights* is a name that is often used to refer to any document that describes the rights of patients in a state or institution (Fig. 3.3). The medical assistant and all employees of the medical office must protect patients' rights (Procedure 3.3).

Another document that is often used to inform patients of what they should expect as far as their rights and responsibilities is The Patient Care Partnership. This document covers what you should expect during your stay in the hospital; high quality hospital care, a clean and safe environment, involvement in your care, protection of your privacy, help when leaving the hospital, and help with your billing claim. The American Hospital Association has developed this document to help explain to patients what they should expect during their stay in a hospital as far as their rights and responsibilities. The Patient Care Partnership document can be viewed at https://www.aha.org/system/files/2018-01/aha-patient-care-partnership.pdf.

Terminating the Provider–Patient Relationship

To end a relationship with a patient, a provider must notify the patient in writing. It is recommended that such a letter be sent via certified mail with return receipt requested. The letter must be dated, must state the reasons for termination of care, and should describe how medical records will be made available. Copies of any correspondence regarding termination and receipts should be kept in the medical record. If the patient notifies the provider by telephone that they wish to terminate the relationship, the provider should send a similar letter as documentation.

WALDEN-MARTIN
FAMILY MEDICAL CLINIC
1234 ANYSTREET ANYTOWN, ANYSTATE 12345
PHONE 123-123-1234 FAX 123-123-5678

Patient Bill of Rights

RIGHTS

1. **Medical Care and Dental Care.** The right to quality care consistent with available resources and accepted standards. The right to refuse treatment to the extent permitted by law and Government regulations, and to be informed of refusal consequences. When concerned about care received, the right to request review of care adequacy.
2. **Respectful Treatment.** The right to considerate and respectful care, with recognition of personal dignity.
3. **Privacy and Confidentiality.** The right, within law and military regulations, to privacy and confidentiality concerning medical care.
4. **Identity.** The right to know, at all times, the identity, professional status, and professional credentials of health care personnel, as well as the name of the health care provider primarily responsible for his or her care.
5. **Explanation of Care.** The right to an explanation concerning diagnosis, treatment, procedures, and prognosis of illness in terms the patient can understand. When it is not medically advisable to give such information to the patient, information should be provided to appropriate family members or, in their absence, another appropriate person.
6. **Informed Consent.** The right to be advised in non-clinical terms of information (significant complications, risks, benefits, and alternative treatments) needed to make knowledgeable decisions on treatment consent or refusal.
7. **Research Projects.** The right to be advised if the facility proposes to perform research associated with care. The right to refuse to participate in any research projects.
8. **Safe Environment**. The right to care and treatment in a safe environment.
9. **Medical Treatment Facility (MTF) or Dental Treatment Facility (DTF) Rules and Regulations.** The right to be informed of facility conduct rules and regulations. The patient should be informed about smoking rules and should expect compliance with those rules from other individuals. Patients are entitled to information about the MTF or DTF mechanism for the initiation, review and resolution of patient complaints.

RESPONSIBILITIES

1. **Providing Information.** The responsibility to provide, to the best of his or her knowledge, accurate and complete information about complaints, past illness, hospitalizations, medications, and other matters relating to his or her health. A patient has the responsibility to let his or her primary health care provider know whether he or she understands the treatment and what is expected of him or her.
2. **Respect and Consideration.** The responsibility for being considerate of the rights of other patients and MTF and DTF health care personnel and for assistance in the control of noise, smoking, and the number of visitors. The patient is responsible for being respectful of the property of other persons and of the facility.
3. **Compliance with Medical Care.** The responsibility for complying with medical and nursing treatment plans, including follow-up care, recommended by health care providers. This includes keeping appointments on time and notifying the MTF or DTF when appointments cannot be kept.
4. **Medical Records**. The responsibility for ensuring that medical records are promptly returned to the medical facility for appropriate filing and maintenance when records are transported by the patients for the purpose of medical appointment or consultation, etc.
5. **MTF and DTF Rules and Regulations.** The responsibility for following the MTF or DTF rules and regulations affecting patient care conduct. Regulations regarding smoking should be followed by all patients.
6. **Reporting of Patient Complaints.** The responsibility for helping the MTF or DTF commander provide the best possible care to all beneficiaries. Patients' recommendations, questions, or complaints should be reported to the patient contact representative.

Fig. 3.3 The Patients' Bill of Rights is found in the Forms Repository Section of the SimChart for the Medical Office.

Common reasons for a provider terminating care of a patient include the following:

- The provider moves.
- The provider retires.
- The provider dies.
- The provider closes the practice for other reasons.
- The patient regularly and continually breaks appointments.
- The patient regularly and continually refuses to follow medical advice.

If a patient can convince a court that they were under the belief that a provider–patient relationship still existed and because of such belief did not seek out another practitioner, and sustained injury, a successful case can be made for **abandonment.** This is rare and should never happen if the provider keeps good written records about any termination notification.

PERSONAL AND PROFESSIONAL LIABILITY

A person is responsible for their actions and may be held liable if those actions injure another person. In daily life we are required to act as a reasonable person would act in the same circumstances. The failure to act—or to refrain from acting—as a reasonable person would act in similar circumstances is called *negligence.*

A common example of negligence relates to a wet floor. If someone washes the floor or spills water on the floor and does not wipe it up, the floor becomes slippery. When an unsuspecting person comes along and is not aware that the floor is wet, that person could slip and be injured. The person responsible for making the floor wet would be expected to know that the wet floor would be slippery and could cause someone to fall. A person who notices the spill would also be expected to know that the wet floor could cause a fall. If a floor has been washed, a sign announcing that the floor is wet is considered adequate warning that individuals should be careful.

If there is no notification and a person falls, is injured, and files a lawsuit, the person who washed the floor or another person with responsibility for public safety who noticed the spill could be found to be negligent and be held responsible (liable) to pay for the injured person's medical care, lost wages, and any other costs caused by the fall on the wet floor.

Standard of Care

A person without any special training is held only to the standard of a "reasonably prudent person." The term **prudent** means careful or using common sense. For instance, any reasonably prudent person is expected to realize that an infant or unconscious person will not be able to remove a heating pad that is too hot. If an infant or unconscious person is burned by a heating pad, the person who placed it will be considered liable and will be responsible for medical bills as well as compensation for pain and suffering.

In general, a medical assistant is held to a professional standard, especially when they are performing procedures that are often done by a licensed health professional. The medical assistant must be especially careful to avoid offering advice or making decisions that may be interpreted as diagnosing illness or prescribing treatment.

If the medical assistant administers medication, they must do so correctly and must follow proper procedures and precautions to protect the patient from injury. A provider must be on the premises (not necessarily in the room) any time medication is given by a medical assistant because in most states the medical assistant can perform the procedure only under the authority and supervision of a provider. It is important for medical assistants to find out what they are legally allowed to do in the state where they work.

In emergency situations, when no qualified professional is available, health care practitioners are expected to give care for which they have been trained but at which they may not be proficient. For instance, any physician would be expected to initiate emergency care for a patient who suddenly went into cardiac arrest, even a specialist such as an ophthalmologist. Patients make an assumption that in a medical office they will receive medical treatment, even in the event of an emergency. All medical office personnel are expected to be able to give advice in an emergency or to activate the local emergency medical system if they cannot handle the situation.

Many or most medical offices train all of their personnel in cardiopulmonary resuscitation (CPR) and first aid. If a medical assistant, secretary, or receptionist tells any patient that a problem is not serious and it is, they may be liable if there is injury to the patient caused by delay of treatment. Failure to respond correctly to an emergency can be considered a "breach of contract" because there is an implied contract between a patient and a medical office that any emergency will be handled by competent staff.

Health professionals are, in general, held to a high standard of care. For physicians and other health professionals, the term **standard of care** defines the level of appropriate care legally required of any other practitioner with the same education and training providing the same care in the same geographic region. In general, if a legal question arises, a medical assistant will be held to the standard of care of the professional who would normally perform the care in question.

For example, if a family practice physician prescribes blood pressure medication, they have to do it as competently as another family practice physician in the same area. If a nurse practitioner prescribes blood pressure medication, they have to meet the same standard as the family practice physician. If a patient sustains injury from taking the medication in either case, the court would look at the appropriateness of the medication for the particular patient, the dose, and the follow-up to see whether either practitioner acted at an acceptable level.

Informed Consent

Consent can be implied by a patient's actions. If a medical assistant says, "Would you please roll up your sleeve so that I can give you an injection?" and the patient does so, the patient has given **implied consent** to the medical assistant to administer the injection. Even though the patient has not verbally agreed, the act of preparing for the injection suggests that the patient is willing to undergo the procedure.

Expressed consent is an agreement using spoken or written words. We know, however, that simply expressing consent does not always represent understanding. Patients today have the legal right to completely understand what will be done to them or for them. For this reason, most medical offices now use written consent forms to obtain informed consent.

Written consent forms are now always used for surgery, for procedures involving entry into a sterile body cavity, for procedures that carry a risk to the patient's health, and for testing for human immunodeficiency virus (HIV), the virus that causes acquired immunodeficiency syndrome (AIDS). Written consent forms are increasingly being used as well for immunizations; treatment with birth control pills; transfusions of blood or blood products, such as plasma; and other treatments and procedures.

Legally it is not the form but the understanding by the person on whom the treatment or procedure will be performed that truly represents consent. It is the responsibility of the person performing the procedure, prescribing the medication, or performing the test or examination to provide the following information to the patient before consent is obtained:

1. The nature of the patient's condition
2. The nature and purpose of the recommended procedure
3. An explanation of risks involved with the procedure
4. Alternative treatments or procedures available
5. The likely outcome of the procedure (prognosis)
6. The risks of declining or delaying the procedure

The explanation must be given in terms the patient can understand, and the patient should be given an opportunity to ask questions regarding the information.

After the consent form has been personalized for the patient and the procedure has been explained, the medical assistant may be asked to obtain the signature. If the medical assistant believes that the patient does not fully understand what they are consenting to, the matter should be referred back to the physician. This is a good example of the medical assistant acting as a liaison between the patient and the physician and being an advocate for the patient. Depending on state law, there may be special consent forms for the release of information about HIV test results and/or treatment, drug and alcohol rehabilitation, services for mental health, or other health-related information.

A patient can rescind (withdraw) the authorization to release information at any time by notifying the medical office in writing.

What Would You Do? What Would You *Not* Do?

Case Study 2

Howard Morton, 72 years old, has come to the office because of severe back pain. After examining him, the physician referred him to an orthopedic surgeon for evaluation. While Vicki is preparing the referral form for Mr. Morton, he says, "If I see an orthopedic surgeon, they are probably going to want to do surgery. Do you think surgery is the best treatment for my kind of problem? What else could I try? Should I see a chiropractor? Or do you think acupuncture might help?" ■

Professional Negligence

Professional negligence is often called **malpractice.** To avoid lawsuits for malpractice, a health professional must be sure that they are acting within the limits of their profession and must act (or refrain from acting) in a given situation as a reasonable and prudent person of the same profession would. When the medical assistant performs procedures that are usually performed by other professionals, such as nurses, the medical assistant will be held to the same standard as the professional who usually performs the procedure. No one always does everything perfectly, and both negligence and malpractice are assumed to be mistakes and unintentional.

Requirements to Prove Professional Negligence

To prove that a professional is guilty of professional negligence and liable for the outcome, four things must be proved by a preponderance of the evidence. This means that they are more likely than not. Sometimes these things are called the *Four Ds of Malpractice*:

1. The person who caused the injury has a *duty* to the person who was injured.
2. The person was *derelict* (neglectful) in performing that duty.
3. The failure to perform the duty was the *direct cause* of the injury and nothing could have intervened.
4. The failure to perform the duty caused *damage* or injury.

In some instances, the plaintiff has no direct knowledge of the incident (e.g., if the plaintiff is under general anesthesia). In such a case a lawsuit may be allowed under the doctrine of ***res ipsa loquitur***, whereby the court assumes that negligence must have occurred because of the type of injury. An example would be if the gallbladder was removed when the patient was scheduled for a hysterectomy.

If a professional does exactly what any other professional would have done and the patient has a poor outcome, the professional is not necessarily negligent. For example, even with the best sterile technique it is possible to get a wound infection. A person with a wound infection must show that proper technique was not used. If the injured person does not follow directions to keep the wound dry and the wound gets infected, the infection might have occurred because the patient did not follow directions.

If someone makes a mistake but there is no injury, the person who makes the mistake will not be liable and will not have to pay any damages. Many mistakes can be corrected if they are reported promptly.

Professional Liability Insurance

To protect against financial loss if the patient sues, physicians usually have professional liability insurance (also called *malpractice insurance*). (See Chapter 49 for a discussion of other types of insurance in the medical office.) This is for two reasons. One is to protect physicians for their own negligent actions, and the second is to protect physicians if they are sued for the negligent actions of their employees while on the job.

If an injury occurs, the law allows the injured person to sue both the person responsible for causing the injury *and that person's employer* provided that the incident occurred at work. This occurs under what is known as the doctrine of *respondeat superior*. The English translation of this Latin term is literally "let the master answer," meaning let the person at the head of the organization answer for the injuries caused by their employees.

This legal doctrine provides an incentive for employers to be sure that their employees are careful and gives the injured person a better chance of collecting damages for any injury. Even if the employee does not have insurance to cover such an incident or enough money to pay the amount received in judgment, the employer ought to have liability insurance. As the number of lawsuits for outpatient care increases, it is recommended that medical assistants carry their own malpractice insurance.

Laws that protect health professionals from being sued for giving emergency care at the scene of an accident are called **Good Samaritan Laws**. These acts vary from state to state and may cover physicians, nurses, emergency medical technicians, anyone certified to perform CPR, and other professionals.

MALPRACTICE LITIGATION

Litigation (the process of taking a lawsuit or criminal case through the courts) is complex. Lawsuits take up a lot of time, even though less than 5% of all lawsuits brought against medical professionals or medical institutions ever reach the stage of going to trial. The best defense against lawsuits is to provide competent care with excellent documentation.

If there is a trial, the court may issue a **subpoena**, a court order that requires an individual to be present to testify during some part of the trial process. A physician or nurse may provide a deposition before the actual trial, which is legal testimony given under oath to an officer of the court. To require that the original medical record be present, the court will issue a **subpoena *duces tecum***, a court order requiring that documents (or other material evidence) be made available. An employee of the health care facility should bring the original paper medical record to court each day that it is required and be present wherever the medical record is at all times. Electronic health records (EHRs) contain more detailed patient information than paper medical records. Electronic tracking data and time stamps of clinical activity and the input of orders can be required by the court in most states. Electronic records contain an *audit trail* or *audit log*, a chronologic record that provides evidence of the sequence of activities that have occurred within the record. The printed version of the electronic record may not accurately reflect the screen seen at the time when information was entered. If a medical office is on notice of a credible probability that it will become involved in litigation, employees must be careful to preserve in the electronic record all information that may be relevant to the lawsuit.

Alternative Dispute Resolution

Instead of a trial, both parties may agree to have their dispute decided by a neutral third party. This process can reduce time, expense, and publicity of a dispute. Such a process may take the form of mediation or arbitration.

Mediation uses a facilitator to help two parties in conflict settle their differences. This can be done in different ways, and if no settlement is reached, either party may find recourse in the court system.

Arbitration is a process whereby a neutral party settles the dispute. The arbitration can be either binding or nonbinding.

In nonbinding arbitration, the parties do not have to accept the decision and one party can proceed with a court case. In binding arbitration, the parties agree at the beginning to be bound by the decision of the arbitrator or arbitrators.

Various organizations provide lists of arbitrators, and depending on the circumstances and applicable state law, the parties in arbitration either select a mutually acceptable arbitrator or are assigned one from a list prepared during the arbitration process.

Arbitration is not common in malpractice cases; it is far more common in commercial contract and labor contract disputes.

TORT DEFENSES

There are various defenses to torts including *privilege* (special permission due to institutional policy or legal precedent), consent, self-defense or the defense of others, contributing to an injury, and failing to follow medical advice (thus becoming responsible for any negative outcome). In a case of negligence or malpractice, each state defines a time limit (usually 1 to 3 years) during which a lawsuit must be initiated (called the **statute of limitations**). After this time limit, no lawsuit can be brought. Although state law can vary, the statute of limitations usually begins at one of three points:

1. When the injury occurred.
2. When the individual first realized that an injury had occurred; for instance, if a hemostat is left in the body during surgery, the statute of limitations begins to run when the instrument is discovered on a radiograph taken at a later date for another reason.
3. When a minor reaches the age of majority or some other specific age (such as 21).

What Would You Do? What Would You *Not* Do?

Case Study 3

While walking down the hall to call the next patient, Vicki notices a large wet area on the linoleum floor of the hall. She gets several dry paper towels and goes to clean up the spill. Just as she bends over to wipe up the water, the physician comes out of examination room 4. He looks at the open door of his other examination room and, noticing that it is empty, says, "Where's my next patient? And can you take an ECG on the patient in room 4 right away?" ■

FEDERAL AND STATE LAWS AFFECTING THE MEDICAL OFFICE

CONTROLLED SUBSTANCES AND PRESCRIPTIONS

Controlled Substances

The **Drug Enforcement Administration (DEA)** enforces the Controlled Substances Act of 1970. A **controlled substance** is a drug that has a potential for addiction and/or abuse. Providers who prescribe controlled substances must register with the DEA and renew their registration every year, but the provider's DEA number should not be preprinted on prescription forms. The DEA updates the five schedules of controlled substances annually. Schedule I controlled substances have the highest potential for abuse and currently have no accepted medical use in the United States, whereas Schedule V controlled substances have the lowest potential for abuse. The specific medications are discussed in more detail in Chapter 26.

Federal law requires that controlled substances be stored away from other medications in a sturdy, locked cabinet. It is recommended to use a double-locked box or drawer—a box or drawer with an outer lock or key and an inner compartment that also has a lock or key. A physician may not legally obtain Schedule I controlled substances unless they are participating in an authorized experiment. Schedule II controlled substances are ordered from a manufacturer or a distributor with federal triplicate order form DEA Form 222. Schedule III through V controlled substances do not require the special triplicate form; however, they do require that invoices and packing slips be kept for 2 years.

If controlled substances are kept in a medical office, an inventory sheet must be maintained. The controlled substance stock should be counted daily and verified by a second person. The two people must sign the inventory sheet. Every 2 years, a record of daily inventory of controlled substances must be submitted to the DEA. If controlled substances must be discarded or destroyed, two witnesses must sign the inventory sheet. If any controlled substances are stolen, local police must be alerted immediately.

Prescribing, dispensing, and/or administering controlled substances also requires documentation. States vary on what paperwork is necessary; some require a special narcotic prescription form for Schedule II prescriptions. Any physician copies of controlled substance prescription forms should be kept in a secure, fireproof safe or other storage unit. If controlled substances are administered or dispensed only rarely, records can be kept in the patients' records and made available to DEA investigators.

A medical assistant must know the legal requirements regarding controlled substances that have been set by the DEA and the state in which they work. Some states allow physicians to write prescriptions for medical marijuana, but federally this is still considered illegal. Different states also have different limits regarding the amount of opioids that a physician can prescribe. A medical assistant will often be responsible for flagging the physician's DEA registration renewal date as well as for providing security and inventory record keeping for all controlled substances. A medical assistant may also be responsible for properly disposing of expired controlled substances and keeping records. In some states medical assistants are not permitted to administer controlled substances even if they are allowed to administer other medications.

Prescriptions

Federal law also identifies drugs that require a prescription. A **prescription** is an order from a physician or other licensed health care provider to a pharmacist to dispense a supply of medication. Individual states have different regulations within a set of federal guidelines. The medical assistant must know the laws of the state in which they work.

To prevent theft or alteration of written prescriptions, it is recommended that providers adhere to the following recommendations related to written prescriptions:

1. Store all prescription blanks in a safe place where they cannot be stolen and keep the number of prescription pads in use to a minimum.
2. Write out the actual amount prescribed in words in addition to the number. This makes it more difficult to alter the amount.
3. Use prescription blanks only for writing prescriptions and not for notes.
4. Do not sign prescription blanks in advance.
5. Use tamper-resistant prescription pads.

The physician may also write on the prescription whether a generic substitute may be provided. Different states have different laws regarding substitution of a generic preparation for a brand-name drug.

Electronic prescriptions are sent directly by the physician or other authorized provider to a pharmacy or mail-order pharmacy through a prescription program or the EHR. Usually, the prescription function is limited to individuals with prescribing privileges. In most states it is now allowed to prescribe controlled substances electronically in addition to ordinary prescriptions. Both provider and pharmacy must follow state guidelines to avoid prescription drug misuse, abuse, and diversion.

FEDERAL AND STATE LAWS PROTECTING EMPLOYEES

Hiring and Firing

A person who works for an organization that has more than 15 employees is protected by federal Equal Opportunity Employment laws (Title VII of the Civil Rights Act of 1964) and the federal Age Discrimination in Employment Act of 1967. These laws make it illegal for a company to discriminate in hiring practices on the basis of race, sex, religion, national origin, or age. Title VII also protects employees from discrimination based on sexual orientation or gender identity. Complaints about discrimination in hiring are submitted to the federal Equal Employment Opportunity Commission (EEOC).

Employment policies must treat employees equally and cannot discriminate against any category of employees by paying one group (such as men) more than another group for the same duties. During an interview for employment, the interviewer may not ask questions related to race, sex, religion, national origin, or age unless it relates to legal age for employment or serving alcoholic beverages.

Preemployment Testing

Preemployment testing is allowed only to determine if the potential employee has the skills and abilities to perform a specific job. If keyboarding is included in the job description, the employer may administer a keyboarding test to test a candidate's qualifications for the position. This also applies to any testing done before an individual with a disability is hired.

Preemployment drug tests have been ruled legal for any position. However, random drug tests while on the job are usually legal only if the demands of public safety outweigh the employee's right to privacy. Some health care facilities perform drug tests on all new employees.

The Americans With Disabilities Act and Its Amendments

The Americans with Disabilities Act (ADA) of 1990 discusses the need for employers to make "reasonable accommodations" for any individual with a physical or mental disability who is otherwise qualified to perform the tasks necessary in the job. The law also deals with the necessity of making public accommodations accessible to disabled individuals. The EEOC also hears complaints about possible failure to comply with the workplace portions of the ADA.

The Americans with Disabilities Act Amendments Act (ADAAA) was enacted in 2008 to make it easier for an individual to establish that they have a disability within the meaning of the law. Any substantial limitation in performing a major life activity (and this is intended to be interpreted broadly) would make it possible for an individual to require a reasonable accommodation. Previously it was required that an individual be severely or significantly restricted.

Occupational Safety and Health Act of 1970

The Occupational Safety and Health Administration (OSHA) was created by the Occupational Safety and Health Act of 1970 to be the federal agency responsible for the physical protection of employees in the workplace. OSHA regulates all workplace environments but has two specific functions related to the medical office. The Bloodborne Pathogens Standard relates to preventing exposure to pathogens that cause disease. This standard is discussed in detail in Chapter 17. OSHA also regulates the exposure of employees to hazardous chemicals in the workplace and requires employers to inform employees of the hazards of any chemicals used. See Chapter 18 for a discussion of the newest Hazard Communication Standard information. The 1988 Clinical Laboratory Improvement Amendments, which regulate office laboratories, are discussed in detail in Chapter 29.

Family and Medical Leave Act

The Family and Medical Leave Act of 1993 (FMLA) applies to employers with 50 or more employees. Under FMLA, employees are entitled to up to 12 weeks of unpaid leave annually to accommodate a serious health crisis of any family member or the birth or adoption of a child. The employee must notify the employer before the beginning of the leave as to how much of the leave they intend to take. After the employee returns, they must be given back the former job and seniority status.

Sexual Harassment

Sexual harassment is defined as any unwanted physical or verbal sexual attention from anyone an individual interacts with on the job that causes that individual to fear reprisal if the attention is refused. Sexual harassment is not flirting. Flirting occurs when both parties engage in actions or verbal exchanges intended to attract or compliment the other. Harassment occurs when one party (most often but not necessarily a man) engages another party in unwanted comments or physical contact of a sexual nature. If a comment or attention is unwanted, it should be clearly stated to the offending party. Sometimes individuals hesitate to "hurt the other person's feelings" or are uncomfortable speaking out, and communication is unclear.

Minimum Wage and Overtime

The federal Fair Labor Standards Act regulates the minimum wage, although some states have a higher minimum wage than that set under federal law. The Fair Labor Standards Act also requires overtime pay of 1.5 times the employee's regular rate of pay for time worked beyond 40 hours in 1 week. Professional and supervisory employees are exempt from the law. Registered nurses and office managers are considered professional employees but medical assistants are not and are covered by the overtime rules.

Employee Retirement Income Security Act

The Employee Retirement Income Security Act of 1974 (ERISA) regulates employee benefit plans, including managed care health plans, pension plans, and other employee benefits. ERISA sets minimum standards for pension plans to prevent unfair denial of pension rights. Under ERISA, employee health plans cannot use health status or medical condition to deny certain employees the right to insurance.

Genetic Information Nondiscrimination Act

The Genetic Information Nondiscrimination Act of 2008 prohibits the use of genetic information in health insurance and employment. Employers may not use an individual's genetic information to make hiring, firing, job placement, or promotion decisions. In addition, health insurers are prohibited from denying coverage to a healthy individual or charging higher premiums based on a genetic predisposition to develop a disease in the future.

HEALTH INSURANCE PORTABILITY AND ACCOUNTABILITY ACT

The Health Insurance Portability and Accountability Act of 1996 (HIPAA) provides legislation related to several aspects of health insurance, the privacy of patient information, and standards for filing health insurance claims electronically. This act has several sections.

Health Insurance Availability and Coverage

The first part deals with health insurance availability and coverage. It provides specific regulations for group health insurance plans to prevent eligibility rules that exclude patients with certain diagnoses or genetic conditions or require such patients to pay higher premiums.

Privacy Rule

The HIPAA Privacy Rule (one part of the law) went into effect in 2003. This rule provides patients with control over the use and disclosure of their health information. The Privacy Rule contains provisions that describe how personal health information may be used, stored, maintained, or transmitted electronically. In addition, it describes how patients must be informed of their right to control their health information.

1. The medical office must inform patients in writing how their protected health information (PHI) will be used by the medical office. This document is called a *Notice of Privacy Practices* (NPP). PHI includes written, oral, and electronic health information that contains data through which the patient can be identified, such as the Social Security number, name, and telephone number. Patients must sign to indicate that they have received a notice regarding privacy protection.
2. A patient's written consent is not required for the use or disclosure of PHI if the purpose of disclosure is medical treatment, payment, or health care operations. Therefore, individuals who are involved in caring for the patient (including medical assistants and medical assisting students) may have access to PHI.
3. Patients have the right to access their medical records and to request changes to the records if they believe they are inaccurate.
4. The medical office must have procedures in place to prevent unnecessary or inappropriate access to PHI, including request forms for information; procedures to prevent unauthorized individuals from viewing records, appointment books, computer screens, or other material that might contain PHI; and procedures for storing and destroying records containing PHI so that no unauthorized access occurs.
5. Patients have a right to request an accounting of the transfer of their information for purposes other than treatment, payment, or health care operations.
6. The medical office must have written agreements with each outside agency that handles PHI—such as medical laboratories, transcription services, law and accounting firms, software and hardware consultants, and billing services—to ensure that these other agencies handle PHI in accordance with the HIPAA Privacy Rule.
7. All employees must be trained in the privacy and security of PHI.

Transaction and Code Set Rule

The Transaction and Code Set Rule prescribes electronic data interchange standards for structuring information that must be used for Medicare and Medicaid insurance claims. Providers that file Medicare claims electronically must adhere to these electronic data interchange standards.

Security Rule

The Security Rule complements the Privacy Rule by setting standards to maintain the security of personal health information that is transmitted electronically. It identifies administrative, physical, and technical security safeguards for electronic protected health information (EPHI). The final compliance date was April 21, 2006.

Other Provisions

The Unique Identifiers Rule established a new provider identification number called the *National Provider Identifier* (NPI), a 10-digit identification number issued to each provider by the Centers for Medicare and Medicaid Services (CMS). The NPI replaced other physician insurance identification numbers but not the DEA number or state physician license number.

The final part of HIPAA is the Enforcement Rule, which describes penalties for violating HIPAA rules.

PATIENT SAFETY AND QUALITY IMPROVEMENT ACT

The Patient Safety and Quality Improvement Act of 2005 (PSQIA) was passed to encourage the reporting of adverse events, near misses, and unsafe conditions and decrease the number of preventable medical errors. It went into effect in January 2009. In addition to setting up Patient Safety Organizations (PSOs), the act also defines requirements for reporting events that threaten patient safety and patient safety work products (e.g., data, reports, and records assembled to report to a PSO) and the confidentiality protections for patients related to the patient safety evaluation system. Common formats for reporting various types of events have been developed for hospitals and will be developed in the future for ambulatory settings. Many states have passed specific laws defining mandated reports.

HEALTH INFORMATION TECHNOLOGY FOR ECONOMIC AND CLINICAL HEALTH ACT

The Health Information Technology for Economic and Clinical Health (HITECH) Act, part of the American Recovery and Reinvestment Act of 2009, includes incentives to encourage adoption of EHRs by physicians and health care facilities and to create a national health care infrastructure. This act also includes a 1% reduction in the Medicare fee schedule if an EHR has not been adopted by 2015.

To continue to protect the individual's right to privacy in the face of increased sharing of health care data, this act also increases the security provisions of HIPAA and adds increased financial penalties for privacy violations. It requires notification of patients for unauthorized use and unencrypted disclosure of PHI; breaches involving more than 500 patients must be reported to federal agencies and sometimes local media. Privacy requirements are imposed directly on business associates, whereas formerly, health care providers were required to have contracts with business associates. Business associates also become liable for financial penalties for privacy violation.

MANDATORY REPORTING

For public health reasons and the good of society as a whole, providers are required to make certain reports, usually to a state or local agency. Some are required by law and cannot be refused because the patient does not want the information released.

1. Records of births, stillbirths, and deaths.
2. Reports must be made to the medical examiner or coroner (the name depends on the state) for certain types of deaths that may indicate suspicious circumstances or may be a result of a crime. The medical examiner then decides whether to investigate.
3. Infectious disease cases have to be reported to the local board of health. Each state has a list of reportable diseases, including diseases that pose a public health risk such as rabies, measles, and AIDS. Dog bites and human bites must usually also be reported.
4. Injuries that may have occurred as a result of violence must be reported to the police. Sometimes a patient asks that the report not be made. Even if the injured person does not intend to press charges, the injury must still be reported. If there is a likely need for evidence to be collected from the injured person (e.g., in the case of a rape), the person should be directed to an emergency department, which would have personnel trained in the procedure.
5. Possible abuse or neglect must be reported to the police or a particular state agency, depending on state law. Suspicion does not have to be backed up with evidence. Certain professions are mandated (legally required) to report, especially child abuse or elder abuse. Physicians and nurses are always required to make such reports; in some states, medical assistants, as allied health care professionals, are also included in the list of those required to make reports.
6. Crimes that occur in the office—such as burglary, theft (especially theft of narcotics), and criminal assault—must be reported to the police.
7. Various other reports are mandated by the states. Some states require reports of seizures (a symptom of epilepsy) to the department of motor vehicles, and some states require that all cancer cases treated by health professionals be reported to a state cancer registry.

Failure to make a mandated report is a crime. When a report is required by law, the patient should be informed why the report is required and to whom the report will be made (Procedure 3.4).

STATE REGULATION OF HEALTH OCCUPATIONS

The laws that regulate the practice of medicine are called *medical practice acts*; in general, they contain the following two elements:

- Definition of the practice of medicine.
- Limitation to qualified practitioners by **licensure**—the process by which the state examines a person's qualifications and issues a license to practice medicine. All states require a license to practice medicine, although a physician may practice in certain federal facilities and agencies with a license from a different state than the one in which the facility is located. Practicing medicine without a license is a criminal act.

Physicians can also be licensed in most states if they have held a medical license in another state for more than 5 to 10 years. This is called **reciprocity** or *reciprocal licensing*.

Revoking or Suspending a Physician's License

A physician licensing board can revoke or suspend a physician's license for conviction of a crime, unprofessional activity, and physical or mental incapacity, including alcoholism, drug abuse, and senility. If the physician is convicted of a crime, the seriousness and nature of the crime will influence the physician licensing board's decision about the length of time the person's license may be suspended.

Similar laws govern the licensure and revocation of licenses for such professionals as registered nurses, nurse practitioners, and physician assistants. These laws clarify what the member of the profession can and cannot do.

FACILITY LICENSING AND ACCREDITATION

State Requirements

Each state requires certain types of health care facilities to obtain a license. This gives the state oversight into the activities of the facility and allows for on-site surveys to maintain quality standards. A list of these types of facilities can be found in Box 3.3. Physicians' offices are usually not included, but if laboratory testing is done in the office, it may be necessary to get a license or certificate of waiver for the laboratory depending on the type of testing being done. Health insurance companies and HMOs are also licensed by the state, which sets certain requirements for their business operations.

Federal Requirements

In addition to state licensure, health care facilities that bill Medicare and Medicaid for services fall under CMS oversight and are responsible for meeting all regulatory standards.

The CMS also participates with state and private agencies to regulate clinical laboratories and determine compliance with regulations for quality assurance. This is discussed in more detail in Chapter 29.

Voluntary Accreditation

Many health care facilities—including hospitals, ambulatory surgical centers, clinical laboratories, health clinics, and physicians' offices—seek accreditation by independent accrediting agencies as a means of improving health care and maintaining high standards. Accreditation may also be a means of complying with regulations for state licensure and regulations of the CMS.

BOX 3.3 List of Health Care Facilities That May Be Licensed by the State

- Ambulatory surgical centers
- Blood banks
- Clinics or community clinics
- Commercial independent laboratories
- Substance abuse treatment facilities
- End-stage renal disease centers
- Health departments
- Home health agencies
- Hospices
- Hospitals
- Intermediate care facilities
- Nursing homes
- Physician's office laboratories
- Pregnancy counseling centers

The Joint Commission (formerly the Joint Commission on Accreditation of Healthcare Organizations [JCAHO]) was originally established in 1951 to accredit hospitals, rehabilitation centers, and nursing homes. In recent years it has expanded its activities to accredit almost all kinds of health care facilities, including clinics and physicians' offices. To become accredited, the health care facility must prepare a report demonstrating compliance with all standards of the Joint Commission. This is followed by a survey visit with follow-up to improve in any areas of weakness that might be found during that visit.

The Accreditation Association for Ambulatory Health Care (AAAHC) performs a similar type of accreditation for most types of ambulatory health care facilities.

What Would You Do? What Would You *Not* Do? RESPONSES

Case Study 1
Page 36

What Did Vicki Do?

- ❑ Told Denise that she would have to point out the burn to the physician because he had to be sure it was healing properly.
- ❑ Told Denise that she would have to tell the physician what Denise had said about the burn.
- ❑ Explained that burning someone with a cigarette is not acceptable behavior and encouraged Denise to discuss the incident with the physician or another adult.
- ❑ Asked Denise if her boyfriend had hurt her any other time.

What Did Vicki Not Do?

- ❑ Did not tell Denise that she had to break up with her boyfriend immediately.
- ❑ Did not agree to hide the information about the burn from the physician.
- ❑ Did not promise that the physician would not tell her parents.
- ❑ Did not discuss Denise's burn or explanation for it with anyone other than the physician.

Case Study 2
Page 45

What Did Vicki Do?

- ❑ Told Mr. Morton that the orthopedic surgeon specializes in musculoskeletal conditions and does not always recommend surgery.
- ❑ Asked Mr. Morton if he questioned the physician about other kinds of treatments.
- ❑ Asked Mr. Morton if he wanted her to complete the referral and make the appointment.
- ❑ Reported to the physician whether Mr. Morton refused the referral.
- ❑ Asked Mr. Morton whether he needed more time to speak to the physician.

Continued

What Would You Do? What Would You *Not* Do? RESPONSES—cont'd

What Did Vicki Not Do?

- ❑ Did not make recommendations about other types of treatment for back pain.
- ❑ Did not give an opinion about the benefits of one type of procedure compared with another.
- ❑ Did not promise that the orthopedic surgeon would not want to do surgery.
- ❑ Did not tell Mr. Morton that the physician should have done a better job of explaining possible treatments.

Case Study 3

Page 47

What Did Vicki Do?

- ❑ Told the physician politely that she had to finish cleaning up the spill in the hall because someone might otherwise slip and fall.
- ❑ Worked as quickly as possible to dry the floor of the hall and then call the next patient.
- ❑ Asked the physician if he wanted to talk to the next patient before she took the vital signs.
- ❑ Obtained the electrocardiogram (ECG) for the patient in room 4 after calling and preparing the physician's next patient.

What Did Vicki Not Do?

- ❑ Did not leave the spilled water on the floor while she called the next patient and performed the ECG.
- ❑ Did not ask whether the physician thought that she could do two things at once.
- ❑ Did not go around the office later trying to find out who spilled water without cleaning it up.

TERMINOLOGY REVIEW

Key Term	Word Parts	Definition
Abandonment		Failure to continue to provide medical care to a patient without proper notification.
Act		A bill or measure that has become law. Often refers to legislation with several parts.
Advocate		A person who intercedes on another person's behalf.
Arbitration		A formal process whereby the parties to a dispute agree to submit to the decision of a neutral party.
Autonomy		Ability to make independent decisions without constraint or coercion by others.
Beneficence		Acting in the best possible way; performing good deeds.
Civil law		Law that regulates relationships and interactions between individuals and groups.
Cloning		Producing genetically identical cells or individuals artificially.
Controlled substance		A drug that has the potential for addiction or abuse.
Crime		An offense in violation of a law that prohibits or requires certain behavior.
Criminal law		Law that regulates offenses against the public welfare.
Defendant		The person or group against which an action is brought in a court of law.
Do-not-resuscitate (DNR) order		A medical order signed by a physician that relieves health care personnel from the obligation to resuscitate a patient who stops breathing or whose heart stops.
Drug Enforcement Administration (DEA)		The federal agency that enforces the Controlled Substances Act of 1970.
Duty		Commitment to act in a certain way.
Emancipated minor		A person younger than 18 years of age with the rights of an adult, including the ability to consent to medical care.
Ethics		The branch of knowledge that deals with standards of behavior or beliefs.
Expressed consent		Agreement using spoken or written words.
Felony		A serious crime punishable by death or imprisonment.
Fidelity		Faithfulness.
Fraud		Intentional deception resulting in injury or loss.
Gene therapy		Giving patients new genes or parts of genes to treat a disease or condition.
Genetic engineering		Making, altering, or repairing genetic material.
Health care proxy		A legal document that names an agent to make decisions about a person's medical care if they become unable to make such wishes known.
Implied consent		Indication of agreement indicated by actions instead of words.
Informed consent		Agreement to a medical procedure based on understanding of the procedure and its possible consequences and effects.
Liability		Legal responsibility.

TERMINOLOGY REVIEW—cont'd

Key Term	Word Parts	Definition
License		Official permission to perform an activity or practice a profession.
Licensure		The process by which the state examines qualifications and gives permission to an individual or organization to engage in a profession or business.
Litigation		The process of taking a lawsuit through the courts.
Living will		A legal document that specifies the kind of medical treatment a patient wants or does not want if they become incapacitated.
Locum tenens		A person who performs the duties of another on a temporary basis.
Malpractice		Negligence by a professional.
Mature minor		An individual younger than 18 years of age with the maturity to provide informed consent for certain medical procedures.
Mediation		Negotiation by a third party to help two parties resolve a dispute.
Medical durable power of attorney		A written authorization to make health care decisions for a specified individual that is in effect if the individual becomes incapacitated.
Misdemeanor		A less serious crime, punishable by a fine or imprisonment for less than 1 year.
Morals		Beliefs about what is right and wrong.
Negligence		Failure to act (or to refrain from acting) as a reasonably prudent person would in similar circumstances.
Nonmalfeasance		Ethical concept requiring that an action do no harm or do less harm than good.
Patient incompetence		Legal inability to consent to medical treatment decisions.
Plaintiff		The person or group that makes the complaint in a lawsuit.
Prescription		An order to a pharmacist to dispense a supply of a medication.
Prudent		Using care or common sense.
Reciprocity		Automatic issuing of a license in one state to the holder of a license in another state.
Res ipsa loquitur		A legal doctrine that assumes negligence because of the type of injury.
Respondeat superior		A legal doctrine making an employer liable for the negligent acts of employees.
Right		A claim that is expected to be honored.
Standard of care		Level of appropriate care required of a health professional.
Statute of limitations		A law limiting the time period for beginning a lawsuit.
Stem cells		Cells that have the capacity to develop into various types of body tissue.
Subpoena		A court order for a witness to appear and give testimony.
Subpoena *duces tecum*		A court order to produce documents or records.
Tort		An injury or wrong against a person or property that does not involve breach of contract.
Veracity		Truthfulness.

PROCEDURE 3.1 Separating Personal and Professional Ethics

Outcomes

1. Develop a plan for the separation of personal and professional ethics.
2. Recognize the impact that personal ethics and morals have on the delivery of health care.

Equipment/Supplies:

- Paper
- Pen
- Computer and printer
- Blank index cards

1. **Procedural Step.** Research one of the following ethical issues: abortion, stem cell research, genetic engineering, cloning, refusing or withholding treatment, and physician-assisted suicide.
2. **Procedural Step.** Identify conflicting values related to the ethical issue you have chosen and determine your own personal beliefs related to this ethical issue.

Continued

PROCEDURE 3.1 Separating Personal and Professional Ethics—cont'd

Principle. Analysis of ethical issues enables a person to identify their personal values and beliefs.

3. **Procedural Step.** Write a summary of the ethical issue, your personal position on the issue, and the reasons for your position. Share this information with a group of your classmates.
4. **Procedural Step.** Imagine a possible situation involving a patient who has made a different choice from yours as related to this ethical issue and describe the situation on an index card.
   Principle. Different ethical values and beliefs must be respected to demonstrate sensitivity to patients' rights.
5. **Procedural Step.** Role-play an interaction between yourself and the patient in which you maintain a professional demeanor.
6. **Procedural Step.** Participate in a group discussion in which you identify specific requirements for professionalism when there is a conflict between your personal beliefs and patients' needs or rights.
   Principle: Professional ethics places patients' rights above personal ethical beliefs and values.
7. **Procedural Step.** Write a short description of the effect that personal ethics may have on professional behavior and the delivery of health care. Relate this to the conflict you identified earlier and describe the potential impact on the health care provided to the patient.
   Principle. Planning for the separation of personal and professional ethics increases a medical assistant's ability to respond in a professional way.
8. **Procedural Step.** Hand in your report to the instructor.

PROCEDURE 3.2 Demonstrating Appropriate Response to Ethical Issues

Outcome Demonstrate appropriate responses to ethical issues

Equipment/Supplies:

- Paper
- Pen
- Computer and printer
- Blank index cards

1. **Procedural Step.** Make a list of at least three examples of ethical issues that might arise in a medical practice affecting the medical assistant. Describe why these issues create ethical but not legal issues. Create a scenario related to one of these ethical issues and summarize it on an index card.
   Principle. Some activities are legal but not considered ethical for a health professional.
2. **Procedural Step.** Role-play your situation related to an ethical issue with a classmate demonstrating the professional and ethically appropriate response. Then role-play the classmate's situation. Discuss other possible responses and distinguish ethical from unethical responses.
   Principle. As a professional, a medical assistant is expected to behave ethically as well as to adhere to any laws affecting the situation.
3. **Procedural Step.** Write a brief description of your role play explaining why your actions were ethical. Hand in your examples, index card, and description of your behavior to your instructor.

PROCEDURE 3.3 Incorporating the Patients' Bill of Rights

Outcomes

1. Apply the Patients' Bill of Rights as it relates to choice of treatment, consent for treatment, and refusal of treatment.
2. Apply Health Insurance Portability and Accountability Act (HIPAA) rules relating to privacy.
3. Demonstrate sensitivity to patient rights.

Equipment/Supplies:

- Paper
- Pen
- Computer and printer
- Role-play cards (from instructor)

1. **Procedural Step.** Make a list identifying policies or procedures a medical office should have in place to protect patients' rights related to choice of treatment, consent for treatment, refusal of treatment, and privacy. Use Fig. 3.3 (or print a copy of the Patients' Bill of Rights from SimChart for the Medical Office) and identify a policy or procedure for each right and responsibility. Also include ways in which patient privacy should be protected.
   Principle. Patient rights are protected by moral obligation and sometimes also by federal and/or state law.
2. **Procedural Step.** Include specific examples of ways a medical assistant should behave to preserve patient rights related to choice of treatment, consent for treatment, and refusal of treatment. Describe how a medical assistant should respond if a patient refuses to undergo a diagnostic test or treatment. Give specific examples.
3. **Procedural Step.** Working with one or more classmates and using index cards of situations obtained from your instructor, role-play activities to identify how the Patients' Bill of Rights can be applied to personal practice. During your role play, demonstrate sensitivity to patients' rights. Role-play at least one activity related to consent for or refusal of treatment. Role-play at least one activity related to HIPAA and confidentiality.
   Principle. Medical assistants must apply legal and ethical principles to their personal practice.
4. **Procedural Step.** Write a short summary of your role play, including a description of how you demonstrated sensitivity to patients' rights. Hand in your written list, examples, and summary of your role play to your instructor.

PROCEDURE 3.4 Reporting Illegal Activities and Complying With Public Health Statutes

Outcomes

1. Perform compliance reporting based on public health statutes.
2. Report illegal activities in the health care setting.

Equipment/Supplies:

- Paper
- Computer with internet capability
- Printer

1. **Procedural Step.** Do research using the internet and make a written list of federal, state, and/or local agencies to report each of the following:
   a. Theft or diversion of controlled substances
   b. Wounds or injuries that might be the result of criminal activity or reportable abuse
   c. Public health threats (e.g., communicable diseases, animal bites)
2. **Procedural Step.** Print at least one report form from a government agency.
3. **Procedural Step.** Make a table with two columns identifying specific reportable conditions or actions and the agency (or agencies) to which they must be reported.
4. **Procedural Step.** Discuss in writing the rights of a patient when a legal report is mandated.
   Principle: Patients have a right to know how and why information about them is reported to a public agency.
5. **Procedural Step.** Role-play making a verbal report of an illegal activity and a public health threat.
6. **Procedural Step.** Hand in your list, table, and sample report form to your instructor.

4 Interacting with Patients

Check out the Evolve site at http://evolve.elsevier.com/Bonewit/today to access additional interactive activities and exercises to help you study and prepare for success.

LEARNING OBJECTIVES

Communicating With Patients

1. Describe the steps in the communication process.
2. Differentiate between verbal and nonverbal communication.
3. List several types of nonverbal communication.
4. Identify and describe factors that can interfere with effective communication.
5. Explain the elements of active listening.
6. Describe the effect of assertive, aggressive, and passive behaviors on communication.
7. Describe how eye contact can have different meanings based on cultural background.
8. Give examples of techniques that encourage a patient to continue speaking.
9. Explain how to overcome sensory and language barriers to communication.
10. Describe ways to evaluate if communication has been effective.

Establishing Relationships to Meet Patient Needs

11. List factors that affect patient expectations of health care.
12. Explain the levels of Maslow's hierarchy of needs.
13. Correlate the existence of unmet needs to types of patient behavior in the health care setting.
14. List several ways to establish caring relationships with patients.
15. Describe the importance of maintaining appropriate self-boundaries.
16. Explain the role of empathy in the relationship between the medical assistant and patients.
17. Describe how the medical assistant can handle common emotional responses to illness.
18. Clarify how empathy helps improve the relationship between the medical assistant and the patient.
19. Describe ways to support the terminally ill patient in all stages of the grieving process.
20. Demonstrate respect for cultural and ethnic diversity in approaching patients and families.

PROCEDURES

Demonstrating effective and respectful verbal and nonverbal communication.

Maintaining boundaries and demonstrate respect for boundaries in communication.

CHAPTER OUTLINE

KEY TERMS

active listening
anxiety
body language
chronic
closed questions
denial
ego defense mechanism
empathy
hierarchy (HIGH-er-ark-ee)
hospice (HOSS-piss)
judgmental
nonverbal
open questions
oral
paraphrasing
physiologic
projection
reflecting
self-actualization
summarizing
sympathy
terminal phase
verbal
webcam

INTRODUCTION TO COMMUNICATION

To respond to a patient effectively, the medical assistant must be able to communicate effectively. Major components of health care include reducing a patient's fear and anxiety and helping the patient understand how to promote health and manage illness. To assess a patient's perception of their health status, the medical assistant must be effective at both sending and receiving messages.

COMMUNICATING WITH PATIENTS

Fig. 4.1 outlines the basic model of communication. A sender sends a message to a receiver. The message can be **verbal**, meaning that spoken or written words are used to send the message. It can also be **nonverbal**, meaning that the message is expressed without words through body language, facial expression, and other means. Most messages are sent using a combination of verbal and nonverbal communication. The *feedback* from the receiver to the sender, also verbal or nonverbal, helps the sender decide whether to initiate a new message, expand on the original message, or clarify the message.

VERBAL AND NONVERBAL COMMUNICATION

Verbal communication is either **oral** (spoken) or written. Written communication has traditionally been thought of as more formal than oral conversation—a letter rather than a phone call. Today, however, with the increasing use of e-mail, written communication may be as informal as oral communication.

Nonverbal communication refers to information that is received from body language. **Body language** is the way a

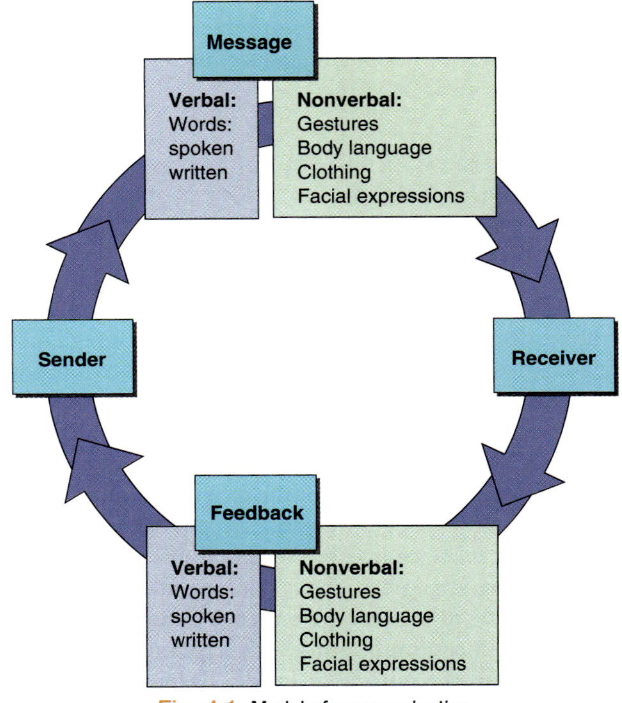

Fig. 4.1 Model of communication.

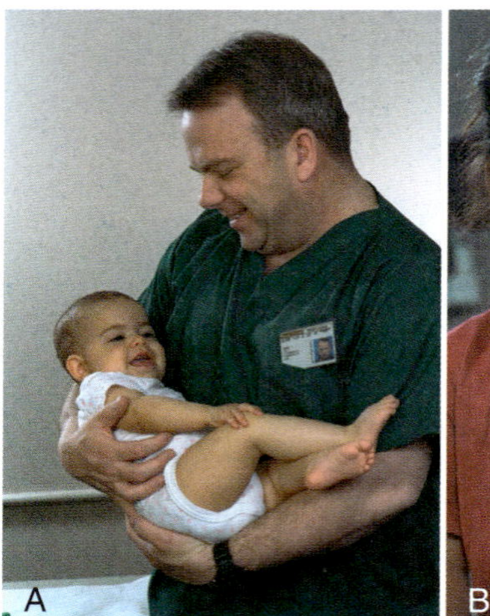
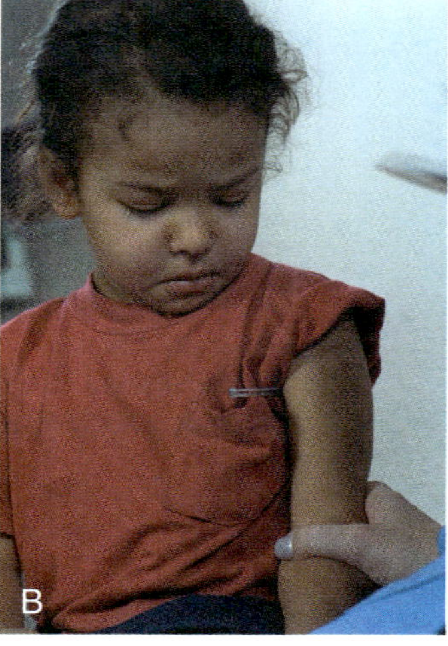
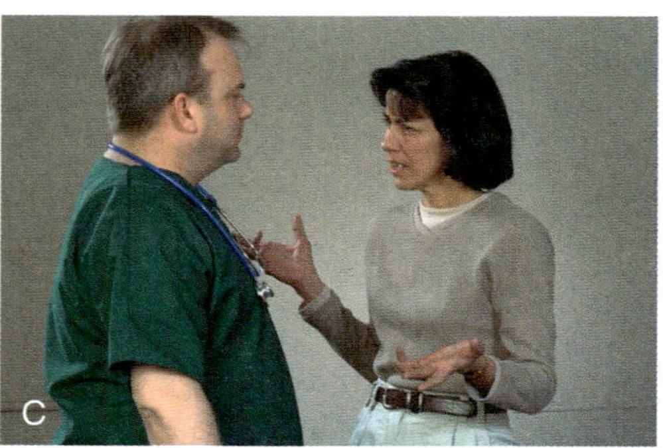

Fig. 4.2 Most adults can easily identify the people in these photographs as expressing (A) pleasure; (B) uncertainty or lack of confidence; (C) confusion.

person's body signals feelings or emotions. For example, arms folded across the chest and a rigid posture may signal anger. Nonverbal communication also includes the secondary communication that occurs during oral conversation. Secondary communication consists of tone of voice, voice pitch, voice volume, and voice quality. Nonverbal communication often provides more information than the words themselves (Fig. 4.2).

The response to a simple question such as "How are you feeling today, Mr. Jackson?" may consist only of the words "All right." The quality of the voice—pinched, pained, flat, excited, spoken with a deep sigh—gives more information than the words about Mr. Jackson's physical condition and his state of mind than the actual verbal response.

Other types of nonverbal communication include facial expression, body position, and gestures used while speaking. These are known as *nonverbal cues.*

INTERFERENCE WITH COMMUNICATION

Numerous elements can interfere with communication between the sender and receiver. An analogy for interference is listening to the radio. The radio station can be thought of as the sender of a message. The message is sent through radio signals. Any number of outside elements can interfere with the radio station's signal to the receiver, such as a storm that causes electrical interference in the atmosphere, air traffic controllers switching to a radio frequency that interferes with the broadcast frequency, or the receiver driving through a tunnel or over a bridge with steel suspension. In addition, interference can be caused by elements inside the receiver, such as having strong emotions, thinking about something else, or needing to concentrate on driving carefully.

Similarly, in communicating with a patient, interference can come from the outside or inside. Examples of outside interference include a distracting environment, noise, and lack of privacy during communication. Examples of inside interference include fatigue, fear, pain, anxiety, anger, or being preoccupied with something else. All of these factors can cause the message to be diluted, changed, or not completely understood by the receiver. Other barriers arise because understanding or senses are impaired.

The ability to identify a patient's strong emotions or feelings from the nonverbal cues exhibited by the patient may cross cultural boundaries. For example, infants and children from all cultures cry when they receive immunizations. The ability of the medical assistant or a patient to interpret subtle feelings or gestures, however, does not typically cross cultural boundaries. For example, shaking the head from side to side does not always mean "no." In some cultures, it may mean "yes," or it may be used to express other meanings such as an acknowledgement that the listener has heard what was said.

Individuals who come from different cultures also have a different idea of personal space and may interpret physical touch in a different way. Cultural sensitivity is especially important if communication is to be effective. Nonverbal communication that is accepted in the sender's culture, such as smiling, looking straight into the speaker's eyes, or lightly touching someone's shoulder to show concern, may create interference if the gesture has a different significance in the listener's culture. The medical assistant should learn as much as possible about cultural or ethnic differences, especially for those groups that are frequent patients of the medical practice where the medical assistant works.

First impressions based on personal appearance may influence the way an individual is addressed. For example, it is easy to assume that an individual who looks homeless, who is dressed in dirty clothing, or who has a strong body odor is also uneducated. In the same way, individuals who are dressed in expensive suits often are treated with great respect. Other social issues may also provoke emotional responses in health care providers. Even if a medical assistant disapproves of the lifestyle of patients who are homosexual or transgender, for example, it is important to respond to each patient as an individual.

Communication with Different Age Groups

When working in an area like family care you often encounter a wide age range of patients. That means that you would need to have a wide range of communication skills. No matter what area you work in, knowing how to communicate with the age group you will most likely encounter is a valuable skill. Let's take a look at the different generations and their preferred communication styles:

- *Gen Alpha (2013–2025)* – This is our youngest generation, and we need to know that they are very tech savvy and it is their preferred mode of communication. Yet, in health care we need to communicate with them in an in-person setting some of the time. It is important to engage them in our conversation about their health, as appropriate. Keeping things short and to the point is going to work best for them.
- *Gen Z (1996–2012)* – This generation prefers to not use their phones for making calls, like setting up appointments. It is important for the healthcare facility to have other options for them for doing things, like setting up appointments online. For that appointment time this generation likes to have one-on-one type conversations so you will likely get the information you need from them when they are in the office for an appointment.
- *Millennials (1981–1996)* – This generation would prefer to never talk on the phone. If it is necessary, they would prefer a text to let them know that you need to talk to them and then let them call you back. They would appreciate having a virtual visit if it is appropriate, but understand if they need to come in.
- *Gen X (1965–1980)* – This generation doesn't mind phone calls and very much appreciates emails. They are also less app friendly than the later generations so the best form of communication would be a phone call. They do not mind coming in for an appointment, but they should not be kept waiting for an extended period of time.
- *Baby Boomers (1946–1964)* – This generation prefers face-to-face or talking over the phone. You would see this generation typically making their appointments over the phone and wanting to see the provider face-to-face to talk about their particular health issues.

LISTENING SKILLS

Good listening skills are major components of good communication. Some health professionals are naturally better listeners than others, but listening skills can be learned and practiced.

The most important listening skill is known as *active listening.* **Active listening** means being "in the moment" and paying close attention to what is being said without thinking about anything else. Focusing all the attention on the sender of the message is important. To receive a message clearly, the listener cannot allow emotions or thoughts to interfere with the sender's message.

What a sender says will naturally trigger a response. Letting go of the urge to respond verbally, take over the conversation, and express one's own views is important. By focusing on the sender, the medical assistant will not be tempted to let their own mental responses become spoken responses. It will also prevent the medical assistant from focusing on their mental responses, thereby preventing messages from the sender from being received clearly.

Additional guidelines for the medical assistant to demonstrate good listening techniques include the following:

1. Checking to make sure the patient's interpretation of a message is correct. This may involve asking the patient to repeat what has been said by rephrasing a question.
2. Listening for feelings. Medical assistants should be alert for key words or themes the patient uses frequently to describe their medical condition. These can be important clues to the patient's emotional state. The medical assistant should also be aware of changes in their own feelings. The medical assistant's emotions may mirror the emotions of patients. For example, if the medical assistant begins to get impatient or aggravated with a patient, it may be a clue that the patient is upset or angry.
3. Being observant while listening. The patient's facial expressions, body language, tone of voice, and other nonverbal cues can tell a lot about what the patient is feeling.
4. Being patient and listening completely. Patients should be allowed to "tell their story" in their own time and in their own way. Interruption interferes with this process. Although there are questions that need to be asked, the medical assistant should introduce questions in a way that interferes as little as possible with the patient's natural storytelling flow.

Effects of Assertive, Aggressive, and Passive Behaviors on Communication

Assertive behavior includes actions such as stating opinions and standing up for oneself in a calm and positive way. A medical assistant may act assertively while still being respectful of others. Assertive behavior actually facilitates effective communication because it allows the medical assistant to be genuine and express real opinions so that problems can be resolved. Aggressive behavior, on the other hand, ignores the opinions of others and includes measures to attack, belittle, or shame another person. It impedes effective communication and often disrupts relationships. Passive behavior includes complaining to others (instead of the person who needs to hear a complaint), avoiding situations and problems, and using indirect statements to avoid confrontation. Passive behavior causes communication to be ineffective; problems are not discussed or resolved. Sometimes passive individuals use indirect measures to express their displeasure such as procrastinating, misplacing important materials, or insulting others in subtle ways. In this case the behavior is called passive–aggressive, and communication is also usually ineffective. The recipient becomes upset or angry rather than being encouraged to deal directly with a problem.

NONVERBAL MEASURES TO FACILITATE COMMUNICATION

In the United States, eye contact is important (Fig. 4.3). Maintaining eye contact is a sign of interest and involvement. However, being aware that in many cultures it is not respectful to look directly at older people is important. This is especially true in Asian and Native American cultures. Many Latinos also do not look directly at a person they respect, such as a teacher or a provider.

If the patient looks away and the medical assistant continues to seek eye contact, the patient may perceive this as aggression. Maintaining eye contact with someone who is culturally uncomfortable with that nonverbal communication creates a barrier between the two individuals.

For the most part, control of body language is unconscious. Therefore it is important for the medical assistant to be aware of the patient's nonverbal messages. Being alert to the patient's body language allows the medical assistant to notice when a patient feels uncomfortable or anxious. When a patient's words and body language do not match, the body language is usually a more genuine reflection of the patient's feelings.

Touching a person, even gently, can also be interpreted in many different ways. Moving closer can indicate interest, but it may also be viewed as aggressive. Many adults do not like to be touched by people they do not know well.

Cultural sensitivity is extremely important. For example, some Asians do not like to have their heads or their children's heads touched. This may present a problem when the medical assistant must measure the head circumference of an Asian infant. If this occurs, the medical assistant should stress to the infant's parent in a reassuring tone of voice that measuring head circumference is an important health assessment procedure and that there is no disrespect intended by the action.

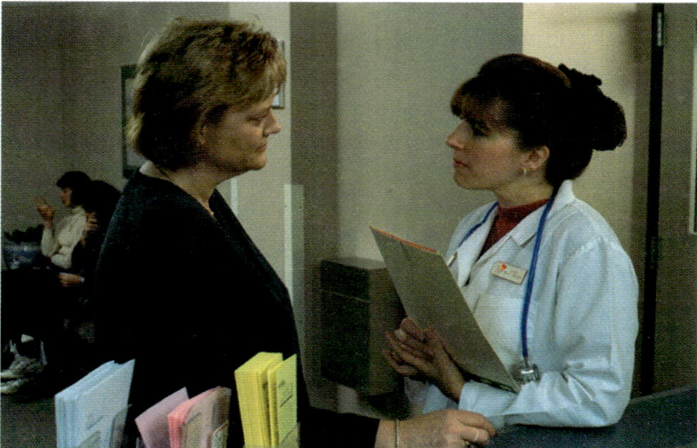

Fig. 4.3 Photograph showing a comfortable talking distance and eye contact that is typical for the United States.

A gentle pat on the shoulder can be reassuring to a patient, but it is important to notice if the patient becomes tense or appears uncomfortable when touched. If the medical assistant steps back, the patient will usually relax. In the United States, people normally maintain a distance of about 3 to 4 feet for conversation with others, but in other cultures, this comfort zone varies. If a patient is standing too close for comfort, before responding, the medical assistant should consider the patient's cultural or ethnic background. This allows a choice between a response that sets limits for the patient and a response that gives information about typical conversational distance in the United States.

If the medical assistant must penetrate the patient's personal comfort zone for a procedure, it may help make a statement that prepares the patient for movement into the patient's personal space. For example, when applying a sterile dressing to a wound, the medical assistant might say, "I'm going to have to move in now so I have a better view of the area."

What Would You Do? What Would You *Not* Do?

Case Study 1

Nancy Walker, the medical assistant, has called Jennifer Boland, a 32-year-old married mother of three, from the waiting room. Nancy notices that Jennifer is not looking at her, but the patient cooperates with getting her weight and vital signs. When Nancy asks the reason for today's visit, it seems to take Jennifer a long time to answer. She picks at the sleeve of her jersey and finally says in a low voice that she is afraid she might be pregnant. Her voice cracks a little, and then she wipes one of her eyes. ■

INTERVIEWING TECHNIQUES

Closed Questions

Two types of questions can be used in conducting a patient interview. These include closed questions and open questions. **Closed questions** are questions that can be answered with one word (e.g., yes or no) or a short answer (e.g., I was born on January 16, 1985). Closed questions are especially effective when the medical assistant needs to obtain specific information.

Examples of closed questions include the following:

- What is your date of birth?
- Who referred you to our office?
- Have you taken any medication for your pain?
- What medications are you currently taking?

Open Questions

Open questions consist of questions that encourage the patient to open up and talk. Examples of open questions include the following:

- What brings you to see the doctor today?
- Can you describe your pain?
- What has been going on with you since you were last here?
- How has your appetite changed over the past few months?

Open questions help the patient do the following:
- Identify what is important
- Express feelings
- Relay perceptions

Open questions are particularly effective in allowing the patient to describe a problem in their own words and explain how the patient feels about the problem. Because of this, open questions should be used to obtain a patient's chief complaint and conduct a patient interview. In using open questions, it is important for the medical assistant to employ active listening techniques.

If the medical assistant asks primarily closed questions, the patient may fail to give important details or mention other problems. If the medical assistant asks directly if the patient has been following a special diet or taking prescribed medication, the patient may feel pressure to agree, even if this has not always been the case. When a patient is encouraged to talk freely, a more realistic picture may emerge.

Keeping the Conversation Going

On occasion the medical assistant will need to employ techniques to keep a conversation going with a patient. For example, the medical assistant may need additional information from a patient, but the patient stops talking. When this occurs, the medical assistant should employ techniques that encourage the patient to continue speaking without steering the conversation in a particular direction. A useful technique in such a situation is to ask the patient an open question; however, "why" questions should not be used. Examples of "why" questions include the following:
- Why aren't you taking your medication?
- Why aren't you following your diet?

"Why" questions tend to make people defensive. Rather than having the patient justify their actions, it is important to identify the underlying reasons as to why the patient did not take the medication or stay on the diet. Effective questions that keep the conversation flowing without making a patient defensive include the following:
- How do you set up your meals and snacks?
- What problems are you having taking your medication?
- What do you think about having to take medication at school?

In answering these questions, the patient may provide clues as to the underlying reasons for not staying with the prescribed treatment plan.

Drawing Patients Out

Active listening includes techniques to draw a patient out and/or clarify what a patient is saying. This is especially important when the patient is trying to cope with strong feelings about their medical problems. Refer to Table 4.1 for a listing of communication techniques that demonstrate active listening.

Table 4.1 Communication Techniques That Demonstrate Active Listening

Technique	Description	Example
Using open questions	Asking questions that do not expect a particular answer, especially a yes or no answer.	*Medical assistant:* "What's been going on lately?" "How would you describe your stomach pain?"
Repeating or rephrasing	Saying the same thing as the patient, either as a statement or a question, to encourage agreement, disagreement, or clarification.	*Patient:* "It feels like someone is stabbing me in the side." *Medical assistant:* "Like a knife in your side…"
Translating a nonverbal message into words	Translating the patient's nonverbal expression of emotion into a verbal expression.	*Patient:* Throws hands up and lets them fall into their lap. *Medical assistant:* "It looks like you feel overwhelmed."
Reflecting	**Reflecting** is turning a question or statement around to reflect back to the patient; this gives the patient confidence to continue.	*Patient:* "Would you have this surgery if you were me?" *Medical assistant:* "What do you think about having the surgery?"
Paraphrasing and summarizing	**Paraphrasing** puts the patient's statement into the medical assistant's own words; **summarizing** restates the meaning but may leave out some of the details. The purposes are to validate that the medical assistant has understood and to encourage clarification.	*Medical assistant:* "So for the past week the pain has been getting steadily more intense and more frequent, and since this morning it hasn't let up at all."
Providing silence	Simply waiting for the patient to continue; allows the patient to choose whether to continue or choose a new topic.	(Silence)
Verbalizing the implied	Saying what the patient seems to mean but has not expressed.	*Patient:* "Usually I don't mind coming to see Dr. Hughes." *Medical assistant:* "But you didn't want to come today…"
Asking for clarification	Asking for more detail or a clearer statement; lets the patient know that the medical assistant has not understood and may show the patient how to make the message clearer.	*Medical assistant:* "It's not clear to me how often you have been taking this medication. Do you take it before every meal, or just when you are at home?"

Styles of Communication

Communication is most effective when all contributors are clear, direct, and respectful in their communication. For a variety of reasons, individuals may hold back and not participate completely, or be too active and disregard the feelings of others when communicating. Passive communication occurs when an individual avoids expressing feelings even in response to hurtful or anger-inducing situations. Passive communicators do not stand up for themselves and tend to try to keep the peace at all costs. The opposite type of communicator is aggressive in interactions with others. Aggressive communicators express their feelings and opinions as if they were more important than those of other speakers. They may not give others a chance to speak, and they may interrupt and criticize others. They tend to blame others instead of taking responsibility for their own behavior. Some individuals have characteristics of both types of communication. Passive–aggressive communication is a style in which a person appears passive on the surface but acts in an unfriendly way later or is sarcastic and exhibits facial expressions that do not match the underlying feelings of anger. The most respected style of communication is assertive communication, by which individuals clearly state their opinions and feelings and advocate for their rights without violating the rights of others. To be assertive, an individual must own their feelings and behavior, while still maintaining self-control. Assertive communicators listen without interrupting but state their needs clearly and respectfully.

Avoiding Responses That Inhibit Communication

The medical assistant should avoid communication techniques that exhibit disapproval or blame as well as statements that are challenging or not genuine. If a patient feels that the medical assistant is not really listening, does not understand their point of view, or does not validate emotions, the patient may become defensive or stop speaking altogether. The medical assistant's ability to demonstrate acceptance of strong emotions experienced by the patient is especially important.

When a patient expresses concerns, it is tempting to try to reassure the patient. For example, a patient might express anxiety about the results of a diagnostic test. If the medical assistant reassures the patient that the results will probably be normal, the fact that the patient is worried is not validated and the reassurance implies that the patient's worry is unreasonable or unacceptable. If the medical assistant confirms that it is difficult to wait for test results, the patient is more likely to feel that their feelings have been accepted.

Because the medical assistant's job is to make the person feel comfortable, it is important to avoid being too casual or familiar with a patient. If a subject is sensitive, but it is important to ask about it, the medical assistant can do so in a somewhat tentative way to make it easier for the patient to reply. The medical assistant can identify what the patient might be feeling, but the patient will not always agree. Many people are not always aware of their feelings and may deny feelings that they are communicating nonverbally. This should be respected. Others are only too glad to have their feelings recognized.

Medical assistants should express themselves honestly, without being **judgmental**, which means critical or negative. They can disagree with what a patient is saying, especially if that disagreement will get the patient to elaborate on what is being said. But they should not argue because arguing sets up a competitive situation. Because the medical assistant represents medical authority, the patient can easily feel threatened and unworthy.

The responses that should be avoided are summarized in Table 4.2.

Table 4.2 Responses That Inhibit Communication

Technique	Description	Example
Offering false reassurance	Telling the patient that everything will be all right; implies that the patient should not feel anxiety or concern. Especially inappropriate when the medical assistant does not know what will happen.	"Don't worry; your husband will come through this with flying colors."
Disapproving, blaming	Making a negative value judgment about the patient's thinking or behavior; by implying or stating that a patient is responsible for their health problem, the medical assistant encourages the patient to defend against attack rather than establishing trust.	"You shouldn't be smoking, you know. No wonder you have trouble breathing."
Challenging	Insisting that the patient prove a statement or belief.	"Just show me something in writing that says people should never take a bath."
Defending	Protecting oneself or someone else from criticism (implies that the patient does not have the right to have a different opinion).	"Dr. Lawler's patients never have to wait very long."
Asking for explanations of feelings or behavior	Because patients often don't know why they feel or act as they do, asking why may be frustrating and cause them to become defensive.	"Why don't you stick to your diet?" "Why are you angry?"
Belittling or negating feelings	Acting as if feelings are less intense than they are or not even present; this implies that the patient's feelings are not real or not justified	"You're really making a big deal out of a little cut."

BARRIERS TO EFFECTIVE COMMUNICATION

Impaired Level of Understanding

Occasionally a patient with an impaired level of understanding visits the medical office. When this occurs, the medical assistant needs to simplify their method of speaking. The medical assistant should use short sentences and simple words. Speaking slowly in a normal speaking tone is important. Raising one's voice does not help in this situation. The tone of voice should express concern and empathy without being condescending or implying that the patient is not intelligent. Strong and constant eye contact also helps the patient to focus.

It may be necessary to say the same thing more than once, either by repeating it or by saying the same thing in a different way. In addition, gestures and demonstration help reinforce the information.

Those with limited understanding of medical information need constant reassurance. This includes children, the elderly (especially those with some degree of dementia), and those who are mentally disabled. Giving a direct and complete explanation at the patient's level of understanding is important. Even young children need to be informed about what is going to be done to them. For instance, if the medical assistant is going to draw blood, it is not enough to say, "I'm going to draw your blood. It's going to hurt for just a moment."

It may be necessary to say something like, "I'm going to use this needle to take some blood from your arm. I'm going to put it through the skin, into where your blood is. It will feel kind of like someone is pinching you, but only for a second. Then I'll put a Band-Aid on it, and it will stop bleeding."

After an explanation to an individual with impaired understanding, the medical assistant should ask the patient to repeat the explanation back in their own words. If the patient simply repeats a small part of the explanation, communication may have been ineffective. If the medical assistant explains a procedure such as a colonoscopy, for example, they should then ask the patient, "Can you tell me what a colonoscopy is?" An answer that may indicate lack of understanding is, "It's when they do a colonoscopy." The medical assistant can then make another attempt to provide a simple explanation.

A young child or an individual with an impaired level of understanding cannot give informed consent. This must be obtained from an individual who can legally give informed consent for the impaired patient before the medical assistant can proceed.

Sight Impaired

Many degrees of vision loss exist. Total blindness is the complete inability to perceive light and form. *Legally blind* is a term used to describe individuals whose vision cannot be corrected beyond 20/200 in the better eye. This means that with glasses, at 20 feet the person sees the same as or less than a person with normal vision sees at 200 feet. A person may be called *sight impaired* if their vision is better than 20/200 but they still have low vision or a decreased field of vision.

It is important for the medical assistant to be verbally descriptive when working with a patient with impaired vision. The medical assistant should use touch and guidance when escorting patients who cannot see to walk safely from the waiting room to the examination room and also when helping them around the examination room. Patients with impaired vision usually prefer to take the medical assistant's arm and follow their movements, rather than vice versa. To explain exactly where things are, a clock image sometimes helps. Saying that the examination table is at 3 o'clock tells a blind patient that the examination table is on the right, directly to the side.

Hearing Impaired

The term *deaf* is usually used when individuals cannot hear well enough to use the sense of hearing to process information. However, there are many more individuals whose hearing is impaired than those who are deaf, especially in certain tone ranges or when sound is not loud enough.

Special techniques should be used with patients who are hearing impaired. The medical assistant should get that patient's attention, speak clearly, slowly, and in short sentences. The medical assistant's voice should be slightly louder than normal, but not so loud that it loses clarity or sounds like shouting. Eye contact is also important when communicating with a hearing-impaired patient. Even if the hearing-impaired patient does not lip-read, most people who lose their hearing learn how to associate facial expression and mouth shape with words they know and recognize.

When beginning a conversation with a hearing-impaired patient, it may be necessary to touch the person gently to get their attention. If the patient is wearing a hearing aid, it may be helpful to ask if the hearing aid has been working well for them.

Sign language is often used to communicate with the deaf. Hand and finger positions represent letters or words. Several different systems exist, but American Sign Language is the recognized language in the United States.

Because each sign can represent an entire word, a person who uses sign language may be able to communicate as fast as, or faster than, a person who is speaking. Sign language has its own structure and grammar system, so it takes considerable practice to become fluent. A patient who uses sign language to communicate is usually accompanied by an interpreter. If the patient does not have an interpreter, the law requires the office to provide one. Sign language interpretation can be provided by an interpreter. It can also be provided by setting up a video relay service account. Video service links the deaf patient with a sign language interpreter. When a sign language interpreter's services are being used, it is important that the medical assistant maintain eye contact with the patient. Hearing-impaired and deaf patients are able to obtain information from facial expressions and body language. They may also be able to read lips.

Language Barriers

A language barrier interferes with communication when two people speak different languages. Depending on the patient's ability with English, this interference may vary from slight to severe.

The best way to work around language barriers is with translation assistance. It is preferred to use trained medical interpreters or translators whenever possible. When scheduling an appointment for a patient with a language barrier, the medical assistant should arrange translation assistance at the same time. Sometimes a patient with a language barrier brings a child to translate. The medical assistant should be aware that children are the least reliable interpreters because they have a tendency to skip over medical words they do not understand or cannot translate without realizing that important information may be lost. It may also be embarrassing for a patient to discuss certain medical problems if a child is translating for them. Some facilities require a trained or certified medical interpreter for the health care provider, even if a family member is also present and translating for the patient.

When conversing with a patient through an interpreter, the medical assistant should speak to the patient and not to the interpreter. The medical assistant should allow the interpreter to translate a sentence before going on to the next sentence. The medical assistant should speak slowly and carefully, using simple terms and short sentences. Many people who do not feel comfortable speaking English can still understand much of what is said to them in English.

If the patient is comfortable working with a computer or hand-held device, a translating application could be used. As of this date the top medical translation apps include: Systran, Pairaphrase, MediBabble, VerbalCare, and ITranslate. The electronic health record used by the healthcare facility may have a translating app already for use.

At times, the medical assistant may need to improvise when working with a patient with a language barrier. This may be required during the following circumstances: the office does not have translation services, the interpreter is busy, or the patient's family member is translating but the patient wants to converse with the medical assistant in private. In these situations, the medical assistant should use gestures and mime to convey their ideas.

Translation assistance is required before a patient with a language barrier gives written consent to an invasive procedure or minor office surgery. The law states that a patient must be fully informed as to the nature of their surgery or procedure. Consent forms are usually written in English, but the verbal explanation of the procedure needs to be in a language the patient understands well. If a practice has a large number of non–English-speaking patients, it is a good idea to have routine consent forms and instructional materials translated and available.

Telephone and video translation services can be purchased from several companies. Telephone translation assistance allows the patient, medical assistant, and/or physician to speak to the interpreter via a speakerphone. A video translation service requires a computer, a **webcam** (small video camera attached to the computer), and a speakerphone, and allows all parties to see one another during the conversation.

What Would You Do? What Would You *Not* Do?

Case Study 2

When Nancy calls Harold Underwood, a 67-year-old man, from the waiting room, he does not answer until she has repeated his name three times. Because he is a new patient, Nancy introduces herself. He says that he has moved into senior housing nearby so that he can be close to his daughter. Nancy finds that she has to repeat all instructions, and she notices that Harold is wearing a hearing aid in his left ear. When she asks him if he needs help to step up to sit on the examination table, he looks at her blankly. ■

UNDERSTANDING AND MEETING THE NEEDS OF PATIENTS

PATIENT EXPECTATIONS OF HEALTH CARE

Patient expectations depend on many factors including unmet needs and experiences the person has had in the past. Previous interactions with health care facilities also shape a patient's expectations. For example, if there is a long waiting time, a patient who has always had to spend 30 to 40 minutes in the waiting room will be less upset than a patient who is used to being seen within 10 minutes.

Patients usually want to be seen by a physician within a reasonable amount of time, and they hope that the physician will "fix" whatever is wrong. Patients do not expect to have long-term problems. They want to be treated as if they were cars and physicians were mechanics—"fix what's broken and get me back on the road of life!"

In addition, people expect physicians to take care of them when they are really sick and not fuss too much over them when they are, in general, well. People certainly do not want physicians to nag them about changing their lifestyle to improve their health. But physicians are much more likely today to bring up lifestyle issues, such as eating healthy foods in reasonable portions, not smoking, reducing alcohol intake, exercising, and using seat belts. Physicians are well aware that a healthy lifestyle can reduce the amount and intensity of medical care a person needs in the future.

Patients are sometimes so wrapped up in their primary concern—to get relief from pain or other symptoms—that they have difficulty accepting that physicians are often looking for the cause of their illness, not just to alleviate symptoms. This can cause a lot of frustration for patients, especially if no significant relief can be given or if the physician does not seem to think that alleviating the symptoms would be appropriate.

A common example of this is a viral illness such as the common cold. A patient may have a fever, muscle aches, weakness, vomiting, and diarrhea. Once the physician establishes that the patient does not have a more serious condition, the physician may recommend only rest, fluids, and over-the-counter medications (e.g., acetaminophen or ibuprofen for fever reduction and relief of soreness). This plan of treatment can be frustrating for a patient who wants to feel better and have a speedy recovery.

HOW BASIC NEEDS AFFECT THE BEHAVIOR OF PATIENTS

Maslow's Hierarchy of Needs

Abraham Maslow was an American psychiatrist. In his book *Motivation and Personality* he defined what has come to be known as "Maslow's hierarchy of needs." A **hierarchy** is an arrangement in order of importance. Maslow describes human needs as a hierarchy with the most important needs at the lowest level. The image of a pyramid is often used to depict this visually, as shown in Fig. 4.4. On the bottom of the pyramid (Level 1) are the **physiologic** needs. These are the basic biologic needs for survival, which include oxygen, water, food, excretion, sleep, shelter, and sexual expression.

On the next level of the pyramid (Level 2) are the needs for safety and security. Level 2 needs include avoiding harm, attaining physical safety, and the emotional security that comes with freedom from fear and anxiety.

On the middle level of the pyramid (Level 3) are the needs for love and belonging. Level 3 needs include both receiving and giving personal affection, companionship with another individual, and identification with a group.

On the fourth level of the pyramid (Level 4) are the needs for esteem and recognition. Level 4 needs include self-esteem, the respect of others in one's peer group, success in work, and prestige in the community.

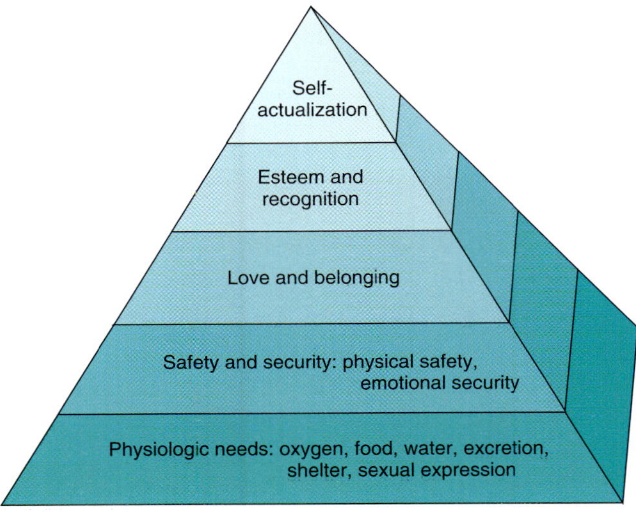

Fig. 4.4 Maslow's hierarchy of needs.

Finally, at the pyramid's pinnacle (Level 5) is the need for **self-actualization**. This is the fulfillment of each individual's potential.

Effects of Unmet Needs During Illness

Understanding that an individual cannot step up to the next level on Maslow's pyramid until their needs have been fully met at the current level is important. An individual's current level may shift several times, even in the course of a day, as different needs are experienced. An individual moves up or down the pyramid depending on what needs are currently unmet. Only when lower-level needs are met will the person be able to devote a significant amount of energy or concern to needs that are higher on the pyramid. In fact, a person has all the needs (outlined on the pyramid) all the time but becomes aware of higher-level needs only once the lower-level needs have been met.

This has a number of implications for how patients relate to the medical care they receive.

Many patients who come to the medical office are struggling to meet basic needs because they are ill. Health care professionals must recognize any difficulties in that area.

Health and happiness require more than just meeting basic needs, however. Part of the role of health professionals is to foster the meeting of needs beyond physiologic needs. For example, intervening for an abused child or battered woman helps meet needs for safety and security, as well as some sense of love and belonging, through knowledge that someone cares. Teaching patients how to manage a **chronic** disease—one that continues to exist over time—helps a person's self-esteem by making the person feel competent in self-care.

Another area in which understanding the hierarchy of needs helps in the health care setting includes learning to recognize situations when attention-getting behavior by patients might be an attempt to satisfy needs for love and belonging, or for esteem and recognition. When people are ill, their usual means for meeting their attention needs (both for love and belonging, as well as esteem and recognition) may be interrupted.

Medical assistants must be able to recognize that they cannot meet all of a patient's needs. For example, the medical assistant is not a close friend and should not attempt to be one, but by recognizing when a patient feels a loss in this area, the medical assistant helps the person to identify their feelings and to cope with whatever need is not being met.

Five Stages of Grief

When working in health care we may find that many of our patients are dealing with grief. It could be from their own personal diagnosis or about someone who is close to them. The diagnosis could be life-threatening or it might be something that will change their life or that of someone close to them. Dr. Elisabeth Kubler-Ross defined five stages of grief: denial, anger, bargaining, depression, and acceptance. Dr. Kubler-Ross has stated that this is not a linear process, meaning that not all people will go through the stages in the same fashion. She also states that everyone will go through all of the stages. It is important to understand that someone who is grieving may go through some or all of the stages at some point during their grieving process. We may encounter someone who is going through these stages. Below is a short description of each of the five stages of grief:

- *Denial* – rejecting the idea that a person is gone or that the medical condition is as bad as it is. They may even deny that they have the condition.
- *Anger* – expressed by patients as they concede that they or a loved one have an actual problem. The anger can be expressed at the providers, but it could also be expressed towards others that they are close to. It could also be expressed as towards themselves.
- *Bargaining* – the patient is trying to take control of the situation. The bargain could be offered in a rational way, such as following all of the provider's orders in turn for a good result, or it could be completely irrational, such as looking for a magical treatment to cure the problem.
- *Depression* – including symptoms such as sadness and fatigue. This is sometimes the easiest to deal with. As caregivers we have seen depression for many reasons, and we feel more comfortable in this situation.
- *Acceptance* – the person has recognized that this is a difficult situation or diagnosis and is no longer working against it. They may accept that this is the last step and may be more accepting of care that is offered instead of always looking for the next new thing.

DEVELOPMENTAL STAGES

A patient's developmental level also affects their relationship with health care providers. The sociologist Erik Erikson identified eight stages of psychosocial development through the life cycle with a challenge for the individual at each stage. Mastery of the challenge would strengthen the individual's development and prepare them to meet the challenges of each subsequent state. Although individuals do not all pass through the stages at the same rate, they are helpful for understanding the challenges and pitfalls of the life cycle (Table 4.3).

The task of infancy is to develop a sense of trust that the infant's basic needs will be met and a hope for the future. The task of a toddler is to develop a sense of self with a certain amount of self-control. Skills that reflect this are toilet training and the ability to tolerate frustration for short periods. The task of a preschool-age child is to develop the ability to explore and act independently. During the grade-school years, children develop self-confidence and the ability to devote themselves to school or sports. In adolescence, social relationships develop along with greater tolerance for differences among people. As a young adult, a person becomes more aware of the requirements for successful intimate relationships and develops closer friendships and/or romantic relationships. In the adult years, people find satisfaction in work or family responsibilities and anxiety about meeting responsibilities may result when they are diagnosed with serious illness. The challenge in the final stage of life is to remain engaged and feel satisfied with one's life, even in the face of physical and mental decline.

ESTABLISHING CARING RELATIONSHIPS

A patient who visits the medical office is often fragile, emotionally as well as physically. Illness interrupts an individual's daily routine and threatens self-concept and self-esteem. A patient who is ill often has a difficult time meeting their physiologic needs. One of the primary roles of a medical assistant is to create and maintain a caring relationship with the patient. The medical assistant is often the patient's earliest, most frequent, and most consistent point of contact with the medical office.

Empathy

To meet a patient's needs, the medical assistant must first be able to identify the patient's feelings. In addition, the medical assistant must be able to understand those feelings, not in an intellectual way but in an emotional way. This understanding is called empathy. **Empathy** is the capacity to make an emotional connection with another person's feelings without allowing the emotional connection to

Table 4.3 Erikson's Stages of Psychosocial Development

Developmental Stage	Approximate Age	Developmental Task	Examples
Infancy	0–2 years	Trust versus mistrust	Crying, being comforted
Toddlerhood	2–4 years	Autonomy versus shame and doubt	Toilet training, getting dressed
Preschool Age	4–5 years	Initiative versus guilt	Exploring, using tools
School Age	6–12 years	Industry versus inferiority	School, sports
Adolescence	13–19 years	Identity versus role confusion	Social relationships
Young Adult	20–25 years	Intimacy versus isolation	Romantic relationships
Adulthood	26–64 years	Generativity versus stagnation	Job or profession, family
Old Age	65 and older	Integrity versus despair	Reflection on life

become overpowering. Empathy is often contrasted with sympathy. **Sympathy** is defined as experiencing the same emotions as another. Sympathy is often accompanied by a feeling of pity.

Empathy is more objective than sympathy. Experiencing empathy requires a person to retain perspective and have confidence that strong emotions are not dangerous. The medical assistant must be sensitive to the feelings patients have when they go through the medical office routine. It is important for the medical assistant to be constantly aware that strong emotions may arise when individuals experience a threat such as an illness. By showing empathy to patients, a medical assistant can support them more effectively (Procedure 4.1).

Expression of Caring

Caring can be expressed through words and body language. The medical assistant expresses caring through words, by drawing patients out and letting them tell their stories in their own ways, in their own time. This was described earlier in this chapter in the section on *Interviewing Techniques*. The medical assistant should accept and validate a patient's feelings. Patients benefit by being acknowledged and having someone else accept them.

Caring can also be expressed nonverbally through body language and through the way a medical assistant positions himself or herself during conversations with patients (Fig. 4.5). The medical assistant should be positioned at the patient's eye level and at a distance of no more than 3 to 4 feet. If the medical assistant stands while the patient sits at a lower level, the patient may feel intimidated or inferior. Typically, the patient sits on the exam table while the medical assistant stands, which has both at almost equal height. If the patient is more comfortable sitting in the examining room chair, the medical assistant can sit on the physician's stool, which again puts both at about equal height. This is much more friendly than if the medical assistant stands while the patient sits in the chair.

Maintaining eye contact and lightly touching the patient, if it seems appropriate, also communicate interest and caring.

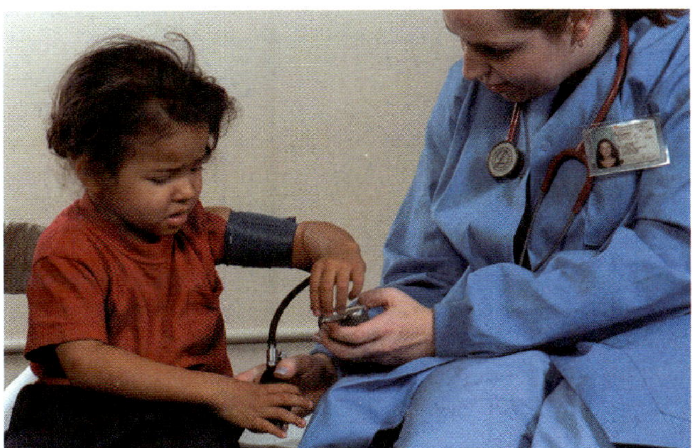

Fig. 4.5 Allowing a preschool child to handle and use the blood pressure cuff may prevent anxiety by giving the child a sense of control.

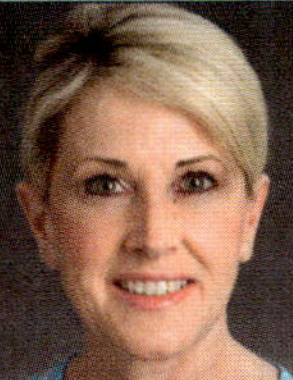

Putting It All Into Practice

My name is Nancy Walker, and I have been working for an oncologist for the past 5 years. Our patients have many different types of cancer and are at many different stages of their diseases. One thing that they all have in common is that they need a lot of emotional support. We provide this primarily by keeping the lines of communication open. We try to create an atmosphere where patients feel able to discuss whatever is on their minds. Some patients never say the word "cancer," and they talk about future plans as if they will be in the peak of health. Other patients are amazingly open and frank, even if they have not responded well to treatment. One patient told me that this is the only place she can talk about dying because her husband and her daughter become so emotional that she feels she has to spare them. We do not push patients to talk about anything they are uncomfortable with, but we do make time if patients want to talk about their feelings. The physicians also refer our patients to support groups or counselors because they believe that it is equally important to manage a patient's emotions and physical symptoms. ■

Value of Effective Relationships With Patients

The medical assistant is often the patient's most frequent, and long-term, point of contact with the medical office. A medical assistant who gets to know a patient well can be of invaluable assistance to both the patient and the physician, through trust established over time.

The experience of being understood and cared for is one of the most important steps in beginning to heal or cope effectively with illness, especially if the patient has a chronic illness. Ideally, each professional with whom the patient comes in contact at the office will convey this sense, but it is most important for those who are performing procedures. If the patient feels understood, they will also develop trust and be able to relax during procedures. This makes the procedure easier and less painful for the patient. It also makes it easier for the medical assistant to perform the procedure.

SELF-BOUNDARIES

Self-boundaries or personal boundaries include physical, mental, and spiritual guidelines or limits that a person uses to define how close other people can come without posing a threat to personal integrity. Self-boundaries indicate a sense of being separate from others instead of defined and controlled by others. The medical assistant and other health professionals allow others to maintain the personal physical space that is necessary for them to feel comfortable, and they do not allow others to intrude into their own physical space. They should also have a clear sense of their own responsibility and the right to decide how to behave based on clear moral and ethical principles without intruding into the personal space of others.

It is not uncommon to encounter individuals with mental boundaries that are too weak or too strong. A person who is very unsure about their boundaries goes along with their companions and is easily manipulated. The opposite type of person maintains rigid control, refuses to be influenced, and usually keeps others at a distance so that no one can get close. Either of these types of individuals may be totally self-absorbed, seeing themselves as the center of the universe and treating others as if their only function is to meet the individual's needs.

When interacting with an individual who does not respect physical or emotional boundaries, it is important for the medical assistant to recognize what is happening and take appropriate steps to maintain self-boundaries. If possible, this should be done in a straightforward way without acting upset or angry. For example, a patient may act as if they are a good friend of the medical assistant or flirt with the medical assistant and ask for a cell phone number or a date. Initially most medical assistants would offer excuses not to comply. If the patient continues to ask for a telephone number, for example, the medical assistant may state calmly that they do not give their cell phone number to patients (Procedure 4.2). To maintain a professional relationship, the medical assistant should always avoid sharing too much personal information, spending time with patients outside the professional relationship, performing or accepting personal favors, or abusing the relationship in any other way.

EMOTIONAL RESPONSES TO ILLNESS

Guilt

Patients may feel guilt about their illness. The amount of guilt they feel varies from one patient to another. The amount of guilt that a patient is willing to express, as opposed to the amount that is repressed, varies from one patient to the next. It is important to foster effective coping mechanisms (such as frank discussion and realistic planning) when patients experience guilt or other negative feelings.

Some individuals engage in behaviors that are known to be risky to health, such as cigarette smoking, drinking, and drug abuse. These patients sometimes feel guilty about a respiratory disease, but others may display a devil-may-care attitude about their disease. People often know intellectually that their high-calorie, high-fat diet or sedentary lifestyle predisposes them to certain illnesses or conditions. Smokers, for example, have been bombarded with scientifically valid information for almost 40 years about the link between smoking and heart disease, lung cancer, and chronic obstructive pulmonary disease. Yet many of these individuals continue established habits without an outward sense of guilt. It seems as though they have convinced themselves that their risky behavior is not the cause of their disease or that they are somehow immune to the consequences of their behavior. These behaviors are nonadaptive coping mechanisms.

On the other hand, patients with conditions totally out of their control may experience guilt. For example, someone with pancreatic cancer might say that he could have avoided the disease if he had taken better care of himself, eaten a healthy diet, or gotten more exercise.

As with other emotions, the medical assistant should accept and validate a patient's description of their feelings. If the patient's previous behavior is partially responsible for current medical problems, the patient requires support and acceptance. If it is unlikely that previous behavior is related to the medical problem, the medical assistant can encourage the patient to discuss the causes of their condition with the physician.

Loss of Control

When people are ill, they often have a feeling of a loss of control. This is especially true if they have sought medical care for their condition. In addition to physiologic changes that may be unwelcome, they feel unable to control their schedule and/or environment. Some decisions are made for them. They have to take off their clothes. People get physically close to them and sometimes even touch them. People tell them to do things they do not want to do. They are anxious and become defensive. The medical assistant should respond to the patient's irritation with patience and kindness. It is important to give the patient choices and make every effort to accommodate the patient's wishes.

Anxiety

Anxiety is a response to a perceived threat. A person who is moderately to severely anxious is not able to converse coherently and will not pick up nonverbal cues that they would normally notice. When working with a patient who is anxious, the medical assistant must first get the person's attention, slow down the conversation, and then help the person to focus on the conversation in order to encourage adaptive coping. It is important to validate the patient's concern, which reduces their anxiety level. This allows the patient's energy to be channeled in a more productive way. When patients are anxious, they may not remember what they are told. The medical assistant can help the patient by creating memory aids. For example, the medical assistant can prompt the patient to record a follow-up appointment in their appointment calendar. It is also a good idea to write the instructions down or provide the patient with a preprinted instruction sheet.

Severe anxiety can be medically problematic. Physical symptoms occur with a full-blown anxiety attack, often termed a *panic attack.* An overly anxious person hyperventilates, has an extremely rapid heart rate, and becomes unresponsive. Some people experience numbness in their fingers and toes; others feel a sensation of fullness in their ears. Some people become intensely fearful and have an overpowering sense of dread.

An anxiety attack must be dealt with as a medical issue first. Helping the patient acknowledge the anxiety is important. Acknowledging anxiety helps a person gain control. In addition, having strong emotions accepted by another person decreases the sense of fear that many people have about their emotions. If the patient is breathing rapidly, the medical assistant should encourage the patient to breathe in through the nose and out through the mouth while taking slow, deep breaths.

If possible, the medical assistant should encourage the patient to validate that anxiety is present without minimizing its significance. If the patient has not experienced severe anxiety before, they may not realize the effects it can cause. The medical assistant can explain that any physical symptoms are the result of anxiety and stay with the patient until the symptoms begin to subside. With most patients, the symptoms begin to diminish after 1 or 2 minutes. After the person has returned to a level of relative calm, it may be possible to discuss how the person handles anxiety. The physician may also refer the patient to a counselor to work on strategies to manage it.

What Would You Do? What Would You *Not* Do?

Case Study 3

Julie Ann Reynolds is a 20-year-old patient who comes to the office and describes four or five recent episodes of shortness of breath, palpitations, faintness, sweating, and nausea. She states that she has just started taking classes at a local university after transferring from a community college. The episodes have occurred mainly in the car on the way to school or shortly after arrival. She says that on one occasion her heart was beating so fast that she had to pull her car over and wait for about 10 minutes before she felt well enough to drive. She says that she has never had a heart problem, but now she is afraid that there is something wrong with her heart. She also says that her mother is worried about her and has suggested that she get an electrocardiogram and other tests because she might have a serious medical condition. ■

Anger

Anger is a natural response to a perceived threat. Anger is often a subconscious response, which means that the patient is unaware of its cause, its intensity, or even its presence. A patient may express anger at a target that did not actually cause the angry feeling. Anger can also escalate quickly if it triggers an angry response from another individual. When dealing with an angry patient, the medical assistant needs to identify the emotion without feeling attacked. If possible, the medical assistant should help the angry person identify the true source of their anger.

Anger is one of the more difficult of the incapacitating emotions to deal with. Anger tests a medical assistant's empathy and ability to put aside private issues to help patients. The first instinct is to defend oneself against a perceived attack by the angry patient, but this is counterproductive. It is more effective to respond with calmness and control using a quiet voice. Accepting that a patient is angry is not the same as allowing the patient to threaten office staff or other patients. It is perfectly acceptable to set personal boundaries by telling the patient that they are acting inappropriately, that they are making it difficult for other patients, or that shouting will not be tolerated. To protect the confidentiality of the patient who is temporarily out of control, the medical assistant should escort the patient to a private area. It is also appropriate for the medical assistant to request assistance from the office manager in dealing with an angry patient. Sometimes anger, like electricity, loses intensity when the connection is broken.

HIGHLIGHT on Ego Defense Mechanisms

An **ego defense mechanism** is an unconscious mental process that offers psychological protection. Everyone uses defense mechanisms at some time or another to protect against being overwhelmed by painful feelings. Although people are sometimes aware of using these mechanisms, usually they operate on an unconscious level—that is, people are not aware that they are disguising or blocking emotions or impulses.

Everyone tends to use defense mechanisms that have been effective in the past to reduce stress or anxiety. When a person first encounters a situation that would provoke strong feelings, such as a diagnosis of serious illness, a defense mechanism such as **denial** helps them avoid feeling overwhelmed and unable to cope. Denial is unconsciously refusing to acknowledge something that is difficult to accept. People say things like, "It doesn't seem real to me" or "This must be a mistake."

Denial allows the truth to penetrate gradually so the person has a chance to get used to the threat, to seek privacy to experience intense emotion, and to avoid total disorientation. However, if a person continues to use denial without attempting to accept the situation, negative consequences may occur.

The person may not take appropriate actions to respond to illness. Friends and family may respond negatively to the person's perceived lack of responsibility. And the person may miss the opportunity to grow and strengthen their sense of self-worth and ability to cope with adversity.

If a medical assistant can identify a patient's defense mechanisms and coping patterns, they can gain a better understanding of the patient's underlying fears and concerns. The medical assistant can try to respond to these concerns but should not directly challenge the defenses or label them.

When defense mechanisms are attacked, it takes more energy to defend against threatening emotions. On the other hand, accepting defenses tends to promote a feeling of being understood and may decrease the need for rigidity in the defenses.

Example

Mr. Sykes has had to wait for about 45 minutes past his appointment time to see Dr. Lopez. When Kathy, the medical assistant, takes him back to the examination room, he says, "I think you should know that some of the people in the waiting room are really upset about how long they have been waiting."

Kathy may suspect that this is an example of **projection**—unconsciously identifying thoughts or feelings as originating in someone else when they really are one's own thoughts and feelings. She can be helpful to Mr. Sykes by responding in a way that reassures him that it is understandable for a person to be upset

Continued

HIGHLIGHT on Ego Defense Mechanisms—cont'd

when there is an unusually long wait. Responses that are not helpful (because they reinforce Mr. Sykes's fear that it would be dangerous to express a negative emotion directly) are as follows:

1. Making it seem as though Mr. Sykes is overreacting and should not feel upset ("Oh, it hasn't been that long.")
2. Labeling or challenging the defense mechanism ("Do you always project your own feelings on people around you?")
3. Defending the physician or office staff ("Dr. Lopez has been very busy with several sick patients.")
4. Talking negatively about the patients in the waiting room ("Some people are never happy, no matter how quickly they are seen.")

In the accompanying box is a list of several other ego defense mechanisms, with examples that might occur in a medical office. Remember that using defense mechanisms usually helps people adapt to stressful situations. ■

Other Ego Defense Mechanisms

Selective inattention	Failing to hear or pay attention to information that may provoke anxiety	A patient says he was told that his cancer will definitely be cured if he has the primary tumor removed.
Regression	Returning to the emotional adjustment of an earlier stage of growth and development	An ill person who could be independent asks for assistance with personal hygiene.
Depersonalization	Removing feeling from something that is perceived as stressful	A medical assistant who is assisting with a lumbar puncture on a young child experiences the child as looking like a toy or doll.
Rationalization	Assigning logical reasons or excuses for actions that may have been motivated by self-interest or other emotions the person does not wish to acknowledge	A patient might justify not telling the physician that he smokes by saying to himself, "The doctor isn't interested because he didn't ask about it."
Repression	Unconsciously excluding unacceptable ideas, impulses, or emotions from awareness	A diabetic patient who hates finger sticks often forgets to test her blood sugar.
Suppression	Deciding to put uncomfortable or painful thoughts out of awareness	A patient says, "I don't want to think about my surgery until the day before."
Displacement	Shifting an emotion or behavior from the original object to a more acceptable substitute	A medical assistant who has just been given a poor evaluation is extremely rude to the next person she talks to on the telephone.
Undoing	An attempt to make amends for a feeling or behavior that makes a person feel guilty	A patient notices that she hates the medical assistant's hairstyle and hair color. Immediately she tells the medical assistant that she has beautiful eyes.
Compensation	Attempting to overcome a real or perceived handicap by developing some other ability or trait	A person who thinks that she isn't very intelligent in school always offers to help the teacher.

THE GRIEVING PROCESS

Any time a disease causes actual or potential loss, including loss of function as well as loss of life, both the patient and family go through a fairly predictable sequence of stages called the *grieving process.* This process was described in detail by the spiritual author Elisabeth Kübler-Ross in relation to individuals with a terminal illness. The **terminal phase** is defined as when the patient is not expected to live longer than 6 months. People go through this sequence over varying lengths of time and may move from one stage to another out of the order presented here. Although the process is individual, it is important to know that even a dying person can come to a type of acceptance, and after death has occurred, there is a time when the grieving relatives and friends will again be able to engage in loving and fulfilling relationships.

The following five steps are those described by Kübler-Ross for the patient with a terminal illness:

1. *Denial.* This is the initial response to knowledge that one has a terminal illness. It is a state of shock and disbelief. Most people simply deny the idea. Denial can be useful; it can provide a period of time to find a way to deal with death or disability. If a patient is using denial, the medical assistant should remember that this is a defense against unmanageable anxiety. The medical assistant should listen to the patient actively, without confronting unrealistic statements. Acceptance of the patient's need to deny reality provides support for a patient to accept at their own pace. The patient and family will start to accept reality when they are ready to handle the strong emotions.
2. *Anger.* Frustration and anger usually follow denial. The patient is in the "Why me?" mode. The illness seems

unfair, and the patient may respond by being belligerent, uncooperative, and critical of those around them. Health care providers may become targets of this anger and criticism. The medical assistant must keep in mind that any such display of anger is not directed at them personally but toward the situation and circumstances over which the patient has no control.

3. *Bargaining.* In this stage, which usually follows anger closely, the patient may try to give something up to gain more time. Most bargaining is done between the patient and their personal concept of God. If bargaining is verbalized, the medical assistant should be accepting of the patient's wish to make a bargain that will reverse their condition or prolong their life.
4. *Depression.* The patient recognizes the facts that cannot be denied and becomes depressed. Most people become silent at this stage and prefer to be alone. The patient who is withdrawn is more difficult to deal with than the person who is openly angry. In this situation, a medical assistant needs to be available and present with the patient for companionship and to provide a nonjudgmental listening ear. The medical assistant should always strive to maintain communication with a patient in the depression stage. Counseling and support groups may be appropriate referrals for both patients and family members in this stage.
5. *Acceptance.* Some people find a degree of peace within themselves when they accept their imminent death. They willingly stop resisting death and rest quietly. This is seldom seen by professionals who work in medical offices, because those who reach this stage may be in a hospital, in a hospice center, or at home. The dying person may want loved ones present at death and may not interact with others at all. Most people fear dying alone and want the comfort of having someone, preferably a loved one, present in the final moments.

A dying person has a number of fears, such as fear of the unknown, fear of pain, and fear of helplessness. It is a challenge for all health care professionals to accept the difficult feelings of fear.

Listening closely to the patient allows the medical assistant to help the patient respond to all hints of deterioration, as well as actual problems, as soon as they become apparent. The patient may need to be seen by several health care professionals while receiving additional care at home. The medical assistant can be helpful by being aware of community resources and by communicating the needs of the patient and their family to the doctor. This requires knowledge of insurance benefits and of the types of insurance the office accepts, as well as other sources of funding assistance the patient may be able to obtain.

A patient whose condition has stabilized or whose active treatment has ended but who still requires pain relief, nursing care, and/or comfort measures must receive them at home, in a nursing home, in a rehabilitation center, or in a hospice center. A **hospice** is an organization that provides comfort, pain relief, and personal care for dying patients.

Most hospices provide nursing care, nursing assistants, and volunteers to visit terminal patients in their homes, working with the families to increase the individual's comfort once active treatment is no longer effective or desired. There are also some hospice centers, which provide centralized care. In some areas a patient can receive similar services from home health care agencies and visiting nurse associations.

The medical assistant may serve as a patient navigator or liaison to obtain appropriate referrals from the doctor and assist the patient and/or family to locate providers of needed services. Communication on this level must be two-way; if a patient is being seen by visiting nurses, hospice, or other health professionals, the medical assistant may be the person who facilitates communication between the doctor and these other parties.

CULTURAL INFLUENCES AFFECTING HEALTH CARE

Patients often come from cultures that have some level of distrust of Western scientific medicine and/or strong belief in their own medical traditions. In addition to seeking care from a physician, these patients may complement their care by visiting traditional practitioners. In many traditional practices, religion and medicine are tightly interwoven. Both patients and practitioners hope to affect health by influencing spirits or gods in the unseen world. People from many cultures believe in the effectiveness of sacred words, tattoos, or amulets (objects worn to prevent injury or evil), as well as specific rituals that may involve chanting, fire, or even animal sacrifice.

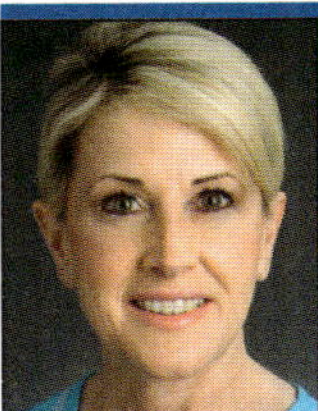

Memories *from* Practicum

Nancy Walker: I did my practicum in the adult medicine area of a clinic in a large metropolitan area. We had several African patients who came to our area as refugees from Somalia. If they were recent immigrants, we had to explain many things about our clinic to them because they were not familiar with preventative care from their own country. The female patients were modest; they did not shake hands with male physicians and avoided undressing for examinations. We tried to assign them to female practitioners, if possible, and everyone in the office learned to adapt procedures by having the patient remove the minimum possible amount of clothing. For example, the physicians usually listened to a female patient's heart and respirations just by placing the stethoscope under her clothing. One of these patients told me that some offices were not as accepting of their customs as we were. She said that it is considered immodest for a woman to remove clothing in front of any male, even a physician. She told me that if she had to do it, she would just stay sick. ■

Causes of Illness

Many cultures distinguish between illness caused by bad spirits or evil people and illness with physiologic origins. It is important to not ridicule these theories if patients believe them. When patients feel that health professionals do not respect their beliefs, they may not follow recommendations or return for follow-up care. An open attitude and the willingness to listen to the patient's beliefs are required to establish a relationship of trust with the patient.

Fundamentals of scientific medical practice—such as frequent handwashing to remove invisible organisms, taking medicine when one does not feel ill, and causing pain to healthy children by giving them immunizations—may be foreign to certain traditional practices.

Treatments and Traditional Practices

When patients have beliefs that do not correspond to those of the health care team, it is important to keep the lines of communication open. Patients need to be able to discuss other treatments that are being used. They also need to understand the importance of the treatments being offered by scientific medicine so that they can comply with standard medical treatment regimens in addition to their traditional practices.

As a general rule, the health care team should accept any traditional practice that is not dangerous. For example, some patients from Cambodia and other parts of Southeast Asia believe that rubbing the skin with the side of a coin dipped in a camphor preparation is a treatment for colds and headaches. This treatment leaves bruises on the skin but does not cause breaks in the skin. A child with bruises from this type of treatment is not a victim of child abuse, but the bruises might look like abuse. The medical assistant should learn about traditional treatments used by patients in the practice where they work.

One area in which family and cultural traditions may be strong relates to diet and herbal preparations. In many traditions, certain diseases and conditions are considered "hot" and others are considered "cold." The patient may be advised to either eat or avoid certain foods or to take certain herbal preparations to restore balance. If the patient can describe traditional treatments, it will be easier for the physician to identify any practices that might be harmful or that might interfere with prescribed medical treatments.

Behavioral Requirements

In some cultures there are specific behavioral requirements for women and men. There may be cultural norms requiring women to have a male escort when they leave their homes. In some cultures the oldest male in the family must make important decisions. For some individuals there are also cultural requirements prohibiting the removal of clothing, jewelry, and head coverings, even for medical examinations. Medical assistants must learn about cultural norms and respond with acceptance and sensitivity. If necessary, adaptations must be made so that the patient is not forced to violate personal standards.

What Would You Do? What Would You *Not* Do? RESPONSES

Case Study 1

Page 60

What Did Nancy Do?

- ❑ Maintained a warm and accepting posture and a friendly tone of voice.
- ❑ Used an open response to encourage Jennifer to say more about how she feels about possibly being pregnant.
- ❑ Identified verbally that Jennifer seemed a little upset.

What Did Nancy Not Do?

- ❑ Did not immediately congratulate Jennifer or respond as if this was good news.
- ❑ Did not immediately assume a businesslike tone of voice and ask closed questions to obtain information.
- ❑ Did not act as if the patient had nothing on her mind.
- ❑ Did not appear to be in a hurry to finish the interview.

Case Study 2

Page 64

What Did Nancy Do?

- ❑ Made sure that Harold was looking at her when she spoke to him.
- ❑ Spoke clearly and a little more slowly than usual, using a strong voice.
- ❑ Asked Harold if his hearing aid was working well for him.
- ❑ Used gestures to reinforce her directions.
- ❑ Used short sentences.
- ❑ Repeated instructions or questions as needed.

What Did Nancy Not Do?

- ❑ Did not shout.
- ❑ Did not express impatience in her tone of voice or body language.
- ❑ Did not speak in long, complicated sentences.
- ❑ Did not turn away from the patient and keep talking.
- ❑ Did not drop her voice at the end of sentences.

Case Study 3

Page 69

What Would You Do? What Would You *Not* Do? RESPONSES—cont'd

What Did Nancy Do?

- ❑ Expressed to Julie Ann that these symptoms are upsetting.
- ❑ Agreed that it was a good decision to see the doctor.
- ❑ Asked Julie Ann to describe the emotions she was experiencing during these episodes.
- ❑ Maintained an open, friendly, and calm demeanor during the interview.

What Did Nancy Not Do?

- ❑ Did not try to identify the cause of the episodes for Julie Ann.
- ❑ Did not rush through the interview so that the patient would be ready for the physician quickly.
- ❑ Did not say, "It's probably just anxiety."
- ❑ Did not say that there was probably nothing seriously the matter with Julie Ann.

TERMINOLOGY REVIEW

Key Term	Word Parts	Definition
Active listening		Paying close attention to a speaker without thinking of anything else.
Anxiety		A vague, unpleasant emotion of fear or dread often accompanied by restlessness or nervousness.
Body language		Communication that is expressed through facial expressions, body position, muscle activity, and other nonverbal means.
Chronic		Existing over a long period of time.
Closed questions		Questions that anticipate a yes or no or a short answer.
Denial		Failure to acknowledge the reality of a situation.
Ego defense mechanism		Unconscious mental process that offers psychological protection.
Empathy		Objective awareness and sensitivity to the feelings and emotions of others.
Hierarchy		Classified according to rank or importance.
Hospice		An organization that manages care for dying patients including comfort, pain relief, and personal care.
Judgmental		Critical or negative; making judgments about what is good or bad based on a personal opinion.
Nonverbal	*non-:* not *verbum:* word *-al:* pertaining to	Communication that occurs without words, such as through body posture or facial expression.
Open questions		Questions that could have a variety of answers and encourage a personal response.
Oral	*os* (gen. *oris*): mouth *-al:* pertaining to	Spoken; pertaining to the mouth.
Paraphrasing		A restatement of the words of another, often to clarify meaning.
Physiologic	*physis:* nature *logia:* study *-ic:* pertaining to	Pertaining to body processes.
Projection		Experiencing one's own emotions as those of another.
Reflecting		Expressing the meaning and emotion of another's words back to the person.
Self-actualization		The fulfillment of each individual's potential.
Summarizing		Expressing the most important points of a conversation or written document.
Sympathy		Feeling the same emotions as another.
Terminal phase		The last stage of illness, usually used when death is expected to occur within 6 months.
Verbal	*verbum:* word *-al:* pertaining to	Using words to communicate.
Webcam		Small video camera attached to a computer that allows video to be transmitted on the Internet.

PROCEDURE 4.1 Demonstrating Effective and Respectful Verbal and Nonverbal Communication

Outcomes

1. Responds to nonverbal communication
2. Demonstrates nonverbal communication, empathy, and active listening when communicating with patients, family and staff

Equipment/Supplies:

- Index cards with situations
- Paper
- Pen
- Computer and printer

1. **Procedural Step.** Working in groups of three, role-play three situations in which one person plays a medical assistant, one person plays a patient with a terminal illness, and one person plays a family member. The medical assistant should demonstrate empathy and active listening toward the patient and family member.
2. **Procedural Step.** After each role play, describe the nonverbal communication of the "patient" and the "medical assistant," and evaluate the effectiveness of communication.
   Principle: Nonverbal communication is an important part of every interaction.
3. **Procedural Step.** Role-play an additional situation in which a "medical assistant" and "another staff person" disagree and discuss how each displayed active listening and empathy toward the other.
   Principle: The ability to listen closely to and identify with the feelings of another person (empathy) enhances communication, even if the two people disagree strongly.
4. **Procedural Step.** Write a short description of the nonverbal communication that occurred during the role-play situations, and discuss the messages communicated nonverbally. Include ways that empathy is communicated both verbally and nonverbally. Include examples of active listening. Explain how important it is to communicate nonverbally in an effective way. If there were places where nonverbal communication was not effective in the role-play situations, describe them.
5. **Procedural Step.** Hand in the description of the role play and discussion to your instructor.

PROCEDURE 4.2 Maintaining Boundaries and Demonstrating Respect for Boundaries in Communications

Outcomes

1. Demonstrates the principles of self-boundaries
2. Demonstrates respect for individual diversity, including: (a) gender, (b) race, (c) religion, (d) age, (e) economic status, (f) appearance

Equipment/Supplies:

- Paper
- Pen
- Computer and printer

1. **Procedural Step.** Create three situations in which a medical assistant is taking vital signs for each of the following patients:
   a. An indigent person with strong body odor and an undiagnosed skin condition
   b. An 80-year-old Hispanic woman who is hard of hearing and speaks poor English
   c. A woman from Ethiopia who does not look at the medical assistant and whose husband speaks for her and says she will not undress
2. **Procedural Step.** Write dialog including actions of all individuals for a short scene for each situation.
3. **Procedural Step.** Write an analysis of each situation explaining how the appearance of the patient, self-boundaries, and/or personal bias with respect to gender, race, religion, age, appearance, and economic status may influence the interaction. Identify your own biases as honestly as possible.
4. **Procedural Step.** Explain how a medical assistant should protect their own and patients' self-boundaries and demonstrate respect for individual diversity in each of the situations described.
   Principle. Patients are entitled to considerate and respectful care according to the Patients' Bill of Rights.
5. **Procedural Step.** Role-play each scene with a classmate and demonstrate respect for individual diversity with respect to gender, race, religion, age, economic status, and appearance.
6. **Procedural Step.** Hand in your situations and discussion to your instructor.

Introduction to Anatomy and Physiology

 Check out the Evolve site at http://evolve.elsevier.com/Bonewit/today to access additional interactive activities and exercises to help you study and prepare for success.

LEARNING OBJECTIVES

1. Explain why it is important for the medical assistant to be knowledgeable about anatomy and physiology.
2. Explain the relationship between anatomy and physiology.
3. State the six levels of organization within the human body.
4. List the 11 organ systems of the body and describe the function of each.
5. Describe homeostasis and its importance to the human body.
6. Explain how the body maintains homeostasis through use of a negative feedback system.
7. List the four criteria used to describe the anatomic position.
8. Identify body planes, body regions, and relative positions using anatomic terms.
9. Distinguish between the dorsal body cavity and the ventral body cavity, and list the subdivisions of each cavity.
10. Describe the cell membrane.
11. Describe the composition of the cytoplasm.
12. Describe the components of the nucleus and state the function of each component.
13. Identify, describe, and state the function of each of the cytoplasmic organelles.
14. Explain how the cell membrane regulates the composition of the cytoplasm.
15. Describe the various mechanisms that result in the transport of substances across the cell membrane.
16. List the phases of a cell cycle and describe the events that occur in each phase.
17. Explain the difference between mitosis and meiosis.
18. List the four main types of tissue found in the body.
19. Describe the various types of epithelial tissue in terms of structure, location, and function.
20. Describe the general characteristics of connective tissue.
21. List three types of connective tissue cells and state the function of each.
22. Describe the features and location of the various types of connective tissue.
23. Explain the differences among skeletal muscle, smooth muscle, and cardiac muscle in terms of structure, location, and control.
24. State the two categories of cells in nerve tissue and explain their function.

CHAPTER OUTLINE

KEY TERMS

active transport (AK-tiv TRANS-port)
anatomic position (an-ah-TOM-ik poh-ZIH-shun)
axon (AKS-on)
chondrocytes (KON-droh-sytes)
collagenous fibers (koh-LAJ-eh-nuss FYE-burs)
cutaneous membrane (kyoo-TAY-nee-us MEM-brayn)
cytokinesis (sye-toh-kih-NEE-sis)
dendrites (DEN-drytes)
diffusion (dif-YOO-zhun)
elastic fibers (ee-LAS-tick FYE-burs)
erythrocytes (ee-RITH-roh-sytes)
fibroblasts (FYE-broh-blasts)
histology (hiss-TAHL-oh-jee)
homeostasis (hoh-mee-oh-STAY-sis)
human anatomy (ah-NAT-o-mee)
human physiology (fiz-ee-AHL-oh-jee)
leukocytes (LOO-koh-sytes)
macrophages (MAK-roh-fay-jes)
mast cells (MAST SELLS)
meiosis (mye-OH-sis)
meninges (meh-NIN-jeez)
mitosis (mye-TOH-sis)
mucous membranes (MYOO-cus MEM-brayns)
negative feedback (NEG-ah-tiv FEED-bak)
neuroglia (noo-ROG-lee-ah)
neurons (NOO-rons)
osmosis (os-MOH-sis)
osteocytes (AH-stee-oh-sytes)
passive transport (PASS-iv TRANS-port)
pericardium (pair-ih-KAR-dee-um)
peritoneum (pair-ih-toe-NEE-um)
phagocytosis (fag-oh-sye-TOH-sis)
pinocytosis (pin-oh-sye-TOH-sis)
pleura (PLOO-rah)
serous membranes (SEER-us MEM-brayns)
synovial membranes (sih-NOH-vee-al MEM-brayns)
thrombocyte (THROM-boh-syte)
tissue (TISH-yoo)

A BRIEF SUMMARY OF MEDICAL HISTORY

Studies of illness and aging of the human body are major components in the field of medicine. The study of "modern" medicine began in the 5th century BCE.

Hippocrates, who was born in approximately 460 BCE on the Greek island of Cos, is recognized as the "Father of Medicine." After his death, all the existing writings on medicine were gathered into a work called the *Hippocratic Collection* and attributed to him whether he wrote them or not. The Hippocratic Oath, which is still in use today, is from the *Collection.* Hippocrates concluded that illness had rational explanations instead of being caused by evil spirits or disfavor of the gods. This freed medicine from superstition and allowed for scientific study.

Leonardo da Vinci advanced the understanding of human anatomy by carefully dissecting corpses and making detailed anatomic drawings during the 15th century. William Harvey published *An Anatomical Essay on the Motion of the Heart and Blood in Animals* in 1628, detailing how blood was pumped from the heart throughout the body and then returned to the heart and recirculated. Shortly after this, Robert Hooke invented a primitive microscope. A Dutch cloth merchant, Antony van Leeuwenhoek, by grinding his own glass lenses, greatly improved the microscope's design and magnification. Using his new and improved microscope, van Leeuwenhoek discovered blood cells in 1670. He also observed bacteria, yeast cells, spermatozoa, and protozoa. The microscope allowed capillaries to be observed, thus showing the link between arteries and veins and confirming Harvey's theory of blood circulation.

Edward Jenner, an English microbiologist, is known as the "Father of Immunology." He observed that people who had contracted cowpox seemed immune to the deadly smallpox. He theorized that deliberately infecting people with cowpox would protect them from smallpox. He tested his theory on a young boy in 1796 and then demonstrated that the lad was indeed immune to smallpox.

William Beaumont, while serving as an army post surgeon, treated a patient who had been blasted by a musket at close range. The resulting large wound affected part of his lung, two ribs, and his stomach. Beaumont treated the wounds but was unable to get the hole in the stomach to completely close; repeated bandaging was required to prevent food and drink from coming out. Recognizing this as an opportunity to study the digestion process, he tied small pieces of food with silk string and dangled them through the hole in the patient's stomach, then removed the items at 1-hour intervals. He published his observations in 1833.

Medicine truly came of age during the second half of the 19th century. Louis Pasteur and Robert Koch established the germ theory of disease. Florence Nightingale showed the importance of hygiene and sanitation in reducing hospital infections. Sir Humphry Davy discovered the anesthetic properties of nitrous oxide, and Joseph Lister pioneered the use of carbolic acid as an antiseptic to clean wounds and surgical instruments. His antiseptic technique reduced deaths from infection after surgery from about 60% to under 4%. Then in 1895 a German scientist named Wilhelm Roentgen discovered x-rays. Medicine has never been the same since.

The 20th century continued to build on all these discoveries. The pharmaceutical industry mushroomed with the development of thousands of new medicines. Vaccines were developed to prevent polio, measles, mumps, and many other diseases. Cardiac pacemakers and defibrillators were invented. Medical imaging advanced with the development of computed tomography (CT), magnetic resonance imaging (MRI), positron emission tomography (PET), ultrasound, and many other techniques. Numerous advances occurred in surgery, including open-heart surgery and organ transplants. Radiation therapy and chemotherapy for the treatment of cancer were developed. Kidney dialysis machines were invented, and hospital intensive care units (ICUs) were established to better treat very ill patients. In the latter part of the 20th century, a Swedish neurosurgeon, Lars Leksell, developed the Gamma Knife. This is a radiologic technique used to treat tumors in the brain that are not amenable to conventional surgery.

The beginning of the 21st century brought the development of the da Vinci Surgical System, a robotic system that uses a minimally invasive approach. The da Vinci System translates the surgeon's movements into micromovements of the instruments through small incisions. The result is a minimally invasive procedure with less pain, less blood loss, shorter hospital stays, and quicker recovery than with other surgical methods. The list of medical advances goes on and on and is added to every year.

THE HUMAN BODY

The human body is an awesome masterpiece. Imagine billions of microscopic parts, each with their own identity, working together in an organized manner for the benefit of the total being. The human body is more complex than the greatest computer, yet it is personal. The study of the human body is as old as history itself because people have always had an interest in how the body is put together, how it works, why it becomes defective (illness), and why it wears out (aging).

The study of the human body is essential for those planning a career in health sciences, just as knowledge about automobiles is necessary for those planning to repair them. How can you fix an automobile if you do not know how it is put together or how it works? How can you help fix a human body if you do not know how it is put together or how it works?

ANATOMY AND PHYSIOLOGY

Human anatomy is the study of the shape and structure of the human body and its parts. It encompasses a wide range of topics, including the development and microscopic organization of structures, the relationship between structures, and the interrelationship between structure and function. Gross human anatomy deals with the large structures of the human body that can be seen through normal dissection. Microscopic anatomy deals with the smaller structures and fine detail that can be seen only with the aid of a microscope.

Human physiology is the scientific study of the functions or processes of the human body. It answers how, what, and why anatomic parts work. Anatomy and physiology are interrelated because structure and function are always closely associated. The function of an organ, or how it works, depends on how it is put together. Conversely, the anatomy or structure provides clues to understanding how it works. The structure of the hand, with its long, jointed fingers, is related to its function of grasping things. The heart is designed as a muscular pump that can contract to force blood into the blood vessels. By contrast, lungs are made of a thin tissue and function to exchange oxygen and carbon dioxide between the outside environment and the blood. Imagine what would happen if the heart were made of thin tissue and the lungs were made of thick muscle. Structure and function are always related.

LEVELS OF ORGANIZATION

Among the most outstanding features of the complex human body are its order and organization—how all the parts, from tiny cells to visible organs, work together to make a functioning whole. The organizational scheme of the body has six levels (Fig. 5.1).

Starting with the simplest and proceeding to the most complex, the six levels of organization are chemical, cellular, tissue, organ, body system, and total organism. The structural and functional characteristics of all organisms are determined by their chemical makeup.

Chemical Level

The *chemical level* deals with the interactions of atoms, such as hydrogen and oxygen, and their combinations into molecules, such as water. Molecules contribute to the makeup of a cell, which is the basic unit of life.

Cells

Cells, discussed later in this chapter, are the basic living units of all organisms. Estimates indicate that there are about 75 trillion dynamic, living cells in the human body. These cells represent a variety of sizes, shapes, and structures and provide a vast array of functions.

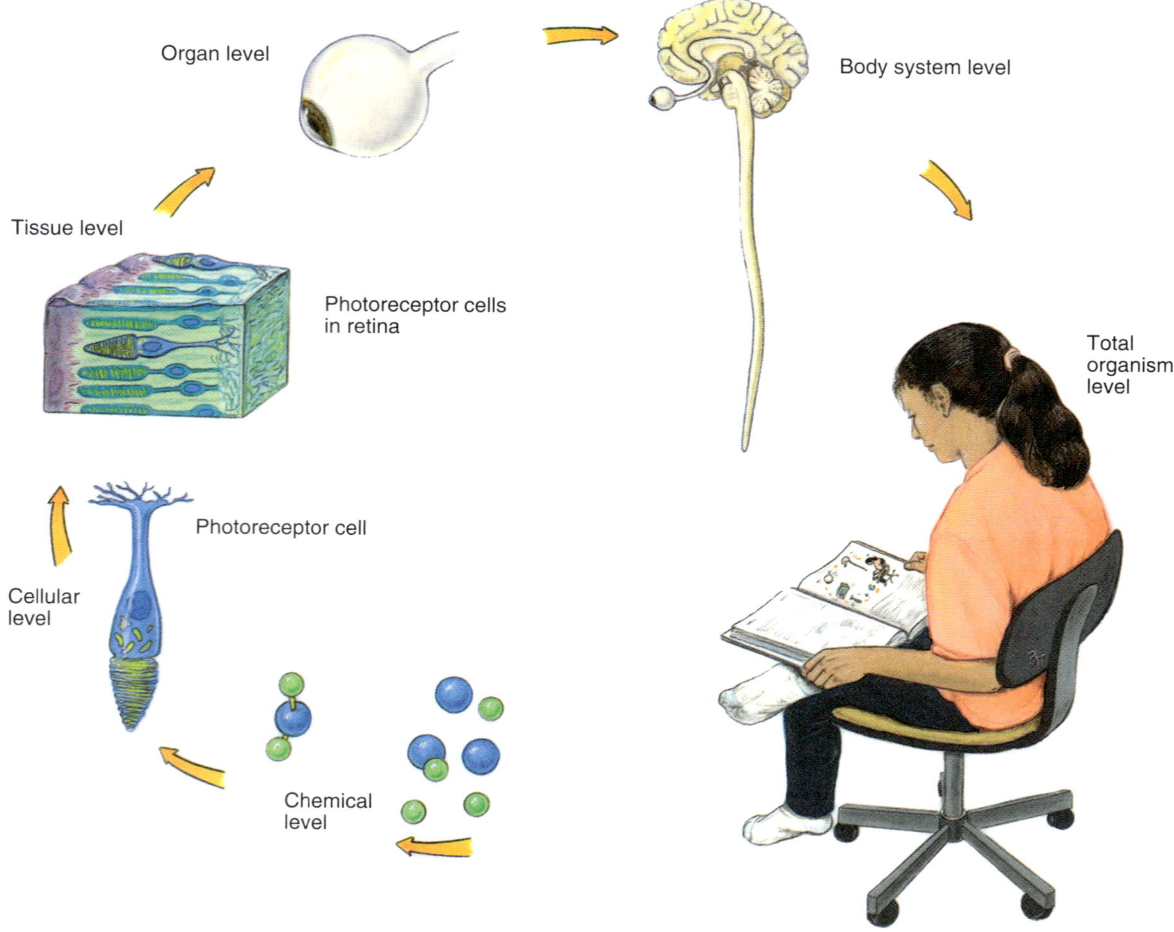

Fig. 5.1 Organizational scheme of the body. From simple to complex, the levels are chemical, cellular, tissue, organ, body system, and total organism. (From Applegate E: *The anatomy and physiology learning system*, ed 4, St. Louis, 2011, Saunders.)

Tissues

Cells with similar structure and function are grouped together as *tissues*. All of the tissues of the body are grouped into four main types: epithelial, connective, muscle, and nervous. The tissue level of organization is discussed later in this chapter.

Organs

An organ is made up of two or more types of tissue that form a more complex structure and work together to perform one or more functions. Examples of organs include the skin, heart, ear, stomach, and liver.

Body Systems

A *body system* consists of several organs that work together to accomplish a set of functions. Some examples of body systems include the nervous system, the digestive system, and the respiratory system.

Total Organism

Finally, the most complex of all the levels is the *total organism*, which is made up of several systems that work together to maintain life.

ORGAN SYSTEMS

The human body has 11 major organ systems, each with specific functions. All of the organ systems are interrelated and work together to sustain life. Each system is described briefly here and then in more detail in later chapters. The organ systems are illustrated and summarized in Table 5.1.

Integumentary System

Integument means skin. The integumentary system consists of the skin and the various accessory organs associated with it. These accessories include hair, nails, sweat glands, and sebaceous (oil) glands. The components of the integumentary

Table 5.1 Organ Systems of the Body

Integumentary System	Skeletal System	Muscular System
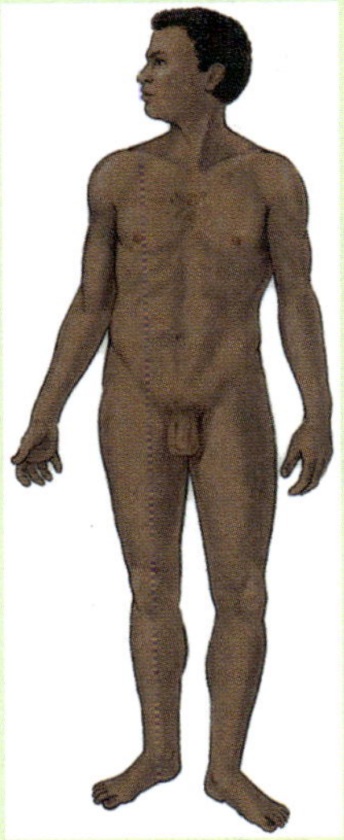	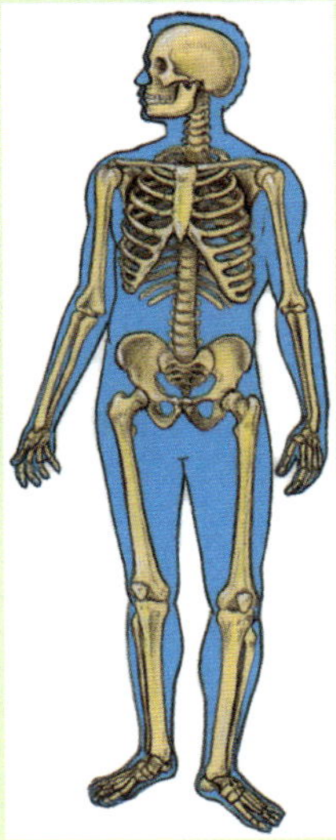	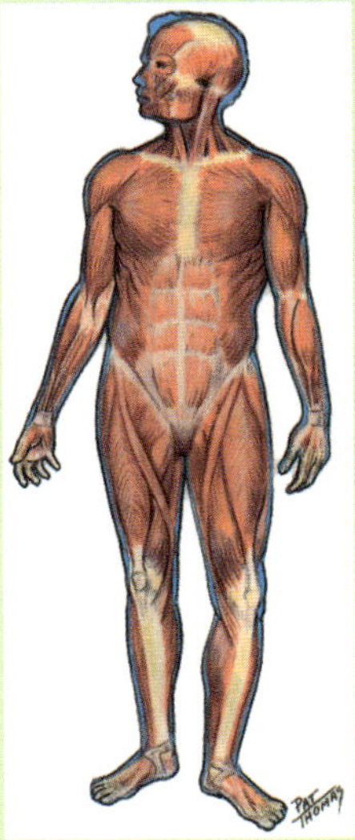
Components: Skin, hair, nails, sweat, sebaceous glands	**Components:** Bones, cartilage, ligaments	**Components:** Muscles
Functions: Covers and protects body; regulates temperature	**Functions:** Provides body framework and support; protects; attaches muscles to bones; provides calcium storage	**Functions:** Produces movement; maintains posture; provides heat
Nervous System	**Endocrine System**	**Cardiovascular System**
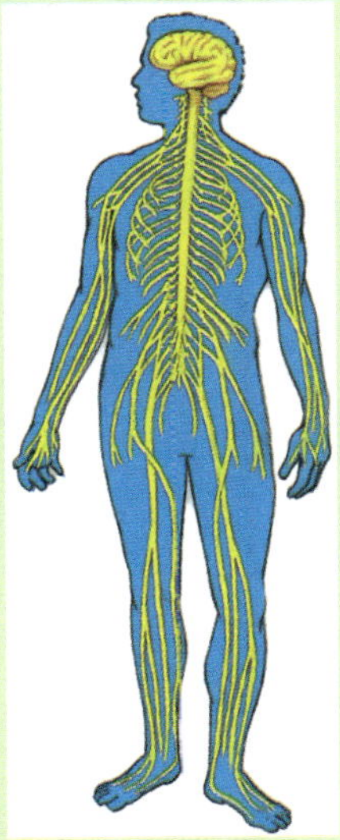	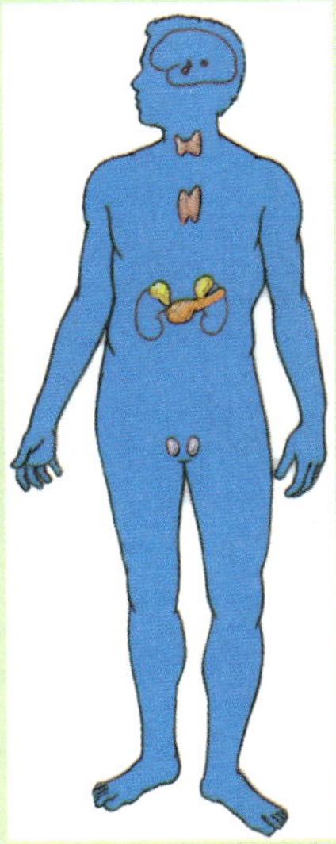	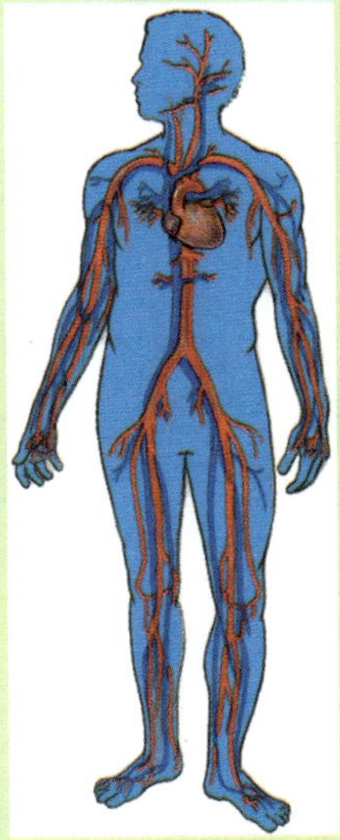
Components: Brain, spinal cord, nerves, sense receptors	**Components:** Pituitary, adrenal, thyroid, other ductless glands	**Components:** Heart, blood vessels, blood
Functions: Coordinates body activities; receives and transmits stimuli	**Functions:** Regulates metabolic activities and body chemistry	**Functions:** Transports material from one part of the body to another; defends against disease

Continued

Table 5.1 Organ Systems of the Body—cont'd

Lymphatic System	Digestive System	Respiratory System
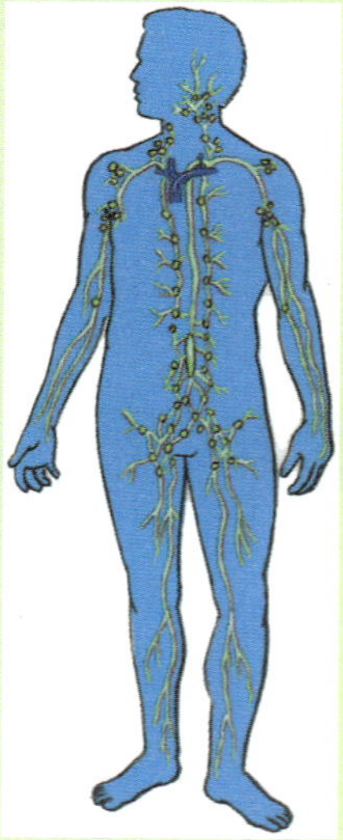	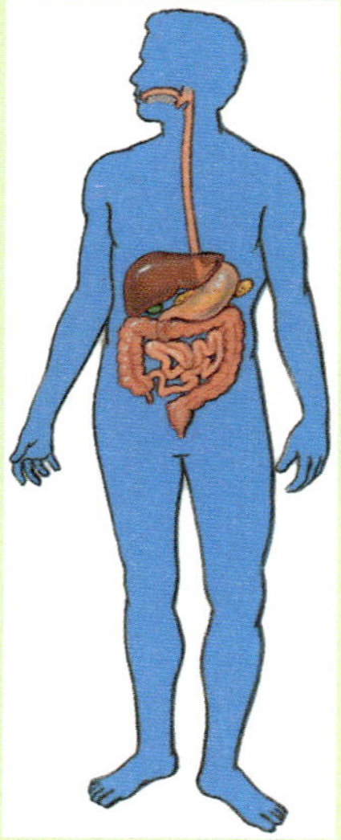	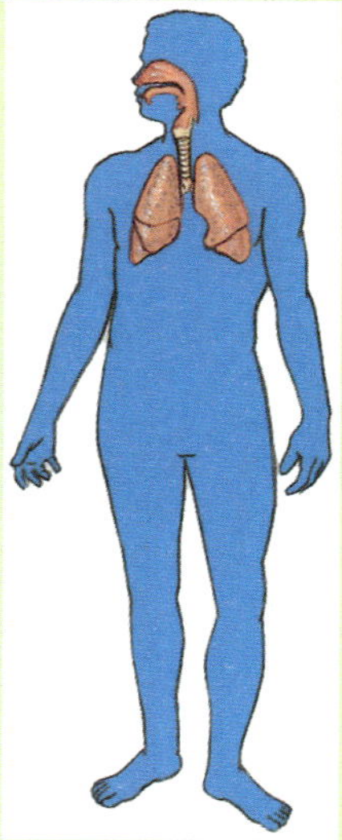
Components: Lymph, lymph vessels, lymphoid organs	**Components:** Mouth, esophagus, stomach, intestines, liver, pancreas	**Components:** Air passageways, lungs
Functions: Returns tissue fluid to the blood; defends against disease	**Functions:** Ingests and digests food; absorbs nutrients into blood	**Functions:** Exchanges gases between blood and external environment
Urinary System	**Reproductive System**	
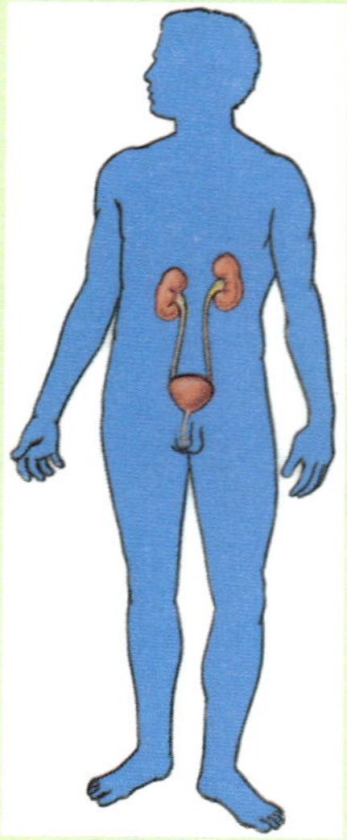	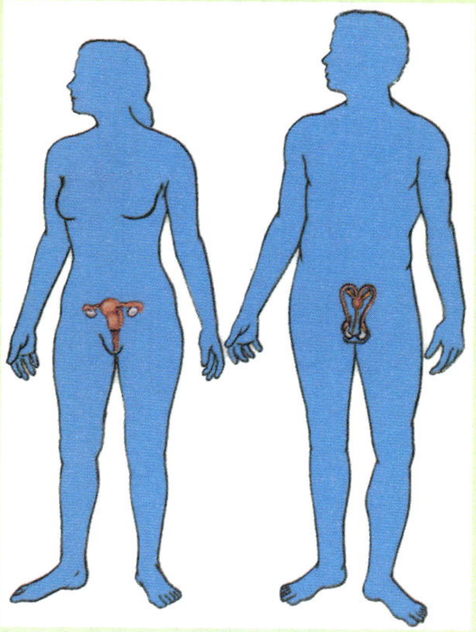	
Components: Kidneys, ureters, urinary bladder, urethra	**Components:** Testes, ovaries, accessory structures	
Functions: Excretes metabolic wastes; regulates fluid balance and acid–base balance	**Functions:** Forms new individuals to provide continuation of the human species	

From Applegate E: *The anatomy and physiology learning system*, ed 4, St. Louis, 2011, Saunders.

system protect the underlying tissues from injury, protect against water loss, contain sense receptors, help in temperature regulation, and synthesize chemicals to be used in other parts of the body.

Skeletal System

The skeletal system forms the framework of the body and protects underlying organs, such as the brain, lungs, and heart. The skeletal system consists of bones and joints along with ligaments and cartilage that bind the bones together. Bones serve as attachments for muscles and act with the muscles to produce movement. Tissues within bones produce blood cells and store inorganic salts containing calcium and phosphorus.

Muscular System

Muscles are the organs of the muscular system. As muscles contract, they create the forces that produce movement and maintain posture. Muscles can store energy in the form of glycogen and are the primary source of heat within the body.

Nervous System

The nervous system consists of the brain, spinal cord, and associated nerves. These organs work together to coordinate body activities. Nerve cells, or **neurons**, are specialized to transmit impulses from one point to another. In this way, body parts can communicate with one another and with the outside environment. Some nerve cells have special endings called *sense receptors* that detect changes in the environment.

Endocrine System

The endocrine system includes all the glands that secrete chemicals known as *hormones*. Hormones travel through the blood and act as messengers to regulate cellular activities. The endocrine and nervous systems work together to coordinate and regulate body activities to maintain a proper balance. The nervous system typically acts quickly, whereas the endocrine system acts slowly but with a more sustained effect. The endocrine system also regulates reproductive functions in both males and females.

Cardiovascular System

The cardiovascular system consists of the blood, heart, and blood vessels. The blood transports nutrients, hormones, and oxygen to tissue cells and removes waste products such as carbon dioxide. Certain cells within the blood known as *white blood cells* defend the body against disease. The heart acts as a pump to create the forces necessary to maintain blood pressure and to circulate the blood. The blood vessels serve as hollow tubes for the flow of blood.

Lymphatic System

The lymphatic system consists of a series of vessels that transport a fluid called *lymph* from the tissues back into the blood. In addition to lymph, the system includes lymph nodes and lymphoid organs, such as the tonsils, spleen, and thymus, that filter the lymph to remove foreign particles as a protection against disease. Lymphoid organs also function in the body's defense mechanism by enhancing the activities of cells that inactivate specific pathogenic agents. The lymphatic system is sometimes considered to be a part of the cardiovascular system.

Digestive System

The organs of the digestive system include the mouth, pharynx, esophagus, stomach, small intestine, and large intestine (colon), which make up the digestive tract. Accessory organs of this system include the teeth, tongue, salivary glands, liver, gallbladder, and pancreas. The functions of this system are to ingest food, process it into molecules that can be used by the body, and then eliminate the residue.

Respiratory System

The respiratory system brings oxygen, in the form of air, into the lungs; removes the carbon dioxide; and provides a membrane for the exchange of these gases between the blood and lungs. The system consists of the nasal cavities, pharynx, larynx, trachea, bronchi, and lungs.

Urinary System

The kidneys, ureters, urinary bladder, and urethra make up the urinary system. The kidneys remove various waste materials from the blood and help to regulate the fluid level and chemical content of the body. The waste product of kidney function is urine, which is transported through the ureters and urethra. The urinary bladder serves as a reservoir or storage area for the urine.

Reproductive System

The purpose of the reproductive system is the production of new individuals. The primary organs of the system are the gonads, which produce the reproductive cells. These include the ovaries in the female and the testes in the male. In addition to gonads, there are accessory glands, supporting structures, and duct systems for the transport of the reproductive cells. In the female the reproductive system produces ova or eggs, receives sperm from the male, and provides for the support and development of the embryo and fetus. The male reproductive system is concerned with the production and maintenance of sperm and the transfer of these cells to the female.

HOMEOSTASIS

Homeostasis refers to the constant internal environment that must be maintained for the cells of the body. The word is derived from two Greek words: *homeo*, which means "alike" or "the same," and *stasis*, which means "always" or "staying." Putting these together, the word *homeostasis* means "staying the same." When the body is healthy, the internal environment always stays the same. It remains stable within a limited normal range.

Everyone is familiar with aspects of the external environment—whether it is cold or hot, humid or dry, smoggy or clear. The internal environment is not quite as obvious. It involves the tissue fluid that surrounds and bathes every cell of the body. Normal functional activities of the cell depend on the internal environment being maintained within a limited normal range. The chemical content, volume, temperature, and pressure of the fluid must stay the same, regardless of external conditions, so that the cell can function properly. If the conditions in the tissue fluid deviate from normal, mechanisms respond that try to restore conditions to normal. If the mechanisms are unsuccessful, the cell malfunctions and dies. This leads to illness and disease. Ultimately the goal of medical treatment is to restore homeostasis.

Negative and Positive Feedback

Any condition or stimulus that disrupts the homeostatic balance in the body is a *stressor.* When a stressor causes internal conditions to deviate from normal, all the body systems work to bring conditions back to the normal range. This is usually accomplished by a **negative feedback** mechanism in which a stimulus initiates reactions that reduce the stimulus. This mechanism works similarly to a thermostat connected to a furnace and an air conditioner. When the temperature in the room decreases (stressor) below the thermostat setting (normal), the sensing device in the thermostat detects the change and causes the furnace to add heat to the room. When the room becomes too warm, the furnace stops, and the air conditioner begins to cool the room. Negative feedback mechanisms do not prevent variation, but they keep variation within a normal range.

An example of a physiologic negative feedback mechanism in the human body involves blood pressure. When blood pressure decreases below normal, body sensors detect the deviation and initiate changes that bring the pressure back within the normal range. When the pressure increases above normal, changes occur to decrease the pressure to normal. Variations in blood pressure occur, but homeostatic mechanisms keep them within the limits of a normal range.

The nervous and endocrine systems work together to control homeostasis, but all the organ systems in the body help maintain the normal conditions of the internal environment. The brain contains centers that monitor temperature, pressure, volume, and the chemical conditions of body fluids. Endocrine glands secrete hormones in response to deviations from normal conditions, and these hormones affect other organs. The changes required to bring conditions back to the normal range are mediated by various organ systems. Good health depends on homeostasis. Illness results when the negative feedback mechanisms that maintain homeostasis are disrupted. Medical therapy attempts to assist the negative feedback process to restore balance, or homeostasis.

ANATOMIC TERMS

Certain basic terms need to be understood if one is to communicate effectively in the health care profession. In other words, you have to speak the language. This section explains some basic terms that relate to the anatomy of the body. They are used to describe directions and regions of the body.

Anatomic Position

If directional terms are to be meaningful, there must be some knowledge of the beginning position. If you give a person directions to go somewhere, you must have a starting reference point. When using directions in anatomy and physiology, it is assumed that the body is in **anatomic position**. In this position, the body is standing erect, the face is forward, and the arms are at the sides with the palms and toes directed forward. Fig. 5.2 illustrates the body in anatomic position. It is important for medical assistants to understand anatomic positioning because all patient documentation is done as if the patient were in anatomic position.

Directions in the Body

Directional terms are used to describe the relative position of one part to another. Note that in the following list of directional terms, the two items in each pair of terms are opposites.

Superior means that a part is above another part, or closer to the head. The nose is superior to the mouth. *Inferior* means that a part is below another part, or closer to the feet. The heart is inferior to the neck.

Anterior (or ventral) means toward the front surface. The heart is anterior to the vertebral column. *Posterior* means that a part is toward the back. The heart is posterior to the sternum.

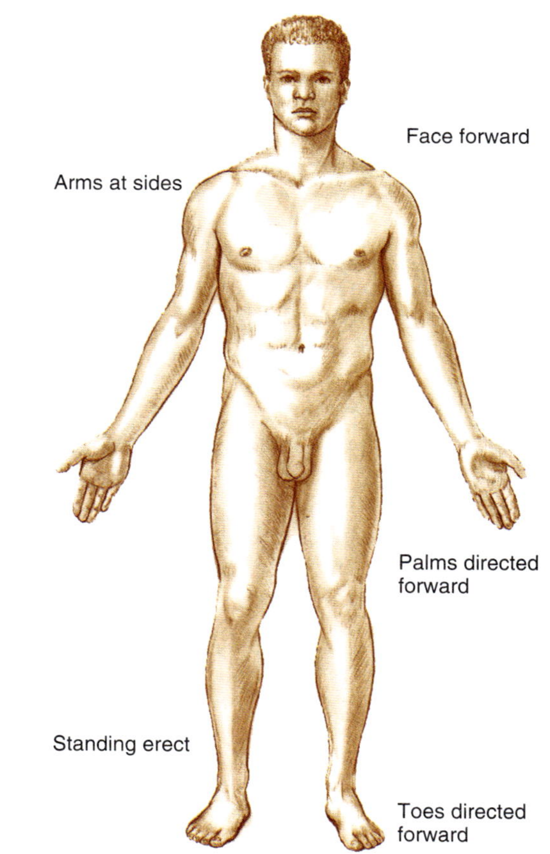

Fig. 5.2 The body in anatomic position. (From Applegate E: *The anatomy and physiology learning system*, ed 4, St. Louis, 2011, Saunders.)

Medial means toward, or nearer, the midline of the body. The nose is medial to the ears. *Lateral* means toward, or nearer, the side, away from the midline. The ears are lateral to the eyes.

Proximal means that a part is closer to a point of attachment, or closer to the trunk of the body, than another part. The elbow is proximal to the wrist. The opposite of proximal is *distal*, which means that a part is farther away from a point of attachment than is another part. The fingers are distal to the wrist.

Superficial means that a part is located on or near the surface. The superficial (or outermost) layer of the skin is the epidermis. The opposite of superficial is *deep*, which means that a part is away from the surface. Muscles are deep to the skin.

Visceral pertains to internal organs or the covering of the organs. The visceral pericardium covers the heart. *Parietal* refers to the wall of a body cavity. The parietal peritoneum lines the wall of the abdominal cavity.

Planes and Sections of the Body

To aid in visualizing the spatial relationships of internal body parts, anatomists use three imaginary planes, each of which is cut through the body in a different direction. Fig. 5.3 illustrates these three planes. These planes are often used to describe surgical incisions and x-ray positions.

The *sagittal* plane refers to a lengthwise cut that divides the body into right and left portions. This is sometimes called a *longitudinal section.* If the cut passes through the midline of the body, it is called a *midsagittal plane*, and it divides the body into right and left halves.

The *transverse plane* or horizontal plane is perpendicular to the sagittal plane and cuts across the body horizontally to divide it into superior and inferior portions. Sections cut this way are sometimes called *cross sections.*

The *frontal plane* divides the body into anterior and posterior portions. It is perpendicular to both the sagittal plane and the transverse plane. This is sometimes called a *coronal plane.*

Body Cavities

Spaces within the body that contain the internal organs or viscera are called *body cavities.* The two main cavities are the *dorsal cavity* and the larger *ventral cavity*, which are illustrated in Fig. 5.4. The dorsal cavity is divided into the *cranial cavity*, which contains the brain, and the *spinal cavity*, which contains the spinal cord. The cranial and spinal cavities join with each other to form a continuous space.

The ventral cavity is much larger than the dorsal cavity and is subdivided into the *thoracic cavity* and the *abdominopelvic cavity.* The thoracic cavity is superior to the abdominopelvic cavity and contains the heart, lungs, esophagus, and trachea. It is separated from the abdominopelvic cavity by the muscular diaphragm. Although there is no clear-cut partition to divide it, the abdominopelvic cavity is separated into the superior *abdominal cavity* and the inferior *pelvic cavity.* The stomach, liver, gallbladder, spleen, and most of the intestines are in the abdominal cavity. The pelvic cavity contains portions of the small and large intestines, the rectum, the urinary bladder, and the internal reproductive organs.

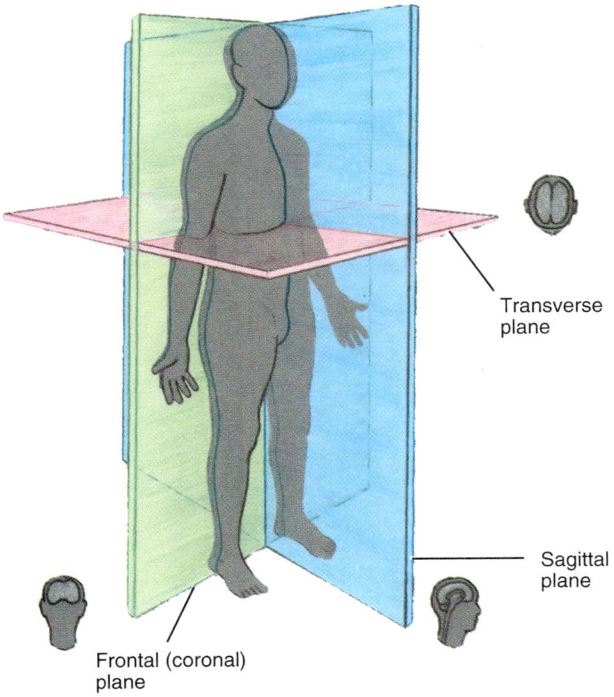

Fig. 5.3 Transverse, sagittal, and frontal planes of the body. (From Applegate E: *The anatomy and physiology learning system*, ed 4, St. Louis, 2011, Saunders.)

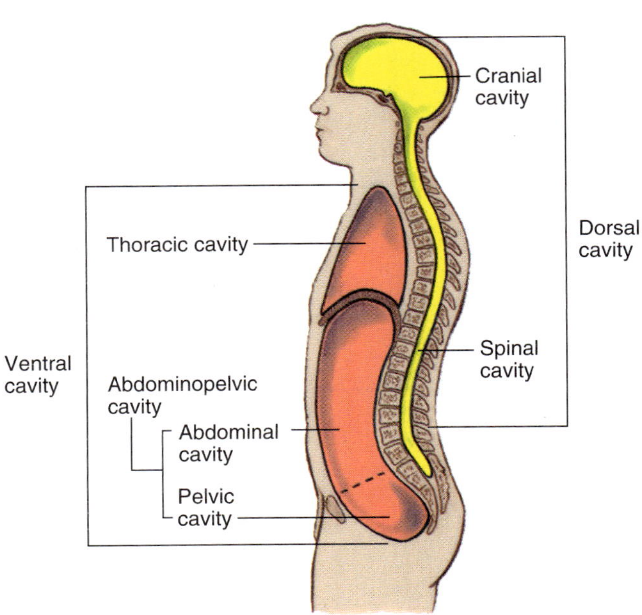

Fig. 5.4 The two major cavities in the body and their subdivisions. (From Applegate E: *The anatomy and physiology learning system*, ed 4, St. Louis, 2011, Saunders.)

To help describe the location of body organs or pain, health care professionals frequently divide the abdominopelvic cavity into regions using imaginary lines. One such method uses the midsagittal plane and a transverse plane that passes through the umbilicus. This divides the abdominopelvic area into four quadrants, illustrated in Fig. 5.5. Another system uses two sagittal planes and two transverse planes to divide the abdominopelvic area into the nine regions illustrated in Fig. 5.6. The three central regions are, from superior to inferior, the *epigastric*, *umbilical*, and *hypogastric* regions. Lateral to these, from superior to inferior, are the right and left *hypochondriac*, right and left *lumbar*, and right and left *iliac* or *inguinal* regions.

Regions of the Body

The body may be divided into the *axial* portion, which consists of the head, neck, and trunk, and the *appendicular* portion, which consists of the limbs. The trunk, or *torso*, includes the thorax, abdomen, and pelvis. In addition to these terms and the nine abdominopelvic regions identified in the previous section, numerous other terms are applied to specific body areas. Some of these are listed in Table 5.2 and are identified in Fig. 5.7.

CELL STRUCTURE AND FUNCTION

STRUCTURE OF THE GENERALIZED CELL

Every individual begins life as a single cell, a fertilized egg. This single cell divides into 2 cells, then 4, 8, 16, and on and on, until the adult human body has an estimated 75 trillion cells. Cells are the structural and functional units of the human body. Homeostasis depends on the interaction between the cell and its environment.

During development, cells become specialized in size, shape, characteristics, and function, resulting in a large variety of cells in the body. For descriptive purposes it is convenient to imagine a typical, generalized cell that contains the components of all the different cell types. Not all the components of a "generalized" cell are present in every cell type, but each component is present in some cells and has its particular function to maintain life. A generalized cell is illustrated in Fig. 5.8, and the structure and functions of the cellular components are summarized in Table 5.3.

Plasma Membrane

Every cell in the body is enclosed by a *plasma (cell) membrane*. The plasma membrane separates the material outside the cell (extracellular) from the material inside the cell (intracellular). If the membrane breaks, the cell dies. The plasma membrane determines what can go into or out of the cell. It is *selectively permeable*, which means that some substances can pass through the membrane but others cannot. The main structural components of the plasma membrane are *phospholipids* and *proteins*.

Cytoplasm

The *cytoplasm* is the gel-like fluid inside the cell. The cytoplasm has numerous small structures, called *organelles*, suspended in it. These organelles, or "little organs," are the functional machinery of the cell, and each organelle type has a specific role in the metabolic reactions that take place in the cytoplasm.

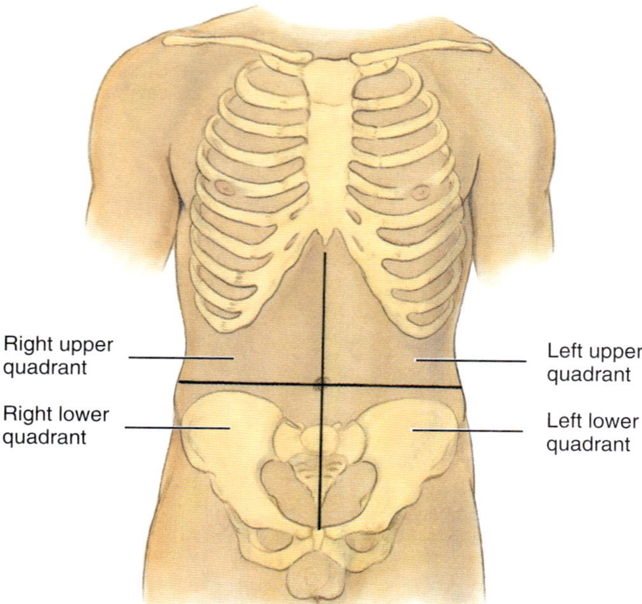

Fig. 5.5 Abdominopelvic quadrants that are formed by a midsagittal plane and a transverse plane through the umbilicus. (From Applegate E: *The anatomy and physiology learning system*, ed 4, St. Louis, 2011, Saunders.)

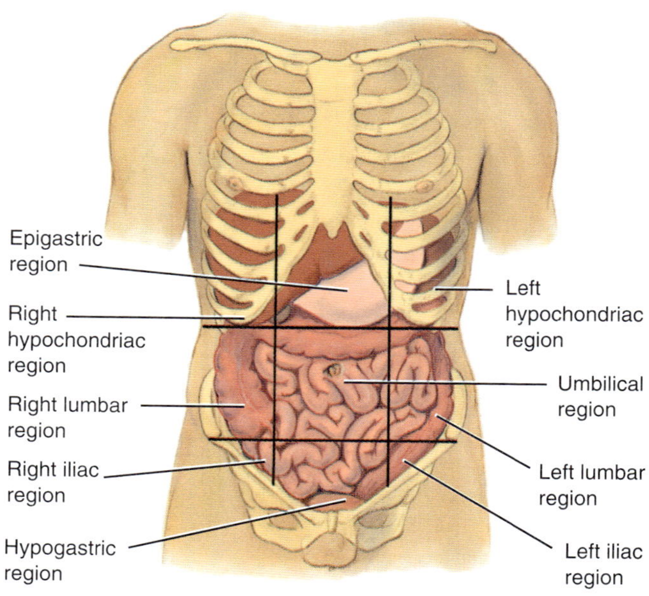

Fig. 5.6 Nine abdominopelvic regions formed by two sagittal planes and two transverse planes. (From Applegate E: *The anatomy and physiology learning system*, ed 4, St. Louis, 2011, Saunders.)

Table 5.2 Body Area Terms

Term	Description
Abdominal (ab-DAHM-ih-nal)	Portion of the trunk between the thorax and pelvis; celiac region
Antebrachial (an-te-BRAY-kee-al)	Region between the elbow and wrist; forearm; cubital region
Antecubital (an-te-KYOO-bih-tal)	Space in front of elbow
Axillary (AK-sih-lair-ee)	Armpit area
Brachial (BRAY-kee-al)	Arm; proximal portion of upper limb
Buccal (BUK-al)	Region of cheek
Buttock (BUT-tuck)	Posterior aspect of lower trunk; gluteal region
Carpal (KAR-pal)	Wrist
Celiac (SEE-lee-ak)	Abdomen
Cephalic (seh-FAL-ik)	Head
Cervical (SER-vih-kal)	Neck region
Costal (KAHS-tal)	Ribs
Cranial (KRAY-nee-al)	Skull
Crural (KROO-rahl)	Portion of lower extremity between knee and foot; leg
Cubital (KYOO-bih-tal)	Forearm; region between elbow and wrist; antebrachial
Cutaneous (kyoo-TAY-nee-us)	Skin
Femoral (FEM-or-al)	Thigh; part of lower extremity between hip and knee
Frontal (FRUN-tal)	Forehead
Gluteal (GLOO-tee-al)	Buttock region
Groin (GROYN)	Depressed region between abdomen and thigh; inguinal
Inguinal (IN-gwih-nal)	Depressed region between abdomen and thigh; groin
Leg (LEG)	Portion of lower extremity between knee and foot; also called the *crural region*
Lumbar (LUM-bar)	Region of lower back and side between lowest rib and pelvis
Mammary (MAM-ah-ree)	Pertaining to the breast
Navel (NAY-vel)	Middle region of the abdomen; umbilical region
Occipital (ahk-SIP-ih-tal)	Lower portion of the back of the head
Ophthalmic (off-THAL-mik)	Pertaining to the eyes
Oral (OH-ral) or (AW-ral)	Pertaining to the mouth
Otic (OH-tik)	Ears
Palmar (PAWL-mar)	Palm of hand
Pectoral (PEK-toh-ral)	Chest region
Pedal (PED-al)	Foot
Pelvic (PEL-vik)	Inferior region of abdominopelvic cavity
Perineal (pair-ih-NEE-al)	Region between anus and pubic symphysis; includes region of external reproductive organs
Plantar (PLAN-tar)	Sole of foot
Popliteal (pop-LIT-ee-al or pop-lih-TEE-al)	Area behind knee
Sacral (SAY-kral)	Posterior region between hip bones
Sternal (STIR-nal)	Anterior midline of the thorax
Tarsal (TAHR-sal)	Ankle and instep of foot
Thigh (THIGH)	Part of lower extremity between hip and knee; femoral region
Thoracic (tho-RAS-ik)	Chest; part of trunk inferior to neck and superior to diaphragm
Umbilical (um-BIL-ih-kal)	Navel; middle region of abdomen
Vertebral (ver-TEE-bral or VER-teh-bral)	Pertaining to spinal column; backbone

From Applegate E: *The anatomy and physiology learning system*, ed 4, St. Louis, 2011, Saunders.

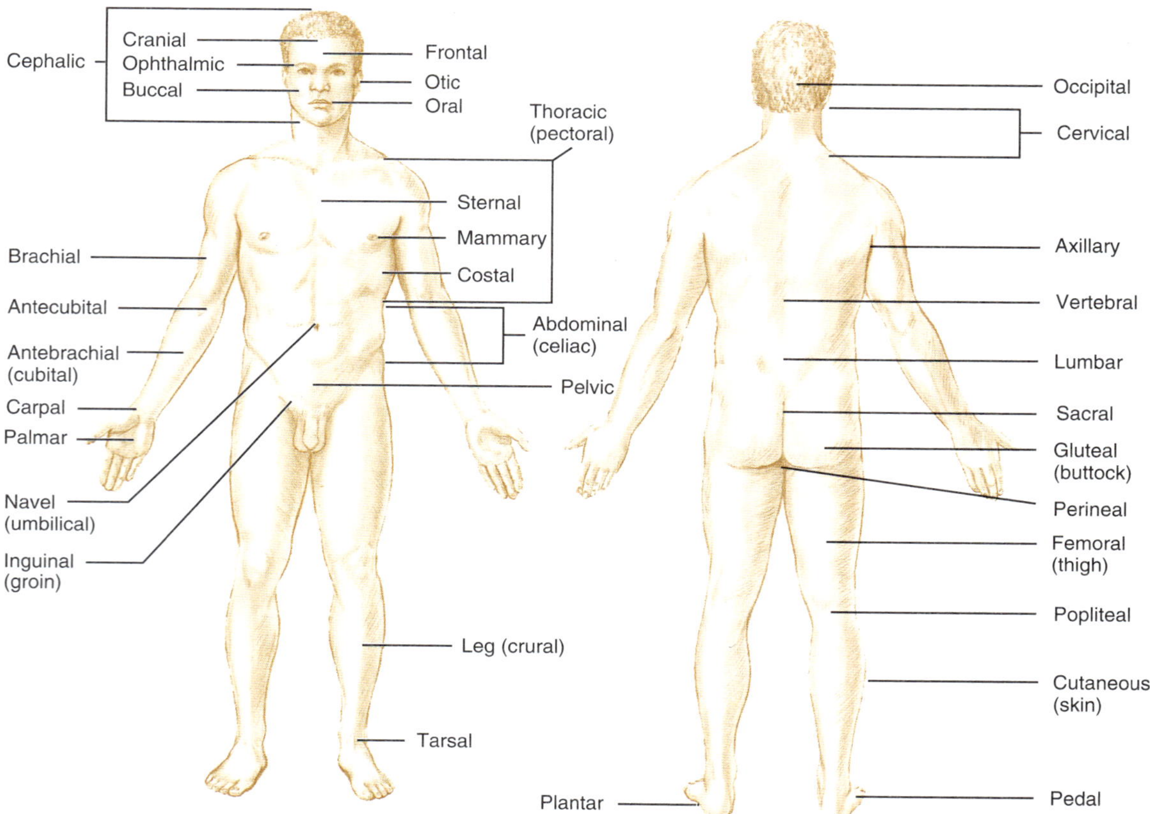

Fig. 5.7 Terms for selected regions of the body. (From Applegate E: *The anatomy and physiology learning system*, ed 4, St. Louis, 2011, Saunders.)

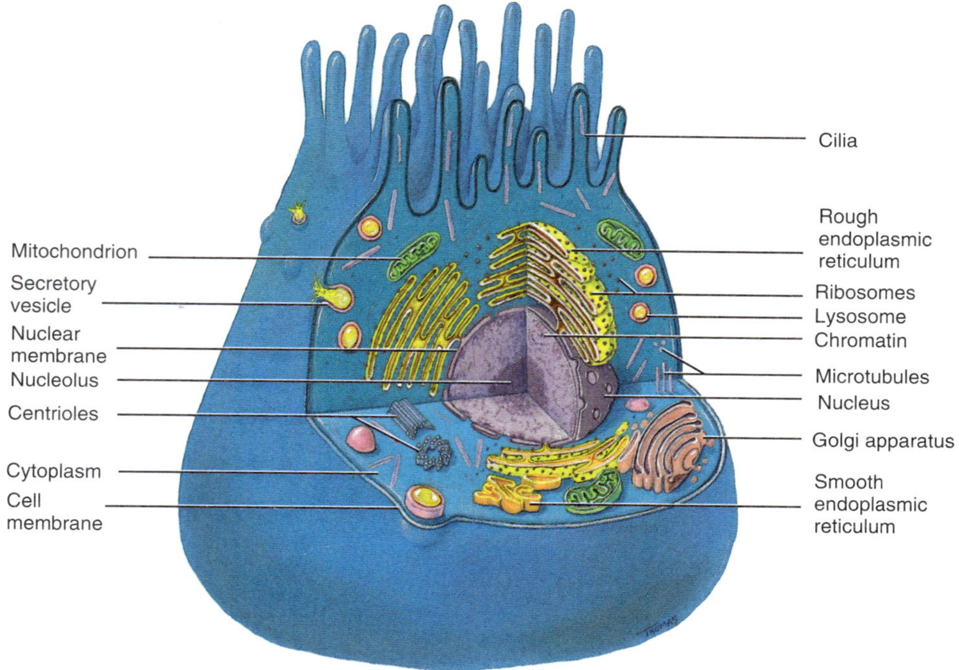

Fig. 5.8 Generalized cell. (From Applegate E: *The anatomy and physiology learning system*, ed 4, St. Louis, 2011, Saunders.)

Table 5.3 Structure and Function of Cellular Components

Component	Structure	Function
Plasma membrane	Bilayer of phospholipid and protein molecules	Maintains integrity of cell; controls passage of materials into and out of cell
Cytoplasm	Water; dissolved ions and nutrients; suspended colloids	Medium for chemical reactions; suspending medium for organelles
Nucleus	Spherical body near center of cell; enclosed in a membrane	Contains genetic material; regulates activities of cell
Nuclear membrane	Double-layered membrane around nucleus; has pores	Separates cytoplasm from nucleoplasm; pores allow passage of material as needed
Chromatin	Strands of DNA in nucleus	Genetic material of cell; becomes chromosomes during cell division
Nucleolus	Dense, nonmembranous body in nucleus; composed of RNA and protein molecules	Forms ribosomes
Mitochondria	Rod-shaped bodies enclosed by a double-layered membrane in cytoplasm; folds of inner membrane form cristae	Major site of adenosine triphosphate synthesis; convert energy from nutrients into a form that is usable by the body
Ribosomes	Granules of RNA in cytoplasm	Protein synthesis
Endoplasmic reticulum	Interconnected membranous channels and sacs in cytoplasm	Transports material through cytoplasm; rough endoplasmic reticulum aids in synthesis of protein; smooth endoplasmic reticulum involved in lipid synthesis
Golgi apparatus	Group of flattened membranous sacs usually near nucleus	Packages products for secretion; forms lysosomes
Lysosomes	Membranous sacs of digestive enzymes in cytoplasm	Digest material taken into cell, debris from damaged cells, worn-out cell components
Cytoskeleton	Protein microfilaments and microtubules in cytoplasm	Provides support for cytoplasm; helps in movement of organelles
Centrioles	Pair of rod-shaped bodies composed of microtubules; located near nucleus at right angles to each other	Distribute chromosomes to daughter cells during cell division
Cilia	Membrane-enclosed bundles of microtubules that extend outward from cell membrane; short and numerous	Move substances across surface of cell
Flagella	Similar to cilia, except usually long and single	Cell locomotion

From Applegate E: *The anatomy and physiology learning system*, ed 4, St Louis, 2011, Saunders.

The cytoplasm is primarily water known as the *intracellular fluid*. About two-thirds of the water in the body is in the cytoplasm of cells. The intracellular fluid contains dissolved electrolytes, metabolic waste products, and nutrients such as amino acids and simple sugars.

Nucleus

The *nucleus* is the control center that directs the activities of the cell. All cells have at least one nucleus at some time during their existence; some, however, such as red blood cells, lose their nucleus as they mature. Other cells, such as skeletal muscle cells, have multiple nuclei.

The nucleus is a relatively large, spherical body that is usually located near the center of the cell (see Fig. 5.8). It is enclosed by a double-layered *nuclear membrane* that separates the cytoplasm of the cell from the *nucleoplasm*, the fluid portion inside the nucleus.

The nucleus contains the genetic material of the cell. In the nondividing cell, the genetic material, deoxyribonucleic acid (DNA), is present as long, slender, filamentous threads called *chromatin* (see Fig. 5.8). When the cell starts to divide or replicate, the chromatin condenses and becomes tightly coiled to form short, rodlike *chromosomes*. Each chromosome, composed of DNA with some protein, contains several hundred genes arranged in a specific linear order. Human cells have 23 pairs of chromosomes that together contain all the information necessary to direct the synthesis of more than 100,000 different proteins.

The *nucleolus* ("little nucleus") appears as a dark-staining, discrete, dense body within the nucleus (see Fig. 5.8). It has no enclosing membrane, and the number of nucleoli may vary from one to four in any given cell. The function of the nucleolus is to produce ribonucleic acid (RNA) and combine it with protein to form ribosomes. Ribosomes function in protein synthesis, as described later in this section. In growing cells and other cells that are making large amounts of protein, the nucleoli are large and distinct.

Cytoplasmic Organelles

Cytoplasmic organelles are "little organs" that are suspended in the cytoplasm of the cell. Each type of organelle has a definite structure and a specific role in the function of the cell.

Mitochondria

Mitochondria (singular *mitochondrion*) are elongated, oval, fluid-filled sacs in the cytoplasm that contain their own DNA and can reproduce themselves (see Fig. 5.8). Enzymes necessary for the production of adenosine triphosphate (ATP) are located inside the mitochondria. ATP is a chemical that stores chemical energy within the cell and provides energy for use by the body cells. Mitochondria could be called the "power plants" of the cell because they convert energy from nutrients into ATP.

Ribosomes

Ribosomes consist of small granules of RNA located in the cytoplasm. The RNA in the ribosomes is from the nucleolus; when fully assembled, ribosomes function in protein synthesis. Some ribosomes are found free in the cytoplasm. These ribosomes function in the synthesis of proteins for use within that same cell. Other ribosomes are attached to the membranes of the endoplasmic reticulum (ER) and function in the synthesis of proteins that are exported from the cell and used elsewhere.

Endoplasmic Reticulum

The *endoplasmic reticulum* (ER) is a complex series of membranous channels extending throughout the cytoplasm. The interconnected membranes form fluid-filled flattened sacs and tubular canals. The membranes are connected to the outer layer of the nuclear membrane, to the inner layer of the cell membrane, and to certain other organelles. The ER provides a path to transport materials from one part of the cell to another.

Some of the membranes of the ER have granular ribosomes attached to the outer surface (see Fig. 5.8). This is called *rough endoplasmic reticulum* (RER) and, because of the ribosomes, it functions in the synthesis and transport of protein molecules. Other portions of the ER lack the ribosomes and appear smooth. This is the *smooth endoplasmic reticulum* (SER), which functions in the synthesis of certain lipid molecules, such as steroids.

Golgi Apparatus

The *Golgi apparatus* is a series of four to six flattened membranous sacs, usually located near the nucleus, and is connected to the ER (see Fig. 5.8). It is the "packaging and shipping plant" of the cell.

Proteins and lipids are carried through the channels of the ER to the Golgi apparatus. Within the Golgi apparatus, the proteins become surrounded by a piece of the Golgi membrane. Then they are pinched off the end of the apparatus to become a *secretory vesicle*, a temporary inclusion in the cytoplasm. The secretory vesicles move to the cell membrane and release their contents to the exterior of the cell.

The Golgi apparatus is especially abundant and well developed in glandular cells that secrete a product, but it also functions in nonsecretory cells. In these cells it appears to package intracellular enzymes in the form of lysosomes. Because of the vesicles pinching off the ends of the flattened membranous sacs, the Golgi apparatus is sometimes described as looking like a stack of pancakes with syrup dripping off the edge.

Lysosomes

Lysosomes are membrane-enclosed sacs of various enzymes that have been packaged by the Golgi apparatus. When cells are damaged, these enzymes destroy the cellular debris. They also function in the destruction of worn-out cell parts. The enzymes break down particles, such as bacteria, that have been taken into the cell. When a white blood cell engulfs bacteria, the enzymes from the lysosomes destroy the bacteria. Lysosomal activity also seems to be responsible for decreasing the size of some body organs at certain periods. Atrophy of muscle because of lack of use, reduction in breast size after breastfeeding, and decrease in the size of the uterus after parturition all seem to be caused by lysosomal function.

Filamentous Protein Organelles

Several types of protein filaments are considered to be cellular organelles. The cytoskeleton and centrioles are in the cytoplasm, but the cilia and flagella project outward, away from the cell surface.

Cytoskeleton

The *cytoskeleton* helps to maintain the shape of the cell. At times it anchors certain organelles in position, but it may also move organelles from one position to another. Some parts of the cytoskeleton may move a portion of the cell membrane, whereas others may move the entire cell. The cytoskeleton also plays a role in muscle contraction.

The cytoskeleton is made up of protein *microfilaments* and *microtubules*. Microfilaments are long, slender rods of protein that support small projections of the cell membrane called *microvilli*. Microtubules are thin hollow cylinders. They are found in centrioles, cilia, and flagella.

Centrioles

A dense area called the *centrosome* is located near the nucleus and contains a pair of *centrioles* (see Fig. 5.8). Each centriole is a nonmembranous rod-shaped structure composed of microtubules. Centrioles function in cell reproduction by aiding in the distribution of chromosomes to the new daughter cells.

Cilia

Cilia are short, cylindric, hairlike processes that project outward from the cell membrane. Each cilium consists of specialized microtubules surrounded by a membrane and anchored under the cell membrane. Cilia create a wavelike motion to move substances across the surface of the cell. They are found in large quantities on the surfaces of cells that line the respiratory tract. Their motion moves mucus, in which particles of dust are embedded, upward and away from the lungs.

Flagella

Similar in structure to cilia, *flagella* are much longer and fewer. In contrast to cilia, which move substances across the surface of the cell, flagella beat with a whiplike motion to move the cell itself. In the human, the tail of the spermatozoon, or sperm cell, is a single flagellum that causes the swimming motion of the cell.

CELL FUNCTIONS

The structural and functional characteristics of different types of cells are determined by the nature of the proteins that are present. Cells of various types have different functions because cell structure and function are closely related. A very thin cell is not well suited for a protective function. Bone cells do not have an appropriate structure for nerve impulse conduction. Just as there are many cell types, there are varied cell functions. The specific functions of cells will become more apparent as the tissues, organs, and systems are studied. This section deals with the more generalized cell functions—the functions that relate to the sustained viability and continuation of the cell itself. These functions include movement of substances across the cell membrane, cell division to make new cells, and protein synthesis.

Movement of Substances Across the Cell Membrane

The cell membrane provides a surface through which substances enter and leave the cell. The cell membrane controls the composition of the cell's cytoplasm by regulating the passage of substances through the membrane. If the membrane breaks, this control is removed and the cell dies. The survival of the cell depends on maintaining the difference between extracellular and intracellular material. Mechanisms of movement across the cell membrane include diffusion, osmosis, filtration, active transport, endocytosis, and exocytosis. These are summarized in Table 5.4.

Diffusion

Diffusion is the movement of substances from a region of high concentration to a region of low concentration. Odors permeate a room because the aromatic molecules diffuse through the air. A crystal of dye will color a whole beaker of water because the dye particles diffuse from the region of high concentration in the dye crystal to regions of low concentration in the water (Fig. 5.9).

In the examples of diffusion cited, there has been no membrane involved. Diffusion can also occur across a membrane as long as the membrane is permeable to the substances involved. For example, oxygen and carbon dioxide are able to diffuse through the cell membrane. When carbon dioxide builds up in the capillaries to a concentration that is higher than in the lungs, the carbon dioxide diffuses into the lungs to be exhaled. Similarly, when the level of oxygen in the capillaries is lower than the level of oxygen in the lungs, oxygen diffuses into the capillaries for distribution to the body cells. In this way, the gases are exchanged between the air and the blood in the lungs, and between the blood and the cells of the various tissues (Fig. 5.10).

Table 5.4 Summary of Membrane Transport Mechanisms

Mechanism	Description
Passive	
Simple diffusion	Molecular movement down a concentration gradient
Osmosis	Movement of solvent toward high solute (low solvent) concentration; requires membrane
Filtration	Movement of solvent using hydrostatic pressure; requires membrane filter
Active	
Active transport	Movement of ions or molecules against a concentration gradient; requires carrier molecule and adenosine triphosphate (ATP)
Phagocytosis	Ingestion of solid particles by creation of vesicles; requires ATP
Pinocytosis	Ingestion of fluid by creation of vesicles; requires ATP
Exocytosis	Secretion of cellular products by creation of vesicles, then liberation of contents to outside of cell; requires ATP

From Applegate E: *The anatomy and physiology learning system*, ed 4, St. Louis, 2011, Saunders.

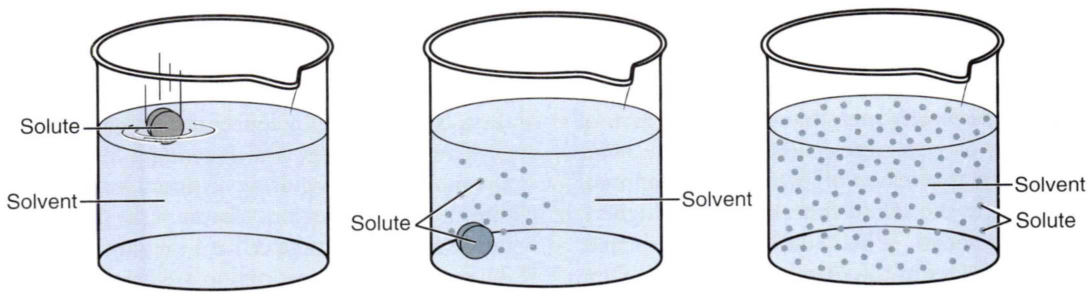

Fig. 5.9 Simple diffusion. Molecules of solute diffuse throughout the solvent until equilibrium exists. (From Applegate E: *The anatomy and physiology learning system*, ed 4, St. Louis, 2011, Saunders.)

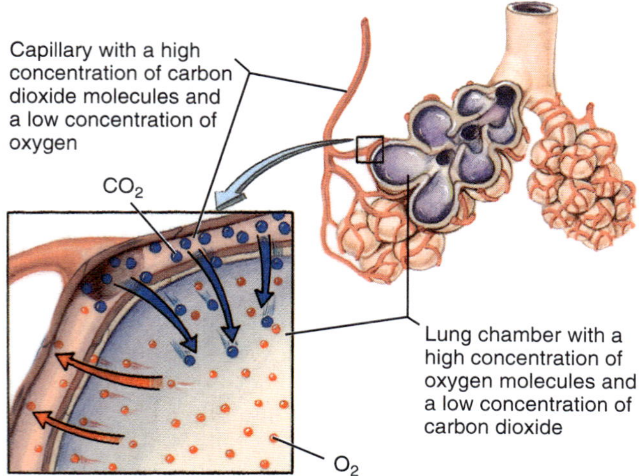

Fig. 5.10 Diffusion of oxygen and carbon dioxide in the lungs. Oxygen moves from the higher concentration in the lung into the lower concentration in the capillary. Carbon dioxide moves in the opposite direction. (From Applegate E: *The anatomy and physiology learning system*, ed 4, St. Louis, 2011, Saunders.)

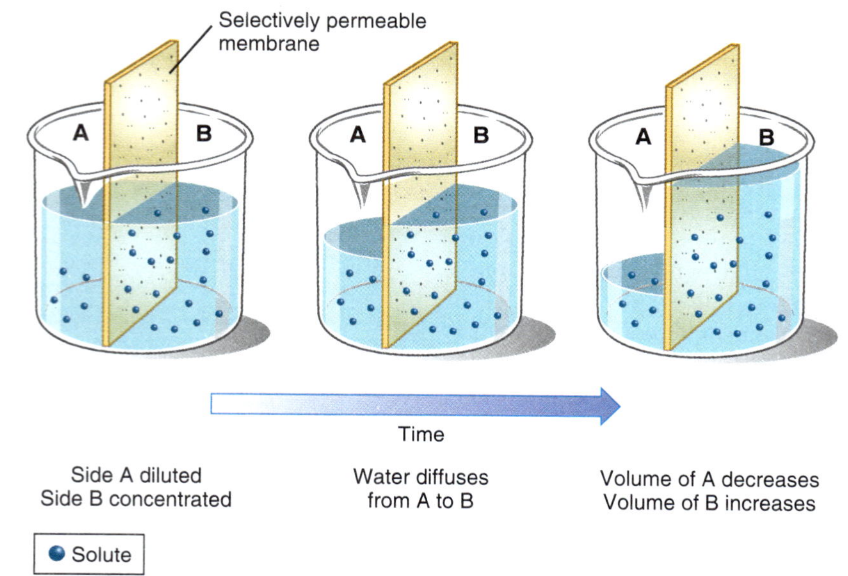

Fig. 5.11 Osmosis. Solvent molecules move across the membrane, but solute molecules do not because the membrane is selectively permeable. (From Applegate E: *The anatomy and physiology learning system*, ed 4, St. Louis, 2011, Saunders.)

Osmosis

Osmosis involves the movement of *solvent* (water) molecules through a *selectively permeable* membrane from a region of higher concentration of water molecules (where the *solute* concentration is lower) to a region of lower concentration of water molecules (where the solute concentration is higher). Fig. 5.11 illustrates osmosis. When equilibrium is reached, the solutions on both sides of the membrane have the same concentration, but the solution that was more concentrated at the start will now have a greater volume. Water molecules continue to pass through the membrane after equilibrium, but because they move in both directions at the same rate, there is no change in concentration or volume.

If a red blood cell, which contains 5% glucose, is placed in a container of 5% glucose solution, water will move in both directions at the same rate because the glucose concentrations inside and outside the cell are the same. Solutions that have the same solute concentration are *isotonic* (Fig. 5.12A).

When a red blood cell is placed in a 10% glucose solution, water will leave the cell (where there are more water molecules)

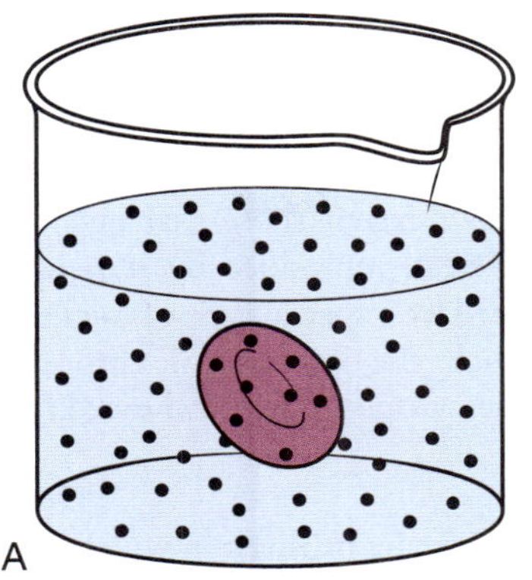

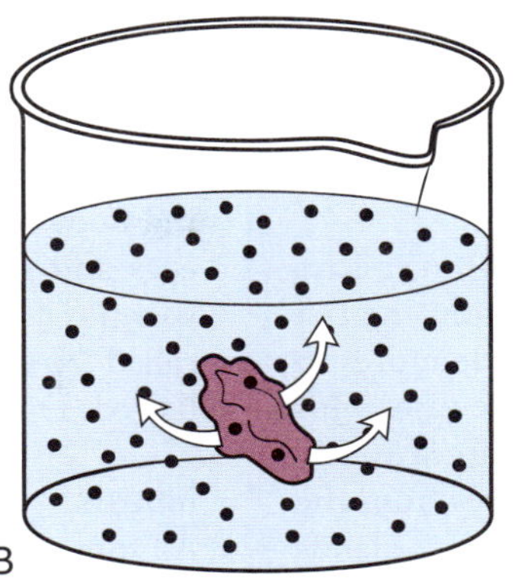

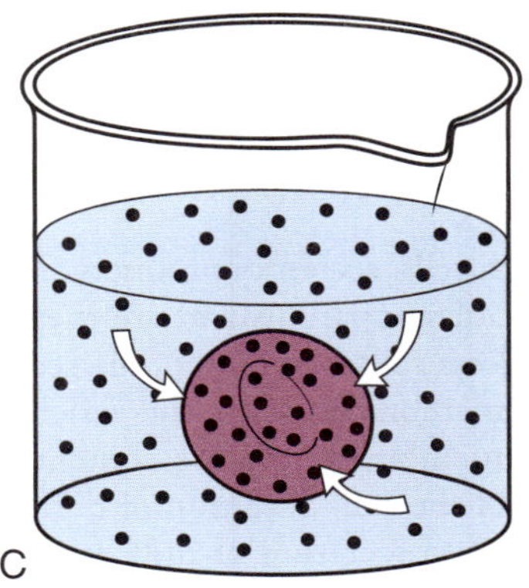

Fig. 5.12 (A) Isotonic solution. The extracellular concentration equals the intracellular concentration and there is no net movement of solvent. (B) Hypertonic solution. The extracellular concentration is greater than the intracellular concentration, and fluid moves from the cell into the surrounding fluid. The cell shrinks (crenates). (C) Hypotonic solution. The extracellular concentration is less than the intracellular concentration, and the solvent moves into the cell. The cell expands. (From Applegate E: *The anatomy and physiology learning system*, ed 4, St. Louis, 2011, Saunders.)

and enter the surrounding fluid (where there are fewer water molecules). When fluid leaves the cells, they will shrink or *crenate.* The 10% glucose solution has a greater solute concentration than the cell. It is *hypertonic* to the cell (see Fig. 5.12B).

When a red blood cell is placed in distilled water, water will enter the cell because there are more water molecules outside the cell than inside. The distilled water has a lower solute concentration than the cell. It is *hypotonic* to the cell. As water enters the cell, it will swell because of the increased volume. If enough water goes into the cell, it may rupture. This is called *lysis.* When this happens to a red blood cell, it is called *hemolysis* (see Fig. 5.12C).

The terms *isotonic*, *hypotonic*, and *hypertonic* are relative. They are used to compare two solutions. A 5% glucose solution is hypertonic to distilled water but hypotonic to a 10% glucose solution.

Filtration

In diffusion and osmosis, particles (whether solute, solvent, or both) pass through a membrane by virtue of their own random movement, which is directed by a difference in concentration. In *filtration*, however, pressure pushes the particles through a membrane. Drip coffee makers, for example, use this principle. Water first drips through the coffee, and then the water and small particles pass through a filter. The large granules of coffee are too big to go through the pores in the filter. The size of the pores determines the size of the particles that can pass through the filter. The pressure is created by the weight of the water on the paper filter.

Contraction of the heart creates pressure in the blood. This fluid pressure or *hydrostatic pressure*, which is greater inside the blood vessels, pushes fluid, dissolved nutrients, and small ions through the capillary walls to form tissue fluid. The large protein molecules and blood cells are unable to pass through the pores in the capillary membrane. Blood is filtered through specialized membranes in the kidney as the initial step in urine formation. Water and small molecules and ions pass through the filtration membrane while blood cells and protein molecules remain in the blood.

Active Transport

In the transport mechanisms discussed thus far, no cellular energy has been involved and the molecules and/or ions have moved from a region of high concentration to one of low concentration. **Active transport** differs from these processes in that it moves molecules and ions "uphill" from an area of lower concentration to an area of higher concentration. To accomplish this, cellular energy is required in the form of ATP. If ATP is not available, active transport ceases immediately. Active transport also uses a carrier molecule.

As a result of active transport, some substances are present in significantly higher concentrations on one side of the cell membrane than on the other. For example, sodium ions are more concentrated outside the plasma membrane than inside the cell. Potassium is just the opposite; its concentration is higher inside the cell. Active transport maintains concentration gradients. Normal **passive transport**, such as diffusion and osmosis, tends to equalize the concentrations on the two sides of the membrane.

Endocytosis

Endocytosis refers to the formation of vesicles to transfer particles and droplets from outside to inside the cell. In this case the material is too large to enter the cell by diffusion or active transport. The process requires energy in the form of ATP. **Phagocytosis**, which means "cell eating," is a form of endocytosis that involves solid material. The cell membrane engulfs a particle to form a vesicle in the cytoplasm. Lysosomes fuse with the vesicle, and the enzymes digest the particle. Certain white blood cells are called *phagocytes* because they engulf and destroy bacteria in this manner. Another form of endocytosis is **pinocytosis** or "cell drinking." It differs from phagocytosis in that the vesicles that are formed are much smaller and their contents are fluids. Pinocytosis is important in cells that function in absorption.

Exocytosis

In certain cells, secretory products are packaged into vesicles by the Golgi apparatus and are then released from the cell by a process called *exocytosis*. The secretory vesicle moves to the cell membrane, where the vesicle membrane fuses with the cell membrane, and the contents are discharged to the outside of the cell. Secretion of digestive enzymes from the pancreas and secretion of milk from the mammary glands are examples of exocytosis. Exocytosis and endocytosis are similar except for working in opposite directions. They are both active processes that require cellular energy (ATP). Exocytosis releases substances to the outside of the cell, and endocytosis transports substances to the inside of the cell.

Cell Division

Cell division is the process by which new cells are formed for growth, repair, and replacement in the body. This process includes division of the nuclear material and division of the cytoplasm. Periods of growth and repair are special periods in the life of an individual when it is obvious that new cells are needed either to increase the number of cells or to repair tissues after an injury. The general maintenance and replacement needs of the body may not be quite as obvious. More than 2 million red blood cells are worn out and replaced in the body every second of every day. Skin cells are continually sloughed off the body's surface and must be replaced. The lining of the stomach is replaced every few days. All cells in the body (somatic cells), except those that give rise to the eggs and sperm (gametes), reproduce by *mitosis*. Egg and sperm cells are produced by a special type of nuclear division called *meiosis*, in which the number of chromosomes is halved. Division of the cytoplasm is called **cytokinesis**.

Mitosis

All somatic cells reproduce by **mitosis**, in which a single cell divides to form two new "daughter cells," each identical to the parent cell. Humans have 23 pairs of chromosomes (or 46 chromosomes) in their cells. Each new cell that forms must also have that same number. For this to occur, events must proceed in an organized manner, chromosome material must replicate exactly, and then the chromosomes must separate precisely so that each new cell receives a set of chromosomes that is a carbon copy of the parent cells. For descriptive purposes, it is convenient to divide the events of mitosis into stages, as illustrated in Fig. 5.13. It is important to remember that the process is a continual one and that there are no starting and stopping points along the way.

Except for size, the two newly formed daughter cells are exact copies of the parent cell. The two daughter cells carry out designated cellular functions and undergo mitosis as needed.

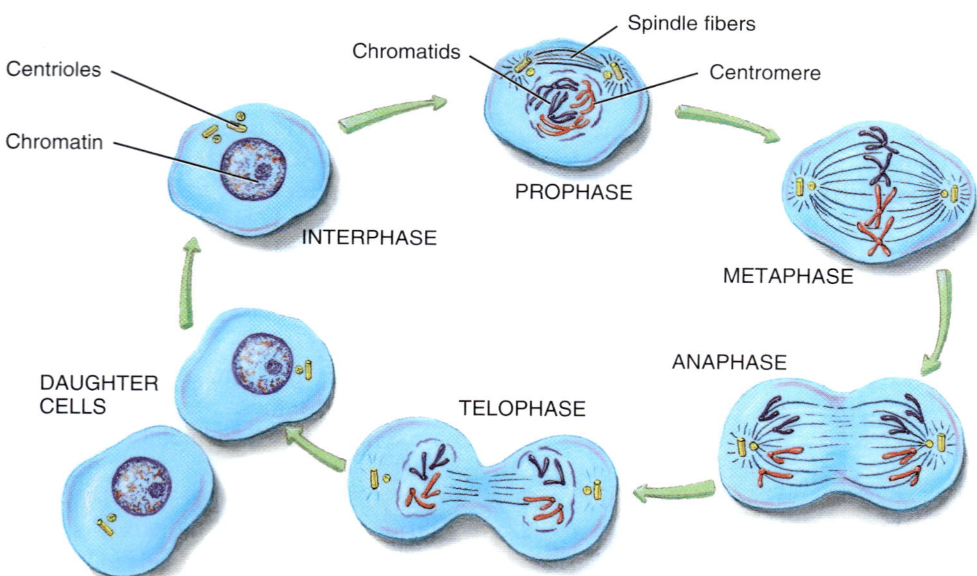

Fig. 5.13 Mitosis. *Interphase* is the period between active cell divisions. During this time the DNA, mitochondria, and centrioles replicate. It is the longest period of the cell cycle. *Prophase* is the first stage in mitosis. The chromatin shortens and thickens to form chromosomes, each with two chromatids connected by a centromere. Spindle fibers form and the nucleolus and nuclear membrane disintegrate. *Metaphase* shows the chromosomes aligned along the center of the cell. *Anaphase* shows the spindle fibers pulling each chromatid of a chromosome to opposite ends of the cell. *Telophase* shows the chromosomes reaching the centrioles at the ends of the cell. A new nuclear membrane and nucleolus form. Cytokinesis occurs. *Daughter cells* are two new interphase cells exactly like the parent cell. (From Applegate E: *The anatomy and physiology learning system*, ed 4, St. Louis, 2011, Saunders.)

Normally, body cells divide at a rate required to replace the dying ones. Normal cells are subject to control mechanisms that prevent overpopulation and competition for nutrients and space. Occasionally a series of events occurs that alters some cells, so they lack the control mechanisms that tell them when to stop dividing. When the cells do not stop their mitotic activity, they form an abnormal growth called a *tumor* or neoplasm.

Meiosis

Meiosis is a special type of cell division that occurs in the production of the gametes, or eggs and sperm. These cells have only 23 chromosomes, one half the number found in somatic cells, so that when fertilization takes place the resulting cell will again have 46 chromosomes, 23 from the egg and 23 from the sperm. Meiosis consists of two cell divisions, but the DNA is replicated only once. The result is four cells, but each one has only 23 chromosomes. Fig. 5.14 compares mitosis and meiosis.

DNA Replication and Protein Synthesis

Proteins that are synthesized in the cytoplasm function as structural materials, enzymes that regulate chemical reactions, hormones, and other vital substances. Because DNA in the nucleus directs the synthesis of the proteins in the cytoplasm, it ultimately determines the structural and functional characteristics of an individual. Whether a person has blue or brown eyes, brown or blond hair, or light or dark skin is determined by the types of proteins synthesized in response to the genetic information contained in the DNA in the nucleus. The portion of a DNA molecule that contains the genetic information for making one particular protein molecule is called a *gene.* If a cell produced for replacement or repair is to function exactly as its predecessor, then it must have the same genes, a carbon copy of the DNA. This is the purpose of DNA replication in cell division.

TISSUES AND MEMBRANES

A **tissue** is a group of cells that have similar structure and that function together as a unit. The microscopic study of tissues is called **histology**. A nonliving material called the *intercellular matrix* fills the spaces between cells. This may be abundant in some tissues and scarce in others. The intercellular matrix may contain special substances, such as salts and fibers, that are unique to a specific tissue and give the tissue distinctive characteristics.

BODY TISSUES

Four main tissue types are found in the body: epithelial, connective, muscle, and nervous. Each is designed for specific functions.

Epithelial Tissue

Epithelial tissues are widespread throughout the body. They form the covering of all body surfaces, line body cavities

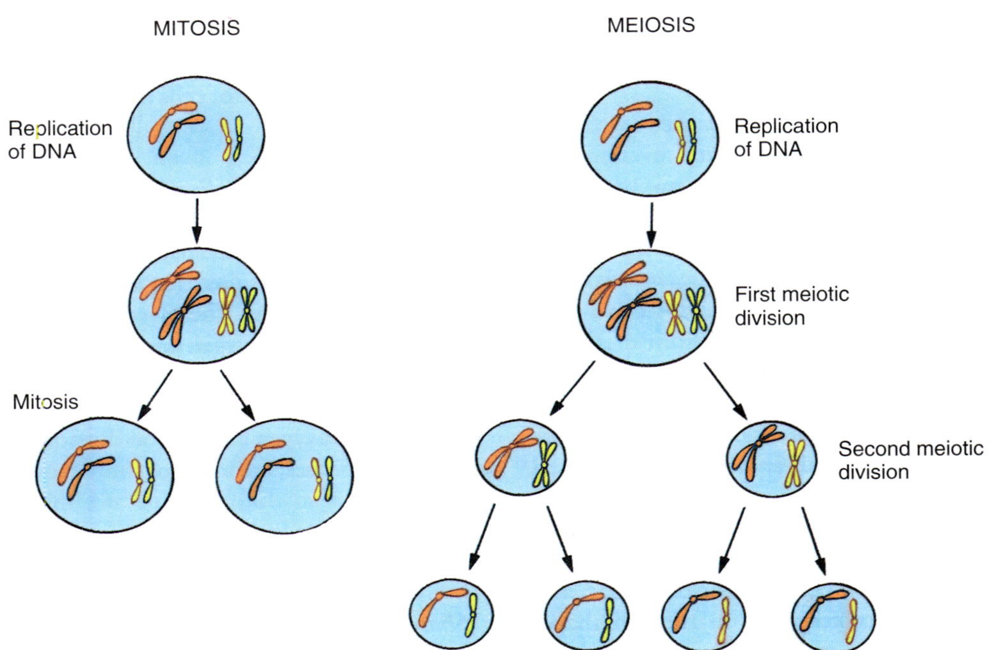

Fig. 5.14 Comparison of mitosis and meiosis. The result of mitosis in humans is two cells, each with 46 chromosomes (23 pairs). Meiosis results in four cells, each with 23 chromosomes. (From Applegate E: *The anatomy and physiology learning system*, ed 4, St. Louis, 2011, Saunders.)

HIGHLIGHT on Cells and Tissues

Congenital Abnormalities

Often, congenital anatomic abnormalities must be surgically repaired so that disruptions in physiology are corrected. For example, a cleft palate (anatomy) is repaired so that food will enter (physiology) the pharynx instead of the nasal cavity. Broken bones (anatomy) are reset so that function (physiology) is restored.

Kidney Dialysis

Normally functioning kidneys remove waste products from the blood. When the kidneys do not function properly, waste molecules can be removed from the blood artificially by a process called *dialysis.* Dialysis is a form of diffusion in which the size of the pores in a selectively permeable membrane separates smaller solute particles from larger solutes. In kidney dialysis, small waste molecules pass through the membrane and are removed from the blood. The protein molecules, which are needed in the blood, are too large to pass through the pores and thus are retained.

Neoplasms

A benign neoplasm consists of highly organized cells that closely resemble normal tissue. In contrast, a malignant neoplasm, or cancer, consists of unorganized and immature cells that are incapable of normal function. These cells may detach from the tumor site and travel in the blood or lymph to another site and establish a new tumor. This is called *metastasis* and is probably the most devastating property of malignant cells. Tumors are named according to the tissue from which they are derived. For example, a benign tumor of glandular epithelial cells is called an *adenoma.* A *lipoma* is derived from fat cells, a *myoma* is formed from muscle tissue, and a *papilloma* may occur on any epithelial surface or lining. Carcinomas are solid cancerous tumors that are derived from epithelial tissue. An adenocarcinoma is a cancerous tumor arising from glandular cells. *Sarcomas* are malignant growths derived from connective tissue cells. Approximately 85% of all malignant neoplasms are carcinomas. These account for approximately 10% of all malignant neoplasms.

Genetic Disorders

Genetic disorders are pathologic conditions caused by mistakes, or mutations, in a cell's genetic code. Mutations may occur naturally, or they may be induced by mutagens, such as radiation and certain chemicals. If the mutations occur in the gametes, the faulty code is passed from one generation to the next. Errors in the genes (DNA) cause the production of abnormal proteins, which result in abnormal cellular function. For example, in sickle cell anemia, a genetic blood disorder, red blood cells have abnormal hemoglobin because there is an "error" in the gene that directs hemoglobin synthesis.

Peritonitis

An inflammation of the serous membranes in the abdominal cavity is called *peritonitis.* This is sometimes a serious complication of an infected appendix. ■

and hollow organs, and are the major tissue in glands. They perform a variety of functions that include protection, secretion, absorption, excretion, filtration, diffusion, and sensory reception.

The cells in epithelial tissue are tightly packed, with little intercellular matrix. Because the tissues form coverings and linings, the cells have one free surface that is not in contact with other cells. Opposite the free surface, the cells are attached to underlying connective tissue by a noncellular *basement membrane.* Because epithelial tissues are typically *avascular* (without blood vessels), they must receive their nutrients and oxygen supply by diffusion from the blood vessels in the underlying tissues. Another characteristic of epithelial tissues is that they regenerate, or reproduce, quickly. For example, the cells of the skin and stomach are continually damaged and replaced, and skin abrasions heal quite rapidly.

Epithelia are classified according to cell shape and the number of layers in the tissue. Classified according to shape, the cells are squamous, cuboidal, or columnar, and the shape of the nucleus corresponds to the cell shape. *Squamous* cells are flat and the nuclei are usually broad and thin. *Cuboidal* cells are cubelike, as tall as they are wide, and the nuclei are spherical and centrally located. *Columnar* cells are tall and narrow, resembling columns, and the nuclei are usually in the lower portion of the cell near the basement membrane. According to the number of layers, epithelia are *simple* if they have only one layer of cells and *stratified* if they have multiple layers. Stratified epithelia are named according to the type of cells at the free surface of the tissue.

Simple Squamous Epithelium

Simple squamous epithelium (Fig. 5.15) consists of a single layer of thin, flat cells that fit closely together with little intercellular matrix. Because it is so thin, simple squamous epithelium is well suited for areas in which diffusion and filtration take place. The alveoli or air sacs of the lungs, where diffusion of oxygen and carbon dioxide gases occurs, are made of simple squamous epithelium. This tissue is also found in the kidney, where the blood is filtered. Capillary walls, where oxygen and carbon dioxide diffuse between the blood and tissues, are made of simple squamous epithelium. Because it is so thin and delicate, this tissue is damaged easily and offers little protective function.

Simple Cuboidal Epithelium

Simple cuboidal epithelium (Fig. 5.16) consists of a single layer of cube-shaped cells. These cells have more volume than squamous cells and also have more organelles. Simple cuboidal epithelium is found as a covering of the ovary, as a lining of kidney tubules, and in many glands, such as the thyroid, pancreas, and salivary glands. In the kidney

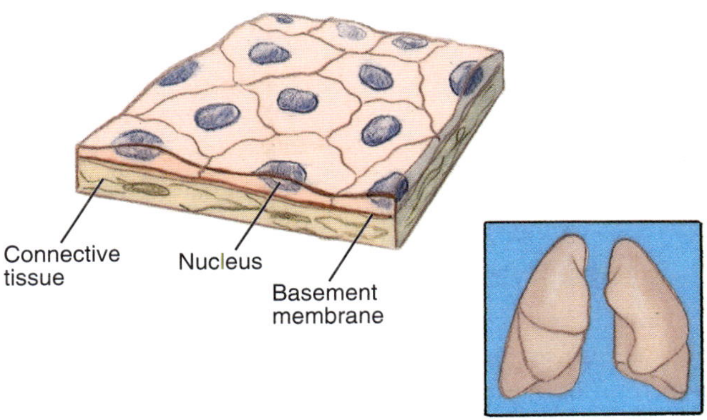

Fig. 5.15 Simple squamous epithelium in the alveoli of the lungs. It is also found in capillary walls and in renal corpuscles of the kidney. (From Applegate E: *The anatomy and physiology learning system*, ed 4, St. Louis, 2011, Saunders.)

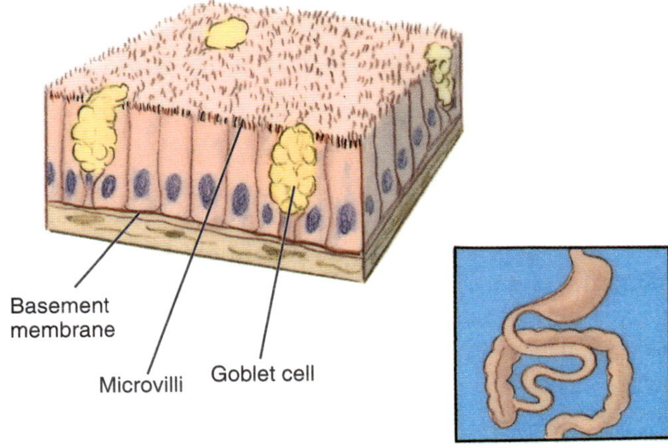

Fig. 5.17 Simple columnar epithelium in the lining of the stomach and intestines. (From Applegate E: *The anatomy and physiology learning system*, ed 4, St. Louis, 2011, Saunders.)

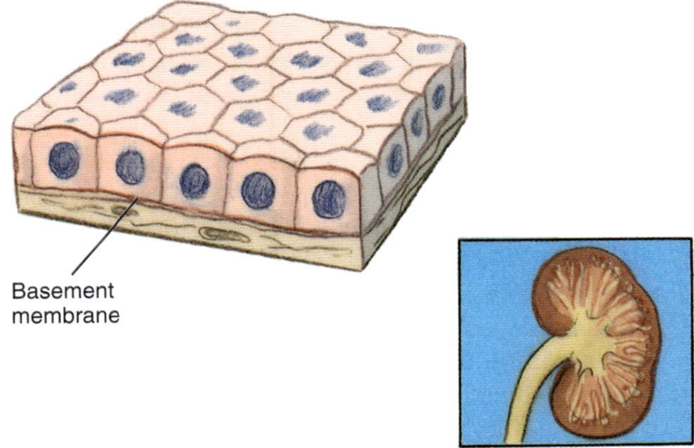

Fig. 5.16 Simple cuboidal epithelium in the kidney tubules. It is also found in many glands and as a covering of the ovary. (From Applegate E: *The anatomy and physiology learning system*, ed 4, St. Louis, 2011, Saunders.)

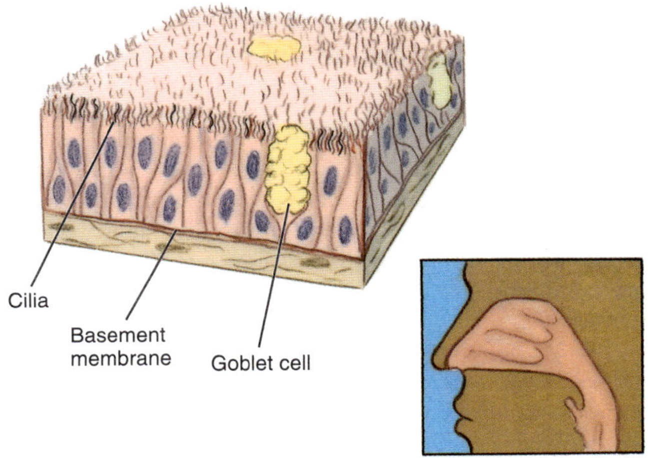

Fig. 5.18 Pseudostratified columnar epithelium in the respiratory tract. It also lines some parts of the male reproductive system. (From Applegate E: *The anatomy and physiology learning system*, ed 4, St. Louis, 2011, Saunders.)

tubules, the tissue functions in absorption and secretion. In glands, simple cuboidal cells form the secretory portions and the ducts that deliver the products to their destination.

Simple Columnar Epithelium

A single layer of cells that are taller than they are wide makes up *simple columnar epithelium* (Fig. 5.17). The nuclei are in the bottom portion of the cell near the basement membrane. Simple columnar epithelium is found lining the stomach and intestines, where it secretes digestive enzymes and absorbs nutrients. Because the cells are taller (or thicker) than either squamous or cuboidal cells, this tissue offers some protection to underlying tissues.

In regions where absorption is of primary importance, such as in parts of the digestive tract, the cell membrane on the free surface has numerous small projections called *microvilli.* Microvilli increase the surface area that is available for absorption of nutrients. *Goblet cells* are frequently interspersed among the simple columnar cells. Goblet cells are flask- or goblet-shaped cells that secrete mucus onto the free surface of the tissue. Cilia may be present to move secretions along the surface.

Pseudostratified Columnar Epithelium

Pseudostratified columnar epithelium (Fig. 5.18) appears to have multiple layers (stratified), but it really does not. This is because the cells are not all the same height. Some cells are short and some are tall, and the nuclei are at different levels. Close examination reveals that all the cells are attached to the basement membrane but that not all cells reach the free surface of the tissue. Cilia and goblet cells are often associated with pseudostratified columnar epithelium. This tissue lines portions of the respiratory tract in which the mucus, produced by the goblet cells, traps dust particles and is then moved upward by the cilia. Pseudostratified columnar epithelium also lines some of the tubes of the male reproductive system. Here the cilia help propel the sperm from one region to another.

Stratified Squamous Epithelium

Stratified squamous epithelium, the most widespread stratified epithelium, is thick because it consists of many layers of cells (Fig. 5.19). The cells on the bottom layer, next to the basement membrane, are usually cuboidal or columnar, and these are the cells that undergo mitosis. As the cells are pushed toward the surface, they become thinner, so the surface cells are squamous. As the cells are pushed farther away from the basement membrane, it is more difficult for them to receive oxygen and nutrients from underlying connective tissue, and the cells die. As cells on the surface are damaged and die, they are sloughed off and replaced by cells from the deeper layers. Because this tissue is thick, it is found in areas in which protection is a primary function. Stratified squamous epithelium forms the outer layer of the skin and extends a short distance into every body opening that is continuous with the skin.

Transitional Epithelium

Transitional epithelium is a specialized type of tissue that has several layers but can be stretched in response to tension. The lining of the urinary bladder is a good example of this type of tissue. When the bladder is empty and contracted, the epithelial lining has several layers of cuboidal cells. As the bladder fills and is distended or stretched, the cells become thinner and the number of layers decreases.

Glandular Epithelium

Glandular epithelium consists of cells that are specialized to produce and secrete substances. Glandular epithelium normally lies deep to the epithelia that cover and line parts of the body. If the gland secretes its product onto a free surface via a duct, it is called an *exocrine gland.* Examples of exocrine glands include sebaceous glands, mammary glands, and salivary glands. If the gland secretes its product directly into the blood, it is a ductless gland, or *endocrine gland.* Endocrine glands are discussed in Chapter 11.

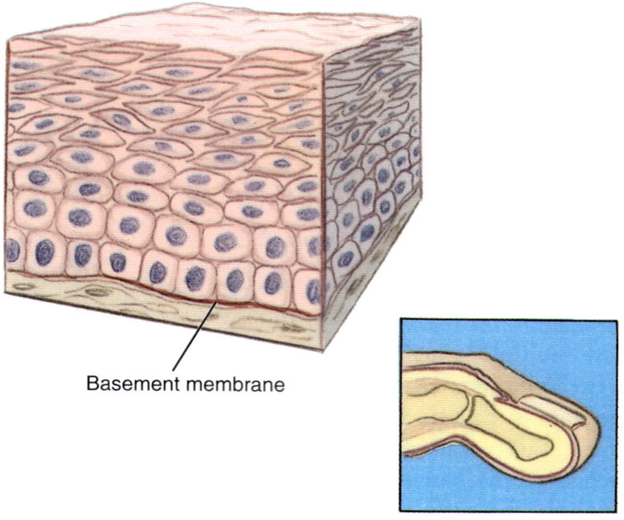

Fig. 5.19 Stratified squamous epithelium from the outer layer of the skin. Note the numerous cell layers and the flattened cells at the surface. (From Applegate E: *The anatomy and physiology learning system*, ed 4, St. Louis, 2011, Saunders.)

Connective Tissue

Connective tissues bind structures together, form a framework and support for organs and the body as a whole, store fat, transport substances, protect against disease, and help repair tissue damage. They occur throughout the body. Connective tissues are characterized by an abundance of intercellular matrix with relatively few cells. Connective tissue cells are able to reproduce but not as rapidly as epithelial cells. Most connective tissues have a good blood supply, but some do not. Examples of connective tissue include adipose tissue, cartilage, and bone.

The intercellular matrix in connective tissue has a gel-like base of water, nonfibrous protein, and other molecules. Various mineral salts in the matrix of some connective tissues, such as bone, make them hard. Two types of fibers, collagenous and elastic, are frequently embedded in the matrix. **Collagenous fibers**, composed of the protein collagen, are strong and flexible but are only slightly elastic. They are able to withstand considerable pulling force and are found in areas in which this is important, such as in tendons and ligaments. When collagenous fibers are grouped together in parallel bundles, the tissue appears white, so they are sometimes called *white fibers.* **Elastic fibers**, composed of the protein elastin, are not very strong, but they are elastic. They can be stretched and will return to their original shape and length when released. Elastic fibers, also called *yellow fibers*, are located where structures are stretched and released, such as the vocal cords.

Numerous cell types are found in connective tissue. Three of the most common are the *fibroblast*, *macrophage*, and *mast cell.* As the name implies, **fibroblasts** produce the fibers that are in the intercellular matrix. **Macrophages** are large phagocytic cells that are able to move about and clean up cellular debris and foreign particles from the tissues. **Mast cells** contain heparin, an anticoagulant, and histamine, a substance that promotes inflammation and that is active in allergies.

Loose Connective Tissue

Loose connective tissue, also called *areolar connective tissue*, is one of the most widely distributed tissues in the body. It is the packing material in the body. It attaches the skin to the underlying tissues and fills the spaces between muscles. Most epithelial tissue is anchored to this tissue by the basement membrane, and the blood vessels in the loose connective tissue supply nutrients to the epithelium above. The matrix is characterized by a loose network of collagenous and elastic fibers. The predominant cell is the fibroblast, but other connective tissue cells are also present (Fig. 5.20).

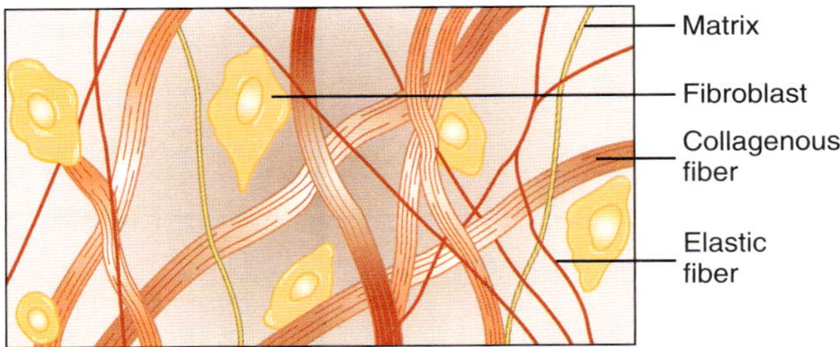

Fig. 5.20 Loose (areolar) connective tissue. Note the fibroblasts and the two types of fibers embedded in a gel-like matrix. (From Applegate E: *The anatomy and physiology learning system*, ed 4, St. Louis, 2011, Saunders.)

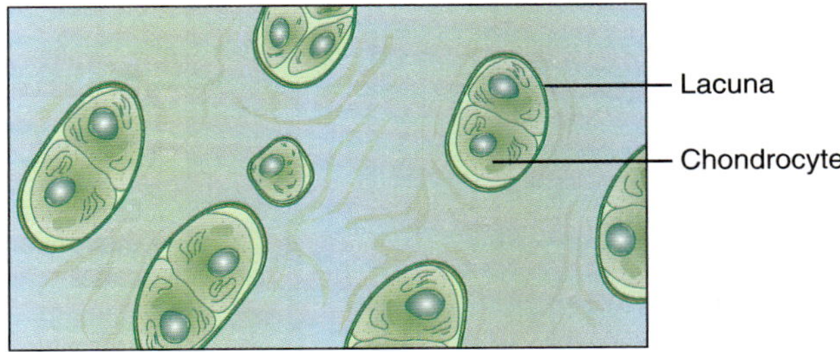

Fig. 5.21 Hyaline cartilage. Note the chondrocytes within the lacunae. (From Applegate E: *The anatomy and physiology learning system*, ed 4, St. Louis, 2011, Saunders.)

Adipose Tissue

Commonly called *fat*, *adipose tissue* is really a specialized form of loose connective tissue in which there is little intercellular matrix. Some of the cells accumulate liquid triglyceride, or fat, droplets. When this happens, the cytoplasm and nucleus are pushed off to one side, and the cells swell and become closely packed together. Fat cells have the ability to take up fat and then release it at a later time. Adipose tissue forms a protective cushion around the kidneys, heart, eyeballs, and various joints. It also accumulates under the skin, where it provides insulation for heat. Adipose tissue is an efficient energy storage material for excess calories.

Dense Fibrous Connective Tissue

Dense fibrous connective tissue is characterized by closely packed parallel bundles of collagenous fibers in the intercellular matrix. There are relatively few cells, and the ones that are present are fibroblasts to produce the collagenous fibers. This is the tissue that makes up *tendons*, which connect muscles to bones, and *ligaments*, which connect bones to bones. Dense fibrous connective tissue has a poor blood supply, and this, along with the relatively few cells, accounts for the slow healing of this tissue.

Elastic Connective Tissue

Elastic connective tissue has closely packed elastic fibers in the intercellular matrix. This type of tissue yields easily to a pulling force and then returns to its original length as soon as the force is released. The vocal cords and the ligaments that connect adjacent vertebrae are composed of elastic connective tissue.

Cartilage

Cartilage has an abundant matrix that is solid, yet flexible, with fibers embedded in it. The matrix contains the protein *chondrin*. Cartilage cells, or **chondrocytes**, are located in spaces called *lacunae* that are scattered throughout the matrix. Typically, cartilage is surrounded by a dense fibrous connective tissue covering called the *perichondrium*. The perichondrium has blood vessels, but they do not penetrate the cartilage itself, and the cells obtain their nutrients by diffusion through the solid matrix. Cartilage heals slowly because there is no direct blood supply, and this also contributes to slow cellular reproduction. Cartilage protects underlying tissues, supports other structures, and provides a framework for attachments.

Hyaline cartilage (Fig. 5.21) is the most common type of cartilage. It has fine collagenous fibers in the matrix and a shiny, white, opaque appearance. It is found at the ends of long bones, in the costal cartilage that connects the ribs to the sternum, and in the supporting rings of the trachea. Most of the fetal skeleton is formed of hyaline cartilage before it is replaced by bone.

Fibrocartilage has an abundance of strong collagenous fibers embedded in the matrix. This allows it to withstand compression, act as a shock absorber, and resist pulling forces. It is found in the intervertebral discs, or pads between the vertebrae; in the symphysis pubis, or pad between the two pubic bones; and between the bones in the knee joint.

Elastic cartilage has numerous yellow elastic fibers embedded in the matrix, which makes it more flexible than hyaline cartilage or fibrocartilage. It is found in the framework of the external ear, the epiglottis, and the auditory tubes.

Bone

Osseous tissue or *bone* is the most rigid of all the connective tissues. Collagenous fibers in the matrix give strength to bone, and its hardness is derived from the mineral salts, particularly calcium, that are deposited around the fibers. Bones form the framework for the body and help protect underlying tissues. They serve as attachments for muscles and act as mechanical levers in producing movement. Bone also contributes to the formation of blood cells and functions as a storage area for mineral salts.

Cylindric structural units, called *osteons* or *haversian systems*, are packed together to form the substance of compact bone (Fig. 5.22). The center or hub of the osteon is a tubular *osteonic* or *haversian canal* that contains a blood vessel. The matrix is deposited in concentric rings called *lamellae* around the canal. **Osteocytes**, or bone cells, are located in lacunae between the lamellae, so they are also arranged in concentric rings. Slender processes from the bone cells extend through tiny tubes in the matrix called *canaliculi* to other cells or to the osteonic canals. This provides a readily available blood supply for the bone cells, which allows a faster repair process for bone than for cartilage.

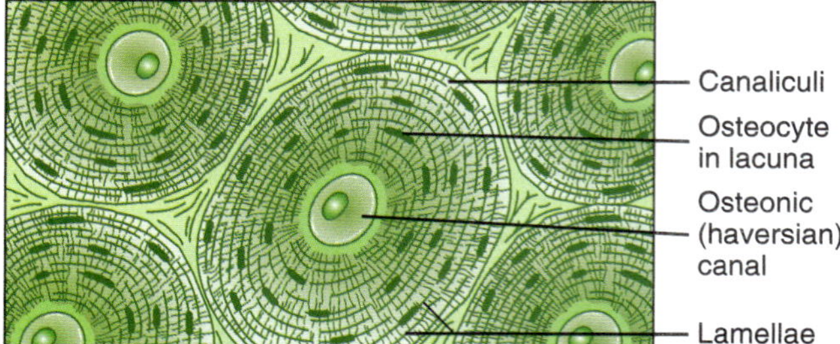

Fig. 5.22 Compact bone (osseous tissue). Note the osteons with a central haversian canal and concentric lamellae of matrix. Canaliculi extend from the osteocytes, which are located within lacunae. (From Applegate E: *The anatomy and physiology learning system*, ed 4, St. Louis, 2011, Saunders.)

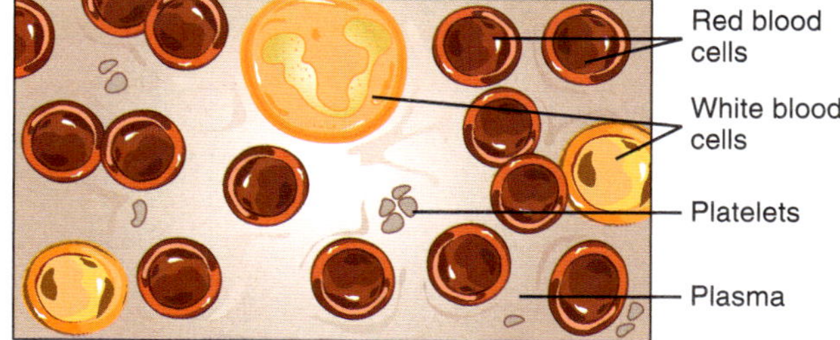

Fig. 5.23 Blood. Note the blood cells and platelets, which are suspended in a liquid plasma. (From Applegate E: *The anatomy and physiology learning system*, ed 4, St. Louis, 2011, Saunders.)

Blood

Blood is a unique connective tissue because it is the only one that has a liquid matrix. It is a vehicle for transport of substances throughout the body. **Erythrocytes**, or red blood cells, and **leukocytes**, or white blood cells, are suspended in a liquid matrix called *plasma* (Fig. 5.23). The red blood cells transport oxygen from the lungs to the tissues. White blood cells are important in fighting disease. Another formed element in the blood is the *platelet*, or **thrombocyte**, which is not actually a cell but a fragment of a giant cell in the bone marrow. Platelets are important in initiating the blood clotting process. Blood is discussed in more detail in Chapter 12.

Muscle Tissue

Muscle tissue is composed of cells that have the special ability to shorten or contract to produce movement of body parts. The tissue is highly cellular and is well supplied with blood vessels. The cells are long and slender, so they are sometimes called *muscle fibers*, and these are usually arranged in bundles or layers that are surrounded by connective tissue. Muscle tissue is of three types: skeletal muscle, smooth muscle, and cardiac muscle.

Skeletal Muscle

Skeletal muscle tissue (Fig. 5.24) is what is commonly thought of as "muscle." It is the meat of animals, and it constitutes about 40% of an individual's body weight. Skeletal muscle cells (fibers) are long and cylindric with many nuclei (multinucleated) peripherally located next to the cell membrane. The cells have alternating light and dark bands that are perpendicular to the long axis of the cell. These bands are a result of the organized arrangement of the contractile proteins in the cytoplasm and give the cell a *striated* appearance. Skeletal muscle fibers are collected into bundles and wrapped in connective tissue to form the muscles, which are attached to the skeleton and which cause body movements when they contract in response to nerve stimulation. Skeletal muscle action is under conscious or voluntary control. Chapter 8 describes skeletal muscles in more detail.

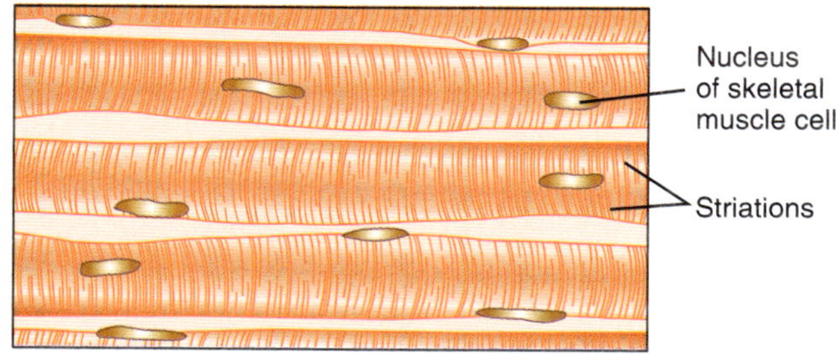

Fig. 5.24 Skeletal muscle. Note the long cylindric fibers with striations. (From Applegate E: *The anatomy and physiology learning system*, ed 4, St. Louis, 2011, Saunders.)

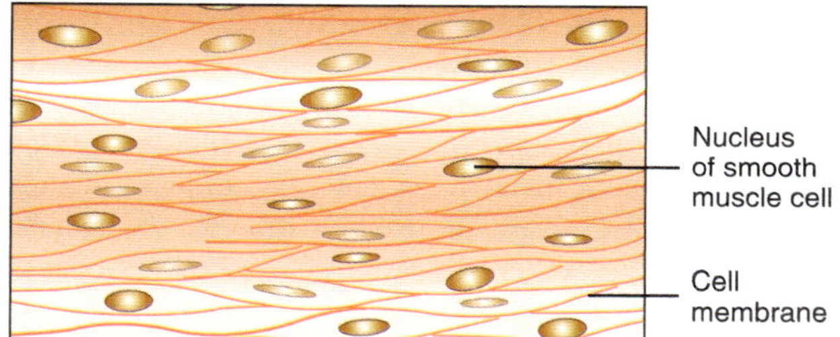

Fig. 5.25 Smooth muscle. Note the spindle-shaped cells with tapered ends. (From Applegate E: *The anatomy and physiology learning system*, ed 4, St. Louis, 2011, Saunders.)

Smooth Muscle

Smooth muscle tissue (Fig. 5.25) is found in the walls of hollow body organs, such as the stomach, intestines, urinary bladder, uterus, and blood vessels. It normally acts to propel substances through the organ by contracting and relaxing. It is called *smooth muscle* because it lacks the striations evident in skeletal muscle. Because it is found in the viscera or body organs, it is sometimes called *visceral muscle*. Smooth muscle cells are shorter than skeletal muscle cells, are spindle-shaped and tapered at the ends, and have a single, centrally located nucleus. Smooth muscle usually cannot be stimulated to contract by conscious or voluntary effort, so it is called *involuntary muscle*.

Cardiac Muscle

Cardiac muscle tissue (Fig. 5.26) is found only in the wall of the heart. The cardiac muscle cells are cylindric and appear striated, similar to skeletal muscle cells. Cardiac muscle cells

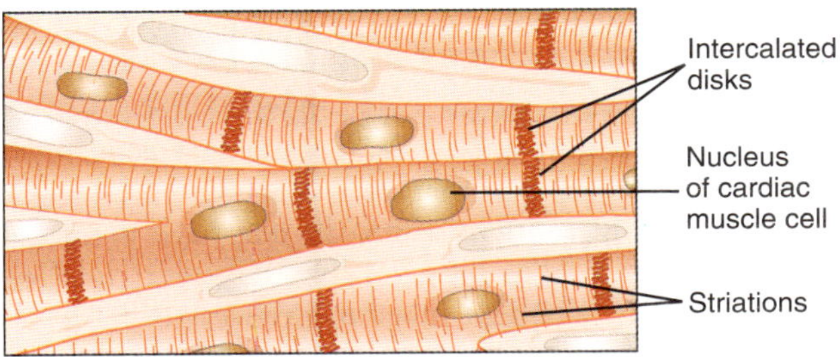

Fig. 5.26 Cardiac muscle. Note the branching striated cells and intercalated disks. (From Applegate E: *The anatomy and physiology learning system*, ed 4, St. Louis, 2011, Saunders.)

are shorter than skeletal muscle cells and have only one nucleus per cell. The cells branch and interconnect to form complex networks. At the point where one cell attaches to another, there is a specialized intercellular connection called an *intercalated disc.* Cardiac muscle appears striated like skeletal muscle, but its contraction is involuntary. It is responsible for pumping the blood through the heart and into the blood vessels.

Nervous Tissue

Nervous tissue is found in the brain, spinal cord, and nerves. It is responsible for coordinating and controlling many body activities. It stimulates muscle contraction, creates an awareness of the environment, and plays a major role in emotions, memory, and reasoning. To do all of these things, cells in nervous tissue need to be able to communicate with one another by way of electrical nerve impulses.

The cells in nervous tissue that generate and conduct impulses are called *neurons* or *nerve cells.* These cells have three principal parts: the dendrites, the cell body, and one axon (Fig. 5.27). The main part of the cell, the part that carries on the general functions, is the *neuron cell body.* **Dendrites** are extensions, or processes, of the cytoplasm that carry impulses to the cell body. An extension or process called an **axon** carries impulses away from the cell body.

Nervous tissue also includes cells that do not transmit impulses but instead support the activities of the neurons. These are the *glial cells*, together termed the **neuroglia**. Supporting, or glial, cells bind neurons together and insulate the neurons. Some are phagocytic and protect against bacterial invasion, whereas others provide nutrients by binding blood vessels to the neurons. Further detail on nerve tissue is presented in Chapter 9.

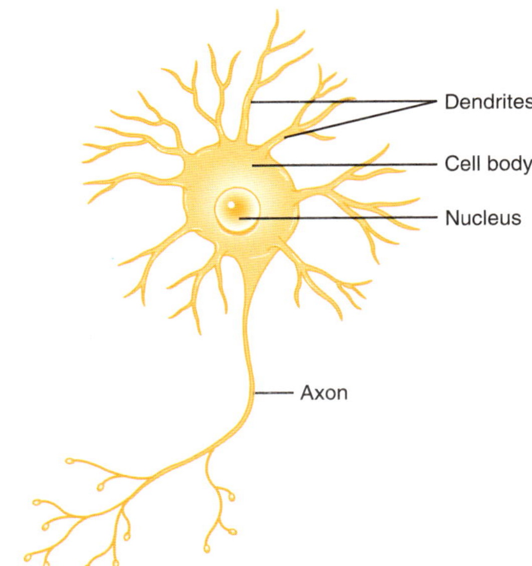

Fig. 5.27 Neuron (nervous tissue). Note the dendrites, axon, and cell body. (From Applegate E: *The anatomy and physiology learning system*, ed 4, St. Louis, 2011, Saunders.)

BODY MEMBRANES

Body membranes are thin sheets of tissue that cover the body, line body cavities, cover organs within the cavities, and line the cavities in hollow organs. By this definition, the skin is a membrane because it covers the body, and indeed, the skin, or integument, is sometimes called the **cutaneous membrane**. This membrane is discussed in Chapter 6. This section examines two epithelial membranes and two connective tissue membranes. Epithelial membranes consist of epithelial tissue and the connective tissue to which it is attached. The two main types of epithelial membranes are the mucous membranes and serous membranes. Connective tissue membranes contain only connective tissue. Synovial membranes and meninges belong to this category.

Mucous Membranes

Mucous membranes are epithelial membranes that consist of epithelial tissue attached to underlying loose connective tissue. These membranes (sometimes called *mucosae*) line the body cavities that open to the outside. The entire digestive tract is lined with mucous membranes. Other examples include the respiratory, urinary, and reproductive tracts. The type of epithelium varies depending on its function. In the mouth the epithelium is of the stratified squamous type for its protection function, but the stomach and intestines are lined with simple columnar epithelium for absorption and secretion. The mucosa of the urinary bladder is transitional epithelium so that it can expand. Mucous membranes get their name from the fact that the epithelial cells secrete mucus for lubrication and protection.

Serous Membranes

Serous membranes line body cavities that do not open directly to the outside, and they cover the organs located in those cavities. A serous membrane, or *serosa*, consists of a thin layer of loose connective tissue covered by a layer of simple squamous epithelium called *mesothelium.* These membranes always have two parts. The part that lines a cavity wall is the *parietal* layer, and the part that covers the organs in the cavity is the *visceral* layer (Fig. 5.28). Serous membranes are covered by a thin layer of *serous fluid* that is secreted by the epithelium. Serous fluid lubricates the membrane and reduces friction and abrasion when organs

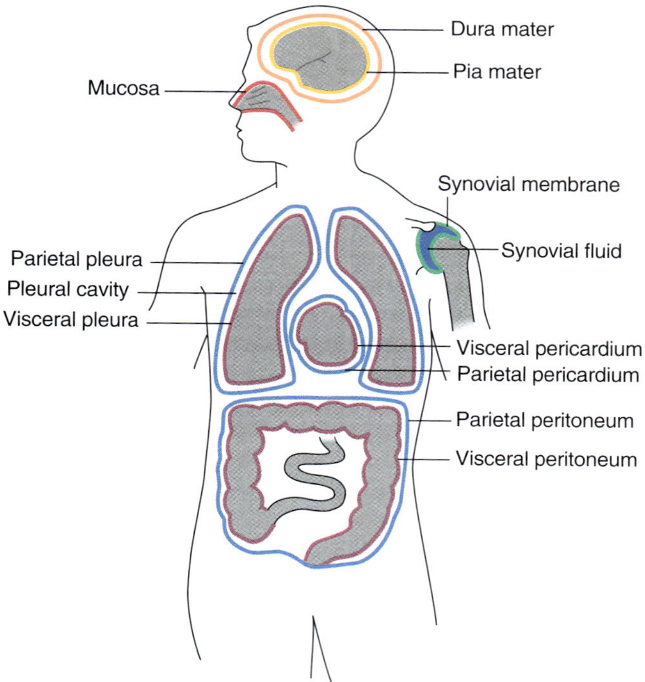

Fig. 5.28 Body membranes. (From Applegate E: *The anatomy and physiology learning system*, ed 4, St. Louis, 2011, Saunders.)

in the thoracic or abdominopelvic cavity move against one another or the cavity wall.

Serous membranes have special names according to their location. The serous membrane that lines the thoracic cavity and covers the lungs is the **pleura**, with the parietal pleura lining the cavity and the visceral pleura covering the lungs. The **pericardium** lines the pericardial cavity and covers the heart. The serous membrane in the abdominopelvic cavity is the **peritoneum**.

Synovial Membranes

Synovial membranes are connective tissue membranes that line the cavities of the freely movable joints such as the shoulder, elbow, and knee. Similar to serous membranes, they line cavities that do not open to the outside. Unlike serous membranes, they do not have a layer of epithelium. Synovial membranes secrete *synovial fluid* into the joint cavity, and this lubricates the cartilage on the ends of the bones so that they can move freely and without friction. In certain types of arthritis, these membranes become inflamed and the fluid becomes viscous. This reduces lubrication and increases friction, and movement becomes difficult and painful.

Meninges

The connective tissue coverings around the brain and spinal cord, within the dorsal cavity, are called **meninges**. They provide protection for these vital structures. Inflammation of the meninges is *meningitis*. Further discussion of the meninges appears in Chapter 9.

HIGHLIGHT on Conditions Affecting Tissues

Adhesion: Abnormal joining of tissues by fibrous scar tissue
Carcinoma: A malignant growth derived from epithelial cells
Lipoma: Benign tumor derived from fat (adipose) cells
Myoma: Benign tumor formed of muscle tissue
Papilloma: Benign epithelial tumor; may occur on any epithelial surface or lining
Sarcoma: A malignant growth derived from connective tissue cells
Scurvy: A condition caused by a deficiency of vitamin C in the diet, which results in abnormal collagen synthesis ■

Genetic Diseases and Disorders

Disease	Signs and Symptoms	Etiology	Diagnosis and Treatment
Angelman syndrome (AS)	The first signs are usually developmental delays observed between 6 and 12 months of age. Other signs may include speech impairment with little or no use of words, movement and balance disorders, frequent laughter and hand flapping, microcephaly, seizures, and an abnormal electroencephalogram (EEG).	The syndrome is most often caused by deletion or inactivation of genes on the maternally inherited chromosome 15.	Confirmation of the diagnosis requires genetic studies of a blood sample from the child. There is no cure for AS. Treatment focuses on managing the signs and symptoms and may include antiseizure medication, physical therapy, speech therapy, and behavioral therapy.
Becker muscular dystrophy (BMD)	Similar to Duchenne muscular dystrophy but later onset and less severe. In general, signs and symptoms appear in the teens or early 20s to mid-20s and include frequent falls, difficulty in running or jumping, waddling gait, difficulty getting up from a lying or sitting position, and large calf muscles.	A mutation in a specific gene on the X chromosome disrupts the synthesis of dystrophin, a protein that helps keep muscle cells intact. In BMD the protein is only partially functional, causing muscles to weaken and degenerate.	Diagnosis involves enzyme tests, electromyography, muscle biopsy, and genetic testing. There is no cure. Treatment focuses on managing the symptoms. Gene therapy may eventually provide a treatment protocol to slow the progression of the disease.

Genetic Diseases and Disorders—cont'd

Disease	Signs and Symptoms	Etiology	Diagnosis and Treatment
Cystic fibrosis (CF)	Secretions such as mucus, sweat, and pancreatic juice, are salty and thick. Thick mucus in the lungs leads to impaired breathing and increased infections. The pancreatic ducts become plugged, which stops the flow of digestive enzymes. Signs and symptoms vary greatly depending on the severity of the disorder.	Caused by mutations in a gene that produces a protein called cystic fibrosis transmembrane conductance regulator (CFTR) that controls the flow of salt and water in and out of the cells. This results in secretions that are thick and salty.	Every state in the United States now routinely screens newborns for cystic fibrosis by testing a blood sample. Older children and adults are diagnosed through a sweat test and genetic testing using DNA. The goals of treatment include preventing and controlling lung infections, loosening and removing mucus from the lungs, preventing and treating intestinal blockage, and providing adequate nutrition.
Down syndrome (DS)	Signs and symptoms include physical growth delays, characteristic facial patterns, and intellectual impairment.	This is the most common chromosomal disorder. It is a genetic disorder caused by the presence of all or part of a third copy of chromosome 21 (trisomy 21).	Screening tests offered as a routine part of prenatal care can indicate likelihood of a Down syndrome baby. Diagnostic tests during pregnancy include amniocentesis and chorionic villus sampling. Diagnosis for newborns depends on chromosomal karyotype. There is no cure. Treatment and medical care are aimed at providing resources for the individual to develop skills as fully as possible.
Duchenne muscular dystrophy (DMD)	Similar to Becker muscular dystrophy but earlier onset and more severe. Signs and symptoms appear when the child begins to walk and include frequent falls, difficulty in running or jumping, waddling gait, difficulty getting up from a lying or sitting position, and large calf muscles. As the disease progresses, the heart and respiratory muscles may weaken, leading to cardiac and respiratory difficulties.	DMD is a severe form of muscular dystrophy that is caused by a total absence of the protein dystrophin, a protein that helps keep muscle cells intact. It is the result of a mutation on the X chromosome. It most commonly occurs in young boys and is characterized by muscle degeneration and weakness.	Diagnosis involves enzyme tests, electromyography, muscle biopsy, and genetic testing. There is no cure. Treatment focuses on managing the symptoms. Gene therapy may eventually provide a treatment protocol to slow the progression of the disease.
Fragile X syndrome (FXS)	The variety and degree of the signs and symptoms depend on the extent of the mutation in the gene, but may include impaired intellectual functioning, distinctive physical features such as large ears and long face, social anxiety, aggressive behavior, language difficulties, and autism-like behavior.	Caused by a mutation in a specific gene on the X chromosome. The mutated gene is unable to direct the synthesis of a protein needed for normal brain development. This is the most commonly known genetic cause of autism spectrum disorder.	Diagnosis is determined by direct analysis of the specific gene site on the X chromosome. Prenatal testing includes amniocentesis and chorionic villus sampling. There is no cure. Early intervention is key to realizing the child's full potential through appropriate education accompanied by behavioral and/or physical therapy as needed.
Huntington disease (HD)	Usually develops in midlife and may include involuntary movements, impairment of voluntary motor skills, cognitive impairment, and psychiatric disorders such as depression, social withdrawal, and bipolar disorder.	An inherited disorder caused by a defect in a single gene that results in the progressive degeneration of brain cells; an autosomal dominant disorder.	Diagnosis is based on medical history, physical examination, evaluation of motor and sensory functions, neurologic testing, psychiatric evaluation, and genetic testing. No treatments can cure or alter the course of the disorder. Medical management is likely to evolve as the condition progresses and may include medications and physical, speech, and/or occupational therapy.

Continued

Genetic Diseases and Disorders—cont'd

Disease	Signs and Symptoms	Etiology	Diagnosis and Treatment
Klinefelter syndrome	Occurs only in males and may not be noticeable until puberty or adulthood. The signs and symptoms are associated with low testosterone levels: less body and facial hair, broad hips, gynecomastia, hypogonadism, and hypospermia.	A condition in which a male has an extra X chromosome (XXY instead of XY). It is caused by an error during meiosis so that the zygote receives an extra X.	Diagnosis can be confirmed by hormone testing and chromosome analysis. Treatment may include testosterone replacement therapy, surgical removal of breast tissue, and fertility treatments.
Noonan syndrome	Unusual facial characteristics, heart defects, short stature, and abnormal bruising or bleeding.	An autosomal dominant congenital disorder that affects both males and females equally. The mutation may be inherited from a parent or occur as a result of a new mutation.	Diagnosis is confirmed by molecular genetic testing. There is no cure. Treatment focuses on controlling the symptoms and complications.
Phenylketonuria (PKU)	Seizures, microcephaly, progressive impairment of cerebral function, hyperactivity, severe learning disabilities, a "musty" odor to sweat and urine.	An autosomal recessive genetic disorder that inhibits the metabolism of the amino acid phenylalanine. As phenylalanine accumulates, it hinders the development of the brain. In PKU, phenylalanine is converted to phenylketones that appear in the urine.	Babies born in the United States and many other countries are screened for PKU soon after birth. Treatment involves controlling phenylalanine through diet. The US Food and Drug Administration (FDA) has approved the drug sapropterin for treatment of PKU. It increases tolerance to phenylalanine in some people.
Sickle cell anemia (SCA)	Major features include fatigue and anemia, dactylitis, bacterial infections, pooling of blood in the spleen, liver congestion, and lung and heart injury. Signs and symptoms are the direct result of lack of oxygen to the organs with impaired circulation.	SCA is a hereditary blood disorder characterized by red blood cells that are rigid and sickle-shaped. The sickling occurs because of a mutation in the gene that codes for hemoglobin. The abnormal red blood cells clump together and block blood flow through the vessels.	Diagnosis can be made by microscopic observation of the abnormally shaped sickle cells and can be confirmed by using hemoglobin electrophoresis. Prenatal diagnosis is possible with use of amniocentesis or chorionic villus sampling. In general, treatment is directed at management and prevention of acute manifestations of the disease and therapies to prevent cells from sticking together. There is no remedy to reverse the condition.
Tay–Sachs disease (TSD)	In the most common form, infantile onset TSD, a baby about 6 months old will begin to show signs of the disorder. The child's body loses function, leading to blindness, deafness, paralysis, and death, usually by age 4.	Rare genetic autosomal recessive disorder passed from parents to child. A fatty substance in the brain accumulates to toxic levels and damages the nerve cells.	Initial testing involves an enzyme assay to determine the activity of hexosaminidase, which is reduced in TSD. This may be followed by molecular analysis. All patients with infantile onset TSD have a "cherry red" macula in the retina. There is no cure. Gene therapy research may eventually lead to a cure or treatment protocol.
Thalassemias	Disruption in normal hemoglobin synthesis causes low hemoglobin levels and a high rate of red blood cell destruction. The result is anemia with fatigue, weakness, jaundice, abdominal swelling, and dark urine.	Caused by hereditary mutations in the DNA of cells that make hemoglobin. There are numerous forms of thalassemia determined by the number of mutations and the part of the hemoglobin molecule that is affected.	Diagnosis is by blood tests that evaluate the quantity and quality of red blood cells and hemoglobin. DNA analysis is also useful. Prenatal testing can be done using amniocentesis or chorionic villus sampling. Treatment depends on the specific type of thalassemia; mild cases may need no treatment, and severe forms may need blood transfusions or a stem cell transplant.

Genetic Diseases and Disorders—cont'd

Disease	Signs and Symptoms	Etiology	Diagnosis and Treatment
Turner syndrome	Lymphedema, short stature, reproductive sterility, amenorrhea, webbed neck, heart problems, horseshoe kidney, defective vision and hearing.	Chromosomal abnormality in females in which all or part of one of the sex chromosomes is missing. In most cases of Turner syndrome, the functional X chromosome comes from the mother. The missing or abnormal chromosome is the result of an error in meiosis in the father.	Prenatal diagnosis is by amniocentesis or chorionic villus sampling. Postnatally, it is often diagnosed subsequent to heart problems associated with the disease. It may go undetected until the changes normally associated with puberty do not occur. Chromosome analysis is the diagnostic test of choice. There is no cure. Treatment is focused on minimizing the symptoms and may include growth hormone and estrogen replacement therapy.

TERMINOLOGY REVIEW

Key Term	Word Parts	Definition
Active transport	*trans-:* across, through	Process that moves substances across or through a membrane and requires cellular energy.
Anatomic position		Standard reference position for the body.
Axon		Efferent process of a neuron.
Chondrocyte	*chondr/o:* cartilage *-cyte:* cell	Cartilage cell.
Collagenous fibers	*-ous:* pertaining to	Strong and flexible connective tissue fibers that contain the protein collagen.
Cutaneous membrane	*cutane/o:* skin -ous: pertaining to	A type of epithelial membrane; skin.
Cytokinesis	*cyt/o:* cell *-kinesis:* movement	Division of the cell at the end of mitosis to form two separate daughter cells.
Dendrites	*dendr-:* tree	Treelike processes of a neuron; efferent processes.
Diffusion		Movement of substances from a region of high concentration to a region of low concentration.
Elastic fibers		Yellow connective tissue fibers that are not particularly strong but can be stretched and will return to their normal shape when released.
Erythrocytes	*erythr/o:* red *cyte:* cell	Red blood cell.
Fibroblast	*fibr/o:* fiber *-blast:* to form, immature cell	Connective tissue cell that produces fibers.
Histology	*-hist/o:* tissues *-logy:* study	Branch of microscopic anatomy that studies tissues.
Homeostasis	*home/o:* sameness, unchanging, constant *-stasis:* to stop, control, place	A normal stable condition in which the body's internal environment remains the same; constant internal environment.
Human anatomy	*anatomy:* structure	Study of human body shape and structure and the relationships of its parts.
Human physiology	*physi/o:* nature, function *-logy:* study	Study of the functions of humans and their separate parts.
Leukocytes	*leuk/o: white* *cyte:* cell	White blood cells.
Macrophage	*macro-:* large *-phage:* eat, swallow	Large phagocytic connective tissue cell that functions in the immune response.
Mast cell		A connective tissue cell that produces heparin and histamine.

Continued

TERMINOLOGY REVIEW—cont'd

Key Term	Word Parts	Definition
Meiosis		Type of nuclear division in which the number of chromosomes is reduced to one half the number found in a body cell; results in the formation of egg or sperm.
Meninges	*Mening/o:* membrane	Connective tissue membranes that cover the brain and spinal cord.
Mitosis		Process by which the nucleus of a body cell divides to form two new cells, each identical to the parent cell.
Mucous membrane		Epithelial membrane that lines body cavities that open directly to the exterior; secretes mucus.
Negative feedback		A mechanism of response in which a stimulus initiates reactions that reduce the stimulus.
Neuroglia	*neur/o:* nerve *-glia:* glue	Supporting cells of nervous tissue; cells in nervous tissue that do not conduct impulses; nerve "glue."
Neuron	*neur/o:* nerve	Nerve cell, including its processes; conducting cell of nervous tissue.
Osmosis		Diffusion of water through a selectively permeable membrane.
Osteocyte	*oste/o:* bone *-cyte:* cell	Mature bone cell.
Passive transport	*trans-:* across, through	Process that moves substances across or through a membrane and does not require cellular energy.
Pericardium	*peri:* around, surrounding *cardi/o:* heart	Membrane that surrounds the heart.
Peritoneum	*periton:* peritoneum	Serous membrane associated with the abdominopelvic cavity.
Phagocytosis	*phag/o:* eat, swallow *-cyt-:* cell *-osis:* condition	Condition of cell eating; a form of endocytosis in which solid particles are taken into the cell.
Pinocytosis	*pin/o:* to drink *-cyt-:* cell *-osis:* condition	Condition of cell drinking; a form of endocytosis in which fluid droplets are taken into the cell.
Pleura	*pleur/o:* pleura	Serous membrane that surrounds the lungs.
Serous membrane	*ser/o: serous, serum*	Epithelial membrane that lines closed body cavities.
Synovial membrane	*synov/o:* synovia	Membrane that lines the cavities of freely movable joints.
Thrombocyte	*thromb/o:* blood clot *cyt/o:* cell	A formed element of the blood that functions in blood clotting; platelet.
Tissue		Group of similar cells specialized to perform a certain function.

Integumentary System

 Check out the Evolve site at http://evolve.elsevier.com/Bonewit/today to access additional interactive activities and exercises to help you study and prepare for success.

LEARNING OBJECTIVES

Describe the structure of the two layers of the skin.
State three names for the layer of tissue that anchors the skin to underlying organs, and describe the structure of this layer.
List three factors that influence skin color.
Describe the structure of hair and nails and their relationship to the skin.
Discuss the characteristics and functions of the various glands associated with the skin.
List and describe four functions of the integumentary system.
Describe ways in which the aging of an individual affects the integumentary system.
Identify pathology related to the integumentary system.

CHAPTER OUTLINE

KEY TERMS

arrector pili (ah-REK-tor PY-lee) muscle
ceruminous glands (see-ROOM-in-us GLANDS)
cutaneous membrane (kyoo-TAY-nee-us MEM-brayn)
dermis (DER-mis)
epidermis (ep-ih-DER-mis)
hypodermis (hye-poh-DER-miss)
keratinization (ker-ah-tin-ih-ZAY-shun)
melanin (MEL-ah-nin)
melanocytes (meh-LAN-oh-sytes)
sebaceous glands (see-BAY-shus GLANDS)
sebum (SEE-bum)
stratum corium (STRAY-tum KOR-ee-um)
stratum corneum (STRAY-tum KOR-nee-um)
subcutaneous layer (sub-kyoo-TAY-nee-us LAY-er)
sudoriferous glands (soo-door-IF-er-us GLANDS)
sweat glands (SWET GLANDS)

INTRODUCTION TO THE INTEGUMENTARY SYSTEM

The skin and the glands, hair, nails, and other structures that are derived from it make up the *integumentary system.* Because it is on the outside of the body, this organ system is our contact with the external environment and is subjected to continual abuse from the environment. However, the skin is resilient and versatile. In general, it quickly repairs itself and continues to perform its many functions year after year.

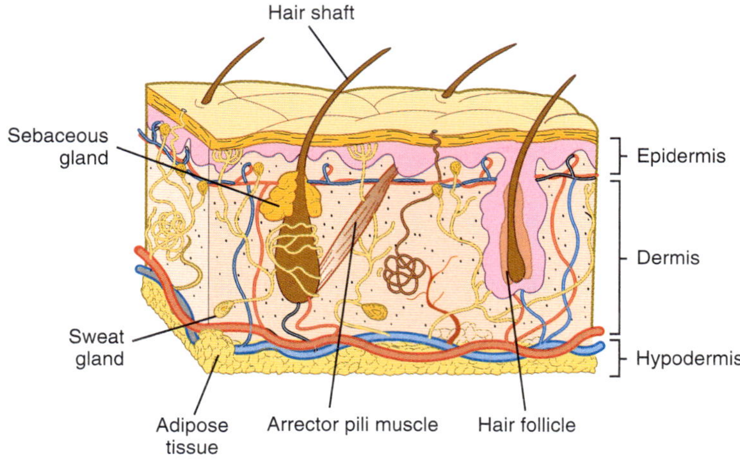

Fig. 6.1 Structure of the skin. Note the epidermis, dermis, and hypodermis. (From Applegate E: *The anatomy and physiology learning system*, ed 4, St. Louis, 2011, Saunders.)

STRUCTURE OF THE SKIN

The skin (sometimes called the **cutaneous membrane**) consists of two distinct layers of tissues. The outer layer is the *epidermis*, and the inner layer is the *dermis*. These are anchored to underlying structures by a third layer, the *hypodermis* or *subcutaneous tissue*.

The structure of the skin is illustrated in Fig. 6.1.

EPIDERMIS

The outer layer of the skin is the **epidermis**. This layer consists of stratified squamous epithelium (see Fig. 6.1). There are no blood vessels present in the epidermis, and the cells receive their nutrients by diffusion from vessels in the underlying tissue. The bottom row of cells in the epidermis is called the *stratum basale*. It consists of actively dividing (mitotic) columnar cells and **melanocytes**. This is the layer next to the basement membrane and closest to the blood supply. As older cells are pushed upward toward the surface by the growing cells next to the basement membrane, they receive fewer nutrients. They also undergo a process called **keratinization**. During keratinization, a protein called *keratin* is deposited in the cell. This causes the chemical composition of the cell to change, and the cell changes shape. By the time the cells reach the surface, they are flat or squamous. They are also dead from lack of nutrients and are sloughed off. They are replaced by other cells that are pushed upward from the stratum basale. About one-fourth of the cells in the stratum basale are melanocytes. Melanocytes are specialized epithelial cells that produce a dark pigment called **melanin**, which is primarily responsible for skin color.

The outermost or surface region of the epidermis is the **stratum corneum**. It makes up about three-fourths of the epidermal thickness and consists of 20 to 30 layers of flattened, dead, completely keratinized cells. The cells in the stratum corneum are continually shed and replaced. About 5 weeks after a cell has been produced in the stratum basale, it is sloughed off the surface of the stratum corneum. The keratin that is present is a tough, water-repellent protein, and its inclusion in the stratum corneum provides protection against water loss from the body.

DERMIS

The **dermis**, or **stratum corium**, is dense connective tissue that is deeper and usually thicker than the epidermis (see Fig. 6.1). Hair, nails, and certain glands (although derived from the stratum basale of the epidermis) are embedded in the dermis. The dermis contains both collagenous and elastic fibers to give it strength and elasticity. If the skin is overstretched, the dermis may be damaged, leaving white scars called *striae*, commonly called "stretch marks." Fibers also form a framework for the numerous blood vessels and nerves that are present in the dermis but generally absent in the epidermis. Many of the nerves in the dermis have specialized endings called *sensory receptors* that detect changes in the environment, such as heat, cold, pain, pressure, and touch. Because there are no nerves in the epidermis, these receptors are the body's contact with the environment.

The upper region of the dermis has numerous *papillae*, or projections, that extend into the epidermis. Blood vessels, nerve endings, and sensory receptors extend into the papillae to bring them into closer proximity to the epidermis and the surface. On the palms, the fingertips, and the soles of the feet, the papillae form distinct patterns or ridges that provide friction for grasping objects. The patterns are genetically determined and are unique for each individual. These are the basis of fingerprints and footprints.

SUBCUTANEOUS LAYER

The **subcutaneous layer** (see Fig. 6.1) is not actually a part of the skin, but it loosely anchors the skin to underlying organs. Because it is beneath the dermis, it is sometimes called the **hypodermis**. It is also referred to as *superficial fascia*. The subcutaneous layer consists largely of loose connective tissue and adipose tissue. The fibers in the loose connective tissue are continuous with those in the dermis, and as a result there is no distinct boundary between the dermis and the subcutaneous tissue.

The adipose tissue in the subcutaneous layer cushions the underlying organs from mechanical shock and acts as a heat insulator in temperature regulation. Fat in the adipose tissue can be mobilized and used for energy when necessary. The distribution of subcutaneous adipose tissue is largely responsible for the differences in body contours between men and women.

SKIN COLOR

Skin color is a result of many factors: some genetic, some physiologic, and some environmental. Basic skin color is caused by the dark pigment *melanin*, produced by the melanocytes in the stratum basale of the epidermis. Everyone has about the same number of melanocytes. The activity of the melanocytes, however, is genetically controlled. Although many genes are responsible for skin color, a single mutation can result in an inability to produce melanin. This results in a condition called *albinism* in which individuals have light skin, white hair, and unpigmented irises in the eyes.

Some people have the yellowish pigment *carotene* in addition to melanin. This gives a yellow tint to the skin. A pinkish tint in the skin is attributable to the blood vessels in the dermis. Ultraviolet light increases melanocyte activity so that more melanin is produced and the skin becomes darker or tanned.

EPIDERMAL DERIVATIVES

Accessory structures of the skin include hair, nails, sweat glands, and sebaceous glands. They are derived from the stratum basale of the epidermis and are embedded in the dermis. Fig. 6.1 illustrates some of the accessory structures associated with the skin.

HAIR AND HAIR FOLLICLES

Hair is found on nearly all body surfaces, but it is absent on the palms of the hands and the soles of the feet. All hair has essentially the same structure. It consists of a shaft and a root that are composed of dead, keratinized epithelial cells. The root is enclosed in a hair follicle that extends through the epidermis and is embedded in the dermis. The function of a hair follicle is to produce or grow hair.

The *shaft* of a hair is that portion that extends beyond the surface of the epidermis. It is the part that you can see. Because it contains no nerves, it can be cut with no sensation of pain. The *root* is the portion of the hair that is below the surface of the skin. It is surrounded by a hair follicle. The shaft and root are continuous and together make up the hair, which is produced by the hair follicle. The outermost covering on a hair is a single layer of overlapping, keratinized cells called the *cuticle*. On the shaft of the hair, the cuticle is exposed to the environment and subjected to abrasion. It tends to wear away at the tip of the shaft. When this happens, the inner portion projects from the tip of the shaft, resulting in "split ends."

The root of a hair is enclosed in a tubular *hair follicle* that is embedded in the dermis. Blood vessels in the dermis provide the blood supply for the epithelial cells of the hair

HIGHLIGHT on the Integumentary System

Skin

For an "average" person, the skin weighs about 5 kg (11 lb), has a surface area of approximately 2 m^2 (21 ft^2), and varies in thickness from 0.05 to 0.4 cm (0.02–0.16 inch).

Acne

Acne is a problem that plagues many teenagers. Increased hormone activity at puberty causes an increase in sebaceous gland activity. Sebum and dead cells may block the hair follicle and form blackheads. Bacteria infect the blocked follicle, and the sebum–dead cell mixture accumulates until the follicle ruptures. This initiates an inflammatory response that soon appears on the surface as a pus-filled pimple.

Adipose Tissue

People who lose weight rapidly may feel cold because they have reduced their adipose insulation.

Blister

A blister is a fluid-filled pocket between the dermis and the epidermis. When the skin is burned or irritated, some plasma escapes from the blood vessels in the dermis and accumulates between the two layers, where it forms the blister.

Dermal Blood Vessels

In people with light skin, when dermal blood vessels dilate and blood flow increases (e.g., during blushing and increased temperature), the skin may be quite red. If the vessels constrict and blood flow decreases, the individual is pale or "white as a sheet."

Dermis

The dermis is the portion of an animal's skin that is used to make leather because the collagen in the dermis becomes tough when treated with tannic acid.

Hair Type

The shape of the hair shaft determines whether hair is straight or curly. If the shaft is round, the hair is straight. If it is oval, the hair is wavy. If it is flat, the hair is curly or kinky. To make their hair curly, individuals often get a "permanent," which flattens the hair. ■

follicle. Stratum basale cells, like those in the skin, provide the mitotic cells that divide and undergo keratinization to produce the hair.

Hair color is determined by the type of melanin produced by the melanocytes in the stratum basale. The shaft of the hair without melanin is clear and transparent. Yellow, brown, and black pigments are present in varying proportions to produce different hair colors. With age, the melanocytes become less active and the hair appears to have less color.

A bundle of smooth muscle cells, called the **arrector pili muscle**, is associated with each hair follicle. Most hair follicles are at a slight angle to the surface of the skin. The arrector pili muscles are attached to the hair follicles in such a way that contraction pulls the hair follicles into an upright position or causes the hair to "stand on end." Contraction of the arrector pili muscles also causes raised areas on the skin, or "goose bumps." Action of the arrector pili muscles is controlled by the nervous system in response to cold and fright.

NAILS

Nails are thin plates of dead stratum corneum that contain a very hard type of keratin and cover the dorsal surfaces of the distal ends of the fingers and toes. Each nail has a *free edge*; a *nail body*, which is the visible portion; and a *nail root*, which is covered with skin. The *eponychium* or *cuticle* is a fold of stratum corneum that grows onto the proximal portion of the nail body. Stratum basale from the epidermis grows under the nail body and is responsible for nail growth. The portion of the body over the growth area appears as a whitish, crescent-shaped area called the *lunula*. Nails appear pink because of the rich supply of blood vessels in the underlying dermis.

GLANDS

The two major glands associated with the skin are the *sebaceous glands* and the *sweat glands* (also called *sudoriferous glands*). A third type, the *ceruminous glands*, are modified sweat glands.

Sebaceous Glands

In general, **sebaceous glands** are associated with hair follicles and are found in all areas of the body that have hair (see Fig. 6.1). Those not associated with hair follicles open directly onto the surface of the skin. The oily secretion, called **sebum**, is transported by a duct into a hair follicle, and from there it reaches the surface of the skin. Sebum functions to keep hair and skin soft and pliable. It also inhibits growth of bacteria on the skin and helps to prevent water loss. Secretory activity of the sebaceous glands is stimulated by sex hormones; consequently, the glands are relatively inactive in childhood, become highly active during puberty, and decrease in activity during old age. Decreased sebum, in part, accounts for the dry skin and brittle hair that are common in older people.

Sweat (Sudoriferous) Glands

Sweat glands (also called **sudoriferous glands**) are widely distributed over the body. They are most numerous in the palms and soles. The glandular portion of a sweat gland is a coiled tube that is embedded in the dermis of the skin, and the duct opens onto the surface of the skin through a *sweat pore* (see Fig. 6.1). The secretion of these glands is primarily water with a few salts. When the body's temperature increases, the glands are stimulated to produce sweat, which evaporates and has a cooling effect. Sweat, or *perspiration*, is also produced in response to nerve stimulation as a result of emotional stress.

Ceruminous Glands

Ceruminous glands are modified sweat glands that are found in the external auditory (ear) canal. They secrete an oily, sticky substance called *cerumen*, or earwax, that is thought to repel insects and trap foreign material.

FUNCTIONS OF THE SKIN

PROTECTION

The skin forms a protective covering over the entire body. The keratin in the cells waterproofs the cells and helps prevent fluid loss from the body. This waterproofing also prevents too much water from entering the body during swimming and bathing. Unbroken skin forms the first line of defense against bacteria and other invading organisms. The oily secretions of the sebaceous glands are acidic and inhibit bacterial growth on the skin. Melanin pigment absorbs light and helps protect underlying tissues from the damaging effects of ultraviolet light. Skin also protects underlying tissues from mechanical, chemical, and thermal injury.

SENSORY RECEPTION

The dermis contains numerous sensory receptors for heat, cold, pain, touch, and pressure. Even though hair itself has no sensory receptors, the movement of hair can be detected by receptors clustered around a hair follicle. The sensory receptors in the dermis relay information about the environment to the brain so that changes can be made to prevent or minimize injury. The sensory receptors are also a means of communication between individuals.

REGULATION OF BODY TEMPERATURE

Normally, body temperature is maintained at 37 °C (98.6° F). It is important that body temperature be regulated because changes in temperature alter the speed of chemical reactions in the body. The skin helps to regulate body temperature in two ways: by dilation and constriction of blood vessels, and by activity or inactivity of the sweat glands. Both of these mechanisms are examples of negative feedback in maintaining homeostasis. Blood vessels dilate and sweat glands become active in response to an increase in body temperature.

Both mechanisms tend to remove heat from the body. In response to cold, blood vessels constrict and sweat glands are inactive to conserve body heat. The adipose tissue in the subcutaneous layer also helps by acting as an insulator.

SYNTHESIS OF VITAMIN D

Vitamin D is required for calcium and phosphorus absorption in the small intestine. The calcium and phosphorus are essential for normal bone metabolism and muscle function. Skin cells contain a precursor molecule that is converted to vitamin D when the precursor is exposed to ultraviolet rays in sunlight. It takes only a small amount of ultraviolet light to stimulate vitamin D production, so this should not be used as an excuse to expose the skin to sun unnecessarily and to risk the damage that may result.

AGING OF THE INTEGUMENTARY SYSTEM

As the skin ages, the number of elastic fibers decreases and adipose tissue is lost from the dermis and subcutaneous layer. This causes the skin to wrinkle and sag. Loss of collagen fibers in the dermis makes the skin more fragile and makes it heal more slowly. Mitotic activity in the stratum basale slows so that the skin becomes thinner and appears more transparent. Reduced sebaceous gland activity causes dry, itchy skin. Loss of adipose tissue in the subcutaneous layer and reduced sweat gland activity lead to an intolerance to cold and susceptibility to heat. The ability of the skin to regulate temperature is reduced. There is a general reduction in melanocyte activity, which decreases protection from ultraviolet light, resulting in increased susceptibility to sunburn and skin cancer. Some melanocytes, however, may increase melanin production, resulting in "age spots."

Despite all the creams and "miracle" lotions, there is no known way to prevent skin from aging. Good nutrition and cleanliness may slow the aging process. Because skin that is exposed to sunlight ages more rapidly than unexposed skin, one of the best ways to slow the aging process is to avoid exposure by wearing protective clothing and by using sunblock whenever possible.

Common Pathology of the Integumentary System

Disease	Signs and Symptoms	Etiology	Diagnosis and Treatment
Alopecia	Absence of hair from skin areas where it normally grows.	May be caused by chemotherapy, injury, or disease. Baldness may be hereditary.	Diagnosis is evident by lack of hair. Medications may help prevent further hair loss. Hair transplants are sometimes indicated.
Cellulitis	Affected area appears swollen and red and feels hot.	Infection of connective tissue with severe inflammation of the dermis and subcutaneous layers of the skin. Caused by bacteria, usually *Streptococcus* or *Staphylococcus*, entering the skin by way of a cut or abrasion.	Diagnosis is by physical examination. Blood tests and a wound culture may be useful. Treatment includes resting the affected area. Cutting away dead tissue may be necessary. Oral antibiotics are usually prescribed.
Dermatitis	Affected area exhibits a red, itchy rash. In some forms, blisters may develop; in others, oily scales may appear.	Inflammation of a region of the skin; commonly an allergic reaction to a specific allergen such as poison ivy.	Diagnosis is by examination. Treatment is typically with moisturizers and steroid creams.
Eczema	Skin shows red, itching, vesicular lesions that may crust over.	Inflammatory skin disease believed to be the result of a combination of hereditary and environmental factors.	Diagnosis is by examination of the skin. Treatment aims to heal the affected skin and to prevent recurrence of the symptoms; may include mild soap and moisturizers, hydrocortisone, and antihistamines. Good skin care is the key for controlling eczema.
Impetigo	Superficial skin infection characterized by vesicles, pustules, and crusted-over lesions, usually on the face.	Highly contagious skin disorder caused by staphylococcal or streptococcal bacteria. Most common in children.	Diagnosis is by examination of the distinctive sores. Antibiotics are usually prescribed. Mild cases may be treated with bactericidal ointment.

Continued

Common Pathology of the Integumentary System—cont'd

Disease	Signs and Symptoms	Etiology	Diagnosis and Treatment
Tinea	Red scaly patches on the skin.	A fungal infection of the skin. Caused by dermatophytes, a type of fungus. Growths on the dead keratinized cells of the skin multiply in warm, damp environments on the body and can be transmitted by touch. Common forms are ringworm, athlete's foot, and jock itch.	Diagnosis is by examination. Treatment includes thoroughly washing and drying the affected area and applying antifungal creams, powders, or sprays.
Urticaria	Skin rash notable for pale red, raised, itchy bumps; commonly called *hives.*	Many different substances in the environment may cause urticaria, including medications, food, and physical agents.	Diagnosis is by examination. Treatment includes avoiding the triggers that cause the outbreaks. Acute episodes may be relieved by antihistamines and hydrocortisone. There are no guaranteed means of controlling attacks.
Warts	The appearance of small, rough skin growths resembling cauliflower.	Caused by human papilloma virus infection of the squamous epithelium.	Diagnosis is by examination. Treatments and procedures associated with wart removal include the use of salicylic acid and cryosurgery.
Decubitus ulcers	Localized open sores on the skin.	Caused by pressure being applied to soft tissue resulting in completely or partially obstructed blood flow. Typically occurs over a bony prominence; commonly called *bedsores.*	Diagnosis is by examination. Treatment involves removing the pressure from the affected areas. Patients with pressure ulcers should not lie or sit on them. In most cases, necrotic tissue should be removed.
Psoriasis	Skin disease characterized by red, scaly patches that usually itch.	In general, considered a genetic disease thought to be triggered or influenced by environmental factors.	Diagnosis is by examination. Treatment includes topical agents for mild disease, phototherapy for moderate disease, and prescribed systemic agents for severe disease.
Skin cancer, basal cell	Typically appears as a waxy bump or a skin sore that does not heal within 2 months while increasing in size.	Damage to the DNA of basal cells is a result of ultraviolet B (UVB) exposure from sunlight or tanning beds.	Early diagnosis by examination and a biopsy by a trained medical professional are vital. Treatments include surgical excision, liquid nitrogen freezing, electrodessication, and curettage.
Skin cancer, melanoma	A skin mole with the following characteristics: *Asymmetry*—irregular shape *Border*—rough, irregular *Color*—nonuniform *Diameter*—more than ¼ inch	Probably caused by excessive exposure to UVB rays from sunlight or tanning beds.	Early diagnosis by examination and a biopsy by a trained medical professional are vital. Treatments include surgery and radiation therapy.
Skin cancer, squamous cell	A firm lump on the skin with a rough, scaly or crusty surface.	Typically caused by excessive exposure to UVB rays from sunlight or tanning beds.	Early diagnosis by examination and a biopsy by a trained medical professional are vital. Treatments include Mohs surgery, radiation therapy, excision, and cryosurgery.

TERMINOLOGY REVIEW

Key Term	Word Parts	Definition
Arrector pili muscle	*pil/o:* hair	Muscle associated with hair follicles.
Ceruminous glands	*cerumin/o:* cerumen	Glands in the ear canal that produce cerumen or ear wax.
Cutaneous membrane	*cutane/o:* skin	Another name for the skin.
Dermis	*derm/o:* skin	Inner layer of the skin that contains the blood vessels, nerves, glands, and hair follicles.
Epidermis	*epi-:* above, upon *-derma:* skin	Outermost layer of the skin.
Hypodermis	*hypo:* below, under *-derma:* skin	Below the skin; a sheet of areolar connective tissue and adipose beneath the dermis of the skin.
Keratinization	*kerat/o:* hard, horny tissue *-ation:* process, condition	Process by which the cells of the epidermis become filled with keratin and move to the surface where they are sloughed off.
Melanin	*melan/o:* black	A dark brown or black pigment found in parts of the body, especially skin and hair.
Melanocytes	*melan/o:* black *cyte:* cell	Cells that produce the dark or black pigment melanin.
Sebaceous glands	*seb/o:* sebum *-ous:* pertaining to	Oil glands of the skin that produce sebum or body oil.
Sebum	*seb/o:* oil	Oily secretion from sebaceous glands.
Stratum corium	*strat:* layer	Another name for the dermis, a layer of the skin.
Stratum corneum	*strat: layer* *corne/:* dead, flattened, scaly	Outermost layer of the epidermis; consists of flattened, dead, keratinized cells.
Subcutaneous layer	*sub-:* under, below *cutane/o:* skin *-ous:* pertaining to	A sheet of areolar connective tissue and adipose tissue beneath the dermis of the skin; also called *hypodermis* or *superficial fascia.*
Sudoriferous glands	*sud-:* sweat *-ous:* pertaining to	Glands in the skin that produce perspiration; also called *sweat glands.*
Sweat glands		Glands in the skin that produce perspiration; also called *sudoriferous glands.*

Skeletal System

 Check out the Evolve site at http://evolve.elsevier.com/Bonewit/today to access additional interactive activities and exercises to help you study and prepare for success.

LEARNING OBJECTIVES

1. List and describe five functions of the skeletal system.
2. Explain the difference between compact and spongy bone.
3. Classify bones according to size and shape.
4. Identify the general features of a long bone.
5. Explain the process by which long bones grow in length.
6. Explain the difference between the axial and appendicular skeletons.
7. Identify the bones of the skull.
8. Identify the structural features of vertebrae.
9. List and describe the divisions of the vertebral column.
10. Describe the structural features of the sternum and ribs.
11. Identify the parts of the pectoral girdle.
12. Identify the bones of the upper extremities.
13. Identify the parts of the pelvic girdle.
14. Identify the bones of the lower extremities.
15. List and describe the different types of joints.
16. Describe ways in which the aging of an individual affects the skeletal system.
17. Identify pathology related to the skeletal system.

CHAPTER OUTLINE

KEY TERMS

amphiarthroses (am-fee-ahr-THROH-sseez)
appendicular skeleton (ap-pen-DIK-yoo-lar SKEL-eh-ton)
appositional growth (ap-poh-ZISH-un-al GROWTH)
articular cartilage (ahr-TIK-yoo-lar KAR-tih-layj)
articulation (ahr-TIK-yoo-lay-shun)
axial skeleton (AK-see-al SKEL-eh-ton)
diaphysis (dye-AF-ih-sis)
diarthroses (dye-ahr-THROH-seez)
endosteum (end-AH-stee-um)
epiphyseal line (ep-ih-FIZ-ee-al LINE)
epiphyseal plate (ep-ih-FIZ-ee-al PLATE)
epiphysis (ee-PIF-ih-sis)
hematopoiesis (hee-mat-oh-poy-EE-sis)
osteoblasts (AH-stee-oh-blasts)
osteoclasts (AH-stee-oh-clasts)
osteocytes (AH-stee-oh-sytes)
osteogenesis (AH-stee-oh-jen-eh-sis)
osteon (AH-stee-ahn)
pectoral girdle (PEK-toh-ral GIR-dull)
pelvic girdle (PEL-vik GIR-dull)
periosteum (pair-ee-AH-stee-um)
sutures (SOO-chers)
synarthroses (sin-ahr-THROH-seez)

INTRODUCTION TO THE SKELETAL SYSTEM

The skeletal system consists of the bones and the cartilage, ligaments, and tendons associated with the bones. It accounts for about 20% of the body weight. Bones are rigid structures that form the framework for the body. People often think of bones as dead, dry, inert pipes and plates because that is how they are seen in the laboratory. In reality, the living bones in our bodies contain active tissues that consume nutrients, require a blood supply, use oxygen and discharge waste products in metabolism, and change shape or remodel in response to variations in mechanical stress. The skeletal system is strong but lightweight. It is well adapted for the functions it must perform. It is a masterpiece of design.

OVERVIEW OF THE SKELETAL SYSTEM

FUNCTIONS OF THE SKELETAL SYSTEM

The skeletal system gives form and shape to the body. Without the skeletal components, we would appear as big "blobs" inefficiently "oozing" around on the ground. In addition to contributing to shape and form, our bones perform several other functions and play an important role in homeostasis.

Support

Bones provide a rigid framework that supports the soft organs of the body. Bones support the body against the pull of gravity, and the large bones of the lower limbs support the trunk when standing.

Protection

The skeleton protects the soft body parts. The fused bones of the cranium surround the brain to make it less vulnerable to injury. The vertebrae surround and protect the spinal cord. The bones of the rib cage help protect the heart and lungs in the thorax.

Movement

Bones provide sites for muscle attachment. Bones and muscles work together as simple mechanical lever systems to produce body movement.

Storage

The intercellular matrix of bone contains large amounts of calcium salts, the most important being calcium phosphate. Calcium is necessary for vital metabolic processes. When blood calcium levels decrease below normal, calcium is released from the bones so that there will be an adequate supply for metabolic needs. When blood calcium levels are increased, the excess calcium is stored in the bone matrix. Storage and release are dynamic processes that go on almost continually.

Blood Cell Formation

Blood cell formation, called *hematopoiesis*, takes place mostly in the red marrow of bones. Red marrow is found in the cavities of most bones in an infant. With age, it is largely replaced by yellow marrow for fat storage. In the adult, red marrow is limited to the spongy bone in the skull, ribs, sternum, clavicles, vertebrae, and pelvis. Red marrow functions in the formation of red blood cells, white blood cells, and blood platelets.

STRUCTURE OF BONE TISSUE

There are two types of bone tissue: compact and spongy. As the names imply, the two types differ in density, or how tightly the tissue is packed together. Three types of cells contribute to bone homeostasis: **osteoblasts**, **osteoclasts**, and **osteocytes**. Osteoblasts are bone-forming cells, osteoclasts resorb or break down bone, and osteocytes are mature bone cells. An equilibrium between osteoblasts and osteoclasts maintains bone tissue.

Compact Bone

The microscopic unit of compact bone is known as the **osteon** (haversian system). The osteon consists of a central canal called the *osteonic* (haversian) *canal*, which is surrounded by concentric rings (lamellae) of hard, calcified matrix. Between

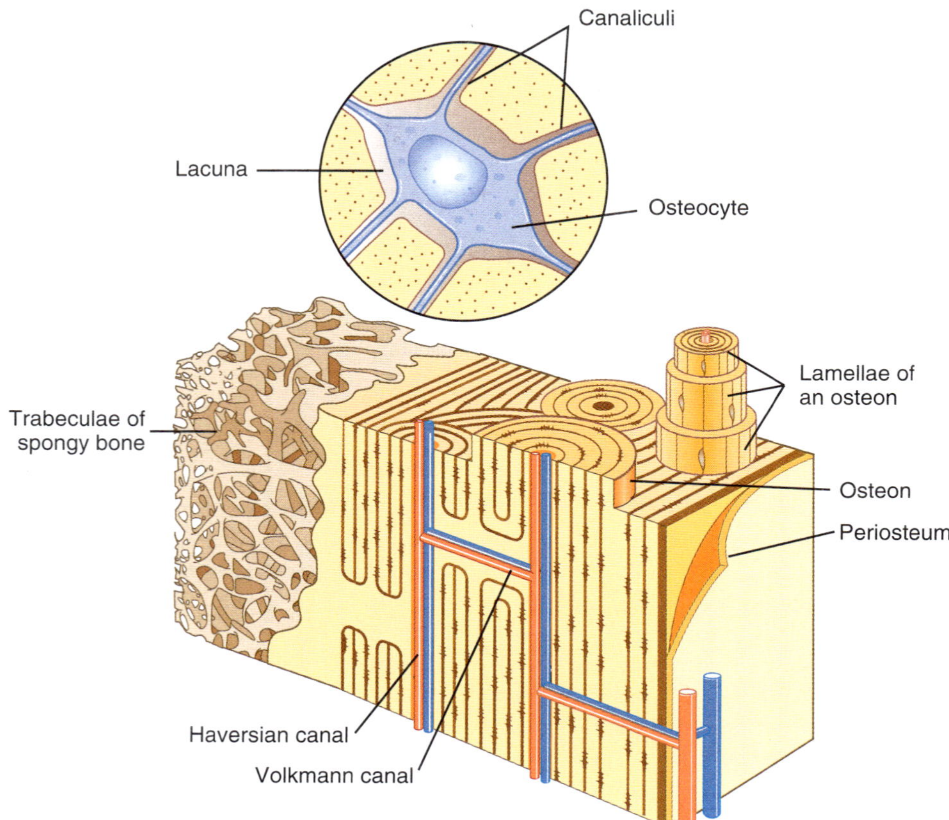

Fig. 7.1 Structure of compact and spongy bone. Note the osteons packed together for compact bone and trabeculae of spongy bone. (From Applegate E: *The anatomy and physiology learning system*, ed 4, St. Louis, 2011, Saunders.)

the rings of matrix, the bone cells (osteocytes) are located in spaces called *lacunae.* Small channels (*canaliculi*) radiate from the lacunae to the osteonic (haversian) canal to provide passageways through the hard matrix. In compact bone the haversian systems are packed tightly together to form what appears to be a solid mass. The osteonic canals contain blood vessels that are parallel to the long axis of the bone. These blood vessels interconnect, by way of perforating (Volkmann) canals, with vessels on the surface of the bone. The microscopic structure of compact bone is illustrated in Fig. 7.1.

Spongy (Cancellous) Bone

Spongy (cancellous) bone is lighter and less dense than compact bone (see Fig. 7.1). Spongy bone consists of plates and bars of bone adjacent to small, irregular cavities that contain red bone marrow. The plates of bone are called *trabeculae.* The canaliculi, instead of connecting to a central haversian canal, connect to the adjacent cavities to receive their blood supply. It may appear that the trabeculae are arranged in a haphazard manner, but they are organized to provide maximum strength in the same way that braces are used to support a building. The trabeculae of spongy bone follow the lines of stress and can realign if the direction of stress changes.

CLASSIFICATION OF BONES

Bones come in a variety of sizes and shapes. Bones that are longer than they are wide are called *long bones.* They consist of a long shaft with two bulky ends or extremities. They are primarily compact bone but may have a large amount of spongy bone at the ends. Examples of long bones are those in the thigh, leg, arm, and forearm.

Short bones are roughly cube-shaped with vertical and horizontal dimensions approximately equal. They consist primarily of spongy bone, which is covered by a thin layer of compact bone. Examples of short bones include the bones of the wrist and ankle.

Flat bones are thin, flattened, and often curved. They are usually arranged like a sandwich with a middle layer of spongy bone called the *diploë.* The diploë is covered on each side by a layer of compact bone; these layers are called the *inner* and *outer tables.* Most of the bones of the cranium are flat bones.

Bones that are not in any of the previously mentioned three categories are classified as *irregular bones.* They are primarily spongy bone that is covered with a thin layer of compact bone. The vertebrae and some of the bones in the skull are irregular bones.

GENERAL FEATURES OF A LONG BONE

Most long bones have the same general features, which are illustrated in Fig. 7.2.

Diaphysis: The shaft of a long bone is called the **diaphysis**. It is formed from relatively thick compact bone that surrounds a hollow space called the *medullary cavity.*

Medullary cavity: In adults the medullary cavity contains yellow bone marrow, so it is sometimes called the *yellow marrow cavity.*

Epiphysis: At each end of the diaphysis, there is an expanded portion called the **epiphysis**. The epiphysis is spongy bone covered by a thin layer of compact bone. The end of the epiphysis, where it meets another bone, is covered by hyaline cartilage, called the **articular cartilage**. This provides smooth surfaces for movement in the joints. In growing bones, there is an **epiphyseal plate** of hyaline cartilage between the diaphysis and epiphysis. Bones grow in length at the epiphyseal plate. Growth ceases when the cartilaginous epiphyseal plate is replaced by a bony epiphyseal line.

Periosteum: Except in the region of the articular cartilage, the outer surface of long bones is covered by a tough, fibrous connective tissue called the **periosteum**. The periosteum is richly supplied with nerve fibers, lymphatic vessels, blood vessels, and osteoblasts.

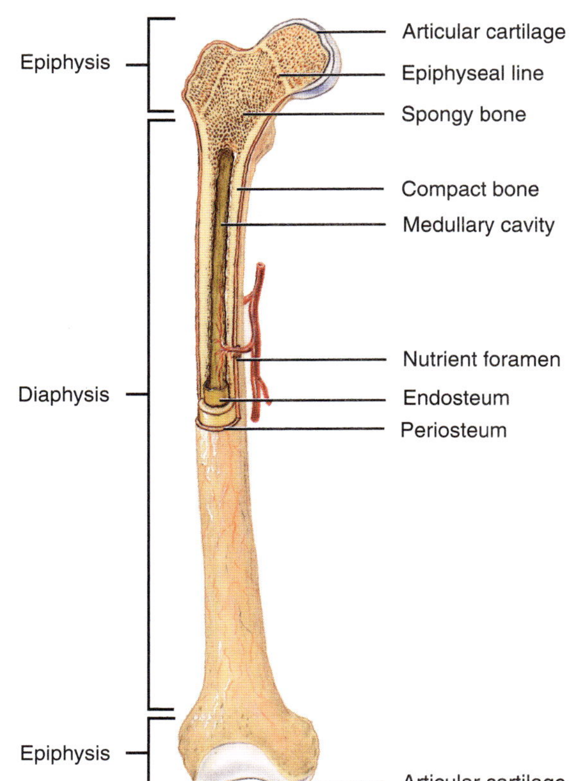

Fig. 7.2 General features of long bones. (From Applegate E: *The anatomy and physiology learning system*, ed 4, St. Louis, 2011, Saunders.)

Nutrient foramina: Blood vessels enter the diaphysis of the bone through small openings called *nutrient foramina.*

Endosteum: The surface of the medullary cavity is lined with a thinner connective tissue membrane, the **endosteum**, which contains osteoclasts.

In addition to the general features that are present in most long bones, all bones have surface markings and characteristics that make a specific bone unique. Bones have holes, depressions, smooth facets, lines, projections, and other markings. These usually represent passageways for vessels and nerves, points of articulation with other bones, or points of attachment for tendons and ligaments.

BONE DEVELOPMENT AND GROWTH

The terms **osteogenesis** and *ossification* are often used synonymously to indicate the process of bone formation. Parts of the skeleton form during the first few weeks after conception. By the end of the eighth week after conception, the skeletal pattern is formed in cartilage and connective tissue membranes, and ossification begins. Bone development continues throughout adulthood. Even after adult stature has been attained, bone development continues for repair of fractures and for remodeling to meet changing lifestyles. Three types of cells are involved in the development, growth, and remodeling of bones. *Osteoblasts* are bone-forming cells; *osteocytes* are mature bone cells; and *osteoclasts* break down and reabsorb bone.

BONE GROWTH IN LENGTH

Bones grow in length at the *epiphyseal plate* located between the diaphysis and epiphysis of a long bone. The hyaline cartilage in the region of the epiphyseal plate next to the epiphysis continues to grow by mitosis. The chondrocytes in the region next to the diaphysis age and degenerate. Osteoblasts move in and ossify the matrix to form bone. This process continues throughout childhood and adolescence until the cartilage growth slows and finally stops. When cartilage growth ceases, usually in the early 20s, the epiphyseal plate completely ossifies so that only a thin **epiphyseal line** remains and the bones can no longer grow in length. Bone growth occurs under the influence of growth hormone from the anterior pituitary gland and sex hormones from the ovaries and testes.

Even though bones stop growing in length in early adulthood, they can continue to increase in thickness or diameter throughout life in response to stress from increased muscle activity or to weight gain. The increase in diameter is called **appositional growth**. Osteoblasts in the periosteum form compact bone around the external bone surface. At the same time, osteoclasts in the endosteum break down bone on the internal bone surface, around the medullary cavity. These two processes together increase the diameter of the bone and at the same time keep the bone from becoming excessively heavy and bulky.

DIVISIONS OF THE SKELETON

The typical adult human skeleton consists of 206 named bones. For convenience, the bones of the skeleton are grouped in two divisions, as illustrated in Fig. 7.3. The 80 bones of the **axial skeleton** form the vertical axis of the body. They include the bones of the head, vertebral column, ribs, and breastbone or sternum. The **appendicular skeleton** consists of 126 bones and includes the free appendages and their attachments to the axial skeleton. The free appendages are the upper and lower extremities, or limbs, and their attachments are called *girdles*. Table 7.1 lists the named bones of the body by category.

BONES OF THE AXIAL SKELETON

The axial skeleton, with 80 bones, is divided into the skull, hyoid, vertebral column, and rib cage.

SKULL

The skull has 28 bones, as illustrated in Figs. 7.4 and 7.5. Eight of these are interlocked to form the *cranium*, which houses the brain. The anterior aspect of the skull, the face, consists of 14 *facial bones*. The remaining six bones are the *auditory ossicles*, tiny bones in the middle ear cavity. With the exception of the lower jaw, or mandible, and the auditory ossicles, the bones in the skull are tightly interlocked along irregular lines called **sutures**. Some of the bones in the skull contain *sinuses*, which are air-filled cavities lined with mucous membranes. The sinuses help to reduce the weight of the skull. The paranasal sinuses are arranged around the nasal cavity and drain into it.

Cranium

Frontal Bone

The frontal bone forms the anterior portion of the skull above the eyes (forehead). The paranasal *frontal sinuses* are cavities in the frontal bone.

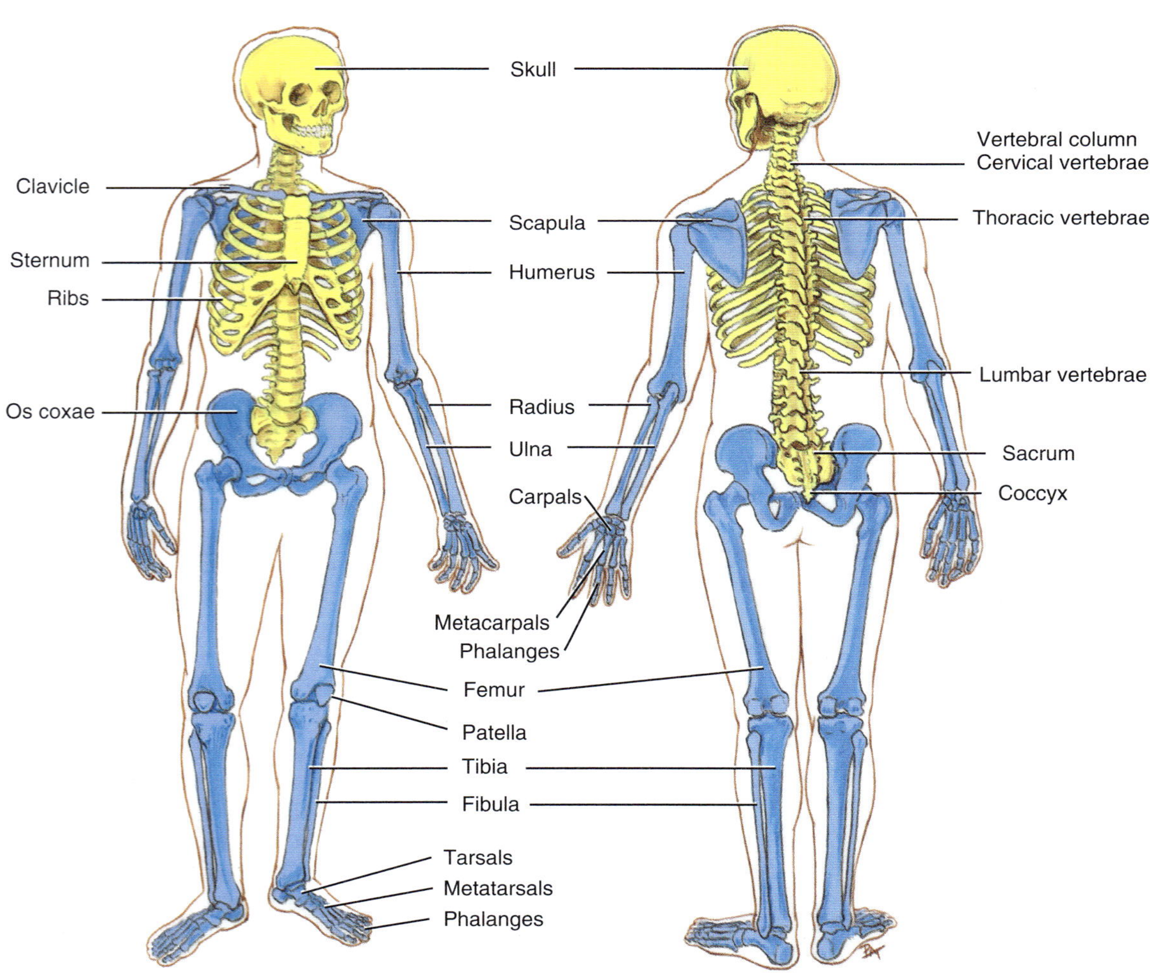

Fig. 7.3 Divisions of the skeleton with major bones identified. *Yellow*, axial skeleton. *Blue*, appendicular skeleton. (From Applegate E: *The anatomy and physiology learning system*, ed 4, St. Louis, 2011, Saunders.)

Table 7.1 Names of Bones of the Body Listed by Category

Bones	Number	Bones	Number
Axial Skeleton (80 Bones)		Thoracic cage	25
Skull (28 Bones)		Sternum (1)	
Cranial bones	8	Ribs (24)	
Parietal (2)		**Appendicular Skeleton (126 Bones)**	
Temporal (2)		Pectoral girdles	4
Frontal (1)		Clavicle (2)	
Occipital (1)		Scapula (2)	
Ethmoid (1)		Upper extremity	60
Sphenoid (1)		Humerus (2)	
Facial bones	14	Radius (2)	
Maxilla (2)		Ulna (2)	
Zygomatic (2)		Carpals (16)	
Mandible (1)		Metacarpals (10)	
Nasal (2)		Phalanges (28)	
Palatine (2)		Pelvic girdle	2
Inferior nasal concha (2)		Coxal, innominate, or hip bones (2)	
Lacrimal (2)		Lower extremity	60
Vomer (1)		Femur (2)	
Auditory ossicles	6	Tibia (2)	
Malleus (2)		Fibula (2)	
Incus (2)		Patella (2)	
Stapes (2)		Tarsals (14)	
Hyoid	1	Metatarsals (10)	
Vertebral column	26	Phalanges (28)	
Cervical vertebrae (7)			
Thoracic vertebrae (12)			
Lumbar vertebrae (5)			
Sacrum (1)			
Coccyx (1)			

From Applegate E: *The anatomy and physiology learning system*, ed 4, St. Louis, 2011, Saunders.

Parietal Bones

The two parietal bones form most of the superolateral aspect of the skull.

Occipital Bone

The single occipital bone forms most of the posterior part of the skull. The *foramen magnum* is a large opening on the lower surface of the occipital bone. The spinal cord passes through this opening. *Occipital condyles* are rounded processes on each side of the foramen magnum. They articulate with the first cervical vertebra.

Temporal Bones

The two temporal bones, one on each side of the head, form parts of the sides and base of the cranium. Near the inferior margin of the temporal bone, there is an opening, the *external auditory meatus*, which is a canal that leads to the middle ear. Just anterior to the external auditory meatus, the temporal bone articulates with the mandible to form the *temporomandibular joint* (TMJ). Posterior and inferior to each external auditory meatus, there is a rough protuberance, the *mastoid process*. The mastoid process contains air cells that drain into the middle ear cavity.

Sphenoid Bone

The sphenoid bone is an irregularly shaped bone that spans the entire width of the cranial floor. It is wedged between other bones in the anterior portion of the cranium. The sphenoid bone contains paranasal *sphenoid sinuses.*

Ethmoid Bone

The ethmoid bone is located anterior to the sphenoid bone and forms most of the bony area between the nasal cavity and the orbits. The ethmoid bone contains many small, paranasal *ethmoidal sinuses.*

Facial Bones

The 14 facial bones form the basic framework and shape of the face. They also provide attachments for the muscles that control facial expression and move the jaw for chewing. All facial bones except the vomer and mandible are paired. Facial bones are illustrated in Figs. 7.4 and 7.5.

Maxillary Bones

The maxillary bones, or *maxillae*, form the upper jaw and the anterior part of the hard palate or roof of the mouth. Each maxilla has a large paranasal *maxillary sinus.* These are the largest of all the paranasal sinuses.

HIGHLIGHT on the Skeletal System

Epiphyseal plate: The epiphyseal plates of specific long bones ossify at predictable times. Radiologists frequently can determine a young person's age by examining the epiphyseal plates to see whether they have ossified. A difference between bone age and chronologic age may indicate some type of metabolic dysfunction.

Sinus problems: The bones with paranasal sinuses are the frontal, the sphenoid, the ethmoid, and the two maxillae. The sinuses are lined with mucous membranes that are continuous with the nasal cavity. Allergies and infections cause inflammation of the membranes, which results in sinusitis. The swollen membranes may reduce drainage from the sinuses so that pressure within the cavities increases, resulting in sinus headaches.

Soft spots: The bones in the skull of a newborn are not completely joined together but are separated by fibrous membranes. The six large areas of membranes are called *fontanels*, or soft spots. The anterior fontanel is on the top of the head, at the junction of the frontal and parietal bones. The posterior fontanel is at the junction of the occipital and parietal bones. On each side of the head there is a mastoid (posterolateral) fontanel near the mastoid region of the temporal bone and a sphenoid (anterolateral) fontanel just superior to the sphenoid bone.

Abnormal spinal curvatures: An abnormally exaggerated lumbar curvature is called lordosis, or swayback. This is often seen in pregnant women as they adjust to their changing center of gravity. An increased roundness of the thoracic curvature is kyphosis, or hunchback. This is frequently seen in elderly people. Abnormal side-to-side curvature is scoliosis. Abnormal curvatures may interfere with breathing and other vital functions.

Yes and no: The atlas holds up the skull and permits you to nod "yes." The axis allows you to rotate your head from side to side to indicate "no."

Marrow biopsy: The sternum is frequently used for a red marrow biopsy because it is accessible. The sample for biopsy is obtained by performing a sternal puncture, in which a large needle is inserted into the sternum to remove a sample of red bone marrow.

Fractured clavicle: The clavicle is the most frequently fractured bone in the body because it transmits forces from the arm to the trunk. The force from falling on the shoulder or outstretched arm is often sufficient to fracture the clavicle.

Pelvic outlet and childbirth: The female pelvis is shaped to accommodate childbearing. Because the fetus must pass through the pelvic outlet, the physician carefully measures this opening to make sure there is enough room. The distance between the two ischial spines is a good indication of the size of the pelvic outlet. If the opening is too small, a cesarean delivery is indicated.

Broken hip: Elderly people, particularly those with osteoporosis, are susceptible to "breaking a hip." The femur is a weight-bearing bone, and when it is weakened, it cannot support the weight of the body and the neck of the femur fractures under the stress. Instead of saying, "Grandma fell and broke her hip," often it is more appropriate to say, "Grandma broke her hip, then fell." ■

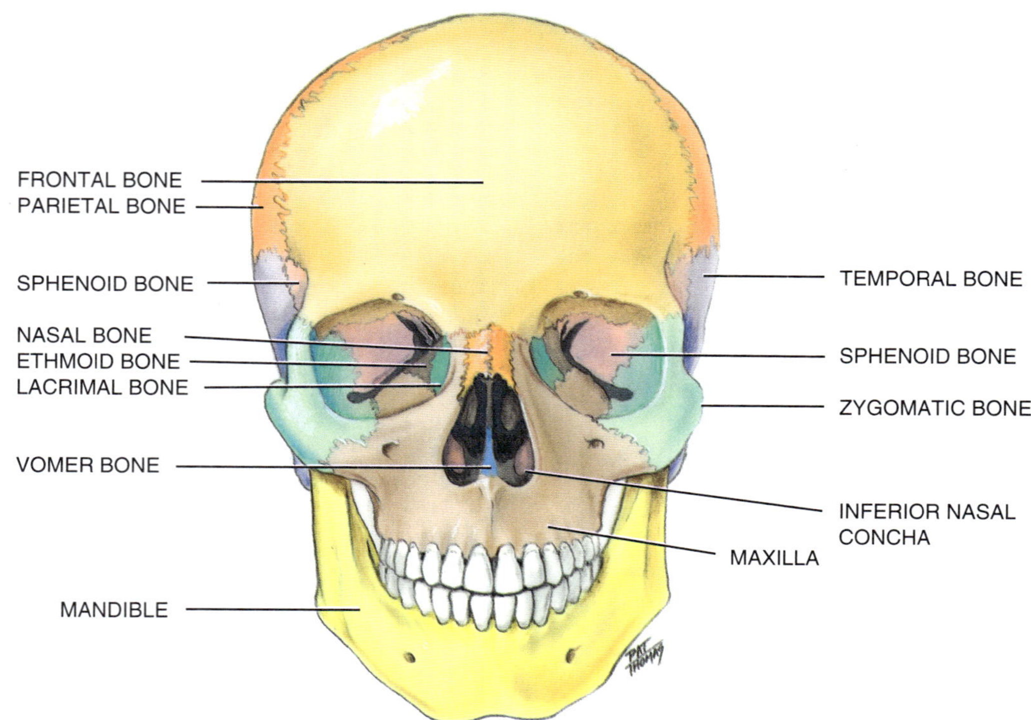

Fig. 7.4 Skull, anterior view. (From Applegate E: *The anatomy and physiology learning system*, ed 4, St. Louis, 2011, Saunders.)

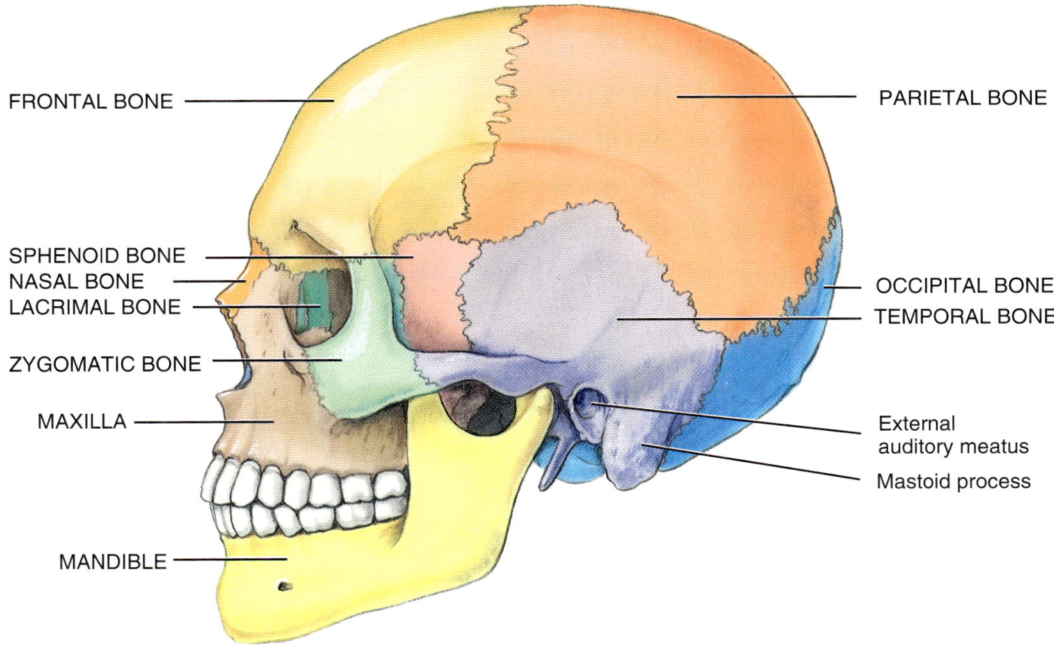

Fig. 7.5 Skull, lateral view. (From Applegate E: *The anatomy and physiology learning system*, ed 4, St. Louis, 2011, Saunders.)

Palatine Bones

The palatine bones are behind, or posterior to, the maxillae and form the posterior portion of the hard palate.

Nasal Bones

The two nasal bones are small rectangular bones that form the bridge of the nose.

Lacrimal Bones

The small, thin lacrimal bones are located in the medial walls of the orbits, between the ethmoid bone and the maxilla. Each one has a small *lacrimal groove* that is a pathway for a tube that carries tears from the eyes to the nasal cavity.

Zygomatic Bones

The zygomatic bones, also called *malar* bones, form the prominences of the cheeks.

Inferior Nasal Conchae

The inferior nasal conchae are thin, curved bones that are attached to the lateral walls of the nasal cavity and project into the nasal cavity.

Vomer

The thin, flat vomer is in the inferior portion of the midline in the nasal cavity. It forms part of the *nasal septum.*

Mandible

The mandible is the lower jaw. It articulates with the temporal bone to form the *temporomandibular joint.*

Auditory Ossicles

Three tiny bones form a chain in each middle ear cavity in the temporal bone. These are the *malleus*, *incus*, and *stapes.* These bones transmit sound waves from the tympanic membrane, or eardrum, to the inner ear, where the sound receptors are located.

HYOID BONE

The hyoid bone is not really part of the skull, so it is listed separately. It is a U-shaped bone in the neck, suspended under the mandible. It is unique because it is the only bone in the body that does not articulate directly with another bone. It functions as a base for the tongue and as an attachment for several muscles associated with swallowing.

VERTEBRAL COLUMN

The vertebral column extends from the skull to the pelvis and contains 26 bones called *vertebrae* (singular, *vertebra*). The bones are separated by pads of fibrocartilage called *intervertebral discs.* The discs act as shock absorbers and allow the column to bend. Normally there are four curvatures, illustrated in Fig. 7.6, that increase the strength and resilience of the column. They are named according to the region in which they are located. The *thoracic* and *sacral curvatures* are concave anteriorly and are present at birth. The *cervical curvature* develops when an infant begins to hold his or her head erect. The *lumbar curvature* develops when an infant begins to stand and walk. Both the cervical and lumbar curvatures are convex anteriorly.

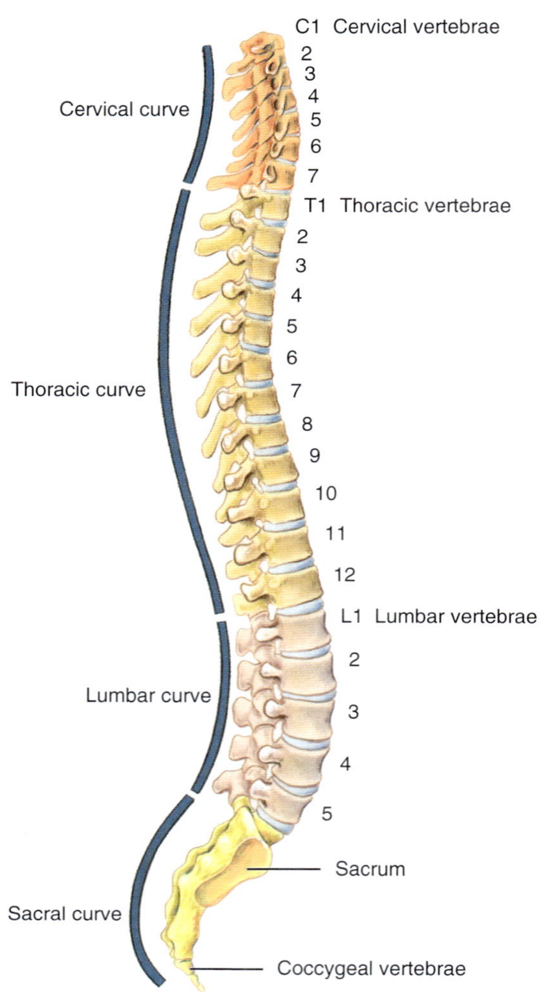

Fig. 7.6 Curvatures of the vertebral column. The thoracic and sacral curvatures are concave anteriorly, and the cervical and lumbar curvatures are convex anteriorly. (From Applegate E: *The anatomy and physiology learning system*, ed 4, St. Louis, 2011, Saunders.)

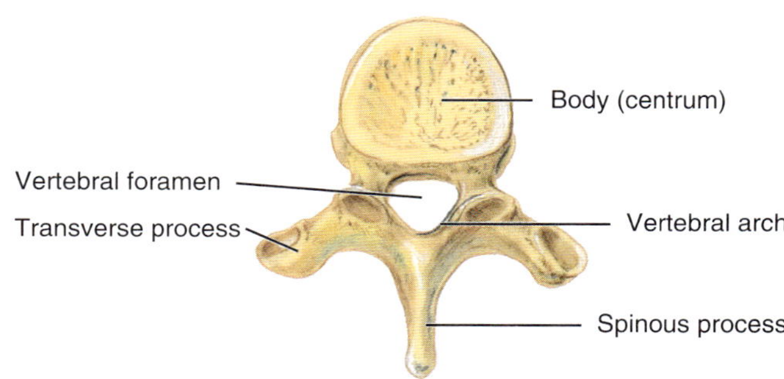

Fig. 7.7 General features of vertebrae, viewed from above. (From Applegate E: *The anatomy and physiology learning system*, ed 4, St. Louis, 2011, Saunders.)

General Structure of Vertebrae

All vertebrae have a common structural pattern, illustrated in Fig. 7.7, although there are variations among them. The thick anterior, weight-bearing portion is the *body* or *centrum.* The posterior curved portion is the *vertebral arch.* The vertebral arch and body surround a central large opening, the *vertebral foramen.* When all the vertebrae are stacked together in a column, the vertebral foramina make a canal that contains the spinal cord. *Transverse processes* project laterally from the vertebral arch, and in the posterior midline there is a *spinous process.* These processes are places for muscle attachment. The spinous processes can be felt as bony projections along the midline of the back.

Composition of the Vertebral Column

The seven *cervical vertebrae* are designated C1 through C7. The 12 *thoracic vertebrae* are designated T1 through T12. Five *lumbar vertebrae*, designated L1 through L5, make up the part of the vertebral column in the small of the back. The lumbar vertebrae have large, heavy bodies because they support most of the body weight and have many back muscles attached to them.

The *sacrum* is a triangular bone just below the lumbar vertebrae. In the child there are five separate bones, but these fuse to form a single bone in the adult. The sacrum articulates with the pelvic girdle laterally, at the *sacroiliac joint*, and forms the posterior wall of the pelvic cavity.

The *coccyx*, or tailbone, is the last part of the vertebral column (Fig. 7.8). A child has four (the number varies from three to five) separate small bones, but these fuse to form a single bone in the adult.

THORACIC CAGE

The thoracic cage, or bony thorax, protects the heart, lungs, and great vessels. It also supports the bones of the shoulder girdle and plays a role in breathing. The components of the thoracic cage are the thoracic vertebrae dorsally, the ribs laterally, and the sternum and costal cartilage anteriorly.

Sternum

The *sternum*, or breastbone, is in the anterior midline (see Fig. 7.8). An important anatomic landmark, the *jugular (suprasternal) notch* is an easily palpable, central indentation in the superior margin of the sternum. The superior portion of the sternum articulates with the clavicles and the first two pairs of ribs. The body of the sternum has notches along the sides where it attaches to the cartilage of the third through seventh ribs.

Ribs

Twelve pairs of *ribs*, illustrated in Fig. 7.8, form the curved, lateral margins of the thoracic cage. One pair is attached to each of the 12 thoracic vertebrae. The upper seven pairs of ribs are called *true*, or *vertebrosternal, ribs* because they attach to the sternum directly by their individual *costal cartilage.* The lower five pairs of ribs are called *false ribs*

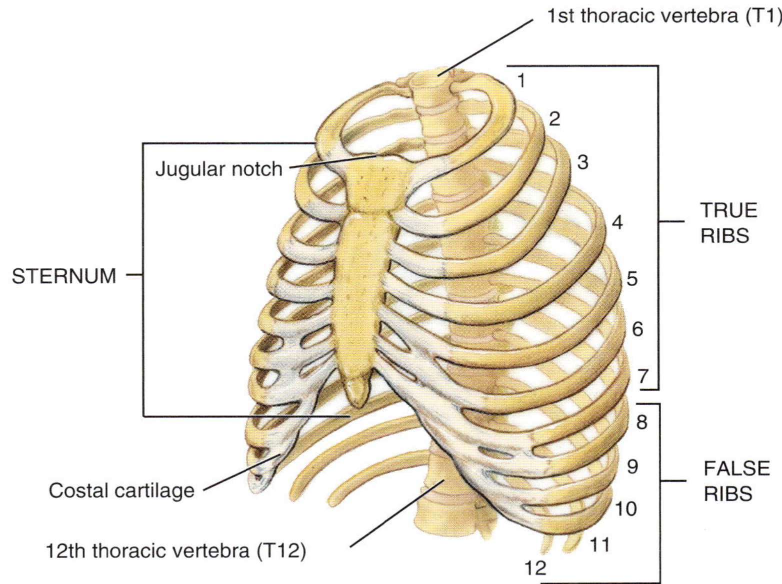

Fig. 7.8 Thoracic cage. (From Applegate E: *The anatomy and physiology learning system*, ed 4, St. Louis, 2011, Saunders.)

because their costal cartilage does not reach the sternum directly. The first three pairs of false ribs reach the sternum indirectly by joining with the cartilage of the ribs above. These are called *vertebrochondral ribs.* The bottom two rib pairs have no anterior attachment and are called *vertebral ribs* or *floating ribs.*

BONES OF THE APPENDICULAR SKELETON

The 126 bones of the appendicular skeleton are suspended from two yokes or girdles that are anchored to the axial skeleton. They are additions or appendages to the axis of the body. The appendicular skeleton is designed for movement. If a portion of the appendicular skeleton is immobilized for a period of time, movement can be awkward.

PECTORAL GIRDLE

Each half of the **pectoral girdle**, or *shoulder girdle*, consists of two bones: an anterior *clavicle* and a posterior *scapula.* The bones of the pectoral girdle, illustrated in Fig. 7.9, form the connection between the upper extremities and the axial skeleton. The clavicles and scapulae, with their associated muscles, also form the shoulder.

The *clavicle* is commonly called the *collarbone.* It is an elongated, S-shaped bone that articulates proximally with the manubrium of the sternum. The distal end articulates with the scapula.

The *scapula*, commonly called the *shoulder blade*, is a thin, flat triangular bone on the posterior surface of the thoracic wall. It articulates with the clavicle and the humerus. The *acromion process* of the scapula forms the point of the shoulder. On the lateral margin of the scapula there is a shallow depression, the *glenoid cavity* (fossa), where the head of the humerus connects to the scapula. The clavicle and scapula provide attachments for numerous muscles.

UPPER EXTREMITY

The upper extremity (limb) consists of the bones of the arm, forearm, and hand.

Arm

The arm, or *brachium*, is the region between the shoulder and the elbow. It contains a single long bone, the *humerus*, illustrated in Fig. 7.10. The *head* is the large, smooth, rounded end that fits into the scapula. The deltoid muscle attaches to the humerus along the shaft of the humerus. At the distal end, on the posterior surface, there is a depression, the *olecranon fossa*, where the ulna fits with the humerus to form the hinged elbow joint. Two smooth, rounded projections are evident on the distal end of the humerus. The capitulum is on the lateral side and articulates with the radius of the forearm. The trochlea is on the medial side and articulates with the ulna of the forearm.

Forearm

The forearm, or *antebrachium*, is the region between the elbow and wrist. It is formed by the *radius* on the lateral side and the *ulna* on the medial side when the forearm is in anatomic position. When the hand is turned so that the palm faces backward, the radius crosses over the ulna. The radius and ulna are illustrated in Fig. 7.11.

The radius has a circular, disclike *head* on the proximal end. This articulates with the capitulum of the humerus.

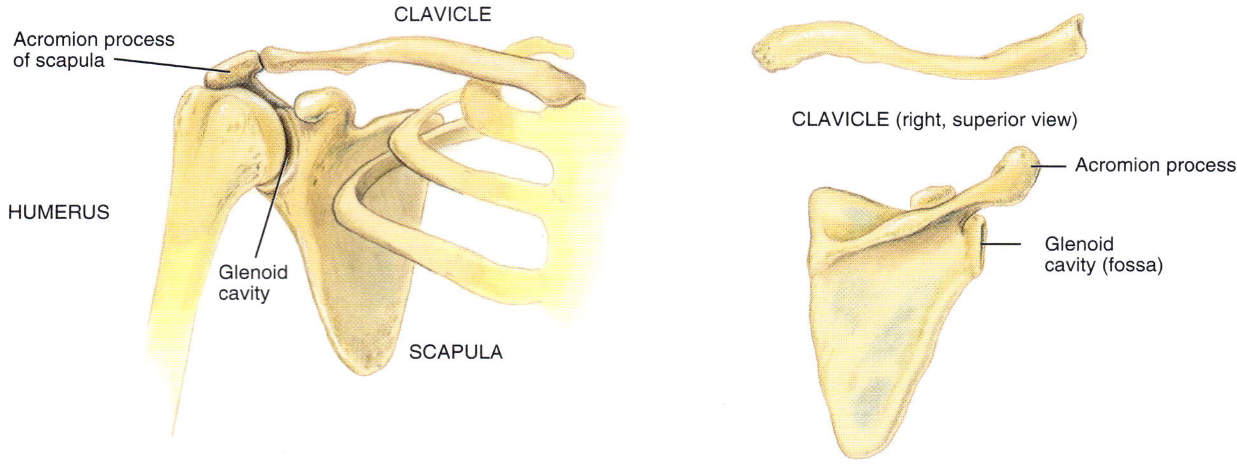

Fig. 7.9 Components of the pectoral girdle: clavicle and scapula. (From Applegate E: *The anatomy and physiology learning system*, ed 4, St. Louis, 2011, Saunders.)

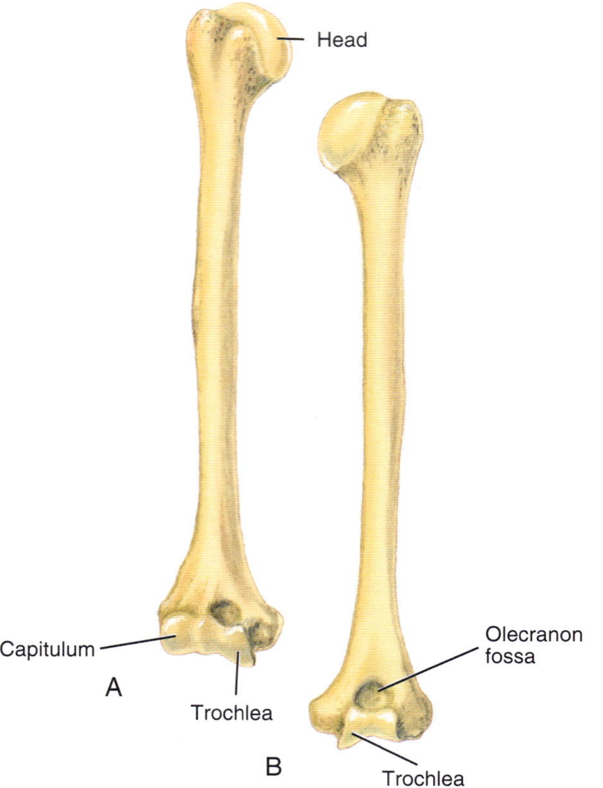

Fig. 7.10 Humerus. (A) Anterior view. (B) Posterior view. (From Applegate E: *The anatomy and physiology learning system*, ed 4, St. Louis, 2011, Saunders.)

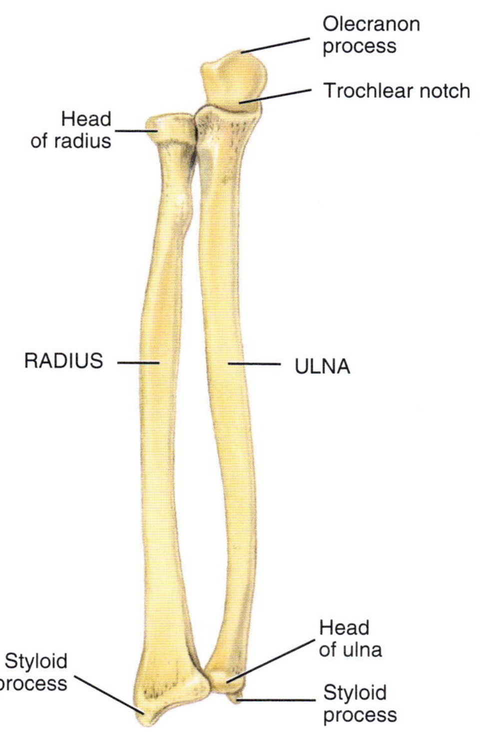

Fig. 7.11 Radius and ulna, anterior view. The radius is on the lateral side, and the ulna is the medial bone. (From Applegate E: *The anatomy and physiology learning system*, ed 4, St. Louis, 2011, Saunders.)

On the distal end, the prominent marking is the *styloid process*, a pointed projection on the lateral side.

The proximal end of the ulna has a wrenchlike shape, with the opening of the wrench being the *trochlear notch*, or semilunar notch. The projection at the upper end of the notch is the *olecranon process*, which fits into the olecranon fossa of the humerus and forms the bony point of the elbow. The *head* is at the distal end, and on the medial side of the head the pointed *styloid process* serves as an attachment point for ligaments of the wrist.

Hand

The hand, illustrated in Fig. 7.12, is composed of the wrist, palm, and five fingers. The wrist, or *carpus*, contains eight small *carpal bones*, tightly bound by ligaments. The palm of the hand, or *metacarpus*, contains five *metacarpal bones*, one in line with each finger. These bones are not named but are numbered one through five starting on the thumb side. The 14 bones of the fingers are called *phalanges*. Some people refer to these as *digits*. Three phalanges are in each finger (a proximal, middle, and distal phalanx) except the thumb, or pollex, which has two. The thumb lacks a middle phalanx. The proximal phalanges articulate with the metacarpals.

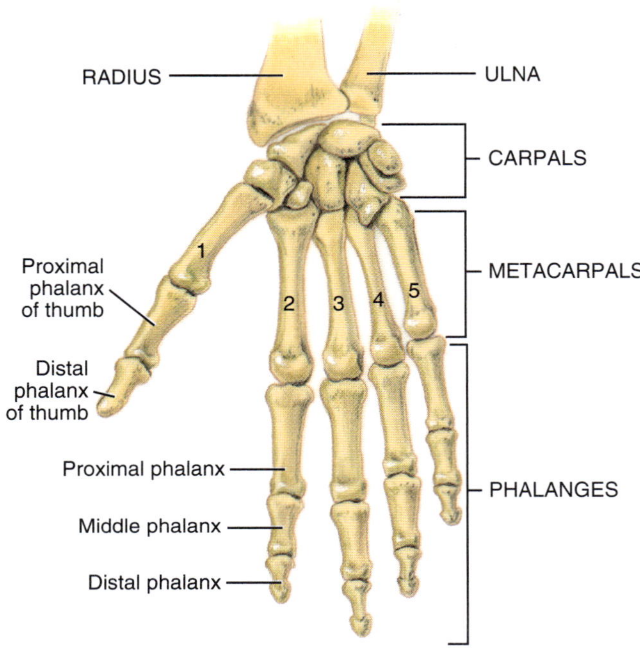

Fig. 7.12 Hand. The carpals form the wrist, the metacarpals form the palm, and the phalanges form the fingers. (From Applegate E: *The anatomy and physiology learning system*, ed 4, St. Louis, 2011, Saunders.)

PELVIC GIRDLE

The **pelvic girdle**, or *hip girdle*, attaches the lower extremities to the axial skeleton and provides a strong support for the weight of the body. It also provides support and protection for the urinary bladder, a portion of the large intestine, and the internal reproductive organs, which are located in the pelvic cavity.

The pelvic girdle consists of two *coxal* (hip) *bones*, illustrated in Fig. 7.13. Anteriorly, the two bones articulate with each other at the *symphysis pubis*; posteriorly, they articulate with the sacrum at the *iliosacral joints.* During childhood, each coxal bone consists of three separate parts: the *ilium*, *ischium*, and *pubis.* In the adult, these bones are firmly fused to form a single bone. Where the three bones meet, there is a large depression, the *acetabulum*, which holds the head of the femur. The *obturator foramen* is a large opening between the pubis and ischium that functions as a passageway for blood vessels, nerves, and muscle tendons.

Together, the sacrum, coccyx, and pelvic girdle form the basin-shaped pelvis. The *false pelvis* (greater pelvis) is surrounded by the flared portions of the ilium bones and the lumbar vertebrae. The *true pelvis* (lesser pelvis) is smaller and inferior to the false pelvis. It is the region below the *pelvic brim*, or *pelvic inlet*, and it is encircled by bone. The large opening at the bottom of this region is the *pelvic outlet.* The dimensions of the true pelvis are especially important in childbirth.

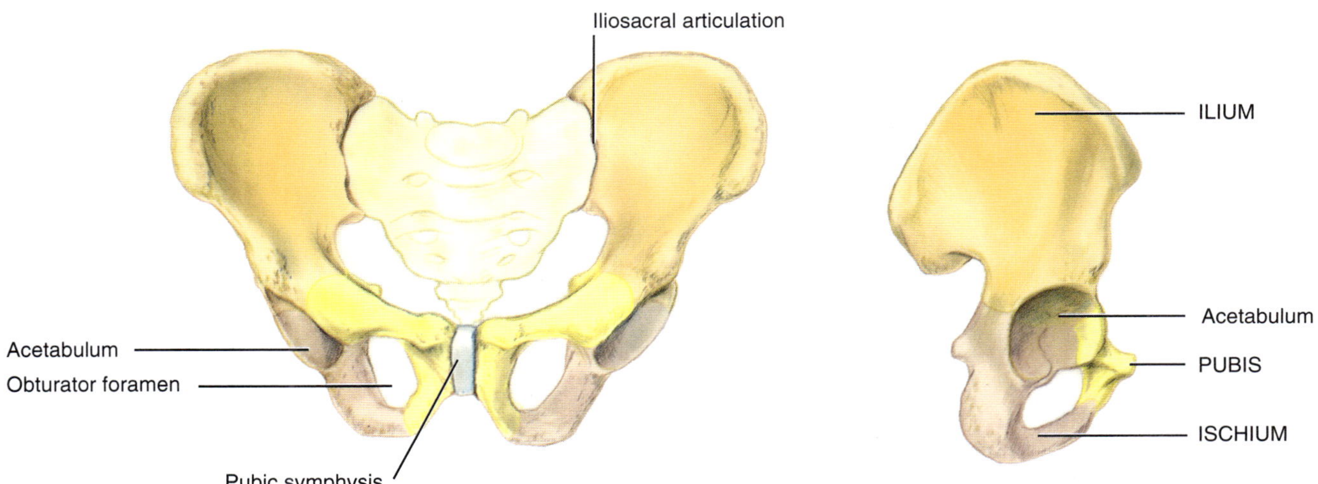

Fig. 7.13 Bones of the pelvic girdle. The right and left ossa coxae form the pelvic girdle. Posteriorly, the two bones are separated by the sacrum. Anteriorly, they meet at the symphysis pubis. (From Applegate E: *The anatomy and physiology learning system*, ed 4, St. Louis, 2011, Saunders.)

LOWER EXTREMITY

The lower extremity (limb) consists of the bones of the thigh, leg, foot, and patella, or kneecap. The lower extremities support the entire weight of the body when we are erect, and they are exposed to tremendous forces when we walk, run, and jump. With this in mind, it is not surprising that the bones of the lower extremity are larger and stronger than those in the upper extremity.

Thigh

The *thigh* is the region from the hip to the knee. It contains a single long bone, the *femur*, illustrated in Fig. 7.14. It is the largest, longest, and strongest bone in the body.

The large, smooth, ball-like *head* of the femur has a small depression called the *fovea capitis*. A ligament attaches here. Prominent projections at the proximal end, the *greater* and *lesser trochanters*, are major sites for muscle attachment. The *neck* is between the head and the trochanters. The distal end is marked by two large, rounded surfaces, the *lateral* and *medial condyles*. These form joints with the bones of the leg. The *intercondylar notch* is a depression between the condyles that contains ligaments associated with the knee joint. On the anterior surface, between the condyles, a smooth *patellar surface* marks the area for the kneecap.

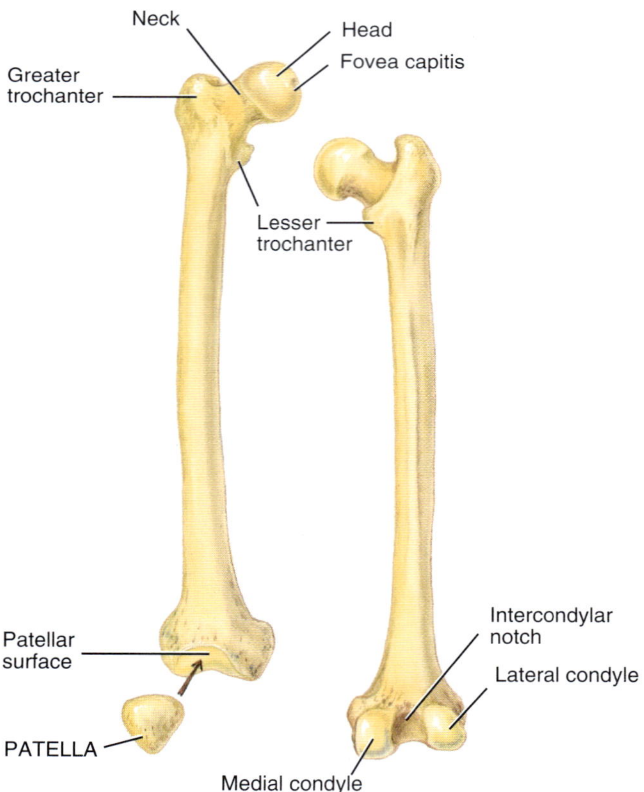

Fig. 7.14 Femur and patella *(right)*. (A) Anterior view. (B) Posterior view. (From Applegate E: *The anatomy and physiology learning system*, ed 4, St. Louis, 2011, Saunders.)

Leg

The *leg* is the region between the knee and the ankle. It is formed by the slender *fibula* on the lateral side and the larger, weight-bearing *tibia*, or shin bone, on the medial side. The tibia articulates with the femur to form the knee joint and with the *talus* (one of the foot bones) to allow flexion and extension at the ankle.

The proximal end of the fibula is the *head*, and the projection at the distal end is the *lateral malleolus*, which forms the lateral bulge of the ankle. The superior surface of the tibia is flattened and smooth, with two slightly concave regions called the *lateral* and *medial condyles*. The condyles of the femur fit into these regions. The *anterior crest* is a sharp ridge on the anterior surface and forms the shin. On the medial side of the distal end, the *medial malleolus* forms the medial bulge of the ankle. Fig. 7.15 illustrates the tibia and fibula.

Foot

The *foot*, illustrated in Fig. 7.16, is composed of the ankle, instep, and five toes. The ankle, or *tarsus*, contains seven *tarsal bones*. These correspond to the carpals in the wrist. The largest tarsal bone is the *calcaneus*, or heel bone. The *talus*, another tarsal bone, rests on top of the calcaneus and articulates with the tibia. The instep of the foot, or *metatarsus*, contains five *metatarsal bones*, one in line with each toe. The distal ends of these bones form the ball of the foot. These bones are not named but are numbered one through five starting on the medial side. The tarsals and metatarsals, together with strong tendons and ligaments, form the arches

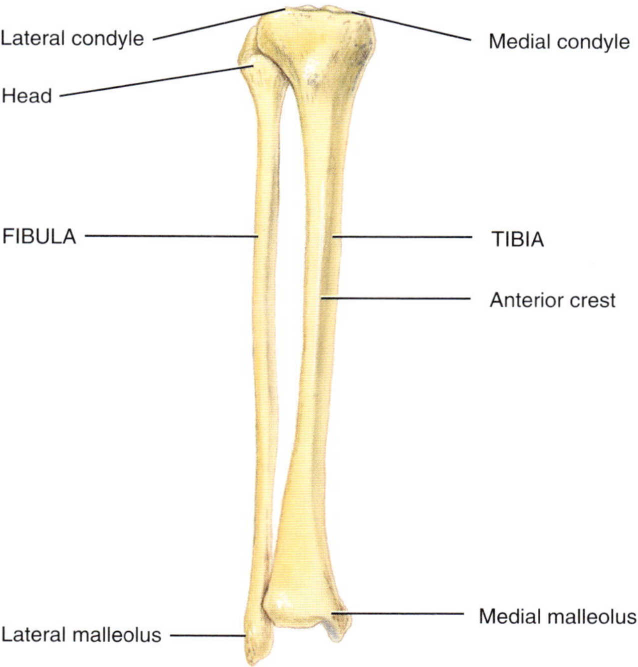

Fig. 7.15 Tibia and fibula, anterior view *(right)*. The fibula is on the lateral side of the leg, and the tibia is on the medial side. (From Applegate E: *The anatomy and physiology learning system*, ed 4, St. Louis, 2011, Saunders.)

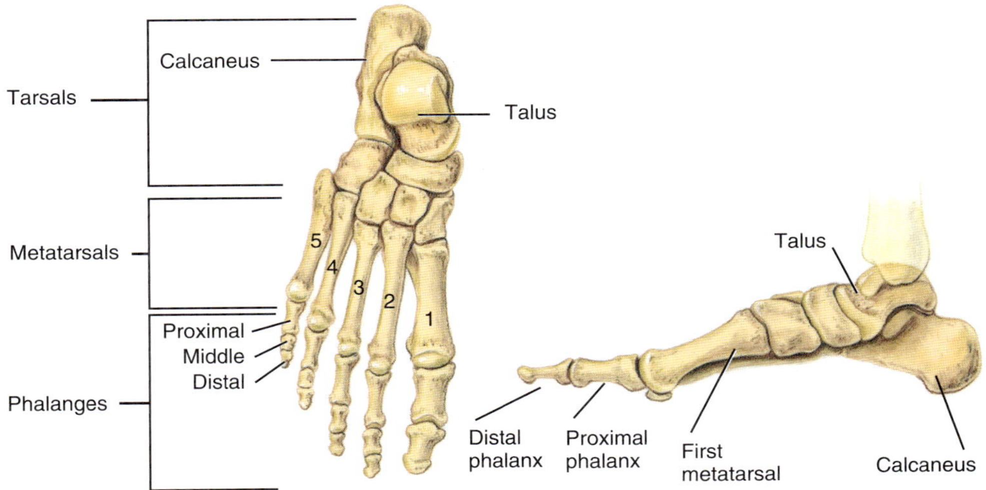

Fig. 7.16 Bones of the foot. (A) Superior view. (B) Lateral view. (From Applegate E: *The anatomy and physiology learning system*, ed 4, St. Louis, 2011, Saunders.)

of the foot. The 14 bones of the toes are called *phalanges*. Three phalanges are in each toe (a proximal, middle, and distal phalanx), except in the great (or big) toe, or hallux, which has only two. The great toe lacks a middle phalanx. The proximal phalanges articulate with the metatarsals.

Patella

The *patella*, or *kneecap*, is a flat, triangular bone enclosed within the major tendon that anchors the anterior thigh muscle to the tibia. It provides a smooth surface for the tendon as it turns the corner between the thigh and leg when the knee is flexed. It also protects the knee joint anteriorly.

ARTICULATIONS

An **articulation**, or joint, is where two bones come together. In terms of the amount of movement that articulations allow, there are three types of joints: immovable, slightly movable, and freely movable.

SYNARTHROSES

Synarthroses are immovable joints. The singular form is *synarthrosis*. In these joints, the bones come in close contact and are separated by only a thin layer of fibrous connective tissue. The *sutures* in the skull are examples of immovable joints.

AMPHIARTHROSES

Slightly movable joints are called **amphiarthroses**. The singular form is *amphiarthrosis*. In this type of joint, the bones are connected by hyaline cartilage or fibrocartilage. The ribs connected to the sternum by costal cartilage are slightly movable joints connected by hyaline cartilage. The symphysis pubis is a slightly movable joint in which there is a fibrocartilage pad between the two bones. The joints between the vertebrae, the intervertebral discs, are also of this type.

DIARTHROSES

Most joints in the adult body are **diarthroses** or freely movable joints. The singular form is *diarthrosis*. In this type of joint, the ends of the opposing bones are covered with hyaline cartilage, the **a***rticular cartilage*, and they are separated by a space called the *joint cavity*. The components of the joints are enclosed in a dense fibrous *joint capsule* (Fig. 7.17).

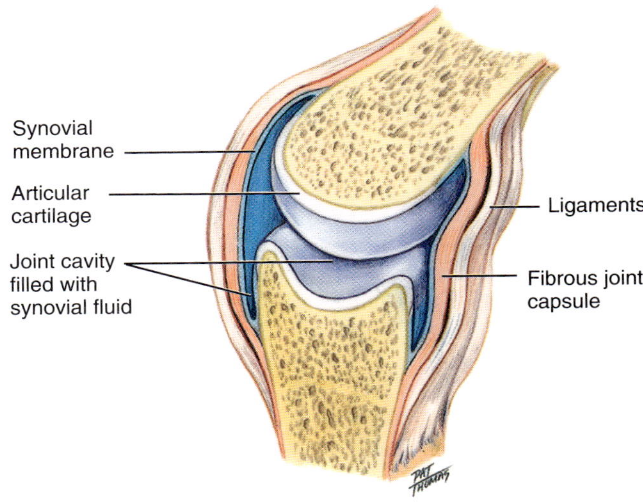

Fig. 7.17 Generalized structure of a synovial joint. (From Applegate E: *The anatomy and physiology learning system*, ed 4, St. Louis, 2011, Saunders.)

The outer layer of the capsule consists of the ligaments that hold the bones together. The inner layer is the *synovial membrane*, which secretes *synovial fluid* into the joint cavity for lubrication. Because all of these joints have a synovial membrane, they are sometimes called *synovial joints.*

Some diarthroses have pads and cushions associated with them. The knee has fibrocartilaginous pads, called *semilunar cartilages* or the *lateral meniscus* and *medial meniscus*, which rest on the lateral and medial condyles of the tibia. The pads help stabilize the joint and act as shock absorbers. *Bursae* are fluid-filled sacs that act as cushions and help reduce friction. Bursae are lined with a synovial membrane that secretes synovial fluid into the sac. They are commonly located between the skin and underlying bone or between tendons and ligaments. Inflammation of a bursa is called *bursitis.*

There are six types of diarthrotic or freely movable joints, based on the shapes of their parts and the types of movement they allow. These are described and illustrated in Fig. 7.18.

AGING OF THE SKELETAL SYSTEM

The major age-related change in the skeletal system is the loss of calcium from the bones. Calcium loss occurs in both men and women, but it starts at an earlier age and is more severe in women. The exact reasons for the loss are unknown and possibly involve a combination of several factors. These may include an imbalance between osteoblast and osteoclast activity, imbalance between calcitonin and parathormone levels, reduced absorption of calcium and/or vitamin D

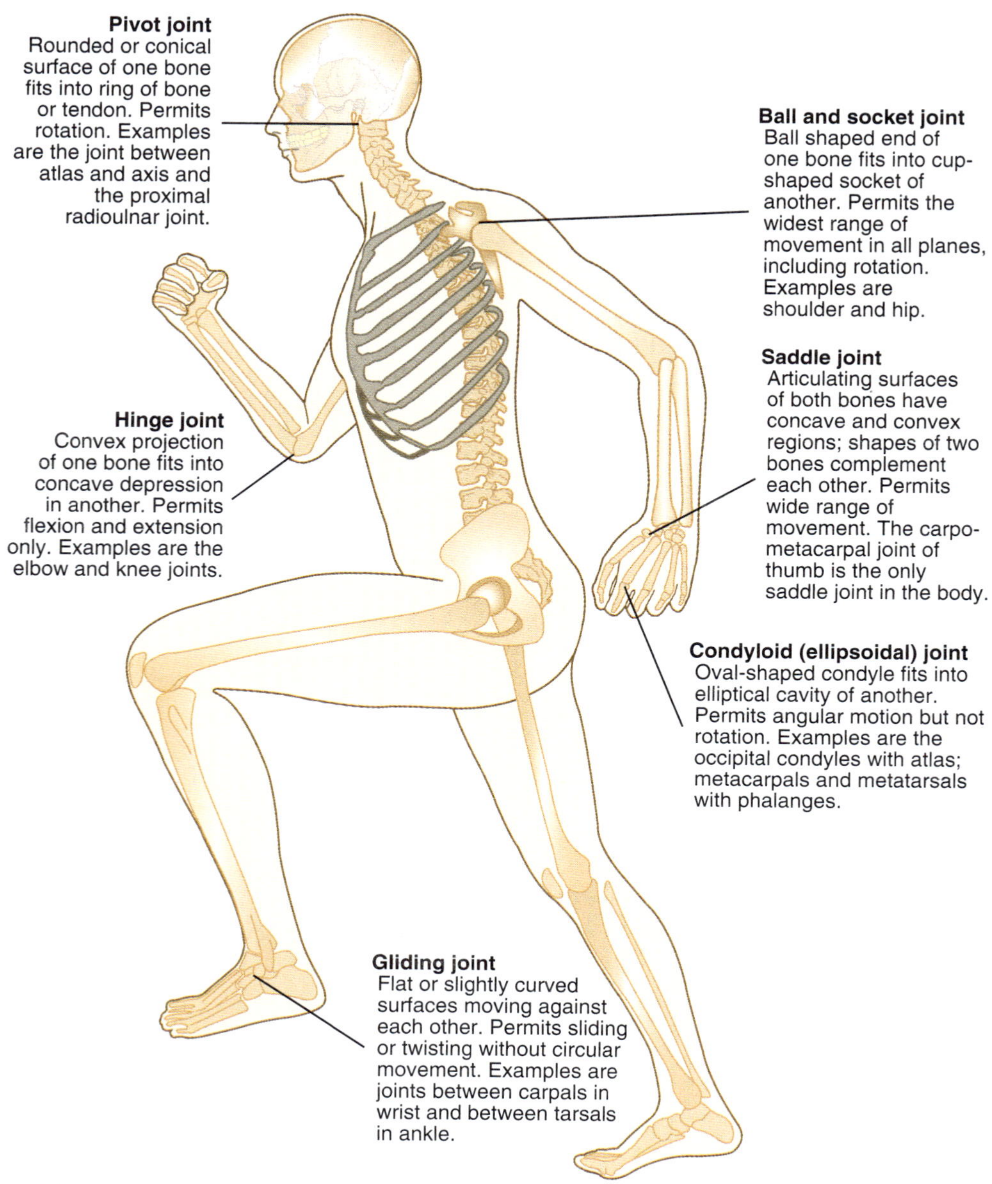

Fig. 7.18 Types of freely movable joints. (From Applegate E: *The anatomy and physiology learning system*, ed 4, St. Louis, 2011, Saunders.)

from the digestive tract, poor diet, and lack of exercise. Whatever the cause, there is no sure way of preventing the loss, but adequate calcium and vitamin D in the diet may help reduce the effects.

Another change with age is a decrease in the rate of collagen synthesis. This means that the bones have less strength and are more brittle. Bones fracture more readily in elderly individuals, and the healing process may be slow or incomplete. Tendons and ligaments become less flexible because of the changes in collagen.

The articular cartilage at the ends of bones tends to become thinner and deteriorates with age. This causes joint disorders that are commonly found in older individuals. People also appear to get shorter as they get older. This is caused partially by loss of bone mass and partially by compression of the intervertebral discs.

Age-related changes in the skeletal system cannot be prevented. An active and healthy lifestyle with appropriate exercise and an adequate diet help reduce the effect of the changes in the skeletal system.

Common Pathology of the Skeletal System

Disease	Signs and Symptoms	Etiology	Diagnosis and Treatment
Sprain	Painful swelling and/or bruising of a joint area with decreased movement ability.	Joint ligament damage caused by the joint being taken beyond its functional range of motion.	Diagnosis is by examination and imaging modalities. Treatment is RICE: *Rest* the sprain. *Ice* should be applied. *Compress* with wraps, immobilize. *Elevate* to minimize swelling.
Strain	Localized stiffness, discoloration, and bruising in the muscle area.	The muscle fibers associated with a joint tear as a result of overstretching.	Diagnosis is by examination and imaging modalities. Treatment is RICE: *Rest* the strain. *Ice* should be applied. *Compress* with wraps, immobilize. *Elevate* to minimize swelling.
Spina bifida	A baby is born with an opening in the back through which the meninges and spinal cord may protrude.	There may be a genetic basis for the condition. It most likely results from the interaction of multiple genes and environmental factors.	Prenatal testing for spina bifida includes blood tests, ultrasound, and amniocentesis. Mild forms may require no treatment. More severe forms require surgery to close the opening. There is no known cure for nerve damage caused by spina bifida.
Osteosarcoma	Recurring limb pain that may be worse at night. If the tumor is large it can appear as a swelling. The affected bone may fracture easily.	Osteoblasts multiply without control and form large tumors in bones.	Diagnosis is by x-ray examination followed by other scan modalities. Current standard treatment uses chemotherapy followed by surgical resection.
Osteoporosis	There are no symptoms. As bone loss becomes more severe, there may be back pain, and bone fractures occur more frequently.	Immobilization and lack of exercise can cause bone loss. Endocrine disorders also may be involved, along with malnutrition and inadequate calcium intake and/or adsorption.	Diagnosis can be made by measuring the bone mineral density. Medications can be used to reduce further bone loss.
Tennis elbow	Pain and swelling at the elbow joint.	Repeated contraction of muscles that control hand and wrist movements cause their proximal attachments on the humerus to become irritated, inflamed, and painful.	Diagnosis is made by clinical signs and symptoms. Minor cases may be treated by simply relaxing the affected arm. Eccentric exercise using a rubber bar may be effective at reducing pain and increasing strength.
Arthritis	Painful inflammation of one or more joints, often accompanied by swelling.	The inflammation is a result of damage to the joint from disease, daily wear and tear on the joint, and/or muscle strains.	Diagnosis is made by clinical examination by an appropriate health professional and may be supported by other tests such as radiology and blood tests. Treatment focuses on relieving pain and reducing swelling.

Continued

Common Pathology of the Skeletal System—cont'd

Disease	Signs and Symptoms	Etiology	Diagnosis and Treatment
Osteoarthritis	Pain during movement, stiffness in the morning or after periods of inactivity, and loss of flexibility.	Characterized by the degeneration of articular cartilage and changes in the synovial membrane.	Diagnosis is based on history, physical examination, and imaging tests. Treatment is aimed at relieving the symptoms.
Rheumatoid arthritis	Tends to first affect the smaller joints such as fingers and toes and then progresses to the knees and hips.	Caused by changes that occur in the connective tissues of the body, especially the joints. It may be an autoimmune disease.	Diagnosis is based on physical examination, blood tests, and imaging modalities. Medications are used to relieve pain, and physical therapy can help maintain flexibility of the joints.
Osteomalacia	Early stages present no symptoms. As the condition progresses, there may be a dull, aching bone pain and muscle weakness. Bones bend easily under stress and become deformed; in childhood this is called *rickets.*	The bones soften because of inadequate amounts of calcium and phosphorus as a result of a lack of vitamin D in the diet. Vitamin D is necessary for the body to absorb the minerals necessary for healthy bones.	Diagnostic techniques include blood and urine tests for levels of calcium, phosphorus, and vitamin D, combined with imaging modalities and a biopsy. Treatment may require vitamin D and calcium or phosphate supplements in the diet. For severe cases injection of large doses of vitamin D may be required.
Osteomyelitis	Tenderness and swelling around the affected bone with fever, fatigue and nausea. If located in the vertebrae, severe back pain is present, especially at night.	Caused by an inflammation of the bone marrow as a result of bacterial infection. The bacteria may enter via the bloodstream, from penetrating trauma, or after internal fixation of fractures.	Diagnosis is based on radiologic results showing a lytic center with a ring of sclerosis. Culture of material taken from a bone biopsy is needed to identify the specific pathogen. Treatment requires prolonged antibiotic therapy.
Dislocation	Difficulty in moving a joint, accompanied by intense pain, joint instability, and deformity of the joint area.	A bone has been dislodged from its joint or socket with the tearing of ligaments, tendons, and the articular capsule.	Diagnosis is by physical examination and imaging modalities. A dislocated joint usually can be successfully returned to its normal position by a trained medical professional.
Gout	A red, tender, hot, swollen joint. The metatarsal-phalangeal joint at the base of the big toe is affected most often.	Caused by an excessive accumulation of uric acid that forms needle-like crystals within the joint.	The disorder is diagnosed by aspiring joint fluid and observing the crystals under the microscope. It can be effectively treated with antiinflammatory drugs and dietary adjustments.
Ankylosing spondylitis	Sacroiliitis is typically the first manifestation, accompanied by a chronic dull pain, felt deep in the lower lumbar or gluteal region, and morning stiffness.	An inflammation causes some of the vertebrae to fuse together. Genetic factors may be involved.	Diagnosis involves imaging tests to observe the changes in the bones and joints. Antiinflammatory drugs are prescribed to relieve pain. Physical therapy may help in maintaining flexibility in the joints.

TERMINOLOGY REVIEW

Key Term	Word Parts	Definition
Amphiarthroses	*arthr/o:* joint *-osis:* condition of	Slightly movable joints; singular, *amphiarthrosis.*
Appendicular skeleton	*appendicul-:* little attachment	Bones that are attached to the body; upper and lower extremities.
Appositional growth		Growth resulting from material being deposited on the surface, such as the growth in diameter of long bones.
Articular cartilage	*artic-:* joint	Thin layer of hyaline cartilage that covers the ends of long bones in joints.
Articulation	*artic-:* joint	A joint; area of contact between two bones.
Axial skeleton		Bones of the head, neck, and trunk.
Diaphysis	*dia-:* through	The long straight shaft of a long bone.
Diarthroses	*arthr/o:* joint *-osis:* condition of	Freely movable joints characterized by a joint cavity; also called a *synovial joint;* singular, *diarthrosis.*
Endosteum	*end/o:* within, inward *oste/o:* bone	Membranous lining of a cavity within a bone.
Epiphyseal line	*epi-:* above, upon, on *-phys:* to grow	The remnant of the epiphyseal plate after the cartilage calcifies and growth ceases.
Epiphyseal plate	*epi-:* above, upon, on *-phys:* to grow	The cartilaginous plate between the epiphysis and diaphysis of a bone; responsible for the lengthwise growth of a long bone.
Epiphysis	*epi-:* above, upon, on	The end of a long bone.
Hematopoiesis	*hem/o:* blood *poie-:* making	Production of blood or its cells.
Osteoblasts	*oste/o:* bone *-blast:* immature cell	Bone-forming cells; immature bone cells.
Osteoclasts	*oste/o:* bone *-clast:* to break	Cells that destroy, break down, or resorb bone tissue.
Osteocytes	*oste/o:* bone *-cyte:* cell	Mature bone cells.
Osteogenesis	*oste/o:* bone *-genesis:* production	Formation of bone; also called *ossification.*
Osteon	*oste/o:* bone	Structural unit of bone; haversian system.
Pectoral girdle	*pect/o:* chest	Attachment for the upper extremities in the chest region; clavicle and scapula.
Pelvic girdle	*pelv:* basin	Attachment for the lower extremities; bones collectively shaped like a basin; ilium, ischium, pubis.
Periosteum	*peri:* around *oste/o:* bone	Tough white outer membrane that covers a bone.
Sutures		Immovable fibrous joints between the flat bones of the skull.
Synarthroses	*syn-:* together *arthr-:* joint *-osis:* condition of	Immovable joints; singular, *synarthrosis.*

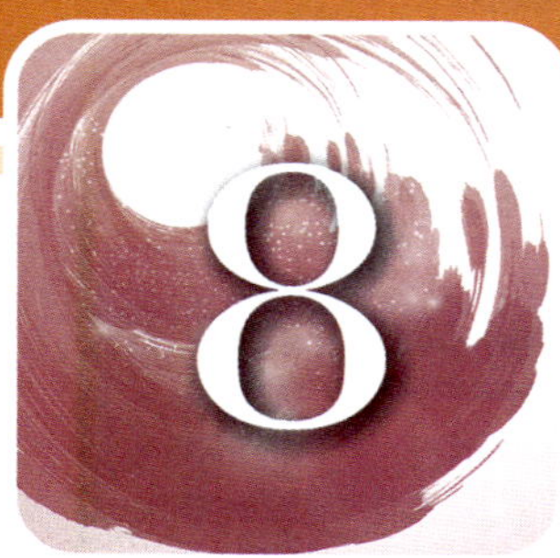

8 Muscular System

Check out the Evolve site at http://evolve.elsevier.com/Bonewit/today to access additional interactive activities and exercises to help you study and prepare for success.

LEARNING OBJECTIVES

1. State the characteristics and functions of muscle tissue.
2. Describe the structure of a skeletal muscle.
3. List and describe the sequence of events involved in the contraction of a skeletal muscle fiber.
4. Explain how energy is provided for a muscle contraction.
5. Describe oxygen debt.
6. Describe and illustrate the movements accomplished by the contraction of skeletal muscle.
7. Identify and describe the major muscles making up the axial skeleton.
8. Identify and describe the major muscles making up the appendicular skeleton.
9. Describe ways in which the aging of an individual affects the muscular system.
10. Identify pathology related to the muscular system.

CHAPTER OUTLINE

KEY TERMS

acetylcholine (ah-see-till-KOH-leen)
acetylcholinesterase (ah-see-till-koh-lin-ES-ter-ase)
antagonists (an-TAG-oh-nists)
aponeurosis (ah-pah-noo-ROE-sis)
contractility (kon-track-TILL-ih-tee)
elasticity (ee-lass-TISS-ih-tee)
epimysium (ep-ih-MYE-see-um)
excitability (eks-eye-tah-BILL-ih-tee)
extensibility (eks-ten-sih-BILL-ih-tee)
insertion (in-SIR-shun)
motor unit (MOH-toar YOO-nit)
neuromuscular junction (noo-roe-MUSK-yoo-lar JUNK-shun)
neurotransmitter (noo-roh-TRANS-mit-ter)
origin (OR-ih-jin)
prime mover (PRYM MOO-ver)
sarcolemma (sar-koh-LEM-mah)
sarcoplasm (SAR-koh-plazm)
synergists (SIN-er-gists)

INTRODUCTION TO THE MUSCULAR SYSTEM

As described in Chapter 5, there are three types of muscle tissue: skeletal, visceral, and cardiac. These are reviewed in Table 8.1. This chapter takes a closer look at skeletal muscle, which makes up about 40% of an individual's body weight. It forms more than 600 muscles that are attached to the bones of the skeleton. Skeletal muscles are under conscious control, and when they contract they move the bones. Skeletal muscles also allow us to smile, frown, pout, show surprise, and exhibit other forms of facial expression.

CHARACTERISTICS AND FUNCTIONS OF THE MUSCULAR SYSTEM

Skeletal muscle has four primary characteristics that relate to its functions:

- **Excitability:** Excitability is the ability to receive and respond to a stimulus. To function properly, muscles have to respond to a stimulus from the nervous system.
- **Contractility:** Contractility is the ability to shorten or contract. When a muscle responds to a stimulus, it shortens to produce movement.
- **Extensibility:** Extensibility means that a muscle can be stretched or extended. Skeletal muscles are often arranged in opposing pairs. When one muscle contracts, the other muscle is relaxed and stretched.
- **Elasticity:** Elasticity is the capacity to recoil or return to the original shape and length after contraction or extension.

Muscle contraction fulfills four important functions in the body:

- Movement
- Posture
- Joint stability
- Heat production

Nearly all movement in the body is the result of muscle contraction. Some exceptions to this are the action of cilia, the motility of the flagella on sperm cells, and the ameboid movement of some white blood cells. The integrated action of joints, bones, and skeletal muscles produces obvious movements such as walking and running. Skeletal muscles also produce more subtle movements that result in various facial expressions, eye movements, and respiration. Posture, such as sitting and standing, is maintained as a result of muscle contraction. The skeletal muscles are continually making fine adjustments that hold the body in stationary positions. Skeletal muscles contribute to joint stability. The tendons of many muscles extend over joints and in this way contribute to joint stability. This is particularly evident in the knee and shoulder joints, where muscle tendons are a major factor in stabilizing the joint. Heat production, to maintain body temperature, is an important by-product of muscle metabolism. Nearly 85% of the heat produced in the body is the result of muscle contraction.

Table 8.1 Summary of Muscle Tissue

Feature	Skeletal	Visceral	Cardiac
Location	Attached to bones	Walls of internal organs and blood vessels	Heart
Function	Produce body movement	Contraction of viscera and blood vessels	Pump blood through heart and blood vessels
Cell shape	Cylindric	Spindle-shaped; tapered ends	Cylindric, branching
Number of nuclei	Many	One	One
Striations	Present	Absent	Present
Type of control	Voluntary	Involuntary	Involuntary

From Applegate E: *The anatomy and physiology learning system*, ed 4, St. Louis, 2011, Saunders.

STRUCTURE OF SKELETAL MUSCLE

A whole skeletal muscle is considered an organ of the muscular system. For example, the biceps brachii muscle is an organ of the muscular system. Each organ or muscle consists of skeletal muscle tissue, connective tissue, nerve tissue, and blood or vascular tissue.

WHOLE SKELETAL MUSCLE

An individual skeletal muscle such as the biceps muscle may consist of hundreds, or even thousands, of muscle cells (fibers) bundled together and wrapped in a connective tissue covering. Each muscle is surrounded by a connective tissue sheath called the **epimysium**. Fascia consists of connective tissue located outside the epimysium. Fascia surrounds and separates the muscles. Skeletal muscle cells (fibers), like other body cells, are soft and fragile. The connective tissue coverings furnish support and protection for the delicate cells and allow them to withstand the forces of contraction. The coverings also provide pathways for the passage of blood vessels and nerves.

SKELETAL MUSCLE FIBERS

Each individual skeletal muscle fiber consists of a single cylindric muscle cell. The cell membrane is called the **sarcolemma**, and the cytoplasm is the **sarcoplasm**. Multiple nuclei are next to the sarcolemma at the periphery of the cell. There are numerous mitochondria to provide the initial energy for contraction. The cells also contain systematically arranged threadlike organelles called *myofilaments* that slide across one another during contraction.

HIGHLIGHT on the Muscular System

Rigor mortis: The term *rigor mortis* means the "stiffness of death." Within a short time of death, the adenosine triphosphate in muscles breaks down. This causes the myofilaments to remain locked in a contracted position and the body becomes rigid. A day or so later, muscle proteins begin to deteriorate and the rigor mortis disappears.

Tetanus: The word *tetanus* is often confusing because it means different things to different people. In reference to muscle contraction, the term denotes a steady contraction of a muscle fiber, without a relaxation phase. The word also refers to a disease, commonly called "lockjaw," that is caused by the bacterium *Clostridium tetani.* The toxin from the bacteria causes nerves to be highly excitable, which in turn causes uncontrollable muscle contractions, or spasms. A third use of the word is to denote a condition caused by a deficiency of calcium ions in the extracellular fluid. The lack of calcium increases nerve excitability with resulting muscle spasms, particularly of the extremities. The word *tetany* is also sometimes used to mean tetanus.

Wryneck: Injury to one of the sternocleidomastoid muscles may result in torticollis, or wryneck. This is characterized by a twisting of the neck and an unnatural position of the head.

Diaphragm: Voluntary forceful contractions of the diaphragm increase intraabdominal pressure to assist in urination, defecation, and childbirth.

Electrical shock: The muscles that flex the fingers and hand are stronger than the extensor muscles. In a normal relaxed position the fingers are slightly flexed because the normal muscle tone is greater in the flexors. Persons who receive a high-voltage electrical shock through the arms flex their hands tightly and "can't let go." All of the flexors and extensors receive the electrical stimulus, but because the flexor muscles are stronger, they contract more forcefully.

Intramuscular injections: The gluteus medius is a common site for intramuscular injections. In general, the injection is given in the center of the upper outer quadrant of the buttock, or gluteal, area. The gluteus medius, rather than the gluteus maximus, is used to avoid damaging the sciatic nerve.

Horseback riding: The adductor muscles in the medial compartment are the horse rider's muscles. These muscles adduct, or press, the thighs together to keep a person on a horse.

Quads: The quadriceps femoris group is a powerful knee extensor that is used in climbing, running, and rising from a chair. ■

NERVE AND BLOOD SUPPLY

Skeletal muscles have an abundant supply of blood vessels and nerves. This is directly related to the primary function of skeletal muscle contraction. Before a skeletal muscle fiber can contract, it must receive an impulse from a nerve cell. Muscle contraction requires adenosine triphosphate (ATP), and blood vessels deliver the necessary nutrients and oxygen to produce it. Blood vessels also remove the waste products that are produced as a result of muscle contraction.

In general, an artery and at least one vein accompany each nerve that penetrates the epimysium of a skeletal muscle. Branches of the nerve and blood vessels follow the connective tissue components of the muscle so that each muscle fiber is in contact with a branch of a nerve cell and with one or more minute blood vessels called *capillaries.*

SKELETAL MUSCLE ATTACHMENTS

In some instances, fibers of the epimysium fuse directly with the periosteum of a bone to form a *direct* attachment. The fleshy part of the muscle is known as the *belly* or *gaster.* More commonly, the connective tissue coverings extend beyond the belly of the muscle to form a thick, ropelike *tendon* or a broad, flat, sheetlike **aponeurosis**. The tendons and aponeuroses form *indirect* attachments from muscles to the periosteum of bones or to the connective tissue of other muscles. Typically, a muscle spans a joint and is attached to bones by tendons at both ends. One of the bones remains relatively fixed or stable, whereas the other end moves as a result of muscle contraction. The fixed or stable end is called the **origin** of the muscle, and the more movable attachment is called the **insertion**.

CONTRACTION OF SKELETAL MUSCLE

Skeletal muscle contraction is the result of a complex series of events based on chemical reactions at the cellular (muscle fiber) level. This chain of reactions begins with stimulation by a nerve cell and ends when the muscle fiber is again relaxed. Contraction of a whole muscle is the result of the simultaneous contraction of many muscle fibers.

STIMULUS FOR CONTRACTION

Skeletal muscles are stimulated to contract by special nerve cells called *motor neurons.* As the axon of the motor neuron penetrates the muscle, the axon branches, so there is an axon terminal for each muscle fiber. A single motor neuron and all the muscle fibers it stimulates make up a **motor unit**. Some motor units include several hundred individual fibers; others contain fewer than 10. Because all the muscle fibers in a motor unit receive a nerve impulse at the same time, all the fibers contract at the same time.

The region in which an axon terminal meets a muscle fiber is called a **neuromuscular junction** or myoneural junction, which is illustrated in Fig. 8.1. The axon terminal does not actually touch the sarcolemma of the muscle cell but fits into a shallow depression in the cell membrane. The fluid-filled space between the axon terminal and sarcolemma is called a *synaptic cleft* (gap). **Acetylcholine** (ACh),

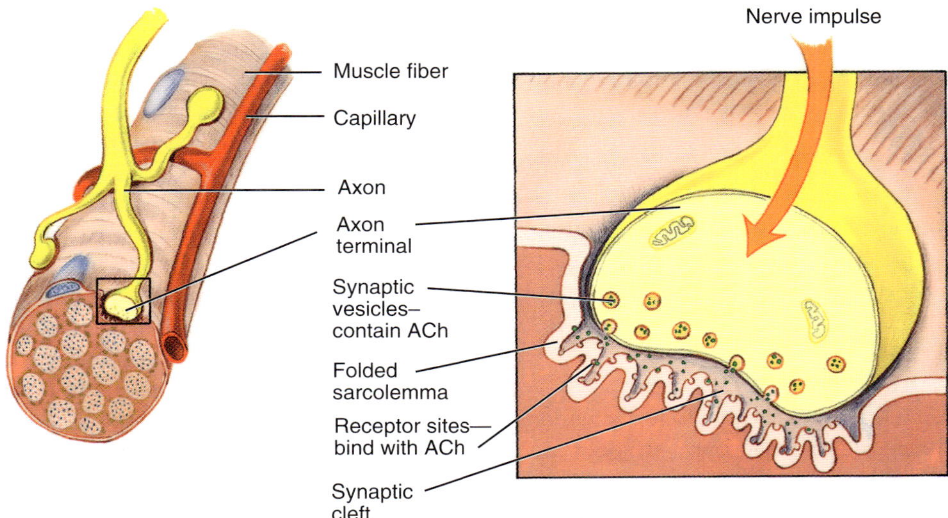

Fig. 8.1 Neuromuscular junction. The axon terminal fits into a depression on the sarcolemma. A nerve impulse travels down the axon to the axon terminal. The impulse causes the synaptic vesicles to release acetylcholine, which diffuses across the synaptic cleft and binds with receptors on the sarcolemma. *ACh*, Acetylcholine. (From Applegate E: *The anatomy and physiology learning system*, ed 4, St. Louis, 2011, Saunders.)

a **neurotransmitter**, is contained within synaptic vesicles in the axon terminal. Receptor sites for the ACh are located on the sarcolemma.

When a nerve impulse reaches the axon terminal, ACh is released. The ACh diffuses across the synaptic cleft and binds with the receptor sites on the sarcolemma. This reaction is the stimulus that causes the myofilaments to slide across one another, resulting in contraction. This is called the *sliding filament theory of contraction*.

The ACh is rapidly inactivated by the enzyme **acetylcholinesterase**. This ensures that one nerve impulse will result in only one contraction of the muscle fiber. Anything that interferes with the production, release, or inactivation of ACh, or its ability to bind with the receptor sites on the sarcolemma, will have an effect on muscle contraction. Muscle relaxant drugs work in this manner.

ENERGY SOURCES AND OXYGEN DEBT

The immediate or initial source of energy for muscle contraction is ATP. Surprisingly, muscles have limited storage facilities for ATP. In working muscles the stored ATP is depleted in about 6 seconds, and new ATP must be regenerated if muscle contraction is to continue.

Creatine phosphate is a unique high-energy compound that is stored in muscles. This compound provides almost instantaneous regeneration of ATP.

This reaction is so effective that there is little change in ATP levels during the initial stages of muscle contraction. Muscles store enough creatine phosphate to regenerate sufficient ATP to sustain contraction for about 10 seconds.

When muscles are actively contracting for extended periods of time, *fatty acids* and *glucose* become the primary energy sources. As ATP and creatine phosphate stores are being used, more ATP is produced from the metabolism of glucose and fatty acids.

If adequate oxygen is available, fatty acids and glucose are broken down in the mitochondria by a process called *aerobic respiration*. The products are carbon dioxide, water, and large amounts of ATP.

When muscles are contracting vigorously for long periods of time, the circulatory system is unable to deliver oxygen fast enough to maintain the aerobic pathways. Processes that do not require oxygen are necessary. Under these conditions, glucose is the primary energy source. If adequate oxygen is not available, glucose is broken down by a process called *anaerobic respiration*. The products of the anaerobic pathway are lactic acid and a small amount of ATP.

Some of the lactic acid accumulates in the muscle and causes a burning sensation. Most of it diffuses out of the muscle and into the bloodstream, which takes it to the liver. Later, when sufficient oxygen is available, the liver converts the lactic acid back to glycogen, the storage form of glucose.

The aerobic pathway produces about 20 times more ATP than the anaerobic pathway. However, the anaerobic pathway provides ATP about two and one-half times faster than the aerobic pathway. Most of the energy for vigorous activity over a moderate period of time comes from anaerobic respiration. Prolonged activities requiring endurance depend on aerobic mechanisms.

Periods of strenuous exercise that require anaerobic mechanisms to regenerate ATP create an *oxygen debt* that must be repaid before equilibrium can be restored. There is an accumulation of lactic acid in the muscle that may cause temporary muscular pain and cramping. The ATP and creatine phosphate in the muscle are depleted and need to be replenished. This additional oxygen is necessary to convert the lactic acid into glycogen, a process that occurs in the liver. Oxygen is also necessary to replenish the ATP and the creatine phosphate in the muscle. Oxygen debt is defined as the additional oxygen that is required after physical activity to restore resting conditions. The debt is paid back by labored breathing that continues after the activity has stopped.

MOVEMENTS

Most intact skeletal muscles are attached to bones by tendons that span joints. When the muscle contracts, one bone (the insertion) moves relative to the other bone (the origin). Frequently muscles work in groups to perform a particular movement. If one muscle has a primary role in providing a movement, it is called a **prime mover**. Muscles that work with, or assist, the prime mover to cause a movement are called **synergists**. Often muscles span more than one joint, and a synergist will stabilize one joint while the prime mover acts on the other joint. For example, the fingers can be flexed to make a fist without bending the wrist because certain muscles fix the wrist in a stabilized position. **Antagonists** are muscles that oppose, or reverse, a particular movement. The biceps brachii muscle on the anterior arm flexes the forearm at the elbow. The triceps brachii muscle on the posterior arm extends the forearm at the elbow. The two muscles are on opposite sides of the humerus and have opposite functions. They are antagonists.

Bones and muscles work together to perform different types of movement at the various joints. Describing muscular action or movement at joints requires a frame of reference and descriptive terminology with definite meaning. Some terms that are commonly used to describe particular movements are defined and illustrated in Fig. 8.2.

SKELETAL MUSCLE GROUPS

The body is composed of more than 600 skeletal muscles. A discussion of each muscle is certainly beyond the scope of this book. Only the more significant and obvious muscles are identified and described here. These are arranged in groups according to location and/or function. If you identify and learn the muscles as group associations, it will make them easier to remember. If you can locate a muscle on your own body, you will be able to contract the muscle and describe its action. Learning anatomy in this manner makes it more meaningful.

NAMING MUSCLES

Most skeletal muscles have names that describe some feature of the muscle. Often several criteria are combined into one name. Associating the muscles' characteristics with their names will help you learn and remember them. The following are some terms relating to muscle features that are used in naming muscles:

- *Size:* vastus (huge); maximus (large); longus (long); minimus (small); brevis (short)
- *Shape:* deltoid (triangular); rhomboid (like a rhombus with equal and parallel sides); latissimus (wide); teres (round); trapezius (like a trapezoid, a four-sided figure with two sides parallel)
- *Direction of fibers:* rectus (straight); transverse (across); oblique (diagonal); orbicularis (circular)
- *Location:* pectoralis (chest); gluteus (buttock or rump); brachii (arm); supra- (above); infra- (below); sub- (under or beneath); lateralis (lateral)
- *Number of origins:* biceps (two heads); triceps (three heads); quadriceps (four heads)
- *Origin and insertion:* sternocleidomastoid (origin on the sternum and clavicle, insertion on the mastoid process); brachioradialis (origin on the brachium or arm, insertion on the radius)
- *Action:* abductor (to abduct a structure); adductor (to adduct a structure); flexor (to flex a structure); extensor (to extend a structure); levator (to lift or elevate a structure); masseter (to chew)

MUSCLES OF THE HEAD AND NECK

Muscles of Facial Expression

Humans have well-developed muscles in the face that permit a large variety of facial expressions. Because these muscles are used to show surprise, disgust, anger, fear, and other emotions, they are an important means of nonverbal communication. The following are some of the muscles used to produce facial expressions.

The *frontalis* lies over the frontal bone of the forehead. It is attached to the soft tissue of the eyebrow; when it contracts, it raises the eyebrows and wrinkles the forehead. The *orbicularis oris* is a sphincter that encircles the mouth. This muscle is used to close the mouth, to form words, and to pucker the lips as in kissing. The *orbicularis oculi* is another sphincter but lies around the eye (oculus). The actions of winking, blinking, and squinting use this muscle. The *buccinator* is the principal muscle in the cheek area and is used to compress the cheek when whistling, sucking, or blowing air out. It is sometimes called the *trumpeter's muscle.* The *zygomaticus* extends from the zygomatic arch to the corners of the mouth. It contracts to raise the corners of the mouth when we smile.

Muscles of Mastication

Four pairs of muscles are responsible for chewing movements or mastication. All of these muscles insert on the mandible, and they are some of the strongest muscles in the body. Two of the muscles, the *temporalis* and *masseter*, are superficial and are identified in Fig. 8.3. The others, the lateral and medial pterygoids, are deep to the mandible and are not shown in the figure. The *temporalis* is the largest of the mastication muscles. As the name implies, it has its origin on the temporal bone. The *masseter* is located along the ramus of the mandible and is a synergist of the temporalis.

Neck Muscles

Only two of the more obvious and superficial neck muscles are considered here. Numerous muscles are associated with the throat, hyoid bone, and vertebral column, a discussion of which is beyond the scope of this text.

The *sternocleidomastoid* muscles ascend obliquely across the anterior neck from the sternum and clavicle to the mastoid process. When both of these muscles contract together, the neck is flexed and the head is bent toward the chest. When one of the muscles contracts, the head turns toward the direction opposite the side that is contracting. When the left

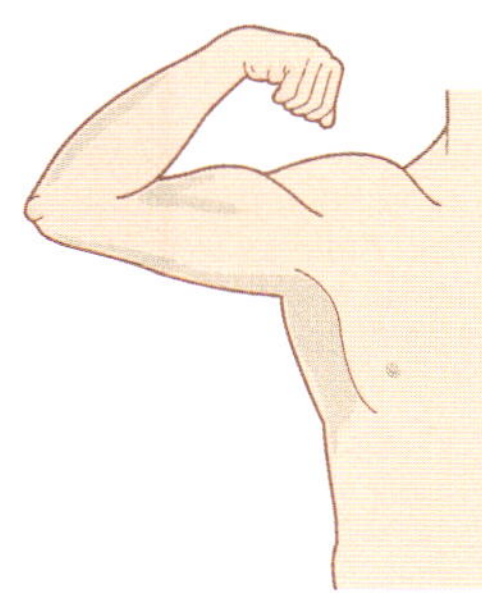

Flexion (FLEK-shun)
Means to bend. Flexion usually brings two bones closer together and decreases the angle between them. Example: bending the elbow or the knee.

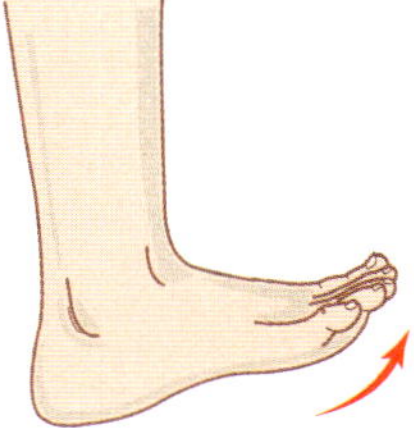

Dorsiflexion (dor-sih-FLEK-shun)
Flexion of the ankle in which the dorsum or top of the foot is lifted upward, decreasing the angle between the foot and leg. Example: standing on your heels.

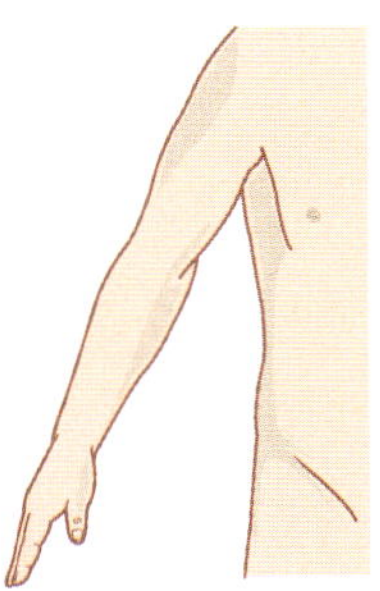

Extension (ek-STEN-shun)
Means to straighten. Extension is the opposite of flexion. It increases the angle between two bones. Example: straightening the elbow or the knee after it has been flexed.

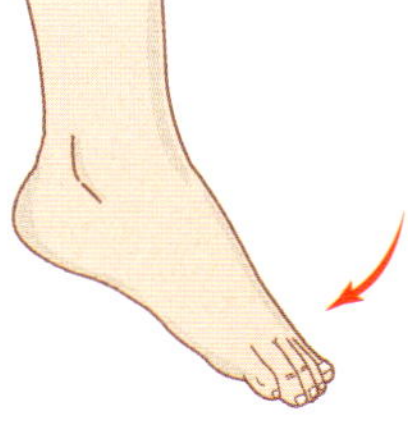

Plantar flexion (PLAN-tar FLEK-shun)
Plantar flexion is movement at the ankle that increases the angle between the foot and leg. Example: standing on your toes.

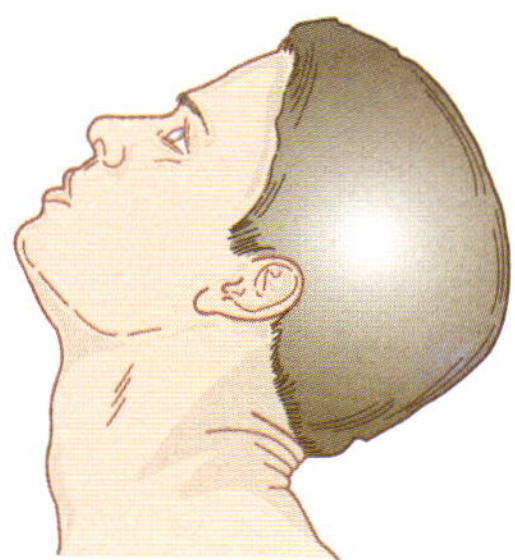

Hyperextension (hye-perk-ek-STEN-shun)
Hyperextension occurs when a part of the body is extended beyond the anatomical position. The joint angle becomes greater than 180°. Example: moving the head backward.

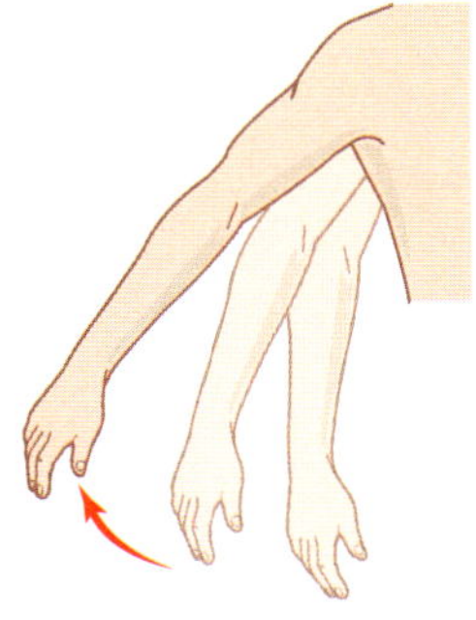

Abduction (ab-DUCK-shun)
Means to take away. Abduction moves a bone or limb away from the midline or axis of the body. Examples: the outward movement of the legs in "jumping jacks," moving the arms away from the body, or spreading the fingers apart.

Fig. 8.2 Types of body movements. (From Applegate E: *The anatomy and physiology learning system*, ed 4, St. Louis, 2011, Saunders.)

Continued

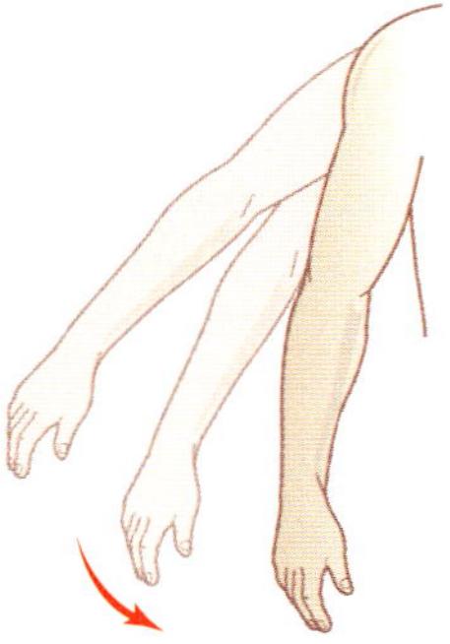

Adduction (ad-DUCK-shun)
Means to bring together. Adduction is the opposite of abduction. It moves a bone or limb toward the midline of the body. Examples: bringing the arms back to the sides of the body after they have been abducted or moving the legs back to anatomical position after abduction.

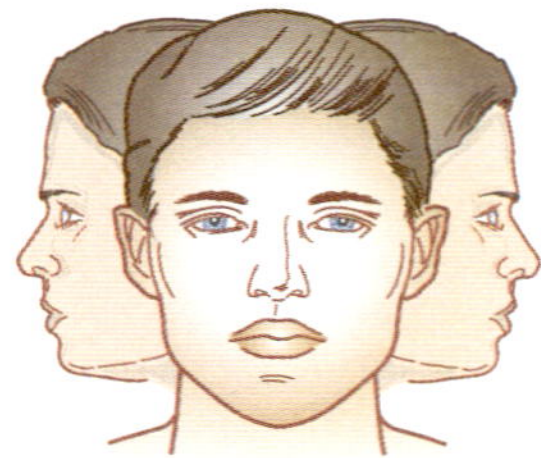

Rotation (roh-TAY-shun)
Rotation is the movement of a bone around its own axis in a pivot joint. Example: shaking your head “no”.

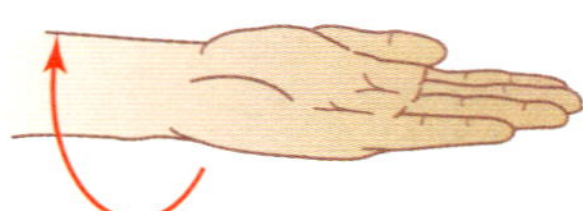

Supination (soo-pih-NAY-shun)
Supination is a specialized rotation of the forearm that turns the palm of the hand forward or anteriorly. If the elbow is flexed, supination turns the palm of the hand upward or superiorly.

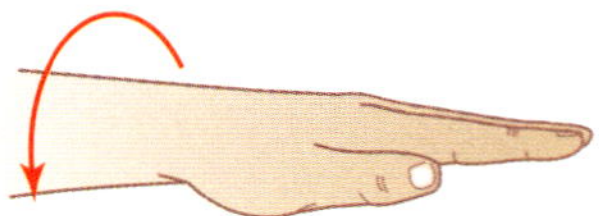

Pronation (proh-NAY-shun)
Pronation is the opposite of supination. It is a specialized rotation of the forearm that turns the palm of the hand backward or posteriorly. If the elbow is flexed, pronation turns the palm of the hand downward or inferiorly.

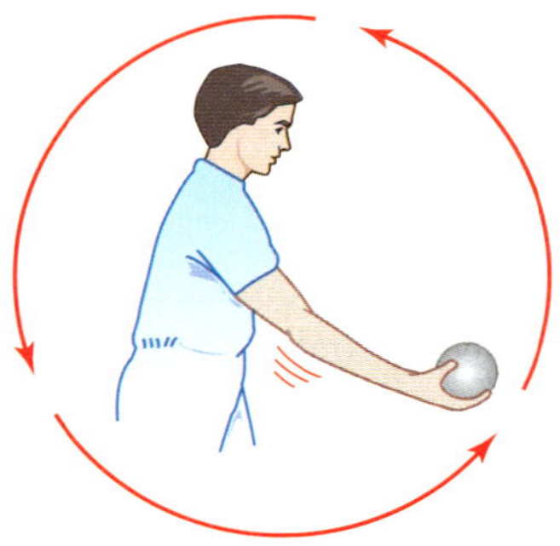

Circumduction (sir-kum-DUCK-shun)
Circumduction is the conelike, circular movement of a body segment. The proximal end of the segment remains relatively stationary while the distal end outlines a large circle. Example: the movement of the arm at the shoulder joint, with the elbow extended, so that the tips of the fingers move in a large circle.

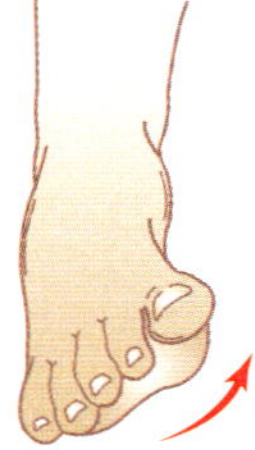

Inversion (in-VER-zhun)
Inversion is the movement of the sole of the foot inward or medially.

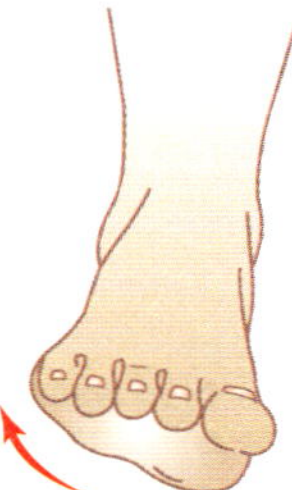

Eversion (ee-VER-zhun)
Eversion is the opposite of inversion. It is the movement of the sole of the foot outward or laterally.

Fig. 8.2, cont’d

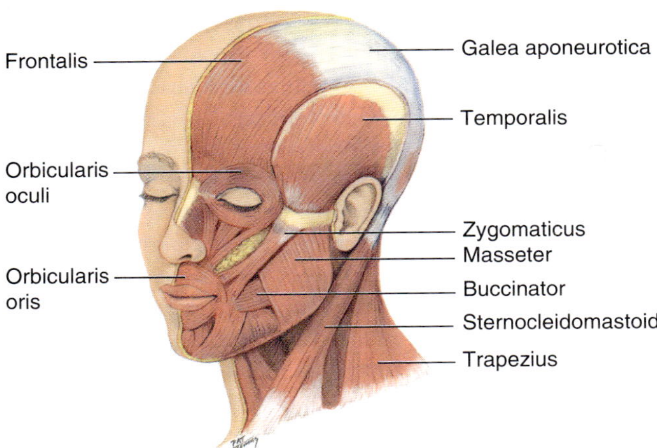

Fig. 8.3 Muscles of the head and neck. (From Applegate E: *The anatomy and physiology learning system*, ed 4, St. Louis, 2011, Saunders.)

muscle contracts, the head turns to the right. A portion of the *trapezius* muscle is in the neck region and moves the head. Each trapezius muscle extends from the occipital bone at the base of the skull to the end of the thoracic vertebrae and also inserts on the scapula laterally. A portion of this muscle extends the head and is antagonistic to the sternocleidomastoid.

MUSCLES OF THE TRUNK

The muscles of the trunk include those that move the vertebral column, the muscles that form the thoracic and abdominal walls, and those that cover the pelvic outlet.

Vertebral Column Muscles

The *erector spinae* group of muscles on each side of the vertebral column is a large muscle mass that extends from the sacrum to the skull. These muscles are primarily responsible for extending the vertebral column to maintain erect posture. Muscle contraction on only one side bends the vertebral column to that side.

Thoracic Wall Muscles

The muscles of the thoracic wall are involved primarily in the process of breathing. The intercostal muscles are located in spaces between the ribs. The *external intercostal muscles* contract to elevate the ribs during the inspiration phase of breathing. The *internal intercostals* contract during forced expiration.

The *diaphragm* is a dome-shaped muscle that forms a partition between the thorax and the abdomen. It has three openings in it for structures that have to pass from the thorax to the abdomen. The diaphragm is responsible for the major movement in the thoracic cavity during quiet, relaxed breathing. When the diaphragm contracts, the dome is flattened. This increases the volume of the thoracic cavity and results in inspiration. When the muscle relaxes, it again resumes its dome shape and decreases the volume of the thoracic cavity, which forces air out during expiration.

Abdominal Wall Muscles

The abdomen, unlike the thorax and pelvis, has no bony reinforcements or protection. The wall consists entirely of four muscle pairs, arranged in layers, and the fascia that envelops them (Fig. 8.4). The aponeuroses of the muscles on opposite sides meet in the anterior midline to form the *linea alba* ("white line"), a band of connective tissue that

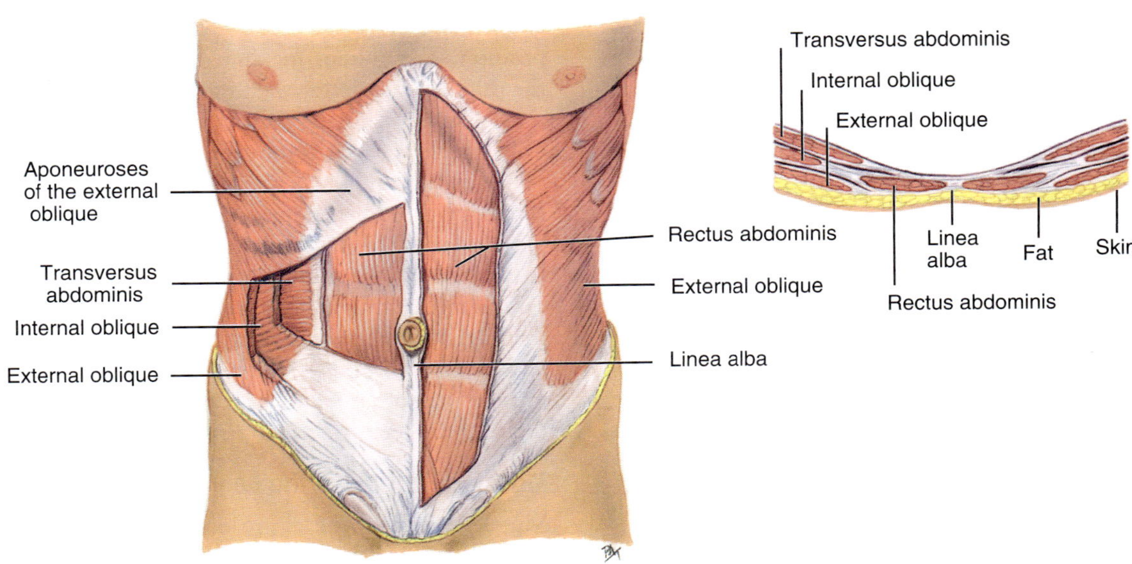

Fig. 8.4 Abdominal wall muscles. (From Applegate E: *The anatomy and physiology learning system*, ed 4, St. Louis, 2011, Saunders.)

extends from the sternum to the pubic symphysis. The outer muscle layer is the *external oblique*. The *internal oblique* lies just underneath it, and the deepest layer of muscle is the *transversus abdominis*. The arrangement of the muscle layers, with the fibers in each layer going in different directions, is similar to the type of construction found in plywood and adds strength to the anterolateral abdominal wall. The fascia of these muscles extends anteriorly to form a broad aponeurosis along much of the anterior aspect of the abdomen. The fascia also envelops the *rectus abdominis* muscle, which runs vertically from the pubic bones to the ribs and the sternum on each side of the midline. All of these muscles compress the abdominal wall and increase intraabdominal pressure. The rectus abdominis also flexes the vertebral column.

Pelvic Floor Muscles

The *pelvic diaphragm* forms the floor of the pelvic cavity. Most of the pelvic diaphragm is formed by the two *levator ani* muscles, which support the pelvic viscera. They resist increased pressure in the abdominopelvic cavity and thus play a role in the control of the urinary bladder and rectum.

MUSCLES OF THE UPPER EXTREMITY

The muscles of the upper extremity include those that attach the scapula to the thorax and in general move the scapula, those that attach the humerus to the scapula and in general move the arm, and those that are located in the arm or forearm and move the forearm, wrist, and hand. Fig. 8.5 illustrates the anterior view of body musculature, and Fig. 8.6 illustrates the posterior view.

Muscles That Move the Shoulder and Arm

The *trapezius* attaches the scapula to the axial skeleton. It is a large superficial triangular muscle of the back. When the trapezius contracts, it adducts and elevates the scapula, as in shrugging the shoulders.

Both the *pectoralis major* and the *latissimus dorsi* muscles attach the humerus to the axial skeleton. The pectoralis major is a superficial muscle on the anterior chest. It has a broad origin on the sternum, costal cartilages, and clavicle, but then the fibers converge to insert on the humerus by way of a short tendon. The primary function of the pectoralis major is to adduct and rotate the arm medially across the chest. The latissimus dorsi is a large, superficial muscle located in the lower back region. It has an extensive origin from the spines of the thoracic vertebrae, ilium, and ribs and then extends upward to insert on the humerus. The latissimus dorsi adducts and rotates the arm medially and lowers the shoulder. It is an important muscle in swimming and rowing motions.

The *deltoid* is a large, fleshy muscle that covers the shoulder and attaches the humerus to the scapula. This muscle abducts the arm to a horizontal position. It is a common site for administering intramuscular injections. Another group of muscles, called the *rotator cuff muscles*, attaches the humerus to the scapula and moves the humerus in various ways. These muscles form a cuff or cap over the proximal humerus. A rotator cuff injury involves damage to one or more of these muscles or their tendons.

Muscles That Move the Forearm and Hand

The muscles that move the forearm are located along the humerus and are divided into anterior and posterior muscle compartments. The *triceps brachii*, the primary extensor of the forearm, is the only muscle in the posterior compartment. As the name implies, it has three heads of origin. The anterior muscle compartment contains the *biceps brachii*, a primary flexor of the forearm.

The 20 or more muscles that cause most wrist, hand, and finger movements are located along the forearm. These muscles are divided into anterior and posterior compartments. Most of the anterior compartment muscles flex the wrist and fingers, whereas the posterior muscles cause extension.

MUSCLES OF THE LOWER EXTREMITY

The muscles of the lower extremity include those that are located in the hip region and in general move the thigh, those that are located in the thigh and move the leg, and those that are located in the leg and move the ankle and foot. See Figs. 8.5 and 8.6 to visualize these muscles.

Muscles That Move the Thigh

The muscles that move the thigh have their origins on some part of the pelvic girdle and their insertions on the femur. The largest muscle mass belongs to the posterior group, the gluteal muscles. The *gluteus maximus* forms the area of the buttocks. The *gluteus medius*, a common site for intramuscular injections, is superior and deep to the gluteus maximus. The *gluteus minimus* is the smallest and deepest of the gluteal muscles and is not illustrated. These muscles abduct the thigh—that is, they raise the thigh sideways to a horizontal position. The gluteus maximus also extends or straightens the thigh at the hip for walking or climbing stairs.

The anterior muscle that moves the thigh is the *iliopsoas*. This muscle is formed from the iliacus, which originates on the iliac fossa, and the psoas, which originates on the lumbar vertebrae. The fibers converge into the iliopsoas and insert on the femur. The iliopsoas flexes the thigh, making it antagonistic to the gluteus maximus.

The medial muscles adduct the thigh—that is, they press the thighs together. This group includes the *adductor longus*, *adductor brevis*, *adductor magnus*, and *gracilis* muscles. These muscles are often called the *horse rider's muscles* because their action keeps the rider on the horse.

Muscles That Move the Leg

Muscles that move the leg are located in the thigh region. The *quadriceps femoris* includes four muscles that are on the anterior and lateral sides of the thigh, namely the *vastus lateralis*, *vastus intermedius*, *vastus medialis*, and *rectus femoris*. As a group, these muscles are the primary extensors of the leg,

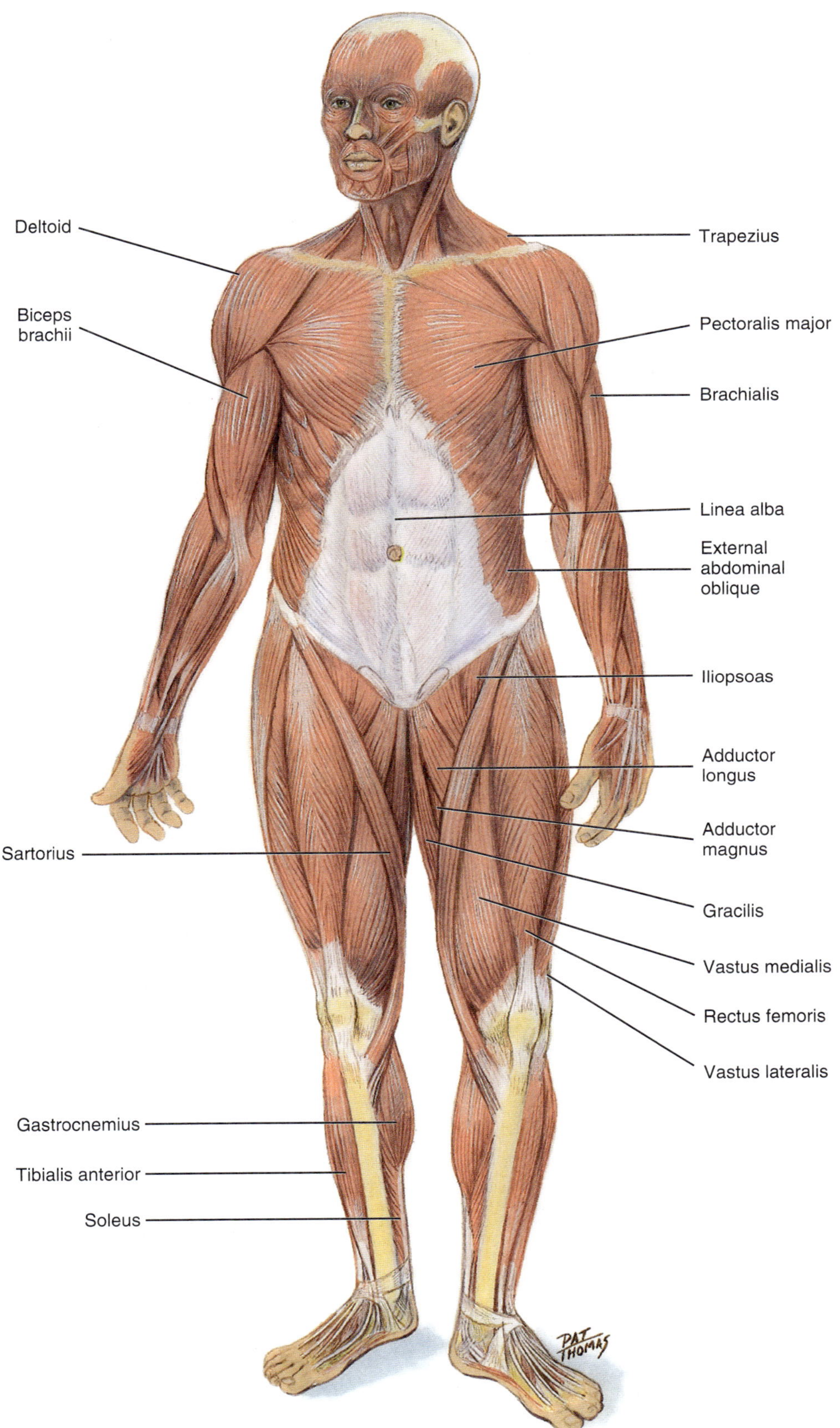

Fig. 8.5 General overview of body musculature. Anterior view. (From Applegate E: *The anatomy and physiology learning system*, ed 4, St. Louis, 2011, Saunders.)

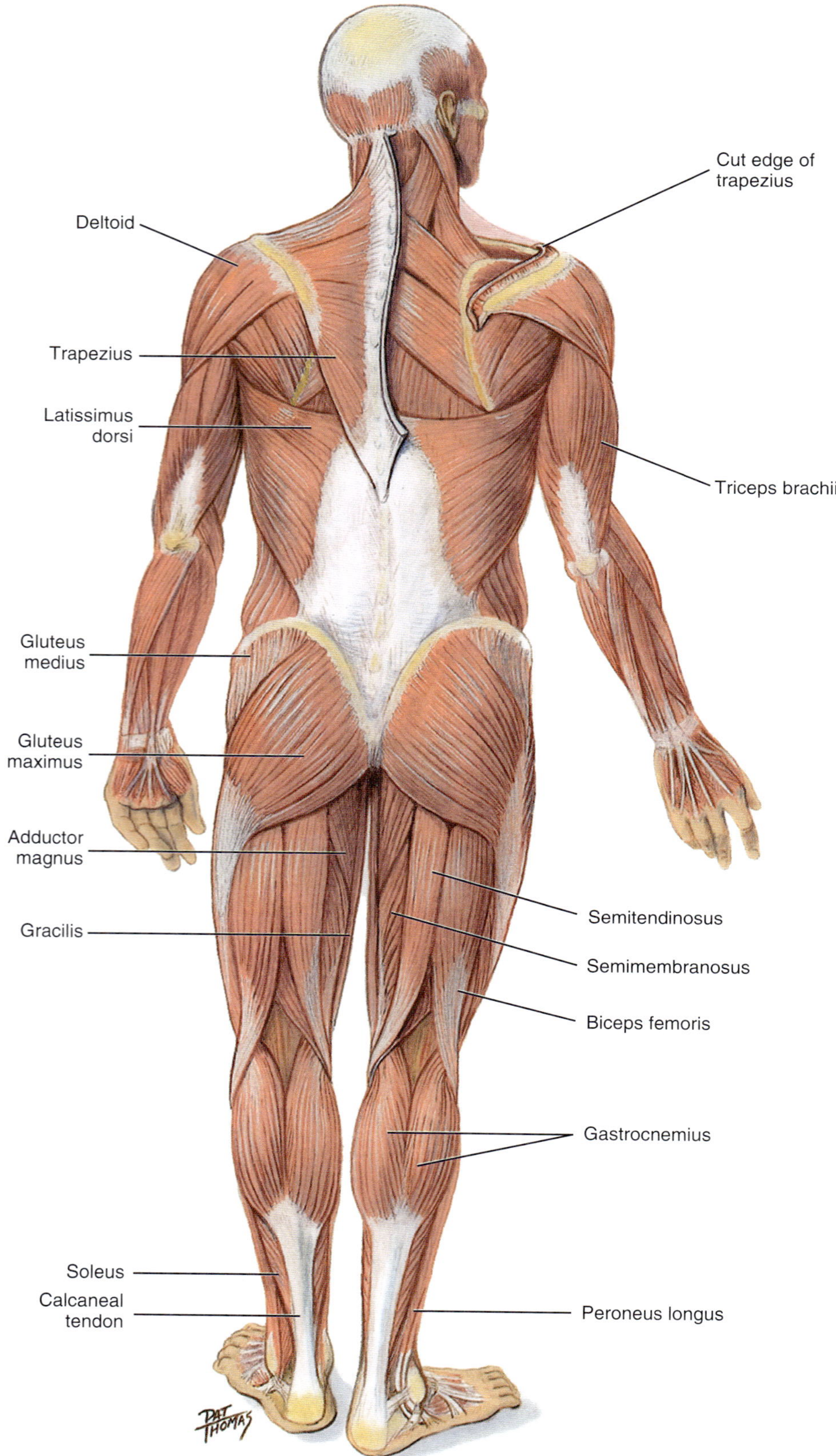

Fig. 8.6 General overview of body musculature. Posterior view. (From Applegate E: *The anatomy and physiology learning system*, ed 4, St. Louis, 2011, Saunders.)

straightening the leg at the knee. The other muscle on the anterior surface of the thigh is the long, straplike *sartorius*, which passes obliquely over the quadriceps group. The sartorius, the longest muscle in the body, flexes and medially rotates the leg when one sits cross-legged.

The posterior thigh muscles are called the *hamstrings*, and they are used to flex the leg at the knee. All have origins on the ischium and insert on the tibia. Because these muscles extend over the hip joint, as well as over the knee joint, they also extend the thigh. The strong tendons of these muscles can be felt behind the knee. These same tendons are present in hogs, and butchers used them to hang the hams for smoking and curing, so they were called "ham strings." The hamstring muscles are the *biceps femoris*, *semimembranosus*, and *semitendinosus*. A "pulled hamstring" is a tear in one or more of these muscles or their tendons.

Muscles That Move the Ankle and Foot

The muscles located in the leg move the ankle and foot and are divided into anterior, posterior, and lateral compartments. The *tibialis anterior* is the primary muscle in the anterior group, and its contraction causes dorsiflexion of the foot. The *peroneus* muscles occupy the lateral compartment of the leg. Contraction of these muscles everts the foot and also helps in plantar flexion. The *gastrocnemius* and *soleus* are the major muscles in the posterior compartment. These two muscles form the fleshy mass in the calf of the leg. They have a common tendon called the *calcaneal tendon* or *Achilles tendon*. These muscles are strong plantar flexors of the foot. They are sometimes called the *toe dancer's muscles* because they allow one to stand on tiptoe. Numerous other deep muscles in the leg cause flexion and extension of the toes.

AGING OF THE MUSCULAR SYSTEM

One of the most obvious age-related changes in skeletal muscles is the loss of muscle mass. This involves a decrease in both the number of muscle fibers and the diameter of the remaining fibers. Once muscle fibers are lost, they cannot be replaced by new ones. Instead, they are replaced by connective tissue, primarily adipose. The number of muscle cells lost depends on several factors, including the amount of physical activity, the nutritional state of the individual, heredity, and the condition of the motor neurons that supply the muscle tissue. There is an age-related loss of motor neurons to skeletal muscle cells, and this is considered an important cause of muscle atrophy. It is probable that exercise enhances the ability of nerves to stimulate muscle fibers and to reduce atrophy.

As muscle mass decreases, there is a corresponding reduction in muscle strength. The amount of strength loss differs, depending to a large extent on the amount of physical activity. There is evidence that the mitochondria function less effectively in nonexercised muscle cells than in exercised cells. When mitochondria are inefficient, lactic acid accumulates, which contributes to muscle weakness.

There is a tendency for the skeletal muscles of older people to be less responsive, or to respond more slowly, than those of younger people. This is because the latent, contraction, and relaxation phases of muscle action all increase in duration. The increase in response time is less in muscles that are used regularly. Continued physical activity and good nutrition are probably the best deterrents to loss of muscle mass and muscle strength and to increased muscle response time.

Common Pathology of the Muscular System

Disease	Signs and Symptoms	Etiology	Diagnosis and Treatment
Myopathy	Muscle weakness with cramps, stiffness, spasms, and tetany.	Myopathy results from several different disease processes. It may result from endocrine, inflammatory, infectious, drug- and toxin-induced, metabolic, and other systemic disorders.	Diagnosis of myopathy is based on symptoms; however, it is important to discover and treat the underlying cause. Treatments for myopathy range from management of the symptoms to very specific cause-targeting treatments. Physical therapy, drug therapy, support bracing, surgery, and massage are all current treatments for this wide variety of conditions.
Myalgia	Muscle pain.	Myalgia without a traumatic history is often the result of a viral infection. It is a symptom of many diseases and disorders. A common cause is the overuse or overstretching of a muscle or group of muscles. It can also be caused by medications or occur as a response to a vaccination.	Diagnosis is based on symptoms; however, it is important to discover and treat the underlying cause. The treatment or management of myalgia differs depending on the underlying causes. Mild cases may be treated with massage, a warm bath, or hot and cold packs. Pain-relieving medications may be required. Muscle relaxants are sometimes helpful.

Continued

Common Pathology of the Muscular System—cont'd

Disease	Signs and Symptoms	Etiology	Diagnosis and Treatment
Myositis	Muscle weakness, swelling, and pain are the common myositis symptoms. Myositis sometimes occurs as part of a systemic infection.	*Myositis* is a general term for inflammation of the muscles. Many such conditions are considered likely to be caused by autoimmune conditions, rather than directly by infection.	Diagnosis is based on symptoms and blood tests. There are two approaches to the treatment of myositis: medical and lifestyle changes. Nonsteroidal antiinflammatory drugs may be used for pain relief. Corticosteroids and other drugs that suppress the immune system may slow down the attack on healthy tissue.
Repetitive stress disorder (RSD)	The symptoms of RSD are pain, tingling, numbness, swelling, redness, loss of flexibility, and muscle weakness.	Conditions associated with RSD include repetitive tasks, forceful exertions, vibrations, mechanical compression, and/or sustained awkward positions.	Usually diagnosed by history and examination. Imaging modalities may be used to rule out other possible causes of the pain. The most-often prescribed treatments for early-stage RSD include drug therapies such as antiinflammatory medications combined with passive forms of physical therapy such as rest, splinting, and massage. Some patients may require more aggressive intervention, including surgery.
Shin splint	Pain along the tibia (shinbone) and mild swelling in the lower leg.	Shin splints are caused by repeated stress of the tibia and the connective tissues that attach muscles to it, especially flexor muscles of the toes.	Usually diagnosed by history and examination. Imaging modalities may be used to rule out other possible causes of the pain. Initial treatment includes rest, ice, and pain medications, which allow the tibia to recover from high levels of stress and reduce the inflammation and pain. Surgery may be performed in more severe cases when more conservative options have been unsuccessful.
Contusion	Typically a moderately large area of the skin that has been darkened as the result of a hit or impact. Commonly called a *bruise*.	A contusion is a hematoma of tissue in which capillaries and sometimes venules are damaged by trauma, allowing blood to enter the surrounding interstitial tissues.	Diagnosis is by examination. Treatment for light bruises is minimal and may include rest, ice, compression, elevation (*RICE*), painkillers, and, later in recovery, light stretching exercises. In most cases hematomas spontaneously resolve, but in cases of large hematomas, the physician may optionally perform a puncture of the hematoma to allow the blood to exit.
Muscular dystrophy	A chronic and progressive weakening of the muscles. There are many forms of the condition, ranging from mild to severe.	Caused by a mutation in one of the genes involved in directing the synthesis of proteins that protect muscle fibers from damage. The mutations may be inherited or occur spontaneously.	Diagnosis depends on patient history, physical examination, muscle enzyme tests, electromyography, muscle biopsy, and genetic testing. At present there is no cure. Treatment is aimed at alleviating the symptoms and complications.
Myasthenia gravis	Notable weakness and rapid fatigue of the skeletal muscles. The first signs occur in the face and throat, such as drooping eyelids and double vision.	Myasthenia gravis occurs when the immune system produces antibodies that block the acetylcholine receptors at the neuromuscular junction.	Diagnosis includes patient history and physical examination, reflex testing, muscle strength, coordination, and balance. Blood analysis may reveal the presence of the antibodies. At present there is no cure. Treatment is aimed at alleviating the symptoms.

Common Pathology of the Muscular System—cont'd

Disease	Signs and Symptoms	Etiology	Diagnosis and Treatment
Poliomyelitis	Flulike symptoms that progress to muscle paralysis. Although approximately 90% of polio infections cause no symptoms at all, affected individuals can exhibit a range of symptoms if the virus enters the bloodstream and affects the nerves. Advanced stages of the disease exhibit muscle weakness and acute flaccid paralysis. Different types of paralysis may occur, depending on the nerves involved.	Poliomyelitis is caused by a contagious enterovirus called the polio virus (PV) that forms colonies in the oropharynx and intestine. Polio is now extremely rare in the Western world because of very effective vaccination programs.	Paralytic poliomyelitis is suspected in individuals experiencing acute onset of flaccid paralysis in one or more limbs with decreased tendon reflexes. Recovery of the virus from a stool sample or throat swab confirms the diagnosis. There is no cure for polio. The focus of modern treatment has been on providing relief of symptoms, speeding recovery, and preventing complications.

TERMINOLOGY REVIEW

Key Term	Word Parts	Definition
Acetylcholine		A neurotransmitter at the neuromuscular junction.
Acetylcholinesterase	*-ase: enzyme*	An enzyme that inactivates acetylcholine.
Antagonists	*anti-:* against	Muscles that have an action opposite to that of the prime mover.
Aponeurosis		A broad flat sheet of connective tissue that connects one muscle to another.
Contractility		The ability of muscle cells to shorten to produce movement.
Elasticity		The ability of tissue to return to its original shape after contraction or extension.
Epimysium	*epi:* above, around *mys:* muscle	Fibrous connective tissue that surrounds a whole muscle.
Excitability		The ability of muscle and nerve tissue to receive and respond to stimuli; also called *irritability.*
Extensibility		The ability of muscle tissue to stretch when pulled.
Insertion		The end of a muscle that is attached to a relatively movable part; the end opposite the origin.
Motor unit		A single neuron and all the muscle fibers it stimulates.
Neuromuscular junction	*neur/o:* nerve	The area of communication between the axon terminal of a motor neuron and the sarcolemma of a muscle fiber; also called a *myoneural junction.*
Neurotransmitter	*neur/o:* nerve *trans-:* across	A chemical substance that is released at the axon terminals to stimulate a muscle fiber contraction or an impulse in another neuron.
Origin		The end of a muscle that is attached to a relatively immovable part; the end opposite the insertion.
Prime mover		The muscle that is mainly responsible for a particular body movement; also called an *agonist.*
Sarcolemma	*sarc/o:* flesh, muscle *lemm-*: peel, rind	Covering of a muscle cell; the muscle cell membrane.
Sarcoplasm	*sarc/o:* flesh, muscle	Cytoplasm of a muscle cell.
Synergist	*syn-:* together *erg/o:* work	Muscles that assist a prime mover but are not capable of producing the movement by themselves; two or more muscles work together to produce a movement.

Nervous System

 Check out the Evolve site at http://evolve.elsevier.com/Bonewit/today to access additional interactive activities and exercises to help you study and prepare for success.

LEARNING OBJECTIVES

1. Describe the organization and functions of the nervous system.
2. Describe the structure and functions of neurons and neuroglia.
3. Explain how an impulse is conducted along the length of a neuron.
4. List and describe the three layers of meninges around the central nervous system.
5. Describe the location, components, and functional areas of the cerebrum, diencephalon, brain stem, and cerebellum.
6. Compare the composition of gray matter and white matter.
7. Explain the function of cerebrospinal fluid.
8. Describe the structure and functions of the spinal cord.
9. Explain the difference in composition of sensory, motor, and mixed nerves.
10. List the 12 cranial nerves and state the function of each.
11. Identify the region of the body that is innervated by each of the following spinal nerve plexuses: cervical, brachial, lumbosacral.
12. Explain the difference between the sympathetic and parasympathetic divisions of the autonomic nervous system.
13. Describe ways in which the aging of an individual affects the nervous system.
14. Identify pathology related to the nervous system.

CHAPTER OUTLINE

KEY TERMS

action potential (ACK-shun po-TEN-shall)
axons (AKS-ons)
basal ganglia (BAY-sal GANG-lee-ah)
brain stem (BRAYN STEM)
central sulcus (SEN-tral SULL-kus)
cerebellum (sair-eh-BELL-um)

cerebrospinal fluid (se-ree-broh-SPY-null FLOO-id)
cerebrum (se-REE-brum)
dendrites (DEN-drytes)
decussation (dee-kuh-SAY-shun)
diencephalon (dye-en-SEF-ah-lon)
myelin (MY-eh-lin)
neurilemma (noo-rih-LEM-mah)
neuroglia (noo-ROG-lee-ah)
neuron (NOO-ron)
neurotransmitters (ne-roh-TRANS-mit-ers)
nodes of Ranvier (nodes of ron-vee-AY)
refractory period (ree-FRAK-toar-ee PEE-ree-od)
saltatory conduction (SAL-tah-toar-ee kon-DUCK-shun)
somatomotor cortex (soh-mat-oh-MOH-ter KOR-tex)
somatosensory cortex (soh-mat-oh-SEN-soar-ee KOR-tex)
synapse (SIN-aps)
threshold stimulus (THRESH-hold STIM-yoo-lus)

INTRODUCTION TO THE NERVOUS SYSTEM

The nervous system is the major controlling, regulatory, and communicating system in the body. It is the center of all mental activity, including thought, learning, and memory. Together with the endocrine system, the nervous system is responsible for regulating and maintaining homeostasis. Through its receptors, the nervous system keeps us in touch with our environment, both external and internal.

Like other systems in the body, the nervous system is composed of organs, principally the brain, spinal cord, nerves, and ganglia. These, in turn, consist of various tissues, including nerve, blood, and connective tissue. Together these carry out the complex activities of the nervous system.

FUNCTIONS OF THE NERVOUS SYSTEM

The various activities of the nervous system can be grouped together as three general functions:

- Sensory functions
- Integrative functions
- Motor functions

Together these functions keep us in touch with our environments, maintain homeostasis, and account for thought, learning, and memory.

Millions of sensory receptors detect changes, called *stimuli*, that occur inside and outside the body. They monitor such things as temperature, light, and sound from the external environment. Inside the body, the internal environment, receptors detect variations in pressure, pH, carbon dioxide concentration, and the levels of various electrolytes. All of this gathered information is called *sensory input.*

Sensory input is converted into electrical signals called *nerve impulses*, which are transmitted to the brain. In the brain, the signals are brought together to create sensations, produce thoughts, or add to memory. Decisions are made each moment on the basis of sensory input. This is called *integration.*

Based on the sensory input and integration, the nervous system responds by sending signals to muscles, causing them to contract, or to glands, causing them to produce secretions. Muscles and glands are called *effectors* because they cause an effect in response to directions from the nervous system. This is the *motor output* or *motor function.*

ORGANIZATION OF THE NERVOUS SYSTEM

There is really only one nervous system in the body, although terminology seems to indicate otherwise. Although each subdivision of the system is also called a "nervous system," all of these smaller systems belong to the single, highly integrated nervous system. Each subdivision has structural and functional characteristics that distinguish it from the others. The nervous system as a whole is divided into two subdivisions: the *central nervous system* (CNS) and the *peripheral nervous system* (PNS) (Fig. 9.1).

CENTRAL NERVOUS SYSTEM

The *brain* and *spinal cord*, located in the dorsal body cavity, are the organs of the CNS. Because they are so vitally important, they are encased in bone for protection. The brain is in the cranial vault, and the spinal cord is in the vertebral canal of the vertebral column. Although considered to be two separate organs, the brain and spinal cord are continuous at the foramen magnum.

PERIPHERAL NERVOUS SYSTEM

The organs of the PNS are the *nerves* and *ganglia.* Nerves are bundles of nerve fibers, much as muscles are bundles of muscle fibers. Cranial nerves (12 pairs) and spinal nerves (31 pairs) extend from the CNS to peripheral organs, such as muscles and glands. Ganglia are collections, or small knots, of nerve cell bodies outside the CNS.

The PNS is further subdivided into an *afferent (sensory) division* and an *efferent (motor) division.* The afferent or sensory division transmits impulses from peripheral organs to the CNS. The efferent or motor division transmits impulses from the CNS out to the peripheral organs to cause an effect or action.

Finally, the efferent or motor division is again subdivided into the *somatic nervous system* and the *autonomic nervous system* (ANS). The somatic nervous system, also called the *somatomotor* or *somatic efferent* nervous system, supplies motor impulses to the skeletal muscles. Because these nerves permit conscious control of the skeletal muscles, the somatic nervous system is sometimes called the *voluntary nervous system.* The ANS, also called the *visceral efferent* nervous system, supplies motor impulses to cardiac muscle,

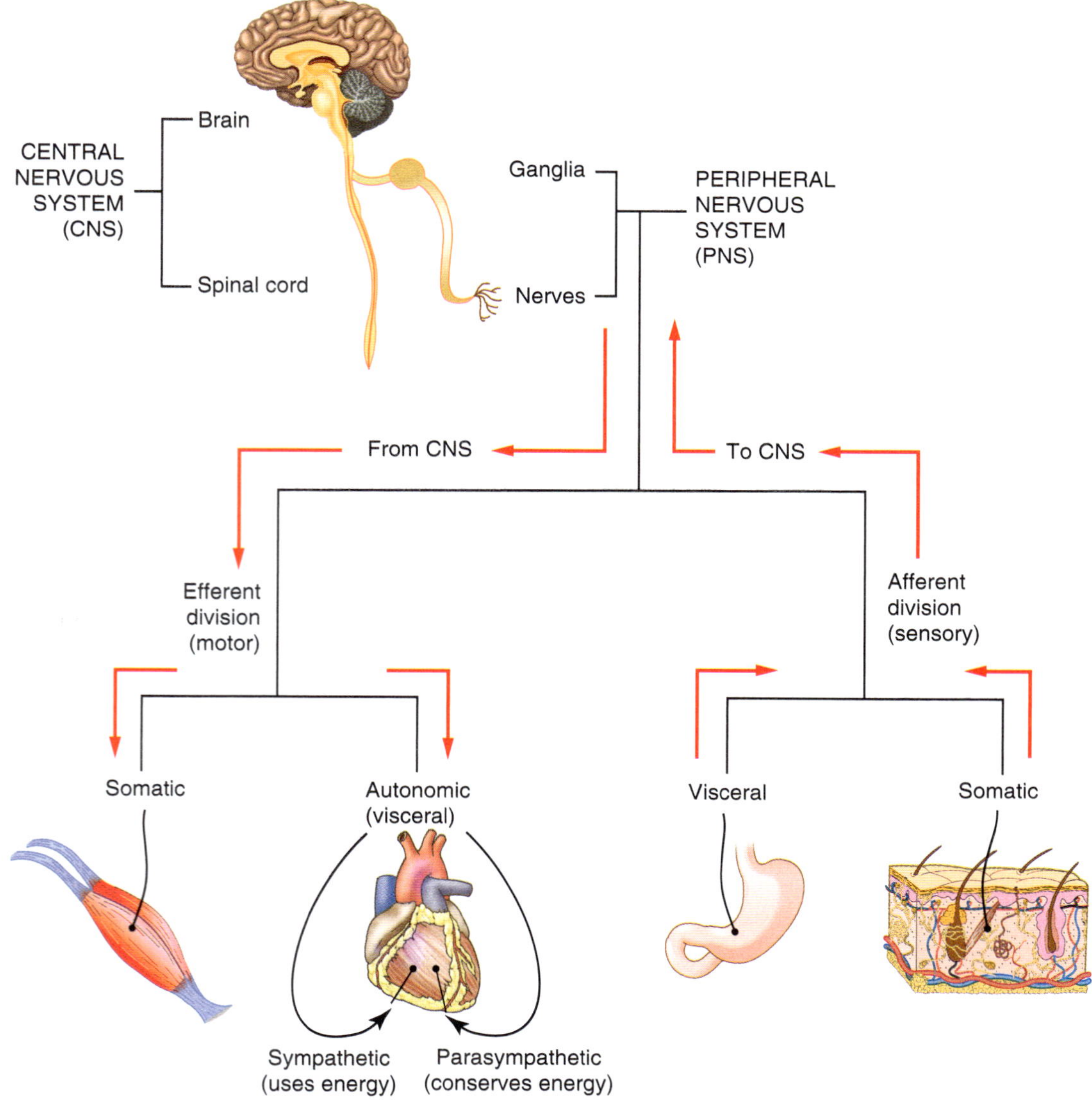

Fig. 9.1 Organization of the nervous system. (From Applegate E: *The anatomy and physiology learning system*, ed 4, St. Louis, 2011, Saunders.)

smooth muscle, and glandular epithelium. It is further subdivided into *sympathetic* and *parasympathetic* divisions. Because the ANS regulates involuntary or automatic functions, it is sometimes called the *involuntary nervous system.*

NERVE TISSUE

Although the nervous system is complex, there are only two main types of cells in nerve tissue. The actual nerve cell is the **neuron**. It is the "conducting" cell that transmits impulses and is the structural unit of the nervous system. The other type of cell is the *neuroglia* or *glial cell.* The word **neuroglia** means "nerve glue." These cells are nonconductive and provide a support system for the neurons. They are a special type of "connective tissue" for the nervous system.

NEURONS

Neurons, or nerve cells, carry out the functions of the nervous system by conducting nerve impulses. They are highly specialized and *amitotic.* This means that neurons do not undergo mitosis, therefore, if a neuron is destroyed, it cannot be replaced.

Each neuron has three basic parts:

- Cell body
- One or more dendrites
- A single axon

Fig. 9.2 illustrates a typical neuron. The main part of the neuron is the *cell body* or *soma.* In many ways the cell body is similar to other types of cells. It has a nucleus with at least one nucleolus and contains many of the typical cytoplasmic organelles. It lacks centrioles, however. Because centrioles function in cell division, the fact that neurons lack these organelles is consistent with the amitotic nature of the cell.

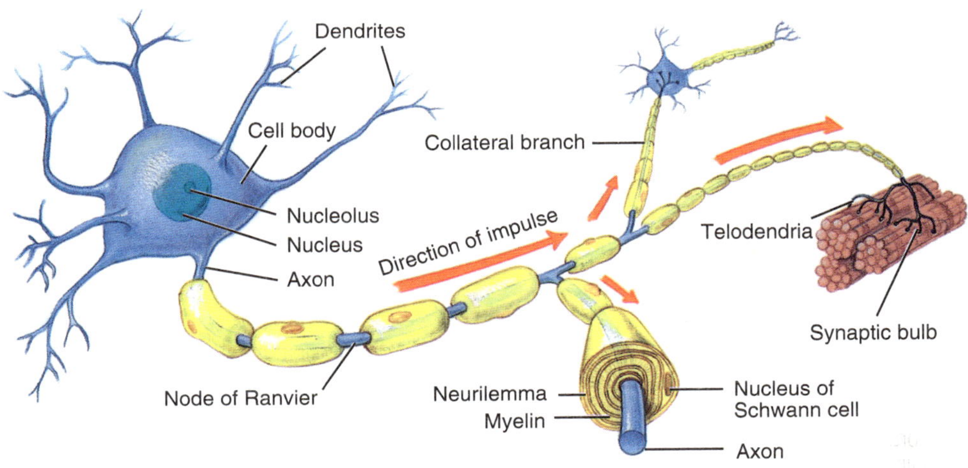

Fig. 9.2 Structure of a typical neuron. (From Applegate E: *The anatomy and physiology learning system*, ed 4, St. Louis, 2011, Saunders.)

Dendrites and **axons** are cytoplasmic extensions, or processes, that project from the cell body. They are sometimes referred to as *fibers*. Dendrites are usually but not always short and branching, which increases their surface area to receive signals from other neurons. The number of dendrites on a neuron varies. They are called *afferent processes* because they transmit impulses to the neuron cell body. Only one axon projects from each cell body. It is usually elongated, and because it carries impulses away from the cell body, it is called an *efferent process*.

An axon may have infrequent branches called *axon collaterals*. Axons and axon collaterals terminate in many short branches or *telodendria*. The distal ends of the telodendria are slightly enlarged to form *synaptic bulbs*. Many axons are surrounded by a segmented white fatty substance called **myelin** or the *myelin sheath*. Myelinated fibers make up the white matter in the CNS, whereas cell bodies and unmyelinated fibers make up the gray matter. The unmyelinated regions between the myelin segments are called the **nodes of Ranvier**. In the PNS the myelin is produced by Schwann cells. The cytoplasm, nucleus, and outer cell membrane of the Schwann cell form a tight covering around the myelin and around the axon itself at the nodes of Ranvier. This covering is the **neurilemma**, which plays an important role in the regeneration of nerve fibers. In the CNS, *oligodendrocytes* produce myelin, but there is no neurilemma, which is why fibers within the CNS do not regenerate. The structure of an axon and its coverings is illustrated in Fig. 9.2.

Functionally, neurons are classified as afferent, efferent, or interneurons (association neurons) according to the direction in which they transmit impulses relative to the CNS (Table 9.1). *Afferent*, or *sensory*, *neurons* carry impulses from peripheral sense receptors to the CNS. They usually have long dendrites and relatively short axons. *Efferent*, or *motor*, *neurons* transmit impulses from the CNS to effector organs, such as muscles and glands.

Table 9.1 Types of Neurons Classified According to Function

Type of Neuron	Structure	Function
Afferent (sensory)	Long dendrites and short axon; cell body located in ganglia in PNS; dendrites in PNS; axon extends into CNS	Transmits impulses from peripheral sense receptors to CNS
Efferent (motor)	Short dendrites and long axon; dendrites and cell body located within CNS; axons extend to PNS	Transmits impulses from CNS to effectors, such as muscles and glands in periphery
Association (interneurons)	Short dendrites; axon may be short or long; located entirely within CNS	Transmits impulses from afferent neurons to efferent neurons

CNS, Central nervous system; *PNS*, peripheral nervous system.

From Applegate E: *The anatomy and physiology learning system*, ed 4, St. Louis, 2011, Saunders.

Efferent neurons usually have short dendrites and long axons. *Interneurons*, or *association neurons*, are located entirely within the CNS, where they form the connecting link between the afferent and efferent neurons. They have short dendrites and may have either short or long axons.

NEUROGLIA

Neuroglial cells do not conduct nerve impulses; instead, they support, nourish, and protect the neurons. They are far more numerous than neurons and, unlike neurons, are capable of mitosis.

HIGHLIGHT on the Nervous System

Brain tumors: Because neurons are not capable of mitosis, primary malignant tumors of the brain are tumors of the glial cells rather than of the neurons themselves. These tumors, called *gliomas*, have extensive roots, making them extremely difficult to remove.

Blood–brain barrier: Neuroglia, particularly astrocytes, form a wall around the outside of the blood vessels in the nervous system. This astrocyte wall plus the blood vessel wall form the blood–brain barrier. Water, oxygen, carbon dioxide, alcohol, and a few other substances are able to pass through this barrier and move between the blood and brain tissue. Other substances, such as toxins, pathogens, and certain drugs, cannot pass through this barrier. This is a protective mechanism to keep harmful substances out of the brain. It has clinical significance because drugs such as penicillin that may be used to treat disorders in other parts of the body have no effect on the brain because they do not cross the blood–brain barrier.

Anesthetics: Some anesthetics produce their effects by inhibiting the diffusion of sodium through the cell membrane, thus blocking the initiation and conduction of nerve impulses.

Meningitis: Meningitis is an acute inflammation of the pia mater and the arachnoid. It is most commonly caused by bacteria. However, viral infections, fungal infections, and tumors may also cause inflammation of the meninges. Depending on the primary cause, meningitis may be mild or it may progress to a severe and life-threatening condition.

Left and right brain: In most people (approximately 90%), the left cerebral hemisphere dominates for language and mathematical abilities. It is the reasoning and analytic side of the brain. The right cerebral hemisphere is involved with motor skills, intuition, emotion, art, and music appreciation. It is the poetic and creative side of the brain. In about 10% of people, these sides are reversed. In some individuals, neither hemisphere dominates. This may result in "confusion" and learning disabilities.

Emotions: The *limbic system* consists of scattered but interconnected regions of gray matter in the cerebral hemispheres and diencephalon. The limbic system is involved in memory and in emotions such as sadness, happiness, anger, and fear. It is our emotional brain.

Hydrocephalus: In hydrocephalus, an obstruction in the normal flow of **cerebrospinal fluid** (CSF) causes the fluid to accumulate in the ventricles. The obstruction may be a congenital defect or an acquired lesion such as a tumor. As the fluid accumulates, it causes the ventricles to enlarge and CSF pressure to increase. When this happens in an infant, before the cranial bones ossify, the cranium enlarges. In an older child or adult, the pressure damages the soft brain tissue.

Lumbar puncture: A lumbar puncture is the withdrawal of a small amount of CSF from the subarachnoid space in the lumbar region of the spinal cord. The extension of the meninges beyond the end of the cord makes it possible to do this without injury to the spinal cord. The needle is usually inserted just above or just below the fourth lumbar vertebra, and the spinal cord ends at the first lumbar vertebra. The CSF that is removed can be tested for abnormal characteristics that may indicate an injury or infection.

Carpal tunnel syndrome: Carpal tunnel syndrome is a common occupational injury to the hand and wrist that is associated with repetitive hand motions. It is also associated with several diseases, including arthritis, diabetes, and gout. Symptoms—which include tingling of the thumb and fingers—result from compression of the median nerve because of inflammation and swelling of the tendons within the carpal tunnel. ■

NERVE IMPULSES

The functional characteristics of neurons are *excitability* and *conductivity*. Excitability is the ability to respond to a stimulus; conductivity is the ability to transmit an impulse from one point to another. All the functions associated with the nervous system—including thought, learning, and memory—are based on these two characteristics. These functional characteristics are the result of structural features of the cell membrane.

RESTING MEMBRANE

A *resting membrane* is the cell membrane of a nonconducting, or resting, neuron. The membrane is impermeable to the passive diffusion of sodium (Na^+) and potassium (K^+) ions. Sodium ions are concentrated in the extracellular fluid, whereas potassium ions are inside the cell. Electrical measurements show the resting membrane to be polarized, with the inside of the membrane more negative than the outside. This is called the resting *membrane potential* and measures about −70 mV.

STIMULATION OF A NEURON

A stimulus is a physical, chemical, or electrical event that alters the permeability of the neuron cell membrane. This allows sodium ions to move inside the cell and potassium ions move to the outside. This ionic movement briefly changes the polarization of the membrane.

This response to a stimulus is called the **action potential**. Electrical measurements show the action potential to peak at approximately +30 mV (Fig. 9.3). At the conclusion of the action potential, the sodium–potassium pump actively transports sodium ions out of the cell and potassium ions into the cell to completely restore resting conditions.

The minimum stimulus necessary to initiate an action potential is called a **threshold stimulus** or *liminal stimulus*. A weaker stimulus, called a *subthreshold (subliminal) stimulus*, does not cause sufficient depolarization to elicit an action potential.

CONDUCTION ALONG A NEURON

Once a threshold stimulus has been applied and an action potential generated, it must be conducted along the total length of the neuron either to an effector or to another neuron.

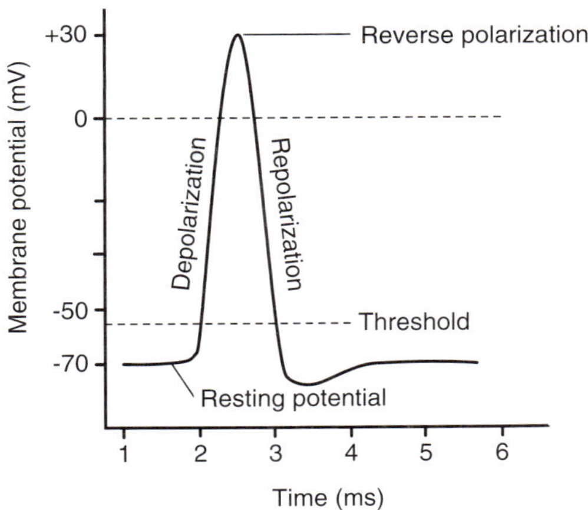

Fig. 9.3 Recording of an action potential. The resting potential is -70 mV and the peak action potential is +30 mV. (From Applegate E: *The anatomy and physiology learning system*, ed 4, St. Louis, 2011, Saunders.)

The threshold stimulus causes a localized action potential on the membrane. The rest of the membrane is in the resting condition. The action potential stimulates the next point. This continues point by point, in domino fashion, along the entire length of the neuron, creating a *propagated action potential*, or *nerve impulse.*

Saltatory Conduction

The conduction described in the previous paragraph is representative of an unmyelinated axon. Because myelin is an insulating substance, it inhibits the flow of current from one point to another. In myelinated fibers, an action potential occurs only at the places where there is no myelin, at the nodes of Ranvier. The action potential "jumps" from node to node. This "jumping" is **saltatory conduction**, which is faster than conduction in unmyelinated fibers.

Refractory Period

The period of time during which a point on the cell membrane is "recovering" from an action potential is called the **refractory period**. That point on the cell membrane cannot respond to a second stimulus, no matter how strong the stimulus.

All-or-None Principle

Nerve fibers obey the *all-or-none principle.* If a threshold stimulus is applied, an action potential is generated and propagated along the entire length of the neuron at maximum strength and speed for the existing conditions. A stronger stimulus does not increase the strength of the action potential or change the rate of conduction. A weaker stimulus is subthreshold and does not evoke an action potential. If a stimulus is at threshold level or greater, an impulse is conducted. If the stimulus is subthreshold, there is no conduction.

CONDUCTION ACROSS A SYNAPSE

A nerve impulse travels along a nerve fiber until it reaches the end of the axon; then it must be transmitted to the next neuron. The region of communication between two neurons is called a **synapse**. This is similar to the neuromuscular junction described in Chapter 8. A synapse has three parts (Fig. 9.4):

- Synaptic knob
- Synaptic cleft
- Postsynaptic membrane

The first neuron, the one preceding the synapse, is called the *presynaptic neuron*; the second neuron, the one following the synapse, is called the *postsynaptic neuron.* Synaptic knobs are tiny bulges at the ends of the telodendria on the presynaptic neuron. Small sacs within the synaptic knobs, called *synaptic vesicles*, contain chemicals known as **neurotransmitters**.

When a nerve impulse reaches the synaptic knob, a series of reactions releases neurotransmitters into the synaptic cleft. The neurotransmitters diffuse across the synaptic cleft and react with receptors on the postsynaptic cell membrane. This is synaptic transmission. To prevent prolonged reactions with the postsynaptic receptors, the transmitters are quickly inactivated by enzymes. One of the best-known neurotransmitters is *acetylcholine*, which is inactivated by the enzyme *cholinesterase.* Table 9.2 lists some of the common neurotransmitters.

In *excitatory transmission*, the neurotransmitter–receptor reaction on the postsynaptic membrane depolarizes the membrane and initiates an action potential. This is excitation or stimulation. Acetylcholine is typically an excitatory neurotransmitter. Some neurotransmitters result in *inhibitory transmission.* In this case, the reaction between the neurotransmitter and the receptor makes it more difficult to generate an action potential. This is inhibition. Gamma-aminobutyric acid (GABA) is an inhibitory neurotransmitter in the CNS.

NEURONAL POOLS

The billions of neurons in the CNS are organized into functional groups called *neuronal pools.* These receive information, process and integrate that information, and then transmit it to some other destination. Neuronal pools are arranged in pathways, or circuits, over which the nerve impulses are transmitted. The simplest pathway is the *simple series circuit* (Fig. 9.5A), in which a single neuron synapses with another neuron, which in turn synapses with another, and so on. Most pathways are more complex. In a *divergence circuit* (see Fig. 9.5B), a single neuron synapses with multiple neurons within the pool. This permits the same information to diverge or go along different pathways at the same time. This type of pathway is important in muscle contraction when many muscle fibers, or even several muscles, must contract at the same time. Another type of pathway is the *convergence circuit* (see Fig. 9.5). In this case, several presynaptic neurons synapse with a single postsynaptic neuron. This accounts for the fact that many different stimuli may have the same ultimate effect. For example, thinking about food, smelling food, and seeing food all have the same effect—the flow of saliva.

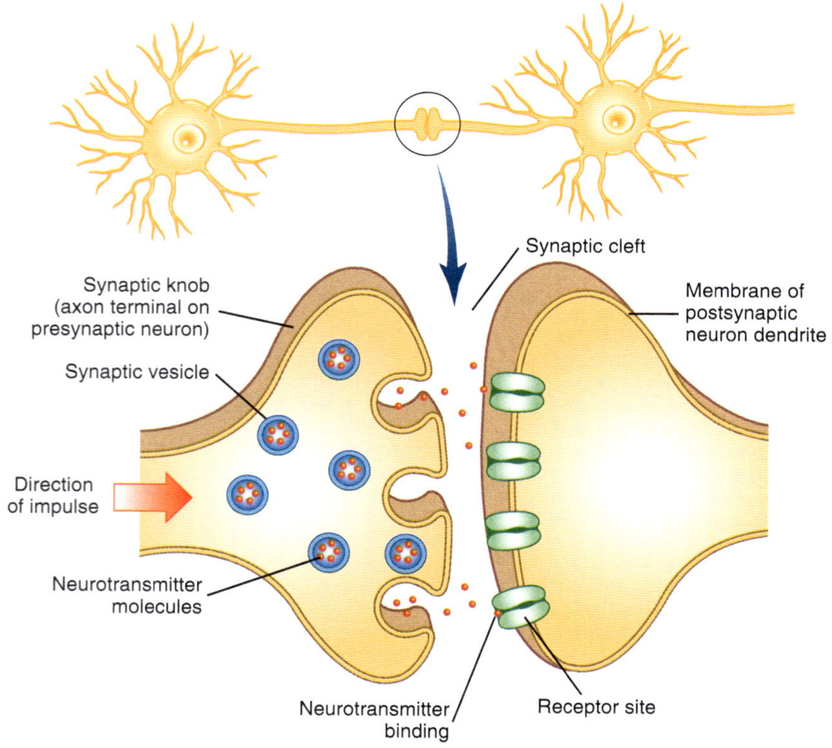

Fig. 9.4 Components of a synapse. The impulse travels from the presynaptic neuron to the postsynaptic neuron. (From Applegate E: *The anatomy and physiology learning system*, ed 4, St. Louis, 2011, Saunders.)

Table 9.2 Some Common Neurotransmitters

Neurotransmitter	Location	Function	Comments
Acetylcholine	CNS and PNS	Generally excitatory but inhibitory to some visceral effectors	Found in skeletal neuromuscular junctions and in many ANS synapses
Norepinephrine	CNS and PNS	May be excitatory or inhibitory depending on receptors	Found in visceral and cardiac muscle neuromuscular junctions; cocaine and amphetamines exaggerate effects
Epinephrine	CNS and PNS	May be excitatory or inhibitory depending on receptors	Found in pathways concerned with behavior and mood
Dopamine	CNS and PNS	Generally excitatory	Found in pathways that regulate emotional responses; decreased levels in Parkinson disease
Serotonin	CNS	Generally inhibitory	Found in pathways that regulate temperature, sensory perception, mood, onset of sleep
Gamma-aminobutyric acid (GABA)	CNS	Generally inhibitory	Inhibits excessive discharge of neurons
Endorphins and enkephalins	CNS	Generally inhibitory	Inhibit release of sensory pain neurotransmitters; opiates mimic effects of these peptides

ANS, Autonomic nervous system; *CNS*, central nervous system; *PNS*, peripheral nervous system.
From Applegate E: *The anatomy and physiology learning system*, ed 4, St. Louis, 2011, Saunders.

REFLEX ARCS

The neuron is the structural unit of the nervous system; the *reflex arc* is the functional unit. The reflex arc is a type of conduction pathway. It is similar to a one-way street because it allows impulses to travel in only one direction. The simplest reflex arc consists of two neurons, but most have three or more neurons in the conduction pathway. Fig. 9.6 illustrates a three-neuron reflex arc. There are five basic components in a reflex arc (Table 9.3):

- Receptor
- Sensory neuron
- Integration center
- Motor neuron
- Effector

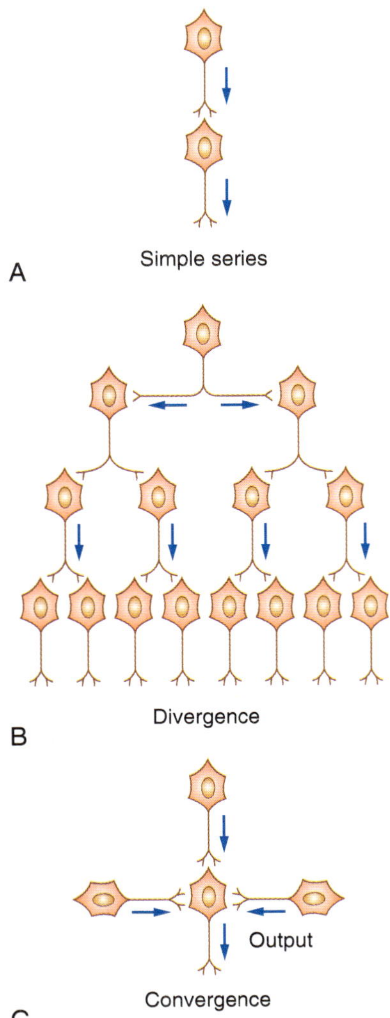

Fig. 9.5 Neuronal pools. (A) Simple series circuit: one neuron synapses with another. (B) Divergence circuit: a single neuron synapses with multiple neurons. (C) Convergence circuit: several neurons synapse with a single postsynaptic neuron. (From Applegate E: *The anatomy and physiology learning system*, ed 4, St. Louis, 2011, Saunders.)

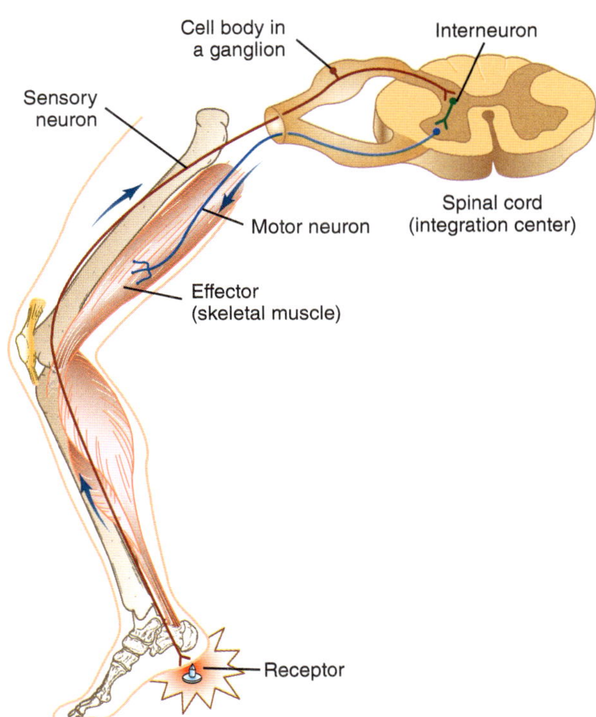

Fig. 9.6 Components of a generalized reflex arc. Note the five components of a reflex arc. (From Applegate E: *The anatomy and physiology learning system*, ed 4, St. Louis, 2011, Saunders.)

A *reflex* is an automatic, involuntary response to some change, either inside or outside the body. Reflexes are important in maintaining homeostasis by making adjustments to heart rate, breathing rate, and blood pressure. Reflexes are also involved in coughing, sneezing, and reactions to painful stimuli. Everyone is familiar with the withdrawal reflex. When you step on a tack or touch a hot iron, you immediately, without conscious thought, withdraw the injured foot or hand from the source of the irritation. Clinicians frequently test an individual's reflexes to determine if the nervous system is functioning properly.

CENTRAL NERVOUS SYSTEM

The CNS consists of the brain and spinal cord, which are located in the dorsal body cavity. These are vital to our well-being and are enclosed in bone for protection. The brain is surrounded by the cranium, and the spinal cord is protected by the vertebrae. The brain is continuous with the spinal cord at the foramen magnum in the occipital bone. In addition to bone, the CNS is surrounded by connective tissue membranes, called *meninges*, and by *CSF*.

MENINGES

Three layers of meninges surround the brain and spinal cord (Fig. 9.7). The outer layer, the *dura mater*, is tough white fibrous connective tissue. It is just inside the cranial bones and lines the vertebral canal. The dura mater contains channels, called *dural sinuses*, that collect venous blood to return it to the cardiovascular system.

The middle layer of meninges is the *arachnoid*, which resembles a cobweb. It is a thin layer with numerous thread-like strands that attach it to the innermost layer. The space under the arachnoid, the *subarachnoid space*, is filled with CSF and contains blood vessels.

The *pia mater* is the innermost layer of meninges. This thin, delicate membrane is tightly bound to the surface of the brain and spinal cord and cannot be dissected away without damaging the surface. It closely follows all surface contours.

BRAIN

The brain is divided into the cerebrum, diencephalon, brain stem, and cerebellum.

Table 9.3 Components of a Reflex Arc

Component	Description	Function
Receptor	Site of stimulus action; receptor end of dendrite or special cell in receptor organ	Responds to some change in internal or external environment
Sensory neuron	Afferent neuron; cell body is in ganglion outside CNS; axon extends into CNS	Transmits nerve impulses from receptor to CNS
Integration center	Always within CNS; in simplest reflexes, it consists of synapse between sensory and motor neurons; more commonly one or more interneurons are involved	Processing center; region in CNS where incoming sensory impulses generate appropriate outgoing motor impulses
Motor neuron	Efferent neuron; dendrites and cell body are in CNS; axon extends to periphery	Transmits nerve impulses from integration center in CNS to effector organ
Effector	Muscle or gland outside CNS	Responds to impulses from motor neuron to produce an action, such as contraction or secretion

CNS, Central nervous system.
From Applegate E: *The anatomy and physiology learning system*, ed 4, St. Louis, 2011, Saunders.

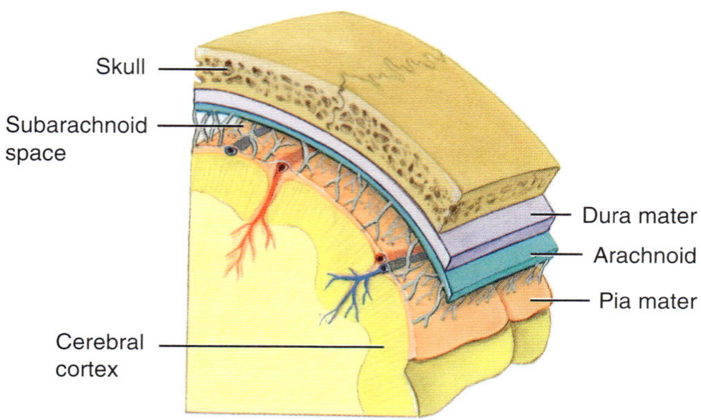

Fig. 9.7 Meninges of the central nervous system. (From Applegate E: *The anatomy and physiology learning system*, ed 4, St. Louis, 2011, Saunders.)

Cerebrum

The largest and most obvious portion of the brain is the **cerebrum**, which is divided by a deep *longitudinal fissure* into two *cerebral hemispheres*. These hemispheres are two separate entities but are connected by an arching band of white fibers, called the *corpus callosum*, which provides a communication pathway between the two halves. The surface of the cerebrum is marked by convolutions, or *gyri*, separated by grooves, or *sulci*. The pia mater closely follows the convolutions and goes deep into the sulci and then up and over the gyri.

Each cerebral hemisphere is divided into five lobes, as illustrated in Fig. 9.8. Four of the lobes have the same name as the bone over them. The *frontal lobe*, under the frontal bone, is the most anterior portion of each hemisphere. The posterior boundary of the frontal lobe is the **central sulcus**. The *parietal lobe* is immediately posterior to the central sulcus, under the parietal bone. The *occipital lobe*, under the occipital bone, is the most posterior portion of the cerebral hemisphere. Laterally, the *temporal lobe* is inferior to the frontal and parietal lobes. The *lateral sulcus* (fissure) separates the temporal lobe from the two lobes that are superior to it. A fifth lobe, the *insula* or *island of Reil*, lies deep within the lateral sulcus. It is covered by parts of the frontal, parietal, and temporal lobes.

The cerebral hemispheres consist of gray matter and white matter. A thin layer of *gray matter*, the *cerebral cortex*, forms the outermost portion of the cerebrum. Gray matter consists of neuron cell bodies and unmyelinated fibers. The *white matter*, which makes up the bulk of the cerebrum, is just beneath the cerebral cortex. White matter comprises myelinated nerve fibers that form communication pathways in the cerebrum.

The cerebral cortex is the neural basis of what makes us "human." It is the center for sensory and motor functions. It is concerned with memory, language, reasoning, intelligence, personality, and all the other factors that we associate with human life. Even though the two cerebral hemispheres are nearly symmetric in structure, they are not always equal in function; instead, there are areas of specialization. However, there is considerable overlap in these regions and no area really works alone; all the areas are dependent on one another for mental "consciousness"—those abilities that involve higher mental processing, such as memory, reasoning, logic, and judgment.

It is possible to identify regions of the cerebral cortex that have specific functions. *Sensory areas* receive information from the various sense organs and receptors throughout the body. The primary sensory area, the **somatosensory cortex,** is located in the *postcentral gyrus* of the parietal lobe, immediately posterior to the central sulcus. This region receives sensory input from sensory receptors in the skin and skeletal muscles. The right side of the somatosensory cortex receives input from the left side of the body and vice versa. *Motor areas* responsible for muscle contraction are located in the frontal lobe. The primary motor area, the **somatomotor cortex**, is in the *precentral gyrus*, immediately anterior to the central sulcus. Neurons in this area allow us to consciously

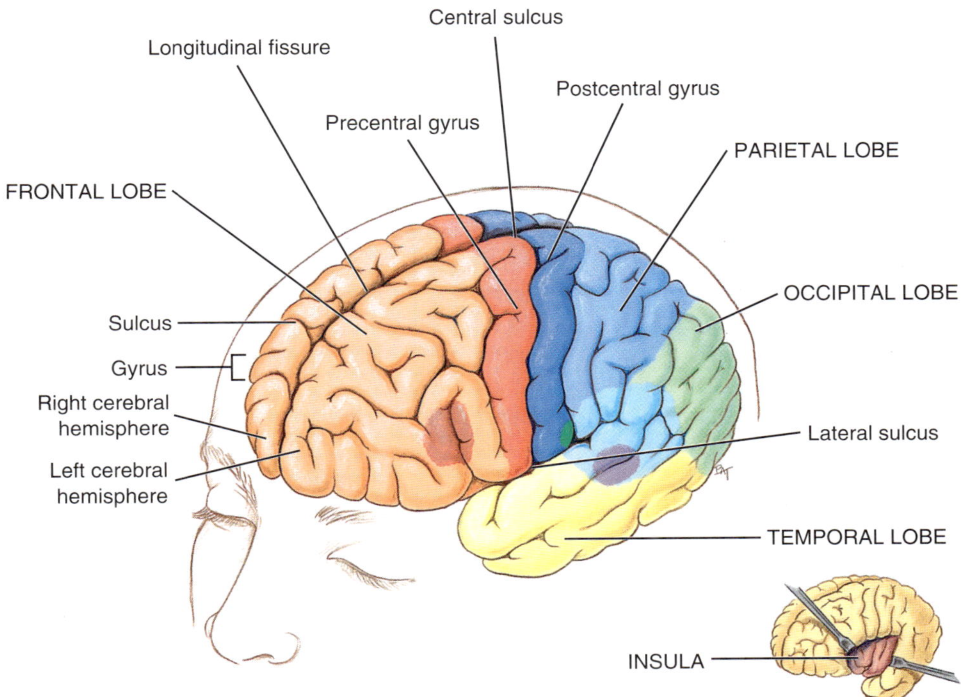

Fig. 9.8 Lobes and landmarks of the cerebrum. (From Applegate E: *The anatomy and physiology learning system*, ed 4, St. Louis, 2011, Saunders.)

control our skeletal muscles. The right primary motor gyrus controls muscles on the left side of the body and vice versa. The primary motor cortex is also highly organized in a manner similar to the primary sensory cortex, with neurons in a specific region responsible for controlling movement in a specific part of the body.

Association areas of the cerebral cortex are involved in the process of recognition. They analyze and interpret sensory information; based on previous experiences, they integrate appropriate responses through the motor areas. Table 9.4 describes some of the specific functional areas of the cerebral cortex.

The **basal ganglia** are functionally related regions of gray matter that are scattered throughout the white matter of the cerebral hemispheres. These regions function as relay stations, or areas of synapse, in pathways going to and from the cortex. The major effects of the basal ganglia are to decrease muscle tone and inhibit muscular activity. Because of these effects, they play an important role in posture and coordinating motor movements. Also, nearly all of the inhibitory neurotransmitter dopamine is produced in the basal ganglia.

Diencephalon

The **diencephalon** is centrally located and is nearly surrounded by the cerebral hemispheres. The regions of the diencephalon are illustrated in Fig. 9.9.

The *thalamus*, about 80% of the diencephalon, consists of two oval masses of gray matter that serve as relay stations for sensory impulses, except those for the sense of smell. These impulses are relayed to the cerebral cortex. The thalamus channels the impulses to the appropriate region of the cortex for discrimination, localization, and interpretation.

The *hypothalamus* is a small region below the thalamus. It plays a key role in maintaining homeostasis because it regulates many visceral activities. The hypothalamus also serves as a link between the nervous and endocrine systems because it regulates secretion of hormones from the pituitary gland. A slender stalk, the *infundibulum*, extends from the floor of the hypothalamus to the pituitary gland and acts as a connector between the two structures. Functions of the hypothalamus include the following:

- Regulates and integrates the ANS
- Regulates emotional responses and behavior
- Regulates body temperature
- Regulates food intake
- Regulates water balance and thirst
- Regulates endocrine system activity

The *epithalamus* is the most superior portion of the diencephalon. The *pineal gland*, or *pineal body*, extends from its posterior margin. This small gland is involved with the onset of puberty and rhythmic cycles in the body. It is similar to a biologic clock.

Brain Stem

The **brain stem** is the region between the diencephalon and the spinal cord. It consists of three regions:

- Midbrain
- Pons
- Medulla oblongata

Regions of the brain stem are illustrated in Fig. 9.9.

Table 9.4 Functional Regions of the Cerebral Cortex

Functional Region	Location	Description	Comments
Primary sensory cortex (somatosensory cortex)	Postcentral gyrus in parietal lobe	Receives sensory input from receptors in skin and skeletal muscles	Functions in sensations of temperature, touch, pressure, pain
Primary visual cortex	Posterior region of occipital lobe	Receives sensory input from retina of eye	Perceives current visual image
Auditory cortex	Superior margin of temporal lobe, along lateral sulcus	Receives auditory impulses related to pitch, rhythm, and loudness from inner ear	Allows the hearing of "sounds"
Olfactory cortex	Medial aspect of temporal lobe	Receives input from olfactory (smell) receptors in nasal cavity	Permits perception of different odors
Gustatory cortex	Parietal lobe where it is overlapped by temporal lobe	Receives input from taste buds on tongue	Permits perception of different tastes
Primary motor cortex (somatomotor cortex)	Precentral gyrus in frontal lobe	Initiates efferent action potentials that control voluntary movements	Permits skeletal muscle contraction
Premotor cortex	Anterior to primary motor cortex in frontal lobe	Controls learned motor skills that involve skeletal muscles, either simultaneously or sequentially	Examples of learned motor skills are playing piano, typing, writing
Broca area (motor speech area)	Inferior portion of frontal lobe in one hemisphere, usually the left	Programs and coordinates muscular movements necessary to articulate words	Person with injury in this area is able to understand words but is unable to speak because of inability to coordinate muscles necessary to form words
Prefrontal cortex	Anterior portion of frontal lobes	Involved with thought, reasoning, intelligence, judgment, planning, conscience	This area is well developed only in humans
Gnostic area (general interpretation area)	Region where parietal, temporal, and occipital lobes meet; found in one hemisphere (usually the left)	Integrates sensory interpretations from adjacent association areas to form thoughts; then transmits signals for appropriate responses	Stores complex memory patterns; allows person to recognize words and arrange them appropriately to express thoughts or to read and understand written ideas

From Applegate E: *The anatomy and physiology learning system*, ed 4, St. Louis, 2011, Saunders.

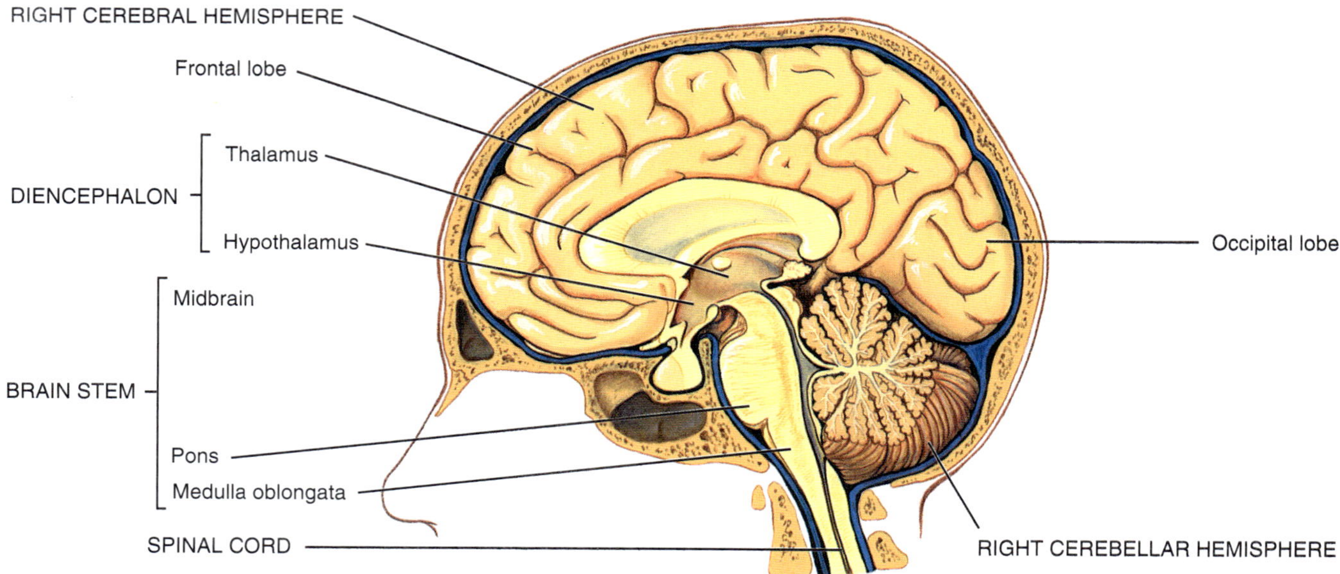

Fig. 9.9 Midsagittal section of the brain showing the major portions of the diencephalon, brain stem, and cerebellum. (From Applegate E: *The anatomy and physiology learning system*, ed 4, St. Louis, 2011, Saunders.)

The *midbrain* is the most superior portion of the brain stem, the region next to the diencephalon. It consists of bundles of myelinated fibers that contain the voluntary motor tracts descending from the cerebral cortex. The *pons* is the bulging middle portion of the brain stem. This region primarily consists of nerve fibers that form conduction tracts between the higher brain centers and the spinal cord. Four cranial nerves originate in the pons. It also contains the *pneumotaxic* and *apneustic areas*, which help regulate breathing movements.

The *medulla oblongata*, or simply *medulla*, extends inferiorly from the pons. It is continuous with the spinal cord at the foramen magnum. All the ascending (sensory) and descending (motor) nerve fibers connecting the brain and spinal cord pass through the medulla. Most of the descending fibers cross over from one side to the other. In other words, fibers descending on the left side cross over to the right and vice versa. This is called **decussation**. Because the fibers decussate, or cross over, the brain controls motor functions on the opposite side of the body. The medulla contains three vital centers that control visceral activities. The *cardiac center* adjusts the heart rate and contraction strength to meet body needs. The *vasomotor center* regulates blood pressure by effecting changes in blood vessel diameter. The *respiratory center* acts with the centers in the pons to regulate the rate, rhythm, and depth of breathing. Other centers are involved in coughing, sneezing, swallowing, and vomiting.

Cerebellum

The **cerebellum**, the second largest portion of the brain, is located below the occipital lobes of the cerebrum. It consists of two *cerebellar hemispheres* connected in the middle by a structure called the *vermis.*

Like the cerebrum, the cerebellum consists of white matter surrounded by a thin layer of gray matter, the *cerebellar cortex.* Because the surface convolutions are less prominent in the cerebellum than in the cerebrum, the cerebellum has proportionately less gray matter.

Bundles of myelinated nerve fibers form communication pathways between the cerebellum and other parts of the CNS.

The cerebellum functions as a motor area of the brain that mediates subconscious contractions of skeletal muscles necessary for *coordination, posture*, and *balance.* The cerebellum coordinates skeletal muscles to produce smooth muscle movement rather than jerky, trembling motion. When the cerebellum is damaged, movements such as running, walking, and writing become uncoordinated. Posture is dependent on muscle tone, which is mediated by the cerebellum. Impulses from the inner ear concerning position and equilibrium are directed to the cerebellum, which uses that information to maintain balance.

VENTRICLES AND CEREBROSPINAL FLUID

A series of interconnected, fluid-filled cavities are found within the brain. These cavities are the *ventricles* of the brain, and the fluid is *cerebrospinal fluid* (CSF). The *lateral ventricles* in the cerebrum are the largest of these cavities. One lateral ventricle exists in each cerebral hemisphere. The CSF is a clear fluid that forms as a filtrate from the blood in specialized capillary networks, the *choroid plexus*, within the ventricles of the brain. It circulates through the ventricles and the central canal of the spinal cord and surrounds the brain in the subarachnoid space. From the subarachnoid space, CSF carrying waste products is returned to the blood. In addition to providing support and protection for the CNS, the CSF helps to nourish the brain and maintain constant ionic conditions for the brain and spinal cord as well as providing a pathway for the removal of waste products.

SPINAL CORD

The *spinal cord*, illustrated in Fig. 9.10, extends from the foramen magnum at the base of the skull to the level of the first lumbar vertebra, a distance of about 43 to 46 cm (approximately 17 to 18 inches). The cord is continuous with the medulla oblongata at the foramen magnum. Distally, it terminates in the *conus medullaris.* Like the brain, the spinal cord is surrounded by bone, meninges, and CSF. The spinal dura is separated from the vertebral bones by an *epidural space.* The meninges extend beyond the end of the spinal cord, down to the upper part of the sacrum. From

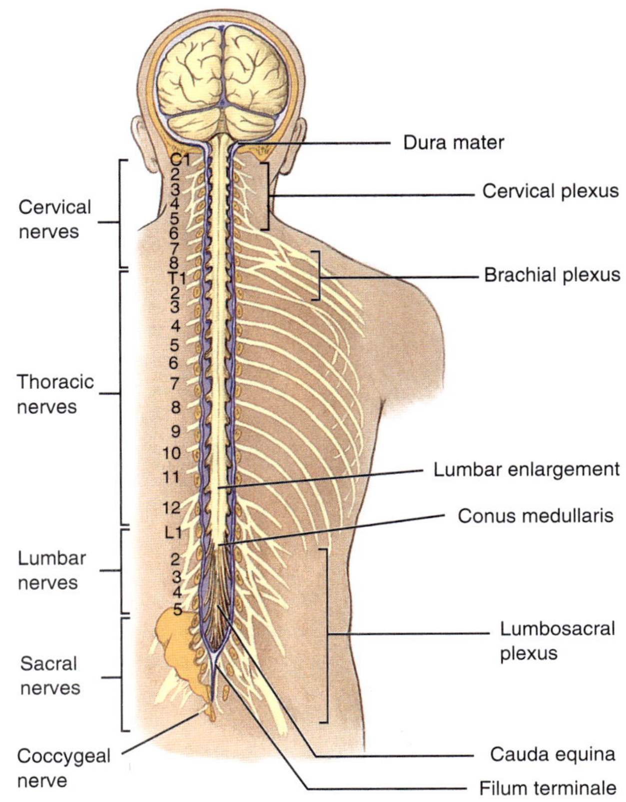

Fig. 9.10 Gross anatomy of the spinal cord. (From Applegate E: *The anatomy and physiology learning system*, ed 4, St. Louis, 2011, Saunders.)

there, a fibrous cord of pia mater, the *filum terminale*, extends down to the coccyx, where it is anchored.

The spinal cord is divided into 31 segments, with each segment giving rise to a pair of spinal nerves. At the distal end of the cord, many spinal nerves extend beyond the conus medullaris to form a collection that resembles a horse's tail. This is the *cauda equina*. There are two enlargements in the cord, one in the cervical region and one in the lumbar region. The *cervical enlargement* gives rise to the nerves that supply the upper extremity. Nerves from the *lumbar enlargement* supply the lower extremity.

In cross section, the spinal cord appears oval (Fig. 9.11). Peripheral white matter surrounds a core of gray matter that resembles a butterfly, or the letter H. The gray matter contains the terminal portions of sensory neuron axons, entire interneurons, and the dendrites and cell bodies of motor neurons. The central connecting bar between the two large areas of gray matter is the *gray commissure*. This surrounds the *central canal*, which contains CSF. The white matter that surrounds the gray matter contains longitudinal bundles of myelinated nerve fibers, called *nerve tracts*.

The spinal cord has two main functions. It is a conduction pathway for impulses going to and from the brain, and it serves as a reflex center. The conduction pathways that carry sensory impulses from body parts to the brain are called *ascending tracts*. Pathways that carry motor impulses from the brain to muscles and glands are *descending tracts*.

In addition to serving as a conduction pathway, the spinal cord functions as a center for spinal reflexes. The reflex arc, described earlier in this chapter and illustrated in Fig. 9.6, is the functional unit of the nervous system. Reflexes are responses to stimuli that do not require conscious thought; consequently they occur more quickly than reactions that require thought processes. For example, with the withdrawal reflex, the reflex action withdraws the affected part before one is aware of the pain. Many reflexes are mediated in the spinal cord without going to the higher brain centers. Table 9.5 describes some clinically significant reflexes.

PERIPHERAL NERVOUS SYSTEM

The PNS consists of the nerves that branch out from the brain and spinal cord. These nerves form the communication network between the CNS and the remainder of the body. The PNS is further subdivided into the *somatic nervous system* and the *ANS*. The somatic nervous system consists of nerves that go to the skin and muscles and is involved in conscious activities. The ANS consists of nerves that connect the CNS to the visceral organs such as the heart, stomach, and intestines. It mediates unconscious activities.

STRUCTURE OF A NERVE

A nerve contains bundles of nerve fibers, either axons or dendrites, surrounded by connective tissue. *Sensory nerves* contain only afferent fibers—long dendrites of sensory neurons. *Motor nerves* have only efferent fibers—long axons of motor neurons. *Mixed nerves* contain both types of fibers.

CRANIAL NERVES

Twelve pairs of cranial nerves, illustrated in Fig. 9.12, emerge from the inferior surface of the brain. All of these nerves

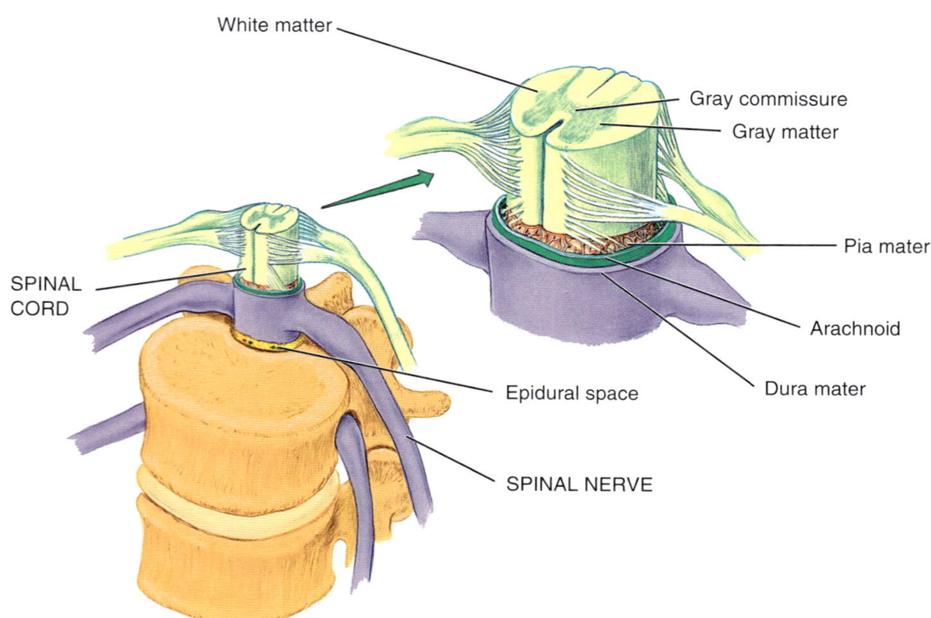

Fig. 9.11 Cross section of the spinal cord. (From Applegate E: *The anatomy and physiology learning system*, ed 4, St. Louis, 2011, Saunders.)

Table 9.5 Some Clinically Significant Reflexes

Reflex	Description	Indications
Patellar (knee-jerk reflex)	Stretch reflex; two-neuron path; reflex hammer strikes patellar tendon just below knee; receptors in quadriceps femoris muscle are stretched; reflex results in immediate "kick"	Reflex is blocked by damage to nerves involved and by damage to lumbar segments of spinal cord; also absent in people with chronic diabetes mellitus and neurosyphilis
Achilles tendon (ankle-jerk reflex)	Stretch reflex; two-neuron path; reflex hammer strikes Achilles tendon just above heel; gastrocnemius and soleus muscles contract to plantar flex foot	Weak or no reflex action indicates damage to nerves involved or to L5–S2 segments of spinal cord; also absent in chronic diabetes, neurosyphilis, and alcoholism
Abdominal	Stroking lateral abdominal wall produces reflex action that compresses abdominal wall and moves umbilicus toward stimulus	Absent in lesions of peripheral nerves, in lesions in thoracic segments of spinal cord, and in multiple sclerosis
Babinski	Lateral sole of foot is stroked from heel to toe; positive sign results in dorsiflexion of big toe and spreading of other toes; negative sign results in toes curling under with a light inversion of foot	Positive Babinski sign is normal in children younger than 18 months of age; negative sign is normal after 18 months of age; if motor tracts in spinal cord are damaged, positive Babinski sign reappears

From Applegate E: *The anatomy and physiology learning system*, ed 4, St. Louis, 2011, Saunders.

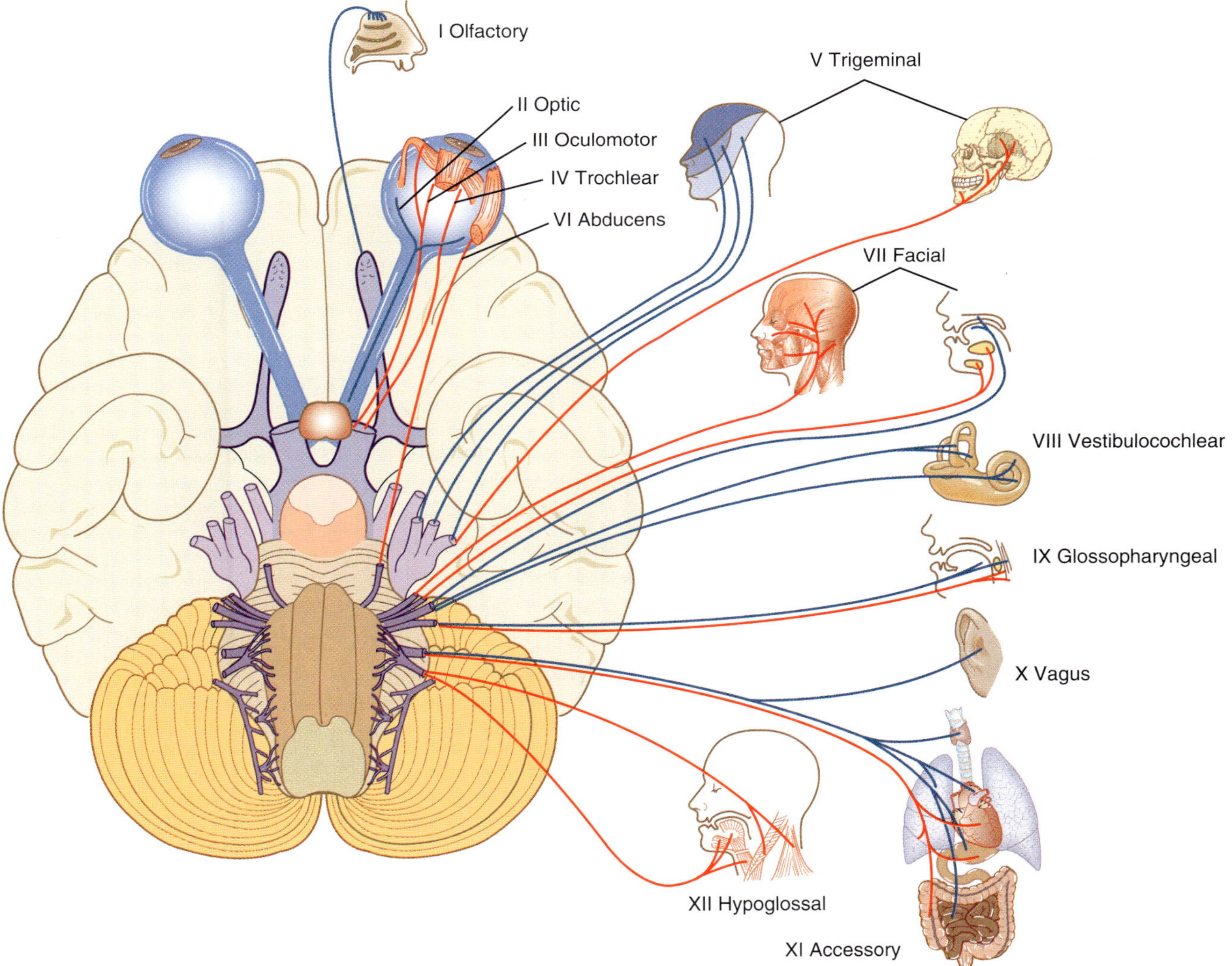

Fig. 9.12 Cranial nerves. The red lines indicate motor function and the blue lines indicate sensory function. (From Applegate E: *The anatomy and physiology learning system*, ed 4, St. Louis, 2011, Saunders.)

except the vagus nerve innervate structures in the head, neck, and facial region. The vagus nerve, cranial nerve X, has numerous branches that supply the viscera.

The cranial nerves are designated both by name and by Roman numerals, according to the order in which they appear on the inferior surface of the brain. Most of the nerves have both sensory and motor components. Three of the nerves (I, II, VIII) are associated with the special senses of smell, vision, hearing, and equilibrium and have only sensory fibers. Five other nerves (III, IV, VI, XI, XII) are primarily motor in function but do have some sensory fibers for proprioception. The remaining four nerves (V, VII, IX, X) consist of significant amounts of both sensory and motor fibers. Table 9.6 itemizes the cranial nerves.

SPINAL NERVES

Thirty-one pairs of spinal nerves emerge laterally from the spinal cord. Each pair of nerves corresponds to a segment of the cord, and the nerves are named accordingly. This means there are *eight cervical nerves* (C1 to C8), *12 thoracic nerves* (T1 to T12), *five lumbar nerves* (L1 to L5), *five sacral nerves* (S1 to S5), and *one coccygeal nerve* (Co).

Each spinal nerve is connected to the spinal cord by a *dorsal root* and a *ventral root*. The dorsal root has only sensory fibers, and the ventral root has only motor fibers. The two roots join to form the spinal nerve just before the nerve leaves the vertebral column. Because all spinal nerves have both sensory and motor components, they are all mixed nerves.

Immediately after they leave the vertebral column, the spinal nerves divide into several branches that provide the nerve supply to the muscles and the skin of the body wall. In the thoracic region, the main portions of the nerves go directly to the thoracic wall, where they are called *intercostal nerves*. In other regions, the main portions of the nerves form complex networks called *plexuses* (see Fig. 9.10). In the plexus, the fibers are sorted and recombined so that the fibers associated with a particular body part are together even though they may originate from different regions of the cord. The *cervical plexus* is located in the neck and sends nerves to the skin and muscles of the neck, shoulder, and diaphragm. The *brachial plexus* is deep to the clavicle and innervates the skin and muscles of the upper extremities. The *lumbosacral plexus* is in the lumbar region of the back. Nerves from this plexus go to the skin and muscles of the lower abdominal wall, the lower extremities, the buttocks, and the external genitalia.

Table 9.6 Summary of Cranial Nerves

Number	Name	Type	Function
I	Olfactory	Sensory	Sense of smell
II	Optic	Sensory	Vision
III	Oculomotor	Primarily motor	Movement of eyes and eyelids
IV	Trochlear	Primarily motor	Movement of eyes
V	Trigeminal	Mixed	
	Ophthalmic branch		Sensory fibers from cornea, skin of nose, forehead, and scalp
	Maxillary branch		Sensory fibers from cheek, nose, upper lip, and teeth
	Mandibular branch		Sensory fibers from skin over mandible, lower lip, and teeth
			Motor fibers to muscles of mastication
VI	Abducens	Primarily motor	Eye movement
VII	Facial	Mixed	Sensory fibers from taste receptors on anterior two-thirds of tongue
			Motor fibers to muscles of facial expression, lacrimal glands, and salivary glands
VIII	Vestibulocochlear	Sensory	Hearing and equilibrium
IX	Glossopharyngeal	Mixed	Sensory fibers from taste receptors on posterior one third of tongue
			Motor fibers to muscles used in swallowing and to salivary glands
X	Vagus	Mixed	Sensory fibers from pharynx, larynx, esophagus, and visceral organs
			Somatic motor fibers to muscles of pharynx and larynx
			Autonomic motor fibers to heart, smooth muscles, and glands to alter gastric motility, heart rate, respiration, and blood pressure
XI	Accessory	Primarily motor	Contraction of trapezius and sternocleidomastoid muscles
XII	Hypoglossal	Primarily motor	Contraction of muscles of tongue

From Applegate E: *The anatomy and physiology learning system*, ed 4, St. Louis, 2011, Saunders.

AUTONOMIC NERVOUS SYSTEM

General Features

The ANS is a visceral efferent system, which means it sends motor impulses to the visceral organs. It functions automatically and continuously, without conscious effort, to innervate smooth muscle, cardiac muscle, and glands. It is concerned with heart rate, breathing rate, blood pressure, body temperature, and other visceral activities that work together to maintain homeostasis.

The ANS has two parts: the *sympathetic division* and the *parasympathetic division* (Table 9.7). Many visceral organs are supplied with fibers from both divisions *(dual innervation)*. In this case, one stimulates and the other inhibits. This antagonistic functional relationship serves as a balance to help maintain homeostasis.

Sympathetic Division

The sympathetic division, illustrated in Fig. 9.13, is concerned primarily with preparing the body for stressful or emergency situations. Sometimes called the *fight-or-flight system*, it is an energy-expending system. It stimulates the responses that are necessary to meet the emergency and inhibits the visceral activities that can be delayed momentarily. For example, during an emergency the sympathetic system increases breathing rate, heart rate, and blood flow to skeletal muscles. At the same time it decreases activity in the digestive tract because that is not necessary to meet the emergency.

The sympathetic preganglionic fibers arise from the thoracic and lumbar regions of the spinal cord; thus the sympathetic division is sometimes called the *thoracolumbar division.*

Parasympathetic Division

The parasympathetic division is most active under ordinary, relaxed conditions (see Fig. 9.13). It also brings the body's systems back to a normal state after an emergency by slowing the heart and breathing rates, decreasing blood pressure, decreasing blood flow to skeletal muscles, and increasing digestive tract activity. Sometimes called the *rest-and-repose system*, it is an energy-conserving system.

The parasympathetic preganglionic fibers arise from the brain stem and sacral region of the spinal cord; thus the parasympathetic division is sometimes called the *craniosacral division.*

AGING OF THE NERVOUS SYSTEM

Aging of the nervous system is of major importance because changes in this system affect organs in other systems and can cause disturbances of many bodily functions. For example, changes in nerves decrease stimulation of skeletal muscle, which contributes to muscle atrophy with age. Because of its widespread consequences, aging of the nervous system is one of the most distressing aspects of growing old.

Like other cells, nerve cells are lost as a person ages, even in the absence of disease processes. Because neurons are amitotic, those that are lost are not replaced. Loss of neurons is largely responsible for the decrease in brain mass that occurs with aging. Fortunately, the brain has a large reserve

Table 9.7 Comparison of Sympathetic and Parasympathetic Actions on Selected Visceral Effectors

Visceral Effectors	Sympathetic Action	Parasympathetic Action
Pupil of eye	Dilates	Constricts
Lens of eye	Lens flattens for distance vision	Lens bulges for near vision
Sweat glands	Stimulates	No innervation
Arrector pili muscles of hair	Stimulates contraction; goose bumps	No innervation
Heart	Increases heart rate	Decreases heart rate
Bronchi	Dilates	Constricts
Digestive glands	Decreases secretion of digestive enzymes	Increases secretion of digestive enzymes
Digestive tract	Decreases peristalsis	Increases peristalsis
Digestive tract sphincters	Stimulates—closes sphincters	Inhibits—opens sphincters
Blood vessels to digestive organs	Constricts	No innervation
Blood vessels to skeletal muscles	Dilates	No innervation
Blood vessels to skin	Constricts	No innervation
Adrenal medulla	Stimulates secretion of epinephrine	No innervation
Liver	Increases release of glucose	No innervation
Urinary bladder	Relaxes bladder and closes sphincter	Contracts bladder and opens sphincter

From Applegate E: *The anatomy and physiology learning system*, ed 4, St. Louis, 2011, Saunders.

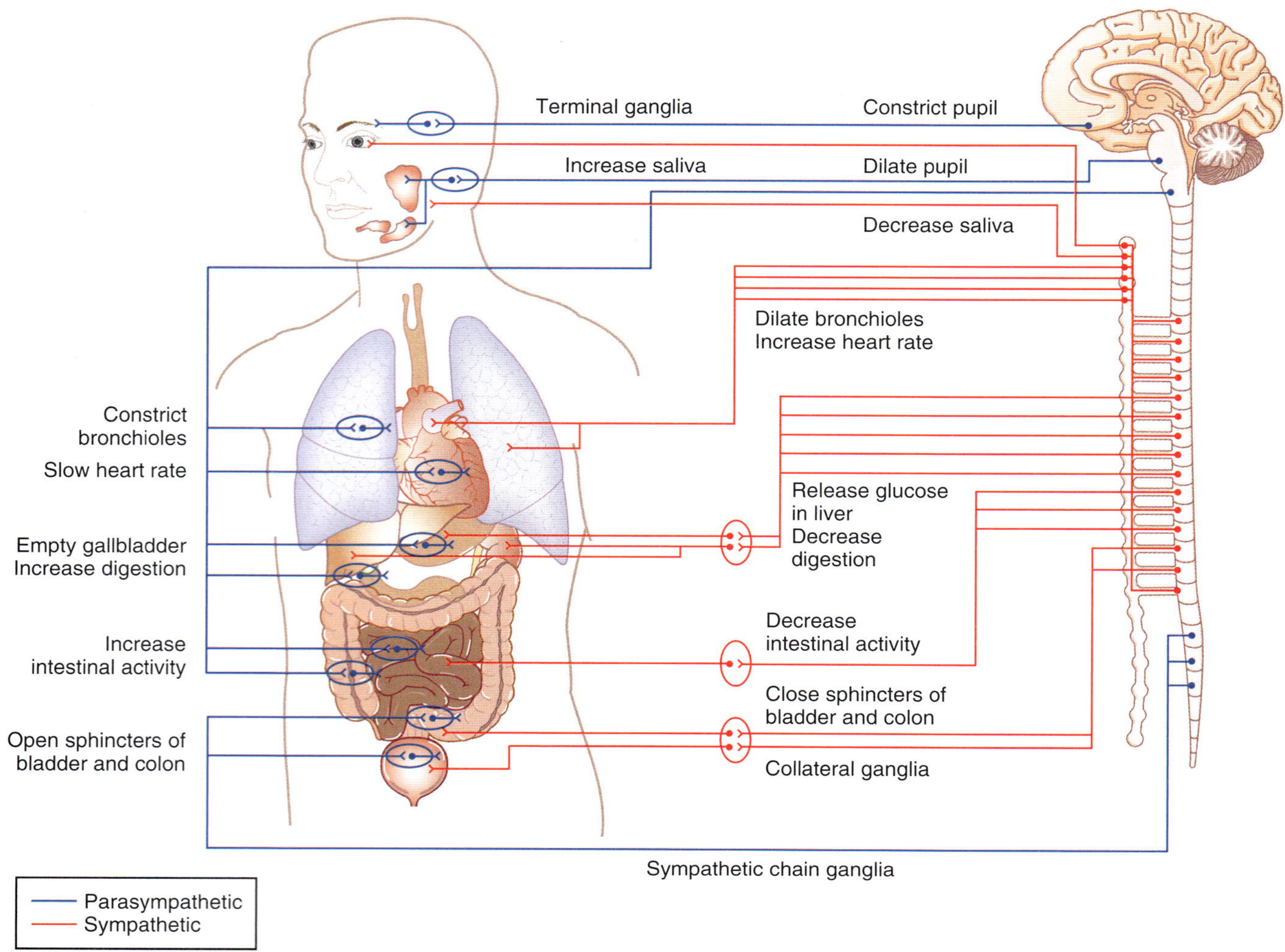

Fig. 9.13 Structure and function of autonomic nervous system. The red lines indicate the sympathetic division and the blue lines indicate parasympathetic innervations. Note the location of the ganglia for each division. (From Applegate E: *The anatomy and physiology learning system*, ed 4, St. Louis, 2011, Saunders.)

supply of neurons, many more than are necessary to carry out its functions, so the decrease in neuron number alone is not devastating. The loss of neurons is not constant in all areas of the brain. For example, about 25% of the specialized cells in the cerebellum, which are responsible for coordinated movements, are lost during aging. This may affect balance and cause difficulty in coordinating fine movements. In other areas of the brain, the number of neurons remains essentially constant throughout life.

It is generally accepted that there is a decline in intelligence with aging, and this is thought to be associated with the loss of neurons. However, it is important to remember that there are wide variations in individuals regarding changes in intellect with age. Because a person is old does not mean that person is "dumb." Many elderly people retain a keen intellect until death. Along with the decline in intelligence, there may be a general decline in memory. Again, this varies from person to person. In general, short-term memory seems to be affected more than long-term memory. Intellect and memory appear to be retained better in people who remain mentally and physically active.

Another change observed in older people is a decrease in the rate of impulse conduction along an axon and across a synapse. A reduction in the amount of myelin around the axon probably accounts for the diminished conduction rate along the axon. Decreases in the quantity of neurotransmitter and in the number of receptor sites cause slower conduction across the synapses. These factors contribute to the slower reflexes and the longer time required to process information that are observed in many elderly people.

Common Pathology of the Nervous System

Disease	Signs and Symptoms	Etiology	Diagnosis and Treatment
Hydrocephalus	Signs and symptoms vary with age of onset. Infants: unusually large head and bulging fontanels. Toddlers: headache, blurred vision, poor coordination. Adults: distorted vision, poor coordination and balance, memory loss.	Caused by an accumulation of CSF in the brain as a result of overproduction, reduced absorption into the blood, or blockage in the pathway of flow. The accumulation of CSF increases pressure on the brain and destroys brain tissue.	Diagnosis is based on physical examination, neurologic examination, and brain imaging techniques. The most common treatment is the surgical insertion of a shunt system to increase the drainage of CSF.
Carpal tunnel syndrome	Tingling or numbness in the fingers and hand; weakness in the wrist and hand.	The condition is caused by compression of the median nerve as it passes through the carpal tunnel in the wrist.	Diagnosis is based on history, physical examinations, x-ray studies, EMG, and nerve conduction studies. Treatment begins with rest and ice for the affected wrist; wrist splinting and drugs to reduce inflammation and swelling may be beneficial. In severe cases, surgery may be necessary to relieve the pressure on the median nerve.
Dementia	A widespread group of disorders characterized by damage to nerve cells in the brain resulting in memory loss, impaired judgment or language, inability to perform daily activities, easily becoming disoriented, inability to reason, paranoia, and agitation. Some forms are progressive.	There are numerous causes including accumulation of toxic substances in the brain and reduced blood supply to the brain; it may also be secondary to other conditions.	Diagnosis is difficult. The health care professional may use a combination of medical history, physical examination, cognitive and neuropsychologic tests, brain scans, and laboratory tests. Most types of dementia cannot be cured. Treatment protocols focus on managing the symptoms.
Alzheimer disease	The most common form of progressive dementia. Signs and symptoms include memory loss, impaired judgment or language, inability to perform daily activities, easily becoming disoriented, inability to reason, paranoia, and agitation.	Caused by a progressive destruction of brain cells. Hallmark abnormalities in the brain include plaques of protein fragments called *β-amyloid*, tangles of protein fragments called *τ*, and a loss of connections among brain cells.	Diagnosis is difficult. The health care professional may use a combination of medical history, physical examination, cognitive and neuropsychologic tests, brain scans, and laboratory tests. Treatment protocols focus on managing the symptoms and keeping the individual comfortable and physically healthy.
Epilepsy	Seizures of epilepsy can produce symptoms such as temporary confusion, staring spells, uncontrollable jerking movements of the arms and legs, loss of consciousness or awareness, and psychic symptoms. Focal seizures originate in one area of the brain; generalized seizures involve all areas of the brain.	Epilepsy is a CNS disorder in which the nerve cell activity in the brain is disturbed. In about half of the cases, there is no identifiable cause. In the other half, there may be genetic factors, head trauma, brain tumor or stroke, infectious diseases, prenatal injury, or developmental disorders.	Diagnosis is based on medical history, neurologic examination, blood tests, EEG, and a variety of imaging modalities. Many patients can be treated with antiseizure medications. Others may require surgery.
Bell palsy	Paralysis of the muscles on one side of the face with sagging of the mouth on the affected side; difficulty making facial expressions.	Caused by neuropathy of cranial nerve VII; cause of the neuropathy unknown; may be result of a viral infection.	No specific diagnostic test for Bell palsy; health professional may order EMG or an imaging scan. Many cases resolve spontaneously. Treatment options include corticosteroids, antiviral drugs, and physical therapy to restore muscle function.
Cerebral concussion	Symptoms range from mild to severe and may include fuzzy or blurry vision, headache, dizziness, nausea and vomiting, sensitivity to light or noise, sleep disturbances, and inability to concentrate.	Caused by a traumatic blow to the head that causes the brain to impact against the skull.	Diagnosis is based on physical and neurologic findings. Initial treatment consists of observation to make sure the condition does not become more serious. Physical and cognitive rest usually allows the condition to resolve within 7–10 days.

Continued

Common Pathology of the Nervous System—cont'd

Disease	Signs and Symptoms	Etiology	Diagnosis and Treatment
Sciatica	Pain that radiates from the lumbar spine to the buttocks and down the back of the leg to the foot; varies from a mild ache to a sharp, burning type of pain.	Occurs when the sciatic nerve becomes pinched or compressed from a herniated disc, bone spur, or tumor.	For a diagnosis, the health professional will test muscle strength and reflexes. If the pain is severe and persists, imaging scans may be used. Treatment, if necessary, may include muscle relaxants, anti-inflammatory drugs, and physical therapy. In some cases injections of corticosteroids may be recommended.
Neuralgia	Sharp, shocking pain that follows the path of a nerve; increased sensitivity to the skin along the path of the nerve; weakness or paralysis of the muscles supplied by the nerve; nerve pain.	Causes include chemical irritation, renal insufficiency, infections, trauma, and pressure on a nerve; in many cases the cause is unknown.	No specific tests for neuralgia. Diagnosis depends on history and physical examination; blood tests, EMG, and MRI may help locate the underlying cause of the pain. Pain relievers may help reduce the pain. Treatment should attempt to reverse or control the underlying cause of the pain.
Cerebral palsy	Signs and symptoms usually appear during infancy or early childhood and may include exaggerated reflexes, abnormalities in muscle tone, abnormal posture, tremors or involuntary movements, unsteadiness in walking, and stiff muscles.	Caused by an abnormality or disruption in brain development, usually in utero. The trigger for the disruption is unknown but may include mutations, fetal stroke, infant infections, lack of oxygen during a difficult delivery, or traumatic head injury.	The child is usually referred to a pediatric neurologist for diagnosis. A combination of medical history, physical examination, brain scans, and EEG is used. A cerebral palsy patient requires long-term care by a team of health professionals including physical therapists, occupational therapists, and speech therapists. Medications may lessen the muscle rigidity. Severe contractures may require surgery.
Cerebrovascular accident (CVA)	Symptoms depend on the area of the brain affected. A convenient system is FAST: *F*acial muscle weakness, *A*rm droop, *S*peech abnormalities, *T*ime to rush to the emergency room.	Most common brain disorder; may be caused either by a decrease in blood supply to the brain (ischemic) or rupture of a blood vessel in the brain (hemorrhagic). Risk factors include hypertension, elevated blood lipids, and diabetes mellitus. Commonly called a *stroke*.	Diagnosis involves a neurologic examination, CT and/or MRI scans, Doppler ultrasound, and arteriography. Treatment options depend on the type and severity of the CVA. For the ischemic type, intervention restores blood flow; for the hemorrhagic type it may be necessary to reduce the pressure on the brain. Long-term stroke rehabilitation attempts to help patients return to normal life as much as possible.
Tic douloureux (trigeminal neuralgia)	Characterized by unilateral, intense, sharp, stabbing pain most commonly felt in the cheek, nose, upper lip, and upper teeth. A muscle spasm accompanies the pain.	Pain is caused by irritation of the trigeminal nerve (V), possibly by a blood vessel pressing on the nerve or other injury.	Diagnosis is based on symptoms, physical and neurologic examinations, and possibly CT and/or MRI scans. There is no specific test to confirm a diagnosis. Treatment options include medications that decrease the ability of the trigeminal nerve to fire off the impulses that cause the pain; muscle relaxants; and narcotic pain relievers. If medications are not effective, surgical procedures on the trigeminal nerve may be necessary.
Reye syndrome (RS)	Disorientation, lethargy, weakness or paralysis in arms and legs, and personality changes; may progress to a coma. Occurs primarily in children.	Exact cause is unknown. Seems to be triggered by use of aspirin to treat a viral illness, particularly influenza and chickenpox, especially in children with an underlying disorder in fatty acid metabolism. Exposure to toxins such as insecticides, herbicides, and paint thinner may be a contributing factor.	There is no specific test for RS. Screening for RS usually begins with blood and urine tests and tests for disorders in fatty acid oxidation. Treatment includes intravenous fluids, diuretics, antiseizure medications, and medications to prevent bleeding.

Common Pathology of the Nervous System—cont'd

Disease	Signs and Symptoms	Etiology	Diagnosis and Treatment
Transient ischemic attack (TIA)	Temporary cerebral dysfunction of sudden onset and short duration; like a stroke but with no permanent damage. Symptoms include weakness of facial and arm muscles, altered speech, blurred vision, and dizziness or loss of balance or coordination.	Common causes are blood clots and atherosclerosis that disrupt blood flow to the brain.	Because TIA is of short duration, diagnosis is based on medical history. The physician will use blood tests and imaging tests to determine underlying cause. Treatment is aimed at correcting the abnormality that caused the TIA and preventing a stroke. Antiplatelet drugs (aspirin) and anticoagulants may suffice. Other options are angioplasty and carotid endarterectomy.
Shingles	Blisters and pain spread over the skin in a bandlike pattern that follows the path of affected nerves.	Caused by the varicella zoster (herpes zoster) virus, the same virus that causes chickenpox. After causing chickenpox, the virus lies dormant for years, only to reappear as shingles. The cause for reappearance is unknown but may be a result of lowered immunity.	Diagnosis is based on history, location of pain, and pattern of rash or blisters. There is no cure. Antiviral medications speed healing and reduce complications. Pain relievers help alleviate the pain.
Multiple sclerosis	Signs and symptoms include numbness or weakness in the extremities, double vision or total loss of vision, slurred speech, fatigue, dizziness, tremors, and a lack of coordination. There is progressive loss of function with periods of remission.	Progressive destruction of the myelin sheaths of the neurons in the CNS. Cause of destruction is unknown, but evidence suggests that the disease may be an autoimmune disorder. Destruction of myelin interferes with the neuron's ability to conduct impulses.	Diagnosis is based on medical history and physical examination. Blood tests, CSF analysis, and imaging scans may be used to rule out other conditions. There is no cure. Treatment focuses on managing the symptoms and slowing the progression of the disorder. Corticosteroids reduce the inflammation during attacks; immunosuppressants slow the progress; physical therapy and muscle relaxants reduce muscle stiffness.
Parkinson disease	Signs and symptoms include tremors, altered speech patterns, lack of facial expression, cognitive impairment, dysphagia, and emotional disorders. Occurs more frequently in men than in women. Signs and symptoms become more pronounced as disease progresses.	Neurons in the basal ganglia do not produce enough of the inhibitory transmitter dopamine, allowing excess excitatory signals to certain voluntary muscles. The reason for the lack of dopamine is unknown.	No specific test for Parkinson disease. Neurologist relies on the signs and symptoms, medical history, and physical examination. Other tests may be used to eliminate other conditions. There is no known cure, but levodopa and dopamine agonists may help control symptoms.
Amyotrophic lateral sclerosis (ALS)(Lou Gehrig disease)	Characterized by progressive muscular weakness and atrophy with spasticity and exaggerated reflexes. Early signs are muscle twitching in arms and legs; slurred speech. Eventually, there is inability to control muscles needed to move, speak, eat, and breathe.	Results from a degeneration of motor neurons in the CNS. The cause is unknown. Suggested causes are gene mutation, a chemical imbalance in the system that is toxic to neurons, and an autoimmune response.	No specific test that will confirm a diagnosis. Neurologist relies on a combination of signs and symptoms, medical history, physical examination, EMG, and nerve conduction studies. Treatment focuses on slowing the progress of the disease and managing complications. Medications may provide relief from symptoms; physical therapy addresses the mobility problems; breathing exercises may help when the respiratory muscles are involved. There is no known cure, and the disease eventually leads to death.

CSF, Cerebrospinal fluid; *CNS*, central nervous system; *CT*, computed tomography; *EEG*, electroencephalography; *EMG*, electromyography; *MRI*, magnetic resonance imaging.

TERMINOLOGY REVIEW

Key Term	Word Parts	Definition
Action potential	*act-:* motion	A nerve impulse; a rapid change in membrane potential that involves depolarization and repolarization.
Axons		The efferent processes of neurons that carry impulses away from the cell bodies.
Basal ganglia	*gangli-:* knot	Paired regions of gray matter located within the white matter of the cerebrum.
Brain stem		The portion of the brain, between the diencephalon and spinal cord, that contains the midbrain, pons, and medulla oblongata.
Central sulcus	*sulc-:* furrow, ditch	The groove or furrow between the frontal and parietal lobes of the cerebrum; also called the *fissure of Rolando.*
Cerebellum	*cerebell/o:* cerebellum	Second largest part of the human brain, located posterior to the pons and medulla oblongata and involved in the coordination of muscular movements.
Cerebrospinal fluid	*cerebr/o:* cerebrum	A fluid, similar to plasma, that fills the subarachnoid space around the brain and spinal cord and is in the ventricles of the brain.
Cerebrum	*cerebr/o:* cerebrum	The largest and uppermost part of the human brain; concerned with consciousness, learning, memory, sensations, and voluntary movements.
Dendrites	*dendr-:* tree	The branching (treelike) afferent processes of a neuron that receive impulses from other neurons and transmit them to the cell body.
Decussation		A crossing over; usually refers to motor fibers that cross over to the opposite side in the medulla oblongata.
Diencephalon	*cephal/o:* head	Part of the brain between the cerebral hemispheres and the midbrain; includes the thalamus and hypothalamus.
Myelin		White fatty substance that surrounds many nerve fibers.
Neurilemma	*neur/o:* nerve *-lemma:* sheath, covering	The layer of cells that surrounds a nerve fiber in the peripheral nervous system and in some cases produces myelin; also called *Schwann sheath.*
Neuroglia	*neur/o:* nerve *gli/a:* glue	Supporting cells of nervous tissue; cells in nervous tissue that do not conduct impulses.
Neuron	*neur/o:* nerve	Nerve cell including its processes; conducting cell of nervous tissue.
Neurotransmitters	*neur/o:* nerve	A chemical substance that is released from axon terminals to stimulate muscle fiber contraction or an impulse in another neuron.
Nodes of Ranvier		Short spaces between segments of myelin in a myelinated nerve fiber.
Refractory period		Time during which an excitable cell cannot respond to a stimulus that is usually adequate to initiate an action potential.
Saltatory conduction	*-tion:* process of	Process in which a nerve impulse travels along a myelinated nerve fiber by jumping from one node of Ranvier to the next.
Somatomotor cortex	*somat/o:* body	The primary motor area of the brain; located in the precentral gyrus; transmits motor impulses to the body.
Somatosensory cortex	*somat/o:* body	The primary sensory area of the brain; located in the postcentral gyrus; receives sensory impulses from the body.
Synapse	*syn-:* together, with	The region of communication between two neurons.
Threshold stimulus		Minimum level of stimulation that is required to start a nerve impulse or muscle contraction; also called *liminal stimulus.*

The Senses

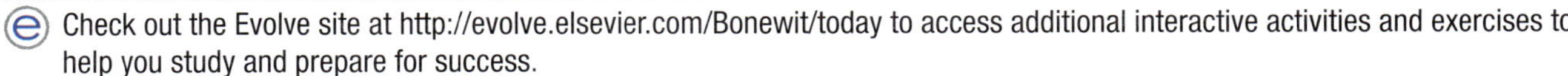

Check out the Evolve site at http://evolve.elsevier.com/Bonewit/today to access additional interactive activities and exercises to help you study and prepare for success.

LEARNING OBJECTIVES

1. Explain the difference between general senses and special senses, and give examples of each.
2. List and describe the five groups of sense receptors.
3. Identify the sense receptors for touch, pressure, proprioception, temperature, and pain.
4. List and identify the location of the four different taste sensations.
5. Locate the sense receptors for smell and trace the impulse pathway to the cerebral cortex.
6. Describe the structure of the eye and explain the function of each structure.
7. Explain how light is focused on the retina.
8. Explain the function of the rods and cones, photoreceptor cells in the retina.
9. Explain how nerve impulses for sight are initiated in response to light.
10. Describe the structure of the ear and explain the function of each structure.
11. Explain how nerve impulses for hearing are initiated in response to sound waves.
12. Explain the difference between static and dynamic equilibrium.
13. Explain how impulses for static and dynamic equilibrium are initiated.
14. Describe ways in which aging affects the senses.
15. Identify pathology related to the senses.

CHAPTER OUTLINE

KEY TERMS

accommodation (ah-kahm-oh-DAY-shun)
bulbus oculi (BUL-bus AHK-yoo-lye)
chemoreceptor (kee-moh-ree-SEP-tor)
cochlea (KOK-lee-ah)
crista ampullaris (KRIS-tah amp-yoo-LAIR-is)
general senses (JEN-er-uhl SEN-sez)
gustatory sense (GUS-tah-toar-ee SENS)
lacrimal apparatus (LACK-rih-mal ap-pah-RAT-us)
macula lutea (MACK-yoo-lah LOO-tee-ah)
mechanoreceptors (mek-ah-noh-ree-SEP-tors)

nociceptors (noh-see-SEP-tors)
olfaction (ohl-FAK-shun)
otoliths (OH-toe-liths)
photoreceptors (foh-toh-ree-SEP-tors)
proprioception (proh-pree-oh-SEP-shun)
refraction (ree-FRAK-shun)
rhodopsin (roe-DOP-sin)
sensory adaptation (SEN-soh-ree add-dap-TAY-shun)
special senses (SPESH-uhl SEN-sez)
thermoreceptors (ther-moh-ree-SEP-tors)

INTRODUCTION TO THE SENSES

Sensory perception depends on receptors that respond to various stimuli. When a stimulus triggers an impulse in a receptor, the action potentials travel to the cerebral cortex, where they are processed and interpreted. Only after this has occurred is a particular sensation perceived. Some senses—such as pain, touch, pressure, and proprioception—are widely distributed in the body. These are called **general senses**. Other senses—such as taste, smell, hearing, and sight—are called **special senses** because their receptors are localized in a particular area.

RECEPTORS AND SENSATIONS

Although there are many different kinds of sense receptors, they can be grouped into five types. The basis for these receptor types is the kind of stimulus to which they are sensitive or for which they have a low threshold. The five types of receptors are chemoreceptors, mechanoreceptors, nociceptors, thermoreceptors, and photoreceptors (Table 10.1).

Perceived sensation occurs only after impulses have been interpreted by the brain. Steps involved in sensory perception include the following:

First there is a *stimulus*.

1. A *receptor* detects the stimulus and creates an action potential.
2. The action potential (impulse) is *conducted* to the central nervous system (CNS).
3. Within the CNS, the impulse is *translated* into information.
4. Information is *interpreted* in the CNS into an awareness or perception of the stimulus.

The impulses from all the receptors are alike. The difference in perception is where they are interpreted in the brain. For example, all impulses going to one particular region are interpreted as sound, whereas those going to another region are interpreted as taste. As the brain interprets a sensation, it projects that sense back to its original source so that the "feeling" seems to come from the receptors that are stimulated. This projection allows us to locate the source of the stimulus.

Some sense receptors undergo **sensory adaptation** when they are continually stimulated. They develop a decreased sensitivity to a continued stimulus and trigger impulses only if the strength of the stimulus is increased.

Table 10.1 Types of Sense Receptors

Receptor	Stimulus	Example
Chemoreceptors	Changes in chemical concentration of substances	Taste and smell
Mechanoreceptors	Changes in pressure or movement in fluids	Proprioceptors in joints, receptors for hearing and equilibrium
Nociceptors	Tissue damage	Pain receptors
Thermoreceptors	Changes in temperature	Heat and cold
Photoreceptors	Light energy	Vision

From Applegate E: *The anatomy and physiology learning system*, ed 4, St. Louis, 2011, Saunders.

GENERAL SENSES

General senses, or *somatic senses*, are those that are found throughout the body. They are associated with the visceral organs as well as the skin, muscles, and joints; they include touch, pressure, proprioception, temperature, and pain.

TOUCH AND PRESSURE

As a group, the receptors for touch and pressure are **mechanoreceptors**, which are sensitive to forces that deform or displace tissues. They are widely distributed in the skin. Three of the mechanoreceptors involved in touch and pressure are free nerve endings, Meissner corpuscles, and pacinian corpuscles.

Free nerve endings are the dendritic ends of sensory neurons that are interspersed among the cells in epithelial tissue. They do not have a connective tissue covering. They are important in sensing objects, such as clothing, that are in continuous contact with the skin. *Meissner corpuscles* consist of the ends of sensory nerve fibers surrounded by connective tissue and are specific in localizing tactile sensations. They are located in the dermal papillae, just beneath the epidermis, where they are important in sensing light-discriminative touch stimuli. *Pacinian corpuscles* are called *lamellated corpuscles* because several layers of connective tissue surround the nerve endings. These are common in deeper dermis and subcutaneous tissues, tendons, and ligaments. They are stimulated by heavy pressure.

PROPRIOCEPTION

Proprioception is the sense of position or orientation. It allows us to sense the location and rate of movement of one body part relative to another. *Golgi tendon organs*, found at the junction of a tendon with a muscle, and *muscle spindles*, located in skeletal muscles, are important mechanoreceptors for proprioception.

TEMPERATURE

Thermoreceptors are located immediately under the skin and are widely distributed throughout the body. They are most numerous on the lips and are least numerous on some of the broad surfaces of the trunk. Thermoreceptors include at least two types of free nerve endings that are sensitive to temperature changes. In general, there are up to 10 times more *cold receptors* in a given area than *heat receptors*. Extremes in temperature stimulate pain receptors. A person determines gradations in temperatures by the degree of stimulation of each type of receptor. Extreme cold and extreme heat feel almost the same—both are painful—because the pain receptors are being stimulated. Thermoreceptors are strongly stimulated by abrupt changes in temperature and then fade after a few seconds or minutes. In other words, thermoreceptors show rapid *sensory adaptation*.

PAIN

The sense of pain is initiated by **nociceptors**, which are free nerve endings that are stimulated by tissue damage. They are widely distributed throughout the skin and in the tissues of the internal organs. The nervous tissue of the brain has no pain receptors; however, other tissues in the head, including the meninges and blood vessels, have an abundant supply. Pain receptors have a protective function because pain is usually perceived as unpleasant and is a signal to locate and remove the source of the tissue damage. Nociceptors usually do not adapt and may continue to send signals after the stimulus has been removed.

GUSTATORY SENSE

The **gustatory sense**, or *taste*, is one of the special senses. As previously explained, the senses of taste, smell, hearing, and sight are called *special senses* because their receptors are localized in a particular area.

The organs of taste, the *taste buds*, are localized in the mouth region, primarily on the surface of the tongue, where they lie along the walls of projections called *papillae* (Fig. 10.1).

The receptors belong to the **chemoreceptor** category because they are sensitive to chemicals in the food we eat. For these chemicals to be detected by a chemoreceptor, they must be dissolved in water.

Within the taste bud, specialized epithelial cells called *gustatory cells* or *taste cells* are interspersed with supporting cells and nerve fibers (see Fig. 10.1). The entire taste bud opens to the surface through a *taste pore*. Tiny *taste hairs* project from the taste cells through the taste pore, and it is these hairs on the taste cells that function as the receptors.

Although all the taste receptors appear to be alike, there are at least four different types, each one sensitive to a

HIGHLIGHT on the Senses

Odors: Nearly everyone is familiar with sensory adaptation in the sense of smell. A particular odor becomes unnoticed after a short time, even though the odor molecules are still present in the air, because the system quickly adapts to the continued stimulation. Odors have the quality of being interpreted as pleasant or unpleasant. Because of this, the sense of smell is as important as taste in the selection of food. For example, a person who has become sick after eating a certain type of food is often nauseated by the smell of that same food on a later occasion.

Cold adaptation: When a person first enters a cool swimming pool on a hot day, they experience an abrupt change in temperature; therefore the cold receptors are strongly stimulated and there is a feeling of discomfort. After a brief time, the receptors adapt, the stimulation fades, and the cool water feels comfortable.

Headache: If there are no pain receptors in the nervous tissue of the brain, what are headaches? Headaches are a type of referred pain, pain that is referred to the surface of the head from deeper structures. The pain stimuli may originate in the meninges or blood vessels within the cranium. Other pain stimuli may originate outside the cranium from muscular spasms, the nasal sinuses, or the eyes.

Bitter taste: The taste receptors with the highest degree of sensitivity are those that are stimulated by bitter substances, and a highly intense bitter taste usually causes a person to reject that substance. This is probably an important protective mechanism because many of the deadly toxins found in poisonous plants have an intensely bitter taste.

Blinking: The eye blinks 6 to 30 times a minute. Blinking stimulates the lacrimal glands to secrete a sterile fluid, or "tears," and helps move the fluid across the eyes.

Corneal transplant: The cornea was one of the first organs transplanted. Surgical removal of deteriorating corneas and replacement with donor corneas is a common medical procedure for several reasons. The cornea is readily accessible and relatively easy to remove. The tissue is avascular, so there is no bleeding problem or difficulty in establishing circulatory pathways. Corneas are less active than other tissues immunologically and are less likely to be rejected. Long-term success after corneal implant surgery is excellent.

Pupil size: In addition to regulating the amount of light that enters the eye, pupillary reflexes may also reflect interest or emotional state. For example, frequently the pupils dilate during problem solving or when the subject is appealing. If the subject is boring or repulsive, the pupils constrict. ■

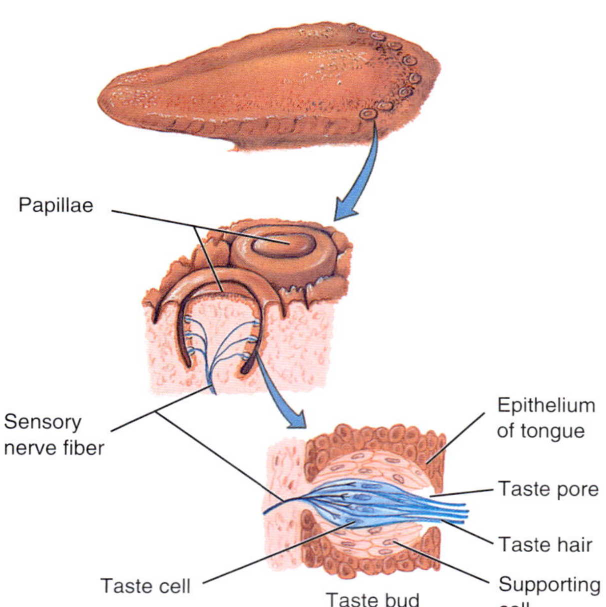

Fig. 10.1 Taste buds on the papillae of the tongue. The taste hairs on taste (gustatory) cells are the receptors for taste. (From Applegate E: *The anatomy and physiology learning system,* ed 4, St. Louis, 2011, Saunders.)

particular kind of stimulus. Consequently there are four different taste sensations: salty, sweet, sour, and bitter.

When the taste hairs, are stimulated, an impulse is triggered on a nearby nerve fiber. Impulses from the anterior two-thirds of the tongue travel along the *facial nerve*, and those from the posterior one-third travel along the *glossopharyngeal nerve*. The impulses are interpreted in the sensory cortex on the parietal lobe of the cerebrum, near the lateral sulcus.

OLFACTORY SENSE

The receptors for **olfaction** (sense of smell) are neurons in the *olfactory epithelium* of the nasal cavity. The *olfactory neurons* are concentrated in the superior region of the cavity. These neurons have long cilia that extend to the surface and project into the nasal cavity. They are believed to be the sense receptors of the neuron.

Like those for taste, the olfactory receptors are *chemoreceptors*. They are stimulated by chemicals dissolved in liquids. In this case, airborne molecules responsible for odors dissolve in the fluid on the surface of the olfactory epithelium and then bind to the receptors and trigger impulses. Axons from the olfactory neurons pass through foramina in the ethmoid bone and enter the olfactory bulb of the olfactory nerve (cranial nerve I). Here they synapse with association neurons that conduct the impulses to the olfactory cortex in the temporal lobe, where they are interpreted.

The senses of taste and smell are closely related and complement each other. They often have a combined effect when they are interpreted in the cerebral cortex. This implies that part of what we "taste" is really smell. Also, part of what we "smell" is taste, because some airborne molecules move from the nose down to the mouth and stimulate taste buds.

VISUAL SENSE

Most of us consider vision to be one of the most important senses we have. The eyes, which contain the **photoreceptors**, are the organs of vision. They are protected by a bony socket and assisted in their function of vision by accessory structures that protect and move them.

PROTECTIVE FEATURES AND ACCESSORY STRUCTURES OF THE EYE

Only a small portion of the eye is visible from the exterior. Most of it is surrounded by a protective bony orbit, or socket, that is formed by portions of seven cranial bones (frontal, lacrimal, ethmoid, maxilla, zygomatic, sphenoid, and palatine). The eye also contains fat, various connective tissues, blood vessels, and nerves.

Eyebrows help to keep perspiration, which can be an irritant, out of the eyes. Eyelids function to open and close the eye and to keep foreign objects from entering it. The muscles associated with the eyelids are the *orbicularis oculi*, which is a sphincter that closes the eye, and the *levator palpebrae superioris*, which elevates the eyelid to open the eye. The *conjunctiva*, a thin mucous membrane, lines the eyelid and then folds back to cover the anterior part of the eyeball except for the central portion, which is the cornea. Mucus from the conjunctiva helps keep the eye from drying out. Eyelashes line the margin of the eyelid and help trap foreign particles. Sebaceous glands associated with the eyelashes secrete an oily fluid that helps lubricate the region. Inflammation of the sebaceous glands is called a *stye*.

The **lacrimal apparatus**, shown in Fig. 10.2, consists of the *lacrimal gland* and various ducts. The *lacrimal gland* is located in the superior and lateral region of the orbit. Tears produced by the lacrimal gland flow through lacrimal ducts and across the surface of the eye to the medial side, where they drain into two small lacrimal canals. From the lacrimal canals, the tears flow into the lacrimal sac and then into the nasolacrimal duct, which opens into the nasal cavity. Tears moisten, lubricate, and cleanse the anterior surface of the eye. Tears also contain an enzyme (lysozyme) that helps destroy bacteria and prevent infections.

STRUCTURE OF THE EYEBALL

The eyeball, or **bulbus oculi**, is somewhat spherical, is 2 to 3 cm in diameter, and has an anterior bulge. It is surrounded by orbital fat within the orbital cavity. Fig. 10.3 illustrates the structure of the bulbus oculi.

The wall of the eyeball is made up of three concentric layers or coats called *tunics*. The outermost layer is the *fibrous tunic*. It consists of the white opaque *sclera* and the transparent *cornea*. The sclera, the white part of the eye, covers the posterior five-sixths of the eyeball, and the muscles that move the eye are attached to it. The transparent cornea, which covers the anterior one-sixth of the eyeball, is the "window" of the eye. It helps focus the light rays that enter the eye.

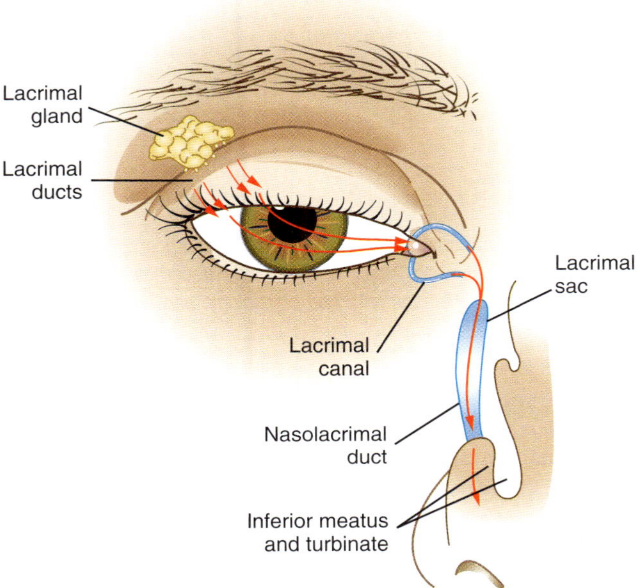

Fig. 10.2 Lacrimal apparatus of the eye. (From Applegate E: *The anatomy and physiology learning system*, ed 4, St. Louis, 2011, Saunders.)

The middle layer of the eyeball is the *vascular tunic*. It consists of the *choroid*, *ciliary body*, and *iris*. The choroid is a highly vascular brown-pigmented layer located between the sclera and the retina in the posterior portion of the eye. It is the largest part of the middle tunic and lines most of the sclera, although it is only loosely connected to the fibrous coat and can be stripped away easily. The choroid is, however, firmly attached to the retina. The brown pigment in the choroid absorbs excess light rays that might interfere with vision. The blood vessels nourish the interior of the eye. Anteriorly, the choroid is continuous with the *ciliary body*. Numerous finger-like ciliary processes within the ciliary body secrete aqueous humor, a fluid in the anterior portion of the eye. The ciliary body also contains the ciliary muscle. Suspensory ligaments connect the ciliary body to the transparent biconvex lens of the eye. When the ciliary muscle contracts, the suspensory ligaments relax and the lens bulges to allow focusing for close vision. The iris is the conspicuous colored portion of the eye. It is a doughnut-shaped diaphragm with a central aperture called the *pupil*. The iris contains two groups of smooth muscles: a radial group and a circular group. When the radial muscles contract, the pupil dilates; when the circular group contracts, the pupil gets smaller. These muscles of the iris continually contract and relax to change the size of the pupil, which regulates the amount of light entering the eye.

The innermost coat of the eyeball is the *nervous tunic*, or retina, which is found only in the posterior portion of the eye. It ends at the posterior margin of the ciliary body. The *retina* contains several layers. The outer layer is deeply pigmented and firmly attached to the choroid. The layer next to the pigmented layer contains the *rods and cones*, which

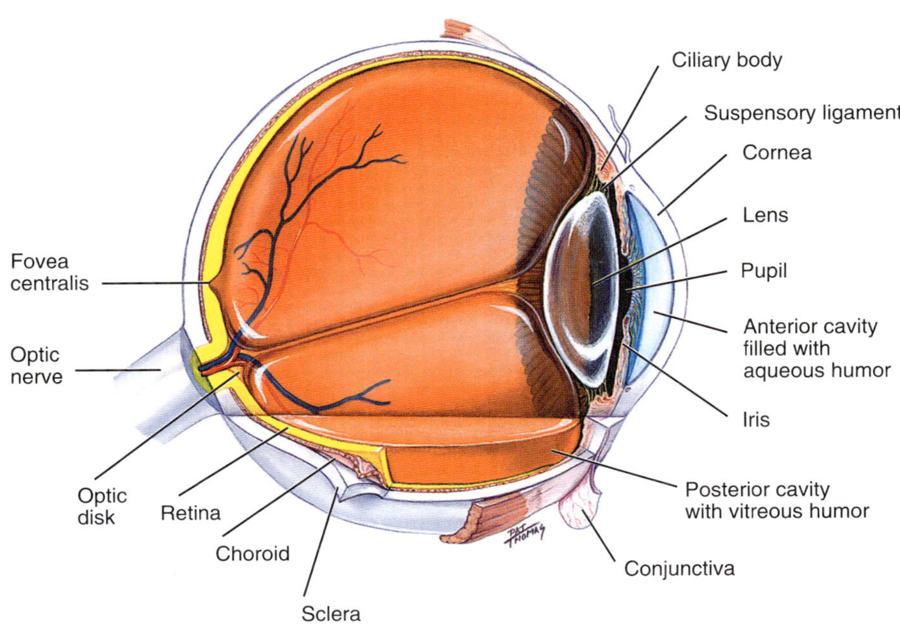

Fig. 10.3 Anatomy of bulbus oculi or eyeball. (From Applegate E: *The anatomy and physiology learning system*, ed 4, St. Louis, 2011, Saunders.)

are the photoreceptor cells. Other layers consist of bipolar neurons and ganglion cells. The axons of the ganglion cells converge to form the optic nerve, which penetrates the tunics at the *optic disc* and passes through the apex of the orbital cavity to reach the brain. Because there are no photoreceptor cells in the optic disc, it is commonly referred to as the "blind spot" of the eye. Just lateral to the optic disc, near the center of the retina, is a yellow spot called the **macula lutea**. The region of the retina that produces the sharpest image is a depression, the *fovea centralis*, in the center of the macula lutea.

The lens, suspensory ligaments, and ciliary body form a partition that divides the interior of the eyeball into two cavities. The space anterior to the lens, between the cornea and the lens, is the *anterior cavity* and is filled with *aqueous humor*, secreted by the ciliary body. Aqueous humor helps to maintain the shape of the anterior part of the eye and nourishes the structures in that region. It is largely responsible for the internal pressure of the eye. The aqueous humor circulates through the anterior cavity and then is reabsorbed into blood vessels at the junction of the sclera and the cornea. The *posterior cavity*, between the lens and the retina, is filled with the colorless, transparent, gel-like *vitreous humor*, which presses the retina firmly against the wall of the eye, supports the internal parts of the eye, and helps to maintain the eye's shape.

PATHWAY OF LIGHT AND REFRACTION

Vision depends on light rays. When a person sees an object, light rays from the object enter the eye. Light rays have two important properties—they travel in a straight line and they can be bent. When light rays travel from one substance to another that has a different optical density, the rays bend. The bending of light rays so they can be focused on the retina is called **refraction**. When light rays hit a concave surface, they scatter or diverge. When the rays meet a convex surface, they get closer together or converge. The eyes have four refractive surfaces and media. In a normal eye, the cornea, aqueous humor, lens, and vitreous humor bend the light rays so that they focus on the retina. The image that forms on the retina is upside down and backward (Fig. 10.4), but the brain turns it around and interprets the image in the correct position.

When an object is at least 20 feet away, the normal relaxed eye is able to focus the image on the retina. When the object is closer than 20 feet, the eye must make adjustments to focus the image. The primary adjustment for close vision is changing the shape of the lens with the *ciliary muscle*. For distance vision, the ciliary muscle is relaxed, the suspensory ligaments are taut, and the lens is flat. When the eyes adapt for close vision, illustrated in Fig. 10.5, the ciliary muscle contracts, the suspensory ligaments become loose or relaxed, and the lens bulges or becomes more convex. The closer the object, the more the light rays have to bend to focus and the greater the curvature of the lens. These adjustments are called **accommodation**.

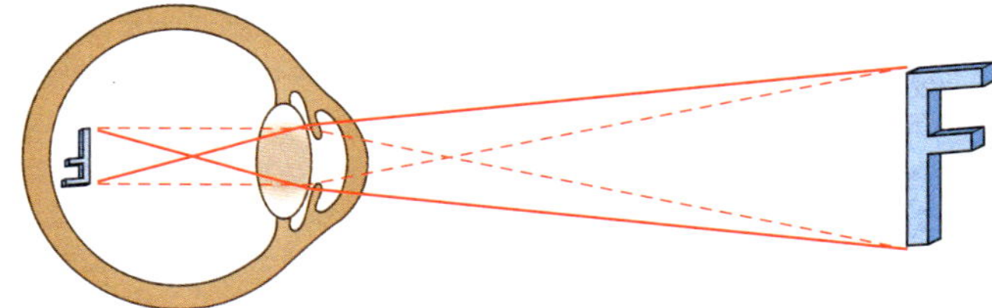

Fig. 10.4 Formation of images on the retina. The image on the retina is upside down and backward. (From Applegate E: *The anatomy and physiology learning system*, ed 4, St. Louis, 2011, Saunders.)

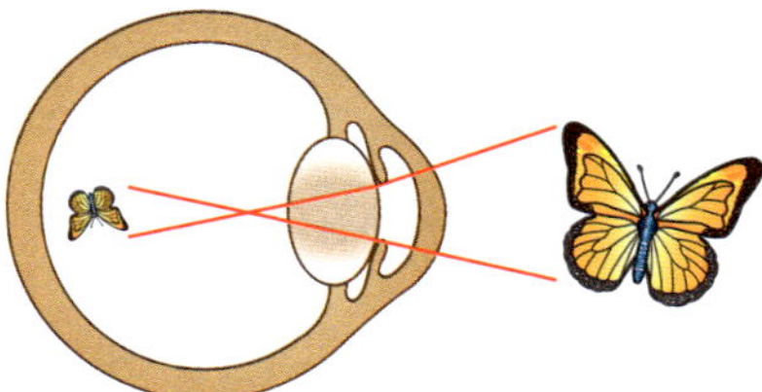

Fig. 10.5 Accommodation for close vision. The ciliary muscles contract, the suspensory ligaments relax, and the lens becomes more convex. (From Applegate E: *The anatomy and physiology learning system*, ed 4, St. Louis, 2011, Saunders.)

PHOTORECEPTORS

The retina contains two kinds of photoreceptor cells: rods and cones. *Rods* are thin cells with slender, rod-like projections and are sensitive to dim light. Even though rods are much more numerous than cones, they are absent in the fovea centralis and their number increases in proportion to the distance away from the fovea centralis. Many rods synapse with a single sensory fiber (convergence); thus vision with rods lacks fine detail. *Cones*, the receptors for color vision and visual acuity, are located primarily in the fovea centralis. They are thicker cells with short, blunt projections. Cones exhibit less convergence than rods, so in addition to color, cones provide sharpness and fine detail. Table 10.2 compares the rods and cones.

Rods contain a substance called **rhodopsin** (visual purple) that is very light sensitive. When even small amounts of light focus on the rods, rhodopsin breaks down into its component parts—opsin (a protein) and retinal (retinene), a derivative of vitamin A. This reaction triggers a nerve impulse. Rhodopsin is resynthesized from opsin and retinal to prepare the rods for receiving subsequent stimuli. The more rhodopsin there is in the rods, the greater the sensitivity to light. In bright light, nearly all the rhodopsin in the rods is decomposed. After entering a dimly lit area, it takes some time for the eyes to adapt to the dim light. During this period, rhodopsin is regenerated in the rods so that they become more sensitive.

Cones function similarly to rods. Light-sensitive pigments break down into component parts, and the reaction triggers nerve impulses. Three different types of cones exist, each with a different visual pigment. All the pigments contain retinal, but the protein portion is different. One type responds best to green light, another responds best to blue light, and a third type responds best to red light. The perceived color of an

Table 10.2 Comparison of Rods and Cones

Feature	Rods	Cones
Shape	Long, slender projections	Short, thick projections
Location	None in fovea centralis; increase in density away from fovea centralis	Concentrated in fovea centralis; decrease in density away from fovea centralis
Quantity	More numerous than cones	Less numerous than rods
Convergence	High degree of convergence	Less convergence
Pigments	Single pigment, rhodopsin	Three pigments, one each for red, green, blue
Functions	Black and white vision; dim light; night vision; vision lacks detail	Color vision; bright light; precise vision with fine detail

From Applegate E: *The anatomy and physiology learning system*, ed 4, St. Louis, 2011, Saunders.

object depends on the quantity and combination of cones that are stimulated. If all the pigments are stimulated, the person senses white. If none are stimulated, the person senses black.

VISUAL PATHWAY

Visual impulses generated in the rods and cones of the retina leave the eyes in the axons that form the optic nerves. Just anterior to the pituitary gland, these nerves form an X-shaped structure, the *optic chiasm*. Within the optic chiasm, the axons from the medial portion of each retina cross over to enter the *optic tract* on the opposite side (Fig. 10.6). The right optic tract contains the fibers from the lateral portion of the right eye and the medial portion of the left eye. The left optic tract contains the fibers from the lateral portion of the left eye and the medial portion of the right eye. The optic tracts lead to the *thalamus*, where they synapse with neurons that carry the impulses to the visual cortex of the occipital lobes. Because some of the fibers cross over to the other side in the optic chiasm, each occipital lobe receives an image of the entire object from each eye but from slightly different perspectives. This enables vision in three dimensions.

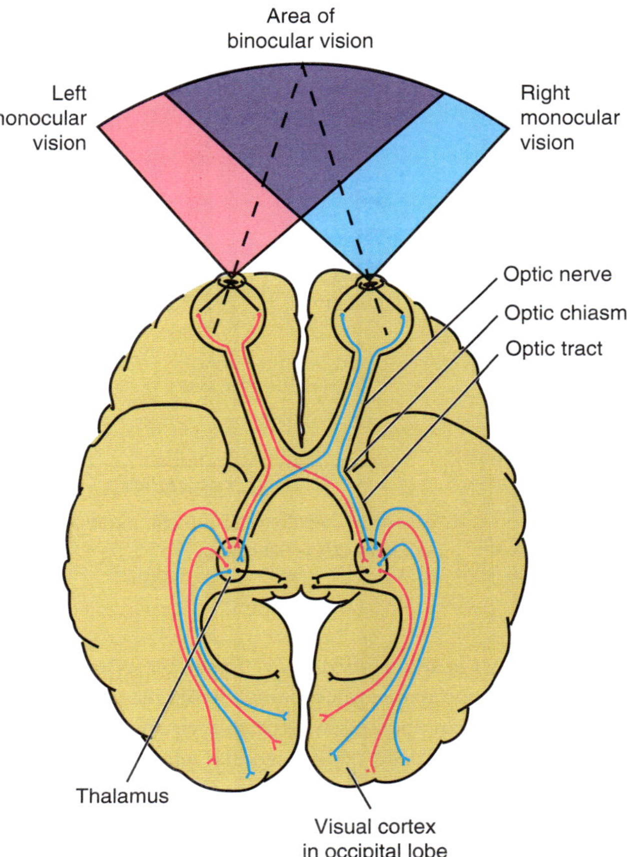

Fig. 10.6 Visual pathway. The optic nerves converge at the optic chiasma, where some axons cross to the opposite side. Impulses then travel to the thalamus, then to the visual cortex of the occipital lobe, where they are interpreted. (From Applegate E: *The anatomy and physiology learning system*, ed 4, St. Louis, 2011, Saunders.)

AUDITORY SENSE

The ear is the organ of hearing (auditory or acoustic organ). It is also the organ for the sense of equilibrium, which is covered later in this chapter. The receptors for hearing, located within the ear, are mechanoreceptors. Physical forces in the form of sound vibrations are responsible for initiating impulses that are interpreted as sound.

STRUCTURE OF THE EAR

The "ears" on the sides of the head are only a portion of the actual organ of hearing. A large part of the organ, actually the most important part, lies hidden from view and protected in the temporal bone. Anatomically, the organ of hearing is divided into the external ear, middle ear, and inner ear. The anatomy of the ear is illustrated in Fig. 10.7.

External Ear

The *external ear* consists of an auricle and the external auditory canal. The *auricle* is the fleshy part of the external ear that is visible on the side of the head and surrounds the opening into the external auditory meatus. The auricle collects sound waves and directs them toward the auditory canal.

The *external auditory canal* is an S-shaped tube, about 2.5 cm long, that extends from the auricle to the *tympanic membrane*. The skin that lines the external auditory canal has numerous hairs and *ceruminous glands*, which secrete a waxy substance called *cerumen*. The hairs and cerumen help prevent foreign objects from reaching the eardrum. The external ear ends at the tympanic membrane.

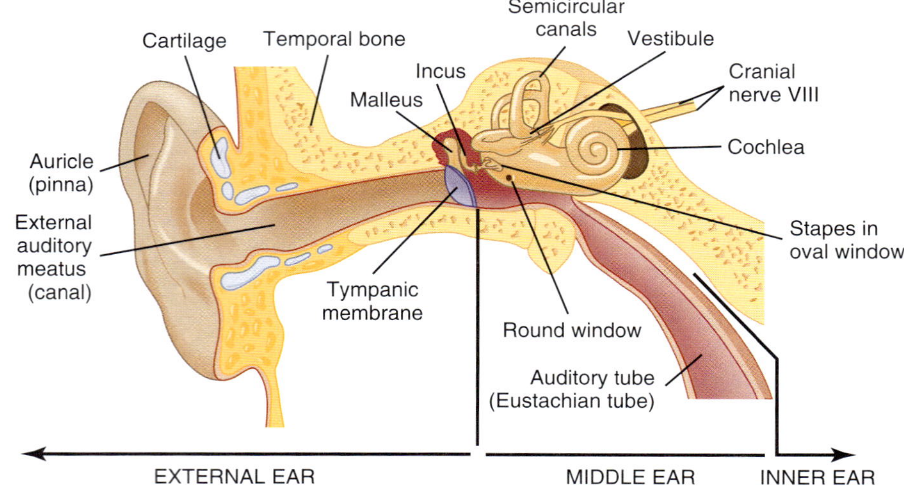

Fig. 10.7 Anatomy of the ear. (From Applegate E: *The anatomy and physiology learning system*, ed 4, St. Louis, 2011, Saunders.)

Middle Ear

The *middle ear* is an air-filled cavity in the temporal bone. It begins at the tympanic membrane, contains the auditory ossicles, and has an opening into the eustachian tube. The *oval window* and the *round window* in the medial wall of the middle ear connect the middle ear with the inner ear. The oval window is closed by the stapes, one of the bones in the middle ear. The round window is closed by a membrane.

The *tympanic membrane*, or eardrum, is a thin membrane that separates the external ear from the middle ear. Sound waves cause the tympanic membrane to vibrate.

An *auditory tube* (Eustachian tube) connects each middle ear with the throat. Its purpose is to equalize the pressure between the outside air and the middle ear cavity, a condition necessary for normal hearing. Throat infections may spread to the middle ear through the auditory tube.

The *auditory ossicles* are three tiny bones: the malleus (hammer), incus (anvil), and stapes (stirrup). These bones are linked by tiny ligaments and form a bridge across the space of the tympanic cavity. The malleus is attached to the tympanic membrane, and the stapes is attached to the oval window between the middle ear and the inner ear. The incus is between the malleus and stapes. When the tympanic membrane vibrates, the ossicles transmit the vibrations across the middle ear to the oval window, which transfers the motion to the fluids in the inner ear. This fluid motion excites the receptors for hearing.

Inner Ear

The *inner ear* consists of a series of interconnecting chambers in the temporal bone. It is divided into the vestibule, semicircular canals, and cochlea. The vestibule and semicircular canals function in the sense of equilibrium. The cochlea functions in the sense of hearing.

The **cochlea** is the coiled portion of the inner ear. It encloses the *organ of Corti*, which contains the receptors for sound. The organ of Corti consists of supporting cells and hair cells (Fig. 10.8). The hair cells are specialized sensory cells that have hair-like projections extending from their free surface. The tips of these projections contact a gelatinous *tectorial membrane* that extends over them. Hair cells have no axons, but they are surrounded by sensory nerve fibers that form the *cochlear branch* of the *vestibulocochlear nerve* (cranial nerve VIII).

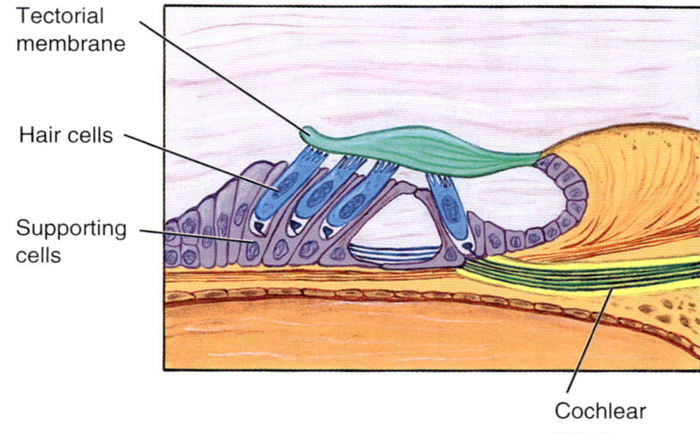

Fig. 10.8 Organ of Corti enlarged to show the hair cells and tectorial membrane. (From Applegate E: *The anatomy and physiology learning system*, ed 4, St. Louis, 2011, Saunders.)

PHYSIOLOGY OF HEARING

Sound travels through the atmosphere in waves of alternating compressions and decompressions of molecules. Low-pitched tones create low-frequency sound waves; high-pitched tones create high-frequency sound waves. An individual with normal hearing should be able to hear the frequencies of normal speech, which range from 300 to 4000 vibrations per second. Hearing is most acute with frequencies between 2000 and 3000 vibrations per second.

Initiation of Impulses

The process of hearing begins when sound waves enter the external auditory canal. As the waves travel through the external ear, they hit the tympanic membrane and cause it to vibrate. Because the malleus is attached to the membrane, the vibrations are transferred from the tympanic membrane to the malleus, then to the incus, and then to the stapes. This creates vibrations in the membrane of the oval window. Movement of the oval window passes the vibrations to the inner ear.

The vibrations cause the organ of Corti to move and the hairs on the hair cells rub against the tectorial membrane. As the hairs contact the membrane, they bend, and this mechanical deformation initiates the nerve impulses that result in hearing. The following list summarizes the sequence of events in the initiation of auditory impulses:

1. The tympanic membrane vibrates in response to sound waves.
2. The malleus, incus, and stapes transfer vibrations to the oval window membrane.
3. Movement from the oval window starts oscillations within the cochlea.
4. As the cochlea moves, the hairs on the hair cells in the organ of Corti rub against the tectorial membrane and bend.
5. Bending of the hairs on the hair cells stimulates the formation of impulses.
6. Impulses are transmitted to the auditory cortex of the temporal lobe by the cochlear branch of cranial nerve VIII, the vestibulocochlear nerve.

Pitch and Loudness

Hair cells in the organ of Corti have varying sensitivities to different frequencies. Pitch is detected by the portion of the organ of Corti that vibrates in response to the sound and the sensitivity of the hair cells.

Loudness is determined by the intensity of the sound waves. Loud sounds create a greater magnitude of oscillation than low-level sounds. This means that more hair cells are stimulated and more impulses travel to the auditory cortex.

SENSE OF EQUILIBRIUM

The sense of equilibrium is a combination of two different senses: the sense of *static equilibrium* and the sense of *dynamic equilibrium.* Static equilibrium is involved in evaluating the position of the head relative to gravity. It occurs when the head is motionless or moving in a straight line. Dynamic equilibrium occurs when the head is moving in a rotational or angular direction.

STATIC EQUILIBRIUM

The organs of static equilibrium are located in the *vestibule* portion of the inner ear. The vestibule is divided into two portions: the *utricle* and the *saccule*. Each of these contains a small structure called a *macula*, which is the organ of static equilibrium. The macula consists of sensory hair cells similar to those in the organ of Corti and supporting cells. The projections, or hairs, of the hair cells are embedded in a gelatinous mass that covers the macula. Grains of calcium carbonate, called **otoliths**, are embedded on the surface of the gelatinous mass.

When the head is in an upright position, the hairs are straight. When the head tilts or bends forward, the otoliths and the gelatinous mass move in response to gravity. As the gelatinous mass moves, it bends some of the hairs on the receptor cells. This action initiates an impulse that travels to the CNS by way of the vestibular branch of the vestibulocochlear nerve. The CNS interprets the information and sends motor impulses out to appropriate muscles to maintain balance.

DYNAMIC EQUILIBRIUM

The sense organs for dynamic equilibrium, the equilibrium of rotational or angular movements, are located in the *semicircular canals.* Three semicircular canals, positioned at right angles to one another, exist in three different planes (see Fig. 10.7). At the base of each canal, near where it attaches to the utricle, there is a swelling called the *ampulla.* The sensory organs of the semicircular canals are located within the ampullae. Each of these organs, called a **crista ampullaris**, contains sensory hair cells and supporting cells. The crista ampullaris is covered by a dome-shaped gelatinous mass called the *cupula*. The hairs of the hair cells are embedded in the cupula.

When the head turns rapidly, the semicircular canals move with the head but the cupula tilts to one side. As the cupula tilts, it bends some of the hairs on the hair cells, which triggers a sensory impulse. Because the three canals are in different planes, their cristae are stimulated differently by the same motion. This creates a mosaic of impulses that are transmitted to the CNS on the vestibular branch of the vestibulocochlear nerve. The CNS interprets the information and initiates appropriate responses in order to maintain balance. The cerebellum is particularly important in mediating the sense of balance and equilibrium.

AGING OF THE SENSES

As the body ages, a general decline in all of the special senses occurs. The most significant changes in the eye occur in the lens. It tends to become thicker and less elastic, which makes it less able to change shape to accommodate for near vision. This condition, called *presbyopia* or farsightedness of aging, is probably the most common age-related dysfunction of the eye. The lens also tends to become cloudy or opaque, forming cataracts. About 90% of people older than age 70 have some degree of cataract formation; however, it is not always significant enough to affect vision. The cornea tends to become more translucent and less spherical, which contributes to an increase in *astigmatism* in older people. Older people require more light to see well because atrophy of the muscles in the iris reduces the ability of the pupil to dilate and decreases the amount of light that reaches the retina. The chemical processes that rebuild the visual pigment, rhodopsin, are slower in older people, so dark adaptation takes longer and is not as complete as in young people. These changes in the eye may make it more difficult for older people to read and fill out forms correctly, especially if the forms are printed in small type and the individual is reading in dim light.

Most age-related changes in the external ear and middle ear have little effect on hearing. A buildup of cerumen, or earwax, in the external ear may contribute to hearing loss in the low-frequency range. The joints between the auditory ossicles in the middle ear may become less movable, which interferes with the transmission of sound waves to the inner ear, but in general it is not clinically significant. Most of the gradual loss of hearing that usually begins by the age of 40 is a result of degeneration of the receptor cells in the spiral organ of Corti in the inner ear. Another factor is the decrease in the number of nerve fibers in the vestibulocochlear nerve. The reduction in fibers in the cochlear branch contributes to hearing loss. A decrease in vestibular fibers affects balance and equilibrium. Age-related changes in the ear may make it more difficult for individuals to hear verbal instructions and other communication correctly, especially if there is background noise.

Taste and smell, both chemical senses, show a decline with age; however, the mechanism is unclear. Diminished perception may be caused by degeneration of the receptor cells, by changes in the way the impulses are processed in the brain, or by other factors. It is likely that decreases in sensory perception result from a combination of several factors. Whatever the cause, deterioration in the sense of taste may make food unappetizing. Loss in the sense of smell may lead to an inability to detect harmful odors such as smoke and gas.

Common Pathology of the Senses

Disease	Signs and Symptoms	Etiology	Diagnosis and Treatment
Nyctalopia	Difficulty seeing in low light; commonly known as *night blindness.*	Night blindness may exist from birth or may develop later because of injury or malnutrition. The most common cause is retinitis pigmentosa, a disorder in which the rod cells in the retina gradually lose their ability to respond to the light.	Treatment depends on the cause of the nyctalopia and may be as simple as increasing vitamin A in the diet. If the cause is cataracts, cataract surgery is indicated. There is no cure for retinitis pigmentosa.
Presbycusis	Progressive difficulty hearing sounds as a person ages. Over time, the detection of high-pitched sounds becomes more difficult, and speech perception is affected.	There are four pathologic types of presbycusis: sensory, characterized by degeneration of organ of Corti; neural, characterized by degeneration of cells of spiral ganglion; strial or metabolic, characterized by atrophy of stria vascularis in the cochlea; and cochlear conductive, caused by stiffening of the basilar membrane.	Diagnosis is based on medical history and a physical examination of the ear canal and eardrum, along with audiometry tests. Devices such as hearing aids and cochlear implants may help improve the hearing of some elderly patients.
Presbyopia	Progressive difficulty in focusing on close objects as a person ages.	Thought to be caused by a loss of elasticity in the lens and/or weakness in the ciliary muscles of the eye.	Corrective lenses provide vision correction, often with varifocal or bifocal lenses to eliminate the need for a separate pair of reading glasses.
Myopia	Distant objects appear very blurry and out of focus, but close objects may be in focus; commonly called *nearsightedness.*	Myopia is a condition of the eye in which the light rays do not directly focus on the retina but tend to focus in front of it. Caused by too much curvature in the cornea and/or lens.	Diagnosis is determined with an eye examination performed by an eye specialist. The condition is normally treated through the use of corrective lenses, such as glasses or contact lenses. It may also be corrected by refractive surgery.
Hyperopia	Distant objects may be in focus, but close objects are blurry and out of focus; commonly called *farsightedness.*	Hyperopia is a condition of the eye in which the light that comes in does not directly focus on the retina but tends to focus behind it. Caused by too little curvature in the cornea and/or lens for accommodation.	Diagnosis is determined with an eye examination performed by an eye specialist. The condition is normally treated through the use of corrective lenses, such as glasses or contact lenses. It may also be corrected by refractive surgery.

Common Pathology of the Senses—cont'd

Disease	Signs and Symptoms	Etiology	Diagnosis and Treatment
Conjunctivitis	Red eye, swelling of the conjunctiva, and watering of the eyes are symptoms common to all forms of conjunctivitis; commonly called *pink eye.*	Conjunctivitis, when caused by an infection, is most commonly caused by a virus. Bacterial infections, allergies, other irritants, and dryness are also common causes. Both bacterial and viral infections are contagious and passed from person to person, but they can also spread through contaminated objects or water.	Differential diagnosis is necessary to determine the underlying cause of the conjunctivitis, which often resolves without treatment. Antibiotics may be prescribed. Conjunctivitis caused by chemicals is treated by irrigation with Ringer lactate or saline solution.
Strabismus	Fuzzy or unclear vision and headaches from eyestrain.	Strabismus is a disorder in which the two eyes do not work together. It may be classified based on the time of onset: congenital, acquired, or secondary to another pathologic process. It may be unilateral if one eye consistently deviates, or alternating if either of the eyes can be seen to deviate. To avoid double vision, the brain may adapt by ignoring one eye.	Tests are performed to determine how much the eyes are out of alignment. Strabismus is usually treated with a combination of eyeglasses, vision therapy, and surgery, depending on the underlying reason for the misalignment.
Sensorineural deafness	Inability to hear normal sounds or to comprehend what is being said.	Sensorineural deafness is a type of hearing loss in which the root cause lies in the vestibulocochlear nerve, the inner ear, or central processing centers of the brain. It can be mild, moderate, or severe, including total deafness. The great majority of cases are caused by abnormalities in the hair cells of the organ of Corti in the cochlea.	A differential diagnosis is required to determine if the condition is acquired or congenital. Sensorineural hearing loss can be treated with hearing aids or cochlear implants, which stimulate cochlear nerves directly.
Tinnitus	A ringing or buzzing sound in the ears when no sound is present.	Tinnitus is not a disease but a condition that can result from a wide range of underlying causes. The most common cause is noise-induced hearing loss. Other causes include neurologic damage, physical and emotional stress, foreign objects in the ear, nasal allergies that prevent fluid drainage, and wax buildup.	Specialized tests are performed to diagnose tinnitus. Some of these tests measure the specific features of the tinnitus itself. They may include x-ray examination, audiograms, tinnitus pitch or loudness match, and residual inhibition. At present there are no medications that are effective for tinnitus.
Vertigo	A feeling of dizziness, loss of balance, and lightheadedness.	Vertigo is caused by problems with the inner ear or vestibular system. Any cause of inflammation—such as the common cold, influenza, and bacterial infections—may cause transient vertigo if it involves the inner ear.	Vertigo is classified as either peripheral or central, depending on the location of the dysfunction of the vestibular pathway. It can also be caused by psychological factors. Definitive treatment depends on the underlying cause of vertigo; there are many treatment modalities.

Continued

Common Pathology of the Senses—cont'd

Disease	Signs and Symptoms	Etiology	Diagnosis and Treatment
Macular degeneration	Loss of central vision and eventual blindness.	The exact cause of macular degeneration is unknown, but smoking, obesity, unhealthy diet, cardiovascular disease, and elevated cholesterol appear to be risk factors. It usually affects older adults and causes a loss of vision in the center of the visual field because of damage to the macula. Macular degeneration by itself will not lead to total blindness. There are two types, wet and dry. Dry is more common.	It is important to have periodic eye examinations in which an ophthalmologist examines the retina. A special type of angiogram may be used to observe the blood vessels in back of the eye to see if they are leaking fluid. At present there is no cure for macular degeneration. Medications may be prescribed to manage the condition, and vision assist devices are available to help an individual with visual tasks.
Glaucoma	A gradual and progressive visual field loss ending in blindness.	Glaucoma is one of the leading causes of blindness in the United States. It is a group of eye conditions that are characterized by increased intraocular pressure resulting in a loss of peripheral vision.	Diagnosis is based on an increase in intraocular pressure, tests for optic nerve damage, and visual field tests to detect peripheral vision loss. The focus of treatment is to lower the intraocular pressure, typically with eye drops.
Detached retina	The disorder is accompanied by peripheral flashes of light, an increase in the number of floaters, and a feeling of heaviness in the eye followed by a dense shadow that slowly progresses toward the central vision. Straight lines suddenly appear curved.	The sensory portion of the retina breaks away the underlying pigmented layer and the cells lose their oxygen supply. Detachment occurs when fluid accumulates beneath the retina, usually through small holes and tears.	Diagnosis is based on a visual examination of the retina with an ophthalmoscope and ultrasonography to create an image of the retina. Surgery is used to repair the holes and tears in the retina and to reattach it. The appearance of sudden flashes of light or a shower of floaters is a medical emergency.
Ménière disease	Spontaneous episodes of dizziness, ringing in the ear, fluctuating hearing loss, and a feeling of pressure in the ear.	Ménière disease is a chronic disorder of the inner ear caused by an abnormal volume or composition of the endolymph in the inner ear.	Diagnosis is based on physical examination and medical history, hearing assessment, and tests for balance. There is no known cure. The symptoms may be managed with motion sickness medications, diuretics, and hearing aids.
Otitis media	Patient experiences ear pain, often accompanied by fever and an upper respiratory tract infection.	*Otitis media* is the medical term for a middle ear infection. The common cause is blockage of the eustachian tube. Because of such blockage, the air volume in the middle ear is trapped and parts of it are slowly absorbed by the surrounding tissues, leading to a mild vacuum in the middle ear.	As its typical symptoms overlap with other conditions, clinical history alone is not sufficient to predict whether acute otitis media is present; it has to be complemented by visualization of the tympanic membrane. Oral and topical painkillers are effective to treat the pain caused by otitis media.

TERMINOLOGY REVIEW

Key Term	Word Parts	Definition
Accommodation		Mechanism that allows the eye to focus at various distances, primarily achieved by changing the curvature of the lens.
Bulbus oculi	*oculo:* eye	The eyeball.
Chemoreceptor	*chemo:* chemical	A sensory receptor that detects the presence of chemicals; responsible for taste, smell, and monitoring of the concentration of certain chemicals in body fluids.
Cochlea	*coch-:* snail	Spiral or snail-shaped portion of the inner ear.
Crista ampullaris		Receptor organ located within the ampulla of the semicircular canals; functions in dynamic equilibrium.
General senses		Senses that are located throughout the body; somatic senses.
Gustatory sense	*gust-:* taste	Sense of taste.
Lacrimal apparatus	*lacr-:* tears	The structures that produce and convey tears.
Macula lutea	*macul-:* spot, depression *lute-*: yellow	Yellowish depression on the retina.
Mechanoreceptors	*mechano:* mechanical	Sensory receptors that respond to a bending or deformation of the cell; examples include receptors for touch, pressure, hearing, and equilibrium.
Nociceptors	*noci:* causing harm or damage *-ceptor:* receptor	Sensory receptors that respond to tissue damage; pain receptors.
Olfaction	*olfacto: smell*	Sense of smell.
Otoliths	*oto: ear* *lith: stone*	Little stones of calcium carbonate in the macula of the inner ear.
Photoreceptors	*photo:* light	Sensory receptors that detect light; located in the retina of the eye.
Proprioception	*proprio:* one's own *-ceptor:* receptor	The sense of body position and movements; responds to stimuli originating within an organism or muscle.
Refraction		The bending of light as it passes from one medium to another.
Rhodopsin	*rhodo:* red	Photosensitive pigment in the rods; also called *visual purple.*
Sensory adaptation		Phenomenon in which some receptors respond when a stimulus is first applied but decrease their response if the stimulus is maintained; receptor sensitivity decreases with prolonged stimulation.
Special senses		Senses with receptors localized in a particular area; taste, smell, vision, hearing, and equilibrium.
Thermoreceptors	*thermo:* heat	Sensory receptors that detect changes in temperature.

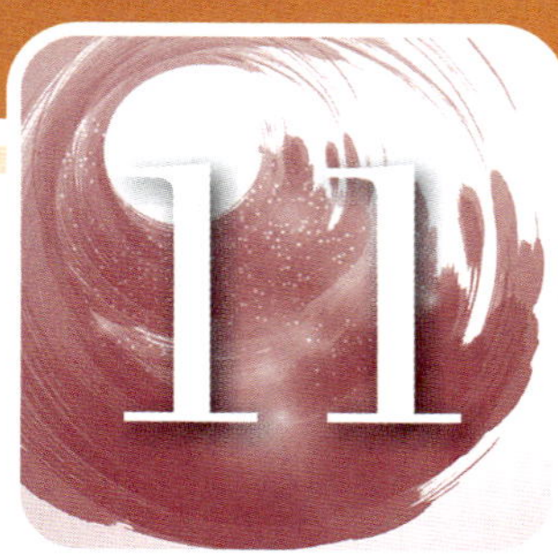

Endocrine System

 Check out the Evolve site at http://evolve.elsevier.com/Bonewit/today to access additional interactive activities and exercises to help you study and prepare for success.

LEARNING OBJECTIVES

1. Compare the actions of the nervous system and the endocrine system.
2. Compare the major chemical classes of hormones.
3. Discuss the general mechanisms of hormone action.
4. Identify the major endocrine glands—pituitary gland, thyroid gland, parathyroid glands, adrenal glands, pancreas, gonads, pineal gland, thymus—and discuss their hormones and function.
5. Describe ways in which the aging of an individual affects the endocrine system.
6. Identify pathology related to the endocrine system.

CHAPTER OUTLINE

KEY TERMS

adenohypophysis (add-eh-noe-hye-PAH-fih-sis)
androgens (AN-droh-jenz)
circadian rhythms (sir-KAY-dee-an RIH-thimz)
endocrine glands (EN-doh-krin GLANDS)
endocrinology (en-doh-krih-NOLL-oh-jee)
estrogens (ESS-troh-jenz)
exocrine glands (EKS-oh-krin GLANDS)
glucocorticoids (gloo-koh-KOR-tih-koyds)
gonadocorticoids (go-nad-oh-KOR-tih-koyds)
hormones (HOAR-mohnz)
mineralocorticoids (min-er-al-oh-KOR-tih-koyds)
neurohypophysis (noo-roh-hye-PAH-fih-sis)
pinealocytes (PIE-nee-al-oh-cytes)
progesterone (proh-JESS-ter-ohn)
target tissue (TAR-get TISH-yoo)

INTRODUCTION TO THE ENDOCRINE SYSTEM

The endocrine system is composed of the endocrine glands, which secrete hormones into the blood. Unlike the organs in other systems, endocrine glands are scattered throughout the body. In addition, they are small and unimpressive; however, as you study this chapter, you will discover that they are extremely important. The study of endocrine glands and hormones is called **endocrinology**.

COMPARISON OF THE ENDOCRINE AND NERVOUS SYSTEMS

The endocrine system, along with the nervous system, functions in the regulation of body activities. The nervous system acts through electrical impulses and neurotransmitters to cause muscle contraction and glandular secretion. The effect is of short duration, measured in seconds, and localized. The endocrine system acts through chemical messengers called **hormones** that influence growth, development, and metabolic activities. The action of the endocrine system is measured in minutes, hours, or weeks and is more generalized than the action of the nervous system.

COMPARISON OF EXOCRINE AND ENDOCRINE GLANDS

The two major categories of glands in the body are exocrine and endocrine. **Exocrine glands** have ducts that secrete their products onto a surface or cavity. These have a variety of functions and include the sweat, sebaceous, and mammary glands and the glands that secrete digestive enzymes. The **endocrine glands** do not have ducts to carry their product to a surface. They are called *ductless glands*. The word *endocrine* is derived from the Greek terms *endo*, meaning "within," and *krine*, meaning "to separate or secrete." The secretory products of endocrine glands are called *hormones* and are secreted directly into the blood and then carried throughout the body, where they influence only those cells that have receptor sites for that hormone. Other cells are not affected. Endocrine glands have an extensive network of blood vessels, and organs with the richest blood supply include some of the endocrine glands, such as the thyroid and adrenal glands.

CHARACTERISTICS OF HORMONES

Each hormone produced in the body is unique. Each one is different in its chemical composition, structure, and action. In spite of the differences, there are similarities in these molecules.

CHEMICAL NATURE OF HORMONES

Chemically, hormones may be classified as either *proteins* or *steroids*. All of the hormones in the human body, except the sex hormones and those from the adrenal cortex, are proteins or protein derivatives. This means that their fundamental building blocks are amino acids. Protein hormones are difficult to administer orally because they are quickly inactivated by the acid and pepsin in the stomach (e.g., insulin). These hormones are usually administered by injection. Sex hormones and those from the adrenal cortex are steroids, which are lipid derivatives. These lipid-soluble hormones may be taken orally.

MECHANISM OF HORMONE ACTION

Hormones are potent substances. This means that small amounts of a hormone may have profound effects on metabolic processes. Hormones are carried by the blood throughout the entire body, yet they affect only certain cells. The specific cells that respond to a given hormone have receptor sites for that hormone. This is sort of a lock-and-key mechanism. If the key fits the lock, the door will open. If a hormone fits the receptor site, there will be an effect (Fig. 11.1). If a hormone and a receptor site do not match, then there is no reaction. All the cells that have receptor sites for a given hormone make up the **target tissue** for that hormone. In some cases the target tissue is localized in a single gland or organ. In other cases the target tissue is diffuse and scattered throughout the body so that many areas are affected. Hormones bring about their characteristic effects on target cells by modifying cellular activity.

ENDOCRINE GLANDS AND THEIR HORMONES

The organs of the endocrine system are the glands that secrete hormones. Fig. 11.2 illustrates that the eight major endocrine glands are scattered throughout the body; however, they are still considered to be one system because they have similar functions, similar mechanisms of influence, and many important interrelationships.

Some glands also have nonendocrine regions that have functions other than hormone secretion. The pancreas is one of these glands. It has a major exocrine portion that secretes digestive enzymes and an endocrine portion that secretes hormones. The ovaries and testes secrete hormones and also produce the ova and sperm. Some organs, such as the stomach, intestines, and heart, produce hormones, but their primary function is not hormone secretion. These organs are discussed in more detail in the chapters dealing with their predominant function. Table 11.1 summarizes the major endocrine glands and their hormones.

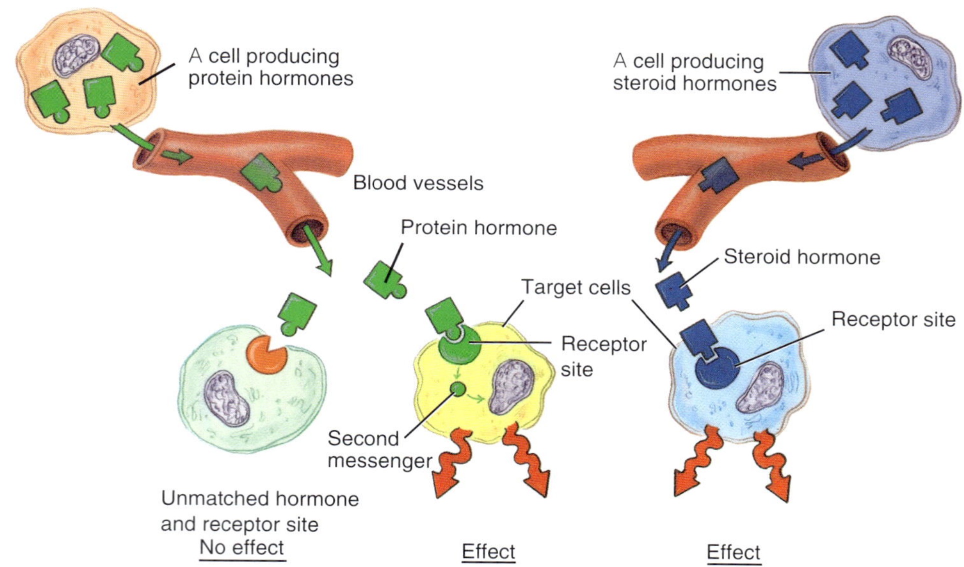

Fig. 11.1 Hormone-receptor action. There must be a match between hormone and receptor. Receptors for protein hormones are on the cell surface. Receptors for steroid hormones are inside the cell. (From Applegate E: *The anatomy and physiology learning system*, ed 4, St. Louis, 2011, Saunders.)

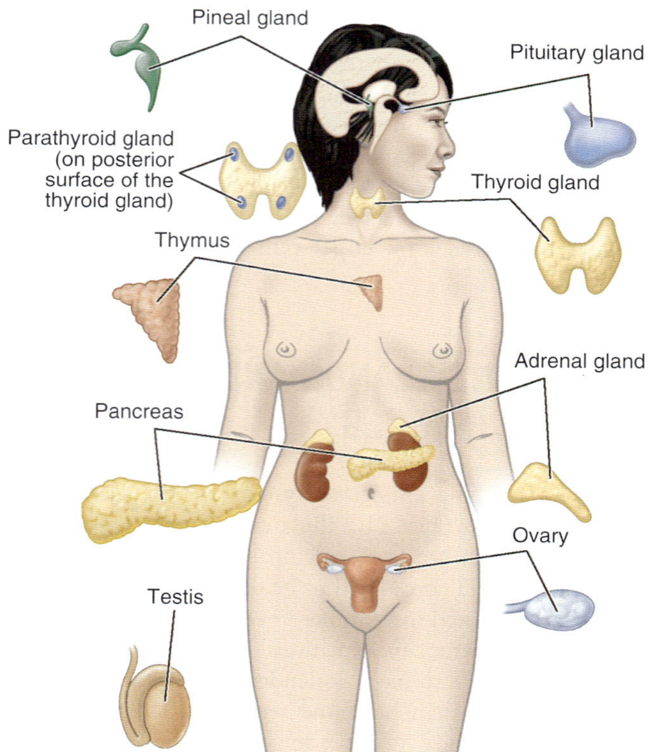

Fig. 11.2 Major endocrine glands. (From Applegate E: *The anatomy and physiology learning system*, ed 4, St. Louis, 2011, Saunders.)

PITUITARY GLAND

The *pituitary gland* or *hypophysis* is a small gland approximately 1 cm in diameter, or about the size of a pea. The gland is connected to the hypothalamus of the brain by a slender stalk called the *infundibulum*. The gland has two distinct regions. The anterior portion is called the **adenohypophysis**. The posterior region is called the **neurohypophysis**. Table 11.1 and Fig. 11.3 summarize the hormones from the pituitary gland.

Hormones of the Anterior Lobe (Adenohypophysis)

Growth Hormone

Growth hormone (GH) stimulates the growth of bones, muscles, and other organs by promoting protein synthesis. This hormone dramatically affects the appearance of an individual because it influences height. If there is too little of the hormone in a child, that person may become a pituitary dwarf of normal proportions but small stature. An excess of the hormone in a child results in exaggerated bone growth, and the individual becomes exceptionally tall or a giant. After ossification is complete and an increase in bone length is no longer possible, excess GH causes an enlargement in the diameter of the bones. The result is a condition called *acromegaly* in which the bones of the hands and face become abnormally large.

Thyroid-Stimulating Hormone

Thyroid-stimulating hormone (TSH), or thyrotropin, causes the glandular cells of the thyroid to secrete thyroid hormone. When there is a hypersecretion of TSH, the thyroid gland enlarges and secretes too much thyroid hormone. Hyposecretion of TSH results in atrophy of the thyroid gland and too little hormone.

Adrenocorticotropic Hormone

Adrenocorticotropic hormone (ACTH) reacts with receptor sites in the cortex of the adrenal gland to stimulate the secretion of cortical hormones, particularly cortisol. ACTH also

Table 11.1 Principal Endocrine Glands and Their Hormones

Gland	Hormone	Target Tissue	Principal Actions
Anterior lobe of pituitary	Growth hormone (GH)	Most tissues in body	Stimulates growth by promoting protein synthesis
	Thyroid-stimulating hormone (TSH)	Thyroid gland	Increases secretion of thyroid hormone; increases size of thyroid gland
	Adrenocorticotropic hormone (ACTH)	Adrenal cortex	Increases secretion of adrenocortical hormones, especially glucocorticoids, such as cortisol
	Follicle-stimulating hormone (FSH)	Ovarian follicles in females; seminiferous tubules of testis in males	Follicle maturation and estrogen secretion in females; spermatogenesis in males
	Luteinizing hormone (LH); also called interstitial cell–stimulating hormone (ICSH) in males	Ovary in females, testis in males	Ovulation; progesterone production in females; testosterone production in males
	Prolactin	Mammary gland	Stimulates milk production
Posterior lobe of pituitary	Antidiuretic hormone (ADH)	Kidney	Increases water reabsorption (decreases water lost in urine)
	Oxytocin	Uterus; mammary gland	Increases uterine contractions; stimulates ejection of milk from mammary gland
Thyroid gland	Thyroxine and triiodothyronine	Most body cells	Increases metabolic rate; essential for normal growth and development
	Calcitonin	Primarily bone	Decreases blood calcium by inhibiting bone breakdown and release of calcium; antagonistic to parathyroid hormone (PTH)
Parathyroid gland	PTH or parathormone	Bone, kidney, digestive tract	Increases blood calcium by stimulating bone breakdown and release of calcium; increases calcium absorption in digestive tract; decreases calcium lost in urine
Adrenal cortex	Mineralocorticoids (aldosterone)	Kidney	Increases sodium reabsorption and potassium excretion in kidney tubules; secondarily increases water retention
	Glucocorticoids (cortisol)	Most body tissues	Increases blood glucose levels; inhibits inflammation and immune response
	Androgens and estrogens	Most body tissues	Secreted in small amounts so that effect is generally masked by hormones from ovaries and testes
Adrenal medulla	Epinephrine, norepinephrine	Heart, blood vessels, liver, adipose	Helps cope with stress; increases heart rate and blood pressure; increases blood flow to skeletal muscle; increases blood glucose level
Pancreas (islets of Langerhans)	Glucagon	Liver	Increases breakdown of glycogen to increase blood glucose levels
	Insulin	General, but especially liver, skeletal muscle, adipose	Decreases blood glucose levels by facilitating uptake and use of glucose by cells; stimulates glucose storage as glycogen and production of adipose
Testes	Testosterone	Most body cells	Maturation and maintenance of male reproductive organs and secondary sex characteristics
Ovaries	Estrogens	Most body cells	Maturation and maintenance of female reproductive organs and secondary sex characteristics; menstrual cycle
	Progesterone	Uterus and breast	Prepares uterus for pregnancy; stimulates development of mammary gland; menstrual cycle
Pineal gland	Melatonin	Hypothalamus	Inhibits gonadotropin-releasing hormone, which consequently inhibits reproductive functions; regulates daily rhythms, such as sleep and wakefulness

From Applegate E: *The anatomy and physiology learning system*, ed 4, St. Louis, 2011, Saunders.

HIGHLIGHT on the Endocrine System

Antidiuretic hormone (ADH): Ingestion of alcoholic beverages inhibits ADH secretion and results in increased urine output. Certain drugs, called *diuretics*, counteract the effects of ADH and result in fluid loss. These drugs are sometimes prescribed for patients with high blood pressure or those with edema caused by congestive heart failure, because the drugs have the effect of removing fluid from the body.

Thyroid function: When thyroxine and triiodothyronine, with their incorporated iodine, are released into the blood, more than 99% combines with plasma proteins. This iodine is called *protein-bound iodine* (PBI). The amount of PBI can be measured by a laboratory procedure and is widely used as a test of thyroid function.

Cortisone: Persons with inflamed joints often receive injections of a pharmaceutic glucocorticoid, cortisone, to relieve the pain and inflammation. Over-the-counter creams and ointments containing hydrocortisone are available to relieve the itching and inflammation of rashes.

Gonadocorticoids: Tumors that result in hypersecretion of gonadocorticoids may have dramatic effects in prepubertal boys and girls. There is a rapid onset of puberty and sex drive in males. Females develop the masculine distribution of body hair, including a beard, and the clitoris enlarges to become more like a penis.

Hypoglycemia: Hyperinsulinism is usually caused by an overdose of insulin. The result is hypoglycemia, or a low blood sugar level. The low blood sugar stimulates the secretion of glucagon, epinephrine, and growth hormone (GH), which causes anxiety, nervousness, tremors, and a feeling of weakness. Insufficient glucose levels in the brain lead to disorientation, convulsions, and unconsciousness. Death can occur quickly unless the blood glucose level is raised. The early symptoms can be treated easily by eating sugar.

Melatonin: Melatonin production appears to be related to the amount of light that enters through the eye. People who work at night and sleep during the day have a reversed cycle of melatonin production. The high melatonin levels occur during the day while they are asleep, and the low levels are at night when they are working and light is entering the eye. ■

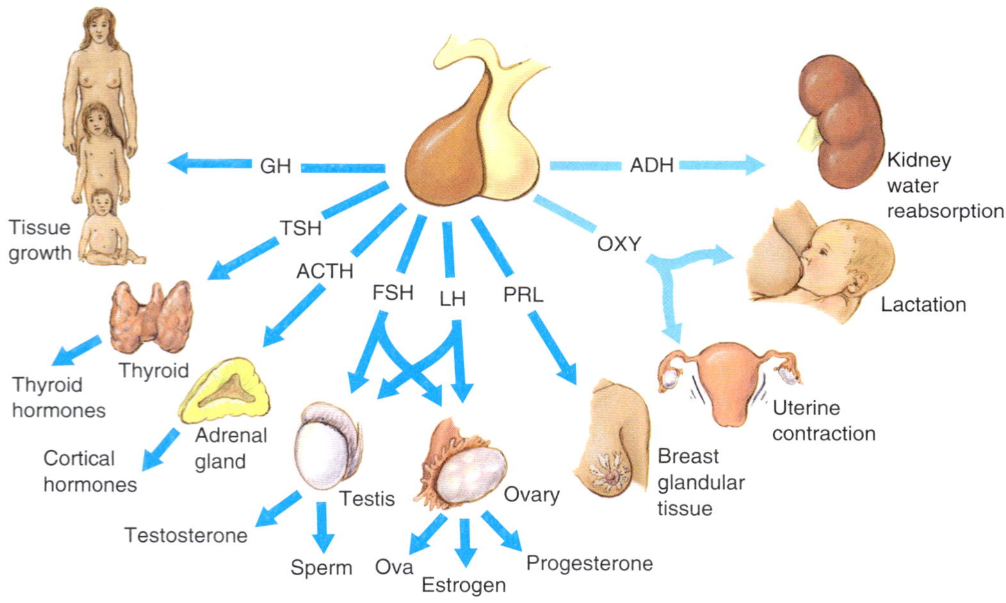

Fig. 11.3 Effects of hormones from the pituitary gland. *ACTH,* Adrenocorticotropic hormone; *ADH,* antidiuretic hormone; *FSH,* follicle-stimulating hormone; *GH,* growth hormone; *LH,* luteinizing hormone; *PRL,* prolactin; *OXY,* oxytocin; *TSH,* thyroid-stimulating hormone. (From Applegate E: *The anatomy and physiology learning system*, ed 4, St. Louis, 2011, Saunders.)

affects the melanocytes in the skin and increases pigmentation. Hypersecretion and hyposecretion of ACTH are reflected in the activity of the adrenal cortex.

Gonadotropic Hormones

Gonadotropic hormones react with receptor sites in the gonads—ovaries and testes—to regulate the development, growth, and function of these organs. Follicle-stimulating hormone (FSH) stimulates the development of eggs or ova in the ovaries and of sperm in the testes. In addition, it stimulates estrogen production in the female. Luteinizing hormone (LH) causes ovulation and the production and secretion of progesterone and estrogen. In the male, LH is sometimes called *interstitial cell–stimulating hormone* (ICSH) because it stimulates the interstitial cells of the testes to produce and secrete the male sex hormone testosterone. Without FSH and LH, the ovaries and testes decrease in size, ova and sperm are not produced, and sex hormones are not secreted.

Prolactin

Prolactin (PRL), or lactogenic hormone, promotes the development of glandular tissue in the female breast during pregnancy and stimulates milk production after the birth of the infant. This hormone does not cause the milk to be ejected from the breast. A hormone from the posterior pituitary and other neural influences are responsible for the ejection of the milk.

Hormones of the Posterior Lobe (Neurohypophysis)

Antidiuretic Hormone

Antidiuretic hormone (ADH) promotes the reabsorption of water by the kidney tubules, with the result that less water is lost as urine. This mechanism conserves water for the body. Insufficient amounts of ADH cause excessive water loss in the urine. Large amounts of a dilute urine are produced. This condition is called *diabetes insipidus*. ADH, especially in large amounts, also causes blood vessels to constrict, which increases blood pressure. For this reason, ADH is sometimes called *vasopressin*.

Oxytocin

Oxytocin (OXY) causes contraction of the smooth muscle in the wall of the uterus. It also stimulates the ejection of milk from the lactating breast. A commercial preparation of this hormone, *Pitocin*, is sometimes used to induce labor.

THYROID GLAND

The thyroid gland is a vascular organ that is located in the neck (see Fig. 11.2). It consists of two lobes, one on each side of the trachea, just below the larynx or voice box. The two lobes are connected by a narrow band of tissue called the *isthmus*.

Thyroxine and Triiodothyronine

Approximately 95% of the active thyroid hormone is thyroxine, and the remaining 5% is triiodothyronine. Both of these require iodine for their synthesis. The iodine is actively transported into the thyroid gland, and then it is incorporated into the hormone molecules.

If there is an iodine deficiency, the thyroid cannot make sufficient hormones. This stimulates the thyroid gland to increase in size in a vain attempt to produce more hormones. However, it cannot produce more hormones because it does not have the necessary raw materials, namely, iodine. This type of thyroid enlargement is called *simple goiter*. The use of iodized salt has reduced the incidence of simple goiter.

Thyroxine and triiodothyronine help to regulate the metabolism of carbohydrates, proteins, and lipids in the body. They do not have a single target organ; instead, they affect most of the cells in the body. Thyroid hormones increase the rate at which cells release energy from carbohydrates, enhance protein synthesis, are necessary for normal growth and development, and stimulate the nervous system.

Calcitonin

Calcitonin is secreted by the thyroid gland and reduces the calcium level in the blood. If the blood calcium level becomes too high, calcitonin is secreted until the calcium ion level decreases to normal.

PARATHYROID GLANDS

Four small masses of epithelial tissue are embedded in the connective tissue capsule on the posterior surface of the thyroid glands. These are the parathyroid glands, and they secrete parathyroid hormone (PTH). PTH is the most important regulator of blood calcium levels. The hormone is secreted in response to low blood calcium levels, and its effect is to increase those levels. PTH is antagonistic to calcitonin from the thyroid gland. Calcitonin reduces blood calcium levels, and PTH increases blood calcium. The two hormones work together to maintain calcium homeostasis.

ADRENAL (SUPRARENAL) GLANDS

The adrenal, or suprarenal, glands are paired, with one gland located near the upper portion of each kidney. The glands are embedded in the fat that surrounds the kidneys. Each gland is divided into an outer region called the *adrenal cortex* and an inner region called the *adrenal medulla* (Fig. 11.4).

Hormones of the Adrenal Cortex

The adrenal cortex consists of three different regions, with each region producing a different group or type of hormones. Chemically, all the cortical hormones are steroids.

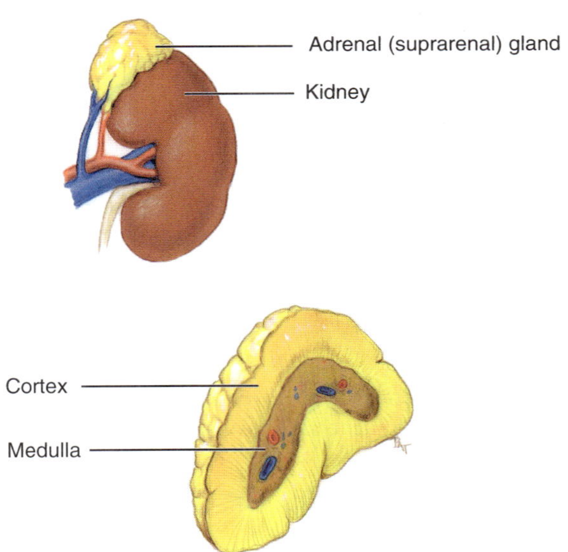

Fig. 11.4 Adrenal gland. The cortex produces mineralocorticoids, glucocorticoids, and gonadocorticoids. The medulla produces epinephrine and norepinephrine. (From Applegate E: *The anatomy and physiology learning system*, ed 4, St. Louis, 2011, Saunders.)

Mineralocorticoids are secreted by the outermost region of the adrenal cortex. As a group, these hormones help to regulate blood volume and the concentration of mineral electrolytes in the blood. The principal mineralocorticoid is *aldosterone*, which primarily affects the kidneys. In general, the primary effect of aldosterone is to conserve sodium ions and water in the body and to eliminate potassium ions. The levels of sodium and potassium ions are important in maintaining blood pressure, nerve impulse conduction, and muscle contraction. **Glucocorticoids** are secreted by the middle region of the adrenal cortex. The principal glucocorticoid is *cortisol*. The overall effect of the glucocorticoids is to increase blood glucose levels. This helps to maintain appropriate blood glucose levels between meals. In times of prolonged stress, cortisol is secreted in greater than normal amounts to help increase glucose levels to provide energy to respond to the stress. Cortisol also helps to counteract the inflammatory response. For this reason it may be used clinically to reduce the inflammation in certain allergic reactions, bursitis and arthritis, infections, and some types of cancer.

Gonadocorticoids, or sex hormones, are the third group of steroids secreted by the adrenal cortex. These are secreted by the innermost region. Male hormones, **androgens,** and female hormones, **estrogens,** are secreted in minimal amounts in both sexes by the adrenal cortex, but their effect is usually masked by the hormones from the testes and ovaries. In females the masculinization effect of androgen secretion may become evident after menopause, when estrogen levels from the ovaries decrease.

Hormones of the Adrenal Medulla

The adrenal medulla secretes two hormones: *epinephrine* (adrenaline) and *norepinephrine* (noradrenaline). Approximately 80% of the medullary secretion is epinephrine. These two hormones are secreted in response to stimulation by sympathetic nerves, particularly during stressful situations. Epinephrine, a cardiac stimulator, and norepinephrine, a vasoconstrictor, together cause increases in heart rate, the force of cardiac muscle contraction, and blood pressure. They divert blood supply to the skeletal muscles and decrease the activity of the digestive tract, dilate the bronchioles and increase the breathing rate, and increase the rate of metabolism to provide energy. They prepare the body for strenuous activity and are sometimes called the *fight-or-flight hormones*. Their effect on the body is similar to effects of the sympathetic nervous system but lasts up to 10 times longer because the hormones are removed from the tissues slowly. The effects of epinephrine are summarized in Fig. 11.5.

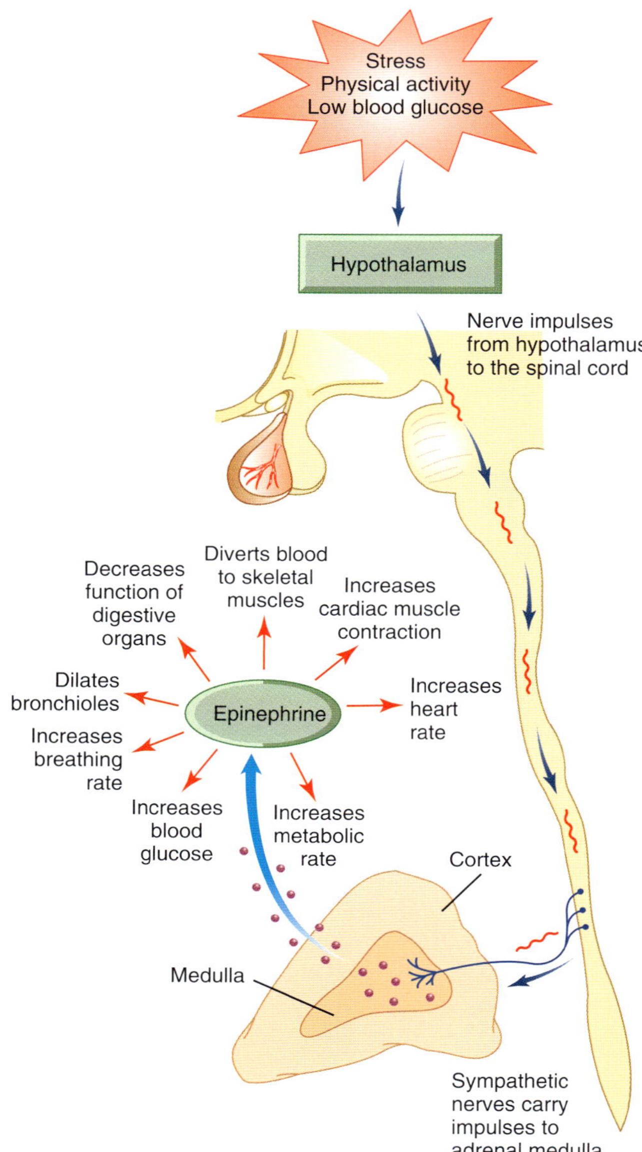

Fig. 11.5 Epinephrine—its effects and control of its secretion. (From Applegate E: *The anatomy and physiology learning system*, ed 4, St. Louis, 2011, Saunders.)

PANCREAS—ISLETS OF LANGERHANS

The pancreas is a long, soft organ that lies transversely along the posterior abdominal wall, posterior to the stomach, and extends from the region of the duodenum to the spleen. This gland has an exocrine portion that secretes digestive enzymes that are carried through a duct to the duodenum, and an endocrine portion that secretes hormones into the blood. The endocrine portion consists of more than 1 million small groups of cells, called *pancreatic islets* or *islets of Langerhans*, which are interspersed throughout the exocrine tissue. The pancreatic islets contain α cells that secrete the hormone *glucagon* and β cells that secrete the hormone *insulin*. Both of these hormones have a role in regulating blood glucose levels.

α Cells in the pancreatic islets secrete the hormone glucagon in response to a low concentration of glucose in the blood. Glucagon's principal action is to raise blood glucose levels to prevent hypoglycemia from occurring between meals or when glucose is being used rapidly. β Cells in the pancreatic islets secrete the hormone insulin in response to a high concentration of glucose in the blood. The action of insulin is the opposite of, or antagonistic to, the action of glucagon. Insulin decreases the blood glucose concentration. Hypoactivity of insulin may be caused by insufficient insulin secretion, insufficient receptor sites on target cell membranes, or defective receptor sites that do not recognize insulin. These dysfunctions lead to diabetes mellitus, which is characterized by abnormally high blood glucose levels.

Maintaining blood glucose levels within a normal range is important because this is the primary source of energy for the nervous system. If blood glucose levels fall too low, the nervous system does not function properly. If blood glucose levels become too high, the kidneys produce large quantities of urine, and dehydration may result.

GONADS (TESTES AND OVARIES)

The gonads, the primary reproductive organs, are the testes in the male and ovaries in the female. These organs are responsible for producing the sperm and ova, but they also secrete hormones and are considered to be endocrine glands. A brief description of their endocrine functions is given here. Information regarding reproductive functions and a more thorough discussion of the hormones appear in Chapter 16.

Testes

Male sex hormones, as a group, are called *androgens*. The principal androgen is *testosterone*, which is secreted by the testes. A small amount is also produced by the adrenal cortex. Production of testosterone begins during fetal development, continues for a short time after birth, nearly ceases during childhood, and then resumes at puberty. This steroid hormone is responsible for the following:

- Growth and development of the male reproductive structures
- Increased skeletal and muscular growth
- Enlargement of the larynx, accompanied by voice changes
- Growth and distribution of body hair
- Increased male sexual drive

Ovaries

Two groups of female sex hormones are produced in the ovaries: the *estrogens* and *progesterone*. These steroid hormones contribute to the development and function of the female reproductive organs and sex characteristics. At the onset of puberty, estrogens promote the following:

- Development of the breasts
- Distribution of fat evidenced in the hips, legs, and breasts
- Maturation of reproductive organs, such as the uterus and vagina

Progesterone causes the uterine lining to thicken in preparation for pregnancy. Together, progesterone and estrogens are responsible for the changes that occur in the uterus during the female menstrual cycle.

PINEAL GLAND

The *pineal gland*, also called *pineal body* or *epiphysis cerebri*, is a small cone-shaped structure that extends posteriorly from the third ventricle of the brain. The gland consists of portions of neurons, neuroglial cells, and specialized secretory cells called **pinealocytes**. The pinealocytes synthesize the hormone *melatonin* and secrete it directly into the cerebrospinal fluid, which takes it into the blood. Melatonin secretion is rhythmic in nature, with high levels secreted at night and low levels secreted during the day.

The function of the pineal gland and melatonin in humans has been the subject of controversy and speculation for centuries. Even the ancient Greeks wrote about it. Evidence accumulated during the 1980s indicates that melatonin has a regulatory role in sexual and reproductive development. Melatonin acts on the hypothalamus to inhibit gonadotropin-releasing hormone (GnRH), which then inhibits gonadal development.

Another function of melatonin involves the organization and regulation of **circadian rhythms,** or daily changes in physiologic processes that follow a regular pattern. An example of this is the sleepiness–wakefulness cycle. Increased plasma melatonin levels, which occur at night, are associated with sleepiness. The hormone also seems to play a role in hunger-satiety cycles, mood changes, and jet lag. The high nighttime level of melatonin seems to be a mechanism to "reset" the biologic clock daily.

THYMUS GLAND

The thymus gland is located near the midline, posterior to the sternum and slightly superior to the heart. Through the production of the hormone *thymosin*, the thymus gland assists in the development of certain blood cells that help to protect the body against foreign organisms. In this way the thymus gland plays an important role in the body's immune mechanism.

AGING OF THE ENDOCRINE SYSTEM

With age, most endocrine glands show some degree of glandular atrophy, with increased amounts of fibrous tissue and fat deposits. However, the glands remain responsive to stimulation and secrete adequate amounts of hormones. Exceptions to this generalization are the gonads, which are discussed in Chapter 16. There is some evidence of a decline in the rate of hormone secretion, but this may be caused by changes in the target tissues that decrease the cellular need for the hormone. There is also evidence of a reduction in target-tissue receptor sites or in their sensitivity. Whatever the reason for the decline in hormone secretion, it is accompanied by a decreased rate of metabolic destruction so that the blood levels of circulating hormones remain relatively constant throughout senescence. There is no evidence that age-related structural changes in endocrine glands have functional significance or contribute to the overall aging process.

Common Pathology of the Endocrine System

Disease	Signs and Symptoms	Etiology	Diagnosis and Treatment
Myxedema	Thickening and swelling of the skin, lethargy, weight gain, fatigue, depression, sensitivity to cold.	The condition is caused by a deficiency of thyroid hormone in the adult (hypothyroidism).	Diagnosis is based on medical history, physical examination, and thyroid function tests. It is more common in women than men. Myxedema can be treated with thyroid replacement hormones.
Progeria	Symptoms resemble normal human aging but occur in young children; wrinkled face, baldness, large head.	The condition is caused by a gene mutation resulting in unstable cells that lead to the aging process.	Diagnosis is suspected according to signs and symptoms, such as skin changes, abnormal growth, and loss of hair. A genetic test for mutations can confirm the diagnosis of progeria. No treatment has proven effective.
Cushing syndrome	Excessive deposition of fat in the subscapular area and face; commonly called *moon face.*	Typically caused by overuse of oral corticosteroid medications. In a minority of cases, the cause is a hypersecretion of glucocorticoids from the adrenal cortex that may be the result of a tumor.	Diagnosis includes indications of high blood pressure, loss of muscle mass, glucose intolerance, and weight gain. Treatment is directed at reducing the levels of glucocorticoids with medications.
Type 1 diabetes mellitus	Symptoms include excessive thirst, frequent urination, and extreme hunger. There also may be weight loss, fatigue, blurred vision, sores that heal slowly, erectile dysfunction, and numbness in feet and hands.	Type 1 diabetes is a chronic condition in which the β cells of the pancreatic islets produce little or no insulin. Also called *insulin-dependent diabetes mellitus* (IDDM) or *juvenile-onset diabetes mellitus.*	Diagnosis relies on various blood tests to evaluate glucose metabolism. Treatment protocol includes monitoring blood sugar levels, taking insulin, exercising regularly, maintaining an optimum weight, and eating a healthy diet. There is no cure.
Type 2 diabetes mellitus	Symptoms include excessive thirst, frequent urination, and extreme hunger accompanied by fatigue, blurred vision, infections that heal slowly, erectile dysfunction, and numbness in the feet and hands.	In this type, the receptors for insulin become resistant so the hormone has a reduced effect. Excess weight and inactivity appear to be contributing factors. Also called non–insulin-dependent diabetes mellitus (NIDDM) or adult-onset diabetes mellitus.	Diagnosis relies on various blood tests to evaluate glucose metabolism. Many individuals are able to manage type 2 diabetes with a healthy diet and regular exercise, whereas others need some form of insulin therapy. There is no cure.
Diabetes insipidus	Patient experiences extreme thirst and produces a large quantity of urine.	Diabetes insipidus occurs when the body is unable to regulate fluids. In the central type, there is damage to the posterior pituitary gland that disrupts the normal production and release of antidiuretic hormone (ADH). In the nephrogenic type, the kidney tubules do not respond to ADH.	Diagnosis is confirmed by a water deprivation test and urinalysis. The central type can be treated with synthetic ADH. The nephrogenic type is managed by a low-salt diet and drinking only sufficient water to avoid dehydration. Complications that may arise from all types are dehydration and electrolyte imbalance.
Hyperthyroidism	Symptoms include sudden weight loss, rapid heartbeat, increased appetite, anxiety, tremor, sweating, frequent bowel movements, and an enlarged thyroid gland.	There are several causes of hyperthyroidism. Most often, the thyroid gland is overproducing thyroid hormone.	Diagnosis is based on a physical examination, blood tests, radioactive iodine uptake test, and thyroid scans. Treatment may involve antithyroid drugs and oral radioactive iodine.
Graves disease	The thyroid significantly enlarges, with increased heartbeat, muscle weakness, disturbed sleep, tremor, weight loss, anxiety, and irritability. It can also cause the eyes to bulge.	Graves disease is caused by a malfunction in the body's disease-fighting immune system that disrupts the normal regulation of the thyroid, resulting in an overproduction of thyroid hormones (hyperthyroidism).	Diagnosis is usually made on the basis of symptoms, although thyroid hormone tests may be useful. The primary treatment goals are to inhibit the overproduction of thyroid hormones and to block the hormonal effects on the body. Protocols include radioactive iodine therapy, antithyroid medications, beta-blockers, and surgery.

Common Pathology of the Endocrine System—cont'd

Disease	Signs and Symptoms	Etiology	Diagnosis and Treatment
Addison disease	The symptoms develop slowly and may include muscle weakness and fatigue, weight loss, decreased appetite, skin darkening, low blood pressure, salt craving, low blood sugar, nausea, joint pain, and depression.	Addison disease results when the adrenal glands produce insufficient amounts of the hormone cortisol (adrenal insufficiency). This may occur because of damaged cells in the adrenal cortex (primary renal insufficiency) or because of inadequate amounts of adrenocorticotropic hormone (ACTH) from the pituitary gland (secondary renal insufficiency). Cortisol influences the body's ability to convert food fuels into energy, plays a role in the inflammatory response, and helps the body respond to stress. Aldosterone from the adrenal may also be involved.	Diagnosis is based on several tests, including blood levels of sodium, potassium, cortisol, and ACTH. Computed tomography (CT) may be used to check the size of the adrenal glands. Treatment involves hormone replacement therapy to correct the levels of steroid hormones the body is not producing.

TERMINOLOGY REVIEW

Key Term	Word Parts	Definition
Adenohypophysis	*aden/o*: gland *hypo-*: beneath, below *-physis*: to grow	Anterior portion of the pituitary gland; the gland that grows below the brain.
Androgens	*andr/o*: male, maleness	Steroid hormones that promote male characteristics.
Circadian rhythms		Biologic clock or a person's 24-hour rhythm such as a natural sleep-wake cycle.
Endocrine glands	*endo-*: in, within *-crine*: to secrete	Glands that secrete their products directly into the blood; opposite of exocrine glands.
Endocrinology	*endo-*: in, within *-crine*: to secrete *-ology*: study	Study of the endocrine glands.
Estrogens		Group of hormones that stimulate the development of female secondary sex characteristics.
Exocrine glands	*exo-*: out, away from *-crine*: to secrete	Glands that secrete their products onto a surface or cavity through ducts; opposite of endocrine glands.
Glucocorticoids	*gluc/o*: sugar *cortic-*: outer region, cortex	Hormones from the adrenal cortex that raise blood sugar levels.
Gonadocorticoids	*gonad/o*: gonad, primary sex organ *cortic-*: outer region, cortex	Sex hormones secreted by the adrenal cortex.
Hormones	*hormon/o*: hormone	Substances secreted by endocrine glands.
Mineralocorticoids	*mineral/o*: pertaining to minerals *cortic-*: outer region, cortex	A group of hormones secreted by the adrenal cortex that regulates electrolyte balance in the body.
Neurohypophysis	*neur/o*: nerve *hypo-*: beneath, below *-physis*: to grow	Posterior portion of pituitary gland; the gland that grows beneath the brain and contains axons of neurons.
Pinealocytes	*-cyte*: cell	Secretory cells of the pineal gland; secrete melatonin.
Progesterone	*pro-*: prepares, for, promotes *-gest-*: pregnancy	A hormone secreted by the ovaries that causes the uterine lining to thicken in preparation for pregnancy and then maintains pregnancy.
Target tissue		A tissue (cells) that responds to a particular hormone because it has receptor sites for that hormone.

12 Circulatory System

 Check out the Evolve site at http://evolve.elsevier.com/Bonewit/today to access additional interactive activities and exercises to help you study and prepare for success.

LEARNING OBJECTIVES

1. Describe the size and location of the heart.
2. Identify the layers of the heart wall, and state the type of tissue in each layer.
3. Label a diagram of the heart, including the chambers, valves, and associated vessels.
4. Trace the pathway of blood flow through the heart.
5. Describe the components and function of the conduction system of the heart.
6. Summarize the events of a cardiac cycle, and correlate the heart sounds heard with these events.
7. Describe the physical characteristics and functions of blood.
8. Identify the composition of blood plasma.
9. Identify the formed elements of the blood.
10. State the function of each formed element in blood.
11. Describe the life cycle of an erythrocyte.
12. List and describe the five types of leukocytes.
13. Explain the blood clotting mechanism of the body.
14. Explain the basis of blood types.
15. Describe the structure and function of arteries.
16. Describe the structure and function of capillaries.
17. Describe the structure and function of veins.
18. State three functions of the lymphatic system.
19. Describe the origin and circulation of lymph.
20. Name four groups of lymphatic organs.
21. Distinguish between first line and second line barriers in nonspecific resistance.
22. State the two characteristics of specific defense mechanisms, and identify the two principal cells involved in specific resistance.
23. Briefly describe the mechanism of cell-mediated immunity, and list four subgroups of T cells.
24. Briefly describe the mechanism of antibody-mediated immunity, and list two subgroups of B cells.
25. Give examples of active natural immunity, active artificial immunity, passive natural immunity, and passive artificial immunity.
26. Describe ways in which the aging of an individual affects the circulatory system.
27. Identify pathology related to the circulatory system.

CHAPTER OUTLINE

KEY TERMS

agranulocytes (ay-GRAN-yoo-loh-sytes)
antibodies (AN-tih-bahd-eez)
antibody-mediated immunity (AN-tih-bahd-ee ih-MYOO-nih-tee)
antigens (AN-tih-jenz)
atria (AY-tree-ah)
atrioventricular valves (ay-tree-oh-ven-TRIK-yoo-lar VALVES)
cardiac cycle (KAR-dee-ak SYE-kul)
cell-mediated immunity (SELL MEE-dee-ate-ed ih-MYOO-nih-tee)
coagulation (koh-ag-yoo-LAY-shun)
conduction myofibers (kon-DUCK-shun my-o-FYE-bers)
diapedesis (dye-ah-peh-DEE-sis)
diastole (dye-AS-toh-lee)
endocardium (end-oh-KAR-dee-um)
epicardium (eh-pih-KAR-dee-um)
erythrocytes (ee-RITH-roh-sytes)
erythropoiesis (ee-rith-roh-POY-ee-sis)
erythropoietin (ee-rith-roh-POY-ee-tin)
granulocytes (GRAN-yoo-loh-sytes)
hematopoiesis (hee-ma-to-poy-EE-sis)
hemocytoblast (hee-moh-SYTE-oh-blast)
hemoglobin (hee-moh-GLOH-bin)
hemostasis (hee-moh-STAY-sis)
immunoglobulins (ih-myoo-noh-GLAHB-yoo-lins)
leukocytes (LOO-koh-sytes)
macrophages (MACK-roh-fayj-es)
megakaryocytes (meg-ah-KAIR-ee-oh-sytes)
myocardium (my-oh-KAR-dee-um)
nonspecific defense mechanisms (non-speh-SIF-ik dee-FENS MECK-ah-nizms)
pericardial cavity (pair-ih-KAR-dee-ull CAV-ih-tee)
pericardium (pair-ih-KAR-dee-um)
pulmonary circulation (PULL-mon-air-ee sir-kyoo-LAY-shun)
renal erythropoietic factor (REE-null ee-rith-roh-POY-eh-tic FACK-tor)
resistance (ree-SIS-tans)
right lymphatic duct (RYTE lim-FAT-ik DUKT)
semilunar valves (seh-mee-LOO-nar VALVES)
specific defense mechanisms (speh-SIF-ik dee-FENS MECK-ah-nizms)
susceptibility (sus-sep-tih-BILL-ih-tee)
systemic circulation (sis-TEM-ik sir-kyoo-LAY-shun)
systole (SIS-toh-lee)
thoracic duct (tho-RAS-ik DUKT)
thrombocytes (THROM-boh-sytes)
ventricles (VEN-trih-kulls)

INTRODUCTION TO THE CIRCULATORY SYSTEM

The circulatory system is made up of the heart, blood, and blood vessels in the cardiovascular component, and the lymph, lymphatic vessels, and lymphatic organs in the lymphatic component. In the cardiovascular component, a central pump, the heart, provides the force to move the blood through a system of blood vessels that extend throughout the body. Blood is the primary transport medium that is responsible for meeting the demands of the cells. The lymphatic system may be included with the circulatory system because it has a fluid (lymph) that flows (circulates) through a system of vessels and then drains into venous blood. The lymphatic system also has a major role in the body's defense against disease or immunology. This chapter focuses on the components that make up the circulatory system: heart, blood, blood vessels, lymph, lymphatic vessels, and lymphatic organs. At the end of the chapter, there is a discussion of the body's defense mechanisms and immunity.

HEART

The heart is a muscular pump that provides the force necessary to circulate the blood to all the tissues in the body. Its function is vital because to survive, the tissues need a continuous supply of oxygen and nutrients, and metabolic waste products must be removed. Deprived of these necessities, cells soon undergo irreversible changes that lead to death. Although blood is the transport medium, the heart is the organ that keeps the blood moving through the vessels. The normal adult heart pumps approximately 5 L of blood every minute throughout life. If it loses its pumping effectiveness for even a few minutes, the individual's life is jeopardized.

OVERVIEW OF THE HEART

Form, Size, and Location of the Heart

Knowledge of the heart's position in the thoracic cavity is important in hearing heart sounds, obtaining electrocardiograms (ECGs), and performing cardiopulmonary resuscitation (CPR). The heart, illustrated in Fig. 12.1, is located in the thoracic cavity between the two lungs. It is posterior to the sternum and anterior to the vertebral column, and it rests on the diaphragm. Approximately two-thirds of the heart mass is to the left of the body's midline, and one-third is to the right. The *apex*, or pointed end of the heart, extends downward to the level of the fifth intercostal space. The opposite end, the *base*, is larger and less pointed than the apex and has several large vessels attached to it. Its most superior portion is at the level of the second rib. The size of the heart varies with the size of the individual. On average, it is approximately 9 cm wide and 12 cm long, which is about the size of a closed fist.

Coverings of the Heart

The heart is enclosed by a loose-fitting, double-layered sac called the **pericardium** or *pericardial sac*. The outer layer of the pericardium consists of tough, white fibrous connective tissue and is called the *fibrous pericardium*. The fibrous pericardium is lined with a serous membrane called the *parietal pericardium*. Where the pericardium is attached to the vessels at the base of the heart, the parietal pericardium reflects onto the surface of the heart to form the *visceral pericardium*. The small space between the parietal and visceral layers of the pericardium is the **pericardial cavity**. It contains a thin layer of serous fluid that reduces friction between the membranes as they rub against each other during heart contractions.

STRUCTURE OF THE HEART

Layers of the Heart Wall

The heart wall is formed by three layers of tissue: an outer epicardium, a middle myocardium, and an inner endocardium. The **epicardium** (which is the same as the visceral pericardium) consists of a serous membrane. It is a thin protective layer that is firmly anchored to the underlying muscle. Blood vessels that nourish the heart wall are located in the epicardium.

The thick middle layer is the **myocardium**. It forms the bulk of the heart wall and is composed of cardiac muscle tissue. Refer to Chapter 5 for a review of the different types of muscle tissue. Contraction of the myocardium provides the force that ejects blood from the heart and moves it through the vessels.

The inner lining of the heart wall is the **endocardium**. Its smooth surface permits blood to move easily through the heart. The endocardium also forms the valves of the heart and is continuous with the lining of the blood vessels. Fig. 12.2 illustrates the layers of the heart wall.

Chambers of the Heart

The internal cavity of the heart is divided into four chambers (Fig. 12.3): right atrium, right ventricle, left atrium, and left ventricle.

The two **atria** are thin-walled chambers that receive blood from the veins. The two **ventricles** are thick-walled chambers that forcefully pump blood out of the heart. Differences in thickness of the heart chamber walls are caused by variations in the amount of myocardium present, which reflects the amount of force each chamber is required to generate.

The *right atrium* receives deoxygenated blood from the superior vena cava and the inferior vena cava. The superior

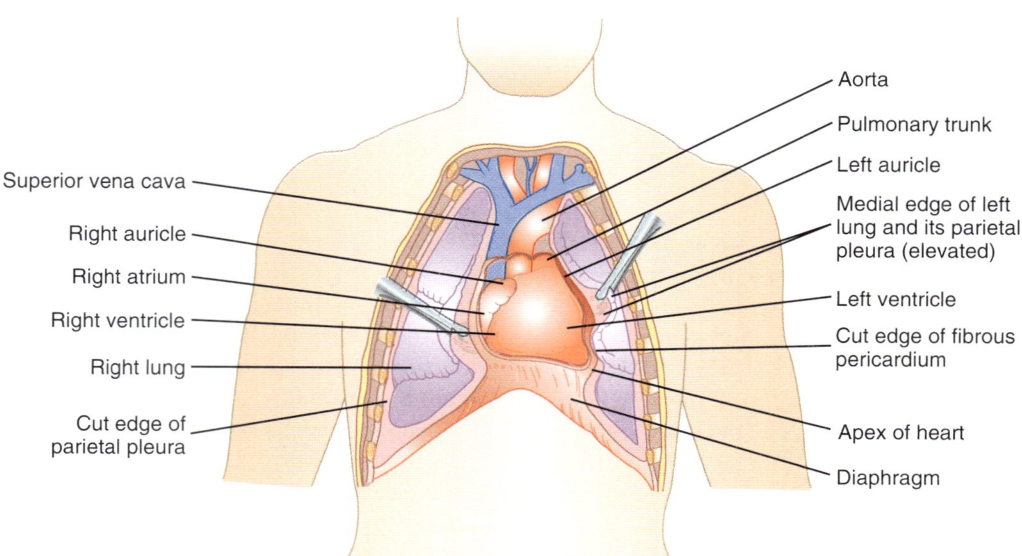

Fig. 12.1 Frontal view of the mediastinum, showing the position of the heart. (From Applegate E: *The anatomy and physiology learning system*, ed 4, St. Louis, 2011, Saunders.)

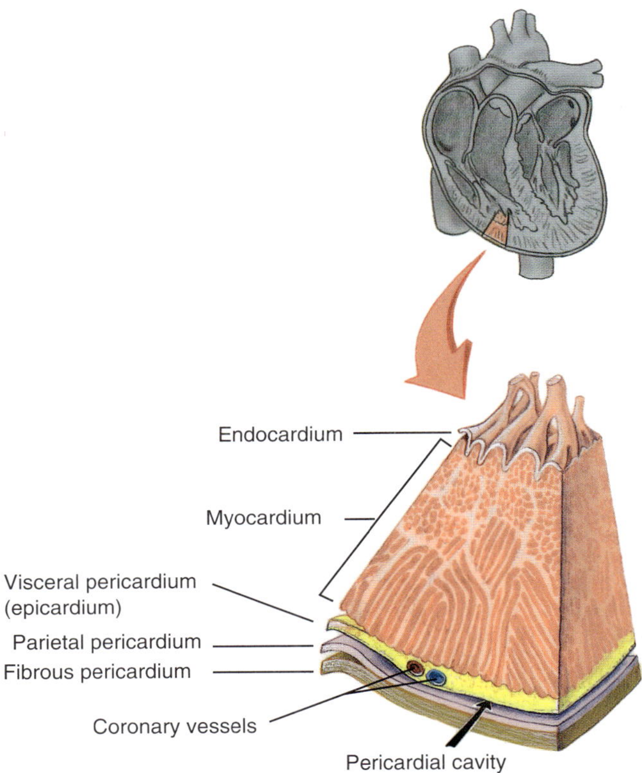

Fig. 12.2 Layers of the heart wall. (From Applegate E: *The anatomy and physiology learning system*, ed 4, St. Louis, 2011, Saunders.)

vena cava returns blood to the heart from the head, neck, and upper extremities. The inferior vena cava returns blood to the heart from the thorax, abdomen, pelvis, and lower extremities. The *left atrium* receives oxygenated blood from the lungs through four pulmonary veins, two on the right and two on the left. Because the atria are "receiving" chambers rather than "pumping" chambers, their myocardium is relatively thin. The right and left atria are separated by a partition called the *interatrial septum*. A thin region, the fossa ovalis, is found in the interatrial septum. This represents an opening, the foramen ovale, that is present between the atria in the fetal heart.

The *right ventricle* receives blood from the right atrium and pumps it out to the lungs, where it picks up a new supply of oxygen. The *left ventricle* receives blood from the left atrium and pumps it out to the tissues of the whole body. The ventricles are "pumping" chambers, and this is reflected by a thick myocardium. Because the left ventricle pumps blood to the whole body and the right ventricle sends blood only to the lungs, the left ventricle has to generate a lot more pumping force than the right ventricle. This is reflected in the fact that the left ventricular wall has a thicker myocardium than the right. Both ventricles hold about the same volume of blood. The thick, muscular partition between the right and left ventricles is the *interventricular septum*.

Valves of the Heart

Pumps need a set of valves to keep the fluid flowing in one direction, and the heart is no exception. The heart has two

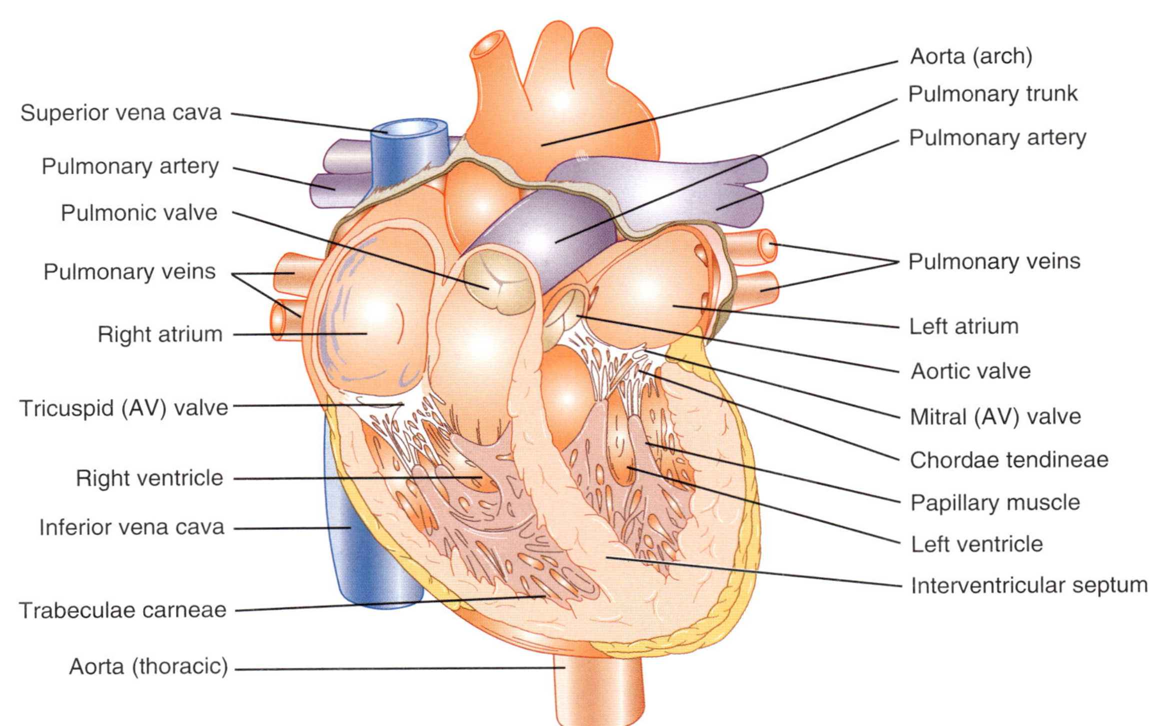

Fig. 12.3 Internal view of the heart showing the chambers and valves. (From Applegate E: *The anatomy and physiology learning system*, ed 4, St. Louis, 2011, Saunders.)

types of valves that keep the blood flowing in the correct direction. The valves between the atria and ventricles are called **atrioventricular (AV) valves**. The valves at the base of the large vessels leaving the ventricles are called **semilunar (SL) valves**.

Atrioventricular Valves

The AV valves permit the flow of blood from the atria into the corresponding ventricle. They also prevent the backflow of blood from the ventricles into the atria. Each valve consists of a fibrous connective tissue ring and double folds of endocardium that form the cusps of the valve. The valve cusps are attached to the ventricles by connective tissue strings called *chordae tendineae* (see Fig. 12.3). As blood returns to the atria, it pushes the valve cusps open and the blood flows into the ventricles. When the ventricles contract, the force of the blood against the cusps causes them to close and prevents the backward flow of blood into the atria.

The AV valve between the right atrium and right ventricle has three cusps and is called the *tricuspid valve.* The valve between the left atrium and left ventricle has only two cusps and is called the *bicuspid*, or *mitral, valve* (see Fig. 12.3).

Semilunar Valves

The SL valves are located at the bases of the large vessels that carry blood from the ventricles (see Fig. 12.3). Each valve consists of three cuplike cusps. Contraction of the ventricles increases the pressure of the blood so that it pushes the valves open and the blood leaves the heart. As the ventricles relax and pressure decreases, the blood starts to flow back down the large vessels toward the ventricles. When the blood flows toward the ventricles, it enters the "cups" of the valve cusps. This closes the opening of the valves and prevents the flow of blood back into the ventricles.

The valve at the exit of the right ventricle is in the base of the pulmonary trunk and is called the *pulmonary SL valve.* The valve at the exit of the left ventricle is in the base of the ascending **aorta**. It is called the *aortic SL valve* (see Fig. 12.3).

Pathway of Blood Through the Heart

Although it is convenient to describe the flow of blood through the right side of the heart and then through the left side, it is important to realize that both atria contract at the same time and that both ventricles contract at the same time. The heart functions as two pumps, one on the right and one on the left, that work simultaneously. The "right pump" pumps the blood to the lungs (**pulmonary circulation**) at the same time that the "left pump" pumps blood to the rest of the body (**systemic circulation**). The sequence in which the chambers contract is described in more detail with the cardiac cycle.

The arrows in Fig. 12.4 depict the direction in which blood flows through the heart. Venous blood from the systemic circulation is relatively low in oxygen and high in carbon dioxide content. This blood enters the *right atrium* through the superior vena cava and inferior vena cava. It then flows through the *tricuspid valve* into the *right ventricle.*

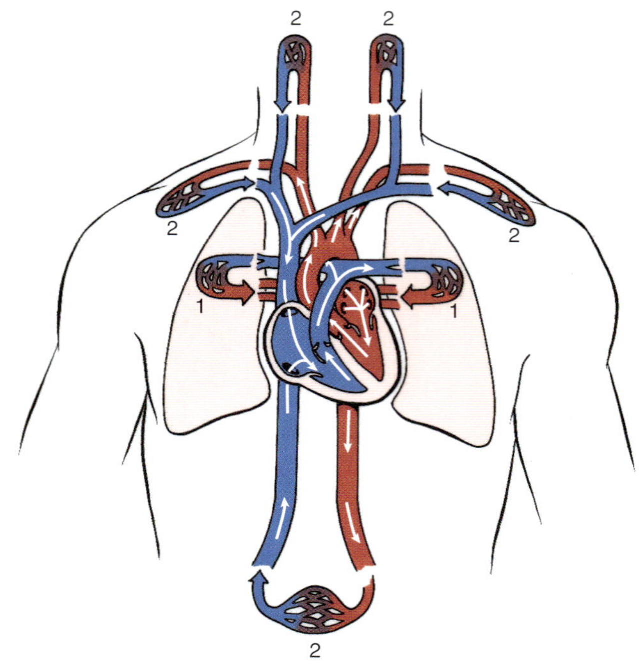

Fig. 12.4 Pathway of the blood through the heart: Superior vena cava and inferior vena cava → Right atrium → Tricuspid valve → Right ventricle → Pulmonary semilunar (SL) valve → Pulmonary trunk → Pulmonary arteries → Capillaries of lungs → Pulmonary veins → Left atrium → Bicuspid valve → Left ventricle → Aortic SL valve → Ascending aorta → Systemic circulation. (From Applegate E: *The anatomy and physiology learning system*, ed 4, St. Louis, 2011, Saunders.)

From the right ventricle, it passes through the *pulmonary SL valve* into the *pulmonary trunk* and then into the *pulmonary arteries.* The *pulmonary arteries* carry the blood to the *lungs.* In the lungs the blood releases carbon dioxide and picks up a new supply of oxygen. *Pulmonary veins* then carry the blood to the *left atrium.* From the left atrium, the blood flows through the *bicuspid valve* into the *left ventricle.* The blood then flows through the *aortic SL valve* into the *ascending aorta.* Oxygen-rich blood flowing into the aorta is distributed to all parts of the body through the systemic circulation.

Blood Supply to the Myocardium

The myocardium of the heart wall is working muscle that needs a continuous supply of oxygen and nutrients to function with efficiency. Unlike skeletal muscle, cardiac muscle cannot build up an oxygen debt to be repaid at a later time. It needs a continuous oxygen supply or it dies. For this reason, cardiac muscle has an extensive network of blood vessels to bring oxygen to the contracting cells and to remove waste products.

Right and left coronary arteries branch from the ascending aorta just distal to the aortic SL valve. These vessels have numerous branches. Blood flow through the coronary arteries is greatest when the myocardium is relaxed. When the ventricles contract, they compress the arteries, which reduces the flow.

PHYSIOLOGY OF THE HEART

The work of the heart is to pump blood to the lungs through the pulmonary circulation and to the rest of the body through the systemic circulation. This is accomplished by contraction and relaxation of the cardiac muscle in the myocardium.

Conduction System

An effective cycle for productive pumping of blood requires that the heart be synchronized accurately. Both atria need to contract simultaneously, followed by contraction of both ventricles. Contraction of the chambers is coordinated by specialized cardiac muscle cells that make up the conduction system of the heart.

Components of the Conduction System

Sinoatrial Node

The conduction system includes several components (Fig. 12.5). The first part of the conduction system is the *sinoatrial (SA) node*, which is located in the right atrium, near the entrance of the superior vena cava. Without any neural stimulation, the SA node rhythmically initiates impulses 70 to 80 times per minute. Because it establishes the basic rhythm of the heartbeat, it is called the "pacemaker" of the heart. The impulses from the SA node rapidly travel throughout the atrial myocardium and cause the two atria to contract simultaneously. At the same time, the impulses reach the second part of the conduction system.

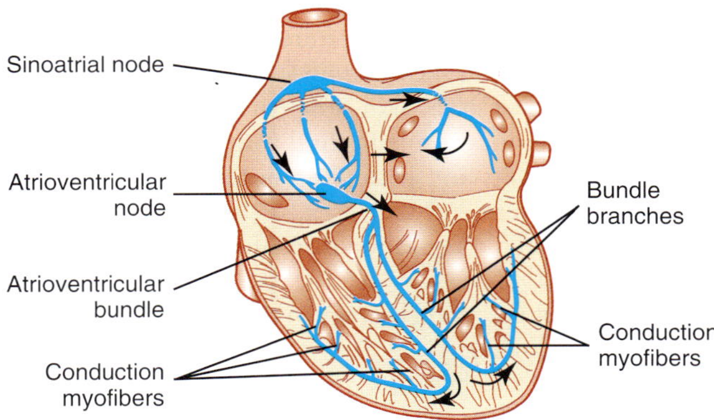

Fig. 12.5 Conduction system of the heart. Impulses travel from the sinoatrial node (pacemaker) → Atrioventricular (AV) node → AV bundle → Right and left bundle branches → Conduction myofibers → Myocardium. (From Applegate E: *The anatomy and physiology learning system*, ed 4, St. Louis, 2011, Saunders.)

Atrioventricular Node

The AV node, the second part of the conduction system, is located in the floor of the right atrium, near the interatrial septum. The cells in the AV node conduct impulses more slowly than do other parts of the conduction system, so there is a brief delay as the impulses travel through the node. This allows time for the atria to finish their contraction phase before the ventricles begin contracting.

Atrioventricular Bundle, Bundle Branches, and Conduction Myofibers

From the AV node, the impulses rapidly travel through the *AV bundle* (bundle of His) to the *right* and *left bundle branches*. The bundle branches extend along the right and left sides of the interventricular septum to the apex. These branch profusely to form **conduction myofibers** (Purkinje fibers), which transmit the impulses to the myocardium. The AV bundle, bundle branches, and conduction myofibers rapidly transmit impulses throughout all the ventricular myocardium so that both ventricles contract at the same time. As the ventricles contract, blood is forced out through the SL valves into the pulmonary trunk and the ascending aorta. After the ventricles complete their contraction phase, they relax and the SA node initiates another impulse to start another cardiac cycle.

Cardiac Cycle

The **cardiac cycle** refers to the alternating contraction and relaxation of the heart chambers during one heartbeat (Fig. 12.6). The two atria contract at the same time; then they relax while the two ventricles simultaneously contract. The contraction phase of the chambers is called **systole;** the relaxation phase is called **diastole**. When the terms *systole* and *diastole* are used alone, they refer to action of the ventricles.

With a heart rate of 75 beats/min, one cardiac cycle lasts 0.8 second. The cycle begins with *atrial systole*, when both atria contract (see Fig. 12.6). During this time, the AV valves are open, the ventricles are in diastole, and blood is forced into the ventricles. Atrial systole lasts for 0.1 second; then the atria relax for the remainder of the cycle, 0.7 second. This is *atrial diastole*.

When the atria finish their contraction phase, the ventricles begin contracting. *Ventricular systole* lasts for 0.3 second. Pressure in the ventricles increases as they contract. This closes the AV valves and opens the SL valves, and blood is forced into the pulmonary trunk and ascending aorta, which carry blood away from the heart. During this time the atria are relaxed and are filling with blood that is returned through the venae cavae and pulmonary veins. After ventricular systole, when the ventricles relax, the SL valves close, the AV valves open, and blood flows from the atria into the ventricles. This is *ventricular diastole*. All chambers are in simultaneous diastole for 0.4 second. Approximately 70% of ventricular filling occurs during this period. The remaining blood enters the ventricles during atrial systole.

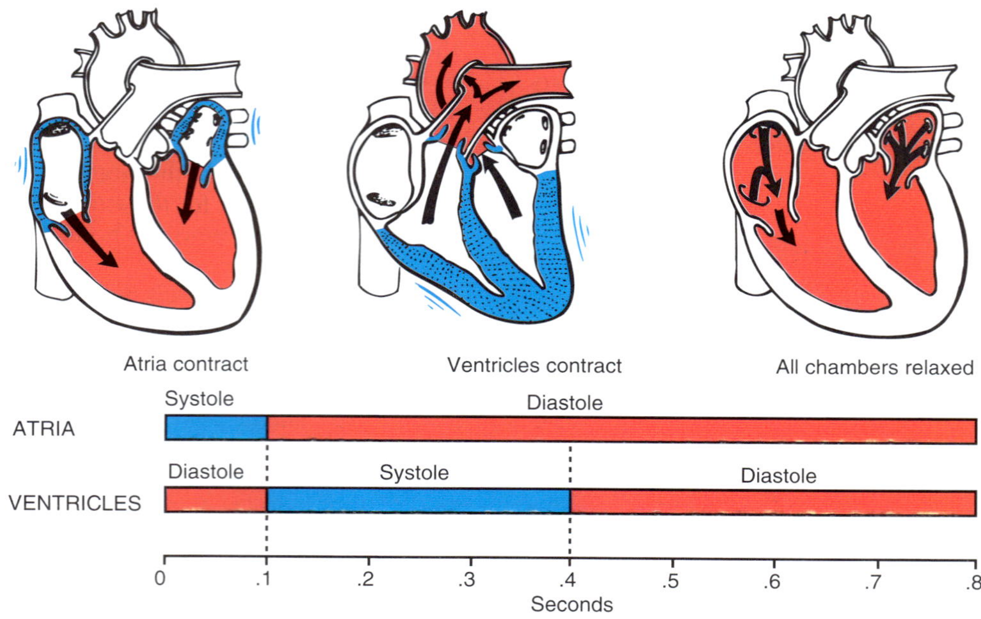

Fig. 12.6 Cardiac cycle. Atrial systole is followed by ventricular systole. All chambers are simultaneously in diastole for one half of the cycle. (From Applegate E: *The anatomy and physiology learning system*, ed 4, St. Louis, 2011, Saunders.)

Heart Sounds

The sounds associated with the heartbeat are caused by the closure of the valves of the heart. A stethoscope is used to listen to these sounds, usually described as *lubb-dupp*. The first heart sound, the *lubb*, is caused by closure of the AV valves. The second heart sound, the *dupp*, is caused by closure of the SL valves. It has a higher pitch than the first heart sound. There is a pause between the *dupp* of the first beat and the *lubb* of the second beat when the entire heart is resting. Therefore the sequence is *lubb-dupp*, pause, *lubb-dupp*, pause, *lubb-dupp*, pause, and so on. Abnormal heart sounds, called *murmurs*, are caused by faulty valves.

BLOOD

The body consists of active cells that need a continuous supply of nutrients and oxygen. Metabolic waste products need to be removed from the cells for maintenance of a stable cellular environment. Blood is the primary transport medium responsible for meeting these cellular demands.

FUNCTIONS AND CHARACTERISTICS OF BLOOD

Blood is one of the connective tissues and is the only liquid tissue in the body. As a connective tissue, it consists of cells and cell fragments (*formed elements*) suspended in an intercellular matrix (**plasma**). The total blood volume in an average adult is 4 to 5 L in women and 5 to 6 L in men. It accounts for approximately 8% of the total body weight. Blood is slightly heavier and four to five times more viscous than water. It is slightly alkaline, with a normal pH range of 7.35 to 7.45.

The activities of the blood may be categorized as *transportation*, *regulation*, and *protection*. These functional categories overlap and interact as the blood carries out its role in providing suitable conditions for cellular functions. The following activities of blood are transport functions:

- It carries oxygen and nutrients to the cells of the body.
- It transports carbon dioxide and nitrogenous wastes from the tissues to the lungs and kidneys, where these wastes can be removed from the body.
- It carries hormones from the endocrine glands to the target tissues.

The following activities of blood are in the regulation category:

- It helps regulate body temperature by removing heat from active areas, such as skeletal muscles, and transporting it to other regions or to the skin, where it can be dissipated.
- It plays a significant role in fluid and electrolyte balance because the salts and plasma proteins contribute to the osmotic pressure.
- It functions in pH regulation through the action of buffers in the blood.

Functions of the blood that are in the protection category include the following:

- Its clotting mechanisms prevent fluid loss through hemorrhage when blood vessels are damaged.
- Certain cells in the blood, the phagocytic white blood cells (WBCs), help to protect the body against microorganisms that cause disease by engulfing and destroying the agent.
- Antibodies in the plasma help to protect against disease by their reactions with offending agents.

HIGHLIGHT on the Circulatory System

Blood doping: Blood doping is a practice reportedly used by some athletes to improve their endurance for aerobic activities such as running, swimming, and cycling. A few weeks before a competition, blood is drawn from the athlete and the red blood cells (RBCs) are separated and frozen. Normal **hematopoiesis** replaces the lost RBCs and brings the blood cell count back to normal. Then, just before the competition, the frozen RBCs are thawed and injected into the athlete. This creates an artificial polycythemia. The idea is that the additional RBCs are able to deliver more oxygen to the muscles and improve aerobic endurance. Whether this occurs is questionable, and the practice is not without danger. All blood transfusions carry some risk. Furthermore, the additional cells increase the viscosity or thickness of the blood and put a strain on the heart.

Damaged heart valves: Sometimes disease processes damage the heart valves so that they are unable to function properly. Incompetent valves permit a backflow of blood, and the heart has to pump the same blood over and over to get it into the vessels. In valvular stenosis, the valves are stiff and have narrow openings. The heart has to work harder to pump blood out through the small opening. Defective heart valves may result in abnormal heart sounds. For example, if the atrioventricular valves are faulty, a hissing sound may be heard between the first and second heart sounds.

Rising rapidly and dizziness: Sometimes there is a feeling of dizziness when rising rapidly from lying down to a standing position. This is because the body has not had time to respond to the decrease in blood pressure caused by the downward pull of gravity on the blood. The dizziness is a signal that the brain is not receiving enough blood.

Hole in the heart: When the foramen ovale between the two atria fails to close after birth, the result is an interatrial septal defect. Because pressure in the right atrium is lower than in the left, blood flows from the left atrium back into the right atrium without going through the systemic circulation. This defect overloads the pulmonary circulation and puts a strain on the heart as it attempts to pump enough blood to maintain adequate supplies to the body tissues.

Coronary artery blockage: If a branch of a coronary artery becomes blocked, blood supply to that region of the heart is cut off and the muscle cells in that area die because of lack of oxygen. This is a myocardial infarction (MI), also called a *coronary* or a *heart attack*. The extent of the damage and chances of recovery depend on the location of the blockage and the length of time that elapses before medical intervention occurs.

Heart enzymes: When heart muscle is damaged, the dying cells release enzymes into the bloodstream. These enzymes can be measured and are useful in confirming an MI. The enzymes assayed are creatine kinase (CK) and lactate dehydrogenase (LDH).

Dysrhythmias: Variations in normal contraction patterns are called *dysrhythmias* (arrhythmias). One type of dysrhythmia occurs when a conduction myofiber or heart muscle cell independently depolarizes to threshold and triggers a premature heart contraction. The cell responsible for the premature contraction is called an *ectopic focus.* Sometimes ectopic foci form feedback loops within the conduction system, causing myocardial contractions to occur at a rapid rate. If not treated properly, this often leads to ventricular tachycardia, fibrillation, and death.

Smoking: Approximately 20% of a cigarette smoker's hemoglobin is nonfunctional for transporting oxygen because it is bound to carbon monoxide from the cigarette smoke.

Varicose veins: Varicose veins are veins that are twisted and dilated with accumulated blood. These frequently occur in the legs. Conditions that hinder venous return, such as pregnancy, obesity, and standing for long periods of time, allow blood to accumulate in the veins of the extremities. This stretches the veins, so the valve flaps no longer overlap and they permit the backflow of blood. Superficial veins are more susceptible because they receive less support from surrounding tissue.

Sunbathing: When a person remains in the sun for an extended period, the cutaneous blood vessels dilate to bring more blood to the skin's surface, which helps keep the body cool. This action decreases the amount of blood in other parts of the body and may diminish the blood supply to the brain. If someone is sunbathing and stands up abruptly, they may feel dizzy. This is because the blood momentarily remains in the dilated cutaneous vessels instead of returning to the heart. This causes a decrease in blood pressure. The dizziness is a signal that the brain is not receiving enough oxygen.

Lymphatic system and cancer: The lymphatic system is one route by which cancer cells can spread from a primary tumor site to other areas of the body. As the cells travel with the lymph, they pass through the lymph nodes, where the lymph is filtered. At first, this traps the cancer cells within the lymph node, and the cells are destroyed. Eventually, the number of cancer cells may overwhelm the filtration ability of the lymph nodes and some of the cells pass through the nodes to establish secondary tumors.

Spleen: The spleen is a rather soft and fragile organ, and although it is somewhat protected by the ribs, it is often ruptured in abdominal injuries. Because the spleen is a reservoir for blood, this results in severe internal hemorrhage and shock, which may lead to death if it is not stopped. A splenectomy, surgical removal of the spleen, may be necessary to stop the bleeding. ■

COMPOSITION OF BLOOD

When a sample of blood is spun in a centrifuge, the cells and cell fragments are separated from the liquid part of the blood (Fig. 12.7). Because the *formed elements* are heavier than the liquid, they are packed in the bottom of the tube by the centrifugal force. The straw-colored liquid on the top is the *plasma.* Fig. 12.7 illustrates that the plasma accounts for approximately 55% of the blood volume and RBCs (*erythrocytes*) make up the remaining 45% of the volume. The WBCs (*leukocytes*)and platelets form a thin white layer, called the "buffy coat," between the plasma and RBCs.

Plasma

Plasma, the liquid portion of the blood, is approximately 90% water. The remaining portion consists of more than 100 different organic and inorganic solutes dissolved in the water. Because plasma is a transport medium, its solutes are continuously changing as substances are added or removed by the cells. With a healthy diet, the plasma is normally in a state of dynamic balance that is maintained by various homeostatic mechanisms.

Plasma Proteins

Plasma proteins are the most abundant of the solutes in the plasma. These proteins normally remain in the blood and interstitial fluid and are not used for energy. The three major classes of plasma proteins are albumins, globulins, and fibrinogen.

Albumins account for approximately 60% of the plasma proteins. Albumin molecules are produced in the liver and are the smallest of the plasma protein molecules. Because they are so abundant, they contribute to the osmotic pressure of the blood and play an important role in maintaining fluid balance between the blood and interstitial fluid. If the osmotic pressure of the blood decreases, fluid moves from the blood vessels into the interstitial spaces, which results in edema. This also decreases blood volume and in severe cases may reduce blood pressure. When blood osmotic pressure increases, fluid moves from the interstitial spaces into the blood vessels and increases blood volume. This increases blood pressure and decreases the amount of water available to the cells.

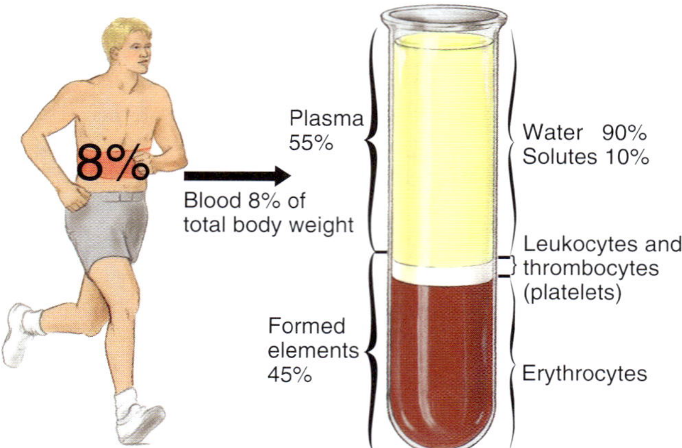

Fig. 12.7 Composition of the blood. (From Applegate E: *The anatomy and physiology learning system*, ed 4, St. Louis, 2011, Saunders.)

Globulins account for approximately 36% of the plasma proteins. Three types of globulins exist: α, β, and γ.

The α- and β-globulins are produced in the liver and function in transporting lipids and fat-soluble vitamins in the blood. γ-Globulins are the **antibodies** that function in immunity. These are produced in lymphoid tissue.

The remaining 4% of the plasma proteins consists of *fibrinogen*, which is the largest of the plasma protein molecules. It is produced in the liver and functions in blood clotting. During the clotting process, a series of reactions converts the soluble fibrinogen into insoluble fibrin, which forms the foundation of a blood clot. When blood clots in a test tube, the liquid that remains is called *serum.* It is similar to plasma but has no fibrinogen because the fibrinogen is converted to fibrin.

Other Solutes

Although protein molecules are the most abundant of the solutes in the plasma, there are additional solutes that play a significant role in homeostasis. Urea and uric acid are waste products of protein metabolism and may become toxic if allowed to accumulate. They are transported, as solutes in plasma, to the kidneys for excretion. The simple molecules that are the end products of digestion are transported as solutes in the plasma. Other plasma solutes include the respiratory gases, oxygen and carbon dioxide, and electrolytes that are important in muscle contraction, nerve impulse conduction, and pH of body fluids.

Formed Elements

The formed elements are cells and cell fragments suspended in the plasma. The three classes of formed elements are the **erythrocytes**, or RBCs; the **leukocytes**, or WBCs; and the **thrombocytes**, or platelets.

The production of these formed elements, or blood cells, is called *hematopoiesis* (*hemopoiesis*). Before birth, hematopoiesis occurs primarily in the liver and spleen. After birth, most production is limited to the red bone marrow in specific regions of the body, but some WBCs are produced in lymphoid tissue. All types of formed elements develop from a single cell type. The precursor cell, or stem cell, is called a **hemocytoblast**. Seven different cell lines develop from the hemocytoblast. Fig. 12.8 illustrates the formed elements.

Erythrocytes

Characteristics and Functions

Erythrocytes, or RBCs, are the most numerous of the formed elements. The normal RBC range for a woman is 4 to 5.5 million RBCs/mm^3 of blood. The normal RBC range for a man is 4.5 to 6.2 million RBCs/mm^3 of blood.

Erythrocytes are tiny biconcave discs approximately 7.5 μm in diameter. They are thin in the middle and thicker around the periphery. The shape of the RBC provides a combination

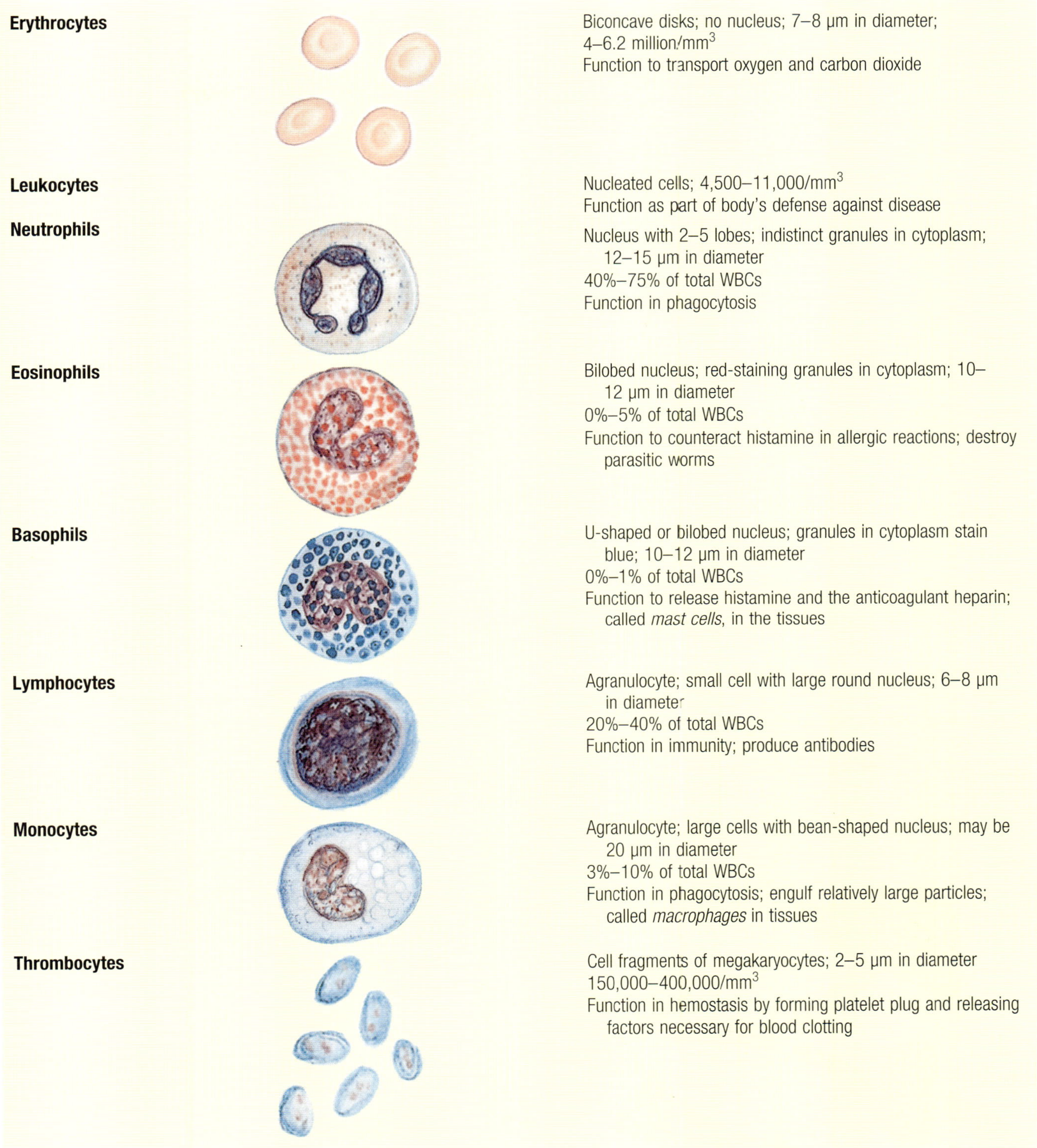

Fig. 12.8 Formed elements in the blood. *WBCs*, White blood cells. (From Applegate E: *The anatomy and physiology learning system*, ed 4, St. Louis, 2011, Saunders.)

of flexibility for moving through tiny capillaries along with a maximum surface area for the diffusion of gases. Mature RBCs are anucleate, meaning they do not have a nucleus. During development the nucleus is lost from the cell, presumably to give the cell more room for hemoglobin. Because the mature cells are anucleate, they cannot undergo mitosis, which means that replacement cells have to develop from the stem cells. The primary function of erythrocytes is to transport oxygen and, to a lesser extent, carbon dioxide. This function is directly related to the **hemoglobin** within the RBC.

Production of Erythrocytes

Erythrocyte production, specifically called **erythropoiesis**, is regulated by a negative feedback mechanism that uses the hormone **erythropoietin** to stimulate erythrocyte production (Fig. 12.9). The liver produces erythropoietin in an inactive form and secretes it into the blood. The kidneys produce **renal erythropoietic factor** (REF), which activates the erythropoietin. When blood oxygen concentration is low, the kidneys release REF into the blood, which activates the erythropoietin, which then stimulates the red bone marrow to produce RBCs. The additional RBCs combine with oxygen to increase the blood oxygen concentration. As blood oxygen concentration increases, levels of REF and active erythropoietin decrease and RBC production decreases. This is an example of negative feedback.

Iron, vitamin B_{12}, and folic acid are essential to normal RBC production. The iron is necessary for the synthesis of normal hemoglobin. Iron deficiency anemia results when there is a lack of iron in the diet. This results in a reduced amount of hemoglobin, which decreases the blood's oxygen-carrying capacity. All cells in the body require vitamins B_{12} and folic acid for normal formation. This is especially significant in erythrocytes because of the large numbers produced every day. Certain cells in the stomach produce *intrinsic factor*, which is a factor necessary for the absorption of vitamin B_{12} in the intestines. Without intrinsic factor, vitamin B_{12} (even though present in the diet) cannot be absorbed. This results in a condition known as *pernicious anemia.*

Destruction of Erythrocytes

Normal erythrocytes live for approximately 120 days. During this time they travel thousands of miles as they circulate throughout the body. Normally the erythrocytes have a flexible cell membrane that allows them to bend and squeeze through the capillaries. However, as they age, their membrane loses its elasticity and becomes fragile. When they are defective or worn out, **macrophages**, which are phagocytic cells in the spleen and liver, remove them from circulation, and they are replaced by an equal number of new cells. Under typical conditions, more than 2 million erythrocytes are destroyed and replaced every second. Bilirubin, a yellow pigment, is a by-product of RBC destruction. It becomes a part of bile and is secreted by the liver.

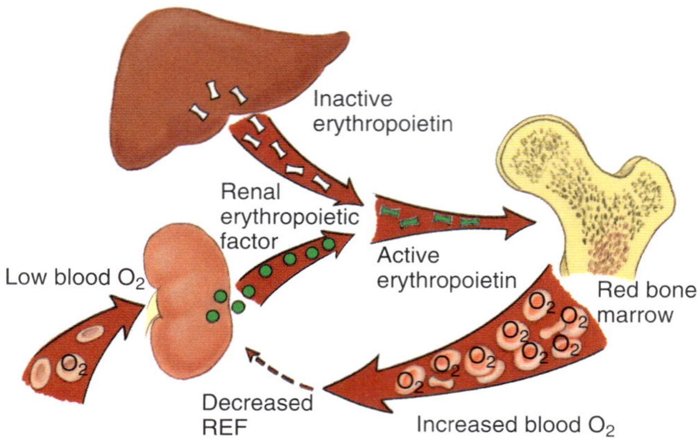

Fig. 12.9 Regulation of erythrocyte production. The liver secretes inactive erythropoietin into the blood. In response to low blood O_2, the kidneys release renal erythropoietic factor (*REF*) into the blood. This activates the erythropoietin, which stimulates the bone marrow to produce red blood cells. (From Applegate E: *The anatomy and physiology learning system*, ed 4, St. Louis, 2011, Saunders.)

Leukocytes

Characteristics and Functions

The function of leukocytes is to defend the body against disease. In general, *leukocytes* (WBCs) are larger than erythrocytes, but they are fewer in number. A normal WBC count ranges from 4500 to 11,000/mm^3. All leukocytes are derived from hemocytoblast stem cells (see Fig. 12.8), but they do not lose their nuclei or accumulate hemoglobin during development. The lack of hemoglobin makes them appear pale in contrast to erythrocytes.

Even though they are considered to be blood cells, leukocytes do most of their work in the tissues. They use the blood as a transport medium. Some are phagocytic, others produce antibodies, some secrete histamine and heparin, and others neutralize histamine. Leukocytes are able to move through the capillary walls into the tissue spaces, a process called **diapedesis**. In the tissue spaces they provide a defense against organisms that cause disease.

Types of Leukocytes

Blood contains two main groups of leukocytes. The cells that develop granules in the cytoplasm are called **granulocytes**, or granular leukocytes, and those that do not have granules are called **agranulocytes**, or nongranular leukocytes. *Neutrophils*, *eosinophils*, and *basophils* are granular leukocytes. *Monocytes* and *lymphocytes* are nongranular leukocytes. Because WBCs are clear and colorless, they must be stained first with an appropriate dye (usually Wright stain) before they can be identified under the microscope. The nucleus, cytoplasm, and any granules in the cytoplasm take on the characteristic color of their cell type, which aids in proper identification. The five types of WBCs are described here, along with their reactions to Wright stain.

Neutrophils are the most common type of leukocyte and make up 40% to 75% of the total number of WBCs. They are characterized by a purple, multilobed nucleus (usually three to five lobes) and many fine granules in the cytoplasm that stain a violet-pink. Neutrophils are the first leukocytes to respond to tissue damage, by engulfing bacteria by phagocytosis. The number of neutrophils increases during acute infections.

Eosinophils make up 0% to 5% of the WBCs. They are characterized by a segmented nucleus, usually of no more than two lobes. Large granules found in the cytoplasm stain a bright reddish orange. Eosinophils neutralize histamine, and their number increases during allergic reactions. They also destroy parasitic worms.

Basophils are the least numerous of the leukocytes. The normal range for basophils is 0% to 1% of the WBCs. A basophil is about the same size as an eosinophil and has an S-shaped nucleus. The cytoplasm has large, coarse granules that stain a dark bluish-black and almost completely obscure the details of the nucleus. In the tissues, basophils secrete histamine and heparin. Histamine dilates blood vessels to increase blood flow to damaged tissues. It also dilates blood vessels in allergic reactions. Heparin is an anticoagulant that inhibits blood clot formation.

Lymphocytes account for 20% to 40% of the WBCs in the blood. Lymphocytes have a large round or slightly indented nucleus that stains a deep purplish-blue. A small rim of sky-blue cytoplasm around the nucleus contains few or no granules. Lymphocytes are involved with the immune system and the production of antibodies. An increase in lymphocytes usually occurs with certain viral diseases, including infectious mononucleosis, mumps, chickenpox, rubella, and viral hepatitis.

Monocytes are the largest of the WBCs and make up 3% to 10% of the leukocytes in the blood. Monocytes have a U-shaped or kidney-shaped nucleus surrounded by abundant cytoplasm that stains grayish-blue. When monocytes leave the blood and enter the tissues, they are called *macrophages*. In damaged tissues, the macrophages engulf bacteria and cellular debris to finish the cleanup process started by the neutrophils.

Thrombocytes

Thrombocytes, or *platelets*, are not complete cells but small fragments of large cells called **megakaryocytes**. Megakaryocytes develop from hemocytoblasts in the red bone marrow. Platelets are one-third to one-half the size of an erythrocyte, and an average platelet count ranges from 150,000 to 400,000 platelets/mm^3 of blood.

Thrombocytes become sticky and clump together to form platelet plugs that close breaks and tears in blood vessels. They also initiate the formation of blood clots.

HEMOSTASIS

Blood vessels that are torn or cut permit blood to escape into the surrounding tissues or to the outside of the body. This has damaging effects on the tissues and, in cases of excessive blood loss, may result in death. Whenever blood vessels are injured, several reactions occur that attempt to minimize blood loss and tissue damage. The stoppage of bleeding is called **hemostasis**. It includes three separate but interrelated processes: vascular constriction, platelet plug formation, and coagulation.

Vascular Constriction

The first response to blood vessel injury is contraction of the smooth muscle in the vessel walls. This creates a *vascular constriction* that restricts the flow of blood through the opening in the blood vessel. The initial constriction lasts for only a few minutes but allows enough time for the other aspects of hemostasis to begin. As platelets accumulate at the site of the injury, they secrete serotonin, a chemical that stimulates smooth muscle contraction and prolongs the vascular constriction.

Platelet Plug Formation

Normally platelets do not stick to one another or to the lining of blood vessel walls. When the lining of the blood vessel breaks, the underlying connective tissue is exposed. The connective tissue attracts platelets and they accumulate in the damaged region, where they adhere to the connective tissue and to one another. This creates a mass of platelets, a *platelet plug*, that obstructs the tear in the vessel. Normal daily activities create numerous tears in minute blood vessels, and these are closed by platelet plugs so that there is no blood loss or damage to surrounding tissues.

Coagulation

The third and most effective mechanism in hemostasis is the formation of a blood clot, or **coagulation**. The blood contains factors called *procoagulants* that promote clotting. It also contains *anticoagulants*, which inhibit clotting. Normally the anticoagulants predominate and override the procoagulants so that the blood remains fluid and does not clot. When vessels are damaged, the procoagulants increase their activity, which results in the formation of a clot.

The formation of a blood clot involves a complex series of chemical reactions and includes numerous clotting factors that are present in the plasma. Even though it is a complex process, it can be summarized in three main steps, as illustrated in Fig. 12.10.

1. Platelets and damaged tissues release chemicals that initiate a series of reactions that result in the formation of *prothrombin activator*.
2. In the presence of calcium ions and prothrombin activator, *prothrombin* in the plasma is converted from an inactive form to active *thrombin*.
3. Thrombin, in the presence of calcium ions, acts as an enzyme to convert inactive and soluble *fibrinogen* into active and insoluble *fibrin*. The fibrin threads form a mesh that adheres to the damaged tissue and traps blood cells and platelets to form the clot.

Platelets and all the necessary clotting factors must be available for successful clot formation. The liver produces most of the clotting factors, and many of them require vitamin K for their synthesis. Numerous reactions in the clotting process also require calcium ions. A low platelet count (thrombocytopenia), deficiency of vitamin K or calcium, and liver dysfunction can impair the clotting process.

After a clot has formed, the fibrin strands contract. This process, called *clot retraction*, causes the clot to condense or shrink. Clot retraction pulls the edges of the damaged tissue closer together, reduces the flow of blood to the area, reduces the probability of infection, and enhances healing. Fibroblasts migrate into the clot and form fibrous connective tissue that repairs the damaged area. As healing occurs, the clot is dissolved by a process called *fibrinolysis*.

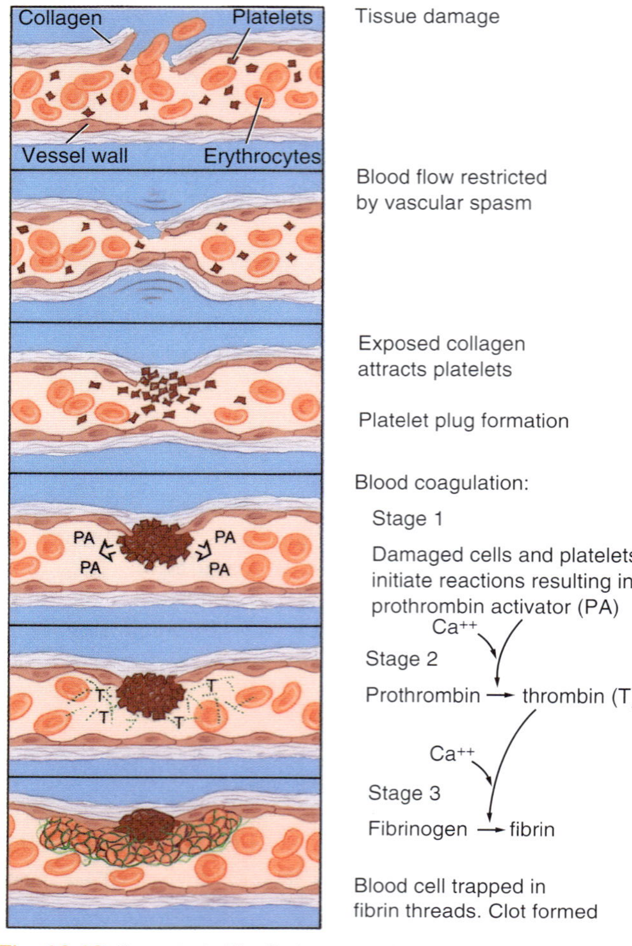

Fig. 12.10 Hemostasis. The first response to vessel injury is a vascular spasm. This is followed by platelet plug formation. The third and most effective mechanism of hemostasis is the formation of a blood clot. (From Applegate E: *The anatomy and physiology learning system*, ed 4, St. Louis, 2011, Saunders.)

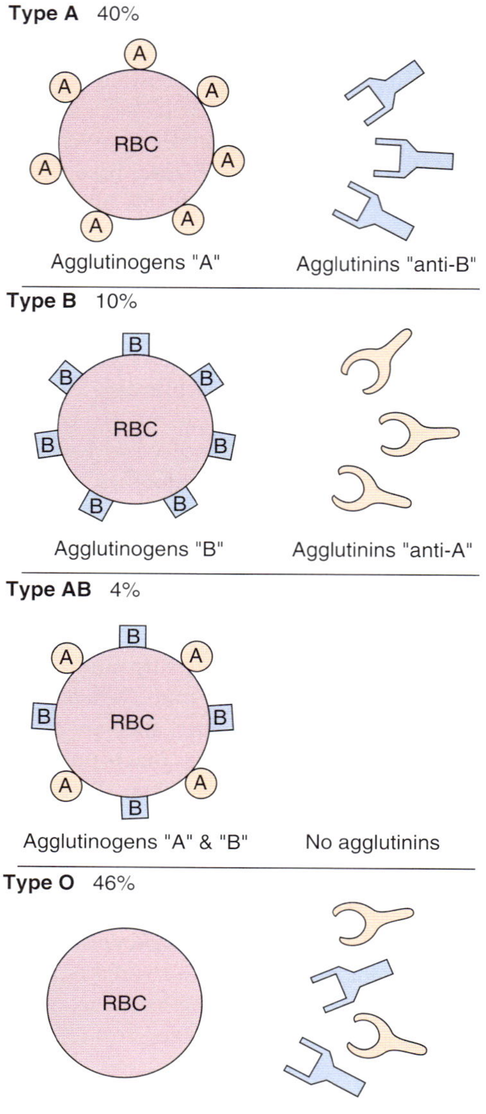

Fig. 12.11 Agglutinogens (antigens) and agglutinins (antibodies) involved in the ABO blood groups. *RBC*, Red blood cell. (From Applegate E: *The anatomy and physiology learning system*, ed 4, St. Louis, 2011, Saunders.)

BLOOD TYPES

ABO Blood Groups

The ABO blood groups are based on the presence or absence of certain antigens called *agglutinogens* on the surface of the RBC membrane. These antigens, A and B, are inherited; consequently, blood types are also inherited. Type A blood has type A antigen; type B blood has type B antigen; type AB blood has both type A and type B antigens; and type O blood has neither type A nor type B antigen (Fig. 12.11). Certain blood antibodies called *agglutinins* develop in the plasma shortly after birth. Specifically, a person with type A blood develops B antibodies; a person with type B blood develops A antibodies; a person with type AB blood develops neither A nor B antibodies; and a person with type O blood develops both A and B antibodies (see Fig. 12.11).

Blood types are important in transfusions. If the blood types are different, the antibodies of the recipient may react with the antigens of the donor and cause hemolysis in the blood. Fig. 12.12 illustrates agglutination (clumping of the red blood cells) and hemolysis.

Rh Blood Groups

Even after the ABO blood groups were well established and accurate blood typing procedures had been developed, there were still unexplained cases of transfusion reactions. This led to more research, which led to the discovery of the *Rh factor*, so named because it was first studied in the rhesus monkey.

People are Rh positive (Rh+) if they have Rh antigens on the surface of their RBCs. Approximately 85% of people are Rh+. The other 15% do not have the Rh antigens and are Rh negative (Rh−). The presence or absence of Rh

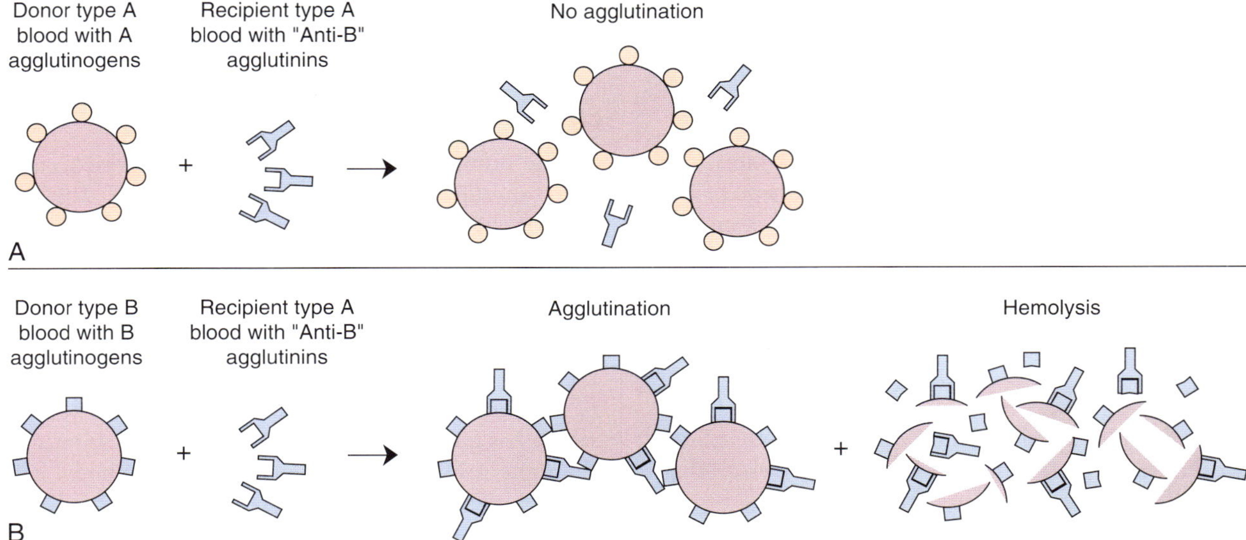

Fig. 12.12 Agglutination reactions. (A) Type A donor and type A recipient results in no agglutination. (B) Type B donor and type A recipient results in agglutination and hemolysis. (From Applegate E: *The anatomy and physiology learning system*, ed 4, St. Louis, 2011, Saunders.)

antigens is an inherited trait. Normally, neither Rh+ nor Rh− individuals have Rh antibodies. If an Rh− person is exposed to Rh+ blood, either through a blood transfusion or by transfer of blood between a mother and fetus, the Rh− individual develops Rh antibodies. If that individual is exposed to Rh+ blood a second time, a transfusion reaction results. When transfusions are given, it is necessary to match both the Rh type and the ABO type.

BLOOD VESSELS

Blood vessels are the channels through which blood is distributed to body tissues. The vessels make up two closed systems of tubes that begin and end at the heart (Fig. 12.13). One system, the *pulmonary vessels*, transports blood from the right ventricle to the lungs and back to the left atrium. The other system, the *systemic vessels*, carries blood from the left ventricle to the tissues in all parts of the body and then returns the blood to the right atrium. Based on their structure and function, blood vessels are classified as arteries, capillaries, or veins.

CLASSIFICATION AND STRUCTURE OF BLOOD VESSELS

Arteries

Arteries carry blood away from the heart. Pulmonary arteries transport blood from the right ventricle to the lungs. This blood has a low oxygen content. Systemic arteries transport oxygenated blood from the left ventricle to the body tissues. Blood is pumped from the ventricles into large elastic arteries that branch repeatedly into smaller and smaller arteries

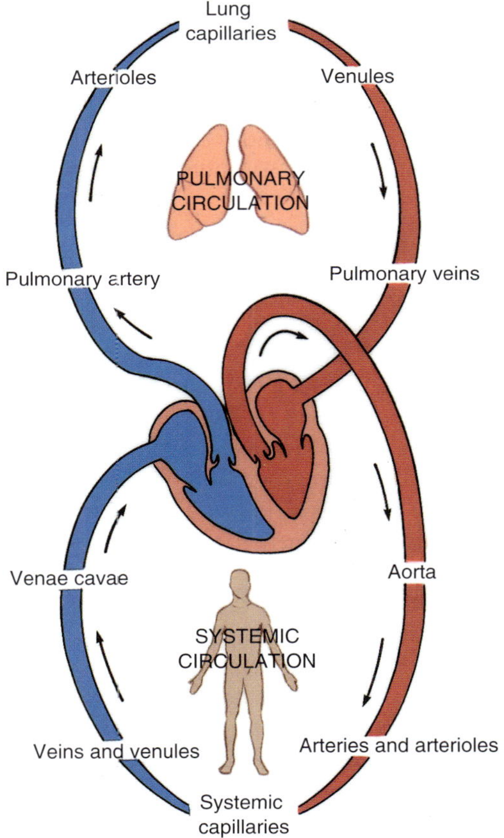

Fig. 12.13 Scheme of circulation. In pulmonary circulation, arteries take blood from the right ventricle to the lungs, and veins return the blood to the left atrium. In systemic circulation, arteries take blood from the left ventricle to the body tissues, and veins return the blood to the right atrium. (From Applegate E: *The anatomy and physiology learning system*, ed 4, St. Louis, 2011, Saunders.)

until the branching results in microscopic arteries called *arterioles*. The arterioles play a key role in regulating blood flow into the tissue capillaries. Approximately 10% of the total blood volume is in the systemic arterial system at any given time.

The wall of an artery consists of three layers. The innermost layer is the *tunica intima* (also called *tunica interna*). The middle layer is the *tunica media*, which consists of smooth muscle and is usually the thickest layer. It not only provides support for the vessel but also changes vessel diameter to regulate blood flow and blood pressure. The outermost layer is the *tunica externa* or *tunica adventitia.*

Capillaries

Capillaries are the smallest and most numerous of the blood vessels. They form the connection between the vessels that carry blood away from the heart (arteries) and the vessels that return blood to the heart (veins). They are the continuation of the smallest arterioles. Arterioles are the smallest vessels that have three distinguishable layers in their wall. When the arterioles branch into capillaries, the middle and outer layers of the wall disappear so that the capillary wall is only a thin endothelium consisting of one cell layer. This thin wall permits the exchange of materials between the blood in the capillary and the adjacent tissue cells. This exchange is the primary function of capillaries.

The diameter of a capillary is so small that erythrocytes must pass through the capillaries in single file. This slows the blood flow to allow ample time for the transport of substances across the capillary endothelium.

Veins

Veins carry blood toward the heart. After blood passes through the capillaries, it enters the smallest veins, called *venules.* From the venules, it flows into progressively larger and larger veins until it reaches the heart. In the pulmonary circuit, the pulmonary veins transport blood from the lungs to the left atrium of the heart. This blood has a high oxygen content because it has just been oxygenated in the lungs. Systemic veins transport blood from the body tissues to the right atrium of the heart. This blood has a reduced oxygen content because the oxygen has been used for metabolic activities in the tissue cells.

The walls of veins have the same three layers as the arteries. Although all the layers are present, there is less smooth muscle and connective tissue. This makes the walls of veins thinner than those of arteries. This is related to the fact that blood in the veins has less pressure than blood in the arteries. Because the walls of the veins are thinner and less rigid than those of arteries, veins can hold more blood. Almost 70% of the total blood volume is in the veins at any given time. Medium and large veins have *venous valves* that help to keep the blood flowing toward the heart. These are similar to the SL valves associated with the heart. Venous valves are especially important in the arms and legs, where they prevent the backflow of blood in response to the pull of gravity.

CIRCULATORY PATHWAYS

The blood vessels of the body are functionally divided into two distinct circuits: the pulmonary circuit and the systemic circuit.

The pump for the pulmonary circuit, which circulates blood through the lungs, is the right ventricle. The left ventricle is the pump for the systemic circuit, which provides the blood supply for the tissue cells of the body.

Pulmonary Circuit

The pulmonary circuit takes blood from the right side of the heart to the lungs and then returns it to the left side of the heart (see Figs. 12.4 and 12.13). Oxygen-poor blood, which has increased levels of carbon dioxide, is returned to the right atrium from the tissue cells of the body. It passes through the tricuspid valve into the right ventricle. During ventricular systole, the blood is ejected through the pulmonary SL valve into the pulmonary trunk, which divides into the right and left pulmonary arteries. Each pulmonary artery enters a lung and repeatedly divides into smaller and smaller vessels until they become capillaries. The capillaries of the lungs form networks that surround the air sacs, or alveoli, of the lungs. Here CO_2 diffuses from the capillary blood into the alveoli of the lungs, and O_2 diffuses from the alveoli into the blood. The newly oxygenated blood enters pulmonary venules, which form progressively larger veins, until two pulmonary veins emerge from each lung and carry the blood to the left atrium. In the pulmonary circuit, the arteries carry deoxygenated blood away from the heart and the veins carry oxygenated blood to the heart.

Systemic Circuit

The systemic circulation provides the functional blood supply to all body tissues. It carries oxygen and nutrients to the cells and picks up carbon dioxide and waste products. Systemic circulation carries oxygenated blood from the left ventricle, through the arteries, to the capillaries in the tissues of the body. The major systemic arteries are illustrated in Fig. 12.14. From the tissue capillaries, the deoxygenated blood returns through a system of veins to the right atrium of the heart. The major systemic veins are illustrated in Fig. 12.15.

LYMPHATIC SYSTEM

The lymphatic system has three primary functions. It returns excess interstitial fluid to the blood to maintain homeostasis between the fluid in the blood and the fluid that surrounds tissue cells. The second function deals with the absorption of fats and fat-soluble vitamins. These substances are absorbed from the intestinal tract into specialized lymph capillaries. The third function of the lymphatic system is defense against invading microorganisms and disease.

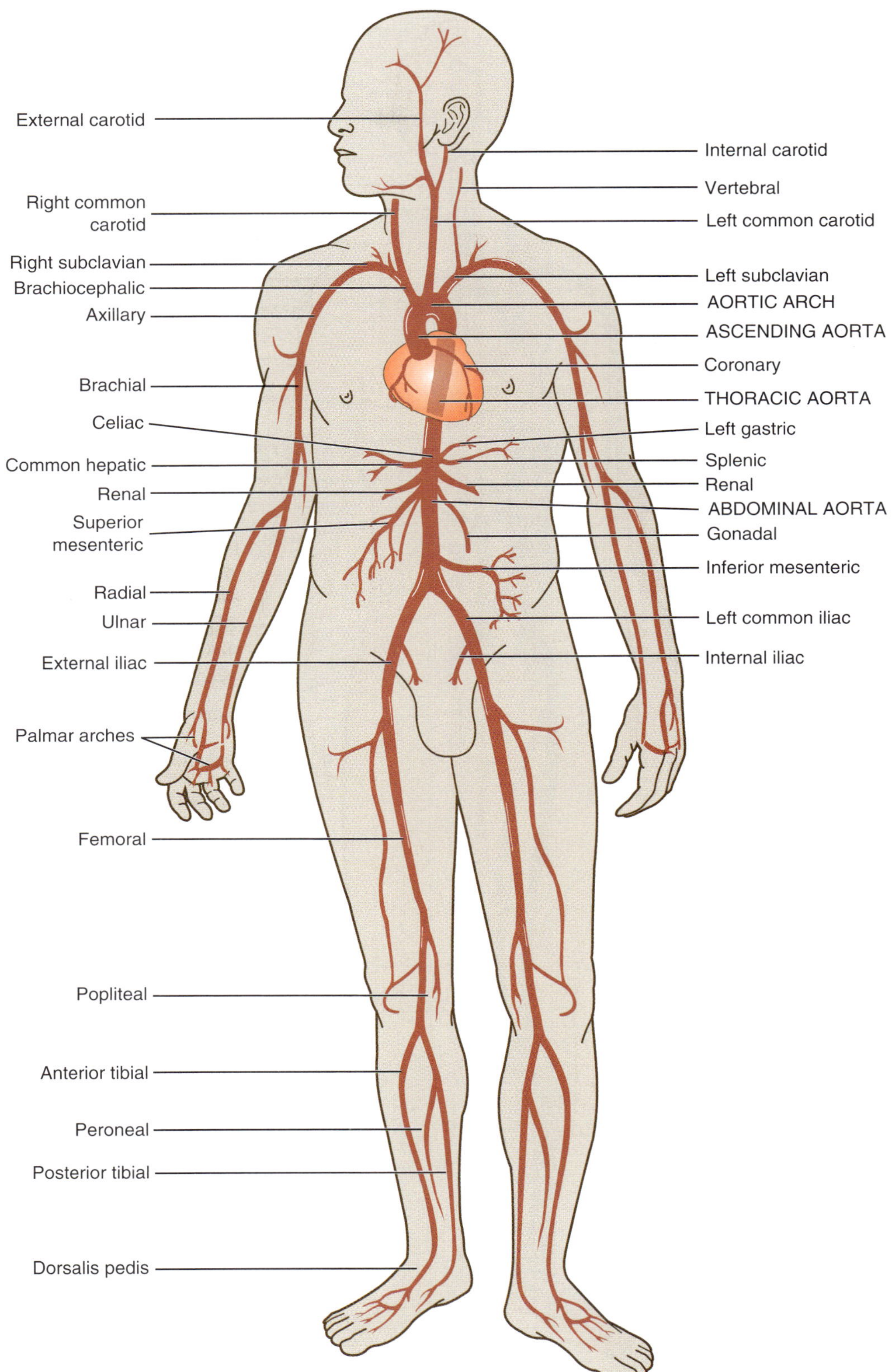

Fig. 12.14 Major systemic arteries. (From Applegate E: *The anatomy and physiology learning system*, ed 4, St. Louis, 2011, Saunders.)

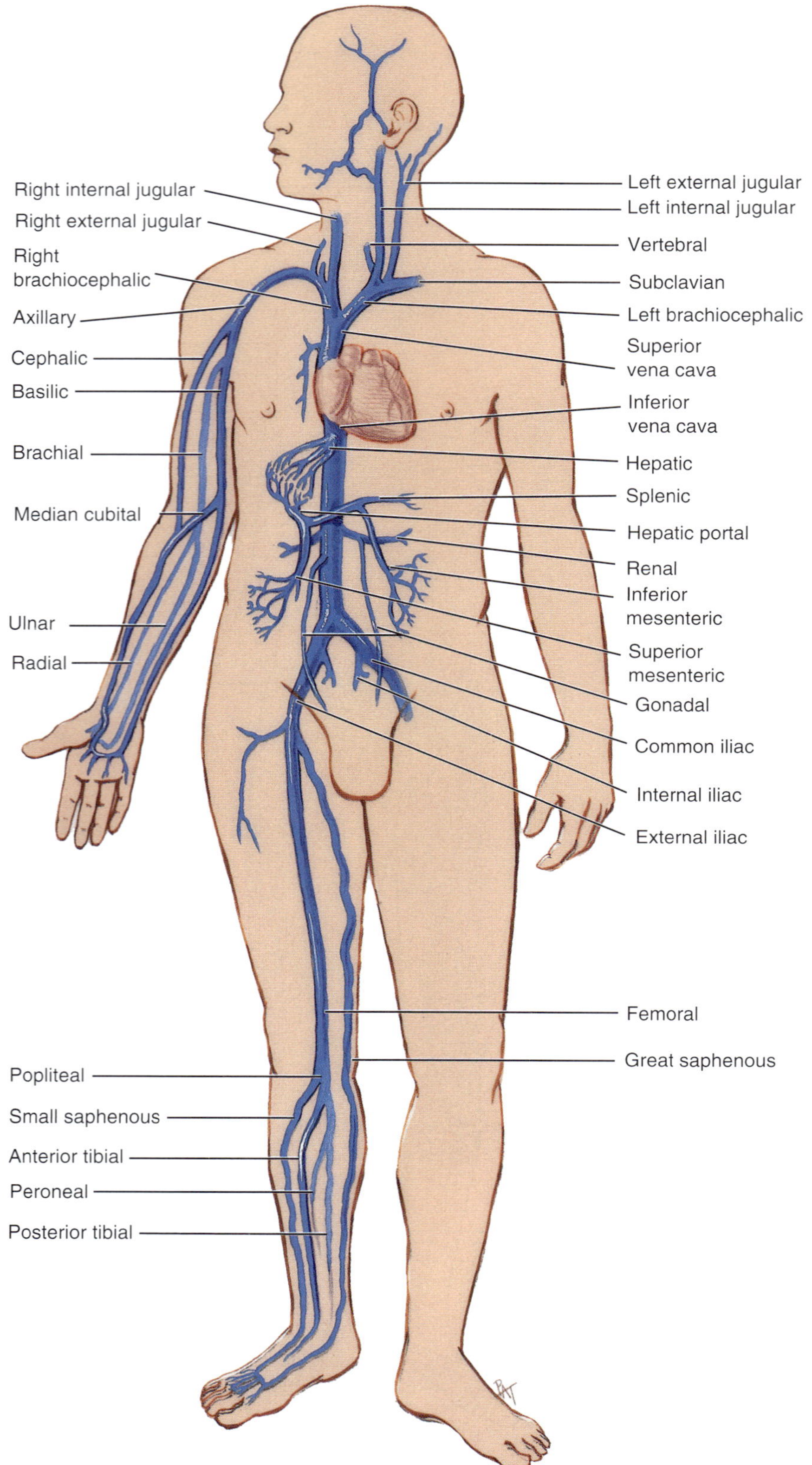

Fig. 12.15 Major systemic veins. (From Applegate E: *The anatomy and physiology learning system*, ed 4, St. Louis, 2011, Saunders.)

LYMPH

The fluid in the lymphatic vessels is called *lymph*. It is similar in composition to blood plasma and is derived from it. At the arteriole end of a capillary, some of the plasma escapes from the blood vessel and enters the tissue spaces. Approximately 90% of this fluid reenters the venule end of the capillary. The remaining 10% remains in the tissue spaces as interstitial fluid. As the fluid accumulates, it is picked up by tiny lymph vessels and becomes lymph. This transition of fluid from blood plasma to interstitial fluid to lymph and eventually back to the blood prevents edema and helps to maintain blood volume, plasma protein concentration, and blood pressure.

LYMPHATIC VESSELS

Lymphatic vessels carry fluid away from the tissues and return it to the venous system. The smallest lymphatic vessels are the lymph capillaries, which are small blind-ended sacs intertwined with the blood capillaries in the tissue spaces. These tiny lymph capillaries merge to form larger and larger vessels until the lymph enters the two lymphatic ducts. The **right lymphatic duct** receives lymph from the upper right quadrant of the body and empties into the right subclavian vein. The **thoracic duct** drains lymph from the remaining three quadrants of the body and empties into the left subclavian vein. Lymph nodes that filter the lymph are located along the various vessels of the lymphatic system. Like veins, the walls of lymph vessels are thin and have valves. Because there is no pump to provide pressure, the flow of lymph is sporadic and sluggish. The force to create pressure gradients for flow must come from external sources such as skeletal muscle contraction and respiratory movements. Anything that interferes with the flow of lymph, such as an obstruction or surgical ligation, may cause tissue fluid to accumulate, resulting in edema.

LYMPHATIC ORGANS

Lymphatic organs are characterized by clusters of lymphocytes and other cells, such as macrophages, with a meshlike framework of connective tissue fibers. When the body is exposed to foreign substances, the lymphocytes proliferate then enter the blood and travel to the site of the foreign substance. This is part of the body's immune response that attempts to destroy the invading agent. The lymph nodes, tonsils, spleen, and thymus are lymphatic organs.

Lymph nodes are small bean-shaped structures that are located along the lymphatic vessels. The primary function of lymph nodes is to filter the lymph as it flows through the vessels so that the lymph is cleansed by lymphocytes and macrophages before it enters the blood. Even though lymph nodes are widely distributed in the body, there are three superficial regions where they tend to cluster. These are the *inguinal nodes* in the groin region, the *axillary nodes* in the armpit, and the *cervical nodes* in the neck. These are illustrated in Fig. 12.16. There are no lymph nodes in the central nervous system.

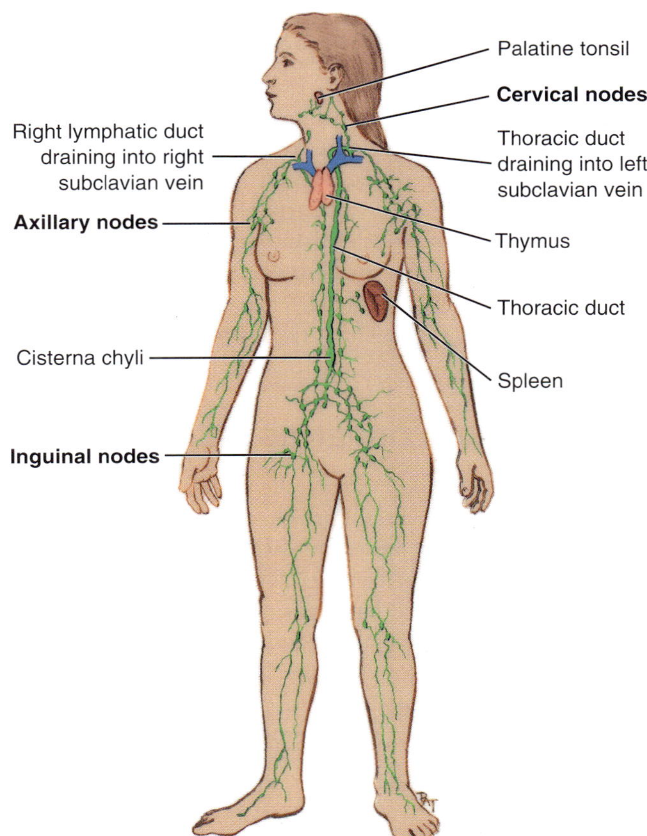

Fig. 12.16 Location of the clusters of superficial lymph nodes. (From Applegate E: *The anatomy and physiology learning system*, ed 4, St. Louis, 2011, Saunders.)

Tonsils are clusters of lymphatic tissue just under the mucous membrane of the nose, mouth, and throat. The *pharyngeal tonsils* are near the opening of the nasal cavity in the pharynx. These are sometimes called *adenoids*. The *palatine tonsils* are located near the opening of the oral cavity into the pharynx. These are the ones commonly referred to as "tonsils." The *lingual tonsils* are located near the base of the tongue. Lymphocytes and macrophages in the tonsils help to protect against pathogens that may enter the body through the nose and mouth.

The *spleen* is located in the upper left quadrant of the abdominal cavity, just under the diaphragm and behind the stomach. It is the largest lymphatic organ. The spleen filters blood in much the same way as a lymph node filters lymph. Lymphocytes and macrophages react with pathogens in the blood and attempt to destroy them. The spleen also acts as a reservoir for blood and destroys old, worn-out erythrocytes.

The *thymus* is a soft, two-lobed organ that is located anterior to the ascending aorta and posterior to the sternum. It is relatively large in infants and children, but after puberty it begins to decrease in size so that in older adults it is quite small. The primary function of the thymus is the maturation of special lymphocytes called *T lymphocytes*. It also produces the hormone *thymosin*, which stimulates the maturation of lymphocytes in other lymphatic organs.

RESISTANCE TO DISEASE

To remain healthy, the body must counteract the effects of pathogens and other harmful substances. This ability is called **resistance**, and the lack of resistance is **susceptibility**. Resistance is dependent on a variety of defense mechanisms. **Nonspecific defense mechanisms** act against all harmful agents; **specific defense mechanisms** are effective against only certain agents. Specific defense mechanisms provide *immunity.* All defense mechanisms act together to maintain a healthy body.

NONSPECIFIC DEFENSE MECHANISMS

Nonspecific mechanisms provide the initial defense against invading agents regardless of their nature. Barriers against entry into the body present the first line of nonspecific defense. Intact or unbroken skin and mucous membranes are effective mechanical barriers against entry. The motion of fluids such as tears, saliva, and urine flushes invading agents away before they can enter the body. Lysozymes in tears and saliva, sebaceous secretions on the skin, and hydrochloric acid in the stomach provide chemical deterrents against invasion. If pathogens succeed in passing through the first line barriers, then nonspecific second line barriers attempt to destroy the invading agents. The second line barriers include chemicals such as interferon and complement, phagocytosis, and inflammation. Specific defense mechanisms provide the third line of defense, or immunity, against microbial invasion. The primary cells involved in immunity are lymphocytes and macrophages. Fig. 12.17 provides an overview of defense mechanisms.

SPECIFIC DEFENSE MECHANISMS

In contrast to the nonspecific nature of the first two lines of defense, *specific defense mechanisms* are programmed to be selective and act against specific pathogens. This characteristic is called *specificity*. The second characteristic of immunity is *memory.* Once the body has been exposed to a particular invading agent, the system "remembers" it and launches a quicker attack when the agent enters the body again.

For the immune system to function properly, lymphocytes must recognize the difference between "self" and "non-self." During development, lymphocytes are programmed to recognize the proteins and other large molecules that belong to the body. Molecules that are not recognized as "self" are

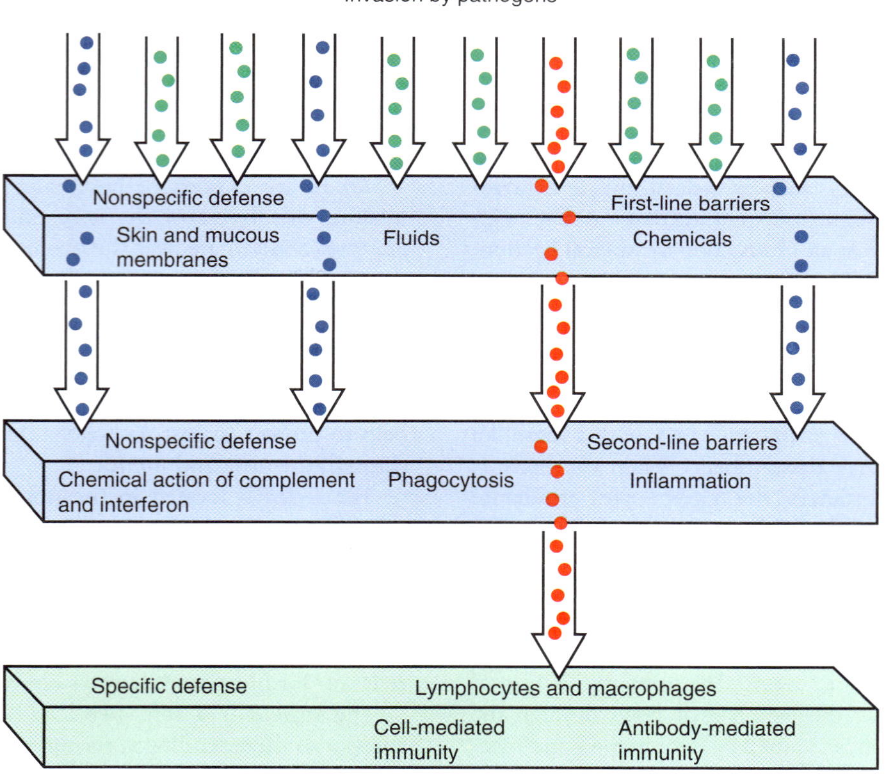

Fig. 12.17 Overview of defense mechanisms. Pathogens that are stopped from entering the body by the first line barriers of nonspecific defense are represented by green dots. Others get through the first line barriers but are stopped by nonspecific second line barriers. These pathogens are represented by blue dots. Those that penetrate nonspecific defense mechanisms are subject to specific defense mechanisms. These pathogens are represented by the red dots. (From Applegate E: *The anatomy and physiology learning system*, ed 4, St. Louis, 2011, Saunders.)

interpreted as "non-self," and the immune system attempts to destroy them. These "non-self" molecules are called **antigens** and are usually proteins or large polysaccharide molecules on the surface of the cell membrane. Usually the antigens that cause problems are foreign molecules that originate outside the body, but occasionally the body fails to recognize its own molecules and triggers an immune response against self. This is the basis of autoimmune diseases.

As indicated earlier in this chapter, lymphocytes develop from hemocytoblasts in the bone marrow. During fetal development, immature lymphocytes are released into the blood. Some of these immature cells go to the thymus where they acquire the ability to distinguish between self and non-self molecules. These become *T lymphocytes* or *T cells*. Differentiated T cells leave the thymus, enter the blood, and are distributed to lymphoid tissue, especially lymph nodes where they are responsible for **cell-mediated immunity**. Approximately 70% of the circulating lymphocytes are T cells. Developing lymphocytes that differentiate in some place other than the thymus are called *B lymphocytes* or *B cells*. These cells also are distributed to lymphoid tissue and are responsible for **antibody-mediated immunity**, or *humoral immunity*. B cells account for approximately 30% of circulating lymphocytes.

CELL-MEDIATED IMMUNITY

In cell-mediated immunity, T cells directly attack invading antigens. It is most effective against virus-infected cells, cancer cells, foreign tissue cells (transplant rejection), fungi, and protozoan parasites. When a foreign antigen enters the body, it is phagocytized by a macrophage, which presents it to a T cell with receptors for that specific antigen. This activates the T cell, and it divides to produce four clones: *killer T cells* that directly destroy the cells with the offending antigen; *helper T cells* that stimulate B cells and promote the immune response; *suppressor T cells* that inhibit B cells and the immune response; and *memory T cells* that promote a faster and more intense response on subsequent exposure to the same antigen. Fig. 12.18 illustrates the mechanism of cell-mediated immunity.

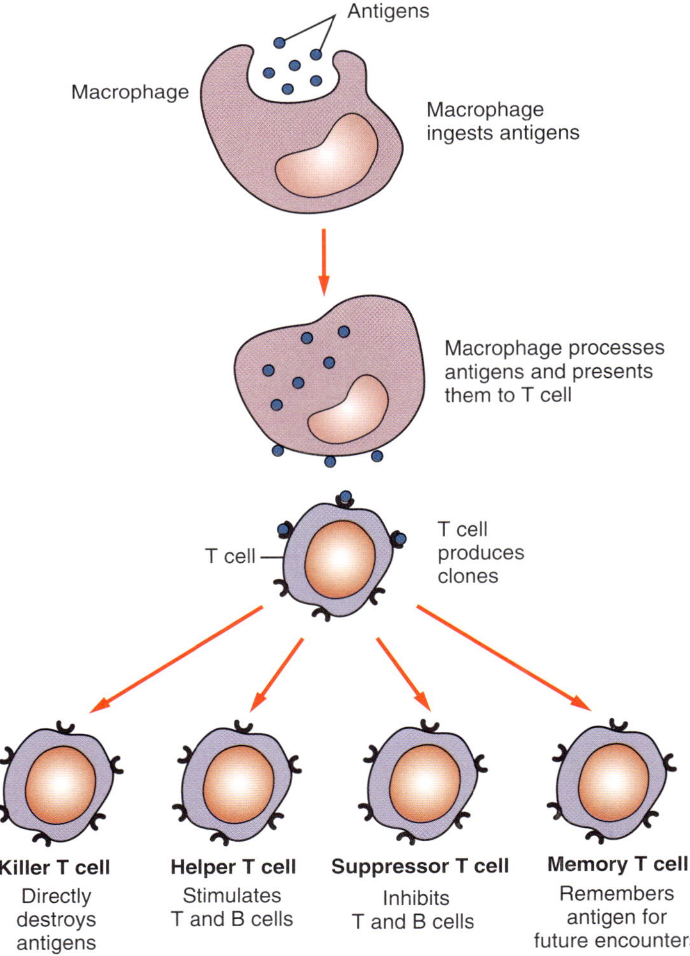

Fig. 12.18 Cell-mediated immunity. Macrophage ingests antigens, processes them, and presents them to the T cell. The T cell produces four clones. (From Applegate E: *The anatomy and physiology learning system*, ed 4, St. Louis, 2011, Saunders.)

ANTIBODY-MEDIATED IMMUNITY

In antibody-mediated immunity, B cells are responsible for the production of *antibodies* that inactivate the invading antigens. Because antibodies are found in body fluids, this type of immunity is sometimes called humoral immunity. Antibody-mediated immunity is most effective against bacteria, viruses that are outside body cells, and toxins. It is also involved in allergic reactions. Like T cells, each type of B cell can respond to only one specific type of antigen. There must be a match between the receptor on the B cell and the antigen. When a foreign antigen enters the body, a macrophage engulfs and processes it, then presents it to specific B cells and helper T cells with receptors for that specific antigen. This activates the cells, and the helper T cells further stimulate the B cells to divide and form two clones: *plasma cells* that produce antibodies, and memory B cells that promote a faster and more intense response on subsequent exposure to the same antigen. Fig. 12.19 illustrates the mechanism of antibody-mediated immunity.

All antibodies have a similar structure, but one part of the molecule differs so that each antibody is capable of reacting with only a specific antigen. Antibodies belong to a class of proteins called *globulins*, and because they are involved in immune reactions, they are called **immunoglobulins**, abbreviated Ig. There are five types of immunoglobulins: IgA, IgG, IgM, IgE, and IgD. IgG immunoglobulins are called *γ-globulins*. Each class of immunoglobulin has a specific role in immunity. These are summarized in Table 12.1.

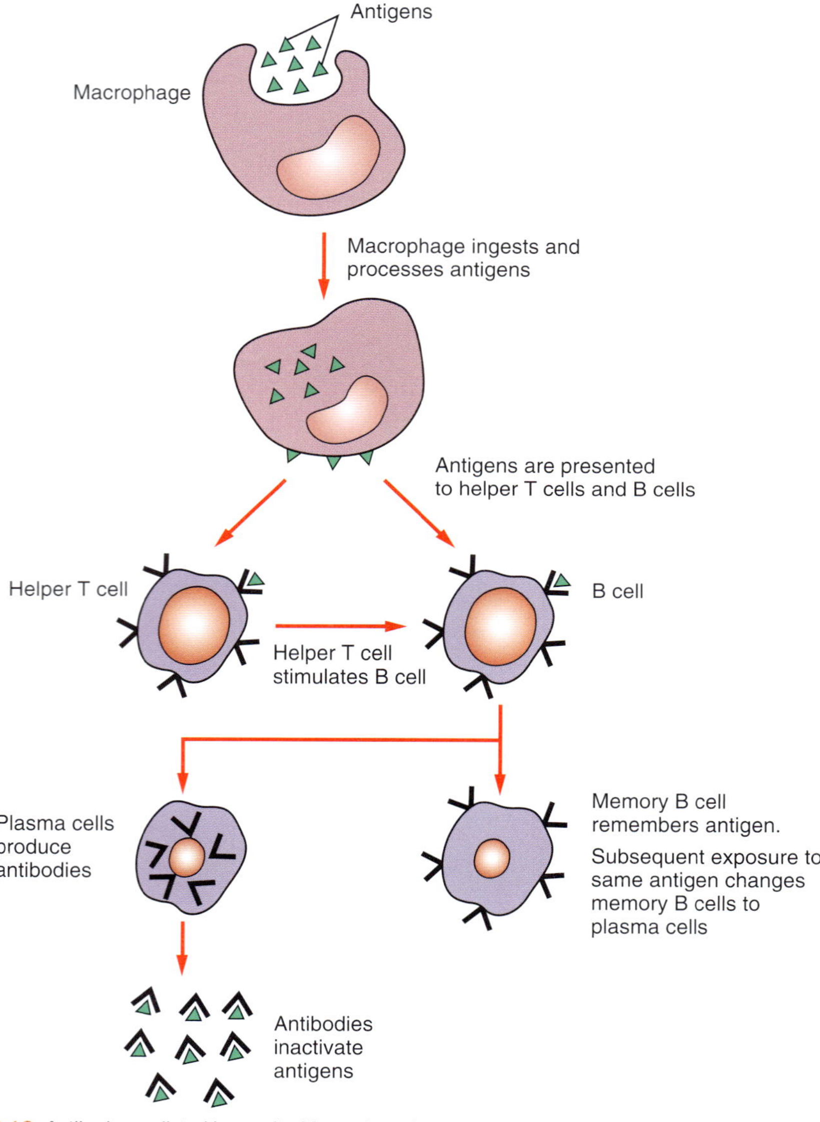

Fig. 12.19 Antibody-mediated immunity. Macrophage ingests and processes antigen, then presents it to helper T cells and B cells. Helper T cells stimulate B cells to divide and produce two clones consisting of memory B cells and plasma cells. Plasma cells produce antibodies that inactivate the antigen. (From Applegate E: *The anatomy and physiology learning system*, ed 4, St. Louis, 2011, Saunders.)

Table 12.1 Classes of Antibodies

Class	Percentage of Total	Location	Function
IgG	75%–85%	Blood plasma	Major antibody in primary and secondary immune responses; inactivates antigen; neutralizes toxins; crosses placenta to provide immunity for newborn; responsible for Rh reactions
IgA	5%–15%	Saliva, mucus, tears, breast milk	Protects mucous membranes for body surfaces; provides immunity for newborn
IgM	5%–10%	Attached to B cells; released into plasma during immune response	Causes antigen to clump together; responsible for transfusion reactions in ABO blood typing system
IgD	0.2%	Attached to B cells	Receptor sites for antigens on B cells; binding with antigen results in B cell activation
IgE	0.5%	Produced by plasma cells in mucous membranes and tonsils	Binds to mast cells and basophils, causing release of histamine; responsible for allergic reactions

From Applegate E: *The anatomy and physiology learning system*, ed 4, St. Louis, 2011, Saunders.

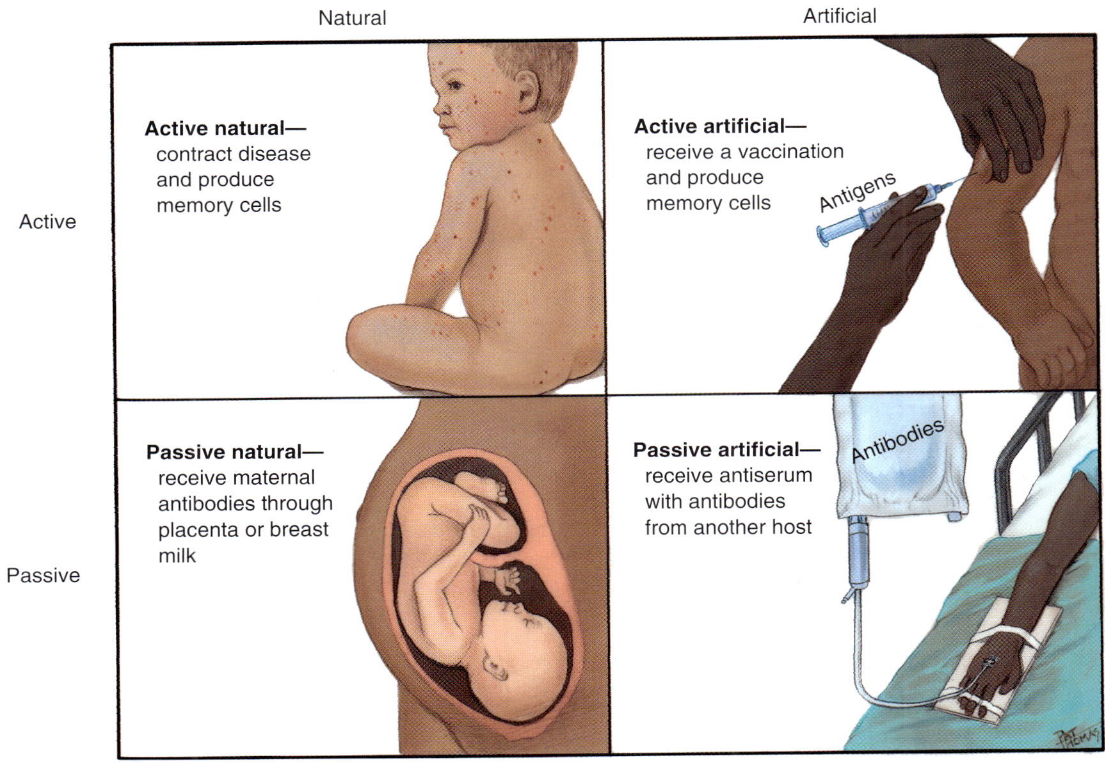

Fig. 12.20 Acquired immunity. (From Applegate E: *The anatomy and physiology learning system*, ed 4, St. Louis, 2011, Saunders.)

ACQUIRED IMMUNITY

There are four ways to acquire immunity. The terms *active* and *passive* refer to whose immune system responds to an antigen. Active immunity occurs when an individual's own body responds and produces memory cells. Passive immunity results when the immune agents develop in another person (or animal) and are transferred to an individual who was not previously immune. The terms *natural* and *artificial* refer to how the immunity is obtained. Natural immunity occurs when the immunity is acquired through normal everyday living without any deliberate action. Artificial immunity results when some deliberate action is taken, such as a vaccination. Combining these terms gives four types of acquired immunity: active natural immunity, active artificial immunity, passive natural immunity, and passive artificial immunity. These four types of immunity are summarized in Fig. 12.20.

AGING OF THE CIRCULATORY SYSTEM

Numerous "age-related" changes occur in the heart. How many of these are caused by an actual aging process and how many are caused by other factors are questions worth considering. Is it possible to lessen the effects of aging by adjusting lifestyle? Cardiac changes that were once thought to be the result of aging are currently believed to be the consequence of a sedentary lifestyle that many consider their "reward" after retirement. Other cardiac changes are caused by a lifetime of habits that, although enjoyable at the time, take their toll later in life. It is difficult to isolate the aging process of the heart because it is so closely related to diet, exercise, and disease processes, but even when these factors are excluded, a clinical pattern of cardiac aging emerges.

In the absence of cardiovascular disease, the heart, particularly the left ventricle, tends to become slightly smaller in elderly people. This results partially from a decrease in the number and size of cardiac muscle cells, and partially from the reduced demands placed on it by decreasing physical activity. However, because of cardiovascular disease, the heart is often enlarged.

A general thickening of the endocardium and valves of the heart occurs as part of the aging process. The valves tend to become more rigid and incompetent. Thus heart murmurs are detected more frequently in the elderly. Structural changes also occur throughout the conduction system as conducting myofibers are replaced with fibrous tissue. Usually this does not alter the resting pulse rate, but there is a greater-than-normal increase in heart rate in response to activity. Dysrhythmias are also more frequent.

Numerous disease processes that occur more frequently in the aging individual have an effect on the heart. Most notable of these is arteriosclerosis, or hardening of the arteries. This puts additional stress on the heart and aggravates the normal age-related changes. Although some degree of arteriosclerosis is probably inevitable in the aging process, a significant amount of vascular disease can be prevented by a proper diet, regular walking or other aerobic exercise, and the elimination of cigarette smoking. In other words, lifestyle probably has more effect on the cardiovascular system than aging.

Common Pathology of the Circulatory System

Disease	Signs and Symptoms	Etiology	Diagnosis and Treatment
Acquired immunodeficiency syndrome (AIDS)	Immune system is badly damaged, making an individual vulnerable to infections and opportunistic illnesses. The helper T cell (CD4) number falls to less than 200 cells/mm^3 in the blood.	Cause is the human immunodeficiency virus (HIV). AIDS is the final stage in the course of the disease.	Diagnosis relies on the HIV enzyme-linked immunosorbent assay (ELISA) and the HIV Western blot test. The helper T cell (CD4) number is less than 200 cells/mm^3 in the blood. Early stages of HIV may be treated with antiretroviral therapy (ART). There is no cure. By the time HIV has progressed to AIDS, life expectancy is approximately 3 years.
Anemia	Fatigue and lethargy, pale skin, dizziness, cold hands and feet, headache, irregular heartbeat.	Most common cause is blood loss; dysfunction in syntheses of hemoglobin; excessive destruction of red blood cells.	Typically diagnosed by a routine blood test, but further testing may be necessary to determine underlying cause. Treatment depends on underlying cause. May need to replace blood cells through transfusion or increase iron or vitamin K in the diet.
Anemia, iron deficiency	Fatigue and lethargy, pale skin, dizziness, cold hands and feet, headache, irregular heartbeat.	Deficiency of iron in the diet, blood loss, ulcers, cancer, prolonged use of aspirin.	Typically diagnosed by a routine blood test, but further testing may be necessary to determine underlying cause. Common treatments are to replace blood cells through transfusion and increase iron in the diet.
Anemia, pernicious	Fatigue and lethargy, pale skin, dizziness, cold hands and feet, headache, irregular heartbeat.	Lack of intrinsic factor from the parietal cells in the stomach interferes with the absorption of vitamin B_{12}, which is necessary for production of healthy red blood cells. The most likely cause of the parietal cell dysfunction is an autoimmune response.	Diagnosis is made by use of a combination of medical history, physical examination, and blood tests. Treatment is aimed at restoring vitamin B_{12} levels, usually through pills or injections.

Common Pathology of the Circulatory System—cont'd

Disease	Signs and Symptoms	Etiology	Diagnosis and Treatment
Angina pectoris	Chest pain.	Reduced blood flow to the cardiac muscle.	Some of the tests used to diagnose angina are the electrocardiogram (ECG), stress test, echocardiogram, nuclear stress test, coronary angiography, cardiac magnetic resonance imaging (MRI), and computed tomography (CT). Treatment aims to restore blood flow through rest, angioplasty, stents, or coronary artery bypass grafting (CABG).
Atherosclerosis	In the heart, chest pain; in the brain, transient ischemic attacks (TIAs); in the arms and legs, peripheral artery disease (PAD); in the kidneys, kidney dysfunction.	Specific type of arteriosclerosis (hardening of the arteries) in which fatty deposits narrow the lumen of the vessels. May be caused by high blood pressure, high cholesterol, high triglycerides, smoking, diabetes, infections from other diseases.	Diagnosis is based on physical examination, medical history, blood tests, Doppler ultrasound, ECG, stress test, angiogram, CT, and/or MRI. Treatment options include a healthy diet, exercise regimen, cholesterol medications, beta-blockers, angiotensin-converting enzyme (ACE) inhibitors, antiplatelet medications (blood thinners), diuretics, and calcium channel blockers. In some patients, angioplasty and stents, endarterectomy, or bypass surgery may be necessary.
Cardiomyopathy	Chest pain, dyspnea, peripheral edema, ECG abnormalities.	Causes include ischemia, drug and alcohol toxicity, or certain infections. May be secondary to other conditions such as diabetes mellitus, acromegaly, and muscular dystrophy.	Diagnosis is based on a combination of medical history, blood tests, physical examination, ECG, echocardiogram, cardiac cauterization and biopsy, and cardiac MRI. Treatment depends on the type of cardiomyopathy and condition of the disease but may include one of more of the following: pacemakers, defibrillators, left ventricular assist devices (LVADs), and ablation. Some patients may require a heart transplant.
Congestive heart failure (CHF)	Fatigue, lethargy, peripheral edema, dyspnea.	Heart's pumping ability is impaired; may be caused by coronary artery disease, high blood pressure, cardiomyopathy, valvular disease, or heart defects.	Diagnosis is based on medical history and physical examination; procedures that may aid in diagnosis include ECG, chest x-ray examination, blood tests, and echocardiography. Treatment goal is to have the heart beat more efficiently. Specific treatment depends on underlying cause but may include weight loss, exercise program, and controlling high blood pressure. ACE inhibitors and beta-blockers help heart to beat more effectively.
Coronary artery disease (CAD)	Chest pain, dyspnea, arrhythmias, fatigue.	Coronary arteries become narrow or blocked because of the accumulation of fatty deposits in the wall. Risk factors include high blood pressure, high cholesterol, high triglycerides, smoking, diabetes, lack of exercise, and obesity.	Diagnosis is based on physical examination, medical history, blood tests, echocardiography, nuclear imaging, cardiac CT, stress tests, and heart cauterization. Treatment options include aspirin, beta-blockers, calcium channel blockers, and angioplasty and stents. Bypass surgery may be necessary in some cases. The best treatment is prevention by maintaining a healthy lifestyle, controlling high blood pressure, cholesterol levels, and diabetes.
Hemophilia	Excessive bleeding and frequent bruising.	The cause is an absence of clotting factors in the blood as a result of a gene defect of the X chromosome.	Diagnosis is based on family history, physical examination, and blood tests. Primary treatment is replacement therapy in which clotting factors are slowly infused into a vein.

Continued

Common Pathology of the Circulatory System—cont'd

Disease	Signs and Symptoms	Etiology	Diagnosis and Treatment
Hodgkin lymphoma	Swelling of lymph nodes, fatigue, fever and chills, night sweats, weight loss, dyspnea, loss of appetite, and itching.	Occurs when a B cell develops a mutation in its DNA. Mutation causes a large number of abnormal B cells to accumulate in the lymphatic system, where they crowd out healthy cells.	Diagnostic tools include physical examination, blood tests, imaging tests, lymph node biopsy, and bone marrow testing. Treatment modalities include chemotherapy, radiation therapy, and stem cell transplant.
Hypertension	Typically is asymptomatic.	No identifiable cause for primary (essential) hypertension; secondary hypertension may be caused by kidney disease, tumors of the adrenal gland, or thyroid dysfunction.	Systolic pressure above 140 mm Hg and diastolic pressure greater than 90 mm Hg is typically considered hypertension. Treatment may include lifestyle changes to include a healthy diet and exercise. Medications that lower blood pressure include diuretics, beta-blockers, ACE inhibitors, and calcium channel blockers.
Infectious mononucleosis	Fever, sore throat, swollen lymph nodes, fatigue.	Epstein–Barr virus (EBV) spread through saliva.	Diagnosis is primarily from observation of symptoms. Differential tests may be used to distinguish it from cytomegalovirus and *Toxoplasma gondii* infections. The condition is usually self-limiting and little treatment is required. Medications may be used to reduce pain and fever.
Leukemia	Swollen lymph nodes, frequent nosebleeds, bleeding from the gums or rectum, frequent bruising, heavy menstrual bleeding, fever, loss of appetite, fatigue.	Leukemia occurs when the bone marrow starts to produce an abundance of abnormal white blood cells. Cause is unclear. Risk factors include exposure to high levels of radiation and toxic chemicals.	Diagnostic tools include medical history, physical examination, blood tests, bone marrow aspiration and biopsy, and lymph node biopsy. The treatment goal is to destroy leukemia cells and allow normal cells to form in the bone marrow. Treatment modalities depend on the type of leukemia but may include chemotherapy, radiation therapy, corticosteroids, and stem cell transplant.
Mitral valve prolapse	Most individuals have no symptoms. When symptoms occur, they may include chest pain, shortness of breath, swelling in the legs and feet, and heart palpitations.	In most patients the cause of mitral valve prolapse is unknown. During ventricular systole a portion of the mitral valve slips backward, allowing some of the blood to flow back into the left atrium instead of exiting the heart through the aorta (mitral regurgitation). Common cause of heart murmurs.	Heart murmurs and abnormal heart sounds heard through a stethoscope may indicate mitral valve prolapse. Diagnosis can be confirmed with echocardiography. Treatment usually is not necessary. Severe cases of mitral regurgitation may benefit from surgery to repair or replace the faulty valve.
Multiple myeloma	No symptoms in the early stages. May progress to include bone pain, weakness and fatigue, weight loss, opportunistic infections, and kidney problems.	The underlying cause is unknown. Plasma cells multiply abnormally within the bone marrow. These release unhealthy levels of immunoglobulin into the blood, which accumulates to cause organ damage, bone lesions, and red blood cell dysfunction, resulting in anemia.	Diagnosis is based on blood and urine tests, imaging tests, and bone marrow biopsy. Treatment modalities may include chemotherapy, radiation therapy, and stem cell transplant.
Myocardial infarction (MI)	Acute chest pain, nausea, vomiting, profuse sweating, heartburn or indigestion.	The typical cause is atherosclerosis in which a coronary artery becomes occluded so that cardiac muscle becomes ischemic and dies.	Diagnosis confirmed by ECG and blood tests to assay for enzymes that are released into the blood by dying heart muscle. The typical treatment protocol is fibrolytic agents, diagnostic angiogram, percutaneous coronary intervention (PCI; also called *stenting*). Some cases may require CABG.

Common Pathology of the Circulatory System—cont'd

Disease	Signs and Symptoms	Etiology	Diagnosis and Treatment
Non-Hodgkin lymphoma	Swollen lymph nodes, weight loss, fever, and night sweats.	Cause is unknown. Occurs when the body produces too many T cell and B cell lymphocytes. Risk factors include medications that suppress the immune system, toxic chemicals, and some viral or bacterial infections.	Diagnosis relies on physical examination, medical history, blood tests, chest x-ray examination, CT and/or positron emission tomography (PET) scan, lymph node and bone marrow biopsies. Treatment depends on the type and stage of the lymphoma, its growth rate, and patient's age and health. Modalities include chemotherapy, radiation therapy, drugs to enhance the immune system, and stem cell transplant.
Peripheral arterial disease (PAD)	Leg pain when walking or climbing stairs; leg numbness; sores on the toes, feet, or legs that do not heal; coldness in lower leg or foot; shiny skin on the legs; change in the color of the legs.	Most frequent cause is atherosclerosis that narrows the blood vessels supplying the legs and reduces blood flow to the legs.	Diagnostic tools include physical examination, ankle-brachial index (ABI) to compare blood pressure in the ankle with blood pressure in the arm, ultrasound, angiography, and blood tests. Many patients can be treated with lifestyle changes including diet and exercise. Others may require medications to alleviate pain, prevent blood clots, lower cholesterol, and lower blood pressure. Angioplasty or bypass grafting may be necessary in severe cases.
Polycythemia	Weakness, fatigue, headache, joint pain, dizziness.	In primary polycythemia, a gene mutation results in abnormally high production of red blood cells. In secondary polycythemia, the cause is hypoxia as a result of chronic obstructive pulmonary disease (COPD), chronic heart disease, or renal hypoxia. Temporary polycythemia may occur at high altitudes.	Usually detected by routine blood tests that evaluate hemoglobin, hematocrit, and red blood cell concentration. Other tests may be needed to determine the underlying cause. For primary polycythemia, treatment is phlebotomy and antiplatelet agents. For secondary polycythemia, treatment is directed at the underlying cause.
Rheumatic heart disease (RHD)	Fatigue, lethargy, peripheral edema, dyspnea. Signs and symptoms are caused by heart failure resulting from failure of heart valves to open and close properly.	RHD is caused by faulty mitral and/or aortic valves as a result of endocarditis secondary to rheumatic fever. There may be either stenosis so the valves do not open or regurgitation because the valves do not close.	Diagnosis is based on medical history, chest x-ray examination and/or MRI, echocardiogram, and ECG. Many patients require no treatment. If valve damage is severe, valvuloplasty or valve replacement may be necessary.
Shock	Cool and clammy skin, weak and rapid pulse, nausea, lack of brilliance in eyes, feelings of weakness and confusion.	Trauma, heart failure, bleeding, dehydration, infection, severe allergic reactions. Shock is a life-threatening medical condition as a result of insufficient blood flow through the body.	Diagnosis is based on signs and symptoms. Treatment: call 911 immediately. Administer intravenous fluids to raise blood pressure. Medications such as epinephrine, norepinephrine, and dopamine raise blood pressure. After the patient's condition has been stabilized, treat the underlying cause.
Systemic lupus erythematosus (SLE)	Fever, malaise, joint pain, myalgia, fatigue. There may be skin rash, photosensitivity, mucous membrane ulcers, arthritis, pleuritis or pericarditis, kidney abnormalities, seizures, blood count abnormalities, and antinuclear antibodies in the blood. These are intermittent, and not all are present in any one individual.	SLE is an autoimmune connective tissue disease that can affect any part of the body. There is no single cause. Triggers include heredity, viruses, ultraviolet light, and drugs.	Diagnosis depends on physical examination and blood tests. There is no cure. Treatment is directed at relieving symptoms. Some patients may be treated with immunosuppressants.

Continued

Common Pathology of the Circulatory System—cont'd

Disease	Signs and Symptoms	Etiology	Diagnosis and Treatment
Thrombophlebitis	Redness, swelling, pain, and warmth in the affected area.	Occurs when a blood clot (thrombus) blocks one or more veins, usually in the leg, with subsequent inflammation of the vessel. May be near the surface or deep within the muscles (deep vein thrombosis [DVT]).	Diagnosis is based on patient history, examination, blood tests, ultrasound, and CT scans. Treatment involves application of heat to the affected area, elevation of the leg, and antiinflammatory drugs. Blood thinning and clot dissolving medications, compression stockings, varicose vein stripping, and insertion of a filter in the inferior vena cava (IVC) to trap emboli before they reach the lungs or heart may be necessary.

TERMINOLOGY REVIEW

Key Term	Word Parts	Definition
Agranulocytes	*a:* without *granul/o:* granules *cyte:* cell	White blood cells that lack granules in the cytoplasm.
Antibodies	*anti:* against	Substances produced by the body that inactivate or destroy other substances that are introduced into the body; immunoglobulins.
Antibody-mediated immunity		Immunity that is the result of B cell action and the production of antibodies; also called *humoral immunity.*
Antigens		Substances that trigger an immune response when they are introduced into the body.
Atria (singular atrium)		Thin-walled chambers of the heart that receive blood from veins.
Atrioventricular valves	*atri/o:* atrium *ventricul/o:* ventricle	Valves between the atria and the ventricles in the heart.
Cardiac cycle		A complete heartbeat consisting of contraction and relaxation of both atria and both ventricles.
Cell-mediated immunity		Immunity that is the result of T cell action.
Coagulation	*coagul/o:* clotting *-tion:* process	The process of blood clotting.
Conduction myofibers	*my/o:* muscle	Cardiac muscle cells specialized for conducting action potentials to the myocardium; part of the conduction system of the heart; also called *Purkinje fibers.*
Diapedesis	*dia-:* through	The process by which white blood cells squeeze between the cells in a vessel wall to enter the tissue spaces outside the blood vessel.
Diastole		Relaxation phase of the cardiac cycle; opposite of systole.
Endocardium	*endo:* within *card/i:* heart *-um:* tissue	The thin, smooth inner lining of each chamber of the heart.
Epicardium	*epi:* around, outside *card/i:* heart *-um:* tissue	The outer layer of the heart wall; the visceral pericardium.
Erythrocytes	*erythr/o:* red *-cyte:* cell	Red blood cells.
Erythropoiesis	*erythr/o:* red *-poieses:* formation	The process of red blood cell formation.
Erythropoietin	*erythr/o:* red *-poietin:* substance that forms	A hormone released by the kidneys that stimulates red blood cell production.
Granulocytes	*granul/o:* granules *-cyte:* cell	White blood cells that develop granules in the cytoplasm.

TERMINOLOGY REVIEW—cont'd

Key Term	Word Parts	Definition
Hematopoiesis	*hemat/o:* blood *-poieses:* formation	Blood cell production, which occurs in the red bone marrow; also called *hemopoiesis.*
Hemocytoblast	*hem/o:* blood *-cyt-:* cell *-blast:* to form	A stem cell in the bone marrow from which the blood cells arise.
Hemoglobin	*hem/o:* blood *-globin:* protein	The iron-containing protein in red blood cells that is responsible for the transport of oxygen.
Hemostasis	*hem/o:* blood *-stasis:* control	The control or stoppage of bleeding.
Immunoglobulins	*immun/o:* immunity or protection *globulin:* a class of protein	Substances produced by the body that inactivate or destroy other substances that are introduced into the body; antibodies.
Leukocytes	*leuk/o:* white *-cyt-:* cell	White blood cells.
Macrophages	*macr/o:* large *-phag-:* to eat, devour	Large phagocytic connective tissue cell that functions in immune responses; name given to a monocyte after it leaves the blood and enters the tissues.
Megakaryocytes	*mega:* large *kary/o:* nucleus *cyte:* cell	A large cell that contributes to the formation of platelets.
Myocardium	*my/o:* muscle *card/i-:* heart *-um:* tissue	Middle layer of the heart wall; composed of cardiac muscle tissue.
Nonspecific defense mechanisms		Body's ability to counteract all types of harmful agents.
Pericardial cavity	*peri:* around *card/i:* heart	Small space around the heart, between the parietal pericardium and visceral pericardium, that contains a small amount of serous fluid for lubrication.
Pericardium	*peri:* around *card/i:* heart	Membrane that surrounds the heart; usually refers to the pericardial sac.
Pulmonary circulation	*pulmon-:* lung	The pathway that takes blood from the right side of the heart to the lungs and then returns it to the left side of the heart.
Renal erythropoietic factor	*ren/o:* kidney *erythr/o:* red *poie:* formation of blood cells	A substance produced by the kidneys that activates erythropoietin to stimulate the production of red blood cells.
Resistance		Body's ability to counteract the effects of pathogens and other harmful agents.
Right lymphatic duct		The collecting duct of the lymphatic system that collects lymph from the upper right quadrant of the body.
Semilunar valves		Valves between the ventricles of the heart and the vessels that carry blood away from the ventricles; also pertains to the valves in veins.
Specific defense mechanisms		Activities of the body that counteract only certain types of harmful agents.
Susceptibility		Lack of resistance to disease.
Systemic circulation		Pathways that transport blood from the left side of the heart to all parts of the body and return the blood to the right atrium; excludes pulmonary circulation.
Systole		Contraction phase of the cardiac cycle; opposite of diastole.
Thoracic duct		The primary collecting duct of the lymphatic system that collects lymph from all regions of the body except the upper right quadrant.
Thrombocytes	*thromb/o:* clot *-cyte:* cell	A class of formed elements of the blood; function in blood clotting; also called *platelets.*
Ventricles		Pumping chambers of the heart; right ventricle pumps blood to the lungs and left ventricle pumps blood into systemic circulation.

13 Respiratory System

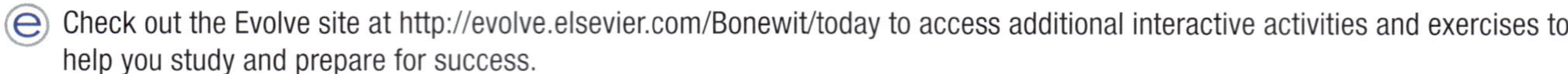

Check out the Evolve site at http://evolve.elsevier.com/Bonewit/today to access additional interactive activities and exercises to help you study and prepare for success.

LEARNING OBJECTIVES

1. List and describe the structures of the upper respiratory tract.
2. List and describe the structures of the lower respiratory tract.
3. Explain what occurs during inhalation and exhalation.
4. Explain the difference between external respiration and internal respiration.
5. Explain how respiration is regulated by the brain.
6. Identify factors that influence breathing.
7. Describe ways in which the aging of an individual affects the respiratory system.
8. Identify pathology related to the respiratory system.

CHAPTER OUTLINE

KEY TERMS

alveoli (al-VEE-oh-lie)
bronchi (BRON-kye)
bronchial tree (BRONG-kee-al TREE)
external respiration (eks-TER-nal res-per-RAY-shun)
fauces (FAW-seez)
internal respiration (in-TER-nal res-per-RAY-shun)
laryngopharynx (lah-rin-joh-FAIR-inks)
larynx (LAIR-inks)
lower respiratory tract (LOW-er RES-per-ah-tor-ee TRACT)
nasopharynx (nay-zoh-FAIR-inks)
oropharynx (ohr-oh-FAIR-inks)
pharynx (FAIR-inks)
pleura (PLOO-rah)
pleural cavity (PLOO-ral CAV-ih-tee)
respiration (res-per-RAY-shun)
respiratory membrane (RES-per-ah-tor-ee MEM-brayn)
surfactant (sir-FAK-tant)
trachea (TRAY-kee-ah)
upper respiratory tract (UP-per RES-per-ah-tor-ee TRACT)
ventilation (ven-tih-LAY-shun)

INTRODUCTION TO THE RESPIRATORY SYSTEM

When the respiratory system is mentioned, people usually think of breathing, but this is only one of the activities of the respiratory system. The cells in the body need a continuous supply of oxygen for the metabolic processes that are necessary to maintain life. The respiratory system works with the circulatory system to provide this oxygen and to remove the waste products of metabolism which consists primarily of carbon dioxide. The respiratory system also helps to regulate the pH of the blood.

FUNCTIONS AND OVERVIEW OF RESPIRATION

Respiration is the sequence of events that results in the exchange of oxygen and carbon dioxide between the atmosphere and the body cells. Every 3 to 5 seconds, nerve impulses stimulate the breathing process, or **ventilation**, which moves air through a series of passages into and out of the lungs. After this there is an exchange of gases between the lungs and the blood. This is called **external respiration**. The blood transports the gases to and from the tissue cells. The exchange of gases between the blood and tissue cells is known as **internal respiration**.

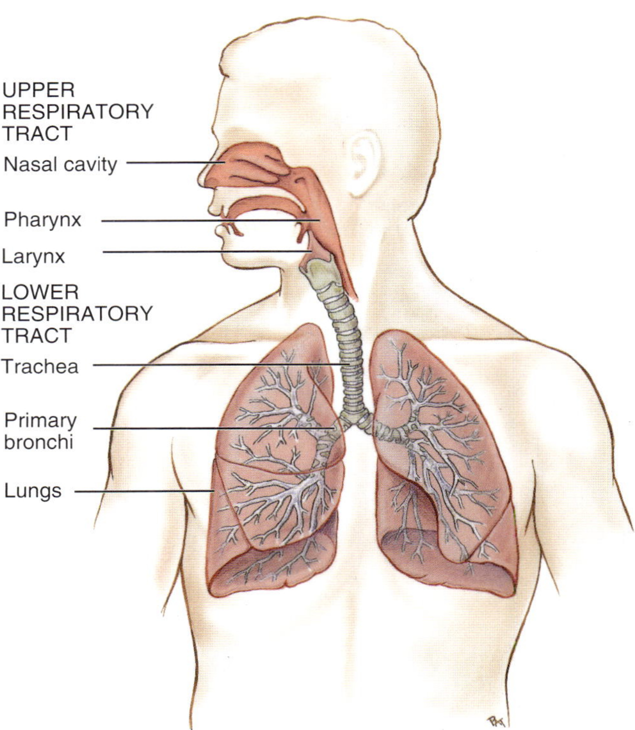

Fig. 13.1 Conducting passages of the respiratory system. The upper respiratory tract includes the nose, pharynx, and larynx. The lower respiratory tract consists of the trachea, bronchial tree, and lungs. (From Applegate E: *The anatomy and physiology learning system,* ed 4, St. Louis, 2011, Saunders.)

VENTILATION

Ventilation, or breathing, is the movement of air through the conducting passages between the atmosphere and the lungs.

CONDUCTING PASSAGES

The conducting passages are divided into the **upper respiratory tract** and the **lower respiratory tract** (Fig. 13.1). The upper respiratory tract includes the nose, pharynx, and larynx. The lower respiratory tract consists of the trachea, bronchial tree, and lungs. These passageways open to the outside and are lined with mucous membrane. In some regions the membrane has hairs that help to filter the air. Other regions have cilia to propel mucus.

Nose and Nasal Cavities

The framework of the nose consists of bone and cartilage. Two small nasal bones and extensions of the maxillae form the bridge of the nose, which is the bony portion. The remainder of the framework is cartilage. This is the flexible portion. Connective tissue and skin cover the framework.

The interior chamber of the nose is the nasal cavity (Fig. 13.2). It is divided into two parts by the nasal septum. Air enters the nasal cavity from the outside through two openings—the nostrils, or external nares. The openings from the nasal cavity into the pharynx are the internal nares. The *palate* forms the floor of the nasal cavity and separates the nasal cavity from the oral cavity. The anterior portion of the palate is called the *hard palate* because it is supported by bone. The posterior portion has no bony support, so it is called the *soft palate.* The soft palate terminates in a projection called the *uvula*, which helps to direct food into the oropharynx.

Nasal conchae are bony ridges that project into the nasal cavity (see Fig. 13.2). The three nasal conchae increase the surface area of the nasal cavity to warm and moisten the air inhaled through the nose. The nasal conchae also help to direct air flow through the nasal cavity. Dust and other particles in the air tend to become trapped in the mucous membrane around the nasal conchae.

Paranasal sinuses are air-filled cavities in the frontal, maxillae, ethmoid, and sphenoid bones. These sinuses surround the nasal cavity and open into it. They reduce the weight of the skull, produce mucus, and influence voice quality by acting as resonating chambers. The sinuses are lined with mucous membrane that produces mucus, which drains into the nasal cavity. During infections and allergies, the membranes in the passages that drain the sinuses become inflamed and swollen. The swelling may block the passages and cause the mucus to accumulate in the sinuses. As the mucus accumulates, pressure within the sinuses increases, resulting in a sinus headache.

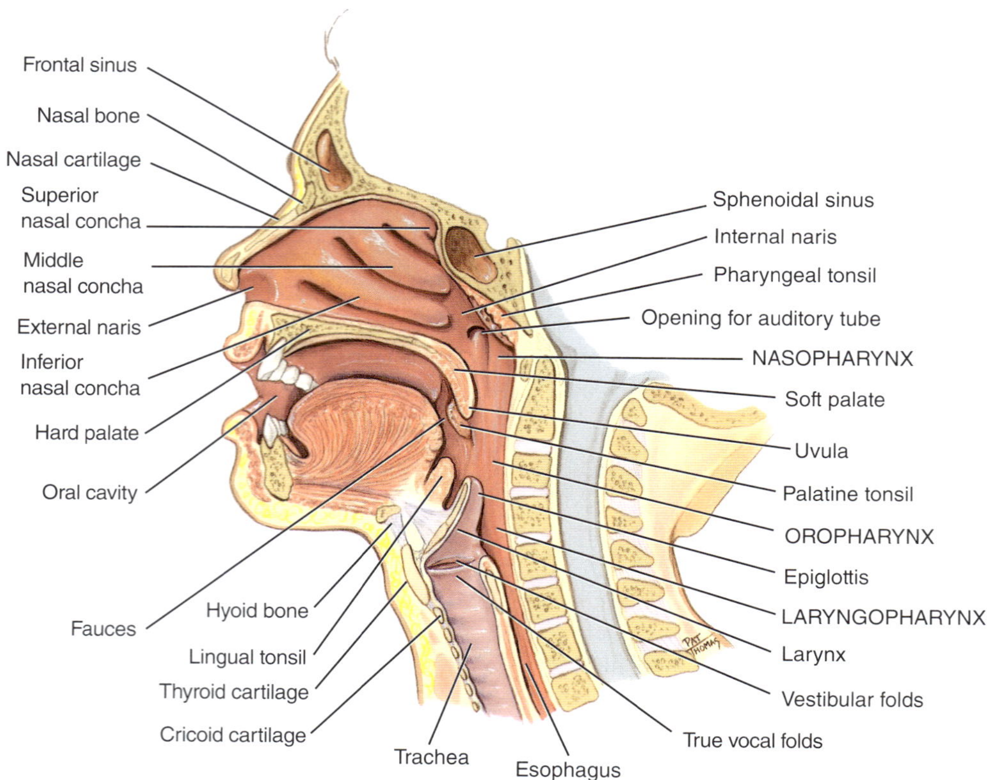

Fig. 13.2 Features of the upper respiratory tract. The upper respiratory tract includes the nose, pharynx, and larynx. (From Applegate E: *The anatomy and physiology learning system*, ed 4, St. Louis, 2011, Saunders.)

As air passes through the nasal cavity, it is filtered, warmed, and moistened. Goblet cells in the mucous membrane produce mucus, which traps microorganisms, dust, and other foreign particles. Cilia attached to the epithelium propel the mucus with the trapped particles toward the pharynx, where it is swallowed. Acid in the gastric juice destroys most of the microorganisms that are swallowed. An extensive capillary network under the mucous membrane warms and moistens the air before it reaches the rest of the respiratory tract.

Pharynx

The **pharynx**, commonly called the *throat*, is a passageway approximately 13 cm long. It serves both the respiratory and digestive systems by receiving air from the nasal cavity and air, food, and water from the oral cavity. Inferiorly, it opens into the larynx and esophagus. The pharynx is divided into three regions according to location: nasopharynx, oropharynx, and laryngopharynx (see Fig. 13.2).

The **nasopharynx** is the portion of the pharynx that is posterior to the nasal cavity and extends to the uvula. Air enters this region from the nasal cavity through the internal nares. The mucous membrane in the nasopharynx is similar to the lining of the nasal cavity. The *auditory* (eustachian) *tubes* from the two middle ear cavities open into the nasopharynx. The auditory tubes help to equalize the air pressure on both sides of the tympanic membrane. Collections of lymphoid tissue, called *pharyngeal tonsils* (or *adenoids*), are located in the posterior wall of the nasopharynx.

The **oropharynx** is the portion of the pharynx that is posterior to the oral cavity. It receives air, food, and water from the oral cavity. During swallowing, the soft palate and uvula move upward to prevent the material from going into the nasopharynx. The opening between the oral cavity and oropharynx is called the **fauces**. The fauces is bordered by masses of lymphoid tissue called *tonsils*. The *palatine tonsils* are in the lateral walls of the oropharynx, adjacent to the fauces. The *lingual tonsils* are located on the surface of the posterior portion of the tongue, also in the region of the fauces. The tonsils in the pharynx function in immune responses and help to prevent infections.

The most inferior portion of the pharynx is the **laryngopharynx** (see Fig. 13.2). It is posterior to the larynx and is continuous with the esophagus.

Larynx

The **larynx**, commonly called the *voice box*, is the passageway for air between the pharynx and the trachea. It is approximately 5 cm long and formed by nine pieces of cartilage that are connected to one another by muscles and ligaments.

The three largest cartilaginous portions of the larynx are the thyroid cartilage, cricoid cartilage, and epiglottis (see Fig. 13.2). The *thyroid cartilage* forms a projection in the neck called the *Adam's apple.* The projection is more pronounced in males than in females. The *cricoid cartilage* forms the base of the larynx and is attached to the trachea. The *epiglottis* is a long, leaf-shaped structure. During swallowing, the epiglottis covers the opening into the larynx to prevent food and water from entering the trachea.

The larynx houses two pairs of ligaments. The upper pair are the *vestibular folds*, or *false vocal cords.* They work with the epiglottis to prevent particles from entering the lower respiratory tract. The lower pair are the *true vocal cords*, which function in sound production. Muscles control the length and tension of the true vocal cords. They are relaxed during normal breathing. When the vocal cords are under tension, exhaled air moving past them causes them to vibrate and produce sound. The length of the vocal cords determines the pitch of the sound, and the force of the moving air regulates the loudness. The opening between the true vocal cords is the *glottis*, which leads to the trachea.

Trachea

The **trachea** is commonly called the *windpipe.* It consists of a tube that extends from the larynx and into the mediastinum, where it divides into the right and left **bronchi** (Fig. 13.3). It is approximately 12 to 15 cm long. The walls of the trachea are supported by 15 to 20 C-shaped pieces of hyaline cartilage that hold the trachea open despite the pressure changes that occur during breathing. The posterior open part of the C-shaped cartilage is closed by smooth muscle and connective tissue and is next to the esophagus. During swallowing, the esophagus bulges into the soft part of the trachea.

The mucous membrane that lines the trachea is ciliated epithelium, similar to that in the nasal cavity and nasopharynx. Goblet cells located in the mucous membrane produce mucus that traps airborne particles and microorganisms. The cilia propel the mucus upward, where it is either swallowed or expelled. Continued irritation from cigarette smoke and other air pollutants damages the cilia, and the mucus with the trapped particles is not removed. Microorganisms thrive in the accumulated mucus, which results in respiratory infections. Irritation and inflammation of the mucous membrane stimulate the cough reflex.

Bronchi and Bronchial Tree

In the mediastinum the trachea divides into the right and left primary bronchi. After the bronchi enter the lungs, they branch several times into smaller and smaller passages to form the **bronchial tree** (see Fig. 13.3). The primary bronchi divide to form secondary (lobar) bronchi. The branching continues until the pathway terminates in clusters of tiny air sacs called **alveoli**.

The alveoli consist primarily of simple squamous epithelium, which permits rapid diffusion of oxygen and carbon dioxide. Exchange of gases between the air in the lungs and the blood in the capillaries occurs across the walls of the alveoli.

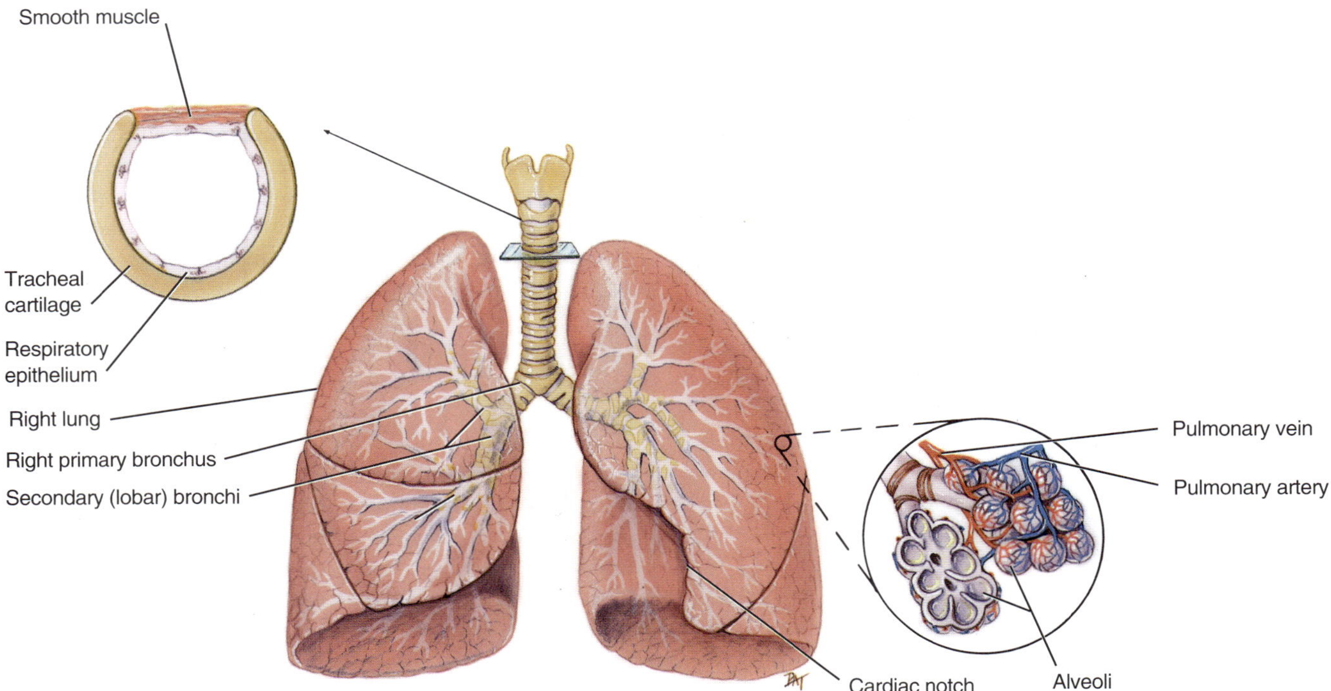

Fig. 13.3 Features of the lower respiratory tract. The lower respiratory tract includes the trachea, bronchial tree, and lungs. Note the C-shaped cartilage ring of the trachea at the upper left and the clusters of alveoli in the lower right. (From Applegate E: *The anatomy and physiology learning system*, ed 4, St. Louis, 2011, Saunders.)

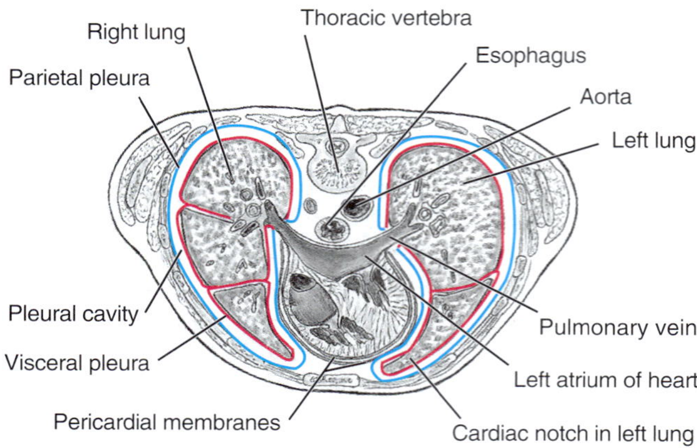

Fig. 13.4 Features of the lungs and pleura. Note the three lobes in the right lung and two lobes in the left lung. *Red* indicates visceral pleura, and *blue* indicates parietal pleura. (From Applegate E: *The anatomy and physiology learning system*, ed 4, St. Louis, 2011, Saunders.)

Lungs

The two lungs occupy most of the space in the thoracic cavity (Fig. 13.4). The lungs are soft and spongy because they are mostly air spaces surrounded by the alveolar cells and elastic connective tissue. The right and left lungs are separated from each other by the mediastinum, which contains the heart. Each lung is roughly cone shaped, rests on the diaphragm, and extends upward just above the midpoint of the clavicle.

The right lung is shorter, is broader, and has a greater volume than the left lung. It is divided into three lobes (superior, middle, and inferior) by two fissures. The left lung is longer and narrower than the right lung. It has an indentation, called the *cardiac notch*, on its medial surface for the apex of the heart. The left lung is divided into two lobes by a single fissure.

Each lung is enclosed by a double-layered serous membrane called the **pleura** (see Fig. 13.4). The *visceral pleura* is firmly attached to the surface of the lung. The visceral pleura is continuous with the *parietal pleura*, which lines the wall of the thorax. The small space between the visceral and parietal pleurae is the **pleural cavity**. It contains a thin film of serous fluid that is produced by the pleura. The fluid acts as a lubricant to reduce friction as the two layers slide against each other.

MECHANICS OF VENTILATION

Pulmonary ventilation is commonly referred to as *breathing.* It is the process of air flowing into the lungs during inhalation and out of the lungs during **exhalation**. Air flows because of pressure differences between the atmosphere and the gases inside the lungs. Under normal conditions, the average adult takes 12 to 20 breaths/min. A breath is one complete respiratory cycle that consists of one inhalation and one exhalation. The amount of air that is exchanged during one cycle varies with age, sex, size, and physical condition.

Inhalation

Inhalation (or *inspiration*) is the process of taking air into the lungs. It is the active phase of ventilation because it is the result of muscle contraction. In normal, quiet breathing, the primary muscle involved in inhalation is the dome-shaped diaphragm. When the diaphragm contracts, it drops, or becomes flatter. This increases the size (volume) of the thoracic cavity. When the thoracic volume increases, the pressure within the lungs decreases to less than atmospheric pressure. This causes air to flow from the region of higher atmospheric pressure outside the body into the region of lower pressure within the lungs. Air continues to flow into the lungs until the pressure equals atmospheric pressure.

Exhalation

Exhalation (or *expiration*) is the process of letting air out of the lungs during the breathing cycle. When the diaphragm relaxes, the volume of the thoracic cavity decreases to its normal resting size. This decrease in lung volume causes an increase in the pressure of the lungs. Air now flows from the region of higher pressure within the lungs to the region of lower atmospheric pressure outside the body until the two pressures are equal.

As air leaves the lungs during exhalation, the alveoli become smaller. The interior surfaces of the alveoli are coated with a thin layer of fluid. The fluid molecules are attracted to one another, which tends to cause the surfaces to adhere to each other. This makes it harder to inflate the lungs during inhalation and creates a tendency for the lungs to collapse. Normally this is prevented by a substance called **surfactant**. Surfactant is a substance that is produced by certain cells within the lung tissue and reduces the attraction between the fluid molecules. Without surfactant, the alveoli collapse and become nonfunctional.

RESPIRATION

EXTERNAL RESPIRATION

External respiration is the exchange of oxygen and carbon dioxide between the lungs and the blood in the surrounding capillaries. Oxygen diffuses from the alveoli of the lungs into the blood, and carbon dioxide diffuses from the blood into the air in the alveoli. The surfaces in the lungs where diffusion occurs constitute the **respiratory membrane**. The rate of gaseous exchange across the respiratory membrane depends on the surface area of the membrane, thickness of the membrane, solubility of the gas, and difference in pressure of the gas on the two sides of the membrane.

HIGHLIGHT on the Respiratory System

Rhinitis: Rhinitis is an inflammation of the nasal mucosa, accompanied by excessive production of mucus. It can be caused by cold viruses, certain bacteria, and allergens.

Pharyngitis and laryngitis: Inflammation of the pharynx, or a sore throat, is pharyngitis. Inflammation of the vocal cords is laryngitis. The inflammation may be caused by overuse of the voice, infection with bacteria or viruses, or inhalation of irritating particles. Laryngitis results in hoarseness or an inability to speak above a whisper.

Tracheotomy: A tracheotomy is the creation of an opening into the trachea through the neck and insertion of a tube to facilitate passage of air or removal of secretions.

Respiratory obstruction: Foreign objects that become lodged in the larynx or trachea are usually expelled by coughing. If a person cannot speak or make a sound because of the obstruction, it means that the airway is completely blocked. This is a life-threatening situation. The Heimlich maneuver is a procedure in which the air in the person's own lungs is used to forcefully expel the object.

Bronchoscopy: Bronchoscopy is a procedure in which a fiberoptic bundle is inserted into the trachea and directed along the conducting passageways to the smaller bronchi. This allows direct visualization of the inside of the bronchi and collection of specimens for cytologic and bacterial studies.

Pleurisy: Pleuritis, or pleurisy, is an inflammation of the pleura and is often painful because the sensory nerves in the parietal pleura are irritated. As the condition progresses, the permeability of the membrane changes, which results in an accumulation of fluid in the pleural cavity, making breathing difficult.

Surfactant: Surfactant is not produced until the late stages of fetal life. Newborns who are born prematurely may not have enough surfactant, and the forces of surface tension collapse the alveoli. The newborn must reinflate the alveoli with each breath, which requires tremendous energy. The lack of surfactant accounts for many of the signs and symptoms of infant respiratory distress syndrome (IRDS). The condition is treated by using positive-pressure respirators that maintain pressure within the alveoli to keep them inflated. ■

INTERNAL RESPIRATION

Internal respiration is the exchange of gases between the tissue cells and the blood in the tissue capillaries. After the blood picks up oxygen in the lungs, the blood returns to the left side of the heart, which pumps it to the tissue capillaries. The oxygen is given off to the tissue cells, and the carbon dioxide is picked up by the blood to be transported as a waste product to the lungs.

REGULATION OF RESPIRATION

The normal breathing rate in adults averages 12 to 20 breaths/min. The rate is higher, up to 40 breaths/min, in children. The basic rate is established by the respiratory center in the brain stem, but environmental conditions and emotions influence variations in the rate.

RESPIRATORY CENTER

Groups of neurons in the *pons* and *medulla oblongata* (regions of the brain stem) make up the *respiratory center.* This center controls the rate and depth of breathing and contains both inhalation and exhalation areas. The inhalation area sends impulses along the *phrenic nerve* to the diaphragm. This causes the diaphragm to contract, and inhalation results. The inhalation neurons fatigue quickly and quit sending impulses to the diaphragm. When the impulses cease, the muscles of the diaphragm relax and exhalation occurs. When forceful exhalation is needed, the exhalation area of the brain sends impulses to the intercostal muscles. If the respiratory center in the brain stem is damaged, the impulses cease and breathing stops. Death will occur within a few minutes unless artificial breathing mechanisms are applied.

FACTORS THAT INFLUENCE BREATHING

Even though the respiratory center establishes the basic rhythm of breathing, it is influenced by factors that cause variations in the rate and depth of breathing.

Chemoreceptors

Chemoreceptors in the medulla are sensitive to changes in carbon dioxide concentrations in the blood and cerebrospinal fluid. They are not sensitive to changes in oxygen levels. If carbon dioxide concentrations increase, the receptors stimulate the respiratory center to increase the rate and depth of breathing. This decreases the concentrations back to normal levels. In contrast, low carbon dioxide levels decrease the rate and depth of breathing. Breathing may even stop for brief periods of time until concentrations increase to normal levels.

Stimulus From Higher Brain Centers

Impulses from higher brain centers may override the respiratory center temporarily. These impulses may be either voluntary or involuntary; however, the voluntary controls are limited. For example, if you try to voluntarily hold your breath, you can do so for only a limited time. When carbon dioxide levels reach a certain critical point, the impulses from the higher brain centers are ignored and the respiratory center resumes regular breathing.

Involuntary impulses from higher brain centers may stimulate rapid breathing in response to emotions, such as anxiety or excitement. Chronic pain also may result in involuntary stimulation from the higher brain centers. In contrast, sudden pain or sudden cold may cause a gasp or a momentary cessation of breathing.

Temperature

An increase in body temperature caused by a fever or strenuous physical exercise increases the breathing rate. The increased body temperature is associated with increased metabolism, which uses more oxygen and generates more carbon dioxide. When body temperature decreases, metabolic rate diminishes and breathing rate also decreases.

NONRESPIRATORY AIR MOVEMENTS

In addition to normal air movements that occur during breathing and result in pulmonary ventilation, there are a number of modifications called *nonrespiratory air movements*. Some of these are reflexes that clear air passages, others are voluntary, and some express emotions. These nonrespiratory air movements are outlined in Table 13.1.

Table 13.1 Nonrespiratory Air Movements

Movement	Description
Sneezing	Spasmodic contraction of exhalation muscles that forces air through nose and mouth.
Coughing	Long inhalation followed by closure of glottis; then a strong exhalation forces glottis open and sends a blast of air through upper respiratory tract.
Sighing	Long inhalation followed by a shorter but forceful exhalation.
Hiccupping	Spasmodic contraction of diaphragm followed by sudden closure of glottis to produce a sharp sound.
Crying	An inhalation followed by many short exhalations; glottis remains open and vocal cords vibrate; usually accompanied by tears and characteristic facial expressions.
Laughing	Same basic movements as crying but facial expressions differ; may be indistinguishable from crying.
Yawning	A deep inhalation through a widely opened mouth.

From Applegate E: *The anatomy and physiology learning system*, ed 4, St. Louis, 2011, Saunders.

AGING OF THE RESPIRATORY SYSTEM

Various harmful substances, including cigarette smoke, air pollution, and pathogens, continually bombard the respiratory system and take their toll. There is no way to avoid all of these irritants except to stop breathing! Some irritants, such as cigarette smoke, can be decreased, but others are inescapable.

Because of the continual contact between the respiratory system and the environment, it is difficult to distinguish between the changes in the tissues of the breathing apparatus, including the lungs, that are the result of aging and those that are the result of disease or other factors outside the body. Modifications in the lining of the respiratory tract probably are caused by environmental rather than solely aging-related factors. Long-term exposure to irritants results in deterioration of the cilia, which hinders their cleansing action and movement of mucus. As a consequence, the occurrence of emphysema and chronic bronchitis increases with age. Diminishing effectiveness of the immune system makes the elderly more susceptible to pneumonia and other microbial diseases. However, excluding external influences, there are changes that take place as a result of "normal" aging.

In general, one of the most common signs of respiratory aging is when a person is unable to maintain the same level of physical activity that was experienced in younger years. This is a gradual decline and may not be noticeable until phrases such as "I used to be able to..." become part of the conversation. The cardiovascular and muscular systems have an effect on endurance, and the skeletal system has an effect on thoracic volume, but the major change is a decreased ability of the respiratory system to acquire and deliver oxygen to the blood.

The impairment in oxygen delivery is the result of structural changes that take place in the respiratory tissues. One type of change is a loss of elasticity in the tissues of the respiratory system. The cartilage in the walls of the trachea and bronchi undergoes a progressive calcification. Smooth muscle fibers in the bronchioles are replaced by fibrous tissue, so they are less able to stretch and contract. Modifications in lung tissue cause the alveoli to lose some of their elastic recoil. The cumulative effect of these changes is a gradual decrease in respiratory volume and capacity and an increase in the volume of residual air in the lungs. Another change is deterioration of the walls between adjacent alveoli. This increases the size of each individual alveolus, but reduces the total surface area of the respiratory membrane for diffusion of gases. A lower percentage of the oxygen in alveolar air is able to diffuse into the lung capillaries. These changes result in a decreased ability to acquire and deliver oxygen to the blood, which reduces the capacity for physical activity.

Common Pathology of the Respiratory System

Disease	Signs and Symptoms	Etiology	Diagnosis and Treatment
Acute respiratory distress syndrome (ARDS)	After an acute lung injury, patient experiences difficulty in breathing, low blood pressure, rapid breathing, and shortness of breath.	ARDS typically occurs in people who are already critically ill or who have had traumatic injuries, such as a pulmonary contusion, aspiration of gastric contents, multiple blood transfusions, or drug overdose. Fluid buildup in the alveoli prevents oxygen from passing into the bloodstream.	An arterial blood gas analysis and chest x-ray examination provide the diagnosis. The overall goal is to maintain acceptable gas exchange. ARDS is typically treated with oxygen therapy, mechanical ventilation, and the administration of antibiotics.
Asthma	Wheezing, shortness of breath, chest tightness, and coughing.	An asthma attack is preceded by airway inflammation, causing the lining of the air passages to swell and the muscles surrounding the airways to tighten. This reduces the amount of air that can pass through the airways. Triggers for the attack are varied and include pollen, pet hair, mold, dust mites, tobacco smoke, air pollution, and many other irritants.	Pulmonary function tests measure how well the lungs are functioning and are used to diagnose and manage asthma. Several types of medications may be prescribed, some inhaled and some taken as pills. All asthma attacks require treatment with a quick-acting inhaler such as albuterol.
Bronchitis	Shortness of breath, often accompanied by fever, chills, fatigue, coughing, and/or the production of mucus (sputum).	Bronchitis may be acute or chronic. Acute bronchitis is usually caused by viruses similar to the cold and flu viruses. Chronic bronchitis is typically the result of smoking. Initially it can be difficult to distinguish the signs and symptoms of bronchitis from those of a common cold.	During a physical examination, a health professional will use a stethoscope to listen closely to lung sounds. A chest x-ray examination and/or pulmonary function tests may be required. Sputum analysis may be needed. Most cases of acute bronchitis resolve without medical treatment. Chronic bronchitis may benefit from pulmonary rehabilitation.
Chronic obstructive pulmonary disease (COPD)	Common signs and symptoms of COPD include chest tightness, a cough that produces mucus, shortness of breath with activity, and wheezing during breathing.	Smoking is the primary cause of COPD. It can also be caused by air pollution and occupational exposures. It is a disease that blocks airflow in and out of the lungs. It usually is a combination of chronic bronchitis and emphysema.	A key factor in diagnosis is the patient history. Pulmonary function tests, along with x-ray examination and computed tomography (CT) scans, confirm and evaluate the progression of the disease. Treatment aims to slow the progress and relieve the symptoms. Medications and oxygen therapy may be needed. The most essential step in treatment is to stop smoking.
Croup	Croup is characterized by a barking cough, hoarseness, and strained breathing, which usually worsens at night. It is more common in children.	Croup is caused by a virus and is an infection of the upper airway which obstructs breathing. It is the result of inflammation around the vocal cords, trachea, and bronchial tubes.	Croup is typically diagnosed by observing breathing patterns, listening to chest sounds, and examining the throat. Sometimes x-ray studies or other tests are used to rule out other possible illnesses. Aggressive treatment is rarely needed. If symptoms persist, a type of steroid to reduce inflammation in the airway may be prescribed.
Emphysema	The main symptom of emphysema is shortness of breath, which usually begins gradually but continues to get worse until breathing is difficult even at rest.	The main cause of emphysema is long-term exposure to tobacco smoke. It may also be caused by other airborne irritants. The alveoli at the end of the airways in the lungs are damaged or destroyed and unable to adequately function in oxygen and carbon dioxide exchange.	A variety of tests may be required to diagnose emphysema, including imaging with x-rays and CT scans, blood laboratory analysis, and lung function evaluation. It cannot be cured, but treatments may relieve symptoms and slow the progression of the disease. Depending on the severity, inhaled steroids, bronchodilators, and/or antibiotics may be prescribed. Pulmonary rehabilitation may be required.

Continued

Common Pathology of the Respiratory System—cont'd

Disease	Signs and Symptoms	Etiology	Diagnosis and Treatment
Laryngitis	Laryngitis symptoms may include hoarseness, a weak voice, a tickling sensation with rawness of the throat, and a dry cough.	Laryngitis may be acute or chronic. Causes of acute laryngitis include viral infections and vocal strain from yelling. Chronic laryngitis may be caused by inhaled irritants such as tobacco smoke, acid reflux, chronic sinusitis, or excessive alcohol use.	Diagnosis involves examining the vocal cords with a laryngoscope and may include a biopsy of tissue for examination under a microscope. Sometimes, corticosteroids help to reduce vocal cord inflammation.
Lung cancer	Lung cancer typically does not produce signs and symptoms in the early stages. Symptoms typically occur only when the disease is advanced and may include a cough that does not go away, shortness of breath, coughing up blood, chest pain, and wheezing.	Smoking causes the majority of lung cancers. It is believed that smoking causes lung cancer by damaging the DNA in the cells that line the lungs. The mutated abnormal cells proliferate to form malignant tumors.	The diagnosis of lung cancer may require various tests, including x-ray and CT scans, sputum cytology, and tissue biopsy with a bronchoscope. Treatment options typically include one or more of the following: surgery, chemotherapy, radiation therapy, or targeted drug therapy.
Pharyngitis	Pharyngitis is an inflammation of the throat. The throat may be sore, dry, and/or scratchy, accompanied by sneezing, runny nose, cough, headache, fatigue, fever, and chills.	Most cases are caused by an infectious organism, either a virus or a bacterium, acquired from close contact with an infected individual. Like many types of inflammation, pharyngitis can be acute (a condition that is characterized by a rapid onset and typically a relatively short course) or chronic.	Diagnosis is by physical examination of the throat and checking for swollen lymph nodes. The examination may include a throat swab to rule out a streptococcal infection. If the pharyngitis is caused by a bacterial infection, antibiotics may be prescribed. If the cause is a virus, home care can help to relieve symptoms.
Pleurisy	Symptoms of pleurisy include chest pain that worsens with breathing, coughing, or sneezing. It may also include shortness of breath and sometimes a cough with fever.	Pleurisy occurs when the pleura around the lung becomes irritated and inflamed. As a result, the two layers of the pleural membrane rub against each other like two pieces of sandpaper, producing pain during breathing.	Diagnosis is by physical examination of the chest with a stethoscope. Various imaging modalities may be used to observe the pleural space. A blood test may identify an infection. The outcome of pleurisy treatment depends on the seriousness of the underlying disease. If the condition that caused pleurisy is diagnosed and treated early, there is likely to be a full recovery.
Pneumoconiosis	Pneumoconiosis, in early stages, may not show any symptoms. When symptoms develop, they include a dry cough, wheezing, and shortness of breath with exercise. As the disease progresses, breathing can become extremely difficult.	Pneumoconiosis is a lung condition that is caused by inhaling particles of mineral dust, usually while working in a high-risk, mineral-related industry. The damaging particles may be asbestos, silica, coal dust, or other agents. At first, the irritating material triggers lung inflammation, causing areas of the lung to be damaged. Over time, these areas can form tough, fibrous tissue that is not effective for oxygen and carbon dioxide exchange.	Diagnosis is based on patient history, physical examination, x-ray films, CT scans, and pulmonary function tests. The outlook for this disease depends on the specific type of pneumoconiosis, the length of exposure to mineral dust, the level of exposure, and whether the patient is a smoker. Medications may be prescribed to make breathing easier.

Common Pathology of the Respiratory System—cont'd

Disease	Signs and Symptoms	Etiology	Diagnosis and Treatment
Pneumonia	Symptoms of pneumonia include fever, cough with fluid, chest pain, shortness of breath, fatigue, muscle aches, headache, nausea, vomiting, and/or diarrhea.	Pneumonia is caused by infections primarily with bacteria or viruses in the air and is classified by the type of infectious agent. Conditions and risk factors that predispose to pneumonia include smoking, immunodeficiency, alcoholism, COPD, chronic kidney disease, and liver disease.	Diagnosis starts with the patient history and physical examination. Chest x-ray films can confirm the presence of pneumonia and determine the extent and location of the infection. Blood tests, pulse oximetry, and a sputum test may be ordered. Oral antibiotics, rest, simple analgesics, and fluids usually suffice for complete resolution. Antibiotics, antiviral medications, and fever reducers may be prescribed.
Pneumothorax	The primary symptoms of a pneumothorax include sudden chest pain and shortness of breath.	A pneumothorax is an abnormal collection of air or gas in the pleural space that separates the lung from the chest wall, often causing the lung to collapse. It can be caused by a puncture trauma to the chest or by rupture of numerous alveoli.	Diagnosis of pneumothorax by physical examination is difficult. A chest x-ray examination or CT scan is usually needed to confirm its presence. The goal in treating a pneumothorax is to relieve the pressure on the lung, allowing it to reexpand, and to prevent recurrences. Often it is self-resolving. A needle may be used to withdraw air from the pleural space. Occasionally surgery is required to close the wound in the chest wall.
Pulmonary edema	The primary symptom of pulmonary edema is difficulty breathing, but signs and symptoms may also include coughing up blood, a feeling of suffocation, and chest pain.	Pulmonary edema is a condition caused by excess fluid in the lungs. This fluid collects in the alveoli of the lungs, making it difficult to breathe. It is often the result of high pressures within the pulmonary circulation caused by congestive heart failure.	Because pulmonary edema requires prompt treatment, initial diagnosis is based on the symptoms, a physical examination, electrocardiogram, and a chest x-ray examination. Providing oxygen therapy is the first step in the treatment of pulmonary edema. Diuretics may be prescribed to reduce the amount of fluid in the lungs, and medications that increase the effectiveness of the heart may reduce the pulmonary hypertension.
Rhinitis	Symptoms of rhinitis include sneezing, coughing, runny nose, watery eyes, and pressure in the ears.	Rhinitis is irritation and inflammation of the mucous membrane inside the nose, accompanied by excessive production of mucus. The most common kind of rhinitis is allergic rhinitis, which is usually triggered by airborne allergens such as pollen and dander. Rhinitis also accompanies viral infections such as cold and flu.	An allergist can diagnose the specific allergens that trigger the illness, or determine if symptoms have nonallergic causes. For allergic rhinitis, intranasal corticosteroids and antihistamines can be used to suppress inflammation and control symptoms.
Tuberculosis (TB)	The general symptoms of TB include fever, chills, night sweats, loss of appetite, weight loss, and fatigue.	TB is a potentially serious infectious disease that mainly affects the lungs. The bacteria that cause TB are spread from one person to another through tiny droplets released into the air via coughs and sneezes.	Diagnosis of active TB is based on chest x-ray films as well as microscopic examination and microbiologic culture of body fluids. Medications are the cornerstone of TB treatment. But treating TB takes much longer than treating other types of bacterial infections.

TERMINOLOGY REVIEW

Key Term	Word Parts	Definition
Alveoli	*alveol-:* tiny cavity	Microscopic dilations of terminal bronchioles in the lungs, where diffusion of gases occurs; air sacs in the lungs.
Bronchi	*bronchi-:* air passages	The airways that are formed when the trachea branches.
Bronchial tree	*bronchi-:* air passages	The bronchi and all their branches that function as passageways between the trachea and the alveoli.
External respiration		Exchange of gases between the lungs and the blood.
Fauces		Opening from the oral cavity into the oropharynx.
Internal respiration		Exchange of gases between the blood and tissue cells.
Laryngopharynx	*laryng/o-:* larynx	Portion of the pharynx that is behind the larynx and extends from the level of the hyoid bone to the lower margin of the larynx.
Larynx		Passageway for air between the pharynx and trachea; commonly called the *voice box*.
Lower respiratory tract		Portion of the respiratory tract that is inferior to the larynx; includes the trachea, bronchial tree, and lungs.
Nasopharynx	*nas/o:* nose	Portion of the pharynx that is posterior to the nasal cavities; extends from the base of the skull to the uvula.
Oropharynx	*or/o:* mouth	Portion of the pharynx that is posterior to the oral cavity; extends from the uvula to the hyoid bone.
Pharynx	*pharyn/o:* pharynx	Passageway for air and food; extends from the base of the skull to the larynx and esophagus; throat.
Pleura	*pleur/o:* ribs	Serous membrane that lines the ribs (parietal layer) and surrounds the lungs (visceral layer).
Pleural cavity	*pleur/o:* ribs, pleura	The small space between the parietal and visceral layers of the pleura.
Respiration	*respir/o:* breath	Exchange of oxygen and carbon dioxide between the atmosphere and the body cells.
Respiratory membrane		Any surface in the lungs where diffusion occurs; consists of the layers that the gases must pass through to get into or out of the alveoli.
Surfactant		A substance, produced by certain cells in lung tissue, that reduces surface tension between fluid molecules that line the respiratory membrane and helps keep the alveolus from collapsing.
Trachea		Passageway for air that extends inferiorly to the carina where it branches into the bronchi; commonly called the *windpipe*.
Upper respiratory tract		Portion of the respiratory tract that includes the nose, pharynx, and larynx.
Ventilation		Movement of air into and out of the lungs; breathing.

14 Digestive System

Check out the Evolve site at http://evolve.elsevier.com/Bonewit/today to access additional interactive activities and exercises to help you study and prepare for success.

LEARNING OBJECTIVES

1. Identify the components of the digestive tract and the accessory organs.
2. List six functions of the digestive system.
3. Describe the general histology of the four layers in the digestive tract wall.
4. Describe the features and function of the oral cavity, teeth, pharynx, and esophagus.
5. List and describe the location of the three salivary glands.
6. Explain the function of saliva.
7. Describe the structure and features of the stomach and its role in digestion.
8. Describe the structure and features of the small intestine and its role in digestion and absorption.
9. Describe the structure, features, and function of the large intestine.
10. Describe the structure and function of the liver, gallbladder, and pancreas.
11. Explain how substances are absorbed into the body through the small intestine.
12. Describe ways in which the aging of an individual affects the digestive system.
13. Identify pathology related to the digestive system.

CHAPTER OUTLINE

KEY TERMS

absorption (ab-SOARP-shun)
chyme (KYME)
defecation (def-eh-KAY-shun)
deglutition (dee-gloo-TISH-un)
fauces (FAW-seez)
gastric juice (GAS-trik JOOS)
gastrin (GAS-trin)
gingiva (JIN-jih-vah)
hydrolysis (hy-DRAHL-ih-sis)
ileocecal valve (ill-ee-oh-SEE-kul VALVE)
lower esophageal sphincter (LOW-er ee-SAHF-oh-jeel SFINK-ter)
mastication (mas-tih-KAY-shun)
mesentery (MEZ-en-tair-ee)
palate (PAL-at)
peristalsis (pair-ih-STALL-sis)
plicae circulares (PLY-kee sir-kyoo-LAIR-eez)
pyloric sphincter (py-LOR-ik SFINK-ter)
rugae (ROO-jee)
teniae coli (TEE-nee-aye KOH-lye)

INTRODUCTION TO THE DIGESTIVE SYSTEM

The digestive system includes the *digestive tract* and its *accessory organs* (Fig. 14.1). The function of the digestive system is to process food into molecules that can be absorbed and used by the cells of the body. Food is broken down, bit by bit, until the molecules are small enough to be absorbed and the waste products are eliminated. The digestive tract (also called the *alimentary canal* or *gastrointestinal [GI] tract*) consists of a long, continuous tube that extends from the mouth to the anus. It includes the mouth, pharynx, esophagus, stomach, small intestine, and large intestine. The tongue and teeth are accessory structures located in the mouth. The salivary glands, liver, gallbladder, and pancreas are not part of the digestive tract but are major accessory organs that have a role in digestion. These secrete fluids into the digestive tract.

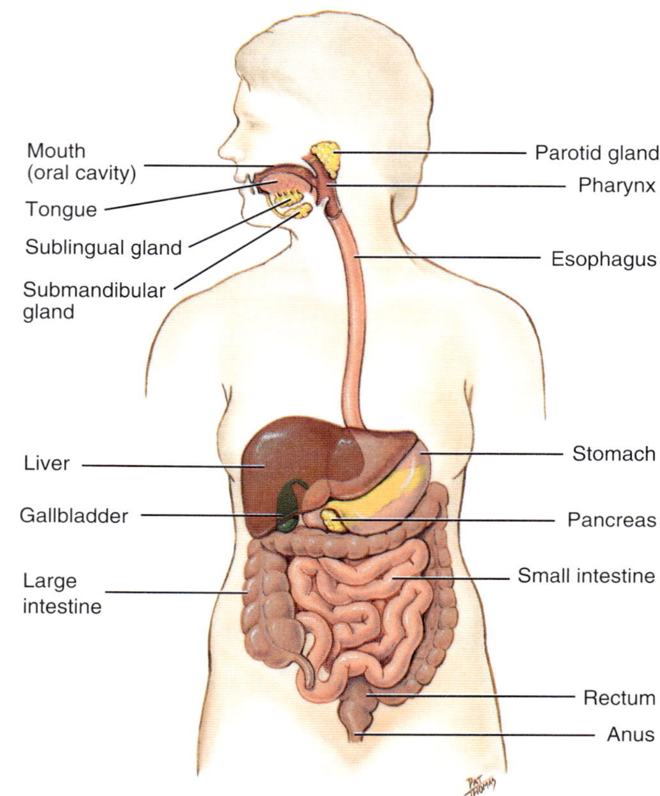

Fig. 14.1 Organs of the digestive system. (From Applegate E: *The anatomy and physiology learning system*, ed 4, St. Louis, 2011, Saunders.)

FUNCTIONS OF THE DIGESTIVE SYSTEM

Food undergoes three types of processes in the body:

- Digestion
- Absorption
- Metabolism

Digestion and absorption occur in the digestive tract. After the nutrients have been absorbed, they are available to all cells in the body and are used by the cells in metabolism.

The digestive system prepares nutrients for use by the body's cells through the following six activities:

- Ingestion—The first activity of the digestive system is to take in food. This process is called *ingestion.* Ingestion has to take place before anything else can happen.
- Mechanical digestion—The large pieces of food that are ingested have to be broken into smaller particles that can be acted on by various enzymes. This is called *mechanical digestion.* Mechanical digestion begins in the mouth with chewing, or **mastication**, and continues with churning and mixing actions in the stomach.
- Chemical digestion—The complex molecules of carbohydrates, proteins, and fats are transformed by chemical digestion into smaller molecules that can be absorbed and used by the cells. Chemical digestion uses water to break down the complex molecules. This process is known as **hydrolysis**. Digestive enzymes speed up the hydrolysis process, which is otherwise slow.
- Movements—After ingestion and mastication, the food particles move from the mouth into the pharynx and then into the esophagus. This movement is called **deglutition**, or swallowing. Mixing movements occur in the stomach as a result of smooth muscle contraction. These repetitive contractions mix the food particles

with enzymes and other fluids. The movements that propel the food particles through the digestive tract are called **peristalsis**. These are rhythmic waves of contractions that move the food particles through the various regions in which mechanical and chemical digestion take place.
- Absorption—The simple molecules that are produced from chemical digestion pass through the lining of the small intestine into the blood. This process is called **absorption**.
- Elimination—The food molecules that cannot be digested need to be eliminated from the body. The removal of indigestible wastes through the anus, in the form of feces, is **defecation**.

GENERAL STRUCTURE OF THE DIGESTIVE TRACT

The digestive tract is a long, continuous tube that is approximately 9 m (30 ft) in length. It opens to the outside at both ends, through the mouth at one end and through the anus at the other. Although there are variations in each region, the basic structure of the wall is the same throughout the entire length of the tube.

The wall of the digestive tract has four layers (Fig. 14.2): mucosa, submucosa, muscular layer (muscularis), and serous layer (serosa).

MUCOSA

The *mucosa*, or mucous membrane layer, is the innermost layer of the wall. It lines the lumen of the digestive tract. The mucosa consists of epithelium, an underlying loose connective tissue layer, and a thin layer of smooth muscle. In certain regions the mucosa develops folds that increase the surface area. Certain cells in the mucosa secrete mucus, digestive enzymes, and hormones. Ducts from other glands pass through the mucosa to the lumen of the digestive tract.

SUBMUCOSA

The *submucosa* is a thick layer of loose connective tissue that surrounds the mucosa. This layer also contains blood and lymphatic vessels, nerves, and some glands. Abundant blood vessels supply necessary nourishment to the surrounding tissues. Blood and lymph carry away absorbed nutrients that are the end products of digestion. The nerves in the submucosa form a network called the *submucosal plexus* that provides autonomic nerve impulses to the muscle layers of the digestive tract.

MUSCULAR LAYER

The *muscular layer* (labeled *muscularis* in Fig. 14.2) consists of two layers of smooth muscle. The inner circular layer has fibers arranged in a circular manner around the circumference of the tube. When these muscles contract, the diameter of the tube is decreased. In the outer longitudinal layer, the fibers run lengthwise along the long axis of the tube. When these fibers contract, their length decreases and the tube shortens. A network of autonomic nerve fibers, called the *myenteric plexus,* exists between the circular and longitudinal muscle layers. The myenteric plexus, along with the submucosal plexus, is important for controlling the movements and secretions of the digestive tract. In general, parasympathetic impulses stimulate movement and secretion in the GI tract, and sympathetic impulses inhibit these activities.

SEROSA OR ADVENTITIA

The fourth and outermost layer in the wall of the digestive tract is called the *adventitia* if it is above the diaphragm and the *serosa* if it is below the diaphragm. The adventitia is composed of connective tissue. The serosa, which is below the diaphragm, has a layer of epithelium covering the connective tissue. It is actually the visceral peritoneum and secretes serous fluid for lubrication. The serous fluid allows the abdominal organs to move smoothly against one another without friction.

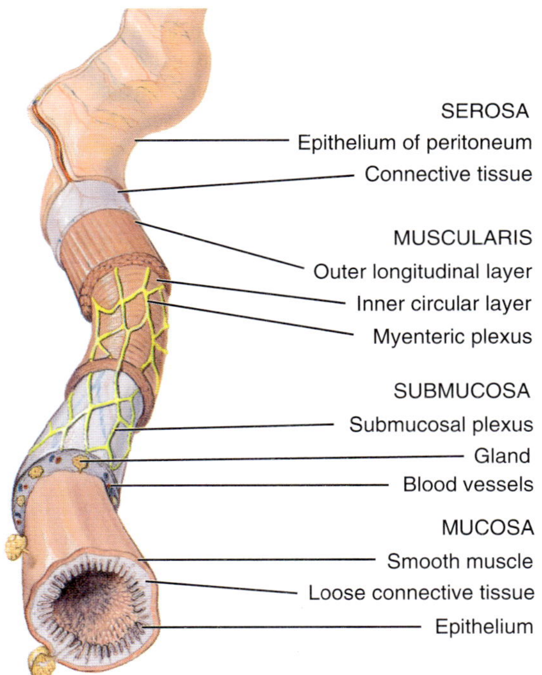

Fig. 14.2 Basic histology of the digestive tract. Progressing from the inner to outer, the tissue layers of the digestive tract are the mucosa, submucosa, muscularis, and serosa (adventitia if above the diaphragm). (From Applegate E: *The anatomy and physiology learning system*, ed 4, St. Louis, 2011, Saunders.)

HIGHLIGHT on the Digestive System

Cold sores: Cold sores, or fever blisters, are small fluid-filled blisters that itch and are painful, usually appearing around the lips and in the mouth. They are caused by recurring infections with the herpes simplex virus. After the initial infection, the virus remains dormant in a cutaneous nerve until it is activated by stress, fever, or ultraviolet radiation.

Cleft palate: Cleft palate is a condition in which the bones in the hard palate do not fuse completely during prenatal development. This leaves an opening between the nasal and oral cavities. An infant with this problem has difficulty creating enough suction for proper feeding. Cleft palate can usually be corrected surgically.

Tongue-tied: A person with a short lingual frenulum is said to be "tongue-tied." The movement of the tongue is abnormally limited, which causes difficulties in speech. Surgically cutting the frenulum corrects this problem.

Wisdom teeth: The third molars are the last teeth to erupt. These are sometimes called "wisdom teeth" because they usually erupt between the ages of 17 and 25 years, when one is supposed to be wise. These teeth may remain embedded in the jawbone. If this happens, they are said to be impacted. In some cases, wisdom teeth are absent altogether.

Gingivitis: Gingivitis is an inflammation of the gingiva, or gum. The gums become sore and red and may bleed. This condition is reversible if it is not neglected and if corrective action is taken. Periodontal disease results when gingivitis is neglected and bacteria invade the bone around the tooth. This is a major cause of tooth loss in adults.

Cavities: Caries, or dental cavities, are caused by the demineralization of the teeth resulting from the action of bacteria that live in the mouth. The bacteria metabolize sugars in the mouth, producing acids that dissolve the calcium salts of the tooth. If the bacteria reach the pulp cavity, it is necessary to perform a root canal procedure. In this procedure, the pulp cavity with its nerve is destroyed, and the cavity is completely filled with a solid filling material.

Mumps: Mumps is a viral infection of the parotid glands. The infection causes inflammation in the gland, which makes opening the mouth and chewing difficult. If the disease occurs in postadolescent males, the infection may spread to the testes, which in severe cases may result in sterility.

Bad breath: Halitosis, commonly called "bad breath," results from an overabundance of bacteria in the mouth. In some cases it may be caused by poor oral hygiene. In others, it may be caused by a disease process that reduces the secretion of saliva for cleansing the mouth and moving food particles to the pharynx for swallowing. As a result, some food particles remain in the mouth and decompose, which provides a growth medium for the bacteria.

Lactose intolerance: Lactose intolerance is caused by a deficiency of the intestinal enzyme lactase, which acts on lactose, a sugar found in milk. When people with lactose intolerance drink milk, this sugar is not digested properly. Bacterial action on the undigested sugar causes gas and a bloated feeling. The undigested lactose also prevents absorption of water from the small intestine, which leads to diarrhea. The solution to this problem is to avoid milk and milk products.

Appendicitis: Appendicitis is an inflammation that sometimes occurs when infectious material becomes trapped inside the appendix. If the inflamed appendix ruptures and releases the infectious contents into the abdominal cavity, the peritoneum may become involved, resulting in a potentially life-threatening inflammation of the peritoneum, called *peritonitis.* Treatment for appendicitis is usually the surgical removal of the appendix.

Borborygmus: Borborygmus is the rumbling noise caused by the propulsion of gas through the intestines. ■

COMPONENTS OF THE DIGESTIVE TRACT

MOUTH

The mouth, or *oral cavity,* is the first part of the digestive tract. It is adapted to perform the following: receive food by ingestion; break it into small particles by *mastication*; and mix it with saliva. The lips, cheeks, and palate form the boundaries of the mouth. The oral cavity contains the teeth and tongue and receives the secretions from the salivary glands.

Lips and Cheeks

The *lips* and *cheeks* help to hold food in the mouth and keep it in place for chewing. They are also used in the formation of words for speech. The lips contain numerous sensory receptors that are useful for judging the temperature and texture of foods. The cheeks form the lateral boundaries of the oral cavity. The main components of the cheeks are the *buccinator muscle* and other muscles of facial expression. On the outside, the muscles are covered by skin and subcutaneous tissue.

Palate

The **palate** is the roof of the oral cavity. It separates the oral cavity from the nasal cavity. The anterior portion, the *hard palate,* is supported by bone. The posterior portion, the *soft palate,* is skeletal muscle and connective tissue. The soft palate ends in a projection called the *uvula.* During swallowing, the soft palate and uvula move upward to direct food away from the nasal cavity and into the oropharynx.

Tongue

The largest and most movable organ in the oral cavity is the *tongue.* Most of the tongue consists of skeletal muscle. The major attachment for the tongue is the posterior region, or root, which is anchored to the hyoid bone. The anterior portion of the tongue is relatively free but is connected to the floor of the mouth, at the midline, by a membranous fold of tissue called the *lingual frenulum.* The dorsal surface of the tongue is covered by tiny projections called *papillae.* The papillae provide friction for manipulating food in the mouth, and they also contain the taste buds (see Chapter 10). The *lingual tonsils* are embedded in the posterior surface of the tongue. The lingual tonsils provide a defense against bacteria that enter the mouth.

The muscles in the tongue allow the tongue to perform the following: manipulate the food in the mouth for mastication; move the food around to mix it with saliva; shape it into a ball-like mass called a *bolus;* and direct it toward the pharynx for swallowing. It is a major sensory organ for taste and is one of the major organs used in speech.

Teeth

Two different sets of teeth develop in the mouth. The first set begins to appear at approximately 6 months of age and continues to develop until about $2^1/_2$ years of age. This set is known as the *primary teeth.* The primary teeth contain 10 teeth in each jaw for a total of 20 teeth. Fig. 14.3A illustrates the types of primary teeth. Starting at 6 years of age, the primary teeth begin to fall out and are replaced by the *permanent teeth.* This set contains 16 teeth in each jaw for a total of 32 teeth. These teeth are illustrated in Fig. 14.3B.

Different teeth are shaped to handle food in different ways. The *incisors* are chisel shaped and have sharp edges for biting food. *Cuspids (canines)* are cone shaped and have points for grasping and tearing food. *Bicuspids (premolars)* and *molars* have flat surfaces with rounded projections for crushing and grinding. Note the location of each type of tooth in Fig. 14.3.

Although the different types of teeth have different shapes, each tooth has three parts: crown, neck, and root.

The *crown* is the visible portion of the tooth, covered by enamel. The *root* is the portion that is embedded in the sockets (alveolar processes) of the mandible and maxilla. The *neck* is a small region in which the crown and root meet and is adjacent to the **gingiva**, or gum.

The central core of a tooth is the *pulp cavity.* It contains the *pulp*, which consists of connective tissue, blood vessels, and nerves. In the root the pulp cavity is called the *root canal.* Nerves and blood vessels enter the root of the tooth through an *apical foramen.* The pulp cavity is surrounded by *dentin*, which forms the bulk of the tooth. Dentin is a living cellular substance similar to bone. In the root the dentin is surrounded by a thin layer of calcified connective tissue called *cementum*, which attaches the root to the periodontal ligaments. The ligaments have fibers that firmly anchor the

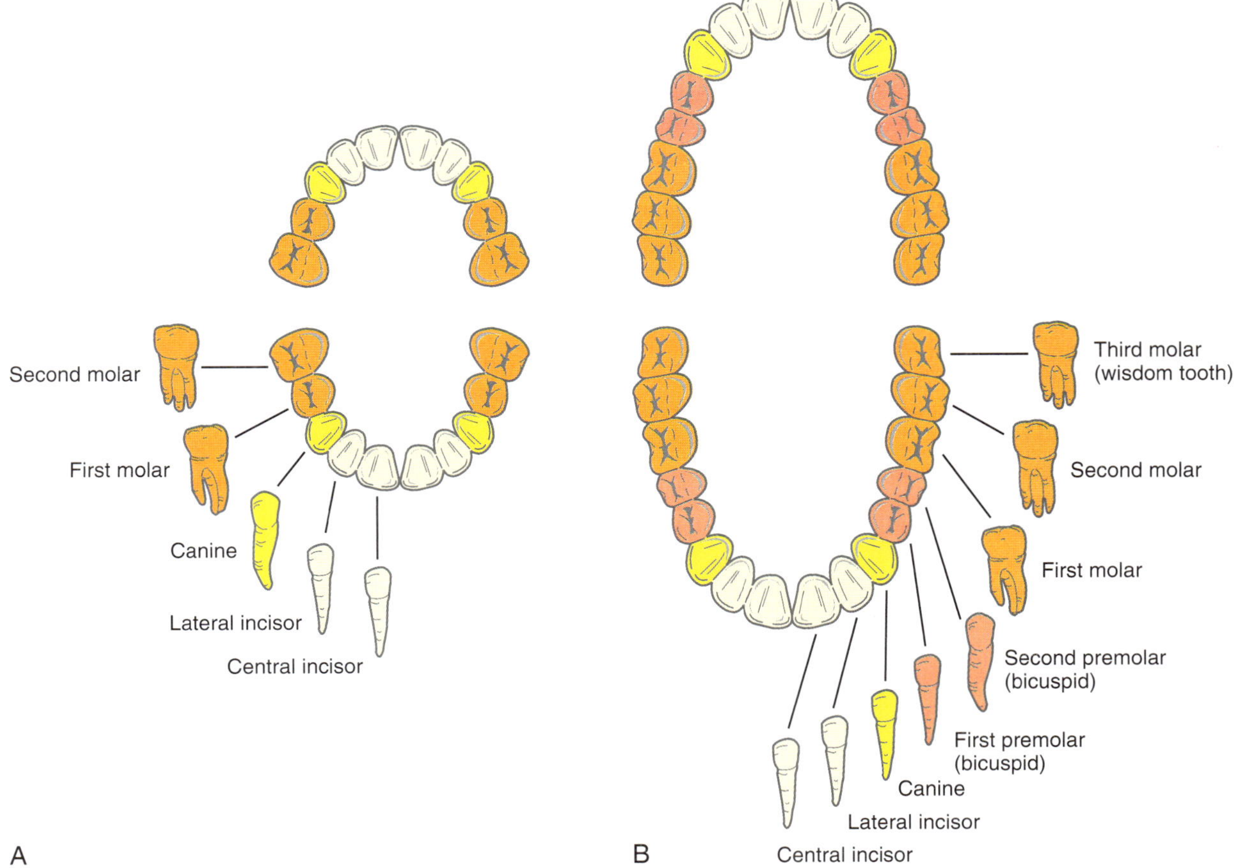

Fig. 14.3 Primary (A) and permanent (B) teeth. The deciduous dentition on the left has 20 teeth. The permanent dentition on the right contains 32 teeth. (From Applegate E: *The anatomy and physiology learning system*, ed 4, St. Louis, 2011, Saunders.)

root in the alveolar process (socket). Enamel surrounds the dentin in the crown of the tooth; it is the hardest substance in the body. Fig. 14.4 shows a longitudinal section of a tooth and illustrates the major features.

Salivary Glands

Three pairs of salivary glands secrete saliva into the oral cavity. The saliva is mixed with food during mastication (Fig. 14.5). The *parotid glands* are the largest of the salivary glands. One gland is located on each side of the head just in front of the ear. *Submandibular glands* are located on the floor of the mouth. Small *sublingual glands* are also located in the floor of the mouth, anterior to the submandibular glands, and under the tongue.

Saliva contains water, mucus, and the enzyme *amylase*. Functions of saliva include the following:

- It has a cleansing action on the teeth.
- It moistens and lubricates food during mastication and swallowing.
- It dissolves certain molecules so that foods can be tasted.
- It begins the chemical digestion of starches.

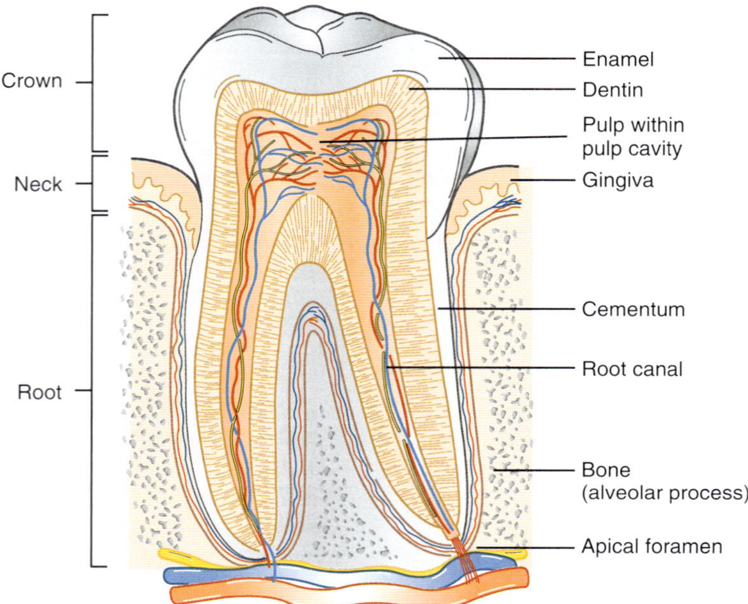

Fig. 14.4 Longitudinal section of a tooth. (From Applegate E: *The anatomy and physiology learning system*, ed 4, St. Louis, 2011, Saunders.)

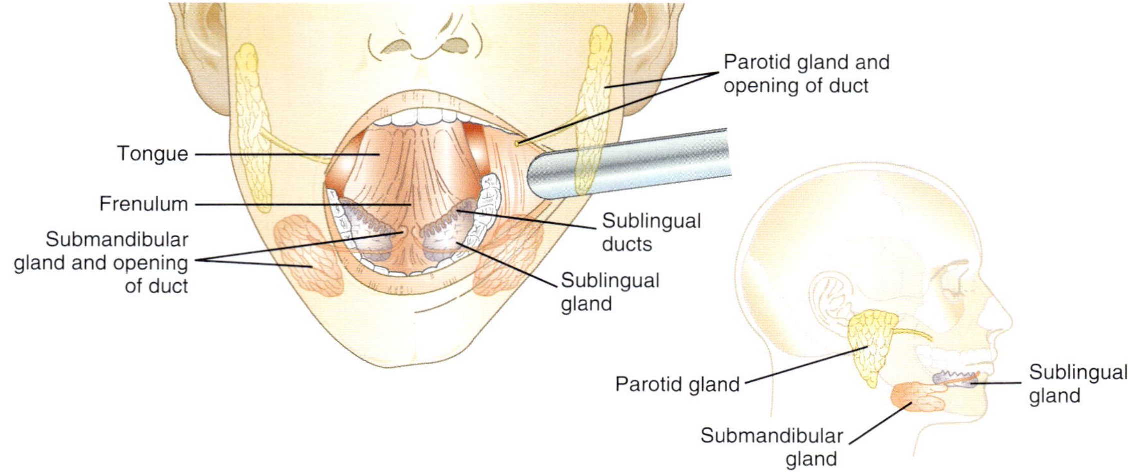

Fig. 14.5 Locations of the salivary glands. (From Applegate E: *The anatomy and physiology learning system*, ed 4, St. Louis, 2011, Saunders.)

PHARYNX

The *pharynx* is a passageway that connects the nasal and oral cavities to the larynx and esophagus (see Fig. 13.2). It serves both the respiratory and digestive systems as a channel for air and food. The upper region is the *nasopharynx* and is posterior to the nasal cavity. It contains the *pharyngeal tonsils*, also known as the *adenoids*. The nasopharynx functions as a passageway for air but has no function in the digestive system. The middle region posterior to the oral cavity is the *oropharynx*. This is the region food enters when it is swallowed. The opening from the oral cavity into the oropharynx is called the **fauces**. Masses of lymphoid tissue, the palatine tonsils, are near the fauces. The lower region of the pharynx is the *laryngopharynx*. The laryngopharynx opens into both the esophagus and the larynx.

Food is forced into the pharynx by the tongue. When food reaches the opening (fauces), sensory receptors around the fauces respond and initiate an involuntary swallowing reflex. Peristaltic movements propel the food from the pharynx into the esophagus.

ESOPHAGUS

The *esophagus* is a collapsible muscular tube, approximately 25 cm (10 inches) long, and it serves as a passageway for food between the pharynx and stomach. It lies behind the trachea and in front of the vertebral column. It passes through an opening in the diaphragm and then empties into the stomach. The mucosa has glands that secrete mucus to keep the lining of the esophagus moist and well lubricated. This eases the passage of food through the esophagus. The **lower esophageal sphincter** (sometimes called the *cardiac sphincter*) controls the movement of food between the esophagus and the stomach.

STOMACH

The stomach receives food from the esophagus and is located in the upper left quadrant of the abdomen. Its capacity varies; in the adult it averages approximately 1.5 L, although in some individuals it may hold up to 4 L.

Structure

The *stomach* is divided into the cardiac, fundus, body, and pyloric regions (Fig. 14.6). The *cardiac region* is a small region around the opening from the esophagus. The *fundus* is the most superior region. It balloons above the cardiac region to form a temporary storage area. The *body* is the main portion of the stomach. The body of the stomach curves to the right, creating two curvatures. The *lesser curvature* is concave and the *greater curvature* is convex. As the body approaches the exit from the stomach, it narrows into the *pyloric region*. A circular band of smooth muscle forms the **pyloric sphincter**, which acts as a valve between the stomach and small intestine.

The muscular layer in the wall of the stomach provides mixing movements to mix the food with enzymes and other fluids. When the stomach is empty, the mucosa and submucosa exhibit longitudinal folds, called **rugae**. These folds allow the stomach to expand, and, as it fills, the rugae become less apparent.

Gastric Secretions

The mucosal lining of the stomach contains numerous *gastric glands*. The gastric glands open to the surface of the mucosa through tiny holes called *gastric pits*. Four different

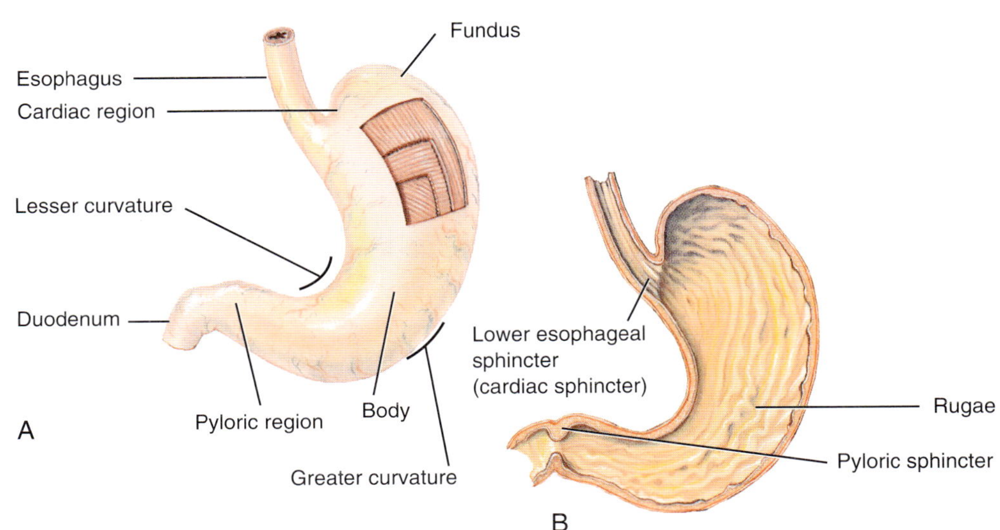

Fig. 14.6 Features of the stomach. (A) External view. (B) Internal view. Note the rugae. (From Applegate E: *The anatomy and physiology learning system*, ed 4, St. Louis, 2011, Saunders.)

types of cells make up the gastric glands: mucous cells, parietal cells, chief cells, and endocrine cells.

Exocrine gastric glands are composed of mucous cells, parietal cells, and chief cells. The secretions of the exocrine gastric glands make up the **gastric juice**. Approximately 2 to 3 L of gastric juice are produced every day. The products of the endocrine cells are secreted directly into the bloodstream and are not a part of the gastric juice.

Mucous cells produce two types of mucus in the stomach. One type is thick and alkaline and forms a protective coating for the stomach lining. The other type is thin and watery. It mixes with the food and creates a fluid medium for chemical reactions. *Parietal cells* secrete hydrochloric acid and intrinsic factor. The hydrochloric acid kills bacteria and provides an acidic environment for the action of enzymes in the stomach. Intrinsic factor aids in the absorption of vitamin B_{12}. *Chief cells* secrete pepsinogen. Pepsinogen is an inactive form of the enzyme pepsin. Hydrochloric acid converts the inactive pepsinogen into the active enzyme pepsin, which begins the chemical digestion of proteins.

The *endocrine cells* secrete the hormone **gastrin**, which functions in the regulation of gastric activity. Table 14.1 summarizes the various cells and secretions of the gastric glands.

The churning action of the muscles in the stomach wall breaks the food particles of the bolus that was swallowed into smaller sizes and mixes them with the gastric juice. This produces a semifluid mixture called **chyme**, which leaves the stomach through the pyloric sphincter and enters the small intestine.

Regulation of Gastric Secretions

The regulation of gastric secretions is accomplished through neural and hormonal mechanisms. Gastric juice is produced all the time, but the amount varies based on certain factors. Regulation of gastric secretions may be divided into cephalic, gastric, and intestinal phases.

The *cephalic phase* begins when an individual thinks pleasant thoughts about food or sees, smells, or tastes food. This phase anticipates food and prepares the stomach to receive it by increasing the secretion of gastric juice. The *gastric phase* accounts for more than two-thirds of the gastric juice secretion. The gastric phase begins when food reaches the stomach. The presence of food in the stomach and the distention of the stomach wall stimulate reflexes that result in gastrin secretion. Gastrin, in turn, stimulates the secretion of gastric juice, which contains hydrochloric acid and pepsinogen. The hydrochloric acid acidifies the stomach contents and activates the pepsinogen into pepsin, which breaks down proteins.

The passage of chyme through the pyloric sphincter into the first part (duodenum) of the small intestine triggers the *intestinal phase* of regulation. Distention and the presence of acid chyme in the duodenum stimulate the secretion of intestinal hormones, which in turn inhibit gastric secretions. These inhibitory responses help to prevent excess acid chyme from entering the small intestine. The intestinal phase regulates the entry of chyme into the small intestine.

Table 14.1 Secretions of Gastric Glands

Cell Type	Secretion	Function
Mucous cells	Mucus (thick, alkaline)	Protects stomach lining
	Mucus (thin, watery)	Medium for chemical reactions
Parietal cells	Hydrochloric acid	Kills bacteria; activates pepsinogen
	Intrinsic factor	Absorption of vitamin B_{12}
Chief cells	Pepsinogen (active form is pepsin)	Begins digestion of proteins into polypeptides
Endocrine cells	Gastrin (a hormone)	Stimulates gastric gland secretion

From Applegate E: *The anatomy and physiology learning system*, ed 4, St. Louis, 2011, Saunders.

Stomach Emptying

Peristalsis in the stomach pushes chyme toward the pyloric region. As the chyme accumulates, the pyloric sphincter relaxes and a small amount of chyme is pumped into the small intestine. The rate at which the stomach empties depends on the nature of the contents and the receptivity of the small intestine. The stomach is usually empty within 4 hours after a meal. Liquids tend to pass through the stomach quickly. Solids stay in the stomach until they are well mixed with gastric juice. Carbohydrates move through rather quickly, proteins take a little longer, and fatty foods may stay in the stomach as long as 4 to 6 hours.

SMALL INTESTINE

The small intestine is approximately 2.5 cm (1 inch) in diameter and 6 m (20 ft) long. It extends from the pyloric sphincter to the **ileocecal valve**, where it empties into the large intestine. The function of the small intestine includes the following: finishing the process of digestion; absorbing the nutrients; and passing the residue on to the large intestine. The liver, gallbladder, and pancreas are accessory organs of the digestive system that are closely associated with the small intestine. These are described later in this chapter.

Structure

The small intestine follows the general structure of the digestive tract in that the wall has four layers: mucosa, submucosa, smooth muscle, and serosa. The mucosa and submucosa have circular folds, called **plicae circulares**, which increase the surface area for absorption (Fig. 14.7). Fingerlike extensions of the mucosa, called *villi*, project from the circular folds, and this further increases the surface area. Each villus surrounds a blood capillary network and a lymph capillary, or *lacteal*. These function in the absorption of nutrients. *Intestinal glands* extend downward between adjacent villi. The surface epithelium on the villi has tiny

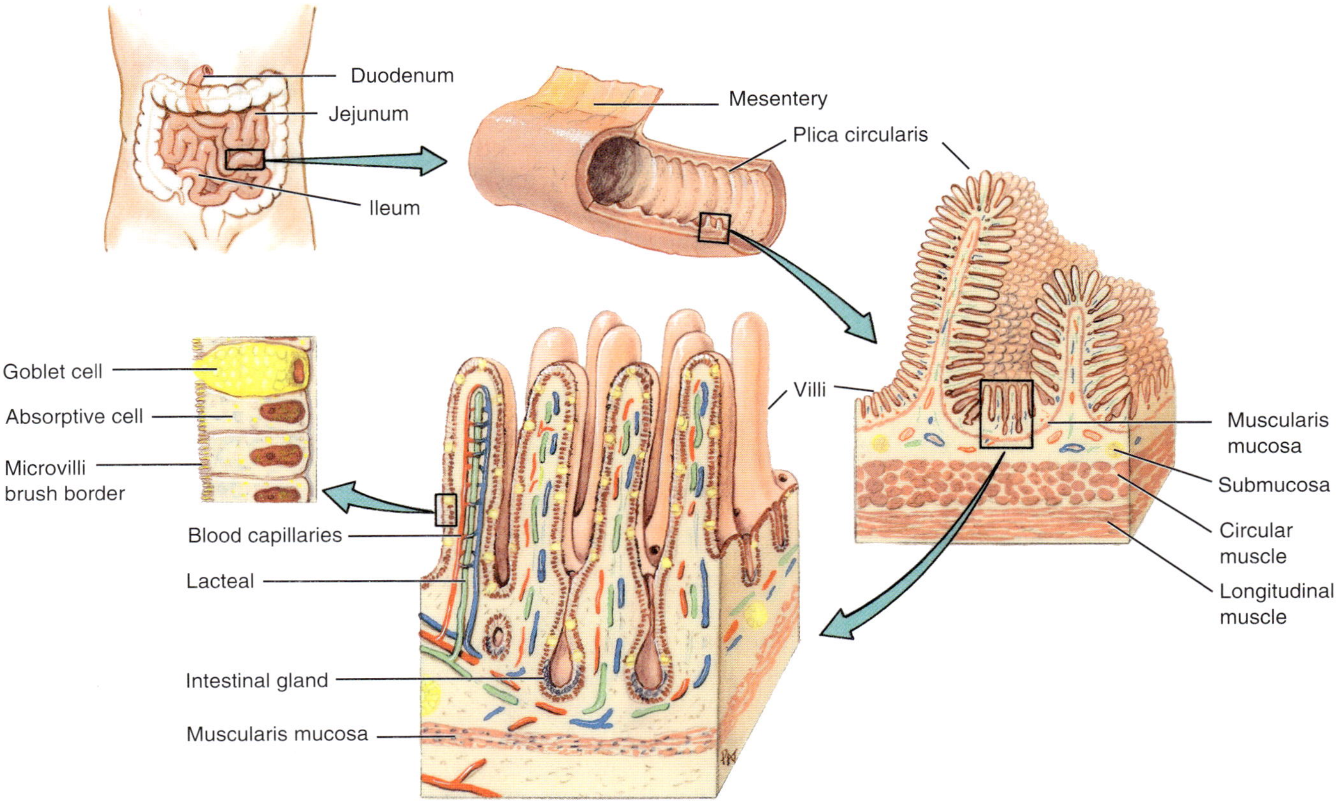

Fig. 14.7 Wall of the small intestine. (From Applegate E: *The anatomy and physiology learning system*, ed 4, St. Louis, 2011, Saunders.)

hairlike cytoplasmic extensions, called *microvilli*, that form a *brush border*, which again increases surface area.

Although the structure is similar throughout, the length of the small intestine is divided into three regions: duodenum, jejunum, and ileum.

The *duodenum* is the first part and is approximately 25 cm (10 inches) long. It begins at the pyloric sphincter and continues in a C-shaped curve to the jejunum. The duodenum receives the chyme from the stomach and secretions from the liver and pancreas.

The second portion of the small intestine is the *jejunum*, which is approximately 2.5 m (8 ft) long. This is continuous with the third portion, the *ileum*, which is approximately 3.5 m (11.5 ft) long. No distinct separation exists between the jejunum and ileum. They are similar in structure and are suspended from the abdominal wall by a fold of peritoneum, called **mesentery**. There is a gradual decrease in the number and length of the villi and an increase in the number of goblet cells in the mucosa from the beginning of the jejunum to the terminal portion of the ileum.

Secretions of the Small Intestine

Intestinal glands secrete large amounts of watery fluid that is neutral or slightly alkaline in pH. It keeps the chyme in a liquid form and provides both an appropriate environment for the many chemical reactions of digestion and a fluid medium for the absorption of nutrients. The fluid is readily reabsorbed by the capillaries in the microvilli.

Mucus is secreted by the wall of the small intestine. The alkaline mucus protects the intestinal wall from the acid chyme and digestive enzymes.

Digestive enzymes are located in the microvilli of the mucosal epithelial cells. These enzymes include the following: *peptidase*, which acts on segments of proteins called *peptides; maltase*, *sucrase*, and *lactase*, which act on disaccharides (double sugars); and an *intestinal lipase*, which acts on neutral fats. *Enterokinase*, although not actually a digestive enzyme, is produced by the mucosal epithelial cells. This enzyme activates a protein-splitting enzyme from the pancreas.

In addition to mucus and digestive enzymes, intestinal cells secrete at least two hormones—secretin and cholecystokinin. *Secretin* stimulates the pancreas to secrete a fluid that has a high bicarbonate ion concentration. This fluid helps to neutralize chyme so that the intestinal enzymes can function. *Cholecystokinin* stimulates the release of bile from the gallbladder and the secretion of digestive enzymes from the pancreas. It also inhibits gastric motility and secretions.

The most important factor for regulating secretions in the small intestine is the presence of chyme. This is largely a local reflex action in response to chemical and mechanical irritation from the chyme and in response to distention of the intestinal wall. This is a direct reflex action; thus the greater the amount of chyme, the greater the secretion.

LARGE INTESTINE

The *large intestine* is larger in diameter (6.25 cm or 2.5 inches) than the small intestine but is only approximately 1.5 m (5 ft) long (Fig. 14.8). It begins at the ileocecal junction, where the ileum enters the large intestine, and ends at the anus. The ileocecal junction has a circular band of smooth muscle fibers—the ileocecal sphincter—and a valve—the ileocecal valve.

Characteristics

The wall of the large intestine has the same types of tissue that are found in other parts of the digestive tract, but there are some distinguishing characteristics. The mucosa has large numbers of goblet cells but does not have any villi. The longitudinal muscle layer, although present, is incomplete. The longitudinal muscle is limited to three distinct bands, called **teniae coli**, that run the entire length of the colon. Contraction of the teniae coli exerts pressure on the wall and creates a series of pouches, called *haustra*, along the colon. *Epiploic appendages*, pieces of fat-filled connective tissue, are attached to the outer surface of the colon.

Regions of the Large Intestine

The large intestine consists of the cecum, colon, rectum, and anal canal (see Fig. 14.8).

Cecum

The *cecum* is the proximal portion of the large intestine. It is a blind pouch that extends from the ileocecal junction. The *vermiform appendix* is attached to the cecum. In humans the appendix has no function in digestion but does contain some lymphatic tissue.

Colon

The *colon* is the longest portion of the large intestine and is divided into ascending, transverse, descending, and sigmoid portions. The *ascending colon* begins at the ileocecal junction and travels upward on the right side, until it reaches the liver. Here it turns to the left, becomes the *transverse colon*, and continues across the abdomen toward the spleen on the left side. Here the colon turns sharply downward and travels along the posterior abdominal wall as the *descending colon*. The descending colon makes an S-shaped curve, called the *sigmoid colon*, and then becomes the rectum. The curve between the ascending and transverse portions is the hepatic flexure. The curve between the transverse and descending portions is the splenic flexure.

Rectum

The *rectum* continues from the sigmoid colon to the anal canal and has a thick muscular layer.

Anal Canal

The last 2 to 3 cm (1 inch) of the digestive tract make up the *anal canal*, which opens to the outside at the *anus*. The mucosa of the anal canal is folded to form longitudinal anal columns. The smooth muscle layer is thick and forms the *internal anal sphincter* at the superior end of the anal canal. This sphincter is under involuntary control. At the inferior end of the anal canal is the *external anal sphincter*. This sphincter is composed of skeletal muscle and is under voluntary control.

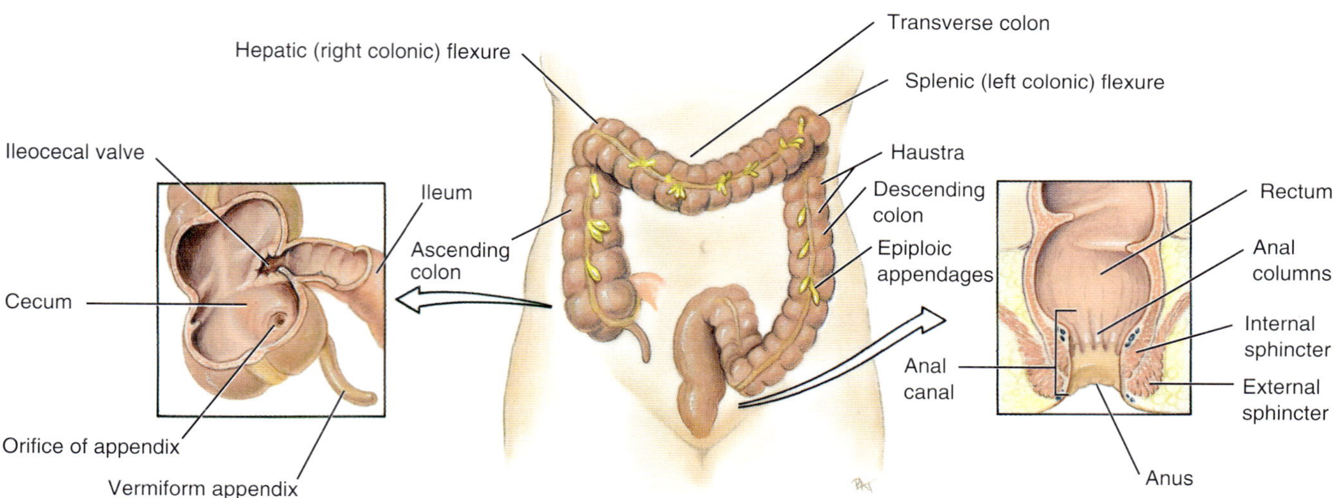

Fig. 14.8 Features of the large intestine. (From Applegate E: *The anatomy and physiology learning system*, ed 4, St. Louis, 2011, Saunders.)

Functions of the Large Intestine

The large intestine produces no digestive enzymes. Chemical digestion is completed in the small intestine before the chyme reaches the large intestine. There are no villi for the absorption of nutrients. This process is also accomplished in the small intestine. The primary functions of the large intestine are the absorption of fluid and electrolytes and the elimination of waste products.

The chyme that enters the large intestine contains materials that were not digested or absorbed in the small intestine—water, electrolytes, and bacteria. Some of the water and electrolytes are absorbed in the cecum and ascending colon. Although the quantity is relatively small, this absorptive function of the large intestine is important in maintaining fluid balance in the body. The residue that remains from the chyme becomes the feces.

The large intestine has the same types of mixing and peristaltic movements as occur in other parts of the digestive tract, but they are more sluggish and occur less frequently. They are more likely to occur after a meal as a result of reflexes initiated in the small intestine. As the rectum fills with feces, the defecation reflex is triggered and the waste products are eliminated.

The only secretory product in the large intestine is mucus from the numerous goblet cells. The mucus protects the intestinal wall against abrasion and irritation from the chyme. It also helps to hold the particles of fecal matter together.

ACCESSORY ORGANS OF DIGESTION

The salivary glands, liver, gallbladder, and pancreas are not part of the digestive tract, but they have a role in digestive activities and are considered accessory organs. Because the salivary glands are so closely associated with the mouth and their primary function is performed in the mouth, they are considered part of the oral cavity. The liver and pancreas have functions in addition to digestion, and the gallbladder is closely related to the liver; thus these three organs are described as separate accessory organs in this section.

LIVER

The *liver* is a large, reddish-brown organ. It is the largest gland in the body and is located in the right hypochondriac and epigastric regions of the abdomen, just beneath the diaphragm.

Structure of the Liver

The *liver* is divided into two major lobes and two minor lobes. The *falciform ligament* attaches the liver to the abdominal wall and separates the right lobe from the left lobe. Two additional small lobes are evident on the visceral surface: the caudate lobe and the quadrate lobe (Fig. 14.9). The *porta* is also on the visceral surface. The porta is where the hepatic artery and hepatic portal vein enter the liver and where the hepatic ducts exit.

The substance of the liver is divided into functional units called *liver lobules.* A liver lobule consists of *hepatocytes* (liver cells) that radiate outward from the *central vein* like spokes of a wheel. Tiny channels, called *bile canaliculi*, are interwoven with the liver cells and carry the bile that is produced by the hepatocytes toward the periphery of the lobule. Bile canaliculi merge to form larger right and left hepatic ducts. These two ducts combine to form the *common hepatic duct*, which transports bile out of the liver. The plates of hepatocytes are separated from one another by venous channels, called *sinusoids*, which carry blood from the periphery of the lobule toward the central vein. The sinusoids are lined with special phagocytic cells, called *Kupffer cells*, that

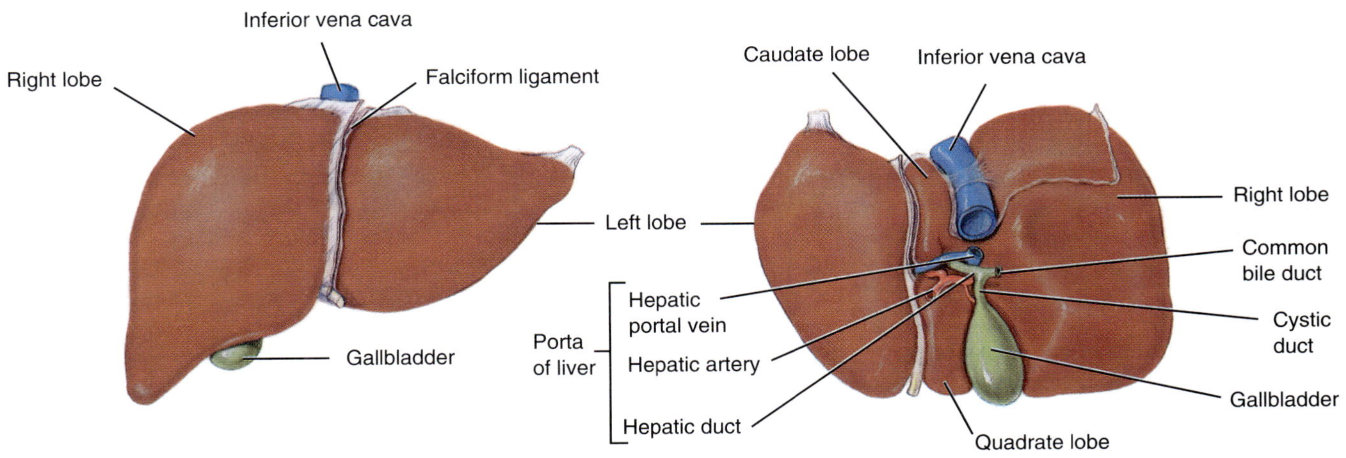

Fig. 14.9 Features of the liver. (From Applegate E: *The anatomy and physiology learning system,* ed 4, St. Louis, 2011, Saunders.)

remove foreign particles from the blood as it flows through the sinusoids. *Portal triads*, which consist of a branch of the hepatic portal vein, a branch of the hepatic artery, and a branch of a hepatic duct, are located around the periphery of the lobule.

Blood Supply to the Liver

The liver receives blood from two sources. Freshly oxygenated blood is brought to the liver by the *common hepatic artery.* Blood that is rich in nutrients from the digestive tract is carried to the liver by the *hepatic portal vein.* Venous blood from the hepatic portal vein and arterial blood from the hepatic arteries mix together as the blood flows through the sinusoids toward the central vein. The central veins of the liver lobules merge to form larger *hepatic veins* that drain into the inferior vena cava.

Functions of the Liver

The liver has a wide variety of functions, many of which are vital to life. Hepatocytes (liver cells) perform most of the functions attributed to the liver, but the phagocytic Kupffer cells that line the sinusoids are responsible for cleansing the blood. Liver functions include the following:

- *Secretion:* The liver produces and secretes bile.
- *Synthesis of bile salts:* Bile salts are produced in the liver and facilitate fat digestion and the absorption of fats and fat-soluble vitamins.
- *Synthesis of plasma proteins:* The liver synthesizes albumin, fibrinogen, globulins, and clotting factors.
- *Storage:* The liver stores glucose in the form of glycogen and also stores iron and vitamins A, B_{12}, D, E, and K.
- *Detoxification:* The liver alters the chemical composition of toxic compounds to make them less harmful. It also changes the configuration of certain drugs, such as penicillin, and excretes them in the bile to remove them from the body.
- *Excretion:* Hormones, drugs, cholesterol, and bile pigments from the breakdown of hemoglobin are excreted in the bile.
- *Carbohydrate metabolism:* The liver has a major role in maintaining blood glucose levels. It removes excess glucose from the blood and converts it to glycogen for storage; it breaks down glycogen into glucose when more is necessary; and it converts noncarbohydrate molecules into glucose.
- *Lipid metabolism:* The liver functions in the breakdown of fatty acids, in the synthesis of cholesterol and phospholipids, and in the conversion of excess carbohydrates and proteins into fats.
- *Protein metabolism:* The liver converts certain amino acids into different amino acids as needed for protein synthesis. It also converts ammonia, produced in the breakdown of proteins, into urea, which is less toxic and can be excreted in the bile.
- *Filtering:* The phagocytic Kupffer cells that line the sinusoids remove bacteria, damaged red blood cells, and other particles from the blood.

Bile

Approximately 1 L of *bile*, a yellowish-green fluid, is produced by liver cells each day. Bile is slightly alkaline, with a pH of 7.6 to 8.6, so it helps to neutralize the acid chyme. The main components of bile are water, bile salts, bile pigments, and cholesterol. The bile salts are useful secretory products of the liver, but the bile pigments and cholesterol are waste products excreted in the bile and eliminated from the body.

Bile salts function in the digestion of fats. They act as emulsifying agents that break large fat globules into tiny fat droplets. This increases the surface area of the fat and allows for more efficient enzyme action in fat digestion. Bile salts also facilitate the absorption of fat-soluble vitamins and the end products of fat digestion.

Bile pigments are produced in the breakdown of hemoglobin from damaged red blood cells. They are responsible for the color of the urine and feces. The principal bile pigment is *bilirubin.* Cholesterol is a product of lipid metabolism. Bile salts act on cholesterol to make it soluble; then it is excreted in the bile.

GALLBLADDER

The *gallbladder* is a pear-shaped sac that is attached to the liver by the cystic duct (see Fig. 14.9). The *cystic duct* joins the *hepatic duct* from the liver to form the *common bile duct.* The common bile duct empties into the duodenum. When the gallbladder contracts, bile is ejected from the gallbladder into the cystic duct.

The principal functions of the gallbladder are to store and concentrate bile. Bile is continuously produced by the liver and then travels through the hepatic duct and common bile duct to the duodenum. There is a *hepatopancreatic sphincter* (*sphincter of Oddi*) where the common bile duct enters the duodenum. If the small intestine is empty, the sphincter is closed and the bile backs up through the cystic duct into the gallbladder for concentration and storage until it is needed. When chyme with fatty contents enters the duodenum, the hormone *cholecystokinin* stimulates the gallbladder to contract and the sphincter of Oddi to open. This permits bile to flow from the gallbladder, through the cystic duct and common bile duct, and then into the duodenum.

PANCREAS

The *pancreas* is an elongated and flattened organ that is located along the posterior abdominal wall. One end of the pancreas, the head, is on the right side within the curve of the duodenum; the other end, the tail, is on the left side next to the spleen.

The pancreas has both endocrine and exocrine functions. The endocrine portion consists of the scattered *islets of Langerhans*, which secrete the hormones insulin and glucagon into the blood. These hormones and their functions are discussed in Chapter 11. The exocrine portion is the major part of the gland. It consists of *pancreatic acinar cells*, which secrete digestive enzymes into tiny ducts interwoven between the cells. These tiny ducts merge to form the main *pancreatic duct*, which extends the full length of the pancreas and empties into the duodenum. The pancreatic duct usually joins the common bile duct to form a single point of entry into the duodenum. Both ducts are controlled by the hepatopancreatic sphincter (sphincter of Oddi).

Pancreatic juice has a high concentration of bicarbonate ions and contains digestive enzymes that act on carbohydrates, proteins, and lipids. *Pancreatic amylase* acts on starch and other complex carbohydrates to break them into simpler sugars called *disaccharides*. Protein-splitting enzymes from the pancreas include *trypsin*. This enzyme breaks the proteins into shorter chains of amino acids, called *peptides*. Like other enzymes that act on proteins, trypsin is secreted in an inactive form, *trypsinogen*. This is activated by enterokinase when it reaches the duodenum. The pancreas also secretes *peptidase enzymes* that break peptides into amino acids. *Pancreatic lipase* breaks fats into fatty acids and monoglycerides.

Pancreatic secretion of digestive juice is regulated by the nervous system and by hormones. When parasympathetic impulses from the nervous system stimulate secretion of gastric juice, some impulses go to the pancreas and stimulate the secretion of pancreatic juice. When acid chyme enters the duodenum, the intestinal mucosa produces the hormone *secretin*, which travels in the blood to the pancreas. Secretin stimulates the pancreas to produce a fluid that has a high concentration of bicarbonate ions to neutralize the acids in the duodenum. Proteins and fats in the chyme stimulate the intestinal mucosa to secrete the hormone *cholecystokinin*, which causes the gallbladder to contract and also travels in the blood to the pancreas. This hormone stimulates the pancreas to produce a pancreatic juice that is rich in digestive enzymes. These digestive enzymes travel through the pancreatic duct to the duodenum, where they perform their actions.

CHEMICAL DIGESTION

Chemical digestion breaks down large complex molecules into smaller molecules that can be absorbed by the cells of the intestinal mucosa. The reactions in chemical digestion are *hydrolysis* reactions, which use water to split molecules. These reactions proceed at a slow rate. The purpose of the various digestive enzymes is to speed up the hydrolysis reactions of chemical digestion. The enzymes do not alter the reactions; they just make them occur more rapidly. Table 14.2 reviews the hormones and digestive enzymes that are discussed in previous sections of this chapter.

CARBOHYDRATE DIGESTION

Starches and other complex carbohydrates are first broken down into disaccharides, or double sugars, by the action of salivary amylase and pancreatic amylase. The disaccharides *sucrose*, *maltose*, and *lactose* are the result of this stage of digestion. Sucrase, maltase, and lactase—enzymes from the small intestine—act on the disaccharides to convert them to monosaccharides, or simple sugars, that can be absorbed. The digestion of maltose yields two molecules of glucose; sucrose produces one molecule of glucose and one of fructose; lactose yields one molecule each of glucose and galactose. The end products of complete carbohydrate digestion are the monosaccharides *glucose*, *fructose*, and *galactose*.

PROTEIN DIGESTION

The first digestive enzyme to act on proteins is pepsin in the stomach. Pepsin is secreted by the gastric glands in an inactive form, pepsinogen, which is activated by hydrochloric acid. When chyme reaches the duodenum, trypsin from the pancreas acts on the proteins. Trypsin is secreted in the inactive form, trypsinogen, which is activated by enterokinase in the small intestine. Pepsin and trypsin break down proteins into shorter chains of amino acids called *peptides*. Peptidase enzymes from the small intestine

Table 14.2 Enzymes and Hormones of the Digestive System

Secretion	Source	Action
Enzymes		
Amylase	Salivary glands Pancreas	Digestion of complex carbohydrates into disaccharides
Pepsin	Stomach	Digestion of proteins into polypeptides
Sucrase Maltase Lactase	Small intestine	Digestion of disaccharides into glucose, fructose, and galactose
Peptidase	Small intestine Pancreas	Digestion of peptides into amino acids
Lipase	Small intestine Pancreas	Digestion of fats into monoglycerides and fatty acids
Enterokinase	Small intestine	Activates trypsinogen
Hormones		
Gastrin	Stomach	Stimulates activity of gastric glands
Secretin	Small intestine	Stimulates pancreas to secrete bicarbonate ions to neutralize acid chyme
Cholecystokinin	Small intestine	Stimulates gallbladder to contract and release bile; stimulates pancreas to secrete digestive enzymes

From Applegate E: *The anatomy and physiology learning system*, ed 4, St. Louis, 2011, Saunders.

and pancreas break the peptide bonds to produce *amino acids.* The amino acids are the absorbable end products of protein digestion.

LIPID DIGESTION

The small intestine is the only place in which lipid (fat) digestion occurs, because the necessary enzymes are produced by the pancreas and enter the small intestine through the pancreatic duct. Triglycerides are the most abundant dietary fats. Fat molecules tend to attract one another to form large globules, which reduces the surface area for enzyme action. After the fats enter the duodenum, they are emulsified by bile. Emulsification does not break any chemical bonds, but it reduces the attraction between molecules so that they disperse. Pancreatic lipases act on the surfaces of the emulsified fat droplets. Lipase action breaks two fatty acid chains from the triglyceride molecules, yielding *monoglycerides* and *free fatty acids.*

ABSORPTION

Approximately 10 L of food, beverage, and secretions enter the digestive tract every day. Usually less than 1 L enters the large intestine. The other 9 L or more are absorbed in the small intestine. Absorption takes place along the entire length of the small intestine, but most of it occurs in the jejunum. By the time the chyme reaches the distal part of the ileum and large intestine, all that remains are some water, indigestible materials, and bacteria.

AGING OF THE DIGESTIVE SYSTEM

Throughout life the digestive system normally functions day after day with relatively few problems. There may be an occasional episode of GI tract inflammation, called *gastroenteritis,* caused by eating something that "doesn't agree," by irritation from excessively spicy foods, or by eating food that is contaminated by bacteria or toxins. Appendicitis tends to be fairly common in teenagers, but the prevalence decreases with age because the opening into the appendix tends to become smaller and possibly eventually closes. Ulcers and gallbladder problems are associated with middle age, often considered to be the high-stress time of life. Most of the difficulties in the digestive system before old age are caused by external problems rather than by structural changes within the system itself.

Structural changes in the digestive system occur as part of the normal aging process. These changes affect the overall operation of the system and may influence the nutritional state of the aging individual. In the mouth, teeth may become loose as a result of periodontal disease and have to be extracted. Because of dental problems, chewing may be uncomfortable. Salivary glands decrease their production of saliva, which reduces the salivary cleansing action and leads to a dry mouth (xerostomia). Thus food is not adequately moistened for chewing and swallowing. Taste sensations diminish, partially because there is less saliva to dissolve the taste particles and partially because there are fewer taste receptors. Loneliness and the problems in the oral cavity associated with aging may make eating a chore rather than a pleasure.

The mucosa in the stomach and intestines undergoes some atrophy with advancing age. In the stomach this may lead to a deficiency in hydrochloric acid and gastric juice for digestion. Pernicious anemia may develop because there is a lack of intrinsic factor from the gastric mucosa. In the small intestine, mucosal atrophy may lead to fewer enzymes and shorter villi; however, this does not appear to impair digestion and absorption in normal healthy people. The wall of the large intestine becomes thinner and weakens. This makes older people more susceptible to diverticulosis, in which the wall bulges outward to form balloonlike pockets. Constipation is a common complaint in the elderly; however, statistically, there seems to be no basis for it. This is more likely caused by lifestyle and habits rather than by structural changes in the digestive system.

Although structural and functional changes take place in the digestive system as part of the aging process, digestion and absorption are not altered noticeably in healthy older persons. A balanced diet, exercise, and a positive outlook on life will keep the digestive system in good working order for a long time.

Common Pathology of the Digestive System

Disease	Signs and Symptoms	Etiology	Diagnosis and Treatment
Anorexia	Extreme weight loss, thin appearance, abnormal blood count, fatigue, insomnia, dehydration, osteoporosis, and obsession with weight, exercise, and calorie intake.	An eating disorder. Exact cause is unknown. It is probably a combination of biologic, psychological, and environmental factors.	Criteria for diagnosis are refusal to maintain a body weight that is at or above minimum normal, intense fear of gaining weight, denying the seriousness of low body weight, and the absence of menstrual periods for at least 3 consecutive cycles. Treatment involves medical care to restore body weight combined with psychotherapy.

Common Pathology of the Digestive System—cont'd

Disease	Signs and Symptoms	Etiology	Diagnosis and Treatment
Appendicitis	Pain in the lower right abdomen, loss of appetite, nausea and/or vomiting, abdominal swelling, fever.	Occurs when the opening (cecum) into the appendix becomes blocked. Bacteria inside the appendix multiply rapidly and cause inflammation. A ruptured appendix is a medical emergency because the bacteria can diffuse throughout the abdomen, causing extensive peritonitis.	Diagnosis relies on patient history, blood and urine tests, and imaging techniques. Treatment is surgical removal of the appendix (appendectomy).
Bulimia	Characterized by binge eating and purging. Signs and symptoms include chronic gastric reflux, dehydration, electrolyte imbalance, esophagitis, depression, low self-esteem, and obsession with weight and calorie intake.	An eating disorder. Exact cause is unknown but probably includes environmental factors in the form of social expectations, genetic predisposition, and psychological factors.	Diagnosis relies on physical examination, blood and urine tests, and psychological evaluation. Diagnostic criteria include repeated binging; getting rid of extra calories by vomiting, use of laxatives or diuretics, or excessive exercise; binging and purging at least twice per week for at least 3 months; excessive importance of body weight and shape to feelings of self-esteem. Treatment of choice is cognitive-behavioral therapy to break the binge–purge cycle, solve emotional issues, and change attitudes about weight, diet, and body shape.
Caries	Dental caries (cavities) may present no signs or symptoms in the early stages. As decay continues, there may be sensitivity to heat and cold, and finally a toothache begins.	Caries is the result of poor dental care. Acids from oral bacteria slowly erode the enamel of the teeth until a cavity forms.	Diagnosis is made by a dentist who uses direct observation and dental x-rays. Once a cavity has developed, the dentist may fill it with an amalgam. Prevention is the best treatment. Routine prophylactic dental care and good dental hygiene are the keys to healthy teeth.
Celiac disease	Anemia, diarrhea, gas and bloating, weight loss, fatigue.	Exact cause is unknown, but evidence indicates genetic factors may be involved. Gluten triggers an immune response that damages the small intestine and interferes with the absorption of nutrients.	Physical examination, medical history, blood tests, antibody tests, and endoscopy are used in diagnosis. Treatment is to avoid eating gluten in any form. Nutritional supplements may be necessary.
Cholecystitis	Pain in upper right abdomen, nausea, vomiting, fever, and abdominal bloating.	Inflammation of the gallbladder is most often caused by gallstones that block the cystic duct.	Ultrasound and/or computed tomography (CT) scan are used to confirm diagnosis. Common treatment is surgical removal of the gallbladder (cholecystectomy).
Cholelithiasis (gallstones)	May be asymptomatic for years. When one or more become lodged in a duct, symptoms appear, including sudden and intense pain in upper right abdomen often accompanied by nausea and vomiting.	Cholelithiasis occurs when cholesterol and other substances in the bile precipitate and form crystals in the gallbladder. These may aggregate to form stones.	Diagnosis relies on patient history, abdominal ultrasound, and CT scans. The most reliable treatment, when necessary, is surgery to remove the gallbladder (cholecystectomy).
Cirrhosis	Signs and symptoms are directly related to liver functions and include bruising and bleeding, accumulation of toxins in the blood, jaundice, malnutrition, portal hypertension, splenomegaly, esophageal varices, dilated periumbilical veins, ascites.	The most common causes of cirrhosis are chronic alcohol abuse, hepatitis B, and hepatitis C.	Tests and procedures used to diagnose cirrhosis include liver function tests; imaging procedures such as ultrasound, CT, and magnetic resonance imaging (MRI); and liver biopsy. Treatment protocols are directed at the underlying cause. The goals of treatment are to slow the development of scar tissue and to prevent or alleviate the symptoms.

Continued

Common Pathology of the Digestive System—cont'd

Disease	Signs and Symptoms	Etiology	Diagnosis and Treatment
Cleft palate or lip	Split or opening in the roof of the mouth (palate) or in the upper lip.	Cause is unknown; probably has genetic and environmental factors. Birth defect that occurs early in pregnancy. Smoking and diabetes in the mother appear to increase the risk.	During pregnancy, ultrasound can detect the deformity. After birth the condition is obvious. Treatment is plastic surgery to close the openings.
Cold sores (fever blisters)	Small blisters on the lip, often red, swollen, and sore.	Caused by the herpes simplex virus (HSV), which enters through a break in the skin around the mouth; spread by coming in contact with infected fluid such as saliva.	The occurrence of the blisters is diagnostic. Sores are usually self-resolving within a few days, but skin creams may relieve the discomfort. The virus cannot be "cured"; it remains in the body. Recurrent outbreaks can be minimized by avoiding triggers such as stress.
Colitis	Inflammation of the lining of the colon with abdominal pain, diarrhea, fever, bloating, and blood in feces.	May be caused by bacterial invasion of the lining, loss of blood supply to the colon, or inflammatory bowel disease.	Diagnostic tools include patient history and physical examination, blood tests, urinalysis, and colonoscopy. Treatment is directed at the underlying cause of the inflammation.
Colorectal cancer	May be several years before symptoms develop and then they are nonspecific: fatigue, irregular bowel habits, blood in feces, abdominal pain, cramps, bloating, and weight loss.	Cause is unknown but risk factors include high-fat diet, family history of colorectal cancer, and inflammatory bowel disease.	Diagnosis is by colonoscopy and/or lower gastrointestinal (GI) series (barium enema). Treatment depends on the stage: early stages may be treated by surgery alone; more advanced cancer may require chemotherapy. Early detection through screening is a key factor.
Crohn disease	A type of inflammatory bowel disease; not limited to colon, may affect any part of the digestive tract and may extend into the deeper tissues of the tract. Signs and symptoms are nonspecific: diarrhea, abdominal pain, cramps, ulcers, loss of appetite, weight loss, malnutrition, fever, fatigue, and blood in feces.	Cause is unknown, but heredity and altered immune response seem to be involved. Risk factors include family history and cigarette smoking.	Diagnostic tools include fecal occult blood test, colonoscopy, sigmoidoscopy, and CT and/or MRI scans. There is no cure. Treatment is directed at managing symptoms and may include antiinflammatory medications, immunosuppressants, and antibiotics.
Diverticulosis	Characterized by pouch-like herniations through the muscular wall of the colon; usually asymptomatic unless they become inflamed (diverticulitis), which may cause symptoms of pain in the lower left abdomen, fever and chills, and nausea and vomiting.	Cause is not completely understood. It occurs when high pressure inside the colon pushes against weak areas in the colon wall. Studies have shown links between diverticulosis and obesity, lack of exercise, and smoking.	Diverticulosis is usually discovered during screening such as colonoscopy and needs no treatment. Diverticulitis is usually treated with oral antibiotics.
Dumping syndrome	Abdominal cramps, nausea, diarrhea	Dumping syndrome occurs when stomach contents move into the small intestine too rapidly. Most likely to develop after stomach surgery.	A gastric emptying test measures how quickly food moves into the small intestine. Alterations in diet may be sufficient treatment. For some individuals, medications may slow the passage of food from the stomach. As a last resort, a feeding tube may be necessary.

Common Pathology of the Digestive System—cont'd

Disease	Signs and Symptoms	Etiology	Diagnosis and Treatment
Gastroenteritis	Commonly called ***stomach flu***, signs and symptoms include watery diarrhea, abdominal cramps, nausea and vomiting, and fever.	Viruses and/or bacteria are the most common cause of the inflammation in the stomach and small intestine.	Usually is self-limiting, and no tests are needed for diagnosis. Patients should have plenty of fluids to prevent dehydration. In some cases, medications may be necessary to stop the diarrhea and vomiting.
Gastroesophageal reflux disease (GERD)	Heartburn, nausea after eating, difficulty swallowing, regurgitation of stomach contents.	Stomach contents leak back into the esophagus because the lower esophageal sphincter (LES) does not close properly and the stomach acid damages the esophageal lining. Risk factors include obesity, pregnancy, hiatal hernia, use of alcohol, smoking, certain foods and medications.	If symptoms are severe, tests to measure the amount of acid in the esophagus and/or upper endoscopy may be necessary. Treatment involves lifestyle changes, antacids for short-term relief, avoiding foods and medications that trigger reflux. If the condition cannot be controlled, surgery to strengthen the LES may be necessary.
Gingivitis	Inflammation of gum tissue evidenced by red, swollen, tender gums, bleeding during brushing, and bad breath (halitosis).	Plaque is the cause of gingivitis. Plaque creates small pockets of bacteria around the teeth resulting in inflammation of the gums. Risk factors include hormonal changes, illnesses, some medications, diabetes, smoking, human immunodeficiency virus and acquired immunodeficiency syndrome (HIV/AIDS), poor oral hygiene, and a family history of dental disease.	Dentists usually diagnose gingivitis based on symptoms and examination of the oral cavity. Treatment involves removing all traces of plaque and tartar, proper oral hygiene, and regular professional dental checkups and cleaning.
Hemorrhoids	Swollen veins around the anus (external) or in the lower rectum (internal); also called ***piles***. Signs and symptoms include itching, discomfort, or pain around the anus; painful bowel movements; blood on tissue after bowel movement.	The cause is increased pressure in the lower rectum. Risk factors include straining during bowel movements, sitting for long periods, chronic diarrhea or constipation, obesity, pregnancy, and a low-fiber diet.	Diagnosis is by visual examination of the area around the anus and a digital rectal examination. Treatments at home are often sufficient, including sitting in a warm water bath, applying creams to relieve itching, and increasing dietary fiber. The doctor may use rubber band ligation or sclerotherapy as a treatment. As a last resort, surgery to remove the hemorrhoids (hemorrhoidectomy) may be advised.
Hepatitis	Swelling and inflammation of the liver; signs and symptoms may be subtle and include fatigue, flulike symptoms, dark urine, pale feces, abdominal pain, loss of appetite, jaundice, and weight loss.	Five types of viral hepatitis, each caused by a different virus. Hepatitis A virus (HAV) is transmitted through contaminated food or water; hepatitis B virus (HBV) through puncture wounds or contact with infectious body fluids; hepatitis C virus (HCV) through direct contact with body fluids, usually through injection drugs or sexual contact. Hepatitis D virus (HDV) occurs in conjunction with hepatitis B and is uncommon in the United States; hepatitis E virus (HEV) is waterborne and occurs in areas of poor sanitation; uncommon in the United States. Nonviral hepatitis may be caused by excessive alcohol consumption, exposure to poisons, overuse of certain medications, and an inappropriate reaction by the immune system.	Diagnosis is by palpation of the liver, liver biopsy, liver function tests, ultrasound, and blood tests. Treatment depends on the type of hepatitis.

Continued

Common Pathology of the Digestive System—cont'd

Disease	Signs and Symptoms	Etiology	Diagnosis and Treatment
Hiatal hernia	By itself, a hiatal hernia causes no symptoms. When symptoms do occur, they are usually due to GERD and include heartburn, chest pain, burping, nausea, vomiting, and large amounts of saliva in the mouth.	A hiatal hernia occurs when a portion of the stomach pushes upward through the diaphragm into the mediastinum. In general, this happens if the diaphragm opening is too large or the surrounding muscle is too weak.	Most cases are discovered during a test or procedure to determine the cause of heartburn; may include barium x-rays, CT scan, and endoscopy. Treatment is aimed at minimizing acid reflux and may include antacids and medications to reduce acid production.
Inflammatory bowel disease (IBD)	A group of inflammatory conditions of the small intestine and colon. Crohn disease and ulcerative colitis are the most common forms. Signs and symptoms are nonspecific: diarrhea, abdominal pain, cramps, ulcers, loss of appetite, weight loss, malnutrition, fever, fatigue, and bloody diarrhea.	Cause is unknown, but heredity and altered immune response seem to be involved.	Diagnostic tools include fecal occult blood test, colonoscopy, sigmoidoscopy, and CT and/or MRI scans. There is no cure. Treatment is directed at managing symptoms and may include antiinflammatory medications, immunosuppressants, and antibiotics.
Irritable bowel syndrome (IBS)	Common disorder of the colon characterized by chronic abdominal pain, bloating, and alterations of bowel habits.	IBS has no known cause; disruptions in the muscle activity and nerve supply of the colon may have a role in the condition. Certain foods, stress, hormone fluctuations, and other illnesses may aggravate the condition.	Diagnosis is based on symptoms and tests to rule out other conditions. Treatment focuses on the relief of symptoms. Dietary adjustments and medications may be advised.
Lactose intolerance	Abdominal pain, gas, bloating, diarrhea, rumbling sounds in the abdomen after eating dairy products.	Occurs when the small intestine does not produce enough lactase enzyme to digest the lactose sugar in milk and dairy products.	Diagnosis is based on symptoms and confirmed by a lactose tolerance test. Treatment involves avoiding the consumption of lactose-containing dairy products or taking lactase supplements.
Leukoplakia	Thick white patches on the tongue and the mucosa of the mouth.	Exact cause is unknown, but evidence suggests the condition results from irritants such as tobacco, whether smoked or chewed, excessive alcohol use, or rough places on the teeth.	A biopsy of the patches confirms the diagnosis. A biopsy may find changes that indicate oral cancer. Treatment is to remove the source of the irritation. Surgical removal may be necessary in some cases.
Malabsorption syndrome	Malabsorption syndrome is an inability of the small intestine to absorb nutrients into the bloodstream. Signs and symptoms vary according to the nutrients not being absorbed, but usually there will be chronic diarrhea, abnormal stools, weight loss, and gas.	Causes include the absence of certain digestive enzymes, lactose intolerance, celiac disease, short bowel syndrome, genetic diseases, and certain medications.	Diagnosis is based on the presence of fat in the feces (steatorrhea). Treatment depends on the cause but may include dietary changes and nutritional supplements.

Common Pathology of the Digestive System—cont'd

Disease	Signs and Symptoms	Etiology	Diagnosis and Treatment
Mumps	Also called ***epidemic parotitis;*** most obvious sign is swelling of the parotid glands, which may be accompanied by fever, headache, and muscle aches. Postpubescent males may develop orchitis. In rare cases mumps may lead to hearing loss.	A contagious disease caused by the mumps virus, it was common until mumps vaccination became routine.	Diagnosis is by physical examination and possibly a blood test to detect mumps antibodies. Mumps is usually self-resolving within 2 weeks and no treatment is necessary.

TERMINOLOGY REVIEW

Key Term	Word Parts	Definition
Absorption		The passage of digestive end products from the gastrointestinal tract into the blood or lymph.
Chyme		The semifluid mixture of food and gastric juice that leaves the stomach through the pyloric sphincter.
Defecation		The expulsion of indigestible wastes, or feces, through the anus.
Deglutition		The process of swallowing.
Fauces		Opening from the oral cavity into the oropharynx.
Gastric juice	*gastr/o:* stomach	The secretions of the exocrine gastric glands.
Gastrin	*gastr/o:* stomach	Hormone secreted by the endocrine glands in the stomach.
Gingiva	*gingiv/o:* gums	Soft tissue that covers the alveolar processes of the mandible and maxillae; also called *gums.*
Hydrolysis	*hydr/o:* water *-lysis:* breaking apart	Chemical breakdown of complex molecules by the addition of water.
Ileocecal valve	*ile/o:* ileum *-cec-:* cecum	The valve between the small intestine and large intestine.
Lower esophageal sphincter		Valve between the esophagus and stomach.
Mastication		The process of chewing.
Mesentery		Extensions of peritoneum that are associated with the intestine.
Palate		Roof of the mouth; separates the oral cavity from the nasal cavity.
Peristalsis	*-stalsis:* contraction	Rhythmic contractions of the intestine that move food along the digestive tract.
Plicae circulares		Circular folds in the mucosa and submucosa of the small intestine.
Pyloric sphincter		Valve between the stomach and first part of the small intestine.
Rugae		Longitudinal folds in the mucosa of the stomach.
Teniae coli	*col-:* colon or large intestine	Bands of longitudinal muscle fibers in the large intestine.

Urinary System

Check out the Evolve site at http://evolve.elsevier.com/Bonewit/today to access additional interactive activities and exercises to help you study and prepare for success.

LEARNING OBJECTIVES

1. State six functions of the urinary system.
2. Describe the location and structural features of the kidneys.
3. Label the parts of a nephron.
4. State the two parts of the juxtaglomerular apparatus.
5. Describe the location, structure, and function of the ureters, urinary bladder, and urethra.
6. List and describe the three steps in urine formation.
7. Identify the hormones that affect kidney function, and explain how they do so.
8. Explain the function of renin.
9. Describe ways in which the aging of an individual affects the urinary system.
10. Identify pathology related to the urinary system.

CHAPTER OUTLINE

KEY TERMS

detrusor muscle (dee-TROO-sor MUH-sull)
erythropoietin (ee-rith-roh-poy-EE-tin)
glomerular capsule (gloh-MER-yoo-lar KAP-sool)
glomerular filtration (gloh-MER-yoo-lar fil-TRAY-shun)
glomerulus (gloh-MER-yoo-lus)
juxtaglomerular apparatus (juks-tah-gloh-MER-yoo-lar ap-pah-RAT-us)
micturition (mik-too-RISH-un)
nephrons (NEFF-rahns)
nephron loop (NEFF-rahn LOOP)
renal corpuscle (REE-nal KOAR-pu-sell)
renal cortex (REE-nal KOAR-teks)
renal medulla (REE-nal meh-DOO-lah)
renal pelvis (REE-nal PELL-vis)
renal tubule (REE-nal TOOB-yool)
renin (REE-nin)
trigone (TRYE-goan)
tubular reabsorption (TOOB-yoo-lar ree-ab-SORP-shun)
tubular secretion (TOOB-yoo-lar see-KREE-shun)
ureter (yoo-REE-ter)
urethra (yoo-REE-thrah)
urinary bladder (YOO-rin-air-ee blad-der)

INTRODUCTION TO THE URINARY SYSTEM

The overall function of the urinary system is to maintain the volume and composition of body fluids within normal limits. The urinary system accomplishes this by excreting the waste products that accumulate as a result of cellular metabolism. Because of this, the urinary system is sometimes referred to as the *excretory system*. Although the urinary system has a major role in excretion, other organs contribute to the excretory function. Some waste products, such as carbon dioxide and water, are excreted by the lungs through the respiratory system. The skin excretes wastes through the sweat glands. The liver and intestines excrete bile pigments that result from the destruction of hemoglobin. The major task of excretion, however, still belongs to the urinary system. If the urinary system fails, the other organs cannot take over and compensate adequately. In addition to eliminating waste products, the urinary system maintains an appropriate fluid volume. It does this by regulating the amount of water that is excreted in the urine. Other functions of the urinary system include regulating the concentrations of various electrolytes in the body fluids and maintaining normal pH of the blood.

In addition to maintaining fluid balance in the body, the urinary system controls red blood cell production by secreting the hormone **erythropoietin**. The urinary system also plays a role in maintaining normal blood pressure by secreting the enzyme **renin**.

COMPONENTS OF THE URINARY SYSTEM

The urinary system consists of the kidneys, ureters, urinary bladder, and urethra. The kidneys produce the urine. The ureters transport the urine away from the kidneys to the urinary bladder. The urinary bladder stores the urine until it is excreted from the body. The urethra is a tubular structure that carries the urine from the urinary bladder to the outside of the body. The components of the urinary system are illustrated in Fig. 15.1.

KIDNEYS

The *kidneys* are the primary organs of the urinary system. They are the organs that filter the blood, remove the wastes from the blood, and excrete the wastes into the urine. They are the organs that perform the functions of the urinary system. The other components of the urinary system are accessory structures to help eliminate the urine from the body.

Location

The kidneys are located between the twelfth thoracic and third lumbar vertebrae, one on each side of the vertebral column. The right kidney is usually slightly lower than the left because the liver displaces it downward. The kidneys are partially protected by the lower ribs and lie in shallow depressions against the posterior abdominal wall behind the peritoneum (retroperitoneal). Each kidney is held in place by connective tissue, called *renal fascia*.

A thick layer of adipose tissue surrounds each kidney. This is called *perirenal fat*, and it helps to protect the kidney. A tough, fibrous connective tissue encases each kidney and is called the *renal capsule*. The renal capsule provides support for the soft tissue that is inside.

Macroscopic Structure

In the adult, each kidney is approximately 3 cm thick, 6 cm wide, and 12 cm long (1.2 × 2.5 × 5 inches). The kidney is bean-shaped with an indentation, called the *hilum*. The hilum leads to a large cavity within the kidney called the *renal sinus*. The *ureter* and *renal vein* leave the kidney at the hilum, and the *renal artery* enters the kidney at the hilum.

The macroscopic internal structure of the kidney is illustrated in Fig. 15.2. The outer, reddish region is the **renal cortex**. The renal cortex surrounds a darker reddish-brown region called the **renal medulla**. The renal medulla consists of a series of *renal pyramids*. The renal pyramids appear striated because they contain straight tubular structures and blood vessels. The wide bases of the pyramids are adjacent to the cortex. The pointed ends of the pyramids, called *renal papillae*, are directed toward the center of the kidney. Portions of the renal cortex extend into the spaces between adjacent pyramids to form *renal columns*. The cortex and medulla make up the functional tissue of the kidney.

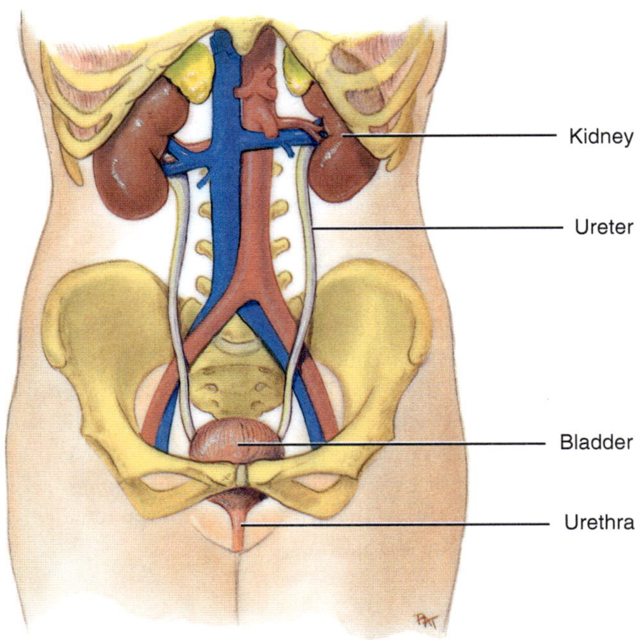

Fig. 15.1 Components of the urinary system. (From Applegate E: *The anatomy and physiology learning system*, ed 4, St. Louis, 2011, Saunders.)

HIGHLIGHT on the Urinary System

Hangover: Alcohol inhibits the secretion of antidiuretic hormone, so when people drink alcohol, they experience diuresis, or excessive urination. Experts believe that the dehydration caused by diuresis contributes to "hangover" symptoms.

Nephrons: The number of nephrons does not increase after birth. Growth of the kidney occurs from enlargement of the individual nephrons. When nephrons are damaged, they are not replaced.

Nephroptosis: Nephroptosis, commonly referred to as a *floating kidney*, occurs when the kidney is no longer held in place by the renal fascia and it drops out of its normal position. This may make the kidney more vulnerable to injury if it is no longer protected by the ribs. Another danger is that the ureter may become twisted and block the flow of urine. Nephroptosis occurs more frequently in horseback riders, truck drivers, and people who ride motorcycles.

Uremia: When the kidneys do not function properly and fail to remove the waste products from the blood, uremia may result. Uremia is a condition in which there is a toxic level of urea in the blood.

Urinary incontinence: Urinary incontinence is the inability to control urination and to retain urine in the bladder. Temporary incontinence may result when the muscles around the bladder and urethra become weakened and lose muscle tone. This is sometimes caused by stretching of the muscles during childbirth. Because these muscles help restrict the outlet of the bladder, their weakness contributes to a leakage of urine. A cough or sneeze may increase pressure within the bladder sufficiently to force urine to escape. Permanent incontinence is usually caused by damage to the central nervous system or by extensive damage to the bladder or urethra.

Urinary tract infection (UTI): UTIs occur more frequently in women than in men because of differences in the urethra. In females the urethral opening is in close proximity to the anal opening, which gives intestinal bacteria easier access to the urethra. The female urethra is short, which allows any infection to spread to the urinary bladder. An infection of the urethra is called *urethritis*, and an infection of the urinary bladder is called *cystitis*. ■

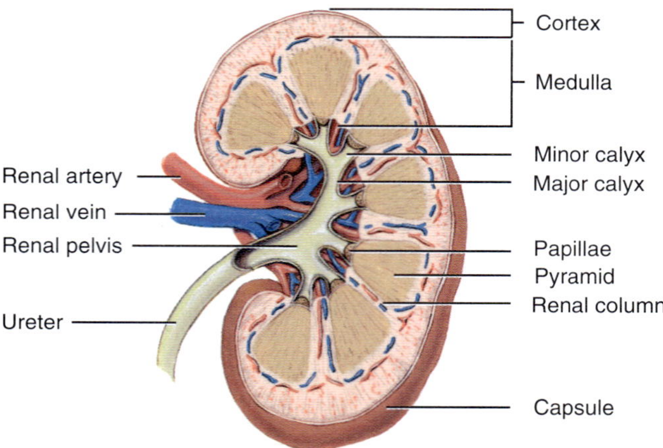

Fig. 15.2 Coronal (frontal) section through the kidney. (From Applegate E: *The anatomy and physiology learning system*, ed 4, St. Louis, 2011, Saunders.)

The central region of the kidney contains the **renal pelvis**, a large cavity that collects the urine as it is produced. The periphery of the renal pelvis is interrupted by cuplike projections called *calyces*. A *minor calyx* surrounds the renal papillae of each pyramid and collects urine from that pyramid. Several minor calyces converge to form a *major calyx*. From the major calyces, the urine flows into the renal pelvis and from there into the ureter.

Nephrons

Each kidney contains more than 1 million functional units, called **nephrons**, located in the cortex and medulla. The nephron is where the blood is filtered and urine is formed. A nephron consists of a renal corpuscle and a renal tubule (Fig. 15.3).

The **renal corpuscle** consists of the **glomerulus** and the **glomerular capsule** (Bowman capsule). The glomerulus is a cluster of capillaries. Blood enters the glomerulus through an *afferent arteriole* and is filtered. The blood then leaves the glomerulus through an *efferent arteriole* (Fig. 15.4). As the blood is filtered, the filtrate enters the glomerular capsule, which continues as the renal tubule. Renal corpuscles are located in the cortex of the kidney and give it a granular appearance.

The **renal tubule**, which carries fluid away from the glomerular capsule, consists of a proximal convoluted tubule, a nephron loop (Henle loop), and a distal convoluted tubule.

The first portion of the tubule, located in the cortex, is highly coiled and is known as the *proximal convoluted tubule*. Next the tubule straightens and dips into the medulla, makes a U-turn, and ascends back toward the cortex. This forms the **nephron loop** (Henle loop). The portion of the loop that descends from the proximal convoluted tubule into the medulla is the *descending limb*, and the part that ascends back toward the cortex is the *ascending limb*. The final region of the tubule, which is also coiled and found in the cortex, is known as the *distal convoluted tubule* (see Fig. 15.4).

Collecting Ducts

Urine passes from the distal convoluted tubules of the nephrons into *collecting ducts*. These straight tubules, with the nephron loops and blood vessels, give the renal medulla its striated appearance. Fluid flows from the collecting ducts into the minor calyces that surround the renal papillae.

Juxtaglomerular Apparatus

The ascending limb of the nephron loop, in the region where it continues into the distal convoluted tubule, comes into contact with the glomerular afferent arteriole of the

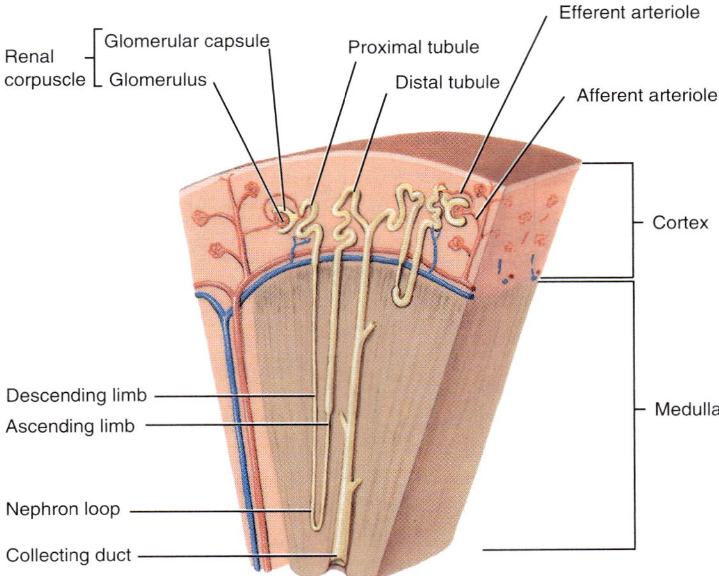

Fig. 15.3 A section of a kidney showing the structures in the cortex and those in the medulla. The renal pyramids in the medulla contain the nephron loops and collecting ducts. (From Applegate E: *The anatomy and physiology learning system,* ed 4, St. Louis, 2011, Saunders.)

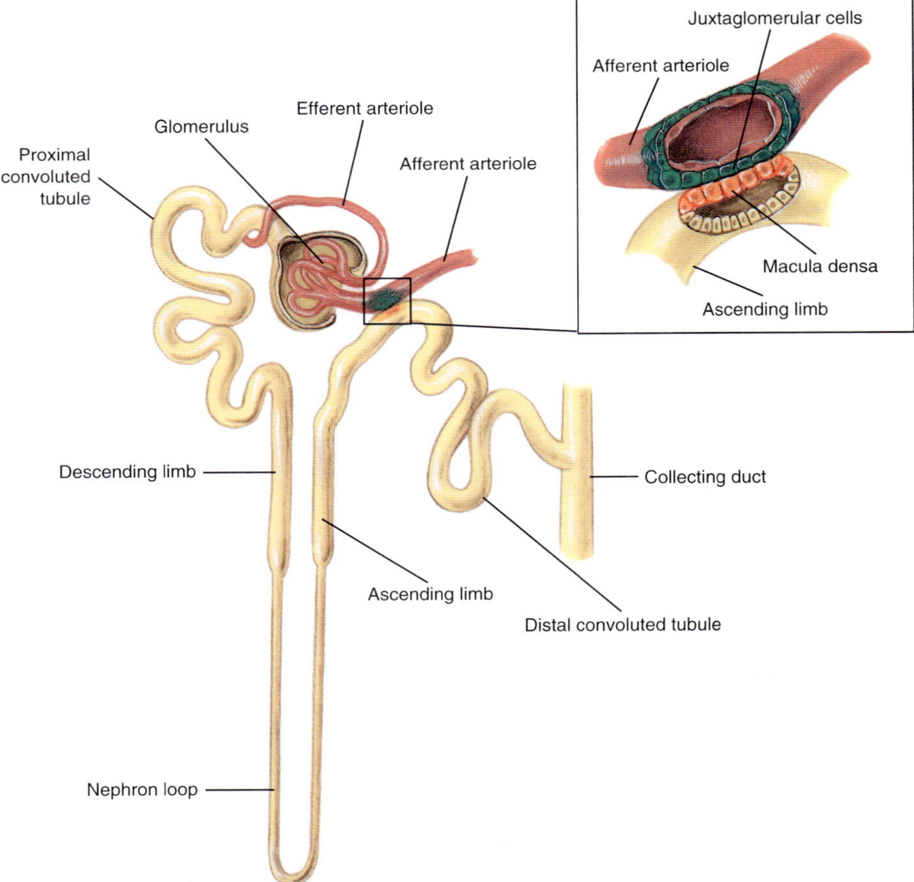

Fig. 15.4 Juxtaglomerular apparatus and its relationship to the nephron. The juxtaglomerular apparatus is in the boxes. In the region of contact, the cells of the ascending limb are modified to form the macula densa, and the cells of the afferent arteriole are modified to form the juxtaglomerular cells. Together, these modified regions are the juxtaglomerular apparatus. (From Applegate E: *The anatomy and physiology learning system*, ed 4, St. Louis, 2011, Saunders.)

same nephron (see Fig. 15.4). In the region of contact, the cells of the ascending limb are modified to form the *macula densa,* and those in the afferent arteriole are modified to form the *juxtaglomerular cells.* The macula densa monitors sodium chloride concentration in the urine and also influences the juxtaglomerular cells. In the afferent arteriole, the juxtaglomerular cells produce the enzyme renin, which has a role in the regulation of blood pressure. Together, the macula densa and juxtaglomerular cells make up the **juxtaglomerular apparatus**.

Blood Flow Through the Kidney

Blood flows through the kidneys at an approximate rate of 1200 mL/min. This is about one-fourth of the total cardiac output. Blood is brought to the kidneys by the renal arteries, which are branches from the abdominal aorta. The blood flows through the arteries of the kidney until it enters the afferent arterioles. Each of these tiny vessels continues into a glomerulus, where the blood is filtered. The blood leaves the glomerulus through an efferent arteriole and enters a series of veins. The renal vein exits the kidney and takes blood to the inferior vena cava.

URETERS

Each **ureter** is a small tube, about 25 cm (10 inches) long, that carries urine from the renal pelvis to the urinary bladder. It descends from the renal pelvis and enters the urinary bladder on the posterior inferior surface.

The wall of the ureter consists of three layers (Fig. 15.5). The outer layer is a supporting layer of fibrous connective tissue known as the *fibrous coat.* The middle layer is known as the *muscular coat.* It consists of smooth muscle. The main function of this layer is peristalsis to propel the urine through the ureter. The inner layer is the *mucosa.* This layer secretes mucus, which coats and protects the surface of the cells.

URINARY BLADDER

The **urinary bladder** is located in the pelvic cavity and is a temporary storage reservoir for urine (see Fig. 15.5). The size and shape of the urinary bladder vary with the amount of urine it contains and with the pressure from surrounding organs.

The inner lining of the urinary bladder consists of a *mucous membrane.* When the bladder is empty, the mucosa has numerous folds called *rugae.* The rugae allow the bladder to expand as it fills. The next layer is the *muscularis,* which is composed of smooth muscle. The smooth muscle fibers in the muscular layer are interwoven in all directions, and collectively these are called the **detrusor muscle**. Contraction of this muscle expels urine from the bladder.

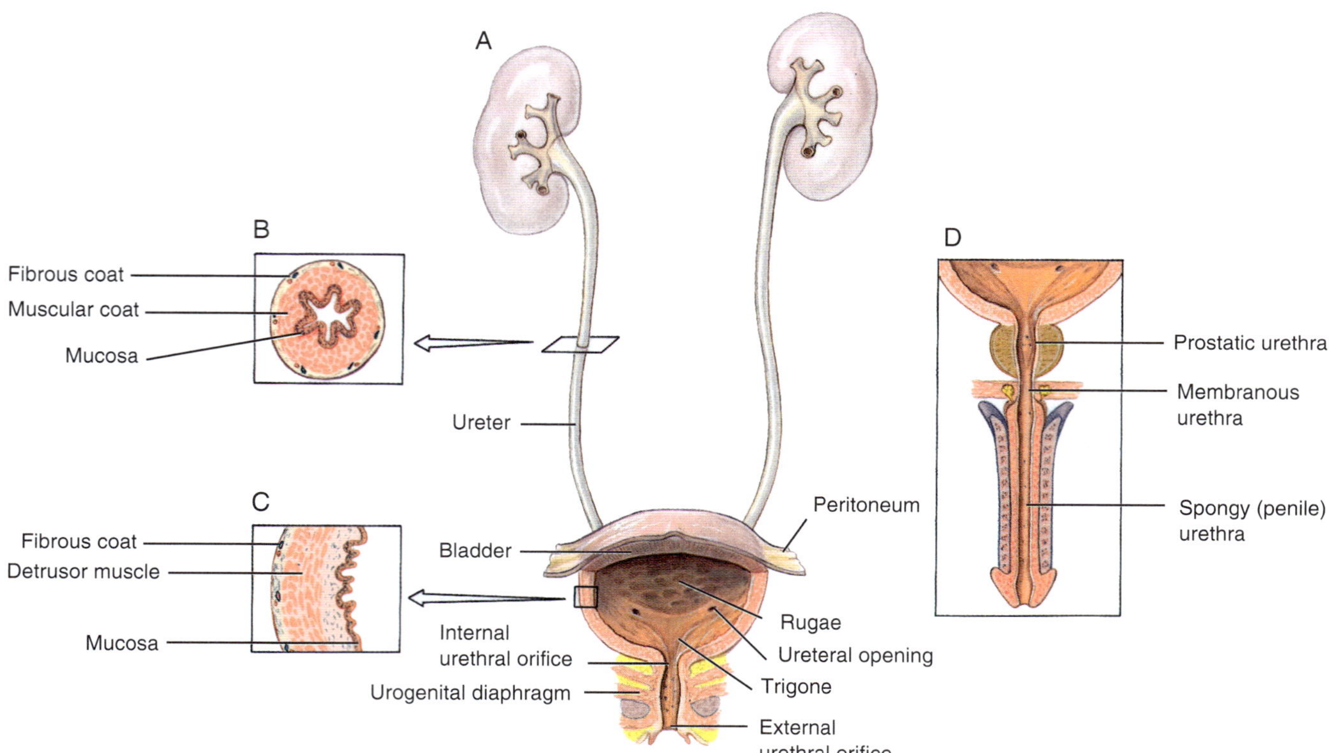

Fig. 15.5 Ureter, urinary bladder, and urethra. (A) Urinary tract. (B) Cross section through the ureter. (C) Cross section of the bladder wall. (D) Regions of the male urethra. (From Applegate E: *The anatomy and physiology learning system*, ed 4, St. Louis, 2011, Saunders.)

A triangular area, called the **trigone**, is formed by three openings in the floor of the urinary bladder. Two of the openings are from the ureters and form the base of the trigone. Small flaps of mucosa cover these openings and act as valves that allow urine to enter the bladder but prevent it from backing up from the bladder into the ureters. The third opening, at the apex of the trigone, is the opening into the urethra. A band of the detrusor muscle encircles this opening to form the *internal urethral sphincter.*

URETHRA

The final passageway for the flow of urine is the **urethra**. The urethra consists of a thin-walled tube that conveys urine from the floor of the urinary bladder to outside of the body (see Fig. 15.5). The opening to the outside is known as the *external urethral orifice.*

The beginning of the urethra, where it leaves the urinary bladder, is surrounded by the *internal urethral sphincter.* This sphincter is smooth (involuntary) muscle. Another sphincter, the *external urethral sphincter*, is skeletal (voluntary) muscle and encircles the urethra where it passes through the pelvic floor. These two sphincters control the flow of urine through the urethra.

In females the urethra is short, only 3 to 4 cm (about $1^1/_2$ inches) long. The external urethral orifice opens to the outside just anterior to the opening for the vagina.

In males the urethra is much longer, about 20 cm (7 to 8 inches) in length, and transports both urine and semen. The first part of the male urethra passes through the prostate gland and is called the *prostatic urethra.* The second part is a short region that penetrates the pelvic floor and enters the penis. This short region is known as the *membranous urethra.* The third part of the male urethra is the longest region and is called the *spongy urethra.* This portion of the urethra extends the entire length of the penis, and the external urethral orifice opens to the outside at the tip of the penis.

URINE FORMATION

The work of the kidneys, performed by the nephrons, is to maintain the volume and composition of body fluids, regulate the pH of the blood, and remove waste products from the blood. The result of this work is the formation of urine. As urine is excreted to the outside of the body, it carries with it the wastes, excess water, and excess electrolytes. At the same time, the kidneys conserve other electrolytes to maintain the appropriate balance. The formation of urine involves glomerular filtration, tubular reabsorption, and tubular secretion, which are illustrated in Fig. 15.6.

GLOMERULAR FILTRATION

The first step in the formation of urine is **glomerular filtration**. During this process, blood plasma leaves the glomerulus and enters the glomerular capsule. The force that moves the fluid across the membrane is *filtration pressure*, and the fluid that enters the capsule is the *filtrate.*

Blood flows through the kidneys at an average rate of 1200 mL/min. As the blood passes through the glomeruli, about 19% of the plasma enters the glomerular capsule as filtrate. This is equivalent to forming filtrate at a rate of 125 mL/min, or 180 L (45 gallons) per day. This is the total value for all the nephrons in both kidneys. The filtration membrane acts as a barrier that prevents blood cells and protein molecules from entering the glomerular capsule; therefore they are absent from the filtrate.

TUBULAR REABSORPTION

If the volume and composition of the filtrate in the glomerular capsule are compared with the volume and composition of urine, it is obvious that changes occur after filtration. First of all, about 180 L (45 gallons) of filtrate are formed in a 24-hour period. This volume is reduced to 1 to 2 L of urine. Glucose is present in the filtrate but normally absent in the urine. Urea and uric acid are present in higher concentrations in the urine than in the filtrate.

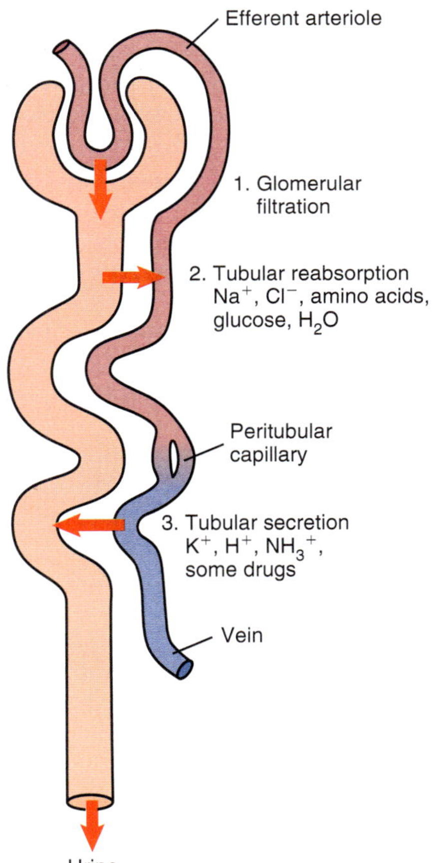

Fig. 15.6 Steps in urine formation. Urine consists of the substances that enter the tubules in glomerular filtration, minus substances that are reabsorbed in the tubules, plus substances that are secreted into the tubules. (From Applegate E: *The anatomy and physiology learning system*, ed 4, St. Louis, 2011, Saunders.)

Tubular reabsorption is the first process that changes the volume and composition of the filtrate. Tubular reabsorption is the movement of substances from the filtrate in the renal tubules into the blood. Only about 1% of the filtrate remains in the tubules and becomes urine. In general, water and other substances that are useful to the body such as glucose and sodium are reabsorbed from the renal tubules back into the blood. Wastes such as urea and uric acid remain in the filtrate and are excreted in the urine.

TUBULAR SECRETION

The final process in the formation of urine is tubular secretion. **Tubular secretion** is the movement of substances from the blood into the renal tubules. Most of these substances are waste products of cellular metabolism that become toxic if allowed to accumulate in the body. Tubular secretion is the method by which some drugs, such as penicillin, are removed from the body. The tubular secretion of hydrogen ions plays an important role in regulating the pH of the blood. Other molecules and ions that may enter the filtrate by tubular secretion include potassium ions, creatinine, and histamine.

The final product, urine, produced by the nephrons of the kidney, consists of the substances that are filtered, minus the substances that are reabsorbed in the tubules, plus the substances that are added by tubular secretion. If kidney function is impaired by disease or injury, dialysis may be necessary to maintain body fluid composition. Dialysis is a procedure used to separate waste material from the blood and to maintain fluid, electrolyte, and acid–base balance in the body.

REGULATION OF URINE CONCENTRATION AND VOLUME

The concentration and volume of urine depend on conditions in the internal environment of the body. Cells in the hypothalamus are sensitive to changes in the composition of the blood and initiate appropriate responses that affect the kidneys. If the concentration of solutes in the blood increases above normal, the kidneys excrete a small volume of concentrated urine. This conserves water in the body and gets rid of solutes to restore the blood to normal. If the blood solute concentration decreases below normal, the kidneys conserve solutes and get rid of water by producing large quantities of dilute urine. Urine production plays an important role in maintaining homeostasis of blood concentration and volume. By regulating blood volume, the kidneys also play a role in regulating blood pressure because volume is directly related to pressure.

Under average conditions, the kidneys produce about 1500 mL of urine in a 24-hour period, but the volume may vary from 1 to 2 L. The pH may vary from 4.6 to 8, with an average of about 6. This means that urine is usually slightly acidic but may become alkaline under certain conditions such as vegetarian diets.

Three hormones—*aldosterone*, *antidiuretic hormone (ADH)*, and *atrial natriuretic hormone*—influence urine concentration and volume. Aldosterone, secreted by cells of the adrenal cortex, acts on the kidney tubules to increase the reabsorption of sodium. When sodium is reabsorbed, water follows by osmosis. This reduces urine output.

ADH is produced by cells in the hypothalamus and is released from the posterior lobe of the pituitary gland. ADH makes the kidney tubules more permeable to water. When ADH is present, more water is reabsorbed, which reduces the volume of urine and makes it more concentrated. Water is conserved in the body. In the absence of ADH, the tubules are less permeable to water and there is less reabsorption. This results in large quantities of dilute urine, and water is lost from the body.

Special cells in the heart produce a hormone called *atrial natriuretic hormone*, or *atriopeptin*, which is secreted when the atrial cells are stretched. This hormone promotes the excretion of sodium and water by acting directly on the kidney tubules and by inhibiting the secretion of ADH, renin, and aldosterone. The result of atrial natriuretic hormone is a decrease in both blood volume and blood pressure.

Renin is an enzyme that is produced by the juxtaglomerular cells in the kidney in response to low blood pressure or decreased blood sodium concentration. Renin promotes the production of *angiotensin II* in the blood. Angiotensin II is a powerful vasoconstrictor, a substance that increases the blood pressure. Angiotensin II also stimulates the adrenal gland to secrete aldosterone, which acts on the kidney tubules to conserve sodium and water. This increases blood volume and consequently increases blood pressure.

MICTURITION

Micturition, commonly called *urination* or *voiding*, is the act of expelling urine from the bladder. The bladder can hold up to a liter of urine, but normally when it contains 200 to 400 mL, stretch receptors in the bladder wall trigger impulses that initiate the *micturition reflex*. This is an automatic and involuntary response that is coordinated in the spinal cord. Impulses are transmitted along parasympathetic nerves to the detrusor muscle. Even though the micturition reflex is involuntary, it can be inhibited or stimulated by higher brain centers.

It is desirable to completely empty the bladder when urinating. Residual urine is what remains in the bladder if an individual is unable to completely empty the bladder. This may be indicative of a pathologic condition such as a UTI or, in males, an enlarged prostate.

AGING OF THE URINARY SYSTEM

Some of the more obvious and familiar aging changes occur in the urinary bladder and urethra. Muscles in the walls of these structures tend to weaken and become less elastic with age. As a person ages, the bladder is unable to expand or contract as much as in younger people. This reduces the capacity of the bladder and makes it more difficult to completely empty it during urination. Awareness of the need to urinate, which usually occurs when the bladder is half full in younger people, may be delayed in the elderly until the bladder is nearly full. The external urethral sphincter also weakens, which adds to the problems.

Several anatomic changes occur in the kidneys as a person ages, and these changes are reflected in their related functions. There is a general atrophy of nephrons so that by the age of 80, the kidney is about 80% of its young but mature size. Some of the remaining glomeruli are modified, and this, along with the decrease in number, results in a decreased glomerular filtration rate so that the blood is not filtered as quickly as before.

The tubules also undergo changes as a person ages. In general, the tubule walls thicken, which makes them less able to reabsorb water to form concentrated urine. The collecting ducts are less responsive to ADH, and this, along with a diminished thirst mechanism, may result in dehydration. The ability to reabsorb glucose and sodium is also diminished. The tubules become less efficient in the secretion of ions and drugs. They have a diminished ability to compensate for drastic changes in acid–base balance. Drugs that are normally eliminated from the body by tubular secretion may accumulate to toxic levels because they are not cleared from the blood as quickly as they are in younger people.

Amazingly, even with the changes caused by aging, the kidneys of elderly persons are capable of maintaining relatively stable balances in the blood and body fluids under normal conditions. However, their ability to compensate for drastic changes and abnormal conditions is diminished.

Common Pathology of the Urinary System

Disease	Signs and Symptoms	Etiology	Diagnosis and Treatment
Acute renal failure	Symptoms of acute renal failure may include decreased urine output, fluid retention, fatigue, drowsiness, shortness of breath, confusion, and nausea.	Acute kidney failure occurs when the kidneys suddenly become unable to filter waste products from the blood, allowing dangerous levels of toxic wastes to accumulate. It may occur when there is direct damage to the kidneys or from other causes.	Diagnosis is based on observation of the urine output, **urinalysis**, blood tests, and imaging diagnostics. Treatment for acute kidney failure involves identifying the illness or injury that originally damaged the kidneys and correcting it. Often, medications are prescribed to restore normal function. In severe cases, hemodialysis may be required.
Chronic renal failure	Chronic renal failure is initially without specific symptoms. As the disease progresses, blood pressure increases and waste products accumulate in the blood, resulting in a general ill feeling and fatigue.	Chronic renal failure is a medical condition in which the kidneys fail to adequately filter waste products from the blood. The three most common causes of chronic renal failure are diabetes mellitus, hypertension, and glomerulonephritis.	It is important to differentiate between acute and chronic renal failure. Sometimes it is necessary to treat for acute failure until it can be determined to be chronic. Controlling blood pressure will slow further kidney damage. Ultimately, frequent hemodialysis is indicated.
Bladder cancer	Blood or blood clots in the urine, pain during urination, need for frequent urination, urinary tract infections, pain in the lower back.	It is not always clear what causes bladder cancer. Bladder cancer develops when cells in the bladder begin to grow abnormally. It has been linked to smoking, parasitic infection, radiation, and chemical exposure.	Diagnosis may be based on laboratory and imaging tests, sometimes using a dye to highlight the kidneys, ureters, and bladder. The bladder can be visually examined and tissue removed for biopsy by cystoscopy. There are many treatment options, including radiation therapy, biologic therapy, chemotherapy, and surgery.
Kidney cancer	Blood in the urine, back pain, abdominal swelling, swelling of the veins around a testicle, flank pain, and weight loss.	Kidney cancer starts in the lining of the kidney tubules. It occurs most often in men aged 50–70. It is not clear what causes the DNA mutation that results in renal cell carcinoma, but some of the risk factors are dialysis treatments, high blood pressure, polycystic kidney disease, and smoking.	Diagnosis is based on symptoms, imaging scans, blood chemistry, IVP, and renal arteriography. Surgery to remove all or part of the kidney is recommended. This may include removing the bladder, surrounding tissues, or lymph nodes. A cure is unlikely unless all of the cancer can be removed.

Continued

Common Pathology of the Urinary System—cont'd

Disease	Signs and Symptoms	Etiology	Diagnosis and Treatment
Cystitis	Burning sensation when urinating, persistent urge to urinate, passing small amount of urine, blood in the urine, discomfort in the pelvic area, and fever.	Cystitis is an inflammation of the bladder usually caused by a UTI and involving *Escherichia coli* bacteria. It may also be caused by an infection in a kidney.	Diagnostic tools include urine analysis, cystoscopy, and imaging tests. Antibiotics are the first line of treatment for cystitis caused by bacteria.
Cystocele	Discomfort when coughing, lifting, or straining; repeated bladder infections; a bulge of tissue that protrudes through the vaginal wall or opening; pain or urinary leakage during sexual intercourse.	Cystocele occurs when the supporting tissue between the female bladder and vaginal wall weakens and stretches, allowing the bladder to bulge into the vagina. It can be caused by obesity, heavy lifting, or childbirth.	Diagnosis is based on history, pelvic examination, urinalysis, and bladder emptying tests. Treatment may include a ring (pessary) inserted into the vagina to support the bladder, and estrogen therapy. In some cases, surgery is necessary.
Glomerulonephritis	Foamy, pink or brown urine with red blood cells. High blood pressure, fluid retention, fatigue.	Glomerulonephritis is an inflammation of the glomeruli in the kidneys. Glomeruli remove waste products from the bloodstream and pass them in the urine. Glomerulonephritis may develop after a strep throat infection, or from bacterial, viral, or HIV infections.	Diagnosis is based on urinalysis, blood tests, and imaging examinations. In general, the goal of treatment is to protect the kidneys from further damage. Controlling blood pressure is vital.
Hydronephrosis	Common symptoms include flank pain, abdominal mass, nausea and vomiting, urinary tract infection, fever, painful urination, increased urinary frequency, and increased urinary urgency.	Hydronephrosis describes the situation in which the urine collecting system of the kidney is dilated. This may be a normal variant or it may be the result of an underlying illness or medical condition. It can be caused by an obstruction to the free flow of urine from the kidney, sometimes called a ***kidney stone.***	Diagnosis begins with patient history and physical examination. Often, laboratory tests of the urine and blood are required. Treatment of hydronephrosis focuses on the removal of the obstruction and drainage of the urine that has accumulated behind the obstruction.
Interstitial cystitis	Chronic pelvic pain, persistent urge to urinate frequently, pain when bladder is full, pain during sexual intercourse.	Interstitial cystitis is a chronic condition causing frequent painful urination. The exact cause is unknown but may relate to a defect in the protective lining of the bladder.	Diagnosis is based on medical history including a bladder diary, pelvic examination, urinalysis, cystoscopy, and bladder biopsy. Treatment includes physical therapy, nerve stimulation, and oral medications.
Nephroptosis	Asymptomatic in most patients. Some may feel pain when standing that subsides when lying down, along with nausea and chills.	Nephroptosis, also known as ***floating kidney***, occurs when a kidney falls from its normal location into the pelvis. It is usually a congenital defect but also can be caused by a hard blow to the abdomen or by lifting a heavy object.	Diagnosis is based on physical examination and imaging studies, including intravenous urography. Usually no treatment is necessary. In some cases, laparoscopic nephropexy surgery is performed.
Nephrotic syndrome	Foamy urine, fluid retention, swelling around the eyes, ankles, and feet. Usually accompanied by high blood pressure.	Nephrotic syndrome is a kidney disorder that causes the kidney to excrete too much protein in the urine. It is usually caused by damage to glomeruli in the kidneys.	Diagnosis includes urinalysis, blood tests, and kidney biopsy. Drugs called *angiotensin-converting enzyme inhibitors* reduce blood pressure and also reduce the amount of protein released in urine.
Neurogenic bladder	Urinary incontinence, small volume during voiding, dribbling, loss of sensation of bladder fullness, urinary tract infections.	Neurogenic bladder is a condition in which a person lacks bladder control because of a brain, spinal cord, or nerve injury.	Urinary incontinence is diagnostic. Because neurogenic bladder involves the nervous system and bladder, a variety of tests are conducted to determine their status. Catheterization is often necessary. Sometimes a stoma is created to bypass the urethra.

Common Pathology of the Urinary System—cont'd

Disease	Signs and Symptoms	Etiology	Diagnosis and Treatment
Peyronie disease	Penis has a curvature during an erection; a lump of scar tissue may be present under the skin of the penis, and erections are painful.	Peyronie disease normally results from repeated injury to the penis. During healing, a lump of scar tissue forms.	Physical examination is usually sufficient to identify the condition. Interferon, a type of protein that disrupts the production of fibrous tissue and helps break it down, may provide improvement.
Polycystic kidney disease	Blood in urine, high blood pressure, back pain, headaches, abdominal extension, frequent urination, kidney stones, UTIs.	Polycystic kidney disease is an inherited disorder in which clusters of cysts develop within the kidneys. As the cysts accumulate fluid, they can become very large and destroy functioning kidney tissue.	Ultrasound, CT, and MRI examinations detect the size and number of cysts. Medications are prescribed to control blood pressure and pain. Diet and lifestyle changes are often recommended. Dialysis and/or kidney transplant may be necessary as the disease progresses.
Pyelonephritis	Back pain, fever, chills, malaise, nausea, blood in urine, cloudy urine, urination pain, increased urination frequency and urgency.	Pyelonephritis is the result of a urinary tract infection that progresses to involve the upper urinary system. Kidney stones may contribute to the condition.	Diagnosis starts with a physical examination including checking the area over the kidneys for tenderness. Urinalysis and blood tests are required. If kidney stones are suspected, imaging tests are ordered. The condition is treated with antibiotics.
Renal calculi	Severe waves of back and side pain, pain on urination, dark or foul-smelling urine, nausea, frequent urination, fever, chills.	Renal calculi, known as *kidney stones*, are hard crystalline deposits that precipitate from the urine. They occur when the urine contains too much of substances that form crystals. Passing a kidney stone can be very painful.	Diagnosis relies on blood, urine, and imaging tests. Passed stones may be analyzed to determine composition. Drinking large amounts of water can help flush out the system. Pain relievers are often needed. Large stones may be broken up with shock wave lithotripsy.
Uremia	Abdominal pain, dry mouth, easy bruising, edema, confusion, excessive thirst, fatigue, skin pallor, low blood pressure, tremors, nausea, weakness, tachycardia.	In uremia, BUN is elevated because of the kidney's failure to remove the substances. This may be caused by any condition that damages the kidneys.	Patient history is required to determine if condition is chronic or acute. Diagnosis is based on the blood's basic metabolic panel, showing BUN, creatinine, potassium, phosphate, calcium, and sodium levels. The ultimate treatment for uremia is dialysis.
Urethritis	*For men:* Painful or difficult urination, blood in urine or semen, discharge from penis, frequent urination, swelling of penis, pain with ejaculation. *For women:* Burning pain during urination, abdominal pain, fever, chills, pelvic pain, frequent urination.	Urethritis is inflammation of the urethra. It may be caused by a bacterial or viral infection. It can also be caused by an injury or by sensitivity to chemicals used in spermicides.	*For men:* The medical examination includes the abdomen, bladder area, penis, and scrotum. *For women:* The medical examination includes evaluation of abdominal, pelvic, and urethral tenderness. Urinalysis and blood chemistry tests are performed. The goals of treatment are to eliminate the cause of infection and lessen symptoms.
Urinary incontinence	The primary symptom is the leakage of urine.	Urinary incontinence is the loss of bladder control resulting in the leakage of urine. It may be triggered by coughing, sneezing, or lifting. In some cases the urge to urinate is so sudden that the patient is unable to reach a toilet.	Diagnosis begins with urinalysis, medical history, and physical examination. A postvoid residual measurement may be performed. Kegel exercises to strengthen the muscles that control urination may be suggested as treatment.
Urinary tract infection (UTI)	Persistent urge to urinate, burning sensation during urination, strong-smelling cloudy urine, pelvic or rectal pain.	A UTI is an infection in some part of the urinary system. The most common infecting agent is *E. coli.* Catheterization or the use of spermicides increases the risk of infection.	Diagnostic procedures include urinalysis, laboratory cultures of tract bacteria, IVP, and other imaging modalities. For patients with recurrent infections, a course of antibiotics is effective.

Continued

Common Pathology of the Urinary System—cont'd

Disease	Signs and Symptoms	Etiology	Diagnosis and Treatment
Vesicoureteral reflux	Constipation, high blood pressure, protein in urine, and for children, bedwetting.	Vesicoureteral reflux is the abnormal flow of urine from the bladder back up the ureters. It is often caused by a urinary blockage, typically a UTI that causes swelling in a ureter.	Urinalysis can show the presence of a UTI. Ultrasound studies of the kidney and bladder can detect abnormalities. A voiding cystourethrogram can determine bladder emptying problems. Severe cases may require surgery to repair the valve between the bladder and ureter.

BUN, Blood urea nitrogen; *CT*, computed tomography; *HIV*, human immunodeficiency virus; *IVP*, intravenous pyelogram; *MRI*, magnetic resonance imaging; *UTI*, urinary tract infection.

TERMINOLOGY REVIEW

Key Term	Word Parts	Definition
Detrusor muscle		The smooth muscle in the wall of the urinary bladder.
Erythropoietin	*erythr/o:* red	A hormone released by the kidneys that stimulates red blood cell production.
Glomerular capsule		Double-layered epithelial cup that surrounds the glomerulus in a nephron; also called *Bowman capsule.*
Glomerular filtration		The movement of blood plasma across the filtration membrane in the renal corpuscle.
Glomerulus		Cluster of capillaries in the nephron through which blood is filtered.
Juxtaglomerular apparatus	*juxta-:* near to	Complex of modified cells in the afferent arteriole and the ascending limb and distal tubule in the kidney; helps regulate blood pressure by secreting renin; consists of the macula densa and juxtaglomerular cells.
Micturition	*mict-:* to pass	Act of expelling urine from the bladder; also called *voiding* or *urination.*
Nephrons	*nephr/o:* kidney	Functional units of the kidney consisting of a renal corpuscle and a renal tubule.
Nephron loop	*nephr/o:* kidney	The hairpin loop of the renal tubule that extends into the renal pyramids.
Renal corpuscle	*ren/o:* kidney	Portion of the nephron where filtration occurs; consists of the glomerulus and glomerular capsule.
Renal cortex	*ren/o:* kidney	Outer portion of the kidney that appears granular.
Renal medulla	*ren/o:* kidney	Inner portion of the kidney consisting of renal pyramids.
Renal pelvis	*ren/o:* kidney	Large cavity in the central region of the kidney that collects the urine as it is produced.
Renal tubule	*ren/o:* kidney	Tubular portion of the nephron that carries the filtrate away from the glomerular capsule toward the collecting duct site where tubular reabsorption and secretion occur.
Renin	*ren/o:* kidney	An enzyme secreted by the kidneys that functions in blood pressure regulation by stimulating the formation of angiotensin.
Trigone	*tri-:* three	Triangular area in the floor of the urinary bladder formed by the openings for the urethra and the two ureters.
Tubular reabsorption		The movement of substances from the filtrate in the renal tubules back into the blood in response to the body's needs during urine formation.
Tubular secretion		The movement of substances from the blood into the renal tubules in response to the body's needs during urine formation.
Ureter	*-ur-:* urine	Tubular structure that carries urine from the renal pelvis to the urinary bladder.
Urethra	*-ur-:* urine	Passageway that conveys urine from the urinary bladder to the exterior.
Urinary bladder	*-ur-:* urine	Storage reservoir for urine; located in the pelvic cavity.

Reproductive System

Check out the Evolve site at http://evolve.elsevier.com/Bonewit/today to access additional interactive activities and exercises to help you study and prepare for success.

LEARNING OBJECTIVES

1. Distinguish between primary and secondary reproductive organs.
2. Describe the location and structure of each component of the male reproductive system.
3. Explain the process by which spermatids become mature sperm.
4. Trace the pathway of sperm from the testes to the outside of the body.
5. Outline the physiologic events in the male sexual response.
6. Describe the roles of gonadotropin-releasing hormone (GnRH), follicle-stimulating hormone (FSH), luteinizing hormone (LH), and testosterone in male reproductive functions.
7. Identify each component of the female reproductive system, including the mammary glands.
8. Describe oogenesis.
9. Describe the development of ovarian follicles.
10. Outline the physiologic events in the female sexual response.
11. Describe the roles of GnRH, FSH, LH, estrogen, and progesterone in female reproductive functions.
12. Describe what happens in each phase of the ovarian and uterine cycles, when each phase occurs, and how the cycles interact.
13. Describe the three stages of prenatal development.
14. Distinguish between developmental age and clinical age in prenatal development.
15. Identify five features of fetal circulation that are different from postnatal circulatory pathways.
16. Identify the three stages of labor and describe the events that occur in each stage.
17. Identify the two hormones responsible for lactation and describe the function of each.
18. Name and describe the six periods of postnatal development.
19. Describe ways in which the aging of an individual affects the reproductive system.
20. Identify pathology related to the reproductive system.

CHAPTER OUTLINE

KEY TERMS

clinical age (KLIN-ih-kull AGE)
corpora cavernosa (KOR-por-ah kav-er-NOH-sah)
corpus albicans (KOR-pus AL-bih-kans)
corpus luteum (KOR-pus LOO-tee-um)
corpus spongiosum (KOR-pus spun-jee-OH-sum)
developmental age (dee-VEL-op-men-tul AGE)
ductus deferens (DUCK-tus DEFF-er-enz)
embryonic period (em-bree-ON-ik PEER-ee-ud)
endometrium (end-oh-MEE-tree-um)
epididymis (ep-ih-DID-ih-mis)
fetal period (FEE-tal PEER-ee-ud)
gametes (GAM-eets)
gestation (jes-TAY-shun)
gonads (GO-nads)
interstitial cells (in-ter-STISH-al SELZ)
lactation (lak-TAY-shun)
menarche (meh-NAHR-kee)
myometrium (my-oh-MEE-tree-um)
oogenesis (oh-oh-JEN-eh-sis)
oogonia (oh-oh-GO-nee-ah)
ovarian cycle (oh-VAIR-ee-an SYE-kul)
ovarian follicles (oh-VAIR-ee-an FAHL-ih-kuls)
parturition (par-too-RIH-shun)
perimetrium (pair-ih-MEE-tree-um)
postnatal development (POST-nay-tal dee-VELL-op-ment)
preembryonic period (pree-em-bree-AHN-ik PEER-ee-ud)
prenatal development (PREE-nay-tal dee-VELL-op-ment)
seminiferous tubules (seh-mih-NIFF-er-us TOOB-yools)
spermatogenesis (spur-mat-oh-JEN-eh-sis)
spermatogonia (spur-mat-oh-GOH-nee-ah)
spermiogenesis (spur-mee-oh-JEN-eh-sis)
stratum basale (STRAY-tum BAY-sah-lee)
stratum functionale (STRAY-tum FUNK-shun-al-ee)
uterine cycle (YOO-ter-in SYE-kul)
uterine tubes (YOO-ter-in TOOBS)
vulva (VUL-vah)
zygote (ZYE-goht)

INTRODUCTION TO THE REPRODUCTIVE SYSTEM

The major function of the reproductive system is to produce offspring. The reproductive system is responsible for the following four functions:

- To produce egg and sperm cells
- To transport and sustain the egg and sperm cells
- To nurture the developing offspring
- To produce hormones

These functions are divided between the primary reproductive organs and the secondary (or accessory) reproductive organs. The primary reproductive organs are called **gonads**. They include the ovaries and testes. These gonads are responsible for producing the egg and sperm cells, known as **gametes**. They are also responsible for producing hormones that function in the maturation of the reproductive system and the development of sexual characteristics. The hormones also play important roles in regulating the normal physiology of the reproductive system. All other organs, ducts, and glands in the reproductive system are considered secondary, or accessory, reproductive organs. These structures transport and sustain the gametes and nurture the developing offspring.

MALE REPRODUCTIVE SYSTEM

The male reproductive system produces, sustains, and transports sperm; introduces the sperm into the female vagina; and produces hormones. Fig. 16.1 illustrates the organs of the male reproductive system.

TESTES

The *testes* (or *testicles*) are the male gonads. The testes begin their development high in the abdominal cavity, near the kidneys. During the last 2 months before birth, or shortly after birth, the testes descend into the *scrotum*. The scrotum is an external pouch of skin and subcutaneous tissue that contains the testes. It is located below the abdomen and behind the penis. The location of the testes outside the abdominal cavity may make them vulnerable to injury. However, this location provides a temperature about 3°C below normal body temperature. This lower temperature is necessary for the production of viable sperm. There is a vertical septum, or partition, of subcutaneous tissue in the center of the scrotum that divides it into two parts, each containing one testis. Smooth muscle fibers, called the *dartos muscle*, are located in the subcutaneous tissue. The dartos muscle contracts to give the scrotum its wrinkled appearance. When this muscle is relaxed, the scrotum is smooth. Another muscle known as the *cremaster muscle* is located in the spermatic cord. The cremaster controls the position of the scrotum and testes. When it is cold or a man is sexually aroused, this muscle contracts to pull the testes closer to the body for warmth.

Structure

Each testis is an oval structure about 5 cm long and 3 cm in diameter (Fig. 16.2). A tough, white fibrous connective tissue capsule, known as the *tunica albuginea*, surrounds each testis. The tunica albuginea extends inward to form *septa* that partition the testis into *lobules*. Each testis contains about 250 lobules. Each lobule contains one to four tightly coiled **seminiferous tubules** in which sperm are produced. The seminiferous tubules converge into a series of duets that exit

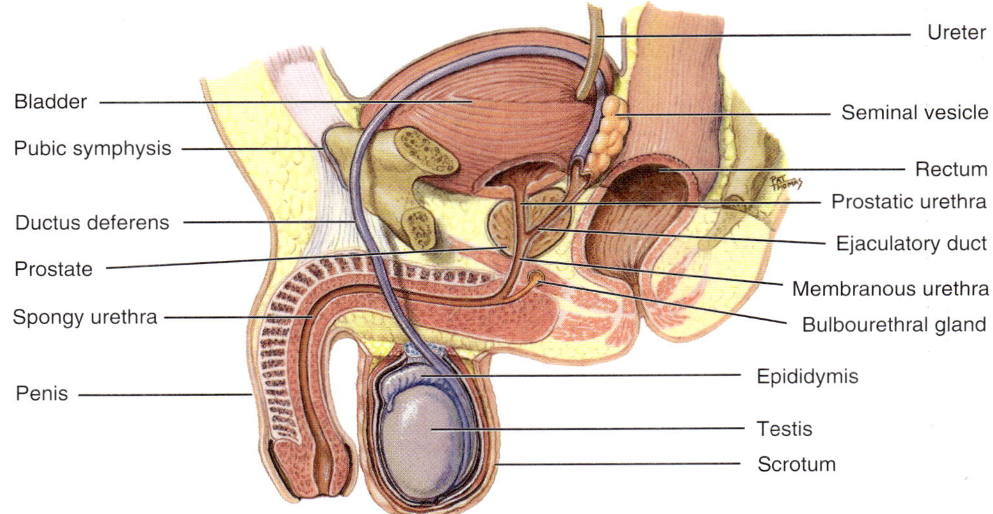

Fig. 16.1 Structures in the male reproductive system. The testes are the primary reproductive organs in the male. The ducts and glands are accessory organs. (From Applegate E: *The anatomy and physiology learning system,* ed 4, St. Louis, 2011, Saunders.)

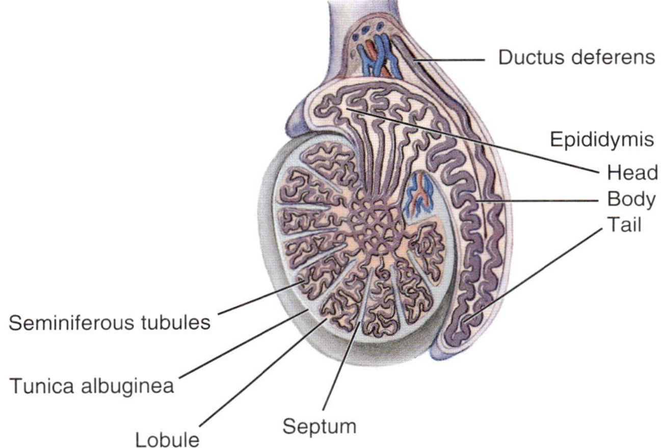

Fig. 16.2 Sagittal section of a testis. (From Applegate E: *The anatomy and physiology learning system*, ed 4, St. Louis, 2011, Saunders.)

the testes and enter the epididymis. **Interstitial cells** (cells of Leydig) are located between the seminiferous tubules within a lobule. Interstitial cells produce male sex hormones.

Spermatogenesis

Sperm are produced within the seminiferous tubules. The process of sperm formation is **spermatogenesis**, a form of meiosis. The seminiferous tubules are packed with cells in various stages of spermatogenesis (Fig. 16.3). Interspersed with these cells are large cells that extend from the periphery of the tubule to the lumen. These large cells are the *supporting cells* (Sertoli cells), which support and nourish the other cells.

Early in embryonic development, *primordial germ cells* enter the testes and differentiate into **spermatogonia**. Spermatogonia (singular, spermatogonium) are immature cells that remain dormant until puberty. These cells are located around the periphery of the seminiferous tubules. They are diploid cells, meaning that they contain 46 chromosomes (23 pairs). At puberty, hormones stimulate these immature cells to begin dividing by mitosis. Some of the daughter cells produced by mitosis remain at the periphery of the seminiferous tubules as spermatogonia. Others are pushed toward the lumen and undergo some changes to become *primary spermatocytes.* Because they are produced by mitosis, primary spermatocytes are diploid and have 46 chromosomes.

Each primary spermatocyte goes through the first meiotic division (meiosis I) to produce two *secondary spermatocytes.* In the second meiotic division (meiosis II), each secondary spermatocyte divides to produce two *spermatids.* As a result of the two meiotic divisions, each primary spermatocyte produces four spermatids (Fig. 16.4). During spermatogenesis there are two cellular divisions but only one replication of DNA, so each spermatid has 23 chromosomes (haploid), one from each pair in the original primary spermatocyte. Each successive stage in spermatogenesis is pushed toward the center of the seminiferous tubule. This results in the more immature cells being at the periphery, and the more differentiated cells being nearer the center (see Fig. 16.3).

Spermatogenesis (and oogenesis in the female) differs from mitosis (review Chapter 5) because the resulting cells have only half the number of chromosomes as the original cell. When the sperm cell nucleus unites with an egg cell nucleus, the full number of chromosomes is restored. If sperm and egg cells were produced by mitosis, then each successive generation would have twice the number of chromosomes as the preceding one.

The final step in the development of sperm is called **spermiogenesis**. In this process, the spermatids formed

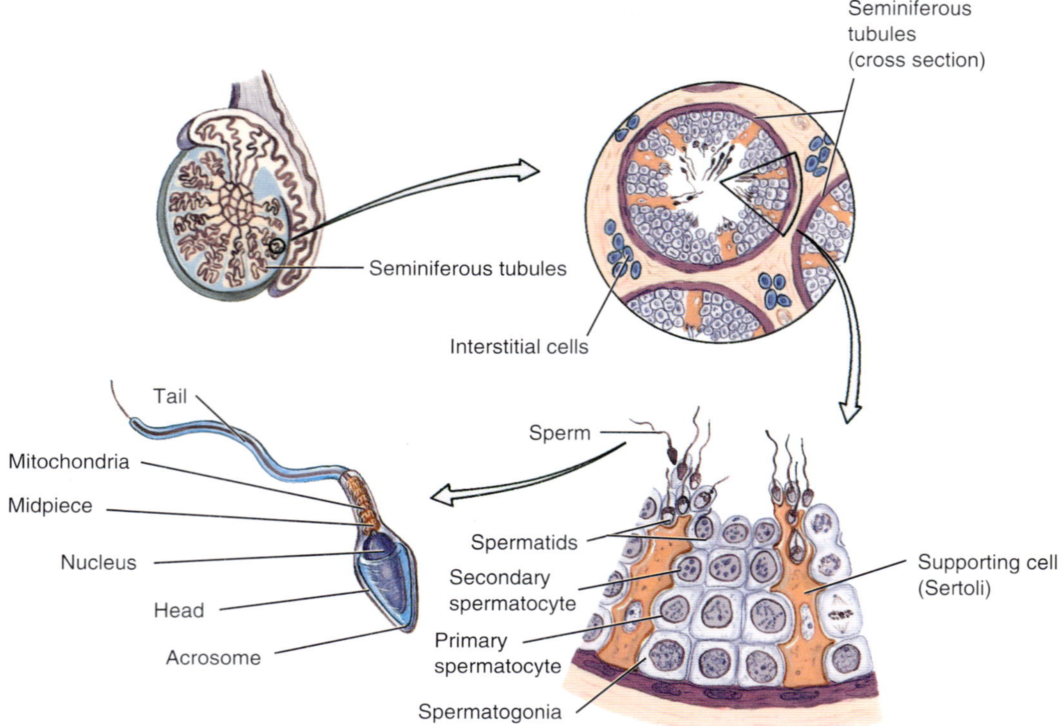

Fig. 16.3 Cross section of a seminiferous tubule showing the different cell types. Interstitial cells that produce testosterone are between the seminiferous tubules. Spermatids in the lumen become sperm by a process called spermiogenesis. (From Applegate E: *The anatomy and physiology learning system*, ed 4, St. Louis, 2011, Saunders.)

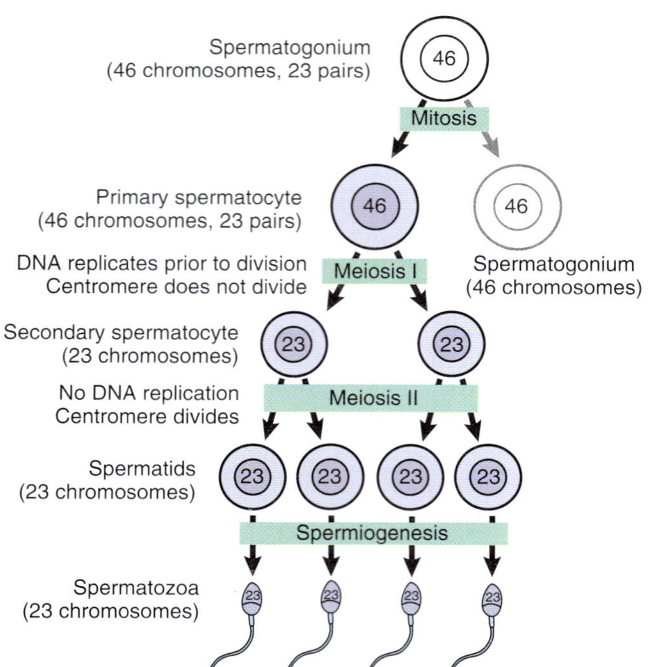

Fig. 16.4 Spermatogenesis. Each primary spermatocyte yields four spermatids by meiosis. (From Applegate E: *The anatomy and physiology learning system*, ed 4, St. Louis, 2011, Saunders.)

from spermatogenesis become mature spermatozoa, or sperm. The mature sperm cell has a head, midpiece, and tail (see Fig. 16.3). The head contains the 23 chromosomes surrounded by a nuclear membrane. The tip of the head is covered by an *acrosome.* The acrosome contains enzymes that help the sperm penetrate the female gamete. The midpiece contains mitochondria that provide adenosine triphosphate (ATP). The tail, also called the *locomotor region*, is a typical flagellum for locomotion. The sperm are released into the lumen of the seminiferous tubule, where they leave the testes and enter the epididymis. In the epididymis the sperm undergo final maturation and become capable of fertilizing a female gamete.

Sperm production begins at puberty and continues throughout the life of a male. The entire process, beginning with a primary spermatocyte, takes about 74 days. After ejaculation, the sperm can live for about 48 hours in the female reproductive tract.

DUCT SYSTEM

Sperm cells pass through a series of ducts to reach the outside of the body. After they leave the testes, the sperm pass through the epididymis, ductus deferens, ejaculatory duct, and urethra.

Epididymis

Sperm leave the testes through a series of ducts that enter the **epididymis** (see Fig. 16.2). The epididymis is a long tube that is tightly coiled to form a comma-shaped organ. When the sperm leave the testes, they are immature and incapable of fertilizing ova. They complete their maturation process and become fertile as they move through the epididymis. Mature sperm are stored in the lower portion of the epididymis.

Ductus Deferens

The **ductus deferens** (also called *vas deferens*) is a tube that is continuous with the epididymis (see Fig. 16.2). The ductus deferens enters the abdominopelvic cavity, then descends along the posterior wall of the bladder toward the prostate gland (see Fig. 16.1). Sperm are stored in the ductus deferens, near the epididymis, and peristaltic movements propel the sperm through the ductus deferens and into the ejaculatory duct.

The proximal portion of the ductus deferens is a component of the *spermatic cord*, which contains vascular and neural structures that supply the testes. The spermatic cord contains the ductus deferens, testicular artery and veins, lymph vessels, testicular nerve, cremaster muscle (which elevates the testes for warmth and at times of sexual stimulation), and a connective tissue covering.

Ejaculatory Duct

Each ductus deferens joins a duct from an adjacent seminal vesicle to form a short *ejaculatory duct* (see Fig. 16.1). Each ejaculatory duct passes through the prostate gland and empties sperm and fluid from a seminal vesicle into the urethra.

Urethra

The *urethra* extends from the urinary bladder to the external urethral orifice at the tip of the penis. It is a passageway for sperm and fluids from the reproductive system and for urine from the urinary system. While reproductive fluids are passing through the urethra, sphincters contract tightly to keep urine from entering the urethra.

The male urethra is divided into three regions (see Fig. 16.1). The *prostatic urethra* is the portion that passes through the prostate gland. It receives the ejaculatory duct and numerous ducts from the prostate gland. The next portion, the *membranous urethra*, is a short region that passes through the pelvic floor. The longest portion is the *penile urethra* (also called *spongy urethra*), which extends the length of the penis and opens to the outside at the external urethral orifice. The ducts from the bulbourethral glands open into the penile urethra.

ACCESSORY GLANDS

The accessory glands of the male reproductive system include the seminal vesicles, prostate gland, and bulbourethral glands. These glands secrete fluids that enter the urethra.

Seminal Vesicles

The paired *seminal vesicles* are saclike glands located between the urinary bladder and the rectum (see Fig. 16.1). Each gland has a short duct that joins with the ductus deferens to form an ejaculatory duct. The ejaculatory ducts empty into the urethra. The seminal vesicles secrete a fluid that is viscous and contains fructose. The fructose provides an energy source for the spermatozoa.

Prostate

The *prostate gland* is a firm, dense structure that is located just inferior to the urinary bladder (see Fig. 16.1). It is about the size of a walnut and encircles the urethra as it leaves the urinary bladder. Numerous short ducts from the prostate gland empty into the prostatic urethra. The secretions of the prostate are thin, milky colored, and alkaline. They enhance the motility of the sperm.

Bulbourethral Glands

The paired *bulbourethral (Cowper) glands* (see Fig. 16.1) are small, about the size of a pea, and are located near the base of the penis. A short duct from each gland enters the penile urethra. In response to sexual stimulation, the bulbourethral glands secrete an alkaline, mucus-like fluid. This fluid performs the following functions: neutralizes the acidity of the urine residue in the urethra; helps to neutralize the acidity of the vagina; and provides some lubrication for the tip of the penis during intercourse.

Seminal Fluid

Seminal fluid (or *semen*) consists of a slightly alkaline (pH 7.5) mixture of sperm cells and secretions from the accessory glands. Secretions from the seminal vesicles make up about 60% of the semen. Most of the remaining semen consists of secretions from the prostate gland. Spermatozoa and secretions from the bulbourethral glands contribute only a small volume to the semen.

The volume of semen in a single ejaculation varies from 1.5 mL to 6 mL. There are usually between 50 and 150 million sperm per milliliter of semen. Sperm counts below 10 to 20 million per milliliter usually cause fertility problems. Although only one spermatozoon actually penetrates and fertilizes an ovum, it takes several million spermatozoa in an ejaculation to ensure that fertilization will take place.

PENIS

The *penis* is the male copulatory organ located in front of the scrotum. The penis functions in transferring sperm to the vagina. It consists of three columns of erectile tissue that are wrapped in connective tissue and covered with skin (Fig. 16.5). There are two dorsal columns known as the **corpora cavernosa**. A single, midline ventral column surrounds the urethra and is called the **corpus spongiosum**.

The penis has a root, body, and glans penis. The root of the penis attaches it to the pubic arch. The body (or shaft)

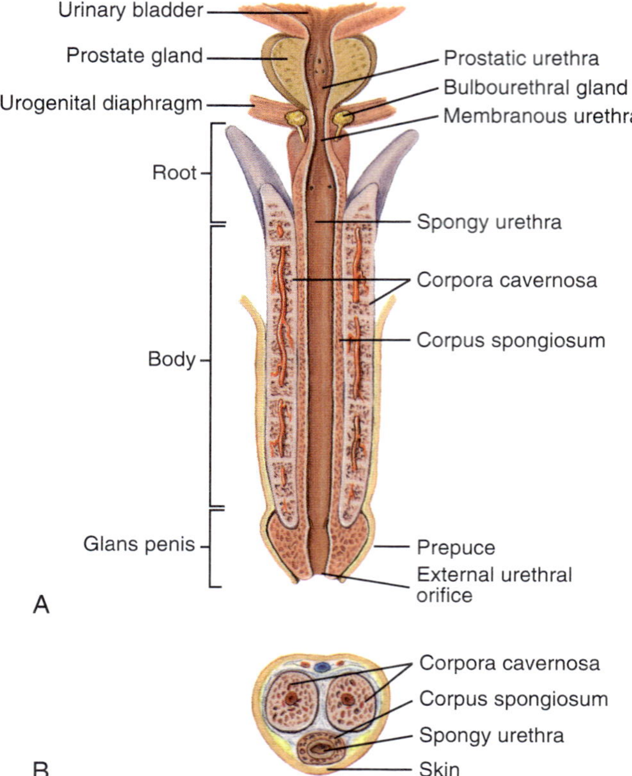

Fig. 16.5 Structure of the penis. (A) Longitudinal section. (B) Cross section. Note that the penis has three regions: root, body, and glans penis. There are two dorsal columns of corpora cavernosum and a ventral column of corpus spongiosum. (From Applegate E: *The anatomy and physiology learning system*, ed 4, St. Louis, 2011, Saunders.)

of the penis is the visible, pendant portion. The *corpus spongiosum* expands at the end of the penis to form the glans penis. The urethra opens through the external urethral orifice at the tip of the glans penis. A loose fold of skin, called the *prepuce*, or foreskin, covers the glans penis.

MALE SEXUAL RESPONSE

In the absence of sexual arousal, the erectile tissue of the penis contains only a small volume of blood, causing the penis to be flaccid. During sexual excitement, arterioles that supply blood to the erectile tissue dilate. As a result, the spaces in the erectile tissue become engorged with blood, causing the penis to enlarge and become rigid. This is called *erection* and is necessary to allow the penis to enter the vagina. The erection reflex may be initiated by stimuli such as anticipation, memory, and visual sensations. It may also be the result of stimulation of touch receptors on the glans penis and skin of the genital area. Emotions and thoughts can inhibit erection.

Continued sexual stimulation causes the reflexes that promote an erection to become more and more intense until a level is reached that prompts a surge of impulses to the genital organs. These impulses stimulate rhythmic contractions of the epididymides, vasa deferentia, and ejaculatory ducts. The impulses also cause contractions of the accessory glands. This results in *emission*, which is the forceful discharge of semen into the urethra. *Ejaculation* immediately follows emission and is the forceful expulsion of semen from the urethra to the exterior. Concurrently with emission and ejaculation, the sphincters of the urinary bladder constrict to prevent semen from entering the bladder and to inhibit the flow of urine from the bladder.

The rhythmic muscle contractions of ejaculation are accompanied by feelings of intense pleasure, increased heart rate, elevated blood pressure, and increased respiration. Together, these physiologic activities are referred to as *climax* or *orgasm*. This is quickly followed by relaxation, and blood leaves the penis so that it becomes flaccid. After orgasm, there is a latent period, lasting from several minutes to several hours, during which another erection is impossible.

HORMONAL CONTROL

The hypothalamus, anterior pituitary, and testes have significant roles in the hormonal control of male reproductive functions. Puberty in males usually begins at ages 10 to 12 and continues until ages 16 to 18. During this period the male reproductive organs become sexually mature. The sequence of events that triggers the onset of puberty is unknown. It begins when certain unknown stimuli cause the hypothalamus to start secreting *gonadotropin-releasing hormone* (GnRH), which enters the blood and goes to the anterior pituitary gland.

In response to GnRH, the anterior pituitary secretes *luteinizing hormone* (LH) and *follicle-stimulating hormone* (FSH). LH promotes the growth of the interstitial cells in the testes and stimulates the cells to secrete *testosterone.* FSH acts with testosterone to stimulate spermatogenesis in the seminiferous tubules. Fig. 16.6 summarizes the hormonal control of testicular functions.

Male sex hormones are collectively called *androgens.* The most abundant androgen is testosterone. Before birth, testosterone from the adrenal cortex stimulates the development of the male reproductive organs. Between birth and puberty, testosterone levels are low. Then at puberty, under the influence of LH, the interstitial cells begin secreting high levels of testosterone. The adrenal cortex continues to secrete small amounts of androgens. The increase in testosterone levels at puberty promotes the maturation of the male reproductive organs, stimulates spermatogenesis, and promotes the development of the male secondary sex characteristics.

After puberty, testosterone production is controlled by a negative feedback mechanism that involves the hypothalamus (see Fig. 16.6). High blood testosterone levels inhibit GnRH. This removes the stimulus for LH, which reduces the testosterone level back to normal. Testosterone production continues from puberty throughout the rest of a man's life, although there is some decline in quantity in old age.

HIGHLIGHT on the Male Reproductive System

Undescended testicles: The condition in which the testes do not descend into the scrotum is called *cryptorchidism. Crypt* means "hidden" and *orchid* refers to the testis, so the term literally means "hidden testis." Cryptorchidism results in sterility if it is not corrected before puberty because the cooler temperature of the scrotum is necessary for sperm production.

Vasectomy: A vasectomy is a surgical procedure, usually accomplished through a tiny incision in the scrotum, that severs the vas deferens. A bilateral vasectomy results in sterility because it interrupts the pathway of the sperm to the outside of the body.

Enlarged prostate gland: Benign prostatic hyperplasia is a common condition in older men. In this condition, the prostate enlarges and compresses the urethra, making urination difficult. This situation results in urine retention in the bladder, which makes the individual more susceptible to urinary tract infections.

Circumcision: Circumcision is the surgical removal of the prepuce of the penis. Sometimes this is done to correct phimosis, a condition in which the prepuce is too tight and obstructs urine flow. In certain cultures, circumcision is performed as a religious rite or an ethnic custom. For others, it is a matter of family preference. The medical benefits of circumcision are a subject of debate in the medical community. Some believe it is practical for hygienic reasons. Evidence indicates that circumcision may reduce the risk of penile cancer. ■

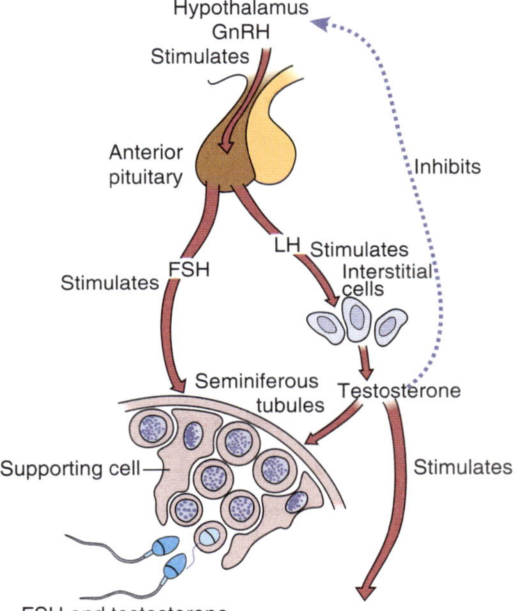

Fig. 16.6 Hormonal regulation of testicular function. *FSH*, Follicle stimulating hormone; *GnRH*, gonadotropin-releasing hormone; *LH*, luteinizing hormone. (From Applegate E: *The anatomy and physiology learning system*, ed 4, St. Louis, 2011, Saunders.)

FEMALE REPRODUCTIVE SYSTEM

The organs of the female reproductive system perform the following functions: produce and sustain the female sex cells (*egg cells*, or *ova*); transport these cells to a site where they may be fertilized by sperm; provide a favorable environment for the developing offspring; move the offspring to the outside at the end of the development period; and produce the female sex hormones. The female reproductive system includes the ovaries, uterine tubes, uterus, vagina, accessory glands, and external genital organs (Fig. 16.7).

OVARIES

The primary reproductive organs in the female are the paired *ovaries*. Each ovary is a solid, ovoid structure about the size and shape of an almond (approximately 3.5 cm long, 2 cm wide, and 1 cm thick). The ovaries are located in shallow depressions, called *ovarian fossae*, one on each side of the uterus. They are held loosely in place by peritoneal ligaments.

Structure

The ovaries are covered on the outside by a layer of epithelium called *germinal (ovarian) epithelium* (Fig. 16.8) and a dense connective tissue capsule known as the *tunica albuginea*. The substance of the ovaries is indistinctly divided into an outer cortex and an inner medulla. The cortex appears denser and more granular because of the presence of numerous **ovarian follicles** in various stages of development. Each of the follicles contains a female germ cell known as an *oocyte*. The medulla consists of loose connective tissue with abundant blood vessels, lymphatic vessels, and nerve fibers.

Oogenesis

Female sex cells (or gametes) develop in the ovaries by a form of meiosis called **oogenesis**. The sequence of events in oogenesis is similar to the sequence in spermatogenesis, but the timing and final result are different (Fig. 16.9). Early in fetal development, primitive germ cells in the ovaries differentiate into **oogonia** (singular, oogonium). The oogonia divide rapidly to form thousands of cells that have a full complement of 46 chromosomes (23 pairs). Oogonia then enter a growth phase, enlarge, and become *primary oocytes*.

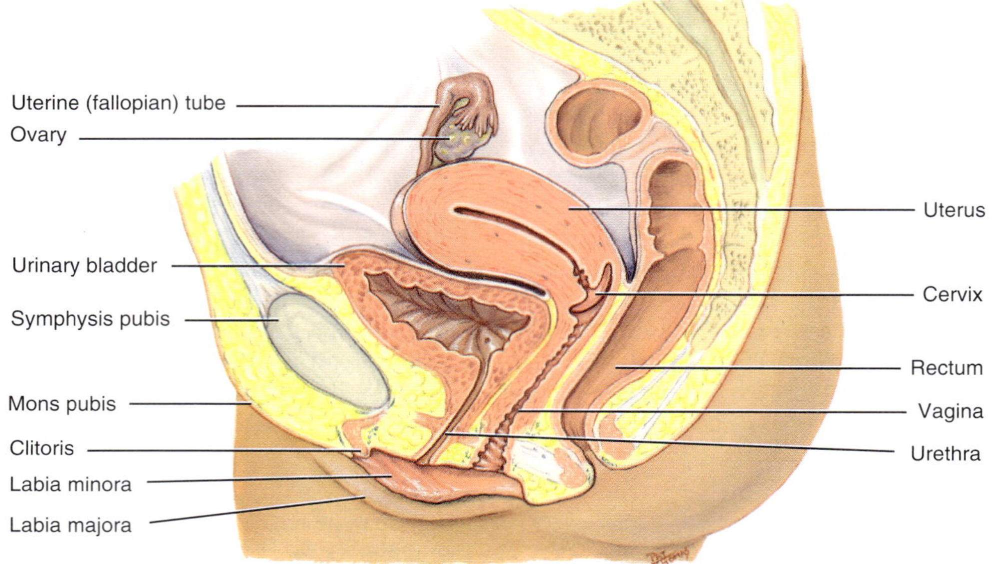

Fig. 16.7 Organs of the female reproductive system. (From Applegate E: *The anatomy and physiology learning system*, ed 4, St. Louis, 2011, Saunders.)

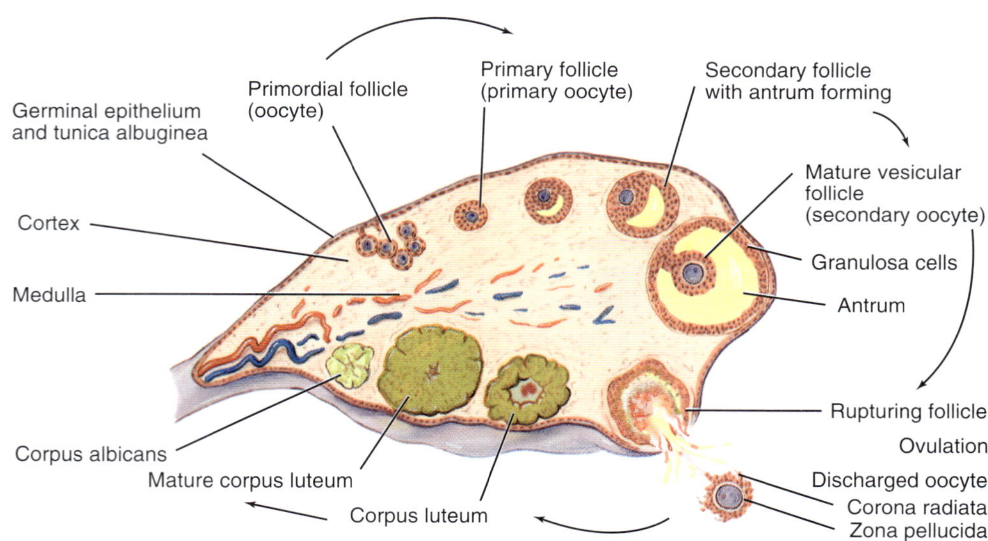

Fig. 16.8 Structure of an ovary illustrating the stages in follicle development and corpus luteum formation. (From Applegate E: *The anatomy and physiology learning system*, ed 4, St. Louis, 2011, Saunders.)

The primary oocytes (with 46 chromosomes) replicate their DNA and begin the first meiotic division. This process stops in prophase, and the cells remain in this suspended state until puberty. Many of the primary oocytes degenerate before birth. Even with this decline, the two ovaries together contain approximately 700,000 oocytes at birth. This is the lifetime supply, and no more will develop. This is quite different than in the male, in whom spermatogonia and primary spermatocytes continue to be produced throughout the reproductive lifetime. By puberty the number of primary oocytes has further declined to about 400,000.

Beginning at puberty, several primary oocytes start to grow again each month. One of the primary oocytes seems to outgrow the others, and it resumes meiosis I. The other cells degenerate. The large cell undergoes an unequal division so that nearly all the cytoplasm, the organelles, and half the chromosomes go to one cell, which becomes a *secondary oocyte*. The remaining half of the chromosomes go to a smaller cell called the *first polar body*. The secondary oocyte begins the second meiotic division, but the process stops in metaphase. At this point, ovulation occurs. If fertilization occurs, meiosis II continues. Again,

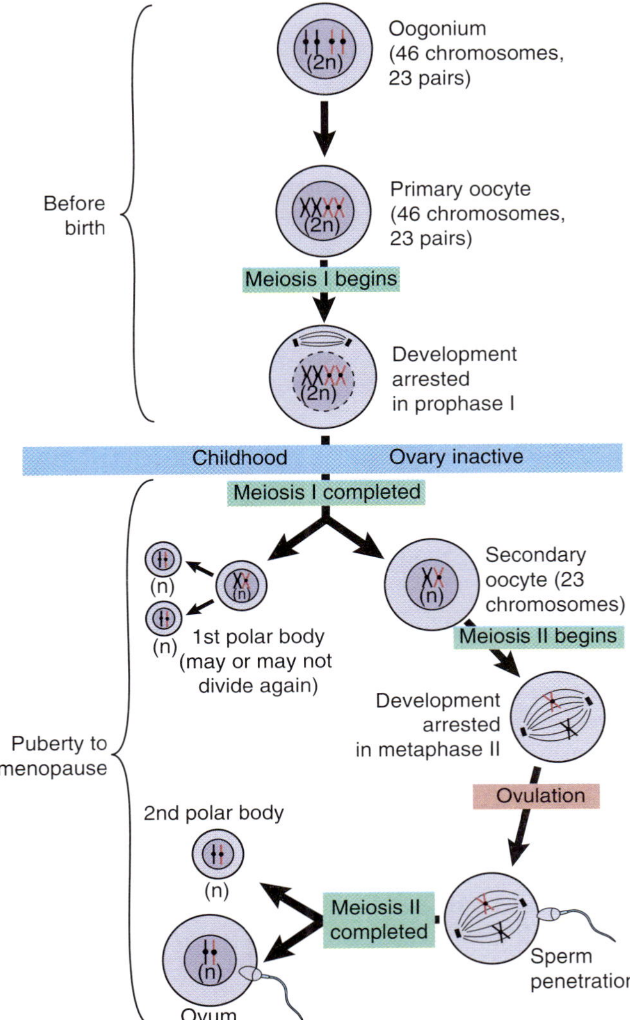

Fig. 16.9 Oogenesis. The first meiotic division is interrupted in prophase before birth and does not resume until after puberty. The second meiotic division is interrupted in metaphase and does not resume unless a sperm penetrates the cell. (From Applegate E: *The anatomy and physiology learning system*, ed 4, St. Louis, 2011, Saunders.)

this is an unequal division, with all of the cytoplasm going to the ovum, which has 23 single-stranded chromosomes. The smaller cell from this division is a *second polar body.* The first polar body also usually divides in meiosis II to produce two even smaller polar bodies. If fertilization does not occur, the second meiotic division is never completed and the secondary oocyte degenerates. Here again, there are obvious differences between the male and female. In spermatogenesis, four functional spermatozoa develop from each primary spermatocyte. In oogenesis, only one functional fertilizable cell develops from a primary oocyte. The other three cells are polar bodies and they degenerate.

Ovarian Follicle Development

An ovarian follicle consists of a developing oocyte surrounded by one or more layers of cells called *follicular cells.* While the oocyte is progressing through meiosis, corresponding changes are taking place in the follicular cells (see Fig. 16.8). *Primordial follicles,* which consist of a primary oocyte surrounded by a single layer of flattened cells, develop in the fetus and are the stage that is present in the ovaries at birth and throughout childhood.

Beginning at puberty, FSH stimulates changes in the primordial follicles. The follicular cells become cuboidal, the primary oocyte enlarges, and a *primary follicle* is created. The follicles continue to grow under the influence of FSH, and the follicular cells proliferate to form several layers of *granulosa cells* around the primary oocyte. Most of these primary follicles degenerate along with the primary oocytes within them, but usually one continues to develop each month. The granulosa cells start secreting estrogen. In addition, a cavity known as the *antrum* forms within the follicle. When the antrum starts to develop, the follicle becomes a *secondary follicle.* The granulosa cells also secrete a substance that forms a clear membrane, known as the *zona pellucida,* around the oocyte. After about 10 days of growth the follicle is a mature vesicular (graafian) follicle, which forms a "blister" on the surface of the ovary. It contains a secondary oocyte ready for ovulation.

Ovulation

Ovulation occurs when the mature follicle at the surface of the ovary ruptures and releases the secondary oocyte into the peritoneal cavity. The ovulated secondary oocyte is ready for fertilization. It is still surrounded by the zona pellucida and a few layers of cells called the *corona radiata.* If it is not fertilized, the secondary oocyte degenerates in a couple of days. If a spermatozoon passes through the corona radiata and zona pellucida and enters the cytoplasm of the secondary oocyte, the second meiotic division resumes to form a polar body and a mature ovum.

After ovulation, the portion of the follicle that remains in the ovary enlarges and is transformed into a **corpus luteum** (see Fig. 16.8). The corpus luteum is a glandular structure that secretes progesterone and some estrogens. Its fate depends on whether fertilization occurs. If fertilization does not take place, the corpus luteum remains functional for about 10 days and then begins to degenerate into a **corpus albicans.** This structure is primarily scar tissue, and its hormone output ceases. If fertilization occurs, the corpus luteum persists. The corpus luteum continues its hormone functions until the placenta develops sufficiently to secrete the necessary hormones. Again, the corpus luteum ultimately degenerates into a corpus albicans; it just remains functional for a longer period of time.

GENITAL TRACT

Uterine Tubes

There are two **uterine tubes** (also called *fallopian tubes*). Each tube is about 4 cm long and about 1 cm in diameter, and extends laterally from the upper portion of the uterus

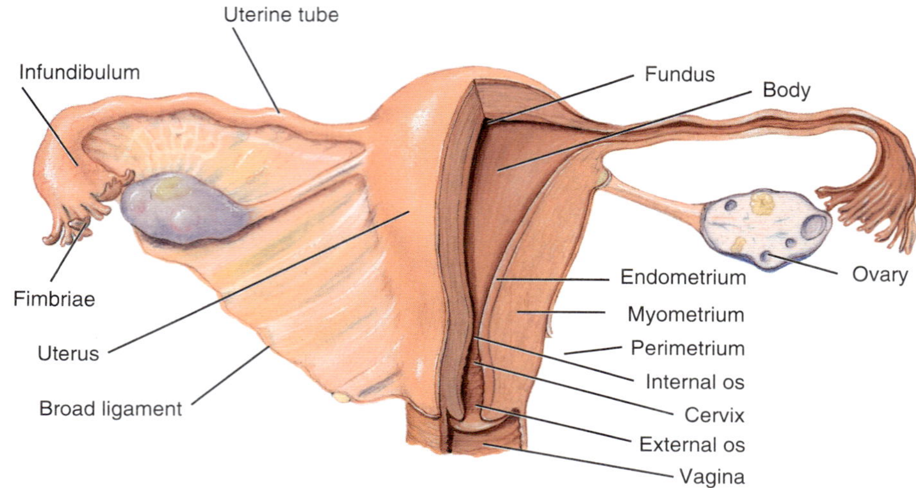

Fig. 16.10 Uterus and uterine tubes. (From Applegate E: *The anatomy and physiology learning system*, ed 4, St. Louis, 2011, Saunders.)

to the region of the ovary on that side (Fig. 16.10). One tube is associated with each ovary. The end of the tube near the ovary expands to form a funnel-shaped *infundibulum*, which is surrounded by finger-like extensions called *fimbriae*. Because there is no direct connection between the infundibulum and the ovary, the oocyte enters the peritoneal cavity before it enters the uterine tube. At the time of ovulation, the fimbriae increase their activity and create currents in the peritoneal fluid that help propel the oocyte into the uterine tube. Once inside the uterine tube, the oocyte is moved along by the rhythmic beating of cilia on the epithelial lining and by the peristaltic action of the smooth muscle in the wall of the tube. The journey through the uterine tube takes about 7 days. Because the oocyte is fertile for only 24 to 48 hours, fertilization usually occurs in the uterine tube.

Uterus

The *uterus* is a muscular organ that receives the fertilized oocyte and provides an appropriate environment for the developing offspring. It is located in the pelvic cavity, between the rectum and urinary bladder (see Fig. 16.7). Before the first pregnancy, the uterus is about the size and shape of a pear, with the narrow portion directed inferiorly. After childbirth the uterus is usually larger, and then it regresses after menopause.

The upper, bulging surface of the uterus, above the entrance of the uterine tubes, is known as the *fundus* (see Fig. 16.10). The large main portion of the uterus is the *body*. The narrow region of the uterus that is directed into the vagina is the *cervix*. The opening between the body and cervix is known as the *internal os*, and the opening from the cervix into the vagina is the *external os*. Several ligaments hold the uterus in place. The largest of these is the *broad ligament*, which drapes over the uterus like a sheet and extends laterally to the lateral pelvic wall. The broad ligament also encloses the uterine tubes.

The wall of the uterus consists of perimetrium, myometrium, and endometrium. The outer serous layer is known as the **perimetrium**. The thick middle layer is known as the **myometrium**. The myometrium consists of smooth muscle and makes up the bulk of the uterine wall. The inner layer is called the **endometrium**. It is a mucous membrane that is subdivided into two regions. The **stratum functionale** of the endometrium is the portion that is sloughed off during menstruation. The deeper, thinner **stratum basale** is more constant and provides the materials to rebuild the stratum functionale after menstruation.

Vagina

The *vagina* is a fibromuscular tube, about 10 cm long, that extends from the cervix of the uterus to the outside. It is located between the rectum and urinary bladder. The vagina provides a passageway for menstrual flow to reach the outside, receives the penis and semen during sexual intercourse (coitus), and serves as the birth canal during the birth of a baby. The smooth muscle and mucosal lining of the vaginal wall are capable of stretching to accommodate the erect penis and to permit passage of a baby. The opening of the vagina to the outside is known as the *vaginal orifice*. The vaginal orifice may be incompletely covered by a thin fold of mucous membrane called the *hymen*.

EXTERNAL GENITALIA

The external genitalia are accessory structures of the female reproductive system that are outside the vagina. They are also referred to as the **vulva**. The external genitalia include the labia majora, mons pubis, labia minora, clitoris, and glands within the vestibule (Fig. 16.11).

The *labia majora* are two large fat-filled folds of skin that enclose the other external genitalia. Anteriorly the labia majora merge to form the *mons pubis*. The mons pubis is a rounded elevation of fat that overlies the pubic symphysis.

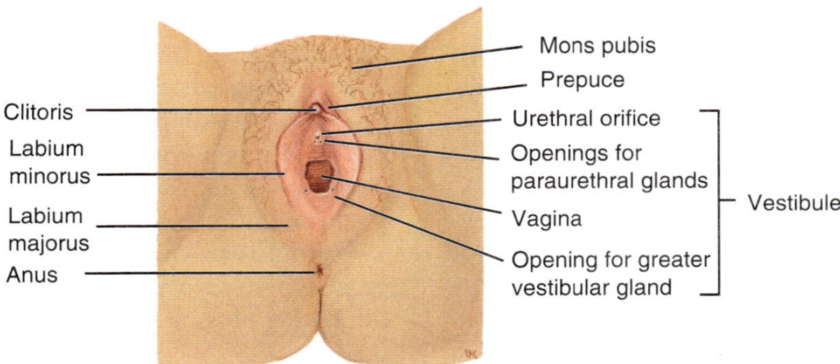

Fig. 16.11 Female external genitalia. The area between the two labia minora is the vestibule. (From Applegate E: *The anatomy and physiology learning system*, ed 4, St. Louis, 2011, Saunders.)

After puberty the mons pubis and labia majora are covered with coarse pubic hair. The *labia minora* are two smaller folds of skin medial to the labia majora.

The area between the two labia minora is called the *vestibule.* At the anterior end of the vestibule (where the two labia minora meet), there is a small mass of erectile tissue called the *clitoris.* The clitoris becomes erect in response to sexual stimulation. The labia minora merge and form a hood over the clitoris, known as the *prepuce.* Posterior to the clitoris, the urethra and vagina open into the vestibule. *Paraurethral glands* open into the vestibule on each side of the urethral orifice. These glands secrete mucus. The *greater vestibular glands* (Bartholin glands) open into the vestibule next to the vaginal orifice. These glands produce a mucus-like secretion for lubrication during sexual intercourse.

FEMALE SEXUAL RESPONSE

The female sexual response is similar to that of the male and consists of erection and orgasm. The body's responses to sexual stimuli produce increased blood flow to the erectile tissue in the clitoris, the vaginal mucosa, breasts, and nipples. The clitoris and nipples become rigid and erect. The breasts and vaginal mucosa enlarge. Glands in the cervix and the vestibular glands secrete fluids that lubricate the vaginal mucosa and aid the entry of the penis.

With continued stimulation, the female response culminates in orgasm. This is accompanied by rhythmic contractions of the uterus and muscles of the pelvic floor. This helps the movement of sperm through the uterus toward the uterine tubes. The rhythmic muscle contractions are accompanied by feelings of intense pleasure, increased heart rate, elevated blood pressure, and increased respiration rate. This is followed by a general relaxation and feeling of warmth throughout the body.

HORMONAL CONTROL

As in the male, the hypothalamus, anterior pituitary, and gonads secrete hormones that have significant roles in the control of reproductive functions (Fig. 16.12). The

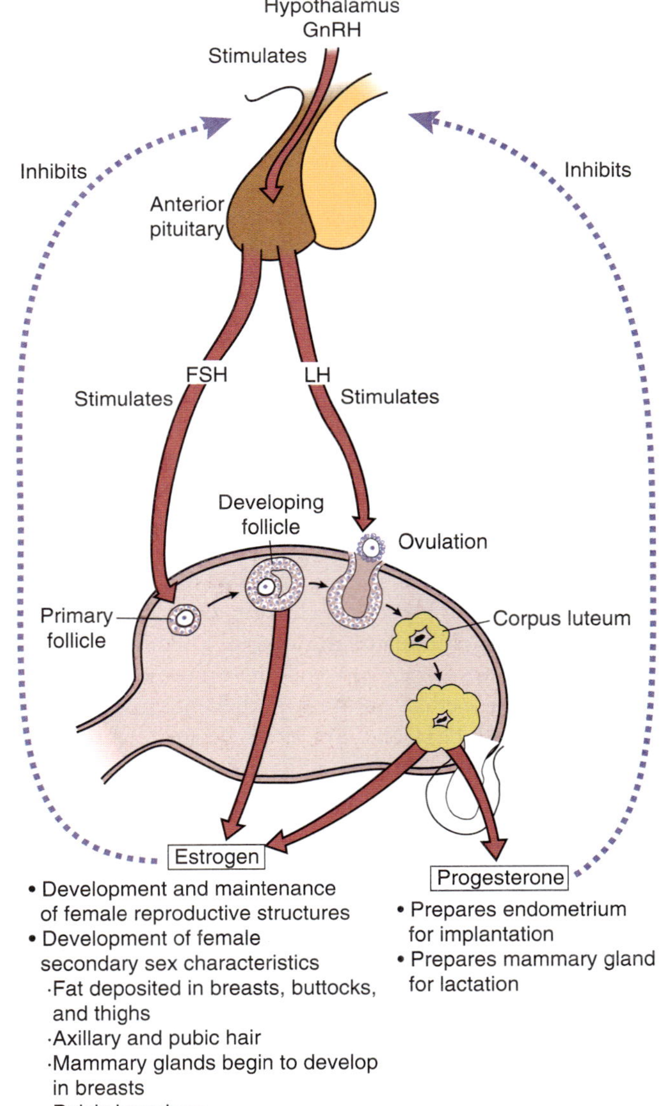

Fig. 16.12 Hormonal regulation of ovarian functions. *FSH*, Follicle stimulating hormone; *GnRH*, gonadotropin-releasing hormone; *LH*, luteinizing hormone. (From Applegate E: *The anatomy and physiology learning system*, ed 4, St. Louis, 2011, Saunders.)

hypothalamus secretes GnRH, the anterior pituitary secretes FSH and LH, and the ovaries secrete the sex hormones *estrogen* and *progesterone.* Unlike in the male, the secretion of these hormones follows monthly cyclic patterns that affect the ovaries and uterus. These cycles, referred to as the **ovarian cycle** and the **uterine cycle** (menstrual cycle), begin at puberty and continue for about 40 years.

At puberty certain stimuli cause the hypothalamus to start secreting GnRH. This hormone enters the blood and goes to the anterior pituitary gland, where it stimulates the secretion of FSH and LH. These hormones, in turn, affect the ovaries and uterus, and the monthly cycles begin. In females the beginning of puberty is marked by the first period of menstrual bleeding, called **menarche**. After this the cycles continue, more or less regularly, until the late 40s or early 50s. At this time the cycles become increasingly irregular until they finally stop. *Menopause* is the cessation of the reproductive cycles.

Ovarian Cycle

The *ovarian cycle* includes the changes that occur within the ovaries as the follicles develop (follicular phase), ovulation occurs (ovulatory phase), and the corpus luteum develops (luteal phase) (Fig. 16.13).

The *follicular phase* of the cycle begins when GnRH from the hypothalamus stimulates increased secretion of FSH from the anterior pituitary. FSH stimulates growth of the ovarian follicles. As the follicles enlarge, estrogen secretion increases. The follicle continues to grow and mature until the middle of the cycle.

The *ovulatory phase* is the result of high levels of estrogen from the mature follicles, which result in a surge of LH. The surge of LH stimulates resumption of meiosis in the oocyte and causes the rupture of the follicle and the release of the oocyte into the peritoneal cavity (ovulation). When the follicle ruptures, estrogen levels decline.

The *luteal phase* occurs when the surge of LH stimulates the development of the corpus luteum from the ruptured follicle. LH also stimulates the corpus luteum to secrete progesterone and some estrogen. These hormones have a negative feedback effect on the hypothalamus and anterior pituitary so that FSH and LH levels decline. As the LH level declines, corpus luteum activity declines, the inhibitory effect is removed, and the cycle starts over.

Uterine (Menstrual) Cycle

The *uterine cycle* (menstrual cycle) reflects changes in the endometrium of the uterus. These changes occur to the thick outer layer of the endometrium, known as the *stratum functionale.* Changes in estrogen and progesterone levels are responsible for the changes in the uterus. The uterine cycle is divided into the menstrual phase, proliferative phase, and secretory phase (see Fig. 16.13).

The *menstrual phase* begins on the first day of the cycle and continues for 3 to 5 days. The thick stratum functionale detaches from the uterine wall and passes through the vagina as the menstrual flow. During this time, follicles are growing in the ovary.

The *proliferative phase* begins with the end of the menstrual phase and lasts for about 8 days. The growing follicles in the ovary secrete increasing levels of estrogen. The estrogen stimulates repair of the endometrium in the uterus. The endometrium thickens, glands develop, and blood vessels grow in the new tissue. Ovulation in the ovary occurs at the end of this uterine phase.

During the *secretory phase*, the corpus luteum secretes progesterone, which stimulates continued growth and thickening of the endometrium. Arteries and glands grow

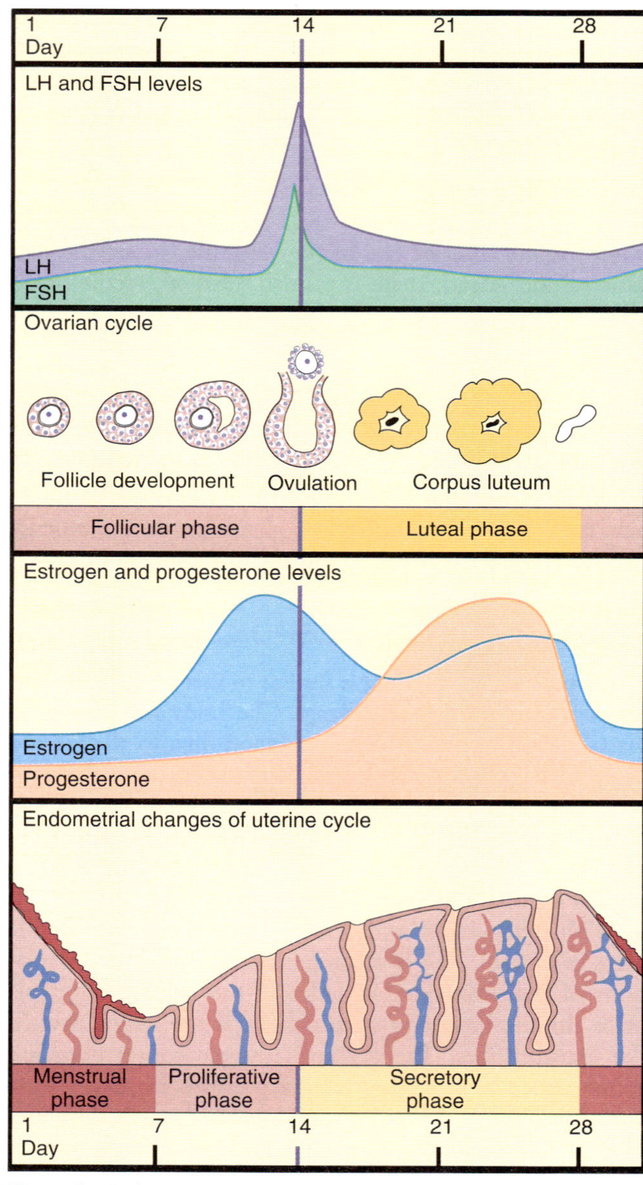

Fig. 16.13 Correlation of events in the ovarian and uterine cycles. The menstrual and proliferative phases of the uterine cycle correspond to the follicular phase of the ovarian cycle. The secretory phase of the uterine cycle corresponds to the luteal phase of the ovarian cycle. Note the relative hormone levels in each phase. *FSH*, Follicle stimulating hormone; *LH*, luteinizing hormone. (From Applegate E: *The anatomy and physiology learning system*, ed 4, St. Louis, 2011, Saunders.)

and enlarge. The glands secrete glycogen, which will nourish a developing embryo if fertilization occurs. If fertilization does not occur, the corpus luteum in the ovary begins to degenerate. This leads to menstruation, and the cycle starts over again.

Menopause

Menopause is the cessation of the female reproductive cycles. Even though menopause is marked by the lack of menstrual cycles, the first changes occur in the ovary. By the age of 45 or 50, ovarian follicles cease responding to FSH and LH from the pituitary gland. As a result, the follicle cells do not produce estrogen and there is no ovulation, no corpus luteum, and no progesterone. Without estrogen and progesterone, the cyclic changes in the uterus stop and menstruation ceases. This is the visible evidence of menopause. As estrogen and progesterone levels decline, FSH and LH increase because of the lack of ovarian hormone feedback. These high levels of pituitary hormones, with the low levels of ovarian hormones, are believed to be responsible for a variety of effects associated with the onset of menopause. Some women experience hot flashes, sweating, depression, headaches, irritability, and insomnia. Many other women experience few, if any, of these.

MAMMARY GLANDS

The *mammary glands* are the organs of milk production. Mammary glands are located in the breast, overlying the pectoralis major muscles. They are present in both sexes but usually functional only in the female.

Each breast has a raised *nipple*, which is surrounded by a circular pigmented area called the *areola*. The nipples are sensitive to touch, and they contain smooth muscle that contracts and causes them to become erect in response to stimulation.

The adult female breast contains 15 to 20 lobes of glandular tissue that radiate around the nipple (Fig. 16.14). The lobes are separated by connective tissue and adipose. The connective tissue helps support the breast. Some bands of connective tissue, called *suspensory* (Cooper) *ligaments*, extend through the breast from the skin to the underlying muscles. The amount and distribution of the adipose tissue determines the size and shape of the breast. Each lobe consists of *lobules* that contain the glandular units. A *lactiferous duct* collects the milk from the lobules within each lobe and carries it to the nipple. Just before the nipple, the lactiferous duct enlarges to form a *lactiferous sinus (ampulla)*, which serves as a reservoir for milk. After the sinus, the duct again narrows and each duct opens independently on the surface of the nipple.

Mammary gland function is regulated by hormones. At puberty, increasing levels of estrogen stimulate the development of glandular tissue in the female breast. Estrogen also causes the breasts to increase in size through the accumulation of adipose tissue. Progesterone stimulates the development of the duct system. During pregnancy these hormones further enhance development of the mammary glands. Prolactin from the anterior pituitary stimulates the production of milk within the glandular tissue, and oxytocin causes the ejection of milk from the glands.

HIGHLIGHT on the Female Reproductive System

Ovarian cancer: Carcinomas of the ovary account for more deaths than do cervical and uterine cancers together. Because there are no screening tests and few symptoms in the early stages, ovarian carcinomas are usually in an advanced stage when they are discovered. Surgery, radiation therapy, and chemotherapy are used as therapeutic measures.

Tubal ligation: Tubal ligation is a surgical procedure in which the uterine tubes are burned or severed and tied off. This is a permanent method of birth control because sperm are unable to reach the egg for fertilization. The technique involves making a small incision in the abdomen and inserting a small tube through which the ligation instruments can be introduced.

Mittelschmerz: Mittelschmerz is a term to describe one-sided lower abdominal pain, which may switch sides from one month to another, at or around the time of ovulation. The pain is usually described as sharp or cramping and lasts from 24 to 48 hours. There is no known prevention, and treatment consists of analgesics.

Fibrocystic disease: Fibrocystic disease is a common benign condition of the breast. Small sacs of tissue and fluid develop in the breast tissue and the patient notices lumps in the breast, often associated with premenstrual tenderness. Mammography and surgical biopsy may be indicated to differentiate between fibrocystic disease and carcinoma of the breast. ■

DEVELOPMENT

Development is a continuous process that starts with fertilization (conception) and ends with death. Birth is an awesome event that divides the total span of development into two portions. It is the culmination of 38 weeks of **prenatal development** within the uterus. The period of **postnatal development** begins with birth and lasts until death.

Fertilization, or conception, is the union of the sperm cell nucleus with an egg cell nucleus. The resulting cell is called a **zygote**. Because the egg cells are fertile for only about 24 hours, fertilization usually occurs in the uterine tube near the infundibulum. The zygote is the first cell of the future offspring and has a full

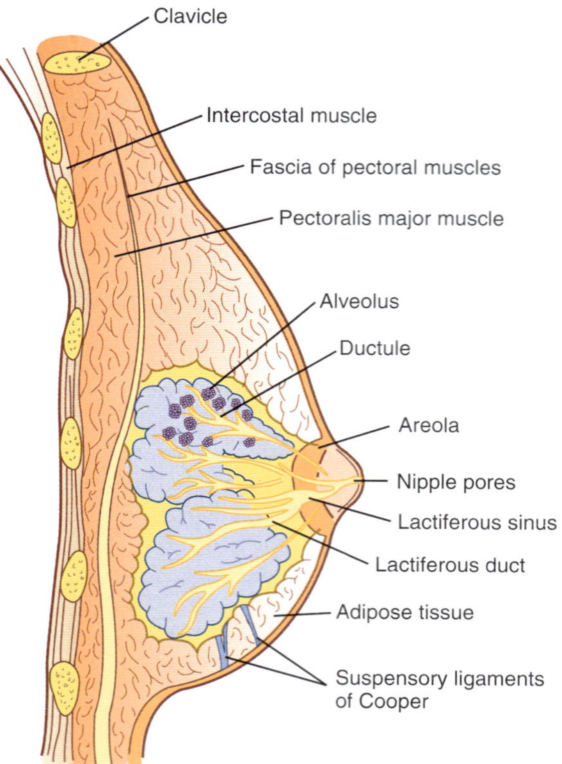

Fig. 16.14 Breast and mammary glands. (From Applegate E: *The anatomy and physiology learning system*, ed 4, St. Louis, 2011, Saunders.)

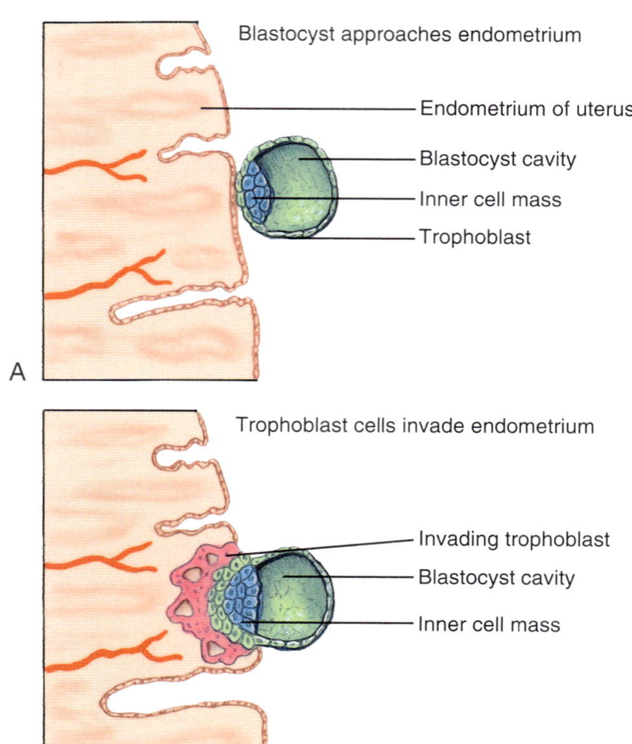

Fig. 16.15 Process of implantation. (A) Blastocyst approaches the endometrium. (B) Trophoblast cells invade the endometrium. (From Applegate E: *The anatomy and physiology learning system*, ed 4, St. Louis, 2011, Saunders.)

complement of 46 chromosomes: 23 from the sperm and 23 from the egg.

PRENATAL DEVELOPMENT

The period of prenatal development, or pregnancy, is referred to as **gestation**. Embryologists describe the timing of events in prenatal development by using the term **developmental age**, which begins at fertilization. The medical community uses **clinical age**, which begins at the date of the last menstrual period (LMP). Developmental age is 2 weeks less than clinical age. In humans, the normal gestation period for developmental age is 266 days from fertilization to the birth of the infant. The normal gestation period for clinical age is 280 days from the beginning of the LMP to the birth of the infant. Prenatal development is divided into preembryonic, embryonic, and fetal periods.

The **preembryonic period** lasts for about 2 weeks after fertilization. During this time the zygote undergoes numerous cell divisions and moves through the uterine tube into the cavity of the uterus. By the 7th day after fertilization (21st day of a menstrual cycle), the zygote has developed into a hollow mass of cells called a *blastocyst*. The cavity is called the *blastocele*, the flattened cells around the cavity make up the *trophoblast*, and the mass of cells on one side is the *inner cell mass*. The blastocyst approaches the endometrium, usually high in the uterus, and attaches to it. This begins the process of *implantation* (Fig. 16.15). The trophoblast cells secrete enzymes that erode the endometrium to form a hole, and the blastocyst "burrows" into the thick endometrial tissue. The blastocyst saves itself from being aborted by secreting *human chorionic gonadotropin* (HCG), a hormone that causes the corpus luteum to remain functional and secrete progesterone to maintain the endometrium. Pregnancy tests are based on the presence of HCG in the blood or urine because it is not produced in a woman unless she is pregnant.

The **embryonic period** lasts from the beginning of the third week to the end of the eighth week. The developing offspring is called an *embryo* during this time. Significant changes during this 6-week period include the formation of the *placenta* and all of the *organ systems*. The placenta is a highly vascular disc that develops from both embryonic and maternal tissue. It is usually formed and fully functioning by the end of the embryonic period. After the infant is born, the placenta is expelled from the uterus as part of the afterbirth. By diffusion of substances across the membranes, the placenta functions as a nutritive, respiratory, and excretory organ for the fetus. It also secretes hormones and thus functions as a temporary endocrine gland. The formation of body organs and organ systems is called *organogenesis*. The skin, one of the earliest organs to develop, forms during the third week. By the end of the fourth week, the heart is pumping blood to all parts of the embryo. By the end of the eighth week, all the main internal body organs are

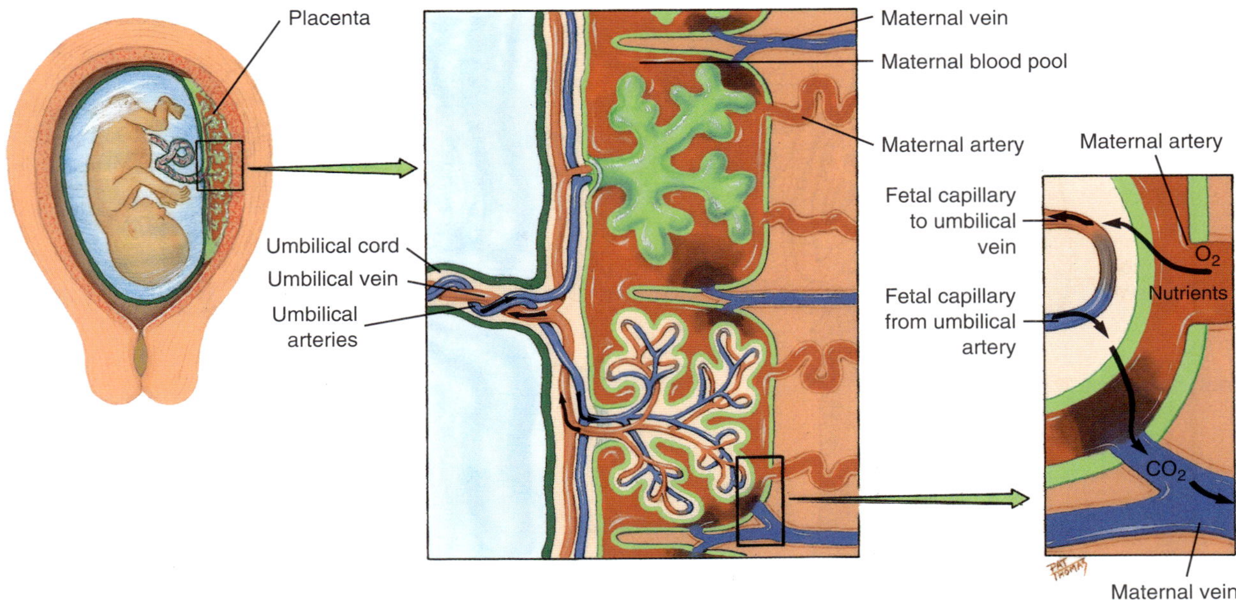

Fig. 16.16 Structural features of the placenta and exchange of nutrients and gases between maternal and fetal blood. (From Applegate E: *The anatomy and physiology learning system*, ed 4, St. Louis, 2011, Saunders.)

established and the embryo has a humanlike appearance, even though it is only about 25 mm (1 inch) long and weighs about 1 gram.

The **fetal period** of development starts at the beginning of the ninth week and lasts until birth. The developing offspring is called a *fetus* during this time. Because all the organ systems are formed during the embryonic period, the fetus is less vulnerable than the embryo to malformations caused by radiation, viruses, and drugs. The fetal period is a time of growth and maturation.

The fetus obtains oxygen and nutrients from maternal circulation and also depends on maternal circulation to remove carbon dioxide and other wastes. This exchange occurs through the placenta, which is attached to the uterine wall of the mother and connected to the umbilicus (navel) of the fetus by the umbilical cord (Fig. 16.16). The umbilical cord contains two umbilical arteries and one umbilical vein. Umbilical arteries, branches of the fetal internal iliac arteries, carry blood that is loaded with carbon dioxide and waste products from the fetus to the placenta where they diffuse into the maternal blood. At the same time, oxygen and nutrients diffuse from maternal blood into the umbilical vein, which carries them to fetal circulation. Normally, membranes within the placenta keep the fetal and maternal blood from actually mixing. Because the fetal liver and lungs are immature and nonfunctional, there are special adaptations in fetal circulation that permit most of the blood to bypass these organs. These adaptations are the *ductus venosus*, which is between the umbilical vein and inferior vena cava and bypasses the immature liver; the *foramen ovale*, which is an opening in the interatrial septum that allows blood to bypass pulmonary circulation; and the *ductus arteriosus*, which is a shunt between the pulmonary trunk and aorta to bypass the lungs. Fig. 16.17 illustrates fetal circulation and Table 16.1 provides a summary of the specialized structures. At or shortly after birth, when the lung and liver functions are established, the adaptations in the fetal circulatory pathway are no longer necessary, and changes occur that make the structures nonfunctional. The circulatory pathway becomes like that of an adult.

PARTURITION AND LACTATION

Parturition refers to the birth of an infant, and *labor* is the process by which forceful contractions expel the fetus from the uterus. The onset of *true labor* is characterized by rhythmic contractions, dilation of the cervix, and a discharge of bloody mucus from the cervix and vagina. The onset of labor appears to be the interaction of progesterone, estrogen, oxytocin, and prostaglandins. Labor is divided into three periods: the dilation stage, expulsion stage, and placental stage. These are illustrated in Fig. 16.18. The *dilation stage* begins with the onset of true labor and lasts until the cervix is fully dilated to a diameter of 10 cm. This is the longest stage and may last 24 hours or longer. The *expulsion stage* lasts from full dilation of the cervix until the delivery of the fetus. This stage usually lasts less than an hour. The final stage is the *placental stage*. Usually within 10 or 15 minutes after the delivery of the fetus, the placenta separates from the uterine wall and forceful contractions expel the placenta and attached membranes as the afterbirth. The contractions also constrict the torn blood vessels to prevent hemorrhage. Normally less than half a liter of blood is lost during delivery.

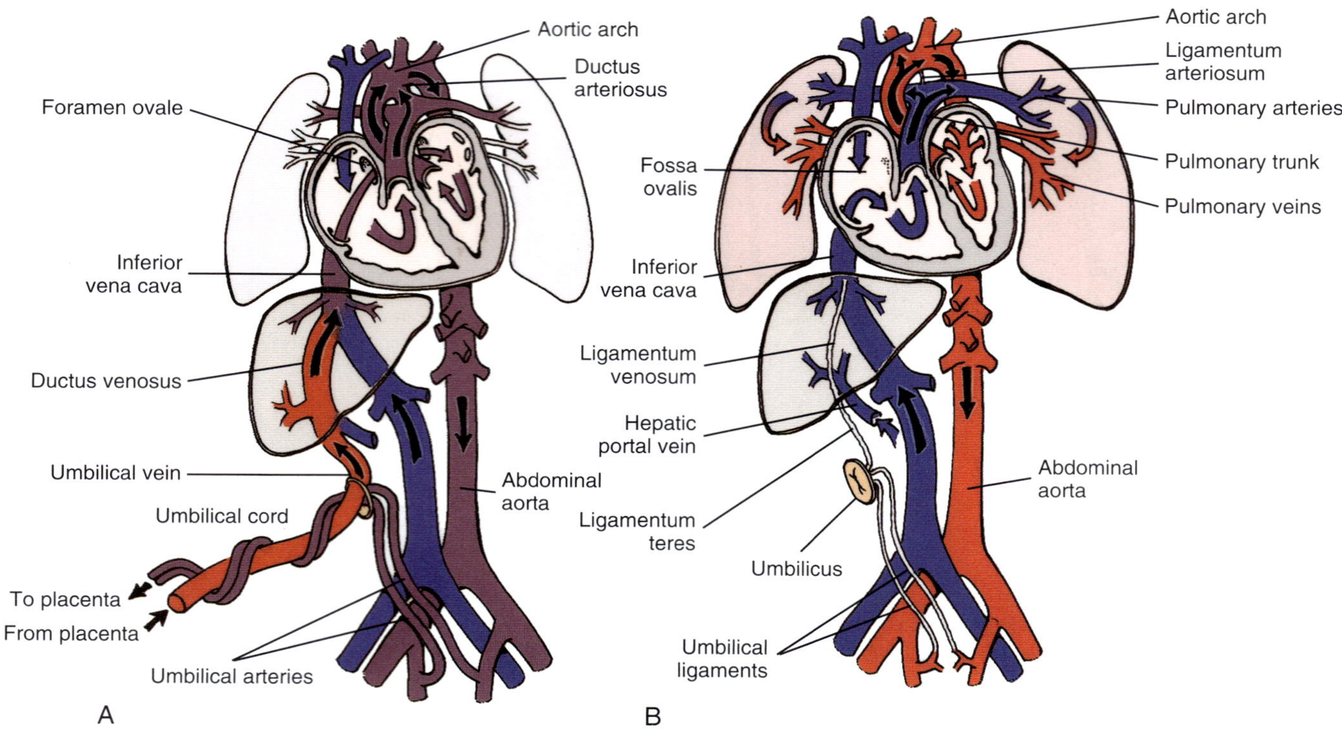

Fig. 16.17 Circulation patterns before and after birth. (A) Fetal circulation. (B) Circulation after birth. Before birth, the two umbilical arteries transport blood to the placenta and a single umbilical vein returns blood from the placenta to the fetus. The ductus venosus bypasses the nonfunctional fetal liver. The ductus arteriosus and foramen ovale permit blood to bypass the lungs, which are nonfunctional. After birth, the circulatory patterns change to include the liver and lungs. (From Applegate E: *The anatomy and physiology learning system*, ed 4, St. Louis, 2011, Saunders.)

Table 16.1 Summary of Special Features in Fetal Circulation

Feature	Location	Before Birth	After Birth
Umbilical arteries (2)	Umbilical cord	Transport blood from fetus to placenta	Degenerate to become lateral umbilical ligaments
Umbilical vein (1)	Umbilical cord	Transports blood from placenta to fetus	Becomes ligamentum teres (round ligament) of liver
Ductus venosus	Between umbilical vein and inferior vena cava	Carries blood directly from umbilical vein to inferior vena cava; bypasses liver	Becomes ligamentum venosum of liver
Foramen ovale	Interatrial septum	Allows blood to go directly from right atrium into left atrium to bypass pulmonary circulation	Closes after birth to become fossa ovalis
Ductus arteriosus	Between pulmonary trunkand aorta	Permits blood in pulmonary trunk to go directly into descending aorta and bypass pulmonary circulation	Becomes a fibrous cord; ligamentum arteriosum

From Applegate E: *The anatomy and physiology learning system,* ed 4, St. Louis, 2011, Saunders.

Lactation refers to the production of milk by the mammary glands and the ejection of the milk from the breast. Prolactin is the most important hormone that stimulates the production of milk. Prolactin levels increase during pregnancy; however, the hormone's activity is inhibited by the estrogen and progesterone from the placenta. After parturition, when the placenta is expelled, this inhibition is removed and milk production begins. The infant's suckling stimulates the release of oxytocin from the posterior pituitary gland. Oxytocin causes the ejection of milk from the breast.

POSTNATAL DEVELOPMENT

Development after birth is called **postnatal development** and lasts from parturition until death. It is divided into the neonatal period, infancy, childhood, adolescence, adulthood, and senescence.

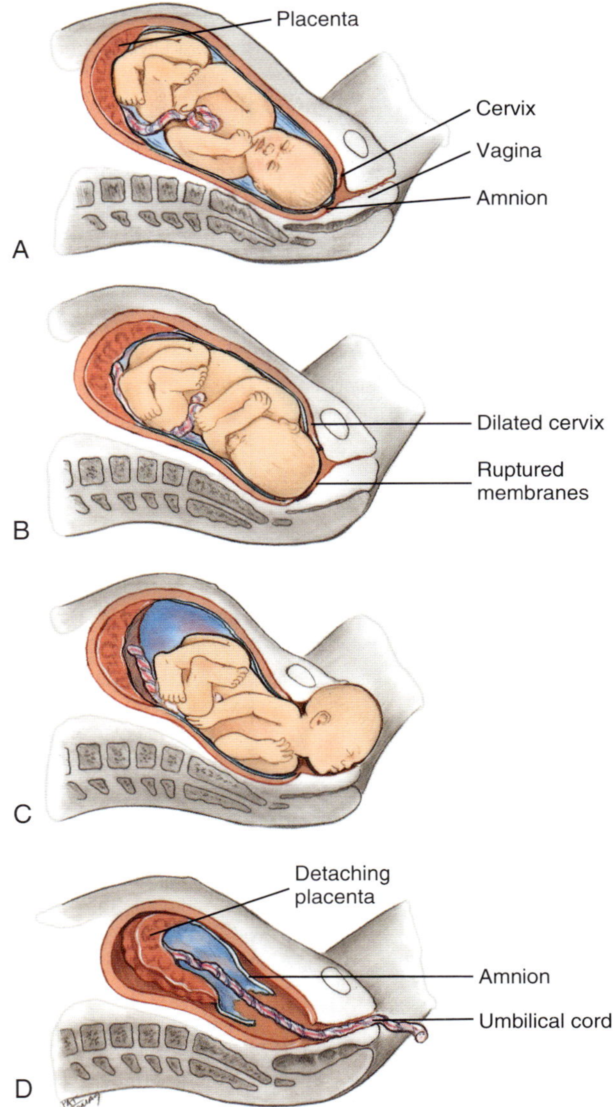

Fig. 16.18 Three stages of labor. (A) Before labor begins. (B) Dilation stage begins with onset of true labor and lasts until the cervix is fully dilated. (C) Expulsion stage is from full cervical dilation until delivery of the fetus. (D) Placental stage lasts from delivery of the fetus until the placenta and extraembryonic membranes are expelled. (From Applegate E: *The anatomy and physiology learning system*, ed 4, St. Louis, 2011, Saunders.)

The *neonatal period* encompasses the first 4 weeks after parturition. During this time the baby is called a *neonate.* This period is critical because the neonate has to make numerous adjustments to life outside the uterus, including changes in respiration and in the circulatory pathways. Temperature-regulating mechanisms and the immune system are not yet fully developed, so the neonate is vulnerable to environmental temperature changes and infections.

Infancy lasts from the end of the first month until the end of the first year. Many developmental changes occur during this time. There is an increase in the production of myelin within the nervous system, and this results in improved muscle coordination. The baby learns to sit, crawl, stand, and walk during this period. Teeth begin to erupt, and the baby starts to communicate by smiling, laughing, and making sounds.

Childhood lasts from the end of the first year until puberty. Bone ossification is rapid. Growth is rapid and then slows until puberty, then increases again. Deciduous teeth are shed and replaced by permanent teeth. Language skills develop, motor coordination becomes more refined, and intellect develops.

Adolescence lasts from puberty until adulthood. The individual becomes capable of reproduction during this time. Secondary sex characteristics appear. The adolescent shows increasing levels of motor skills, intellectual ability, and emotional maturity.

Adulthood is the period between adolescence and senescence. The beginning and ending of adulthood are somewhat vague. In general, adulthood is characterized by a maintenance of existing body tissues so that the body remains unchanged anatomically and physiologically for many years.

Senescence is the period of older adulthood that ends in death; the transition from adulthood to senescence is vague. This period is marked by degenerative changes that make the body less capable of coping with the demands placed on it. Changes related to aging and senescence occur in all body systems; however, the rate at which they occur varies from system to system and from individual to individual. Even though there are degenerative changes in all body systems, death usually results from cardiovascular disorders, failure of the immune system, or disease processes that affect vital organs.

AGING OF THE REPRODUCTIVE SYSTEM

Men normally do not experience a sudden decline in reproductive function comparable to menopause in women. Instead, they experience a gradual and subtle decline over many years. After age 50, men have some testicular atrophy, partially caused by a decrease in the size of the seminiferous tubules and partially as a result of a reduction in the number of interstitial cells. These changes are accompanied by a decline in sperm and testosterone production. Both the seminal vesicles and the prostate show a decrease in secretory activity, which results in a reduction in the volume of semen. The portion of the prostate gland that surrounds the urethra often enlarges and may constrict the urethra, making urination difficult. The penis may undergo some atrophy and become smaller with age. The blood vessels and erectile tissue in the penis become less elastic, which hinders the ability to attain an erection. Although there is a general decline in the aging male reproductive system, many men are capable of achieving erection and ejaculation into old age.

After menopause, there is a gradual decline in the female reproductive system. Most of the changes are believed to be caused by the reduction in estrogen. The ovaries undergo progressive atrophy. The uterus becomes smaller, and fibrous connective tissue replaces much of the myometrium. The vagina becomes narrower and shorter, and its walls become thin and less elastic. Glands that lubricate the vagina reduce their secretory activity, and the vagina becomes dry. The vaginal secretions that remain are less acidic, which makes older women more susceptible to vaginal infections. The external genitalia and mammary glands undergo atrophic changes. The lack of estrogen also affects nonreproductive organs. This is particularly true in the case of bone metabolism, which is indicated by the increased prevalence of osteoporosis in postmenopausal women. There is also increased cardiovascular disease.

Estrogen replacement therapy is prescribed for many women to combat osteoporosis and other effects of menopause. However, there is controversy about the risks involved with this treatment, particularly the risks of uterine and breast cancer. Consideration should be given to the risks and benefits before beginning estrogen replacement therapy. Current practice often involves prescription of progesterone in conjunction with estrogen, which seems to reduce some of the risks.

There is a growing awareness that elderly people have sexual needs and enjoy sexual relations. Although age-related physical and hormonal changes that take place in the reproductive system may alter these needs and sexual functioning, studies demonstrate that sexuality remains important to many older people.

Common Pathology of the Reproductive System

Disease	Signs and Symptoms	Etiology	Diagnosis and Treatment
Abruptio placentae	Also called *placental abruption*; premature separation of placenta from the uterine wall. Signs and symptoms include bleeding, uterine contractions, and fetal distress.	Exact cause is unknown. Risk factors include maternal hypertension, maternal trauma, cigarette smoking, cocaine use, alcohol consumption, and blood clotting disorders.	Diagnosis is based on symptoms combined with ultrasound, fetal monitoring, and blood tests. Treatment includes intravenous (IV) fluids and blood transfusion if bleeding has been severe. An emergency cesarean section may be needed. If the baby is very premature and there is little separation, mother may be kept on bed rest for several days.
Benign prostatic hypertrophy(BPH)	Also called *benign prostatic hyperplasia;* especially common; estimated that 90% of men over age of 70 have some degree of BPH. Symptoms include difficulty in urinating, dribbling at the end of urination, and being unable to completely empty the bladder.	Symptoms occur when the prostate enlarges and compresses the urethra enough to interfere with urine flow. The reason for the hypertrophy is unknown.	Diagnosis is based on medical history, physical examination, digital rectal examination (DRE), and urinalysis. Other tests may be required to rule out other conditions such as prostate cancer and infections. Medications may be sufficient for mild to moderate symptoms. The standard surgical procedure is transurethral resection of the prostate (TURP).
Cancer, breast	Lump or mass in the breast tissue, tenderness in the breast, skin changes in the breast, and changes in the nipple.	Cause is unknown. Occurs when some cells in the breast begin growing abnormally to accumulate and form a mass. Cells may spread to nearby lymph nodes and to other parts of the body. A family history of breast cancer increases the risk.	Diagnosis is based on a breast examination, mammogram, breast ultrasound, and biopsy of the tumor. Treatment involves surgical removal of either the tumor and a small amount of breast tissue (lumpectomy) or the entire breast (mastectomy). Depending on the type of breast cancer and the stage, further treatment by radiation therapy, chemotherapy, or hormone therapy may be necessary.
Cancer, cervical	Early cervical cancer usually produces no signs or symptoms; later stages may cause abnormal vaginal bleeding or other vaginal discharge and pelvic pain.	Occurs when healthy cells undergo a genetic mutation that turns them into abnormal cells that grow and multiply out of control. The accumulating cells form a tumor that can spread to nearby tissues, or pieces can break off and spread to other parts of the body. The cause of the mutation is unknown, but various strains of human papillomavirus (HPV) appear to have a role in many cases.	Diagnosis is accomplished by visual examination of the cervix (colposcopy) and by a cytologic examination of a tissue sample for abnormal cells. Imaging modalities are used to determine the stage of the cancer. Treatment depends on the stage and personal preference. Treatment options include surgery, radiation, and chemotherapy. Early detection through a Papanicolaou (Pap) smear and/or HPV DNA test is key to successful treatment.

Common Pathology of the Reproductive System—cont'd

Disease	Signs and Symptoms	Etiology	Diagnosis and Treatment
Cancer, ovarian	Early ovarian cancer is usually asymptomatic. Advanced cancer symptoms are non-specific. They include abdominal bloating or swelling, weight loss, discomfort in the pelvic area, changes in bowel habits, and a frequent need to urinate.	As with most other cancers, there is no specific known cause. A genetic mutation turns normal healthy cells into rapidly growing cancer cells of the ovary. The accumulating cancer cells form a tumor that may spread to surrounding tissue and to other parts of the body.	Diagnosis is based on a pelvic examination, imaging tests, blood tests, and a biopsy. Treatment is a combination of surgery and chemotherapy.
Cancer, uterine	Vaginal bleeding after menopause, an abnormal discharge from the vagina, pelvic pain, and pain during intercourse.	As with most other cancers, there is no specific known cause. A genetic mutation turns normal healthy uterine cells into rapidly growing cancer cells. The accumulating cancer cells form a tumor that may spread to surrounding tissue and to other parts of the body.	There are no screening methods for uterine cancer. Diagnosis is by pelvic examination, transvaginal ultrasound, hysteroscopy, and tissue biopsy. Treatment depends on characteristics of the cancer and the stage. The recommended treatment is surgery to remove the uterus (hysterectomy). Usually the uterine tubes and ovaries are also removed (salpingo-oophorectomy). Additional treatments are radiation therapy, chemotherapy, and hormone therapy.
Cancer, prostate	Prostate cancer may cause no symptoms and go undetected in the early stages. As it progresses, it produces a lump on the surface of the gland. There may be difficulty in urinating, some discomfort in the pelvic region, blood in the urine and/or semen, and erectile dysfunction.	The initial cause is unknown. A mutation in a few cells, usually in one of the secretory glands of the prostate, causes them to become abnormal. These cells grow rapidly and also destroy normal cells. The accumulating abnormal cells form a tumor that may invade surrounding tissue.	Diagnosis is based on DRE, prostate-specific antigen (PSA) test, and tissue biopsy of the prostate. Imaging techniques are useful to determine the stage of the cancer and how far it has spread, then treatment protocols may be established. Options include surgery to remove the prostate (prostatectomy), radiation therapy, chemotherapy, and hormone therapy.
Cancer, testicular	Lump in either testicle, feeling of heaviness in scrotum, sudden collection of fluid in scrotum, pain or discomfort in scrotum. Signs and symptoms usually affect only one side.	As with most other cancers, there is no specific known cause. A genetic mutation turns normal healthy cells into rapidly growing cancer cells. The accumulating cancer cells form a tumor that may spread to surrounding tissue and to other parts of the body. Nearly all testicular cancers begin in the germ cells.	Most men discover the lump in the testicle themselves. Ultrasound and blood tests help determine if the lump is cancer. Typically, the testicle is surgically removed (orchiectomy) and cells examined to confirm diagnosis. Computed tomography (CT) and blood tests determine the type and stage. Surgical removal is usually sufficient for early stage cancer. More advanced stages may require radiation therapy and chemotherapy.
Candidiasis	Vaginal itching, burning sensation when urinating, white vaginal discharge.	Caused by an overgrowth of the fungal microorganism *Candida albicans.*	Testing a sample of the vaginal discharge confirms diagnosis. Over-the-counter and prescription medications are usually sufficient treatment.
Cryptorchidism	Absence of one or both testicles in the scrotum.	Cause is unknown. The testicles develop in the abdominal cavity, then shortly before birth they descend into the scrotum. For some reason, one (or both) may not descend all the way. The condition will cause sterility if not corrected.	Not finding a testicle in the scrotum is sufficient for diagnosis. A minor surgical procedure will correct the problem.

Continued

Common Pathology of the Reproductive System—cont'd

Disease	Signs and Symptoms	Etiology	Diagnosis and Treatment
Ectopic pregnancy	Often the first indication is abdominal or pelvic pain and light vaginal bleeding. Severe pain and bleeding indicate a crisis.	The zygote implants somewhere other than the uterine wall, often in the uterine tubes. Risk factors include a history of pelvic inflammatory disease (PID), sexually transmitted disease (STD), a previous ectopic pregnancy, or scarring from previous pelvic surgery.	Diagnosis is based on physical examination and ultrasound. The embryo or fetus cannot develop outside the uterus, so an ectopic pregnancy must be terminated. The early stages of pregnancy can be terminated using medications. A ruptured uterine tube is a medical crisis and requires emergency surgery.
Endometriosis	Pelvic pain associated with menstruation (dysmenorrhea), pain with intercourse, pain with bowel movements and urination, infertility.	Endometriosis occurs when pieces of endometrial tissue grow in places other than the lining of the uterus; usually on the ovaries, intestines, or pelvic wall. The cause is unknown, but it is most likely the result of retrograde menstruation when pieces of endometrium pass through the uterine tubes into the pelvic cavity instead of passing out of the uterus with the menstrual flow.	A pelvic examination, ultrasound, and laparoscopy may be used in diagnosis. Treatment consists of pain medications and possibly hormone therapy or laparoscopic surgery.
Erectile dysfunction, impotence	Inability to develop or maintain an erection of the penis during sexual activity.	Male sexual arousal is a complex interaction of many factors; consequently, dysfunction has numerous causes. Most causes are physical secondary to other health conditions—for example, heart disease, atherosclerosis, diabetes, and treatment for prostate cancer; other causes may be psychological, such as depression, anxiety, and stress.	The condition is not difficult to diagnose, but it may be difficult to determine the underlying cause. A variety of medications are available to promote an erection. If these are insufficient, penis pumps and penile implants are available; if the difficulty is of a psychological nature, then counseling may be recommended.
Fibrocystic disease	Lumps in the breast, aches in the breast, tenderness of breast tissue, thickened areas of breast tissue, cysts.	Exact cause is unknown.	Tests are used to differentiate between fibrocystic disease and breast cancer. These include a clinical breast examination, mammography, ultrasound, fine needle aspiration of fluid in cysts, and breast biopsy. Mild symptoms usually require no treatment. If the cysts are large and painful, fine needle aspiration to remove the fluid will reduce the size. Rarely is surgery necessary.
Genital herpes	Pain, itching, and sores in the genital area. The initial infection may produce flulike symptoms.	Caused by the herpes simplex virus. It is a common STD spread by sexual contact.	The physician can usually diagnose by looking at the sores but may test a sample from the sores for confirmation. There is no cure. Once the virus is present in the body, it remains there, but it may remain dormant until a recurrent outbreak. Medications can prevent or shorten outbreaks.
Genital warts	Small flesh-colored or pink growth in the genital area, itching and discomfort in the genital area, and bleeding during intercourse.	Genital warts are caused by HPV, which is easily transmitted by sexual contact.	Diagnosis is by visual examination. A mild acetic acid solution may be used to whiten the warts to make them more visible. Usually no treatment is needed. If the warts are causing discomfort, there are medications to relieve an outbreak. There is no cure. Once the virus is present in the body, it remains there.

Common Pathology of the Reproductive System—cont'd

Disease	Signs and Symptoms	Etiology	Diagnosis and Treatment
Gonorrhea	Many patients have no symptoms. For men, symptoms may include painful urination, puslike discharge from the tip of the penis, and pain or swelling in the testicles. For women, there may be painful urination, vaginal discharge, abdominal or pelvic pain, and vaginal bleeding. The disease can also affect the rectum, eyes, throat, and joints.	Gonorrhea is an STD caused by the bacterium *Neisseria gonorrhoeae.* Babies can be infected during childbirth.	Diagnostic tools include a urine test to detect bacteria in the urethra and a swab of the affected area to detect the bacteria. This is a bacterial disease, so antibiotics are an effective treatment.
Gynecomastia	Enlarged breast gland tissue, breast tenderness, feelings of embarrassment.	Gynecomastia is enlarged breast tissue in boys or men, caused by an imbalance of the hormones estrogen and testosterone. It also occurs in Klinefelter syndrome.	Diagnosis is by physical examination with careful evaluation of breast tissue, assisted by blood tests, imaging scans, biopsies, and mammograms. If the condition is very bothersome, surgery may be required to remove the breast tissue.
Hypospadias	Hooded appearance of the penis with a downward curve, abnormal spraying during urination.	Hypospadias is a condition in which the opening of the urethra is on the underside of the penis instead of at the tip. It is a congenital defect that may be inherited.	Hypospadias may be diagnosed by physical appearance. In some cases, treatment involves surgery to reposition the urethral opening and to straighten the shaft of the penis if necessary.
Inguinal hernia	A bulge in the pubic bone area with an aching sensation; pain when lifting, coughing, or bending over; and weakness or pressure in the groin.	In an inguinal hernia, a portion of the intestines protrudes through a weak point of the abdominal wall. If the intestine becomes trapped in the abdominal wall, its blood supply may be cut off. This is called a *strangulated hernia.*	An inguinal hernia can usually be diagnosed with only a physical examination. An enlarged or painful hernia will usually require surgery to relieve discomfort and prevent serious complications.
Mastitis	Breast tenderness and swelling, pain while breast feeding, skin redness, fever, malaise.	Mastitis is a breast tissue infection. It may be caused by a blocked milk duct or by bacteria entering the breast.	Mastitis diagnosis is based on patient history and physical examination, looking for a tender wedge-shaped area on the breast that points toward the nipple. Treatment is with antibiotics and pain relievers.
Ovarian cysts	Menstrual irregularities, pelvic pain at the start and end of the period, pain during bowel movements, nausea, breast tenderness.	Most ovarian cysts develop from the follicles that develop each month. For some unknown reason, some of the follicles may continue to grow and form fluid-filled cysts on the surface of the ovary instead of degenerating with the monthly cycle. Typically, ovarian cysts cause little or no discomfort and are harmless. Cysts that have ruptured can lead to severe pain and internal bleeding.	An ovarian cyst diagnosis may be achieved with pelvic ultrasound or laparoscopy. The physician may suggest removal of a large cyst if it is growing or persists through two or three menstrual cycles. Cysts that cause pain or other symptoms may also be removed.
Placenta previa	Vaginal bleeding without pain during the second half of pregnancy is the main sign of placenta previa.	Placenta previa is an obstetric complication in which the placenta is inserted partially or wholly over the cervix. The exact cause is unknown. It has been suggested that it may be the result of irregularities in the vascularization of the endometrium.	Placenta previa can be diagnosed with ultrasound. If the patient has little or no bleeding, bed rest at home may be recommended. If the bleeding is heavy, a cesarean delivery is scheduled for as soon as the baby can be delivered safely.

Continued

Common Pathology of the Reproductive System—cont'd

Disease	Signs and Symptoms	Etiology	Diagnosis and Treatment
Polycystic ovary syndrome (PCOS)	Infertility, infrequent or prolonged menstrual periods, facial hair, cysts of the ovaries, obesity, pelvic pain, depression, sleep apnea.	PCOS is a varied disorder of uncertain cause. There is strong evidence that it is a genetic disease. The condition name comes from the appearance of the ovaries, which contain numerous small cysts.	There is no single test for diagnosing PCOS. Medical history, physical examination, pelvic examination, blood tests, and vaginal ultrasound are typical procedures. There is no cure for PCOS. Management includes lifestyle modifications, use of birth control pills, and fertility medications.
Preeclampsia and eclampsia	Increase in blood pressure, signs of kidney problems, severe headaches, blurred vision, abdominal pain, nausea, decreased urine output, edema, shortness of breath.	Preeclampsia is a disorder in pregnancy in which the patient has high blood pressure and proteinuria. The exact cause of preeclampsia is unknown. During pregnancy, new blood vessels develop to provide blood to the placenta. In women with preeclampsia, these blood vessels do not seem to develop properly, limiting the blood flow.	Preeclampsia is diagnosed when a pregnant woman's blood pressure abruptly increases. The only known definitive treatment for preeclampsia is delivery of the fetus and placenta. Women with severe hypertension during pregnancy should receive treatment with antihypertensive agents. Eclampsia is the development of convulsions in a patient with preeclampsia.
Syphilis	The first sign of syphilis is a small sore, called a *chancre,* that appears at the spot where the bacteria entered the body. A few weeks later a rash appears. If untreated the disease enters a latent stage.	Syphilis is an STD that can have very serious complications when left untreated. It is caused by the spirochete *Treponema pallidum.*	A blood test can be used to test for syphilis. Syphilis can be cured with the proper antibiotics, but it is important to receive treatment at the first sign of the chancre.
Trichomoniasis	Most infected people do not have symptoms. When symptoms appear, they can range from mild irritation to severe inflammation and include a foul-smelling vaginal discharge in women; a discharge from the urethra in men; redness, burning, and itching in the genital area; and painful urination or intercourse. Pregnant women with trichomoniasis are more likely to have their babies prematurely.	Trichomoniasis is a common STD caused by a protozoan parasite, *Trichomonas vaginalis.* Although symptoms of the disease vary, most women and men who have the parasite are not aware that they are infected. The parasite is passed from an infected person to an uninfected person during sex.	Trichomoniasis is diagnosed by collecting a specimen and visually observing the trichomonads via a microscope. It can be cured with a single dose of antibiotic medication.

TERMINOLOGY REVIEW

Key Term	Word Parts	Definition
Clinical age		Method of timing in development that begins with the last menstrual period; 2 weeks more than developmental age.
Corpora cavernosa	*corpor/o-:* body *cav/o-:* hollow, cavity	Two dorsal columns of erectile tissue found in the penis.
Corpus albicans	*corp/o-:* body *alb/o-:* white	Scar tissue in the ovary that forms when the corpus luteum degenerates.
Corpus luteum	*corp/o-:* body *lute/o-:* yellow	The yellow structure that develops from the mature follicle after ovulation.
Corpus spongiosum	*corp/o-:* body	Ventral column of erectile tissue found in the penis.

TERMINOLOGY REVIEW —cont'd

Key Term	Word Parts	Definition
Developmental age		Method of timing in development that begins with fertilization; 2 weeks less than clinical age.
Ductus deferens	*duct/o-:* to lead or carry	Tubular structure that is continuous with the epididymis; it transports sperm from the epididymis to the ejaculatory duct.
Embryonic period	*embry/o-:* embryo	Stage of development that lasts from the beginning of the third week until the end of the eighth week after fertilization; period during which the organ systems develop in the body.
Endometrium	*endo-:* in; within *metri/o-:* uterus	Innermost mucous membrane layer of the uterine wall.
Epididymis		Tightly coiled tubule along the posterior margin of each testicle; functions in the maturation and storage of sperm.
Fetal period		Stage of development that starts at the beginning of the ninth week after fertilization and lasts until birth.
Gametes		Sex cells: sperm and ova.
Gestation	*gest/o-:* pregnancy	Time of prenatal development; pregnancy.
Gonads		Primary reproductive organs; organs that produce the gametes: testes in the male and ovaries in the female.
Interstitial cells	*inter-:* between	Cells between the seminiferous tubules in the testes; produce testosterone; also called *cells of Leydig.*
Lactation	*lact/o-:* milk	Milk production and ejection from the mammary glands.
Menarche	*men/o-:* menses; menstruation *-arche:* beginning	First period of menstrual bleeding at puberty.
Myometrium	*my/o-:* muscle *-metri-:* uterus	Thick middle layer of the uterus; it is composed of smooth muscle.
Oogenesis	*oo-:* egg, ovum *-genesis:* producing, forming	Process of meiosis in the female in which one ovum and three polar bodies are produced from one primary oocyte.
Oogonia	*oo-:* egg, ovum *-gon-:* seed	Stem cells that give rise to ova or egg cells.
Ovarian cycle	*ovario: ovary*	Monthly cycle of events that occur in the ovary from puberty to menopause; occurs concurrently with the uterine cycle.
Ovarian follicles	*ovario*: ovary	Oocytes surrounded by one or more layers of cells within the ovaries.
Parturition	*partum:* birth; labor	Act of giving birth to an infant.
Perimetrium	*peri-:* around *metri/o-:* uterus	Outermost layer of the uterus.
Postnatal development	*-nat/i-:* birth	Development that begins with birth and lasts until death.
Preembryonic period	*pre-:* before; in front of *embry/o:* embryo	First 2 weeks after fertilization; period of cleavage, implantation, and formation of primary germ layers.
Prenatal development	*pre-:* before; in front of *nat/i-:* birth	Development within the uterus.
Seminiferous tubules	*semin/i:* semen; seed *tub/o-:* tube	Tightly coiled structures within which sperm are produced in the testes.
Spermatogenesis	*spermat/o:* spermatozoa, sperm cells	Process of meiosis in the male in which four spermatids are produced from one primary spermatocyte.
Spermatogonia	*spermat/o:* spermatozoa, sperm cells *-gon-:* seed	Stem cells that give rise to sperm cells.
Spermiogenesis	*spermi/o:* spermatozoa, sperm cells *-genesis:* producing, forming	Morphologic changes that transform a spermatid into a mature sperm.
Stratum basale	*strat-:* layer	Bottom layer of the endometrium that is responsible for rebuilding the stratum functionale after menstruation.
Stratum functionale	*strat-:* layer	Portion of the endometrium that is sloughed off during menstruation.

Continued

TERMINOLOGY REVIEW —cont'd

Key Term	Word Parts	Definition
Uterine cycle	*uter/o:* uterus, womb	Monthly cycle of events that occur in the uterus from puberty to menopause; also called the *menstrual cycle;* occurs concurrently with the ovarian cycle.
Uterine tubes	*uter/o:* uterus	The tubes that extend laterally from the upper portion of the uterus to the region of the ovaries; also called *fallopian tubes* or *oviducts.*
Vulva	*vulv/o-:* vulva	Collective term for the external accessory structures of the female reproductive system; also called the *pudendum.*
Zygote	*zyg/o-:* union; pair; tied together	The single diploid cell that is a fertilized ovum.

Medical Asepsis and the OSHA Standard

Check out the Evolve site at http://evolve.elsevier.com/Bonewit/today to access additional interactive activities and exercises to help you study and prepare for success.

LEARNING OBJECTIVES

Microorganisms and Medical Asepsis

1. Define microorganism and give examples of types of microorganisms.
2. Explain the difference between a nonpathogen and a pathogen.
3. Define medical asepsis.
4. List the six basic requirements for growth and multiplication of microorganisms.
5. Outline the infection cycle, including the following:
   - List examples of the means of entry of pathogens into the body.
   - List and describe the means of transmission of pathogens from one person to another.
   - List examples of the means of exit of pathogens from the body.
6. List and explain the protective mechanisms the body uses to prevent the entrance of microorganisms.
7. Explain the difference between resident flora and transient flora.
8. State when each of the following is performed: handwashing, antiseptic handwashing, and use of an alcohol-based hand sanitizer.
9. Explain the difference between surgical gloves and exam gloves and when each should be worn.
10. State the advantages and disadvantages of the following types of gloves: latex, nitrile, and vinyl.
11. Explain why it is important to wear the correct size gloves.
12. Explain the purpose of a mask.
13. List and describe the three different types of masks used in the medical office.
14. List the guidelines that should be followed when using a mask.
15. Identify medical aseptic practices that should be followed in the medical office.

OSHA Bloodborne Pathogens Standard

16. Explain the purpose of the Occupational Safety and Health Administration (OSHA).
17. List and describe the elements that must be included in the OSHA exposure control plan.
18. Explain the purpose of the following OSHA requirements: labeling requirements and sharps injury log.
19. List the steps that must be performed following an exposure incident.
20. Define and provide examples of each of the following: engineering controls, work practice controls, personal protective equipment, and housekeeping procedures.
21. Identify the guidelines for use of personal protective equipment.

PROCEDURES

Handwashing.
Application of an alcohol-based hand sanitizer.
Determination of glove size.
Application and removal of disposable exam gloves.
Application and removal of a mask.

Adhere to the OSHA Bloodborne Pathogens Standard.

LEARNING OBJECTIVES

Regulated Medical Waste

22. List examples of regulated medical waste (RMW) and explain how to discard each type of waste.
23. Explain how to handle and dispose of RMW.

Bloodborne Diseases

24. Explain the differences between acute and chronic hepatitis B.
25. Explain the difference between acute and chronic hepatitis C.
26. List the means of transmission for hepatitis B and C.
27. Describe the treatment for hepatitis B and C.
28. Explain what occurs when HIV gains entrance into the body.
29. List the means of transmission for HIV.
30. List and describe the three types of HIV tests.
31. Describe the treatment for HIV-infected individuals.

PROCEDURES

Prepare RMW for pickup by a medical waste service.

CHAPTER OUTLINE

INTRODUCTION TO MEDICAL ASEPSIS AND THE OSHA STANDARD
MICROORGANISMS AND MEDICAL ASEPSIS
Growth Requirements for Microorganisms
INFECTION CYCLE
Components of the Infection Cycle
Infectious Agent
Reservoir Host
Portal of Exit
Mode of Transmission
Portal of Entry
Susceptible Host
Protective Mechanisms of the Body
MEDICAL ASEPSIS IN THE MEDICAL OFFICE
Hand Hygiene
Hand Hygiene Techniques
Medical Gloves
Glove Categories
Glove Sizing
Glove Guidelines
Masks
Types of Masks
Mask Guidelines
Infection Control
OSHA BLOODBORNE PATHOGENS STANDARD
Purpose of the Standard
OSHA Terminology
Components of the OSHA Standard
Exposure Control Plan
Labeling Requirements
Communicating Hazards to Employees
Record Keeping
Control Measures
Engineering Controls
Work Practice Controls
Personal Protective Equipment
Housekeeping Procedures
Hepatitis B Vaccination
REGULATED MEDICAL WASTE
Handling Regulated Medical Waste
Disposal of Regulated Medical Waste
BLOODBORNE DISEASES
Hepatitis B
Acute Hepatitis B
Chronic Hepatitis B
Transmission
Hepatitis B Vaccine
Treatment
Hepatitis C
Transmission
Treatment
HCV Testing Recommendations
Acquired Immunodeficiency Syndrome
Transmission
HIV Testing
Types of Tests
Treatment

KEY TERMS

acute infection
aerobe (AIR-obe)
anaerobe (AN-er-obe)
antiseptic
barrier protection
bloodborne disease
bloodborne pathogens
chronic infection
cilia (SIL-ee-ah)
contagious
contaminated
decontamination
exposure incident
hand hygiene
infection
infectious agent
infectious disease
medical asepsis
microorganism (MYE-kroe-OR-gan-iz-um)
nonintact skin
nonpathogens (non-PATH-oh-jen)

occupational exposure
opportunistic (OP-pore-tune-IS-tik) infection
optimum (OP-tuh-mum) growth temperature
other potentially infectious materials (OPIM)
parenteral (pare-EN-ter-al)
pathogen (PATH-oh-jen)
personal protective equipment
pH (PEE-AYCH)
regulated medical waste
reservoir host
resident flora (FLOE-ruh)
sharps
susceptible host
transient (TRAN-zee-ent) flora

INTRODUCTION TO MEDICAL ASEPSIS AND THE OSHA STANDARD

Medical asepsis and infection control are crucial in preventing the spread of disease. The medical assistant should always practice good medical aseptic techniques to provide a safe and healthy environment in the medical office. The Occupational Safety and Health Administration (OSHA) Bloodborne Pathogens Standard is important for infection control. This standard is required by the federal government to reduce the exposure of employees to infectious diseases. This chapter presents a thorough discussion of medical asepsis, infection control, the OSHA Bloodborne Pathogens Standard, and the bloodborne diseases that pose the greatest threat to the medical assistant.

MICROORGANISMS AND MEDICAL ASEPSIS

Microorganisms are tiny living plants or animals that cannot be seen with the naked eye, but instead must be viewed with the aid of a microscope. Common types of microorganisms include bacteria, viruses, fungi, protozoa, and parasites. Most microorganisms are harmless and do not cause disease. They are termed **nonpathogens.** Other microorganisms, known as **pathogens**, are harmful to the body and can cause disease.

In the medical office, practices must be employed to inhibit the growth and hinder the transmission of pathogenic microorganisms to prevent the spread of infection. These practices are known as *medical asepsis.* **Medical asepsis** means that an object or area is clean and free from disease-producing microorganisms (pathogens). Nonpathogens would still be present on a clean or medically aseptic object or surface, but all the pathogens would have been eliminated.

GROWTH REQUIREMENTS FOR MICROORGANISMS

For microorganisms to survive, certain growth requirements must be present in the environment, as follows:

1. *Proper nutrition.* Microorganisms that use inorganic or nonliving substances as sources of food are known as *autotrophs.* Microorganisms that use organic or living substances for food are known as *heterotrophs.*
2. *Oxygen.* Most microorganisms need oxygen to grow and multiply and are termed **aerobes.** Other microorganisms, known as **anaerobes**, grow best in the absence of oxygen.
3. *Temperature.* Each microorganism has a temperature at which it grows best, known as the **optimum growth temperature.** Most microorganisms grow best at 98.6°F (37°C), the human body temperature.
4. *Darkness.* Microorganisms grow best in darkness.
5. *Moisture.* Microorganisms need moisture for cell metabolism and to carry away wastes.
6. *pH.* The **pH** is the degree to which a solution is acidic or basic. Most microorganisms prefer a neutral pH. If the environment of the microorganisms becomes too acidic or too basic, they die.

If growth requirements are taken away from the environment of pathogenic microorganisms, they are unable to survive. Eliminating these conditions is one way to reduce the growth and transmission of pathogens in the medical office.

INFECTION CYCLE

Infection is the condition in which the body, or part of it, is invaded by a pathogen. In order for a pathogen to survive and spread disease, a continuous cycle must be followed; this is known as the *infection cycle* (Fig. 17.1). For an infection cycle to continue, pathogens must be able to leave an infected individual and survive transmission in the environment and then enter a noninfected individual where they grow and multiply. If the cycle is interrupted at any point, the pathogens die, and the cycle is broken. The medical assistant has a responsibility to help break this cycle in the medical office by practicing good techniques of medical asepsis. These techniques are discussed in the next section of this chapter.

COMPONENTS OF THE INFECTION CYCLE

The infection cycle is made up of six components linked together. Each of these components is described below.

1. Infectious Agent

An **infectious agent** is a pathogen capable of causing an infectious disease. Infectious agents are divided into groups and include bacteria, viruses, fungi, protozoa, and parasites. An **infectious disease** is a disease caused by the entrance into the body of an infectious agent where it grows and multiplies resulting in harmful effects to the host. Many infectious diseases are contagious. A **contagious disease** refers to a disease that is capable of being transmitted directly or indirectly from one person to another.

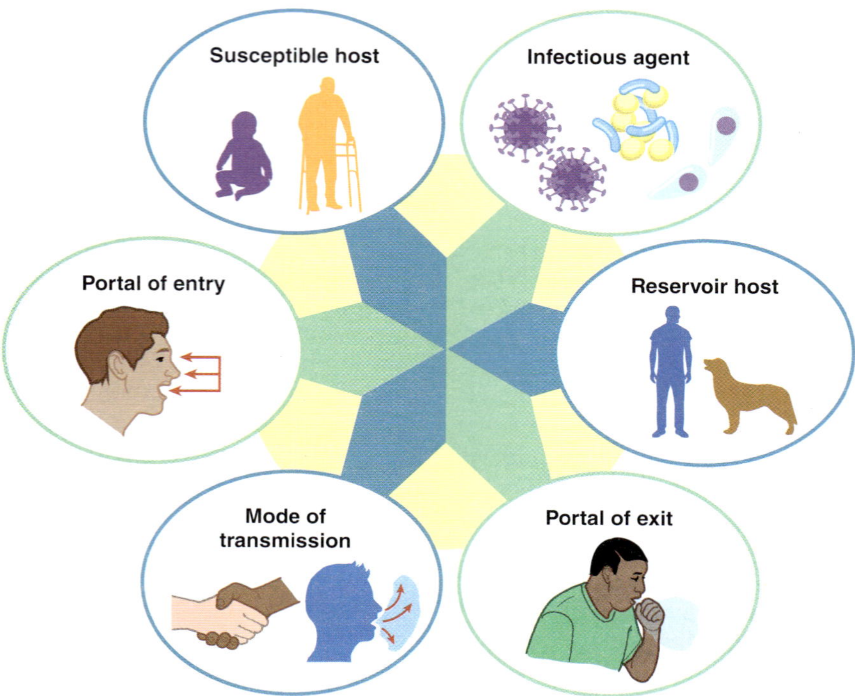

Fig. 17.1 The infection cycle.

2. Reservoir Host

The **reservoir host** is the location in which an infectious agent lives and usually grows and multiplies. Reservoir hosts include humans, animals, and the environment (e.g., soil, water, food). Many of the common infectious diseases have human reservoirs from which an infectious agent is transferred to a noninfected individual. Infectious diseases transmitted from human-to-human include influenza, COVID-19, sexually transmitted infections (STIs), and streptococcal infections. An example of an infectious disease that does not have a human reservoir is tetanus. The causative agent of tetanus is a bacterium known as *Clostridium tetani* which uses soil as its reservoir host and is spread from the soil to a human.

3. Portal of Exit

The portal of exit is the route from which an infectious agent leaves a reservoir host. For humans, the portal of exit includes the respiratory tract through coughing and sneezing; the gastrointestinal tract through fecal material, vomiting, and diarrhea; the genitourinary tract through sexual intercourse; and the skin through open wounds.

4. Mode of Transmission

The mode of transmission is the mechanism by which an infectious agent is spread to a susceptible host. To continue the infection cycle, the infectious agent must be transmitted from a portal of exit of a reservoir host to a portal of entry of a susceptible host. The two main categories of transmission include *direct transmission* and *indirect transmission* which can be further divided into subcategories which are discussed next.

Direct Transmission

Direct transmission involves the spread of an infectious disease through *direct contact transmission* or *droplet transmission*. With direct transmission, the infectious agent infects a susceptible host shortly after leaving the reservoir host. For direct transmission to occur, the reservoir host must be in close proximity with the susceptible host. Direct transmission includes the following subcategories.

Direct Contact Transmission

Direct contact transmission occurs when an infected individual has direct bodily contact with a susceptible host allowing the infectious agent to pass directly from an infected person to a noninfected person.

Direct contact transmission may occur through skin-to-skin contact such as touching an open wound that is infected. It may occur through kissing, which is the mode of transmission for mononucleosis. It may also occur through sexual intercourse, which is the mode of transmission for most STIs, such as chlamydia and gonorrhea.

Droplet Transmission

Droplet transmission is the primary mode of transmission for respiratory infections. Respiratory droplets consist of secretions of mucus and saliva that are exhaled by both healthy individuals and those with infectious respiratory diseases. Droplet transmission occurs when infectious agents carried by respiratory droplets are transmitted from an infected person to a noninfected person. Millions of respiratory droplets loaded with infectious agents are expelled into the air each time an infected individual breathes, speaks,

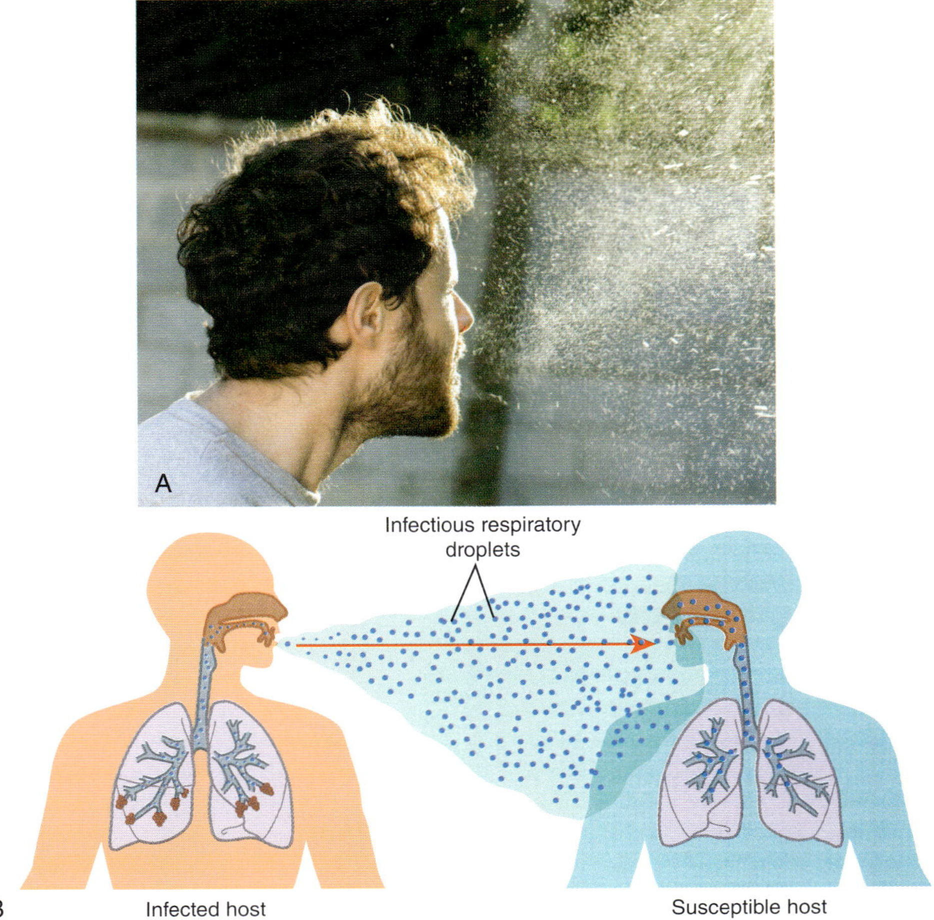

Fig. 17.2 (A) Millions of respiratory droplets are expelled into the air when an individual sneezes. (B) Droplet transmission occurs when infectious respiratory droplets are transmitted from an infected host to a susceptible host. (A, from iStock.com/pabst_ell.)

coughs, sneezes, sings, or shouts (Fig. 17.2A). These infectious droplets travel a short distance from the infected host where they can be inhaled into the respiratory tract by a susceptible host (Fig. 17.2B). The infectious droplets can also be deposited on the mucosal surfaces of the eyes, nose, or mouth of a susceptible host. The size of a respiratory droplet is larger than 5 micrometers in diameter.

Respiratory droplets are large and cannot usually travel more than 6 feet (2 meters) after leaving an infected host, with most droplets traveling less than 3 feet (1 meter). Because of this, droplet transmission requires close proximity between an infected individual and a noninfected individual. Droplet transmission is the primary mode of transmission for the following infectious diseases: common cold, influenza, RSV (respiratory syncytial virus) infection, and COVID-19 (coronavirus disease of 2019).

Respiratory droplets are too large to be airborne for very long and rapidly fall downward through the force of gravity, after being expelled from an infected host. The infectious droplets land on inanimate (nonliving) surfaces and contaminate them. The contaminated surface might then be touched by a susceptible host and transferred to a portal of entry of the host. This type of indirect transmission is known as *fomite transmission*, which is discussed in more detail in the next section.

Indirect Transmission

Indirect transmission is the spread of an infectious disease through microscopic airborne particles (droplet nuclei), contaminated surfaces, vehicles, and vectors. Indirect transmission requires an intermediatory between the portal of exit and the portal of entry for the infectious agents to continue the infection cycle, such as a doorknob contaminated with influenza viruses. With indirect transmission, the infected individual does not need to be in close proximity to the susceptible host for transmission to occur. Indirect transmission includes the subcategories listed and described next.

Airborne Transmission

Airborne transmission (also known as *aerosol transmission*) occurs when an infectious agent is transmitted from an infected host to a susceptible host on tiny airborne particles that float through the air. These microscopic airborne particles (also known as *aerosols*) result when some of the large respiratory

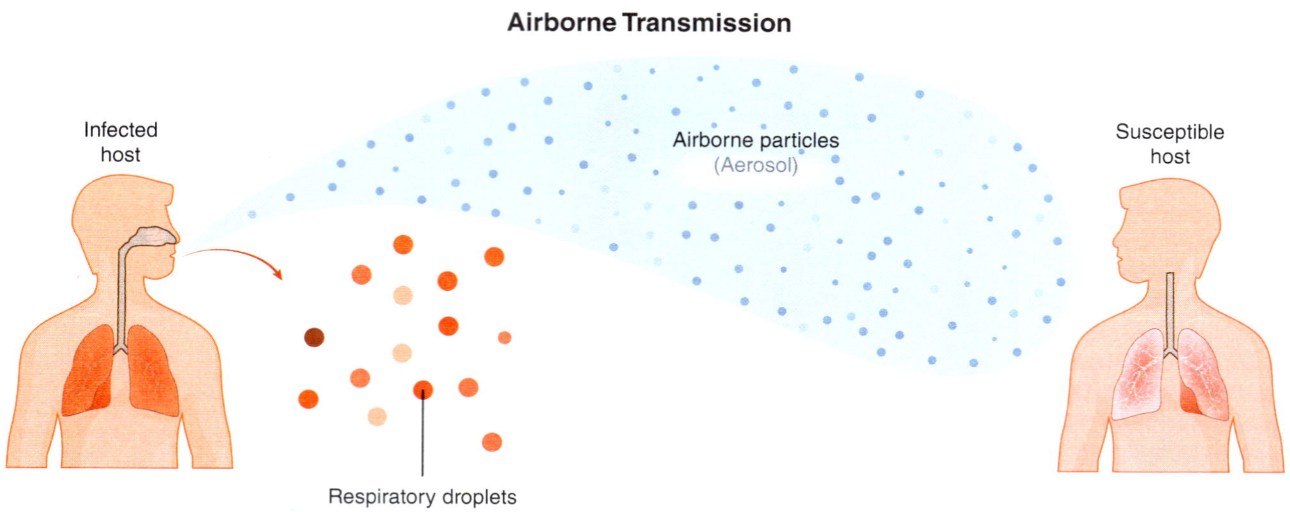

Fig. 17.3 Airborne transmission occurs when infectious agents are transmitted from an infected host to a susceptible host on tiny airborne particles. (Modified from Robinson DS: *Modern dental assisting*, ed 14, St. Louis, 2024, Elsevier.)

droplets in the air evaporate and dry out leaving microscopic airborne particles known as *droplet nuclei*; each droplet nuclei measures 5 micrometers or less. Because droplet nuclei are so tiny and lightweight, they can remain suspended in the air for longer periods of time and can travel greater distances than respiratory droplets (Fig. 17.3). In fact, infectious droplet nuclei can remain suspended in the air even after the infected person has left the area. As an example, measle viruses can remain suspended in the air for up to 18 hours after an infected person exhales them.

Infectious droplet nuclei suspended in the air can be inhaled into the respiratory tract by a susceptible host. This can occur over a short distance or a long distance, however the risk of transmission is greater when the susceptible host is in close proximity to the infected individual. The further the droplet nuclei travel from the infected individual, the lower the risk of infection.

The infectious droplet nuclei continue to float in the air and eventually settle on inanimate surfaces and contaminate them. The contaminated material may then be transferred to a portal of entry of a susceptible host through *fomite transmission* (discussed in more detail in the next section).

Because of their small size, infectious droplet nuclei are more likely to be inhaled deeply into the lower respiratory tract of a susceptible host than larger infectious respiratory droplets. In the lower respiratory tract, droplet nuclei can infect the lungs and alveolar tissue which may result in a serious illness such as pneumonia. Rooms that are poorly ventilated allow droplet nuclei to float in the air for a longer period of time; on the other hand, droplet nuclei scatter quickly if they are floating in an outdoor setting.

There are a limited number of diseases spread through airborne transmission; examples include tuberculosis, chickenpox (varicella), and measles (rubeola). Recent studies show that airborne transmission of COVID-19 may occur under certain conditions. These include being in a crowded indoor space with poor ventilation for a long period of time, especially if people are shouting, singing, coughing, or sneezing.

Fomite Transmission

Fomite transmission occurs indirectly when infectious droplets travel from an infected host to an inanimate surface (or fomite) and then are transmitted to a portal of entry of a susceptible host (Fig. 17.4). A *fomite* is defined as any inanimate surface or object that is likely to become contaminated with an infectious agent, such as a doorknob. The most common means of transmitting an infectious agent from a fomite to a susceptible host is through hand contact of a susceptible host with a fomite (Fig. 17.4B). For example, if a contaminated fomite is touched by a susceptible host followed by the host touching their eyes, nose, or mouth, the infectious agent can be transferred to the susceptible host and possibly result in an infectious disease. Infectious diseases that can be spread through fomite transmission include the common cold, influenza, and gastroenteritis.

Fomites include surfaces that are frequently touched by people, such as furniture, handrails, doorknobs, elevator buttons, computer keyboards, touch screens, mobile phones, faucet handles, light switches, countertops, and toilet seats. Some examples of fomites in the medical office include waiting room furniture and toys, examining tables, stethoscopes, electronic thermometers, blood pressure cuffs, and items that are not properly sterilized (e.g., operating scissors).

The length of time that an infectious agent can survive outside of a host on a fomite depends primarily on the type of infectious agent. Some pathogens can survive for only minutes, whereas others are hardier and can survive for days, weeks, or even months. HIV is extremely fragile in nature and dies almost instantly outside of the body. The influenza virus can survive on a fomite for up to 48 hours. Cold-causing rhinoviruses typically survive for only a day

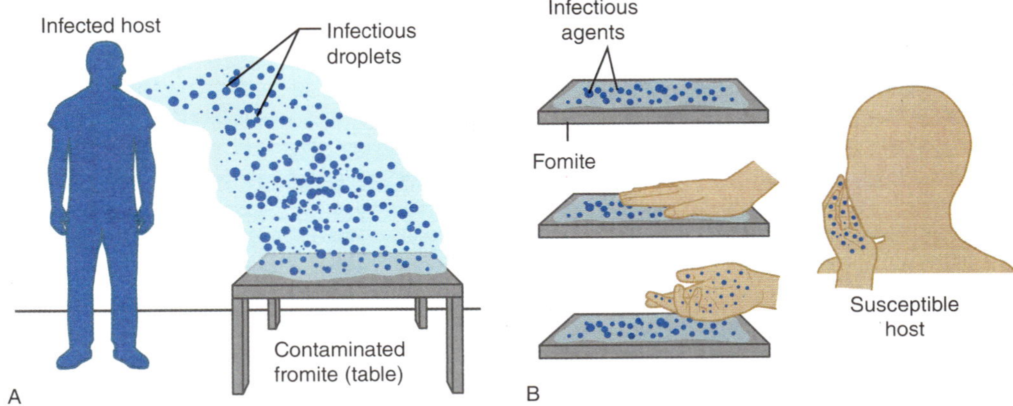

Fig. 17.4 Fomite transmission. (A) Infectious droplets travel from an infected host to a fomite. (B) The infectious agents are transmitted by hand contact to a susceptible host.

on a fomite. Infectious agents that can survive for a longer period of time include the hepatitis B virus, which can survive on a fomite for up to a week, and the rotavirus, which can survive on a fomite for up to 2 months.

Other Modes of Transmission

Vehicle-Borne Transmission

Vehicle-borne transmission occurs indirectly when infectious agents travel from an infected host to a susceptible host by way of a vehicle such as food, water, and soil. The vehicle provides an environment in which the infectious agent grows and multiplies or produces a toxin. Infectious diseases transmitted by vehicles include tetanus, hookworm, botulism, and *Escherichia coli* (*E. coli*) food poisoning.

Food is often a vehicle of transmission for pathogens of the gastrointestinal tract and upper respiratory tract. This is why transparent shields are often placed above food trays in a restaurant to prevent pathogens expelled through coughs and sneezes from contaminating the food.

Vector-Borne Transmission

Vector-borne transmission occurs indirectly when infectious agents travel from an infected host to a susceptible host by way of a vector. A *vector* is an organism that does not cause the disease itself but transmits infectious agents from one host to another. Vectors feed on infected hosts such as humans, animals, and birds. Vectors then harbor the infectious agents within their bodies and transmit them to susceptible human hosts, usually through a bite. Examples of vectors include mosquitos, ticks, fleas, and mites. Infectious diseases transmitted though vectors include Lyme disease, malaria, yellow fever, the plague, and typhus fever.

5. Portal of Entry

The portal of entry is the route by which infectious agents enter a host. Infectious agents often use the same portal to enter a host as they used to exit the reservoir host, which includes the respiratory tract, the gastrointestinal tract, the genitourinary tract, and the skin through open wounds. Infectious agents can also enter a host through a sharps injury, such as accidentally being stuck by a contaminated needle after administering an injection.

6. Susceptible Host

A **susceptible host** is the one who is capable of being infected by a pathogen. An infectious disease does not occur automatically when pathogens enter the body of a person whose immune system is functioning normally. Many times, individuals exposed to infectious agents never develop the infection. An individual must be susceptible to the infectious agent for an infection to occur. This means that the resistance or ability to fight off disease by the host is low.

Factors that contribute to low resistance and increased susceptibility to developing an infectious disease include:

- Poor health
- Poor hygiene
- Poor nutrition
- Illness
- Stress
- Younger children and elderly
- Immunocompromised

PROTECTIVE MECHANISMS OF THE BODY

The body has protective mechanisms in the form of physical and chemical barriers that help prevent the entrance of pathogens. These mechanisms are known as the *first line of defense* of the body; they help break the infection cycle and include the following.

1. The skin is the body's most important defense mechanism; it serves as a protective barrier against the entrance of pathogens.
2. The mucous membranes of the body, which line the nose and throat and respiratory, gastrointestinal, and genital tracts, help protect the body from invasion by pathogens.

3. Mucus and cilia in the nose and respiratory tract fight off pathogens. Mucus traps pathogens that enter the the respiratory tract and cilia removes them from the body. **Cilia** are slender hairlike projections attached to the epithelium of the respiratory tract. Cilia constantly beat in a wave-like motion to propel mucus with trapped pathogens toward the mouth. After reaching the mouth, the mucus is either swallowed or coughed up which results in the removal of the pathogens from the body.
4. Coughing and sneezing help force pathogens from the body.
5. Lysozyme is an enzyme present in tears, saliva, and sweat that destroys bacteria that attempt to enter the body.
6. Urine and vaginal secretions are acidic. Pathogens cannot grow in an acidic environment.
7. The stomach secretes hydrochloric acid, which helps in the process of digestion. This acidic environment discourages the growth of pathogens that enter the stomach.

BOX 17.1 CDC Guidelines for Hand Hygiene in Health Care Settings

Wash Hands with Soap and Water

- When the hands are visibly soiled
- After caring for a person with known or suspected infectious diarrhea
- After known or suspected exposure to spores (e.g. *B. anthracis, C. difficile* outbreaks)
- Before eating
- After using the restroom

Apply an Alcohol-Based Hand Sanitizer (or Wash Hands)

- Immediately before touching a patient
- Before performing an aseptic task or handling invasive medical devices
- Before moving from work on a soiled body site to a clean body site on the same patient
- After touching a patient or the patient's immediate environment
- After contact with blood, body fluids or contaminated surfaces as long as the hands are not visibly soiled
- Immediately after glove removal

MEDICAL ASEPSIS IN THE MEDICAL OFFICE

There are many important medical aseptic practices employed in the medical office to break the infection cycle and prevent the spread of infection. The most important of these practices are hand hygiene and the use of medical gloves and masks, which are each discussed in this section.

HAND HYGIENE

Hand hygiene refers to the process of cleansing or sanitizing the hands. Hand hygiene is considered the most important medical aseptic practice for preventing the spread of infection. According to the World Health Organization (WHO), appropriate hand hygiene can prevent up to 50% of avoidable infections acquired during healthcare delivery.

Specific techniques for sanitizing the hands in the medical office include the following:

- Handwashing with plain soap and water
- Handwashing with an antimicrobial soap and water
- Applying an alcohol-based hand sanitizer

The CDC has established recommendations for hand hygiene in health care settings. The purpose of these guidelines is to promote improved hand hygiene practices and to reduce transmission of pathogenic microorganisms to patients and employees in health care settings. The CDC guidelines for hand hygiene as they apply to the medical office are outlined in Box 17.1.

Resident and Transient Flora

Microorganisms residing on the skin can be classified into the following categories: resident flora and transient flora. **Resident flora** (also known as *normal flora*) normally resides and grows in the epidermis and deeper layers of the skin known as the *dermis*. Resident flora is usually harmless and nonpathogenic. Because resident flora is attached to the deeper skin layers, it is difficult to remove from the skin.

Transient flora lives and grows on the superficial skin layers, or epidermis. It is picked up on the hands during daily activities. In the medical office, this may include contact with an infected patient, contaminated equipment, or contaminated surfaces. Transient flora is often pathogenic, but because it is attached loosely to the skin, it can be removed easily from the hands with proper hand hygiene techniques.

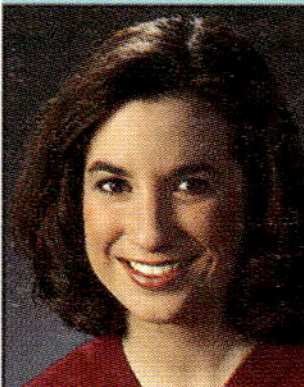

Putting It All Into Practice

My name is Jennifer, and I work for a large group of physicians in a multispecialty clinic. I work in both the front and back areas of the office. I really enjoy experiencing all these areas of the office, and I definitely never get bored.

The most interesting experience I have had as a practicing medical assistant is seeing the impact that I make in patients' lives. They rely on you and look to you first for help in their health care situation. You are most often the first person they come into contact with within the office, and they look to you for understanding and empathy. Patients who come to your office on a regular basis see you as a kind of family member. They appreciate a familiar face and a smile. Most often, you are the individual giving patients instructions concerning laboratory testing they will be having or medication they will be taking. Patients truly do count on your knowledge and assistance throughout their course of care. I was genuinely surprised at what an impact I could have on others. ■

Hand Hygiene Techniques

Hand hygiene techniques are essential in preventing the spread of disease in the medical office. It is important to follow the hand hygiene procedures exactly to ensure the removal of dirt and transient flora from the hands.

Handwashing

Handwashing refers to washing the hands with plain soap and water. Plain soap is available as a liquid or a solid bar and contains agents that help break down and emulsify dirt and oil present on the skin so it can be carried away. Soap sanitizes the hands through the physical removal of dirt and transient flora. It is important to use adequate friction during handwashing to ensure the removal of all transient flora. The CDC recommends that the hands be rubbed together vigorously for at least 20 seconds, making sure to cover all surfaces and to focus on the fingertips and fingernails. Procedure 17.1 outlines the handwashing procedure.

The CDC hand hygiene guidelines recommend that handwashing be performed when the hands are visibly soiled with dirt or body fluids, before eating, and after using the restroom (see Box 17.1). If the hands are not visibly soiled, the CDC recommends that an alcohol-based hand sanitizer, rather than handwashing, be used to sanitize the hands. This is because repeated handwashing tends to dry out the hands, leading to irritation, chapping, and dermatitis.

Antiseptic Handwashing

Washing the hands with an antimicrobial skin cleanser is termed *antiseptic handwashing.* Antimicrobial skin cleansers are available as a liquid or a solid bar. They contain an **antiseptic,** which is an agent that functions to kill or inhibit the growth of microorganisms (Fig. 17.5A). Antiseptic handwashing sanitizes the hands through mechanical scrubbing action and through the action of the antiseptic. Proper handwashing with an antimicrobial skin cleanser removes all soil and transient flora from the hands. Most antimicrobial skin cleansers also deposit an antibacterial film on the skin that discourages bacterial growth. The medical assistant should perform antiseptic handwashing before performing a sterile procedure or assisting with minor office surgery. An example of a common antiseptic contained in antimicrobial skin cleansers is chlorhexidine gluconate; brand names include Hibclens and DynaHex.

Alcohol-Based Hand Sanitizers

CDC guidelines recommend the use of an alcohol-based hand sanitizer (ABHS) for cleansing the hands when they are not visibly soiled. ABHSs, also known as *alcohol-based hand rubs,* consist of 60% to 95% alcohol (isopropanol or ethanol) and come in the forms of gels, foams, and sprays (Fig. 17.5B). Studies have shown that ABHSs are more effective than plain soap and water handwashing in removing transient flora and reducing bacterial counts on the hands. The advantages that ABHSs offer over traditional handwashing are as follows:

- ABHSs are usually more accessible than sinks.
- ABHSs do not require rinsing and hand drying with a towel.

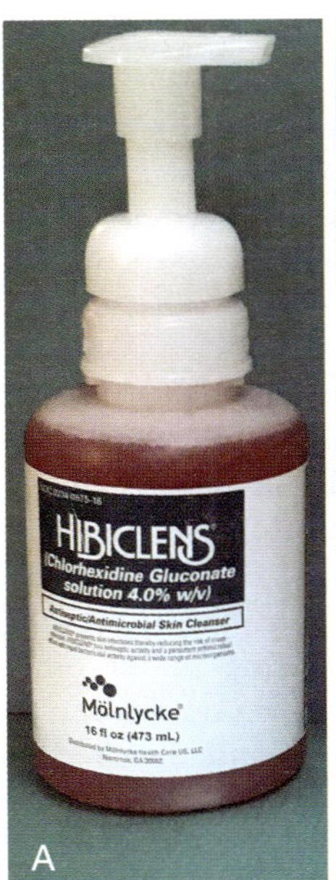

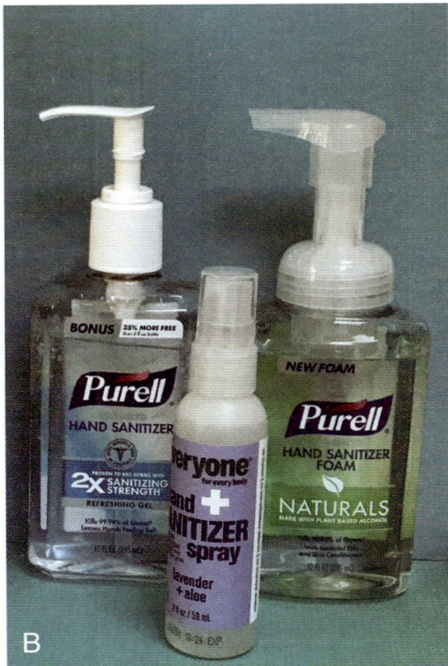

Fig. 17.5 (A) Antimicrobial skin cleanser. (B) Alcohol-based hand sanitizers.

- Less time is required to perform hand hygiene. It takes approximately 30 seconds to sanitize the hands with an ABHS compared with 1 to 2 minutes to perform proper handwashing.
- ABHSs are less damaging to the skin, resulting in less dryness and irritation. Most ABHSs contain emollients, which help prevent the skin of the hands from over drying. As the alcohol dries in the ABHS, protective fats and oils remain on the hands.

The disadvantage of ABHSs is that they cause a brief stinging sensation if applied to broken skin, such as a cut or abrasion on the hand. Because ABHSs are made up of 60% or more alcohol, they should be stored in a cool, well-ventilated place. They should not be stored near heat or ignition sources such as heating vents or wall outlets. Procedure 17.2 describes the proper steps for sanitizing the hands with an ABHS.

MEDICAL GLOVES

Medical gloves are essential in protecting health care workers and patients from infectious diseases. Gloves provide a physical barrier to protect against infection; this is known as **barrier protection**. The CDC recommends that medical gloves be worn when the health care worker is likely to come in contact with blood and other potentially infectious materials (OPIM); mucous membranes or nonintact skin; when performing vascular access procedures; and when handling or touching contaminated surfaces or items.

Medical gloves consist of a durable layer of material that forms a physical barrier between the health care worker's hands and the patient and/or contaminants. The glove material must be flexible, free from holes, breaches and cracks, and strong enough to prevent breakage during normal use.

Glove Categories

There are two categories of gloves used in the medical office: surgical gloves and exam gloves. The type of glove used depends on the procedure being performed. In general, surgical gloves are used for sterile procedures while exam gloves are used for aseptic procedures.

Surgical Gloves

Surgical gloves are disposable and sterile, meaning they are free of all microorganisms. They are designed to fit each hand separately and are manufactured to a higher standard than exam gloves to offer superior comfort, fit, strength, and flexibility. Surgical gloves are used by the medical assistant to perform sterile procedures (e.g., sterile dressing change) and to assist the provider during minor office surgery. They help prevent the patient from developing an infection following a sterile procedure and also reduce the risk of exposure of the medical assistant to blood and body fluids. Surgical gloves are discussed in more detail in Chapter 25: Minor Office Surgery.

Exam Gloves

Exam gloves are disposable, nonsterile, and ambidextrous, meaning the same design is used for both hands. They are used to protect against infection when performing certain procedures such as administering an injection, performing a venipuncture, or performing a urinalysis. Exam gloves are also worn to protect the medical assistant from pathogens when handling or touching contaminated surfaces or items such as cleaning up a blood spill or sanitizing contaminated instruments. Procedure 17.3 presents the proper method for applying and removing disposable exam gloves.

Types of Exam Gloves

There are three types of exam gloves commonly used in the medical office. They are categorized by the material making them up and include latex, nitrile, and vinyl.

1. Latex Gloves

Latex gloves are made from natural rubber latex (NRL), which is a milky liquid that is extracted from rubber trees. Latex gloves offer many advantages. They are highly durable and flexible, provide a high level of touch sensitivity, offer good barrier protection and are cost-effective. Latex gloves fit like a second skin which makes them comfortable to wear for an extended period.

The primary disadvantage of latex gloves is that they can cause an allergic reaction in individuals with a hypersensitivity to latex. A mild allergic reaction to latex causes the following symptoms: redness of the skin, urticaria (hives), and itching (Fig. 17.6). A more severe allergic reaction causes sneezing, itchy red eyes, runny nose, and asthma symptoms (shortness of breath, coughing, and wheezing). Symptoms typically begin within minutes after contact with the latex.

Anyone with frequent exposure to latex, such as a health care worker, is at a greater risk for developing a hypersensitivity to latex. The incidence of latex allergy in the general population tends to be low (1% to 6%), however the risk for health care workers developing a hypersensitivity to latex ranges from 8% to 12%. Because of this, most medical offices now use latex-free gloves. This protects both health care workers and patients with a hypersensitivity to latex.

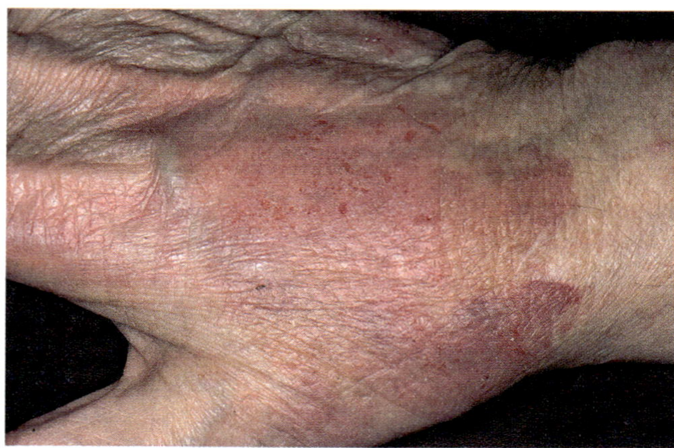

Fig. 17.6 Latex glove allergy. (From Goodman CC: *Pathology: implications for the physical therapist*, ed 3, St. Louis, 2010, Saunders.)

2. Nitrile Gloves

Nitrile gloves are made from a synthetic rubber that does not contain latex. They are highly durable, have a comfortable fit, offer excellent resistance to punctures, provide good barrier protection, and have a long shelf life. Based on these qualities, nitrile gloves are an ideal alternative when latex allergies are a concern. The primary disadvantage of nitrile gloves is that they are more expensive than either latex or vinyl gloves.

3. Vinyl Gloves

Vinyl gloves are made of polyvinyl chloride and were the first latex-free alternative to become available for health care workers with a latex allergy. They are easy to put on and take off and are low in cost. However, vinyl gloves have some disadvantages. They are not as elastic and flexible as latex and nitrile gloves. This causes them to fit loosely resulting in less comfort and dexterity when performing procedures. Vinyl gloves are also not as durable as other types of gloves, making them susceptible to tearing and puncturing when put under stress. Because of this, the barrier protection of vinyl gloves is not as reliable as latex and nitrile gloves. Based on these disadvantages, it is recommended that vinyl gloves be used for short-term procedures in which the medical assistant is not likely to come into contact with blood, or OPIM.

Glove Sizing

Gloves are required for many procedures performed in the medical office. To ensure adequate barrier protection when wearing gloves, it is essential that the medical assistant determine their correct glove size. Gloves that fit correctly feel comfortable and allow the medical assistant to perform procedures in the same way the procedures could be performed with the bare hands. Gloves that are too small may rip as they are applied or may become uncomfortable to wear. Gloves that are too large may make it difficult to perform procedures because the excess material will get in the way.

Surgical gloves are sized more precisely than exam gloves because they are usually worn for a longer period to perform procedures requiring exceptional dexterity. Surgical gloves are sized in numerical sizes that range from 5.5 to 9.0. Exam gloves are sized in lettered sizes and come in the following sizes: XS, S, M, L, XL.

Glove size is determined through a two-part process. The circumference of the widest part of the dominant hand is first measured to obtain an individual's approximate glove size. Next, the fit of the gloves in the approximate size is assessed to determine the exact glove size for that individual. The correct glove size may end up being a size larger or smaller than the approximate size obtained through the hand measurement. This is because glove size can vary based on certain factors, such as the shape of the hand, shape and length of the fingers, material making up the glove, and the brand of the glove. The procedure for determining glove size is presented in Box 17.2.

BOX 17.2 Determination of Glove Size

1. Remove all rings. Extend the dominant hand. The dominant hand is preferred because the muscles in this hand are more developed resulting in a larger measurement than the nondominant hand.
2. Measure the circumference in inches of the widest part of the palm of your dominant hand by placing a cloth tape measure around the hand just below your knuckles. A cloth tape measure should be used because it will not stretch during the measurement. *(Note: It may be easier to ask another individual to perform this step of the procedure.)*

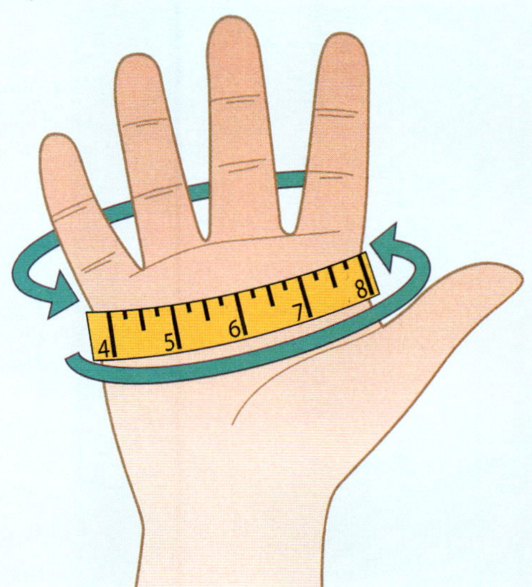

3. Determine your approximate glove size as follows:
   A. **Surgical gloves:** Round the hand measurement to the nearest whole or half-inch and convert it to a decimal number (For example 7¼ inches is rounded to 7½ inches and converted to 7.5; therefore, 7.5 is the approximate glove size).
   B. **Exam gloves:** Round the number to the nearest whole inch. Translate this number to the appropriate letter size using the General Exam Glove Sizing Chart provided here. (For example, 7½ inches is rounded to 8 inches which translates to an M glove size).
   (Note: If the manufacturer includes a brand-specific sizing chart on their glove box or on their website it should be used instead of the General Chart.)
4. Don a pair of gloves in the approximate size determined through the hand measurement.
5. Perform the following assessment to determine your correct glove size:
   A. **Correctly Fitted Gloves:**
   If the fit of your gloves meets these criteria, this is your correct glove size.
   - The gloves are snug on your hand without restricting movements.
   - The gloves are comfortable and fit like a second skin.
   - You can move your fingers normally without stretching the gloves too much as you move and flex your fingers.

   B. **Gloves Are Too Large:**
   If your gloves are too large, one or more of the criteria listed below will be evident. Obtain the next size smaller and repeat the assessment. If necessary, repeat this step until you have determined your correct glove size.
   - When applying the gloves, they do not have to stretch very much to fit your hands.
   - Wrinkles are observed around your palms and the rest of the glove bunches up around your wrists.
   - Your fingertips do not reach the end of the gloves leaving material dangling at the end of each finger.

   C. **Gloves Are Too Small:**
   If your gloves are too small, one or more of the criteria listed below will be evident. Obtain the next size larger and repeat the assessment. If necessary, repeat this step until you have determined your correct glove size.
   - When applying the gloves, they must stretch significantly for your hands to fit inside.
   - The fingertips of the gloves press against your fingers and may even puncture through the gloves.
   - The gloves are uncomfortable, and movements are stifled by the gloves.

General Chart: Exam Glove Sizing

Hand Measurement (in inches)	Exam Glove Size
6	XS
7	S
8	M
9	L
10	XL

Glove Guidelines

The medical assistant should adhere to the following glove guidelines to ensure proper barrier protection:

1. Wear the correct size glove to ensure a snug and comfortable fit and to avoid hand fatigue.
2. Wear gloves if contact with blood or OPIM, mucous membranes, and nonintact skin could occur.
3. Keep fingernails trimmed short (less than ¼ inch long) to reduce the risk of tearing the gloves during application and use.
4. If gloves become contaminated, torn, or punctured, replace them as soon as practicable.
5. Remove gloves after caring for a patient. Do not wear the same pair of gloves for the care of more than one patient.
6. Sanitize the hands after removing gloves regardless of whether or not the gloves are visibly contaminated. Pathogens may gain access to the medical assistant's hands through small defects in the gloves or by contamination of the hands during glove removal.
7. Do not store gloves in areas where there are extremes in temperatures (e.g., near a heater or an air conditioner). These conditions can cause deterioration of the gloves resulting in glove defects which, in turn, may not provide adequate barrier protection.

MASKS

In the medical office, disposable masks are an important means of protecting medical assistants and patients from infectious respiratory diseases spread through respiratory droplets and airborne particles. Masks provide a physical barrier over the mouth and nose that greatly reduces the number of pathogens inhaled or exhaled. This lessens the risk of infectious disease transmission between infected and noninfected individuals. Masks also protect the medical assistant from splashes and sprays of blood and body fluids. Since the COVID-19 pandemic, many medical offices now require patients to wear a mask during their office visits, especially if they are exhibiting signs or symptoms of illness.

The effectiveness of a mask depends on the thickness of the mask and the fit of the mask. Masks that consist of three or more layers are more effective in filtering pathogens than those made up of only one or two layers. It is important that the mask fits properly on the wearer's face. It should completely cover the mouth and nose and be held securely in place on the face with elastic head straps, ear loops, or other means. Most disposable masks have a flexible metal nosepiece or nose strip along the top of the mask to mold the mask to the bridge of the nose. This prevents air that may contain infectious agents from leaking in or out of the top of the mask. It also prevents fogging of eyeglasses.

Types of Masks

There are several different types of disposable masks used in the medical office. Each type covers the wearer's mouth and nose but offers a different level of protection based on the design of the mask. Masks used in the medical office are categorized below by their level of protection starting with the highest level of protection.

1. N95 mask
2. KN95 mask
3. Medical mask

N95 Mask

An N95 mask (also known as an *N95 respirator*) is a mask that offers the highest level of protection (Fig. 17.7A). An N95 mask filters out both large respiratory droplets and microscopic airborne particles (droplet nuclei). In fact, when worn correctly, an N95 mask filters out 95% or more of all airborne particles. If the medical assistant also needs protection from splashes and sprays of blood and body fluids, an *N95 surgical mask* should be used. A N95 surgical mask looks identical and functions the same as an N95 mask but is also fluid resistant.

An N95 mask is disposable and typically consists of five layers of material made up of polypropylene fibers. Polypropylene is a durable plastic that is breathable, water-resistant, lightweight and is a good filter of airborne contaminants.

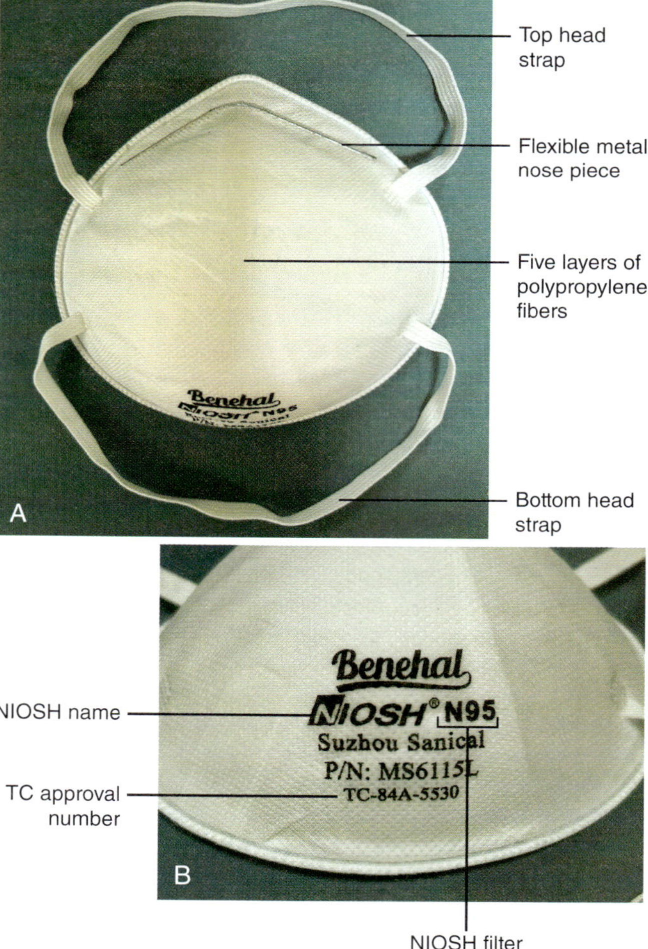

Fig. 17.7 (A) N95 mask. (B) NIOSH approval information.

Depending on the brand, an N95 mask may come in only one size, or have sizes ranging from small to large.

A proper fit is essential to ensure the high level of protection offered by an N95 mask. An N95 mask is designed with two elastic head straps and a flexible metal nosepiece along the top of the mask. These features function in forming a tight seal between the edges of the mask and the wearer's face. This ensures that almost all the inhaled and exhaled air is directed through the filter layers of the mask with minimal air leakage around the edges of the mask.

An N95 mask should feel snug to the wearer with no visible gaps along the edges of the mask. Gaps prevent a good seal which allows airborne particles to leak in and out around the edges of the mask. Gaps can be caused by jewelry, eyeglasses, facial hair, scalp hair and clothing. Most gaps can be eliminated by removing or adjusting the obstruction causing the gap. Facial hair causing gaps (e.g., beard) should be trimmed or removed (if possible) until a tight seal is attained. Each time an N95 mask is applied, a *seal check* should be performed to determine if the mask fits properly. The procedures for the application and removal of a flat-fold and cup N95 mask and the procedure for performing a seal check are outlined in Box 17.3.

BOX 17.3 Application of an N95 Mask

1. Pull back your hair (if needed) and secure it with a hair band so that it does not become tangled in the head straps of the mask. If you wear glasses, remove them.
2. Sanitize your hands.
3. Remove an N95 mask from the box and unfold it, if needed.
4. Inspect the mask for manufacturing defects such as tears and holes and damage to the head straps and nosepiece. If defects are present, replace the mask with a new one.
5. Cup the mask in one hand, with the flexible metal nosepiece resting near your fingertips.
6. Position the head straps facing towards the floor so they hang freely below your hand and are not tangled or twisted.

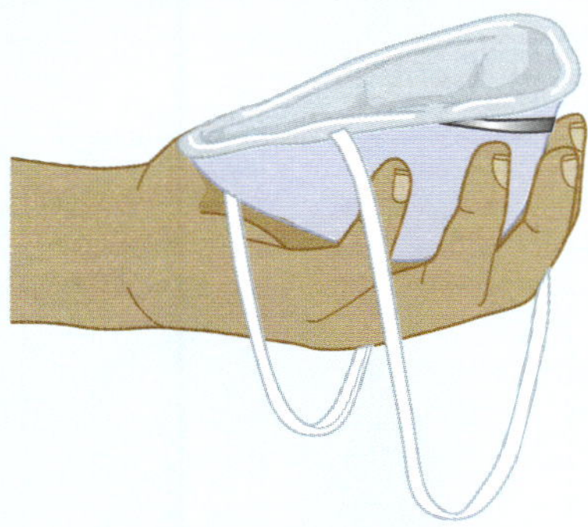

7. Place the mask over your nose and mouth with the bottom of the mask under your chin and the nosepiece positioned over the bridge of your nose.
8. While holding the mask in place, pull the top strap over your head with your free hand and position it at the crown of your head.

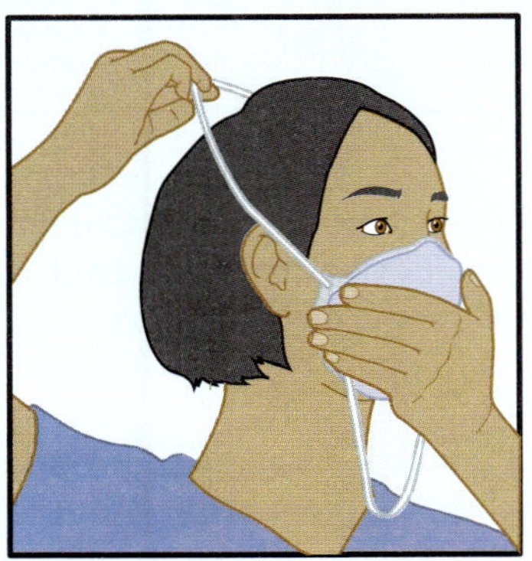

9. Continue to hold the mask in place and pull the bottom strap over your head and position it around your upper neck and below your ears. The bottom strap should be worn under (not over) your hair.

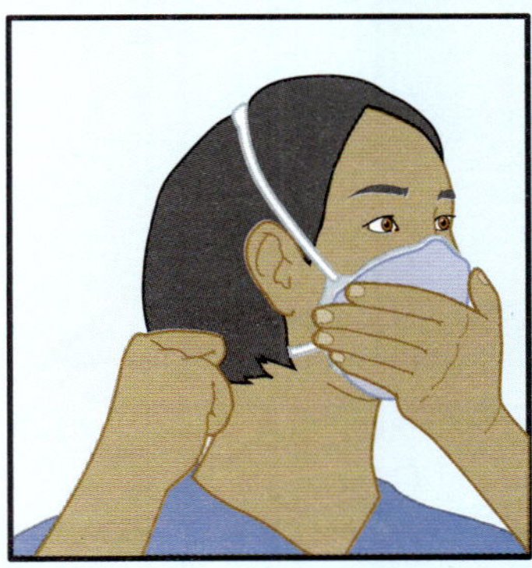

10. Adjust the straps to lie flat around your head, making sure they are not overlapping, tangled, or twisted.
11. Adjust the mask using both hands to make sure it is correctly positioned under your chin with the nosepiece over the bridge of the nose.
12. Use the first two fingertips of both hands to firmly mold the nosepiece to conform to the shape of your nose bridge. Start at the center of the nosepiece and press inwards while moving your fingertips down both sides of the nosepiece. Repeat this step, as needed, to ensure a good seal. Pinching the nosepiece with only one hand is not recommended as it may result in an inadequate seal around the nose area.

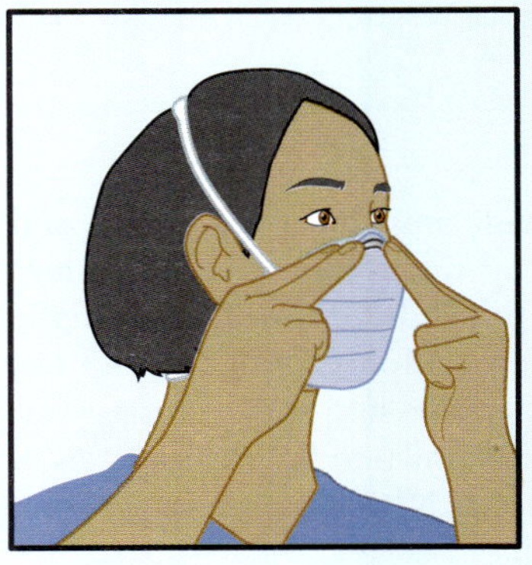

Continued

BOX 17.3 Application of an N95 Mask—cont'd

13. If you wear glasses, put them back on, making sure to position them over (not under) the top of the mask.
14. Use a mirror to check the placement of the mask and further adjust the mask, as needed, to ensure a snug fit. Check for gaps between the edges of the mask and your face and eliminate them if present.

Perform a Seal Check

1. Place both hands over your mask, covering as much surface area as possible.
2. Inhale quickly and then forcefully exhale. If your mask fits properly, it will bulge slightly upon exhalation and warm air will be felt coming out the front of the mask.

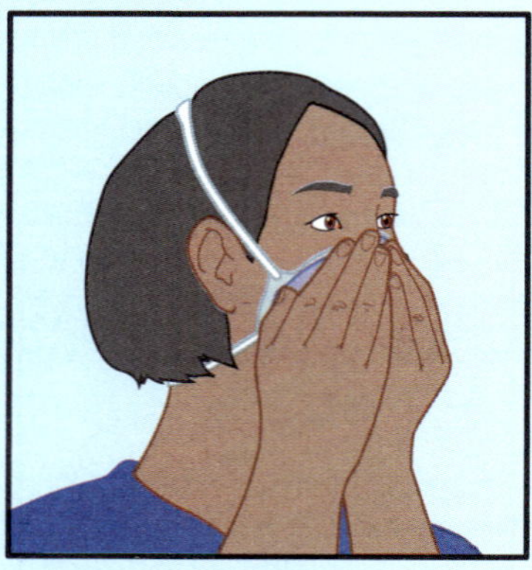

3. Cup your hands around the outside edges of the mask and continue to inhale and exhale.
4. Feel for air leakage around the edges of the mask during exhalation. If air leakage is felt, readjust the straps making sure they are positioned correctly at the crown of your head and around your upper neck.
5. Feel for air leakage around the nosepiece during exhalation. If air leakage is felt (or your glasses fog up), remold the nosepiece to the bridge of your nose using additional pressure.
6. Interpret the seal check results:
   a. If no air leakage is felt, you have performed a successful seal check and your mask fits properly.
   b. If air leakage is felt, the mask does not fit properly. Readjust your mask and repeat the seal check procedure. If air leakage still occurs, try a different shape or size of mask until one is found that provides a tight seal.

Removal of an N95 Mask

1. If you wear glasses, remove them.
2. Sanitize your hands.
3. Tilt your head slightly forward during mask removal. Grasp the bottom strap of the mask on each side with your hands. Pull the bottom strap outward from the head and then lift the strap over your head without touching the mask. Let go of the bottom strap of the mask. *(Note: Only the head straps should be touched during mask removal to prevent coming in contact with any infectious contaminants that may be on the mask.)*

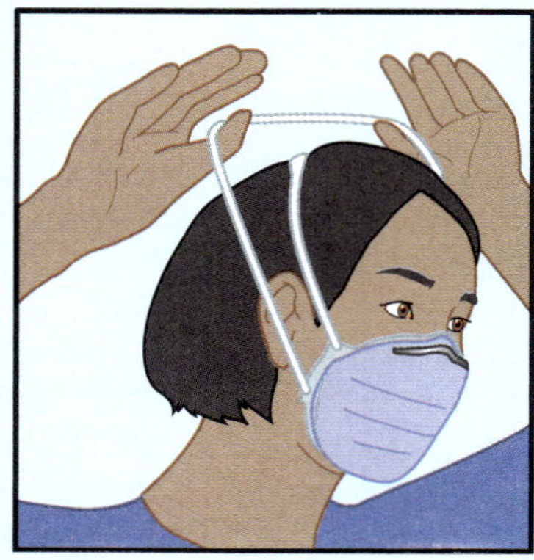

4. Grasp the top strap of the mask on each side with your hands. Pull the top strap outward from the head and then slowly and carefully lift the strap over your head. Continue to hold onto the top strap and allow the mask to fall forward away from your face.

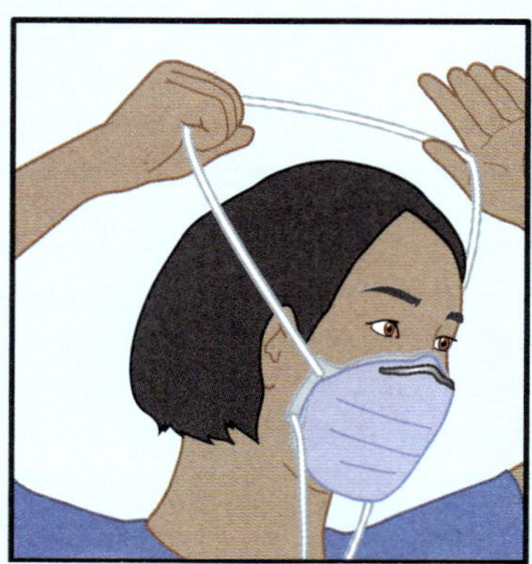

5. Immediately dispose of the mask by the top strap in a waste receptacle making sure not to touch the mask.
6. Sanitize your hands and, if needed, put your glasses back on.

An N95 mask must meet the quality and performance standards set by the National Institute for Occupational Safety and Health (NIOSH) which is a division of the Centers for Disease Control (CDC). NIOSH tests and certifies N95 masks to make sure they filter out at least 95% of airborne particles down to 0.3 micrometers in diameter. An N95 mask that has NIOSH approval will have the NIOSH name in capital block letters, the NIOSH filter designation (N95), and the TC (testing and certification) approval number printed on the outside of the mask (Fig. 17.7B).

KN95 Mask

A KN95 mask (also known as a *KN95 respirator*) is a disposable mask intended to provide the same level of protection

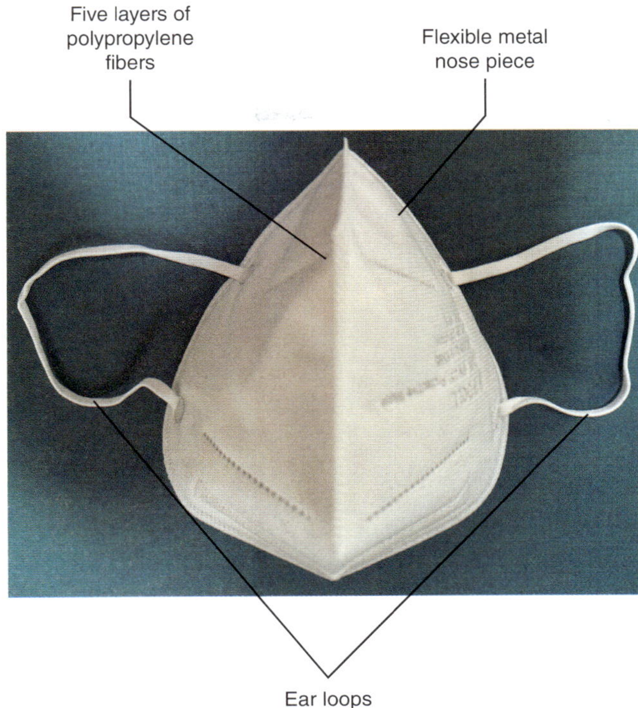

Fig. 17.8 KN95 mask.

as an N95 mask; however, KN95 masks are not NIOSH approved. This is because KN95 masks are manufactured outside the United States and follow different regulatory structures which tend to be less stringent than those set forth by NIOSH. This may result in a K95 mask not providing the same level of protection as an N95 mask. In addition, a KN95 mask usually attaches to the head with ear loops rather than head straps (Fig. 17.8). This prevents a KN95 mask from sealing as tightly to the contours of the face as the head straps of an N95 mask. As with an N95 mask, a KN95 mask consists of five layers of polypropylene fibers and has a flexible metal nosepiece along the top of the mask to mold the mask to the bridge of the nose.

A KN95 mask is applied in a similar manner as an N95 mask except for the steps involved in securing the mask to the face. The KN95 mask is cupped in one hand and placed over the nose and mouth and then secured to the face with ear loops which are placed over the ears one at a time. A KN95 mask is removed following the same procedure used to remove a medical mask (refer to Box 17.4).

Medical Masks

Medical masks (also known as surgical masks) are loose-fitting, disposable masks (Fig. 17.9) that create a physical barrier between the mouth and nose of the wearer and contaminants in the environment. If worn properly, a medical mask can block large-particle respiratory droplets from coughs and sneezes as well as splashes and sprays of blood and body fluids. Unfortunately, medical masks are not designed to provide the wearer with a reliable level of protection against small airborne particles. This is because the mask does not fit tightly against the face resulting in gaps between the mask and the face. These gaps allow small airborne particles, which may carry infectious agents, to enter and leave the mask.

A medical mask is rectangular in shape with pleats. The pleats allow the wearer to expand and curve the mask so that it can cover the area from the chin to the bridge of the nose. A medical mask consists of three layers of polypropylene with the middle layer serving as a filter. The outward facing side of the mask is usually colored (e.g., blue, green, yellow) for ease in identifying the front of the mask. There is a flexible metal nose strip along the top of the mask for molding the mask to the bridge of the nose. This provides a good seal around the nose area. There are two elastic ear loops attached to the four corners of the mask to hold the mask in place on the face. A seal check does not need to be performed with a medical mask since the edges of the mask are not meant to fit tightly against the face. The procedure for application and removal of a medical mask is presented in Box 17.4.

Mask Guidelines

Guidelines that should be followed when using a mask include the following:

1. Choose a mask that provides a level of protection appropriate for your work activities and the environment. For example, the CDC recommends wearing a mask with a high level of protection (N95 mask) when caring for a patient with suspected or confirmed COVID-19.
2. Read the manufacturer's instructions to determine the following: level of protection provided, instructions for use, application and removal procedures, storage conditions, and shelf life.
3. Inspect all parts of the mask before use for damage such as tears and holes. If present, discard the mask and replace it with a new one; a damaged mask may not provide adequate protection.
4. Sanitize your hands before putting on a mask.
5. To prevent fogging of eyeglasses, try pulling the mask further up over your nose and rest your eyeglasses on top of the mask. This blocks air from escaping out of the top of the mask which can cause eyeglasses to fog up. Over-the-counter anti-fogging eyeglass sprays, gels, and wipes are also available which disperse fog droplets on eyeglasses.
6. Do not pull the mask up on your forehead or down under your nose or chin while wearing it because your mouth and/or nose will no longer be protected from environmental contaminants.
7. Remove and replace your mask if it becomes damaged or deformed; no longer forms an effective seal to the face; becomes damp or visibly dirty; breathing becomes difficult; or if it becomes contaminated with blood, respiratory or nasal secretions, or other bodily fluids from patients.

BOX 17.4 Application of a Medical Mask

1. Pin back your hair (if needed) so that it is not covering your ears which can interfere with the application of the ear loops. If you wear glasses, remove them.
2. Sanitize your hands.
3. Remove a mask from the box.
4. Inspect the mask for manufacturing defects such as tears or holes and damage to the ear loops and nose strip. If damage is present, replace the mask with a new one.
5. Determine which side of the mask is the front. The colored side of the mask is the front and should face outwards, while the white side is the inside of the mask which touches your face.
6. Determine which side of the mask is the top. This is the edge of the mask where the flexible metal nose strip is located.
7. Hold the mask in front of your face by the ear loops with the colored side facing outward and the nose strip at the top of the mask.
8. Secure the mask to your face by placing the ear loops around your ears.

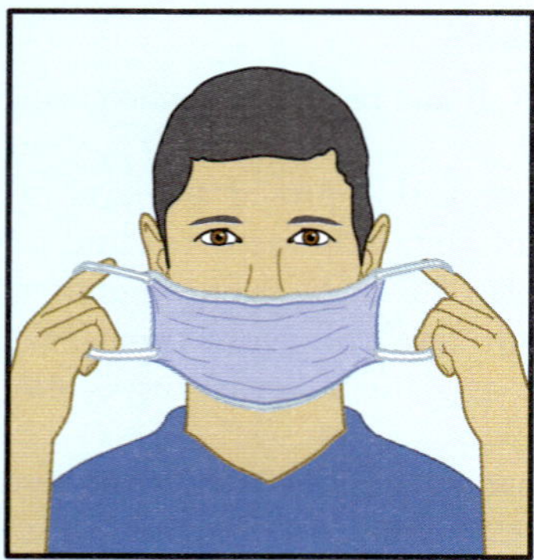

9. Adjust the mask on your face with both hands using the pleats and ear loops to ensure a good fit. The mask should be positioned over your nose and mouth with the bottom of the mask under your chin and the nosepiece positioned over the bridge of your nose. Avoid touching the inside of the mask.
10. Pinch the metal nose strip with the index finger and thumb of one hand to mold it to the bridge of your nose. Repeat this step as many times as necessary to attain a good seal.

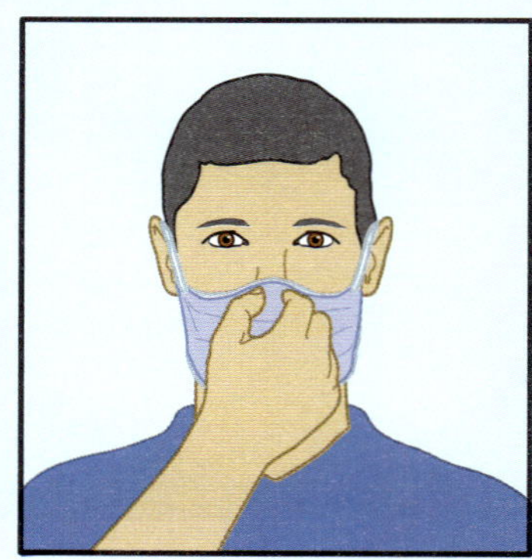

11. If you wear glasses, put them back on making sure to position them over (not under) the top of the mask.

Removal of a Medical Mask

1. If you wear glasses, remove them.
2. Sanitize your hands.
3. Lift the ear loops off the ears at the same time without touching the mask.
4. Remove the mask slowly and carefully from your face using the ear loops.
5. Continue holding the mask by the ear loops and immediately dispose of it in a waste receptacle making sure not to touch the mask
6. Sanitize your hands and, if needed, put your glasses back on.

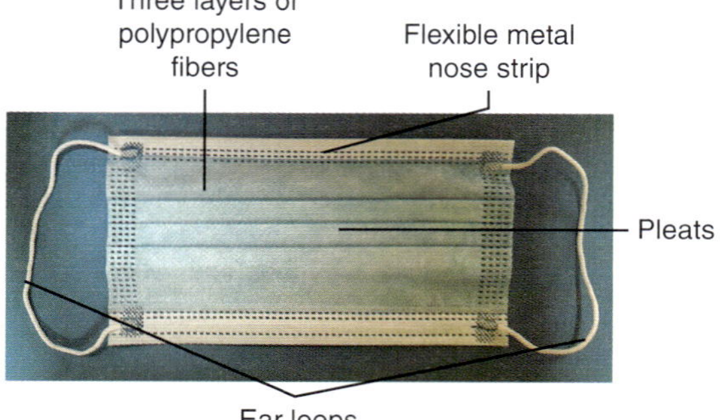

Fig. 17.9 Medical mask.

8. Do not touch your mask or your face while removing your mask.
9. Sanitize your hands immediately after removing the mask.
10. Ideally (as recommended by the CDC), masks used in a health care setting should be discarded after each patient encounter.

INFECTION CONTROL

In addition to hand hygiene and glove and mask protection, other good aseptic practices to control infection in the medical office include the following:

1. Follow the OSHA Bloodborne Pathogens Standard (presented in this chapter).
2. Keep the medical office free from dirt and dust, which can collect and carry pathogens.
3. Ensure that the reception area and examining rooms are well ventilated. Poorly ventilated rooms encourage microorganisms to settle on objects.
4. Keep the reception area and examining rooms bright and airy. Light discourages the growth of microorganisms.
5. Eliminate insects. Insects are a means of transmission of pathogens.
6. Carefully dispose of wastes, such as urine, feces, and respiratory secretions; all wastes should be handled as though they contain pathogens.
7. Do not let soiled items touch your clothing.

8. Avoid coughs and sneezes of patients. Respiratory droplets expelled from the respiratory tract during coughing and sneezing may contain pathogens.
9. Use discretion in the amount of jewelry worn; wear minimal jewelry or no jewelry at all. Pathogens can become lodged in the grooves and crevices of jewelry and serve as a means of transmission of pathogens.
10. Teach patients aseptic practices to control the spread of infection at home.

OSHA BLOODBORNE PATHOGENS STANDARD

PURPOSE OF THE STANDARD

The federal government established the Occupational Safety and Health Administration (OSHA) to assist employers in providing a safe and healthy working environment for their employees. To provide a safe working environment for health care workers, OSHA developed a comprehensive set of regulations known as the *OSHA Occupational Exposure to Bloodborne Pathogens Standard.* These regulations went into effect in 1992 and are designed to reduce the risk to employees of exposure to infectious diseases.

The OSHA Bloodborne Pathogens Standard must be followed by any employee with occupational exposure to pathogens, regardless of the place of employment. In addition to medical assistants, examples of other employees with occupational exposure include providers, nurses, dentists, dental hygienists, medical laboratory personnel, and emergency medical technicians. Employees who may have less obvious occupational exposure are correctional and law enforcement officers, firefighters, hospital laundry workers, morticians, and custodians.

Failure by employers to comply with the OSHA Bloodborne Pathogens Standard could result in a citation carrying a maximum penalty of $7000 for each violation and a maximum penalty of $70,000 for repeat violations.

What Would You Do? What Would You *Not* Do?

Case Study 1

Petra Meyer has come in for her annual gynecologic examination. Because Petra has been feeling tired and run-down, the provider orders blood to be drawn for a complete blood count (CBC) and a comprehensive blood chemistry profile. Petra indicates that she wears latex gloves when house-cleaning to protect her hands from the chemicals in her cleaning solution. Petra says that the last two times she cleaned her house, she experienced redness and itching of her hands along with a runny nose and red itchy eyes. She wants to know if this might be caused by breathing in the cleaning solution or getting some of it on her hands after taking off her gloves. Petra says she also experienced redness and itching of her feet the last time she wore her rubber flip flops. ■

OSHA TERMINOLOGY

The following definitions help clarify terms related to the OSHA Bloodborne Pathogens Standard.

OPIM (Other potentially infectious materials)*:* Body fluids, tissues, and organs from a human that can spread infection which include the following:
- Semen and vaginal secretions
- Cerebrospinal, synovial, pleural, pericardial, peritoneal, and amniotic fluids
- Any body fluid that is visibly contaminated with blood
- Any body fluid that has not been identified
- Saliva in dental procedures
- Any fixed human tissue or organ
- Any cell, tissue, or organ cultures known to be HIV infected

Bloodborne pathogens*:* Pathogenic microorganisms present in human blood that can cause disease in humans. Bloodborne pathogens include, but are not limited to, hepatitis B virus (HBV), hepatitis C virus (HCV), and human immunodeficiency virus (HIV).

Occupational exposure*:* Reasonably anticipated skin, eye, mucous membrane, or parenteral contact with blood or OPIM that may result from the performance of an employee's duties.

Sharps*:* Sharps are objects that can penetrate the skin, including (but not limited to) needles, lancets, scalpels, broken glass, and broken capillary tubes.

Parenteral*:* Piercing of the skin barrier or mucous membranes, such as through needlesticks, human bites, cuts, and abrasions.

Contaminated*:* The presence or reasonably anticipated presence of blood or OPIM on an item or surface.

Decontamination: The use of physical or chemical means to remove, inactivate, or destroy bloodborne pathogens on a surface or item to the point where they are no longer capable of transmitting infectious particles, and the surface or item is rendered safe for handling, use, or disposal.

Nonintact skin*:* Skin that has a break in its surface. It includes, but is not limited to, skin with dermatitis, abrasions, cuts, burns, hangnails, chapping, and acne.

Exposure incident*:* A specific eye, mouth, or other mucous membrane, nonintact skin, or parenteral contact with blood or OPIM that results from the performance of an employee's duties.

COMPONENTS OF THE OSHA STANDARD

The OSHA Occupational Exposure to Bloodborne Pathogens Standard is presented in the following text as it pertains to the medical office. The OSHA Standard includes the following categories:
- Exposure control plan
- Labeling requirements
- Communication of hazards to employees
- Record keeping

Exposure Control Plan

The OSHA Standard requires that the medical office develop an exposure control plan (ECP). The ECP is a written document stipulating the protective measures that must be followed in that medical office to eliminate or minimize employee exposure to bloodborne pathogens and OPIM. The ECP must be made available for review by all medical office staff. The ECP must include the following sections:

1. *Exposure Determination.* The purpose of this section of the ECP is to identify employees who must receive OSHA Standard training, PPE, hepatitis vaccination, and other protections required by the OSHA Bloodborne Pathogens Standard. The exposure determination must include (1) a list of all job classifications in which *all* employees are likely to have occupational exposure, such as providers, medical assistants, and laboratory technicians, and (2) a list of job classifications in which only *some* employees have occupational exposure, such as custodians. For the second classification of jobs, the determination must include a list of tasks in which occupational exposure may occur, such as emptying the trash or disinfecting a laboratory counter.
2. *Method of Compliance.* The method of compliance section of the ECP must document the specific health and safety control measures that are taken in the medical office to eliminate or minimize the risk of occupational exposure. These measures are extremely important in reducing the risk of infectious disease for the medical assistant and are discussed in greater detail later in this section (see the section on *Control Measures*).
3. *Postexposure Evaluation and Follow-up Procedures.* The postexposure evaluation and follow-up section must specify the procedures to follow in the event of an exposure incident in the medical office, including the method of documenting and investigating an exposure incident and the postexposure evaluation, medical treatment, and follow-up that would be made available to the employee (Box 17.5).

OSHA requires employers to review and update their ECP at least annually to ensure that the plan remains current with the latest information on eliminating or reducing exposure to bloodborne pathogens. The ECP also must be updated whenever necessary to reflect new or modified tasks and procedures performed in the medical office that affect occupational exposure.

BOX 17.5 OSHA Postexposure Evaluation and Follow-up Procedures

An exposure incident is a specific eye, nose, mouth, or other mucous membrane, nonintact skin, or parenteral contact with blood or other potentially infectious materials that results from an employee's duties. In the event of an exposure incident involving bloodborne pathogens or other potentially infectious materials (OPIM), OSHA requires the following steps to be performed:

1. Perform initial first aid measures immediately (e.g., wash a needlestick injury thoroughly with soap and water).
2. Document the route of exposure and the conditions and circumstances of the exposure incident. This includes such information as the engineering controls, the work practice controls, and PPE being used at the time of the incident.
3. Identify and document the source individual (unless the employer can establish that identification is not feasible or is prohibited by state or local law). A *source individual* is any person, living or dead, whose blood or OPIM may be a source of occupational exposure to the health care worker.
4. Obtain consent to test the source individual's blood. Test it as soon as possible to determine hepatitis B virus (HBV), hepatitis C virus (HCV), and human immunodeficiency virus (HIV) infectivity. The following guidelines apply to this requirement:
   - If consent is not obtained, the employer must document that legally required consent cannot be obtained.
   - If the source individual's consent is not required by law, the source individual's blood (if available) must be tested and the results documented.
   - If the source individual is already known to be infected with HBV, HCV, or HIV, testing does not need to be repeated.
5. Provide the exposed employee with the source individual's test results. Inform the employee of applicable laws and regulations concerning disclosure of the identity and infectious status of the source individual.
6. Obtain consent to test the employee's blood. Collect and test the blood of the employee as soon as possible for HBV, HCV, and HIV.
7. When medically indicated, provide the employee with appropriate postexposure prophylaxis, as recommended by the U.S. Public Health Service.

Labeling Requirements

The OSHA Bloodborne Pathogens Standard requires that containers and appliances containing biohazardous materials be labeled with a *biohazard warning label.* The biohazard warning label must be fluorescent orange or orange red in color and must contain the biohazard symbol and the word *BIOHAZARD* in a contrasting color (Fig. 17.10A).

A warning label must be attached to the following: (1) containers of regulated medical waste; (2) refrigerators and freezers used to store blood and OPIM; and (3) containers and bags used to store, transport, or ship blood or OPIM (Fig. 17.10B). Red biohazard bags or red sharps containers may be substituted for biohazard warning labels. The labeling requirement is designed to alert employees to possible exposure, particularly in situations in which the nature of the material or contents is not readily identifiable, such as blood or OPIM.

Communicating Hazards to Employees

According to the OSHA Standard, employers must ensure that all medical office employees with risk of occupational exposure participate in a training program. This program must present the ECP for the medical office while focusing on the measures that employees are to take for their safety.

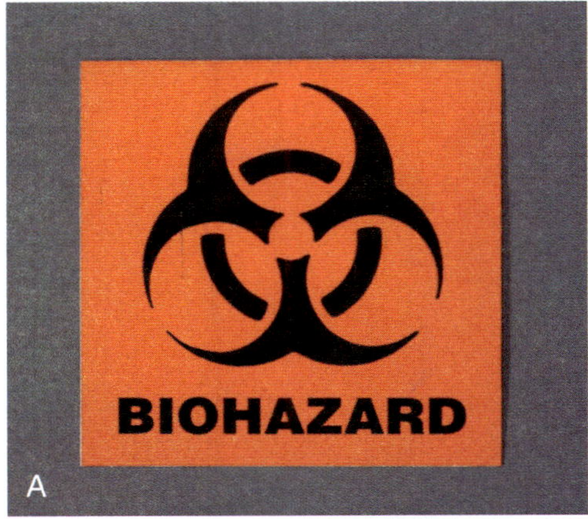

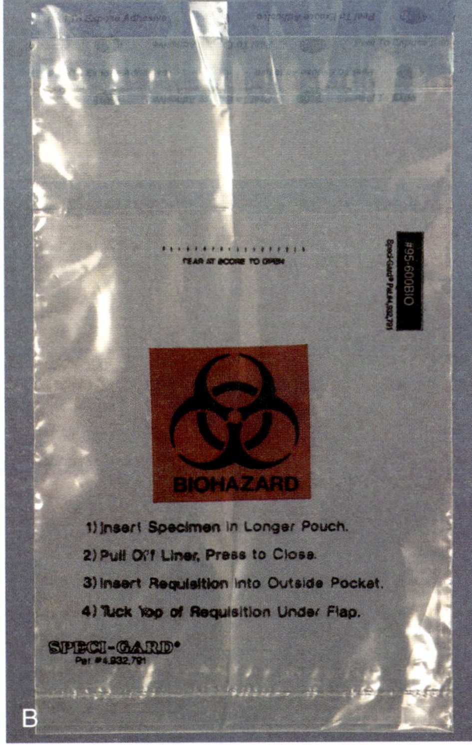

Fig. 17.10 (A) Biohazard warning label. (B) Biohazard bag used to hold and transport blood or other potentially infectious materials.

Training must be provided at the time an employee is initially assigned to tasks in which occupational exposure may occur and at least annually thereafter.

The employer must maintain records of the training sessions, which must include presentation dates, content of the sessions, names and qualifications of the trainers, and names and job titles of employees who attended. These records must be maintained for 3 years from the date of the training session.

Record Keeping

The OSHA Bloodborne Pathogens Standard requires that the following records be maintained:

1. *OSHA Medical Record.* The OSHA Standard requires that the employer maintain an accurate OSHA record of every medical office employee at risk for occupational exposure. These records must be kept confidential except for review by OSHA officials and as required by law. The OSHA medical record must include the following: employee's name; hepatitis B vaccination status, including dates of vaccination; results of any postexposure examinations, medical testing, and follow-up procedures; and a written evaluation of any exposure incident along with a copy of the exposure incident report.
2. *Sharps Injury Log.* Employers with more than 10 employees at risk for occupational exposure are required to maintain a log of injuries from contaminated sharps. The log must be maintained in a way that protects the confidentiality of injured employees (e.g., removal of personal identification). The purpose of the log is to help employers and employees keep track of all needlestick injuries. This tracking helps in identifying problem areas that need attention or any ineffective devices that need to be replaced. The sharps injury log must contain the following information:
   - Type and brand of device involved in the injury
   - Location of the incident (i.e., work area)
   - Explanation of how the incident occurred

CONTROL MEASURES

Specific health and safety control measures are required by the OSHA Standard to eliminate or minimize the risk of occupational exposure in the medical office. These measures are divided into five categories: engineering controls, work practice controls, personal protective equipment, housekeeping, and hepatitis B vaccination.

Engineering Controls

The medical office must use engineering controls to eliminate or minimize the risk of occupational exposure. *Engineering controls* include all control measures and devices that isolate or remove the bloodborne pathogens hazard from the workplace. They are considered a first line of defense for avoiding exposure to bloodborne pathogens and OPIM. Engineering controls must be examined and maintained or replaced as required to ensure their effectiveness. Examples of engineering controls include readily accessible handwashing facilities, safer medical devices, biohazard sharps containers, and biohazard bags.

Safer Medical Devices

Safer medical devices are an example of an engineering control. A *safer medical device* is a device that, based on reasonable judgment, would make an exposure incident involving a contaminated sharp less likely. *Reasonable judgment* refers to the judgment of the health care worker who would be using the device.

Safer medical devices include sharps with engineered sharps injury protection and needleless systems. A *sharp with engineered sharps injury protection (SESIP)* is a nonneedle sharp or a needle device with a built-in safety feature

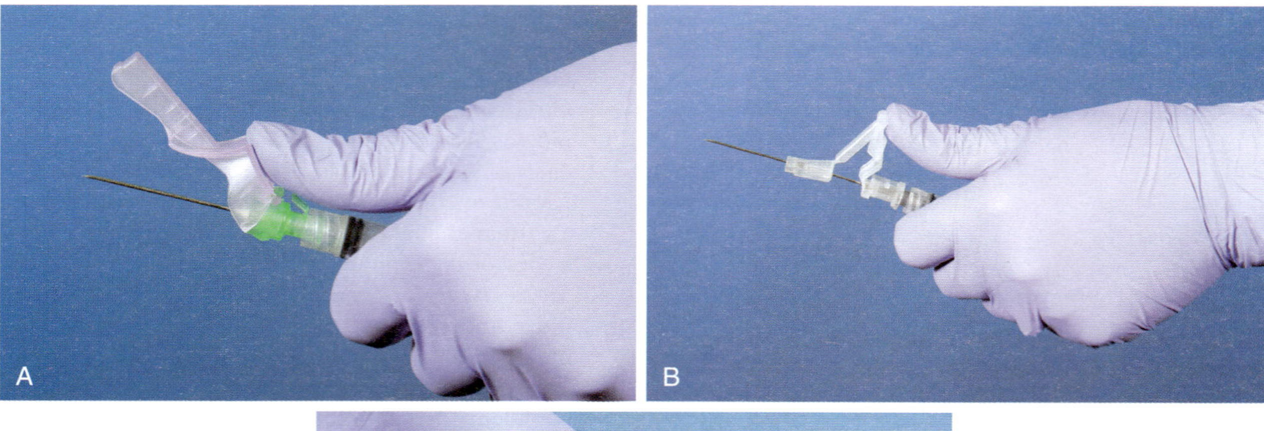

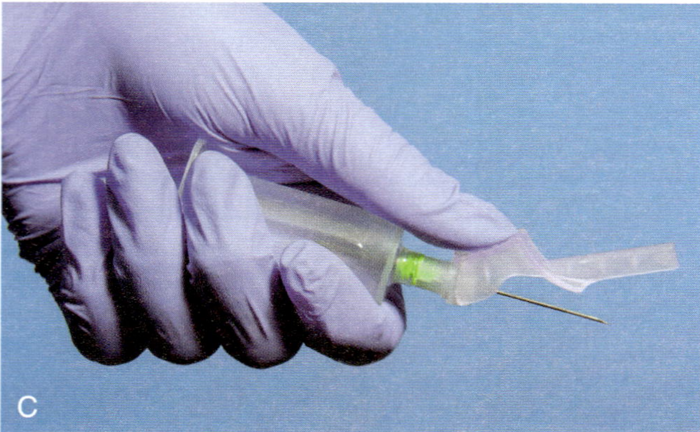

Fig. 17.11 (A, B) Safety-engineered syringes. (C) Safety-engineered phlebotomy device.

used for procedures that involve the risk of sharps injury. Examples of SESIPs include safety-engineered syringes and phlebotomy devices (Fig. 17.11).

Work Practice Controls

Work practice controls are controls that reduce the likelihood of an exposure incident by altering the manner in which the technique is performed. It is important that the medical assistant consistently adhere to these safety rules, which include the following:

1. Perform all procedures involving blood or OPIM in a manner that minimizes splashing, spraying, spattering, and generation of droplets of these substances.
2. Observe warning labels on biohazard containers and appliances. Bags or containers that bear a biohazard warning label or are color-coded red indicate that they hold blood or OPIM. Refrigerators, freezers, and other appliances that contain hazardous materials also must bear a biohazard warning label.
3. Bandage cuts and other lesions on the hands before gloving.
4. Sanitize the hands after removing gloves, regardless of whether or not the gloves are visibly contaminated.
5. If your hands or other skin surfaces come in contact with blood or OPIM, thoroughly wash the area as soon as possible with soap and water.
6. If your mucous membranes (e.g., eyes, mouth, nose) come in contact with blood or OPIM, flush them with water as soon as possible.
7. Do not break or shear contaminated needles.
8. Do not remove, recap, or bend a contaminated needle. (*Note:* Sterile needles may be recapped, such as after the withdrawal of medication from a vial or ampule.)
9. Immediately after use, place contaminated sharps in a puncture-resistant, leakproof container that is appropriately labeled or color-coded red to alert employees that the contents are hazardous. *Contaminated sharps* are contaminated objects that can penetrate the skin, including (but not limited to) contaminated needles, lancets, scalpels, broken glass, and capillary tubes.
10. Do not eat, drink, smoke, apply cosmetics or lip balm, or handle contact lenses in areas where you may be exposed to blood or OPIM.
11. Do not store food or drinks in refrigerators, freezers, or cabinets or on shelves or countertops where blood or OPIM are present.
12. Place blood specimens or OPIM in containers that prevent leakage during collection, handling, processing, storage, transport, or shipping. Ensure that the containers are closed before they are stored, transported, or shipped, and are labeled or color-coded for easy identification.
13. Before any equipment that might be contaminated is serviced or shipped for repair or cleaning, such as a centrifuge, it must be inspected for blood or OPIM. If such material is present, the equipment must be decontaminated. If it cannot be decontaminated, it must be

appropriately labeled to indicate clearly the contamination site, to enable those coming into contact with the equipment to take appropriate precautions.

14. If you are exposed to blood or OPIM, perform first aid measures immediately (e.g., wash a needlestick injury thoroughly with soap and water). After taking these measures, report the incident to your provider-employer as soon as possible so that postexposure procedures can be instituted (see Box 17.5). The most obvious exposure incident is a needlestick, but any eye, mouth, or other mucous membrane, nonintact skin, or parenteral contact with blood or OPIM constitutes an exposure incident and should be reported.

Personal Protective Equipment

The OSHA Standard specifies that personal protective equipment (PPE) must be used in the medical office whenever occupational exposure remains after engineering and work practice controls have been instituted. **Personal protective equipment** is specialized clothing or equipment worn by an employee for protection against a hazard. In the health care setting, PPE protects an individual from contact with blood and OPIM. Examples of PPE include gloves, masks, chin-length face shields, protective eyewear, laboratory coats, and gowns. The type of protective equipment appropriate for a given task depends on the degree of exposure that is anticipated, as outlined here:

1. Wear gloves when it is reasonably anticipated that your hands will have contact with blood and OPIM, mucous membranes, or nonintact skin; when performing vascular access procedures; and when handling or touching contaminated surfaces or items. Gloves cannot prevent a needlestick or other sharps injury, but they can prevent a pathogen from entering the body through a break in the skin, such as a cut, abrasion, burn, or rash.
2. Wear chin-length face shields or masks in combination with eye-protection devices whenever splashes, spray, spatter, or droplets of blood or OPIM may be generated, posing a hazard through contact with the eyes, nose, or mouth (e.g., removing a stopper from a tube of blood, transferring serum from whole blood).
3. Wear appropriate protective clothing, such as gowns, aprons, and laboratory coats, when gross contamination can reasonably be anticipated during performance of a task or procedure (e.g., laboratory testing procedures). The type of protective clothing needed depends on the task and degree of exposure anticipated.

Personal Protective Equipment Guidelines

Certain guidelines must be followed when using PPE:

1. PPE must not allow blood or OPIM to pass through or reach the skin, underlying garments (e.g., scrubs, street clothes, undergarments), eyes, mouth, or other mucous membranes under normal conditions of use and for the duration of time the protective equipment is used.
2. The employer must provide appropriate PPE at no cost to the health care worker. The employer is responsible for ensuring that the equipment is available in appropriate sizes, is readily accessible, and is used correctly. In addition, the employer must ensure that the equipment is cleaned, laundered, repaired, replaced, or disposed of as necessary to ensure its effectiveness.

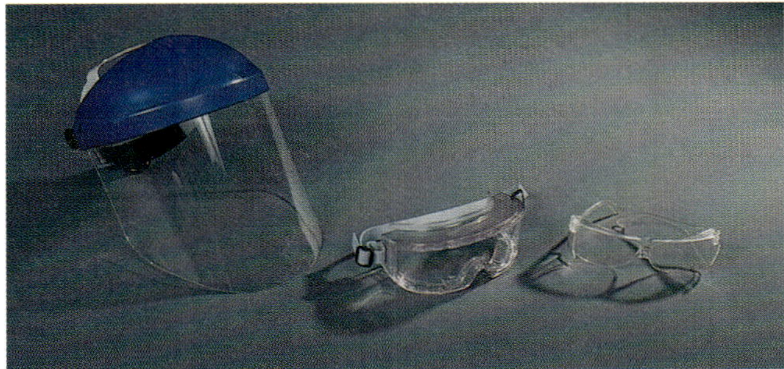

Fig. 17.12 Examples of eye-protection devices. *Left,* Face shield; *center,* safety goggles; *right,* safety glasses with solid side shields.

3. If the medical office utilizes latex gloves, latex-free alternatives must be provided for employees who are allergic to latex gloves. Examples of alternatives include nitrile and vinyl gloves.
4. If gloves become contaminated, torn, or punctured, replace them as soon as practical.
5. All eye-protection devices must have solid side shields; chin-length face shields, safety goggles, and safety glasses with solid side shields are acceptable (Fig. 17.12). Standard prescription eyeglasses are unacceptable as eye protection devices.
6. If a garment (e.g., laboratory coat) is penetrated by blood or OPIM, it must be removed as soon as possible and placed in an appropriately designated container for washing.
7. All PPE must be removed before you leave the medical office.
8. When protective equipment (e.g., masks, protective eyewear) is removed, it must be placed in an appropriately designated area or container for disposal, decontamination, washing or storage.
9. Utility gloves may be decontaminated and reused unless they are cracked, peeling, torn, or punctured or no longer provide barrier protection.

Housekeeping Procedures

The OSHA Standard requires that specific housekeeping procedures be followed to ensure that the work site is maintained in a clean and sanitary condition. The medical office must develop and implement a written schedule for cleaning and decontaminating each area where exposure occurs. The cleaning and decontamination method must be specified for each task and should be based on the type of surface to be cleaned, the type of soil present, and the tasks or procedures being performed in that area. Housekeeping procedures include the following:

1. Clean and decontaminate equipment and work surface (e.g., laboratory counter) after completing procedures that involve blood or OPIM. Cleaning is accomplished

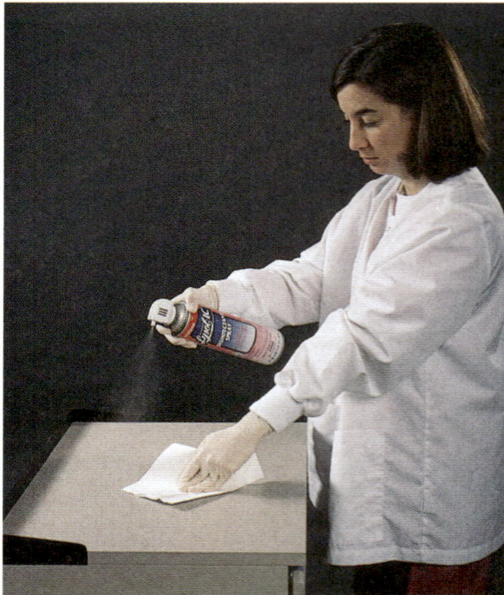

Fig. 17.13 Clean and decontaminate work surfaces with an appropriate disinfectant after completing procedures involving blood and other potentially infectious materials.

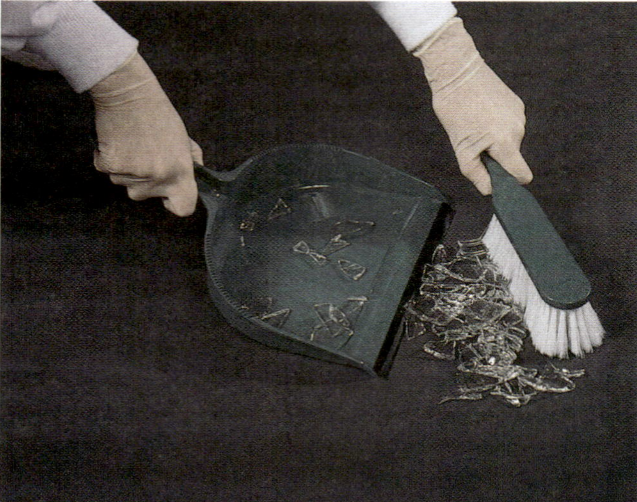

Fig. 17.14 Use mechanical means to pick up broken contaminated glass.

using plain soap, and decontamination is performed using an appropriate disinfectant (Fig. 17.13).

2. Clean and decontaminate all equipment and work surfaces as soon as possible after exposure to blood or OPIM. For decontamination of blood spills, OSHA recommends the use of a 10% solution of sodium hypochlorite (household bleach) in water (1 part bleach to 9 parts water).
3. Do not pick up broken, contaminated glassware with the hands, even if gloves are worn. Use mechanical means, such as a brush and dustpan, tongs, and forceps (Fig. 17.14).
4. Handle contaminated laundry as little as possible and with appropriate PPE. Place all contaminated laundry in leakproof bags that are properly labeled or color-coded.

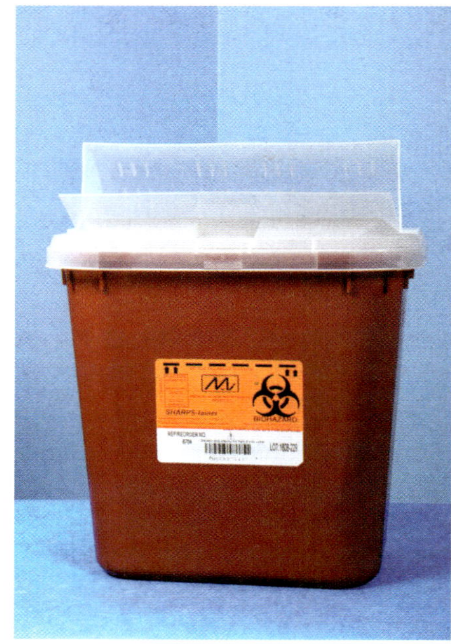

Fig. 17.15 Biohazard sharps container.

Contaminated laundry must not be sorted or rinsed at the medical office.

5. If the outside of a biohazard container becomes contaminated, it must be placed in a second suitable container.
6. Biohazard sharps containers (Fig. 17.15) must be closable, puncture resistant, and leakproof. They must bear a biohazard warning label and must be color-coded red to ensure identification of the contents as hazardous. To ensure effectiveness, the following guidelines must be observed:
   - Locate the sharps container as close as possible to the area of use to avoid the hazard of transporting a contaminated needle through the workplace.
   - Maintain sharps containers in an upright position to keep liquid and sharps inside.
   - Do not reach into a sharps container with your hand.
   - Replace sharps containers on a regular basis, and do not allow them to overfill. (It is recommended that sharps containers be replaced when they are three-quarters full.)

What Would You Do? What Would You *Not* Do?

Case Study 2

Tracy Smith is pregnant and is at the medical office to have her blood drawn for a prenatal profile. Tracy says she has been reading information about the hepatitis B vaccine because she knows her baby will be given this vaccine soon after birth. She wants to know why it is recommended that an infant be immunized for hepatitis B. Tracy says that infants are not at risk for contracting hepatitis B because the way it is transmitted is mostly through sexual contact and illegal drug use. ■

HEPATITIS B VACCINE REFUSAL

I understand that due to my occupational exposure to blood or other potentially infectious materials, I may be at risk of acquiring hepatitis B virus (HBV) infection. I have been given the opportunity to be vaccinated with hepatitis B vaccine at no charge to myself. However, I decline hepatitis B vaccination at this time. I understand that by declining this vaccine I continue to be at risk of acquiring hepatitis B, a serious disease. If in the future I continue to have occupational exposure to blood or to other potentially infectious materials and I want to be vaccinated with hepatitis B vaccine, I can receive the vaccination series at no charge to me.

Employee Name (printed)

Employee Signature — Date

Witness Signature — Date

Fig. 17.16 Hepatitis B declination form. This form must be signed by an employee with occupational exposure who declines hepatitis B vaccination.

Hepatitis B Vaccination

The OSHA Standard requires employers to offer the hepatitis B vaccination series free of charge to all medical office personnel who have occupational exposure. The vaccination must be offered within 10 working days of initial assignment to a position with occupational exposure, unless the following factors exist: (1) the individual has previously received the hepatitis B vaccination series, (2) antibody testing has revealed that the individual is immune to hepatitis B, or (3) the vaccine is contraindicated for medical reasons.

Medical office personnel who decline vaccination must sign a hepatitis B waiver form documenting refusal. This form must be filed in the employee's OSHA medical record (Fig. 17.16). Employees who decline vaccination may request the vaccination later; the employer must then provide it, according to the aforementioned criteria.

Approximately 5% of the population does not form antibodies to the hepatitis B vaccine. Because of this, the CDC recommends that an antibody titer test be performed on all health care workers between 1 and 2 months after the last dose of the hepatitis B vaccine. The titer test is performed to determine if the health care worker has developed protective antibodies against HBV and is immune to infection. Health care workers who do not respond to the primary vaccination series, as indicated by a negative titer test, must be revaccinated with a second three-dose vaccination series and then undergo a repeat titer test. If the titer test is still negative, this means that the health care worker probably lacks immunity to HBV infection.

REGULATED MEDICAL WASTE

Regulated medical waste (RMW) is medical waste that may contain infectious materials posing a threat to health and safety.

HANDLING REGULATED MEDICAL WASTE

RMW must be handled carefully to prevent an exposure incident. The OSHA Bloodborne Pathogens Standard outlines specific actions to take when handling RMW, as follows:

1. Separate RMW from the general refuse at its point of origin. In other words, disposable items containing RMW should be placed directly into biohazard containers or bags and should not be mixed with the regular trash (refer to Box 17.6: Guidelines for Discarding Medical Waste in the Medical Office).
2. Ensure that biohazard containers are closable, leakproof, and suitably constructed to contain the contents during handling, storage, and transport. These containers include biohazard bags and sharps containers.
3. To prevent spillage or protrusion of the contents, close the lid of a sharps container before removing it from an examining room. Never open, empty, or clean a contaminated sharps container. If there is a chance of leakage from the sharps container, the medical assistant should place it in a second container that is closable, leakproof, and appropriately labeled or color-coded.
4. Securely close biohazard bags before removing them from the examining room. To provide additional protection, some medical offices double-bag by placing the primary bag inside a second biohazard bag.
5. Transport full biohazard containers to a secure area away from the general public, using PPE (e.g., gloves).

DISPOSAL OF REGULATED MEDICAL WASTE

Each state is responsible for developing policies for disposal of RMW. To avoid noncompliance, it is important for

BOX 17.6 Guidelines for Discarding Medical Waste in the Medical Office

Regular Waste Container

The following items that have been used for health care *are not* considered regulated medical waste and can be discarded in a covered waste container lined with a regular trash bag.

- Disposable drapes
- Disposable patient gowns
- Examining table paper
- Disposable clean or sterile gloves
- Gauze tinged with blood or other body fluids
- Disposable probe covers for thermometers
- Tongue depressors
- Tissues with respiratory secretions
- Disposable ear speculums
- Empty urine containers
- Urine testing strips
- Disposable diapers
- Feminine hygiene products

Biohazard Sharps Container

The following items are sharps. They *are* considered regulated medical waste and must be discarded in a biohazard sharps container.

- Hypodermic syringes and needles
- Venipuncture needles
- Lancets
- Razor blades
- Scalpel blades
- Suture needles
- Blood tubes
- Capillary pipettes
- Microscope slides and coverslips
- Broken glassware

Biohazard Bag Waste Container

The following items *are* considered regulated medical waste. They are not sharps and can be discarded in a covered waste container lined with a biohazard bag.

- Any item saturated or dripping with blood or other potentially infectious materials (OPIM) (e.g., dressings, gauze, cotton balls, paper towels, tissues that are saturated or dripping with blood)
- Any item caked with dried blood or OPIM, such as dressings and sutures
- Disposable clean or sterile gloves contaminated with blood or OPIM
- Disposable vaginal speculums and collection devices (e.g., swabs, spatulas, brushes)
- Tissue or fluid removed during minor office surgery
- Microbiologic waste, such as specimen cultures and collection devices
- Discarded live and attenuated vaccines

Sanitary Sewer

Disposal of small quantities of blood and other body fluids to the sanitary sewer is considered a safe method of disposing of these waste materials. The following fluids can be carefully poured down a utility sink, drain, or toilet. (*Note:* State regulations may dictate the maximum volume allowable for discharge of blood or body fluids into the sanitary sewer.)

- Blood
- Body excretions such as urine
- Body secretions such as sputum

medical office personnel to keep current with the specific RMW policies and guidelines set forth in their state.

Most medical offices use a commercial medical waste service to dispose of RMW. This service is responsible for picking up and transporting the medical waste to a treatment facility for incineration (or other means) to destroy pathogens and render them harmless. The RMW can then be safely disposed of in a sanitary landfill. RMW treatment facilities must be licensed and hold permits issued by the Environmental Protection Agency (EPA), allowing them to dispose of RMW.

A series of steps must be followed for preparing and storing RMW for pickup by the service. Although these steps may vary slightly from state to state, general measures required by most states include the following:

1. Place biohazard bags and sharps containers into a receptacle provided by the medical waste service. The receptacle is usually a cardboard box (Fig. 17.17). The box should be securely sealed with packing tape, and a biohazard warning label must appear on two opposite sides of the box.

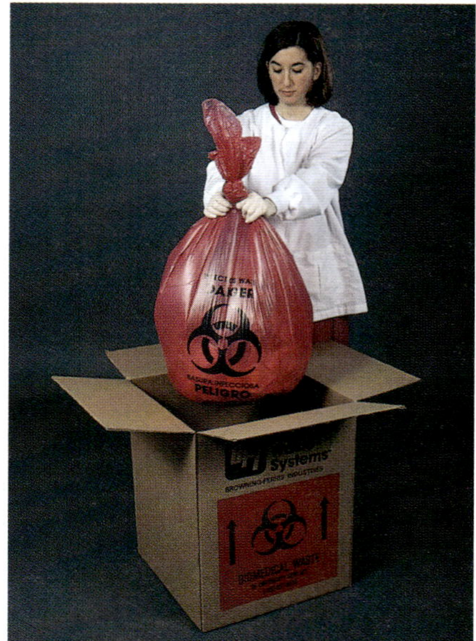

Fig. 17.17 Jennifer places a biohazard bag inside a cardboard box in preparation for pickup by the medical waste service.

2. Store the biohazard boxes in a locked room inside the facility or in a locked collection container outside for pickup by the medical waste service. This step is aimed at preventing unauthorized access to items such as needles and syringes. The RMW storage area should be labeled with one of the following:
   - "Authorized Personnel Only" sign
   - International biohazard symbol
3. Many states require that a tracking record be completed when the RMW is picked up by the medical waste service. This form includes such information as the type and quantity of RMW (weighed in pounds) and where it is being sent. The form must be signed by a representative of the medical waste service and a designated medical office employee. After the RMW has been destroyed at the treatment facility, a record documenting its disposal is transmitted to the medical office.

What Would You Do? What Would You *Not* Do?

Case Study 3

Giles Lee is at the medical office. In 1988, he was in a serious car accident and had to have a blood transfusion. Giles says that he donated blood for the first time 2 months ago. Last week he received a letter saying that the blood he donated tested positive for hepatitis C and that he should see his provider. Giles says that he must have gotten hepatitis C from the blood transfusion he received many years ago. He does not understand how that could have happened because he thought the blood supply was tested for hepatitis C. Giles wants to know why he has not had any symptoms of hepatitis C. and also wants to know if he can give hepatitis C to his wife. ■

BLOODBORNE DISEASES

A **bloodborne disease** is any disease caused by a pathogen that is carried in blood and spread through contact with blood. The most common route of transmission of bloodborne pathogens to a health care worker is through accidental needlesticks and other sharps-related injuries. There are more than 20 bloodborne pathogens that can infect a health care worker. The bloodborne pathogens that are the biggest threats to health care workers include hepatitis B virus (HBV), hepatitis C virus (HCV), and human immunodeficiency virus (HIV), which is discussed in greater detail in this section.

Hepatitis B is much easier to transmit than HIV. After a needlestick exposure to HBV-infected blood, health care workers not immune to hepatitis B have a 6% to 30% chance of developing it. The risk of a hepatitis C infection following a needlestick exposure to HCV-infected blood is approximately 2%. After a needlestick exposure to HIV-infected blood, a health care worker has a 0.3% chance of being infected with HIV and a 0.1% chance of being infected after a mucous membrane exposure of the eyes, nose, or mouth. Studies show that most exposures of health care workers to HBV, HBC, and HIV do not result in infection.

HEPATITIS B

Hepatitis B is an infection of the liver caused by the hepatitis B virus which has the potential to cause serious liver damage. The virus is found in the blood and in certain body fluids (e.g., semen and vaginal secretions) of HBV-infected individuals. The hepatitis B virus is capable of causing both acute and chronic infections. A newly acquired infection is known as an acute infection. An **acute infection** is an infection that develops suddenly and lasts for a short period of time (less than 6 months). A **chronic infection** is an infection that lasts longer than 6 months, develops slowly, and may worsen over an extended period of time. Some acute infections (which include both hepatitis B and C) can persist in the body and then develop into chronic infections.

Acute Hepatitis B

Hepatitis B is classified as acute if the infection lasts for 6 months or less. Many individuals do not experience any symptoms with acute hepatitis B. Individuals who do develop symptoms usually experience them for several weeks, but in some cases, they may continue for as long as 6 months. On average, these symptoms appear 3 months after exposure but can appear any time between 2 and 5 months following exposure. Symptoms of acute hepatitis B are often mild and flulike and may be mistaken for another condition, such as influenza. These mild symptoms usually include fever, fatigue, loss of appetite, and nausea/vomiting.

Because of a lack of symptoms or only mild symptoms, many people with acute hepatitis B do not know they are infected. Some HBV-infected individuals may experience more severe symptoms such as abdominal pain, dark urine, joint pain, and jaundice often prompting them to seek medical care. Many people (especially adults) are able to clear the virus from their system and recover completely. These people become immune to hepatitis B and cannot get infected again.

Chronic Hepatitis B

Individuals unable to fight off acute hepatitis B remain infected and may go on to develop chronic hepatitis B. Infants and young children are more likely to develop a chronic infection, while most adults (95%) are able to fight off the virus and do not develop chronic hepatitis B.

Many individuals with chronic hepatitis B are not aware of being infected. This is because chronic hepatitis B does not typically exhibit any symptoms until it causes serious HBV-related health problems. During the asymptomatic period which may last for decades or more, the virus may slowly damage the liver; in addition, the individual is a carrier for hepatitis B during this time and can infect others. Chronic hepatitis B can eventually lead to serious liver disease which includes cirrhosis, liver cancer, and liver failure.

Transmission

HBV is found in the blood and body fluids of infected individuals and is most commonly transmitted through unprotected sexual contact, sharing needles, syringes, or drug preparation equipment, and perinatally from an infected mother to her infant during birth. Other modes of transmission include direct contact with blood or open sores of an infected individual, getting a tattoo or body piercing with contaminated instruments, and the sharing of items such as razors or toothbrushes with an infected individual. Hepatitis B is not spread by food, water, breastfeeding, sneezing, coughing, hugging, kissing, or sharing eating utensils or drinking glasses.

The most common means of transmitting hepatitis B to a health care worker is through blood and blood components (e.g., plasma and serum) transferred through accidental needlesticks and other sharps-related injuries. The virus is also spread to health care workers, but less effectively, through blood splashes to the eyes, mouth, and nonintact skin. Fortunately, the number of health care workers who contract hepatitis B in the workplace has declined dramatically since the development of the hepatitis B vaccine.

Hepatitis B Vaccine

The best means of preventing hepatitis B is through the administration of the hepatitis B vaccine. The hepatitis B vaccine (Fig. 17.18) is an active immunizing agent, meaning the body is actively stimulated to produce antibodies against HBV. The vaccine is administered intramuscularly in a series of three doses; brand names are Recombivax HB and Engerix-B. After the first dose is administered, the second dose is given 1 month after the first dose, and the third dose is administered 6 months after the first dose (i.e., 0, 1 month, and 6 months). There is a new hepatitis B vaccine available for adults that consist of a series of two doses administered intramuscularly 1 month apart. The brand name of this vaccine is Heplisav-B. The hepatitis B vaccine is well tolerated by most patients. The most common side effect is soreness at the injection site, including induration, erythema, and swelling. Occasionally, a low-grade fever, headache, and dizziness occur.

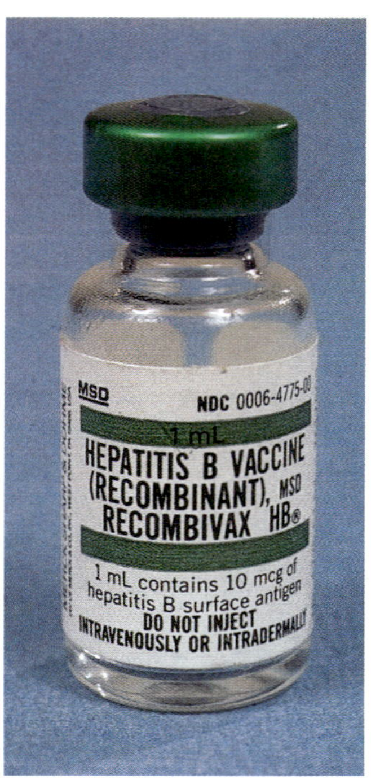

Fig. 17.18 Hepatitis B vaccine.

As previously discussed, the OSHA Standard recommends that all health care workers receive the hepatitis B vaccine as a preventive measure against hepatitis B. Following an exposure incident, a health care worker who has previously been vaccinated probably would not require further treatment.

Treatment

There is no specific treatment for patients diagnosed with acute hepatitis B. In most cases, care is focused on measures to help the body fight off the infection which include a healthy diet, drinking plenty of fluids, and rest. The provider usually orders regular HBV testing to determine if the virus is still in the patient's body.

A patient with acute hepatitis B that goes on to develop a chronic hepatitis B infection can be treated with antiviral medications. These medications slow the replication of the virus and can prevent or delay liver disease; however, they rarely completely rid the body of the virus. Once a patient begins antiviral medication therapy, they must continue it for life. If liver disease develops, treatments are available based upon the type and severity of the liver disease.

HEPATITIS C

Hepatitis C is an infection of the liver caused by the hepatitis C virus that can result in serious liver damage. The virus is found in the blood of an individual infected with hepatitis C. The hepatitis C virus is capable of causing both acute and chronic infections. Most individuals with acute hepatitis C have no symptoms; if symptoms do occur, they typically last 2 weeks to 3 months. The symptoms are usually mild and flulike and very similar to those of acute hepatitis B.

Approximately 15% to 25% of individuals with acute hepatitis C are able to clear the virus from their system within 6 months after infection and recover completely. The remaining 75% to 85% of individuals remain infected and go on to develop chronic hepatitis C. Approximately 20 to 30 years after infection, 10% to 20% of these individuals develop serious liver disease, such as cirrhosis or liver cancer. Ultimately, 1% to 5% of individuals with chronic hepatitis C die from liver failure.

For reasons not yet completely understood, individuals born between 1945 and 1965 (often referred to as "baby boomers") are five times more likely to have chronic hepatitis C as compared with adults born in other years. These HCV-infected baby boomers account for about 75% of all cases of chronic hepatitis C in the United States.

Transmission

An HCV infection can be transmitted when blood from an infected individual enters the bloodstream of a susceptible host. The most common route of transmission is by sharing needles and syringes or drug preparation equipment with an HCV-infected individual. Less commonly, HCV can be transmitted by getting a tattoo or body piercing with HCV-contaminated instruments and from an HCV-infected mother to her infant during birth. Unlike hepatitis B, hepatitis C is rarely transmitted through sexual contact with an HCV-infected individual. Hepatitis C is also not spread by food, water, breastfeeding, sneezing, coughing, hugging, kissing, or sharing eating utensils or drinking glasses.

A test to determine the presence of hepatitis C in blood donations did not exist until 1992. Up until this time, a significant number of people contracted the disease from HCV-infected blood transfusions and organ transplants and are now living with chronic hepatitis C. Routine HCV testing of the U.S. blood supply since 1992 now makes it very rare for someone to contract hepatitis C from a blood transfusion or an organ transplant.

The most common means of transmitting hepatitis C to a health care worker is through HCV-infected blood transferred through accidental needlesticks and other sharps-related injuries. The chance of contracting hepatitis C by a health care worker is much lower than that of contracting hepatitis B.

Treatment

There is no specific treatment for an individual diagnosed with acute hepatitis C. In most cases, care is focused on measures to help the body fight off the infection which include a healthy diet, drinking plenty of fluids, and rest. The provider usually orders regular HCV testing to determine if the virus is still in the body.

The treatment for chronic hepatitis C has evolved substantially since the development of highly effective antiviral medications. Treatment usually involves the daily oral administration of antiviral medications for a period of 8 to 12 weeks. These medications attack the virus and cure the disease in more than 95% of infected individuals, thereby preventing serious liver damage and possible death. Unfortunately, most people with chronic hepatitis C do not know they are infected and therefore, do not receive the needed antiviral medication therapy.

At present, there is no vaccine available to prevent hepatitis C; however, research in this area is ongoing. HCV reinfection can occur in individuals who have been infected with HCV and cleared the virus from their body as well as in individuals who have been cured with antiviral medications. The best way to prevent reinfection is by avoiding high-risk situations and behaviors that can spread the disease, such as injection drug use with contaminated needles and syringes.

HCV Testing Recommendations

Chronic hepatitis C is known as a "silent disease." This is because more than 50% of infected individuals have no symptoms and do not know they are infected; these individuals are also carriers of HCV and can infect others. Individuals with chronic hepatitis C can be infected for years or even decades before symptoms first begin to appear. During this time, the virus may be slowly attacking the liver, eventually resulting in serious liver damage and possible death. To identify individuals with chronic hepatitis C, the CDC recommends a screening test for individuals with a greater risk of being infected with HCV which include:

- Any individual born between 1945 and 1965
- Current or former injection drug users (including those who injected only once many years ago)
- Recipients of blood transfusions or organ transplants prior to July 1992
- Individuals with hemophilia who received clotting factor concentrates made before 1987, when less advanced methods for manufacturing those products were used
- Individuals who received a tattoo or body piercing with contaminated instruments
- Individuals who have undergone long-term hemodialysis treatments
- Health care workers exposed to HCV-infected blood through accidental needlesticks or other sharps injuries or mucous membrane exposure
- People with HIV infection
- Infants born to HCV-infected mothers

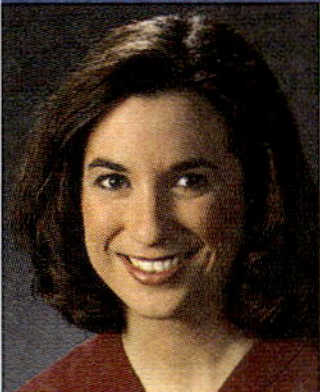

Memories *from* Practicum

Jennifer: As a student, I was extremely nervous to go out on practicum. I was so scared to think that I was actually going to be in a medical office setting and would have to put everything I had learned into practice. Would I remember everything? Would I do something wrong and hurt the patient? It was such an overwhelming feeling! But to my relief, I had a very good experience. The office staff was so friendly and helpful to me, and I surprised myself at how easily everything I had learned stayed with me. It was so exciting to see that I was actually functioning as a team member in the health care field. I could not have had better training. ■

ACQUIRED IMMUNODEFICIENCY SYNDROME

Acquired immunodeficiency syndrome (AIDS) is a chronic disorder of the immune system that eventually destroys the body's ability to fight off infection. AIDS is caused by a retrovirus known as *human immunodeficiency virus (HIV)*. The following description helps to clarify the difference between HIV infection and AIDS. The viral infection of the body with HIV is known as *HIV infection*, whereas *AIDS* is used to refer to the last stage of HIV infection. Simply put,

HIGHLIGHT on Viral Hepatitis A, B, and C

- Hepatitis A, B, and C are infections of the liver caused by three different viruses. They are spread in different ways and can affect the liver differently.
- Hepatitis A is spread through contact with food or water that has been contaminated by an infected individual's stool. Hepatitis B is spread through contact with HBV-infected blood and body fluids and hepatitis C is spread through direct contact with HCV-infected blood.
- Symptoms common to all types of hepatitis include fever, fatigue, loss of appetite, nausea/vomiting, abdominal pain, dark urine, joint pain, and jaundice.
- Hepatitis A, B, and C are designated by the CDC as nationally notifiable diseases. When the provider diagnoses a case of hepatitis A, B, or C, a reportable disease form must be completed and filed with the local public health department.
- There are vaccines to prevent hepatitis A and B, but there is no vaccine to prevent hepatitis C.

Hepatitis B

- It is estimated that 880,000 people in the United States are living with chronic hepatitis B; however, this number may be as high as 2 million people. Many of these individuals do not have symptoms and, therefore, do not know they are infected. These individuals are also carriers of HBV and are capable of transmitting the disease to others.
- Hepatitis B can survive outside the body in a dried state for at least 1 week and still can be capable of causing infection.
- Chronic hepatitis B is often not diagnosed until an HBV-infected individual's blood is screened following a blood donation or when test results are found to be abnormal during routine laboratory testing.
- Every year, approximately 820,000 Americans die as a result of the long-term complications of chronic hepatitis B, such as cirrhosis and liver cancer.
- The most common risk factor among people with new HBV infections is sharing contaminated needles and syringes for injection drug use.
- New hepatitis B infections are highest among adults, ages 30 to 49 years, because many people at risk for infection in this age group have not been immunized with the hepatitis B vaccine.
- Whether or not an individual with acute hepatitis B goes on to develop chronic hepatitis B is related to the age at the time of infection. The younger a person is when infected, the greater the risk of developing a chronic infection. According to the CDC, following infection with acute hepatitis B, chronic infection develops in:
  - 90% of infants infected by their mothers at birth
  - 25% to 50% of young children infected between ages 1 to 5 years
  - 5% of individuals infected as an older child or adult
- Overall, the number of individuals contracting hepatitis B has decreased since the development of the hepatitis B vaccine. As more people become immune to hepatitis B through the immunization of infants, the goal of eliminating hepatitis B in the United States may be realized.

Hepatitis C

- In the United States, chronic hepatitis C is the most common chronic viral infection found in blood and spread through contact with blood.
- Approximately 2.7 to 3.9 million Americans are living with chronic hepatitis C, and most do not have symptoms and therefore do not know they are infected. These individuals are carriers of hepatitis C and can infect others.
- Sharing contaminated needles and syringes for injection drug use is known to play a major role in HCV transmission. According to the CDC, there has been a dramatic increase in new cases of hepatitis C is among young adults between the ages of 18 and 39 years who inject heroin and prescription opioids.
- Chronic hepatitis C is a leading cause of liver cirrhosis and liver transplantation in the United States.
- New screening efforts and effective antiviral treatments for hepatitis C are helping providers identify and cure more people with the disease. As a result, hepatitis C may become less common in the future. Researchers estimate that hepatitis C could be a rare disease in the United States by 2036.

the terms *HIV infection* and *AIDS* refer to different stages of the same disease.

When HIV gains entrance into the body, it begins to attack and destroy certain white blood cells known as *CD4*$^{+}$ *T cells,* which are involved in protecting the body against viral, bacterial, fungal, and protozoal infections. Without treatment, more and more CD4^{+} T cells are destroyed, and the immune system is gradually weakened. After a period of time (without treatment), which typically lasts about 10 years, the body's immune system becomes so weakened by the attack that it is unable to fight off the diseases and infections associated with AIDS. Once an individual reaches the AIDS stage of the infection, life expectancy is about 3 years.

AIDS is characterized by the presence of severe and life-threatening opportunistic infections and unusual cancers that occur as a result of advanced HIV infection and are known as *AIDS-defining conditions*. An **opportunistic infection** is an infection that takes advantage of an opportunity not normally available, such as the weakened immune system of an HIV-infected individual. Opportunistic infections occur more often and are more severe with a weakened immune system than with a healthy immune system. The CDC has developed a list of AIDS-defining conditions; some examples of these include pneumonia, tuberculosis, herpes simplex 1 virus, candidiasis (thrush), salmonella infection, cryptococcal meningitis, toxoplasmosis, cytomegalovirus, anal cancer, and Kaposi sarcoma. Kaposi sarcoma is characterized by slightly

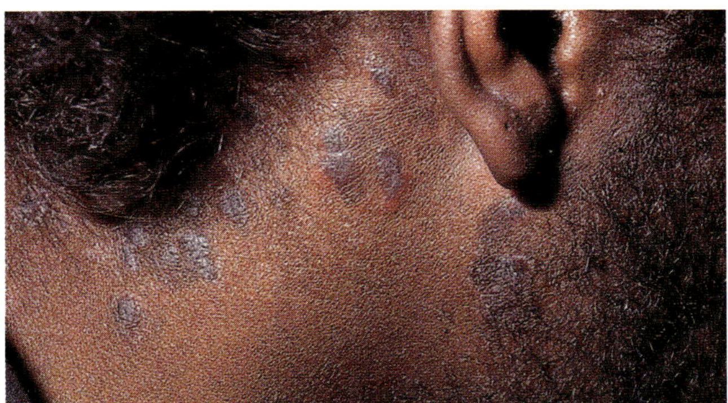

Fig. 17.19 Kaposi sarcoma is an example of an AIDS-defining condition. (From Forbes CD: *Color atlas and text of clinical medicine*, ed 3, St. Louis, 2003, Mosby.)

elevated pink, brown, or reddish-purple blotches or bumps anywhere on the skin (Fig. 17.19).

According to the CDC definition, a patient has AIDS if they have a positive HIV test result and have one or more of the following:

- $CD4^+$ T-cell count below 200 cells/mm^3 (normal $CD4^+$ T-cell count for a healthy individual ranges from 500 to 1500 cells/mm^3
- $CD4^+$ T-cell percentage of total lymphocytes of less than 14%
- Presence of an AIDS-defining condition

Transmission

In the general population, HIV is spread primarily through sexual contact with an infected person and by sharing contaminated needles and syringes for injection drug use with someone who is infected. An untreated HIV-infected mother can transmit the virus to her baby during pregnancy or birth. HIV also can be spread to infants through the breast milk of infected mothers. Because of this, the CDC recommends that HIV testing be included in the routine panel of prenatal screening tests for all pregnant women at the first visit. Treatment of the mother early in the pregnancy can almost completely eliminate transmission of HIV to the fetus.

Scientific evidence shows that HIV is not spread through casual, everyday contact. There is no evidence that HIV is spread by sharing items or facilities such as mobile phones, computer keyboards, food utensils, bedding, doorknobs, and toilet seats. Because HIV is not passed through the air, it is not spread through coughing and sneezing. HIV also is not spread through urine, saliva, tears and sweat, or by shaking hands and hugging, or by mosquitoes, ticks and other blood-sucking insects.

Because HIV is not easily transmitted, the risk to health care workers is quite low. Despite the low risk of infection, the serious nature of HIV infection warrants the use of the OSHA Bloodborne Pathogens Standard by all health care workers. Precautions minimizing the risk of exposure to blood and body fluids also are recommended as a means of protection against other bloodborne pathogens, such as hepatitis B, hepatitis C, and syphilis.

HIV Testing

The only way to know for sure if an individual is infected with HIV is to be tested. The CDC recommends HIV testing for all patients between the ages of 13 and 64 at least once as part of routine health care. Patients should be notified that HIV testing will be performed, however patients have the option of declining the testing (known as *opt-out testing*). The CDC further recommends that individuals at high risk for HIV infection undergo HIV testing at least annually. Examples of high-risk behaviors include having sex with an HIV-infected individual and sharing needles and syringes with an infected person. If the HIV test result is positive, a follow-up test that is more specific is always performed to confirm the test results.

A negative HIV test is not always conclusive for the absence of HIV infection. Once an individual has been infected with HIV, it takes time for the HIV antigens and antibodies to be produced and reach a level that can be detected by HIV tests. The time between HIV infection and when an HIV test can provide an accurate test result is known as the *window period*, which varies from person to person and the type of test being used. If an individual has recently been infected with HIV, the test may yield a false-negative result and the individual should be retested after the window period for that test has been reached.

Types of Tests

Several different types of tests can be used to screen for the presence of HIV. Most tests require a blood specimen obtained through a venipuncture or finger puncture, although some screening tests can be performed on oral fluid. The types of tests used to screen for HIV include the following:

1. *Antibody/Antigen Tests:* Antibody/antigen tests are the most commonly used HIV screening tests ordered by a provider in a medical office setting. The window period needed to provide an accurate test result is between 2 and 6 weeks following exposure. Antigen/antibody tests check for the presence of both HIV antibodies and antigens and are usually performed at an outside medical laboratory with the results being sent to the provider.
2. *Antibody tests:* Antibody tests check the blood only for the presence of HIV antibodies and, because of this, are less sensitive than other types of screening tests. The window period for antibody tests is between 3 and 12 weeks after exposure. The ELISA (enzyme-linked immunosorbent assay) test is usually the first test ordered by the provider to screen for the presence of HIV. Alternatively, rapid CLIA-waived HIV antibody tests are now available that can be performed by the medical assistant in the medical office. The results from a rapid test can be obtained in 30 minutes or less. Brand names of rapid antibody tests include Uni-Gold Recombigen HIV (Trinity Biotech), Clearview HIV (Alere), and OraQuick Advance (OraSure Technologies). Several rapid antibody tests are now

available in drugstores or online and can be performed by an individual at home.
3. *NAT:* The NAT (nucleic acid test) is the most sensitive test and can detect HIV sooner than other types of tests. It uses DNA technology to detect the presence of HIV. The window period for the NAT is 1 to 4 weeks after exposure. This test is expensive and therefore not routinely used for screening individuals for HIV unless they have recently had a high-risk exposure or a possible exposure with early symptoms of HIV.

Treatment

There is no known cure for AIDS and there is no vaccine to prevent HIV infection, however it can be controlled with proper medical care. Powerful antiretroviral medications have been developed that prevent the reproduction of the virus, thereby reducing the viral load and increasing the $CD4^+$ T-cell count. *Viral load* refers to the amount of HIV present in the blood of an infected individual. The daily administration of a combination of these medications is known as *antiretroviral therapy* or *ART*.

If ART is followed as prescribed, HIV-infected patients can get and keep a viral load so low that the virus cannot be detected in their blood, known as an *undetectable viral load*. An undetectable viral load dramatically delays HIV from progressing to full-blown AIDS, thereby allowing patients to live longer and heathier lives. In fact, patients who receive early effective ART following an HIV diagnosis can expect to live a near normal lifespan. An undetectable viral load also makes it virtually impossible to transmit the virus to others. Unfortunately, even with effective medication therapy, HIV cannot be completely eliminated from the body. Once infected, an individual is infected for life; therefore, it is very important that an HIV-infected individual carefully follow their prescribed ART regimen to prevent HIV from reproducing and destroying $CD4^+$ T-cells.

Numerous treatments are available to treat the opportunistic infections and cancers that occur with AIDS. Medications used to treat opportunistic infections include antivirals, antibiotics and antifungal medications. The type of medication used depends on which opportunistic infection has been contracted by the patient.

What Would You Do? What Would You *Not* Do? RESPONSES

Case Study 1

Page 297

What Did Jennifer Do?

- ❑ Told Petra that the physician would need to determine what is causing her symptoms.
- ❑ Documented Petra's symptoms in her medical record. Made sure to document that Petra's symptoms occur after she has contact with rubber latex gloves and rubber flip flops.
- ❑ Used latex-free gloves and tourniquet when drawing Petra's blood.
- ❑ If Petra is diagnosed with a latex allergy, documented this information in her medical record.
- ❑ If instructed to do so by the physician, provided Petra with latex allergy education and guidelines.

What Did Jennifer Not Do?

- ❑ Did not tell Petra that she has a latex allergy, because only the physician is qualified to make a diagnosis.

Case Study 2

Page 302

What Did Jennifer Do?

- ❑ Told Tracy that having her infant immunized for hepatitis B is an investment in her child's future. Explained that her child could come into contact with the virus anytime in their life. Stressed that if a young child becomes infected with hepatitis B, the child has a higher risk of developing chronic hepatitis, which can cause liver problems later in life.
- ❑ Gave Tracy a brochure on hepatitis B to take home.

What Did Jennifer Not Do?

- ❑ Did not needlessly alarm Tracy regarding the complications of hepatitis B.

Case Study 3

Page 305

What Did Jennifer Do?

- ❑ Explained to Giles that the blood supply was not tested for hepatitis C until 1992 because a test to detect the presence of hepatitis C in the blood supply was not developed until then.
- ❑ Told Giles that it is possible for someone to have hepatitis C and not exhibit any symptoms.
- ❑ Told Giles that he should ask the physician his question about giving hepatitis C to others.

What Did Jennifer Not Do?

- ❑ Did not automatically assume that Giles had hepatitis C, because he had not yet been seen by the physician. It would be up to the physician to make a diagnosis of hepatitis C.
- ❑ Did not tell Giles about the serious complications of hepatitis C. If Giles is diagnosed with hepatitis C, it would be the physician's responsibility to relay this information.

TERMINOLOGY REVIEW

Key Term	Word Parts	Definition
Acute infection		An infection that develops suddenly and lasts for a short period of time.
Aerobe	*aer/o:* air	A microorganism that needs oxygen to live and grow.
Anaerobe	*an-:* without *aer/o:* air	A microorganism that grows best in the absence of oxygen.
Antiseptic	*anti-:* against *-septic:* infection	An agent that inhibits the growth of or kills microorganisms.
Barrier protection		A physical barrier that protects against infection.
Bloodborne disease		Any disease caused by a pathogen that is carried in blood and spread through contact with blood.
Bloodborne pathogens	*path/o:* disease *-gen:* producing	Pathogenic microorganisms present in human blood that can cause disease in humans.
Chronic infection		An infection that develops slowly and may worsen over an extended period of time.
Cilia		Slender, hairlike projections attached to the epithelium of the respsiratory tract that constantly beat in a wave-like motion to remove pathogens from the body.
Contagious disease		A disease that is capable of being transmitted directly or indirectly from one person to another
Contaminated		The presence or reasonably anticipated presence of blood or OPIM on an item or surface.
Decontamination		The use of physical or chemical means to remove, inactivate, or destroy bloodborne pathogens on a surface or item to the point where they are no longer capable of transmitting infectious particles, and the surface or item is rendered safe for handling, use, or disposal.
Exposure incident		A specific eye, mouth or other mucous membrane, nonintact skin, or parenteral contact with blood or OPIM that results from the performance of an employee's duties.
Hand hygiene		The process of cleansing or sanitizing the hands.
Infection	*infect-*: to soil or contaminate	The condition in which the body, or part of it, is invaded by a pathogen.
Infectious agent		A pathogen capable of causing an infectious disease.
Infectious disease		An illness caused by the entrance into the body of an infectious agent where it grows and multiplies resulting in harmful effects to the host.
Medical asepsis	*a-:* without *sepsis:* infection	Practices that are employed to inhibit the growth and hinder the transmission of pathogenic microorganisms to prevent the spread of infection.
Microorganism	*micro-:* small *organism:* organism	A microscopic plant or animal.
Nonintact skin		Skin that has a break in its surface.
Nonpathogen	*non-:* not *path/o:* disease *-gen:* producing	A microorganism that is harmless and does not cause disease.
Occupational exposure		Reasonably anticipated skin, eye, mucous membrane, or parenteral contact with blood or OPIM that may result from the performance of an employee's duties.
Opportunistic infection		An infection that takes advantage of an opportunity not normally available such as the weakened immune system of an HIV-infected individual.
Optimum growth temperature		The temperature at which an organism grows best.
Other potentially infectious materials (OPIM)		Body fluids, tissues, and organs from a human that can spread infection.
Parenteral	*para-:* apart from *enter/o:* intestine *-al:* pertaining to	Piercing of the skin barrier or mucous membranes, such as through needlesticks, human bites, cuts, and abrasions.
Pathogen	*path/o:* disease *-gen:* producing	A disease-producing microorganism.

Continued

TERMINOLOGY REVIEW—cont'd

Key Term	Word Parts	Definition
Personal protective equipment		Specialized clothing or equipment worn by an employee for protection against a hazard.
pH		The unit that describes the acidity or alkalinity of a solution.
Regulated medical waste		Medical waste that may contain infectious materials posing a threat to health and safety.
Reservoir host		The location in which an infectious agent lives and usually grows and multiplies.
Resident flora		Harmless, nonpathogenic microorganisms that normally reside on the skin and usually do not cause disease. Also known as *normal flora.*
Sharps		Objects that can penetrate the skin, such as needles and lancets.
Susceptible host		One who is capable of being infected by a pathogen.
Transient flora		Microorganisms that reside on the superficial skin layers and are picked up in the course of daily activities. They are often pathogenic but can be removed easily from the skin by sanitizing the hands.

PROCEDURE 17.1 Handwashing

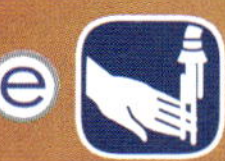

Outcome Perform handwashing.

Equipment/Supplies

- Liquid soap
- Paper towels
- Waste container

1. **Procedural Step.** If wearing a watch, remove it or push it up on the forearm so that the wrist is clear. Avoid wearing rings. If you wear rings, remove all except a plain wedding band and put them in a safe place.
   Principle. Pathogens can lodge in the crevices and grooves of rings.
2. **Procedural Step.** Stand at the sink, making sure clothing does not touch the sink.
   Principle. The sink is considered contaminated, and if the uniform touches the sink, it may pick up microorganisms and transfer them.
3. **Procedural Step.** Turn on the faucets, using a paper towel.
   Principle. The faucets are considered contaminated because they harbor microorganisms.

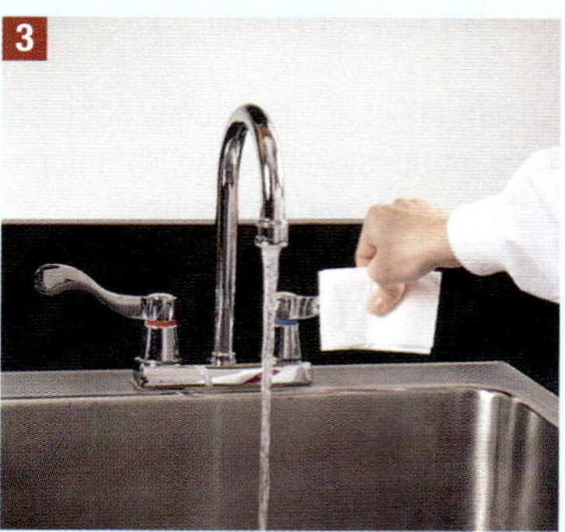

Turn on the faucet using a paper towel.

4. **Procedural Step.** Adjust the water temperature. The water should be warm to make the best suds.
   Principle. Water that is too hot or too cold tends to dry the skin, causing chapping and cracking and making it easy for pathogens to enter the body or be transferred to patients.
5. **Procedural Step.** Discard the paper towel in the waste container.
   Principle. The paper towel is considered contaminated after touching the faucets.
6. **Procedural Step.** Wet the hands and forearms thoroughly with water. The hands should be held lower than the elbows at all times. Do not touch the inside of the sink because it is also contaminated.
   Principle. When you hold your hands lower than the elbows, bacteria and debris are carried away from the arms and body and into the sink.
7. **Procedural Step.** Apply soap to the hands. Apply 1 teaspoon of liquid soap (approximately the size of a nickel) to the palm of one hand.

PROCEDURE 17.1 Handwashing—cont'd

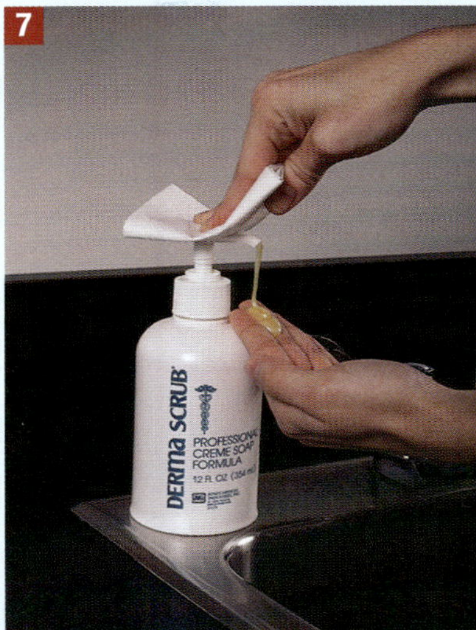

Apply soap to the hands.

8. Procedural Step. Wash the palms and backs of the hands with 10 circular motions. The CDC recommends that the hands be rubbed together vigorously for at least 20 seconds, making sure to cover all surfaces. Use friction along with the circular motions to wash the palm and back of each hand.
Principle. Friction helps to dislodge and remove microorganisms from the hands.

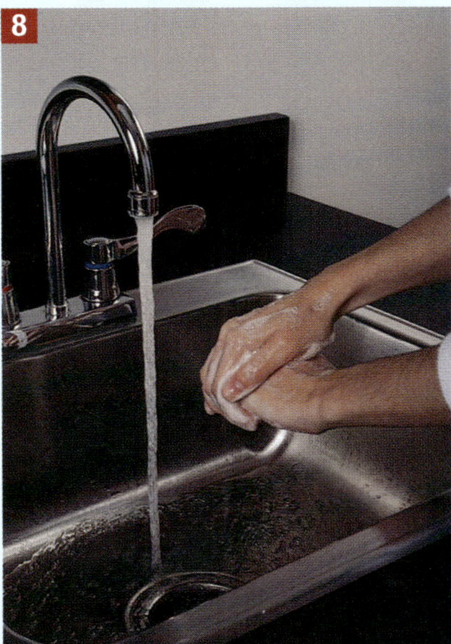

Wash the palms and backs of the hands.

9. Procedural Step. Wash the fingers with 10 circular motions while focusing on the fingertips and fingernails. Interlace the fingers and thumbs and use friction and circular motions while rubbing the fingers back and forth.
Principle. This kind of movement helps remove microorganisms and debris that have accumulated between the fingers.

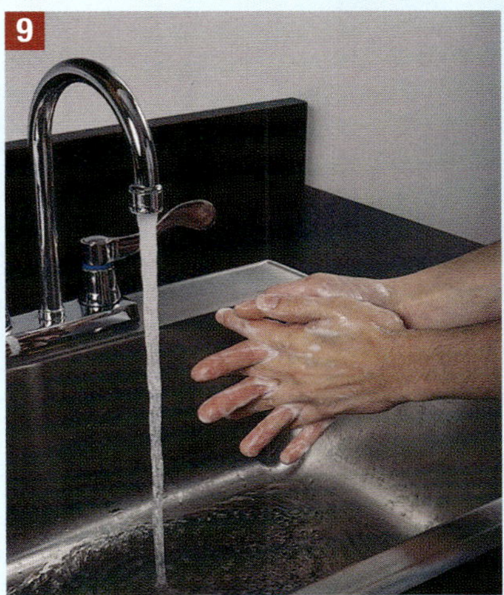

Interlace the fingers and thumbs and use friction.

10. Procedural Step. Rinse well, making sure to hold the hands lower than the elbows.
Principle. Running water helps to rinse away dirt and microorganisms.

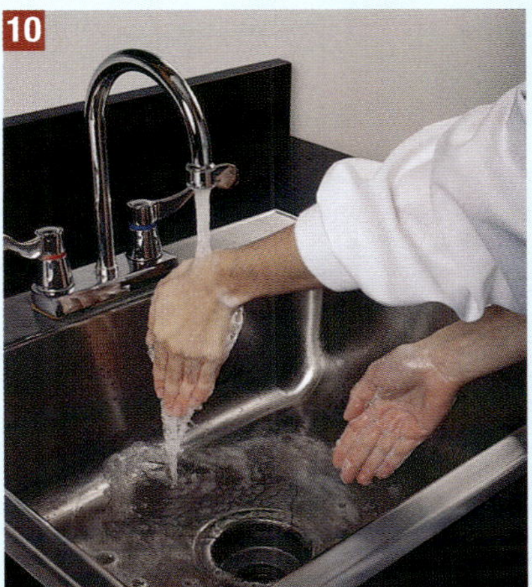

Rinse well, holding the hands lower than the elbows.

Continued

PROCEDURE 17.1 Handwashing—cont'd

11. Procedural Step. Wash the wrists and forearms, using friction along with circular motions.
(*Note:* The hands are washed first because they are the most contaminated; microorganisms and dirt are washed away and do not spread to the wrists and forearms.)

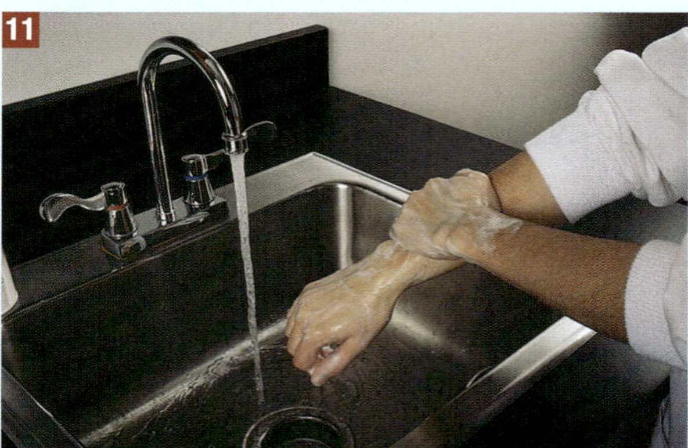

Wash wrists and forearms using friction.

12. Procedural Step. Clean the fingernails with a manicure stick. The fingernails should be cleaned at least once daily, preferably during initial handwashing (i.e., handwashing performed just after arriving at the medical office to begin your day).
Principle. The area under the fingernails is likely to harbor large amounts of microorganisms.

13. Procedural Step. Rinse the arms and hands thoroughly.
Principle. The running water rinses away the dirt and microorganisms.

14. Procedural Step. Repeat the handwashing procedure. For initial handwashing or when the hands come into contact with blood or other potentially infectious materials, the handwashing procedure should be repeated to ensure removal of all pathogens.

15. Procedural Step. Dry the hands gently and thoroughly and discard the paper towel.
Principle. Gently drying the hands prevents them from becoming chapped. Microorganisms can lodge in the crevices of chapped hands. Ensure that the hands are dried completely, because wet skin also may cause chapping.

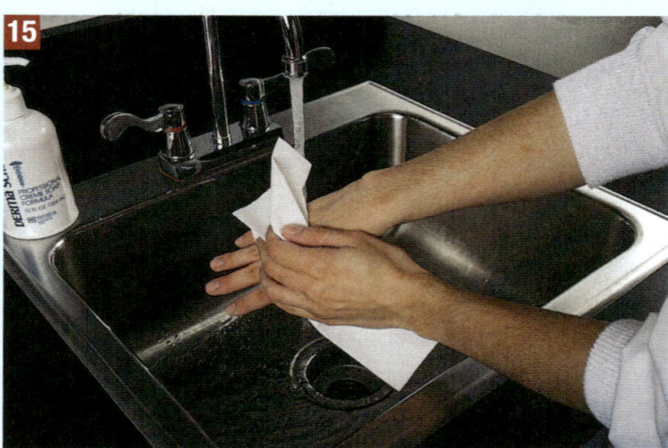

Dry your hands gently and thoroughly.

16. Procedural Step. Turn off the water, using a paper towel, and discard the paper towel in a waste container.
Principle. The faucet is considered contaminated, whereas the hands are medically aseptic or clean.

17. Procedural Step. Do not touch the sink with the bare hands.
Principle. The hands are now medically aseptic, and the sink is considered contaminated.

PROCEDURE 17.2 Applying an Alcohol-Based Hand Sanitizer

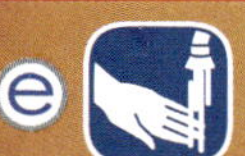

Outcome Apply an alcohol-based hand sanitizer.

Equipment/Supplies

- Alcohol-based hand sanitizer

1. Procedural Step. Inspect the hands to ensure that they are not visibly soiled. Hands that are visibly soiled must be washed with soap and water.
Principle. Alcohol-based hand sanitizers are not intended for the removal of visible soil.

2. Procedural Step. If wearing a watch, remove it or push it up on the forearm. Avoid wearing rings. If you wear rings, remove all except a plain wedding band and put them in a safe place.
Principle. Pathogens can lodge in the crevices and grooves of rings.

PROCEDURE 17.2

PROCEDURE 17.2 Applying an Alcohol-Based Hand Sanitizer—cont'd

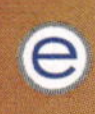

3. Procedural Step. Check the expiration date of the hand sanitizer. Apply the alcohol-based hand sanitizer to the palm of one hand as follows:

a. *Gel:* Apply approximately 1 mL of the gel to the palm of one hand; this amount is approximately equal to the size of a dime.

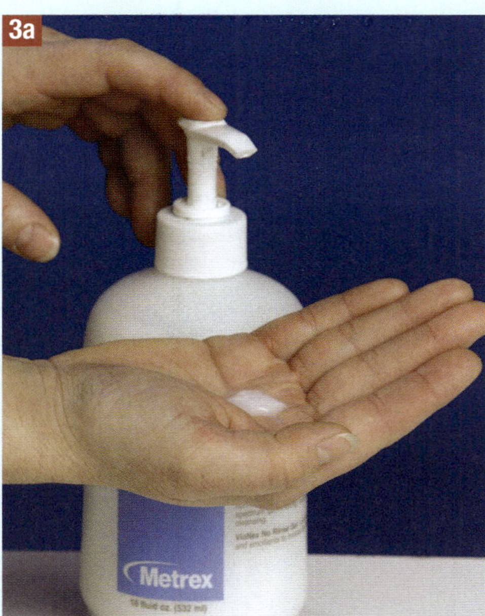

Apply gel equal to the size of a dime.

b. *Foam.* Apply 3 grams of foam to the palm of one hand; this amount is approximately equal to the size of a walnut.

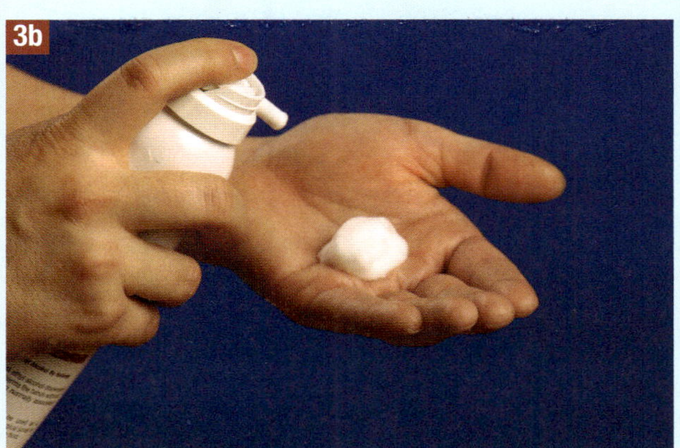

Apply foam equal to the size of a walnut.

Principle. The proper amount of hand sanitizer must be applied to ensure coverage of all surfaces of both hands. Using more than the recommended amount results in a prolonged (and unnecessary) period of time for your hands to dry.

4. Procedural Step. Thoroughly spread the hand sanitizer over all surfaces of both hands (and fingers) up to ½ inch above the wrist. Rub the right palm over the back of the left hand and the left palm over the back of the right hand. Rub palm to palm with the fingers interlaced. Spread the hand sanitizer around and under your fingernails.

Principle. Failure to cover all surfaces can leave areas of the hands contaminated. Microorganisms tend to collect around and underneath the fingernails.

5. Procedural Step. Rub the hands together until they are dry; this usually takes up to 30 seconds. Allow your hands to dry completely before touching anything. The hands are now medically aseptic.

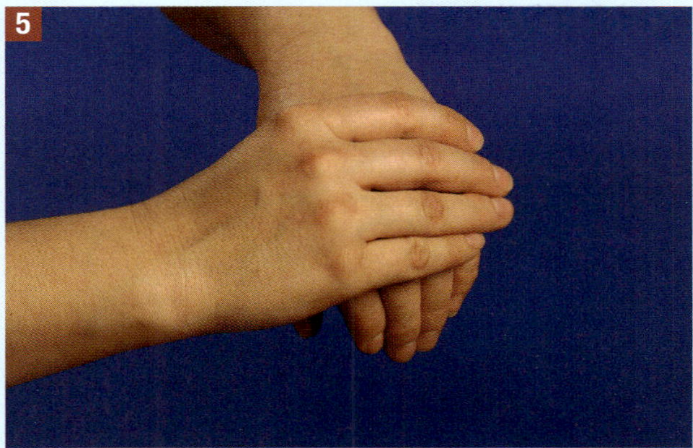

Rub the hands together until they are dry.

Note: After cleaning your hands 5 to 10 times with a hand sanitizer, a buildup of emollients may occur on your hands. The emollients can be easily removed by washing your hands with soap and water.

Principle. If you have applied a sufficient amount of hand sanitizer, it should take up to 30 seconds for your hands to feel dry. Your hands will still feel a little wet at first. Let them dry completely before touching anything.

PROCEDURE 17.3 Application and Removal of Disposable Exam Gloves

Outcome Apply and remove disposable exam gloves.

Equipment/Supplies

- Disposable exam gloves

Applying Disposable Exam Gloves

No special technique is required when disposable exam gloves are applied. This is because the hands are clean, and the gloves are clean; the medical assistant can touch any part of the gloves during application without contaminating them.

1. **Procedural Step.** Remove all rings and sanitize your hands. Handwashing should be performed if the hands are visibly soiled. If this is not the case, use an alcohol-based hand sanitizer to sanitize the hands. Ensure that your hands are completely dry.
   Principle. Rings may cause the gloves to tear. The warm, moist environment inside gloves provides ideal growing conditions for the multiplication of transient microorganisms present on the hands. Sanitizing the hands removes these microorganisms and prevents the transmission of pathogens. Moisture encourages the growth of microorganisms.
2. **Procedural Step.** If needed, determine your glove size (see Box 27.2). Choose your correct glove size. The gloves should fit snugly but not be too tight. Apply the gloves and adjust them so they fit comfortably.
   Principle. If your gloves are too small, they may rip as you are applying them or may become uncomfortable to wear. If they are too large, you may find it difficult to perform your tasks.

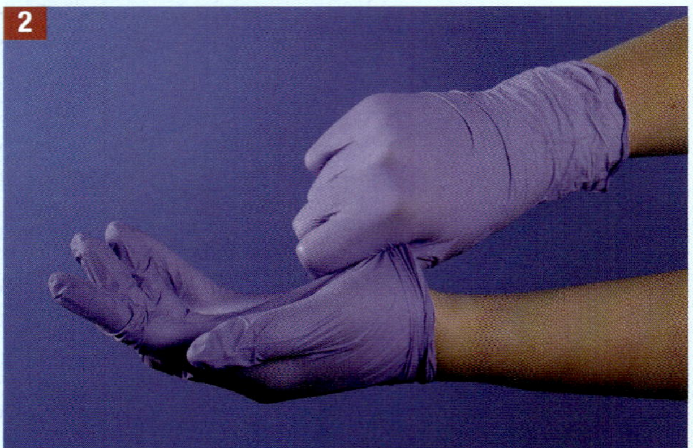

Apply the gloves.

3. **Procedural Step.** Inspect the gloves for tears. If a tear is present, remove the torn glove and apply a new one.

Removing Disposable Exam Gloves

Gloves must be removed in a manner that protects the medical assistant from contaminating their clean hands with pathogens that may be present on the outsides of the gloves. This is accomplished by not allowing the bare hands to come in contact with the outsides of the gloves.

4. **Procedural Step.** Grasp the outside of the left glove 1 to 2 inches from the top with your gloved right hand. (*Note:* It does not matter which glove is removed first. You may start with the right glove if you prefer.)

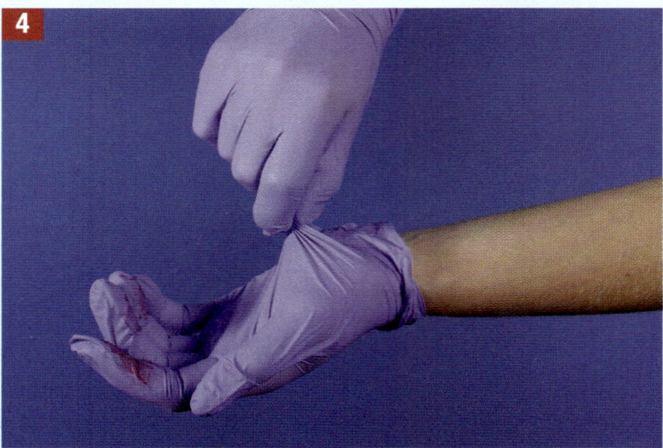

Grasp the glove 1 to 2 inches from the top of the glove.

5. **Procedural Step.** Slowly pull the left glove off the hand. It will turn inside out as it is removed from your hand.
6. **Procedural Step.** Pull the left glove free and scrunch it into a ball with your gloved right hand.

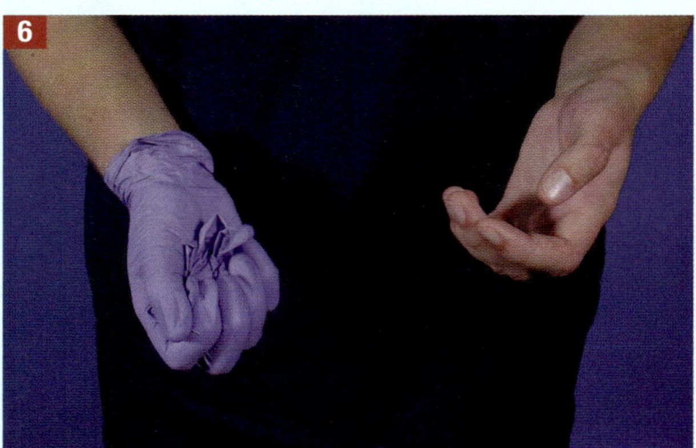

Scrunch the glove into a ball.

PROCEDURE 17.3 Application and Removal of Disposable Exam Gloves—cont'd

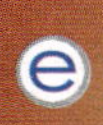

7. Procedural Step. Place the index and middle fingers of the left hand on the inside of the right glove. Do not allow your clean hand to touch the outside of the glove.

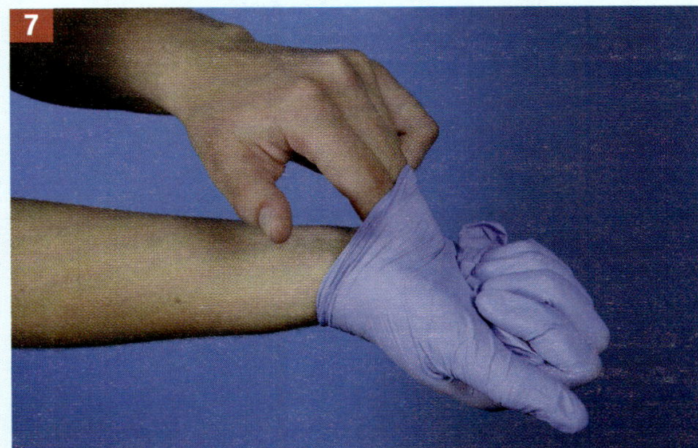

Place the index and middle fingers inside the glove.

8. Procedural Step. Pull the glove off the right hand. It will turn inside out as it is removed from your hand, enclosing the balled-up left glove. Discard both gloves in an appropriate container. If your gloves are visibly contaminated with blood or other potentially infectious materials, discard them in a biohazard waste container. Otherwise, they can be discarded in a regular waste container.

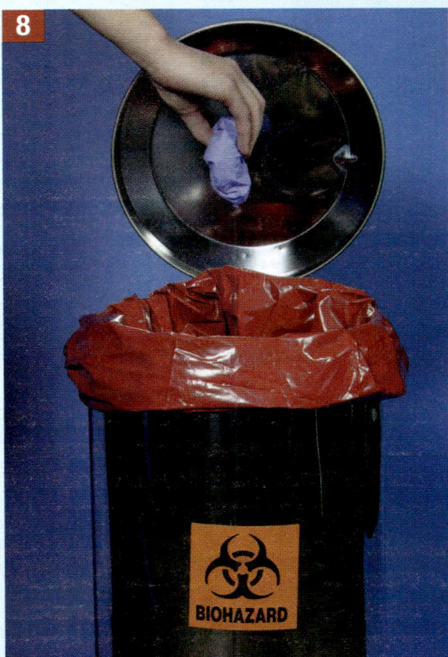

Discard both gloves in an appropriate container.

9. Procedural Step. Sanitize your hands to remove any microorganisms or other contaminants that may have come in contact with your hands during glove removal.

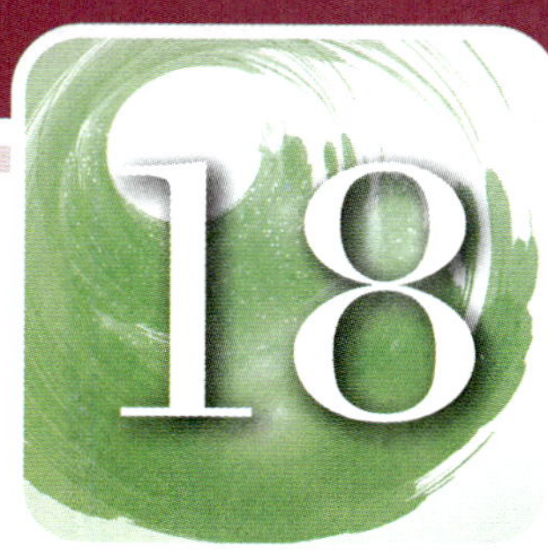

Sterilization and Disinfection

Check out the Evolve site at http://evolve.elsevier.com/Bonewit/today to access additional interactive activities and exercises to help you study and prepare for success.

LEARNING OBJECTIVES/ PROCEDURES

Hazard Communication Standard

1. Explain the purpose of the Hazard Communication Standard.
2. List and describe the information that must be included on a hazardous chemical label.
3. List and describe the information that must be included in a safety data sheet (SDS).

Read and interpret an SDS.

Sanitization

4. State the purpose of sanitization.
5. State the advantages of using an ultrasonic cleaner.
6. List and describe the guidelines for sanitizing instruments.

Sanitize instruments.

Disinfection

7. Describe the three levels of disinfection: high, intermediate, and low.
8. Describe the following: critical item, semicritical item, and noncritical item.
9. List and describe the guidelines for disinfecting items.
10. List and describe the use of disinfectants commonly employed in the medical office.

Sterilization

11. Explain how the autoclave functions to sterilize items.
12. List the components of a sterilization monitoring program.
13. List and describe the various types of sterilization indicators.
14. Identify the advantages of sterilization paper and sterilization pouches.
15. List and describe the guidelines for loading the autoclave.
16. Identify the steps in the autoclave cycle.
17. Explain the importance of drying the sterilized load.
18. Explain how to handle and store sterilized packs and pouches.
19. Identify the daily, weekly, and monthly autoclave maintenance.

Wrap an item with sterilization paper.
Wrap an item with a sterilization pouch.
Sterilize items in an autoclave.

Maintain the autoclave.

Other Sterilization Methods

20. State the primary use of the following sterilization methods: dry heat, ethylene oxide gas, chemicals, and radiation.

CHAPTER OUTLINE

Autoclave
Monitoring Program
Wrap Items
Operate the Autoclave
Handle and Store Wrapped Items
Maintain the Autoclave

Other Sterilization Methods
Dry Heat Oven
Ethylene Oxide Gas Sterilization
Cold Sterilization
Radiation

KEY TERMS

autoclave (AU-toe-klave)
critical item
decontamination
detergent
disinfectant (dis-in-FEK-tant)
hazardous chemical
health hazard
incubate (IN-kyoo-bate)
load
noncritical item
physical hazard
Safety Data Sheet (SDS)
sanitization (san-ih-tih-ZAY-shun)
semicritical item
spore
sterilization (stare-ill-ih-ZAY-shun)

INTRODUCTION TO STERILIZATION AND DISINFECTION

The air and all objects around us contain microorganisms. The medical assistant is responsible for helping to reduce and eliminate microorganisms to prevent the spread of disease. This is accomplished by practicing good techniques of medical and surgical asepsis.

Physical and chemical methods are used to destroy microorganisms in the medical office. The method selected depends on the intended use of the item. Items that penetrate sterile tissue or the vascular system, such as surgical instruments, must be sterilized, typically with the use of an autoclave (physical method). Items that come in contact with the skin, such as stethoscopes, blood pressure cuffs, and percussion hammers, should be disinfected (chemical method).

Sanitization, disinfection, and autoclave maintenance involve the use of hazardous chemicals. It is essential for the medical assistant to know the precautions that are required when working with hazardous chemicals.

DEFINITIONS OF TERMS

Terms that aid in understanding this chapter are listed and defined here.

Sanitization Sanitization is a series of steps designed to remove debris from an item and reduce the number of microorganisms to a safe level. Sanitization removes all organic and inorganic debris from an item, such as blood, body fluids, tissue, and soil. For items that are used in examinations, treatments, and office surgery to be properly sterilized or disinfected, they must first be sanitized.

Decontamination Decontamination refers to the use of physical or chemical means to remove pathogens on an item so that it is no longer capable of transmitting disease; this makes the item safe to handle.

Detergent A detergent is an agent that cleanses by emulsifying dirt and oil.

Disinfectant A disinfectant is an agent used to destroy pathogenic microorganisms; however, it does not kill the resistant spores. The most common disinfectants used in the medical office consist of chemical agents. Chemical disinfectants are used on inanimate objects and surfaces in contrast to antiseptics, which are used on living tissue.

Spore A spore is a hard, thick-walled capsule that some bacteria form by losing moisture and condensing their contents to contain only the essential parts of the protoplasm of the bacterial cell. Spores represent a resting and protective stage of bacteria and are more resistant to drying, sunlight, heat, and disinfectants than vegetative bacteria. Spores cannot reproduce while vegetative bacteria are alive and can reproduce. Favorable conditions cause spores to germinate into vegetative bacteria again, capable of reproducing. Two examples of species of bacteria that form spores are *Clostridium botulinum,* which causes botulism, and *Clostridium tetani,* which causes tetanus.

Sterilization Sterilization is the process of destroying all forms of microbial life, including spores. An item that is *sterile* is free of all living microorganisms and spores. There can be no relative degrees of sterility—an item is either sterile or not sterile. The method most commonly used to sterilize items in the medical office is steam under pressure using an autoclave.

HAZARD COMMUNICATION STANDARD

The Hazard Communication Standard (HCS) is a requirement of OSHA. The purpose of the HCS is to ensure that employees are informed of the hazards associated with chemicals in their workplace and the precautions to take to protect themselves when working with hazardous chemicals. A **hazardous chemical** is any chemical that is a health hazard or a physical hazard. A **health hazard** is defined as the potential of the chemical to cause acute toxicity, skin corrosion or irritation, serious eye damage or irritation, respiratory or skin sensitization, germ cell mutagenicity, cancer, or reproductive toxicity, or is an aspiration hazard. A **physical hazard** is defined as the potential of the chemical to catch fire, explode, or react with other chemicals or materials.

The HCS uses the Globally Harmonized System of Classification and Labeling of Chemicals (GHS) set forth by the United Nations. The GHS is an international standard that provides consistency in the classification and labeling of chemicals. The GHS classifies chemicals according to their health and physical hazards. The GHS also requires the use of a standardized format for container labels and safety data sheets (SDSs).

The GHS enable employees to quickly obtain and more easily understand information regarding the safe handling, use, and disposal of hazardous chemicals. This assists in preventing injury and illness associated with exposure to hazardous chemicals.

In the medical office, sanitization, disinfection, and autoclave maintenance require the use of hazardous chemicals; the medical assistant must have a thorough knowledge of the HCS. The HCS consists of the following components:

- Development of a hazard communication program
- Inventory of hazardous chemicals
- Labeling requirements
- SDS requirements
- Employee information and training

HAZARD COMMUNICATION PROGRAM

As part of the HCS, employers are required to develop a hazard communication program. The hazard communication program consists of a written plan that describes what the facility is doing to meet the requirements of the HCS. The information in the plan must be made available and communicated to all employees who work with hazardous chemicals.

INVENTORY OF HAZARDOUS CHEMICALS

The employer must develop and maintain a list of hazardous chemicals that are used and stored in the workplace. The list must be updated as new chemicals are introduced into the workplace. In the medical office, hazardous chemicals typically include the following:

- Products for sanitization, disinfection, and autoclave maintenance (e.g., chemical disinfectants, instrument cleaners, autoclave cleaners) (Fig. 18.1).
- Chemicals for laboratory testing (e.g., testing reagents, developing solutions, controls)
- Pharmaceutical products such as local anesthetics (e.g., lidocaine [Xylocaine])

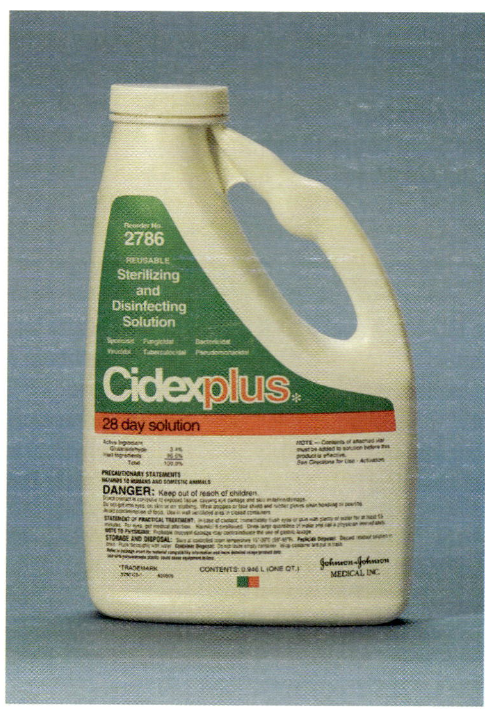

Fig. 18.1 Hazardous chemical used as a disinfectant in the medical office.

- Front office supplies (e.g., copier and printer toners)
- Cleaning products (e.g., drain cleaner, household bleach)

LABELING OF HAZARDOUS CHEMICALS

The HCS requires that a hazardous chemical container be labeled by the manufacturer with a warning to alert the user that the chemical is dangerous. This label must include the possible hazards of the chemical and the steps that can be taken to protect against those risks and must not be removed or defaced. If a label falls off a product or is damaged or obscured, a replacement label must be applied. If a chemical is transferred to a new container, a label with the required information must be attached to the new container.

Container Label Requirements

The HCS requires that manufacturers label their hazardous chemicals according to GHS guidelines. The information on the container label allows the user to determine the hazards of the chemical and how to prevent or lessen exposure to the chemical (Fig. 18.2). Information required on the label of a hazardous chemical container includes the following:

- *Product Identifier:* The product identifier specifies how the chemical is identified. This can be (but is not limited to) the chemical name and the code number or batch number.
- *Supplier Identification:* Supplier information includes the name, address, and telephone number of the chemical manufacturer.

PRODUCT IDENTIFIER
Code: 7489
Product Name: Glutaraldehyde Solution

SUPPLIER IDENTIFICATION
Poston Corporation
2010 East Main Street
Camden, New Jersey 08106
800-249-8240

PRECAUTIONARY STATEMENTS
Do not breathe dust/fumes/gas/mist/vapors/spray
Avoid release to the environment
Wear protective gloves/ eye protection/ face protection
IF ON SKIN: Wash with plenty of soap and water
IF ON EYES: Rinse cautiously with water for several minutes. Remove contact lenses, if present and easy to do. Continue rinsing
IF SWALLOWED: Immediately call a POISON CENTER or doctor/physician

HAZARD PICTOGRAMS

SIGNAL WORD
DANGER

HAZARD STATEMENTS
Toxic if swallowed
May be harmful in contact with skin
Causes skin irritation
Causes serious eye damage
May cause allergy or asthma symptoms or breathing difficulties
May cause respiratory irritation
Very toxic to aquatic life

SUPPLEMENTAL INFORMATION
Storage: Store at room temperature
Disposal: Discard residual solution in drain. Flush thoroughly with water

Expiration Date: 10/15/xx

Fig. 18.2 Hazardous chemical container label following the GHS system.

- *Precautionary Statement(s):* A precautionary statement is a phrase that describes recommended measures to be taken to minimize or prevent adverse effects resulting from exposure to the chemical or improper storage or handling (e.g., wear protective gloves, wear protective eyewear, and wear face protection).
- *Hazard Pictograms:* Hazard pictograms consist of standardized graphic symbols allowing users to quickly identify the types of hazards associated with the chemical. There are eight different pictograms representing the health and physical hazards covered in the GHS (Fig. 18.3).
- *Signal Word:* A signal word indicates the relative degree of severity of the hazardous chemical. There are two signal words under GHS:
  Danger: Denotes a more severe hazard possible
  Warning: Denotes a less serious hazard possible but potentially harmful
- *Hazard Statement(s):* A hazard statement is a phrase that describes the nature and (when appropriate) the degree of hazard associated with the chemical (e.g., toxic if swallowed; causes serious eye damage).
- *Supplementary Information:* The manufacturer may provide additional information such as storage, disposal, and the expiration date of the chemical.

SAFETY DATA SHEETS

A **safety data sheet** (SDS) is a document that provides more detailed information than the container label regarding the chemical, its hazards, and measures to take to prevent injury and illness when handling the chemical (Fig. 18.4). Manufacturers of hazardous chemicals are required to develop and make available an SDS for each hazardous chemical they produce according to GHS guidelines.

The HCS requires that a current SDS be kept on file for each hazardous chemical used or stored in the workplace. In the event of an accidental exposure, information on the SDS must be readily available as a reference for emergency treatment. It is important that the medical assistant thoroughly review the SDS of a hazardous chemical before using it.

If an SDS is missing, it must be replaced. This is accomplished by contacting the manufacturer of the chemical for a replacement or by going to the manufacturer's website; most manufacturers post their SDSs on their websites for easy access.

What Would You Do? What Would You *Not* Do?

Case Study 1

Elba Cordera has brought her daughter Maria in for a well-baby visit. Maria is 9 months old and is just starting to crawl. Mrs. Cordera is taking precautions to baby-proof her house to protect Maria from accidents. Mrs. Cordera wants to know how to tell whether a cleaning product is poisonous. She also wants to know what she should do if Maria gets into a cleaning product and spills it on herself or swallows it. ■

Safety Data Sheet Requirements

The GHS guidelines require that the information on an SDS of a hazardous chemical (see Fig. 18.4) be presented using a standardized 16-section format that follows a specified sequence as outlined:

1. *Identification:* This section provides information used to identify the hazardous chemical and must include the

PICTOGRAM	MEANING OF PICTOGRAM	TYPE OF HAZARD(S) (Associated with this pictogram)
Health Hazard 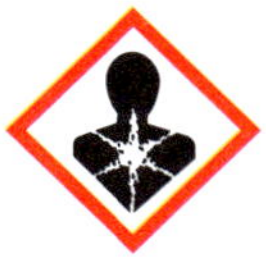	The chemical is a risk to health if used improperly.	• Carcinogen • Mutagenicity • Reproductive Toxicity • Respiratory Sensitizer • Target Organ Toxicity • Aspiration Toxicity
Severe Toxic 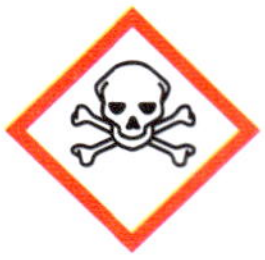	The chemical is a serious health or physical hazard or poison. It will produce adverse effects following a single dose. This pictogram is usually used in combination with the Health Hazard Pictogram.	• Acute Toxicity (fatal or toxic) if inhaled or swallowed, or if it comes in contact with the skin.
Acute Toxic 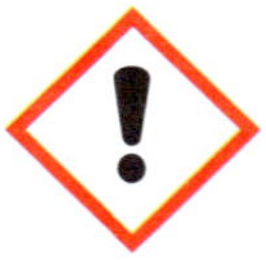	The chemical may cause immediate, serious health effects but it is less severe than the Severe Toxic pictogram (skull and crossbones). This pictogram is usually used in combination with the Health Hazard Pictogram.	• Irritant (skin and eye) • Skin Sensitizer • Acute Toxicity • Narcotic Effects • Respiratory Tract Irritant
Flammable 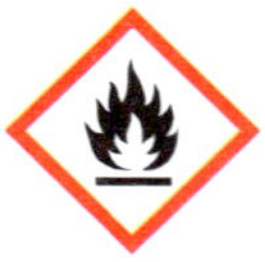	The chemical may burst into flame. Be careful to keep away from ignition sources and combustible materials.	• Flammables • Pyrophorics • Self-Heating • Emits Flammable Gas • Self-Reactive • Organic Peroxides
Corrosive 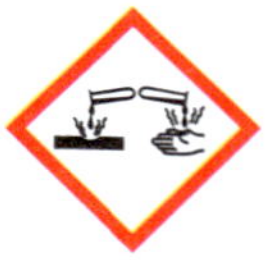	The chemical is a physical or health hazard that can easily damage skin or eyes. Be aware of PPE and storage requirements.	• Skin Corrosion/Burns • Eye Damage • Corrosive to Metals
Oxidizer 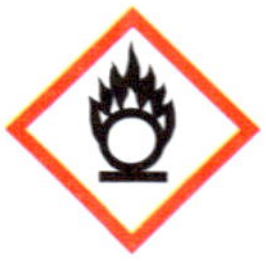	The chemical may cause other materials to ignite or burn faster. It can create an increased fire risk in work or storage environment.	• Oxidizers
Gas Under Pressure 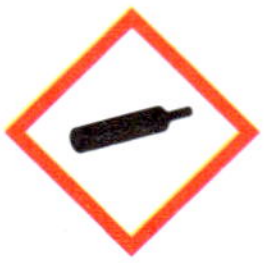	This chemical consists of pressurized gas that would explode, rocket, or damage health if heated, ruptured or leaking.	• Gases Under Pressure
Explosive 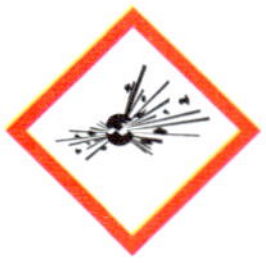	This material can blow up or otherwise create an uncontrolled reaction. Should be treated with extreme caution.	• Explosives • Self-Reactives • Organic Peroxides

Fig. 18.3 GHS Hazard Pictograms. (Pictograms from U.S. Department of Labor, Occupational Safety and Health Administration.)

SAFETY DATA SHEET (SDS)			
SECTION 1: IDENTIFICATION			
Product name:	Glutaraldehyde Solution	**Telephone:**	1 (800) 331-0766
Brand:	Aldecyde	**Emergency phone number:**	1 (800) 773-8690
Manufacturer:	Poston Corporation 2010 East Main Street Camden, New Jersey 08106	**Recommended Use:**	High Level Disinfectant
		Restrictions on Use:	Not recommended for drug, food, or household use.
SECTION 2: HAZARDS IDENTIFICATION			
Hazard Classification			
Acute toxicity, oral:	GHS Category 3	Respiratory sensitization:	GHS Category 1
Skin irritation:	GHS Category 2	Skin sensitization:	GHS Category 1
Serious eye damage:	GHS Category 1	Acute aquatic toxicity:	GHS Category 1
Signal Word			
Danger			

Hazard Statements	
H301	Toxic if swallowed
H313	May be harmful in contact with skin
H315	Causes skin irritation
H318	Causes serious eye damage
H334	May cause allergy or asthma symptoms or breathing difficulties if inhaled
H335	May cause respiratory irritation
H400	Very toxic to aquatic life

Hazard Pictograms

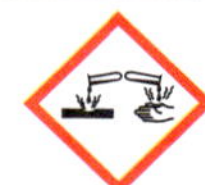

	Precautionary Statements
P260	Do not breathe dust/fumes/gas/mist/vapors/spray
P273	Avoid release to the environment
P280	Wear protective gloves/eye protection/face protection
P302 + P352	IF ON SKIN: Wash with plenty of soap and water
P305 + P351 + P338	IF ON EYES: Rinse cautiously with water for several minutes. Remove contact lenses, if present and easy to do. Continue rinsing.
P310	IF SWALLOWED: Immediately call a POISON CENTER or doctor/physician

SECTION 3: COMPOSITION/INFORMATION ON INGREDIENTS

CAS NUMBER	CHEMICAL NAME OF INGREDIENTS	PERCENT
111-30-8	Glutaraldehyde	2.5
7732-18-5	Water	97.4
7632-00-0	Sodium Nitrite	<1

SECTION 4: FIRST AID MEASURES

Skin Contact: Rinse with water. Remove contaminated clothing and wash before reuse. Consult a physician if skin redness or irritation persist.

Eye Contact: Immediately flush with water for 15 minutes. Seek medical attention.

Inhalation: Remove to fresh air immediately. If experiencing difficulty breathing, seek medical attention.

Ingestion: Call a physician or Poison Control Center immediately. Do not ingest emetic.

SECTION 5: FIRE FIGHTING MEASURES

Suitable Extinguishing Media: Use extinguishing agent which is suitable for the surrounding fire.

Hazardous Combustion Products: Carbon monoxide and carbon dioxide.

Special Protective Equipment for Firefighters: Wear self-contained breathing apparatus for fire fighting if necessary.

Fig. 18.4 Safety data sheet (SDS).

Continued

SAFETY DATA SHEET (SDS)

SECTION 6: ACCIDENTAL RELEASE MEASURES

Personal Precautions: Ventilate area. Avoid breathing vapors or mist. Wear eye and skin protection while handling material for clean-up.

Cleanup Procedures: Contain spill by placing suitable absorbent material around the edges of the spill and work inward. Carefully scoop up into waste container for disposal. Dispose of in accordance with applicable Federal, State and Local regulations.

SECTION 7: HANDLING AND STORAGE

Precautions for Safe Handling: Use in a well-ventilated area. Avoid breathing vapors or mist. Avoid contact with skin, eyes and clothing. Remove contaminated clothing and launder before use.

Conditions for Safe Storage: Store in a cool, dry area (59-86º F) away from direct sunlight or sources of intense heat. Keep container tightly closed when not in use.

SECTION 8: EXPOSURE CONTROLS/PERSONAL PROTECTION

Exposure Control Limits:

PEL: 0.2 ppm
TLV: 0.2 ppm

Engineering Controls and Personal Protective Equipment:

Ventilation: Ensure adequate ventilation.

Respiratory Protection: None normally required for routine use.

Skin Protection: Wear protective chemical resistant gloves. Wear suitable protective clothing.

Eye Protection: Eye protection required.

SECTION 9: PHYSICAL AND CHEMICAL PROPERTIES

APPEARANCE: Bluish-green liquid	BOILING POINT: 212º F
PHYSICAL STATE: Liquid	EVAPORATION RATE: 0.98
ODOR: Sharp odor	VAPOR PRESSURE (mm Hg): 0.20 at 20º C
ODOR THRESHOLD: 0.04 ppm	VAPOR DENSITY (AIR = 1): 1.1
pH: 7.5-8.5	SPECIFIC GRAVITY: 1.004
FREEZING POINT: 32º F	SOLUBILITY IN WATER: Complete (100%)

SECTION 10: STABILITY AND REACTIVITY

STABILITY: Stable under recommended storage conditions.

CONDITIONS TO AVOID: Avoid temperatures above 200º F.

INCOMPATIBILITY (MATERIAL TO AVOID): Strong acids, bases and oxidizing agents.

HAZARDOUS DECOMPOSITION BY PRODUCTS: None

HAZARDOUS POLYMERIZATION: Will not occur

SECTION 11: TOXICOLOGICAL INFORMATION

Acute Health Hazards:

Inhalation: Inhalation of mist or vapors may be severely irritating to the nose, throat and lungs.

Skin Contact: May cause skin irritation. May aggravate pre-existing dermatitis.

Eye Contact: Severe irritant and corrosive to the eyes.

Ingestion: Ingestion of this material may cause oral thrush, nausea, vomiting, epigastric distress, diarrhea, headache, fatigue, dizziness, insomnia, mental confusion, and impairment.

Chronic Health Hazards:

No adverse effects expected based on the available data.

Medical Conditions Aggravated By Exposure:

Inhalation of vapor may cause asthma-like symptoms (chest discomfort and tightness, difficulty with breathing) as well as aggravate pre-existing asthma and inflammatory or fibrotic pulmonary disease.

Carcinogen:

None of the components is listed as a carcinogen or potential carcinogen by NTP, IARC, or OSHA.

SECTION 12: ECOLOGICAL INFORMATION

This product is classified as toxic to the aquatic environment.

Fig. 18.4, cont'd

SAFETY DATA SHEET (SDS)	
SECTION 13: DISPOSAL CONSIDERATIONS	
Container must be triple rinsed and disposed of in accordance with Federal, State, and/or Local regulations. Used solution should be flushed thoroughly with water into sewage disposal in accordance with Federal, State, and/or Local regulations.	
SECTION 14: TRANSPORT INFORMATION	
Restrictions:	None. Not regulated.
UN Number:	None
UN Proper Shipping Name:	N/A
Transport Hazard Class:	N/A
Packing Group Number:	N/A
SECTION 15: REGULATORY INFORMATION	
EPA SARA 311/312 Hazard Classification:	Acute Health, Chronic Health
SECTION 16: OTHER INFORMATION	
Issue Date:	4/28/02
Revision Date:	10/10/2014

Fig. 18.4, cont'd

product name and brand name and the name, address, phone number, and emergency phone number of the manufacturer. This section must also include the recommended use of the chemical and any restrictions on use.

2. *Hazards Identification:* This section includes the hazards of the chemical and the appropriate warning information associated with those hazards and includes the following:
   - Hazard classification of the chemical
   - Signal word
   - Hazard statement(s)
   - Hazard pictograms
   - Precautionary statement(s)
3. *Composition/Information on Ingredients:* This section provides a list of the ingredients in the hazardous chemical.
4. *First-Aid Measures:* This section describes the initial care that an untrained responder can provide to an individual who is exposed to the hazardous chemical. It is subdivided according to the different routes of exposure (e.g., skin contact, inhalation).
5. *Fire-Fighting Measures:* Some hazardous chemicals may cause a fire if used improperly. This section provides recommendations for fighting a fire caused by the chemical, including suitable extinguishing agents.
6. *Accidental Release Measures:* This section provides recommendations on the appropriate response to spills, leaks, or releases of the hazardous chemical including containment and cleanup practices to prevent or minimize exposure to people, properties, or the environment. It also identifies the personal precautions that should be taken during the cleanup such as wearing gloves and protective eyewear.
7. *Handling and Storage:* This section identifies precautions for the safe handling of the hazardous chemical and conditions for the safe storage of the chemical.
8. *Exposure Controls/Personal Protection:* This section indicates the exposure control limits, engineering controls, and personal protective measures that should be used to protect oneself from the hazardous chemical.
9. *Physical and Chemical Properties:* This section lists the physical and chemical properties associated with the hazardous chemical such as appearance, physical state, odor, pH, and boiling point.
10. *Stability and Reactivity:* Some hazardous chemicals react when combined with other chemicals or materials. This section lists the substances and conditions that the chemical should be kept away from to prevent a dangerous reaction.
11. *Toxicological Information:* This section identifies the toxicological effects that can result from overexposure to the hazardous chemical and includes the following:
    - Route of entry, which indicates how the chemical can enter the body, including inhalation, skin contact, eye contact, and ingestion
    - Signs and symptoms of overexposure (e.g., skin irritation, eye damage, lung damage) categorized according to acute and chronic health hazards
    - Medical conditions that are aggravated by exposure to the chemical (e.g., asthma, dermatitis)
    - Indication of whether the chemical has been identified as a potential carcinogen
12. *Ecological Information:* This section provides information to help determine the environmental impact of the hazardous chemical if it were released into the environment.
13. *Disposal Considerations:* This section provides guidance on proper disposal of the hazardous chemical.
14. *Transport Information:* This section provides guidance to suppliers for shipping and transporting the hazardous chemical.
15. *Regulatory Information:* This section identifies the safety, health, and environmental regulations specific

for the hazardous chemical that is not indicated anywhere else on the SDS.

16. *Other Information:* This section includes other important information related to the hazardous chemical such as when the SDS was prepared or when the last known revision was made.

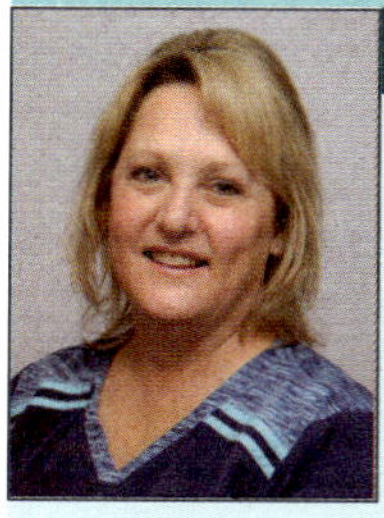

Putting It All Into Practice

My name is Linda, and I work for two physicians in a family practice medical office. As a medical assistant, one of the situations you deal with on an almost-daily basis is drug representatives who come to the office to promote their products. Their job is anything but easy. The waiting and the frequent rejections would make most people think twice before applying for the job.

One winter day, I am sure I made one drug representative really think twice about his career choice. As the representative stopped at our office, he, being a polite young man, let a patient wearing wet, snow-covered boots enter the building first. Trying to make a good impression with a new suit and dress shoes, he soon found himself doing a "Spanish fandango" while trying to maintain his balance and eventually crashed to the floor.

I thought I would help by mopping up the snow-tracked floor. What I did not know was the mop had wax on it. Needless to say, when he returned with the requested drug samples, we were not able to keep him from falling a second time! ■

EMPLOYEE INFORMATION AND TRAINING

The HCS requires that employees be provided with information and training regarding hazardous chemicals in the workplace. The training session must be offered at the time of an employee's initial assignment to a work area where hazardous chemicals are present, and whenever a new chemical hazard is introduced into the work area. The training program must be an ongoing activity, and each training session must be documented.

SANITIZATION

Sanitization consists of a series of steps that remove debris from an item and reduce the number of microorganisms to a safe level (Procedure 18.1). Debris may consist of organic or inorganic material such as blood, body fluids, body tissue, and soil. Debris on the surface of an item can result in incomplete sterilization or disinfection. This is because the debris acts as a physical barrier preventing the physical or chemical agent from reaching the surface of the item to kill microorganisms.

SANITIZING INSTRUMENTS

The items most frequently sanitized in the medical office are medical and surgical instruments. The general steps in the sanitization procedure of instruments are as follows:

1. *Rinse* the instruments immediately after use to prevent debris from drying on the instruments making it harder to remove later.
2. *Decontaminate* the instruments with a chemical disinfectant to remove pathogenic microorganisms making the instrument safe to handle.
3. *Clean* the instruments with an instrument cleaner to remove all organic and inorganic debris. An instrument cleaner contains a detergent and may also be combined with an enzymatic cleaner which can break down organic matter such as blood and tissue.
4. *Thoroughly rinse* the instruments to remove all loosened debris and cleaning solution residue.
5. *Dry* the instruments to prevent stains on the instruments.
6. *Inspect each instrument* for defects and working condition.
7. *Lubricate* hinged instruments to make the instruments function well and last longer.

GUIDELINES FOR SANITIZING INSTRUMENTS

The following guidelines should be followed when sanitizing surgical instruments:

1. *Wear gloves during the sanitization process.* The medical assistant should wear disposable gloves during the entire sanitization procedure. This protects the medical assistant from bloodborne pathogens and other potentially infectious materials. The medical assistant should be especially careful when working with hazardous chemicals and when handling sharp instruments. Heavy-duty utility gloves should be worn over the disposable gloves to provide protection from the irritating effects of chemical agents and accidental punctures or cuts from sharp instruments.
2. *Handle instruments carefully.* Instruments are expensive and delicate, yet durable and can last for many years if handled and maintained properly. Dropping an instrument on the floor or throwing an instrument into a basin may damage it. Instruments should never be piled in a heap because they may become entangled and may be damaged when separated. Keep sharp instruments separate from other instruments to prevent damaging or dulling the cutting edge. Also, keep delicate instruments separate to protect them from damage.
3. *Follow instructions on labels of chemical agents.* Before using a chemical agent (e.g., chemical disinfectant, instrument cleaner), check the expiration date on the container label. Chemicals have a tendency to lose potency over time and should not be used past their expiration date. Thoroughly review the SDS of the chemical agent

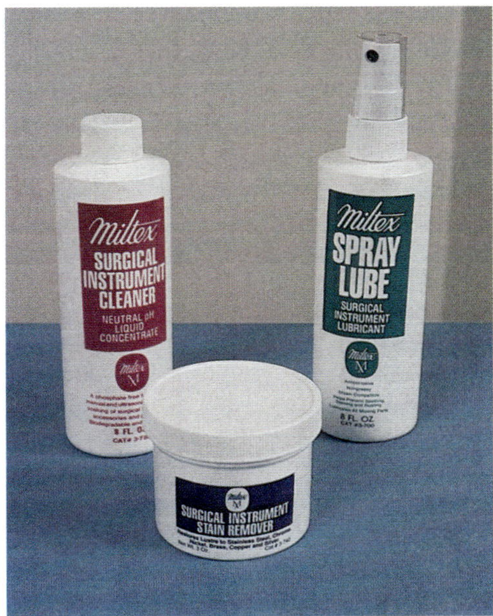

Fig. 18.5 Commercially available instrument cleaners. *Left,* Instrument cleaner; *center,* stain remover; *right,* spray lubricant.

and carefully read the label on the container to determine the use, mixing, storage, and disposal of the chemical agent. Follow the precautions listed on the label regarding personal safety, such as the use of gloves and protective eyewear.

4. *Use a proper cleaning agent.* A low-sudsing instrument cleaner with a neutral pH should be used to clean the instruments. Commercially available instrument cleaners meet these criteria (Fig. 18.5). Instrument cleaners often come in a concentrated form and must be diluted with water before use. Never substitute any other type of cleaner, such as dishwashing soap or laundry detergent; these cleaners may not be low-sudsing or may not have the proper pH for sanitizing instruments. If an instrument cleaner with an alkaline pH is used and is not completely rinsed off, it could leave a residue on the instrument. This could result in an orange-brown stain on the instrument that resembles rust. Using an acidic instrument cleaner also can cause staining and permanent corrosion.
5. *Use proper cleaning devices.* Proper cleaning devices should be used for the manual cleaning of surgical instruments. A stiff nylon brush should be used to clean the surface of the instrument. A stainless-steel wire brush can be used to clean grooves, crevices, or serrations. A stain on an instrument often can be removed by using a commercial instrument stain remover (see Fig. 18.5). Never use steel wool or other abrasives to remove stains because damage to the instrument could occur. Cleaning brushes should be cleaned and decontaminated daily or when heavily soiled. Brushes that show wear should be discarded.
6. *Carefully inspect each instrument for defects and proper working condition.* After cleaning, rinsing, and drying the instrument, it is important to check it for defects and proper working condition as follows:
   - The blades of an instrument should be straight and not bent.
   - The tips of an instrument should approximate tightly and evenly when the instrument is closed.
   - An instrument with a box lock (e.g., hemostatic forceps, needle holders) should move freely but must not be too loose. The pin that holds the box lock together should be flush against the instrument.
   - An instrument with a spring handle (e.g., thumb and tissue forceps) should have sufficient tension to grasp objects tightly.
   - The cutting edge of a sharp instrument should be smooth and devoid of nicks.
   - Scissors should cut cleanly and smoothly. To test for this, the medical assistant should cut into a thin piece of gauze. The scissors are in proper working condition if they cut all the way to the end of the blade without catching on the gauze.
7. *Lubricate hinged instruments.* Lubricate hinged instruments making sure to apply the lubricant only to the moving part of the instrument (e.g., box lock, screw lock). The lubricant makes the instrument function better and last longer. Use a lubricant that can be penetrated by steam, such as a commercial spray lubricant or a lubricant bath (see Fig. 18.5). Lubricate after performing the final rinse (and drying of the instrument); otherwise, the lubricant would be rinsed off the instrument. Never use industrial oils or silicon sprays. These substances are not steam-penetrable and can build up on the instrument, affecting its working condition.

DISINFECTION

Disinfection is the process of destroying pathogenic microorganisms, but it does not kill spores. Disinfection is accomplished in the medical office through the use of liquid chemical agents. Chemical disinfection has been discussed with respect to its role in the sanitization process to decontaminate instruments and make them safe to handle. This section discusses the use of chemical disinfection to disinfect semicritical and noncritical items so they can be used for patient care.

LEVELS OF DISINFECTION

Based on killing action, disinfection can be classified according to three levels.

High-Level Disinfection

High-level disinfection is a process that destroys all microorganisms with the exception of spores. High-level disinfection is used to disinfect semicritical items. A **semicritical**

item is an item that comes in contact with nonintact skin or intact mucous membranes such as a flexible fiberoptic sigmoidoscope. Examples of high-level disinfectants include 2% glutaraldehyde (e.g., Cidex, MetriCide) and orthophthalaldehyde (e.g., Cidex OPA and MetriCide OPA).

Intermediate-Level Disinfection

Intermediate-level disinfection is a process that inactivates tubercle bacilli (the causative agents of tuberculosis), all vegetative bacteria, most viruses, and most fungi, but it does not kill spores. Intermediate-level disinfection is used to disinfect noncritical items. **Noncritical items** are items that come in contact with intact skin but not with mucous membranes, including stethoscopes, blood pressure cuffs, tuning forks, percussion hammers, and crutches. A common intermediate-level disinfectant is isopropyl alcohol, which is frequently used in the form of alcohol wipes.

Low-Level Disinfection

Low-level disinfection is a process that kills most bacteria, some viruses, and some fungi, but it cannot be relied on to kill resistant microorganisms, such as tubercle bacilli, and it cannot kill spores. Low-level disinfectants typically are used to disinfect surfaces such as examining tables, laboratory countertops, walls, furniture, and floors. Low-level disinfectants used in the medical office include sodium hypochlorite (household bleach), phenolics, and quaternary ammonium compounds.

Types of Disinfectants

The disinfectants used most frequently in the medical office are described next. Table 18.1 lists these disinfectants, along with the level of disinfection, common names and uses for each.

Glutaraldehyde

Glutaraldehyde is a high-level disinfectant that has a rapid killing action and is not inactivated by the presence of organic material. Because it does not corrode lenses, metal, or rubber, it is often used for semicritical items that cannot be exposed to heat, such as flexible fiberoptic sigmoidoscopes. It is also used to decontaminate surgical instruments during the sanitization procedure to make them safe to handle. Brand names for glutaraldehyde include Cidex and MetriCide.

Glutaraldehyde is a highly toxic hazardous chemical and can cause harm to the body if not handled properly. When working with glutaraldehyde, the medical assistant must work in an area that is well ventilated. Utility gloves and protective eyewear must be worn to protect oneself from the irritating effects of this chemical (Fig. 18.6). If the hands or any other part of the body comes in contact with glutaraldehyde, the area should be rinsed thoroughly under running water.

Alcohol

Alcohol is frequently used as a disinfectant in the medical office. The two most common types are *ethyl alcohol* and *isopropyl alcohol.* The disinfecting action of alcohol is increased by the presence of water; a 70% solution of alcohol is recommended. Stronger concentrations (95% to 100%) are not as effective. A disadvantage of alcohol is that it tends to dissolve the cement from around the lenses of instruments.

Ethyl alcohol and isopropyl alcohol provide intermediate- to low-level disinfection and can be used to disinfect stethoscopes, blood pressure cuffs, and percussion hammers. Isopropyl alcohol wipes are used to disinfect small surfaces such as the diaphragm of a stethoscope and rubber stoppers on multiple-dose medication vials.

Table 18.1 Disinfectants Used in the Medical Office

Disinfectant	Level of Disinfection	Common Names	Use in the Medical Office
Glutaraldehyde	High-level disinfection	Cidex MetriCide ProCide Omnicide Wavicide	Disinfection of flexible fiberoptic sigmoidoscopes.
Alcohol	Intermediate- to low-level disinfection	Isopropyl alcohol Ethyl alcohol	Disinfection of stethoscopes, blood pressure cuffs, tuning forks, and percussion hammers; isopropyl alcohol wipes are used to disinfect rubber stoppers of multiple-dose medication vials.
Chlorine and chlorine compounds	Intermediate-level disinfection	Sodium hypochlorite (household bleach)	Recommended by OSHA for decontamination of blood spills.
Phenolics	Low-level disinfection	Carbolic acid Hydroxybenzene Phenic acid Phenyl hydroxide Phenylic acid	Disinfection of walls, furniture, floors, and laboratory work surfaces.
Quaternary ammonium compounds	Low-level disinfection	Benzalkonium chloride	Disinfection of walls, furniture, floors, and laboratory work surfaces.

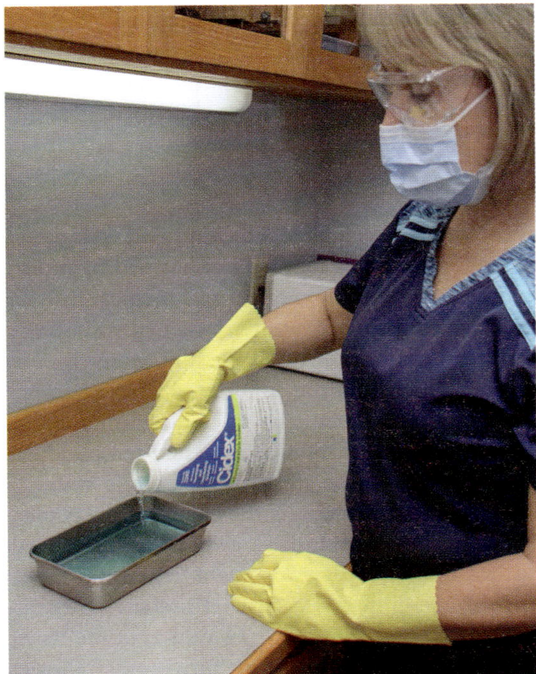

Fig. 18.6 Linda wears utility gloves and protective eyewear to protect her from the irritating effects of glutaraldehyde.

Chlorine and Chlorine Compounds

Chlorine and chlorine compounds are some of the oldest and most used disinfectants. Their most important use is in the chlorination of water. In the medical office, chlorine is used in the form of liquid sodium hypochlorite (household bleach), which is an intermediate level disinfectant. Household bleach inactivates tuberculosis bacteria, hepatitis B and C viruses, HIV, and many bacteria in 10 minutes at room temperature. Because of this, a 10% solution of household bleach in water (i.e., 1 part bleach to 9 parts water) is recommended by OSHA for the decontamination of blood spills. A disadvantage of this disinfectant is that it can irritate skin and mucous membranes and is highly corrosive to metal.

Phenolics

Phenolics are primarily used to disinfect walls, furniture, floors, laboratory work surfaces, and examining tables. This disinfectant is a corrosive poison and tends to be irritating to the eyes and skin. For this reason, gloves and protective eyewear should be worn when working with phenolics in the pure form. Many derivatives of phenolics are commonly used and are usually nonirritating, including Lysol and hexachlorophene.

Quaternary Ammonium Compounds

The quaternary ammonium compounds (often referred to as *quats*) are used in the medical office for the disinfection of noncritical surfaces, such as floors, furniture, and walls in the waiting room and examining rooms.

Guidelines for Disinfection

Certain guidelines should be followed when disinfecting items with a chemical agent.

Observe Safety Precautions

The medical assistant should carefully read the SDS and the container label before using a chemical disinfectant. All safety precautions should be followed when using the chemical to protect against illness or injury from a hazardous chemical.

Properly Prepare and Use the Disinfectant

It is important that the manufacturer's directions on preparation, dilution, and use of the chemical disinfectant be followed carefully. The disinfectant should be prepared exactly as indicated on the container label. Some disinfectants are used at their full strength, whereas others require dilution. Some disinfectants (e.g., glutaraldehyde) require the addition of an activator before they can be used. Properly preparing the disinfectant ensures the destruction of microorganisms. A disinfectant must be applied for a certain length of time to kill microorganisms. The medical assistant must be sure to disinfect for the length of time indicated on the container label.

Properly Store the Disinfectant

Chemical disinfectants should be closed tightly and stored properly under the storage conditions recommended by the manufacturer. Because chemical disinfectants lose their potency over time; the medical assistant should strictly adhere to the manufacturer's recommendations for the shelf life, use life, and reuse life. Each of these terms is defined next as it relates to chemical disinfectants.

Shelf life Shelf life is the length of time a chemical disinfectant may be stored before use and still retain its effectiveness. The shelf life is indicated by an expiration date stamped on the container. The expiration date should always be checked before using the chemical. Outdated disinfectants should not be used.

Use life Some disinfectants must be combined with another chemical to be activated before they are used. Use life is the period of time a disinfecting solution is effective after it has been activated. Cidex Plus (Johnson & Johnson) is effective for 28 days after activation. At the end of this time, any chemical remaining in the container must be discarded. When a chemical disinfectant is activated, the date on which it will expire should be written on the label of the container.

Reuse life Reuse life is the maximum number of days a reusable chemical disinfectant is effective. For example, Cidex Plus can be reused for 28 days to disinfect items. At the end of this time, the disinfectant must be discarded. The name of the disinfectant and the date when the disinfectant must be discarded should be written on an adhesive label and affixed to the container into which the disinfectant will be poured.

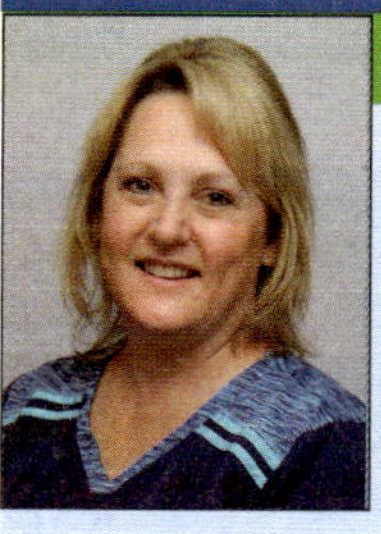

Memories *from* Practicum

Linda: During my practicum experience, I was placed in a pediatrician's office. I wanted to go to a pediatric site because I love being around children. One day I was in the examining room with my patient, a 4-year-old boy who was there with his mother. It was standard procedure at this office to take every patient's temperature. I started getting out our electronic thermometer to take his temperature when I noticed he looked a little frightened. He was looking at the thermometer funny, and he said, "Can you do it in my ear?" I said I was sorry but we didn't have that kind of thermometer. I told him I could do it under his arm or under his tongue. His mom looked at him, and he said, "But I want it in my ear." He finally agreed to let me do it under his arm. When I was finished taking his temperature, he smiled and said, "You are so nice!" ■

STERILIZATION

Sterilization is the process of destroying all forms of microbial life, including spores. An item that is sterile is free of all living microorganisms and spores. Sterilization must be used to process all critical items. A **critical item** is an item that comes in contact with sterile tissue or the vascular system such as surgical instruments.

As previously described, a semicritical item (one that comes in contact with nonintact skin or with intact mucous membranes) can be chemically disinfected with a high-level disinfectant. Most offices prefer instead to sterilize semicritical items (e.g., vaginal specula, nasal specula) in the autoclave. The autoclave provides a convenient, efficient, safe, and inexpensive method for destroying microorganisms. Chemical disinfectants not only are more expensive to use, but also are more hazardous and create problems regarding their proper disposal. The exception is a semicritical item that is heat-sensitive. Flexible fiberoptic sigmoidoscopes would be damaged by the heat of an autoclave and must be chemically disinfected.

STERILIZATION METHODS

Sterilization can be accomplished using physical and chemical methods. The method used to achieve sterility depends primarily on the nature of the item to be sterilized. The most common physical and chemical sterilization methods include the following:

Physical methods:

Autoclave (steam under pressure)
Dry heat oven (hot air)
Radiation

Chemical methods:

Ethylene oxide gas
Cold sterilization (chemical agents)

The most common method for sterilizing items in the medical office is steam under pressure using an autoclave. The autoclave is discussed in detail in this section; the other methods of sterilization are briefly described.

AUTOCLAVE

The **autoclave** is dependable, efficient, and economical and is used to sterilize items that are not harmed by moisture or high temperature such as surgical and medical instruments. An autoclave consists of an outer jacket surrounding an inner sterilizing chamber. Under pressure, water is converted into steam, which fills the inner sterilizing chamber. The pressure plays no direct part in killing microorganisms; rather, it functions to attain a higher temperature than could be reached by the steam from boiling water (212°F [100°C]). As the steam enters the chamber the cooler, drier air present in the chamber is forced out through a valve.

During an autoclave cycle, steam penetrates the articles placed in the chamber. The articles are cooler causing the steam to condense into moisture and transfer its heat to each article, killing all microorganisms and spores present on the article.

For proper sterilization, an autoclave must be operated at a pressure of at least 15 pounds of pressure per square inch (psi) and a temperature of at least 250° F (121°C). Vegetative forms of most microorganisms are killed in a few minutes at temperatures ranging from 130°F to 150°F (54°C to 65°C), but certain spores can withstand a temperature of 240°F (115°C) for longer than 3 hours. No organism, however, can survive direct exposure to saturated steam at 250°F (121°C) for 15 minutes or longer.

The sterilization process using an autoclave is discussed in this section (with the exception of sanitizing items, which was already presented). The sterilization process consists of the following components:

- Monitoring program
- Sanitizing items
- Wrapping items
- Loading the autoclave
- Operating the autoclave
- Handling and storing wrapped items
- Maintaining the autoclave

Monitoring Program

The CDC recommends that medical offices establish and maintain a monitoring program to ensure that autoclaved items are sterile. The monitoring program consists of quality control measures which include the following:

1. Written policies and procedures for each step of the sterilization process.
2. Sterilization indicators to ensure that minimum sterilizing conditions have been achieved.
3. Records for each autoclave cycle, maintained in an autoclave log (Fig. 18.7). Some autoclaves have printers that automatically print out most of this information at the end of the cycle (Fig. 18.8). The information that should

AUTOCLAVE LOG						
Date/Time	**Description of the Load**	**Cycle Time (min)**	**Temperature (° F)**	**Indicator* (+/–)**	**Initials**	**Comments**
7/25/XX 4:00 PM	Surgical instruments	20	250	–	KV	
7/26/XX 3:00 PM	MOS tray setups	30	250	–	KV	

*Indicator Interpretation:
Positive (+): Spores not killed, indicating sterilization conditions have not been met.
Negative (–): Spores killed, indicating sterilization conditions have been met.

Fig. 18.7 Example of an autoclave log.

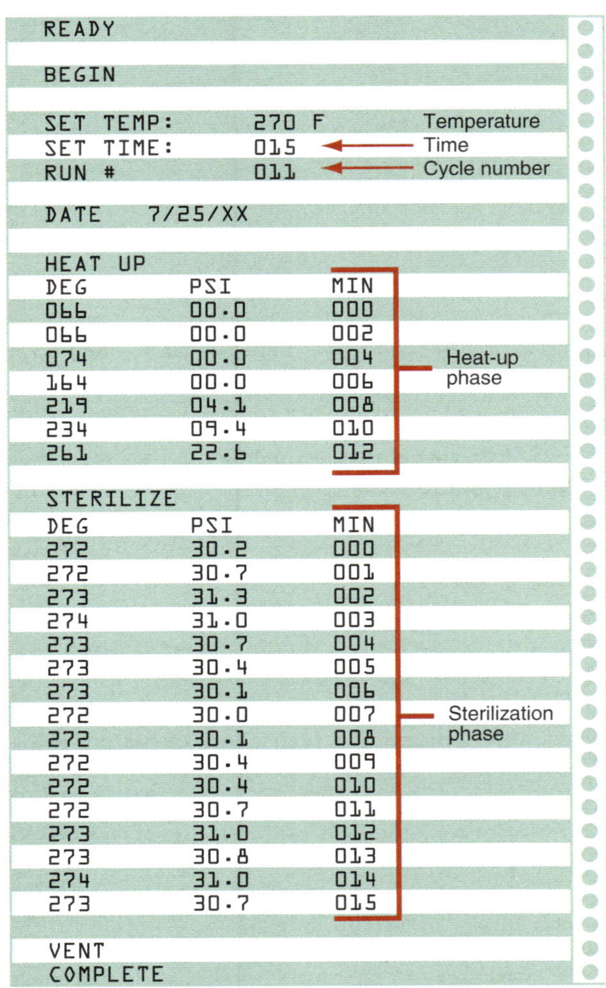

Fig. 18.8 Example of a printout of an autoclave cycle.

be documented for each autoclave cycle includes the following:

- Date and time of the cycle
- Description of the load
- Exposure time
- Exposure temperature and pressure
- Results of the sterilization indicator
- Initials of the operator

Sterilization Indicators

Articles processed in an autoclave must be exposed to steam at a time, temperature, and pressure that will result in sterilization. Sterilization indicators are available to determine the effectiveness of each autoclave cycle and to check against improper wrapping of items, improper loading of the autoclave, and faulty operation of the autoclave.

An item in a wrapped pack is not considered sterile unless the steam has penetrated to the center of the pack, therefore a sterilization indicator should be placed in the center of each pack. The medical assistant should carefully read the instructions that come with the sterilization indicators. The most reliable indicators check for the attainment of the proper temperature and indicate the duration of the temperature.

If an indicator does not change properly, a problem may be present in the sterilization technique or in the working condition of the autoclave. The manufacturer's guidelines for proper sterilization techniques should be reviewed and the items should be resterilized, following these guidelines. If the indicator still does not change properly, the autoclave is in need of repair and should not be used until it has been serviced.

Sterilization indicators should be stored in a cool, dry area. Excessive heat or moisture can damage the indicators. The most common sterilization indicators are chemical indicators and biologic indicators, which are described next.

Chemical Indicators

Chemical indicators are impregnated with a thermolabile dye that changes color when exposed to the sterilization process. If the chemical reaction of the indicator does not show the expected results, the item may not be sterile and must be resterilized. Chemical indicators include autoclave tape and sterilization indicator strips.

Autoclave Tape

Autoclave tape has diagonal lines containing a chemical which changes color (usually from beige to black) if it has been exposed to steam. Autoclave tape is similar to masking tape; however, it is slightly more adhesive which allows it to adhere to a hot, moist pack during the autoclave cycle. The tape is available in a variety of colors, can be written on, and is useful for closing and identifying a wrapped item (Fig. 18.9). Autoclave tape has some limitations as an indicator. Because it is placed on the outside of the pack, it cannot ensure that steam has penetrated to the center of the pack. It also does not ensure that the item has been sterilized; it merely indicates that an item has been in the autoclave and that a high temperature has been attained. This helps to differentiate between processed and unprocessed loads.

Sterilization Indicator Strips

Sterilization indicator strips are commercially prepared strips made of paper or plastic that contain a thermolabile dye and that change color when exposed to steam under pressure for a certain length of time (Fig. 18.10). Most indicator strips are designed to change color after being exposed to a temperature of 250°F (121°C) for 15 minutes. The indicator strip should be placed in the center of the wrapped pack, with the end containing the dye placed in an area of the pack considered to be the hardest for steam to penetrate.

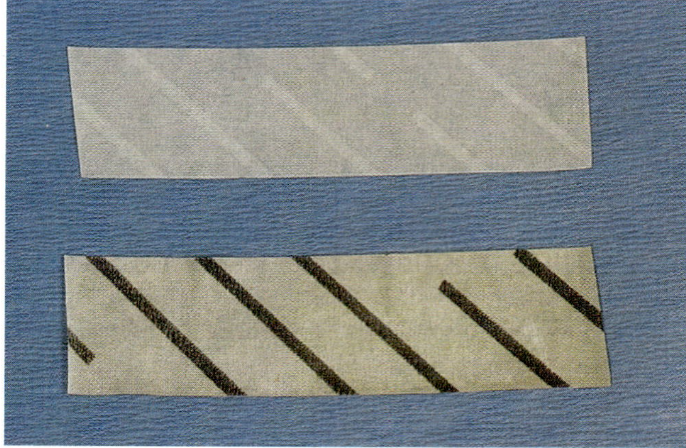

Fig. 18.9 Autoclave tape. *Top*, Autoclave tape as it appears before the sterilization process. *Bottom*, Black diagonal lines appear on the tape indicating the wrapped item has been in the autoclave and subjected to a high temperature.

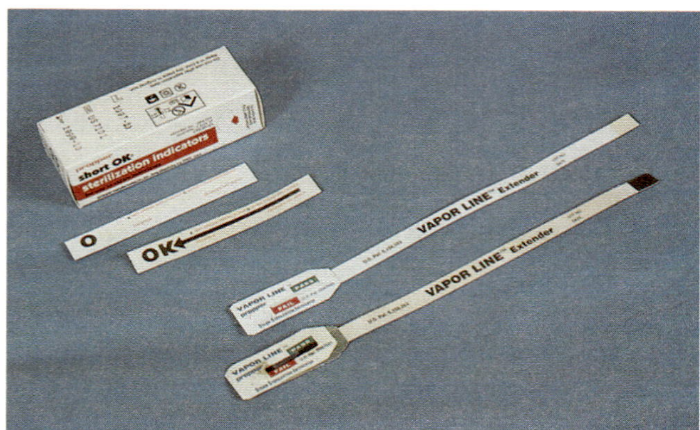

Fig. 18.10 Sterilization indicator strips. Indicator strips contain a thermolabile dye that changes color when exposed to steam under pressure for a certain length of time.

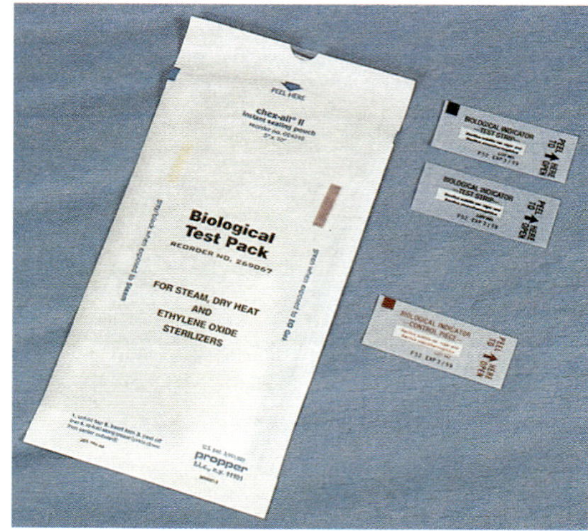

Fig. 18.11 Biologic indicator. A biologic indicator includes two spore tests that are sterilized (*top right*) and one spore control that is not sterilized (*bottom right*).

Biologic Indicators

Biologic indicators are the best means available for determining the effectiveness of the sterilization procedure. The CDC recommends that medical office personnel use a biologic indicator to monitor an autoclave at least once a week.

A biologic indicator is a preparation of bacterial spores. Biologic indicators are commercially available in the form of dry spore strips in small glassine envelopes. Biologic monitoring of an autoclave requires the use of a preparation of spores of *Geobacillus stearothermophilus*, which is a microorganism whose spores are particularly resistant to moist heat and are not harmful to humans.

Each biologic testing unit includes two spore tests that are sterilized and one spore control that is not sterilized (Fig. 18.11). The biologic indicator is placed in the center of two wrapped items. The items are placed in areas of the autoclave that are the least accessible to steam penetration, such as on the bottom tray of the autoclave, near the front of the autoclave, or in the back of the autoclave.

After the indicators have been exposed to sterilization conditions, they must be processed before the results can be obtained. The two methods for processing results are the *in-house method* and the *mail-in method.*

In-House Method

The in-house method involves processing and interpreting the results at the medical office. After sterilization, the sterilized spores are incubated for 24 to 48 hours. **Incubate** means to provide proper conditions for growth and development. If sterilization conditions have been met, the color or condition of the sterilized spores is different from those of the unsterilized control, and the spore test result is interpreted as negative. If sterilization conditions have not been met, the sterilized spores and the unsterilized control display the same color or condition, and the spore test result is interpreted as positive.

Mail-in Method

With this method, the sterilized spores and the unsterilized control are mailed to a processing laboratory. The test is performed by the laboratory, and the results are returned to the medical office.

If spores are not killed in routine spore tests, the autoclave should be checked immediately for proper use and function, and the spore test should be repeated. If the spore test result remains positive, the autoclave should not be used until it is serviced.

Wrap Items

Items to be sterilized in the autoclave must first be thoroughly sanitized (see Procedure 18.1). Next, the items are prepared for autoclaving by wrapping them. The purpose of wrapping items is to protect them from recontamination during handling and storage. Items that are wrapped and handled correctly remain sterile after autoclaving until the package seal is broken.

The wrapping material must be made of a substance that is not affected by the sterilization process and must allow steam to penetrate while preventing contaminants (e.g., dust, insects, microorganisms) from entering during handling and storage. The wrapping material should not tear or puncture easily and should allow the sterilized pack to be opened without contaminating the contents. A wrapper should not be used if it is torn or has a hole. Examples of good wrapping materials for the autoclave include sterilization paper and pouches described as follows.

Sterilization Paper

Sterilization paper is a disposable and inexpensive wrapping material. It consists of square sheets of paper available in various sizes (Fig. 18.12). The most common sizes (in inches) are 12 × 12, 15 × 15, 18 × 18, 24 × 24, 30 × 30, and 36 × 36. An item must be wrapped in such a way that it does not become contaminated when the pack is opened.

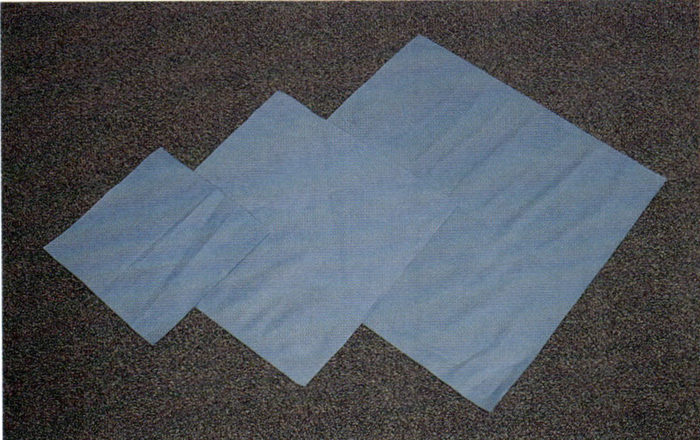

Fig. 18.12 Sterilization wrapping paper. Sterilization wrapping paper consists of square sheets of paper that are available in different sizes.

Autoclave tape is used to seal and label the contents of the pack. After removing a wrapped pack from the autoclave, the medical assistant should check the autoclave tape for the proper color change. If the tape does not change to the appropriate color, the pack must be rewrapped and resterilized.

The proper method for wrapping an instrument using sterilization paper is outlined in Procedure 18.2.

The disadvantage of sterilization paper is that it is difficult to spread open for removal of the contents. It has a "memory" and tends to flip back easily, so it may not open flat to provide a sterile field. (*Memory* is the ability of a material to retain a specific shape or configuration.) Because sterilization paper is opaque, it is not possible to view the contents of the pack before opening it.

Sterilization Pouches

Sterilization pouches consist of a combination of paper and plastic; paper makes up one side of the pouch and a plastic film makes up the other side (Fig. 18.13). Pouches can be labeled on their paper side with their contents and date of sterilization. They are available in various sizes; the most common sizes (in inches) are 3 × 9, 5 × 10, and 7 × 12.

Pouches have a peel-apart seal on one end used to open the pouch for removal of the sterile item inside. The other end of the pouch is open and is used to insert the item into the pouch during the wrapping procedure. Once the item has been inserted, this end is sealed with an adhesive strip or a heat-sealing device. The proper method for wrapping an instrument using a pouch is outlined in Procedure 18.3.

Pouches provide good visibility of the contents on the plastic side. Most manufacturers include a sterilization indicator on the outside of the pouch. After removing a pouch from the autoclave, the medical assistant should check the indicator for the proper color change. If the indicator does not change to the appropriate color (as specified by the manufacturer), the contents of the pouch must be rewrapped and resterilized.

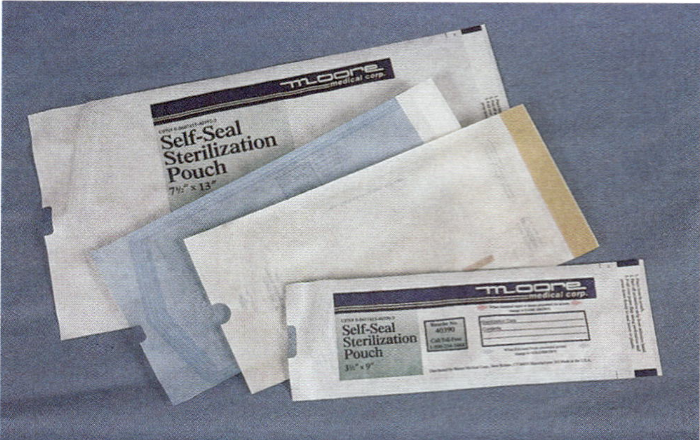

Fig. 18.13 Sterilization pouches. Sterilization pouches consist of a combination of paper and plastic and are available in different sizes.

Load the Autoclave

Before loading the autoclave, the medical assistant should check the level of water in the water reservoir. Distilled water must be used to fill the water reservoir to the proper level. Normal tap water contains minerals which have a corrosive effect on the stainless-steel chamber of the autoclave. Tap water can also cause mineral deposits that prevent valves from opening or closing properly.

For an item to attain sterility, steam must reach all surfaces of an item at a specified time, temperature, and pressure. To accomplish this, wrapped items must be positioned in the autoclave in such a way that allows for the free circulation of steam. Proper positioning also facilitates the drying process. The following guidelines should be followed when loading the autoclave:

1. Small packs are best because steam penetrates them more easily; it takes longer for steam to reach the center of a large pack to ensure sterilization. A pack should be no larger than 12 × 12 × 20 inches.
2. To allow for proper steam circulation, packs should be positioned as loosely as possible inside the autoclave, with approximately 1 to 3 inches between small packs and 2 to 4 inches between large packs. Packs should not be allowed to touch surrounding walls, and at least 1 inch should separate the autoclave trays. Placing the packs too close together interferes with the free circulation of steam within the chamber (Fig. 18.14).
3. Pouches should preferably be positioned vertically on their sides in an autoclave rack to maximize steam circulation and to facilitate the drying process. Pouches can also be placed flat on an autoclave tray. The medical assistant must consult the operating manual accompanying the autoclave to determine the proper placement of pouches on a tray. This is because some types of autoclaves require that the pouches be placed on a tray with the paper side up and the plastic side down. Other types of autoclaves require that the pouches be placed on a tray with the plastic side up and the paper side down.

Operate the Autoclave

The medical assistant must operate the autoclave according to the manufacturer's instructions. The medical assistant should read the operating manual carefully before operating the autoclave for the first time. Thereafter, the manual should be kept in an accessible location so that it is available if needed as a reference. The steps involved in achieving sterilization are known as the *autoclave cycle* and include the following:

1. Water is converted to steam and fills the autoclave chamber.
2. The desired temperature and pressure are reached.
3. The load is sterilized at the proper time, temperature, and pressure.
4. Steam is vented from the chamber.
5. The load is dried.

The proper temperature and pressure must occur during an autoclave cycle to ensure sterilization of the load. A **load** refers to the items being sterilized during an autoclave cycle. The most common sterilization temperature/pressure combinations include 250°F (121°C) at 15 psi and 270°F (132°C) at 27 psi. The sterilizing time is based on the type

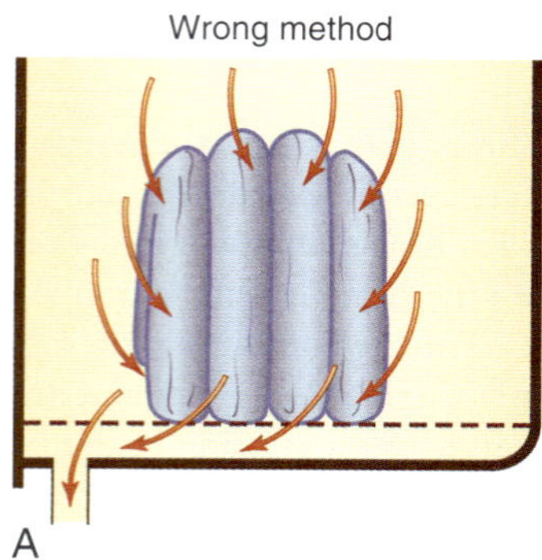

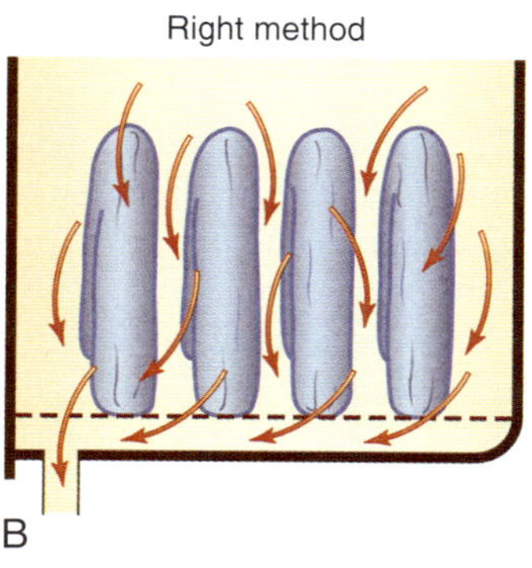

Fig. 18.14 Arrangement of packs in the autoclave. (A) Improper arrangement of packs in the autoclave. This arrangement prevents adequate steam penetration and interferes with proper sterilization. (B) Proper arrangement of packs in the autoclave. The packs are separated from each other, and steam can now penetrate each pack. (Courtesy of and modified from AMSCO/American Sterilizer Company, Erie, PAa.)

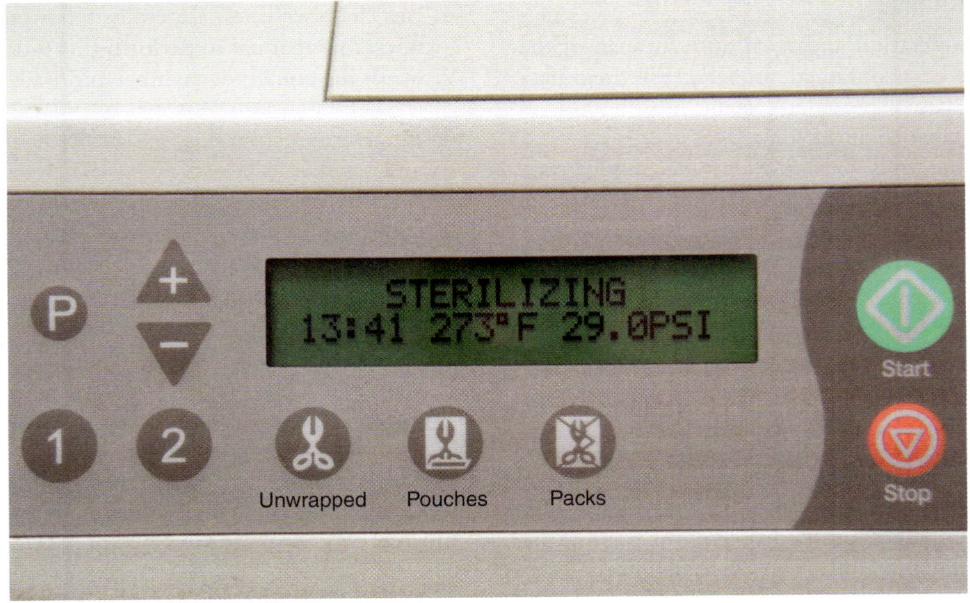

Fig. 18.15 Various autoclave cycles used in the medical office: unwrapped (items), pouches, and packs (items wrapped in sterilization paper).

of load being sterilized. Steam can easily reach the surfaces of hard, nonporous items such as unwrapped instruments (e.g., vaginal specula) to kill microorganisms; these items require a shorter sterilization time. A large minor office surgery pack requires a longer sterilization time because more time is needed for the steam to penetrate to the center of the pack. Sterilizing times typically range from 3 to 30 minutes.

Based on the type of load being sterilized, the medical assistant must select the proper autoclave cycle (Fig. 18.15), which includes one of the following:

- Unwrapped items
- Pouches
- Packs (items wrapped in sterilization paper)

Once the autoclave cycle is selected, the autoclave automatically begins processing the load. Water is converted into steam under pressure and enters the autoclave chamber. After the desired temperature and pressure are attained, the autoclave begins the time countdown. At the end of the countdown, sterilization is achieved. The steam is then automatically vented from the chamber causing the pressure to decrease to zero and the chamber to cool.

The sterilized packs and pouches are moist and must be allowed to dry before they are removed from the autoclave. This is because microorganisms can move quickly through the moisture on a wet wrap contaminating the sterile item inside. After the steam is completely vented from the autoclave the door automatically cracks open approximately ½ inch. This allows moisture on the wet packs and pouches to change from a liquid to a vapor and escape through the crack thus drying the load. The residual heat in the inner chamber also helps dry the load. The load is allowed to dry for 15 to 60 minutes, depending on the type of load. Loads that contain large packs require a longer drying time than loads with smaller packs.

What Would You Do? What Would You *Not* Do?

Case Study 2

Cassie Augusta is in the examining room and is being prepared for the removal of a sebaceous cyst. Cassie is concerned about the instruments that the physician will be using to perform the procedure. She wants to know if they are "safe." Cassie says that her friend Mackenzie got a tattoo several years ago and developed hepatitis C three weeks later. Mackenzie thinks she got hepatitis C from the instruments that were used for her tattoo procedure. Cassie wants to know if it is possible for surgical instruments to give someone hepatitis C. She says she heard that hepatitis can cause liver cancer and wants to know if this is true. Cassie also wants to know if there is a vaccine to prevent hepatitis C. ■

Handle and Store Wrapped Items

Sterilized wrapped items should be handled carefully and as little as possible. If a wrapped item is crushed, compressed, or dropped, the sterility of the contents cannot be assumed, and it must be rewrapped and resterilized. This is known as *event-related sterility,* meaning that a sterile pack or pouch is considered sterile indefinitely unless an event occurs that interferes with the sterility of the item.

Sterilized packs and pouches should be stored in a clean, dry area that is free from dust, insects, and other sources of contamination. Wrapped items should be stored with the most recently sterilized items placed in the back. The medical assistant should carefully inspect each sterilized pack or pouch: before storing it and before using it. If a wrapped item is torn or opened or if it is wet, it is no longer sterile and must be rewrapped and resterilized. Procedure 18.4 outlines a general procedure for sterilizing items in the autoclave.

Maintain the Autoclave

To ensure proper operation and maximum lifespan of the autoclave, it must be maintained properly. The manufacturer's operating manual provides specific information on the care and maintenance of the autoclave.

Safety precautions must be followed when performing maintenance procedures. Before proceeding with maintenance, the autoclave must be cool, the pressure gauge at zero, and the power cord disconnected from the wall socket. Autoclave maintenance should be performed on a daily, weekly, and monthly basis as follows.

Daily Maintenance

1. Wipe the outside of the autoclave with a damp cloth and a mild detergent.
2. Inspect the door gaskets for damage that could prevent a good seal.
3. Clean the rubber gaskets on the inside of the door of the autoclave with a damp cloth (Fig. 18.16).

Weekly Maintenance

1. Drain the water in the reservoir into a container and dispose of it.
2. Clean the inside of the chamber according to the manufacturer's instructions. This usually involves the following steps:
   - Remove the trays and clean the chamber with a soft cloth or a soft brush and an autoclave cleaner. Do not use steel wool, a steel brush, or other abrasive agents because they can damage the chamber.
   - Rinse the chamber thoroughly with distilled water.
   - Thoroughly dry the chamber.
3. Wash the trays with an autoclave cleaner and rinse them thoroughly with distilled water.
4. Refill the water reservoir with distilled water and leave the door open overnight.

Monthly Maintenance

1. Flush the system with an autoclave cleaner to remove any buildup of residue, which could cause corrosion of the chamber lines. Carefully follow the manufacturer's operating manual to perform this procedure.
2. Wash the autoclave chamber and trays with an autoclave cleaner.
3. Remove and clean door gaskets with an autoclave cleaner and a soft brush.
4. Remove and clean filters with an autoclave cleaner and a stiff bristled brush and rinse with distilled water. The filters prevent debris from causing valve failure.
5. Check the pressure relief valve to make sure it is functioning properly. The purpose of the pressure relief valve is to release excessive steam pressure during the autoclave cycle.

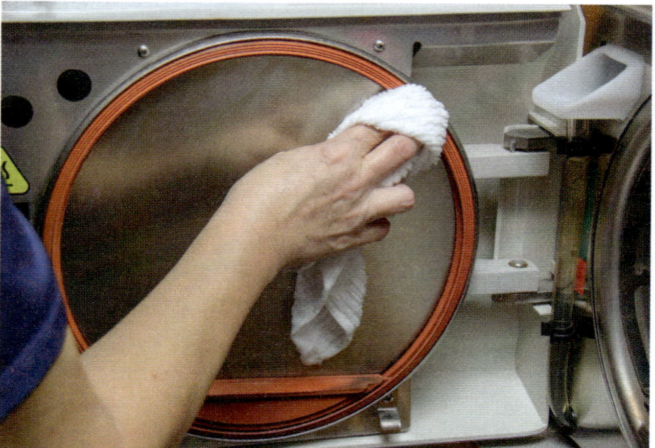

Fig. 18.16 The door gaskets are cleaned with a damp cloth during autoclave maintenance.

OTHER STERILIZATION METHODS

In addition to the autoclave, other methods can be used to sterilize items. These methods are not typically used in the medical office and are discussed only briefly in this chapter.

Dry Heat Oven

Dry heat ovens are used to sterilize items that cannot be penetrated by steam or may be damaged by it. Dry heat is less corrosive than moist heat for instruments with sharp edges; it does not dull their sharp edges. Moist heat sterilization tends to erode the ground-glass surfaces of reusable syringes, whereas dry heat does not.

Dry heat ovens operate similarly to ordinary cooking ovens. A longer exposure period is needed with dry heat because microorganisms and spores are more resistant to dry heat than to moist heat and because dry heat penetrates more slowly and unevenly than moist heat. The most commonly used temperature for dry heat sterilization is 320°F (160°C) for 2 hours or 340°F (170°C) for 1 hour. The recommended wrapping material for dry heat sterilization is aluminum foil because it is a good conductor of heat, and it protects against recontamination during handling and storage. Dry heat sterilization indicators are available to determine the effectiveness of the sterilization process.

Ethylene Oxide Gas Sterilization

Ethylene oxide is a colorless gas that is toxic and flammable. It is used to sterilize heat-sensitive items that cannot be sterilized in an autoclave. After items are sterilized with this gas, they must be aerated to remove the toxic residue of the ethylene oxide.

Ethylene oxide sterilization is a more complex and expensive process than steam sterilization. It frequently is used in the medical manufacturing industry for processing prepackaged, disposable items, such as syringes, sutures, catheters, and surgical packs.

Cold Sterilization

Cold sterilization involves the use of a chemical agent for an extended length of time. Only chemicals that are designated *sterilants* by the EPA (Environmental Protection Agency) can be used for sterilizing items. If a chemical agent holds this status, the word *sterilant* is printed on the front of the container.

The item to be sterilized must be completely submerged in the sterilant for a long period of time (6 to 24 hours depending on the type of sterilant). Prolonged immersion of instruments can damage them. In addition, each time an instrument is added to the sterilant container, the clock must be restarted for the entire amount of time. For these reasons, and because this method involves the use of a hazardous chemical, cold sterilization should be used only when an autoclave, gas, or a dry heat oven is not indicated or is unavailable.

Radiation

Radiation uses high-energy ionizing radiation to sterilize items. Medical manufacturers use radiation to sterilize prepackaged surgical equipment and instruments that cannot be sterilized by heat or chemicals.

What Would You Do? What Would You *Not* Do? RESPONSES

Case Study 1

Page 321

What Did Linda Do?

- ❑ Complimented Mrs. Cordera for her concern and efforts to baby-proof her home.
- ❑ Gave Mrs. Cordera a patient information brochure on baby-proofing the home.
- ❑ Told Mrs. Cordera that she should assume that all cleaning products are poisonous. Showed Mrs. Corder a chemical disinfectant container label and pointed out the information on the label that tells what to do in case of an accidental poisoning.
- ❑ Gave the Poison Help Line number (1-800-222-1222) to Mrs. Cordera and told her that is the fastest way to determine what to do in case of accidental poisoning. Told her to keep this number by her phone.

What Did Linda Not Do?

- ❑ Did not take Mrs. Cordera's question lightly.

Case Study 2

Page 335

What Did Linda Do?

- ❑ Told Cassie that her concern was valid.
- ❑ Told Cassie that hepatitis C can be transmitted through contaminated instruments.
- ❑ Reassured Cassie that surgical instruments used in the medical office are properly sterilized in the autoclave, and includes the use of sterilization indicators to ensure all germs have been killed.
- ❑ Gave Cassie a patient information sheet on hepatitis C. Told her that individuals with chronic hepatitis C can develop liver cancer and that the best way to avoid hepatitis C is through preventative measures and behaviors.
- ❑ Told Cassie that a vaccine is not yet available to prevent hepatitis C, however there are antiviral medications available to treat hepatitis C that are 95% effective.

What Did Linda Not Do?

- ❑ Did not minimize Cassie's concern about contaminated instruments.
- ❑ Did not overly alarm Cassie about the consequences of chronic hepatitis C.

TERMINOLOGY REVIEW

Autoclave	An apparatus for the sterilization of materials, using steam under pressure.
Critical item	An item that comes in contact with sterile tissue or the vascular system.
Decontamination	The use of physical or chemical means to remove pathogens from an item so that it is no longer capable of transmitting disease.
Detergent	An agent that cleanses by emulsifying dirt and oil.
Disinfectant	An agent used to destroy pathogenic microorganisms but not their spores. Disinfectants are usually applied to inanimate objects and surfaces.
Hazardous chemical	Any chemical that is a health hazard or a physical hazard.
Health hazard	The potential of a chemical to cause acute toxicity, skin corrosion or irritation, serious eye damage or irritation, respiratory or skin sensitization, germ cell mutagenicity, cancer or reproductive toxicity, or is an aspiration hazard.
Incubate	To provide proper conditions for growth and development.
Load	The items that are being sterilized in an autoclave.
Noncritical item	An item that comes into contact with intact skin but not with mucous membranes.
Physical hazard	The potential of a chemical to catch fire, explode, or react with other chemicals.
Safety data sheet	A document that provides detailed information on a chemical, its hazards, and measures to take to prevent injury and illness when handling the chemical.
Sanitization	A series of steps designed to removes debris from an item and reduce the number of microorganisms to a safe level
Semicritical item	An item that comes into contact with nonintact skin or intact mucous membranes.
Spore	A hard, thick-walled capsule formed by some bacteria that contains only the essential parts of the protoplasm of the bacterial cell.
Sterilization	The process of destroying all forms of microbial life, including spores.

PROCEDURE 18.1 Sanitization of Instruments

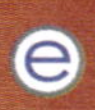

Outcome Sanitize instruments.

Equipment/Supplies

- Sink
- Disposable gloves
- Heavy-duty utility gloves
- Contaminated instruments
- High-level disinfectant and SDS
- Disinfectant container
- Instrument cleaner and SDS
- Basin
- Stiff nylon brush
- Stainless-steel wire brush
- Paper towels
- Cloth towel
- Instrument lubricant

1. **Procedural Step.** Review the SDS for the hazardous chemicals you will be using in the sanitization process.
   Principle. An SDS provides information regarding a chemical agent, its hazards, and measures to take to prevent injury and illness when handling a chemical agent.
2. **Procedural Step.** Apply disposable gloves. Transport the contaminated instruments to the cleaning area as soon as possible after use. The instruments should be carried in a covered basin from the examining room to the cleaning area.
   Principle. Disposable gloves act as a barrier to protect the medical assistant from infectious materials. Transporting contaminated instruments in a covered basin promotes infection control.
3. **Procedural Step.** Apply heavy-duty utility gloves over the disposable gloves.
   Principle. Utility gloves help protect the hands from the irritating effects of chemical solutions.
4. **Procedural Step.** Separate sharp instruments and delicate instruments from other instruments.
   Principle. Separating sharp instruments from others prevents damage to or dulling of the cutting edge of these instruments. Delicate instruments should be separated to protect them from damage.
5. **Procedural Step.** Immediately rinse the instruments thoroughly under warm, not hot, running water (approximately 110°F [44°C]) to remove debris, such as blood, body fluids, and tissue.
   Principle. Rinsing the instruments as soon as possible prevents debris from drying on the instruments, making it difficult to remove later. Hot water may cause coagulation of organic material, making it more difficult to remove.

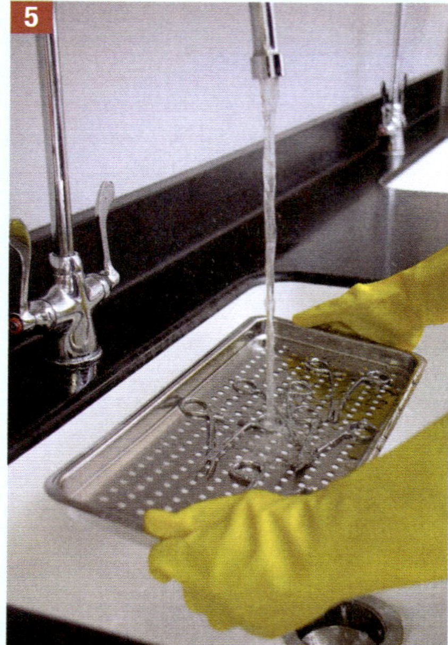

Rinse the instruments under warm water to remove debris.

6. **Procedural Step.** Decontaminate the instruments with a high-level chemical disinfectant as follows:
   a. Select the proper chemical disinfectant (e.g.; glutaraldehyde) and review the SDS for the disinfectant.
   b. Check the expiration date on the container label.
   c. Review and observe all precautionary statements listed on the label of the disinfectant (e.g., Wear protective gloves and protective eyewear).
   d. Read the manufacturer's instructions for the proper activation, dilution, and use of the disinfectant.
   e. Label the container that will hold the disinfectant with the name of the disinfectant and the date when the disinfectant is no longer effective and must be discarded (reuse life).
   f. Pour the chemical into the disinfectant container and immerse the items into the disinfectant. Ensure the items are completely submerged in the disinfectant.
   g. Cover the container and disinfect the items for 10 minutes.

PROCEDURE 18.1 Sanitization of Instruments—cont'd

Principle. Decontamination removes pathogenic microorganisms from the instruments, making them safe to handle. A disinfectant past its expiration date loses its potency and should not be used. The container must be kept covered to prevent the escape of toxic fumes and to prevent evaporation of the disinfectant, which could change its potency.

7. Procedural Step. Clean the instruments.as follows.

a. Obtain the instrument cleaner and check its expiration date.
b. Review and observe all personal safety precautions listed on the label of the instrument cleaner.
c. Prepare the instrument cleaning solution following the manufacturer's directions for proper mixing and use.
d. Remove the items from the disinfectant and place them in the basin containing the instrument cleaner.
e. Use a stiff nylon brush to clean the surface of each instrument. Scrub all parts of the instrument thoroughly. Brush delicate instruments carefully to prevent damaging them.

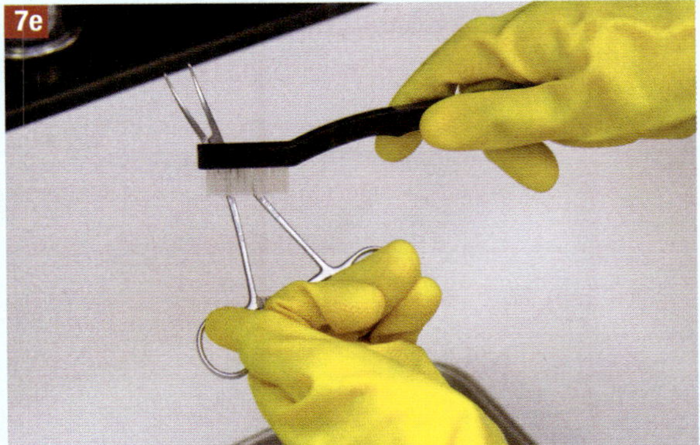
7e

Clean the surface of the instrument with a stiff nylon brush.

f. Use a stainless-steel wire brush to clean grooves, crevices, or serrations where debris such as blood and tissue may collect.

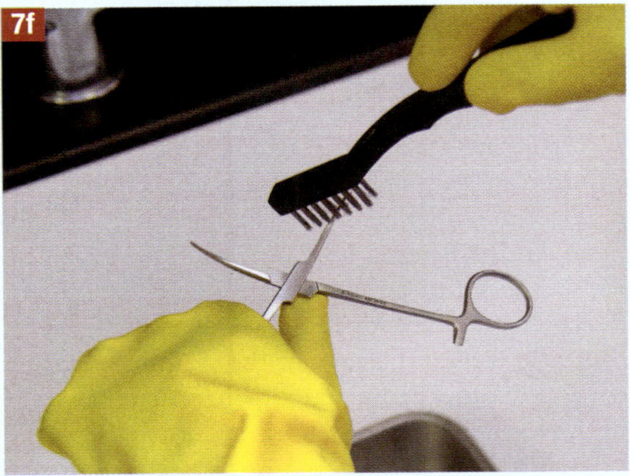
7f

Clean grooves, crevices, or serrations with a wire brush.

g. If there is a stain on the instrument, attempt to remove it with an instrument stain remover.
h. Scrub each instrument until it is visibly clean and free from debris and stains.

Principle. An instrument cleaner past its expiration date loses its potency and should not be used. Taking appropriate precautions with cleaning agents prevents harm to the medical assistant. All debris must be removed from the instruments to ensure proper sterilization.

8. Procedural Step. Rinse each instrument thoroughly with warm, not hot, water (110°F [44°C]) for at least 20 to 30 seconds to remove all traces of the detergent. Open and close hinged instruments while rinsing to ensure the solution is completely rinsed out of every part of the instrument.

Principle. Detergent residue left on the instrument could cause stains, which could build up and interfere with proper functioning of the instrument. Using warm water helps to remove the cleaning solution and facilitates the drying process.

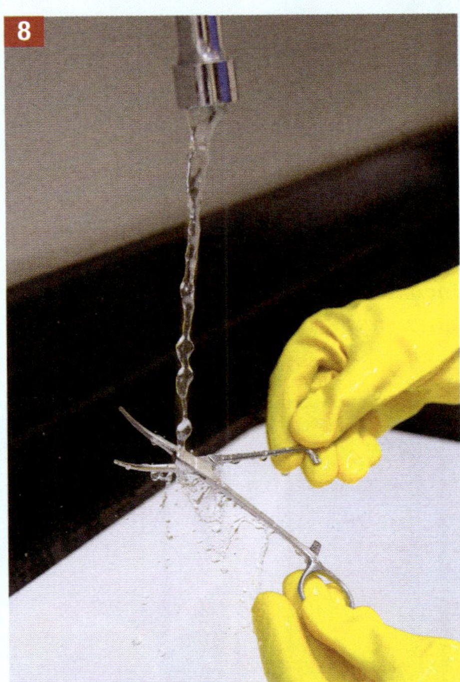
8

Rinse thoroughly with warm water.

9. Procedural Step. Dry each instrument with a paper towel, and place the instrument on a cloth towel for additional air drying.

Principle. If the instrument is not completely dry, stains may occur on the instrument.

Continued

PROCEDURE 18.1 Sanitization of Instruments—cont'd

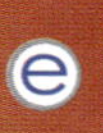

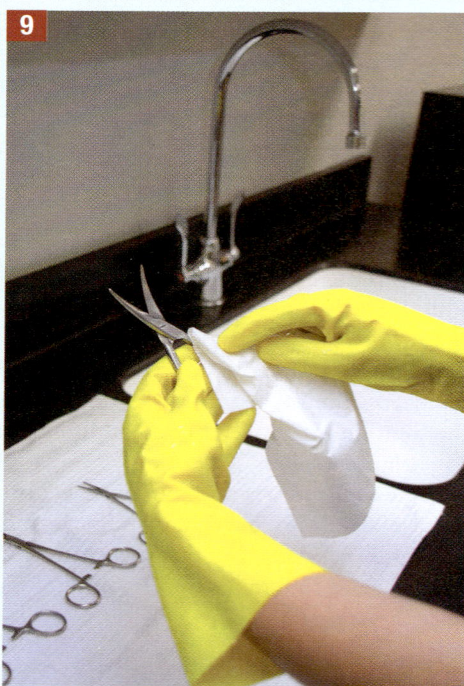

Dry the instrument with a paper towel.

10. Procedural Step. Inspect each instrument for defects and proper working condition. Scissors should cut all the way to the end of a thin piece of gauze without catching. If defects are noted or the instrument is not working properly, it must be discarded or sent to the manufacturer for repair.

Principle. Instruments that have defects or are not in proper working condition are not safe to use during a medical or surgical procedure.

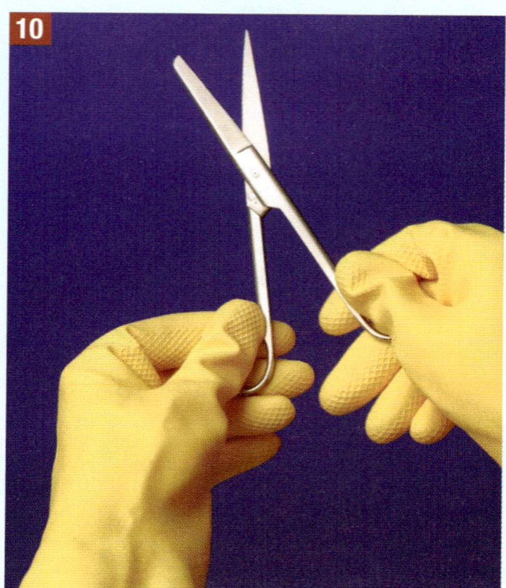

Inspect the instrument for defects and proper working order.

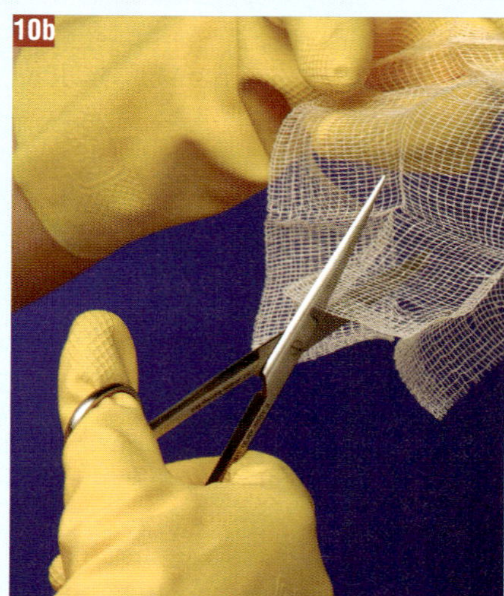

Scissors should cut through gauze without catching.

11. Procedural Step. Lubricate hinged instruments using a steam-penetrable lubricant as follows:

a. Apply the lubricant to a hinged instrument in its open position making sure to apply the lubricant only the moving part of the instrument (e.g., box lock, screw lock).

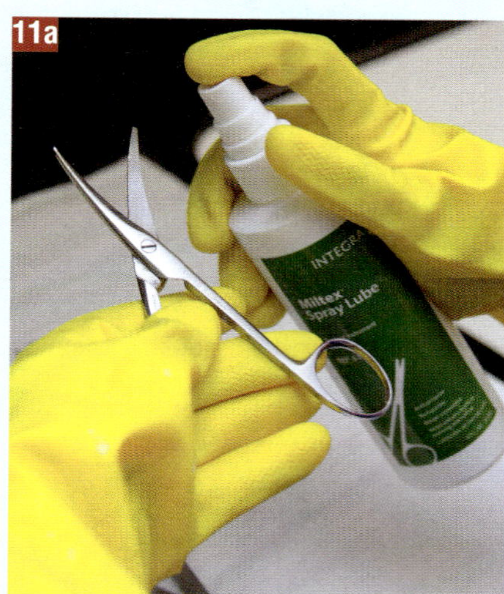

Lubricate hinged instruments.

b. Open and close the instrument after applying the lubricant so it reaches all parts of the hinged area.

c. Place the instrument back on the towel and allow it to air dry. Rinsing or wiping is unnecessary.

Principle. Lubricating an instrument makes it function better and last longer.

12. Procedural Step. Dispose of the cleaning solution according to the manufacturer's instructions. Remove both sets of gloves, and sanitize your hands.

13. Procedural Step. Wrap the instruments and sterilize them in the autoclave.

PROCEDURE 18.2 Wrapping an Instrument Using Sterilization Paper

Outcome Wrap an instrument using sterilization paper.

Equipment/Supplies

- Sanitized instrument
- Appropriate-sized sterilization wrapping paper
- Sterilization indicator strip
- Autoclave tape
- Permanent marker

1. **Procedural Step.** Sanitize your hands.
2. **Procedural Step.** Assemble the equipment. Select the appropriate-sized wrapping paper for the instrument being wrapped. Check the expiration date on the box of sterilization indicators. If the indicator strips are outdated, do not use them.
   Principle. Instruments are wrapped so they are protected from recontamination following sterilization. Outdated indicator strips may not provide accurate test results.
3. **Procedural Step.** Place the wrapping paper on a clean, flat surface. Turn the wrap in a diagonal position to your body so that it resembles a diamond shape.

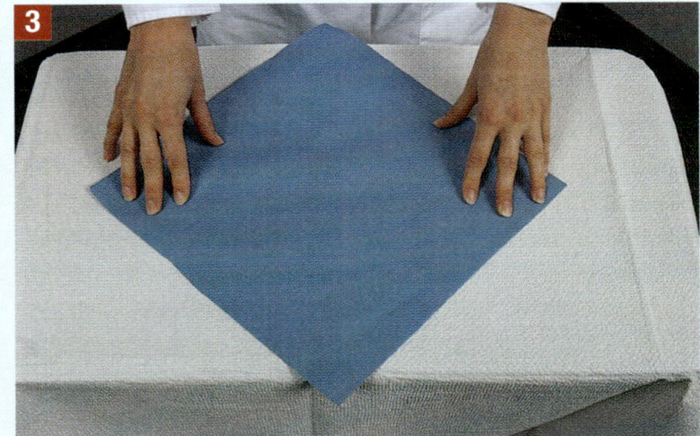

Turn the wrapping paper in a diagonal position.

4. **Procedural Step.** Place the instrument in the center of the wrapping paper with the longest part of the instrument pointing toward the two side corners. If the instrument has a movable joint, place it on the wrap in a slightly open position. If necessary, a gauze square can be used to hold the instrument in an open position.
   Principle. Instruments with movable joints must be in an open position to allow steam to reach all parts of the instrument. If the instrument is in a closed position, heat exposure could cause the instrument to crack at its weakest part, such as the lock area.
5. **Procedural Step.** Place an indicator strip in the center of the wrap next to the instrument.
   Principle. Indicator strips assess the effectiveness of the sterilization process.

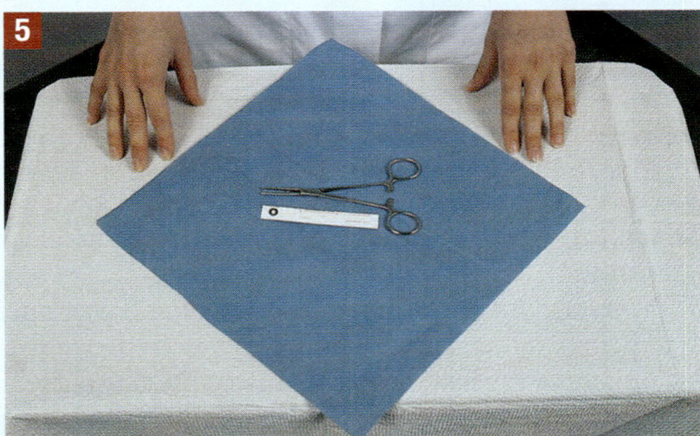

Place an indicator strip in the center of the wrap next to the instrument.

6. **Procedural Step.** Fold the wrapping paper up from the bottom, and double-back a small corner, creating a flap. This flap will later be used to open the sterile pack without contaminating the instrument.

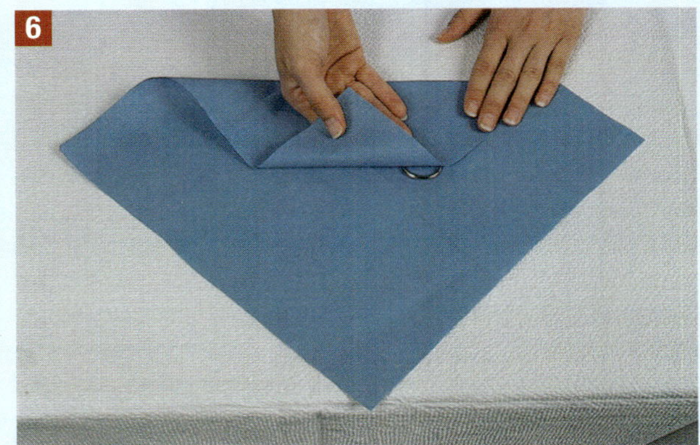

Fold the wrapping paper up from the bottom and double-back a small corner.

7. **Procedural Step.** Fold over one edge of the wrapping paper, and double-back the corner.
8. **Procedural Step.** Fold over the other edge of the wrapping paper, and double-back the corner.

Continued

PROCEDURE 18.2

PROCEDURE 18.2 Wrapping an Instrument Using Sterilization Paper—cont'd

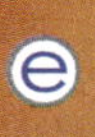

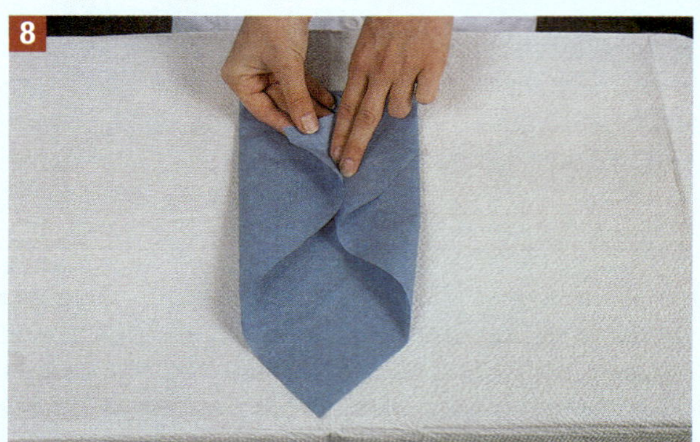

Fold over the other edge of the wrapping paper and double-back the corner.

9. Procedural Step. Fold the wrapping paper up from the bottom, pull the top flap down, and secure it with autoclave tape. Ensure that the pack is firm enough for handling but loose enough to permit proper circulation of steam.

Principle. An instrument must be wrapped properly to permit full penetration of steam and to prevent contaminating it when the pack is opened. Using autoclave tape indicates that the pack has been through the autoclave cycle and prevents mix-ups with packs that have not been processed.

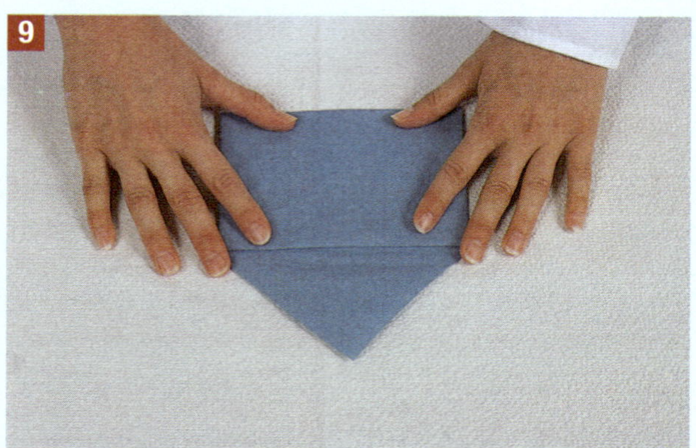

Fold the wrapping paper up from the bottom.

10. Procedural Step. Label the pack according to its contents. Mark the pack with the date of sterilization and your initials.

Principle. Dating the pack helps in ensuring that the most recently sterilized packs are stored behind previously sterilized packs.

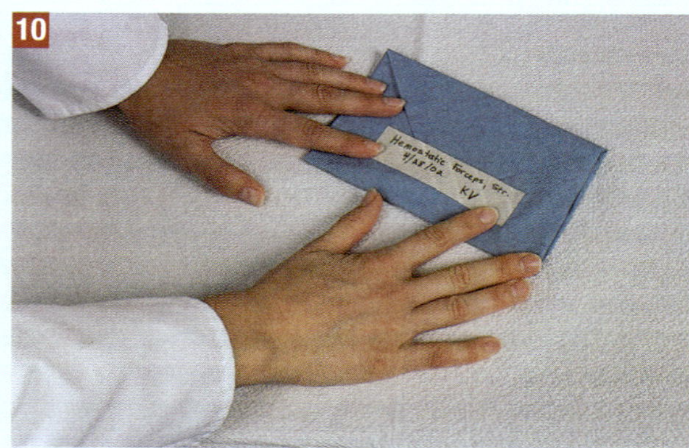

Label and date the pack. Include your initials.

PROCEDURE 18.3 Wrap an Instrument Using a Pouch

Outcome Wrap an instrument using a pouch.

Equipment/Supplies

- Sanitized instrument
- Appropriate-sized sterilization pouch
- Permanent marker

1. **Procedural Step.** Sanitize your hands.
2. **Procedural Step.** Assemble the equipment. Select the appropriate-sized sterilization pouch for the instrument being wrapped. For hinged instruments, use a pouch wide enough so the instrument can be placed in a slightly open position inside the pouch.
   Principle. Instruments are wrapped so they are protected from recontamination following sterilization.
3. **Procedural Step.** Place the pouch on a clean, flat surface.
4. **Procedural Step.** Label the pack according to its contents. Mark the pouch with the date of sterilization and your initials.
   Principle. Dating the pouch helps in ensuring that the most recently sterilized pouches are stored behind previously sterilized pouches.

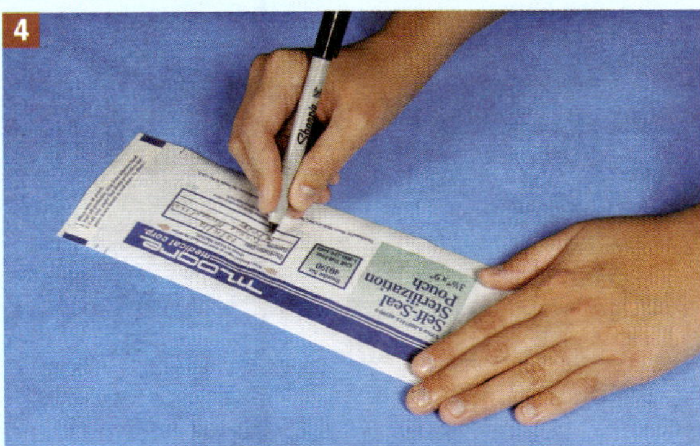

Label and date the pouch. Include your initials.

5. **Procedural Step.** Insert the instrument to be sterilized into the unsealed, open end of the pouch. If the instrument has a movable joint, place it in the pouch in a slightly open position.

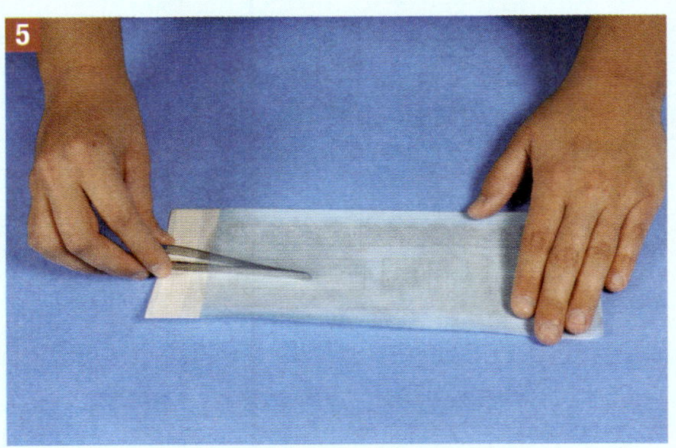

Insert the instrument into the pouch.

6. **Procedural Step.** Seal the open end of the pouch as follows:
   Adhesive Closure. Peel off the paper strip located above the perforated line to expose the adhesive. Fold along the perforated line and press firmly to seal the paper to the plastic. Ensure that the seal is secure by running your fingers back and forth on both sides of the pouch over the entire sealing area.
   Heat Closure. Seal the pouch using a heat-sealing device.

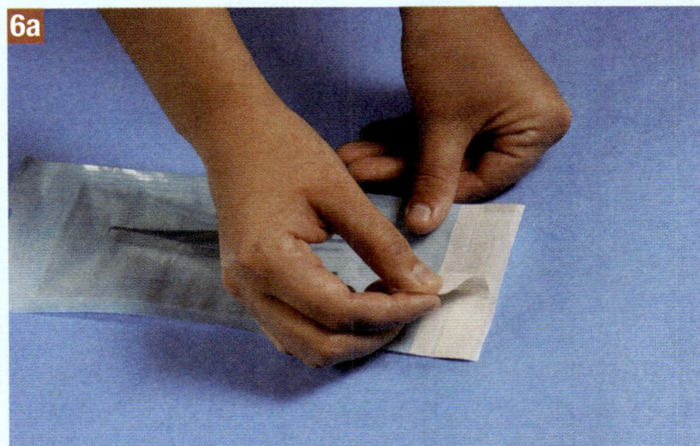

Peel off the paper strip.

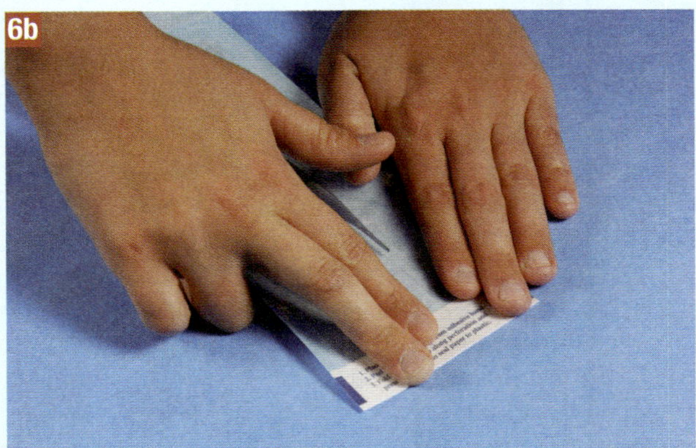

Press firmly to seal the pouch.

7. **Procedural Step.** Sterilize the pouch in the autoclave.

PROCEDURE 18.4 Sterilizing Items in an Autoclave

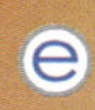

Outcome Sterilize a load in an autoclave.

Equipment/Supplies

- Autoclave and operating manual
- Distilled water
- Wrapped items
- Heat-resistant gloves

1. **Procedural Step.** Assemble the equipment.
2. **Procedural Step.** Check the level of water in the water reservoir and add distilled water, if needed.
   Principle. Distilled water is used to prevent corrosion of the stainless-steel chamber of the autoclave.

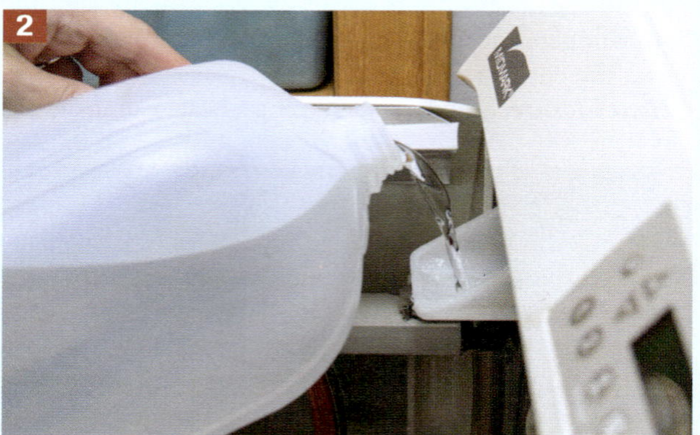

Add distilled water to the water reservoir.

3. **Procedural Step.** Properly load the autoclave following these guidelines:
   a. Place small packs 1 to 3 inches apart, and large packs 2 to 4 inches apart.
   b. Place pouches vertically on their sides in a metal rack to maximize steam circulation and facilitate drying. As an alternative, pouches can be placed flat on an autoclave tray. Consult the operating manual to determine the proper placement of the pouches on a tray. Some types of autoclaves require the pouches to be placed with the paper side up and the plastic side down; while other types require that the pouches be placed with the plastic side up and the paper side down.
   c. Do not allow the wrapped items to touch the chamber walls.
   d. Ensure that at least 1 inch separates the autoclave trays.
   Principle. The autoclave must be loaded properly to ensure proper steam circulation and to facilitate the drying process.

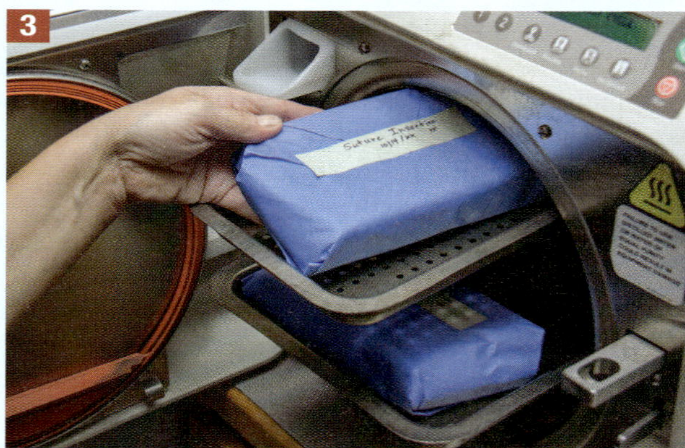

Properly load the autoclave.

4. **Procedural Step.** Operate the autoclave according to the procedure described in the operating manual. A general procedure for autoclave operation is outlined below.
   a. Close and latch the door of the autoclave.
   b. Determine the autoclave cycle according to what is being sterilized as follows:
      - Unwrapped items
      - Pouches
      - Packs (items wrapped in sterilization paper)
   c. Select the desired autoclave cycle by pressing the appropriate button on the autoclave.
   d. Press the start button. A message on the display screen (or indicator light) identifies each stage of the autoclave cycle to tell you what is happening in the autoclave as follows:
      - **Filling:** The chamber fills with water.
      - **Heating:** The temperature and pressure increase until the desired parameters are reached.
      - **Sterilizing:** The load is sterilized at the proper time, temperature, and pressure.
      - **Venting**: Steam vents from the chamber.
      - **Drying**: The door cracks and the load dries.
      - **Ready**: The autoclave cycle is complete and the sterilized load can be removed from the autoclave.

PROCEDURE 18.4 Sterilizing Items in an Autoclave—cont'd

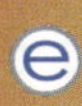

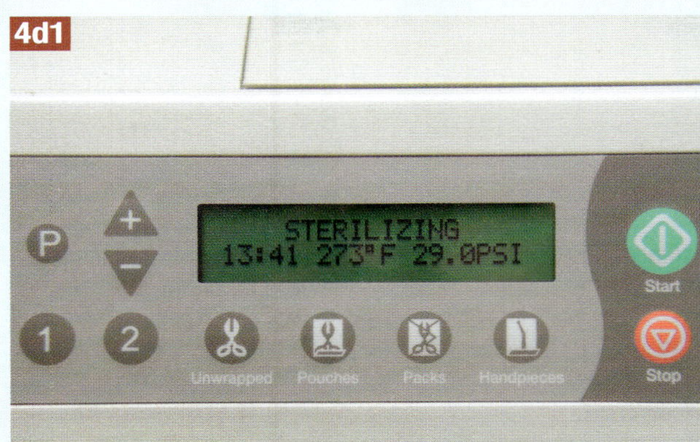

Sterilizing stage.

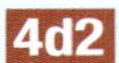

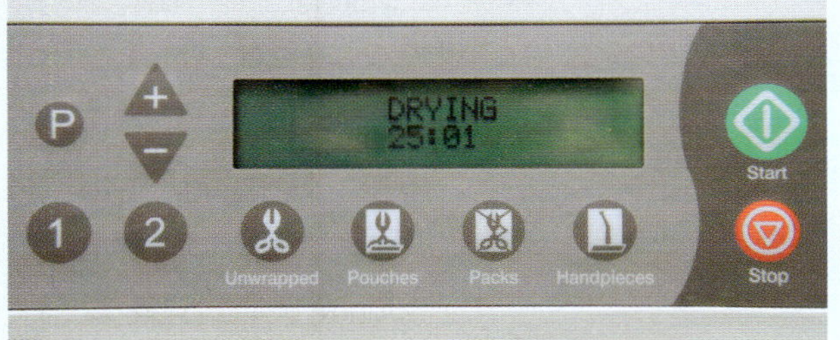

Drying stage.

5. Procedural Step. Turn off the autoclave. Remove the load from the autoclave with heat-resistant gloves. Do not touch the inner chamber of the autoclave with your bare hands.

Principle. Heat-resistant gloves protect the medical assistant's hands when the warm packs and pouches are removed from the autoclave. The chamber of the autoclave is hot and could burn bare skin.

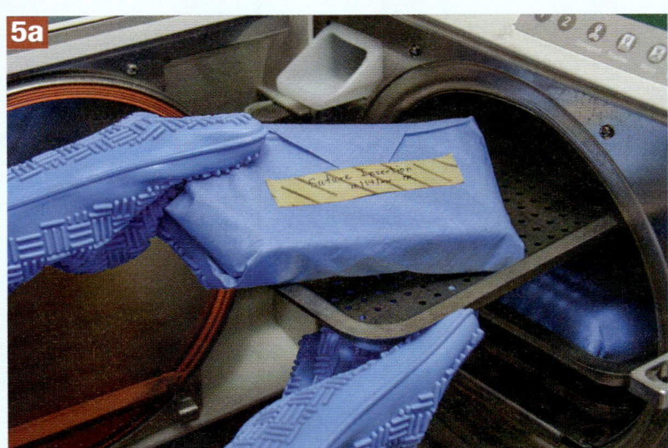

Remove packs from the autoclave.

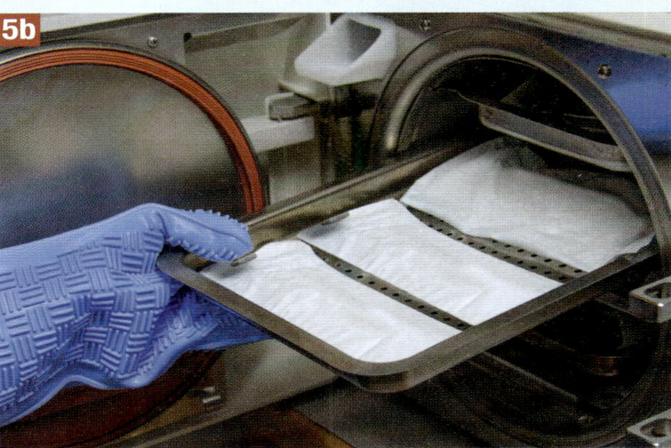

Remove pouches from the autoclave.

6. Procedural Step. Inspect the packs and pouches as you take them out of the autoclave. If a wrapped item shows any damage, such as holes or tears, it should be rewrapped and resterilized.

7. Procedural Step. Check the autoclave tape on the outside of each pack to ensure the proper response has occurred.

Principle. Autoclave tape indicates only that the item has been through the autoclave cycle; it does not ensure that sterilization has taken place. Sterilization is confirmed when the pack is opened for use and the sterilization indicator strip in the center of the pack is checked for its proper response.

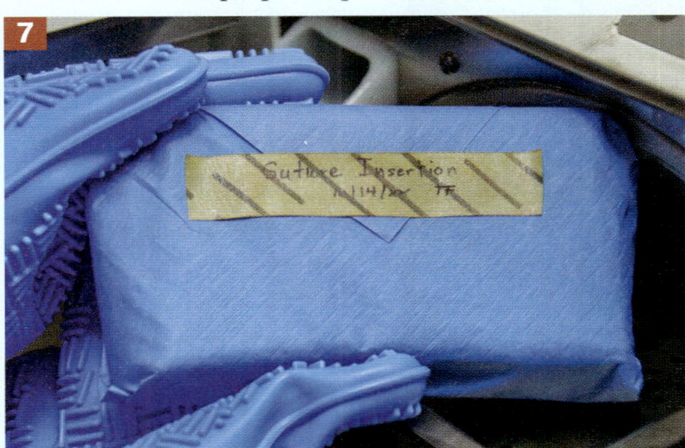

Check the autoclave tape on the outside of the pack.

8. Procedural Step. Document monitoring information in the autoclave log. Include the date and time of the cycle, a description of the load, and the exposure time and temperature. If a biologic indicator has been included in the load, process it according to the medical office policy, and document results on the autoclave log.

9. Procedural Step. Store the wrapped items in a clean, dustproof area with the most recently sterilized items placed behind previously sterilized items.

10. Procedural Step. Maintain appropriate daily care of the autoclave, following the manufacturer's recommendations.

Vital Signs

Check out the Evolve site at http://evolve.elsevier.com/Bonewit/today to access additional interactive activities and exercises to help you study and prepare for success.

LEARNING OBJECTIVES / PROCEDURES

Temperature

1. Define a *vital sign.*
2. Explain the reasons for taking vital signs.
3. Explain how body temperature is maintained.
4. List examples of how heat is produced in the body.
5. List examples of how heat is lost from the body.
6. State the normal body temperature range and the average body temperature.
7. List and explain factors that can cause variation in the body temperature.
8. List and describe the three stages of a fever.
9. List the sites for taking body temperature, and explain why these sites are used.

Measure oral body temperature.
Measure axillary body temperature.
Measure rectal body temperature.
Measure aural body temperature.
Measure temporal artery body temperature.

Pulse

10. Explain the mechanism of pulse.
11. List and explain the factors that affect the pulse rate.
12. Identify a specific use for each of the eight pulse sites.
13. State the normal range of pulse rate for each age group.
14. Explain the difference between pulse rhythm and pulse volume.

Measure radial pulse.
Measure apical pulse.

Respiration

15. Explain the purpose of respiration.
16. State what occurs during inhalation and exhalation.
17. State the normal respiratory rate for each age group.
18. List and explain the factors that affect the respiratory rate.
19. Explain the difference between rhythm and depth of respiration.
20. Describe the character of each of the following abnormal breath sounds: crackles, rhonchi, wheezes, and pleural friction rub.

Measure respirations.

Pulse Oximetry

21. Explain the purpose of pulse oximetry.
22. State the normal oxygen saturation level of a healthy individual.
23. Explain how pulse oximetry results are interpreted.
24. List and describe the functions of the controls, indicators and displays on a pulse oximeter.
25. List and describe factors that may interfere with an accurate pulse oximetry reading.

Perform pulse oximetry.

Blood Pressure

26. Define blood pressure.
27. Identify the blood pressure categories for an adult.
28. List and describe factors that can temporarily affect the blood pressure.
29. List and describe the risk factors that increase the risk of developing primary hypertension.
30. List and describe the categories of hypotension.
31. Identify and describe the different parts of a stethoscope and a sphygmomanometer.
32. Describe the methods for determining proper cuff size.
33. Describe the five phases of the Korotkoff sounds.
34. State the advantages and disadvantages of an automatic blood pressure monitor.
35. Explain how to prevent errors in blood pressure measurement.

Measure blood pressure.
Determine systolic pressure by palpation.

CHAPTER OUTLINE

KEY TERMS

adventitious (ad-ven-TISH-us) sounds
afebrile (uh-FEB-ril)
alveoli (al-VEE-oh-lie)
antecubital (AN-tih-CYOO-bi-tul) space
antipyretic (AN-tih-pye-REH-tik)
aorta (ay-OR-tuh)
apnea (AP-nee-uh)
axilla (aks-ILL-uh)
blood pressure
bounding pulse
bradycardia (BRAY-dee-CAR-dee-uh)
bradypnea (BRAY-dip-NEE-uh)
Celsius (SELL-see-us) scale
conduction (kon-DUK-shun)
convection (kon-VEK-shun)
crisis
cross-contamination
cyanosis (sye-an-OH-sus)
diastole (dye-AS-toh-lee)
diastolic (DYE-uh-STOL-ik) pressure
dyspnea (DISP-nee-uh)
dysrhythmia (dis-RITH-mee-uh)
eupnea (YOOP-nee-uh)
exhalation (EKS-hal-AY-shun)
Fahrenheit (FAIR-en-hite) scale
febrile (FEH-bril)
fever
frenulum linguae (FREN-yoo-lum LIN-gway)
hyperpnea (HYE-perp-NEE-uh)
hyperpyrexia (HYE-per-pye-REK-see-uh)
hypertension (HYE-per-TEN-shun)
hyperventilation (HYE-per-ven-til-AY-shun)
hypopnea (hye-POP-nee-uh)
hypotension (HYE-poe-TEN-shun)
hypothermia (HYE-poe-THER-mee-uh)
hypoxemia (hye-pok-SEE-mee-uh)
hypoxia (hye-POKS-ee-uh)
inhalation (IN-hal-AY-shun)
intercostal (IN-ter-KOS-tul)
Korotkoff (kuh-ROT-kof) sounds
malaise (mal-AYZE)
manometer (man-OM-uh-ter)
orthopnea (orth-OP-nee-uh)
pulse deficit
pulse oximeter
pulse oximetry
pulse pressure
pulse rate
pulse rhythm
pulse volume
radiation (RAY-dee-AY-shun)
SaO_2
sphygmomanometer (SFIG-moe-man-OM-uh-ter)
SpO_2
stethoscope (STETH-uh-skope)
systole (SIS-toh-lee)
systolic (sis-TOL-ik) pressure
tachycardia (TAK-ih-KAR-dee-uh)
tachypnea (TAK-ip-NEE-uh)
thready pulse

INTRODUCTION TO VITAL SIGNS

Vital signs are objective guideposts that provide data to determine a person's state of health. Vital signs include temperature, pulse, and respiration (collectively called *TPR*), and blood pressure. Another indicator of a patient's health status is pulse oximetry. Some providers order this measurement routinely for all patients, while other providers order it only when the patient complains of respiratory problems (e.g., shortness of breath).

The normal ranges of the vital signs are finely adjusted, and any deviation from normal may indicate disease. During the course of an illness, variations in the vital signs may occur. The medical assistant should be alert to any significant changes and report them to the provider because they indicate a change in the patient's condition. When patients visit the medical office, vital signs are routinely checked to establish each patient's usual state of health and to establish baseline measurements against which future measurements can be compared. The medical assistant should have a thorough knowledge of the vital signs and should attain proficiency in taking them to ensure accurate measurements.

General guidelines that the medical assistant should follow when measuring the vital signs are as follows:

1. Be familiar with the normal ranges for all vital signs. Keep in mind that normal ranges vary based on the different age groups (infant, child, adult, elder).
2. Make sure that all equipment for measuring vital signs is in proper working condition to ensure accurate findings.
3. Eliminate or minimize factors that affect the vital signs, such as physical exercise, food and beverage consumption, tobacco use, and emotional states.

TEMPERATURE

REGULATION OF BODY TEMPERATURE

Body temperature is maintained within a fairly constant range by the hypothalamus, which is the heat-regulating center of the body and is located in the brain. The hypothalamus functions as the body's thermostat. It normally allows the body temperature to vary by only about 1° to 2° Fahrenheit (F) throughout the day.

Body temperature is maintained through a balance of the heat produced in the body and the heat lost from the body (Fig. 19.1). A constant temperature range must be maintained for the body to function properly. When minor changes in the temperature of the body occur, the hypothalamus senses this and makes adjustments as necessary to ensure that the body temperature stays within a normal and safe range. If an individual is playing tennis on a hot day, the body's heat-cooling mechanism is activated to remove excess heat from the body through perspiration.

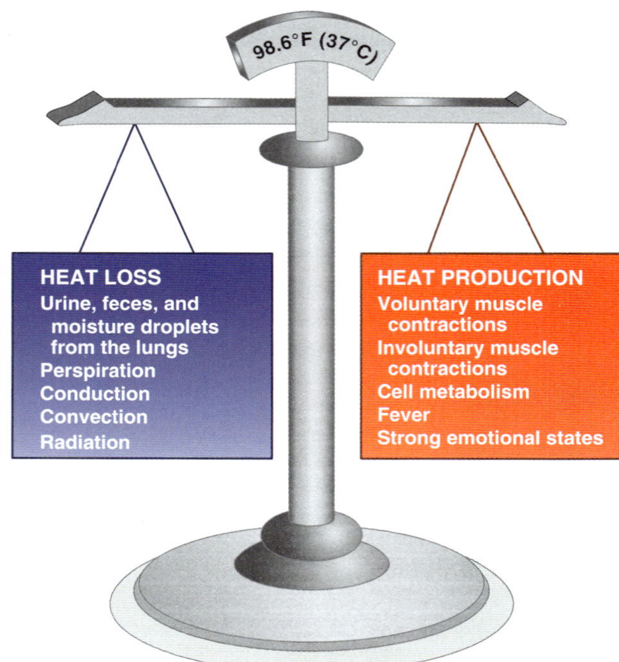

Fig. 19.1 Body temperature represents a balance between the heat produced in the body and the heat lost from the body.

Heat Production

Most of the heat produced in the body is through voluntary and involuntary muscle contractions. Voluntary muscle contractions involve the muscles over which a person has control, for example, the moving of legs or arms. Involuntary muscle contractions involve the muscles over which a person has no control; examples are physiologic processes such as digestion, the beating of the heart, and shivering.

Body heat also is produced by cell metabolism. Heat is produced when nutrients are broken down in the cells. Fever and strong emotional states also can increase heat production in the body.

Heat Loss

Heat is lost from the body through the urine, feces, and in water vapor during exhalation. Perspiration also contributes to heat loss. Perspiration is the excretion of moisture through the pores of the skin. When the moisture evaporates, heat is released and the body is cooled.

Radiation, conduction, and convection all cause loss of heat from the body. **Radiation** is the transfer of heat in the form of waves; body heat is continually radiating into cooler surroundings. **Conduction** is the transfer of heat from one object to another by direct contact; heat can be transferred by conduction from the body to a cooler object it touches. **Convection** is the transfer of heat through air currents; cool air currents can cause the body to lose heat. These processes are illustrated in Fig. 19.2.

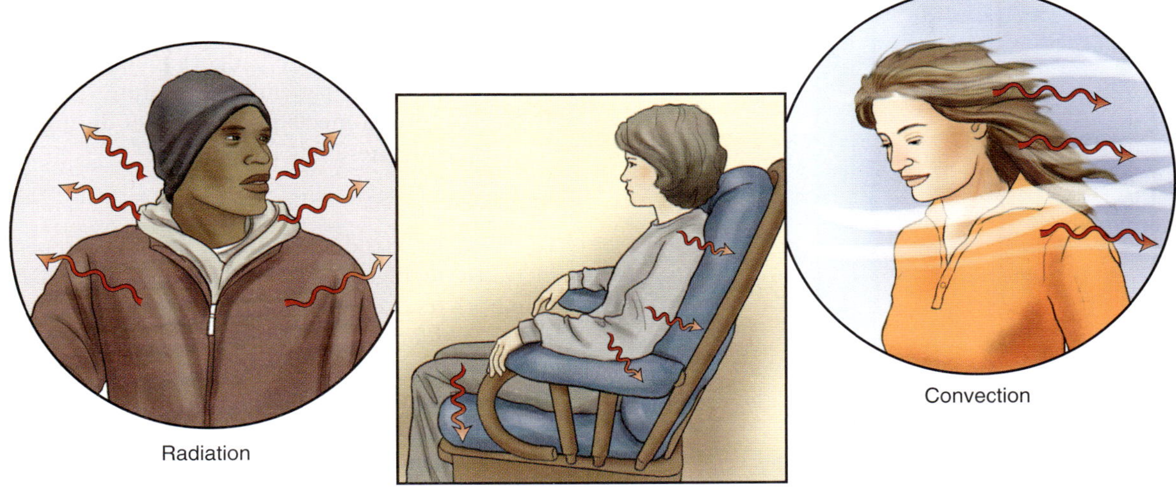

Fig. 19.2 Heat loss from the body. With **radiation,** the body gives off heat in the form of waves to the cooler outside air. With **conduction,** the chair becomes warm as heat is transferred from the individual to the chair. With **convection,** air currents move heat away from the body.

BODY TEMPERATURE RANGE

The purposes of measuring body temperature are to establish the patient's baseline temperature and to monitor an abnormally high or low body temperature. The normal body temperature range is 97°F to 99°F (36.1°C to 37.2°C), the average temperature being 98.6°F (37°C). Body temperature is usually documented using the Fahrenheit system of measurement. Table 19.1 lists comparable **Fahrenheit** and **Celsius** temperatures and explains how to convert temperatures from one scale to the other.

Alterations in Body Temperature

A body temperature greater than 100.4°F (38°C) indicates a **fever,** or *pyrexia.* When an individual has a fever, the heat the body is producing is greater than the heat the body is losing. A fever can be caused by many medical conditions, ranging from non-serious to life-threatening. A body temperature measurement between 99°F (37.2°C) and 100.4°F (38°C) is known as a *low-grade fever.* A temperature reading greater than 106°F (41.1°C) is known as **hyperpyrexia.** Hyperpyrexia is a serious condition, and a temperature greater than 108°F (42.2°C) is generally fatal.

A body temperature less than 97°F (36.1°C) is classified as **hypothermia.** This means that the heat the body is losing is greater than the heat it is producing. A person usually cannot survive with a temperature below 70°F (21°C). Terms used to describe alterations in body temperature are illustrated in Fig. 19.3.

Variations in Body Temperature

During the day-to-day activities of an individual, normal body temperature may fluctuate. The body temperature

Table 19.1 Equivalent Fahrenheit and Celsius Temperatures

Fahrenheit	Celsius
93.2	34
95	35
96.8	36
97.7	36.5
98.6	37
99.5	37.5
100.4	38
101.3	38.5
102.2	39
104	40
105.8	41
107.6	42
109.4	43
111.2	44

Temperature Conversion

1. *Celsius to Fahrenheit:* To convert Celsius to Fahrenheit, multiply by 9/5 and add 32:

$$°F = (°C \times 9/5) + 32$$

2. *Fahrenheit to Celsius:* To convert Fahrenheit to Celsius, subtract 32 and multiply by 5/9:

$$°C = (°F - 32) \times 5/9$$

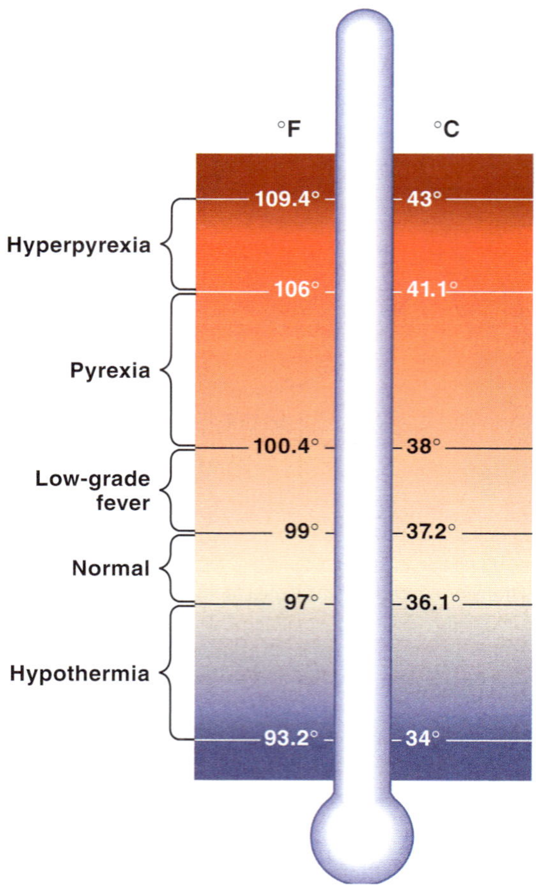

Fig. 19.3 Terms that describe alterations in body temperature (adult oral temperature).

rarely stays the same throughout the course of a day. The medical assistant should take the following points into consideration when evaluating a patient's temperature.

1. *Age.* Infants and young children normally have a higher body temperature than adults because their thermoregulatory system is not yet fully established. Elderly individuals usually have a lower body temperature owing to factors such as loss of subcutaneous fat, lack of exercise, and loss of thermoregulatory control.
2. *Diurnal variations.* During sleep, body metabolism slows down, as do muscle contractions. The body's temperature is lowest in the morning before metabolism and muscle contractions begin increasing.
3. *Emotional states.* Strong emotions such as extreme anger and crying can increase the body temperature. This is important to consider when working with young children, who frequently cry during examination procedures or when they are ill.
4. *Environment.* Cold weather tends to decrease the body temperature, whereas hot weather increases it.
5. *Exercise.* Vigorous physical exercise causes an increase in voluntary muscle contractions, which elevates the body temperature.
6. *Patient's normal body temperature.* Some patients normally run a low or high temperature. The medical assistant should review the patient's temperature recordings before taking the patient's temperature.
7. *Pregnancy.* Cell metabolism increases during pregnancy, and this elevates body temperature.

Fever

Fever, or pyrexia, denotes that a patient's temperature has increased to higher than 100.4°F (38°C). An individual who has a fever is said to be **febrile;** one who does not have a fever is **afebrile.**

Fever is a common symptom of illness, particularly inflammation and infection. When there is an infection in the body, the invading pathogen functions as a *pyrogen,* which is any substance that produces fever. Pyrogens reset the hypothalamus, causing the body temperature to increase to above normal. Fever is not an illness itself, but rather a sign that the body may have an infection. Most fevers are self-limited, that is, the body temperature returns to normal after the disease process is complete.

Stages of a Fever

A fever can be divided into the following three stages:

1. The *onset* is when the temperature first begins to increase. This increase may be slow or sudden, the patient often experiences coldness and chills, and the pulse and respiratory rate increase.
2. During the *course of a fever*, the temperature rises and falls in one of the following three fever patterns: continuous, intermittent, or remittent. Fever patterns are described and illustrated in Table 19.2. During this stage the patient has an increased pulse and respiratory rate and feels warm to the touch. The patient also may experience one or more of the following: flushed appearance, increased thirst, loss of appetite, headache, and malaise. **Malaise** refers to a vague sense of body discomfort, weakness, and fatigue.
3. During the *subsiding stage,* the temperature returns to normal. It can return to normal gradually or suddenly (known as a **crisis**). As the body temperature is returning to normal, the patient usually perspires and may become dehydrated.

ASSESSMENT OF BODY TEMPERATURE

Assessment Sites

There are five sites for measuring body temperature: mouth, axilla, rectum, ear, and forehead. The locations in which temperatures are taken should have an abundant blood supply so that the temperature of the entire body is obtained, not the temperature of only a part of the body. In addition, the site must be as closed as possible to prevent air currents from interfering with the temperature reading. The site chosen for measuring a patient's temperature depends on the patient's age, condition, and state of consciousness; the type of thermometer available; and the medical office policy.

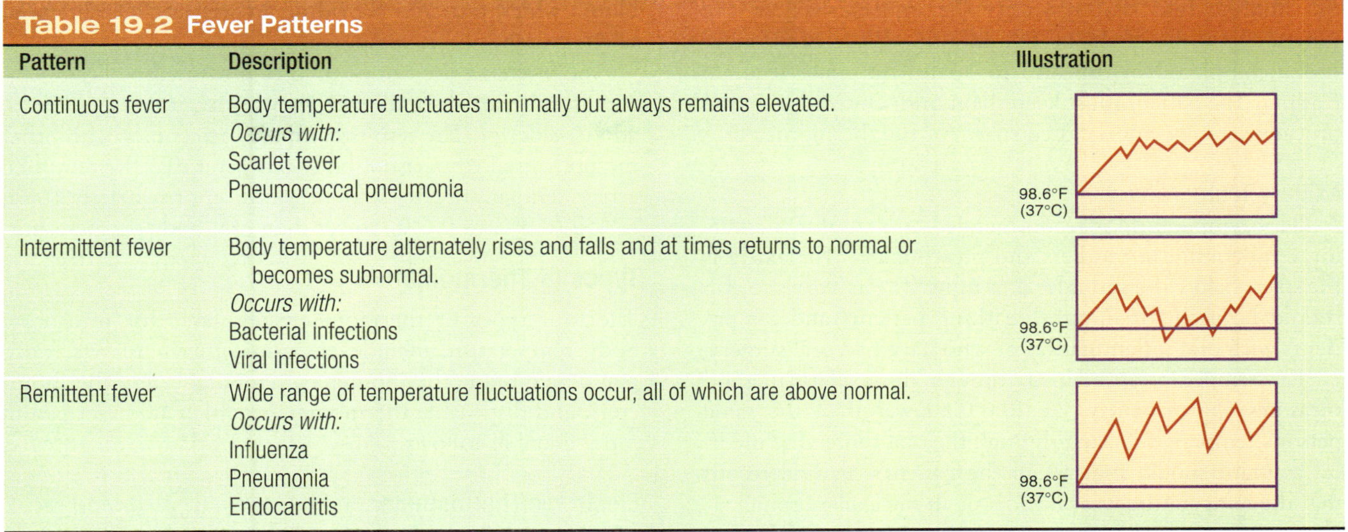

Table 19.2 Fever Patterns

Pattern	Description	Illustration
Continuous fever	Body temperature fluctuates minimally but always remains elevated. *Occurs with:* Scarlet fever Pneumococcal pneumonia	98.6°F (37°C)
Intermittent fever	Body temperature alternately rises and falls and at times returns to normal or becomes subnormal. *Occurs with:* Bacterial infections Viral infections	98.6°F (37°C)
Remittent fever	Wide range of temperature fluctuations occur, all of which are above normal. *Occurs with:* Influenza Pneumonia Endocarditis	98.6°F (37°C)

HIGHLIGHT on Fever

Although most fevers indicate an infection is present, not all do. Noninfectious causes of fever include heatstroke, drug hypersensitivity, neoplasms, and central nervous system damage.

A fever usually is not harmful if the temperature remains below 102°F (38.9°C). Research suggests that fever may serve as a defense mechanism to destroy pathogens that are unable to survive above the normal body temperature range.

The level of the fever is not related to the seriousness of the infection. A patient with a temperature of 104°F (40°C) may not be any sicker than a patient with a temperature of 102°F (38.9°C).

In children, fever often is one of the first signs of illness and has a tendency to become highly elevated. In contrast, in elderly patients, fever may be elevated to only 1°F to 2°F above normal, even with a severe infection.

During a fever, the body's basal metabolism increases by 7% for each degree of temperature elevation. Heart and respiratory rates also increase to meet this metabolic demand.

Chills during a fever result when the hypothalamus has been reset at a higher temperature. In an attempt to reach this temperature, involuntary muscle contractions (chills) occur, which produce heat, causing the temperature of the body to increase. After the higher temperature has been reached, the chills subside, and the individual then feels warm.

Increased perspiration during a fever occurs when the hypothalamus has been reset at a lower temperature, for example, after an individual takes an **antipyretic** medication (drug that reduces fever) or after the cause of the fever has been removed. To cool the body and reach this lower temperature, the body perspires, often profusely; profuse perspiration is known as *diaphoresis*. ■

Putting It All Into Practice

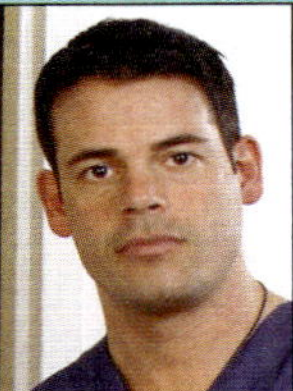

My name is Sergio, and I am a Registered Medical Assistant. I work in a large clinic that is associated with a medical school. At present, I work in the family medicine department, but I also have worked in dermatology and internal medicine. Family medicine is the area I enjoy most because of the wide variety of tasks that are performed. There is rarely a dull moment.

I focus primarily on clinical medical assisting. Taking vital signs is a big part of my job responsibilities. It is routine at my clinic to take the weight, TPR, blood pressure, and pulse oximetry of every patient seen at the clinic, no matter what the reason for their visit. I assist the provider with various procedures, examinations, and minor office surgery, and I administer injections, run electrocardiograms, and perform various laboratory tests.

Taking vital signs and height and weight on young children can be very challenging at times. Some children start to cry as soon as they are put on the scale. I try to calm the child as much as possible, and for good behavior, I give a lot of praise. Stickers also are a great reward for cooperative behavior. Usually when young children understand that they can trust you, they are not as frightened by the experience. It is rewarding when a child learns not to be afraid of being evaluated for routine vital signs. ■

Oral Temperature

The oral method is a convenient and one of the most common means for measuring body temperature. When the medical assistant documents a temperature, the provider assumes it has been taken through the oral route unless otherwise noted. There is a rich blood supply under the tongue in the area on either side of the **frenulum linguae**, which is the midline fold that connects the undersurface of the tongue with the floor of the mouth. The thermometer should be placed in this area to obtain the most accurate reading. The patient must keep the mouth closed during the procedure to provide a closed space for the thermometer.

Axillary Temperature

Axillary temperature is recommended as a site for measuring temperature in toddlers and preschoolers. The **axilla** is the space below the shoulder or armpit. The axillary site also should be used for mouth-breathing patients and for patients with oral inflammation or who have had oral surgery.

The temperature obtained through the axillary method measures approximately 1°F (0.6°C) lower than the same person's temperature taken through the oral route. The medical assistant should indicate in the patient's medical record that the temperature was taken through the axillary route.

Rectal Temperature

The rectal temperature provides an extremely accurate measurement of body temperature because few factors can alter the results. The rectum is highly vascular and, of the five sites, provides the most closed cavity. The temperature obtained by the rectal route measures approximately 1°F (0.6°C) higher than the same person's temperature taken by the oral route. The medical assistant should indicate in the patient's medical record if the temperature has been taken rectally.

In general, the rectal method is used for infants and young children, unconscious patients, and mouth-breathing patients and when greater accuracy in body temperature is desired. The rectal site should not be used with newborns because of the danger of rectal trauma.

Aural Temperature

The aural (ear) site is used with the tympanic membrane thermometer. The ear provides a closed cavity that is easily accessible. Tympanic membrane thermometers provide instantaneous results, are easy to use, and are comfortable for the patient. They make it easier to measure the temperature of children between the ages of 6 months and 6 years, uncooperative patients, and patients who are unable to have their temperatures taken orally. The aural site should not be used for children under 6 months of age because their ear canals are too narrow for proper positioning of the thermometer. The aural temperature reading measures approximately 0.5°F to 1°F (0.3°C to 0.6°C) higher than oral body temperature.

Forehead Temperature

The temporal artery is a major artery of the head that runs laterally across the forehead and down the side of the neck. In the area of the forehead, the temporal artery is located approximately 2 mm below the surface of the skin. Because the temporal artery is located so close to the skin surface and is easily accessible, the forehead provides an ideal site for obtaining a body temperature measurement. In addition, the temporal artery has a constant steady flow of blood, which assists in providing an accurate measurement of the patient's body temperature.

The forehead site can be used to measure body temperature in individuals of all ages (newborns, infants, children, adults, elderly). The results compare in accuracy with other methods used to measure body temperature. The temporal artery temperature reading measures approximately 0.5°F to 1°F (0.3°C to 0.6°C) lower than oral body temperature.

Types of Thermometers

The four types of thermometers available for measuring body temperature include electronic thermometers, tympanic membrane thermometers, temporal artery thermometers, and disposable thermometers, which are described in more detail as follows.

Electronic Thermometer

An electronic thermometer can be used in the medical office to measure body temperature. Electronic thermometers are portable and measure oral, axillary, and rectal temperatures ranging from 84°F to 108°F (28.9°C to 42.2°C).

An electronic thermometer measures body temperature in a brief time—between 4 and 20 seconds depending on the brand of thermometer used. The temperature results are digitally displayed on a liquid crystal diode (LCD) screen. An electronic thermometer consists of interchangeable oral and rectal probes attached to a battery-operated portable unit (Fig. 19.4). The probes are color-coded for ease in identifying them. The oral probe is color-coded with blue on its collar and is used to take oral and axillary temperatures; the rectal probe is color-coded with red on its collar and is used to take rectal temperatures only.

A disposable plastic cover is placed over the probe to prevent the transmission of microorganisms among patients. Depending on the method of taking the temperature, the probe may be inserted into the mouth, axilla, or rectum and is left in place until an audible tone is emitted from the thermometer. When the tone sounds, the patient's temperature in degrees Fahrenheit (or Celsius) is displayed on the screen of the thermometer. The medical assistant ejects the plastic probe cover into a regular waste container.

The casing, probes, and attached cords of the electronic thermometer should be periodically cleaned with a soft cloth slightly dampened with a solution of warm water and a disinfectant cleaner.

Procedures 19.1, 19.2, and 19.3 outline the methods for measuring oral, axillary, and rectal temperatures using an electronic thermometer.

Tympanic Membrane Thermometer

The tympanic membrane thermometer is used at the aural site. The tympanic membrane thermometer functions by detecting thermal energy that is naturally radiated from the body. As with the rest of the body, the tympanic membrane gives off heat waves known as *infrared waves.* The sensor lens of a tympanic thermometer functions like a camera by taking a "picture" of these infrared waves, which are considered

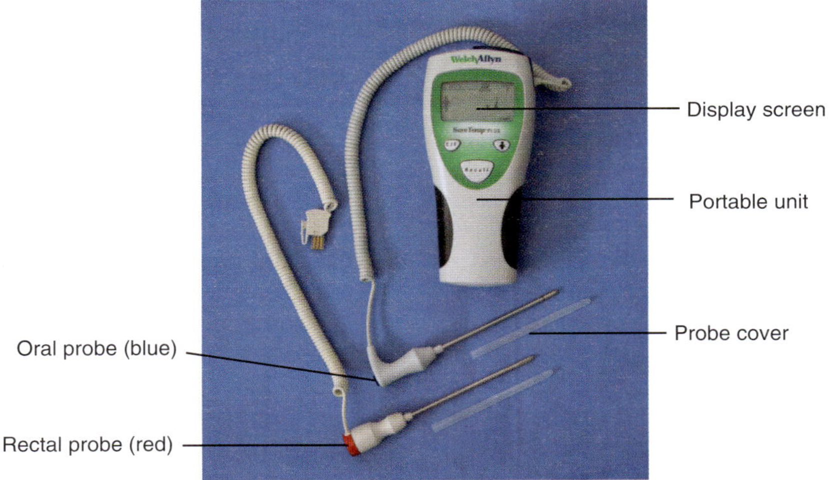

Fig. 19.4 Electronic thermometer.

a documented indicator of body temperature (Fig. 19.5). The thermometer calculates the body temperature from the thermal energy generated by the waves and displays the result on the screen of the thermometer.

The tympanic membrane thermometer is battery operated and consists of a small handheld device with a probe containing a sensor lens (Fig. 19.6). To operate the thermometer, the probe is covered with a disposable soft plastic cover and is placed in the outer third of the external ear canal. An activation button is depressed momentarily, and the results are digitally displayed in 1 to 2 seconds on the screen of the thermometer. The probe cover is ejected into a regular waste container. Additional guidelines for using a tympanic membrane thermometer are presented in Box 19.1. The procedure for taking aural body temperature using a tympanic membrane thermometer is presented in Procedure 19.4.

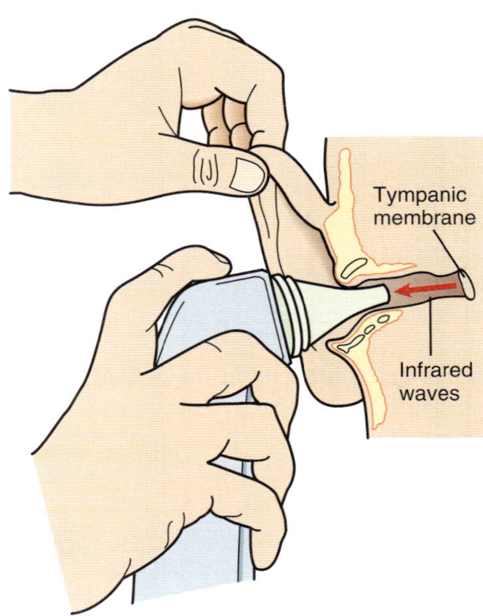

Fig. 19.5 The tympanic membrane thermometer functions by detecting thermal energy that is naturally radiated from the tympanic membrane.

Temporal Artery Thermometer

Use of a temporal artery thermometer is the newest method for assessing body temperature. The temporal artery thermometer is battery operated and consists of a small handheld device with a probe containing a sensor lens.

A temporal artery thermometer works in a similar manner to a tympanic membrane thermometer. The temporal artery gives off infrared waves and the sensor lens captures these thermal waves and calculates the body temperature and digitally displays it on the screen of the thermometer. There are two types of temporal thermometers which include a *contact temporal artery thermometer* (Fig. 19.7A) and a *non-contact temporal artery thermometer* (see Fig. 19.7B). As their names imply, the contact thermometer comes in contact with the patient's skin and the non-contact thermometer does not. A non-contact thermometer poses the lowest risk of cross-contamination between patients among the various types of thermometers. **Cross-contamination** is the process by which microorganisms are unintentionally transferred from one person, object or place to another

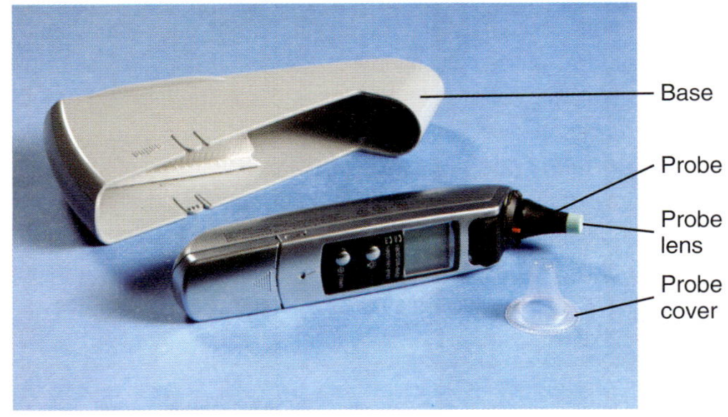

Fig. 19.6 Tympanic membrane thermometer.

BOX 19.1 Guidelines for Using a Tympanic Membrane Thermometer

The following guidelines help ensure accurate aural temperature measurement with a tympanic membrane thermometer.

1. **Determine whether a tympanic thermometer can be used to measure the patient's temperature.** Due to the size of their ear canal, a tympanic thermometer is not recommended for infants under 6 months of age. The tympanic thermometer should not be used on a patient with inflammation of the external ear canal (e.g., otitis externa) or when the ear contains a discharge such as blood or pus. The presence of otitis media and tympanostomy tubes does not significantly affect the temperature reading; a normal amount of cerumen also has no effect. An excessive buildup of cerumen that occludes the ear canal can result in a falsely low temperature reading.
2. **Determine whether external factors are present that may influence the temperature reading.** If any of these factors are present, remove the individual from the situation and wait 20 minutes before taking the temperature. External factors are present in an individual who has been lying on one ear or the other, who has had the ears covered (e.g., hat, earmuffs), who has been exposed to very hot or very cold temperatures, or who has been recently swimming or bathing. If an individual wears hearing aids, remove the hearing device from one ear and wait 20 minutes before taking the temperature in that ear.
3. **Select the temperature measurement system desired.** The temperature of a tympanic membrane thermometer can be displayed in degrees Fahrenheit or degrees Celsius. Follow the manufacturer's instructions to change from one measurement to the other.
4. **Place the probe properly in the patient's ear.** The most important factor in obtaining an accurate temperature is proper placement of the probe in the patient's ear, which is outlined as follows:
   - **Straighten the ear canal.** The ear canal has an S shape that obstructs the view of the tympanic membrane. To obtain an accurate temperature measurement, the ear canal must be straightened before inserting the probe. This allows the probe sensor to obtain a clear picture of the tympanic membrane. In adults and children older than 3 years of age, the canal is straightened by gently pulling the ear auricle upward and backward. In children younger than 3 years of age, the canal is straightened by pulling the ear pinna downward and backward.
   - **Seal the opening of the ear.** The probe must be inserted tightly enough to seal the opening of the ear without causing the patient discomfort. If the probe does not seal the ear canal, cooler external air can cause the thermometer to register a lower temperature.
   - **Correctly position the probe.** Position the tip of the probe toward the opposite temple (approximately midway between the opposite ear and the eyebrow). This allows the sensor to obtain the best possible picture of the tympanic membrane. If the tip is positioned incorrectly, it may be aimed at the ear canal, which results in a falsely low reading.
5. **Verify the accuracy of the temperature reading, if needed.** If you need to take the patient's temperature again, you can use the other ear. There are slight but insignificant differences between temperature readings in the right ear and those in the left ear. Before using the same ear, however, you must wait 2 minutes to allow the aural temperature to stabilize.
6. **Check the probe lens before taking the temperature.** The end of the probe is covered with a lens that is transparent to heat waves. To ensure an accurate temperature measurement, it is extremely important to keep this lens clean, dry, and intact. To protect the lens, always store the thermometer in its storage base when transporting or storing the thermometer. Before taking a temperature, always check to ensure that the lens is shiny and clear. Fingerprints, cerumen, and dust reduce the transparency of the lens, resulting in falsely low temperature readings. If the lens is dirty, it must be cleaned before taking the patient's temperature. If the lens is damaged, the thermometer cannot be used and must be repaired or replaced.
7. **Respond appropriately to digital messages.** A message to alert the user appears on the display screen under the following circumstances:
   - An attempt is made to take a temperature without changing the cover after the last temperature.
   - An attempt is made to take a temperature with no probe cover in place.
   - The ambient (surrounding) temperature is not within the operating range for the thermometer (50°F [10°C] to 104°F [40°C]).
   - The battery is low.
   - The thermometer is in need of repair.
8. **Care for the tympanic thermometer properly.**
   - **Probe lens.** Dust and other minute particles of environmental debris can build up on the probe lens during normal use. The lens should be cleaned as a part of routine maintenance or when it becomes dirty. If the thermometer is placed in the ear without a probe cover, immediately remove the probe and clean the lens. To clean the lens, gently wipe its surface with an antiseptic wipe and allow it to dry. After cleaning, allow at least 5 minutes before taking a temperature.
   - **Thermometer casing.** Clean the casing of the thermometer periodically by wiping it dry with a soft cloth slightly moistened with alcohol. Never submerge the thermometer in water or a cleaning solution. Do not use an abrasive cleaner on the casing, as this could damage the casing.
9. **Store the thermometer properly.** The thermometer must be stored in its storage base to protect the lens from damage and dirt. Store the thermometer in a clean, dry area within a temperature range of 50°F (10°C) to 104°F (40°C). Keep the thermometer away from temperature extremes, which could damage the thermometer.

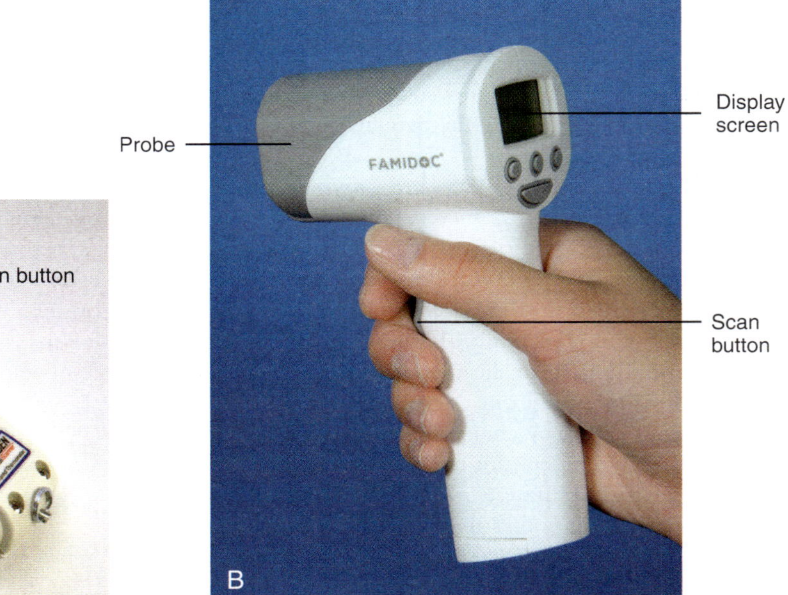

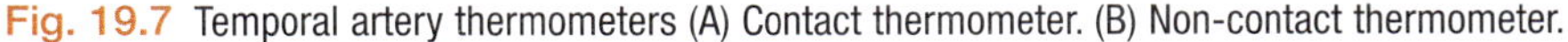

Fig. 19.7 Temporal artery thermometers (A) Contact thermometer. (B) Non-contact thermometer.

which may result in the spread of disease. Guidelines for temporal artery temperature measurement are presented in Box 19.2.

The procedure for measuring body temperature with a contact and non-contact temporal artery thermometer is presented in Procedure 19.5.

Earlobe Temperature Measurement

Sweating of the forehead can cause an inaccurate temporal artery temperature reading. This is because perspiration causes the skin of the forehead to cool, resulting in a falsely low temperature reading. Sweating of the forehead occurs when a patient's fever breaks. It also occurs when a patient's skin is clammy; in this instance, forehead sweating may be present but not readily visible. To avoid this problem, the temperature of the neck area located just behind the earlobe is also measured when taking temperature with a contact temporal artery thermometer.

The area behind the earlobe is less affected by sweating than the forehead. During sweating, the blood vessels behind the earlobe dilate, resulting in a constant, steady flow of blood, which provides an accurate measurement of body temperature. After scanning the forehead with a contact thermometer, the medical assistant should place the probe of the thermometer in the soft depression of the neck just below the mastoid process of the ear. If the patient's forehead has cooled from sweating, the temperature of the neck area behind the earlobe automatically registers as the peak temperature, thereby overriding the forehead temperature.

It is important to note that the area behind the earlobe does not normally provide an accurate body temperature measurement and supersedes the forehead measurement only when the patient is in a diaphoretic state.

BOX 19.2 Temporal Artery Thermometer Guidelines

1. The operating environmental temperature for a temporal artery thermometer is 60°F to 104°F (15.5°C to 40°C).
2. Ensure that the sensor lens is clean and intact. Fingerprints, cerumen, and dust reduce the transparency of the lens, resulting in falsely low temperature readings. The lens is cleaned by gently wiping its surface with an antiseptic wipe or a cotton-tipped swab moistened with alcohol and allowing it to dry. If the sensor lens is damaged, the thermometer cannot be used and must be repaired or replaced.
3. Do not use the thermometer in direct sunlight. Sunlight warms up the forehead leading to a falsely high temperature reading.
4. Ensure that the forehead is exposed to the environment. Anything covering the area to be measured (e.g., hair, hat, wig, bandages) traps body heat, resulting in a falsely high reading.
5. Clean the forehead if sweat is present. Sweat on the forehead can result in a falsely low temperature reading.
6. Do not take temperature over scar tissue, open sores, or abrasions.
7. Do not touch the lens of the probe with your fingers.
8. The temporal artery thermometer should be stored in a clean, dry area. The thermometer must be protected from extremes in temperature, direct sunlight, and dust.
9. The casing of the thermometer should be cleaned periodically with a soft cloth moistened with a solution of warm water and a disinfectant cleaner; never splash water on or immerse the unit in water because this could damage the internal components of the thermometer.

Manufacturers of non-contact temporal artery thermometers do not recommend the use of the earlobe site when measuring a patient's temperature; if sweating of the forehead is present, it should be removed by wiping the forehead with a soft cloth before taking the patient's temperature.

Disposable Thermometer

Disposable single-use thermometers are convenient to use and reduce the likelihood of cross-contamination between patients. They can measure both oral and axillary temperature; brand names for disposable thermometers include Tempa DOT and NexTemp. Disposable thermometers contain chemicals that are heat sensitive. A grid of small chemical dots is located at one end of the thermometer that responds to body heat by changing color. Disposable thermometers have a temperature measuring range from 96°F to 104.8°F and are accurate to within 0.2°F.

Each thermometer comes in its own wrapper. The protective wrapper must be peeled back to expose the handle of the thermometer. The thermometer is removed from the wrapper by pulling on the handle, taking care not to touch the grid of chemical dots (Fig. 19.8A). The thermometer is inserted under the patient's tongue in the pocket located on either side of the frenulum linguae (Fig. 19.8B) and is left in place for the duration of time recommended by the manufacturer (usually 60 seconds). The thermometer is then removed from the patient's mouth and the dots are observed. Each dot represents a different temperature and changes color when the specific temperature is reached for that dot. The temperature result is read accrding to the manufacturer's instructions With the NexTemp disposable thermometer (Fig. 19.8C) a dot turns from green to black when the specific temperature for that dot is reached. The thermometer is read by noting the last black dot on the grid that changed from green to black (Fig. 19.8C). The thermometer is discarded after use in a regular waste container.

Because of their chemical makeup, disposable thermometers should be stored in a cool dry area that is 86°F (30°C) or below and should not be exposed to direct sunlight because heat may cause the thermometer to register a higher temperature.

PULSE

MECHANISM OF THE PULSE

When the left ventricle of the heart contracts, blood is forced from the heart into the **aorta,** which is the major trunk of the arterial system of the body. The aorta is already filled with blood and must expand to accept the blood being pushed out of the left ventricle. This creates a pulsating wave that travels from the aorta through the walls of the arterial system. This wave, known as the *pulse*, can be felt as a light tap by an examiner. The pulse rate is measured by counting the number of taps, or beats, per minute. The **pulse rate**, also known as the heart rate, is defined as the number of times the heart beats in one minute.

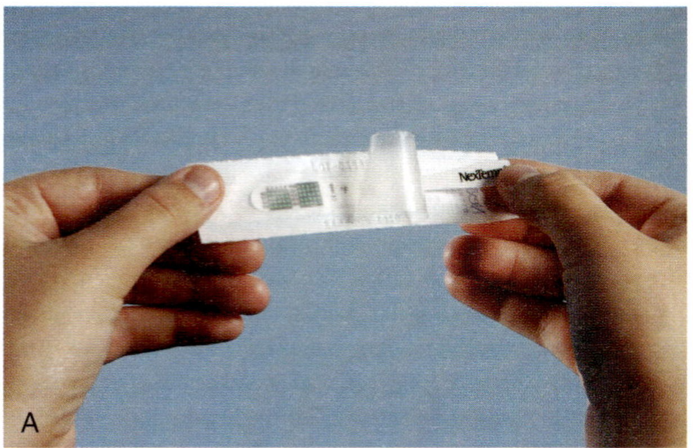

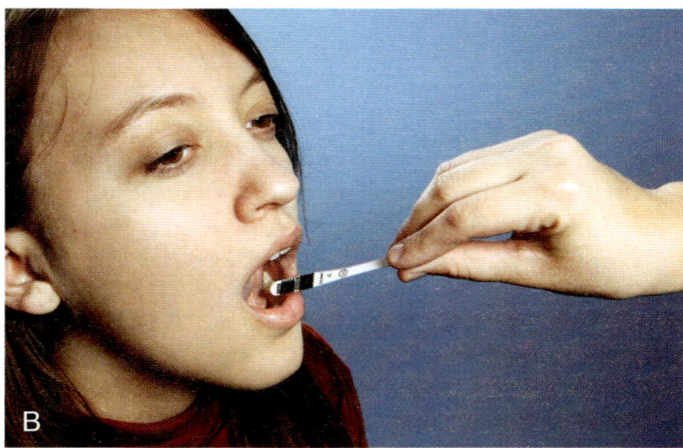

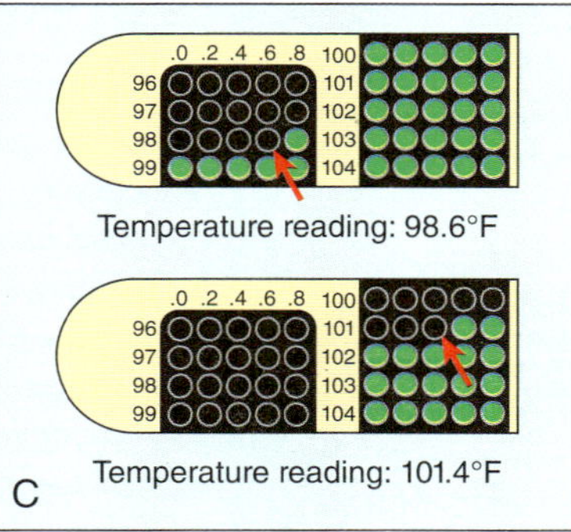

Fig. 19.8 Disposable thermometer. (A) The thermometer is removed from the wrapper by pulling on the handle. (B) The thermometer is inserted under the tongue and is left in place for 60 seconds. (C) The thermometer is read by noting the last black dot on the grid that changed from green to black.

Table 19.3 Pulse Rates of Various Age Groups

Age Group	Pulse Range (beats/min)	Average Pulse (beats/min)
Infant (birth to 1 yr)	120–160	140
Toddler (1-3 yr)	90–140	115
Preschool child (3–6 yr)	80–110	95
School-age child (6–12 yr)	75–105	90
Adolescent (12–18 yr)	60–100	80
Adult (after 18th yr)	60–100	80
Adult (after 60th yr)	67–80	74
Well-trained athletes	40–60	50

Factors Affecting Pulse Rate

Pulse rate (heart rate) can vary depending on many factors. The medical assistant should take each of the following into consideration when measuring pulse:

1. *Age.* The pulse rate varies inversely with age. As age increases, the pulse rate gradually decreases. Table 19.3 lists the pulse rates of various age groups.
2. *Gender.* Women tend to have a slightly faster pulse rate than men.
3. *Physical activity.* Physical activity, such as jogging and swimming, increases the pulse rate temporarily.
4. *Emotional states.* Strong emotional states, such as anxiety, fear, excitement, and anger, temporarily increase the pulse rate.
5. *Metabolism.* Increased body metabolism, such as occurs during pregnancy, increases the pulse rate.
6. *Fever.* Fever increases the pulse rate.
7. *Medications.* Medications may alter the pulse rate. For example, digitalis decreases the pulse rate, and epinephrine increases it.

What Would You Do? What Would You *Not* Do?

Case Study 1

Marcela Mason comes in with Olivia, her 5-year-old daughter. Olivia has had a fever and sore throat for the past 2 days. Sergio takes Olivia's temperature in her left ear with a tympanic membrane thermometer, and it measures 103.3°F. Mrs. Mason says that she has an ear thermometer at home, but when she took Olivia's temperature with it, the readings were always below 97°F. She knew that could not be right because Olivia felt so warm. Mrs. Mason prefers to use her ear thermometer to take Olivia's temperature, but she thinks that it might be broken because of the low readings. ■

Pulse Sites

The pulse is felt most strongly when a superficial artery is held against a firm tissue, such as bone. The locations of sites used for measuring the pulse are shown in Fig. 19.9 and are described next.

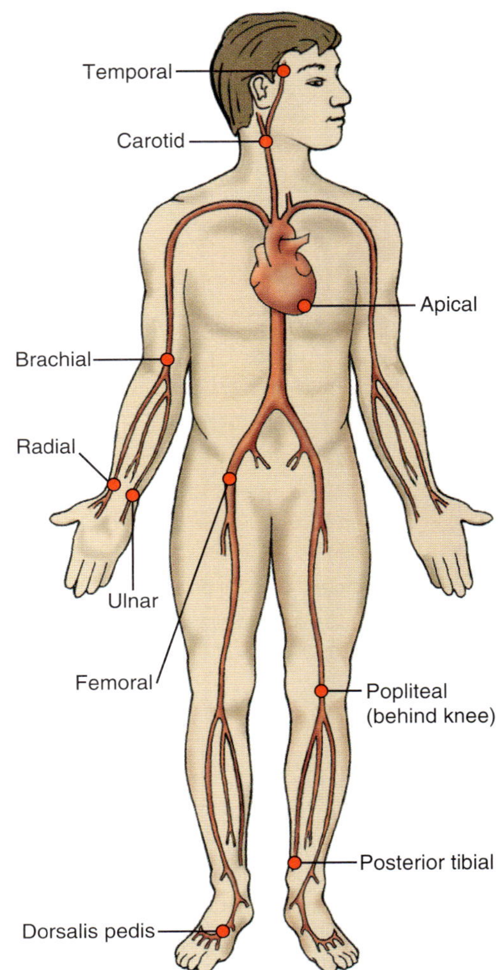

Fig. 19.9 Pulse sites.

Radial

The most common site for measuring the pulse is the radial artery, which is located in a groove on the inner aspect of the wrist just below the thumb. The radial pulse site is easily accessible and can be measured with no discomfort to the patient. This site is also used by individuals at home monitoring their own heart rates, such as athletes, patients taking heart medication, and individuals starting an exercise program. The procedure for measuring radial pulse is outlined in Procedure 19.6.

Apical

The apical pulse has a stronger beat and is easier to measure than the other pulse sites. If the medical assistant is having difficulty feeling the radial pulse, or if the radial pulse is irregular or abnormally slow or rapid, the apical pulse should be taken (Procedure 19.7). The apical pulse site is often used to measure pulse in infants and in children up to 3 years old because the other sites are difficult to palpate accurately in these age groups. The apical pulse is measured using a stethoscope. The chest piece of the stethoscope is placed lightly over the apex of the heart, which is located in

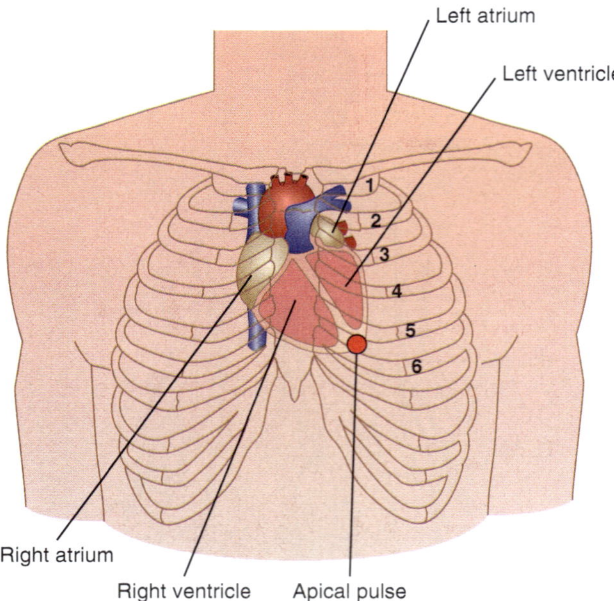

Fig. 19.10 The apical pulse is found over the apex of the heart, which is located in the fifth intercostal space at the junction of the left midclavicular line.

the fifth **intercostal** (between the ribs) space at the junction of the left midclavicular line (Fig. 19.10). A *lub-dup* sound is heard through the stethoscope. The *lub* sound occurs when the cuspid valves of the heart valves of the heart close and the *dup* sound occurs when the semilunar valves of the heart close. Each *lub-dup* is counted as one heartbeat.

Brachial

The brachial pulse site is in the **antecubital space,** which is the space located at the front of the elbow. This site is used to take blood pressure, to measure pulse in infants during cardiac arrest, and to assess the status of the circulation to the lower arm.

Ulnar

The ulnar pulse site is located on the ulnar (little finger) side of the wrist. It is used to assess the status of circulation to the hand.

Temporal

The temporal pulse site is located in front of the ear and just above eye level. This site is used to measure pulse when the radial pulse is inaccessible. It is also an easy access site to assess pulse in children.

Carotid

The carotid pulse site is located on the anterior side of the neck, slightly to one side of the midline, and is the best site to find a pulse quickly. This site is used to measure pulse in children and adults during cardiac arrest. The carotid site also is commonly used by individuals to monitor pulse during exercise.

Femoral

The femoral pulse site is in the middle of the groin. This site is used to measure pulse in infants and children and in adults during cardiac arrest and to assess the status of circulation to the lower leg.

Popliteal

The popliteal pulse site is at the back of the knee and is detected most easily when the knee is slightly flexed. This site is used to measure blood pressure when the brachial pulse is inaccessible and to assess the status of circulation to the lower leg.

Posterior Tibial

The posterior tibial pulse site is located on the inner aspect of the ankle just posterior to the ankle bone. This site is used to assess the status of circulation to the foot.

Dorsalis Pedis

The dorsalis pedis pulse site is located on the upper surface of the foot, between the first and second metatarsal bones. This site is used to assess the status of circulation to the foot.

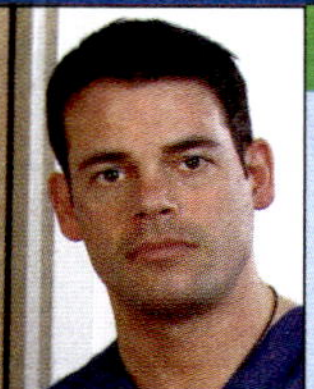

Memories *from* Practicum

Sergio: One experience that really stands out in my memory occurred during my practicum at a family practice medical office. I needed to take the blood pressure of a small 6-year-old boy. After I put the cuff on his arm, his eyes started filling up with tears. I stopped, removed the cuff, and asked him if something was wrong. He said he was afraid that when I started squeezing that thing around his arm, his hand would fall off. I sat down next to him, spent some time talking with him, and reassured him that his hand would be perfectly fine and would not fall off. I put the cuff on my arm and pumped it up to show him that he would be safe. He then agreed to let me take his blood pressure. After I took his blood pressure, he wiggled his hand, gave me a big smile, and said that it didn't hurt at all. That situation made me realize that children may have a lot of fears about what might happen to them at the medical office. Since that experience, I always take the time to explain procedures to children before I perform them. ■

ASSESSMENT OF PULSE

The purpose of measuring pulse is to establish the patient's baseline pulse rate and to assess the pulse rate after special procedures, medications, or disease processes that affect heart functioning. Pulse is measured using palpation at all of the pulse sites except the apical site.

Pulse is palpated by applying moderate pressure with the sensitive pads located on the tips of the three middle fingers. The pulse should not be taken with the thumb because the thumb has a pulse of its own. This could result in measurement of the medical assistant's pulse rather than the patient's pulse.

Excessive pressure should not be applied when measuring pulse because this could obliterate or close off the artery at the pulse site and the pulse may not be felt. It may not be possible to detect the pulse if too little pressure is applied, however. An accurate assessment of pulse includes determinations of the pulse rate, the pulse rhythm, and the pulse volume.

Pulse Rate

The pulse rate is the number of heart pulsations or heartbeats that occur in 1 minute; therefore, pulse rate is measured in beats per minute. Normal pulse rates vary widely in the various age groups, as shown in Table 19.3. For a healthy adult, the normal resting pulse rate ranges from 60 to 100 beats per minute, with the average falling between 70 and 80 beats per minute.

An abnormally fast heart rate of more than 100 beats per minute is known as **tachycardia.** Tachycardia may indicate disease states such as hemorrhaging or heart disease. Tachycardia usually occurs when an individual is involved in vigorous physical exercise or is experiencing strong emotional states.

Bradycardia is an abnormally slow heart rate—less than 60 beats per minute. A pulse rate of less than 60 beats per minute may occur normally during sleep. Trained athletes often have low pulse rates. If a patient exhibits tachycardia or bradycardia during radial pulse measurement, the apical pulse should also be measured.

Pulse Rhythm and Volume

In addition to measuring the pulse rate, the medical assistant should determine the rhythm and volume of the pulse. The **pulse rhythm** denotes the time interval between heartbeats; a normal rhythm has the same time interval between beats and is described as regular. Any irregularity in the heart's rhythm is known as a **dysrhythmia** (also termed *arrhythmia*) and is characterized by unequal or irregular intervals between the heartbeats. If a dysrhythmia is present, the provider may order one or more of the following: an apical-radial pulse, an electrocardiogram, or Holter monitoring.

An *apical-radial pulse* is measured to determine whether a pulse deficit is present. Taking an apical-radial pulse involves measuring the apical pulse at the same time as the radial pulse for a duration of 1 full minute. A **pulse deficit** exists when the radial pulse rate is less than the apical pulse rate. If one medical assistant measures an apical pulse rate of 88 beats per minute while another medical assistant simultaneously measures a radial pulse rate of 76 beats per minute, this results in a pulse deficit of 12 beats. A pulse deficit means that not all of the heartbeats are reaching the peripheral arteries. A pulse deficit is caused by an inefficient contraction of the heart that is not strong enough to transmit a pulse wave to the peripheral pulse site. A pulse deficit frequently occurs with atrial fibrillation, which is a type of dysrhythmia.

The **pulse volume** refers to the strength of the heartbeat. The amount of blood pumped into the aorta by each contraction of the left ventricle should remain constant, making the pulse feel strong and full. If the blood volume decreases, the pulse feels weak and may be difficult to detect. This type of pulse is usually accompanied by a fast heart rate and is described as a **thready pulse.** An increase in the blood volume results in a pulse that feels extremely strong and full, known as a **bounding pulse.**

PATIENT COACHING Aerobic Exercise

Answer questions patients have about aerobic exercise.

What is aerobic exercise?

Aerobic exercise is any type of cardiovascular conditioning. Aerobic means "with oxygen." During aerobic exercise, muscles must work harder which increases the demand for oxygen. This causes the breathing and heart rate to increase to supply the body with enough oxygen. Over time, aerobic exercise strengthens the heart muscle making the heart a more efficient pump resulting in a slower resting heart rate. Aerobic exercise is accomplished through steady, nonstop activity, such as walking, jogging, cycling, or swimming. Each workout should include warm-up and cool-down periods of 5 to 10 minutes. This is needed to prevent muscle or joint injuries.

What are the benefits of an aerobic exercise program?

The benefits of an aerobic exercise program include a lower risk of heart disease and stroke, lowering of the blood pressure, reduction of stress, increased energy, reduction of body fat, better sleep, better bone health, and fewer symptoms of depression and anxiety.

How often should aerobic exercise be performed?

The American Heart Association recommends that healthy adults get at least 150 minutes per week of *moderate-intensity* aerobic activity a week or 75 minutes per week of *vigorous intensity* aerobic activity (or a combination of both), preferably spread out through the week. Exercise intensity refers to how hard the body is working during physical activity. Your health and fitness goals, as well as your current level of fitness, will determine your ideal exercise intensity.

How is exercise intensity measured subjectively?

A subjective measurement of exercise intensity is based upon how you feel during the exercise.

- **Moderate-intensity aerobic exercise.** When you are engaged in moderate-intensity exercise, your heart beats faster and your breathing is heavier, and you can carry on a conversation, but you can't sing. You also develop a light sweat and feel some strain on your muscles. Examples of moderate-intensity exercise include walking at a brisk pace, riding a bike on flat ground, pushing a lawnmower, playing a game of volleyball or badminton, and performing continuous gardening chores (such as weeding and mulching).

Continued

PATIENT COACHING Aerobic Exercise—cont'd

- **Vigorous intensity aerobic exercise.** Vigorous intensity exercise is conducted at a higher intensity level and feels more taxing. During vigorous exercise your heart beats much faster, your breathing is deep and rapid, and you can't say more than a few words without pausing for breath. Examples of vigorous intensity exercise include running/jogging, racquetball or tennis, swimming laps, biking up a hill, and basketball.

How is exercise intensity measured objectively?

Your target heart rate (THR) range offers a more objective way to measure exercise intensity. Your THR range is a safe and effective exercise range that indicates you are exercising at the right level for your age and for what you are trying to accomplish with exercise (e.g., weight loss, improve fitness, train for a competition). Exercising at a level below your THR range does little to promote fitness; exercising at a level above your THR may not be safe. THR range can be determined using a THR online calculator or through the following formulas:

1. **Moderate-intensity aerobic exercise.** Your THR range during moderate-intensity exercise should be 50% to 70% of your maximum heart rate (MHR) which is calculated as follows.
   a. Subtract your age from 220 to determine your MHR, which is the upper limit of what your body can handle during exercise for your age. The MHR of a 40-year-old person is calculated as follows:

      220 − 40 years old = **180** (MHR)

   b. Determine the lower end of your THR range by multiplying your MHR by 0.5. For our example:

      180 × 0.50 = **90** (low end of THR)

   c. Determine the upper end of your THR range by multiplying your MHR by 0.7. For our example:

      180 × 0.70 = **126** (upper end of THR)

   The THR range for moderate-intensity exercise for a 40-year old individual is a heart rate that falls between 90 and 126 beats per minute during physical activity.

2. **Vigorous-intensity aerobic exercise.** Your THR range during vigorous-intensity exercise should be 70% to 85% of your maximum heart rate (MHR), which is calculated as follows:
   a. Determine the lower end of your THR range by multiplying your MHR by 0.7. For our example:

      180 × 0.70 = **126** (low end of THR)

   b. Determine the upper end of your THR range by multiplying your MHR by 0.85. For our example:

      180 × 0.85 = **153** (upper end of THR)

   The THR range for vigorous-intensity exercise for a 40-year-old individual is a heart rate that falls between 126 and 153 beats per minute during physical activity. ■

RESPIRATION

MECHANISM OF RESPIRATION

The purpose of respiration is to provide for the exchange of oxygen and carbon dioxide between the atmosphere and the blood. Oxygen is taken into the body to be used for vital body processes, and carbon dioxide is given off as a waste product.

Each respiration is divided into two phases: **inhalation** and **exhalation** (Fig. 19.11). During inhalation, or inspiration, the diaphragm descends and the lungs expand, causing air containing oxygen to move from the atmosphere into the lungs. Exhalation, or expiration, involves the removal of carbon dioxide from the body. The diaphragm ascends, and the lungs return to their original state so that air containing carbon dioxide is expelled. One complete respiration is composed of one inhalation and one exhalation.

Respiration can be classified as *external* or *internal.* External respiration involves the exchange of oxygen and carbon dioxide between the alveoli and the blood. **Alveoli** (singular, *alveolus*) are thin-walled air sacs in the lungs located at the end of the bronchioles (Fig. 19.12). The blood, located in small capillaries, comes in contact with the alveoli, picks up oxygen, and carries it to the cells of the body. At this point, the oxygen is given off to the cells, and carbon dioxide is picked up by the blood to be transported as a waste product to the lungs. The exchange of oxygen and carbon dioxide between the blood and body cells is known as *internal respiration.*

Control of Respiration

The medulla oblongata, located in the brain, is the control center for involuntary respiration. A buildup of carbon dioxide in the blood sends a message to the medulla, which triggers respiration to occur automatically.

To a certain extent, respiration is also under voluntary control. An individual can control respiration during activities such as singing, laughing, talking, eating, and crying. Voluntary respiration is ultimately under the control of the medulla oblongata. The breath can be held for only a certain length of time, after which carbon dioxide begins to build up in the body, resulting in a stimulus to the medulla that causes respiration to occur involuntarily. Small children may voluntarily hold their breath during a temper tantrum. A parent who does not understand the principles of respiration may be concerned that the child might stop breathing. The medical assistant should be able to explain that involuntary respiration would eventually occur, and the child would resume breathing.

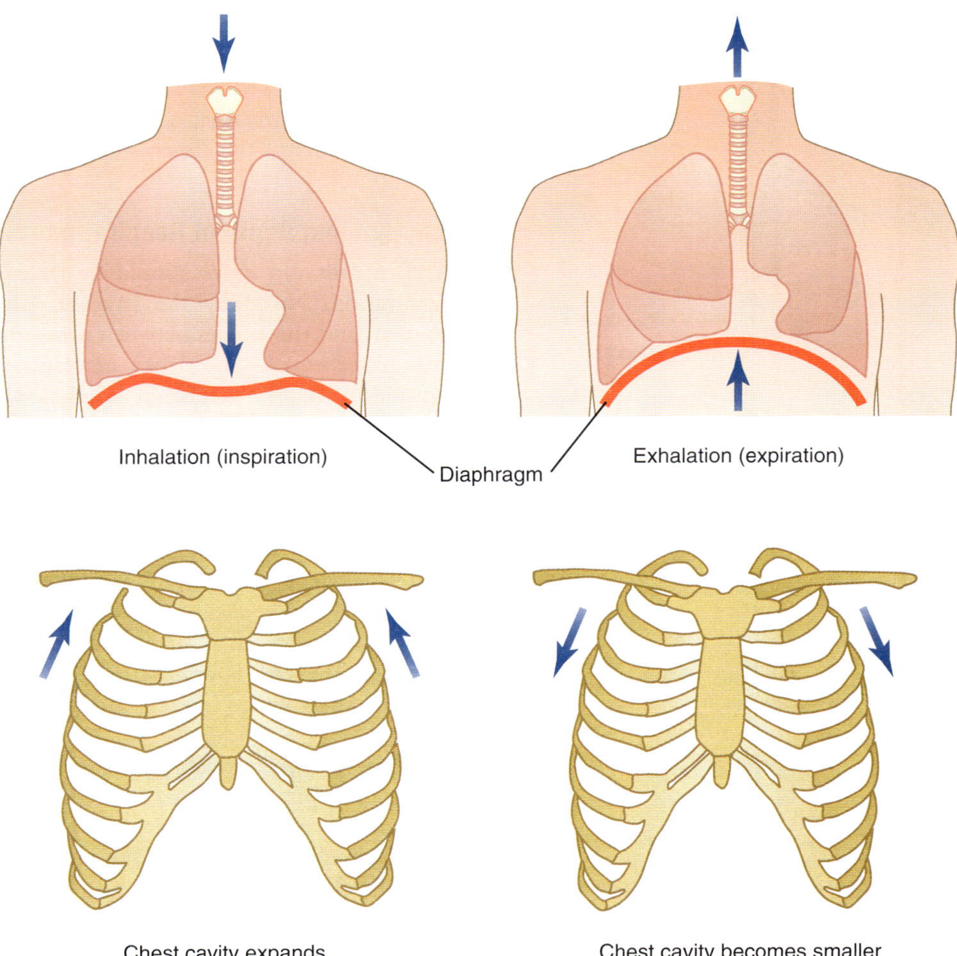

Fig. 19.11 Inhalation and exhalation.

What Would You Do? What Would You *Not* Do?

Case Study 2

Alex Jacoby is 18 years old and a senior in high school. He comes to the office complaining of severe pain in his left shoulder. His vital signs are as follows: temperature 98.5°F, pulse 48 beats per minute, respirations 12 breaths per minute, and blood pressure 108/68 mmHg. Alex is an outstanding competitive swimmer and is currently ranked first in the state in the 100-yard butterfly. Alex has an important swim meet coming up and must do well so that he can get a college athletic scholarship. He says he thinks he can take 2 seconds off his best time at this meet and he doesn't want anything to interfere with that. Alex wants the physician to do whatever she can to make his shoulder better and thinks that a steroid injection and pain pills might be the answer. Alex also wants to know why his pulse rate is so slow. ■

ASSESSMENT OF RESPIRATION

Because an individual can control their respiration, the medical assistant should measure respirations without the patient's knowledge. Patients may change their respiratory rate unintentionally if they are aware that they are being measured. An ideal time to measure respiration is after the pulse is taken. Procedure 19.6 outlines the procedures for taking pulse and respiration in one continuous procedure.

Respiratory Rate

The respiratory rate of a normal healthy adult ranges from 12 to 20 respirations per minute. With most adults, there is a ratio of one respiration for every four pulse beats. If the respiratory rate is 18, the pulse rate would be approximately 72 beats per minute. An abnormal increase in the respiratory rate of more than 20 respirations per minute is referred to as **tachypnea.** An abnormal decrease in the respiratory rate of less than 12 respirations per minute is known as **bradypnea.** When measuring the respiratory rate, the medical assistant should take into consideration the following factors:

1. *Age.* As age increases, the respiratory rate decreases. The respiratory rate of a child would be expected to be faster than that of an adult. Table 19.4 provides a chart of the respiratory rates for various age groups.
2. *Physical activity.* Physical activity increases the respiratory rate temporarily.

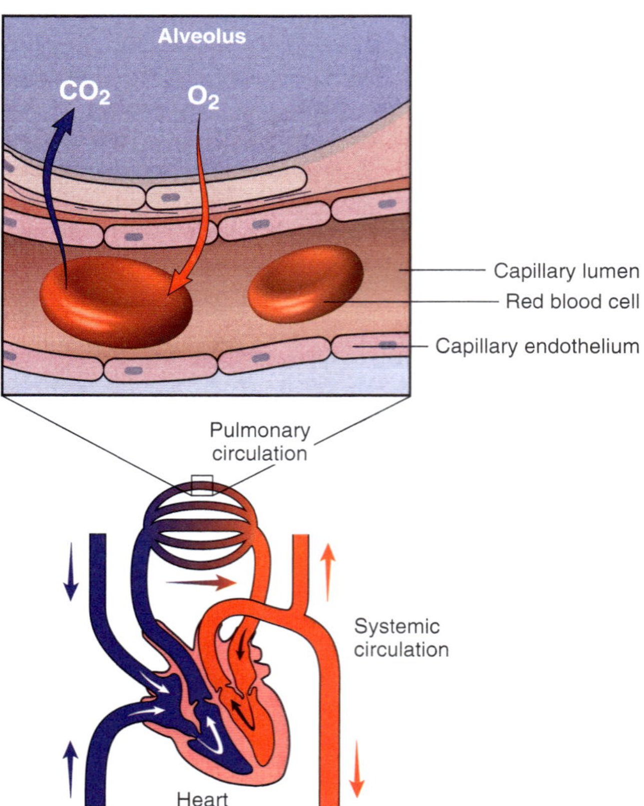

Fig. 19.12 Exchange of oxygen and carbon dioxide between the alveoli of the lungs and the blood.

Table 19.4 Respiratory Rates of Various Age Groups

	Average Respiratory Range, Breaths per Minute	Respiratory Average, Breaths per Minute
Infant (birth to 1 yr)	30–60	35
Toddler (1–3 yr)	24–40	30
Preschool child (3–6 yr)	22–34	25
School-age child (6–12 yr)	18–30	22
Adolescent (12–18 yr)	12–16	16
Adult (after 18th yr)	12–20	16

3. *Emotional states.* Strong emotional states temporarily increase the respiratory rate.
4. *Fever.* A patient with a fever has an increased respiratory rate. One way that heat is lost from the body is through the lungs; a fever causes an increased respiratory rate as the body tries to rid itself of excess heat.
5. *Medications.* Certain medications increase the respiratory rate, and others decrease it. If the medical assistant is unsure of what effect a particular drug may have on the respiratory rate, a drug reference should be consulted, such as the *Prescriber's Digital Reference* (available online).

Rhythm and Depth of Respiration

The *rhythm* and *depth* should be noted when measuring respiration. Normally the rhythm should be even and regular, and the pauses between inhalation and exhalation should be equal. The depth of respiration indicates the amount of air that is inhaled or exhaled during the process of breathing. Respiratory depth is typically described as normal, deep, or shallow and is determined by observing the amount of movement of the chest. For normal respirations, the depth of each respiration in a resting state is approximately the same. Deep respirations are those in which a large volume of air is inhaled and exhaled, whereas shallow respirations involve the exchange of a small volume of air. Normal respiration is referred to as **eupnea.** The rate is approximately 12 to 20 breaths per minute, the rhythm is even and regular, and the depth is normal.

Hyperpnea is an abnormal increase in the rate and depth of respirations. A patient with hyperpnea exhibits a very deep, rapid, and labored respiration. Hyperpnea occurs normally with exercise and abnormally with pain and fever. It also can occur with any condition in which the supply of oxygen is inadequate, such as heart disease and lung disease.

Hyperventilation is an abnormally fast and deep type of breathing that is usually associated with acute anxiety conditions, such as panic attacks. An individual who is hyperventilating is "overbreathing," which usually causes dizziness and weakness.

Hypopnea is a condition in which a patient's respirations exhibit an abnormal decrease in rate and depth. The depth is approximately half that of normal respiration. Hypopnea often occurs in individuals with sleep disorders.

Color of the Patient

The patient's color should be observed while the respiration is being measured. A reduction in the oxygen supply to the tissues results in a condition known as **cyanosis,** which causes a bluish discoloration of the skin and mucous membranes. Cyanosis is first observed in the nail beds and lips because in these areas the blood vessels lie close to the surface of the skin. Cyanosis typically occurs in patients with advanced emphysema and in patients during cardiac arrest.

Respiratory Abnormalities

Apnea is the temporary cessation of breathing. Some individuals experience apnea during sleep; this condition is known as *sleep apnea.* Apnea can be a serious condition if

PATIENT COACHING Chronic Obstructive Pulmonary Disease

Answer questions that patients have about chronic obstructive pulmonary disease (COPD).

What is COPD?
COPD is a chronic airway obstruction that results from emphysema or chronic bronchitis or a combination of these conditions. COPD is a chronic, debilitating, irreversible, and sometimes fatal disease.

How many people have COPD?
More than 16 million Americans have been diagnosed with COPD; however, it is estimated that millions more have the disease but remain undiagnosed. COPD is the third leading cause of death in the United States behind heart disease and cancer. Although COPD is much more common in men than in women, the greatest increase in death rates is occurring in women.

What causes COPD?
Cigarette smoking over a period of many years is the leading cause of COPD. Other causes include air pollution and occupational exposure to irritating inhalants, such as noxious dusts, fumes, and vapors.

What types of tests might the provider order?
Respiratory tests to diagnose COPD include various types of pulmonary function tests. Examples of pulmonary function tests are spirometry, lung volumes, diffusion capacity, arterial blood gas studies, and cardiopulmonary exercise tests.

What treatment might the provider prescribe?
Treatment is focused on improving breathing difficulties and may include bronchodilator drug therapy, breathing exercises, and oxygen therapy.

1. Encourage patients with COPD to comply with the therapy prescribed by the provider.
2. Provide the patient with information about smoking, emphysema, and chronic bronchitis. Educational materials are available from the American Lung Association, the American Heart Association, and the American Cancer Society.

the individual's breathing ceases for more than 4 to 6 minutes because brain damage or death could occur. A patient who is having difficulty breathing or shortness of breath has a condition known as **dyspnea.** Dyspnea may occur normally during vigorous physical exertion and abnormally in patients with asthma and emphysema. A patient with dyspnea may find it easier to breathe while in a sitting or standing position. This state is called **orthopnea** and occurs with disorders of the heart and lungs, such as asthma, emphysema, pneumonia, and congestive heart failure.

Breath Sounds

Breath sounds are caused by air moving through the respiratory tract. Normal breath sounds are quiet and barely audible. Abnormal breath sounds are referred to as **adventitious sounds** and typically signify the presence of a respiratory disorder. The causes and characters of abnormal breath sounds are presented in Table 19.5.

PULSE OXIMETRY

Pulse oximetry is a painless and noninvasive procedure used to measure the oxygen saturation of hemoglobin in arterial blood. Hemoglobin is a complex compound found in red blood cells that functions in transporting oxygen in the body. Pulse oximetry provides information on a patient's cardiorespiratory status—in particular, the amount of oxygen being delivered to the tissues of the body. The procedure for performing pulse oximetry is presented in Procedure 19.8.

A **pulse oximeter** is a device used to measure and display the oxygen saturation of the blood. It is a computerized portable device that consists of a display monitor and a two-sided, clip-on probe (Fig. 19.13). A pulse oximeter also measures the patient's pulse rate in beats per minute. Pulse oximeters can be obtained by individuals over-the-counter or through a provider's prescription for use at home. The measurement of the oxygen saturation of

Table 19.5 Abnormal Breath Sounds

Type	Cause	Character
Crackles* (rales)	Air moving through airways that contain fluid	Dry or wet intermittent sounds that vary in pitch (this sound can be duplicated by rubbing hair together next to ear)
Rhonchi*	Thick secretions, tumors, or spasms that partially obstruct air flow through large upper airways	Deep, low-pitched, rumbling sound more audible during expiration
Wheezes	Severely narrowed airways caused by partial obstruction in smaller bronchi and bronchioles; common symptom of asthma	Continuous, high-pitched, whistling musical sounds heard during inspiration and expiration
Pleural friction rub*	Inflamed pleurae rubbing together	High, grating sound similar to rubbing leather pieces together, heard on inspiration and expiration

*Audible only through a stethoscope.

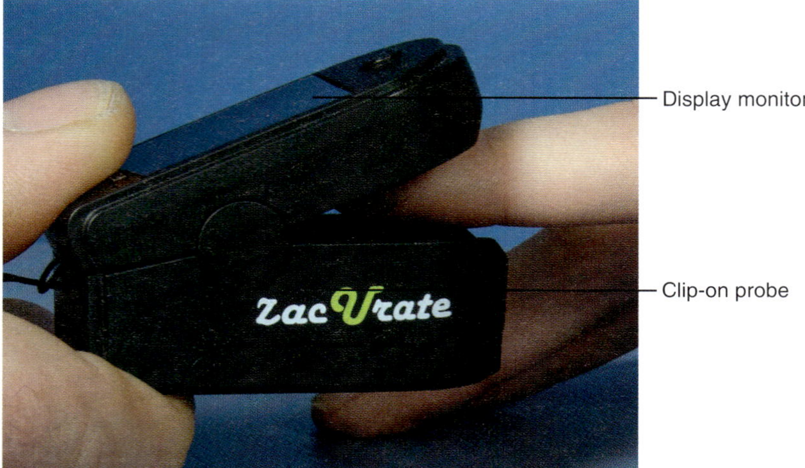

Fig. 19.13 Pulse oximeter.

blood by patients at home has increased substantially as a result of the COVID-19 pandemic.

ASSESSMENT OF OXYGEN SATURATION

The clip-on probe of the pulse oximeter must be attached to a peripheral pulsating capillary bed, such as the tip of a finger. One side of the probe contains a *light-emitting diode (LED)* that transmits infrared light and red light through the capillary bed in the patient's finger to a light detector located on the other side of the probe, known as a *light sensor* (Fig. 19.14).

Hemoglobin that is bright red in color has a high oxygen content *(oxygen rich)* and absorbs more of the infrared light emitted by the LED. Hemoglobin that is dark red in color is low in oxygen *(oxygen poor)* and absorbs more of the red light. The computer of the oximeter compares and calculates the light transmitted from the oxygen-rich hemoglobin and the oxygen-poor hemoglobin and from this ratio is able to determine the oxygen saturation of the patient's hemoglobin. This measurement is converted to a percentage and is displayed as a digital readout on the screen of the monitor. Because the pulse oximeter measures the oxygen saturation of peripheral capillaries, the abbreviation **SpO_2** *(saturation of peripheral oxygen)* is used to document the reading.

A more complete but invasive measurement of oxygen saturation is arterial blood gas analysis, which requires drawing a blood specimen from an artery. The abbreviation for this type of arterial oxygen saturation measurement is ***SaO_2*** *(saturation of arterial oxygen).*

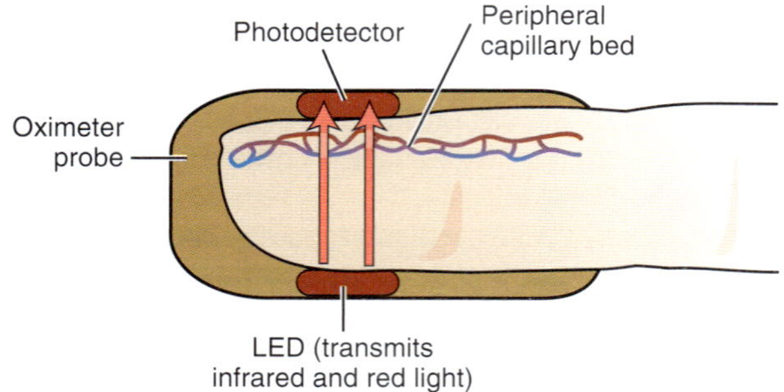

Fig. 19.14 The probe of the pulse oximeter is attached to a peripheral capillary bed in the fingertip. The LED transmits light through the capillary bed to a light sensor located on the other side of the probe to measure the oxygen saturation of hemoglobin.

Interpretation of Results

The pulse oximetry reading represents the percentage of hemoglobin that is saturated (filled) with oxygen. Each molecule of hemoglobin can carry four oxygen molecules. If 100 molecules of hemoglobin were fully saturated with oxygen, they would be carrying 400 molecules of oxygen, and the oxygen saturation reading would be 100%. If these same 100 molecules of hemoglobin were carrying only 360 molecules of oxygen, however, the oxygen saturation reading would be 90%. The more hemoglobin that is saturated with oxygen, the higher the oxygen saturation of the blood.

The oxygen saturation level of most healthy individuals is 95% to 99%. Because the air we breathe is only 21% saturated with oxygen, it is unusual for an individual's hemoglobin to be fully or 100% saturated with oxygen. Patients on supplemental oxygen sometimes have a reading of 100%, however.

An oxygen saturation level of less than 95% typically results in an inadequate amount of oxygen reaching the tissues of the body, although patients with chronic pulmonary disease are sometimes able to tolerate lower saturation levels. Respiratory failure, resulting in tissue damage, usually occurs when the oxygen saturation decreases to a level between 85% and 90%. Cyanosis typically appears when an individual's oxygen saturation reaches a level of 75%, and an oxygen saturation of less than 70% is life-threatening.

A decrease in the oxygen saturation of the blood (less than 95%) is known as **hypoxemia.** Hypoxemia can lead to a more serious condition known as hypoxia. **Hypoxia** is defined as a reduction in the oxygen supply to the tissues of the body, and if not treated it can lead to tissue damage and death. The first symptoms of hypoxia include headache, mental confusion, nausea, dizziness, shortness of breath, tachycardia, and cyanosis. The tissues most sensitive to hypoxia are the brain, heart, pulmonary vessels, and liver.

Purpose of Pulse Oximetry

In the medical office, pulse oximetry is performed on patients complaining of respiratory problems (e.g., dyspnea). A decreased pulse oximetry reading (along with clinical signs and symptoms and further testing) assists in the proper diagnosis and treatment of a patient's condition, which may include drug therapy and oxygen therapy.

Conditions that can cause a decreased SpO_2 value (hypoxemia) include the following:

- Acute pulmonary disease (e.g., pneumonia)
- Chronic pulmonary disease (e.g., emphysema, asthma, bronchitis)
- Cardiac problems (e.g., congestive heart failure, coronary artery disease)

In addition to assisting in the diagnosis of a patient's condition, pulse oximetry is used to assess the following:

- Effectiveness of oxygen therapy
- Patient's tolerance to activity
- Effectiveness of treatment (e.g., bronchodilators)
- Patient's tolerance to analgesia and sedation

In the medical office, pulse oximetry is most often used as a "spot-check" measurement—in other words, as a single measurement of oxygen saturation. Occasionally, pulse oximetry may be used in the medical office for the short-term *continuous monitoring* of a patient experiencing an asthmatic attack or to monitor a patient during minor office surgery.

Components of the Pulse Oximeter

Most medical offices use a handheld pulse oximeter, which is portable, lightweight, and battery operated. This is in contrast to a stand-alone oximeter, which is more apt to be used in a hospital setting for the continuous bedside monitoring of a patient's oxygen saturation level and pulse rate. The two main parts of the pulse oximeter—the monitor and the probe—are described in detail next.

Monitor

The monitor of the pulse oximeter contains controls, indicators, and displays (Fig. 19.15). These may vary slightly depending on the brand of oximeter. Those that are found on most handheld pulse oximeters include the following:

1. *Power-on control.* Turns the oximeter on.
2. *SpO_2% display.* A digital display of the patient's oxygen saturation expressed as a percent. This number is updated with every few pulse beats.

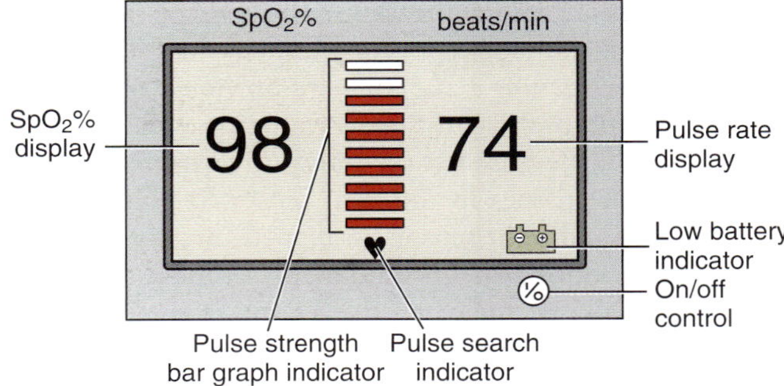

Fig. 19.15 Pulse oximeter monitor: controls, indicators, and displays.

3. *Pulse rate display.* This display indicates the patient's pulse rate in beats per minute. This number is updated with each pulse beat.
4. *Pulse strength bar-graph indicator.* This indicator provides a visual display of the patient's pulse strength at the probe placement site. The pulse strength indicator consists of a segmented display of bars. The pulse strength indicator "sweeps" with each pulse beat, and the stronger the pulse, the more segments that light up on the bar graph.
5. *Battery icon display.* The battery icon is used to warn that the battery is getting low. When the battery icon flickers continuously on the LED screen, the battery is low and needs to be replaced.
6. *Power-on self-test.* When the pulse oximeter is turned on, it will take about 4 to 6 seconds before the results are displayed. It automatically performs a power-on self-test (POST), which takes a few seconds. During the POST, the oximeter checks its internal systems to ensure they are functioning properly. When the POST is completed, the oximeter begins searching for a pulse. It takes several seconds for the oximeter to locate a pulse and to calculate and display the SpO_2 reading. If the oximeter is unable to detect a pulse, or if the pulse is too weak to provide the data needed to calculate oxygen saturation, the oximeter is unable to make a measurement. In this case, the pulse oximeter fails to display the blood oxygen saturation level and/or the pulse rate. If this occurs, the medical assistant should reposition the probe or move the probe to another finger and perform the procedure again.

Clip-On Probe

The clip-on probe must be attached to the patient at a peripheral site that is highly vascular and where the skin is thin. The most common site to apply the probe a probe is the tip of a finger: any finger except for the little finger can be used. Many manufacturers of pulse oximeters recommend the thumb as an application site. Other acceptable probe application sites include the big toe and the earlobe.

Factors Affecting Pulse Oximetry

Although pulse oximetry is an easy procedure to perform, the medical assistant must be aware of certain factors that may interfere with an accurate reading. These factors are listed, along with guidelines for correcting or preventing them.

1. *Incorrect positioning of the probe.* As previously discussed, the oximeter probe consists of two parts: an LED and a light sensor. Because light is transmitted from the LED through the tissues to the light sensor, it is important that LED and light sensor be aligned directly opposite each other during the measurement. In most cases, this automatically occurs when the clip-on probe is applied to the patient's finger. Proper alignment of the probe may be impossible, however, with patients who have very small fingers (e.g., a thin individual and a child) because the probe cannot detect enough blood to make a measurement. To obtain an accurate reading, the probe must be moved to another site, such as the big toe or earlobe.
2. *Fingernail polish or artificial nails.* A dark, opaque coating on the fingernail may result in a falsely low reading. This is because the coating interferes with proper light transmission through the finger. The darker the coating, the more likely that the SpO_2 reading will be affected. Blue, black, and green fingernail polishes tend to cause the most problems. If the patient is wearing dark fingernail polish, it should be removed with acetone or fingernail polish remover. If the patient has long fingernails or artificial fingernails, another site should be used to take the measurement, such as the big toe or earlobe. These situations may obstruct the light sensor and prevent an accurate measurement. Oil, dirt, and grime on the fingertip can also interfere with proper light transmission. If the patient's fingertip is dirty, cleanse the site with soap and water and allow it to dry. Areas with bruises, burns, stains, broken skin, or tattoos should be avoided as a probe placement site. Darkly pigmented skin and jaundice do not usually affect the ability of the oximeter to obtain an accurate reading.
3. *Low pulse bar strength.* The pulse strength bar graph indicator can be used to determine the reliability of a reading. If the height of the pulse bar graph is less than 30%, this indicates signal inadequacy and the displayed SpO_2 and pulse rate readings are potentially incorrect. In this case, the probe should be repositioned on the patient's finger making sure the tip of the finger touches the end of the probe stop and that the LED light and the light sensor are aligned directly opposite to each other.
4. *Poor peripheral blood flow.* A pulse oximeter works best when there is a strong pulse in the finger to which the probe is applied. Poor peripheral blood flow may cause the pulse to be so weak that the oximeter cannot obtain a reading. Conditions resulting in poor blood flow include peripheral vascular disease, vasoconstrictor medications, severe hypotension, and hypothermia. In addition, patients with cold fingers (but who are not hypothermic) may have enough constriction of the peripheral capillaries that it interferes with obtaining a reading. To solve these problems, the medical assistant should ask the patient to warm their hands and fingers by rubbing the hands together. The probe should never be attached to the finger of an arm to which an automatic blood pressure cuff is applied because blood flow to the finger will be cut off when the cuff inflates, resulting in loss of the pulse signal.
5. *Ambient (surrounding) light.* Ambient light shining directly on the probe, such as bright fluorescent light, direct sunlight, or an overhead examination light, may result in an inaccurate reading. This is because some of the ambient light may be picked up by the light sensor and alter the reading. This problem can be corrected by one of the following: turning off the light, moving the patient's hand away from the light source, or covering the probe with an opaque material such as a washcloth.
6. *Finger movement.* Finger movement during the measurement is a common cause of an inaccurate reading. Motion affects the ability of the light to travel from the LED to the light sensor and prevents the probe from picking up the pulse signal. To avoid this problem, it is important that the medical assistant instruct the patient to keep their finger stationary during the procedure. Occasionally, movement of the fingers cannot be eliminated, such as when the patient has tremors of the hands. In these instances, the oxygen saturation level should be measured at a site that is less affected by motion, such as the big toe or the earlobe.

Care and Maintenance

The pulse oximeter should be cleaned periodically using a cloth slightly dampened with a solution of warm water and a disinfectant cleaner. The medical assistant should make sure that the cloth is not too wet to prevent the solution from running into the oximeter, which could damage the internal components.

The inside of the probe also should be disinfected before and after each patient measurement by wiping it thoroughly with an antiseptic wipe and allowing it to dry. The probe should never be soaked or immersed in a liquid solution because this would damage it. The probe is heat sensitive and cannot be autoclaved. The pulse oximeter should be stored at room temperature in a dry environment.

BLOOD PRESSURE

MECHANISM OF BLOOD PRESSURE

Blood pressure is the pressure or force exerted by the circulating blood on the walls of the arteries. Contraction and relaxation of the heart result in two different pressures—systolic pressure and diastolic pressure. Each time the ventricles contract, blood is pushed out of the heart and into the aorta and pulmonary trunk, exerting pressure on the walls of the arteries. This phase in the cardiac cycle is known as **systole,** and it represents the highest point of blood pressure in the body, or the **systolic pressure.** The phase of the cardiac cycle in which the heart relaxes between contractions is referred to as **diastole.** The **diastolic pressure**

(documented during diastole) is lower because the heart is relaxed.

Blood Pressure Measurement

Blood pressure is measured with a **sphygmomanometer**, which is a device that measures the pressure of blood within an artery. There are two types of sphygmomanometers which include the *aneroid* sphygmomanometer and the *digital* sphygmomanometer (more commonly known as an *automatic blood pressure monitor*).

A blood pressure reading consists of two numbers. The top number is the systolic pressure and the bottom number is the diastolic pressure. The standard unit for measuring blood pressure is millimeters of mercury (mmHg). A blood pressure reading of 110/70 mmHg means that there was enough force to raise a column of mercury 110 mm during systole and 70 mm during diastole. These two numbers identify whether a blood pressure reading is healthy or unhealthy. According to the American Heart Association (AHA) normal healthy blood pressure for an adult is a reading less than 120/80 mmHg.

Blood pressure should be taken during every office visit to compare a patient's readings over time. This is a good preventive measure in guarding against problems that may occur as a result of high blood pressure. A single blood pressure reading taken on one occasion does not characterize an individual's blood pressure accurately. An average of two or more blood pressure readings taken on two or more separate office visits is recommended to minimize errors and provide a more accurate measurement.

Blood Pressure Categories

In 2017, the ACC (American College of Cardiology) and the AHA issued new guidelines for the interpretation of blood pressure in adults. The new guidelines are outlined in Table 19.6 and are described below.

Normal: A blood pressure reading of less than 120/80 mmHg is classified as normal.

Elevated: A systolic reading between 120 and 129 mmHg *and* a diastolic reading less than 80 mm Hg is classified as elevated. An *elevated* reading means that an individual has an increased risk of developing high blood pressure. Without lifestyle modifications, an individual with a consistently elevated reading is likely to develop high blood pressure.

High blood pressure: The 2017 ACC/AHA guidelines lowered the threshold for the diagnosis of high blood pressure. This is because scientific studies showed that the risk of some complications of high blood pressure begin to develop at a blood pressure reading lower than previously thought. A systolic reading of 130 mmHg or higher *or* a diastolic reading of 80 mmHg or higher is classified as high blood pressure or *hypertension*. The previous guidelines set the threshold for the diagnosis of high blood pressure at a systolic reading of 140 mmHg or higher *or* a diastolic reading of 90 mmHg or higher. The goal of the new guidelines is to allow for earlier intervention of complications caused by high blood pressure (e.g. cardiovascular disease) much earlier than before.

Factors Temporarily Affecting Blood Pressure

Blood pressure does not remain at a constant level. A number of factors may temporarily affect blood pressure throughout the course of a day. If possible, the medical assistant should make an attempt to reduce or eliminate these factors if present. This helps to ensure an accurate blood pressure reading.

1. *Diurnal variations.* Fluctuations in an individual's blood pressure are normal during the course of a day. Blood pressure is normally lower at night as a result of decreased metabolism and physical activity during sleep. The blood pressure begins to rise several hours before waking. As metabolism and activity increase during the day, the blood pressure continues to rise, usually peaking in the middle of the afternoon. In the later afternoon and evening, the blood pressure begins dropping again. Patients who are self-monitoring their blood pressure at home should measure their blood pressure at the same time of day.

Table 19.6 Categories of Blood Pressure in Adults[a]

Blood Pressure Category[b]	Systolic Blood Pressure (mmHg)		Diastolic Blood Pressure (mmHg)
Normal	Less than 120	*and*	Less than 80
Elevated	120–129	*and*	Less than 80
Hypertension			
Hypertension Stage 1	130–139	*or*	80–89
Hypertension Stage 2	140 or higher	*or*	90 or higher

[a]Individuals with a systolic BP and a diastolic BP in two different categories should be designated to the higher BP category.
[b]Based on an average of two or more readings taken on two or more separate occasions.
Modified from Whelton PK, Carey RM, Aronow WS, et al. 2017 ACC/AHA/AAPA/ABC/ACPM/AGS/APhA/ASH/ASPC/NMA/PCNA Guideline for the Prevention, Detection, Evaluation, and Management of High Blood Pressure in Adults: Executive Summary: A Report of the American College Cardiology/American Heart Association Task Force on Clinical Practice Guidelines. *Hypertension.* 2018;71(6):1269–1324.

2. *Emotional states.* Strong emotional states, such as anger, fear, and excitement, increase the blood pressure. If the medical assistant observes such a reaction, an attempt should be made to calm the patient before taking their blood pressure.
3. *Physical exercise.* Physical activity temporarily increases the blood pressure. To ensure an accurate reading, a patient who has been involved in physical activity should be given an opportunity to rest for 20 to 30 minutes before blood pressure is measured.
4. *Body position.* The blood pressure of a patient who is in a lying or standing position is usually different from that measured when the patient is sitting. For example, the diastolic pressure of an individual in a sitting position is higher than their diastolic pressure in a lying position. A notation should be made in the patient's medical record if the reading was obtained in any position other than sitting, by using the following abbreviations: *L* (lying) and *St* (standing).
5. *Full bladder.* A full bladder can increase the blood pressure as much as 10 to 15 mmHg. To ensure an accurate reading, a patient should be asked to void before blood pressure is measured.
6. *Tobacco use.* Tobacco products (cigarettes, cigars, smokeless tobacco) contain nicotine which temporarily increases the blood pressure. To ensure an accurate reading, patients should not use tobacco products for 30 minutes before having their blood pressure measured.
7. *Medications.* Certain medications may increase or decrease the blood pressure. For example, OTC cold medications that contain decongestants (e.g., phenylephrine, pseudoephedrine) may cause a temporary increase the blood pressure. Because of this, it is important to document all prescription and over-the-counter medications patients are taking in their medical records.
8. *Alcohol and caffeine consumption.* Alcohol and caffeine consumption can cause a temporary increase in the blood pressure. A patient should not consume these substances for at least 30 minutes before having blood pressure measured.
9. *Other factors.* Other factors that may temporarily increase the blood pressure include pain and a recent meal.

Pulse Pressure

The difference between the systolic pressure and the diastolic pressure is known as the **pulse pressure.** It is determined by subtracting the smaller number from the larger. If the blood pressure is 110/70 mmHg, the pulse pressure would be 40 mmHg. A pulse pressure between 30 and 50 mmHg is considered to be within normal range.

HYPERTENSION

High blood pressure or **hypertension** means the force of the circulating blood against the walls of the blood vessels is consistently above normal. Hypertension is the most common cause of cardiovascular disease-related deaths among Americans. It is estimated that 116 million adult Americans have high blood pressure but only 1 in 4 adults (25%) have their high blood pressure under control. The incidence of hypertension in the United States has increased dramatically as a result of a sedentary lifestyle, and an increased incidence of obesity and diabetes.

If hypertension is not brought under control, over time it can cause severe damage to the blood vessels of vital organs, such as the heart, brain, kidneys, and eyes. This damage increases the risk of a heart attack or heart failure, stroke, aneurysm, kidney damage, and damaged vision. Early detection and treatment of high blood pressure can prevent these complications. High blood pressure is often discovered during a routine medical examination or (less commonly) when an individual experiences one of the complications of hypertension caused by damage to a vital organ.

Hypertension Categories

The 2017 ACC/AHA guidelines categorize hypertension into the following stages:

1. *Hypertension Stage 1:* Hypertension stage 1 is defined as a sustained systolic reading between 130 and 139 mmHg, *or* a sustained diastolic reading between 80 and 89 mmHg. At this stage, the provider is likely to prescribe lifestyle modifications and may consider adding blood pressure medication if the patient currently has or is at increased risk for cardiovascular disease.
2. *Hypertension Stage 2:* Hypertension stage 2 is defined as a sustained systolic reading of 140 mmHg or higher, *or* a sustained diastolic reading of 90 mmHg or higher. At this stage, the provider is likely to prescribe a combination of blood pressure medications and lifestyle modifications.

Symptoms

Hypertension is known as a "silent killer" because there are typically few or no warning signs or symptoms until the sustained increase in the blood pressure has caused significant damage to vital organs resulting in serious complications. Without regular blood pressure measurements, an individual with hypertension may go undiagnosed for many years. Symptoms that may indicate the presence of the serious complications of hypertension include one or more of the following: headaches, dizziness, flushed face, fatigue, epistaxis (nosebleed), excessive perspiration, heart palpitations, chest pain, vision problems, shortness of breath, frequent urination, and leg claudication (cramping in the legs with walking).

Primary Hypertension

In 90% to 95% of cases, the precise cause of hypertension is unknown. This type of hypertension is known *primary* or *essential hypertension.* Without treatment, primary hypertension usually worsens over time. Certain factors increase the risk of developing primary hypertension which are listed and described below.

Uncontrollable Risk Factors

- *Heredity.* A family history of high blood pressure increases an individual's risk of developing high blood pressure.
- *Ethnicity.* In the United States, African-Americans tend to develop hypertension more often than individuals of any other racial background.
- *Age.* Blood pressure normally increases as an individual grows older. For example, a healthy 6-year-old child may have a blood pressure reading of 104/68 mmHg, whereas a young, healthy adult may have a blood pressure reading of 118/78 mmHg, and it would not be unusual for a 60-year-old man to have a reading of 134/84 mm Hg. As an individual gets older, there is a loss of elasticity in the walls of the blood vessels, causing this increase in pressure to occur.
- *Gender.* A greater percentage of men (50%) have high blood pressure as compared to women (44%).

Controllable Risk Factors

- *Obesity.* Obesity is one of the biggest risk factors for hypertension, especially in younger people. This is because an increased body mass requires more blood to supply the tissues with oxygen and nutrients. This increased volume of blood circulating through the blood vessels results in an increase in the blood pressure.
- *Sodium intake.* Sodium, found in salt and many processed foods, canned foods, and snack foods, does not cause high blood pressure; however, it can aggravate high blood pressure. As sodium increases in the body, more water is retained by the body to try to balance the sodium concentration. This increases the blood volume which causes an increase in the blood pressure. Most Americans consume more sodium than they need. The current AHA recommendation is to consume no more than 2300 mg of sodium per day (equivalent to 1 teaspoon of salt) while an ideal limit is no more than 1500 mg of sodium per day (equivalent to 2/3 teaspoon of salt).
- *Lack of physical exercise.* Physical activity is important for a healthy heart and circulatory system. A sedentary lifestyle increases the chance of developing high blood pressure.
- *Chronic stress.* Research indicates that individuals under continuous stress tend to develop more heart and circulatory problems than people not under stress, which can result in an increase in the blood pressure.
- *Tobacco use:* Over time, tobacco use may damage the walls of blood vessels which can result in an increase in the blood pressure.
- *Alcohol consumption.* Heavy and regular alcohol consumption can increase blood pressure.

Treatment

Primary hypertension cannot be cured, but treatments are available to bring it under control. These include lifestyle modifications, such as weight reduction; a healthy diet such as the DASH diet (refer to Chapter 35: Nutrition), lowering sodium (salt) intake and increasing potassium intake; regular physical exercise; cessation of tobacco use; limitation or elimination of alcohol consumption; and stress management. If lifestyle modifications alone are not enough, medications are available for reducing blood pressure, allowing the patient to lead a normal, healthy, active life. Treatment for essential hypertension is usually life-long. If the patient discontinues lifestyle modifications or stops taking medication, the blood pressure will increase again.

Secondary Hypertension

While 90% to 95% of individuals with hypertension have primary hypertension, the remaining 5% to 10% of individuals have *secondary hypertension.* This means that the hypertension is secondary to another medical condition and has a known cause.

Conditions that can result in secondary hypertension include chronic kidney disease, adrenal and thyroid disorders, narrowing of the aorta, steroid therapy, oral contraceptives, diabetes, obstructive sleep apnea, and preeclampsia associated with pregnancy. Once the underlying medical condition is treated, the patient's blood pressure usually decreases or even returns to normal

HYPOTENSION

Hypotension or low blood pressure means the pressure of the circulating blood against the walls of the blood vessels is below normal. Hypotension is defined as a blood pressure reading of less than 90/60 mmHg. Hypotension can be temporary or chronic. Chronic hypotension in healthy individuals without any symptoms usually requires no treatment.

Hypotension may occur as a result of a medical condition, especially when the blood pressure drops suddenly or is accompanied by signs and symptoms such as dizziness or lightheadedness, fainting, blurred vision, nausea, fatigue, and lack of concentration. Medical conditions that cause hypotension include pregnancy, dehydration, heart conditions, endocrine disorders, moderate or severe blood loss, anaphylactic shock, and a severe infection of the bloodstream (septicemia).

Categories of Hypotension

Hypotension is divided into the following categories based upon when the blood pressure drops.

1. *Orthostatic hypotension:* Orthostatic hypotension (or postural hypotension) is a drop in blood pressure caused by a sudden change in body position. It occurs most often when an individual is sitting or lying down and then suddenly stands up. After standing up, the patient may experiences dizziness and lightheadedness which is often referred to as "seeing stars." Orthostatic hypotension occurs more often in older adults, especially those on antihypertensive medication and/or diuretics. Orthostatic hypotension can be prevented by using slow and gradual movements when standing up.
2. *Postprandial hypotension:* Postprandial hypotension is a sudden drop in blood pressure that occurs after eating. Older adults, especially those with Parkinson's disease, are more likely to develop this type of hypotension.

3. *Neurally mediated hypotension*: Neurally mediated hypotension may occur after an individual has been standing or exercising for a long period of time, causing dizziness or nausea. It is more commonly seen in children and young adults. Emotionally upsetting or scary events can also cause this type of hypotension.
4. *Severe hypotension:* Severe hypotension can occur with shock and is the most extreme form of hypotension. Shock is caused by the failure of the cardiovascular system to deliver enough blood to the body's vital organs to function properly. Shock causes the blood pressure to drop to a dangerously low level and can be life-threatening if not treated promptly. The organs most affected are the heart, brain, and lungs, which can be irreparably damaged in 4 to 6 minutes. The general signs and symptoms of severe shock are weakness, restlessness, anxiety, disorientation, pallor, cold and clammy skin, rapid breathing, and rapid pulse. If not treated, these symptoms can progress rapidly to a significant drop in the blood pressure, cyanosis, loss of consciousness, and death.

What Would You Do? | What Would You *Not* Do?

Case Study 3

Tyrone Jackson, 45 years old, is at the medical office to have his blood pressure checked. Six months ago, Tyrone started taking a diuretic and an antihypertensive drug prescribed by the physician to reduce his blood pressure. The last documentation in his medical record indicates that Tyrone's blood pressure decreased from 168/112 mmHg to 118/78 mmHg; however, his blood pressure at this visit is 138/98 mmHg. Tyrone says that he has not been very good at following the lifestyle modifications and medication plan prescribed by the physician. He says it is hard to remember to take his blood pressure pills every day. He says that he felt just fine before being put on blood pressure pills, but when he started taking them, he felt awful. He had to urinate more often; when he got up fast, he felt dizzy; and he also has some problems with headaches. Tyrone says that he decided to cut back on his medication to see if these problems got better, and sure enough, they went away altogether. ■

BLOOD PRESSURE MEASUREMENT: MANUAL METHOD

The manual method requires the medical assistant to perform the steps in the blood pressure procedure manually or by hand; this includes inflation and deflation of the cuff of the sphygmomanometer and determining the blood pressure measurement by listening to the sounds produced by the brachial artery (Korotkoff sounds). The equipment needed to measure blood pressure using the manual method includes a stethoscope and an aneroid sphygmomanometer.

Stethoscope

A **stethoscope** is a medical device that amplifies sounds produced by the body and allows a user to hear them. The stethoscope was first introduced in the 1800s by a French physician named René Laennec. This early stethoscope consisted of a simple wooden tube with a bell-shaped opening at one end.

The most common type of stethoscope used in the medical office is the acoustic stethoscope, which consists of the following parts: earpieces, eartubes, tubing, and a chest piece (Fig. 19.16A). The *earpieces* are made of a soft flexible material to provide a comfortable fit. They should fit snugly in the ear canal to provide for effective auscultation and to keep out unwanted sounds. The *eartubes* consist of metal tubes that connect the earpieces to the tubing. The eartubes are angled in a way that allows the earpieces to be directed slightly forward. This allows the earpieces to follow the direction of the ear canal to provide for maximum sound quality. The *tubing* connects the eartubes to the chest piece. The purpose of the *tubing* is to transfer sounds from the chest piece and relay them to the earpieces. The usual length of the tubing on a stethoscope is 12 to 16 inches (30 to 40 cm). This length provides convenience and ease when placing the chest piece over the brachial artery during blood pressure measurement.

Chest Piece

There are two types of chest pieces: a *diaphragm*, which is a large, flat disc, and a *bell*, which has a bowl-shaped appearance and is surrounded by a rubber ring (see Fig. 19.16B). Most health care workers prefer a two-sided chest piece with a diaphragm on one side and a bell on the other side.

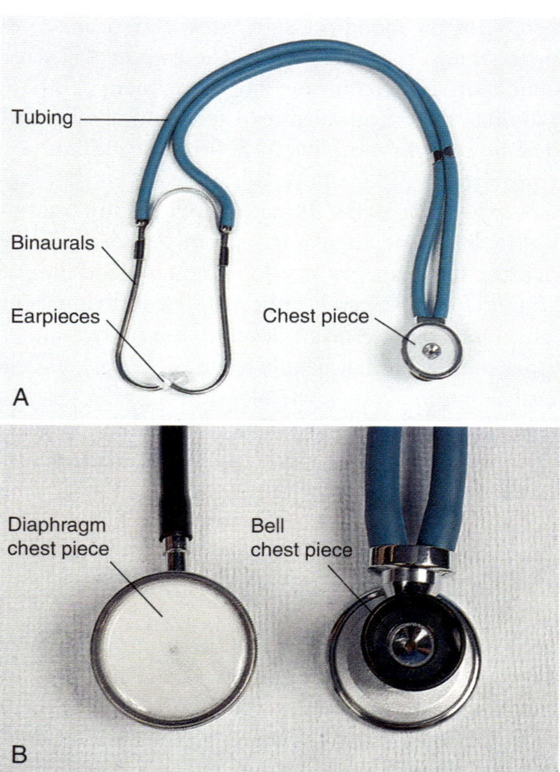

Fig. 19.16 (A) The parts of a stethoscope. (B) Types of chest pieces.

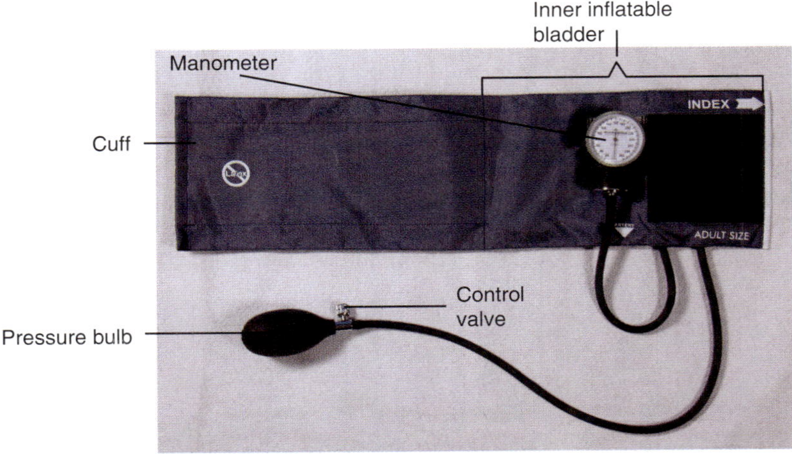

Fig. 19.17 The parts of an aneroid sphygmomanometer.

When using a two-sided chest piece, the medical assistant must ensure that the desired side is rotated into its proper position before use. Failure to do so prevent the medical assistant from hearing sounds through the earpieces.

The diaphragm chest piece is more useful for hearing medium to high-pitched sounds, such as lung and bowel sounds, whereas the bell chest piece is more useful for hearing low-pitched sounds, such as those produced by the heart and vascular system. Studies have shown that the diaphragm and bell provide similar results when measuring blood pressure and therefore, either one can be used for the reliable measurement of blood pressure. Because the diaphragm is easier to hold firmly in place on the patient's arm and covers a larger area, most health care workers use the diaphragm for measuring blood pressure. However, if the medical assistant is having difficulty hearing sounds from the diaphragm when measuring blood pressure, the medical assistant should switch to the bell.

Care and Maintenance

Stethoscopes must be cared for properly to ensure proper functioning and to prevent the transmission of pathogens in the medical office. The earpieces should be removed and cleaned regularly with a cotton-tipped applicator moistened with alcohol to remove cerumen. The chest piece should be cleaned with an antiseptic wipe to remove dirt, dust, lint, and oils. The tubing should be cleaned with a paper towel using an antimicrobial soap and water. Alcohol should not be used to clean the tubing because it can dry out the tubing and cause it to crack over time.

Aneroid Sphygmomanometer

A sphygmomanometer is a device that measures the pressure of blood within an artery. An aneroid sphygmomanometer consists of a **manometer** (for registering pressure), an inner inflatable bladder surrounded by a covering known as the *cuff*, and a pressure bulb with a control valve to inflate and deflate the inner bladder (Fig. 19.17). The manometer consists of a gauge with a round scale which is calibrated in millimeters

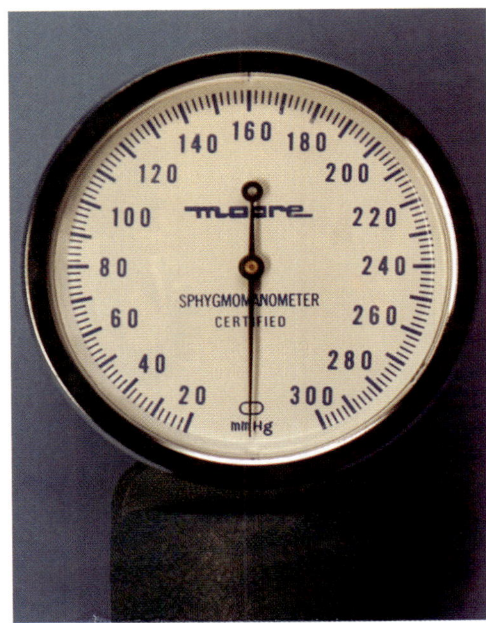

Fig. 19.18 The scale of the gauge of an aneroid sphygmomanometer.

with a needle that points to the calibrations (Fig. 19.18). To ensure an accurate reading, the needle must be positioned initially at zero. At least once a year an aneroid sphygmomanometer should be recalibrated to ensure its accuracy.

Aneroid sphygmomanometers are available in three different designs:

- Portable aneroid sphygmomanometer (see Fig. 19.17)
- Wall-mounted aneroid sphygmomanometer (Fig. 19.19A)
- Mobile floor-stand aneroid sphygmomanometer (see Fig. 19.19B)

Cuff Sizes

Blood pressure cuffs for adults come in a variety of sizes, which include *small adult*, *adult*, *large adult* and *adult thigh* (Fig. 19.20). The adult cuff is typically used for the average-sized adult arm while a small adult cuff is used for

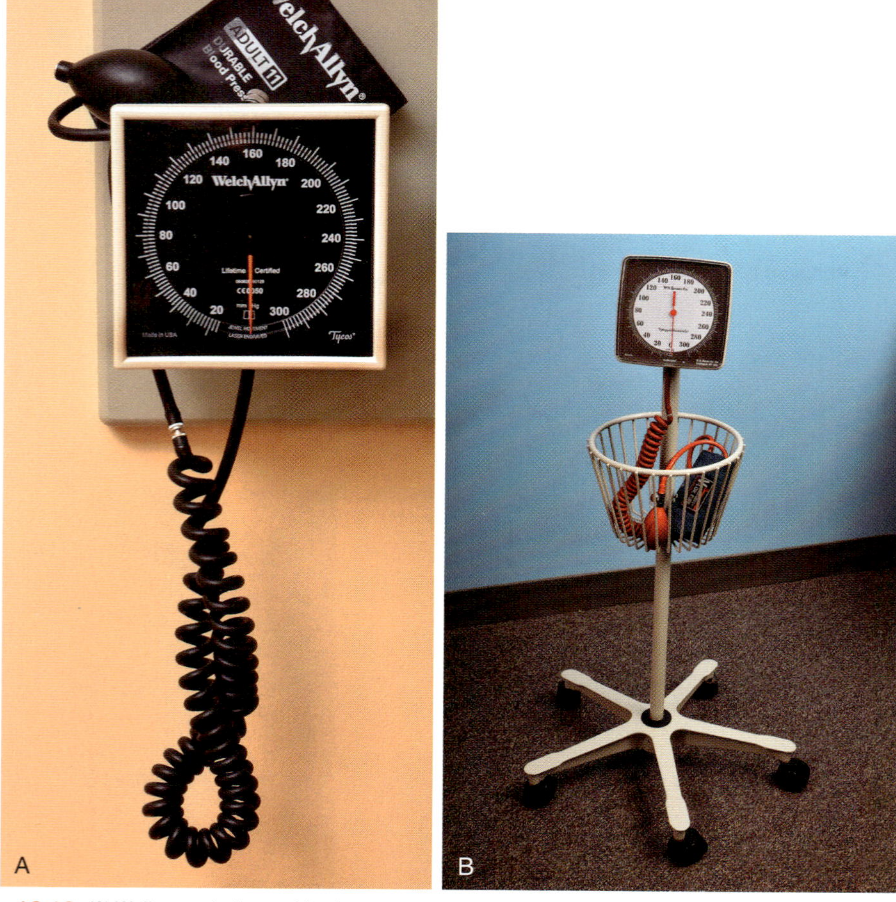

Fig. 19.19 (A) Wall-mounted aneroid sphygmomanometer. (B) Mobile floor-stand aneroid sphygmomanometer. (A, Courtesy of Holzer Health Systems, Athens, OH.)

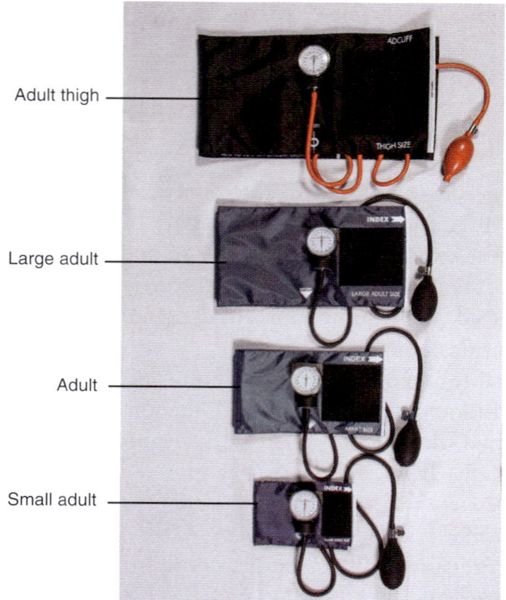

Fig. 19.20 Blood pressure cuffs: small adult, adult, large adult, and adult thigh.

adults with thin arms. The adult thigh cuff is used for taking blood pressure from the thigh or for adults with large arms.

It is essential that the correct cuff size be used to measure blood pressure. If the cuff is too small, the reading may be falsely high, as it would be, for example, when an adult cuff is used on a patient with a large arm. If the cuff is too large, the reading may be falsely low, as it would be when an adult cuff is used on a patient with a thin arm. Prevention of errors is of upmost importance when measuring blood pressure (Box 19.3). Not using the correct cuff size is the most common error made in blood pressure measurement.

In obese patients with an arm circumference greater than 52 cm (20 inches), it may not be possible to fit even an adult thigh cuff around the patient's arm. In this situation the AHA states that the patient's blood pressure can be measured using the forearm and radial artery; however, the AHA further states that this method may result in a falsely high systolic reading. When this method is used, an appropriate-sized cuff should be positioned midway between the elbow and the wrist, with the center of the bladder positioned over the radial pulse. The medical assistant should then place the chest piece of the stethoscope over the radial

BOX 19.3 Prevention of Errors in Blood Pressure Measurement

The following guidelines should be followed to prevent errors in blood pressure measurement:

1. *Instruct the patient* not to consume caffeine or alcohol, use tobacco, or exercise for 30 minutes before blood pressure measurement to prevent a falsely high blood pressure reading.
2. *The patient should be comfortably seated* in a quiet room for at least 5 minutes before blood pressure is taken. Patient anxiety and apprehension caused by being in a medical office setting can temporarily increase the blood pressure reading by as much as 30 mmHg. This is known as the "white coat effect," which refers to the white lab coat worn by the provider.
3. *Position the patient properly.* The patient should be seated in a chair with back support with the legs uncrossed (at the knees) and both feet flat on the floor. If the back is not supported (such as when a patient is seated on an examining table), the diastolic reading can be increased by as much as 6 mmHg. Crossing the legs at the knees can increase the systolic reading by 2 to 8 mmHg. The arm should be positioned at heart level and well supported on a flat surface with the palm facing upward. If the arm is above heart level, the blood pressure reading may be falsely low. If the arm is not supported or is placed below heart level, the blood pressure reading may be falsely high.
4. *Never take blood pressure over clothing.* Taking blood pressure over clothing could result in an inaccurate reading. The patient's sleeve should be rolled up approximately 5 inches above the elbow so that the cuff can be applied to bare skin. If the sleeve is too tight after being rolled up, the arm should be removed from the sleeve. A tight sleeve creates a tourniquet-like effect which causes partial compression of the brachial artery, resulting in a falsely low reading.
5. *Always use the correct cuff size.* Incorrect cuff size is the most common cause of an inaccurate blood pressure measurement. If the cuff is too small, it may come loose as the cuff is inflated, or the reading may be falsely high. If the cuff is too large, the reading may be falsely low.
6.* *Correctly position the cuff.* The center of the inner bladder should be positioned directly above the brachial pulse site with the lower edge of the cuff approximately 1 to 2 inches (2.5 to 5 cm) above the bend in the elbow. Most cuffs are labeled with arrows indicating the center of the bladder for the right and left arms. Centering the inner bladder above the pulse site allows for complete compression of the brachial artery. The cuff should be placed high enough above the bend in the elbow to prevent the diaphragm of the stethoscope from touching it; otherwise, extraneous sounds may be picked up which could interfere with an accurate measurement.
7. *Wrap the cuff snugly around the patient's arm.* The cuff should be snug but not too tight. To assess the appropriate tightness of the cuff, one finger should slip easily under the cuff.
8.* *Position the earpieces so that the sounds can be heard clearly.* The earpieces of the stethoscope should be positioned in the ears with the earpieces directed slightly forward. This allows the earpieces to follow the direction of the ear canal, which facilitates hearing.
9.* *Position the chest piece properly.* The chest piece should be placed firmly, but gently, over the brachial pulse site to assist in transmission of clear and audible sounds. The chest piece should not be allowed to touch the cuff, to prevent extraneous sounds from being picked up, which could interfere with an accurate measurement.
10.* *Rapidly inflate the cuff.* The cuff should be rapidly inflated to a level that is approximately 30 mmHg above the previously measured or palpated systolic pressure. Overinflation of the cuff may result which is uncomfortable for the patient and could result in a falsely high blood pressure reading.
11.* *Release the pressure at a moderate steady rate.* The pressure in the cuff should be released at a rate of 2 to 3 mmHg per second to ensure an accurate blood pressure measurement. Releasing the pressure too slowly is uncomfortable for the patient and could cause a falsely high diastolic reading. Releasing the pressure too quickly could cause a falsely low systolic reading.
12. *Wait before taking blood pressure again.* The medical assistant should wait 1 to 2 minutes before taking blood pressure again in the same arm to allow the blood flow in the brachial artery to return to normal to ensure an accurate reading.
13. *Measure and document the blood pressure in both arms during the initial blood pressure assessment of a new patient.* There may normally be a small difference in blood pressure between the two arms. During return visits, the blood pressure should be measured in the arm with the higher initial reading.

*Applies only to the manual method of measuring blood pressure. (The absence of an asterisk applies to both the manual and automatic methods of measuring blood pressure.)

pulse and should measure the patient's blood pressure using the same technique presented in Procedure 19.9.

Determination of Correct Cuff Size

There are several ways to determine the correct cuff size of a patient to ensure an accurate blood pressure measurement.

1. **Assessment of bladder length and width:** For accurate blood pressure measurement, the cuff size should have an inner bladder length that encircles at least 80% (but not more than 100%) of the arm circumference and a bladder width that is at least 40% of the arm circumference (Fig. 19.21).
2. **Determination of upper mid-arm circumference:** The correct cuff size can be determined based on the circumference of the upper mid-arm which is located midway between the shoulder and elbow (Fig. 19.22A). The circumference of the upper mid-arm should be measured with a flexible centimeter tape measure wrapped evenly around the arm (Fig. 19.22B). The measurement is then compared to a table outlining the cuff sizes and the mid-arm circumference range of each (Table 19.7).
3. **Assessment of Range and Index Lines:** Most blood pressure cuffs are marked with two *range lines* (Fig. 19.23A) and an *index line* located at the end of the

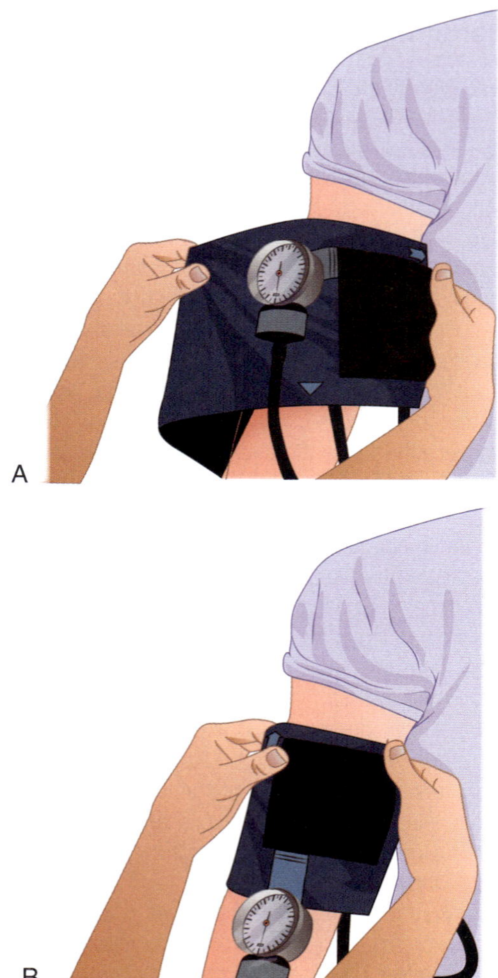

Fig. 19.21 Determination of cuff size using bladder length and width. (A) The inner bladder length should encircle at least 80% of the arm circumference. (B) The bladder width should be at least 40% of the arm circumference.

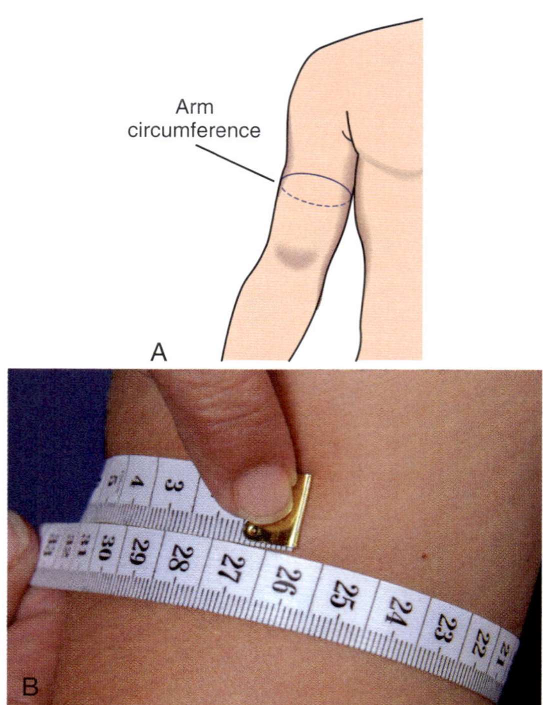

Fig. 19.22 Determination of cuff size using upper mid-arm circumference. (A) Upper mid-arm circumference is located midway between the shoulder and elbow. (B) Upper mid-arm circumference is measured with a centimeter tape measure. The mid-arm circumference of this patient is 25.5 cm which means a small adult BP cuff is required.

Table 19.7 Recommended Cuff Size for Adults

Upper Mid-Arm Circumference Range (cm)	Cuff Size
22 to 26 cm	Small adult
27 to 34 cm	Adult
35 to 44 cm	Large adult
45 to 52 cm	Adult thigh

cuff. When the correct-sized cuff is applied to the patient's arm, the *index line* should fall between the two range lines (see Fig. 19.23B). If the index line does not fall within the range lines, the cuff is not a correct fit for that patient and a larger or a smaller cuff must be used.

Korotkoff Sounds

Korotkoff sounds are used to determine systolic and diastolic blood pressure readings. When the bladder of the cuff is inflated, the brachial artery is compressed so that no audible sounds are heard through the stethoscope. As the cuff is deflated, the sounds become audible until the blood flows freely, at which point the sounds can no longer be heard (Table 19.8). The first clear tapping sound (Phase I) represents the systolic pressure and the point at which the sounds disappear (Phase V) represents the diastolic pressure. The medical assistant should practice listening to these sounds and should be able to identify the various Korotkoff phases.

Procedure 19.9 outlines the procedure for taking blood pressure using an aneroid sphygmomanometer. Procedure 19.10 outlines the procedure for determining systolic pressure by palpation.

BLOOD PRESSURE MEASUREMENT: AUTOMATIC METHOD

Automatic blood pressure monitors are increasingly being used in medical offices to measure blood pressure. The steps in the procedure are performed automatically by the monitor (Procedure 19.11). The equipment for measuring blood pressure using the automatic method includes an automatic blood pressure monitor (also known as a digital sphygmomanometer). Automatic monitors are especially popular for the home monitoring of blood pressure.

Automatic monitors use an electronic pressure sensor to measure oscillations from the wall of the brachial artery as the cuff gradually deflates. An oscillation is a back-and-forth movement that occurs in the brachial artery as the pulse wave travels through it. The point of maximum oscillation corresponds to the mean arterial pressure, which is an overall

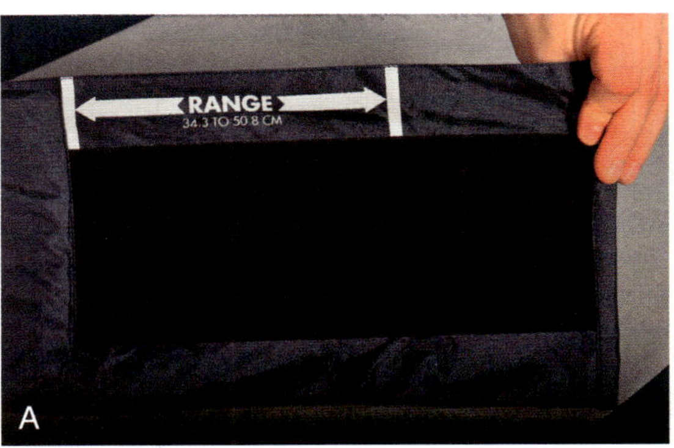

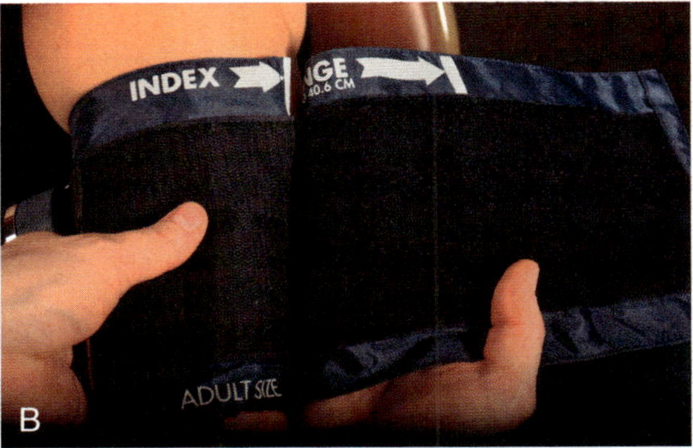

Fig. 19.23 Determination of cuff size using the range and index lines. (A) Range lines on a blood pressure cuff. (B) The index line falls within the range lines, indicating this is the proper-sized cuff for this patient.

index of an individual's blood pressure. A computer in the monitor then uses this information to calculate the systolic blood pressure and the diastolic blood pressure. Results are then digitally displayed on an LED screen. The automatic blood pressure procedure takes approximately 30 seconds to complete from start to finish.

Automatic blood pressure monitors are available in the following designs:

- Portable automatic monitor (Fig. 19.24A)
- Mobile floor-stand automatic monitor (see Fig. 19.24B)

The medical assistant should closely follow the manufacturer's instructions for the particular brand and model of

Table 19.8 Korotkoff Sounds

Phase	Description	Illustration
	Inflation of cuff compresses and closes off brachial artery so that no blood flows through the artery.	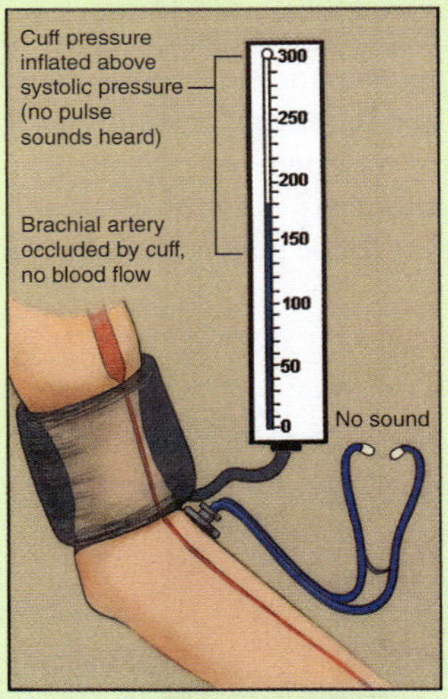 Cuff pressure inflated above systolic pressure (no pulse sounds heard) Brachial artery occluded by cuff, no blood flow 300, 250, 200, 150, 100, 50, 0 No sound
Phase I	First faint but clear tapping sound is heard, and it gradually increases in intensity. First clear tapping sound is documented as the systolic pressure.	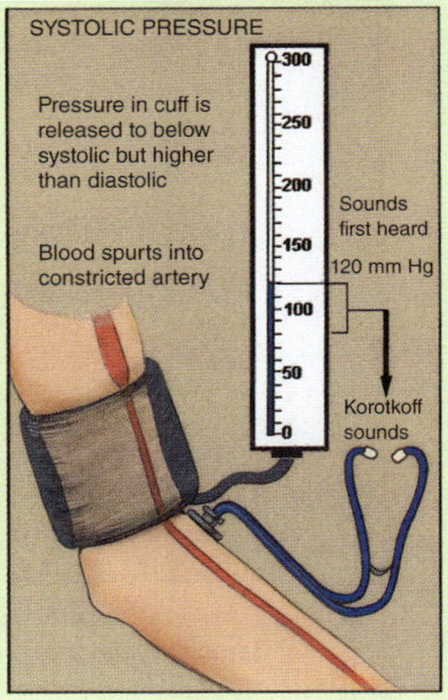 SYSTOLIC PRESSURE Pressure in cuff is released to below systolic but higher than diastolic Blood spurts into constricted artery 300, 250, 200, 150, 100, 50, 0 Sounds first heard 120 mm Hg Korotkoff sounds

Continued

Table 19.8 Korotkoff Sounds—cont'd

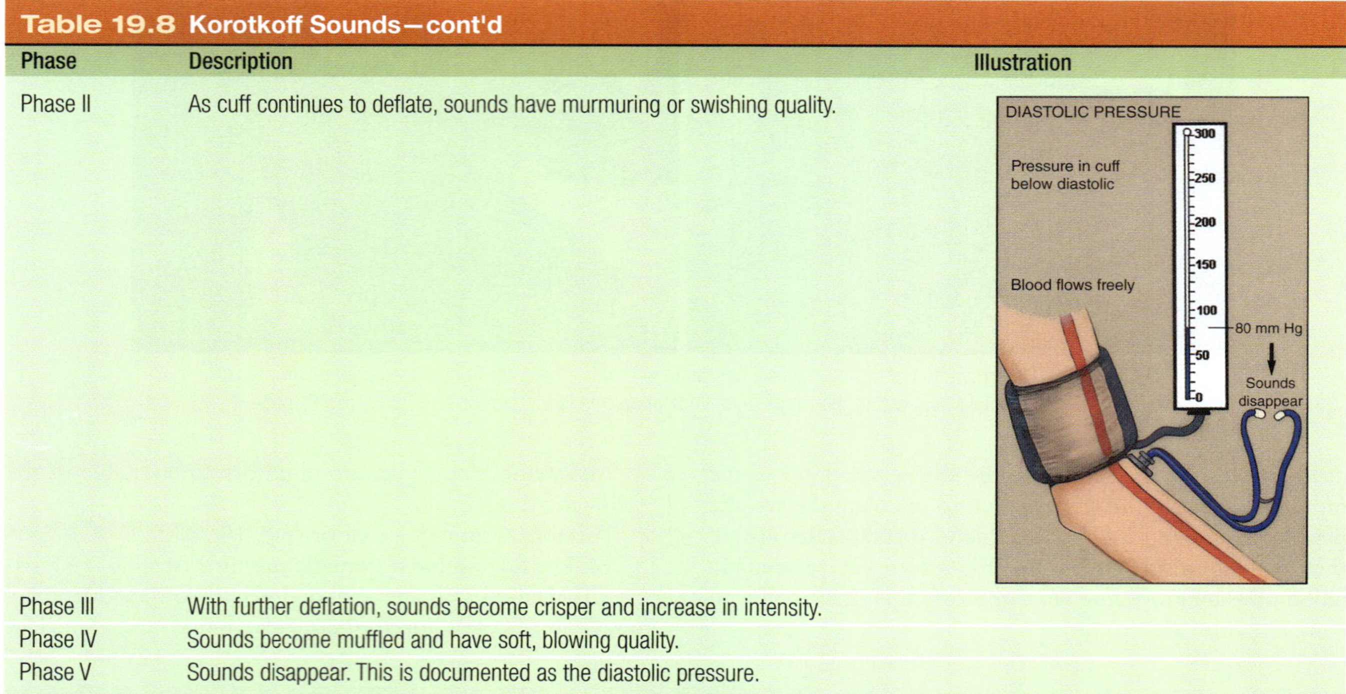

Phase	Description	Illustration
Phase II	As cuff continues to deflate, sounds have murmuring or swishing quality.	
Phase III	With further deflation, sounds become crisper and increase in intensity.	
Phase IV	Sounds become muffled and have soft, blowing quality.	
Phase V	Sounds disappear. This is documented as the diastolic pressure.	

automatic monitor used; these instructions are outlined in the user manual that accompanies the monitor. Many of the guidelines for the accurate measurement of blood pressure using the automatic method are the same as those for the manual measurement of blood pressure (see Box 19.3). The automatic monitor should be calibrated periodically according to the manufacturer's recommendations. Automatic monitors offer certain advantages and disadvantages, described as follows.

Advantages

1. The cuff does not have to be manually inflated and deflated because this function is performed automatically by the monitor.

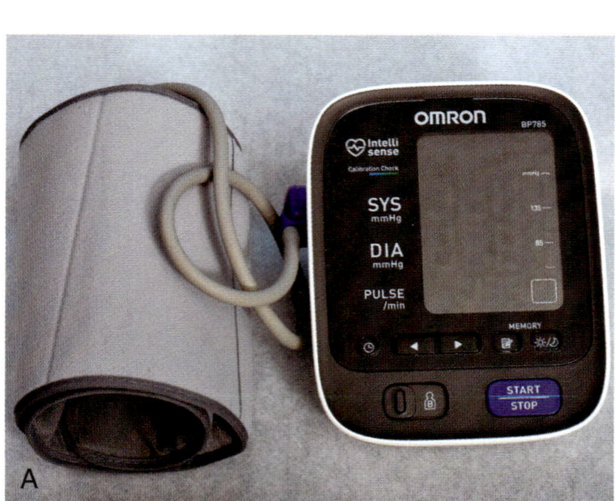

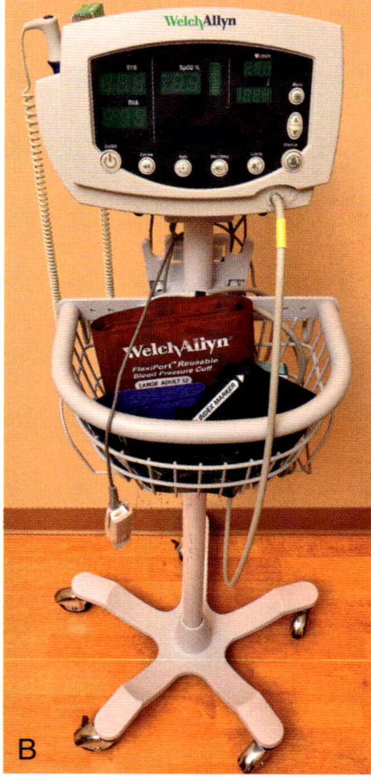

Fig. 19.24 Automatic blood pressure monitors. (A) Portable automatic monitor. (B) Mobile floor-stand automatic monitor (also includes an electronic thermometer and pulse oximeter). (B, Courtesy of Holzer Health Systems, Athens, OH.)

2. A stethoscope and user listening skills are not required to obtain the reading because the electronic pressure sensor in the automatic monitor measures oscillations from the wall of the brachial artery to obtain the reading.
3. Automatic monitors are less susceptible to external environmental noise than are manual monitors.
4. The blood pressure measurement is easy to read because the systolic and diastolic readings are shown on a display screen as a digital readout.
5. Most automatic monitors allow multiple readings to be taken during the measurement procedure. The monitor automatically calculates averages of these values and displays them on the screen of the monitor.
6. Automatic monitors measure the pulse rate, which is displayed on the screen along with the blood pressure measurement.
7. Most automatic monitors come equipped with an internal memory for storing multiple blood pressure measurements.

Disadvantages

1. There are certain conditions that may result in an inaccurate reading with an automatic blood pressure monitor. These include preeclampsia, dysrhythmias (such as atrial fibrillation), arteriosclerosis, and a very weak pulse. If any of these conditions are present, an alternative method of blood pressure measurement should be used.
2. Because the monitor relies on brachial artery oscillations to obtain a reading, stiff arteries (especially in older patients) can interfere with obtaining an accurate reading.
3. Automatic monitors designed for use in a medical office setting are more expensive than manual monitors.

What Would You Do? What Would You *Not* Do? RESPONSES

Case Study 1
Page 357

What Did Sergio Do?
- ❑ Told Mrs. Mason that sometimes ear thermometers can be a little tricky to use.
- ❑ Showed Mrs. Mason how to use the ear thermometer and let her practice by taking Olivia's temperature.
- ❑ Explained how to care for and maintain the ear thermometer to prevent inaccurate readings.

What Did Sergio Not Do?
- ❑ Did not ask Mrs. Mason if she had read the directions that came with her ear thermometer.
- ❑ Did not ask Mrs. Mason why she waited so long to bring Olivia to the office.

Case Study 2
Page 361

What Did Sergio Do?
- ❑ Recognized and congratulated Alex on his swimming achievements.
- ❑ Told Alex that it is normal for his pulse to be that slow because of his athletic training and it shows that he is in good shape.
- ❑ Assured Alex that the physician will do everything she can to help Alex.
- ❑ Stressed to Alex how important it is to follow the physician's advice so that his shoulder heals as soon as possible.

What Did Sergio Not Do?
- ❑ Did not comment on Alex's request for a steroid injection or pain pills. Made sure to document the information so that the physician could handle the situation.
- ❑ Did not criticize Alex for putting a swim meet before his health.

Case Study 3
Page 370

What Did Sergio Do?
- ❑ Empathized with Tyrone about having to remember to take his medication. Suggested that he get a daily pill container to help him remember.
- ❑ Stressed to Tyrone the importance of following his lifestyle modifications and taking his blood pressure medication. Explained to him that high blood pressure is a "silent disease." He may feel fine, but damage to his body organs can still be taking place if he does not follow his treatment plan.
- ❑ Gave Tyrone a brochure about high blood pressure and went over the long-term effects of hypertension and lifestyle modifications that could help lower blood pressure.
- ❑ Encouraged Tyrone to call the office when he experiences side effects from medications because the physician may be able to do something to help.

What Did Sergio Not Do?
- ❑ Did not minimize the importance of following his treatment plan.

TERMINOLOGY REVIEW

Key Term	Word Parts	Definition
Adventitious sounds		Abnormal breath sounds.
Afebrile	*a-:* without	Without fever; the body temperature is normal.
Alveoli	*alveol/o:* air sac	Thin-walled air sacs of the lungs in which the exchange of oxygen and carbon dioxide takes place.
Antecubital space	*ante-:* before cubitum: elbow	The space located at the front of the elbow.

Continued

TERMINOLOGY REVIEW—cont'd

Key Term	Word Parts	Definition
Antipyretic	*anti-:* against *pyr/o:* fever *-ic:* pertaining to	An agent that reduces fever.
Aorta		The major trunk of the arterial system of the body. The aorta arises from the upper surface of the left ventricle.
Apnea	*a-:* without or absence of *-pnea:* breathing	The temporary cessation of breathing.
Axilla		The area under the shoulder or armpit.
Blood pressure		The pressure or force exerted by the circulating blood on the walls of the arteries.
Bounding pulse		A pulse with an increased volume that feels very strong and full.
Bradycardia	brady-: slow cardi/o: heart *-ia:* condition of diseased or abnormal state	An abnormally slow heart rate (less than 60 beats per minute).
Bradypnea	brady-: slow *-pnea:* breathing	An abnormal decrease in the respiratory rate of less than 12 respirations per minute.
Celsius scale		A temperature scale in which the freezing point of water is 0° and the boiling point of water is 100°; also called the *centigrade scale.*
Conduction		The transfer of energy, such as heat, from one object to another by direct contact.
Convection		The transfer of energy, such as heat, through air currents.
Crisis		A sudden falling of an elevated body temperature to normal.
Cross-contamination		The process by which microorganisms are unintentionally transferred from one person, object, or place to another.
Cyanosis	cyan/o: blue *-osis:* abnormal condition	A bluish discoloration of the skin and mucous membranes.
Diastole		The phase in the cardiac cycle in which the heart relaxes between contractions.
Diastolic pressure		The point of lesser pressure on the arterial wall, which is recorded during diastole.
Dyspnea	*dys-:* difficult, painful, abnormal *-pnea:* breathing	Shortness of breath or difficulty in breathing.
Dysrhythmia	*dys-:* difficult, painful, abnormal rhythm: rhythm *-ia:* condition of diseased or abnormal state	An irregular rhythm; also termed *arrhythmia.*
Eupnea	*eu-:* normal, good *-pnea:* breathing	Normal respiration. The rate is 12 to 20 respirations per minute, the rhythm is even and regular, and the depth is normal.
Exhalation	*-ex:* outside, outward	The act of breathing out.
Fahrenheit scale		A temperature scale in which the freezing point of water is 32° and the boiling point of water is 212°.
Febrile		Pertaining to fever.
Fever		A body temperature that is above normal; synonym for *pyrexia.*
Frenulum linguae		The midline fold that connects the undersurface of the tongue with the floor of the mouth.
Hyperpnea	*hyper-:* above, excessive *-pnea:* breathing	An abnormal increase in the rate and depth of respirations.
Hyperpyrexia	*hyper-:* above, excessive *pyr/o:* fever *-ia:* condition of diseased or abnormal state	An extremely high fever.
Hypertension	*hyper-:* above, excessive *-tension:* pressure	The force of the circulating blood against the walls of the blood vessels is consistently above normal.
Hyperventilation	*hyper-:* above, excessive	An abnormally fast and deep type of breathing, usually associated with acute anxiety conditions.

TERMINOLOGY REVIEW—cont'd

Key Term	Word Parts	Definition
Hypopnea	*hypo-:* below, deficient *-pnea:* breathing	An abnormal decrease in the rate and depth of respirations.
Hypotension	*hypo-:* below, deficient *tension:* pressure	The pressure of the circulating blood against the walls of the blood vessels is below normal.
Hypothermia	*hypo-:* below, deficient therm/o: heat *-ia:* condition of diseased or abnormal state	A body temperature that is below normal.
Hypoxemia	*hypo-:* below, deficient *ox/i:* oxygen *-emia:* blood condition	A decrease in the oxygen saturation of the blood. Hypoxemia may lead to hypoxia.
Hypoxia	*hypo-:* below, deficient *ox/i:* oxygen *-ia:* condition of diseased or abnormal state	A reduction in the oxygen supply to the tissues of the body.
Inhalation	*in-:* in, into	The act of breathing in.
Intercostal	*inter-:* between cost/o: rib *-al:* pertaining to	Between the ribs.
Korotkoff sounds		Sounds heard during the measurement of blood pressure that are used to determine the systolic and diastolic blood pressure readings.
Malaise	*-mal:* bad	A vague sense of body discomfort, weakness, and fatigue that often marks the onset of a disease and continues through the course of the illness.
Manometer	*-meter:* instrument used to measure	An instrument for measuring pressure.
Orthopnea	*orth/o:* straight *-pnea:* breathing	The condition in which breathing is easier when an individual is in a sitting or standing position.
Pulse oximeter	*ox/i:* oxygen *-meter:* instrument used to measure	A device used to measure the oxygen saturation of arterial blood.
Pulse oximetry	*ox/i:* oxygen *-metry:* measurement	The use of a pulse oximeter to measure the oxygen saturation of arterial blood.
Pulse pressure		The difference between the systolic and diastolic pressures.
Pulse rhythm		The time interval between heartbeats.
Pulse rate		The number of times the heart beats in one minute; also known as heart rate.
Pulse volume		The strength of the heartbeat.
Radiation		The transfer of energy, such as heat, in the form of waves.
SaO_2 (saturation of arterial oxygen)		Abbreviation for the percentage of hemoglobin that is saturated with oxygen in arterial blood.
Sphygmomanometer	sphygm/o: pulse *-meter:* instrument used to measure	A device that measures the pressure of blood within an artery.
SpO_2 (saturation of peripheral oxygen)		Abbreviation for the percentage of hemoglobin that is saturated with oxygen in arterial blood as measured by a pulse oximeter.
Stethoscope	*steth/o:* chest *-scope:* to view, to examine	An instrument used for amplifying and hearing sounds produced by the body.
Systole		The phase in the cardiac cycle in which the ventricles contract, sending blood out of the heart and into the aorta and pulmonary trunk.
Systolic pressure		The point of maximum pressure on the arterial walls, which is recorded during systole.
Tachycardia	*tachy-:* fast, rapid cardi/o: heart *-ia:* condition of diseased or abnormal state	An abnormally fast heart rate (more than 100 beats per minute).
Tachypnea	tachy-: fast *-pnea:* breathing	An abnormal increase in the respiratory rate of more than 20 respirations per minute.
Thready pulse		A pulse with a decreased volume that feels weak and thin.

PROCEDURE 19.1 Measuring Oral Body Temperature—Electronic Thermometer

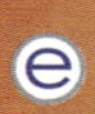

Outcome Measure oral body temperature.

Equipment/Supplies

- Electronic thermometer
- Oral probe (blue collar)
- Plastic probe cover
- Waste container

1. **Procedural Step.** Sanitize your hands and assemble the equipment.
2. **Procedural Step.** Remove the thermometer unit from its storage base and attach the oral (blue collar) probe to it. This is accomplished by inserting the latching plug (at the end of the coiled cord of the oral probe) to the plug receptacle on the thermometer unit until it clicks into place. Insert the probe into the face of the thermometer.
   Principle. The oral probe is color-coded with a blue collar for ease in identifying it.

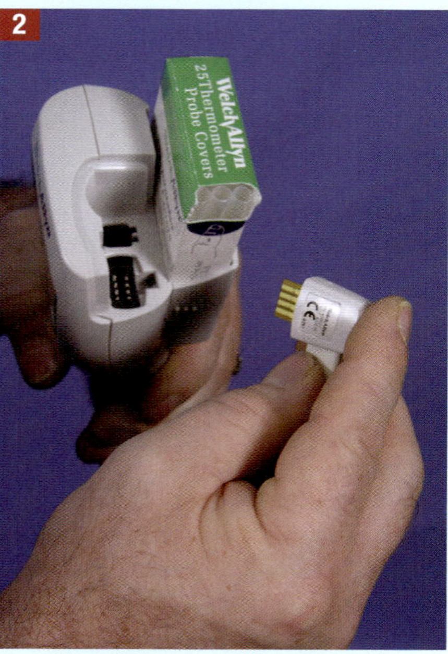

Attach the oral probe to the thermometer.

3. **Procedural Step.** Greet the patient and introduce yourself. Identify the patient and explain the procedure. If the patient has recently ingested hot or cold food or beverages or has been smoking, you must wait 15 to 30 minutes before taking the temperature.
   Principle. Ingestion of hot or cold food or beverages and smoking change the temperature of the mouth, which could result in an inaccurate reading.
4. **Procedural Step.** Grasp the probe by the collar and remove it from the face of the thermometer. Slide the probe into a disposable plastic probe cover until it locks into place.
   Principle. Removing the probe from the thermometer automatically turns on the thermometer. The probe cover prevents the transfer of microorganisms from one patient to another.

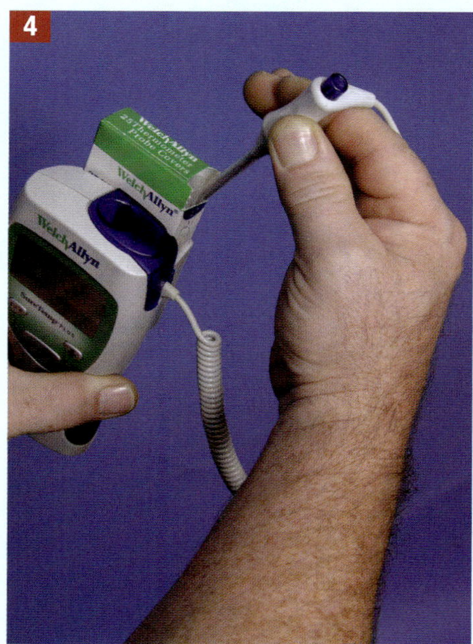

Slide the probe into a probe cover.

5. **Procedural Step.** Take the patient's temperature by inserting the probe under the patient's tongue in the pocket located on either side of the frenulum linguae. Instruct the patient to keep the mouth closed.
   Principle. There is a good blood supply in the tissue under the tongue. The mouth must be kept closed to prevent cooler air from entering and affecting the temperature reading.

PROCEDURE 19.1 Measuring Oral Body Temperature—Electronic Thermometer—cont'd

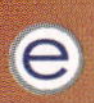

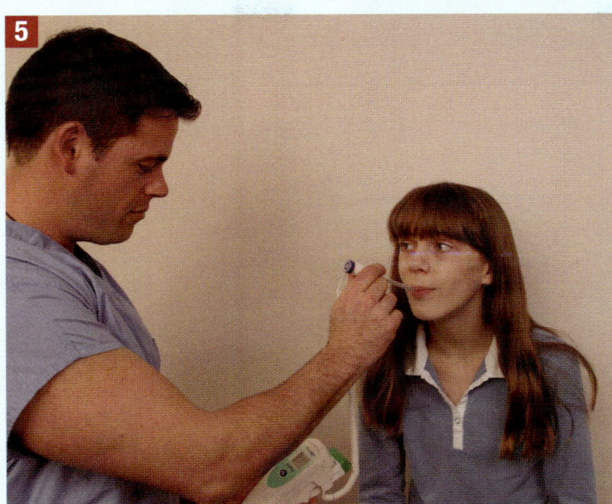

Insert the probe under the patient's tongue.

6. Procedural Step. Hold the probe in place until you hear the tone. At that time, the patient's temperature appears as a digital display on the screen of the thermometer. Make a mental note of the temperature reading. (The temperature indicated on this thermometer is 98.5°F [36.9°C].)

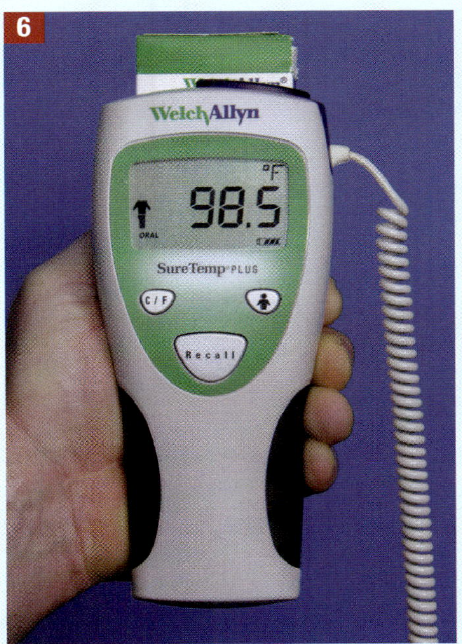

The temperature appears as a digital display on the screen of the thermometer.

7. Procedural Step. Remove the probe from the patient's mouth. Discard the probe cover by firmly pressing the ejection button while holding the probe over a regular waste container. Do not allow your fingers to come in contact with the probe cover.

Principle. The probe cover should not be touched, to prevent the transfer of microorganisms from the patient to the medical assistant. Saliva is not considered regulated medical waste; the probe can be discarded in a regular waste container.

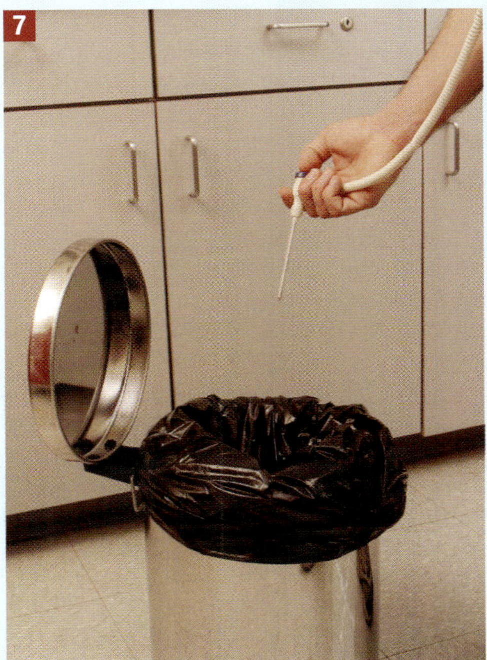

Discard the probe cover by pressing the ejection button.

8. Procedural Step. Return the probe to its stored position in the thermometer unit. Return the thermometer unit to its storage base.

Principle. Returning the probe to the unit automatically turns off and resets the thermometer.

9. Procedural Step. Sanitize your hands.

10. Procedural Step. Document the results in the patient's medical record.

a. *Electronic health record:* In SimChart for the Medical Office, document the temperature reading and site using textboxes, drop-down menus, and/or radio buttons. The temperature can be documented in either Fahrenheit or Celsius, and the software will convert the temperature so that both are displayed (refer to the SimChart example).

Continued

PROCEDURE 19.1

PROCEDURE 19.1 Measuring Oral Body Temperature—Electronic Thermometer—cont'd

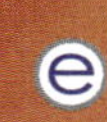

10a

EHR DOCUMENTATION EXAMPLE

Add Vital Signs

Temperature
- Fahrenheit: 98.5 — Site: Oral (-Select-, Forehead, Oral, Rectal, Tympanic)
- Celsius: 36.9

Pulse
- Pulse: — Site: -Select-

Respiration
- Respiration:

Blood Pressure
- Systolic: — Site: -Select-
- Diastolic: — Mode: -Select-
- Position: -Select-

Oxygenation
- Saturation %: — Site: -Select-

Oxygen Delivery: Room Air / Oxygen in Use (Amount in L/min)

b. *Paper-based patient record:* Document the date, the time, and the temperature reading.

Principle. Patient data must be documented properly to aid the provider in the diagnosis and to provide future reference.

10b

DOCUMENTATION EXAMPLE

Date	
10/15/XX	2:15 p.m. T: 98.5° F. ——S. Martinez, RMA

PROCEDURE 19.2 Measuring Axillary Body Temperature—Electronic Thermometer

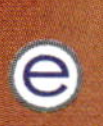

Outcome Measure axillary body temperature. Note: Many of the principles for taking a temperature already have been stated and are not included in this procedure.

Equipment/Supplies

- Electronic thermometer
- Oral probe (blue collar)
- Plastic probe cover
- Waste container

1. **Procedural Step.** Sanitize your hands and assemble the equipment.
2. **Procedural Step.** Remove the thermometer unit from its storage base and attach the oral (blue collar) probe to it. This is accomplished by inserting the latching plug (on the end of the coiled cord of the oral probe) to the plug receptacle on the thermometer unit until it locks into place. Insert the probe into the face of the thermometer.
3. **Procedural Step.** Greet the patient and introduce yourself. Identify the patient and explain the procedure.
4. **Procedural Step.** Remove clothing from the patient's shoulder and arm. Ensure that the axilla is dry. If it is wet, pat it dry with a paper towel or a gauze pad.

PROCEDURE 19.2 Measuring Axillary Body Temperature—Electronic Thermometer—cont'd

Principle. Clothing removal provides optimal exposure of the axilla for proper placement of the thermometer. Rubbing the axilla causes an increase in the temperature in that area owing to friction, resulting in an inaccurate temperature reading.

5. **Procedural Step.** Grasp the probe by the collar and remove it from the face of the thermometer. Slide the probe into a disposable probe cover until it locks into place.
6. **Procedural Step.** Take the patient's temperature by placing the probe in the center of the patient's axilla. Instruct the patient to hold the arm close to the body. Hold the arm in place for small children and other patients who cannot maintain the position themselves.
   Principle. Interference from outside air currents is reduced when the arm is held in the proper position.

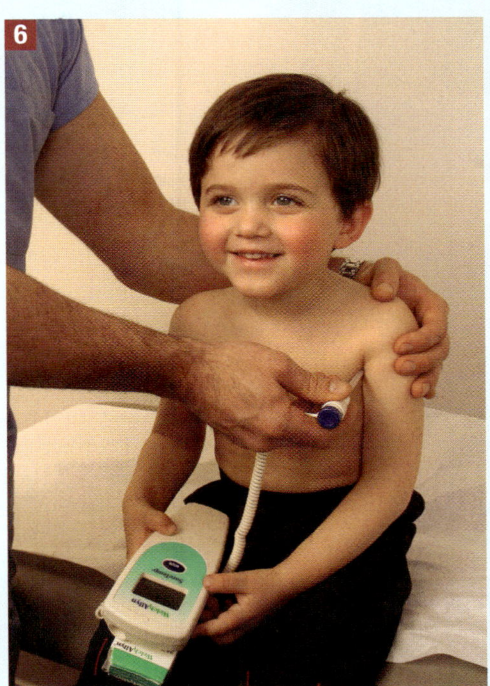

Place the probe in the center of the patient's axilla.

7. **Procedural Step.** Hold the probe in place until you hear the tone. At that time, the patient's temperature appears as a digital display on the screen of the thermometer. Make a mental note of the temperature reading.
8. **Procedural Step.** Remove the probe from the patient's axilla. Discard the probe cover by firmly pressing the ejection button while holding the probe over a regular waste container. Do not allow your fingers to come in contact with the probe cover.
9. **Procedural Step.** Return the probe to its stored position in the thermometer unit. Return the thermometer unit to its storage base.

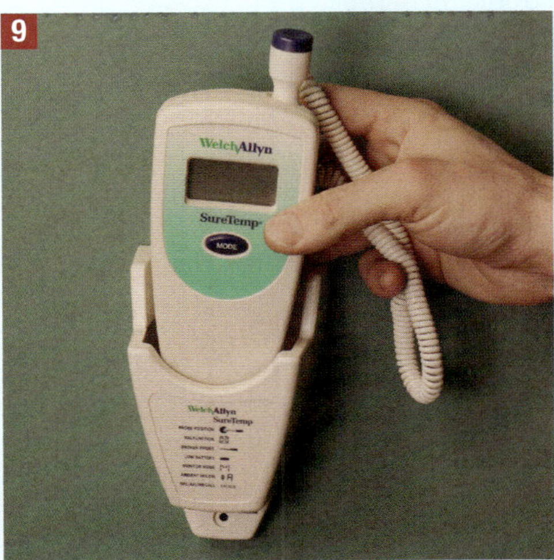

Return the thermometer to its base.

10. **Procedural Step.** Sanitize your hands.
11. **Procedural Step.** Document the results in the patient's medical record.
    a. *Electronic health record:* In SimChart for the Medical Office, document the temperature reading and site using textboxes, drop-down menus, and/or radio buttons. The temperature can be documented in either Fahrenheit or Celsius and the software will convert the temperature so that both are displayed.
    b. *Paper-based patient record:* Document the date, the time, and the axillary temperature reading. The symbol (A) must be documented next to the temperature reading to tell the provider that an axillary reading was taken.

11b DOCUMENTATION EXAMPLE

Date	
10/15/XX	9:30 a.m. T: 97.4° F (A) –S. Martinez, RMA

PROCEDURE 19.3 Measuring Rectal Body Temperature—Electronic Thermometer

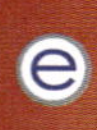  

Outcome Measure rectal body temperature.

Equipment/Supplies

- Electronic thermometer
- Rectal probe (red collar)
- Plastic probe cover
- Lubricant
- Disposable gloves
- Tissues
- Waste container

1. **Procedural Step.** Sanitize your hands and assemble the equipment.
2. **Procedural Step.** Remove the thermometer unit from its storage base. Attach the rectal (red collar) probe to it. This is accomplished by inserting the latching plug (on the end of the coiled cord of the rectal probe) to the plug receptacle on the thermometer unit. Insert the probe into the face of the thermometer.
   Principle. The rectal probe is color-coded with a red collar for ease in identifying it.
3. **Procedural Step.** Greet the patient and introduce yourself. Identify the patient and explain the procedure. If the patient is a child or an adult, provide them with a patient gown. Instruct the patient to remove enough clothing to provide access to the anal area and to put on the gown with the opening in the back. If the patient is an infant, ask the parent to remove the infant's diaper.
   Principle. It is important to explain what you will be doing, because body temperature may be higher in a fearful or apprehensive patient. The patient gown provides the patient with modesty and comfort.
4. **Procedural Step.** Apply gloves. Position the patient. *Adults and children:* Position the patient in the modified left lateral recumbent (Sims) position and drape the patient to expose only the anal area. *Infants:* Position the infant on his or her abdomen.
   Principle. Gloves protect the medical assistant from microorganisms in the anal area and feces. Correct positioning allows clear viewing of the anal opening and provides for proper insertion of the thermometer. Draping reduces patient embarrassment and provides warmth.
5. **Procedural Step.** Grasp the probe by the collar and remove it from the face of the thermometer. Slide the probe into a disposable plastic probe cover until it locks into place. Apply a lubricant to the tip of the probe cover up to a level of 1 inch.
   Principle. A lubricated thermometer can be inserted more easily and does not irritate the delicate rectal mucosa.

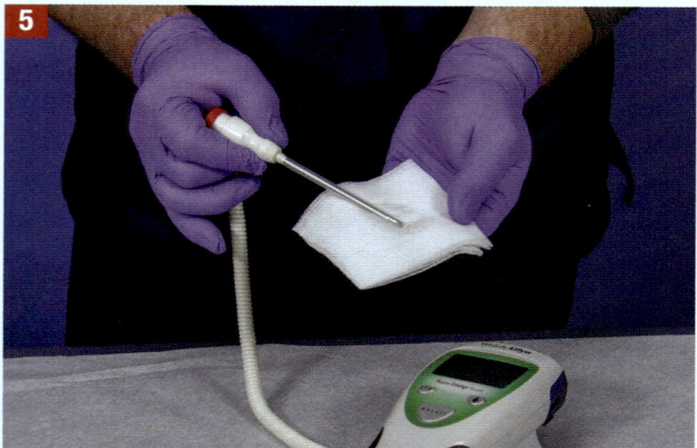

Apply a lubricant to the tip of the probe cover.

6. **Procedural Step.** Instruct the patient to lie still. Separate the buttocks to expose the anal opening, and gently insert the thermometer probe approximately 1 inch into the rectum of an adult, 5/8 inch in children, and 1/2 inch in infants. Do not force insertion of the probe. Hold the probe in place until the temperature registers.
   Principle. The probe must be inserted correctly to prevent injury to the tissue of the anal opening. The probe should be held in place to prevent damage to the rectal mucosa.

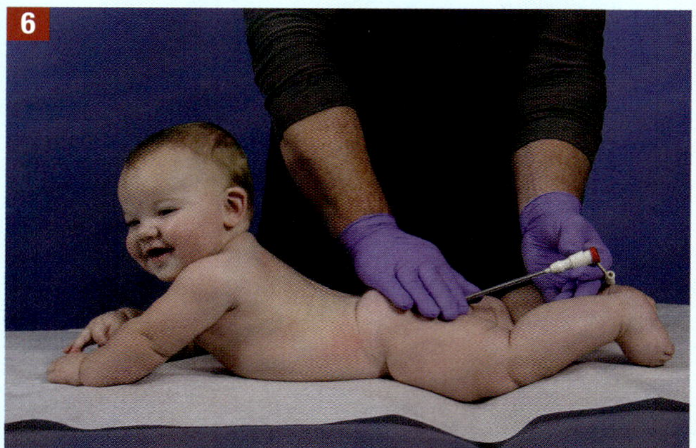

Gently insert the probe into the rectum.

PROCEDURE 19.3 Measuring Rectal Body Temperature—Electronic Thermometer—cont'd

7. **Procedural Step.** Hold the probe in place until you hear the tone. At that time, the patient's temperature appears as a digital display on the screen of the thermometer. Make a mental note of the temperature reading.
8. **Procedural Step.** Gently remove the probe from the rectum in the same direction as it was inserted. Avoid touching the probe cover. Discard the probe cover by firmly pressing the ejection button while holding the probe over a regular waste container. Return the probe to its stored position in the thermometer unit. Return the thermometer unit to its storage base.
   Principle. Fecal material is not considered regulated medical waste; the probe can be discarded in a regular waste container.
9. **Procedural Step.** Wipe the patient's anal area with tissues to remove excess lubricant. Dispose of the tissues in a regular waste container.
   Principle. Wiping the anal area makes the patient more comfortable.
10. **Procedural Step.** Remove gloves and sanitize your hands.
11. **Procedural Step.** Document the results in the patient's medical record.
    a. *Electronic health record:* In SimChart for the Medical Office, document the temperature reading and site using textboxes, drop-down menus, and/or radio buttons. The temperature can be documented in either Fahrenheit or Celsius and the software will convert the temperature so that both are displayed.
    b. *Paper-based patient record:* Document the date, the time, and the rectal temperature reading. The symbol Ⓡ must be documented next to the temperature reading to tell the provider that a rectal reading was taken.

11b

DOCUMENTATION EXAMPLE

Date	
10/15/XX	11:15 a.m. T: 99.8° F Ⓡ — S. Martinez, RMA

PROCEDURE 19.4

PROCEDURE 19.4 Measuring Aural Body Temperature

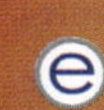
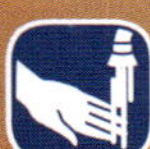

Outcome Measure aural body temperature.

Equipment/Supplies

- Tympanic membrane thermometer
- Probe cover
- Waste container

1. **Procedural Step.** Sanitize your hands and assemble the equipment.
   Principle. Your hands should be clean and free from contamination.
2. **Procedural Step.** Greet the patient and introduce yourself. Identify the patient and explain the procedure.
   Principle. It is important to explain what you will be doing, because body temperature may be higher in a fearful or apprehensive patient.
3. **Procedural Step.** Remove the thermometer from its storage base. Ensure that the sensor lens is clean and intact. If the lens is dirty, gently wipe it with an antiseptic wipe or cotton swab moistened with alcohol and allow it to dry. After cleaning, allow at least 5 minutes before taking the temperature. If the lens is damaged, the thermometer cannot be used and must be repaired or replaced.
   Principle. A dirty sensor lens reduces the transparency of the lens and may result in a falsely low temperature reading.
4. **Procedural Step.** Attach a cover on the probe by pressing the probe tip straight down into the cover box. You will be able to see and feel the cover snap securely into place on the probe. This procedure automatically turns on the thermometer.
   Principle. The probe cover protects the sensor lens and provides infection control. The cover must be seated securely on the probe to activate the thermometer.

Continued

PROCEDURE 19.4 Measuring Aural Body Temperature—cont'd

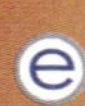

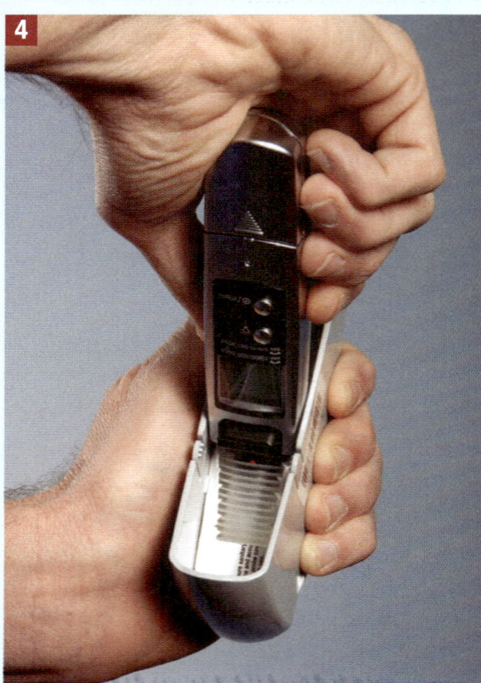

4 Place a cover on the probe.

5. Procedural Step. Pull the probe straight up from the cover box. Look at the display screen to see if the thermometer is ready to use. The °F (or °C) icon flashes when the thermometer is ready to use.

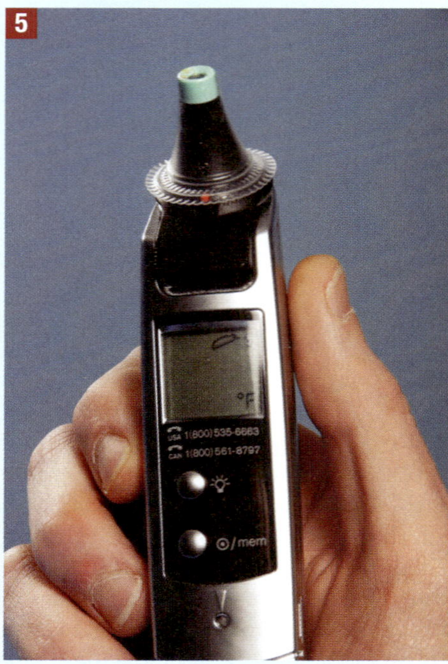

5 Look to see if the thermometer is ready for use.

6. Procedural Step. Hold the thermometer in your dominant hand. If you are right-handed, you should take the temperature in the patient's right ear. If you are left-handed, take the temperature in the patient's left ear.

Principle. Taking the temperature with the dominant hand assists in the proper placement of the probe in the patient's ear.

7. Procedural Step. Straighten the patient's external ear canal with your nondominant hand, as follows:

Adults and children older than 3 years: Gently pull the ear auricle upward and backward.

Children younger than 3 years: Gently pull the ear pinna downward and backward.

Principle. Straightening the ear canal allows the probe sensor to obtain a clear picture of the tympanic membrane, resulting in an accurate temperature measurement.

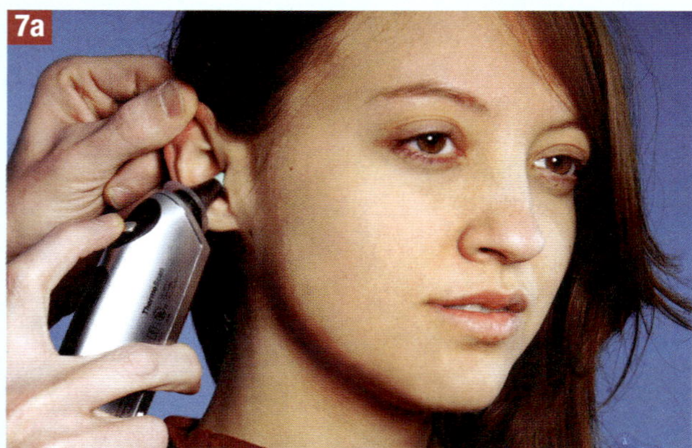

7a Straighten the canal of adults and children older than 3 years by pulling the ear auricle upward and backward.

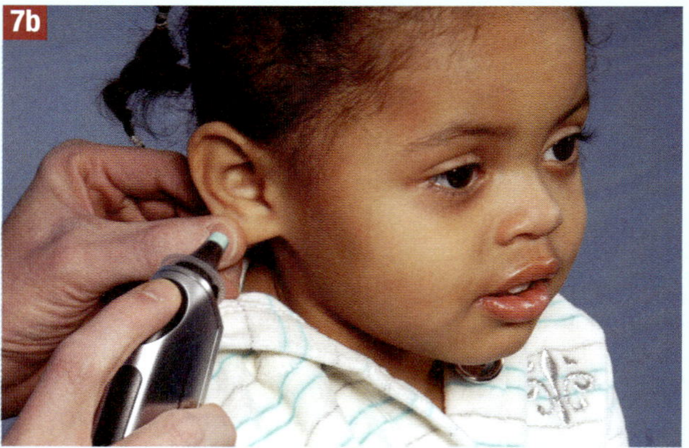

7b Straighten the canal of children younger than 3 years by pulling the ear auricle downward and backward.

8. Procedural Step. Insert the probe into the patient's ear canal tightly enough to seal the opening, but without causing patient discomfort. Point the tip of the probe toward the opposite temple (approximately midway between the opposite ear and eyebrow).

PROCEDURE 19.4 Measuring Aural Body Temperature—cont'd

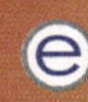

Principle. Sealing the ear canal prevents cooler external air from entering the ear, which could result in a falsely low reading. Correct positioning of the probe optimizes the view of the tympanic membrane by the sensor lens, leading to an accurate temperature reading.

9. **Procedural Step.** Ask the patient to remain still. Hold the thermometer steady, and depress the activation button. Depending on the brand of the thermometer, perform one of the following:
   a. Hold the button down for 1 full second and then release it, or
   b. Hold down the button down until an audible tone is heard.

   Principle. The thermometer cannot take a temperature unless the activation button is depressed for 1 full second. When the button is depressed, the sensor lens scans the thermal energy radiated by the tympanic membrane.

10. **Procedural Step.** Remove the thermometer from the ear canal. Turn the display screen of the thermometer toward you and read the temperature. Make a mental note of the temperature reading. If the temperature seems to be too low, repeat the procedure to ensure that you have used the proper technique. The temperature indicated on this thermometer is 99.8°F (37.7°C). The temperature remains on the display screen for 30 to 60 seconds or until another cover is inserted on the probe (whichever occurs first).

    Principle. Improper technique can result in a falsely low temperature reading.

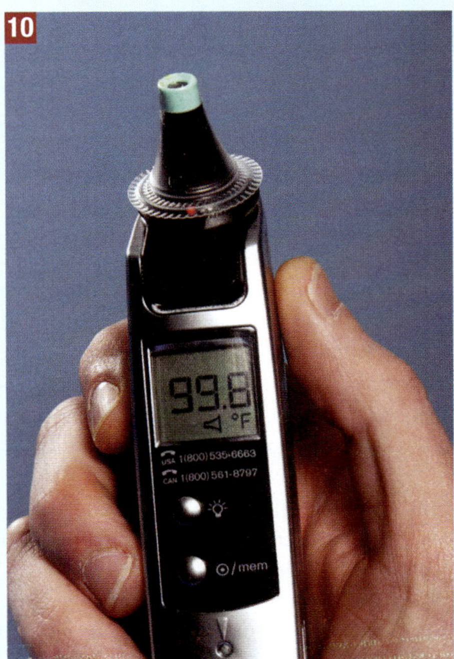

Read the temperature on the display screen.

11. **Procedural Step.** Dispose of the probe cover by ejecting it into a regular waste container. Wipe the sensor lens with an antiseptic.

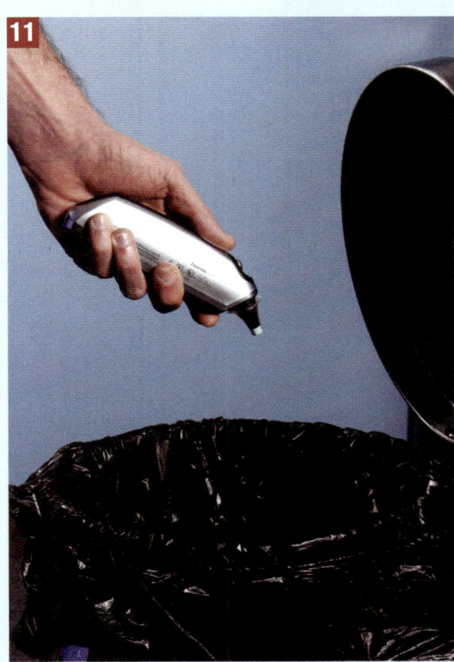

Dispose of the probe cover.

12. **Procedural Step.** Replace the thermometer in its storage base.

    Principle. The thermometer should be stored in its base to protect the sensor lens from damage and dirt.

13. **Procedural Step.** Sanitize your hands.

14. **Procedural Step.** Document the results in the patient's medical record.
    a. *Electronic health record:* In SimChart for the Medical Office, document the temperature reading and site using textboxes, drop-down menus, and/or radio buttons. The temperature can be documented in either Fahrenheit or Celsius and the software will convert the temperature so that both are displayed.
    b. *Paper-based patient record:* Document the date, the time, the aural temperature reading, and which ear was used to take the temperature. Indicating which ear was used alerts the provider that the temperature was taken through the aural route.

14b

DOCUMENTATION EXAMPLE

Date	
10/15/XX	3:00 p.m. T: 99.8° F, (R) ear—S. Martinez, RMA

PROCEDURE 19.5 Measuring Temporal Artery Body Temperature

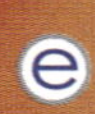

Outcome Measure temporal artery body temperature.

Equipment/Supplies

- Contact temporal artery thermometer and probe cover
- Non-contact temporal artery thermometer
- Antiseptic wipe or cotton swab moistened with alcohol
- Waste container

1. **Procedural Step.** Sanitize your hands and assemble the equipment.
2. **Procedural Step.** Greet the patient and introduce yourself. Identify the patient and explain the procedure.
3. **Procedural Step.** Examine the sensor lens of the thermometer to ensure that the lens is clean and intact, making sure not to touch it with your fingers. If the sensor lens is dirty, clean it with an antiseptic wipe or a cotton swab moistened with alcohol and allow it to dry. If the lens is damaged, the thermometer cannot be used and must be repaired or replaced.
   Principle. A dirty sensor lens reduces the transparency of the lens and may result in a falsely low temperature reading.
4. **Procedural Step.** Place a disposable cover over the probe. If the thermometer does not use disposable covers, clean the sensor lens with an antiseptic wipe or a cotton swab moistened with alcohol, and allow it to dry *(Note: This cleansing step does not need to be performed if it was previously performed in Step 3).*
   Principle. Applying a probe cover or cleaning the probe with an antiseptic prevents cross-contamination.

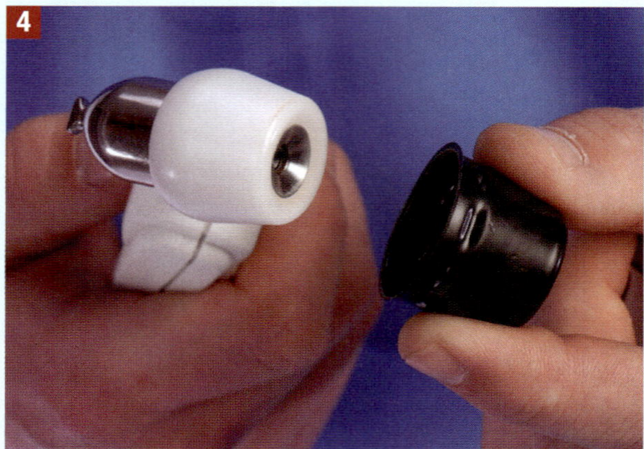

4 Place a disposable probe cover on the thermometer.

Contact temporal artery thermometer measurement

5. **Procedural Step.** Select an appropriate site; the right or left side of the forehead can be used. The site selected should be fully exposed to the environment.
   Principle. The temporal artery is located in the center of the forehead, approximately 2 mm below the surface of the skin.
6. **Procedural Step.** Prepare the patient by brushing away any hair that is covering the side of the forehead to be scanned and the area behind the earlobe on the same side.
   Principle. Hair covering the area to be measured traps body heat, resulting in a falsely high temperature reading.
7. **Procedural Step.** Hold the thermometer in your dominant hand with your thumb on the scan button.
8. **Procedural Step.** Gently position the probe of the thermometer on the center of the patient's forehead, midway between the eyebrow and the hairline.

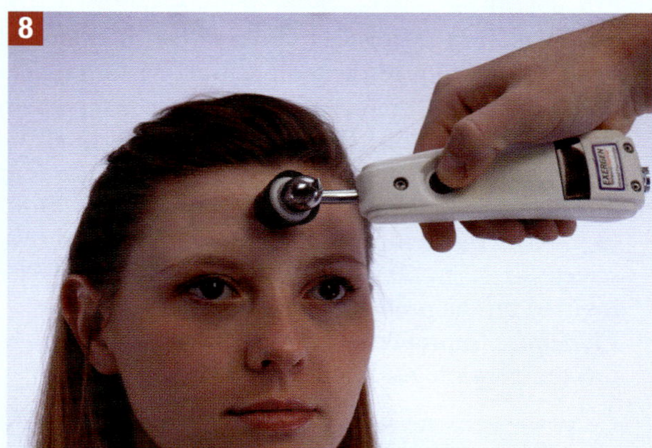

8 Position the probe on the center of the patient's forehead.

9. **Procedural Step.** Depress the scan button, and keep it depressed for the entire measurement.
   Principle. Not keeping the scan button depressed can result in a falsely low temperature reading.
10. **Procedural Step.** Slowly and gently slide the probe straight across the forehead, midway between the eyebrow and the upper hairline. Continue until the hairline is reached. Keep the scan button depressed and the probe flush (flat) against the forehead. During this time, a beeping sound occurs and a red light blinks to indicate that a measurement is taking place. Rapid beeping and blinking indicate a rise to a higher temperature. Slow beeping indicates that the thermometer is still scanning but is not finding a higher temperature.
   Principle. The thermometer continually scans for the peak temperature as long as the scan button is depressed. The probe must be held flat against the forehead to ensure accurate scanning of the temporal artery.

PROCEDURE 19.5 Measuring Temporal Artery Body Temperature—cont'd

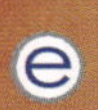

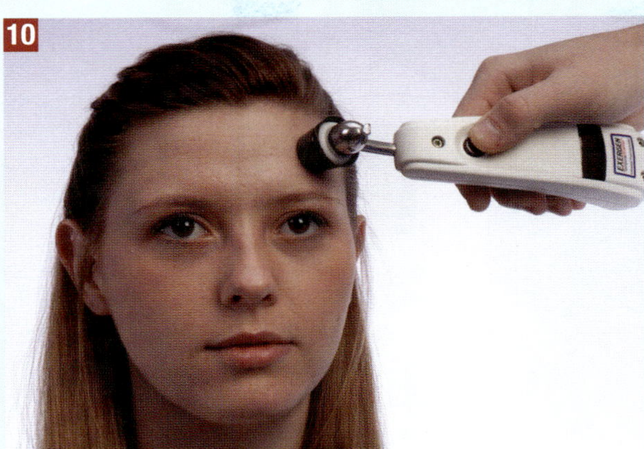

Slowly slide the probe straight across the patient's forehead.

11. Procedural Step. Keeping the button depressed, lift the probe from the forehead, and gently place the probe behind the earlobe in the soft depression of the neck just below the mastoid process. Hold the probe in place for 1 to 2 seconds.

Principle. Taking the patient's temperature behind the earlobe prevents an error in temperature measurement in the event that the patient's forehead is sweating.

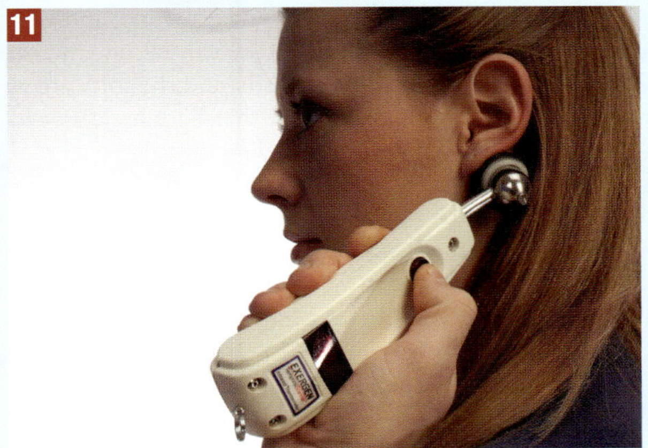

Place the probe behind the earlobe.

12. Procedural Step. Release the scan button, and read the temperature on the screen of the thermometer. Make a mental note of the temperature reading. (The temperature indicated on this thermometer is 99.1°F [37.3°C].) The reading remains on the display screen for approximately 15 to 30 seconds after the scan button is released. The thermometer shuts off automatically after 30 seconds. If the patient's temperature needs to be taken again, wait 60 seconds or use the opposite side of the forehead.

Principle. Taking a measurement cools the skin, and taking another measurement too soon may result in an inaccurate reading.

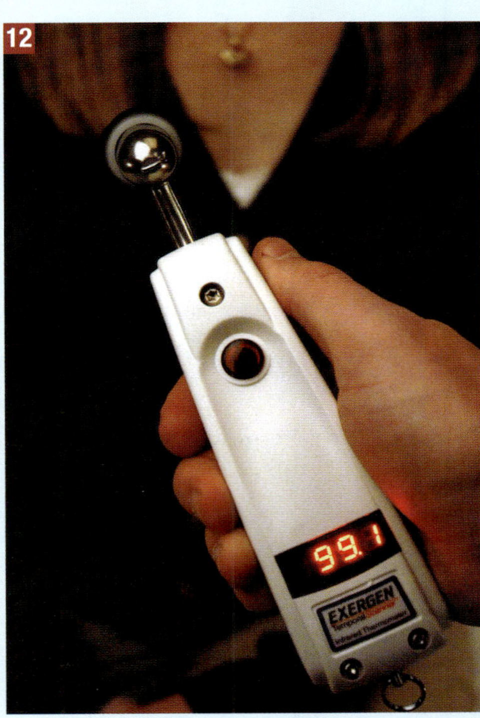

Read the temperature on the display screen.

13. Procedural Step. Dispose of the probe cover by pushing it off the probe with your thumb and ejecting it into a regular waste container. Wipe the sensor lens with an antiseptic wipe.

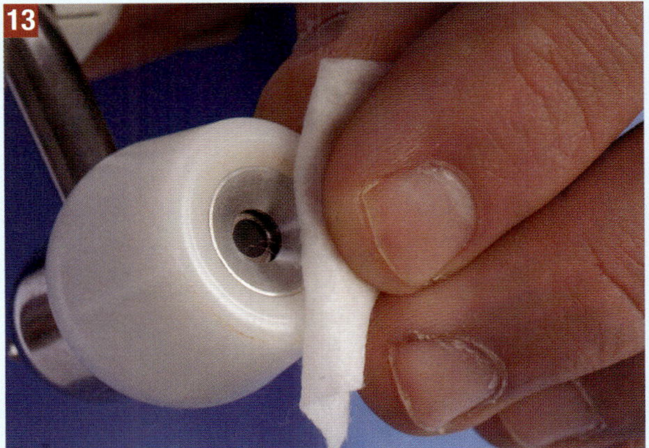

Wipe the probe with an antiseptic wipe.

Continued

PROCEDURE 19.5 Measuring Temporal Artery Body Temperature—cont'd

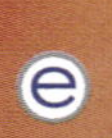

Non-contact temporal artery thermometer measurement

14. **Procedural Step:** Prepare the patient by brushing away any hair covering the forehead. If sweat is present on the patient's forehead, remove it by wiping the forehead with a soft cloth.
    Principle. Sweating of the forehead may result in a falsely low temperature reading.
15. **Procedural Step:** Hold the thermometer in your dominant hand and position the probe of the thermometer 2 inches (5 cm) away from the center of the patient's forehead (between the eyebrows).
    Principle. If the thermometer is positioned more than 2 inches away from the forehead, a falsely low temperature reading may occur.

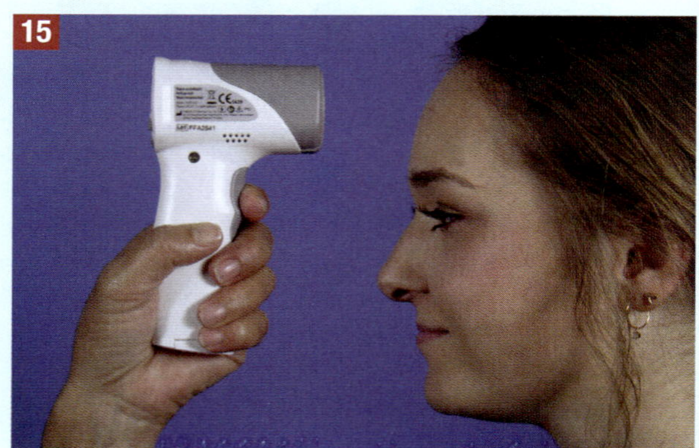

Position the probe of the thermometer.

16. **Procedural Step:** Holding the thermometer steady, press the scan button until an audible tone is heard. Release the scan button and read the temperature on the screen of the thermometer. Make a mental note of the temperature reading. (The temperature indicated on this thermometer is 98.1 °F [36.7 °C].) The reading remains on the display screen for approximately 15 to 30 seconds after the scan button is released. The thermometer shuts off automatically after 30 seconds. If the patient's temperature needs to be taken again, wait 60 seconds.
    Principle. When the scan button is depressed, the sensor lens scans the thermal energy radiated by the temporal artery. Moving the thermometer during the measurement may result in an inaccurate measurement.

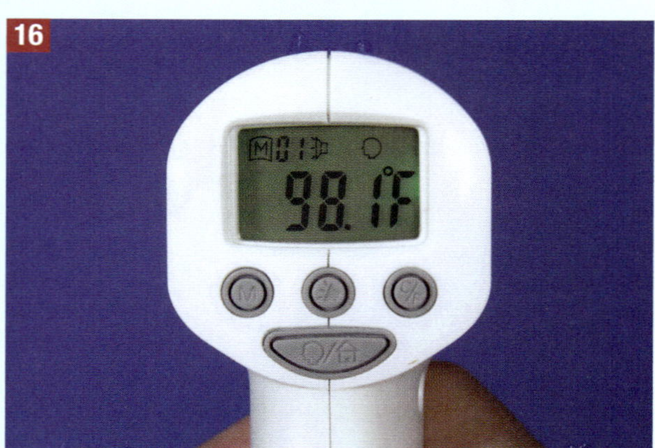

Read the temperature on the display screen.

17. **Procedural Step:** Wipe the sensor lens with a cotton swab moistened with alcohol.

Complete both procedures as follows:

18. **Procedural Step.** Sanitize your hands.
19. **Procedural Step.** Document the results in the patient's medical record.
    a. *Electronic health record:* In SimChart for the Medical Office, document the temperature reading and site using textboxes, drop-down menus, and/or radio buttons. The temperature can be documented in either Fahrenheit or Celsius and the software will convert the temperature so that both are displayed.
    b. *Paper-based patient record:* Document the date, the time, and the temperature reading. The symbol (TA) must be documented next to the temperature reading to tell the provider that a temporal artery reading was taken.

19b

DOCUMENTATION EXAMPLE

Date	
10/15/XX	9:15 a.m. T: 98.1° F (TA)— S. Martinez, RMA

20. **Procedural Step.** Store the thermometer in a clean, dry area.

PROCEDURE 19.6 Measuring Pulse and Respiration

Outcome Measure pulse and respiration.

Equipment/Supplies

- Watch with a second hand

1. **Procedural Step.** Sanitize your hands. Greet the patient and introduce yourself. Identify the patient and explain the procedure. Observe the patient for any signs that might affect the pulse or respiratory rate.
   Principle. Pulse rate can vary according to the factors listed on pages 356–358.
2. **Procedural Step.** Have the patient sit down. Position the patient's arm in a comfortable position. The forearm should be slightly flexed to relax the muscles and tendons over the pulse site.
   Principle. Relaxed muscles and tendons over the pulse site make it easier to palpate the pulse.
3. **Procedural Step.** Place your three middle fingertips over the radial pulse site. Never use your thumb to take a pulse. The radial pulse is located in a groove on the inner aspect of the wrist just below the thumb.
   Principle. The thumb has a pulse of its own; using the thumb results in measurement of the medical assistant's pulse and not the patient's pulse.

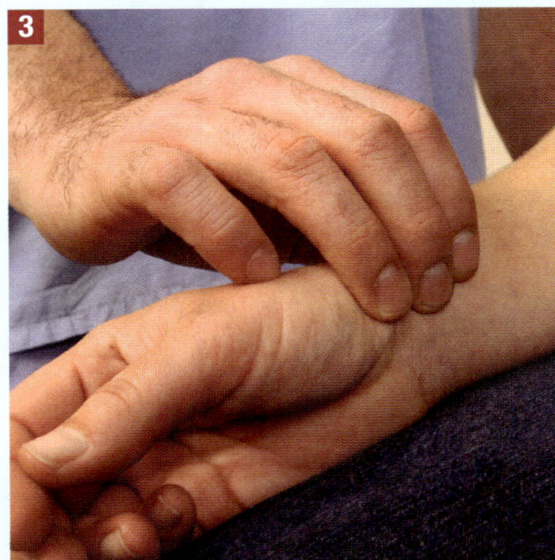

Place the three middle fingers over the radial pulse site.

4. **Procedural Step.** Apply moderate, gentle pressure directly over the site until you feel the pulse. If you cannot feel the pulse, this may be caused by:
   - Incorrect location of the radial pulse: Move your fingers to a slightly different location in the groove of the wrist until you feel the pulse.
   - Applying too much pressure or not enough pressure: Vary the depth of your hold until you can feel the pulse.

   Principle. A normal pulse can be felt with moderate pressure. The pulse cannot be felt if not enough pressure is applied, whereas too much pressure applied to the radial artery closes it off, and no pulse is felt.
5. **Procedural Step.** Count the pulse for 30 seconds and make a mental note of this number. Note the rhythm and volume of the pulse. If abnormalities are present in the rhythm or volume, count the pulse for 1 full minute.
   Principle. A longer time ensures an accurate assessment of abnormalities.

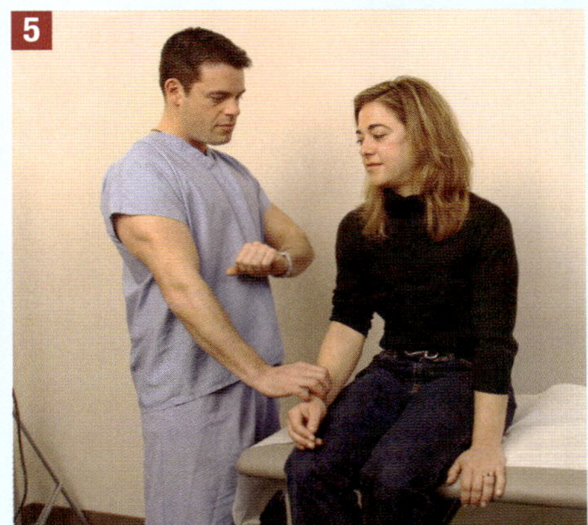

Count the pulse for 30 seconds.

6. **Procedural Step.** After taking the pulse, continue to hold three fingers on the patient's wrist with the same amount of pressure, and measure the respirations. This helps to ensure that the patient is unaware that respirations are being monitored.
   Principle. If the patient is aware that respiration is being measured, the breathing may change.

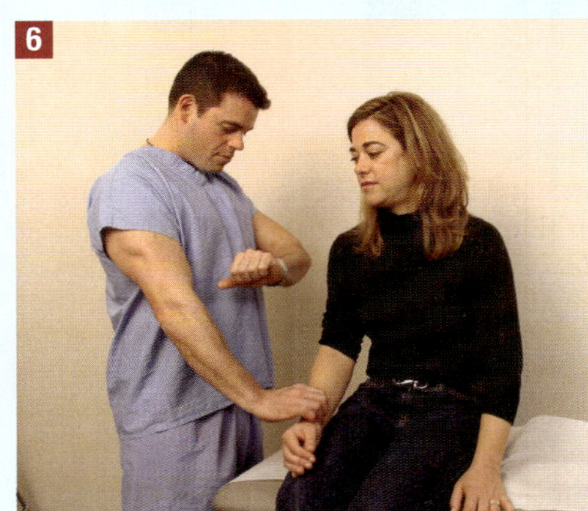

Count the number of respirations for 30 seconds.

Continued

PROCEDURE 19.6 Measuring Pulse and Respiration—cont'd

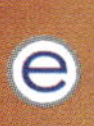

7. **Procedural Step.** Observe the rise and fall of the patient's chest as the patient inhales and exhales.
   Principle. One complete respiration includes one inhalation and one exhalation.
8. **Procedural Step.** Count the number of respirations for 30 seconds and make a mental note of this number; note the rhythm and depth of the respirations. Also observe the patient's color. If abnormalities are present in rhythm or depth, count the respiratory rate for 1 full minute.
9. **Procedural Step.** Sanitize your hands.
10. **Procedural Step.** Document the results in the patient's medical record. If you counted the pulse and respirations for 30 seconds, multiply each of the numbers counted by 2. This will give you the pulse rate and respiratory rate for 1 full minute.
    a. *Electronic health record:* In SimChart for the Medical Office, document the pulse rate, rhythm, volume, and site for taking the pulse; and the respiratory rate, rhythm, and depth using textboxes, dropdown menus, and/or radio buttons.
    b. *Paper-based patient record:* Document the date; the time; the pulse rate, rhythm, and volume; and the respiratory rate, rhythm, and depth.

10b

DOCUMENTATION EXAMPLE

Date	
10/15/XX	2:30 p.m. P: 74. Reg and strong. R: 18.
	Even and reg. ———— S. Martinez, RMA

PROCEDURE 19.7

PROCEDURE 19.7 Measuring Apical Pulse

Outcome Measure apical pulse.

Equipment/Supplies

- Watch with a second hand
- Stethoscope
- Antiseptic wipe

1. **Procedural Step.** Sanitize your hands. Greet the patient and introduce yourself. Identify the patient and explain the procedure. Observe the patient for any signs that might increase or decrease the pulse rate.
2. **Procedural Step.** Assemble the equipment. If the stethoscope's chest piece consists of a diaphragm and a bell, rotate the chest piece to the bell position. Clean the earpieces and chest piece of the stethoscope with an antiseptic wipe.
   Principle. The bell position allows better auscultation of heart sounds. Cleaning the earpieces helps prevent the transmission of microorganisms.
3. **Procedural Step.** Ask the patient to unbutton or remove their shirt. Have the patient sit or lie down (supine).
   Principle. A sitting or supine position allows access to the apex of the heart.
4. **Procedural Step.** Warm the chest piece of the stethoscope with your hands. Insert the earpieces of the stethoscope into your ears, with the earpieces directed slightly forward, and place the chest piece over the apex of the patient's heart. The apex of the heart is located in the fifth intercostal space at the junction of the left midclavicular line.
   Principle. Warming the chest piece reduces the discomfort of having a cold object placed on the chest. In addition, a cold chest piece could startle the patient, resulting in an increase in pulse rate. The earpieces should be directed forward to follow the direction of the ear canal, which facilitates hearing.

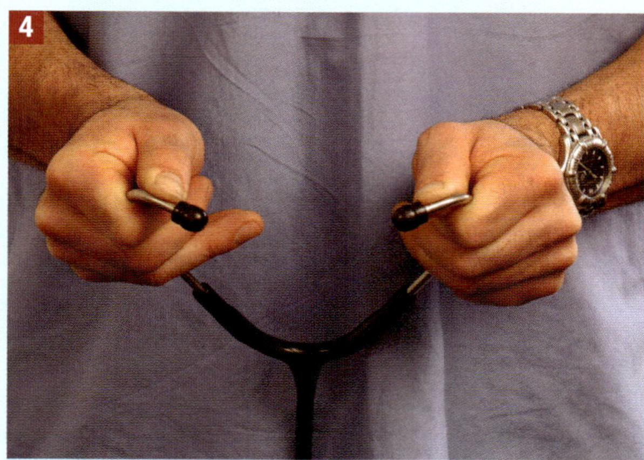

Insert the earpieces into your ears with the earpieces directed slightly forward.

PROCEDURE 19.7 Measuring Apical Pulse—cont'd

5. Procedural Step. Listen for the heartbeat and count the number of beats for 30 seconds (and multiply by 2) if the rhythm and volume are normal or if the apical pulse of an infant or child is being taken. If abnormalities are present in the rhythm or volume, count the pulse for 1 full minute. You will hear a *lub-dup* sound through the stethoscope. This sound is the closing of the valves of the heart. Each *lub-dup* is counted as one beat.

5

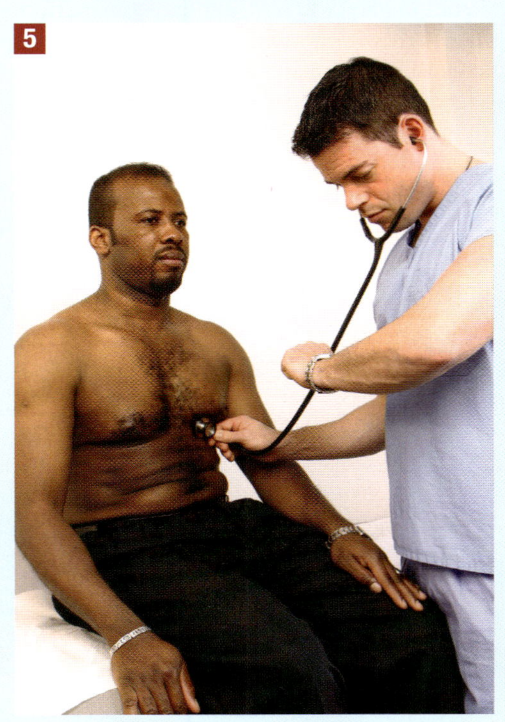

Count the number of beats for 30 seconds, and multiply by 2.

6. Procedural Step. Sanitize your hands.

7. Procedural Step. Document the results in the patient's medical record.

a. *Electronic health record:* In SimChart for the Medical Office, document the rate, rhythm, and volume and the site for taking the pulse using textboxes, drop-down menus, and/or radio buttons.

b. *Paper-based patient record:* Document the date, the time, and the apical pulse rate, rhythm, and volume.

7b

DOCUMENTATION EXAMPLE

Date	
10/15/XX	10:15 a.m. AP: 68. Reg and strong.________
	________ S. Martinez, CMA (AAMA)

8. Procedural Step. Clean the earpieces and the chest piece of the stethoscope with an antiseptic wipe.

PROCEDURE 19.8

PROCEDURE 19.8 Performing Pulse Oximetry

Outcome Perform pulse oximetry.

Equipment/Supplies

- Handheld pulse oximeter
- Antiseptic wipe

1. Procedural Step. Sanitize your hands.

2. Procedural Step. Assemble the equipment. Handle the pulse oximeter carefully, and perform the following:

a. Carefully inspect the probe to ensure it opens and closes smoothly. Inspect the probe windows (LED and light sensor) to ensure they are clean and free of lint.

b. Disinfect the probe windows and surrounding platforms with an antiseptic wipe and allow them to dry.

Continued

PROCEDURE 19.8 Performing Pulse Oximetry—cont'd

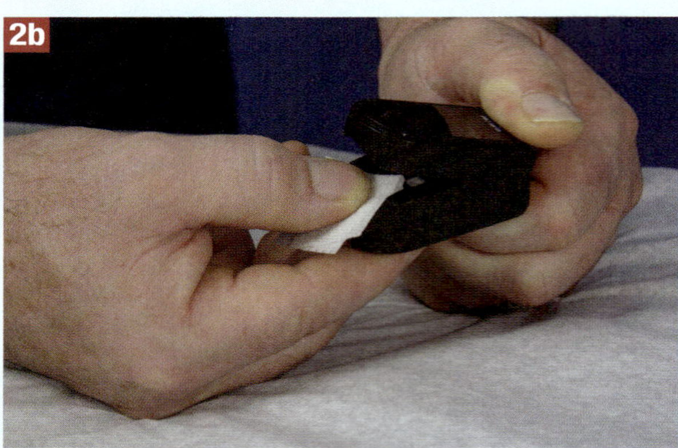
Disinfect the probe with an antiseptic wipe.

Principle. Misuse or improper handling of the pulse oximeter could damage it. Dirt or lint on the probe windows could interfere with proper light transmission, leading to an inaccurate reading. Cross-contamination between patients is prevented by disinfecting the probe.

3. **Procedural Step.** Greet the patient and introduce yourself. Identify the patient and explain the procedure. Explain to the patient that the clip-on probe does not hurt and feels similar to a clothespin attached to the finger.
4. **Procedural Step.** Seat the patient comfortably in a chair with the lower arm firmly supported just below heart level and the palm facing down.
   Principle. Supporting the lower arm helps prevent patient movement during the procedure. Placing the lower arm just below heart level helps to ensure an accurate reading.
5. **Procedural Step.** Select an appropriate finger to apply the probe. Use the tip of the patient's index, middle, ring finger, or thumb. If the patient's fingers are small and the probe cannot seem to be aligned properly, use the big toe or earlobe to take the measurement. If the patient exhibits tremors of the hands, use the earlobe to obtain the reading.
   Principle. The probe must be applied to a peripheral site with thin skin that is highly vascular. Small fingers may not allow for proper positioning of the probe on the finger.
6. **Procedural Step.** Observe the patient's fingernail. If the patient is wearing dark fingernail polish, ask them to remove it with acetone or nail polish remover. If the patient has long nails or is wearing artificial nails, choose another probe site, such as the big toe or earlobe.
   Principle. An opaque coating on the fingernail may interfere with proper light transmission through the finger, leading to an inaccurate reading. Long nails or artificial nails may obstruct the light sensor and prevent an accurate measurement.
7. **Procedural Step.** Check to ensure that the patient's fingertip is clean. If it is dirty, cleanse the site with soap and water, and allow it to dry. Ensure that the patient's finger is not cold. If it is cold, ask the patient to rub their hands together.
   Principle. Oils, dirt, or grime on the finger can interfere with proper light transmission through the finger, leading to an inaccurate reading. Sometimes patients with cold fingers may have enough constriction of the capillaries that it interferes with obtaining a reading.
8. **Procedural Step.** Ensure that ambient light does not interfere with the measurement. Position the probe securely on the fingertip as follows:
   a. Ensure that the probe window is fully covered by placing the finger over the LED window, with the fleshy tip of the finger covering the window. The tip of the finger should touch the end of the probe stop.

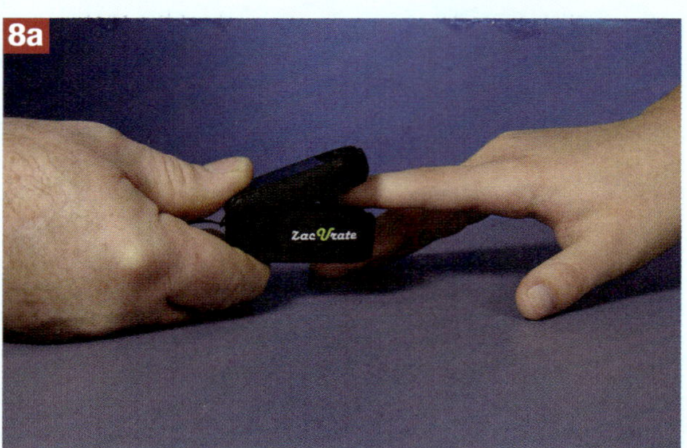

Position the probe securely on the fingertip.

   b. Ensure that the LED and the light sensor are aligned opposite to each other.
   Principle. Ambient light can be picked up by the probe and alter the reading. Proper alignment of the LED and light sensor is necessary for an accurate reading.
9. **Procedural Step.** Instruct the patient to keep their finger stationary and to breathe normally. Turn on the oximeter by pressing the power-on control. Wait while the oximeter goes through its power-on self-test (POST).
   Principle. Finger movement may lead to an inaccurate reading. The monitor automatically conducts a POST to ensure that it is functioning properly.
10. **Procedural Step.** Allow several seconds for the pulse oximeter to detect the pulse and calculate the oxygen saturation of the blood. Ensure that the pulse strength indicator fluctuates with each pulsation and that the pulse signal is strong. If the oximeter is unable to locate a pulse, reposition the probe on the patient's finger or move the probe to another finger, and perform the procedure again.

PROCEDURE 19.8 Performing Pulse Oximetry—cont'd

Principle. The reading takes 4 to 6 seconds to display the results on the screen of the oximeter. The pulse strength indicator provides a quick assessment of pulse quality. If the oximeter is unable to locate a pulse, it will be unable to obtain a reading.

11. Procedural Step. Leave the probe in place until the oximeter displays a reading. Read the oxygen saturation value and pulse rate and make a mental note of these readings. On this pulse oximeter, the oxygen saturation reading is 97% and the pulse rate is 88. If the SpO_2 reading is less than 95%, reposition the probe on the finger or move the probe to a different finger, and perform the procedure again.

Principle. A low SpO_2 reading may be caused by improper positioning of the probe on the finger.

11

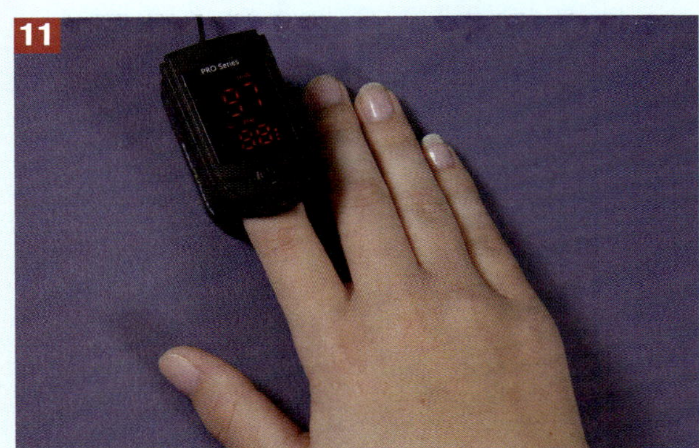

Read the oxygen saturation value and pulse rate.

12. Procedural Step. Remove the probe from the patient's finger. The pulse oximeter will automatically shut down after the finger is removed from the probe.

13. Procedural Step. Sanitize your hands.

14. Procedural Step. Document the results in the patient's medical record.

a. *Electronic health record:* In SimChart for the Medical Office, enter the SpO_2 reading and the pulse rate using textboxes, drop-down menus, and/or radio buttons.

b. *Paper-based patient record:* Document the date, the time, the SpO_2 reading, and the pulse rate.

14b

DOCUMENTATION EXAMPLE

Date	
10/15/XX	2:30 p.m. SpO_2: 97%. P: 75. ————
	———— S. Martinez, RMA

15. Procedural Step. Disinfect the probe with an antiseptic wipe. Properly store the monitor in a clean, dry area.

PROCEDURE 19.8

PROCEDURE 19.9 Measuring Blood Pressure: Manual Method

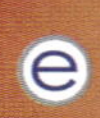

Outcome Measure blood pressure using the manual method.

Equipment/Supplies

- Stethoscope
- Portable aneroid sphygmomanometer
- Antiseptic wipe

1. Procedural Step. Sanitize your hands and assemble the equipment. If the chest piece consists of a diaphragm and a bell, rotate it to the diaphragm position. Clean the earpieces and diaphragm of the stethoscope with the antiseptic wipe.
Principle. The diaphragm must be rotated to the proper position for sound to be heard through the earpieces.

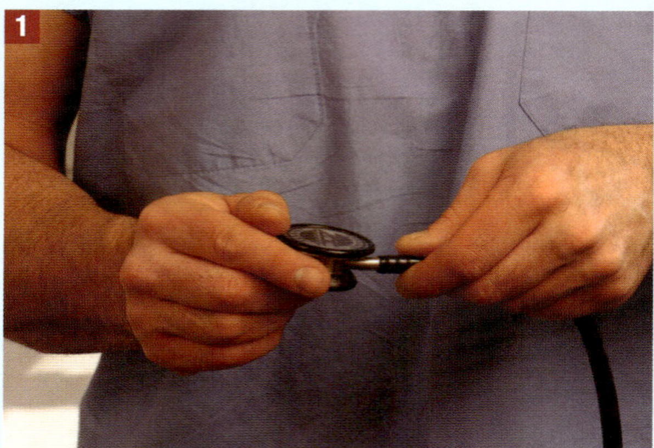

Rotate the chest piece to the diaphragm position.

2. Procedural Step. Greet the patient and introduce yourself. Identify the patient and explain the procedure. Ask the patient to empty the bladder. Observe and question the patient for factors that might influence the blood pressure reading (e.g., emotional states, physical activity). If it is not possible to reduce or eliminate these factors, document them in the patient's medical record.
Principle. A full bladder can increase the blood pressure reading. An inaccurate reading may occur if factors are present that could influence the reading.

3. Procedural Step. Instruct the patient sit quietly in a comfortable position with the legs uncrossed at the knees and the feet flat on the floor. The patient should be allowed to relax in a sitting position for at least 5 minutes before the blood pressure measurement.
Principle. Patient anxiety can cause a significant increase in blood pressure.

4. Procedural Step: Roll up the patient's sleeve approximately 5 inches above the elbow so that the cuff can be applied to bare skin. If the sleeve does not roll up or is too tight after being rolled up, remove the arm from the sleeve. The arm should be positioned at heart level and well supported on a flat surface, with the palm facing upward.
Principle. Clothing can result in an inaccurate blood pressure reading. A tight sleeve causes partial compression of the brachial artery, resulting in an inaccurate reading. Placing the arm above heart level may cause the reading to be falsely low. Not supporting the arm or placing it below heart level and crossing the legs at the knees may cause the reading to be falsely high.

5. Procedural Step. Determine the patient's correct cuff size. Make sure the cuff is completely deflated so that there is no residual air in the bladder of the cuff.
Principle. The correct-sized cuff must be used to ensure an accurate measurement. If the cuff is too small, it may come loose as the cuff is inflated, or the reading may be falsely high. If the cuff is too large, the reading may be falsely low.

6. Procedural Step. Make sure the arm is well extended; locate the brachial pulse with the index and middle fingertips. The brachial pulse is located near the center of the antecubital space but slightly toward the little finger–side of the arm. Center the inner bladder above the brachial pulse site with the lower edge of the cuff approximately 1 to 2 inches (2.5 to 5 cm) above the bend in the elbow. Most cuffs are labeled with arrows indicating the center of the bladder for the right and left arms.
Principle. A well-extended arm allows easier palpation of the brachial pulse. Centering the inner bladder above the pulse site allows complete compression of the brachial artery. The cuff should be placed high enough above the bend in the elbow to prevent the diaphragm of the stethoscope from touching it; otherwise, extraneous sounds may be picked up which could interfere with an accurate measurement,

PROCEDURE 19.9 Measuring Blood Pressure: Manual Method—cont'd

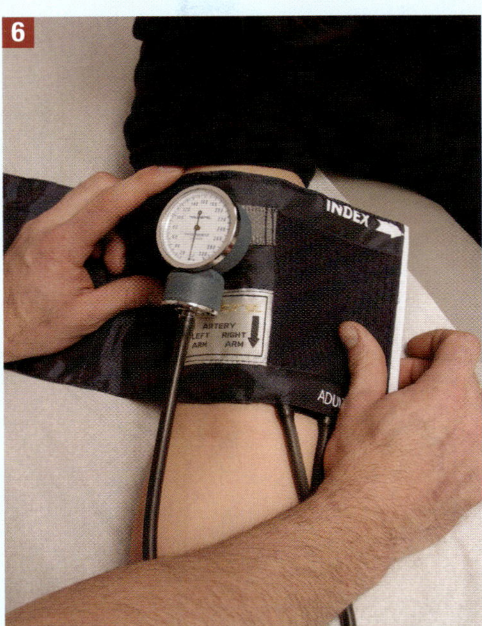

Center the inner bladder above the brachial pulse site.

7. **Procedural Step.** Wrap the cuff smoothly and snugly around the patient's arm and secure the end of it. The cuff should be snug but not too tight. To assess the appropriate tightness of the cuff, one finger should slip easily under the cuff. Position the manometer for direct viewing and at a distance of no more than 3 feet.
   Principle. Applying the cuff properly facilitates the application of equal pressure over the brachial artery. The medical assistant may have trouble seeing the scale on the manometer if it is placed more than 3 feet away.
8. **Procedural Step**. Determine how high to pump the cuff by checking the patient's medical record for the previously measured systolic reading or determine the patient's systolic pressure by palpation (see Procedure 19.10).
9. **Procedural Step.** Instruct the patient to relax as much as possible and not to talk or move during the procedure. Place the earpieces of the stethoscope in your ears, with the earpieces directed slightly forward. During the blood pressure measurement, the tubing of the stethoscope should hang freely and should not be permitted to rub against any object.
   Principle. Patient talking or movement can result in a falsely high reading. The earpieces should be directed forward, permitting them to follow the direction of the ear canal, which facilitates hearing. If the stethoscope tubing rubs against an object, extraneous sounds may be picked up which could interfere with an accurate measurement.
10. **Procedural Step.** Locate the brachial pulse again and place the diaphragm of the stethoscope over the brachial pulse site. The diaphragm should be positioned to make a tight seal against the patient's skin. Do not allow the diaphragm to touch the cuff.
    Principle. Proper positioning of the diaphragm and good contact of the diaphragm with the skin help transmit clear and audible Korotkoff sounds through the earpieces of the stethoscope to ensure an accurate measurement.

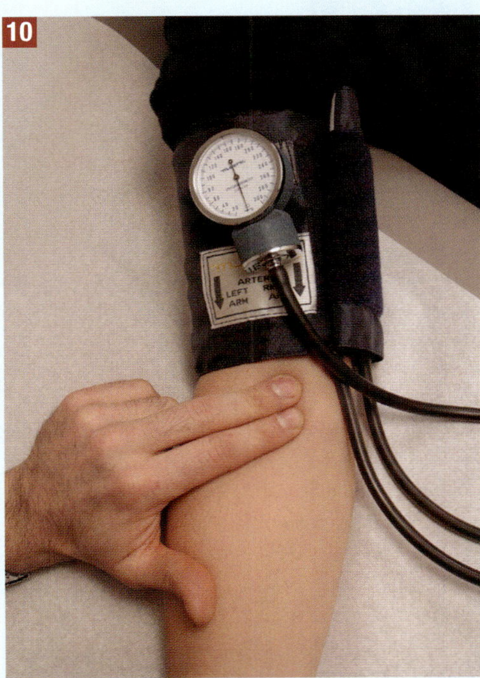

Locate the brachial pulse again before placing the diaphragm over the site.

11. **Procedural Step.** Close the control valve on the bulb by turning the thumbscrew clockwise (to the right) with the thumb and forefinger of your dominant hand until it feels tight but can still be loosened when you need to deflate the cuff. Pump air into the cuff as rapidly as possible to approximately 30 mmHg above the previously measured or palpated systolic pressure. Do not overinflate the cuff.
    Principle. Inflation of the cuff compresses and closes off the brachial artery so that no blood flows through the artery. Overinflation of the cuff is uncomfortable for the patient and may result in a falsely high blood pressure reading.

Continued

PROCEDURE 19.9

PROCEDURE 19.9 Measuring Blood Pressure: Manual Method—cont'd

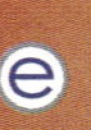

11

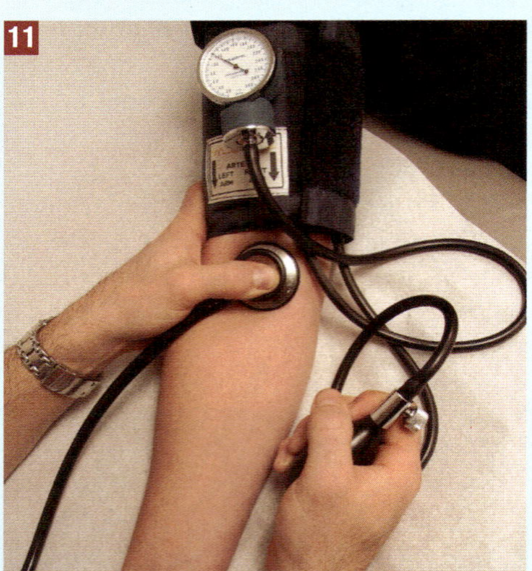

Pump air into the cuff as rapidly as possible.

12. Procedural Step. Release the pressure at a moderately steady rate of 2 to 3 mmHg/sec by slowly turning the thumbscrew counterclockwise (to the left) with the thumb and forefinger. This opens the control valve and allows the air in the cuff to escape slowly. Listen for the first clear tapping sound (phase I of the Korotkoff sounds). This represents the systolic pressure. Note this point on the scale of the gauge.
Principle. Releasing the pressure too slowly is uncomfortable for the patient and could cause a falsely high diastolic reading. Releasing the pressure too quickly could cause a falsely low systolic reading and a falsely high diastolic reading.

12

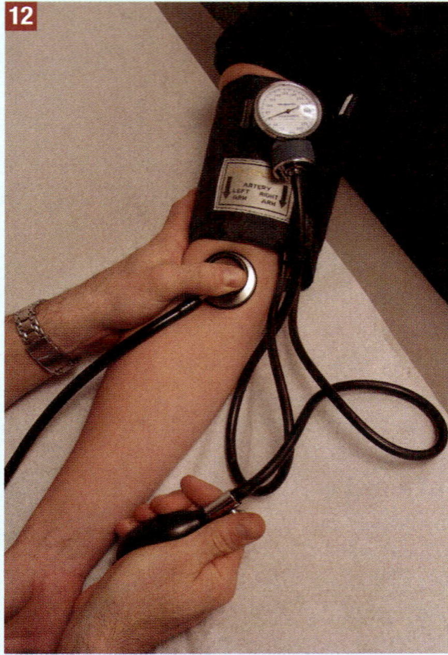

Release the pressure at a moderately steady rate.

13. Procedural Step. Continue to deflate the cuff while listening to the Korotkoff sounds. Listen for the onset of the muffled sound that occurs during phase IV. Continue to deflate the cuff and note the point on the scale of the gauge at which the sound ceases (phase V). This represents the diastolic pressure. Continue to steadily deflate the cuff for another 10 mmHg to ensure that there are no more sounds. Quickly and completely deflate the cuff to zero.

14. Procedural Step. If you are taking two or more blood pressure readings or if you could not obtain an accurate blood pressure reading, wait 1 to 2 minutes before taking another measurement from the same arm.
Principle. Waiting 1 to 2 minutes allows the blood flow in the brachial artery to return to normal.

15. Procedural Step. Remove the earpieces of the stethoscope from your ears, and carefully remove the cuff from the patient's arm.

16. Procedural Step. Sanitize your hands.

17. Procedural Step. Calculate an average of the readings if two or more blood pressure readings were taken. Document the results in the patient's medical record.

a. *Electronic health record:* In SimChart for the Medical Office, enter the blood pressure reading, which arm was used, and what position the patient was in when the blood pressure was taken using textboxes, drop-down menus, and/or radio buttons.

b. *Paper-based patient record:* Document the date, the time, and the blood pressure reading. Make a notation in the patient's medical record if the lying or standing position was used to take blood pressure. Abbreviations that can be used are *L* (lying) and *St* (standing).

17b DOCUMENTATION EXAMPLE

Date	
10/20/XX	2:30 p.m. BP: 106/74.—S. Martinez, RMA

18. Procedural Step. Clean the earpieces and the chest piece of the stethoscope with an antiseptic wipe.

PROCEDURE 19.10 Determining Systolic Pressure by Palpation

Outcome Determine systolic pressure by palpation.

Equipment/Supplies

- Sphygmomanometer

1. **Procedural Step.** Sanitize your hands and assemble the equipment.
2. **Procedural Step.** Locate the brachial pulse with the fingertips. Place the cuff on the patient's arm so that the inner bladder is centered over the brachial pulse site.
3. **Procedural Step.** Wrap the cuff smoothly and snugly around the patient's arm and secure the end of it.
4. **Procedural Step.** Position the manometer for direct viewing and at a distance of no more than 3 feet.
5. **Procedural Step.** Locate the radial pulse with your fingertips.
6. **Procedural Step.** Close the valve on the bulb, and pump air into the cuff until the pulsation ceases.
7. **Procedural Step.** Release the valve at a moderate rate of 2 to 3 mmHg per heartbeat while palpating the artery with your fingertips.
8. **Procedural Step.** Document the point at which the pulsation reappears as the palpated systolic pressure.
9. **Procedural Step.** Deflate the cuff completely and wait 15 to 30 seconds before taking the patient's blood pressure.

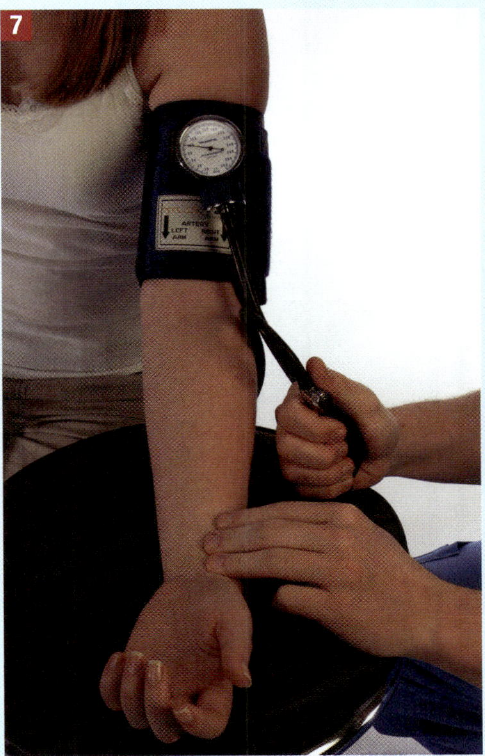

Release the valve while palpating the radial artery.

PROCEDURE 19.11 Measuring Blood Pressure: Automatic Method

Outcome Measure blood pressure using the automatic method.

Equipment/Supplies

- Automatic blood pressure monitor

1. **Procedural Step.** Sanitize your hands and assemble the equipment. Connect the air tube to the monitor by plugging the air plug into the air jack on the monitor.
2. **Procedural Step.** Greet the patient and introduce yourself. Identify the patient and explain the procedure. Ask the patient to empty the bladder. Observe and question the patient for factors that might influence the blood pressure reading (e.g., emotional states, physical activity). If it is not possible to reduce or eliminate these factors, document them in the patient's medical record.
3. **Procedural Step.** Instruct the patient sit quietly in a comfortable position with the legs uncrossed at the knees and the feet flat on the floor. The patient should be allowed to relax in a sitting position for at least 5 minutes before the blood pressure measurement.
4. **Procedural Step:** Using the left arm, roll up the patient's sleeve approximately 5 inches above the elbow so that the cuff can be applied to bare skin. If the sleeve does not roll up or is too tight after being rolled up, remove the arm from the sleeve. The arm should be positioned

Continued

PROCEDURE 19.11 Measuring Blood Pressure: Automatic Method—cont'd

at heart level and well supported on a flat surface, with the palm facing upward.

5. **Procedural Step.** Determine the correct cuff size.
6. **Procedural Step.** Make sure the arm is well extended; locate the brachial pulse with the index and middle fingertips. The brachial pulse is located near the center of the antecubital space but slightly toward the little finger–side of the arm. Position the lower edge of the cuff approximately 1 inch (2.5 cm) above the bend in the elbow with the artery position indicator (consisting of a stripe or an arrow) placed above the brachial pulse site.

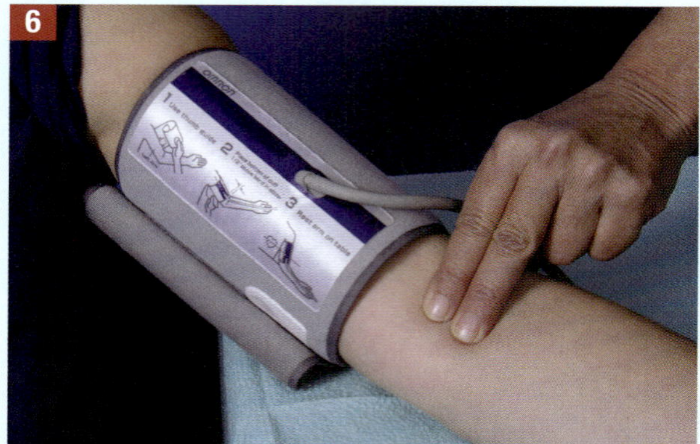

Place the artery position indicator above the brachial pulse site.

7. **Procedural Step.** Wrap the cuff smoothly and snugly around the patient's arm and secure the end of it. The cuff should be snug but not too tight. To assess the appropriate tightness of the cuff, one finger should slip easily under the cuff. Position the display screen for direct viewing and at a distance of no more than 3 feet.

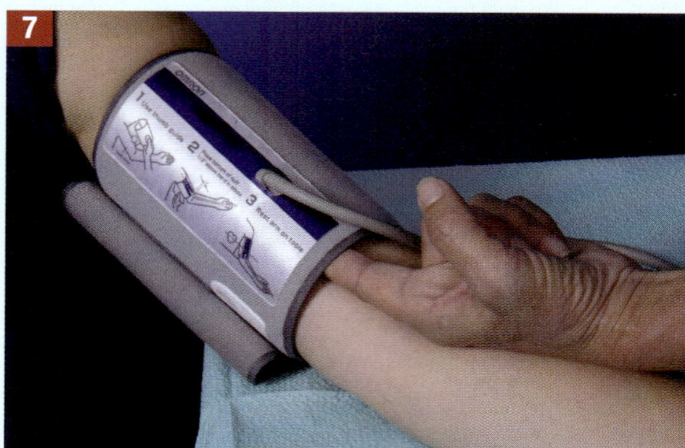

One finger should slip easily under the cuff.

8. **Procedural Step.** Instruct the patient to relax as much as possible and not to talk or move during the procedure. Make sure the patient's arm does not rest on the air tube

   Principle. Talking or moving can result in an error message on the display screen indicating the monitor was unable to obtain a reading. The patient's arm resting on the air tube restricts the flow of air to the cuff.
9. **Procedural Step.** Press the START/STOP button. All symbols temporarily appear on the display screen followed by the automatic inflation of the cuff. The monitor determines how much the cuff should be inflated to reach a pressure that is approximately 30 mmHg above the systolic pressure. Once the electronic pressure sensor has detected the patient's blood pressure reading and pulse rate, the cuff automatically deflates. As the cuff deflates, decreasing numbers appear on the display screen.
10. **Procedural Step.** Following deflation of the cuff, the systolic and diastolic pressures and the pulse rate appear on the display screen. The systolic BP reading on this monitor is 121 and the diastolic BP reading is 76. The pulse rate is 72. Make a mental note of the readings and press the START/STOP button to turn off the monitor.

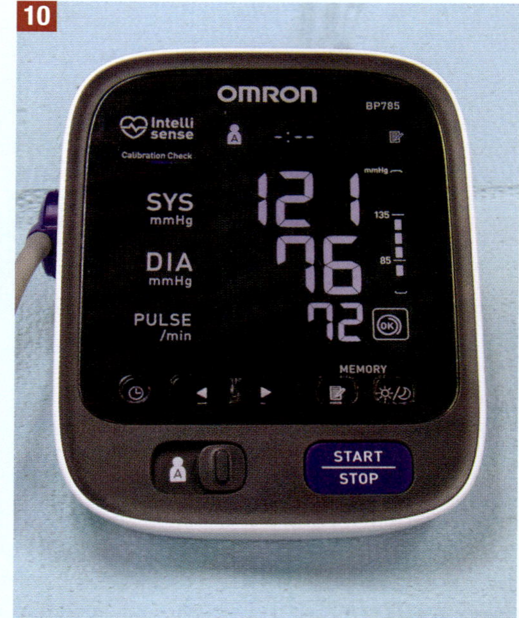

The readings appear on the display screen.

PROCEDURE 19.11

PROCEDURE 19.11 Measuring Blood Pressure: Automatic Method—cont'd

11. **Procedural Step.** Sanitize your hands.
12. **Procedural Step.** Document the results in the patient's medical record.
    a. *Electronic health record:* In SimChart for the Medical Office, enter the blood pressure results including the systolic and diastolic readings, which arm was used, and what position the patient was in when the blood pressure was taken using textboxes, drop-down menus, and/or radio buttons. Also enter the pulse rate.
    b. *Paper-based patient record:* Document the date, the time, and the blood pressure results including the systolic and diastolic readings. Make a notation in the patient's medical record if the lying or standing position was used to take blood pressure. Abbreviations that can be used are *L* (lying) and *St* (standing). Also document the pulse rate.

12b

PPR Documentation Example

Date	
10/20/xx	2:30 p.m. BP: 121/76. Pulse: 72. ______
	______ S. Martinez, RMA

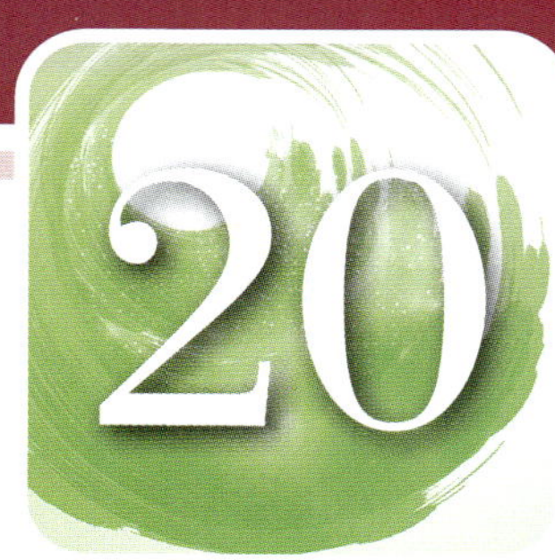

The Physical Examination

Check out the Evolve site at http://evolve.elsevier.com/Bonewit/today to access additional interactive activities and exercises to help you study and prepare for success.

LEARNING OBJECTIVES

Preparation for the Physical Examination

1. Identify the three components of a complete patient examination.
2. List the guidelines that should be followed in preparing the examining room.
3. Identify equipment and instruments used during the physical examination.

Measuring Weight and Height

4. Explain the purpose of measuring weight and height.
5. List the guidelines that should be followed when measuring weight and height.

Body Mechanics

6. Explain the benefits of proper body mechanics.
7. Identify the basic principles that should be followed related to body mechanics.

Positioning and Draping

8. Explain the purposes of positioning and draping.
9. List one use of each patient position.

Wheelchair Transfer

10. Explain the purpose of a wheelchair.
11. Describe the purpose of a transfer belt.

Assessment of the Patient

12. List and define the four techniques of examining the patient.
13. State an example of the use of each examination technique.

Assisting the Provider

14. Describe the responsibilities of the medical assistant during the physical examination.

PROCEDURES

Prepare the examining room.

Operate and care for items used during the physical examination, according to the manufacturers' instructions.

Prepare a patient for a physical examination.

Measure weight and height.

Demonstrate proper body mechanics when standing, sitting, and lifting an object.

Position and drape a patient in each of the following positions:

- Sitting
- Supine
- Prone
- Dorsal recumbent
- Lithotomy
- Modified left lateral recumbent
- Knee–chest
- Fowler

Transfer a patient from a wheelchair to the examining table and back again.

Assist the provider during a physical examination

CHAPTER OUTLINE

KEY TERMS

acute illness
audiometer
auscultation (os-kul-TAY-shun)
body mechanics
chronic illness
clinical diagnosis
diagnosis
differential (diff-er-EN-shul) diagnosis
inspection
mensuration (men-soo-RAY-shun)
palpation (pal-PAY-shun)
percussion (per-KUSH-un)
prognosis
risk factor
screening test
symptom

INTRODUCTION TO THE PHYSICAL EXAMINATION

A complete patient examination consists of three parts: the *health history*, the *physical examination* of each body system, and *laboratory and diagnostic tests.* The provider uses the results to determine the patient's general state of health, to arrive at a diagnosis and prescribe treatment, and to observe any change in a patient's illness after treatment has been instituted.

An important and frequent responsibility of the medical assistant is to assist with a physical examination. Because health-promotion and disease-prevention activities have become an important focus of health care, individuals are becoming more aware of the need for a yearly physical examination to detect early signs of disease and to prevent serious health problems. Also, a physical examination may be a prerequisite for employment, participation in sports, attendance at summer camp, and admission to school. The physical examination is explained in detail in this chapter. Taking the health history, collecting specimens, and performing laboratory and diagnostic tests are discussed in other chapters.

DEFINITIONS OF TERMS

The medical assistant should know and understand the following terms related to the patient examination.

Final diagnosis. Often simply called the **diagnosis**, this term refers to the scientific method of determining and identifying a patient's condition through evaluation of the health history, the physical examination, laboratory tests, and diagnostic procedures. A final diagnosis is crucial because it provides a logical basis for treatment and prognosis.

Clinical diagnosis. The clinical diagnosis is an intermediate step in the determination of a final diagnosis. The clinical diagnosis of a patient's condition is a tenative diagnosis obtained through evaluation of the health history and the physical examination without the benefit of laboratory or diagnostic tests. Laboratory and diagnostic imaging facilities usually require that the clinical diagnosis be entered on request forms; this information assists the facility in correlating data from their test results with the provider's needs. When the provider has analyzed the test results, a final diagnosis can often be established.

Differential diagnosis. Two or more diseases may have similar symptoms. A **symptom** is any change in the body or its functioning that indicates a disease might be present. The differential diagnosis involves determining which of these diseases is producing the patient's symptoms so that a final diagnosis can be established. For example, streptococcal sore throat and pharyngitis have similar symptoms. A differential diagnosis is made by collecting a throat specimen and performing a strep test.

Prognosis. The prognosis consists of the probable course and outcome of a patient's condition and the patient's prospects for recovery.

Risk factor. A risk factor is a physical or behavioral condition that increases the probability that an individual will develop a particular condition; examples are genetic factors, habits, environmental conditions, and physiologic

HIGHLIGHT on Health Screening for Adults

The chance of developing certain diseases is greater at different ages. Periodic health screening is recommended for the detection and early treatment of disease.

Test or Procedure	Gender	Recommended Frequency (for Individuals of Average Risk)
Blood pressure	M and F	Every year beginning at age 3.
Cholesterol levels	M and F	Every 4 to 6 years beginning at age 20.
Cervical cancer screening	F	Every 3 years with a Pap test beginning at age 21 until age 29. Beginning at age 30, preferred screening includes a Pap test and an HPV test every 5 years until age 65.
Blood glucose level	M and F	Every 3 years beginning at age 45.
Testicular self-examination	M	Every month beginning at age 15.
Fecal occult blood test	M and F	Every year beginning at age 45.
Colonoscopy	M and F	Every 10 years beginning at age 45.
Prostate cancer screening	M	Should be offered by a health provider every year beginning at age 50 to men with a life expectancy of at least 10 years.
Chlamydia and gonorrhea	F	Every year for all sexually active women age 25 and younger.
Mammography	F	Women between 40 and 44 years of age should have the choice to start annual breast cancer screening with mammograms if they wish to do so. Women between 45 to 54 years of age should undergo a mammogram every year. Women 55 years of age and older should switch to a mammogram every two years, or choose to continue yearly screening.
Electrocardiogram	M and F	One baseline recording starting at age 40.

conditions. The presence of a risk factor for a certain disease does not mean that the disease will develop; it means only that a person's chances of developing that disease are greater than those of a person without the risk factor. For example, cigarette smoking is a risk factor for developing lung cancer and heart disease. A person who smokes has a higher risk of developing lung cancer than a person who does not smoke or who has stopped smoking.

Screening test. A test performed on a large number of individuals (apparently in good health) for the early detection of a condition before it causes symptoms. Refer to *Highlight on Health Screening* for an outline of screening guidelines for common tests and procedures.

Acute illness. An acute illness is characterized by symptoms that have a sudden and rapid onset, are usually severe and intense, and subside after a relatively short time (6 months or less). They are often caused by viruses and bacteria but can also be caused by injuries or the misuse of drugs. Acute illnesses are usually treatable, or they may go away on their own. Examples of acute illness include the common cold, influenza, strep throat, pneumonia, and broken bones.

Chronic illness. A chronic illness is characterized by symptoms that persist for longer than 6 months and show little change or may worsen over time. Chronic illnesses have a slow progression and last for months, years or even a lifetime. As people get older, they are more likely to develop chronic illnesses. Chronic illnesses cannot usually be cured but they are often manageable. Examples of chronic illnesses include heart disease, diabetes mellitus, hypertension, emphysema, and arthritis.

Therapeutic procedure. A therapeutic procedure is performed to treat a patient's condition with the goal of eliminating it or promoting as much recovery as possible. Examples of therapeutic procedures include administration of medication, ear and eye irrigations, and application of heat and cold.

Laboratory testing. A laboratory test is the clinical analysis and study of a body substance to obtain objective data for the diagnosis, treatment, and management of a patient's condition. Examples of laboratory tests include the hemoglobin test, glucose test, urinalysis, and strep test.

Diagnostic procedure. A diagnostic procedure is a procedure performed to assist in the diagnosis of a patient's condition; examples include electrocardiography, colonoscopy, and mammography.

PREPARATION OF THE EXAMINING ROOM

Proper preparation of the examining room provides a comfortable and healthy environment for the patient and facilitates the physical examination. The following guidelines should be followed in preparing the examining room:

1. Ensure that the examining room is free of clutter and well lit.
2. Check the examining rooms daily to ensure there are ample supplies. Restock supplies that are getting low.
3. Empty waste receptacles frequently.
4. Replace biohazard containers as necessary. When removing biohazard containers from the examining

room (see Chapter 17), follow the OSHA Bloodborne Pathogens Standard.
5. Make sure the room is well ventilated, and install an air freshener to eliminate odors.
6. Maintain room temperatures that are comfortable not only for a fully clothed individual, but also for an individual who has disrobed.
7. Clean and disinfect examining tables, countertops, faucets, and door handles daily.
8. Remove dust and dirt from furniture.
9. Change the examining table paper after each patient by unrolling a fresh length. Check to ensure there is an ample supply of gowns and drapes ready for use.
10. Ensure that the examining room door is closed during the examination to protect patient privacy.
11. Properly clean and prepare equipment, instruments, and supplies used for patient examination. Table 20.1 lists the equipment and supplies, along with their uses, that may be employed during a physical examination.
12. Check equipment and instruments regularly to verify that they are in proper working condition to protect the patient from harm caused by faulty equipment.
13. Make sure equipment and supplies are ready for the examination and arranged for easy access by the provider. Equipment and supplies needed for the physical examination vary according to the type of examination and the provider's preference (Fig. 20.1).
14. Properly operate and care for each piece of equipment and each instrument. The manufacturer provides an operating manual, which should be read carefully and kept available for reference.

PREPARATION OF THE PATIENT

It is the medical assistant's responsibility to prepare the patient for the physical examination. After greeting and escorting the patient to the examining room, the medical assistant should identify the patient by asking the patient to state their full legal name and date of birth. This information should be compared with the demographic data indicated in the patient's medical record. The patient should *not* be asked whether he or she is a certain patient. For example, the patient should not be asked: "Are you Mary Williams?"

Table 20.1 Equipment and Supplies for the Physical Examination

Item	Description and Purpose
Patient examination gown	Gown made of disposable paper or cloth that provides patient modesty, comfort, and warmth.
Drape	A length of disposable paper or cloth to cover a patient or parts of a patient to provide comfort and warmth and reduce exposure.
Sphygmomanometer	Instrument used to measure blood pressure.
Stethoscope	Instrument used to auscultate body sounds, such as blood pressure and lung and bowel sounds.
Thermometer	Instrument used to measure body temperature.
Upright balance scale	Device used to measure weight and height.
Otoscope	Lighted instrument with lens, used to examine external ear canal and tympanic membrane.
Tuning fork	Small metal instrument consisting of stem and two prongs, used to test hearing acuity.
Ophthalmoscope	Lighted instrument with lens, used for examining interior of eye.
Tongue depressor	Flat wooden blade used to depress patient's tongue during examination of mouth and pharynx.
Antiseptic wipe	Disposable pad saturated with antiseptic, such as alcohol, that is used to cleanse skin.
Tape measure	Flexible device calibrated in inches on one side and centimeters on the other side, used to measure patient (e.g., diameter of limb, head circumference).
Percussion hammer	Instrument with rubber head, used for testing neurologic reflexes.
Speculum	Instrument for opening body orifice or cavity for viewing (e.g., ear speculum, nasal speculum, vaginal speculum).
Disposable gloves	Gloves, usually latex, that are worn only once to provide protection from bloodborne pathogens and other potentially infectious materials.
Lubricant	Agent that is applied to provider's gloved hand or to speculum that reduces friction between parts to make insertion easier.
Specimen container	Container in which body specimen is placed for transport to laboratory (after it has been labeled).
Tissues	Used for wiping body secretions.
Cotton-tipped applicator	Small piece of cotton wrapped around the end of a slender wooden stick, used for collection of a specimen from the body.
Overhead examination light	Light mounted on flexible movable stand to focus light on area for good visibility.
Basin	Container in which used instruments are deposited.
Biohazard container	Specially made container used for receiving items that contain infectious waste.
Waste receptacle	Container for used disposable articles that do not contain infectious waste.

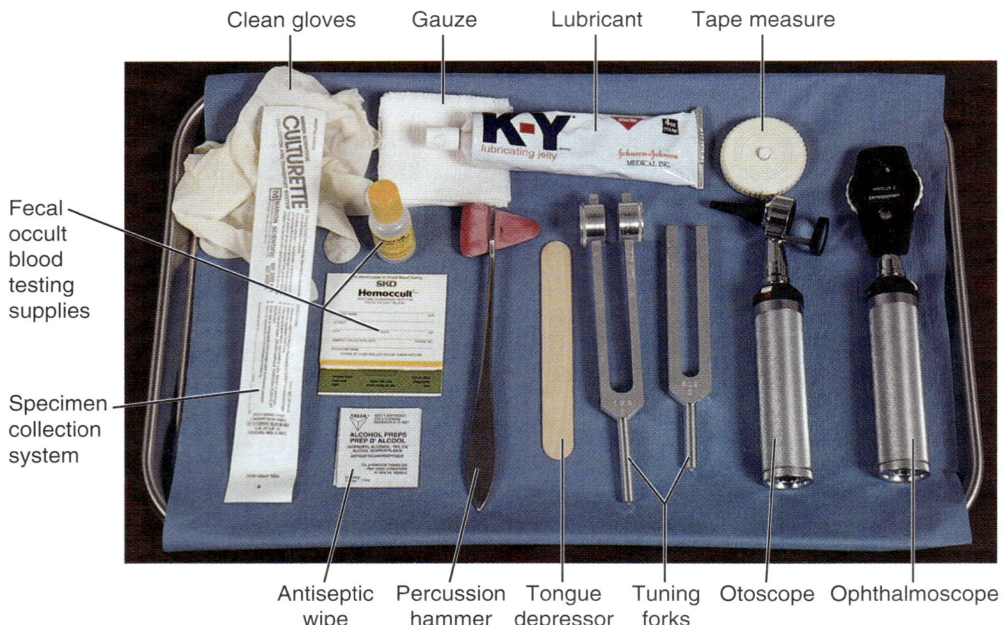

Fig. 20.1 Instruments and supplies used during the physical examination.

The patient may not hear the medical assistant correctly or may not be paying attention and may answer in the affirmative even if they are not that patient. Proper identification is essential to avoid mistaking one patient for another. If the medical assistant performs a procedure on the wrong patient by mistake, he or she could be held liable. The medical assistant then takes vital signs and measures the weight and height of the patient. The results of these procedures are documented in the patient's medical record.

The medical assistant can reduce a patient's apprehension by addressing the patient by their name of choice, by adopting a friendly and supportive attitude, and by speaking clearly, distinctly, and slowly. The medical assistant should explain the purpose of the examination and offer to answer any questions.

The patient should be asked whether they need to void before the examination. An empty bladder makes the examination easier and is more comfortable for the patient. If a urine specimen is needed, the patient is asked to void.

Instructions on disrobing for the examination should be specific so that the patient understands what items of clothing to remove and where to place the clothing. The disrobing area should be comfortable and should provide privacy. It is helpful to have a place for the patient to sit to make it easier to remove clothing and shoes. The area also should be equipped with hooks for hanging clothing. Instructions for putting on the examination gown and for locating the gown opening reduce patient confusion. If the medical assistant senses that the patient will have trouble undressing, assistance should be offered. Elderly and disabled patients sometimes have difficulty removing clothing.

The physical examination is performed with the patient positioned on an examining table, which is specially constructed to facilitate the examination. For safety, it is advisable to help the patient onto and off of the examining table.

HIGHLIGHT on Patient Coaching

The purpose of patient coaching is to help the patient develop habits, attitudes, and skills that enable the individual to maintain and improve his or her own health.

Fact: Patients who are active, informed participants in their health care are more apt to follow the provider's instructions than patients who are passive recipients of medical services.

Action: Provide patients with information on health care. Every patient interaction is an opportunity for teaching.

Fact: Adult learners are goal oriented and performance centered. They need and want information that would assist them in managing and improving their health.

Action: Review the information that you provide to patients, and determine whether it is nice to know or necessary to know. Select subject matter that is practical and useful and relates directly to the patient's needs.

Fact: The more information that is presented, the more the patient is likely to forget. Approximately one half of information presented to the patient is forgotten in the first 5 minutes after the patient receives it.

Action: When teaching, use the following pointers to help patients learn and retain information:

- Keep it short and be specific.

HIGHLIGHT on Patient Coaching—cont'd

- Speak in terms the patient can understand.
- Focus on "how" rather than "why."
- Repeat and reinforce important information.
- Give practical examples, and provide ample time for patient practice.
- Ask for feedback from the patient to determine whether they understand the information.
- Provide the patient with written information.

Fact: Each individual has a distinct style of learning and learns best when using their preferred learning style. The three main learning styles are reading, listening, and doing. People often use more than one style for learning.

Action: Use a variety of teaching strategies to engage the various learning styles of patients. Examples of teaching strategies include explanations, printed handouts, audiovisual aids, demonstrations, and discussions.

Fact: Only two-thirds of patients comply with health care instructions prescribed by the provider. Factors that influence compliance include the patient's adaptation to illness, motivation to change, physical capability, and support systems.

Action: The following help increase patient compliance with prescribed treatment:

- Address the patient by their name of choice. (Keep in mind that some patients object to being called by their first name by strangers.)
- Encourage the patient to take an active role in personal health care.
- Help the patient set goals and objectives for change.
- Encourage care and support from family members.
- Make the patient aware of outside resources.
- Give positive reinforcement when the patient makes healthy changes.

Putting It All Into Practice

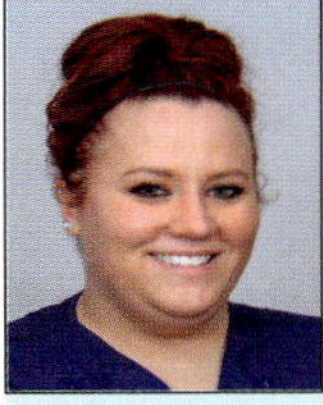

My name is Abby, and I am a certified medical assistant. I work in a medical clinic with a family medicine department of 10 physicians and 10 residents and interns. My duties cover a broad spectrum, from pediatrics to geriatrics, and include prenatal care, allergy injections, minor office surgery, electrocardiograms, colposcopies, immunizations, and wound care.

At our clinic, many of the patients are elderly. I occasionally come across geriatric patients who are not very cooperative and are "set in their ways." One 90-year-old woman, in particular, had a reputation in the office for being cantankerous and difficult to work with. One day when the physician ordered laboratory work on her, I prepared to draw blood from her tiny, frail body, praying that everything would go smoothly. As I helped her up after a successful "stick," she, of all people, reached to give me a hug and said to me, "I like you. That didn't even hurt!" She continued to hold my hand and talk to me as I walked her out of the office. This turned out to be the last time I would see her because she moved out of town, but not out of my heart, leaving a lasting impression on my life. ■

What Would You Do? What Would You *Not* Do?

Case Study 1

Evalyn Auden, 35 years old, is at the medical office. Her husband got a backyard trampoline for their two school-aged children, and she decided to try it out. Evalyn landed wrong on the trampoline and hurt her back and neck. For the past 5 days, she has been having headaches and back pain. Evalyn refuses to have her weight taken because she has gained weight over the past several years and does not want to know how much she's gained. She does not understand why weight has to be taken at an office visit in the first place. Evalyn says that many times when she should go to the doctor, she doesn't, just to avoid being weighed. She says she would not even be here now except that her husband insisted that she come. ■

MEASURING WEIGHT AND HEIGHT

The medical assistant routinely measures the weight and height of many types of patients. The process of measuring the patient is known as **mensuration.** A change in weight may be significant in the diagnosis of a patient's condition and in prescribing the course of treatment. Underweight and overweight patients who follow a diet therapy program should be weighed at regular intervals to determine their progress. Prenatal patients are weighed during each prenatal visit to assist in the assessment of fetal development and of the mother's health.

An adult's weight usually is measured during each office visit; an adult's height is typically measured only during the first visit or when a complete physical examination of the patient is requested. Children are weighed and their height (or length) is measured during each office visit to observe their pattern of growth, identify nutritional problems, and determine medication dosage.

TYPES OF SCALES

There are two types of scales commonly used in the medical office. These include the *balance beam scale* and the *electronic digital scale.* A balance beam scale uses sliding weights that are manually moved on horizontal calibration bars to measure the patient's weight. The patient's height is measured using a sliding vertical calibration rod with a measuring (headpiece) bar. Balance beam scales are quite accurate and do not require a power source. It is important, however, that the medical assistant interpret the calibration markings correctly when measuring weight and height to prevent an error in the measurements. Specific guidelines for using a balance beam scale are presented in Box 20.1. Procedure 20.1 outlines the procedure for measuring height and weight using a balance beam scale.

BOX 20.1 Guidelines for Using a Balance Beam Scale

When using an upright balance scale to measure weight and height, use the following guidelines.

Weight

1. *Locate the scale to provide privacy for the patient.* Place the scale on a hard, level surface in a private location. Many patients are self-conscious about having their weight measured and prefer that it be done in privacy. Do not make weight-sensitive comments during the procedure. This is especially important for patients with eating disorders such as compulsive overeating and anorexia.
2. *Balance the scale before measuring weight.* If the scale is not balanced, the weight measurement will be inaccurate. The scale is balanced when the upper and lower weights are on zero and the indicator point comes to a rest in the center of the balance area.
3. *Ensure an accurate weight measurement.* Always ask the patient to remove their shoes. Measure weight with the patient in normal clothing. Ask the patient to remove heavy outer clothing, such as a sweater or a jacket.
4. *Assist the patient.* Assist the patient onto and off of the scale platform. The scale platform moves slightly and may cause the patient to become unsteady.
5. *Interpret the calibration markings accurately.* The lower calibration bar is divided into 50-lb increments (Fig. 20.2A). The upper calibration bar is divided into pounds and quarter pounds. The longer calibration lines indicate pound increments, and the shorter calibration lines indicate quarter-pound and half-pound increments (Fig. 20.2B).
6. *Determine the patient's weight and document the measurement correctly.* Add the measurement on the lower scale to the measurement on the upper scale. The result should be rounded to the nearest quarter pound. Occasionally the patient's weight may need to be converted to kilograms, which is the metric unit of measurement for weight. This may be required when determining medication dosage. The following formulas are used to convert weight measurements from one system to another.

Weight Conversion

Pounds to kilograms: Divide the number of pounds by 2.2:

$136 \text{ lb} \div 2.2 = 61.8 \text{ kg}$

Kilograms to pounds: Multiply the number of kilograms by 2.2:

$75 \text{ kg} \times 2.2 = 165 \text{ lb}$

Height

1. *Provide for the patient's safety.* Follow the proper procedure when measuring the patient's height. An error in technique could result in injury. If a patient is placed on the scale in a forward position, the measuring bar could fall into the patient's face when they step off of the scale, causing a facial injury.
2. *Interpret the calibration markings accurately.* Depending on the brand of scale, the calibration markings are divided into inches or feet and inches. (Fig. 20.3 is an example of a scale divided into feet and inches.) The calibration rod also is calibrated into centimeters, which is the metric unit of measurement for height. This unit of measurement is not typically used to measure height in the United States.
3. *Read the measurement correctly.* The height measurement is read from the top of the bar down and should be read to the nearest quarter inch. For most patients, you can read the height measurement at the junction of the stationary calibration rod and the movable calibration rod (Fig. 20.4A). If the patient's height is less than the top value of the stationary calibration rod, however, you must read the measurement from the bottom of the bar up directly on the stationary rod. (*Note:* The measuring bar must first be released (Fig. 20.4B) and moved down to the stationary bar.) The highest calibration on the stationary rod of most scales is 50 inches; therefore, patients with a height of 50 inches or less would have their height read directly from the stationary rod (Fig. 20.4C).
4. *Document the height measurement correctly.* Document the height measurement in feet and inches. If the scale is calibrated in inches, convert the reading to feet and inches by dividing the number of inches by 12. A height measurement of 60 inches is documented as 5 feet (60 inches $\div$ 12 = 5). If the patient's height measurement is 64 inches, the results would be documented as 5 feet, 4 inches.

An electronic scale (Fig. 20.5A) automatically measures a patient's weight and may also (automatically) measure a patient's height. The results are displayed digitally on a display screen (Fig. 20.5B). An electronic scale is able to determine a patient's body mass index (BMI) and display it on the screen of the scale (Fig.20-5C). It takes less time to measure weight and height with an electronic scale as compared to a balance beam scale. The weight and height measurements are considered accurate; however, they can sometimes be affected by temperature and humidity. An electronic scale requires a power supply (e.g., battery, AC adapter).

BODY MASS INDEX

The patient's weight and height are used to determine body mass index (BMI). The BMI strongly correlates with the total body fat content in adults and therefore is used as a screening tool to identify patients who may be at risk for health problems associated with being underweight, overweight or obese. Although BMI can be used as an indirect measurement of total body fat content for most adult men and women, it does have some limitations. It may overestimate body fat content in athletes and others who have a muscular build, and it may underestimate body fat content in older individuals who have lost muscle mass.

The BMI can be determined by comparing a patient's weight and height against a BMI table (Fig. 20.6). The BMI can also be determined through the use of a BMI calculator available as part of an electronic health record (EHR) program or an internet BMI-calculator website. For adults 20 years and older, BMI is then interpreted using weight status categories. Adult patients with a BMI

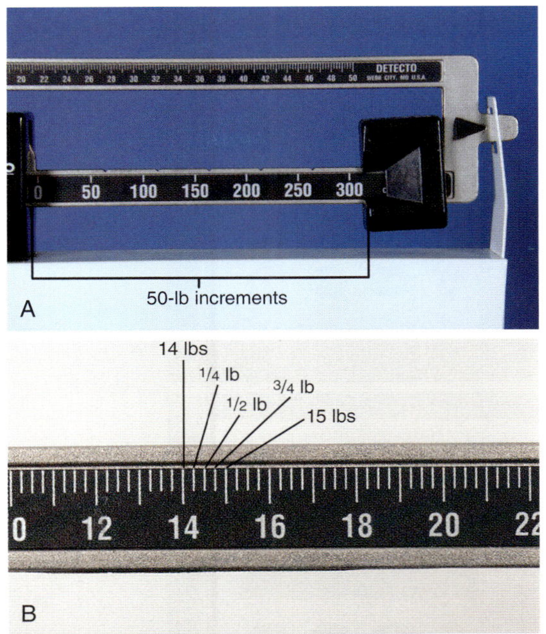

Fig. 20.2 Calibration markings for measuring weight. (A) Lower calibration bar. (B) Upper calibration bar.

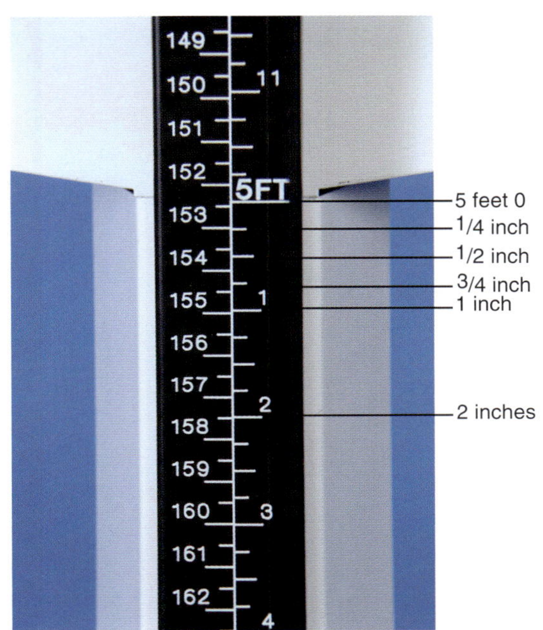

Fig. 20.3 Calibration markings for height.

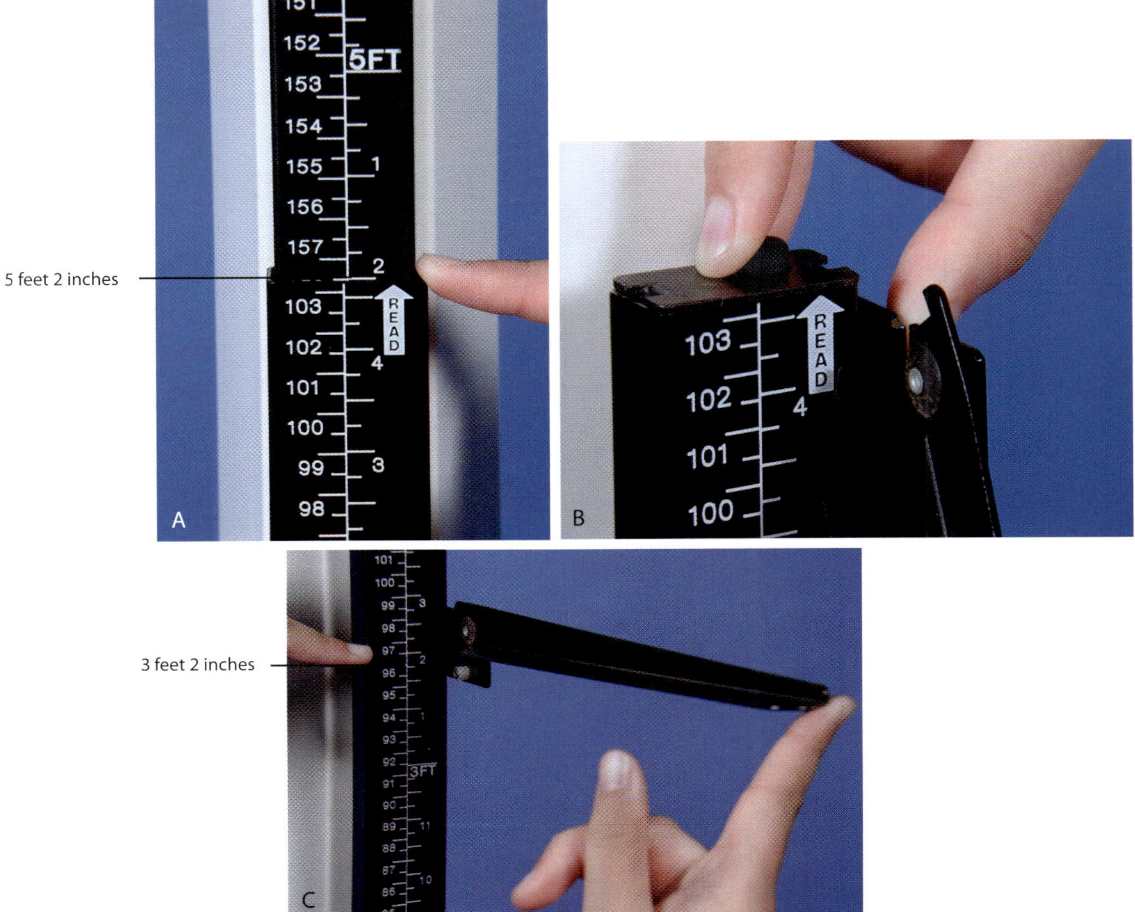

Fig. 20.4 (A) Reading a height measurement. The height measurement in this illustration is 6 feet, 1 inch. (B) Moving the measuring bar. (C) Reading a height measurement on the stationary calibration rod. The height measurement in this illustration is 3 feet, 2 inches.

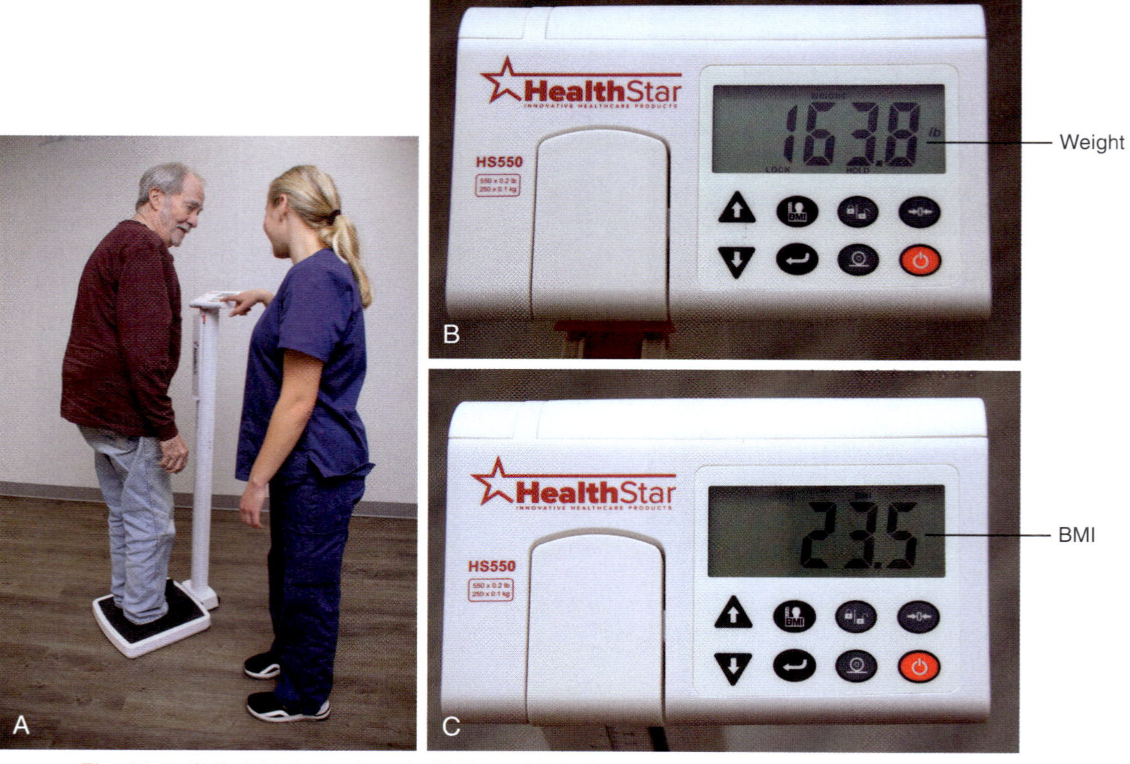

Fig. 20.5 (A) Upright electronic scale. (B) The weight is displayed on the screen of the scale (163.8 pounds). (C) The body mass index (BMI) is calculated using the weight and height measurements and displayed on the screen of the scale (BMI of 23.5).

between 18.5 and 24.9 are considered to be within normal weight. Table 20.2 outlines each of the BMI ranges and the corresponding weight status categories.

What Would You Do? What Would You *Not* Do?

Case Study 2

Karen Steiner drops her 17-year-old daughter, Mikayla, off at the medical office for her sports physical examination. Mikayla is captain of the varsity cheerleading squad and is getting ready to start her senior year in high school. Mikayla's vital signs are normal, and she measures 5 feet, 6 inches tall, weighs 105 pounds, and has a BMI of 16.9. With some reluctance, Mikayla admits that she's been having problems with heartburn, and she's pretty sure she knows what's causing it. She says that she has to keep her weight down for cheerleading, and after eating dinner with her family, she makes herself vomit to get rid of the food in her stomach. Mikayla is not too concerned about doing this because a lot of the popular girls at school are doing the same thing. She says it's the easy way to stay slim, and she would like to lose another 10 pounds before football season starts. Mikayla wants some prescription drug samples to help with the heartburn because the over-the-counter pills that she's been taking are not working anymore. She does not want her parents to know about any of this because she's afraid that they would not understand and might make her drop out of cheerleading. ■

BODY MECHANICS

Daily activities in a medical office sometimes carry the risk of acute or chronic musculoskeletal injury. Because of this, the medical assistant should have a thorough knowledge of the principles of proper body mechanics and know when to use them. **Body mechanics** is the use of the correct muscles to maintain proper balance, posture, and body alignment to accomplish a task safely and efficiently without undue strain on muscles or joints. Proper body mechanics should be used when the medical assistant performs the following: standing, walking, sitting, lifting, positioning a patient on the examining table, and transferring a patient. The medical assistant should also use proper body mechanics at home in their activities of daily living. Using proper body mechanics prevents musculoskeletal strains to the back and other body structures such as the knees, neck, shoulders, and wrists.

The primary benefits of proper body mechanics include the following:

1. Allows an individual to conserve energy, which makes it easier to perform a task
2. Protects the body from injury by reducing stress and strain on muscles, nerves, joints, tendons, ligaments, and soft tissues
3. Helps to maintain proper body control and balance
4. Promotes effective, efficient, and safe movement

Body Mass Index Table 1																
	Healthy Weight						Overweight					Class I Obesity				
BMI	19	20	21	22	23	24	25	26	27	28	29	30	31	32	33	34
Height							Body Weight (pounds)									
4' 10"	91	96	100	105	110	115	119	124	129	134	138	143	148	153	158	162
4' 11"	94	99	104	109	114	119	124	128	133	138	143	148	153	158	163	168
5' 0"	97	102	107	112	118	123	128	133	138	143	148	153	158	163	168	174
5' 1"	100	106	111	116	122	127	132	137	143	148	153	158	164	169	174	180
5' 2"	104	109	115	120	126	131	136	142	147	153	158	164	169	175	180	186
5' 3"	107	113	118	124	130	135	141	146	152	158	163	169	175	180	186	191
5' 4"	110	116	122	128	134	140	145	151	157	163	169	174	180	186	192	197
5' 5"	114	120	126	132	138	144	150	156	162	168	174	180	186	192	198	204
5' 6"	118	124	130	136	142	148	155	161	167	173	179	186	192	198	204	210
5' 7"	121	127	134	140	146	153	159	166	172	178	185	191	198	204	211	217
5' 8"	125	131	138	144	151	158	164	171	177	184	190	197	203	210	216	223
5' 9"	128	135	142	149	155	162	169	176	182	189	196	203	209	246	223	230
5' 10"	132	139	146	153	160	167	174	181	188	195	202	209	216	222	229	236
5' 11"	136	143	150	157	165	172	179	186	193	200	208	215	222	229	236	243
6' 0"	140	147	154	162	169	177	184	191	199	206	213	221	228	235	242	250
6' 1"	144	151	159	166	174	182	189	197	204	212	219	227	235	242	250	257
6' 2"	148	155	163	171	179	186	194	202	210	218	225	233	241	249	256	264
6' 3"	152	160	168	176	184	192	200	208	216	224	232	240	248	256	264	272
6' 4"	156	164	172	180	189	197	205	213	221	230	238	246	254	263	271	279

Body Mass Index Table 2																			
	Class II Obesity					Class III Obesity													
BMI	35	36	37	38	39	40	41	42	43	44	45	46	47	48	49	50	51	52	53
Height						Body Weight (pounds)													
4' 10"	167	172	177	181	186	191	196	201	205	210	215	220	224	229	234	239	244	248	253
4' 11"	173	178	183	188	193	198	203	208	212	217	222	227	232	237	242	247	252	257	262
5' 0"	179	184	189	194	199	204	209	215	220	225	230	235	240	245	250	255	261	266	271
5' 1"	185	190	195	201	206	211	217	222	227	232	238	243	248	254	259	264	269	275	280
5' 2"	191	196	202	207	213	218	224	229	235	240	246	251	256	262	267	273	278	284	289
5' 3"	197	203	208	214	220	225	231	237	242	248	254	259	265	270	278	282	287	293	299
5' 4"	204	209	215	221	227	232	238	244	250	256	262	267	273	279	285	291	296	302	308
5' 5"	210	216	222	228	234	240	246	252	258	264	270	276	282	288	294	300	306	312	318
5' 6"	216	223	229	235	241	247	253	260	266	272	278	284	291	297	303	309	315	322	328
5' 7"	223	230	236	242	249	255	261	268	274	280	287	293	299	306	312	319	325	331	338
5' 8"	230	236	243	249	256	262	269	276	282	289	295	302	308	315	322	328	335	341	348
5' 9"	236	243	250	257	263	270	277	284	291	297	304	311	318	324	331	338	345	351	358
5' 10"	243	250	257	264	271	278	285	292	299	306	313	320	327	334	341	348	355	362	369
5' 11"	240	257	265	272	279	286	293	301	308	315	322	329	338	343	351	358	365	372	379
6' 0"	258	265	272	279	287	294	302	309	316	324	331	338	346	353	361	368	375	383	390
6' 1"	265	272	280	288	295	302	310	318	325	333	340	348	355	363	371	378	386	393	401
6' 2"	272	280	287	295	303	311	319	326	334	342	350	358	365	373	381	389	396	404	412
6' 3"	279	287	295	303	311	319	327	335	343	351	359	367	375	383	391	399	407	415	423
6' 4"	289	295	304	312	320	328	336	344	353	361	369	377	385	394	402	410	418	126	435

Fig. 20.6 Body mass index (BMI) table. To use the table, find the appropriate height in the left-hand column labeled Height. Move across to a given weight (in pounds). The number at the top of the column is the BMI at that height and weight. Pounds have been rounded off. (Data from National Heart, Lung, and Blood Institute, U.S. Department of Health and Human Services.)

HIGHLIGHT on Cultural Diversity

Culture consists of the values, beliefs, and practices of a particular group of people. Culture is deeply rooted and is passed on from one generation to the next through communication. It includes areas such as religion, dietary practices, family lines of authority, family life patterns, beliefs, and health practices.

As the demographics of the United States continue to change, the medical assistant is faced with the challenge of providing care to an increasing number of cultural groups. It is important for the medical assistant to learn as much as possible about the cultural values of patients coming to the medical office. This is known as *cultural awareness* and can be accomplished by carefully observing and listening to patients to acquire knowledge of their cultural values.

Cultural sensitivity is respect and appreciation for cultural diversity, whereas *cultural competence* is understanding and using the cultural background of a patient to assist with the resolution of a problem. Because health practices are part of a patient's culture, changing them may have a negative impact on the patient. Whenever possible, the medical assistant should incorporate factors from a patient's cultural background into the patient' health care.

Guidelines for Achieving Cultural Competence

The following guidelines help the medical assistant in developing cultural awareness and sensitivity and in achieving cultural competence:

1. ***Respect the patient's values, beliefs, and practices.*** Even if you do not agree with them, it is important to respect the patient's right to hold these values and to not dismiss them as strange or odd. Cultural values play an important role in a patient's lifestyle. Patients from some cultures believe that losing blood depletes the body's strength and provides a route for the soul to leave the body. If a blood specimen is needed, these patients may become highly distressed or refuse to have their blood drawn. Members of some cultural groups believe that illness results when the body's natural balance or harmony is disturbed. To restore the balance, alternative forms of medicine, such as herbal remedies and aromatherapy, are used.
2. ***Refrain from cultural stereotypes.*** Not all people of a cultural group have the same beliefs, practices, and values. Assuming that all members of a cultural group are alike is known as *stereotyping* and should be avoided. Just as one would never assume that all people in the United States like hamburgers and baseball, every individual must be approached according to their specific beliefs and practices.
3. ***Address patients appropriately.*** Always address patients by their last names (and Mr., Mrs., Miss, Ms.) unless they give you permission to use other names. In many cultures, using a first name to address anyone other than family or friends is considered disrespectful. Some older people in the United States dislike being called by their first name and feel it shows a lack of respect.
4. **Speak slowly and clearly.** Communicating with a patient may be difficult if the patient has a limited knowledge of English. With these patients, you should speak slowly and clearly in a normal tone and volume of voice. Speaking loudly does not help the patient understand any better and is often offensive to the patient.
5. **Show respect for cultural lines of authority.** In many cultures, respect is given based on age and gender. In certain cultures, elders are considered the holders of the culture's wisdom and are highly respected. In other cultures, youth is valued over age. In certain cultures men dominate, and women have very little status. Because of this, a female patient from this type of culture may not be permitted to give her own health history or to answer questions. In addition, a male patient from this culture may not accept instructions from a female medical assistant.
6. ***Use appropriate eye contact.*** In most cultures, direct eye contact is important and in general shows that the other is attentive and listening. It conveys self-confidence, openness, interest, and honesty, whereas the lack of eye contact may be interpreted as secretiveness, shyness, guilt, or lack of interest. Other cultures consider eye contact impolite or an invasion of privacy; these patients show respect by avoiding direct eye contact.
7. ***Be aware of cultural responses to illness.*** The conditions under which an individual assumes the role of a (sick) patient and the way they perform in that role vary with culture. Individuals of some cultures resist the sick role and blame sickness on external forces as a means of punishment. These individuals may deny their illness and fail to provide much information when the medical assistant takes their symptoms. In other cultures, individuals take an optimistic view of the outcome of health care and because of this are more likely to offer information and to follow the provider's instructions.
8. ***Appreciate and celebrate diversity.*** Learn to appreciate the richness of diversity as an asset, rather than a hindrance to communication and effective interaction with patients.

Studies show that health care workers sustain a significantly higher incidence of back injuries compared with workers in other professions. To help prevent an injury to the back, a primary focus of proper body mechanics is to keep the natural curves of the spine or vertebral column in proper alignment. The vertebral column has four curvatures. These curvatures increase the strength and resilience of the vertebral column and include the cervical curvature, thoracic curvature, lumbar curvature, and sacral curvature (Fig. 20.7). The vertebral column extends from the skull to the pelvis and consists of a series of bones known as *vertebrae.* The vertebrae are separated by shock-absorbing *intervertebral discs* (see Fig. 20.7). These discs allow an individual to bend and twist. Over time, with improper and repeated bending and twisting (especially while carrying an object), the discs can deteriorate, which causes them to narrow, to harden, and even to crack and tear. This condition is known as *degenerative disc disease.* With degenerative disc disease, the discs lose their shock-absorbing ability and cause the patient to experience localized pain and stiffness

Table 20.2 Interpretation of Body Mass Index (BMI)

BMI	Weight Status Category
Less than 16	Severely underweight
16 to 16.9	Moderately underweight
17 to 18.49	Underweight
18.5-24.9	Healthy weight
25-29.9	Overweight
30-34.9	Obese Class I (Moderately obese)
35.0-39.9	Obese Class II (Severely obese)
40 or more	Obese Class III (Very severely obese)

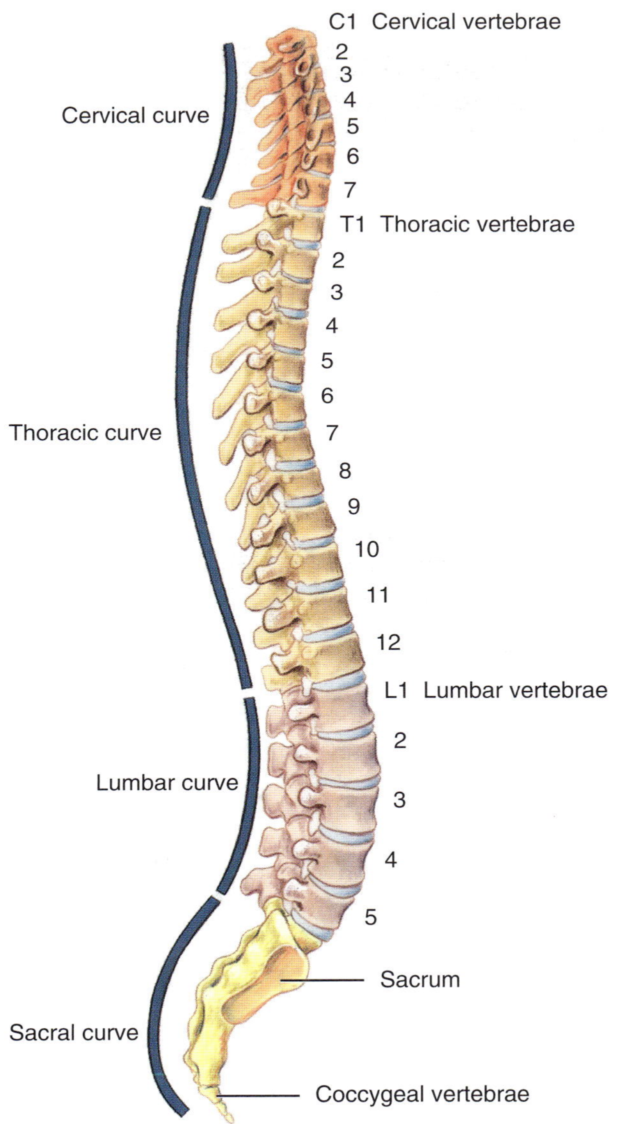

Fig. 20.7 Vertebral column. (From Applegate E: *The anatomy and physiology learning system*, ed 4, St. Louis, 2011, Saunders.)

in the area of disc deterioration. In addition, once a disc is weakened, it can bulge out or rupture; this is known as a *herniated disc.*

PRINCIPLES

There are some basic principles related to proper body mechanics that should be followed:

1. Movements should be smooth and coordinated rather than jerky.
2. Keeping the body in good physical condition through exercising, stretching, and weight training helps to prevent musculoskeletal injury.
3. To avoid straining the back, do not reach for something that is farther than 14 to 18 inches away.
4. Work at a comfortable height that avoids having to bend the neck or back forward to perform the task. People are usually most comfortable working at a height that falls between the waist and elbow levels.
5. If possible, push, pull, or slide an object rather than lifting it. This conserves energy and places less strain on the back.
6. Lighter items should be stored on higher shelves or cabinets, and heavier items should be stored at or below waist level.
7. When an object from an overhead shelf or cabinet needs to be retrieved, use a step stool or chair to come up to the level of the object. Reaching for a stored overhead item can produce strain on the back.
8. When lifting an object or transferring a patient, the large muscles of the arms and legs should be used as much as possible and the back muscles as little as possible. The more muscle groups that are used, the more evenly the weight is distributed over the medical assistant's body, which puts less strain on the back.
9. When transferring a patient, encourage the patient to assist as much as possible.
10. If a patient becomes dizzy or faint or starts to fall during the transfer, do not try to hold the patient in an upright position. Instead, balance yourself with your legs apart to form a wide base of support, and gently and gradually lower the patient to a chair or to the floor.
11. Always ask for assistance if you don't think you can lift a heavy object or transfer a patient.

APPLICATION OF BODY MECHANICS

The medical assistant should practice proper body mechanics when standing, sitting, lifting an object, positioning a patient on the examining table, and transferring a patient from a wheelchair to an examining table and back again, as outlined on the following pages.

Standing

It is important to maintain good posture by positioning the body in the correct standing position as outlined here. This

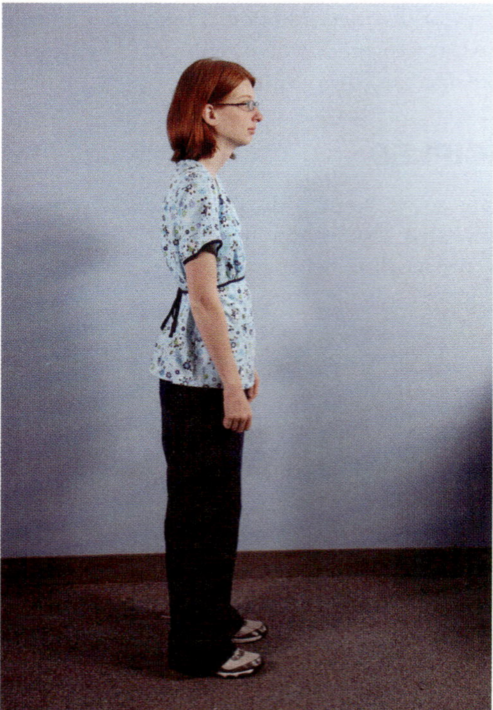

Fig. 20.8 Proper standing position.

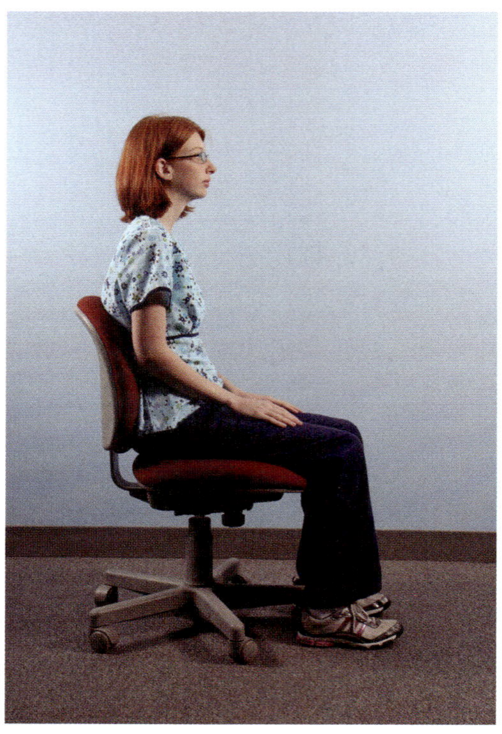

Fig. 20.9 Proper sitting position.

provides the medical assistant with good balance and stability and reduces strain on the back by keeping the vertebral column at its natural alignment.

1. Wear comfortable low-heeled shoes that provide good support.
2. Hold the head erect at the midline of the body, the back as straight as possible with the pelvis tucked inward, the chest forward with the shoulders back, and the abdomen drawn in and kept flat. This helps to maintain appropriate alignment of the vertebral column (Fig. 20.8).
3. The knees should be slightly flexed with the feet pointing forward and parallel to each other about 3 inches apart. This provides a broad base of support and improves balance.
4. The arms should be positioned comfortably at the side, and the weight of the body should be evenly distributed over both feet.

Sitting

The medical assistant should use proper body mechanics when in a sitting position (Fig. 20.9), as follows:

1. Sit in a chair with a firm back.
2. Sit firmly with the back and buttocks supported against the back of the chair; avoid slumping. The body weight should be evenly distributed over the buttocks and thighs.
3. Use a small pillow or a rolled towel to support the lower back.
4. The feet should be flat on the floor, and the knees should be level with the hips.
5. If you need to sit for a prolonged period of time, use a footstool to raise one knee to reduce strain on the back.
6. Take frequent stretch breaks.

Lifting

The following steps outline the procedure for lifting an object while using proper body mechanics:

1. First determine the weight of the object to determine if you can safely lift it. Pushing the object with one foot can help you determine if you can lift it without assistance. Never lift anything heavier than you can easily manage.
2. Stand in front of the object and balance yourself with the feet about 6 to 8 inches apart, toes pointed outward, and one foot slightly forward to provide a wide base of support. Tighten the stomach and gluteal muscles in preparation for lifting the object.
3. To lift the object, always bend the body at the knees and hips (Fig. 20.10A). This helps to maintain your center of gravity and allows the strong muscles of the legs to do the lifting. Never bend from the waist (Fig. 20.10C).
4. Grasp the object firmly with both hands.
5. Keeping the back straight, lift the object smoothly with the leg muscles, not the back muscles (Fig. 20.10B). The muscles of the back are not as strong and are more easily injured than the leg muscles.
6. Hold the object as close to the body as possible and at waist level. This allows the weight of the object to be lifted by the arm and leg muscles rather than the back

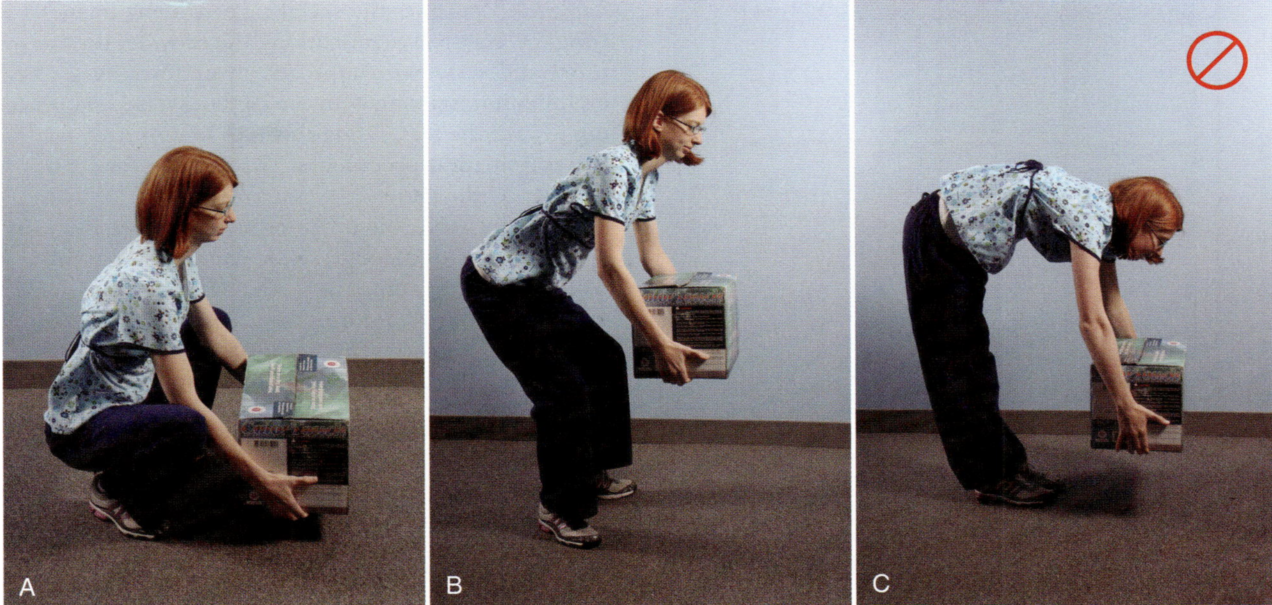

Fig. 20.10 (A) To lift the object, always bend the body at the knees and hips. (B) Lift with the leg muscles, while keeping the back straight. (C) Do not bend from the waist.

muscles. To prevent strain on the back, never lift anything higher than the level of the chest.

7. If you need to turn after lifting the object, don't twist. Turn by pivoting your whole body. Twisting the spine can cause a serious back injury.
8. If you need to carry the object to another location, make sure the area of transport is dry and free of clutter.
9. Lower the object slowly, making sure to bend from the knees to allow the leg muscles to do the work.

POSITIONING AND DRAPING

Correct positioning of the patient facilitates the examination by permitting better access to the part being examined or treated. The basic positions used in the medical office are sitting, supine, prone, dorsal recumbent, lithotomy, modified left lateral recumbent, knee–chest, and Fowler.

The position used depends on the type of examination or procedure to be performed. More than one position may be used to examine the same body part during the physical examination. The sitting and supine positions are both used to examine the chest. It is important to know the correct position for each examination or treatment. When positioning a patient, the medical assistant should explain the position to the patient and assist the patient in attaining it. The medical assistant should make sure to use proper body mechanics when positioning a patient to avoid musculoskeletal injuries.

It is important to take the patient's endurance and degree of wellness into consideration when positioning them. Patients who are weak or ill may be unable to assume a position or may require special assistance in attaining it. Some positions, such as the lithotomy and knee–chest positions, are embarrassing and uncomfortable. A patient should not be kept in these positions any longer than necessary. Some patients (especially the elderly) become dizzy after a time in certain positions, such as the knee–chest position. These patients should be allowed to rest before they get off the examining table. The medical assistant also should assist patients off the examining table to prevent falls.

The patient is draped during positioning to provide for modesty, comfort, and warmth. Only the part to be examined should be exposed. Patient gowns and drapes used in the medical office are usually made of paper but also may be made of cloth. Procedures 20.2–20.9 present proper positioning and draping of the patient.

WHEELCHAIR TRANSFER

A wheelchair is a chair mounted on wheels designed to make mobility easier for individuals who cannot walk or who are having difficulty walking because of illness or disability (e.g., congestive heart failure, severe arthritis). Although some patients who come to the medical office in a wheelchair are able to transfer themselves from a wheelchair to an examining table, others may need assistance. The medical assistant plays an important role in the safe and efficient transfer of a patient from a wheelchair to an examining table and back again.

The Occupational Safety and Health Administration (OSHA) recommends that assistive devices be used whenever possible to transfer patients. A transfer belt (also known as a *gait belt*) is a safety device that is approximately 1½ to

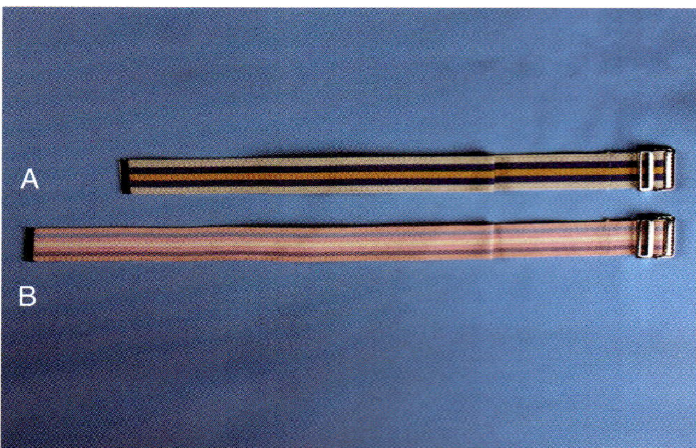

Fig. 20.11 Transfer belts. (A) Transfer belt that is 48 inches in length. (B) Transfer belt that is 60 inches in length.

2 inches wide and 48 or 60 inches long and is made of a durable fiber such as canvas, nylon, or leather (Fig. 20.11). It can be used to assist in the safe transfer of a patient from a wheelchair to an examining table and back again. The transfer belt is wrapped around the patient's waist over their clothing and is securely fastened. The belt provides the medical assistant with a secure grip for holding onto the patient and controlling the patient's movement. This makes the transfer more comfortable for the patient because the medical assistant will not have to grasp the patient around the rib cage or under the axillae to make the transfer. Using a transfer belt also reduces the chance of the medical assistant hurting their musculoskeletal system while transferring a patient. Procedure 20.10 outlines the procedure for transferring a patient from a wheelchair to an examining table and back again using a transfer belt.

It is important for the medical assistant to realize that it may not always be possible to transfer a patient from a wheelchair to the examining table, even with the use of a transfer belt. Before transferring a patient, the medical assistant should carefully assess their ability to make the transfer. There are certain factors that may place undue strain on the medical assistant's musculoskeletal system. These factors include patients who are overweight or patients who have conditions that limit their mobility (e.g., leg paralysis), making it impossible for the patient to assist with the transfer. If factors exist that might cause strain to the medical assistant's musculoskeletal system, the medical assistant should ask for assistance or notify the provider that it is not possible to transfer the patient to the examining table.

ASSESSMENT OF THE PATIENT

The extent of patient assessment during the physical examination depends on the purpose of the examination and the patient's condition. A complete physical examination involves a thorough assessment of all body systems. Table 20.3 outlines the specific assessments included in a complete physical examination. The provider uses an organized and systematic approach in performing a physical examination, starting with the patient's head and proceeding toward the feet. Using this type of approach facilitates the examination process and requires the fewest position changes by the patient.

With an EHR, the provider uses free-text entry, drop-down lists, and check-boxes to enter findings from the physical examination into the computer. The EHR program uses this information to generate the physical examination report. This means that by the end of the examination, the physical examination report is complete, and the provider does not need to dictate their findings at a later time. This alleviates the need for transcribing the provider's dictation into a written report. With a paper-based patient record, the provider documents the results of the physical examination in the patient's medical record, typically on a preprinted form.

Patients who exhibit symptoms of illness usually require only select portions of the physical examination. A patient who comes to the medical office with symptoms of bronchitis usually does not require a complete physical examination; rather, the provider examines the body system that is most likely to be associated with the symptoms. Four assessment techniques are used to obtain information during the physical examination: inspection, palpation, percussion, and auscultation.

INSPECTION

Inspection involves observation of the patient for any signs of disease, and of the four assessment techniques, it is the one most frequently used. Good lighting is important for effective observation. The patient's color, speech, deformities, skin condition (e.g., rashes, scars, warts), body contour and symmetry, orientation to the surroundings, body movements, and anxiety level are assessed through inspection. The medical assistant should develop a high level of detailed observational skills to assist the provider in assessing physical characteristics.

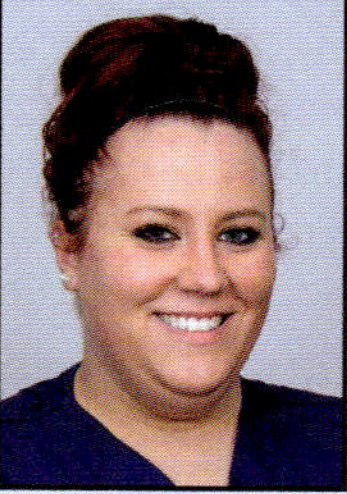

Memories *from* Practicum

Abby: During my practicum at a student health center at a 4-year college, I was responsible for working up patients for gynecologic examinations. The two-piece drapes had the top opening in the front and the bottom opening in the back. After explaining this to an Asian student who spoke very little English, I noticed that she had the openings opposite of what I had explained. I explained again, with words and gestures, that she needed to reverse the openings. To my surprise, she stood up, turned around in a circle, and sat down! ■

Table 20.3 Physician Assessment During the Physical Examination

Body Structure	Assessment	Normal Findings	Abnormal Findings
General appearance	Observation of body build, posture, gait	Good posture and balance Steady gait	Poor posture or balance Unsteady, irregular, or staggering gait
	Determination of weight and height	Weight within ideal range	Patient is overweight or underweight
	Observation of hygiene and grooming	Good hygiene and grooming	Poor hygiene and grooming
	Observation for signs of illness	No signs of illness	Obvious signs of illness
	Observation of attitude, emotional state, mood	Patient speaks clearly and is cooperative	Patient is uncooperative, withdrawn, incoherent, negative, or hostile
Skin	Inspection of skin for color, vascularity, lesions	Smooth, supple, free of blemishes	Blisters, wounds, lesions, rashes, swelling
		No unusual color	Unusual skin color (e.g., flushing, cyanosis, jaundice, pallor)
	Palpation of temperature, moisture, turgor, texture	Warm to touch	Rough, dry, flaky skin Poor skin turgor
Head and neck	Inspection of size, shape, contour of head	Round head with prominences in front and back	Head is asymmetric or of unusual size
	Inspection of hair and scalp	Hair is resilient, evenly distributed, and not excessively dry or oily	Loss of hair Scaliness or dryness of scalp Presence of lice or other parasites
	Palpation of head and neck	No lumps, swelling, tenderness, or lesions of head or neck	Lumps, swelling, tenderness, or lesions of head or neck
Eyes	Evaluation of visual acuity and color vision	Good visual ability with or without glasses or contact lenses	Poor visual acuity or blindness
		Appropriate color perception	Color blindness
	Evaluation of visual field	No visual field loss	Gaps in field of vision
	Inspection of eyelids and eyeballs	Eyes are bright	Dull or glossy eyes
	Inspection of conjunctiva	Pink mucous membranes	Inflamed mucous membranes Excessive tearing Drainage from eyes
	Inspection of eye movements	Eyes move equally in all directions	Drooping eyelids Uncoordinated eye movements
	Tests for pupillary reaction using penlight	Pupils are black, equal in size, react appropriately to light	Dilated, constricted, or unequal pupils
	Inspection of internal eye structures using ophthalmoscope	Reddish-pink retina, even caliber, intact retinal blood vessels	Cloudy lens or narrowed blood vessels
Ears	Test for hearing using tuning fork or audiometer	Good hearing ability	Limited hearing or deafness
	Inspection of size, shape, symmetry of ears	Ears are symmetric and proportionate to head	Ears are asymmetric and not proportionate to the head
	Inspection of external ear canal and tympanic membrane using an otoscope	Cerumen is soft and easily removed	Lesions, redness, or swelling of external ear canal
		No drainage or discomfort Skin of ear canal is intact, pink, warm, and slightly moist	Drainage from ear Pain when ear is moved Impacted cerumen
		Tympanic membrane is pearly gray and semitransparent	Tympanic membrane is red, bulging, or perforated
Nose	Inspection of size, shape, symmetry of nose	Nose is symmetric, straight, not tender	Nose is asymmetric, deformed, flaring, or tender
	Inspection of nostrils using nasal speculum	Septum is intact and midline	Deviation or perforation of septum
		Nasal mucosa is moist and pink	Redness, swelling, polyps, or discharge Nostrils are obstructed
	Test for sense of smell	Correct or very few incorrect responses to odors	Absent, decreased, exaggerated, or unequal responses to test substances

Continued

Table 20.3 Physician Assessment During the Physical Examination—cont'd

Body Structure	Assessment	Normal Findings	Abnormal Findings
Mouth and pharynx	Inspection of lips for contour, color, texture	Pink, moist, soft, smooth lips	Pallor, cyanosis, blisters, swelling, cracking, excessive dryness of lips
	Inspection of mucosa	Pink, moist mucous membranes	Pale or dry mucosa with ulcers or abrasions
	Inspection of gums and palate	Smooth, pink, moist, firm gums Hard palate is firm and white Soft palate is pink and cushiony	Gums are red, bleeding, swollen, tender, spongy, or receding
	Inspection of teeth	Smooth, white enamel; regularly spaced teeth or well-fitting dentures	Missing or loose teeth, dental caries, poor-fitting dentures
	Inspection of tongue	Moist, pink, slightly rough-surfaced tongue	Tongue is dry, furry, smooth, red, or ulcerated
	Inspection of pharynx	Pink and smooth pharynx	Pharynx is red, swollen, or ulcerated
		Tonsils are pink and normal in size	Tonsils are red or swollen
		Gag reflex is present	Absent gag reflex
Arms and hands	Inspection of hands and arms for general appearance	Firm, strong muscles	Muscle weakness, lack of control or coordination
		Normal range of motion in joints	Restricted range of motion
	Palpation of arm muscles	Good muscle control and coordination	
	Palpation for tenderness or lumps	No tenderness or lumps	Tenderness or lumps in hands or arms
	Inspection of fingernails	Colorless nail plate with a convex curve Smooth nail texture	Indentation, infection, brittleness, thickening, or angulation of nails Cyanosis or pallor of nails
Chest and lungs	Inspection of size and shape of chest	Chest is symmetric	Abnormal chest contour
	Assessment of respiratory rate, rhythm, depth Percussion of chest	Normal respiratory rate, rhythm, depth	Labored, slow, rapid, or irregular respirations
	Auscultation of breath sounds	Normal breath sounds	Flat or dull lung sounds Noisy breath sounds
		No cough	Productive or nonproductive cough
	Palpation of ribs	No tenderness of ribs	Tenderness of ribs
Heart	Auscultation of heart sounds	Normal heart sounds	Irregular heartbeats or murmur
	Auscultation of apical pulse, rate, rhythm, volume	Regular, strong heartbeats	Rates slower or more rapid than normal
	Palpation of peripheral pulses	Palpable peripheral pulses	Weak or absent peripheral pulses
	Auscultation of blood pressure	Blood pressure within normal range for age	Low or high blood pressure
	Assessment of peripheral vascular perfusion	Skin is pink, resilient, moist	Cyanosis, pallor, edema
		Immediate return of color to nail beds	Poor capillary filling in nail beds
	Electrocardiogram to assess heart function	Normal heart function	Abnormal electrocardiogram
Breasts	Inspection of size, symmetry, contour	Breasts are round, smooth, symmetric	Retraction, dimpling, redness, or swelling of breasts
	Inspection of nipple	Nipples are round and equal in size, similar in color, appear soft and smooth Areola is round and pink	Bleeding, cracking, discharge, or inversion of nipples
	Palpation of breasts and axillary lymph nodes	No lumps in or tenderness of breasts or axillary lymph nodes	Lumps in or tenderness of breasts or axillary lymph nodes

Table 20.3 Physician Assessment During the Physical Examination—cont'd

Body Structure	Assessment	Normal Findings	Abnormal Findings
Abdomen	Inspection of contour, symmetry, skin condition, integrity	Symmetric contour	Asymmetric contour
		Unblemished skin	Rash or other skin lesions
		Soft abdomen	Abdominal distention
	Auscultation of bowel sounds	Active bowel sounds	Increased, diminished, or absent bowel sounds
	Percussion to assess underlying organs Palpation of underlying organs, tenderness, lumps	Normal position and size of liver and spleen	Tenderness or lumps Enlarged liver or spleen
Genitalia and rectum	Male		
	Inspection of penis and urethra	Penis is smooth	Ulceration or discharge from penis
	Inspection of scrotum and palpation of testes	Testicles are smooth, firm, and movable within scrotal sac Scrotum is symmetric	Lumps or tenderness of scrotum, testes, or prostate gland
	Palpation of rectum and prostate gland	Increased pigmentation in anal area Good anal sphincter tone	Enlarged prostate gland Hemorrhoids or relaxed anal sphincter
	Stool specimen to test for occult blood	Absence of occult blood in stool	Occult blood in stool
	Female		
	Inspection of external genitalia	External genitalia are smooth and without lesions	Ulceration or redness or swelling of external genitalia
	Inspection of vagina and cervix using vaginal speculum	Vaginal mucosa is pink and moist Cervix is pink and smooth	Lacerations, tenderness, redness, or discharge from vagina or cervix
	Specimen collection from vagina and cervix for Pap test	Pap test is normal	Pap test is abnormal
	Bimanual pelvic examination	No tenderness or lumps in uterus and ovaries	Tenderness in or lumps of uterus and ovaries
	Palpation of rectum	Good anal sphincter tone	Hemorrhoids or relaxed anal sphincter
	Stool specimen to test for occult blood	Increased pigmentation in anal area	Occult blood in stool
Legs and feet	Inspection of legs for general appearance and palpation of legs	Firm, strong muscles	Muscle weakness, lack of control or coordination
		Normal range of motion in joints	Restricted range of motion Tenderness or lumps Limp or foot dragging during walking
	Inspection of toenails	Smooth nail texture	Indentation, infection, brittleness, thickening, or angulation of nails
Neurologic	Determination of mental status and level of consciousness	Alert and responds appropriately	Responds inappropriately
		Oriented to person, place, and time	Disoriented
	Determination of sense of pain and touch	Normal responses to pain and touch	Diminished or absent response to stimuli
	Use of percussion hammer to test reflexes	Normal reflexes	Abnormal or absent reflexes

PALPATION

Palpation is the examination of the body using the sense of touch (Fig. 20.12). The provider uses palpation to determine the placement and size of organs; the presence of lumps; and the existence of pain, swelling, or tenderness. Examining the breasts and taking the pulse are performed by palpation. Palpation often helps verify data obtained by inspection. The patient's verbal and facial expressions also are observed during palpation to assist in the detection of abnormalities.

The two types of palpation—light and deep—are categorized by the amount of pressure applied. *Light palpation* of structures is performed to determine areas of tenderness. The fingertips are placed on the part to be examined and are gently depressed approximately ½ inch. *Deep palpation* is used to examine the condition of organs such as those in the abdomen. Two hands are used for deep palpation. One hand is used to support the body from below, and the other hand is used to press over the area to be palpated.

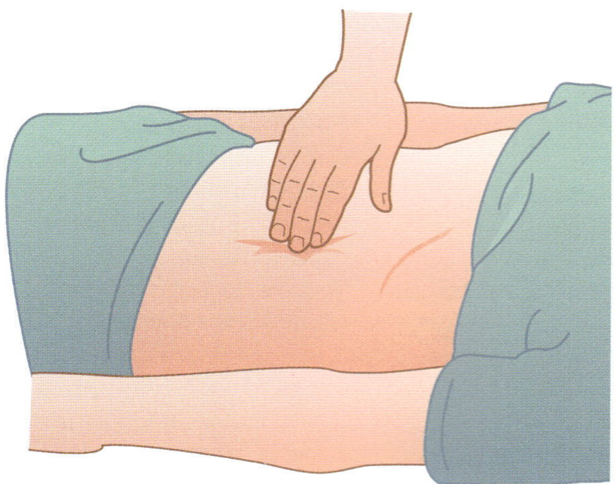

Fig. 20.12 Palpation is examination of the body using the sense of touch.

Deep palpation is used by the provider to perform a bimanual pelvic examination.

PERCUSSION

Percussion involves tapping the patient with the fingers and listening to the sounds produced to determine the size, density, and locations of organs. This technique is often used to examine the lungs and abdomen.

The fingertips are used to produce a sound vibration similar to that of tapping a drumstick on a drum. The non-dominant hand is placed directly on the area to be assessed, with the fingers slightly separated. The dominant hand is used to strike the joint of the middle finger placed on the patient to produce the sound vibration (Fig. 20.13). Structures that are dense, such as the liver, spleen, and heart, produce a dull sound. Empty or air-filled structures, such as the lungs, produce a hollow sound. Any condition that changes the density of an organ or tissue, such as fluid in the lungs, would change the quality of the sound.

AUSCULTATION

Auscultation is an examination technique that involves listening with a stethoscope to the sounds produced within the body. This technique is used to listen to the heart and lungs or to measure blood pressure (manual method). Environmental noise interferes with effective auscultation of body sounds and should be minimized. The diaphragm of the stethoscope chest piece is used to assess high-pitched sounds, such as lung and bowel sounds; the bell of the stethoscope chest piece is used to assess low-pitched sounds, such as those produced by the heart and vascular system. The chest piece should be cleaned with an antiseptic wipe and warmed with the hands before being placed on the patient.

What Would You Do? | What Would You *Not* Do?

Case Study 3

Ben-Yi Sun has brought his father, Chang-Yi Sun, to the medical office. Chang-Yi Sun is 76 years old and lives with Ben-Yi and his family. Because there is a large Asian population in the community, the medical office personnel have learned two things about the Asian culture: (1) They are brought up to respect elders, and elders are always considered first, and (2) Asians have a great respect for harmony. If they do not understand something, they may not admit it to avoid disrupting harmony. Ben-Yi Sun speaks very good English, but his father understands only a few words of English. Chang-Yi Sun has been diagnosed with hypertension, and he needs education about going on a low-sodium diet. He also needs instructions on taking his blood pressure at home and documenting the results. ■

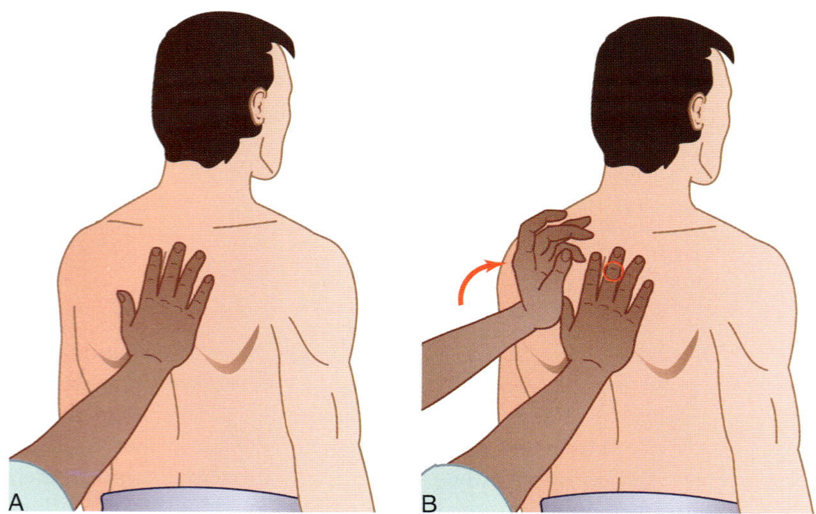

Fig. 20.13 Percussion involves tapping the patient with the fingers. (A) The nondominant hand is placed directly on the area to be assessed, with the fingers slightly separated. (B) The fingers of the dominant hand are used to strike the joint of the middle finger to produce a sound vibration.

ASSISTING THE PROVIDER

During the patient assessment, the medical assistant should assist the provider as required. This includes helping the patient change positions for the provider's examination of different parts of the body, handing the provider instruments and supplies, and reassuring the patient to reduce apprehension. When the examination is completed, the medical assistant should assist the patient off the examining table and provide additional information if needed, such as scheduling a return visit or patient education to promote wellness. Procedure 20.11 describes the procedure for assisting with the physical examination.

What Would You Do? What Would You *Not* Do? RESPONSES

Case Study 1
Page 407

What Did Abby Do?

- ❑ Empathized with Evalyn and told her that a lot of patients feel just like she does about having their weight taken. Explained that the information in her medical record is strictly confidential.
- ❑ Told Evalyn that weight is important so that the physician can properly diagnose and treat her condition, and that medication dosage is often based on a person's weight.
- ❑ Told Evalyn that she could close her eyes while her weight is being measured so that she would not see the reading on the scale.
- ❑ Returned the weights to zero before Evalyn got off the scale.
- ❑ Documented Evalyn's weight in her medical record without telling her the results.
- ❑ Encouraged Evalyn to see the physician when she needs to so that she stays as healthy as possible.

What Did Abby Not Do?

- Did not make any comments about Evalyn's body or weight after weighing her.
- Did not criticize Evalyn for letting her weight stand in the way of coming in when she needed health care.

Case Study 2
Page 410

What Did Abby Do?

- ❑ Listened carefully to Mikayla and showed concern verbally and nonverbally.
- ❑ Carefully documented the information relayed by Mikayla so that the physician would be aware of all aspects of Mikayla's problem.
- ❑ Told Mikayla that she needs to talk to the physician about wanting some medicine for heartburn.
- ❑ Encouraged Mikayla to talk to her parents about what's been going on with her.

What Did Abby Not Do?

- ❑ Did not agree with Mikayla that she needs to lose more weight.
- ❑ Did not make comments about Mikayla being too thin.

Case Study 3
Page 420

What Did Abby Do?

- ❑ Greeted Chang-Yi first before greeting his son.
- ❑ Spoke clearly and slowly to Ben-Yi in a normal tone of voice.
- ❑ Gave them a brochure on low-sodium diets and go over the foods that are low in sodium.
- ❑ Asked Chang-Yi (via Ben-Yi's translating) to indicate the foods he likes that he thinks would be low in sodium. Determined whether these foods are low in sodium.
- ❑ Showed Ben-Yi how to take his father's blood pressure. Had Ben-Yi practice taking his father's blood pressure.
- ❑ Made sure that Chang-Yi and Ben-Yi understood all of the information before they left the office.

What Did Abby Not Do?

- ❑ Be careful not to ignore Chang-Yi.

TERMINOLOGY REVIEW

Key Term	Word Parts	Definition
Acute illness		An illness characterized by symptoms that have a sudden and rapid onset, are usually severe and intense, and subside after a relatively short time (6 months or less).
Audiometer	*audi/o:* hearing *-meter:* instrument used to measure	An instrument used to measure hearing.
Auscultation		The process of listening to the sounds produced within the body to detect signs of disease.
Body mechanics		The use of the correct muscles to maintain proper balance, posture, and body alignment to accomplish a task safely and efficiently without undue strain on any muscle or joint.
Chronic illness		An illness characterized by symptoms that persist for longer than 6 months and show little change or may worsen over time.
Clinical diagnosis		A tentative diagnosis of a patient's condition obtained through evaluation of the health history and the physical examination, without the benefit of laboratory or diagnostic tests.
Diagnosis	*dia-:* through, complete *-gnosis:* knowledge	The scientific method of determining and identifying a patient's condition.
Differential diagnosis		A determination of which of two or more diseases with similar symptoms is producing a patient's symptoms.
Inspection		The process of observing a patient to detect signs of disease.
Mensuration		The process of measuring a patient.
Palpation		The process of feeling with the hands to detect signs of disease.
Percussion		The process of tapping the body to detect signs of disease.
Prognosis	*pro-:* before *-gnosis:* knowledge	The probable course and outcome of a patient's condition and the patient's prospects for recovery.
Risk factor		A physical or behavioral condition that increases the probability that an individual will develop a particular condition.
Screening test		A test performed on a large number of individuals for the early detection of a condition before it causes symptoms.
Symptom		Any change in the body or its functioning that indicates a disease might be present.

PROCEDURE 20.1 Measuring Weight and Height

Outcome Measure weight and height.

Equipment/Supplies

- Balance beam scale
- Paper towel

Weight

1. **Procedural Step.** Sanitize your hands.
2. **Procedural Step.** Check the scale to ensure it is balanced as follows:
   a. Make sure the upper and lower weights are on zero. When the weights are on zero, they are all the way to the left of the calibration bars.

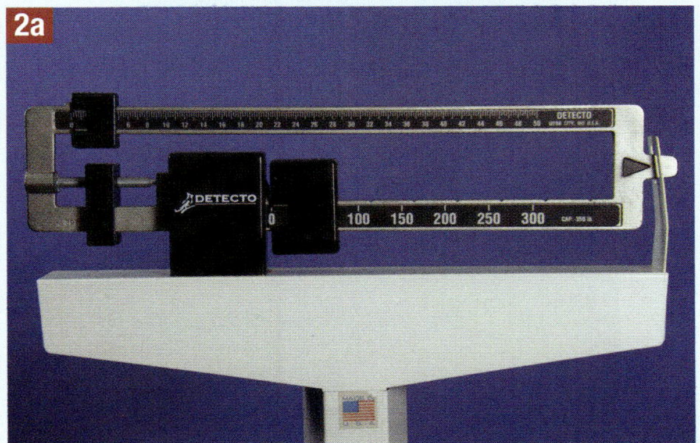

Ensure that the upper and lower weights are on zero.

   b. Look at the indicator point. If the scale is balanced, the indicator point is resting in the center of the balance area.
   c. If the indicator point rests below the center, adjust the screw on the balance knob by turning it clockwise (to the right) until the indicator point rests in the center of the balance area.

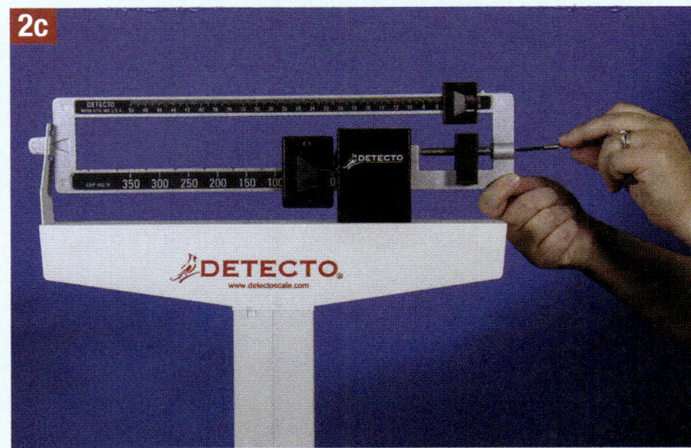

Correct the balance by adjusting the screw on the balance knob.

   d. If the indicator point rests above the center, adjust the screw on the balance knob by turning it counterclockwise (to the left) until the indicator point rests in the center of the balance area.

   Principle. If the scale is not balanced, the weight measurement will be inaccurate.
3. **Procedural Step.** Greet the patient and introduce yourself.
4. **Procedural Step.** Identify the patient and explain to the patient that you will be measuring their height and weight.
5. **Procedural Step.** Instruct the patient to remove shoes and outer clothing such as a jacket or sweater. A good medical aseptic practice is to place a paper towel on the platform of the scale to protect the patient's feet.

   Principle. Removing heavy clothing and shoes allows a more accurate measurement of the patient's weight.
6. **Procedural Step.** Assist the patient onto the scale, and instruct the patient not to move.

   Principle. It is not possible to balance the scale if the patient is moving.
7. **Procedural Step.** Balance the scale as follows:
   a. Move the lower weight to the notched groove that does not cause the indicator point to drop to the bottom of the balance area. Ensure that the lower weight is seated firmly in its groove.
   b. Slide the upper weight slowly along its calibration bar by tapping it gently until the indicator point comes to rest at the center of the balance area.

   Principle. Not seating the lower weight firmly in its groove results in an inaccurate reading.

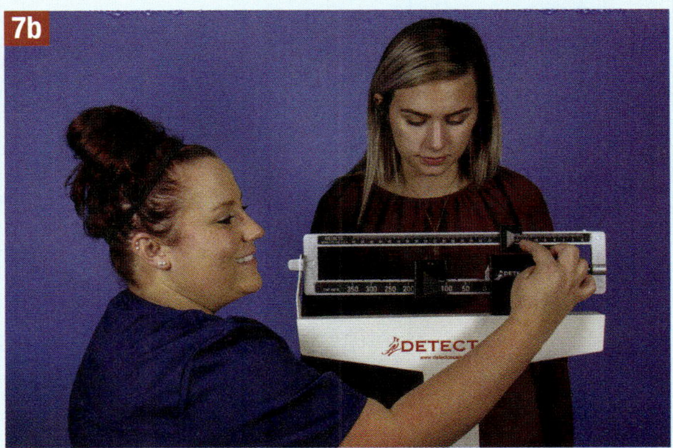

Slide the upper weight by tapping it gently.

PROCEDURE 20.1

Continued

PROCEDURE 20.1 Measuring Weight and Height—cont'd

8. **Procedural Step.** Read the results to the nearest quarter pound by adding the measurement on the lower scale to the measurement on the upper scale. Jot down this value or make a mental note of it.

9. **Procedural Step.** Ask the patient to step off of the scale platform. Provide assistance if needed.

Height

10. **Procedural Step.** Slide the movable calibration rod upward until the measuring bar is well above the patient's apparent height. Open the measuring bar to its horizontal position.

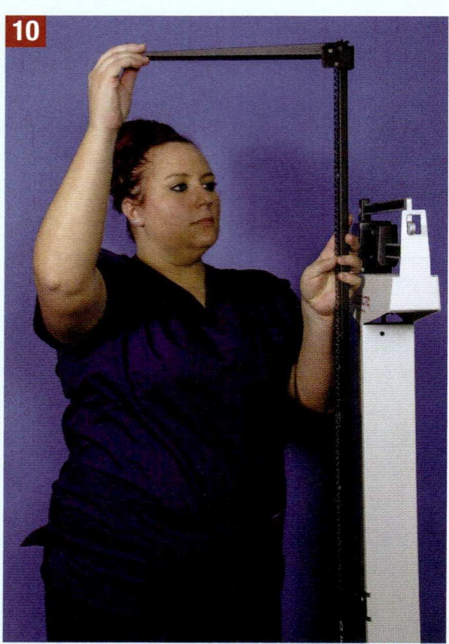

Slide the bar upward until it is well above the patient's height.

11. **Procedural Step.** Instruct the patient to step onto the scale platform with their back to the scale. Provide assistance if needed. Instruct the patient to stand erect and to look straight ahead.
    Principle. Looking straight ahead helps the patient to stand erect and balanced, which ensures an accurate measurement.

12. **Procedural Step.** Carefully lower the measuring bar (keeping it horizontal) until it rests gently on top of the patient's head with the hair compressed. The measuring bar should form a 90-degree angle with the calibration rod.
    Principle. The measuring bar must be at a 90-degree angle to ensure an accurate height measurement.

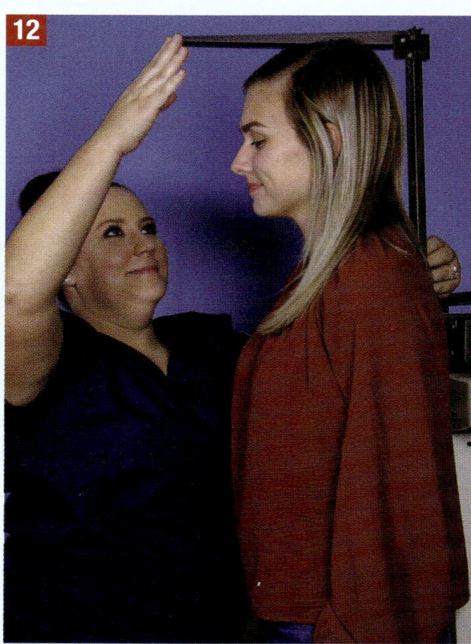

Lower the bar until it rests on top of the patient's head.

13. **Procedural Step.** Keeping the measuring bar in a horizontal position, instruct the patient to step down and put on their shoes. Hold the bar in a horizontal position until the patient has stepped off the scale.

14. **Procedural Step.** Read the height measurement from the top down to the nearest quarter-inch marking at the junction of the stationary calibration rod and the movable calibration rod. (*Note:* If the patient's height is less than the top value of the stationary rod, read the measurement from the bottom up directly on the stationary calibration rod.) Jot down this value or make a mental note of it.

PROCEDURE 20.1 Measuring Weight and Height—cont'd

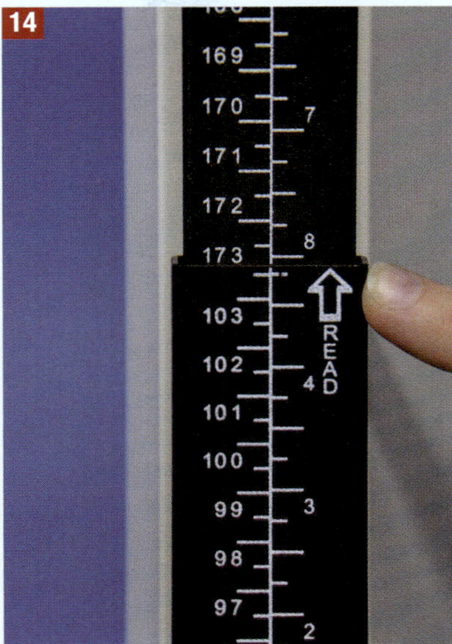

Read the measurement to the nearest ¼-inch marking.

15. **Procedural Step.** Return the measuring bar to its vertical (resting) position, and slide the movable calibration rod to its lowest position. Return the weights to zero.
16. **Procedural Step.** Sanitize your hands.
17. **Procedural Step.** Document the results in the patient's medical record.
    a. *Electronic health record:* In SimChart for the Medical Office, document the patient's weight and height measurements. You will be using textboxes, drop-down menus, and/or radio buttons to enter this information. (*Note:* The EHR automatically calculates and documents the patient's BMI from the weight and height measurements that are entered into the computer.)
    b. *Paper-based medical record:* Document the date and time and the patient's weight and height measurements. The weight should be documented in pounds to the nearest quarter pound, and the height should be documented in feet and inches to the nearest quarter inch. If required by the medical office policy, determine the patient's BMI and document this number following the weight and height measurements.

17b

DOCUMENTATION EXAMPLE

Date	
11/5/XX	10:15 a.m. Wt: 126 1/2 lbs. Ht: 5' 8" BMI: 19.2
	————————A. Erdy, CMA (AAMA)

PROCEDURE 20.2 Sitting Position

Outcome Position and drape a patient in the sitting position.

The sitting position is used to examine the head, neck, chest, and upper extremities and to measure vital signs.

Equipment/Supplies

- Examining table
- Disposable patient gown
- Disposable patient drape

1. **Procedural Step.** Sanitize your hands. Greet the patient and introduce yourself.
2. **Procedural Step.** Identify the patient and explain the type of examination or procedure that will be performed.
3. **Procedural Step.** Provide the patient with a patient gown. Instruct the patient to remove clothing as appropriate for the type of examination being performed and to put on the patient gown with the opening in front.
4. **Procedural Step.** Pull out the footrest of the examining table, and assist the patient into a sitting position. The patient's buttocks and thighs should be firmly supported on the edge of the table.

Continued

PROCEDURE 20.2 Sitting Position—cont'd

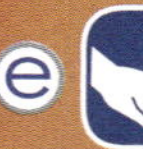
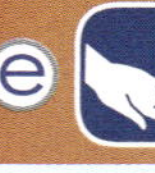

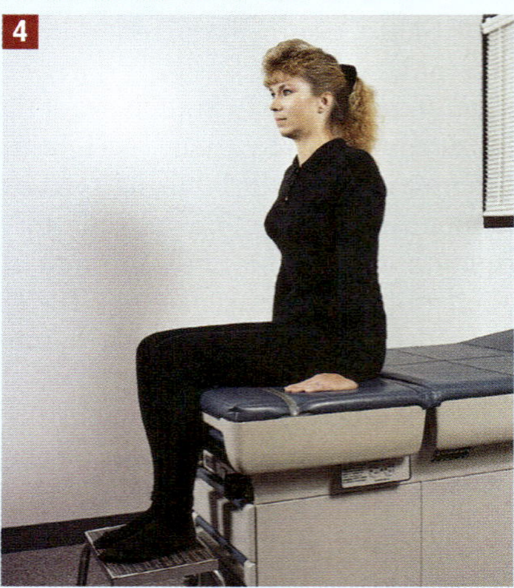

Assist the patient in a sitting position.

5. **Procedural Step.** Place a drape over the patient's thighs and legs to provide warmth and modesty.

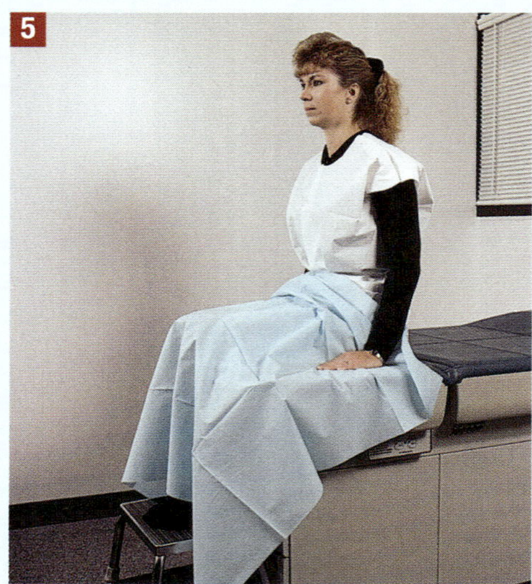

Place the drape over the patient's thighs and legs.

6. **Procedural Step.** After completion of the examination, assist the patient down from the table. Return the footrest to its normal position. Instruct the patient to get dressed. Discard the gown and drape in a waste container.

PROCEDURE 20.3 Supine Position

Outcome Position and drape a patient in the supine position.
The supine position is used to examine the head, chest, abdomen, and extremities.

Equipment/Supplies

- Examining table
- Disposable patient gown
- Disposable patient drape

1. **Procedural Step.** Sanitize your hands. Greet the patient and introduce yourself.
2. **Procedural Step.** Identify the patient and explain the type of examination or procedure that will be performed.
3. **Procedural Step.** Provide the patient with a patient gown. Instruct the patient to remove clothing as appropriate for the type of examination being performed and to put on the patient gown with the opening in front.
4. **Procedural Step.** Pull out the footrest of the examining table, and assist the patient into a sitting position. Place a drape over the patient's thighs and legs.
5. **Procedural Step.** Ask the patient to move back on the table. As the patient is doing this, pull out the table extension while supporting the patient's lower legs.

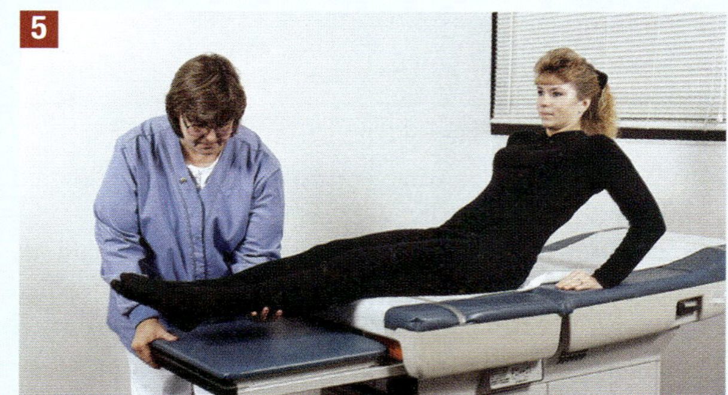

Pull out the table extension while supporting the patient's legs.

PROCEDURE 20.3 Supine Position—cont'd

6. Procedural Step. Ask the patient to lie on their back with the legs together. Provide assistance if needed. The patient's arms may be placed above the head or alongside the body.

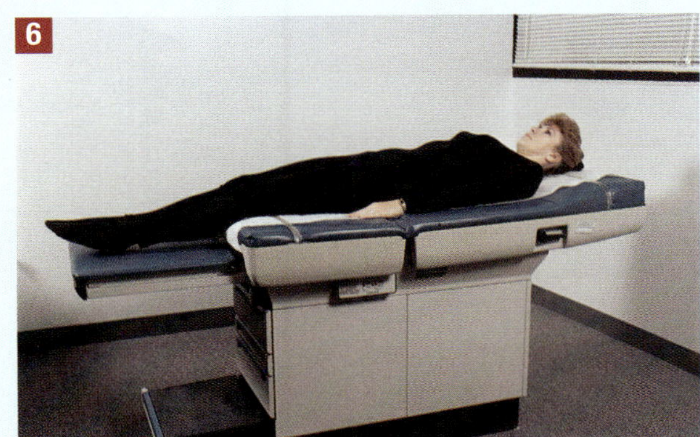
6

Position the patient on the back with the legs together.

7. Procedural Step. Position the drape lengthwise over the patient to provide warmth and modesty. As the provider examines the patient, move the drape according to the body parts being examined.

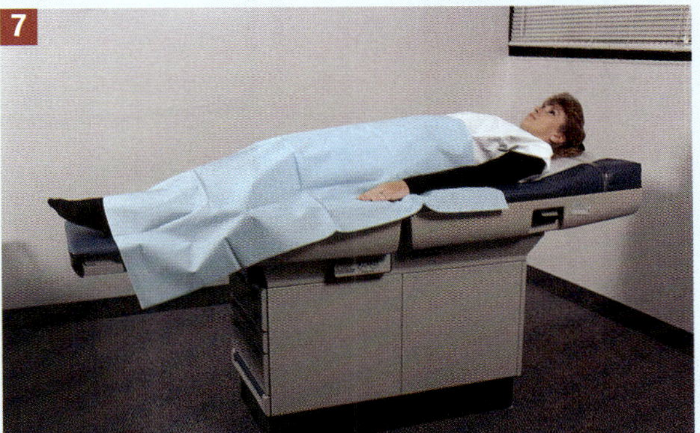
7

Place a drape lengthwise over the patient.

8. Procedural Step. After completion of the examination, assist the patient into a sitting position. Slide the table extension back into place while supporting the patient's lower legs.

9. Procedural Step. Assist the patient down from the table. Instruct the patient to get dressed. Return the footrest to its normal position. Discard the gown and drape in a waste container.

PROCEDURE 20.4 Prone Position

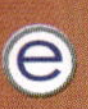
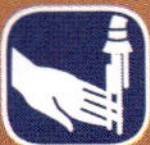

Outcome Position and drape a patient in the prone position.

The prone position is used to examine the back and to assess extension of the hip joint.

Equipment/Supplies

- Examining table
- Disposable patient gown
- Disposable patient drape

1. Procedural Step. Sanitize your hands. Greet the patient and introduce yourself.

2. Procedural Step. Identify the patient and explain the type of examination or procedure that will be performed.

3. Procedural Step. Provide the patient with a patient gown. Instruct the patient to remove clothing as appropriate for the type of examination being performed and to put on the patient gown with the opening in back.

4. Procedural Step. Pull out the footrest of the examining table, and assist the patient into a sitting position. Place a drape over the patient's thighs and legs.

5. Procedural Step. Ask the patient to move back on the table. As the patient is doing this, pull out the table extension while supporting the patient's lower legs.

6. Procedural Step. Ask the patient to lie on their back. Provide assistance if needed. Position the drape lengthwise over the patient.

7. Procedural Step. Ask the patient to turn onto their stomach by rolling toward you. Provide assistance for this step by helping the patient turn and adjusting the drape to provide modesty.

Principle. This step prevents the patient from accidentally rolling off the table.

8. Procedural Step. Position the patient with the legs together and the head turned to one side. The arms can be placed above the head or alongside the body.

Continued

PROCEDURE 20.4 Prone Position—cont'd

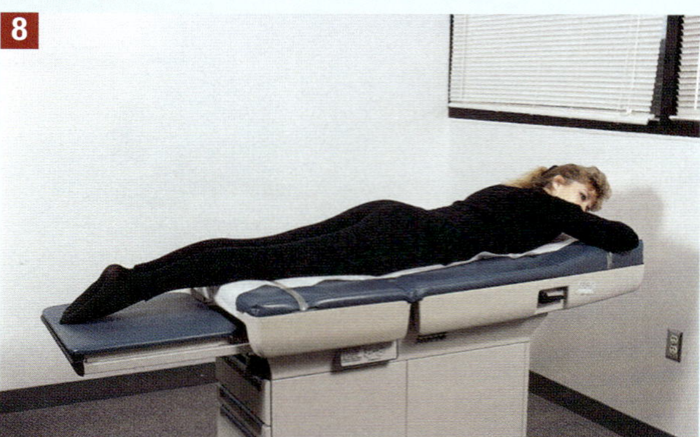

8 Position the patient's legs together with the head turned to one side.

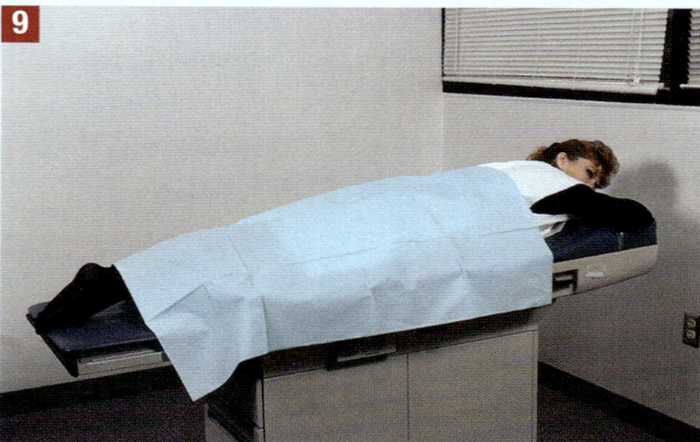

9 Place a drape lengthwise over the patient.

9. **Procedural Step.** Adjust the drape as needed so that it is positioned lengthwise over the patient to provide warmth and modesty. As the provider examines the patient, move the drape according to the body parts being examined.
10. **Procedural Step.** After completion of the examination, ask the patient to turn back over by rolling toward you. Assist the patient into a supine position and then into a sitting position. Slide the table extension back into place while supporting the patient's lower legs.
11. **Procedural Step.** Assist the patient down from the table. Return the footrest to its normal position. Instruct the patient to get dressed. Discard the gown and drape in a waste container.

PROCEDURE 20.5 Dorsal Recumbent Position

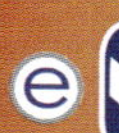

Outcome Position and drape a patient in the dorsal recumbent position.

The dorsal recumbent position is used to perform vaginal and rectal examinations; to insert a urinary catheter; and to examine the head, neck, chest, and extremities of patients who have difficulty maintaining the supine position. The supine position is an uncomfortable position for patients with respiratory problems, back injury, or lower back pain. Bending the legs (rather than lying flat) is more comfortable for these patients and is easier to maintain.

Equipment/Supplies

- Examining table
- Disposable patient gown
- Disposable patient drape

1. **Procedural Step.** Sanitize your hands. Greet the patient and introduce yourself.
2. **Procedural Step.** Identify the patient and explain the type of examination or procedure that will be performed.
3. **Procedural Step.** Provide the patient with a patient gown. Instruct the patient to remove clothing as appropriate for the type of examination being performed and to put on the patient gown with the opening in front.
4. **Procedural Step.** Pull out the footrest of the examining table, and assist the patient into a sitting position. Place a drape over the patient's thighs and legs.
5. **Procedural Step.** Ask the patient to move back on the table. As the patient is doing this, pull out the table extension while supporting the patient's lower legs.
6. **Procedural Step.** Ask the patient to lie on their back. Provide assistance if needed. The arms can be placed above the head or alongside the body. Position the drape diagonally over the patient.
7. **Procedural Step.** Ask the patient to bend the knees and place each foot at the edge of the examining table with the soles of the feet flat on the table. Provide assistance during this step. Push in the table extension and the footrest.

PROCEDURE 20.5 Dorsal Recumbent Position—cont'd

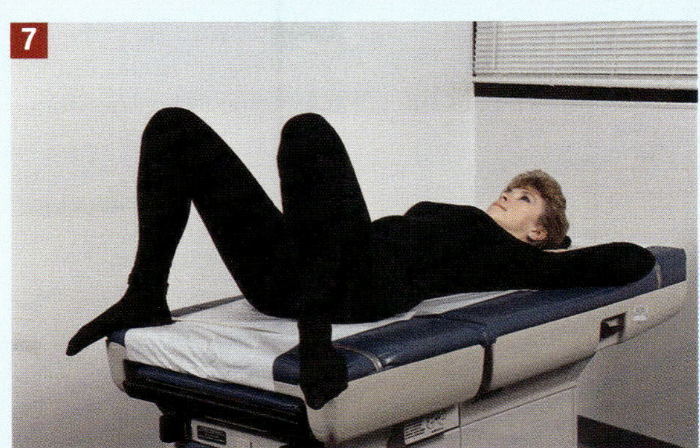

Ask the patient to bend the knees and place each foot at the edge of the examining table.

8. Procedural Step. Adjust the drape as needed to provide the patient with warmth and modesty. The drape should be positioned diagonally, with one corner over the patient's chest; the opposite corner falls between the patient's legs and completely covers the pubic area.

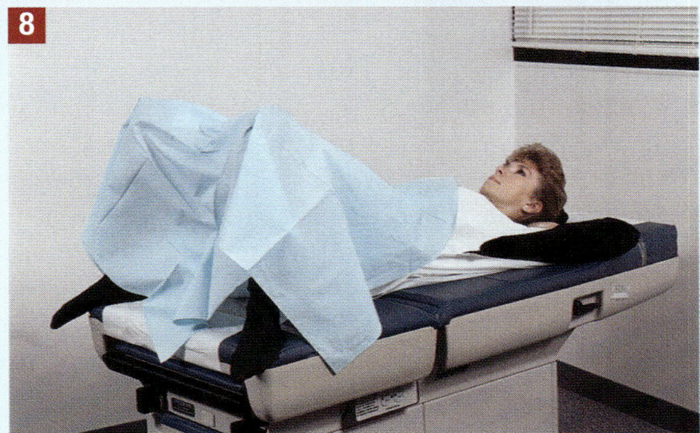

Place a drape diagonally over the patient.

9. Procedural Step. When the provider is ready to examine the genital area, the center corner of the drape is folded back over the abdomen.

10. Procedural Step. After completion of the examination, pull out the footrest and the table extension. Assist the patient into a supine position and then into a sitting position. Slide the table extension back into place while supporting the patient's lower legs.

11. Procedural Step. Assist the patient down from the table. Return the footrest to its normal position. Instruct the patient to get dressed. Discard the gown and drape in a waste container.

PROCEDURE 20.6 Lithotomy Position

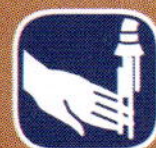

Outcome Position and drape a patient in the lithotomy position.

The lithotomy position is used for vaginal, pelvic, and rectal examinations. The lithotomy position is the same as the dorsal recumbent position except that the patient's feet are placed in stirrups. The lithotomy position provides maximal exposure to the genital area and facilitates insertion of a vaginal speculum. Because this is an uncomfortable position for the patient to maintain, the patient should not be put into this position until just before the examination.

Equipment/Supplies

- Examining table
- Disposable patient gown
- Disposable patient drape

1. Procedural Step. Sanitize your hands. Greet the patient and introduce yourself.

2. Procedural Step. Identify the patient and explain the type of examination or procedure that will be performed.

3. Procedural Step. Provide the patient with a patient gown. Instruct the patient to remove clothing as appropriate for the type of examination being performed and to put on the patient gown with the opening in front. If the patient is wearing socks, tell her that she may keep them on during the procedure.

Principle. Socks help to keep the patient's feet warm after they are placed in the metal stirrups.

4. Procedural Step. Some medical offices use disposable stirrup covers. If this is the case, apply a cover to each stirrup. Pull out the footrest of the examining table, and assist the patient into a sitting position. Place a drape over the patient's thighs and legs.

Continued

PROCEDURE 20.6 Lithotomy Position—cont'd

Principle. Stirrup covers provide a soft, warm, nonslip surface for the patient's feet.

5. **Procedural Step.** When the provider is ready to examine the patient, ask the patient to move back on the table. As the patient is doing this, pull out the table extension while supporting the patient's lower legs.
6. **Procedural Step.** Ask the patient to lie on the back. Provide assistance if needed. The arms can be placed above the head or alongside the body.
7. **Procedural Step.** Position the drape over the patient to provide warmth and modesty. The drape should be positioned diagonally with one corner over the patient's chest and the opposite corner between the patient's feet.
8. **Procedural Step.** Pull out the stirrups and position them at an angle. Position the stirrups so that they are level with the examining table and pulled out approximately 1 foot from the edge of the table. Check to make sure the stirrups are not too far apart or too close together. Lock the stirrups into place.

   Principle. If the stirrups are too far apart, it is uncomfortable for the patient. If the stirrups are too close together, the patient will be unable to move her buttocks to the edge of the table as needed for the examination.
9. **Procedural Step.** Ask the patient to bend the knees and place each foot, one at a time, into a stirrup. Provide assistance during this step. Push in the table extension and the footrest.

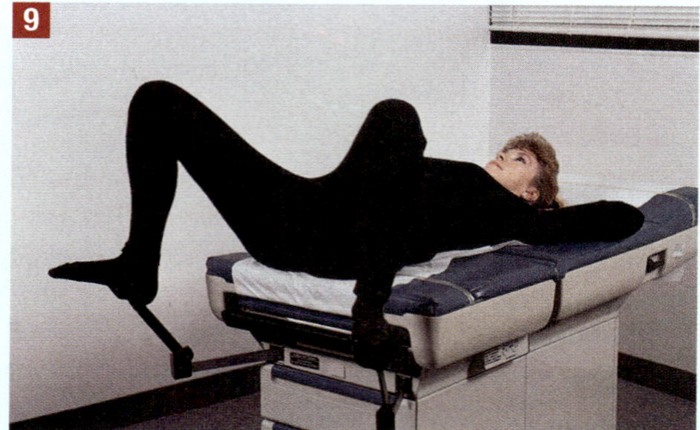

Ask the patient to slide the buttocks to the edge of the table and to rotate the thighs outward.

10. **Procedural Step.** Instruct the patient to slide the buttocks all the way down to the edge of the examining table and to let her legs fall apart as far as is comfortable.

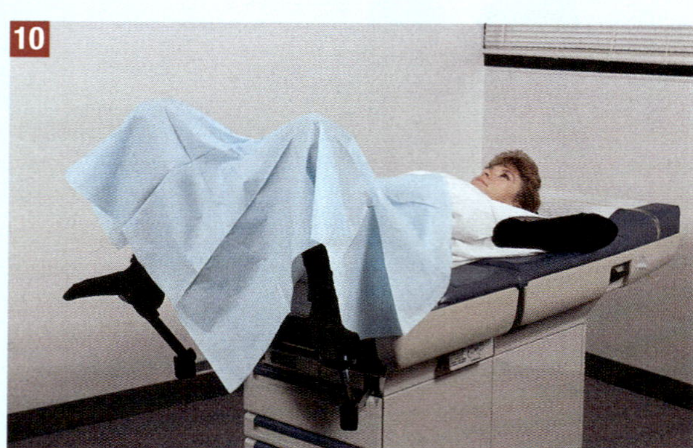

Position the drape diagonally.

11. **Procedural Step.** Reposition the drape as needed so that one corner is over the patient's chest and the opposite corner falls between the patient's legs and completely covers the perineal area. When the provider is ready to examine the genital area, the center corner of the drape is pulled up and folded back over the knees.
12. **Procedural Step.** After completion of the examination, pull out the footrest and table extension. Ask the patient to slide the buttocks back from the end of the table. Lift the patient's legs out of the stirrups at the same time, and place them on the table extension (supine position). Remove the stirrup covers and discard them in a waste container. Return the stirrups to their normal position. Assist the patient into a sitting position. Slide the table extension back into place while supporting the patient's lower legs.

    Principle. Lifting both the patient's legs out of the stirrups at the same time avoids strain on the back and abdominal muscles.
13. **Procedural Step.** Assist the patient down from the table. Return the footrest to its normal position. Instruct the patient to get dressed. Discard the gown and drape in a waste container.

PROCEDURE 20.7 Modified Left Lateral Recumbent Position

Outcome Position and drape a patient in the modified left lateral recumbent position.

The modified left lateral recumbent position(also known as Sims position) is used to examine the vagina and rectum, to measure rectal temperature, to perform a flexible sigmoidoscopy, and to administer an enema.

Equipment/Supplies

- Examining table
- Disposable patient gown
- Disposable patient drape

1. **Procedural Step.** Sanitize your hands. Greet the patient and introduce yourself.
2. **Procedural Step.** Identify the patient and explain the type of examination or procedure that will be performed.
3. **Procedural Step.** Provide the patient with a patient gown. Instruct the patient to remove clothing from the waist down and to put on the patient gown with the opening in back.
4. **Procedural Step.** Pull out the footrest of the examining table, and assist the patient into a sitting position. Place a drape over the patient's thighs and legs.
5. **Procedural Step.** Ask the patient to move back on the table. As the patient is doing this, pull out the table extension while supporting the patient's lower legs.
6. **Procedural Step.** Ask the patient to lie on their back. Provide assistance if needed.
7. **Procedural Step.** Position the drape lengthwise over the patient to provide warmth and modesty.
8. **Procedural Step.** Ask the patient to turn onto the left side. Provide assistance during this step to prevent the patient from accidentally rolling off the table and to adjust the drape to provide modesty. The patient's left arm should be positioned behind the body and the right arm forward with the elbow bent. Assist the patient in flexing the legs. The right leg is flexed sharply, and the left leg is flexed slightly.

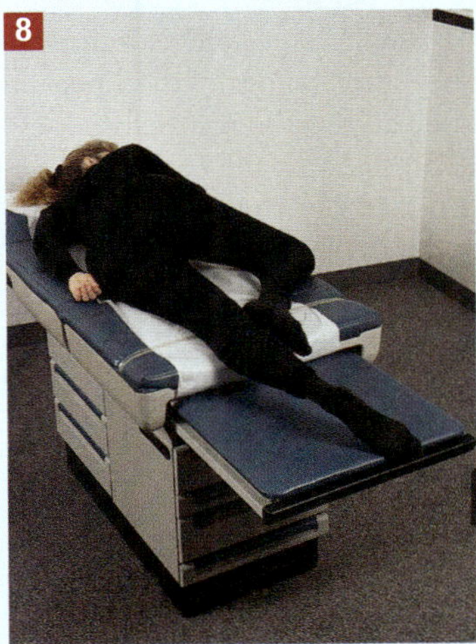

The right leg is flexed sharply and the left leg is flexed slightly.

9. **Procedural Step.** Adjust the drape as needed. When the provider is ready to examine the patient, a small portion of the drape is folded back to expose the anal area.

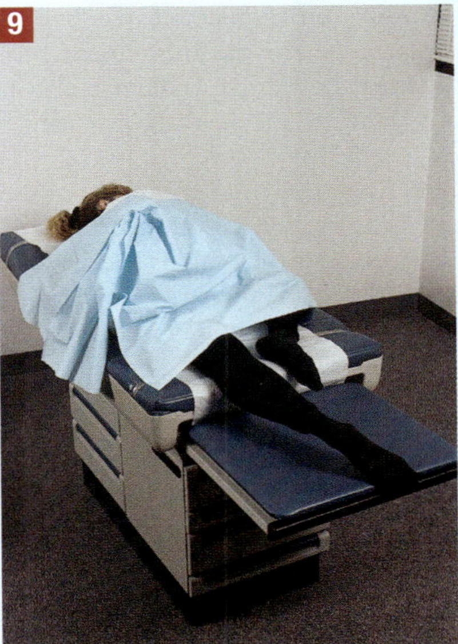

Adjust the drape as needed.

10. **Procedural Step.** After completion of the examination, assist the patient into a supine position and into a sitting position. Slide the table extension back into place while supporting the patient's lower legs.
11. **Procedural Step.** Assist the patient down from the table. Return the footrest to its normal position. Instruct the patient to get dressed. Discard the gown and drape in a waste container.

PROCEDURE 20.8 Knee–Chest Position

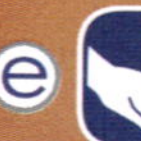

Outcome Position and drape a patient in the knee–chest position.

The knee–chest position is used to examine the rectum and to perform a proctoscopic examination because it provides maximal exposure to the rectal area. This is a difficult position to maintain; the patient should not be put into this position until just before the examination.

Equipment/Supplies

- Examining table
- Disposable patient gown
- Disposable patient drape
- Pillow

1. **Procedural Step.** Sanitize your hands. Greet the patient and introduce yourself.
2. **Procedural Step.** Identify the patient and explain the type of examination or procedure that will be performed.
3. **Procedural Step.** Provide the patient with a patient gown. Instruct the patient to remove clothing from the waist down and to put on the gown with the opening in back.
4. **Procedural Step.** Pull out the footrest of the examining table, and assist the patient into a sitting position. Place a drape over the patient's thighs and legs.
5. **Procedural Step.** Ask the patient to move back on the table. As the patient is doing this, pull out the table extension while supporting the patient's lower legs.
6. **Procedural Step.** Assist the patient into the supine position and then into the prone position, making sure to have the patient roll toward you. Position the drape diagonally over the patient to provide warmth and modesty.
7. **Procedural Step.** Ask the patient to bend the arms at the elbows and rest them alongside the head. Ask the patient to elevate the buttocks while keeping the back straight. The patient's head should be turned to one side, and the weight of the body should be supported by the chest. A pillow under the chest can give additional support and aid in relaxation. The knees and lower legs are separated approximately 12 inches.

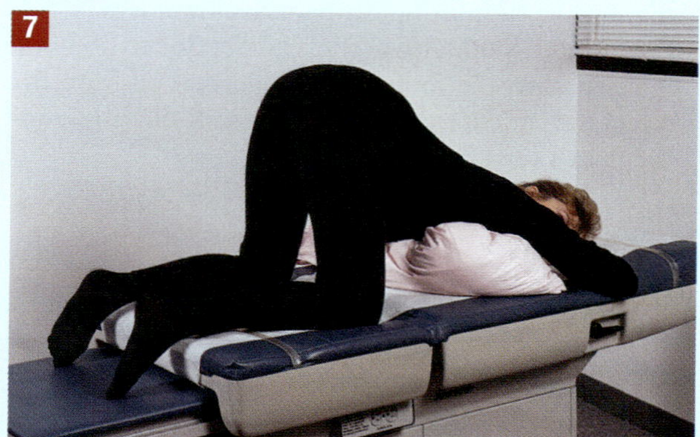

The buttocks are elevated, and the head is turned to one side.

8. **Procedural Step.** Adjust the drape diagonally as needed with one corner over the patient's back and the opposite corner over the buttocks and falling between the patient's legs. When the provider is ready to examine the patient, a small portion of the drape is folded back to expose the anal area.

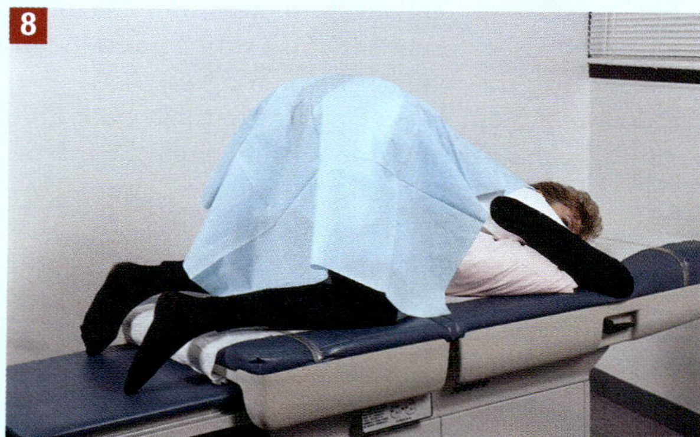

Position the drape diagonally.

9. **Procedural Step.** After completion of the examination, assist the patient into a prone position and then into a supine position. Allow the patient to rest in the supine position before they sit up.
   Principle. Patients (especially elderly ones) frequently become dizzy after being in the knee–chest position and should be allowed to rest before they sit up.
10. **Procedural Step.** Assist the patient into a sitting position. Slide the table extension back into place while supporting the patient's lower legs.
11. **Procedural Step.** Assist the patient down from the table. Return the footrest to its normal position. Instruct the patient to get dressed. Discard the gown and drape in a waste container.

PROCEDURE 20.9 Fowler Position

Outcome Position and drape a patient in the Fowler position.

The Fowler position is used to examine the upper body of patients with cardiovascular and respiratory problems, such as congestive heart failure, emphysema, and asthma. These patients find it easier to breathe in this position than in a sitting or supine position. This position also is used to draw blood from patients who are likely to faint.

Equipment/Supplies

- Examining table
- Disposable patient gown
- Disposable patient drape

1. **Procedural Step.** Sanitize your hands. Greet the patient and introduce yourself.
2. **Procedural Step.** Identify the patient and explain the type of examination or procedure that will be performed.
3. **Procedural Step.** Provide the patient with a patient gown. Instruct the patient to remove clothing as appropriate for the type of examination being performed and to put on the patient gown with the opening in front.
4. **Procedural Step.** Position the head of the table as follows:
   a. For the semi-Fowler position, the table should be positioned at a 45-degree angle.
   b. For the full Fowler position, the table should be positioned at a 90-degree angle.
5. **Procedural Step.** Pull out the footrest of the examining table, and assist the patient into a sitting position. Place a drape over the patient's thighs and legs.
6. **Procedural Step.** Pull out the table extension while supporting the patient's lower legs. Ask the patient to lean back against the table head. Provide assistance during this step.

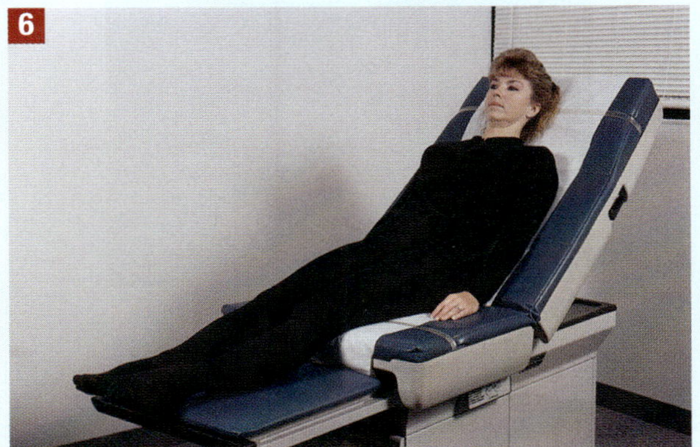

Ask the patient to lean back against the table head.

7. **Procedural Step.** Position the drape lengthwise over the patient to provide warmth and modesty. As the provider examines the patient, move the drape according to the body parts being examined.

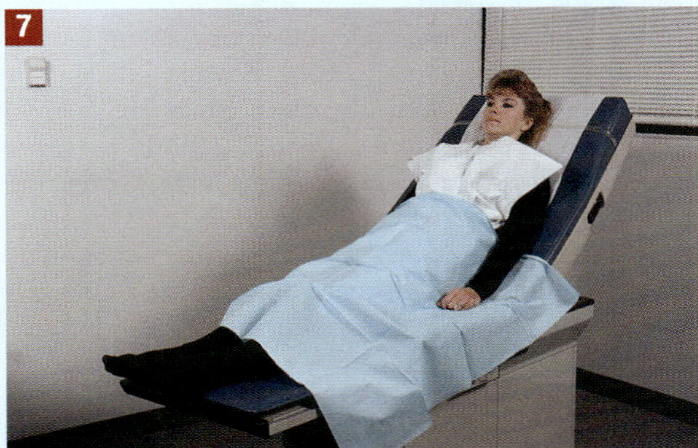

Position the table at a 45-degree angle for the semi-Fowler position.

8. **Procedural Step.** After completion of the examination, assist the patient into a sitting position. Slide the table extension back into place while supporting the patient's lower legs.
9. **Procedural Step.** Assist the patient down from the table. Instruct the patient to get dressed. Return the head of the table and the footrest to their normal positions. Discard the gown and drape in a waste container.

PROCEDURE 20.10 Wheelchair Transfer

Outcome Transfer a patient from a wheelchair to the examining table and from an examining table to a wheelchair.

Equipment/Supplies

- Examining table
- Transfer belt

Transferring the Patient to the Examining Table

1. **Procedural Step.** Sanitize your hands.
2. **Procedural Step.** Greet the patient and introduce yourself. Identify the patient and explain the procedure.
3. **Procedural Step.** Evaluate the patient to determine their mental and physical capabilities to perform the transfer. Determine how heavy the patient is and if they are able to assist in the transfer. Assess whether or not you are able to perform the transfer safely. Do not perform the transfer if you think you may incur a musculoskeletal injury.
4. **Procedural Step.** Wrap the transfer belt snugly around the patient's waist over the patient's clothing with the buckle in front. Securely fasten the belt by threading it through the teeth of the buckle. Put the belt through the other two openings to lock it. The belt should be snug with just enough space between the belt and the patient's clothing to allow your fingers to be inserted comfortably between the belt and the patient's waist.
   Principle. Placing the transfer belt over the patient's clothing prevents abrasions to the patient's skin. The belt must be snug to prevent it from sliding upward on the patient's body.
5. **Procedural Step.** With the patient's stronger side next to the examining table, position the wheelchair at a 45-degree angle to the end of the examining table.

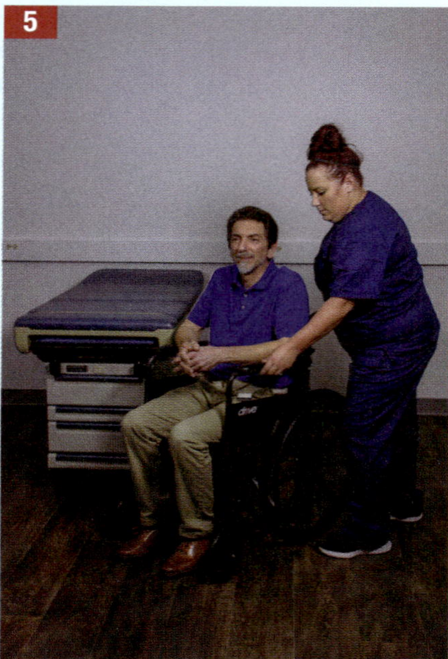

Position the wheelchair at a 45-degree angle.

6. **Procedural Step.** If the examining table is height adjustable, lower it to the same height as the wheelchair or slightly lower. If it is not height adjustable, pull out the footrest of the examining table.
7. **Procedural Step.** Lock the brakes of the wheelchair and fold back the wheelchair footrests.
   Principle. The wheels must be locked to prevent the chair from moving during the transfer. The wheelchair footrests must be out of the way to provide an unobstructed path for making the transfer.

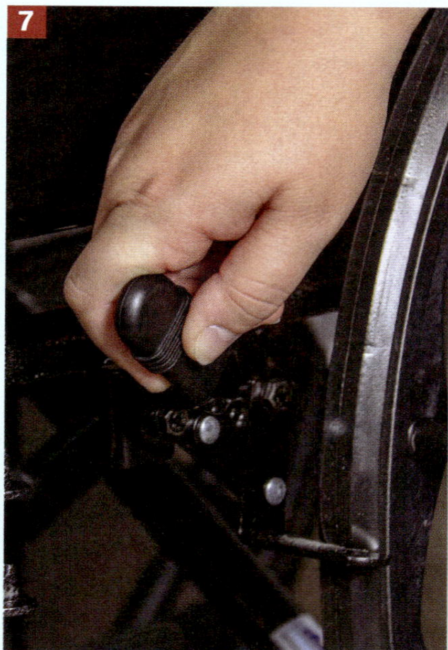

Lock the brakes.

8. **Procedural Step.** Inform the patient of what they will be required to do during the transfer. During the transfer, clearly state in a step-by-step manner what the patient should do. Encourage the patient to help as much as possible during the transfer by using the muscles of their arms and legs.
9. **Procedural Step.** Make sure the patient's feet are positioned flat on the floor.
   Principle. Making sure the patient's feet are flat on the floor provides the patient with balance and stability when they stand.

PROCEDURE 20.10 Wheelchair Transfer—cont'd

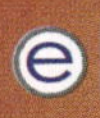

10. **Procedural Step.** Stand in front of the patient with your feet apart about 6 to 8 inches, the toes pointed outward, one foot slightly forward, and the knees bent.
    Principle. This position conserves energy and provides a wide base of support for the transfer.
11. **Procedural Step.** Ask the patient to place their hands on the armrests of the wheelchair and to lean forward.
12. **Procedural Step.** Grasp the transfer belt on either side of the patient's waist using an underhand grasp.
    Principle. The transfer belt provides a secure handle for holding onto the patient and controlling the patient's movement.

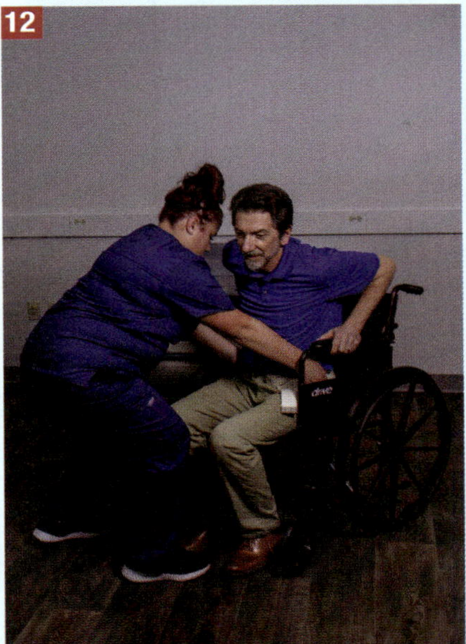

Grasp the transfer belt on either side of the patient's waist.

13. **Procedural Step.** Tighten your abdominal gluteal muscles in preparation for the transfer. Ask the patient to push off the armrests and into a standing position on the count of 3. At the same time, straighten your knees and assist the patient to a standing position by pulling upward on the transfer belt, making sure to keep your back straight.
    Principle. The patient pushing upward with their arm and leg muscles provides an additional lifting force and reduces the chance of straining your back muscles. Lifting the patient using your knees and the transfer belt allows the strong muscles of the legs and arms to do the lifting, rather than the back muscles.
14. **Procedural Step.** Pivot the patient toward the examining table. Position the patient's buttocks and backs of the knees toward the examining table. Instruct the patient to step onto the footrest (backward) one foot at a time.
    Principle. Pivoting prevents twisting of the spine, which can result in a serious back injury.

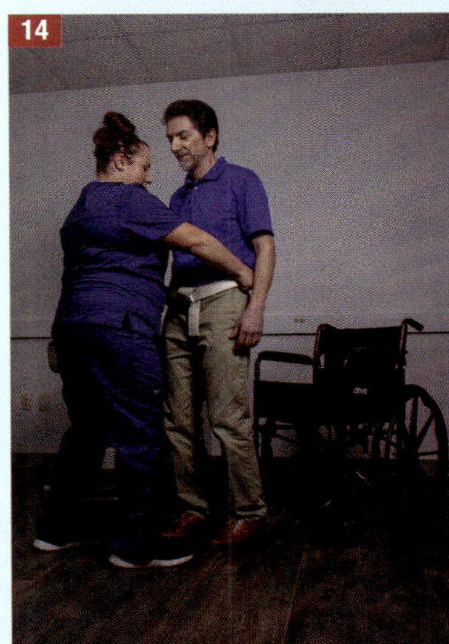

Position the patient toward the table.

15. **Procedural Step.** Gradually lower the patient into a sitting position on the examining table. Make sure the patient's buttocks and thighs are firmly supported on the table. Remove the transfer belt.

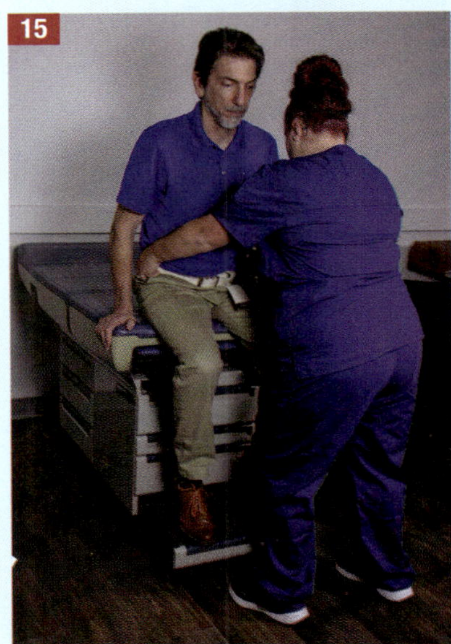

Gradually lower the patient onto the table.

16. **Procedural Step.** Unlock the wheelchair and move it out of the way of the examining table. Push in the footrest of the examining table.
17. **Procedural Step.** Stay with the patient to prevent falls.

Continued

PROCEDURE 20.10 Wheelchair Transfer—cont'd

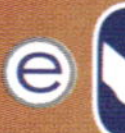

Transferring the Patient to the Wheelchair

1. **Procedural Step.** Wrap the transfer belt snugly around the patient's waist and securely fasten it.
2. **Procedural Step.** Position the wheelchair at a 45-degree angle to the end of the examining table.
3. **Procedural Step.** If the examining table is height adjustable, lower it to the same height as the wheelchair or slightly lower. If it is not height adjustable, pull out the footrest of the examining table.
4. **Procedural Step.** Lock the wheelchair into place and fold back the footrests.
5. **Procedural Step.** Inform the patient of what they will be required to do during the transfer.
6. **Procedural Step.** Stand in front of the patient with the feet apart about 6 to 8 inches, the toes pointed outward, one foot slightly forward, and the knees bent.
7. **Procedural Step.** Ask the patient to place their arms on your shoulders. To prevent a neck injury, do not allow the patient to place their arms around your neck.

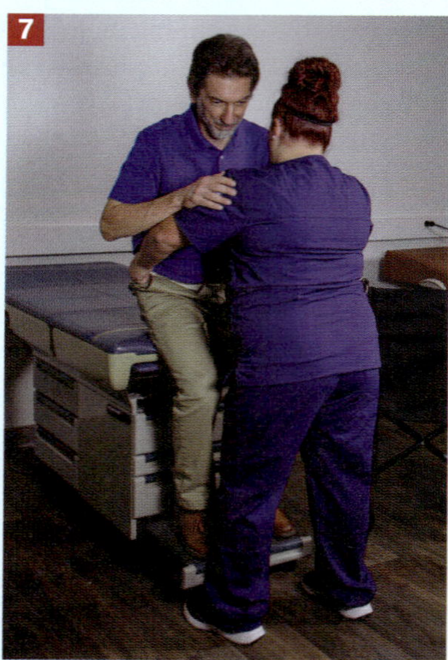

Ask the patient to put their arms on your shoulders.

8. **Procedural Step.** Grasp the transfer belt on either side of the patient's waist using an underhand grasp.
9. **Procedural Step.** Ask the patient to push to a standing position using their thigh and leg muscles on the count of 3. At the same time, straighten your knees and assist the patient to a standing position by pulling upward on the transfer belt.

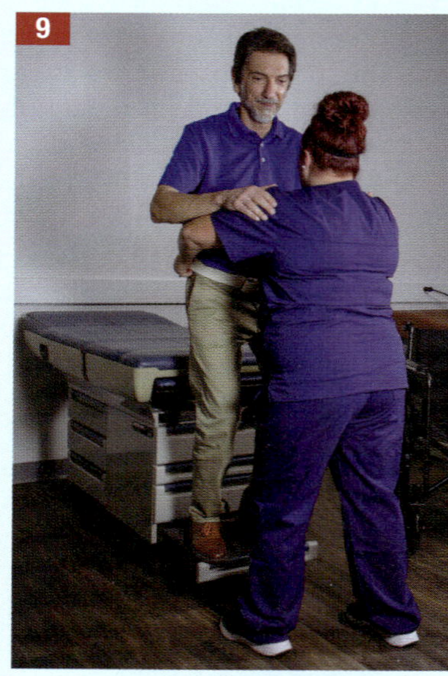

Assist the patient to a standing position.

10. **Procedural Step.** Instruct the patient to step down from the footrest, one foot at a time.
11. **Procedural Step.** Pivot the patient toward the wheelchair. Position the backs of the patient's legs against the seat of the wheelchair.
12. **Procedural Step.** Ask the patient to grasp the armrests of the wheelchair. Bend at your knees and gradually lower the patient into a sitting position in the wheelchair with the patient's buttocks at the back of the chair. Remove the transfer belt and make sure the patient is comfortable.

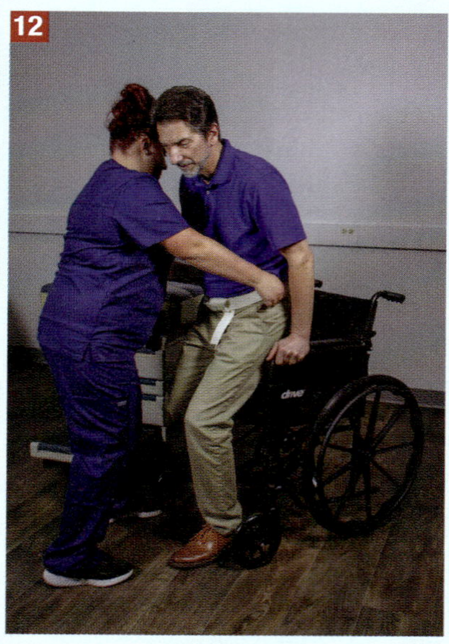

Gradually lower the patient into the wheelchair.

PROCEDURE 20.10 Wheelchair Transfer—cont'd

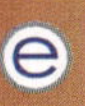

13. **Procedural Step.** Reposition the wheelchair footrests and place the patient's feet in the footrests. Unlock the wheelchair.
14. **Procedural Step.** Push in the footrest of the examining table.

PROCEDURE 20.11 Assisting with the Physical Examination

Outcome Prepare the patient and assist with a physical examination.

Equipment/Supplies

- Examining table
- Equipment for the type of examination to be performed

1. **Procedural Step.** Prepare the examining room. Ensure that the room is clean, free of clutter, and well lit, and that the room temperature is comfortable for the patient.
2. **Procedural Step.** Sanitize your hands.
3. **Procedural Step.** Assemble the equipment according to the type of examination to be performed and the provider's preference. Arrange the instruments and supplies in a neat and orderly manner on a table or tray. Do not allow one item to be placed on top of another.

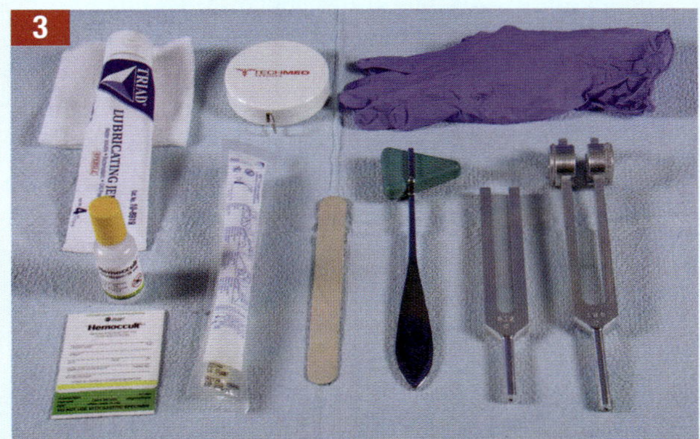

Assemble the equipment.

4. **Procedural Step.** Obtain the patient's medical record. (If an EHR is being used access the computer record for the appropriate patient.) Go to the waiting room and ask the patient to come back to the examining room.
5. **Procedural Step.** Escort the patient to the examining room.
6. **Procedural Step.** Ask the patient to be seated. Greet the patient and introduce yourself using a calm and friendly manner. Identify the patient by their full legal name and date of birth.

   Principle. Identifying the patient correctly avoids mistaking one patient for another. Using a calm and friendly manner helps to put the patient at ease.
7. **Procedural Step.** Seat yourself so that you face the patient at a distance of 3 to 4 feet.
8. **Procedural Step.** Obtain essential information from the patient on allergies, current medications, and symptoms and document this information in the patient's medical record.

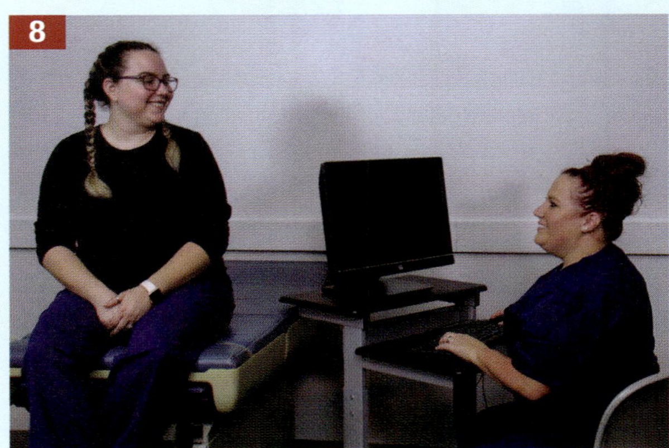

Obtain information from the patient.

9. **Procedural Step.** Measure the weight and height of the patient, and document the results. If required by the medical office policy, determine the patient's BMI and document this number following the weight and height measurements. (*Note:* The EHR automatically calculates and documents the patient's BMI from the weight and height measurements that are entered into the computer.)

Continued

PROCEDURE 20.11 Assisting with the Physical Examination—cont'd

10. **Procedural Step.** Measure the patient's vital signs and document the results.
11. **Procedural Step.** Instruct and prepare the patient for the examination as follows:
    a. Ask the patient whether they need to empty the bladder before the examination. If a urine specimen is needed, the patient will be required to void into a urine container.
    b. Provide the patient with a patient gown. Instruct the patient to remove all clothing and to put on the patient gown. Offer assistance if you sense the patient may have trouble undressing. Leave the room to provide the patient with privacy.

    Principle. An empty bladder makes the examination easier and is more comfortable for the patient.

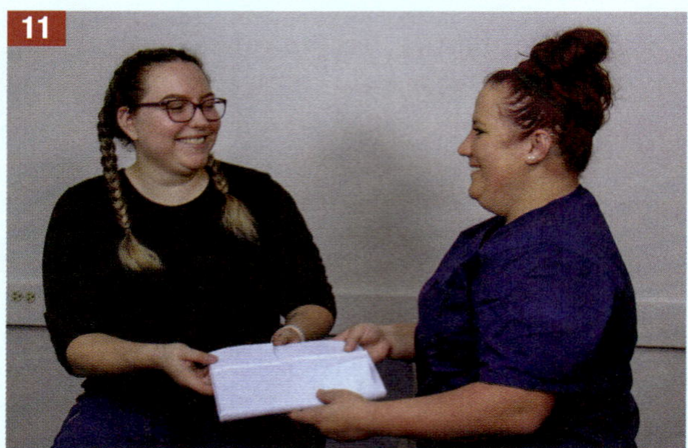

Instruct and prepare the patient for the examination.

12. **Procedural Step.** Check to make sure that the patient is ready to be seen by the provider. Before entering a patient's room, knock lightly on the door to let the patient know that you are getting ready to enter the room. If a patient is ready to be seen, inform the provider. This may be done using a color-coded flagging system mounted on the wall next to the examining room.
13. **Procedural Step.** Make the patient's medical record available to the provider.
14. **Procedural Step.** Assist the provider with examination of the body systems as follows:
    a. Ensure that the patient is positioned correctly in a sitting position on the examining table. This allows the provider to examine the patient's head, eyes, ears, nose, mouth and pharynx, neck, chest, lungs, and heart.
    b. Hand the provider the ophthalmoscope, otoscope, and tongue depressor.
    c. Dim the light when the provider is ready to use the ophthalmoscope. The dim light helps dilate the patient's pupils, providing the provider better visualization of the interior of the eye.
    d. After use, the tongue depressor should be transferred by holding it at the center to prevent contact with the patient's secretions, which may contain pathogens. Dispose of the tongue depressor in a regular waste container.

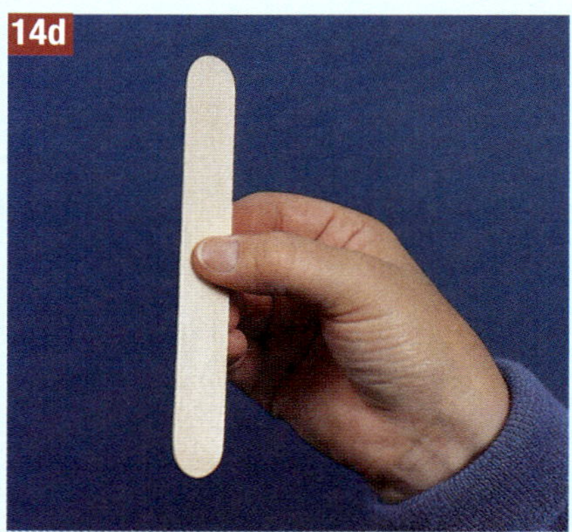

Transfer the tongue depressor by holding it at the center.

    e. Offer reassurance to the patient to reduce apprehension.
15. **Procedural Step.** Position the patient as required for examination of the remaining body systems. Place and drape the patient in the proper position for examination of a particular part of the body using proper body mechanics.
16. **Procedural Step.** Assist and instruct the patient as follows:
    a. Allow the patient to rest in a sitting position on the examining table before they get off of it. Some patients become dizzy after being positioned on the examining table.
    b. Assist the patient off the examining table to prevent falls.
    c. Instruct the patient to get dressed. Provide assistance if needed.
    d. Provide the patient with any necessary instructions, such as patient education and scheduling a return visit. Give instructions involving medical care in terms the patient can understand; do not use medical terms.
    e. Sanitize the hands, and document in their medical record any instructions given to the patient.
    f. Escort the patient to the reception area.
17. **Procedural Step.** Clean the examining room in preparation for the next patient as follows:
    a. Apply gloves and discard the paper on the examining table. Clean and disinfect the table and unroll a fresh length of paper on the table.

PROCEDURE 20.11 Assisting with the Physical Examination—cont'd

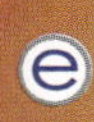

17a

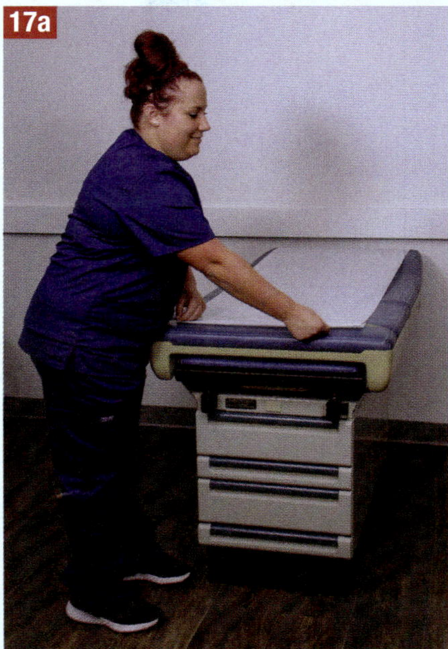

Unroll a fresh length of paper on the table.

b. Discard all disposable supplies into an appropriate waste container.
c. Ensure that there are ample numbers of clean gowns and drapes and other supplies.
d. Remove reusable equipment to a work area for sanitization, sterilization, or disinfection as required by the medical office policy.

17d

DOCUMENTATION EXAMPLE

Date	
11/20/XX	11:30 a.m. CC. Shortness of breath x 2 days.
	T: 98.8° F (TA) P: 78 reg and strong, R: 20
	even and reg, BP: 110/68, Wt: 158, Ht: 5' 6"
	BMI: 25.5 ——— A. Erdy, CMA (AAMA)

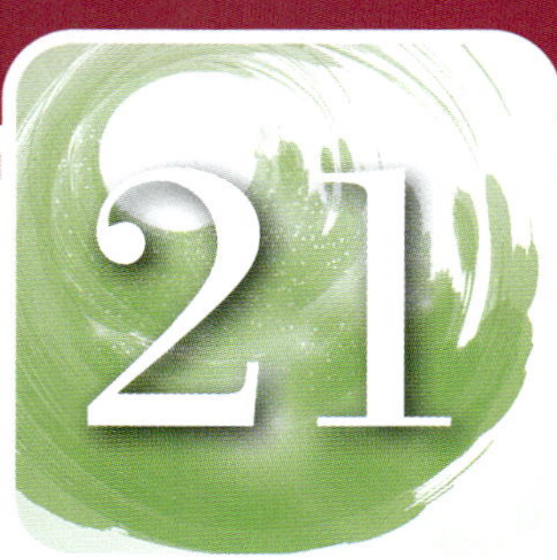

Eye and Ear Assessment and Procedures

Check out the Evolve site at http://evolve.elsevier.com/Bonewit/today to access additional interactive activities and exercises to help you study and prepare for success.

LEARNING OBJECTIVES

The Eye

1. Define visual acuity.
2. State the cause and visual difficulty of each of the following:
   - Myopia
   - Hyperopia
   - Astigmatism
   - Presbyopia
3. State the responsibilities of the following eye specialists: ophthalmologist, optometrist, and optician.
4. Explain the significance of the top and bottom numbers next to each line of letters on the Snellen eye chart.
5. Explain the difference between congenital and acquired color vision deficiencies.
6. State the purpose of an eye irrigation and an eye instillation.

The Ear

7. Identify conditions that may cause conductive and sensorineural hearing loss.
8. List and describe the ways in which hearing acuity can be tested.
9. State the purpose of an ear irrigation and an ear instillation.

PROCEDURES

Assess distance visual acuity.
Assess near visual acuity.
Assess color vision.
Perform an eye irrigation.
Perform an eye instillation.

Perform an ear irrigation.
Perform an ear instillation.

CHAPTER OUTLINE

KEY TERMS

astigmatism (uh-STIG-muh-tiz-em)
audiologist
audiometer (aw-dee-OM-eh-ter)
canthus (KAN-thus)
cerumen
hearing range
hyperopia (HYE-per-OP-ee-uh)
impacted cerumen
instillation (IN-still-AY-shun)
irrigation (EAR-ih-GAY-shun)
myopia (mye-OH-pee-uh)
ophthalmologist
optician
optometrist
otolaryngologist
otologist
otosclerosis
otoscope (AH-toe-skope)
presbycusis
presbyopia (PRESS-bee-OH-pee-uh)
refraction (ree-FRAK-shun)
tympanic membrane (tim-PAN-ik MEM-brane)
visual acuity

INTRODUCTION TO THE EYE

The medical assistant is responsible for performing a variety of assessments and procedures that involve the eye. A visual acuity test is usually part of the routine physical examination. This test is a screening test to detect deficiencies in vision.

The medical assistant may also be responsible for assessing color vision with the use of specially prepared colored plates. As a result of this testing, color blindness can be detected. Color blindness is an inability to distinguish certain colors; the most common problem is with the colors red and green. Color blindness is particularly significant if the patient is involved in an activity that relies on the ability to distinguish colors, such as electronics or interior decorating.

The medical assistant is responsible for performing or teaching the patient to perform eye irrigations and instillations. **Irrigation** is washing a body canal with a flowing solution. **Instillation** is dropping a liquid into a body cavity.

Before beginning a study of this chapter, it is important to thoroughly review the section on the anatomy and physiology of the eye and ear in Chapter 10: The Senses.

EYE SPECIALISTS

Several types of specialists are involved in the care of the eyes. These include the following:

Ophthalmologist: An ophthalmologist is a physician who specializes in diagnosing and treating diseases and disorders of the eye. An ophthalmologist is qualified to prescribe ophthalmic and systemic medications and to perform medical and surgical treatments for eye conditions.

Optometrist: An optometrist is a licensed primary health care provider who has expertise in measuring visual acuity and prescribing corrective lenses for the treatment of refractive errors. An optometrist is also qualified to diagnose and treat disorders and diseases of the eye and to prescribe ophthalmic medications. An optometrist is not a physician and is not permitted to prescribe systemic medications or to perform eye surgery.

Optician: An optician is a technician who fits eyeglasses, contact lenses, and other vision-correcting devices. Opticians cannot perform eye exams or diagnose and treat eye diseases.

VISUAL ACUITY

Visual acuity refers to acuteness or sharpness of vision. A person with normal visual acuity can see clearly and is able to distinguish fine details close up and at some distance.

Errors of refraction are the most common causes of defects in visual acuity (Fig. 21.1). **Refraction** refers to the ability of the eye to bend the parallel light rays coming into it so that they can be focused on the retina. An *error of refraction* means that the light rays are not being refracted or bent properly and are not adequately focused on the retina. A defect in the shape of the eyeball can cause a refractive error. Errors of refraction can be improved with corrective lenses.

A person who is nearsighted has a condition termed **myopia.** The eyeball is too long from front to back, causing the light rays to be brought to a focus in front of the retina. A myopic person has difficulty seeing objects at a distance and may squint and have headaches as a result of eyestrain. Corrective lenses (e.g., eyeglasses, contact lenses) or laser eye surgery can correct this condition, which then allows the light rays to come to a focus on the retina.

A person who is farsighted has a condition known as **hyperopia.** The eyeball is too short from front to back, resulting in a different type of refractive error, in which the light rays are brought to a focus behind the retina. The individual has difficulty viewing objects at a reading or working distance. An individual with hyperopia may experience blurring, headaches, and eyestrain while performing up-close tasks. Corrective lenses can correct this condition by causing the light rays to come to a focus on the retina.

Astigmatism is a refractive error that causes distorted and blurred vision for both near and far objects. A normal cornea has a round or spherical shape and is smooth. With astigmatism, the cornea is curved into an oval shape. This causes the

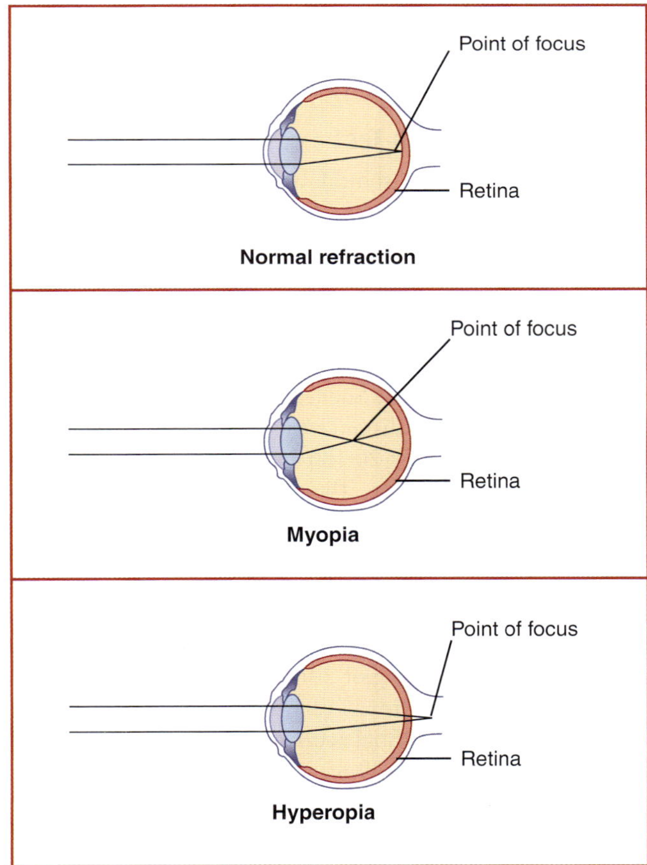

Fig. 21.1 Diagram of normal refraction compared with myopia (nearsightedness) and hyperopia (farsightedness), which are errors of refraction that cause visual defects.

light rays to focus on two different points on the retina, instead of just one, resulting in distorted and blurred vision. Astigmatism often occurs in combination with myopia or hyperopia and can be corrected with corrective lenses.

In most people, a decrease in the elasticity of the lens of the eye begins to occur with aging (usually after age 40 years). This condition, **presbyopia,** results in a decreased ability to focus clearly on close objects.

ASSESSMENT OF DISTANCE VISUAL ACUITY

Myopia can be diagnosed (in combination with other tests) by a distance visual acuity (DVA) test. In the medical office, the Snellen eye chart is most often used. Several types of charts are available. One type is used for school-age children and adults and consists of a chart of letters in decreasing sizes (Fig. 21.2). Another type of chart is used for preschool children, non–English-speaking people, and nonreaders known as the Snellen Big E chart. The Big E chart is composed of the capital letter *E* in decreasing sizes and arranged in different directions (Fig. 21.3). Visual acuity charts with pictures of familiar objects also are available for use with preschool children. Testing with these charts tends to be less accurate than with the Snellen charts. Some children are unable to identify the objects because of lack of recognition, not because of a defect in visual acuity. It is suggested that the Snellen Big E chart be used with preschool children.

Conducting a Snellen Test

The visual acuity test should be performed in a well-lit room that is free of distractions. The test is usually performed at a distance of 20 feet; this can be conveniently marked off in the medical office with paint or a piece of tape so that it does not have to be remeasured every time the test is performed.

Two numbers, separated by a line, appear at the side of each row of letters on the Snellen chart. The number above the line represents the distance (in feet) at which the test is conducted. It is usually 20 feet because most eye tests are conducted at this distance. The number below the line represents the distance from which a person with normal visual acuity can identify the row of letters. The line marked 20/20 indicates normal distance visual acuity, or 20/20 vision. This means a person can identify what he or she is supposed to identify at a distance of 20 feet.

A visual acuity reading of 20/30 means this is the smallest line that the individual can identify at a distance of 20 feet. People with normal acuity would be able to identify this line at a distance of 30 feet.

A visual acuity reading of 20/15 means this is the smallest line that the individual can identify at a distance of 20 feet. It indicates above-average acuity for distance vision. People with normal acuity would be able to identify this line at 15 feet.

The acuity of each eye should be measured separately, traditionally beginning with the right eye. Most providers

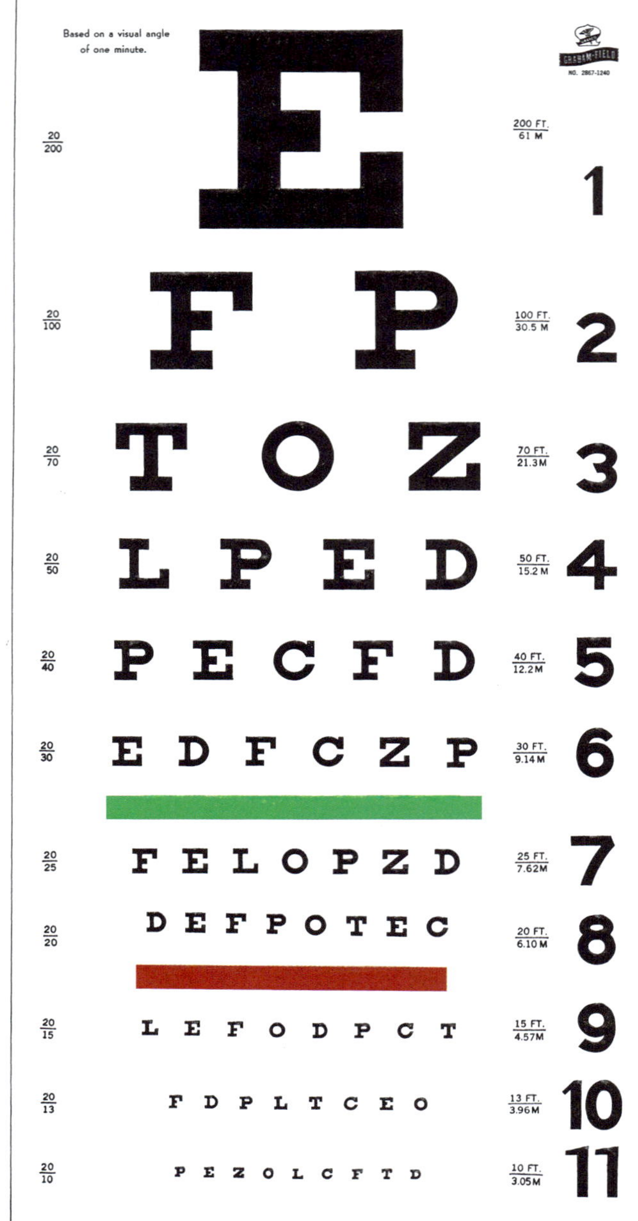

Fig. 21.2 Snellen eye chart consisting of letters in decreasing sizes; this chart is used to measure distance visual acuity.

prefer that patients wear their contact lenses or eyeglasses (except reading glasses) during the test. The medical assistant should document in the patient's medical record if corrective lenses were worn by the patient during the test. An eye occluder should be held over the eye not being tested. The patient's hand should not be used to cover the eye because this may encourage peeking through the fingers, especially in the case of children. The patient should be instructed to leave open the eye not being tested because closing it causes squinting of the eye that is being tested which temporarily improves vision. The procedure for measuring distance visual acuity is outlined in Procedure 21.1.

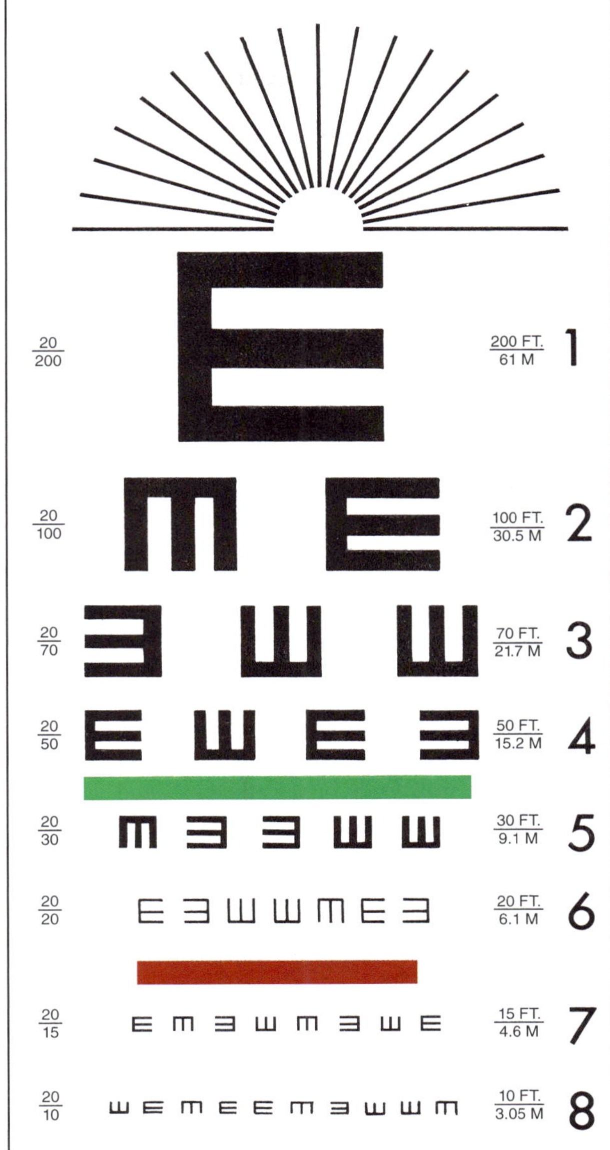

Fig. 21.3 Snellen Big E eye chart consisting of the capital letter *E* in decreasing sizes and arranged in different directions; this chart is used to measure distance visual acuity.

Assessing Distance Visual Acuity in Preschool Children

With minor variations, Procedure 21.1 can be used to test distance visual acuity in preschool children. The Snellen Big E chart is used for this purpose.

Children need a complete and thorough explanation of what is expected of them before beginning the test. Tell the child you will be playing a pointing game. Do not force the child to play the game because the results then tend to be inaccurate. Draw the capital letter *E* on an index card, and teach the child to point in the direction of the open part of the *E* by turning the card in different directions (up, down, to the right, and to the left). Using such phrases as "fingers" or "the legs of the table" to describe the open part of the *E* helps the child understand what is expected (Fig. 21.4). Allow the child to practice the pointing game with the index card until you are sure this level of skill has been mastered. Be sure to praise the child when the correct response is given.

The child might need help holding the eye occluder in place. The aid of another person, such as the parent, would then be required.

ASSESSMENT OF NEAR VISUAL ACUITY

Near visual acuity (NVA) testing assesses the patient's ability to read type at a close distance (i.e., at a reading or working distance); the test results are used to detect hyperopia and presbyopia.

The test is conducted with a card similar to the Snellen eye chart; however, the size of the type ranges from the size of newspaper headlines down to considerably smaller print such as would be found in a telephone directory (Fig. 21.5). The test card is available in a variety of forms, such as printed paragraphs, printed words, and pictures.

The test should be performed in a well-lit room free of distractions. It is conducted with the patient holding the test card at a distance between 14 and 16 inches. If the patient wears reading glasses, they should be worn during the test. The acuity should be measured in each eye separately, traditionally beginning with the right eye. An eye occluder should be held over the eye not being tested. The patient should be instructed to keep the covered eye open because closing it may cause squinting of the eye that is being tested. The patient is asked to read each line of type. During the test, the patient should be observed for unusual symptoms, such as squinting, tilting the head, or watering of the eyes, which may indicate that the patient is having difficulty reading the card. The patient continues until reaching the smallest type that can be read.

The results are documented as the smallest type that the patient could comfortably read with each eye at the distance at which the card was held (i.e., 14 to 16 inches). The documentation is based on the type of test card used to conduct the test. One type of card uses a documentation method similar to that used with the Snellen eye test. For this type of near visual acuity card, the results would be documented as 14/14 for a patient with normal near visual acuity. This means the patient read what was supposed to be read at a distance of 14 inches. Also included in the documentation should be the date and time, corrective lenses worn, and any unusual symptoms exhibited by the patient.

ASSESSMENT OF COLOR VISION

Defects in color vision may be classified as congenital or acquired. *Congenital color vision* deficiencies are more common and refer to a color vision deficiency that is inherited and is present at birth. Congenital color vision deficiencies

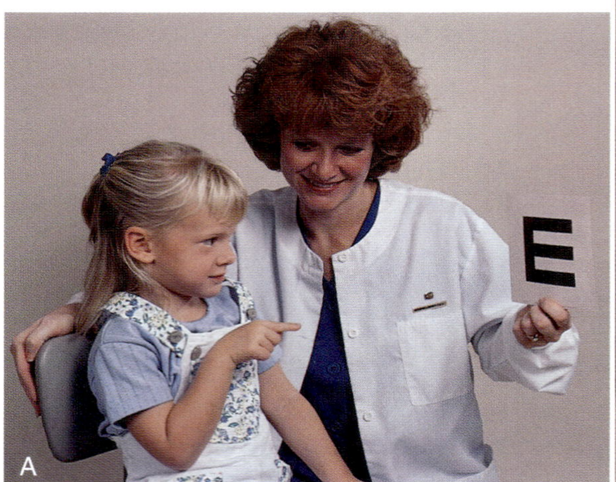

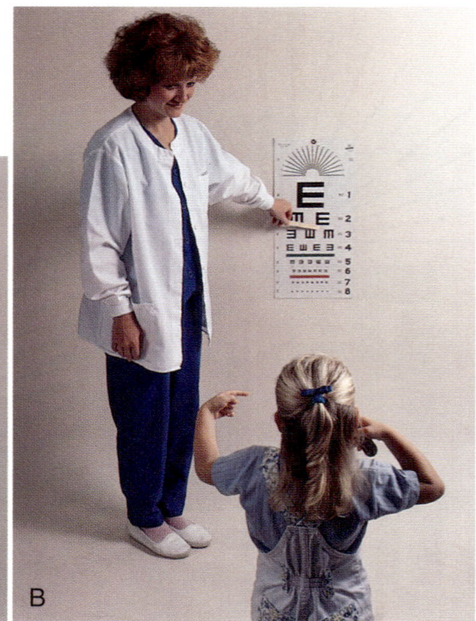

Fig. 21.4 (A) Cammie teaches a preschool child to point in the direction of the open part of the capital letter *E*. (B) Cammie performs the Snellen Big E visual acuity test.

No. 1.
.37M

In the second century of the Christian era, the empire of Rome comprehended the fairest part of the earth, and the most civilized portion of mankind. The frontiers of that extensive monarchy were guarded by ancient renown and disciplined valor. The gentle but powerful influence of laws and manners had gradually cemented the union of the provinces. Their peaceful inhabitants enjoyed and abused the advantages of wealth.

No. 2.
.50M

fourscore years, the public administration was conducted by the virtue and abilities of Nerva, Trajan, Hadrian, and the two Antonines. It is the design of this, and of the two succeeding chapters, to describe the prosperous condition of their empire; and afterwards, from the death of Marcus Antoninus, to deduce the most important circumstances of its decline and fall; a revolution which will ever be remembered, and is still felt by

No. 3.
.62M

the nations of the earth. The principal conquests of the Romans were achieved under the republic; and the emperors, for the most part, were satisfied with preserving those dominions which had been acquired by the policy of the senate, the active emulations of the consuls, and the martial enthusiasm of the people. The seven first centuries were filled with a rapid succession of triumphs; but it was

No. 4.
.75M

reserved for Augustus to relinquish the ambitious design of subduing the whole earth, and to introduce a spirit of moderation into the public councils. Inclined to peace by his temper and situation, it was very easy for him to discover that Rome, in her present exalted situation, had much less to hope than to fear from the chance of arms; and that, in the prosecution of

No. 5.
1.00M

the undertaking became every day more difficult, the event more doubtful, and the possession more precarious, and less beneficial. The experience of Augustus added weight to these salutary reflections, and effectually convinced him that, by the prudent vigor of

No. 6.
1.25M

his counsels, it would be easy to secure every concession which the safety or the dignity of Rome might require from the most formidable barbarians. Instead of exposing his person or his legions to the arrows of the Parthinians, he obtained, by an honor-

No. 7.
1.50M

able treaty, the restitution of the standards and prisoners which had been taken in the defeat of Crassus. His generals, in the early part of his reign, attempted the reduction of Ethiopia and Arabia Felix. They marched near a thou-

No. 8.
1.75M

sand miles to the south of the tropic; but the heat of the climate soon repelled the invaders, and protected the unwarlike natives of those sequestered regions

No. 9.
2.00M

The northern countries of Europe scarcely deserved the expense and labor of conquest. The forests and morasses of Germany were

No. 10.
2.25M

filled with a hardy race of barbarians who despised life when it was separated from freedom; and though, on the first

No. 11.
2.50M

attack, they seemed to yield to the weight of the Roman power, they soon, by a signal

Fig. 21.5 Example of a near visual acuity card.

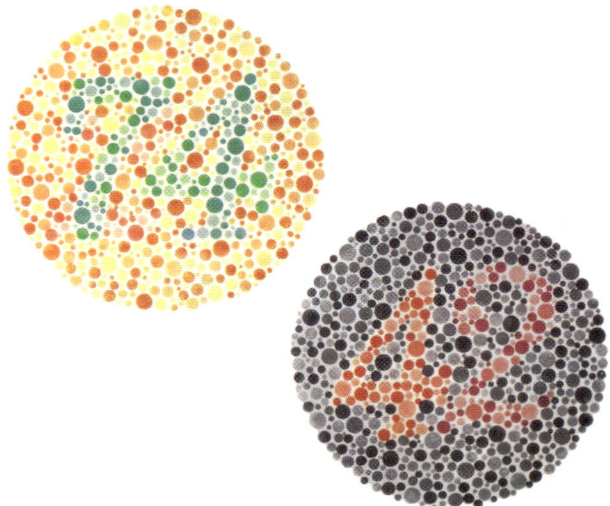

Fig. 21.6 Ishihara test plates. In the upper test plate, a person with normal color vision identifies the number as 74, but a person with a red–green color deficiency identifies it as 21. In the lower test plate, a person with a red color deficiency (protanope) identifies the number as 2, and a person with a green color deficiency (deuteranope) identifies it as 4. A normal-vision person identifies the number as 42. Reproduced plates are not good for testing for color deficiency. (From Isihara J: *Tests for color blindness*, Tokyo, 1920, Kanehara.)

most often affect males. *Acquired color vision* deficiencies refer to a color vision deficiency that is acquired after birth, which may result from disorders of the retina or optic nerve. Color vision tests, such as the Ishihara test (Fig. 21.6), detect congenital color vision deficiencies and are commonly performed in the medical office. A basic screening for color vision can be performed by asking the patient to identify the red and green lines on the Snellen eye chart.

What Would You Do? What Would You *Not* Do?

Case Study 1

Nicole Neason brings her daughter, Haley, to the office for a camp physical. Haley has just completed the fourth grade and is going to summer camp for 2 weeks with Tess, her best friend. Tess wears glasses and Haley thinks they are really cool. She often asks to try on Tess's glasses and wishes she could wear glasses just like her best friend. When Haley is measured for visual acuity, she misses a few letters on the 20/70 line, the 20/50 line, the 20/40 line, and the 20/20 line. She says she cannot identify any of the letters on the 20/15 line. After the examination, Haley wants to know if she's missed enough letters to be able to get glasses. ■

ISHIHARA TEST

The Ishihara test for color vision is a convenient and accurate method to detect congenital color vision deficiencies by assessing an individual's ability to perceive primary colors and shades of color. The most common congenital color vision deficiency is a red-green deficiency. The Ishihara book contains a series of circular plates consisting of colored dots of different sizes. The dots are arranged to form a numeral against a background of similar dots of contrasting colors (see Fig. 21.6). Patients with normal color vision are able to identify the appropriate numeral; however, patients with color vision defects identify the dots either as not forming a number at all or as forming a number different from the one identified by the individual with normal color vision. The first plate in the Ishihara book is a demonstration plate designed to be identified correctly by all individuals (with normal vision and exhibiting color vision deficiencies). The demonstration plate usually consists of the number 12 and is used to explain the procedure to the patient.

The book includes plates with winding colored lines for patients who are unable to identify the numbers by name, such as preschool children and non–English-speaking people. The patient should be asked to trace the line formed by the colored dots using a cotton swab or the eraser end of a pencil. The patient's finger should not be used to do the tracing because over time soiled fingers can degrade the polychromatic plates.

The Ishihara test should be conducted in a quiet room illuminated by natural daylight. If this is not feasible, a room lit with electric light may be used; however, the light should be adjusted to resemble the effect of natural daylight as much as possible. Using light other than just described, such as bright sunlight, may change the appearance of shades of color on the plates, leading to inaccurate test results.

The medical assistant is responsible for performing the color vision test and for documenting results in the patient's medical record. The provider assesses the results to determine whether the patient has a deficiency in color vision.

The Ishihara test presented in this text consists of a book with 14 test plates. *(Note Ishihara books are also available with 10, 24, and 38 test plates.)* Plates 1 through 11 are used to conduct the basic test, and plates 12, 13, and 14 are used to further assess patients who exhibit a color vision deficiency. It is unnecessary to include these plates (12, 13, and 14) in the test of patients who exhibit normal color vision. In interpreting the results, if only 7 or fewer of the 11 Ishihara plates are correctly identified, the patient is identified as having a color vision deficiency. For example, if 5 of the 11 plates are correctly identified, the results are interpreted as a color vision deficiency and the patient would also need to identify plates 12, 13, and 14. On the other hand, if 10 of the 11 plates are correctly identified, the results are interpreted as normal color vision.

If a color vision deficiency is detected, the patient is referred for additional assessment of color vision to an ophthalmologist or optometrist, who would use more precise color vision tests. The procedure for assessing color vision using the Ishihara book of 14 test plates is outlined in Procedure 21.2.

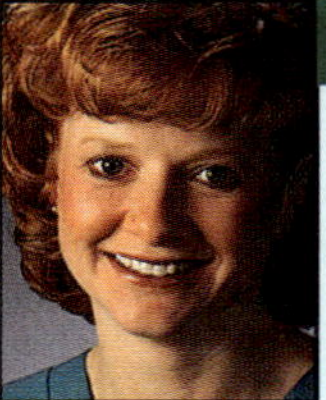

Putting It All Into Practice

My name is Cammie, and I work for an ear, nose, and throat (ENT) surgeon. There are administrative responsibilities in my job; however, the focus is on the clinical aspects, including vital signs measurements, allergy testing, immunotherapy, and assisting with minor office surgeries, such as excision of skin lesions and tympanostomy tube insertions. Over past years in an ENT practice, there have been many challenging and rewarding situations. A recent incident was one that certainly falls into the rewards category.

A young girl came into the office from the emergency department for repair of a facial laceration. It had been quite a day for her, so it was understandable that she was a bit nervous and upset. As the suturing was being performed, she grasped her mother's hand as I tried to discuss interests and school with her. She did fine and was very relieved when the last suture was done.

On her return visit for suture removal, her mother could not accompany her. As I was showing her to the examination room, she quietly asked if I would be in the room. I said, "If you would like, I certainly will." She anxiously nodded yes. As the sutures were removed, she squeezed my hand tighter and tighter. After all of them were out, she first checked her appearance in the mirror, then turned before going out the door and gave me a big hug and a "thank you." Days like this one are truly great rewards and make you feel you really can make a difference in someone's care. ■

EYE IRRIGATION

An eye irrigation involves washing the eye with a flowing solution. Eye irrigations are performed for the following purposes: to cleanse the eye by washing away foreign particles, ocular discharges, or harmful chemicals; to relieve inflammation through the application of heat; and to apply an antiseptic solution. Procedure 21.3 shows how to perform an eye irrigation.

EYE INSTILLATION

An eye instillation involves the dropping of a liquid into the lower conjunctival sac of the eye. Eye instillations are performed to treat eye infections (with medication), to soothe an irritated eye, to dilate the pupil, and to anesthetize the eye during an eye examination or treatment. Medication to be instilled in the eye may come in the form of a liquid, as ophthalmic drops, or as an ophthalmic ointment. Eye drops are usually dispensed in a flexible plastic container with an attached dropper. Eye ointment is dispensed in a small metal tube with a small tip for applying the medication. Procedure 21.4 shows how to perform an eye instillation.

What Would You Do? What Would You *Not* Do?

Case Study 2

Peter Mitchell comes in with his 5-year-old son, Clive. Clive is diagnosed with conjunctivitis (pink eye), and the provider prescribes Polytrim ophthalmic suspension. Mr. Mitchell says that Clive does not cooperate very well when having drops put in his eyes and asks for any ideas that might make it less of an ordeal. Mr. Mitchell has 7-year-old twin girls at home and wants to know what can be done so they don't get pink eye. He asks if it would be all right to instill the drops in the twins' eyes as a preventive measure. ■

PATIENT COACHING Conjunctivitis

Answer questions that patients have about conjunctivitis.

What is conjunctivitis?

Conjunctivitis, often referred to as *pink eye*, is an inflammation of the conjunctiva (see illustration). The conjunctiva is a thin transparent membrane that covers the white of the eye. Conjunctivitis occurs when the conjunctiva becomes infected with a bacterium or virus. Other causes of conjunctivitis include allergies, prolonged wearing of contact lenses, and irritation from wind, dust, and smoke. Conjunctivitis is almost always harmless and clears up by itself within 2 weeks. If it is caused by a bacterium, the provider may prescribe antibiotic eye drops or ointment.

What are the symptoms?

Most types of conjunctivitis are relatively painless. The eye is red or pink because of irritation, and there is a feeling of sandiness or grittiness in the eye. A discharge is usually present, which dries at night when the eyes are closed. This may cause the eyelids to be stuck together in the morning. Other symptoms include tearing, itching, and sensitivity to light.

Is it contagious?

Conjunctivitis caused by a virus or bacterium is highly contagious. It can be spread easily from one eye to another and throughout a family or classroom in a matter of days.

How can its spread be prevented?

The following measures help prevent the spread of conjunctivitis:

- Avoid touching or rubbing the infected eye, which can spread the infection to the other eye or to other people.
- Sanitize your hands frequently with soap, particularly after touching the eyes or face.
- Do not share washcloths, towels, or pillows with anyone.
- Do not wear contact lenses or eye makeup until the conjunctivitis is completely gone.
- Discard eye makeup that was used while you were infected to prevent reinfection.
- Encourage the patient to practice techniques that prevent the spread of conjunctivitis.

PATIENT COACHING Conjunctivitis—cont'd

- If the provider has prescribed eye medication, teach the patient (or parent) the proper procedure for performing an eye instillation.
- Give the patient educational materials on conjunctivitis.

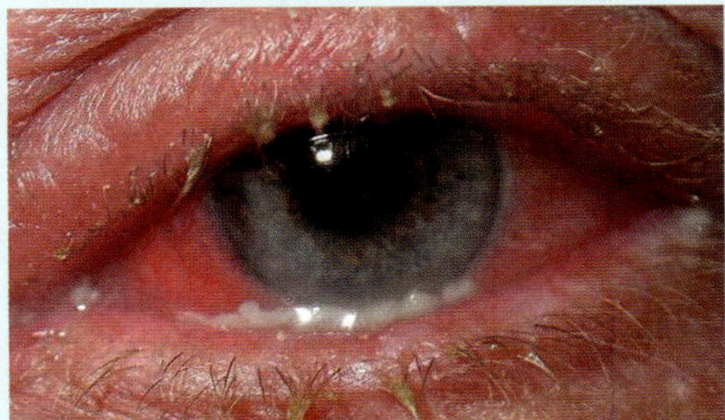

Bacterial conjunctivitis. (From Cuppett M, Walsh KM: *General medical conditions in the athlete*, St. Louis, 2005, Elsevier.)

INTRODUCTION TO THE EAR

The medical assistant is responsible for performing a variety of procedures that involve the ear. Hearing tests also may be part of the routine physical examination. During contact with the patient, the medical assistant should be alert to signs that indicate the patient might be having difficulty hearing what is being said. The medical assistant may be responsible for assisting with hearing acuity tests such as tuning fork tests and audiometry. The medical assistant is also responsible for performing or teaching the patient to perform ear irrigations and instillations.

EAR SPECIALISTS

Several types of specialists are involved in the care of the eyes. These include the following:

Otolaryngologist: An otolaryngologist is a physician who specializes in the diagnosis and treatment of disorders of the ears, nose, and throat (ENT). An otolaryngologist is qualified to prescribe medication and to perform ear, nose, and throat surgery. An otolaryngologist is also known as an ENT physician.

Otologist: An otologist is a physician who can treat more complex ear conditions and perform more complex ear surgeries as compared with an otolaryngologist. An otologist is an otolaryngologist who has completed further training and specializes only in the ear.

Audiologist: An audiologist is a licensed health care professional who evaluates, diagnoses, treats, and manages hearing loss and balance disorders in adults and children. An audiologist can prescribe, fit, and dispense hearing aids and other amplification and hearing assistive devices. Responsibilities of an audiologist include conducting hearing examinations, fitting hearing aids, and monitoring patient use of hearing devices.

ASSESSMENT OF HEARING ACUITY

The assessment of hearing acuity is an integral part of a complete physical examination. It is possible for an individual to have hearing loss and not be aware of it. Early detection and treatment of hearing problems help prevent permanent hearing loss. The number of individuals with a hearing impairment has gradually increased over the past 20 years. Factors that contribute to this increase include an aging population and a noisier environment.

Hearing range describes the range of sound frequencies that can be heard by humans (or animals). Sound frequency or pitch is measured in Hz (hertz) and refers to the number of sound vibrations in a single second. The number of vibrations per second relates to how low- or high-pitched a sound is. If the number of vibrations per second is low, the sound is low-pitched. On the other hand, if the number of vibrations per second is high, the sound is high-pitched. The human ear can hear a wide range of sound frequencies, ranging from 20 Hz (very low-pitched) to 20,000 Hz (very high-pitched). The hearing range of an individual varies based on the following factors: heredity, age, amount of exposure to loud noises, and certain illnesses (e.g., meningitis). For example, because of the normal aging process, 12,000 Hz is difficult for anyone over 50 years of age to hear.

What Would You Do? What Would You *Not* Do?

Case Study 3

Willow Madison brings in her 6-year-old daughter, Jade. For the past 3 days, Jade has been running a fever and has had persistent pain and hearing loss in her left ear. Ms. Madison practices alternative medicine and uses prescription medications as little as possible. She says that she has been trying herbal therapy and aromatherapy to make Jade better, but it does not seem to be helping. Jade is diagnosed with acute otitis media, and the physician prescribes amoxicillin for 10 days. Ms. Madison wants to know if she has to give Jade the amoxicillin for the entire 10 days. She asks if she can stop using it when Jade starts feeling better. Ms. Madison also wants to know if the ear infection will cause a permanent problem with Jade's hearing. ■

TYPES OF HEARING LOSS

Hearing loss is a common health problem affecting millions of individuals. The treatment of hearing loss depends on the type of hearing loss and its cause. There are three types of hearing loss: conductive, sensorineural, and mixed.

Conductive Hearing Loss

Conductive hearing loss (CHL) results when there is a physical interference of the normal conduction of sound waves through the external ear and middle ear. Because of the interference, the amount of sound reaching the inner ear is less than normal, resulting in hearing impairment. With CHL, soft sounds may be hard to hear, and loud sounds may sound muffled.

CHL in the external ear can be caused by a blockage in the external ear canal, such as swelling from external otitis (swimmer's ear), foreign bodies, benign growths such as polyps, and excessive or impacted cerumen.

Cerumen is a yellowish waxy substance secreted by glands in the external ear canal that lubricates and protects the ear canal. **Impacted cerumen** refers to cerumen that is wedged firmly together in the ear canal so as to be immovable. CHL in the middle ear may be caused by serous otitis media (fluid in the middle ear), acute otitis media (infection in the middle ear), or a perforated **tympanic membrane** (eardrum).

The cause of CHL can often be determined by examining the ear with an otoscope. An **otoscope** is an instrument used to examine the external ear canal and tympanic membrane. Hearing is frequently restored by removing the blockage (e.g., impacted cerumen) or treating the disorder (e.g., serous otitis media).

Another cause of CHL is otosclerosis. **Otosclerosis** is an abnormal bone growth in the middle ear. This prevents the three small ear bones located in the middle ear (*malleus*, *incus*, and *stapes*) from vibrating normally in response to sound waves. Mild otosclerosis can be treated with a hearing aid, but surgery is often required in a procedure known as a *stapedectomy*.

Sensorineural Hearing Loss

Sensorineural hearing loss (SNHL) results from damage to the inner ear or the auditory nerve. With this type of hearing loss, sound is conducted normally through the outer ear and middle ear, but because of a problem with the perception of sound waves, a hearing deficit occurs. SNHL is usually irreversible and permanent. Specific causes of SNHL include aging, hereditary factors, loud noise exposure, tumors, infectious diseases (e.g., meningitis, measles, mumps), and ototoxicity caused by certain medications. The most common cause of SNHL in an adult is presbycusis. **Presbycusis** is defined as the gradual loss of hearing in both ears due to the normal aging process. As an individual ages, nerves and sensory receptor cells in the inner ear deteriorate, leading to a gradual loss of hearing. Refer to the *Patient Coaching* box on *Noise-Induced Hearing Loss* for more information on SNHL caused by exposure to loud noises.

Many people with SNHL may benefit from hearing aids and cochlear implants. *Hearing aids* are small electronic devices that amplify sounds to a level that the inner ear can detect. A hearing aid can help people hear better in both quiet and noisy situations. A *cochlear implant* is a small, complex electronic device that can provide a sense of sound to an individual who has a profound hearing loss. A cochlear implant is surgically implanted and works by bypassing damaged portions of the inner ear and directly stimulating the auditory nerve. Once the auditory nerve is stimulated, the sound signals are sent to the brain where the signals are recognized as sound.

Mixed Hearing Loss

A mixed hearing loss is a combination of CHL and SNL. This means that there may be damage to the external or middle ear as well as the inner ear or auditory nerve.

DEGREE OF HEARING LOSS

All types of hearing loss create problems with communication. The degree of hearing loss refers to the severity of the hearing loss. An audiologist is qualified to determine the degree of hearing loss using various hearing tests. The degree of hearing loss can range from mild to profound, described as follows.

Mild Hearing Loss: An individual with mild hearing loss can hear a one-on-one conversation but has difficulty hearing a conversation in a noisy environment such as a restaurant. In addition, it is difficult for the individual to hear quiet or soft sounds, such as a ticking clock or a dripping faucet.

Moderate Hearing Loss: An individual with moderate hearing loss has difficulty understanding speech at a normal volume level without hearing aids. The individual frequently asks people to repeat themselves or to speak louder and higher volumes are also needed for television and radio listening.

Severe Hearing Loss: An individual with severe hearing loss cannot hear normal conversational speech at all without powerful hearing aids. The individual can only hear loud speech when it is shouted directly into their ear.

Profound Hearing Loss: An individual with profound hearing loss does not hear any speech at all and can only hear extremely loud sounds. The individual may rely on lip-reading, gestures, or sign language to communicate. Hearing aids may not be effective, and the individual may need cochlear implants to assist with hearing. (Note: Total hearing loss means that an individual cannot hear any sounds at all).

PATIENT COACHING Noise-Induced Hearing Loss (NIHL)

Answer questions that patients may have on NIHL.

What is NIHL?

NIHL occurs when the tiny and delicate hair cells located in the inner ear become damaged or destroyed due to loud noise. These tiny hair cells are responsible for creating an electrical signal from sound waves entering the ear. The electrical signal is then transmitted to the brain to be interpreted into sound that can be recognized and understood by the listener. Loud noise overstimulates these delicate hair cells which can damage and destroy them. Once hair cells are destroyed, they cannot grow back. Over time, as more and more hair cells are destroyed permanent hearing loss may occur. People of all ages can develop NIHL including children, teens, young adults, mature adults, and older adults.

PATIENT COACHING Noise-Induced Hearing Loss (NIHL)—cont'd

What causes NIHL?

NIHL can be caused by a very loud and sudden exposure to intense noise occurring close to the ears, such as a gunshot, firecracker, or explosion. It can also be caused by continuous and repeated exposure to loud sounds over an extended period of time. NIHL is often seen in individuals who frequently listen to loud music, fire guns without ear protection, or are exposed to loud noise as part of their jobs.

What noises can cause NIHL?

Noises that are too loud and last too long can result in NIHL. The loudness of sound is measured in units called *decibels* (dB). Sounds of less than 75 dB, even after long exposure, are unlikely to cause hearing loss. Normal conversation is approximately 60 dB, and a whisper is 30 dB. Continued exposure to noise louder than 85 dB can gradually cause hearing loss over time. Examples of common noises and the decibel level of each include:

Safe Noise Levels	Decibels
Normal breathing	10
Kitchen appliances	40 to 60
Television (normal volume)	70
Vacuum cleaner	60 to 80
Traffic noises	80

Noise Levels at Risk for NIHL	Decibels
Motorcycle, dirt bikes, and snowmobiles	80 to 110
Music through headphones or earbuds (at max volume)	80 to 120
Shouting in the ear	110
Music concerts and sporting events	120
Chain saw	120
Car stereo (at max volume)	90 to130
Siren	120 to 130
Fireworks	140 to 160
Firearms	140 to 170

What are the symptoms of NIHL?

NIHL can have a significant impact on an individual's quality of life and may lead to avoidance of social situations. Some of the most common symptoms of NIHL include:

- Trouble hearing soft or faint sounds
- Normal conversation sounds are muffled or distorted
- Frequently asking people to repeat what they have said
- Difficulty in following conversations and communicating with friends and family
- A feeling of fullness and pressure in the ears
- Ringing or buzzing in the ears (known as tinnitus)
- A need to increase television volume

Can NIHL be prevented?

Unlike other types of hearing loss, NIHL is completely preventable. Measures to take to prevent NIHL include:

- Knowing which noises are too loud and can cause hearing damage
- Avoid or limit exposure to excessively loud sounds
- Avoid playing music at a loud volume
- Wear hearing protection devices (e.g., earplugs, earmuffs) when involved in an activity with loud noise
- Move away from loud noise if it is not possible to protect the ears from it
- Protect small children from loud noise
- Make friends and family aware of the hazards of loud noise

What is the treatment for NIHL?

In most cases, NIHL is treated with hearing aids. However, if NIHL worsens over time, hearing aids may not provide enough benefit and other options might be recommended such as cochlear implants. ■

HEARING ACUITY TESTS

Numerous tests can be used to assess hearing acuity. Tests range from qualitative tests using a tuning fork to highly specific quantitative tests using an audiometer. It is important to test only one ear at a time because a hearing deficit can exist in one ear only. The ear not being tested should be blocked by an earplug or masked. *Masking* involves the presentation of sound (usually noise) to the ear not being tested so that the patient's response is based only on hearing in the ear being tested.

Tuning Fork Tests

Tuning fork tests provide a general assessment of hearing acuity and may be part of the physical examination. A patient exhibiting a hearing impairment during these tests is referred to an audiologist for further testing and evaluation.

A tuning fork with a frequency of 512 Hz or 1024 Hz is usually used because these frequencies fall within the range of normal speech. The Weber and Rinne tests are the tuning fork tests most commonly performed by the provider; they are used to identify conductive and sensorineural hearing loss.

The *Weber test* is a useful assessment of hearing loss when one ear hears better than the other. The tuning fork is set in vibration, and the base of the fork is placed on the center of the patient's head. The patient is asked to indicate where the sound is heard best. A patient with normal hearing would hear the sound equally in both ears or in the center of the head. Fig. 21.7 illustrates the Weber test and describes the interpretation of results.

The *Rinne test* compares the duration of sound perception by air conduction with that of bone conduction. The tuning fork is set in vibration, and the base of the fork is

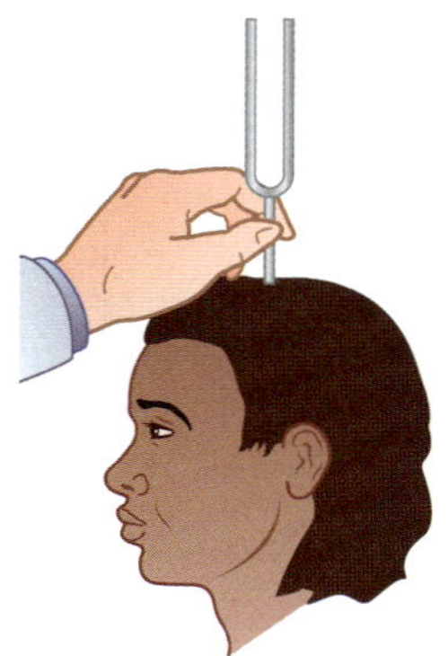

Fig. 21.7 Weber test.

placed against the bone of the mastoid process. The patient is instructed to indicate when the sound is no longer heard. The prongs of the fork (still vibrating) are placed in the air about 1 inch from the opening of the patient's ear canal, and the patient indicates when the sound is no longer heard. An individual with normal hearing is able to hear the sound at least twice as long through air conduction as through bone conduction. Fig. 21.8 illustrates the Rinne test and describes the interpretation of results.

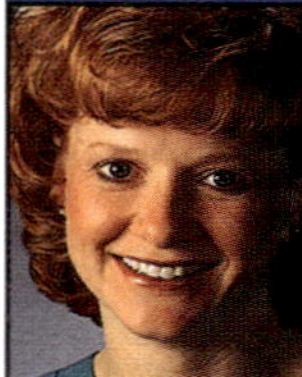

Memories *from* Practicum

Cammie: There is one characteristic that is shared by all patients. I first noticed this during my practicum, and it does not seem to matter what type of practice it is. Patients like to feel special and to be treated that way. They like consistency in their provider and in the office staff, and seeing familiar faces. This is especially hard during practicum. The time spent is too short to truly get to know the patients, but it is a great learning experience.

It is important to observe the staff and patient communication and interaction skills. By doing this, you can decide which ones you admire and those that you do not wish to copy. The following are just a few of the guidelines that have helped me: (1) Call patients by name and be sure that they know your name. (2) Follow through with what you have told patients you will do and keep them updated if circumstances change. (3) Smile, and do not let one patient's negative attitude interfere with your care of others. (4) Take time to listen.

When you do begin your career, it does not take long to get into a routine and to start knowing your patients. When patients see a familiar face, they are more willing to share information that can contribute to improved communication and good health care. ■

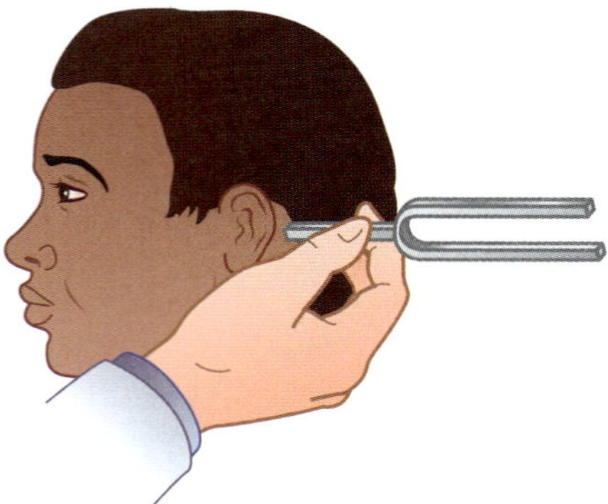

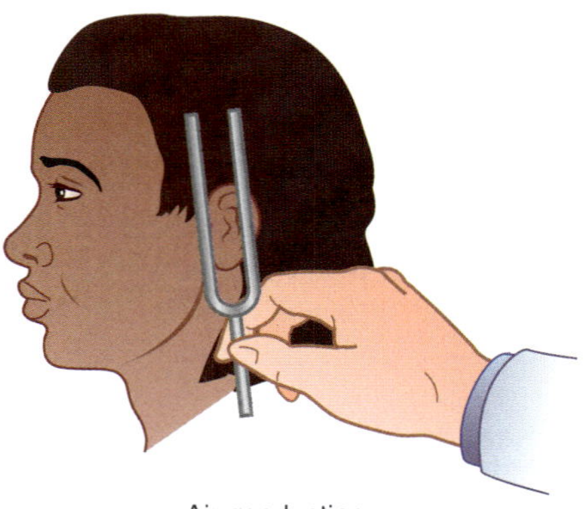

Fig. 21.8 Rinne test.

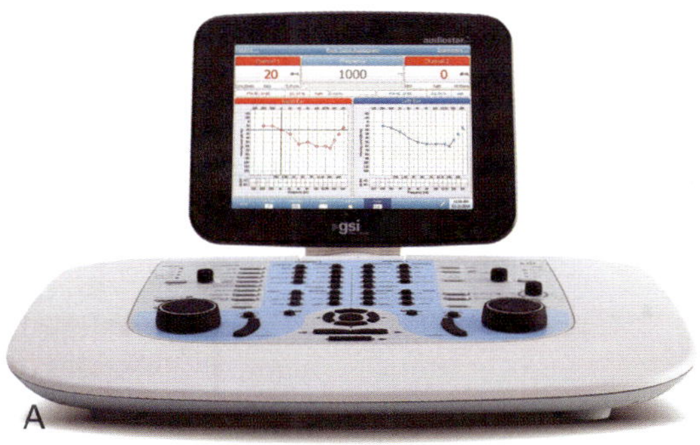

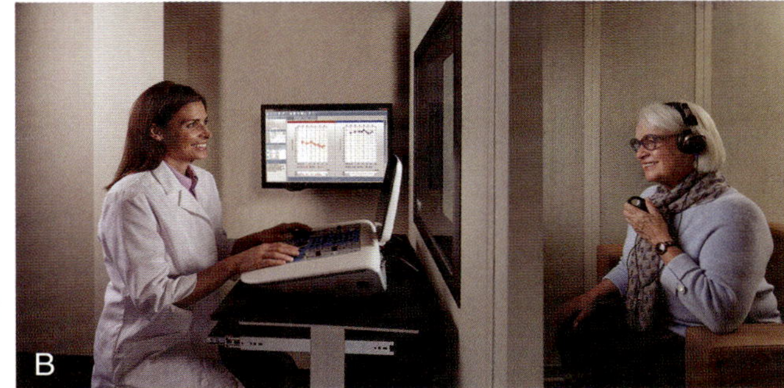

Fig. 21.9 (A) Audiometer. (B) The patient signals when she hears a sound. (A and B, Courtesy of GSI Grason-Stadler.)

Audiometry

Audiometry is the measurement of hearing acuity using a special instrument called an **audiometer** (Fig. 21.9A). An audiometer quantitatively measures hearing for the various frequencies of sound waves. Audiometry is a more specific hearing acuity test because it provides information on how extensive a hearing loss is and which frequencies are involved. It is important that the test be conducted in a quiet room because outside noise may affect the results, especially in the lower frequencies. The patient wears headphones placed snugly over the ears (Fig. 21.9B). The audiometer delivers a single frequency at a time at specific intensities, starting with low-frequency tones of 250 to 500 Hz and going to high-frequency tones of 6000 to 8000 Hz. The patient is asked to signal when a sound is heard so that the patient's hearing threshold for each frequency can be determined. The hearing acuity in each ear is assessed separately, and the results are plotted on a graph known as an *audiogram.*

Tympanometry

Tympanometry is not a hearing test, but it does help determine the cause of hearing loss, so it is presented in this section. The tympanometer consists of an earpiece attached to an electronic device (Fig. 21.10A). The earpiece is placed snugly in the patient's ear, and low-frequency sound waves are directed against the eardrum while pressure is applied in the ear canal (Fig. 21.10B). With a normal ear, the eardrum exhibits mobility in response to the pressure, as indicated on a graphic readout known as a *tympanogram.* If there is fluid in the middle ear, the eardrum does not move but remains stiff, as indicated on the tympanogram. Tympanometry is useful in diagnosing serous otitis media (fluid in the middle ear), which is a common cause of temporary hearing loss in children.

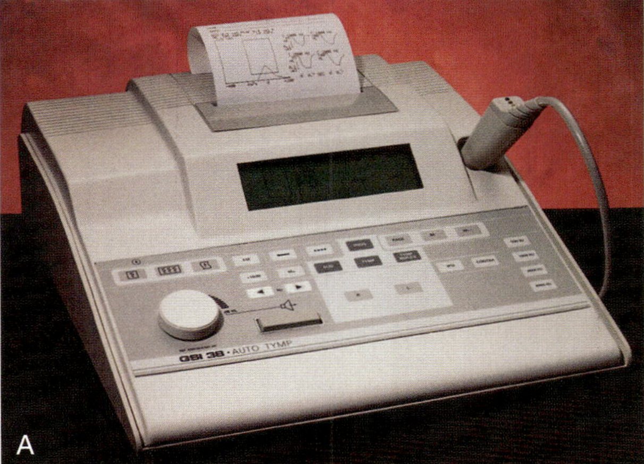

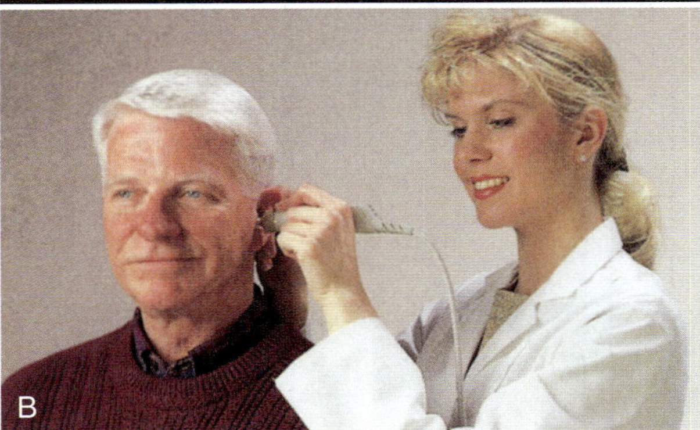

Fig. 21.10 (A) Tympanometer. (B) The earpiece is placed snugly in the patient's ear.

EAR IRRIGATION

An ear irrigation is the washing of the external ear canal with a flowing solution. Ear irrigations are performed for the following purposes: to cleanse the external ear canal to remove cerumen, discharge, or a foreign body; to relieve inflammation by applying an antiseptic solution; and to apply heat to the ear. Before irrigating, impacted cerumen must be softened by instilling warm mineral oil or hydrogen peroxide into the ear canal for 10 to 15 minutes. An ear irrigation should not be performed if the tympanic membrane is perforated because this could result in severe irritation or infection of the middle ear.

Ear irrigations are most commonly performed in the medical office using an Elephant Ear Wash System. Procedure 21.5 outlines the procedure for performing an ear irrigation.

EAR INSTILLATION

An ear instillation involves dropping a liquid into the external ear canal. Ear instillations are performed to soften impacted cerumen, to combat infection with the use of antibiotic ear drops, and to relieve pain. The ear drops are usually dispensed in a flexible plastic container with an attached dropper. Procedure 21.6 shows how to perform an ear instillation.

PATIENT COACHING Acute Otitis Media

Answer questions that patients have about otitis media.

What is otitis media?

An infection of the middle ear is medically referred to as *acute otitis media.* It is an inflammation of the middle ear caused by an infection and can occur in one or both ears. It is common in young children 3 months to 3 years old, but is unusual in adults. Otitis media is not serious if treated promptly and effectively. If not treated, however, otitis media can lead to serious complications, such as acute mastoiditis, meningitis, and permanent hearing loss.

What causes otitis media?

Otitis media is often the result of an upper respiratory infection or allergy that causes the eustachian tube to swell and become blocked. The blockage causes fluid to build up in the middle ear. This fluid is an ideal place for bacteria to grow. If this occurs, the result is acute otitis media.

What are the symptoms of otitis media and how is it diagnosed?

The most common symptoms are intense pain, fever, and temporary hearing loss. Other symptoms may include dizziness, nausea and vomiting, and (if the eardrum ruptures) drainage from the ear. To diagnose otitis media, the provider examines the ears with an otoscope. If otitis media is present, the eardrum is red and swollen (see illustration) as a result of irritation from the infection, and pus and mucus can be seen behind the eardrum.

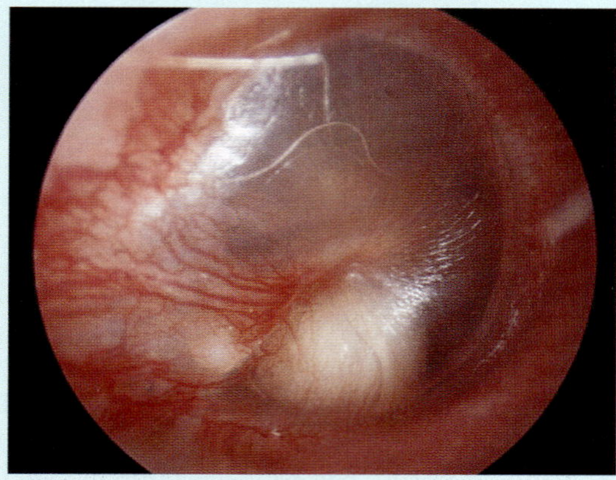

Chronic otitis media. (From Damjanov I, Linder J: *Pathology: a color atlas*, St. Louis, 1999, Mosby.)

How is otitis media treated?

Otitis media is usually treated with an oral antibiotic for 10 to 14 days. It is important to complete the entire prescribed course of antibiotics; otherwise, the infection may recur. The provider also may recommend a decongestant to help open the blocked eustachian tube. After the acute infection is over, fluid may remain trapped in the middle ear. This condition is known as *serous otitis media* (see illustration) and, if not treated, may last for days, weeks, months, or even a year. Although fluid in the middle ear is painless, it may result in a feeling of fullness or pressure in the ears and temporary hearing loss.

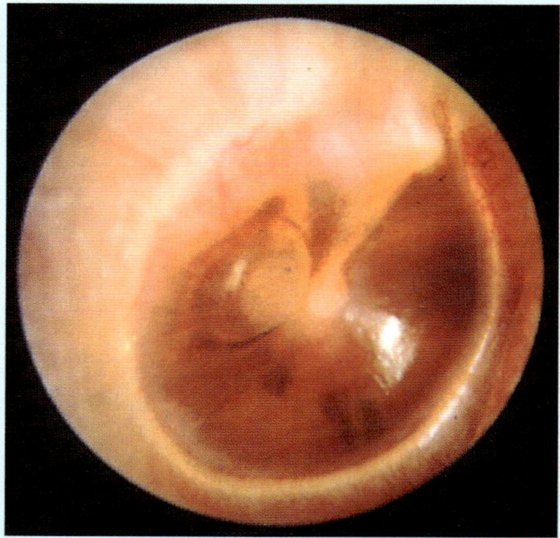

Serous otitis media. (From Swartz MH: *Textbook of physical diagnosis*, ed 5, Philadelphia, 2006, Elsevier.)

Why is otitis media so common in children?

In children, the eustachian tube is positioned horizontally and is shorter and narrower than in adults. When a child has an upper respiratory infection, bacteria can travel easily to the middle ear resulting in otitis media. In addition, swelling from the respiratory infection can block this narrow tube, which causes fluid to build up in the middle ear.

- Encourage the patient to complete the entire prescribed course of antibiotics.
- If the provider has prescribed ear drops, teach the patient (or parent) the proper procedure for performing an ear instillation.
- Encourage early treatment of upper respiratory infections.
- Give the patient educational materials on otitis media. ■

What Would You Do? What Would You *Not* Do? RESPONSES

Case Study 1
Page 445

What Did Cammie Do?
- ❑ Talked with Haley (on her level) about why someone needs to wear glasses.
- ❑ Retested Haley with the Snellen chart to see if she missed the same letters.
- ❑ Tested Haley with the Big E chart to give the physician an additional measurement to assess Haley's visual acuity.
- ❑ Informed the physician of the situation.

What Did Cammie Not Do?
- ❑ Did not tell Haley that she needs glasses.
- ❑ Did not scold Haley for trying to miss letters on the test.

Case Study 2
Page 446

What Did Cammie Do?
- ❑ Gave Mr. Mitchell some suggestions on how to put drops in Clive's eyes so it is less scary. One idea is to have Clive lie down flat and close his eyes. Place the drops in the inner corner of his eye next to the bridge of his nose, letting them make a little lake there. When Clive relaxes and opens his eye, the drops will gently flow into his eye.
- ❑ Talked with Clive (on his level) about why he needs eye drops.
- ❑ Told Mr. Mitchell that the eye drops were prescribed for Clive, and they should be used only for Clive. Told him that if the twins developed conjunctivitis, he should call the office.
- ❑ Gave Mr. Mitchell suggestions for preventing the twins from getting conjunctivitis (not touching the infected eye, frequent handwashing, not sharing toys or towels).

What Did Cammie Not Do?
- ❑ Did not tell Mr. Mitchell to hold Clive down or force the drops into his eyes.
- ❑ Did not tell Mr. Mitchell that he should know better than to think about giving the twins a medication not prescribed for them.

Case Study 3
Page 447

What Did Cammie Do?
- ❑ Explained to Ms. Madison that Jade may begin to feel better after several days of antibiotics, but not all of the germs causing her ear infection will have been killed by then. If she does not give Jade the full course of antibiotics, the infection could come back.
- ❑ Documented all the medications that Ms. Madison has administered to Jade.
- ❑ Gave Ms. Madison a patient information brochure on acute otitis media.
- ❑ Told Ms. Madison that she needs to talk to the physician about her concern regarding hearing loss because the physician is most qualified to answer that question.
- ❑ Encouraged Ms. Madison to bring Jade in sooner when she develops fever and ear pain.

What Did Cammie Not Do?
- ❑ Did not criticize Ms. Madison for waiting so long to bring Jade in.
- ❑ Did not offer a personal opinion about alternative medicine.

TERMINOLOGY REVIEW

Key Term	Word Parts	Definition
Astigmatism	*a-:* without *stigma/a:* point *-ism:* state of	A refractive error that causes distorted and blurred vision for both near and far objects due to a cornea that is oval shaped.
Audiologist	*audi/o:* hearing *-ologist:* one who studies and practices	A licensed health care professional who evaluates, diagnoses, treats, and manages hearing loss and balance disorders in adults and children.
Audiometer	*audi/o:* hearing *-meter:* instrument used to measure	An instrument used to quantitatively measure hearing acuity for the various frequencies of sound waves.
Canthus		The junction of the eyelids at either corner of the eye.
Cerumen		A yellowish waxy substance secreted by glands in the ear canal which functions to lubricate and protect the ear canal. Earwax.
Hearing range		The range of sound frequencies that can be heard by a human.
Hyperopia	*hyper-:* above, excessive *-opia:* vision	A refractive error in which the light rays are brought to a focus behind the retina resulting in difficulty viewing objects at a reading or working distance. Farsightedness.
Impacted cerumen		Cerumen that is wedged firmly together in the ear canal so as to be immovable.

Continued

TERMINOLOGY REVIEW—cont'd

Key Term	Word Parts	Definition
Instillation		The dropping of a liquid into a body cavity.
Irrigation		The washing of a body canal with a flowing solution.
Myopia	*-opia:* vision	A refractive error in which the light rays are brought to a focus in front of the retina resulting in difficulty viewing objects at a distance. Nearsightedness.
Ophthalmologist	*ophthalmo-:* eye *-ologist:* one who studies and practices	A physician who specializes in diagnosing and treating diseases and disorders of the eye.
Optician	*opto-:* vision *-ician:* a person skilled in	A technician who fits eyeglasses, contact lenses, and other vision-correcting devices.
Optometrist	*opto-:* vision *-metrist:* to measure	A licensed primary health care provider who has expertise in measuring visual acuity and prescribing corrective lenses for the treatment of refractive errors.
Otolaryngologist	*ot/o:* ear *-ologist:* one who studies and practices	A physician who specializes in the diagnosis and treatment of disorders of the ear, nose, and throat. (Also known as an ENT physician.)
Otologist	*ot/o:* ear *-ologist:* one who studies and practices	A physician who can treat more complex ear conditions and perform more complex ear surgeries as compared with an otolaryngologist.
Otosclerosis	*ot/o:* ear *-sclerosis:* hardening	An abnormal bone growth in the middle ear.
Otoscope	*ot/o:* ear *-scope:* to view	An instrument used to examine the external ear canal and tympanic membrane.
Presbycusis	*presby-:* aging *-cusis:* hearing	The gradual loss of hearing in both ears due to the normal aging process.
Presbyopia	*presby-:* aging *-opia:* vision	A decrease in the elasticity of the lens that occurs with aging, resulting in a decreased ability to focus on close objects.
Refraction		The deflection or bending of light rays by a lens.
Tympanic membrane	*tympan/o:* eardrum *-ic:* pertaining to	A thin, semitransparent membrane between the external ear canal and the middle ear that receives and transmits sound waves. Also known as the *eardrum.*
Visual acuity		Acuteness or sharpness of vision. A person with normal visual acuity can see clearly and is able to distinguish fine details close up and at some distance.

PROCEDURE 21.1 Assessing Distance Visual Acuity—Snellen Chart

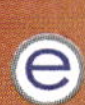

Outcome Assess distance visual acuity.

Equipment/Supplies

- Snellen eye chart
- Eye occluder
- Antiseptic wipe

1. **Procedural Step.** Sanitize your hands.
2. **Procedural Step.** Assemble the equipment. Perform the test in a well-lit room that is free of distractions. Wipe the eye occluder with an antiseptic wipe and allow it to dry completely.
   Principle. The eye occluder should be disinfected before use to prevent the spread of infection.
3. **Procedural Step.** Greet the patient and introduce yourself. Identify the patient and explain the procedure. Explain that the patient will be asked to identify several lines of letters. The patient should not have an opportunity to study or memorize the letters before beginning the test.
4. **Procedural Step.** Determine whether the patient wears corrective lenses (other than reading glasses). If corrective lenses are being worn, tell the patient to keep them on during the test.
5. **Procedural Step.** Ask the patient to stand on the marked line located 20 feet from the chart.

PROCEDURE 21.1 Assessing Distance Visual Acuity—Snellen Chart—cont'd

6. **Procedural Step.** Position the center of the Snellen chart at the patient's eye level. Stand next to the chart during the test to indicate to the patient the line to be identified.
   Principle. Ensure that the chart is at the patient's eye level rather than at your eye level, to provide the most accurate results.
7. **Procedural Step.** Test the acuity of each eye separately. Measure the visual acuity of the right eye first.
   Principle. The medical assistant should establish a pattern of beginning with the same eye (traditionally the right eye) every time the test is performed. This helps to reduce errors during the documentation of results.
8. **Procedural Step.** Ask the patient to cover the left eye with the eye occluder. If eyeglasses are being worn, tell the patient to place the occluder in front of the glasses gently to prevent the glasses from being moved out of their normal position. Instruct the patient to keep the left eye open. During the test, the medical assistant should check to make sure the patient is keeping the left eye open.
   Principle. Eyeglasses moved out of normal position may lead to inaccurate test results. Keeping the left eye open prevents squinting of the right eye, which temporarily improves vision, leading to inaccurate test results.
9. **Procedural Step.** Instruct the patient not to squint during the test because squinting temporarily improves vision. Ask the patient to identify orally one line at a time on the Snellen chart, starting with the 20/70 line (or a line that is several lines above the 20/20 line).
   Principle. It is best to start at a line above the 20/20 line to give the patient a chance to gain confidence and to become familiar with the test procedure.

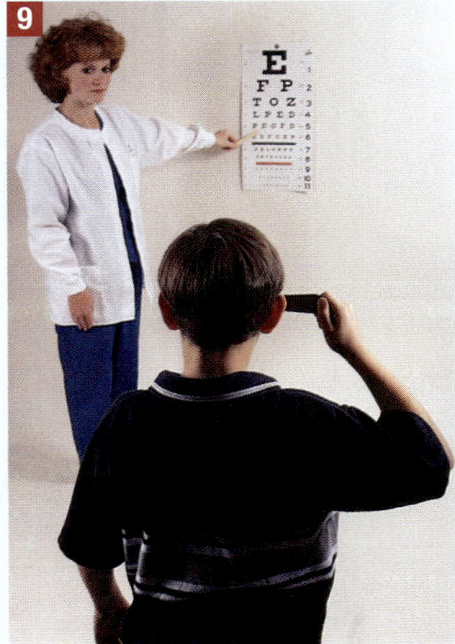

Ask the patient to identify one line at a time.

10. **Procedural Step.** If the patient can identify the 20/70 line, proceed down the chart until reaching the smallest line of letters the patient can identify. If the patient is unable to identify the 20/70 line, proceed up the chart until the smallest line of letters the patient can identify is reached.
11. **Procedural Step.** While the patient is identifying the letters, observe the patient for unusual symptoms, such as squinting, tilting of the head, or watering of the eyes.
    Principle. These symptoms may indicate that the patient is having difficulty identifying the letters.
12. **Procedural Step.** On a small piece of paper, jot down the numbers that are displayed next to the smallest line of letters that the patient can identify. If one or two letters are missed, document the visual acuity with a minus sign next to the bottom number, along with the number of letters missed. If more than two letters are missed, the previous line is documented.
13. **Procedural Step.** Ask the patient to cover the right eye with the eye occluder and to keep the right eye open. Measure the visual acuity in the left eye as described in steps 9 through 12. During the test, check to make sure the patient is keeping the right eye open.
    Principle. Keeping the right eye open prevents squinting of the left eye.

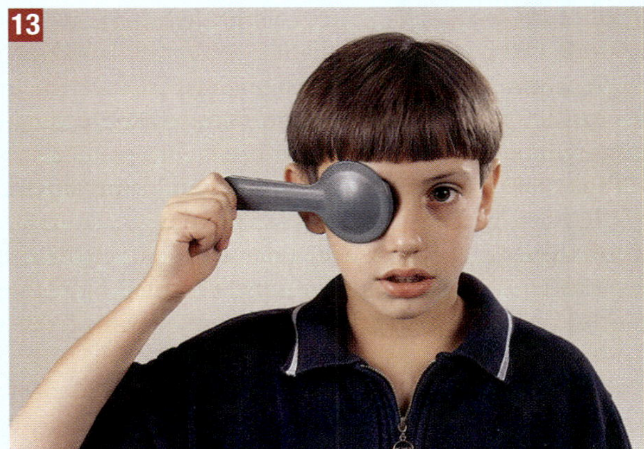

Ask the patient to cover the right eye and to keep the left eye open.

14. **Procedural Step.** Document the procedure in the patient's medical record.
    a. *Electronic health record:* In SimChart for the Medical Office, document the visual acuity results and any unusual symptoms the patient exhibited during the test using the correct radio buttons, drop-down menus, and free text fields. It should also be documented if the patient was wearing corrective lenses

PROCEDURE 21.1

Continued

PROCEDURE 21.1 Assessing Distance Visual Acuity—Snellen Chart—cont'd

during the test and what type of corrective lenses were used (eyeglasses or contact lenses).

b. *Paper-based patient record:* Document the date and time, the name of the test (Snellen test), the visual acuity results, and any unusual symptoms the patient exhibited during the test. Also document whether the patient was wearing corrective lenses during the test. Use the following abbreviations: $\overline{sc}$ for $\overline{cc}$ "without correction" or for "with correction."

14b

DOCUMENTATION EXAMPLE

Date	
11/5/XX	3:30 p.m. Snellen test, $\bar{s}$c: Ⓡ eye: 20/20-1.
	Ⓛ eye: 20/25. Exhibited squinting, Ⓡ eye.
	——————— C. Lindner, CMA (AAMA)

15. **Procedural Step.** Disinfect the eye occluder with an antiseptic wipe and sanitize your hands.

PROCEDURE 21.2 Assessing Color Vision—Ishihara Test

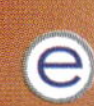

Outcome Assess color vision.

Equipment/Supplies

- Ishihara book
- Cotton swab

1. **Procedural Step.** Sanitize your hands. Assemble the equipment.
2. **Procedural Step.** Conduct the test in a quiet room illuminated by natural daylight.
   Principle. Using unnatural light may change the appearance of the shades of color on the plates, leading to inaccurate test results.
3. **Procedural Step.** Greet the patient and introduce yourself. Identify the patient and explain the procedure. Using the first (practice) plate as an example, instruct the patient to orally identify numbers formed by colored dots. Tell the patient that 3 seconds will be given to identify each plate.
   Principle. The first plate is designed to be identified correctly by all individuals and is used to explain the procedure to the patient.
4. **Procedural Step.** Hold the first color plate 30 inches (75 cm) from the patient, at a right angle to the patient's line of vision. The patient should keep both eyes open during the test.

4

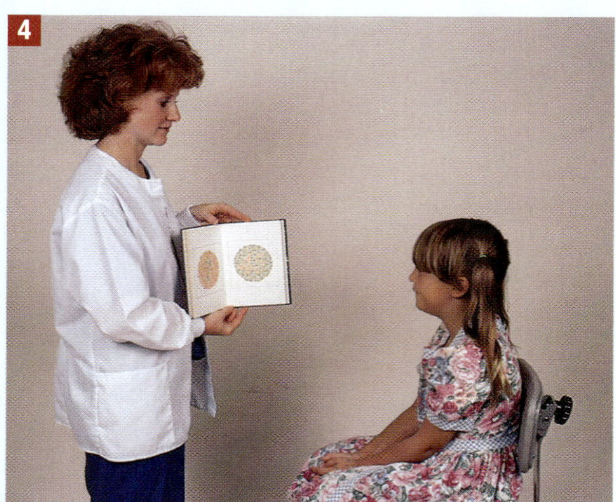

Hold the color plate 30 inches from the patient.

5. **Procedural Step.** Ask the patient to identify the number on the plate. If the plate consists of a traceable winding colored line, ask the patient to trace the line using a

PROCEDURE 21.2 Assessing Color Vision—Ishihara Test—cont'd

cotton swab or the eraser end of a pencil. The patient's finger should not be used to make the tracing.

Principle. The patient's finger should not be used to trace the line because soiled fingers can degrade the plate over time.

6. Procedural Step. Document results after each plate. Continue until the patient has viewed all the plates.

a. *Paper-based patient record:* To document color vision results, use the plate identification number and the number given by the patient. If the patient is unable to identify a number, the mark X should be documented to indicate that the patient could not identify the plate. Examples:

Plate 5: 21. This means the patient identified the number 21 on plate 5 (instead of 74).

Plate 6: X. This means the patient could not identify a number on plate 6.

Plate 11: Traceable. This means that the patient correctly traced a winding line on plate 11.

As you can see from the results of this patient's color vision test, the patient correctly identified more than 7 plates correctly, which indicates normal color vision. Because the patient has normal color vision, the medical assistant did not need to include plates 12, 13, and 14 in the color vision test.

b. *Electronic health record:* In SimChart for the Medical Office, document the color vision results using the correct radio buttons, drop-down menus, and free text fields to indicate the plate identification number and the number given by the patient or to indicate that the patient is unable to identify a number.

Principle. If only 7 or fewer plates are read correctly, the patient is identified as having a color vision deficiency.

6a

DOCUMENTATION EXAMPLE

Plate No.	Normal Person	Results
1	12	12
2	8	8
3	5	5
4	29	29
5	74	21
6	7	X
7	45	45
8	2	2
9	X	X
10	16	16
11	Traceable	Traceable
11/6/XX	10:00 a.m.	
	C. Lindner, CMA (AAMA)	

7. Procedural Step. Complete the documentation entry.

a. *Electronic health record:* In SimChart for the Medical Office, document any unusual symptoms the patient exhibited during the test, such as squinting or rubbing the eyes.

b. *Paper-based patient record:* Document the date and time, the name of the test (Ishihara test), and any unusual symptoms the patient exhibited during the test, such as squinting or rubbing the eyes.

8. Procedural Step. Return the Ishihara book to its proper place. The book of test plates must be stored in a closed position to protect it from light.

Principle. Exposing the plates to excessive and unnecessary light results in fading of the color on the plates.

PROCEDURE 21.3 Performing an Eye Irrigation

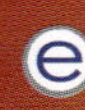

Outcome Perform an eye irrigation.

Equipment/Supplies

- Disposable gloves
- Irrigating solution
- Solution basin
- Bath thermometer
- Disposable rubber bulb syringe
- Basin
- Moisture-resistant towel
- Gauze pads

Continued

PROCEDURE 21.3 Performing an Eye Irrigation—cont'd

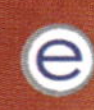 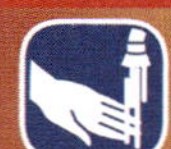 

1. **Procedural Step.** Sanitize your hands.
2. **Procedural Step.** Assemble the equipment. If both eyes are to be irrigated, two sets of equipment must be used to prevent cross-infection from one eye to the other. Normal saline is usually used to irrigate the eye. Perform the following:
   a. Carefully check the label of the irrigating solution three times to make sure you have the correct solution. The first time is after you remove the solution container from the shelf. Compare the label of the solution container with the provider's instructions.
   b. Check the expiration date of the solution.
   c. Warm the irrigating solution to body temperature (98.6°F [37°C]) by placing the solution container in a basin of warm water. Use a bath thermometer to make sure the temperature of the water used to warm the solution does not exceed body temperature.
   d. Check the solution label a second time before pouring the solution.
   e. Pour the solution as follows:
   Palm the label of the container and remove the cap. Place the cap on a flat surface with the open end up. Pour the solution into the basin and replace the cap without contaminating it. Cover the basin to keep the solution warm.
   f. Check the solution label a third time before returning the container to its storage area.

   Principle. The solution label should be carefully checked three times to prevent an error. Outdated solutions may produce undesirable effects and should be discarded. If the solution is too cold or too warm, it will be uncomfortable for the patient. Palming the label prevents solution from dripping on the label and obscuring it or loosening the label. Placing the cap open end up prevents contamination.
3. **Procedural Step.** Greet the patient and introduce yourself. Identify the patient and explain the procedure and the irrigation. If the patient wears eyeglasses or contact lenses, ask the patient to remove them.
4. **Procedural Step.** Position the patient. The patient may be placed in a sitting or lying position. Place a moisture-resistant towel on the patient's shoulder to protect the patient's clothing. Position a basin tightly against the patient's cheek under the affected eye to catch the irrigating solution, and ask the patient to hold it in place. Ask the patient to tilt the head in the direction of the affected eye.

   Principle. The patient is positioned so that the solution flows away from the unaffected eye to prevent cross-infection.
5. **Procedural Step.** Apply disposable gloves. Cleanse the eyelids from inner to outer **canthus** with a moistened gauze pad to remove any discharge or debris on the lids. The inner canthus is the inner junction of the eyelids next to the nose. The outer canthus is the junction of the eyelids farthest from the nose. Normal saline or the solution ordered for the irrigation may be used. Discard the gauze pad after each wipe.

   Principle. The eyelids should be clean to prevent foreign particles from entering the eye during the irrigation. Cleansing from inner to outer canthus prevents cross-infection.

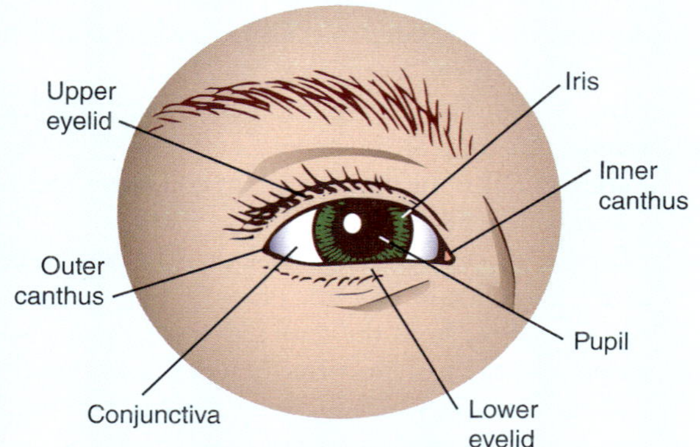

Cleanse the eyelids from inner to outer canthus.

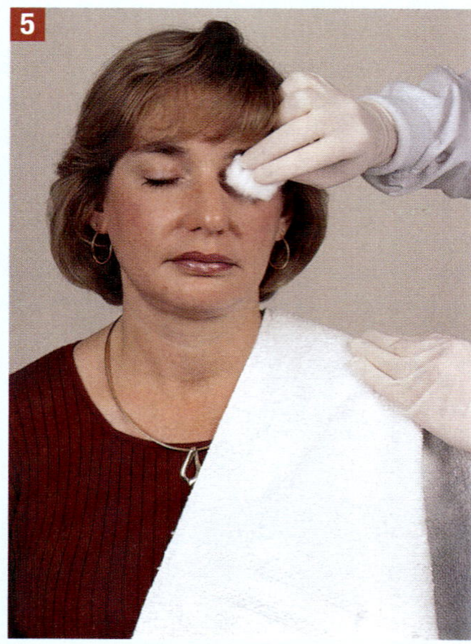

Cleanse the eyelids from inner to outer canthus.

6. **Procedural Step.** Fill the irrigating syringe with the solution by squeezing the bulb and slowly releasing it until the desired amount of solution enters the bulb. Instruct the patient to keep both eyes open and to find a focal point in the room and focus on it.

   Principle. Looking at a focal point helps the patient keep the irrigated eye open during the procedure.

PROCEDURE 21.3 Performing an Eye Irrigation—cont'd

 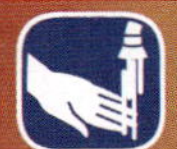 

7. **Procedural Step.** Separate the eyelids with the index finger and thumb to expose the lower conjunctiva and to hold the upper eyelid open.
   Principle. The medical assistant must hold the eye open during the procedure because the patient has a tendency to close it.

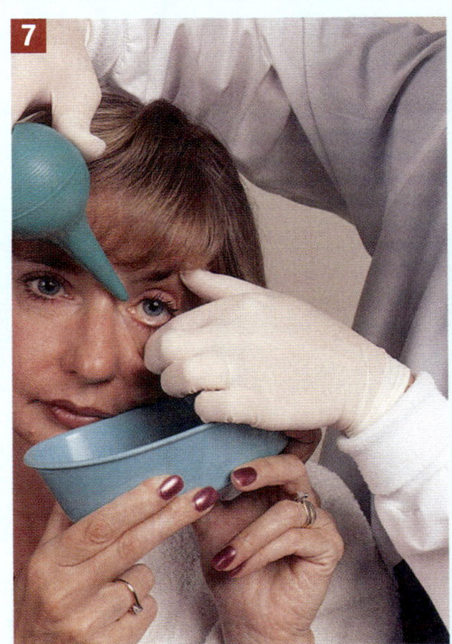

Separate the eyelids and hold the tip of the syringe 1 inch above the eye.

8. **Procedural Step.** Hold the tip of the syringe approximately 1 inch above the eye. Gently release the solution onto the eye at the inner canthus. This allows the solution to flow over the eye at a moderate rate from the inner to the outer canthus. Direct the solution to the lower conjunctiva. To prevent injury, do not allow the tip of the syringe to touch the eye.
   Principle. The solution flows away from the unaffected eye to prevent cross-infection. The cornea is sensitive and can be harmed easily. The irrigating solution must be directed to the lower conjunctiva to prevent injury to the cornea.
9. **Procedural Step.** Refill the syringe, and continue irrigating until the desired results have been obtained or all the solution is used, depending on the purpose of the irrigation.
10. **Procedural Step.** Dry the eyelids from inner to outer canthus with a gauze pad.
11. **Procedural Step.** Remove the gloves, and sanitize your hands.
12. **Procedural Step.** Document the procedure in the patient's medical record.
    a. *Electronic health record:* In SimChart for the Medical Office, document, using the correct radio buttons, drop-down menus, and free text fields, which eye was irrigated; the type, strength, and amount of solution used; and any significant observations and patient reactions.
    b. *Paper-based patient record:* Document the following: the date and time; which eye was irrigated; the type, strength, and amount of solution used; and any significant observations and patient reactions.

12b DOCUMENTATION EXAMPLE

Date	
11/5/XX	10:30 a.m. Irrigated (L) eye c̄ sterile saline
	at 98.6° F. No complaints of discomfort.
	——————— C. Lindner, CMA (AAMA)

13. **Procedural Step.** Remove reusable equipment to a work area for sanitization, sterilization, or disinfection as required by the medical office policy.

PROCEDURE 21.4 Performing an Eye Instillation

Outcome Perform an eye instillation.

Equipment/Supplies

- Disposable gloves
- Ophthalmic drops or ophthalmic ointment as ordered by the provider
- Tissues
- Gauze pads

Continued

PROCEDURE 21.4 Performing an Eye Instillation—cont'd

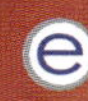

1. **Procedural Step.** Sanitize your hands.
2. **Procedural Step.** Assemble the equipment, and perform the following:
   a. Check the drug label three times to make sure you have the correct medication. The first time should be when you remove the medication from the shelf. The medication label must bear the word *ophthalmic.*
   b. Check the medication label a second time against the provider's instructions. Also check the dose ordered by the provider.
   c. Check the expiration date.
   d. Check the medication label a third time before the cap is removed to instill the medication (as indicated in Procedural Step 5).

   Principle. The drug label should be carefully checked three times to prevent a medication error. Medication not bearing the word *ophthalmic* must never be placed in the eye because it could injure the eye. An outdated medication may produce undesirable effects and should be discarded.
3. **Procedural Step.** Greet the patient and introduce yourself. Identify the patient and explain the procedure and the purpose of the instillation. If the patient wears eyeglasses or contact lenses, ask the patient to remove them.
4. **Procedural Step.** Help the patient into a sitting or supine position.
5. **Procedural Step.** Apply disposable gloves. Prepare the medication.

   Eye drops: If the medication requires mixing, shake the container well. Check the medication label for the third time and remove the cap from the container.

   Eye ointment: Check the medication label for the third time and remove the cap from the tip of the tube.
6. **Procedural Step.** Ask the patient to look up at the ceiling and expose the lower conjunctival sac by using the fingers of the nondominant hand placed over a tissue. The fingers should be placed on the patient's cheekbone just below the eye, and the skin of the cheek should be drawn gently downward.

   Principle. Looking up helps keep the patient from blinking when the drops are instilled.
7. **Procedural Step.** Insert the medication.

   Eye drops: Invert the container and hold the tip of the dropper approximately {1/2} inch above the eye sac. Do not allow the dropper to touch the eye or any other surface. Gently squeeze the container and place the correct number of eye drops in the center of the lower conjunctival sac. Never place the drops directly on the eyeball. Replace the cap on the container.

   Eye ointment: Gently squeeze the tube and place a thin ribbon of ointment along the length of the lower conjunctival sac from inner to outer canthus. Be careful not to touch the tip of the ointment tube to the eye or any other surface. Discontinue the ribbon by twisting the tube. Replace the cap on the tube.

   Principle. Touching the dropper or tip of the tube to the eye (or other surfaces) could injure the eye and contaminate the medication. Placing the medication in the conjunctival sac, rather than directly on the eyeball, is more comfortable for the patient.

7

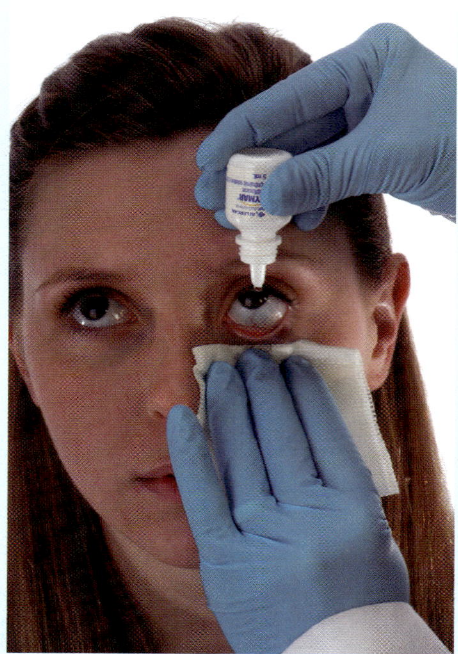

Ask the patient to look up and insert the medication.

8. **Procedural Step.** Ask the patient to close their eyes gently and move the eyeballs. Instruct the patient not to shut the eyes tight or to blink and to keep the eyes closed for 1 to 2 minutes. Tell the patient that the instillation may blur the vision temporarily.

   Principle. Moving the eyeballs helps distribute the medication over the entire eye. Keeping the eyes closed allows the medication to be absorbed. If the eyes are shut tightly or if the patient blinks, the drops or ointment may be pushed out of the eye.
9. **Procedural Step.** Dry the eyelid from inner to outer canthus with a gauze pad to remove excess medication.
10. **Procedural Step.** Remove the gloves and sanitize your hands.
11. **Procedural Step.** Document the procedure in the patient's medical record.
    a. *Electronic health record:* In SimChart for the Medical Office, document, using the correct radio buttons,

PROCEDURE 21.4 Performing an Eye Instillation—cont'd

drop-down menus, and free text fields, the name and strength of the medication, the number of drops or amount of ointment, which eye received the instillation, your observations, and the patient's reaction.

b. *Paper-based patient record:* The medication dosage for eye drops is documented in the number of drops instilled. The documentation should include the date and time, the name and strength of the medication, the number of drops or amount of ointment, which eye received the instillation, your observations, and the patient's reaction.

11b

DOCUMENTATION EXAMPLE

Date	
11/5/XX	2:30 p.m. Atropine sulfate, 1%, 2 drops in each eye.
	Pt states a temporary blurring of vision. ——
	______________ C. Lindner, CMA (AAMA)

12. Procedural Step. Return the medication to its proper storage area.

PROCEDURE 21.5 Performing an Ear Irrigation

Outcome Perform an ear irrigation.

Equipment/Supplies

- Disposable gloves
- Irrigating solution
- Solution basin
- Bath thermometer
- Elephant Ear Wash System
- Ear basin
- Moisture-resistant towel
- Gauze pads
- Ear wick

1. Procedural Step. Sanitize your hands.

2. Procedural Step. Assemble the equipment. If both ears are to be irrigated, two sets of equipment must be used to prevent cross-infection from one ear to the other.

2

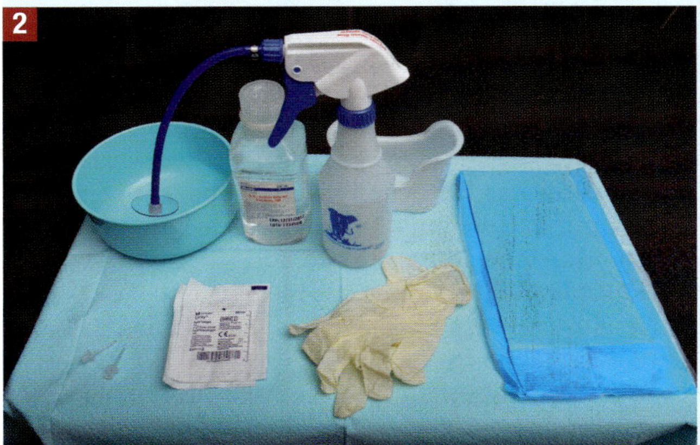

Elephant Ear Wash System setup.

3. Procedural Step: Prepare the irrigating solution:

a. Carefully check the label of the irrigating solution three times to make sure you have the correct solution. The first time is after you remove the solution container from the shelf. Compare the label of the solution container with the provider's instructions.

b. Check the expiration date of the solution.

c. Warm the irrigating solution to body temperature (98.6°F [37°C]) by placing the solution container in a basin of warm water. Use a bath thermometer to make sure the temperature of the water used to warm the solution does not exceed body temperature.

d. Check the solution label a second time before pouring the solution.

e. Palm the label of the container and remove the cap. Place the cap on a flat surface with the open end up. Remove the top of the ear wash spray bottle and pour the solution into the bottle. Replace the top of the spray bottle.

f. Check the solution label a third time before returning the container to its storage area.

Principle. The solution label should be carefully checked three times to prevent an error. An outdated solution may produce undesirable effects. If the solution is too cold or too warm, it might stimulate the inner ear and the patient may become dizzy. Palming the label prevents the solution from dripping on the label and obscuring it or loosening the label. Placing the cap open end up prevents contamination.

Continued

PROCEDURE 21.5 Performing an Ear Irrigation—cont'd

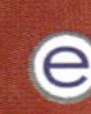

4. **Procedural Step.** Greet the patient and introduce yourself. Identify the patient and explain the procedure. Explain the purpose of performing the irrigation—for example, to remove cerumen. Tell the patient the procedure is not painful; however, a minimal amount of discomfort and occasional dizziness, fullness, and warmth may be felt as the ear solution comes in contact with the tympanic membrane.
5. **Procedural Step.** Position the patient in a sitting position. Place a moisture-resistant towel on the patient's shoulder under the ear to be irrigated to protect clothing and to prevent water from running down the neck. Position a basin tightly against the patient's neck under the affected ear to catch the irrigating solution and ask the patient to hold it in place. Ask the patient to tilt the head in the direction of the affected ear.
   Principle. The patient is positioned so that gravity aids the flow of the solution out of the ear and into the basin.
6. **Procedural Step.** Apply gloves. Cleanse the outer ear with a moistened gauze pad to remove any discharge or debris present. Normal saline or the solution ordered for the irrigation may be used.
   Principle. The outer ear should be clean to prevent foreign particles from entering the ear canal during the irrigation.
7. **Procedural Step.** Twist a disposable tip onto the nozzle of the tubing, making sure to screw it firmly into place.

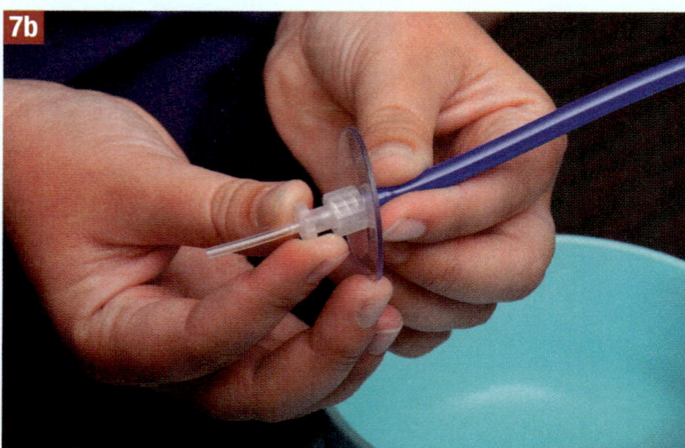

Twist a disposable tip onto the nozzle.

8. **Procedural Step.** Straighten the external ear canal. The canal is straightened by gently pulling the ear upward and backward for adults and children older than 3 years and downward and backward for children 3 years old or younger.
   Principle. Straightening the canal permits the irrigating solution to reach all areas of the canal.
9. **Procedural Step.** Insert the tip of the irrigating device into the ear, but not too deeply.
   Principle. Inserting the tip of the syringe too deeply causes discomfort for the patient and possible injury to the tympanic membrane.
10. **Procedural Step.** Spray the irrigating solution toward the roof of the ear canal by depressing the trigger handle of the Elephant Ear Wash System. Make sure to keep the tubing fairly straight to prevent bending of the tubing. This ensures a good flow of solution into the ear.

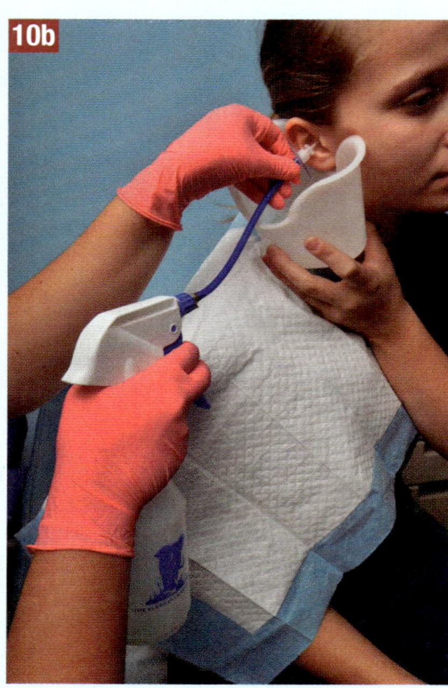

Spray the irrigating solution toward the roof of the ear canal.

   Principle. The tip of the irrigating device should be directed at the roof of the canal to prevent injury to the tympanic membrane and to aid in the removal of foreign particles by allowing the solution to flow down the length of the canal and out the bottom. In addition, severe patient discomfort and dizziness may occur if the solution is injected directly onto the tympanic membrane.
11. **Procedural Step.** Continue irrigating until the desired results have been obtained or all the solution is used, depending on the purpose of the irrigation. Observe the returning solution to note the material present (e.g., cerumen, discharge, a foreign object) and the amount (small, moderate, or large).
12. **Procedural Step.** Dry the outside of the ear with a gauze pad. Have the patient lie on the affected side on the treatment table. Tell the patient that the ear will feel sensitive for a short time. Place a cotton wick loosely in the ear canal for 15 minutes if instructed to do so by the provider.

PROCEDURE 21.5 Performing an Ear Irrigation—cont'd

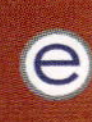  

Principle. Having the patient lie on the affected side allows any solution remaining in the ear canal to drain out. A cotton wick makes the patient's ear feel less sensitive after the irrigation.

13. **Procedural Step.** Remove the gloves and sanitize your hands.
14. **Procedural Step.** Document the procedure in the patient's medical record.
    a. *Electronic health record:* In SimChart for the Medical Office, document, using the correct radio buttons, drop-down menus, and free text fields, which ear was irrigated; the type, strength, and amount of solution used; the amount and type of material returned in the irrigation solution; any significant observations, and patient reactions.
    b. *Paper-based patient record:* Document the following: the date and time; which ear was irrigated; the type, strength, and amount of solution used; the amount and type of material returned in the irrigating solution; any significant observations; and patient reactions.

14b

DOCUMENTATION EXAMPLE

Date	
11/15/XX	2:15 p.m. Irrigated Ⓡ ear c̄ saline, 200 mL
	at 98.6° F. Mod amt of cerumen present in
	returned solution. Cotton wick placed in ear
	canal × 15 min. No complaints of discomfort.
	———————— C. Lindner, CMA (AAMA)

15. **Procedural Step.** Remove equipment to a work area for sanitization, sterilization, disinfection, or disposal as required by the medical office policy.

PROCEDURE 21.6

PROCEDURE 21.6 Performing an Ear Instillation

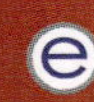  

Outcome Perform an ear instillation.

Equipment/Supplies

- Disposable gloves
- Otic drops
- Gauze pad

1. **Procedural Step.** Sanitize your hands.
2. **Procedural Step.** Assemble the equipment, and perform the following:
    a. Check the drug label three times to make sure you have the correct medication. The first time should be when you remove the medication from the shelf. The medication label must bear the word *otic.*
    b. Check the medication label a second time against the provider's instructions. Also check the dose ordered by the provider.
    c. Check the expiration date.
    d. Check the medication label a third time before the cap is removed to instill the medication (as indicated in Procedural Step 6).

    Principle. The drug label should be carefully checked three times to prevent a medication error. Medication not bearing the word *otic* must never be placed in the ear because it could injure the ear. An outdated medication may produce undesirable effects and should be discarded.
3. **Procedural Step.** Greet the patient and introduce yourself. Identify the patient and explain the procedure and the purpose of the instillation.
4. **Procedural Step.** Position the patient in a sitting position.
5. **Procedural Step.** Warm the drops to body temperature by holding the medication container in the palms of your hands for a few minutes. Do not warm the drops by placing them in hot water.

    Principle. If the drops are too cold or too warm, they might stimulate the inner ear, causing the patient to become dizzy.
6. **Procedural Step.** Apply gloves. If the medication requires mixing, shake the container well. Check the medication label for the third time and remove the cap from the container.
7. **Procedural Step.** Ask the patient to tilt the head in the direction of the unaffected ear. Straighten the external ear canal. The canal is straightened by pulling the ear

Continued

PROCEDURE 21.6 Performing an Ear Instillation—cont'd

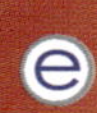  

upward and backward for adults and children older than 3 years and downward and backward for children 3 years old and younger. Gravity aids in the flow of medication into the ear canal.

Principle. Straightening the canal permits the medication to reach all areas of the canal.

8. **Procedural Step.** Invert the container and place the tip of the dropper at the opening of the ear canal. Be careful not to touch the tip of the dropper to the ear. Gently squeeze the container and instill the correct number of drops along the side of the canal. Replace the cap on the container.

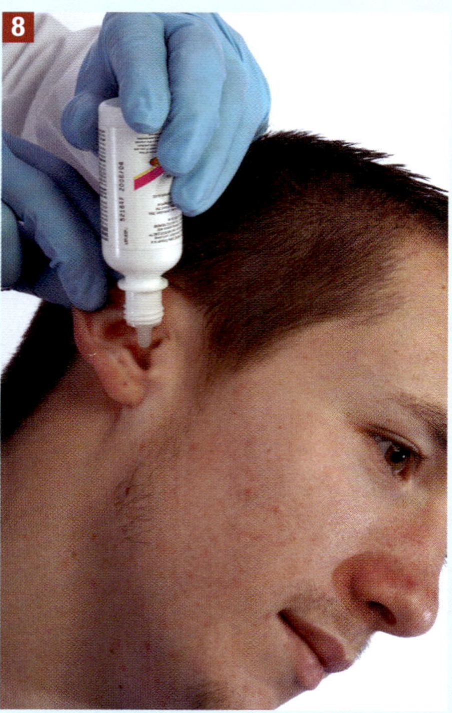

8 Instill the medication along the side of the ear canal.

9. **Procedural Step.** Instruct the patient to lie on the unaffected side for 2 to 3 minutes.

Principle. Lying on the unaffected side prevents the medication from running out and allows complete distribution of the medication.

10. **Procedural Step.** Place a moistened cotton wick loosely in the ear canal for 15 minutes if instructed to do so by the provider.

Principle. The cotton wick prevents the medication from running out when the patient is upright. Moistening the wick prevents the medication from being absorbed by the cotton.

11. **Procedural Step.** Remove the gloves and sanitize your hands.

12. **Procedural Step.** Document the procedure in the patient's medical record.
    a. *Electronic health record:* In SimChart for the Medical Office, document, using the correct radio buttons, drop-down menus, and free text fields, the strength of the medication, the number of drops, which ear received the instillation, and any significant observations, as well as the patient's reaction.
    b. *Paper-based patient record:* Document the date and time, the name and strength of the medication, the number of drops, which ear received the instillation, any significant observations, and the patient's reaction.

12b DOCUMENTATION EXAMPLE

Date	
11/20/XX	9:30 a.m. Auralgan, 2 drops, (R) ear. No
	discharge present. Pt states a relief of pain.
	______________ C. Lindner, CMA (AAMA)

13. **Procedural Step.** Return the medication to its storage area.

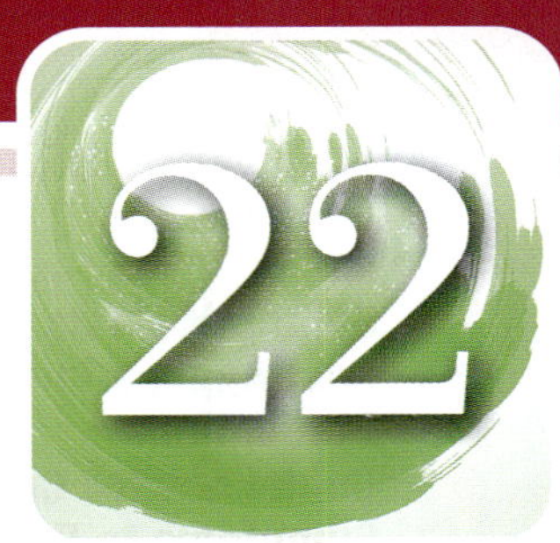

Physical Agents to Promote Tissue Healing

Check out the Evolve site at http://evolve.elsevier.com/Bonewit/today to access additional interactive activities and exercises to help you study and prepare for success.

LEARNING OBJECTIVES

Local Application of Heat and Cold

1. State examples of moist and dry applications of heat and cold.
2. State the factors to consider when applying heat and cold.
3. List the effects of local application of heat, and state reasons for applying heat.
4. List the effects of local application of cold, and state reasons for applying cold.

Casts

1. List reasons for applying a cast.
2. Explain the purpose of each step in the cast application procedure.
3. List the guidelines that should be followed for proper cast care.

Splints and Braces

1. Describe a splint and explain its use.
2. Explain the purpose of a brace.

Ambulatory Aids

1. List factors that are taken into consideration when ambulatory aids are prescribed.
2. Explain the difference between an axillary crutch and a forearm crutch.
3. State conditions that may result when axillary crutches are not fitted properly.
4. List the guidelines that should be followed by the patient to ensure safe use of crutches.
5. State the use of each of the following crutch gaits: four-point gait, two-point gait, three-point gait, swing-to gait, and swing-through gait.
6. List and describe the three types of canes.
7. Identify the patient conditions that warrant the use of a cane or walker.

PROCEDURES

Apply each of the following heat treatments:
- Heating pad
- Hot soak
- Hot compress
- Chemical hot pack
- Gel pack

Apply each of the following cold treatments:
- Ice bag
- Cold compress
- Chemical cold pack
- Gel pack

Assist with the application of a cast.
Assist with the removal of a cast.
Instruct a patient in proper cast care.

Apply a splint following the manufacturer's instructions.
Apply a brace following the manufacturer's instructions.

Measure a patient for axillary crutches.
Instruct a patient in the proper use of crutches.
Instruct a patient in the proper procedure for each of the following crutch gaits:
- Four-point
- Two-point
- Three-point
- Swing-to
- Swing-through

Instruct a patient in the use of a cane.
Instruct a patient in the proper use of a walker.

CHAPTER OUTLINE

KEY TERMS

ambulation (AM-byoo-LAY-shun)
ambulatory
brace
cast
compress (KOM-press)
edema (uh-DEE-muh)
erythema (err-uh-THEE-muh)
exudate (EKS-oo-date)
long arm cast
long leg cast
maceration (mass-er-AY-shun)
orthopedist (OR-thoe-PEE-dist)
short arm cast
short leg cast
soak
splint
sprain
strain
suppuration (SUP-er-AY-shun)

INTRODUCTION TO TISSUE HEALING

Physical agents are often employed in the medical office to promote tissue healing for individuals who experience a disability as a result of injury, disease, or loss of a body part. Physical agents are used therapeutically to improve circulation, provide support, and promote the return of motion so that the individual can perform the activities of daily living. Physical agents frequently used in the medical office include heat and cold applied locally and ambulatory aids, such as crutches, canes, and walkers.

LOCAL APPLICATION OF HEAT AND COLD

The application of heat and cold is used therapeutically to treat conditions such as infection and trauma. The medical assistant is responsible for applying heat and cold therapy and for instructing patients in the procedure for applying heat or cold therapy at home. The medical assistant should have a basic understanding of the physiologic effects of heat and cold on the body and of possible adverse reactions if they are not administered correctly.

Heat and cold can be applied in moist or dry forms. Common applications of dry and moist heat and cold are as follows:

1. *Dry heat:* heating pad, chemical hot pack, gel pack
2. *Moist heat:* hot soak, hot compress
3. *Dry cold:* ice bag, chemical cold pack, gel pack
4. *Moist cold:* cold compress

Heat and cold are applied for short periods (typically 15 to 30 minutes) to produce the desired therapeutic results. The application may be repeated at time intervals specified by the provider. Prolonged application of heat or cold is not recommended because it can result in adverse secondary effects. The type of heat or cold application depends on the purpose of the application, the location and condition of the affected area, and the age and general health of the patient. The provider instructs the medical assistant to apply a heat or cold treatment based on these factors.

Heat and cold receptors in the skin readily adapt to changes in temperature, eventually resulting in diminished heat or cold sensations. The temperature actually remains the same and is providing the intended therapeutic effects. The patient, not perceiving the same degree of temperature, may want to increase the intensity of the application, however, without realizing the inherent dangers. Excessive heat or cold could result in tissue damage. A common example of this situation is a patient who turns up the setting of a heating pad from medium to high when the heating pad no longer feels warm. The medical assistant should fully explain to the patient the necessity of maintaining a safe temperature range during the application.

FACTORS AFFECTING THE APPLICATION OF HEAT AND COLD

Before applying heat or cold, certain factors must be taken into consideration to prevent unfavorable reactions, such as tissue damage. The temperature may need to be adjusted based on the following conditions:

1. *The age of the patient.* Young children and elderly patients tend to be more sensitive to the application of heat or cold.
2. *Location of the application.* Certain areas of the body are more sensitive to the application of heat or cold, especially thin areas of the skin and areas that are usually covered by clothing, such as the chest, back, and abdomen. The skin on the hands and face is not as sensitive

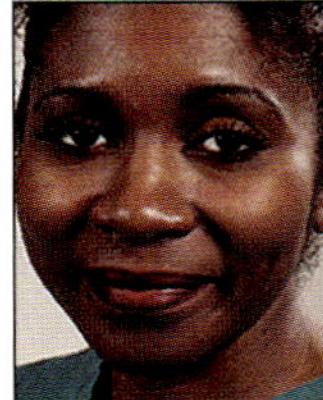

Putting it All into Practice

My name is Marlyne, and I am a Certified Medical Assistant. I work in a community health center. My primary responsibilities are to take patients back to the examination rooms and to prepare them for procedures and treatments. I take the patient's chief complaint and the health history. I greet each patient in a kind and calm way. This helps put the patient at ease before the physician goes into the examining room.

I once worked in a private office with a small waiting room and a narrow hall. One of my regular patients was a healthy 20-year-old man who was confined to a wheelchair by a spinal injury from an automobile accident. He had great difficulty maneuvering his motorized chair in tight spaces, and he felt embarrassed and conspicuous sitting in the middle of the waiting room. I began bringing him through the larger back door into the physician's office, directly into an examination room. Talking about things we had in common, such as interests in sports and movies, made him feel more at ease. By making the situation as easy as possible for him, I was able to help him keep his dignity while not drawing attention to his special needs. ■

and is better able to tolerate temperature change. Broken skin, such as is found with an open wound, is more sensitive to heat and cold and is more prone to tissue damage.

3. *Impaired circulation.* Patients with impaired circulation tend to be more sensitive to heat and cold. This impairment may be at the site of the application or may be a systemic problem involving the entire body that is a result of certain conditions (e.g., peripheral vascular disease, diabetes mellitus, congestive heart failure).
4. *Impaired sensation.* Patients with impaired sensation, such as diabetic patients, must be watched carefully because tissue damage may occur from the application of heat or cold without the patient's awareness.
5. *Individual tolerance to change in temperature.* Some individuals cannot tolerate temperature change as easily as others.

The medical assistant should observe the area to which the heat or cold has been applied before, during, and after treatment for signs indicating that a modification of temperature is needed. The patient should also be asked whether the application feels comfortable or is too hot or too cold. Prolonged erythema or paleness, pain, swelling, and blisters should be reported to the provider.

HEAT

Local Effects of Heat

The application of moderate heat to a localized area of the body for a short time (approximately 15 to 30 minutes) produces *dilation*, or an increase in diameter, of the blood vessels in the area as the body tries to rid itself of excess heat (Fig. 22.1). This results in an increased blood supply to the area, and tissue metabolism increases. Nutrients and oxygen

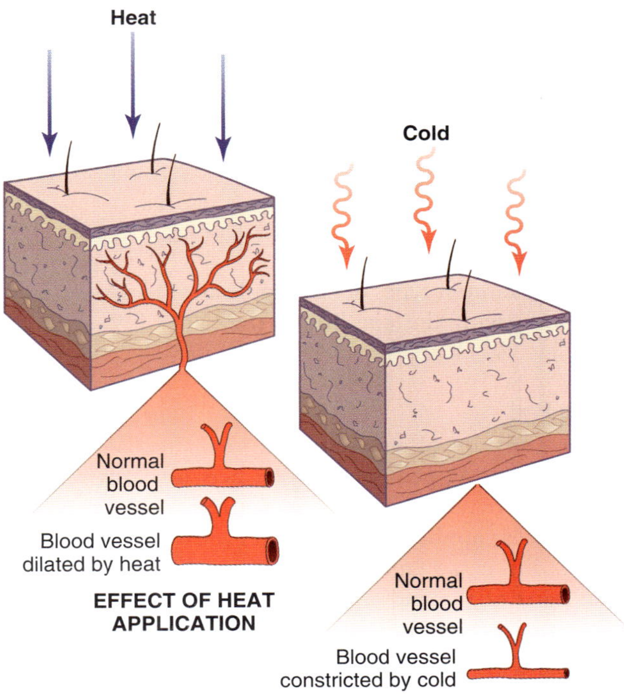

Fig. 22.1 Effects of the local application of heat and cold. (From Wood LA, Rambo BJ: *Nursing skills for allied health services*, vol 2, Philadelphia, 1980, Saunders.)

are provided to the cells at a faster rate, and wastes and toxins are carried away faster. The skin in the area becomes warm and exhibits erythema. **Erythema** is reddening of the skin caused by dilation of superficial blood vessels in the skin.

These physiologic effects of moderate heat applied to a localized area promote healing. Prolonged application of heat (longer than 1 hour) produces secondary effects, however, that reverse this healing process. Blood vessels constrict, and blood supply to the area decreases. The medical assistant must be careful to apply heat for the length of time specified by the provider.

Purpose of Applying Heat

Heat functions in relieving pain, congestion, muscle spasms, and inflammation. Conditions for which the local application of heat is often prescribed are low back pain, arthritis, menstrual cramping, and localized abscesses.

Heat promotes muscle relaxation and is often used for the relief of pain caused by excessive contraction of muscle fibers. **Edema**, or swelling, already present in the tissues can be reduced through the application of heat because the increased blood supply functions to increase the absorption of fluid from the tissues through the lymphatic system.

Heat (usually in the form of a hot compress) can be used to soften exudates. A **compress** is a soft, moist, absorbent cloth that is folded in several layers and applied to a part of the body in the local application of heat or cold.

An **exudate** is a discharge produced by the body's tissues. Exudates may sometimes form a hard crust over an area and require removal. Heat also increases **suppuration**, or the process of pus formation, to help in the relief of inflammation by breaking down infected tissues. Heat is not recommended, however, for the initial treatment of acute inflammation or trauma.

Types of Heat Applications

The most common types of heat applications are described next, along with the conditions they are often used to treat.

Heating Pad

Heating pads are often used to relieve pain and muscle spasms. A heating pad consists of a network of wires that converts electrical energy into heat to provide a constant and even heat application. The wires must not be bent or crushed. This could damage the pad, resulting in overheating of parts of the pad and leading to burns or fire. Pins must not be inserted into the pad as a means of securing it; if a pin comes in contact with a wire, an electric shock could result. To prevent electric hazards, heating pads should not be used over areas that contain moisture, such as wet dressings.

Hot Soak

A **soak** is the direct immersion of a body part in water or a medicated solution. A soak can be applied to an extremity or a part of the torso. Hot soaks are often prepared using a ratio (e.g., two parts water to one part medication), and are used to cleanse open wounds, increase suppuration, increase the blood supply to an area to hasten the healing process, and apply a medicated solution to an area.

Hot Compress

A hot compress is a soft, moist, absorbent cloth, such as a washcloth, that is immersed in a warm solution and applied to a body part. Hot compresses are used to increase suppuration, to improve circulation to a body part to aid in healing, to promote drainage from infection, and to soften exudates. Applying a hot compress to an open wound requires the use of sterile technique.

Chemical Hot Pack

Chemical hot packs are available in a variety of sizes and shapes. When activated, they provide a specific degree of heat for a specific period of time (usually 30 to 60 minutes), as indicated on the package label. A chemical hot pack consists of a vinyl bag containing calcium chloride crystals and a smaller bag (encased in the vinyl bag) containing water. Pressure is applied with the hands to break the inner bag. The water in the inner bag combines with the calcium chloride crystals to produce heat. After using the pack, it should be discarded in an appropriate receptacle. Chemical hot packs should be stored at room temperature and are used as an alternative to a heating pad to relieve pain and muscle spasms.

Procedures 22.1, 22.2, 22.3, and 22.6 present the proper application of heat with a heating pad, a hot soak, a hot compress, and a chemical hot pack.

What Would You Do? What Would You *Not* Do?

Case Study 1

Aaron Collins is at the office. Aaron recently helped a friend move, and the next day he developed intense pain in his lower back. To alleviate the pain, he slept on a heating pad, but when he woke up, his back was red and blistered. Aaron says he turned the setting on the heating pad to high because his back was hurting so much and he thought that it would help his back feel better sooner. Aaron wants to know the best way to apply heat using a heating pad. He also wants to know what he can do to prevent low back pain in the future. ■

COLD

Local Effects of Cold

The application of moderate cold to a localized area produces constriction, or a decrease in diameter, of blood vessels in the area as the body attempts to prevent heat loss (see Fig. 22.1). This constriction leads to decreased blood supply to the area. Tissue metabolism decreases, less oxygen is used, and fewer wastes accumulate. The skin becomes cool and pale. Prolonged application of cold (longer than 1 hour) has a reverse secondary effect. Blood vessels dilate, and tissue metabolism is increased. To prevent secondary effects, the medical assistant must only apply cold for the recommended length of time.

Purpose of Applying Cold

The application of moderate cold for a short time is used to prevent edema (swelling). Cold may be applied immediately after an individual has sustained direct trauma, such as a bruise, minor burn, sprain, strain, joint injury, or fracture. A **sprain** involves trauma to a joint that causes injury to the ligaments while a **strain** is an overstretching of a muscle caused by trauma. The cold limits the accumulation of fluid in the body tissues by constricting blood vessels and reducing the leakage of fluid into the tissues. Through constriction of peripheral blood vessels, cold can be used to control bleeding. Cold temporarily relieves pain through its anesthetic, or numbing, effect, which reduces stimulation of the pain receptors. Cold also slows the movement of blood and tissue fluids in the affected area, resulting in less pressure against pain receptors and therefore less pain. In the early stages of an infection, the local application of cold inhibits the activity of microorganisms. In this way, suppuration is decreased and inflammation is reduced. Cold applications should always be placed in a protective covering because applying cold directly to the skin could result in a skin burn.

Types of Cold Applications

Ice Bag

An ice bag consists of a waterproof bag with a screw-on cap. Before use, it must be filled with small pieces of ice and placed in a protective covering. Ice bags are used to prevent swelling, control bleeding, and relieve pain and inflammation.

Cold Compress

A cold compress is a soft, moist, absorbent cloth, such as a washcloth, that is immersed in a cold solution and applied to a body part. Cold compresses are used to relieve pain and inflammation and to treat conditions such as headache, injury to the eye, and pain after tooth extraction.

Chemical Cold Pack

Chemical cold packs are available in a variety of sizes and shapes. When activated, they provide a specific degree of coldness for a specific period of time (usually 30 to 60 minutes), as indicated on the package label. Most cold packs consist of a vinyl bag of ammonium nitrate crystals. Enclosed in this bag is a smaller vinyl bag of water. The cold pack is activated by applying pressure until the inner bag ruptures. This releases the water into the larger bag, and a chemical reaction occurs between the crystals and the water, producing coldness. These packs are disposable, and when the coldness diminishes, they should be discarded in an appropriate receptacle. Chemical cold packs should be stored at room temperature. They are used as an alternative to ice bags for the local application of cold to prevent swelling, control bleeding, and relieve pain and inflammation.

Procedures 22.4, 22.5, and 22.6 present proper application of cold with an ice bag, a cold compress, and a chemical cold pack.

Table 22.1 Gel Pack Application Guidelines

Gel Pack Heat Therapy

1. A gel pack used for heat therapy should be stored at room temperature.
2. Before heating the pack, the gel should be evenly distributed in the pack and the pack laid flat in a microwave.
3. Microwave the gel pack on high power for the length of time specified in the instructions accompanying the pack (usually 1 minute).
4. Use heat-resistant gloves to remove the gel pack from the microwave.
5. Knead the gel pack using heat-resistant gloves to evenly distribute the heat in the pack.
6. If the pack is too hot, allow it to cool before applying it to the treatment area.
7. If the pack is not hot enough, return it to the microwave and heat the pack in 10-second intervals until it reaches the desired temperature.
8. Make sure to avoid overheating the gel pack to prevent it from swelling up and bursting.
9. Before application to the treatment area, wrap the gel pack in a protective covering such as a dry towel to provide for patient comfort.

Gel Pack Cold Therapy

1. Place the gel pack in the freezer for the length of time specified in the instructions accompanying the pack (usually 1 to 2 hours).
2. The gel pack can be permanently stored in the freezer.
3. Before application to the treatment area, wrap the gel pack in a protective covering such as a dry towel to provide for patient comfort.

GEL PACK

A gel pack consists of a reusable vinyl or nylon bag containing a water-based gel that can be heated or cooled (Fig. 22.2). A gel pack is flexible and molds well to a body area. Gel packs can be used for the local application of heat as an alternative to a heating pad, or for the local application of cold as an alternative to an ice bag. Before using a gel pack, it is important to check it for damage. If the bag is ruptured or leaking, it must be discarded. Depending on the type of application required, the pack should be heated or cooled by carefully following the specific instructions accompanying the pack. General guidelines for the application of a gel pack are outlined in Table 22.1.

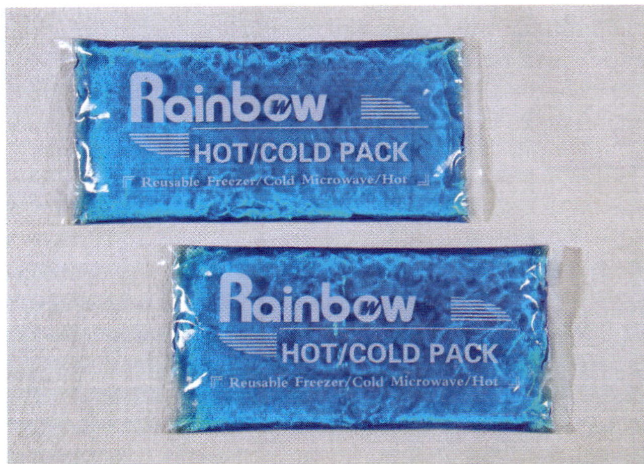

Fig. 22.2 Gel packs.

PATIENT COACHING Low Back Pain

Answer questions patients have about low back pain.

What causes low back pain?

Low back pain is one of the most common health problems in the United States. Approximately 80% of Americans are affected by low back pain at some time during their life. The most frequent cause of low back pain is poor posture and poor body mechanics, which strain the muscles and ligaments that support the back. Most cases of low back pain can be prevented by practicing good body mechanics.

Other causes of low back pain include physical inactivity, excessive body weight, disc damage, osteoarthritis, spondylitis, and congenital deformities.

Continued

PATIENT COACHING Low Back Pain—cont'd

What is the treatment for low back pain?

To treat low back pain caused by strain, the provider may prescribe a combination of one or more of the following: bed rest, local application of heat or cold, massage, medications, back manipulation, use of back-supporting devices, deep-heating treatments such as ultrasound, and exercises to strengthen the supporting structures of the back and prevent the back pain from recurring or becoming chronic.

How can low back pain be prevented?

- Wear comfortable low-heeled shoes that offer good support.
- Maintain correct posture while sitting, standing, and sleeping.
- Never lift anything heavier than you can easily manage. To lift an object, always bend the body at the knees and hips. Never bend from the waist. List the object with the leg muscles and hold it close to the body at waist level. Never lift anything higher than chest level.
- Sit in a chair with a firm back.
- The car seat should be positioned so that the driver's back is straight and the knees are raised.
- Maintain a healthy body weight.

CASTS

A **cast** is a stiff cylindrical casing that is used to immobilize a body part until healing occurs. Casts are applied most often when an individual sustains a fracture (Fig. 22.3). The cast keeps the fractured bones aligned until proper healing occurs. Casts also are used to support and stabilize weak or dislocated joints; to promote healing after a surgical correction, such as knee surgery; and to aid in the nonsurgical correction of deformities, such as congenital dislocation of the hip.

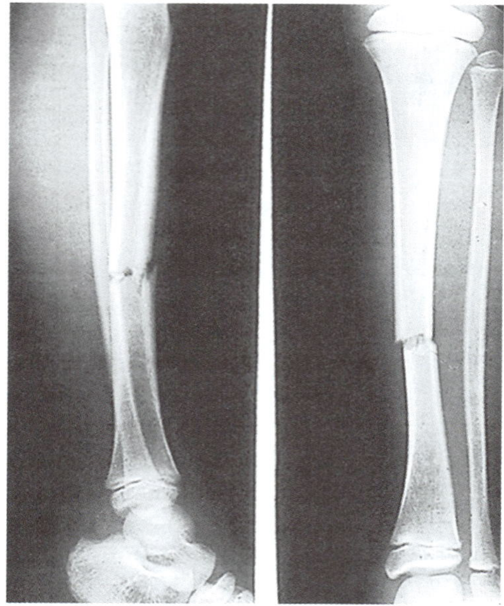

Fig. 22.3 A fracture of the tibia in the left lower leg. (From McRae R, Esser M: *Practical fracture treatment*, ed 4, Philadelphia, 2002, Churchill Livingstone.)

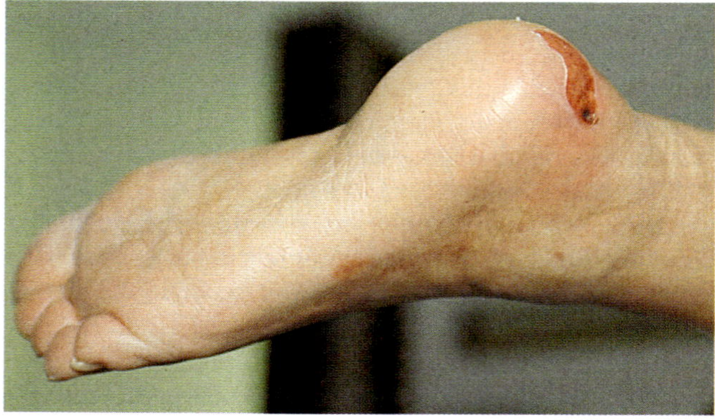

Fig. 22.4 Pressure ulcer.(From Patton KT: *Anatomy and physiology*, ed 9, St. Louis, 2016, Mosby.)

Casts are applied by an orthopedist, also known as an *orthopedic surgeon*. An **orthopedist** is a physician who specializes in the diagnosis and treatment of disorders of the musculoskeletal system. An orthopedist treats patients with deformities, injuries, and diseases of the bones, joints, ligaments, tendons, muscles, nerves, and skin. The role of the medical assistant in cast application is to assemble the equipment and supplies, prepare the patient for the procedure, assist the provider during the application, provide or reinforce cast care instructions, and clean the examining room after the application.

An important goal of cast management is the prevention of pressure areas, which are most apt to occur over bony prominences. A *pressure area* occurs when the cast presses or rubs against the patient's skin and prevents adequate circulation to the area. When this occurs, the patient usually feels a painful rubbing, burning, or stinging sensation under the cast. If permitted to continue, the pressure can cause the skin to break down, leading to the development of a *pressure ulcer* (Fig. 22.4). If not treated, a pressure ulcer progresses from a simple red patch of skin to erosion into the subcutaneous tissue and eventually erosion into the muscle and bone. Deep pressure ulcers often become infected by invading organisms and develop gangrene. It is important to detect the occurrence of a pressure area early so that prompt treatment can be instituted to prevent serious complications.

SYNTHETIC CASTS

Synthetic casts are the most common type of cast used to immobilize a body part. A synthetic cast consists of a knitted fabric tape made of fiberglass, polyester and cotton, or plastic. The tape is impregnated with polyurethane resin that is activated when soaked in water. Of the three kinds of synthetic material, fiberglass is used most often. Synthetic tape comes in different colors and is packaged as an

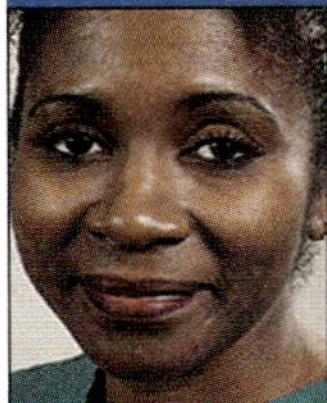

Memories *from* Practicum

Marlyne: At my first practicum site, I was scared to death about having to give injections to small children. I didn't want to hurt them. A 6-month-old infant was brought to the office for her immunizations. My practicum supervisor wanted me to give the injections. The infant was so small, and she was crying before I even gave her the first injection. I knew that when I gave the injection, she was going to cry even more, and that made me feel bad. My supervisor was there with me, and she talked me through it. It turned out that it wasn't as bad as I had thought it would be. My supervisor was very helpful in keeping me calm. After that first experience, I felt much more comfortable when I had to give an injection to a small child. ■

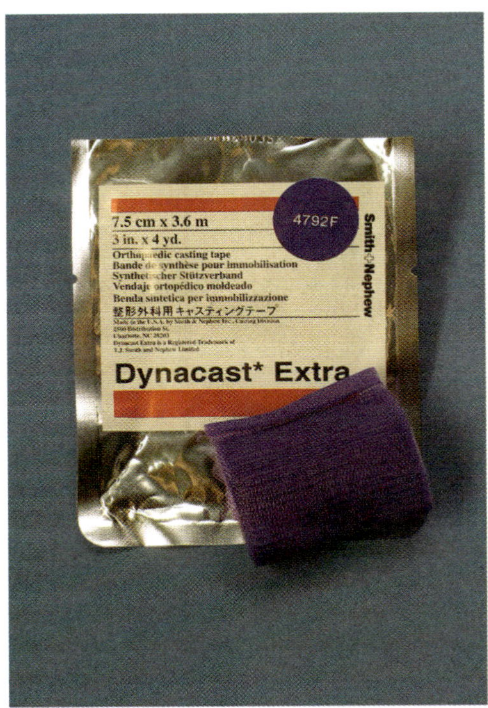

Fig. 22.5 A roll of synthetic tape comes packaged in an airtight pouch.

individual roll in an airtight pouch (Fig. 22.5). Synthetic tape is available in widths ranging from 2 to 8 inches.

CAST APPLICATION

The provider applies the cast so that it fits snugly but still allows adequate circulation necessary for proper healing. Four to six weeks are usually required for the complete healing of a fracture.

Casts are classified according to the body part they cover. The types of casts most frequently applied in the medical office and common uses of each are illustrated and described in Fig. 22.6. The type of cast applied depends on the nature of the patient's injury or condition. A **short arm cast** is used for a fracture of the wrist, and a **long arm cast** is used for a fracture of the distal humerus.

Short Arm Cast

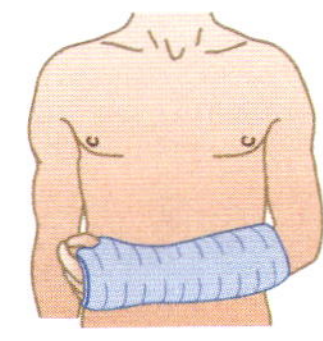

Extends from below the elbow to the base of the fingers

Use:
- Fracture of the distal radius, wrist, or hand
- Postoperative immobilization of the forearm

Long Arm Cast

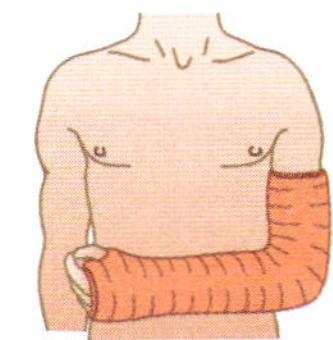

Extends from the upper arm to the base of the fingers, usually with a bend in the elbow

Use:
- Fracture of the distal humerus, forearm, or elbow
- Postoperative immobilization of the elbow and forearm

Short Leg Cast

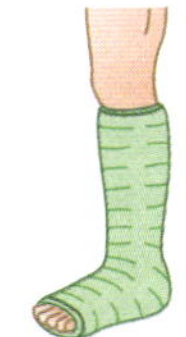

Begins below the knee and extends to the base of the toes

Use:
- Fracture of the distal tibia and fibula, ankle, or foot
- Severe ankle sprain or strain
- Postoperative immobilization of the lower leg, ankle, and foot
- Correction of a deformity

Long Leg Cast

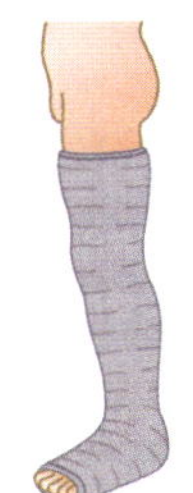

Extends from the thigh to the base of the toes

Use:
- Fracture of the distal femur, knee, or lower leg
- Dislocation or severe sprain of the knee
- Postoperative immobilization of the leg, knee, and ankle

Fig. 22.6 Types of casts.

The following steps are performed in applying a cast:

1. **Inspect the skin.** The area to which the cast is to be applied must be clean and dry. The patient's skin should be inspected for redness, bruises, and open areas. This information should be documented in the patient's medical record because it may assist in evaluating patient complaints after the cast has been applied.
2. **Apply the stockinette.** Before applying the cast, the provider covers the body part with a stockinette (Fig. 22.7). A stockinette consists of a soft, tubular, knitted cotton material that stretches up to three times its original width to accommodate the diameter of the body part. It is put on like a stocking. The purpose of the stockinette is to provide patient comfort and to cover the rough edges at the ends of the cast. Stockinette come in widths ranging from 2 to 12 inches; the width used depends on the diameter of the part to be covered. Typically, a 3-inch width

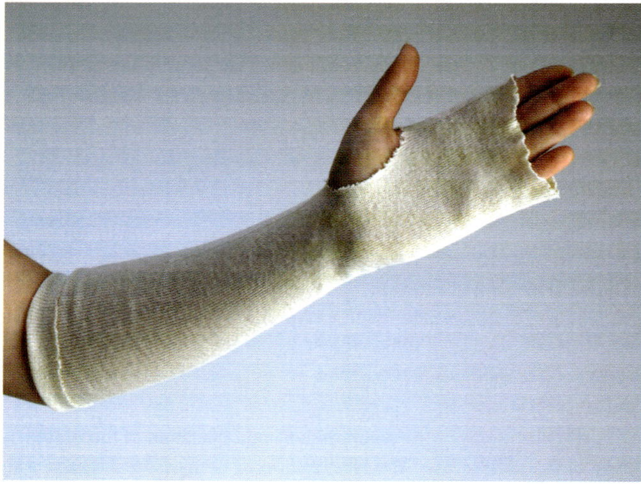

Fig. 22.7 Application of a stockinette.

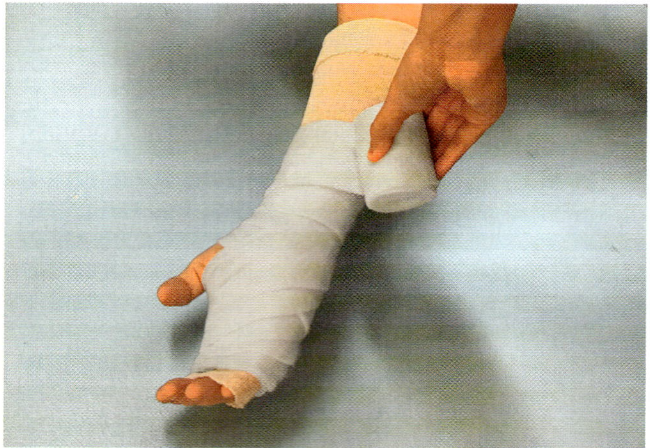

Fig. 22.8 Application of cast padding. (Courtesy 3M Health Care, St. Paul, MN.)

is used for arm casts, a 4-inch width is used for leg casts, and a 10- to 12-inch width is used for body casts.

3. **Apply the cast padding.** Cast padding consists of a soft cotton material that comes in a roll in widths ranging from 2 to 6 inches. The purpose of cast padding is to prevent pressure areas and to shield the patient's skin when the cast is removed. Two or three layers are applied directly over the stockinette, using a spiral turn. Each turn overlaps the preceding one by one-half the width of the roll. Extra layers of padding are applied over bony prominences to prevent pressure areas (Fig. 22.8).
4. **Prepare the synthetic tape.** The roll of synthetic tape is fully immersed in cool, room-temperature water (68°F to 75°F [20°C to 24°C]) for a period of time recommended by the manufacturer. Fiberglass tape is immersed for 5 to 15 seconds. The airtight pouch containing a roll of synthetic tape should remain sealed until just before it is time to immerse the roll in water. This is because air causes the resin in the tape to begin to harden and become rigid, making it unacceptable for use.

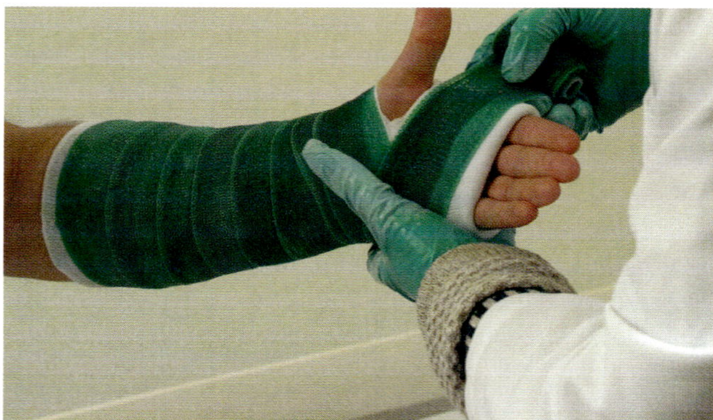

Fig. 22.9 Wrapping the tape over the body part, using a spiral turn.

5. **Apply the cast tape.** The synthetic tape is applied over the cast padding. The provider wears rubber gloves during the procedure to protect the hands from the casting material. The tape is wrapped over the body part, using a spiral turn, until the desired number of layers have been applied (Fig. 22.9). Generally three or four layers are applied for a nonweight-bearing cast (e.g., short arm cast or long arm cast), and five to eight layers are applied for a weight-bearing cast (e.g., **short leg cast** or **long leg cast**).
6. **Allow the cast to dry.** The cast is allowed to dry for a period of time specified by the manufacturer. A fiberglass cast usually dries within 30 minutes. Only when a cast is completely dry does it become hard and inflexible and able to bear weight. The provider usually prescribes a supportive device, such as a sling or crutches, to prevent unnecessary strain and to minimize swelling during the healing process.

PRECAUTIONS

The following precautions should be observed during and after cast application:

- Remove excess casting particles. Remove synthetic casting material with a swab moistened with alcohol or acetone. If cast particles are not removed, they may work their way under the cast, resulting in irritation and infection.
- Before the patient leaves the medical office, the provider checks the circulation, sensation, and movement of the exposed extremity to ensure that the cast is not too tight. The provider also ensures that all joints excluded from the cast are free to move.

GUIDELINES FOR CAST CARE

The medical assistant is often responsible for explaining or reinforcing the guidelines that should be followed by a patient with a cast to promote the healing process. These guidelines are often presented on an instruction sheet that is signed by the patient, with a copy filed in the patient's medical record. Guidelines for cast care include the following:

- Allow the cast to dry before putting any pressure or weight on the cast. Synthetic casts can bear weight approximately 30 minutes to 1 hour after application.

- Elevate the cast above heart level for the first 24 to 48 hours to decrease swelling and pain. This can be accomplished by propping the casted extremity on pillows or some other type of support.
- Gently move the toes or fingers frequently to prevent swelling and joint stiffness and to increase circulation.
- Apply ice to the casted extremity for the first 24 to 48 hours to reduce swelling. Place small pieces of ice in an ice bag with a protective covering, and apply it to the top of the cast directly over the injury. Apply the ice bag as recommended by the provider, which is usually for 15 to 30 minutes every 2 hours.
- Take precautions to prevent dirt, sand, powder, and other foreign particles from becoming trapped under the cast. They can cause irritation to the skin, leading to infection.
- Do not apply powder for itching under the cast. Do not use any object to scratch the skin under the cast. Inserting anything under the cast, such as a pencil, coat hanger, or knitting needle, may cause a break in the skin, which could become infected. Also, the object may become lost in the cast.
- Do not engage in activities that could cause injury because of impairment of your physical abilities (e.g., driving a car).
- Keep the cast dry. When taking a bath or shower, cover the cast with a plastic bag and secure the bag to the skin with waterproof tape. If possible, hang the casted limb over the side of the tub or outside of the shower. Although the material making up a synthetic cast is moisture resistant, the cast padding is not. If a synthetic cast becomes wet, it must be dried as soon as possible to prevent maceration. **Maceration** is the softening and breaking down of the skin, which can lead to infection.
- To dry a wet cast, first blot the outside of the cast with an absorbent towel. This should be followed by the application of a blow dryer on the cool setting using a sweeping motion over the entire cast until it is completely dry. The medium and high settings on the blow dryer should not be used because this amount of heat could burn the patient's skin under the cast.
- Inspect the skin around the cast at regular intervals to check for redness, sores, or swelling.
- Do not trim the cast or break off any rough edges because this may weaken or break the cast. If the surface of the cast has a rough edge, a metal nail file or emery board can be used to smooth it. Notify the provider if the cast becomes loose, broken, dented, or cracked, because the cast may need to be replaced.

SYMPTOMS TO REPORT

The patient should report the following symptoms *immediately* to the provider; they may indicate that the cast is too tight or an infection is developing:

- Increased pain or swelling that does not go away with application of an ice bag, medication, elevation, or rest
- A feeling that the cast is too tight. Slight pressure applied with the thumbnail to the fingernail or toenail should cause it to blanch white, and then when the pressure is released, the nail should immediately return to its normal color. If this does not occur, it could indicate insufficient blood flow to the extremity from a cast that is too tight
- Tingling, numbness, or loss of movement of the fingers or toes
- Coldness, paleness, or blueness of the fingers or toes
- Painful rubbing, burning, or stinging under the cast
- Foul odor or drainage coming from the cast
- Sore areas around the edge of the cast
- Chills, fever, nausea, or vomiting

CAST REMOVAL

The easiest and safest way to remove a cast is to bivalve it – this means cutting the cast into two halves, resulting in an anterior shell and a posterior shell. To bivalve a cast, the provider cuts the entire length of the cast on two opposite sides down to the level of the cast padding. The cuts are made with a cast cutter. A cast cutter is a handheld electric saw with a circular blade that oscillates, which means that the saw vibrates but does not rotate (Fig. 22.10A). The medical assistant should reassure the patient that, although the saw is noisy, only a tickling sensation and some heat are felt from the saw's vibration. After cutting the cast, the provider pries it apart with a cast spreader (Fig. 22.10B). Next, the provider uses bandage scissors to cut through the cast padding and stockinette (Fig. 22.10C). The cast is carefully removed from the patient's extremity.

The skin of the affected extremity typically appears yellow and scaly. The extremity also appears thinner, and the muscles are flabby. The medical assistant should explain to the patient that this is normal and results from lack of use of the extremity. The provider may recommend exercises or physical therapy or both to help the patient regain strength and function of the body part.

What Would You Do? | What Would You *Not* Do?

Case Study 2

Christina Themes calls the office. Two days ago, Christina fell while she was inline skating and broke the radius and ulna of her right arm. The physician applied a long arm fiberglass cast. While at the medical office, Christina received oral and written instructions on how to care for her cast. Christina says that in all the confusion, she misplaced the instructions. She said she didn't want to bother anyone at the office, so she did what she could to make her arm feel better. She says that it didn't work because now her arm is swollen and hurts. She took a bath, and the cast got wet, so she wants to know how to dry it. Christina asks if it would be possible to have one of those removable casts, so she can take it off when she takes a bath. ■

SPLINTS AND BRACES

Along with casts, splints and braces are used to assist in the treatment of fractures. A **splint** is a rigid removable device

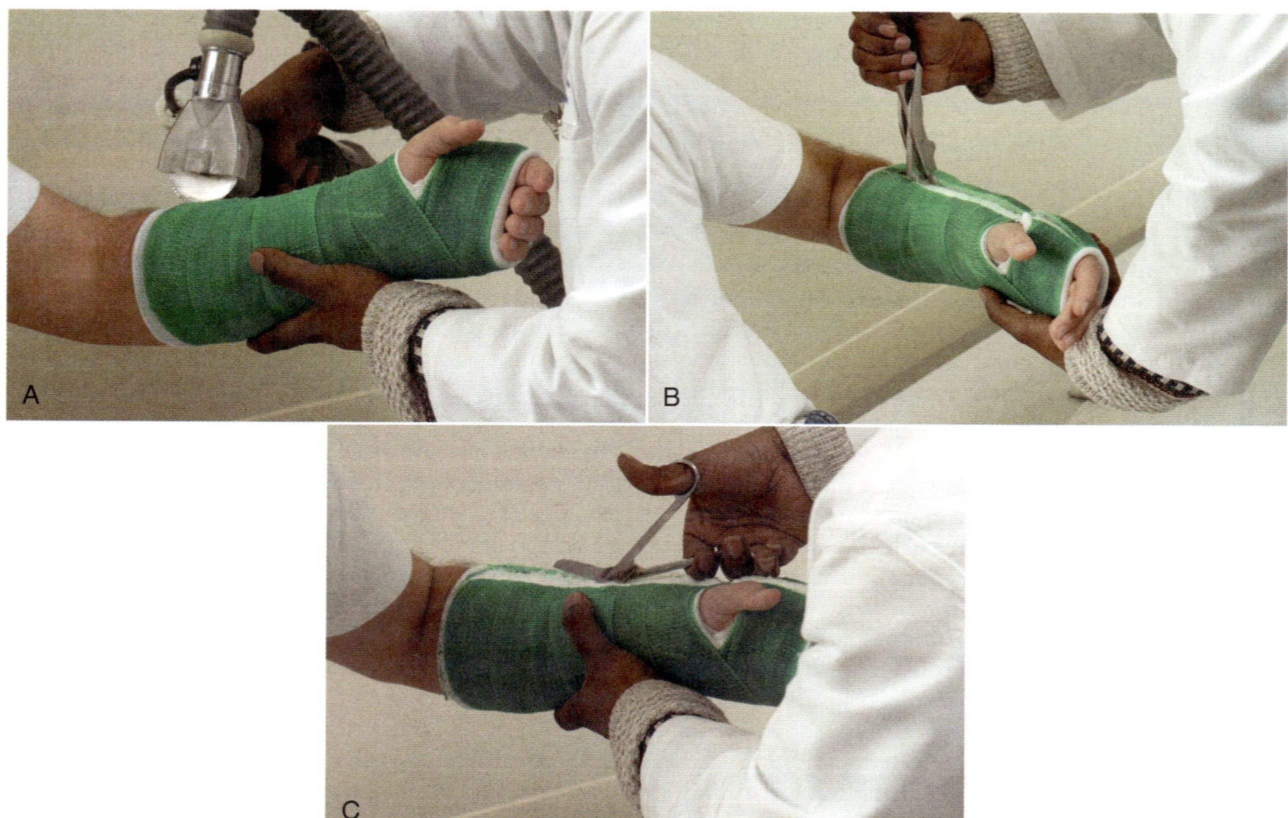

Fig. 22.10 Cast removal. (A) A cast cutter is used to cut the entire length of the cast. (B) The cast is pried open with a cast spreader. (C) Bandage scissors are used to cut through the cast padding and stockinette.

used to support and immobilize a displaced or fractured part of the body. Splints also are commonly used to protect areas that are sprained or strained. Splints are molded to fit specific parts of the body and are well padded to provide patient comfort and to prevent pressure areas. A splint can be custom made by an orthopedist using plaster or fiberglass casting materials. Splints also are commercially available and consist of two parts: a rigid material such as plastic or fiberglass, and straps with Velcro that hold the splint in place (Fig. 22.11).

A splint may be applied initially to a fractured limb because it can be adjusted to accommodate swelling from injuries more easily than a cast. After the swelling subsides, a cast is usually applied. When the fracture is almost healed, the cast may be removed and another splint applied. This allows for bathing of the extremity and easy removal for therapy until the fracture heals completely and the splint is no longer needed.

A **brace** is designed to support a part of the body and hold it in its correct position to allow for functioning of the body part while healing takes place. An example of a brace is a *short leg walker*, which consists of a rigid lightweight frame with a removable padded liner (Fig. 22.12). A short leg walker is often used, instead of a cast, to heal a stable fracture (e.g., stress fracture) of the lower leg. A short leg walker is available in different sizes so it can be properly fitted to extend from just below the patient's knee to the toes. Special fasteners or straps with Velcro are used to hold the walker in place and allow for adjustment of it (see Fig. 22.12). A short leg walker permits walking and standing, which encourage healing. It also can be removed to permit bathing of the leg.

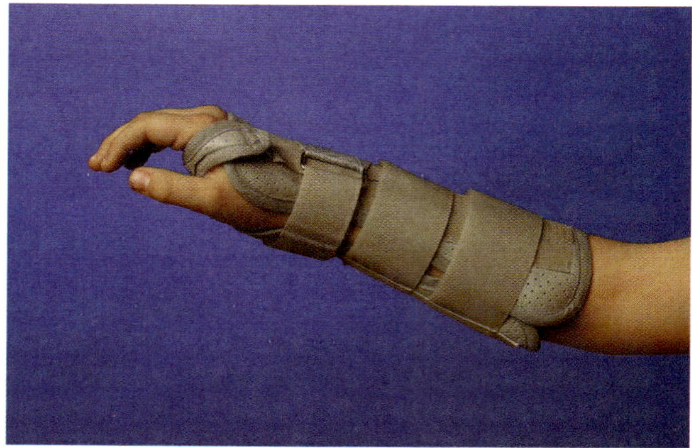

Fig. 22.11 Arm splint.

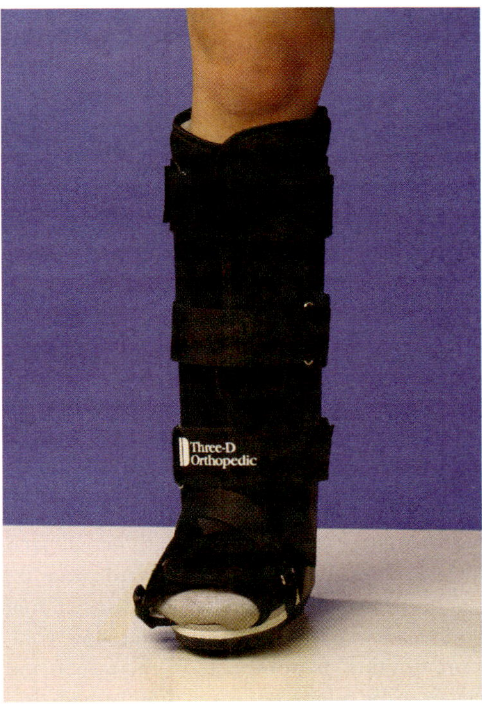

Fig. 22.12 Short leg walker, which is an example of a leg brace.

PATIENT COACHING Cast Care

Coach the patient in the important guidelines of cast care.

- Emphasize the importance of contacting the provider immediately if any signs of circulatory impairment or infection occur.
- If the provider has prescribed cold to reduce swelling, teach the patient the procedure for applying an ice bag to the casted extremity.
- Emphasize the importance of returning to have the cast checked by the provider.
- If the provider prescribes isometric exercises to maintain the muscle tone of the affected extremity, provide the patient with a sheet that illustrates the exercises.
- Provide the patient with printed materials on cast care.

AMBULATORY AIDS

Mechanical assistive devices are used by individuals who require aid in ambulation. The word **ambulation** means walking; patients who are **ambulatory** are able to walk as opposed to being confined to a wheelchair or a bed. Ambulatory aids include crutches, canes, and walkers. The device used depends on factors such as the type and severity of the disability, the amount of support required, and the patient's age and degree of muscular coordination. The ambulatory aid may be prescribed for a temporary condition, such as a fracture, a sprain to a lower extremity, and disability after orthopedic surgery. It also may be prescribed for a long-term condition, such as paralysis, deformity, and permanent weakness of the lower extremities.

CRUTCHES

Crutches are artificial supports that are used by patients requiring assistance in walking as a result of disease, injury, or birth defects of the lower extremities. Crutches function by removing weight from the legs and transferring it to the arms. The two main crutch types are the axillary crutch and the forearm crutch (Fig. 22.13). The axillary crutch and the forearm crutch require rubber tips, which increase surface tension, to prevent the crutches from slipping on the floor.

The *axillary crutch* is used most frequently and is made of tubular aluminum or wood. This type of crutch has a shoulder rest and handgrips and extends from the ground almost to the patient's axilla.

The *forearm crutch* (also known as an *elbow crutch*) consists of a single adjustable tube of aluminum that extends to the forearm. A metal or plastic cuff attached to the crutch fits securely around the patient's forearm, and a handgrip covered with rubber extends from the crutch for weight bearing. The cuff and the handgrip stabilize the patient's

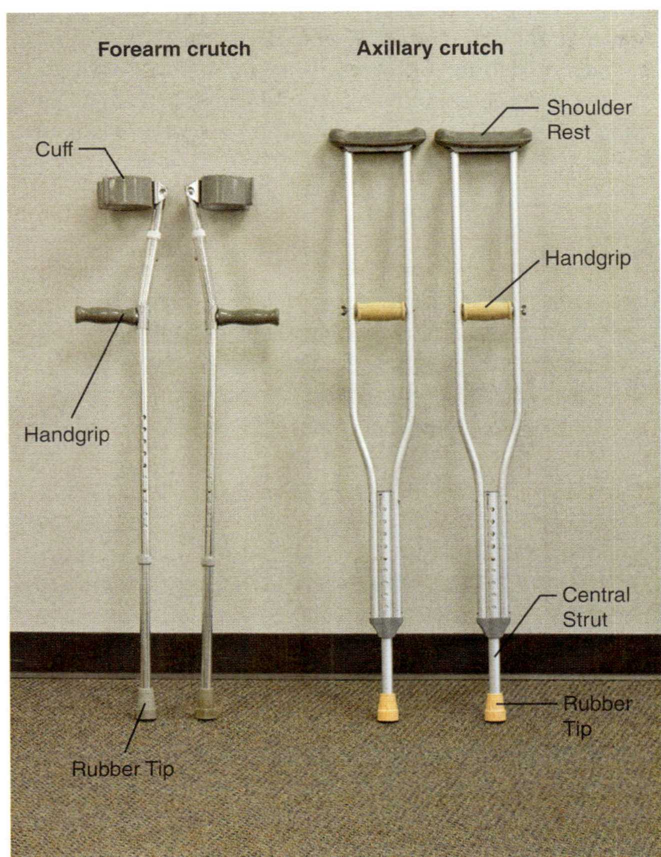

Fig. 22.13 Types of crutches. Forearm crutch is on the left and axillary crutch is on the right. (Modified from Niedzwiecki B, Pepper J, Weaver PA: *Kinn's the medical assistant*, ed 14, St. Louis, 2020, Elsevier.)

wrists to make walking safer and easier. One advantage of the forearm crutch is that the individual can release the handgrip, enabling use of the hand, while the cuff holds the crutch in place. Forearm crutches are used most often by individuals with long-term disabilities such as paraplegia or cerebral palsy.

Axillary Crutch Measurement

The patient must be measured for axillary crutches to ensure the correct crutch length and proper placement of the handgrip. Incorrectly fitted crutches increase the patient's risk of developing back pain, nerve damage, and injuries to the axillae and palms of the hands. Procedure 22.7 presents the correct way to measure a patient for axillary crutches.

If the crutches are too long, the shoulder rests exert pressure on the patient's axillae. This can injure the radial nerve in the brachial plexus, which eventually may lead to *crutch palsy*, a condition of muscular weakness in the forearm, wrist, and hand. In addition, crutches that are too long force the patient's shoulders forward, preventing the patient from pushing their body off the ground. Crutches that are too short force the patient to be bent over and uncomfortable, also making them awkward to use. If the handgrips are too low, pressure is put on the patient's axillae, whereas handgrips that are too high are awkward.

Aluminum crutches consist of aluminum tubes. Spring-loaded pushbuttons on an inner tube "pop out" into holes on an outer tube to allow proper adjustment of the crutch length.

Wooden crutches are made with bolts and wing nuts, which allow proper adjustment of the length and handgrip level.

PATIENT COACHING Crutches

Coach the patient in the guidelines for the proper use of crutches.

- Provide the patient with an exercise sheet that illustrates exercises to strengthen arm muscles before beginning crutch walking.
- Teach the patient the crutch gaits prescribed by the provider, and have the patient demonstrate the gaits before leaving the office.
- Provide the patient with a list of local vendors who provide crutch services, such as repairs and supplies (e.g., rubber tips, crutch pads).
- Provide the patient with printed educational materials on the use of crutches and crutch gaits.

Crutch Guidelines

It is important that the patient receive specific guidelines to ensure safety while using crutches, to prevent injuries and falls. The medical assistant is responsible for instructing the patient in the following guidelines:

1. Wear well-fitting flat shoes with firm, nonskid soles to provide good traction and stability.
2. Use good posture to prevent strain on muscles and joints and to maintain proper body balance.
3. Support your weight with your hands on the handgrips and the axillary pads pressing against the sides of the rib cage. The body weight should not be supported by the axillae because pressure on the axillae may cause crutch palsy.
4. Look ahead when walking, rather than down at your feet.
5. Be aware of the surface on which you are walking. It should be clean, flat, dry, and well lit. Throw rugs and objects serving as obstacles should temporarily be removed from your environment to prevent falls.
6. Keep the crutches about 4 to 6 inches out from the sides of your feet when walking to prevent obstruction of the pathway for the feet.
7. Take steps by moving the crutches forward a safe and comfortable distance, preferably 6 inches. When first learning to use the crutches, take small steps rather than large ones. Do not move forward more than 12 to 15 inches with each step. A greater distance might cause the crutches to slide forward and you to lose your balance.
8. Report tingling or numbness in the upper body to the provider. You might be using the crutches incorrectly, or they might be the wrong size for you.
9. Extra padding can be added to the shoulder rests of your crutches to make them more comfortable. If you do this, ensure that the extra padding does not press against your axillae, but rather against your lateral rib cage. The handgrips also can be padded for increased comfort.
10. To prevent slipping, keep the crutch tips dry to maintain their surface friction. If they become wet, dry them completely before use.
11. Inspect the crutch tips regularly. They should be securely attached. If the crutch tips are worn down, they should be replaced with tips of the proper size.
12. For wooden crutches, periodically check the wing nuts holding the central strut and handgrips in place to ensure that they are tight.

Crutch Gaits

The type of crutch gait used depends on the amount of weight the patient is able to support with one or both legs and the patient's physical condition and muscular coordination. The patient should learn a fast and a slow gait. The faster gait is used for making speed in open areas, and the slower one is used in crowded places. In addition, learning more than one gait reduces patient fatigue because a different combination of muscles is used for each gait. Procedure 22.8 provides guidelines and charts for use in instructing the patient on how to walk with crutches.

CANES

A cane is a lightweight, easily movable device made of aluminum or wood with a rubber tip and is used to help

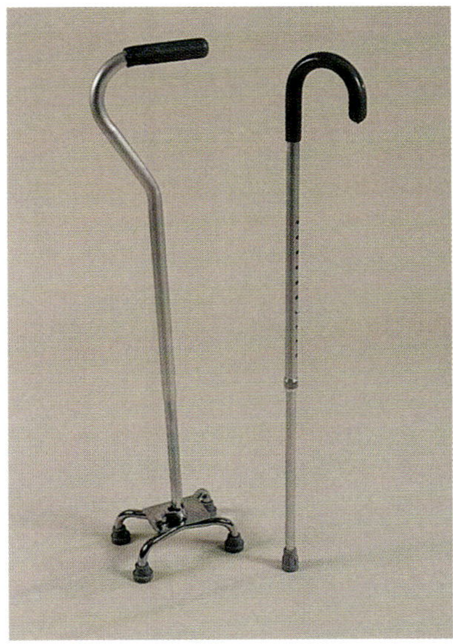

Fig. 22.14 Examples of a quad cane (left) and a standard cane (right). (Courtesy 3M Health Care, St. Paul, MN.)

provide balance and support. Canes are generally used by patients who have weakness on one side of the body, such as patients with hemiparesis, joint disabilities, or defects of the neuromuscular system. The three main types of canes are the *standard cane*, the *tripod cane*, and the *quad cane* (Fig. 22.14). The standard cane provides the least amount of support and is used by patients who require only slight assistance in walking. The tripod and quad canes have three and four legs, respectively, a bent shaft, and a T-shaped handle with grips. They are easier to hold and provide greater stability than a standard cane because of the wider base of support. In addition, multilegged canes are able to stand alone, which frees the arms when the patient is getting up from a chair. The disadvantage of a multilegged cane is that it is bulkier and more difficult to move.

A cane is held on the side of the body opposite the side that needs support (i.e., the strong side of the body). The cane length must be properly adjusted to ensure optimal stability. The cane handle should be approximately level with the greater trochanter, and the elbow should be flexed at a 25- to 30-degree angle. The patient should be instructed to stand erect and not lean on the cane to ensure good balance. Procedure 22.9 presents guidelines on instructing the patient on how to walk with a cane.

WALKERS

A walker is an ambulatory aid consisting of an aluminum frame with handgrips and four widely placed legs with

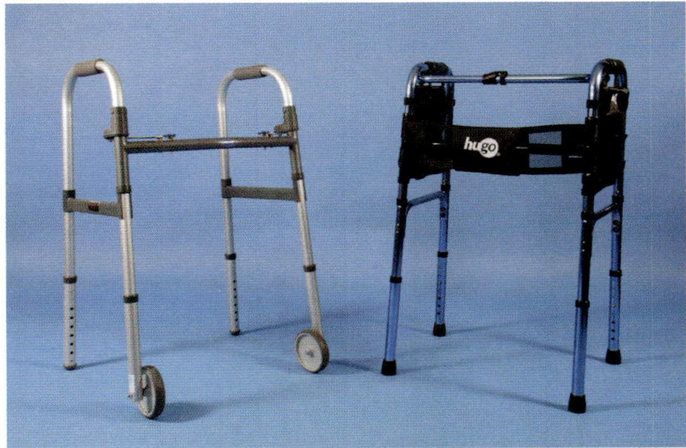

Fig. 22.15 Walkers.

rubber suction tips and one open side (Fig. 22.15). A walker is light and easily movable. Walkers are available with wheels that facilitate movement of the walker. They are also available with a fold-up feature that allows them to be easily transported in a vehicle. For proper ambulation, the walker should extend from the ground to approximately the level of the patient's hip joint. Procedure 22.10 presents guidelines on instructing the patient on how to walk with a walker.

Walkers are used most often by geriatric patients with weakness or balance problems. Walkers also are used during the healing process for patients who have had knee or hip joint replacement surgery. These patients need more help with balance and walking than can be provided by crutches or a cane. Because of its wide base, a walker provides the patient with a great amount of stability and security. Disadvantages of a walker include a slow pace and difficulty in maneuvering the walker in a small room.

What Would You Do? What Would You *Not* Do?

Case Study 3

Thaddeus Bernard calls the office. Thaddeus fractured the femur of his left leg 2 weeks ago in a skiing accident. The physician applied a long leg fiberglass cast, and Thaddeus was properly fitted with aluminum crutches. Thaddeus says that he is having some problems with his crutches. He is complaining of weakness in his forearms and hands and some tingling and numbness in his fingers. He also says that he has bruises under his arms. Thaddeus says that after he got home, his crutches didn't seem to fit right, so he readjusted them. Thaddeus is getting ready to return to college and wants to know the best way to carry his books while using crutches. ■

What Would You Do? What Would You *Not* Do? RESPONSES

Case Study 1
Page 468

What Did Marlyne Do?
- ❑ Empathized with Aaron for being in so much pain.
- ❑ Explained to Aaron that he should never sleep on a heating pad because the heat builds up and causes the type of burn he experienced.
- ❑ Explained to Aaron that it is best to apply heat for 15 to 30 minutes at a time with the pad set no higher than the medium setting. Told him the pad may not feel warm after his body gets used to it, but that it is still helping him. Told Aaron that the high setting could burn his skin.
- ❑ Told Aaron how to prevent low back pain by using good body mechanics, especially during lifting.

What Did Marlyne* Not *Do?
- ❑ Did not criticize Aaron for sleeping on the heating pad or turning the pad to the high setting.

Case Study 2
Page 473

What Did Marlyne Do?
- ❑ Reassured Christina that the medical staff is there to help her, and she should never hesitate to call when she needs information or is having a problem.
- ❑ Asked Christina what she did to try to make her arm feel better and documented this information in her medical record. Checked with the physician to determine whether he wanted to see Christina.
- ❑ Reeducated Christina in proper cast care instructions over the phone and mailed her another cast care instruction sheet.
- ❑ Explained to Christina how to dry her cast properly by first blotting it and then using a hair dryer. Told her that if she is unable to dry her cast completely, she will need to come in to have it replaced.
- ❑ Explained to Christina that the physician applied the type of cast that would best treat her injury and help her to heal.

What Did Marlyne* Not *Do?
- ❑ Did not criticize Christina for waiting so long to call the office.
- ❑ Did not tell Christina it would be a good idea for her to have a "removable cast."

Case Study 3
Page 477

What Did Marlyne Do?
- ❑ Listened carefully and empathetically to Thaddeus's problems with and concerns about his crutches.
- ❑ Explained to Thaddeus that the crutches were adjusted to fit him properly at the office and that some problems may have developed after he readjusted them.
- ❑ Scheduled an appointment for Thaddeus to come in that day so the physician could examine him and his crutches could be checked for proper length.
- ❑ Went over crutch guidelines and crutch gaits with Thaddeus again when he came to the office for his appointment.
- ❑ Told Thaddeus that he should use a backpack to carry his books to keep his hands free to move on his crutches. Stressed that he should keep his backpack as light as possible and keep the weight evenly distributed on his back (i.e., use both straps).

What Did Marlyne* Not *Do?
- ❑ Did not tell Thaddeus to readjust the crutches himself.
- ❑ Did not tell Thaddeus that he should have paid more attention when he was being instructed in crutch guidelines. ■

TERMINOLOGY REVIEW

Medical Term	Word Parts	Definition
Ambulation		Walking or moving from one place to another.
Ambulatory		Able to walk as opposed to being confined to bed or a wheelchair.
Brace		An orthopedic device used to support and hold a part of the body in the correct position to allow for functioning of the body part while healing takes place.
Cast		A stiff cylindrical casing that is used to immobilize a body part until healing occurs.
Compress		A soft, moist, absorbent cloth that is folded in several layers and applied to a part of the body in the local application of heat or cold.
Edema		The retention of fluid in the tissues, resulting in swelling.
Erythema	*hem/o:* blood	Reddening of the skin caused by dilation of superficial blood vessels in the skin.
Exudate		A discharge produced by the body's tissues.
Long arm cast		A cast that extends from the axilla to the fingers of the hand, usually with a bend in the elbow.
Long leg cast		A cast that extends from the midthigh to the toes.
Maceration		The softening and breaking down of the skin as a result of prolonged exposure to moisture.

TERMINOLOGY REVIEW—cont'd

Medical Term	Word Parts	Definition
Orthopedist	*orth/o:* straight *-ist:* specialist	A physician who specializes in the diagnosis and treatment of disorders of the musculoskeletal system, which includes the bones, joints, ligaments, tendons, muscles, and nerves.
Short arm cast		A cast that extends from below the elbow to the fingers.
Short leg cast		A cast that begins just below the knee and extends to the toes.
Soak		The direct immersion of a body part in water or a medicated solution.
Splint		An orthopedic device that is rigid and removable used to support and immobilize a part of the body.
Sprain		Trauma to a joint that causes injury to the ligaments.
Strain		An overstretching of a muscle caused by trauma.
Suppuration		The process of pus formation.

PROCEDURE 22.1 Applying a Heating Pad

Outcome Apply a heating pad.

Equipment/Supplies

- Heating pad with a protective covering

1. **Procedural Step.** Sanitize your hands.
2. **Procedural Step.** Assemble the equipment.
3. **Procedural Step.** Greet the patient and introduce yourself. Identify the patient and explain the procedure. Explain the purpose of the application (e.g., to relieve pain).
4. **Procedural Step.** Place the heating pad in the protective covering.
   Principle. The protective covering provides more comfort for the patient and absorbs perspiration.

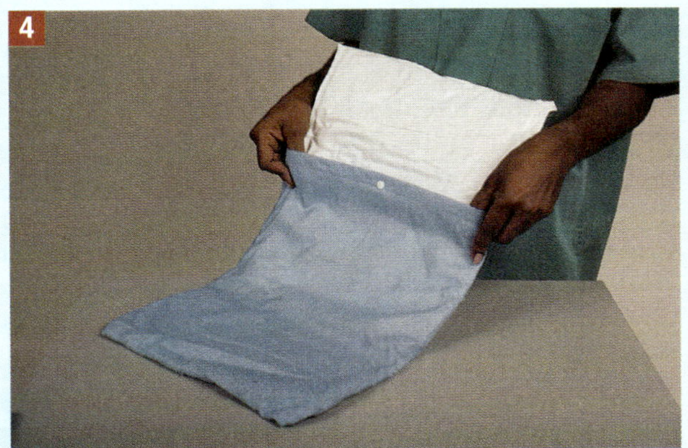

Place the heating pad in a protective covering.

5. **Procedural Step.** Connect the plug to an electric outlet. Set the selector switch at the proper setting, as designated by the provider (usually low or medium).
6. **Procedural Step.** Place the heating pad on the patient's affected body area. Ask the patient how the temperature feels. The heating pad should feel warm but not uncomfortable.
7. **Procedural Step.** Instruct the patient not to lie on the pad or turn the control higher to prevent burns.
   Principle. Lying on the pad causes heat to accumulate and burn the patient. The patient's heat receptors eventually become adjusted to the temperature change, resulting in a decreased heat sensation, and the patient may be tempted to increase the temperature. Turning the control higher results in excessive heat on the patient's skin, which could burn the patient.
8. **Procedural Step.** Check the patient periodically for signs of an increase or decrease in redness or swelling, and ask the patient whether the site is painful. Administer the treatment for the proper length of time as designated by the provider.
9. **Procedural Step.** Sanitize your hands.

Continued

PROCEDURE 22.1 Applying a Heating Pad—cont'd

10. Procedural Step. Document the procedure in the patient's medical record.

a. *Electronic health record (EHR):* Using an EHR such as SimChart for the Medical Office, use the correct radio buttons, drop-down menus, and free text fields to document the method of heat application, the location and duration of the application, the appearance of the application site, and the patient's reaction. Also, document any instructions provided to the patient on applying a heating pad at home.

b. *Paper-based patient record:* Document the date and time, method of heat application (heating pad), temperature setting of the pad, location and duration of the application, appearance of the application site, and the patient's reaction. Also, document any instructions provided to the patient on applying a heating pad at home.

10b

DOCUMENTATION EXAMPLE

Date	
12/10/XX	10:15 a.m. Heating pad on medium setting
	applied to lower back x 20 min. Area appears
	pink following application. Pt states a relief of
	pain and better mobility. Provided
	instructions on the application of a heating
	pad at home.______ M. Cooper, CMA (AAMA)

11. Procedural Step. Properly care for equipment, and return it to its storage location. Also, if the protective covering is disposable, throw it away; if it is reusable, either wash it in the washing machine or sanitize it before reusing it.

PROCEDURE 22.2 Applying a Hot Soak

Outcome Apply a hot soak.

Equipment/Supplies

- Soaking solution ordered by the provider
- Bath thermometer
- Basin
- Bath towels

1. **Procedural Step.** Sanitize your hands.
2. **Procedural Step.** Assemble the equipment. Check the label on the solution container to make sure you have the correct solution as ordered by the provider. Place the solution container in a basin of warm water. Warm the soaking solution to a temperature between 105°F and 110°F (41°C and 44°C).
3. **Procedural Step.** Greet the patient and introduce yourself. Identify the patient and explain the procedure. Explain the purpose of the application (e.g., to apply a medicated solution).
4. **Procedural Step.** Fill the basin one-third to two-thirds full with the warmed soaking solution.
5. **Procedural Step.** Check the temperature of the solution with a bath thermometer. The temperature for an adult should be 105°F to 110°F (41°C to 44°C).
6. **Procedural Step.** Assist the patient into a comfortable position to avoid fatigue and muscle strain. Pad the side of the basin with a towel for the patient's comfort.
7. **Procedural Step.** Slowly and gradually immerse the patient's affected body part in the solution. Ask the patient how the temperature feels.
   Principle. The affected body part should gradually become accustomed to the change in temperature.
8. **Procedural Step.** Test the temperature of the solution frequently. To keep the solution at a constant temperature, remove cooler fluid every 5 minutes and replace it with hot solution. Pour the hot solution in near the edge of the basin by placing your hand between the patient and the solution. Stir the solution as you pour.
   Principle. The solution should be added away from the patient's body part to prevent splashing hot fluid on the patient. Stirring in the solution helps distribute the heat and keep the temperature constant.

PROCEDURE 22.2 Applying a Hot Soak—cont'd

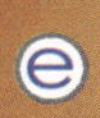

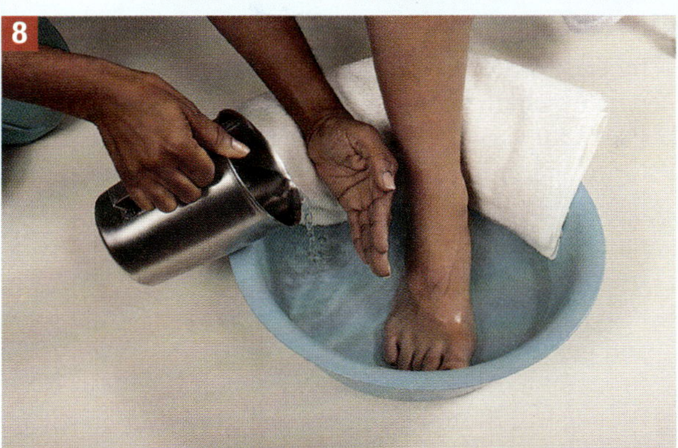
8 Replace cooler solution with hot solution.

9. **Procedural Step.** Check the patient's skin periodically for signs of an increase or decrease in redness or swelling, and ask the patient whether the site is painful. Apply the hot soak for the proper length of time as designated by the provider (usually 15 to 20 minutes).
10. **Procedural Step.** Dry the affected part completely and gently.
11. **Procedural Step.** Sanitize your hands.
12. **Procedural Step.** Document the procedure in the patient's medical record.
    a. *Electronic health record (EHR):* Using an EHR such as SimChart for the Medical Office, use the correct radio buttons, drop-down menus, and free text fields to document the method of heat application, name and strength of the solution, temperature of the soak, location and duration of the application, appearance of the application site, and the patient's reaction.
    b. *Paper-based patient record:* Document the date and time, method of heat application (hot soak), name and strength of the solution, temperature of the soak, location and duration of the application, appearance of the application site, and the patient's reaction.

12b

DOCUMENTATION EXAMPLE

Date	
12/12/XX	1:15 p.m. Normal saline hot soak at 105° F
	applied to Ⓡ ankle x 20 min. Area appears
	pink following application. Pt states less
	stiffness in ankle.__M. Cooper, CMA (AAMA)

13. **Procedural Step.** Properly care for equipment and return it to its storage location.

PROCEDURE 22.3 Applying a Hot Compress

Outcome Apply a hot compress.

Equipment/Supplies

- Solution ordered by the provider
- Bath thermometer
- Basin
- Washcloths
- Waterproof covering
- Towel

1. **Procedural Step.** Sanitize your hands.
2. **Procedural Step.** Assemble the equipment. Check the label on the solution container to make sure you have the correct solution as ordered by the provider. Place the solution container in a basin of warm water. Warm the soaking solution to a temperature between 105°F and 110°F (41°C and 44°C).
3. **Procedural Step.** Greet the patient and introduce yourself. Identify the patient and explain the procedure. Explain the purpose of the application (e.g., to soften an exudate).
4. **Procedural Step.** Fill the basin half full with warmed solution. Check the temperature of the solution with the bath thermometer. The temperature for an adult should be 105°F to 110°F (41°C to 44°C).
5. **Procedural Step.** Completely immerse the compress in the solution. Wring the compress to remove excess moisture. The compress should be wet but not dripping. Apply it lightly at first to the affected site to allow the patient to become used to the heat gradually. You may want to cover the compress with a waterproof cover to help hold in the heat. Ask the patient how the

Continued

PROCEDURE 22.3 Applying a Hot Compress—cont'd

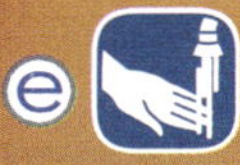

temperature feels. The compress should be as hot as the patient can comfortably tolerate.
Principle. The waterproof cover prevents cool air currents from coming into contact with the compress and reduces the number of times the compress needs to be changed.

5 (1)

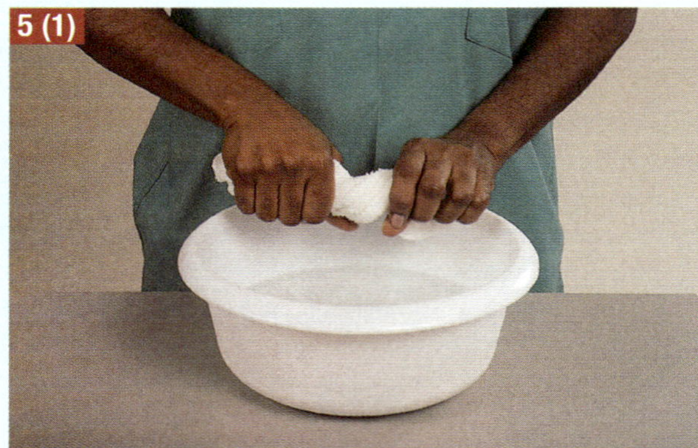

Wring out the compress.

5 (2)

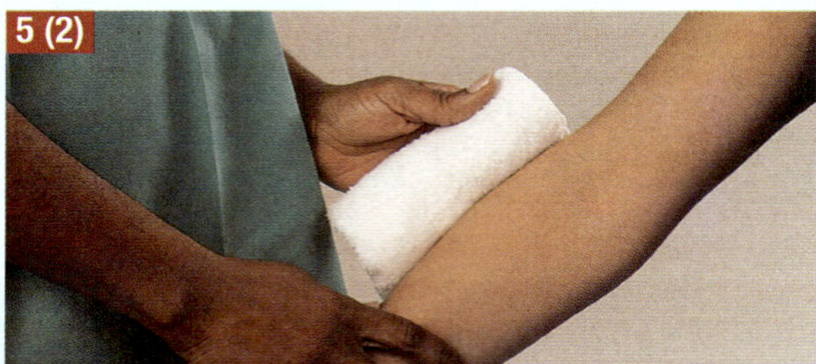

Apply the compress to the affected site.

6. **Procedural Step.** Place additional compresses in the solution so that they are ready for use.
7. **Procedural Step.** Repeat the application of the compress every 2 to 3 minutes for the duration of time specified by the provider (usually 15 to 20 minutes). Check the patient's skin periodically for signs of an increase or decrease in redness or swelling, and ask the patient whether the site is painful.
8. **Procedural Step.** Check the temperature of the solution periodically. Remove cooler fluid and replace it with hot solution if needed. Administer the treatment for the proper length of time as designated by the provider.
9. **Procedural Step.** Dry the affected part thoroughly and gently.
10. **Procedural Step.** Sanitize your hands.
11. **Procedural Step.** Document the procedure in the patient's medical record.
    a. *Electronic health record (EHR):* Using an EHR such as SimChart for the Medical Office, use the correct radio buttons, drop-down menus, and free text fields to document the method of heat application, name and strength of the solution, temperature of the solution, location and duration of the application, appearance of the application site, and the patient's reaction.
    b. *Paper-based patient record:* Document the date and time, method of heat application (hot compress), name and strength of the solution, temperature of the solution, location and duration of the application, appearance of the application site, and the patient's reaction.

11b

DOCUMENTATION EXAMPLE

Date	
12/20/XX	10:30 a.m. Normal saline hot compress at
	110° F applied to Ⓡ forearm x 20 min. No
	complaints of discomfort. ————————
	———————— M. Cooper, CMA (AAMA)

12. **Procedural Step.** Properly care for equipment and return it to its storage location.

PROCEDURE 22.4 Applying an Ice Bag

Outcome Apply an ice bag.

Equipment/Supplies

- Ice bag with a protective covering
- Small pieces of ice (ice chips or crushed ice)

1. **Procedural Step.** Sanitize your hands.
2. **Procedural Step.** Assemble the equipment.
3. **Procedural Step.** Greet the patient and introduce yourself. Identify the patient and explain the procedure. Explain the purpose of applying the ice bag (e.g., to prevent swelling).

PROCEDURE 22.4 Applying an Ice Bag—cont'd

4. **Procedural Step.** Check the ice bag for leakage.
   Principle. A leaking bag would get the patient wet and cause chilling.
5. **Procedural Step.** Fill the bag one-half to two-thirds full with small pieces of ice.
   Principle. Small pieces of ice work better than large pieces because they reduce the air spaces in the bag, resulting in better conduction of cold. In addition, small pieces of ice allow the bag to mold better to the body area.
6. **Procedural Step.** Expel air from the bag by squeezing the empty top half of the bag together and screwing on the stopper.
   Principle. Air is a poor conductor of cold and makes it difficult to mold the ice bag to the body area.

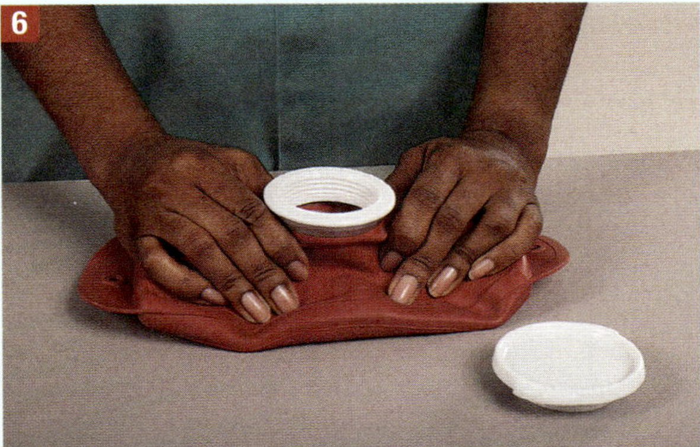

Expel air from the bag.

7. **Procedural Step.** Place the bag in the protective covering.
   Principle. The protective covering provides for patient comfort and absorbs the moisture that condenses on the outside of the bag.
8. **Procedural Step.** Place the bag on the patient's affected body area. Ask the patient how the temperature feels. The application of ice is usually uncomfortable, but most patients tolerate it when they know how much benefit may be derived from it.
   Principle. Individuals vary in their ability to tolerate cold.
9. **Procedural Step.** Check the patient's skin periodically for signs of an increase or decrease in redness or swelling, and ask the patient whether the site is painful. If extreme paleness and numbness or a mottled blue appearance occur at the application site, remove the bag and notify the provider.
10. **Procedural Step.** Refill the bag with ice as necessary, and change the protective covering if needed. Administer the treatment for the proper length of time, as designated by the provider (usually until the area feels numb, approximately 15 to 30 minutes).
11. **Procedural Step.** Sanitize your hands.
12. **Procedural Step.** Document the procedure in the patient's medical record.
    a. *Electronic health record (EHR):* Using an EHR such as SimChart for the Medical Office, use the correct radio buttons, drop-down menus, and free text fields to document the method of cold application, location and duration of the application, appearance of the application site, and the patient's reaction. Also, document any instructions provided to the patient on applying an ice bag at home.
    b. *Paper-based patient record:* Document the date and time, method of cold application (ice bag), location and duration of the application, appearance of the application site, and the patient's reaction. Also, document any instructions provided to the patient on applying an ice bag at home.

12b

DOCUMENTATION EXAMPLE

Date	
12/22/XX	11:30 a.m. Ice bag applied to Ⓡ knee x 20
	min. Pt complained of slight discomfort
	during the application. Area appears less
	swollen following application. Provided
	instructions on the application of an ice bag
	at home.________ M. Cooper, CMA (AAMA)

13. **Procedural Step.** Properly care for the ice bag. Dispose of or launder the protective covering as required. Cleanse the ice bag with a warm detergent solution, rinse thoroughly, and dry by hanging the bag upside down with the top removed. Store the bag by screwing on the stopper, leaving air inside to prevent the sides from sticking together.

PROCEDURE 22.5 Applying a Cold Compress

Outcome Apply a cold compress.

Equipment/Supplies

- Ice cubes
- Basin
- Washcloths
- Towel
- Ice bag

1. **Procedural Step.** Sanitize your hands.
2. **Procedural Step.** Assemble the equipment. Check the label on the solution container to make sure you have the correct solution as ordered by the provider.
3. **Procedural Step.** Greet the patient and introduce yourself. Identify the patient and explain the procedure. Explain the purpose of the application (e.g., to treat an eye injury).
4. **Procedural Step.** Place large ice cubes in the basin. Add the solution until the basin is half full.
   Principle. Using larger pieces of ice prevents them from sticking to the compress and slows the rate at which they melt in the solution.

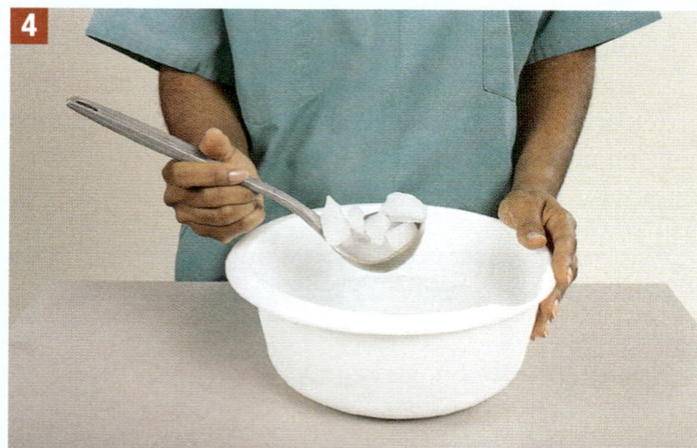

Place large ice cubes in the basin.

5. **Procedural Step.** Completely immerse the compress in the solution. Wring the compress to rid it of excess moisture. The compress should be wet but not dripping. Apply it lightly at first to the affected site to allow the patient to become used to the cold gradually. The compress can be covered with an ice bag to help keep it cold and to reduce the number of times it needs to be changed. Ask the patient how the temperature feels.
6. **Procedural Step.** Place additional compresses in the solution to be ready for use.
7. **Procedural Step.** Repeat the application of the compress every 2 to 3 minutes for the duration of time specified by the provider (usually 15 to 20 minutes). Check the patient's skin periodically for signs of an increase or decrease in redness or swelling, and ask the patient whether the site is painful.
8. **Procedural Step.** Add ice if needed to keep the solution cold. Administer the treatment for the proper length of time designated by the provider.
9. **Procedural Step.** Thoroughly dry the affected part.
10. **Procedural Step.** Sanitize your hands.
11. **Procedural Step.** Document the procedure in the patient's medical record.
    a. *Electronic health record (EHR):* Using an EHR such as SimChart for the Medical Office, use the correct radio buttons, drop-down menus, and free text fields to document the method of cold application, location and duration of the application, appearance of the application site, and patient's reaction.
    b. *Paper-based patient record:* Document the date and time, method of cold application (cold compress), location and duration of the application, appearance of the application site, and patient's reaction.

11b DOCUMENTATION EXAMPLE

Date	
12/27/XX	9:15 a.m. Normal saline cold compress
	applied to bridge of nose x 15 min. Nose
	appears less swollen following application.
	Tolerated application well. ————
	———— M. Cooper, CMA (AAMA)

12. **Procedural Step.** Properly care for equipment, and return it to its storage location.

PROCEDURE 22.6 Applying a Chemical Pack

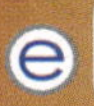

Outcome Apply a chemical cold pack and a chemical hot pack.

Equipment/Supplies

- Chemical cold pack
- Chemical hot pack

The procedure for applying a chemical cold or hot pack is as follows:

1. **Procedural Step.** Assemble equipment. Shake the crystals to the bottom of the bag.

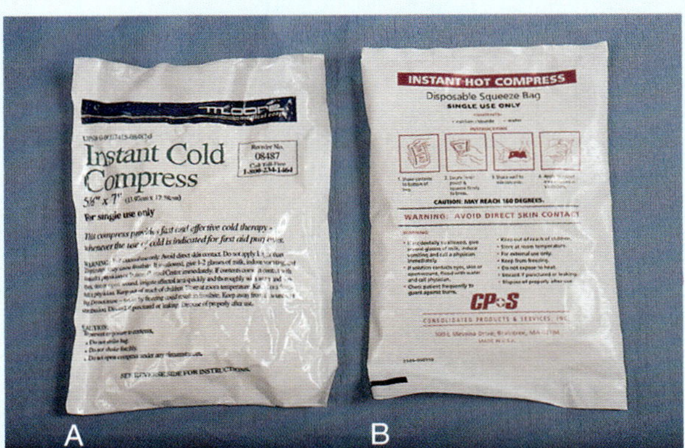

Chemical packs. (A) Chemical cold pack. (B) Chemical hot pack.

2. **Procedural Step.** Squeeze the bag firmly with your hands to break the inner water bag.
3. **Procedural Step.** Shake the bag vigorously to mix the contents.
4. **Procedural Step.** Cover the bag with a protective covering.
5. **Procedural Step.** Apply the bag to the affected area. Check the patient's skin periodically.
6. **Procedural Step.** Administer the treatment for the proper length of time.
7. **Procedural Step.** Discard the bag in an appropriate receptacle.
8. **Procedural Step.** Sanitize your hands.
9. **Procedural Step.** Document the procedure in the patient's medical record.
   a. *Electronic health record (EHR):* Using an EHR such as SimChart for the Medical Office, use the correct radio buttons, drop-down menus, and free text fields to document the method of application (chemical cold or hot pack), location and duration of the application, appearance of the application site, and patient's reaction.
   b. *Paper-based patient record:* Document the date and time, method of application (chemical cold or hot pack), location and duration of the application, appearance of the application site, and patient's reaction.

9b DOCUMENTATION EXAMPLE

Date	
12/28/XX	1:30 p.m. Cold pack applied to (L) knee
	x 20 minutes. Area appears less swollen
	following application. Provided instructions on
	the application of an ice pack at home.
	M.Cooper, CMA(AAMA)

PROCEDURE 22.7

PROCEDURE 22.7 Measuring for Axillary Crutches

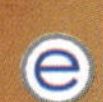

Outcome Measure an individual for axillary crutches.

Equipment/Supplies

- Axillary crutches
- Goniometer

1. **Procedural Step.** Greet the patient and introduce yourself. Identify the patient and inform the patient that you will be performing axillary crutch measurment. Discuss the importance of properly fitted crutches with the patient.

Determining Crutch Length

For you to determine crutch length correctly, the patient must wear shoes while being measured. The measurement is taken while the patient is standing.

Continued

PROCEDURE 22.7 Measuring for Axillary Crutches—cont'd

2. **Procedural Step.** Ask the patient to stand erect.
3. **Procedural Step.** Position the crutches with the crutch tips at a distance of 2 inches (5 cm) in front of and 4 to 6 inches (15 cm) to the side of each foot. (The large dots in the figure represent crutch tips.)

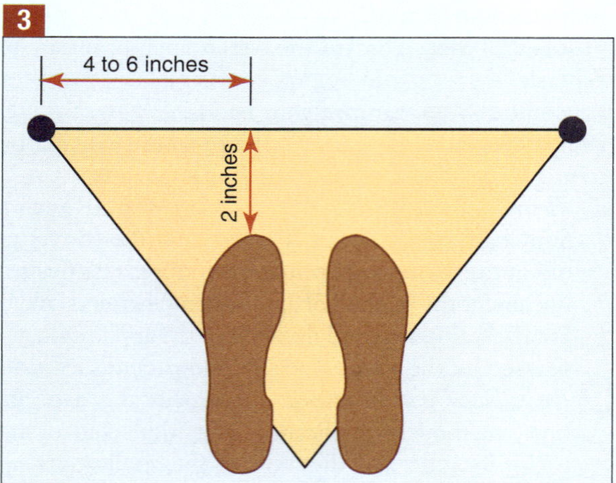

Position for measuring for crutches.

4. **Procedural Step.** Adjust the crutch length so that the shoulder rests are approximately 1½ to 2 inches (about two finger widths) below the axillae.
   - *Aluminum crutches.* The length of the crutch is adjusted by pressing the spring-loaded push button with your thumb and sliding the outer tube upward or downward as necessary to attain the proper length. The spring-loaded button on the inner tube should be allowed to "pop out" into the appropriate hole on the outer tube.
   - *Wooden crutches.* The length of the crutch is adjusted by removing the bolt and wing nut and sliding the central strut (support piece) at the bottom upward or downward as necessary to attain the proper length. The strut is secured by replacing the bolt and securely fastening the wing nut.

Handgrip Positioning

When the crutch length has been adjusted, correct placement of the handgrips must be determined.

5. **Procedural Step.** Ask the patient to stand erect with a crutch under each arm and to support their weight by the handgrips.
6. **Procedural Step.** Adjust the handgrips on the crutches so that the patient's elbow is flexed to an angle of approximately 30 degrees. The handgrip level is adjusted by removing the bolt and wing nut and sliding the handgrip upward or downward, as required. The handgrip is secured by replacing the bolt and tightly fastening the wing nut. The angle of elbow flexion can be verified by using a measuring device known as a goniometer. A goniometer is an instrument that measures the angle of a joint.
7. **Procedural Step.** Check the fit of the crutches. If the crutches are measured correctly, the medical assistant should be able to insert two fingers between the top of the crutches and the axillae when the patient is standing erect with the crutches under the arms.

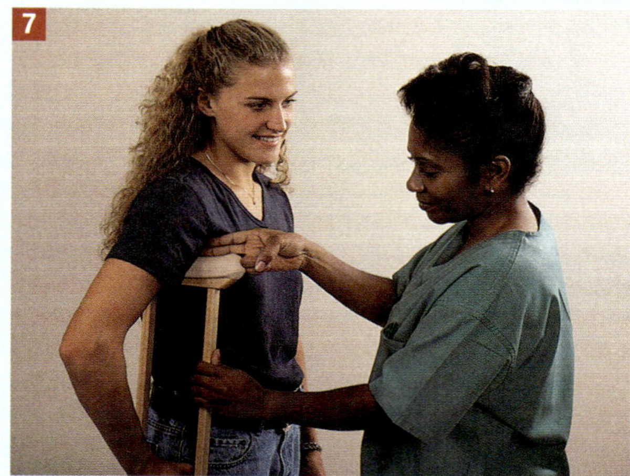

Insert two fingers between the top of the crutch and the axilla.

8. **Procedural Step.** Document the procedure in the patient's medical record.
   a. *Electronic health record (EHR):* Using an EHR such as SimChart for the Medical Office, use the appropriate radio buttons, drop-down menus, and free text fields to document the axillary crutch measurement procedure.
   b. *Paper-based patient record:* Document the date and time and the axillary crutch measurement procedure.

PROCEDURE 22.8 Instructing a Patient in Crutch Gaits

Outcome Instruct a patient in the following crutch gaits: four-point, two-point, three-point, swing-to, and swing-through.

Equipment/Supplies

- Axillary crutches

1. **Procedural Step.** Greet the patient and introduce yourself. Identify the patient and inform the patient that you will be providing instructions for crutch gaits. Discuss the importance of the proper use of crutches with the patient.
2. **Procedural Step.** Instruct the patient in the tripod position as follows:
   a. Stand erect, and face straight ahead.
   b. Place the tips of the crutches 4 to 6 inches (15 cm) in front of the feet and 4 to 6 inches (10 to 15 cm) to the side of each foot. (The large dots in the figure represent crutch tips.)

   Principle: The tripod position is the basic crutch stance used before crutch walking. It provides a wide base of support and enhances stability and balance.

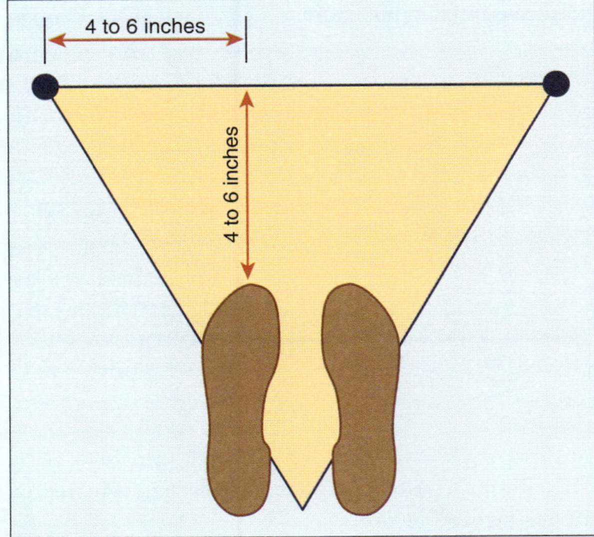

Tripod position

3. **Procedural Step.** Instruct the patient in the four-point gait.

   Four-Point Gait: The four-point gait is a basic and slow gait. To use this gait, the patient must be able to bear considerable weight on both legs. The four-point gait is the most stable and the safest of the crutch gaits because it provides at least three points of support at all times. It is used most often by patients who have leg muscle weakness or spasticity, poor muscular coordination or balance, or degenerative leg joint disease. Instruct the patient in the procedure for the four-point gait, following the steps in the accompanying figure.

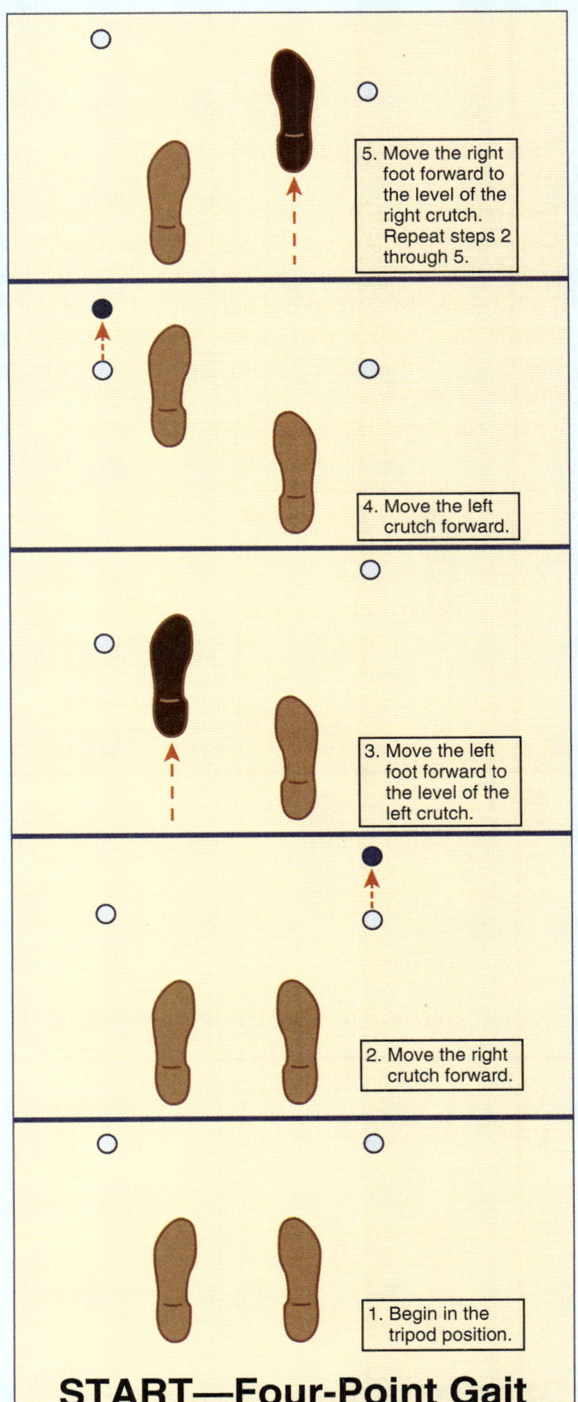

PROCEDURE 22.8

Continued

PROCEDURE 22.8 Instructing a Patient in Crutch Gaits—cont'd

DOCUMENTATION EXAMPLE

Date	
12/15/XX	1:30 p.m. Instructed pt in four-point gait. Pt
	was able to demonstrate four-point gait. ——
	———————— M. Cooper, CMA (AAMA)

4. **Procedural Step.** Instruct the patient in the two-point gait.
   Two-Point Gait: The two-point gait is similar to, but faster than, the four-point gait. This gait requires better balance because only two points support the body at one time. The two-point gait is used when the patient is capable of partial weight bearing on each foot and has good muscular coordination. Instruct the patient in the procedure for the two-point gait, following the steps in the accompanying figure.

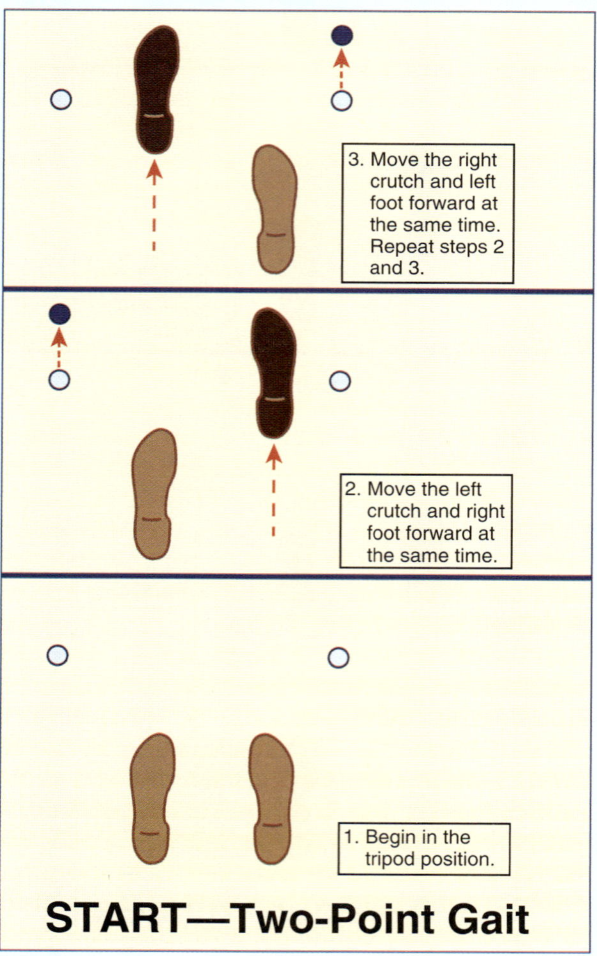

DOCUMENTATION EXAMPLE

Date	
12/16/XX	2:30 p.m. Instructed pt in two-point gait. Pt
	was able to demonstrate two-point gait. ——
	———————— M. Cooper, CMA (AAMA)

5. **Procedural Step.** Instruct the patient in the three-point gait.
   Three-Point Gait: The three-point gait is used by patients who cannot bear weight on one leg. The patient must be able to support their full weight on the unaffected leg. With this gait, the crutches and the unaffected leg alternately bear the patient's weight. This gait is used most often by amputees without a prosthesis, patients with musculoskeletal or soft tissue trauma to a lower extremity (e.g., fracture, sprain), patients with acute leg inflammation, and patients who have had recent leg surgery. To use this gait, the patient must have good muscular coordination and arm strength. Instruct the patient in the procedure for the three-point gait, following the steps in the accompanying figure.

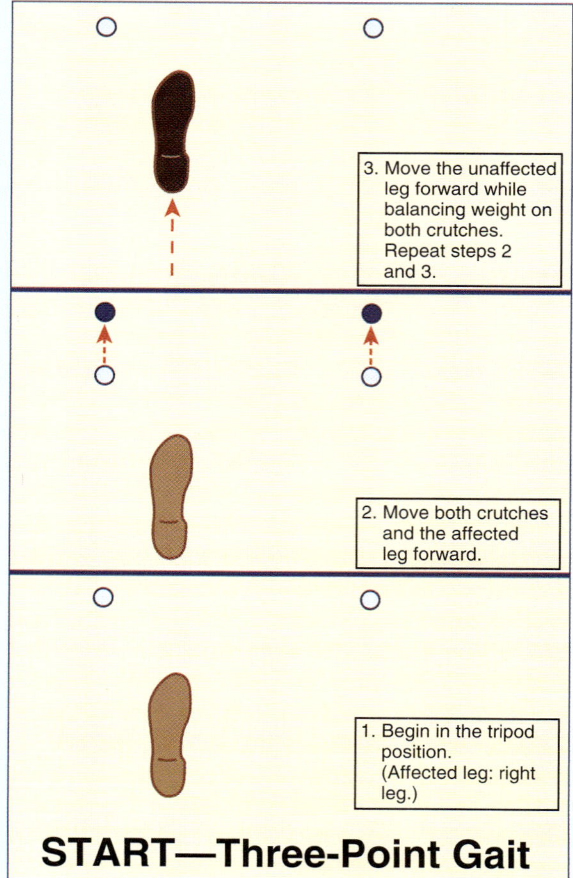

PROCEDURE 22.8 Instructing a Patient in Crutch Gaits—cont'd

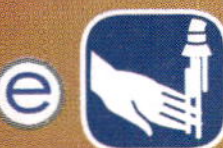

DOCUMENTATION EXAMPLE

Date	
12/17/XX	2:30 p.m. Instructed pt in three-point gait. Pt
	was able to demonstrate three-point gait. ——
	———————— M. Cooper, CMA (AAMA)

6. **Procedural Step.** Instruct the patient in the swing gaits.
Swing Gaits: The swing gaits include the swing-to gait and the swing-through gait and are used by patients with severe lower extremity disabilities, such as paralysis, and by patients who wear supporting braces on their legs. Instruct the patient in the procedures for the swing-to and the swing-through crutch gaits, following the steps in the accompanying figures.

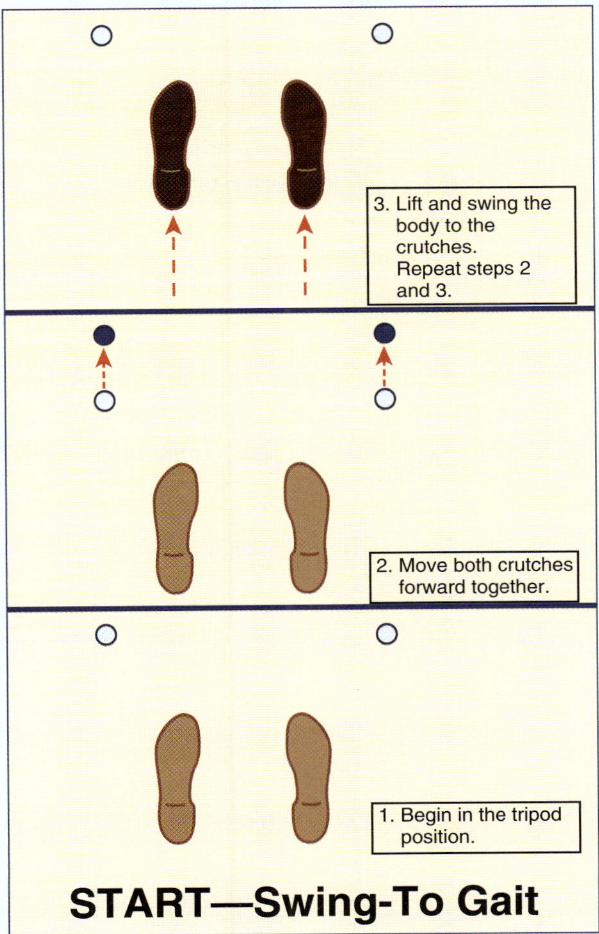

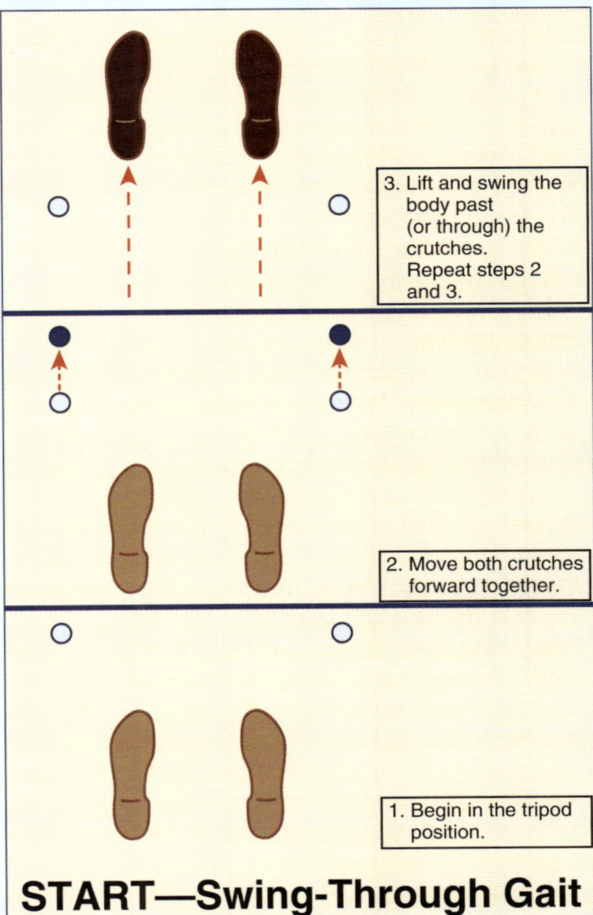

DOCUMENTATION EXAMPLE

Date	
12/18/XX	3:30 p.m. Instructed pt in swing-to and
	swing-through gaits. Pt was able to demon-
	strate swing gaits.—M. Cooper, CMA (AAMA)

7. **Procedural Step.** Document the procedure in the patient's medical record.
   a. *Electronic health record (EHR):* Using an EHR such as SimChart for the Medical Office, use the appropriate radio buttons, drop-down menus, and free text fields to document the type of instructions given to the patient. Document that the patient was able to properly demonstrate the crutch gaits.
   b. *Paper-based patient record:* Document the date and time and the type of instructions given to the patient. Document that the patient was able to properly demonstrate the crutch gaits. See the examples given.

PROCEDURE 22.9 Instructing a Patient in Use of a Cane

Outcome Instruct the patient in the use of a cane.

Equipment/Supplies

- Cane

1. **Procedural Step.** Greet the patient and introduce yourself. Identify the patient and inform the patient that you will be providing instructions on the use of a cane. Discuss the importance of proper cane use with the patient. Instruct the patient as follows:
2. **Procedural Step.** Hold the cane on the strong side of the body (i.e., in the hand opposite the affected extremity).
3. **Procedural Step.** Place the tip of the cane 4 to 6 inches to the side of the foot.
4. **Procedural Step.** Move the cane forward approximately 12 inches (1 foot).
5. **Procedural Step.** Move the affected leg forward to the level of the cane.
6. **Procedural Step.** Move the strong leg forward and ahead of the cane and weak leg.
7. **Procedural Step.** Repeat steps 3 through 5.
   Note: The cane and the affected leg can be moved forward simultaneously (steps 3 and 4); however, the patient has less support with this method.
8. **Procedural Step.** Document the procedure in the patient's medical record.
   a. *Electronic health record (EHR):* Using an EHR such as SimChart for the Medical Office, use the appropriate radio buttons, drop-down menus, and free text fields to document the type of instructions given to the patient. Document that the patient was able to demonstrate proper use of a cane.
   b. *Paper-based patient record:* Document the date and time and the type of instructions given to the patient. Document that the patient was able demonstrate proper use of a cane.

8b

DOCUMENTATION EXAMPLE

Date	
12/20/XX	2:30 p.m. Instructed pt in the procedure for
	using a cane. Pt was able to demonstrate
	proper use of a cane. ___
	M. Cooper, CMA (AAMA)

PROCEDURE 22.10 Instructing a Patient in Use of a Walker

Outcome Instruct the patient in the use of a walker.

Equipment/Supplies

- Walker

1. **Procedural Step.** Greet the patient and introduce yourself. Identify the patient and inform the patient that you will be showing him or her how to use a walker. Discuss the importance of proper walker use with the patient.
   Instruct the patient as follows:
2. **Procedural Step.** Pick up the walker, and move it forward approximately 6 inches.
3. **Procedural Step.** Move the right foot and then the left foot up to the walker.
4. **Procedural Step.** Repeat steps 1 and 2.
5. **Procedural Step.** Document the procedure in the patient's medical record.
   a. *Electronic health record (EHR):* Using an EHR such as SimChart for the Medical Office, use the appropriate radio buttons, drop-down menus, and free text fields to document the type of instructions given to the patient. Document that the patient was able to demonstrate proper use of a walker.
   b. *Paper-based patient record:* Document the date and time and the type of instructions given to the patient. Document that the patient was able to demonstrate proper use of a walker.

5b

DOCUMENTATION EXAMPLE

Date	
12/21/XX	9:30 a.m. Instructed pt in the procedure for
	using a walker. Pt was able to demonstrate
	proper use of a walker. ________________
	M. Cooper, CMA (AAMA)

The Gynecologic Examination and Prenatal Care

 Check out the Evolve site at http://evolve.elsevier.com/Bonewit/today to access additional interactive activities and exercises to help you study and prepare for success.

LEARNING OBJECTIVES

Gynecologic Examination

1. State the purpose of the gynecologic examination.
2. List and define the terms associated with the female reproductive system.

Breast Examination

3. Explain what is assessed during a clinical breast examination.
4. Identify the breast cancer screening guidelines recommended by the American Cancer Society.

Pelvic Examination

5. Explain the purpose of a pelvic examination.
6. List and describe the four parts of the pelvic examination.
7. State the purpose of cervical cancer screening.
8. Identify the cervical cancer screening guidelines recommended by the American College of Obstetricians and Gynecologists.
9. Explain the purpose of the Pap test and the HPV test.
10. List and describe the patient preparation recommended for cervical cancer screening.
11. List and describe each category on a cytology request for a Pap test.
12. List and describe the procedures that may be performed as a result of an abnormal Pap test result.

Gynecologic Infections

13. Identify the symptoms, diagnosis, and treatment of each of the following gynecologic infections:
    - Bacterial vaginosis
    - Vulvovaginal candidiasis
    - Trichomoniasis
    - Chlamydia
    - Gonorrhea
    - Genital herpes
    - Human papillomavirus infection

Prenatal Care

Prenatal Visits

14. Explain the purpose of each part of the prenatal record.
15. List and explain each part of the initial prenatal examination.
16. List and explain the purpose of each prenatal laboratory test.
17. Explain the purpose of return prenatal visits.

PROCEDURES

Coach a patient in breast self-awareness.

Prepare a patient for a gynecologic examination.
Assist the provider with a gynecologic examination.
Complete a cytology requisition form.

Assist in the collection of a specimen for the detection of a vaginal infection or sexually transmitted infection.
Instruct a patient in the procedure for a patient-collected vaginal specimen.

Calculate the expected date of delivery (EDD).
Complete a prenatal health history.
Assist the provider with an initial prenatal examination.

LEARNING OBJECTIVES

18. Explain the purpose of each of the following:
    - Carrier screening
    - First trimester prenatal screening test
    - Noninvasive prenatal test
    - Multiple marker test
    - Obstetric ultrasound scan
    - Amniocentesis
    - Fetal heart rate monitoring

PROCEDURES

Assist the provider with a return prenatal examination.

CHAPTER OUTLINE

INTRODUCTION TO THE GYNECOLOGIC EXAMINATION AND PRENATAL CARE

GYNECOLOGIC EXAMINATION

Terms Related to Gynecology

Breast Examination

Breast Cancer Screening

Pelvic Examination

Inspection of External Genitalia, Vagina, and Cervix

Cervical Cancer Screening

Bimanual Pelvic Examination

Rectal-Vaginal Examination

GYNECOLOGIC INFECTIONS

Vaginal Infections

Bacterial Vaginosis

Vulvovaginal Candidiasis

Trichomoniasis

Sexually Transmitted Infections

Chlamydia

Gonorrhea

Genital Herpes

Human Papillomavirus Infection

PRENATAL CARE

Obstetric Terminology

Prenatal Visits

First Prenatal Visit

Prenatal Record

Initial Prenatal Examination

Return Prenatal Visits

Special Tests and Procedures

Medical Assisting Responsibilities

KEY TERMS

Gynecology

abortion
amenorrhea (AY-men-ah-REE-ah)
cervix (SER-viks)
colposcopy (kol-POS-koe-pee)
cytology (sy-TOL-oh-jee)
dysmenorrhea (DIS-men-ah-REE-ah)
dyspareunia (DIS-pah-ROO-nee-ah)
dysplasia (dis-PLAY-shah)
ectocervix (EK-toe-SER-viks)
endocervix (EN-doe-SER-viks)
external os (eks-TER-nal AHS)
gynecology (gie-nuh-KOL-oh-jee)
menopause (MEN-oh-paws)
menorrhagia (men-uh-RAY-jee-ah)
metrorrhagia (met-ro-RAY-jee-ah)
perimenopause (PEAR-ee-MEN-oh-paws)
perineum (pear-ih-NEE-um)
risk factor
vulva (VUL-va)

Obstetrics

Braxton Hicks contractions (BRAK-stun HIKS con-TRAK-shuns)
dilation (of the cervix) (die-LAY-shun)
effacement (eh-FAYS-ment)
embryo (EM-bree-oh)
engagement
expected date of delivery (EDD)
fetal heart rate
fetal heart tones
fetus (FEE-tus)
fundus (FUN-dus)
gestation (jess-TAY-shun)
gestational age (jess-TAY-shun-al)
infant
multigravida (MUL-tee-GRAV-ih-duh)
multipara (mul-TIH-pear-uh)
nullipara (nul-IH-pear-uh)
obstetrics (ob-STEH-triks)
position
postpartum (poest-PAR-tum)
preeclampsia (PREE-ih-KLAMP-see-ah)
prenatal (pree-NAY-tul)
presentation
primigravida (PRIH-mih-GRAV-ih-duh)
primipara (prih-MIH-pear-uh)
puerperium (PYOO-ur-PEER-ee-um)
quickening
toxemia (tok-SEE-mee-uh)
trimester (try-MES-ter)

INTRODUCTION TO THE GYNECOLOGIC EXAMINATION AND PRENATAL CARE

The medical assistant should have knowledge of gynecology and obstetrics to assist in examinations and treatments in these specialties. Gynecologic examinations are frequently and routinely performed in the medical office. Prenatal care consists of a series of scheduled medical office visits for the promotion of the health of the mother and fetus during the pregnancy. Obtaining the patient's cooperation makes the gynecologic or prenatal examination proceed more smoothly and, as a result, makes the patient feel more comfortable. The medical assistant can help by explaining the purpose of the procedure to the patient. If the patient understands the beneficial results to be derived from the examination, she is more likely to participate as required. For means of convenience, this chapter is divided into two sections: the Gynecologic Examination and Prenatal Care.

GYNECOLOGIC EXAMINATION

Gynecology is the branch of medicine that deals with health maintenance and diseases of the female reproductive system. The gynecologic examination is frequently and routinely performed in the medical office.

The purpose of the gynecologic examination is to assess the health of the female reproductive organs to detect early signs of disease, leading to early diagnosis and treatment. Assisting with a gynecologic examination is usually a routine procedure for the medical assistant; however, the patient may not consider it a routine examination. To reduce apprehension or embarrassment, the medical assistant should fully explain the procedure to the patient and offer to answer any questions.

TERMS RELATED TO GYNECOLOGY

The medical assistant should have a thorough knowledge of the female reproductive system (refer to Fig. 23.1 and Chapter 16), as well as the following terms associated with the female reproductive system:

Amenorrhea Absence or cessation of the menstrual period. Amenorrhea occurs normally before puberty, during pregnancy, and after menopause.

Cervix The lower narrow end of the uterus that opens into the vagina.

Colposcopy Examination of the cervix using a colposcope (a lighted instrument with a magnifying lens).

Dysmenorrhea Pain that is associated with the menstrual period.

Dyspareunia Pain in the vagina or pelvis experienced by a woman during sexual intercourse.

Dysplasia The growth of abnormal cells. Dysplasia is a precancerous condition that may or may not develop into cancer.

Menopause The permanent cessation of menstruation, which usually occurs between the ages of 45 and 55 with an average age of 51.

Menorrhagia Excessive bleeding during a menstrual period, in the number of days, the amount of blood, or both. Also called *dysfunctional uterine bleeding* (DUB).

Metrorrhagia Bleeding between menstrual periods.

Perimenopause Before the onset of menopause, the phase during which a woman with regular periods changes to irregular cycles and increased periods of amenorrhea.

Perineum The external region between the vaginal orifice and the anus in a female and between the scrotum and the anus in a male.

Risk factor Anything that increases an individual's chance of developing a disease. Some risk factors (e.g., smoking) can be avoided, but others cannot (e.g., age and family history).

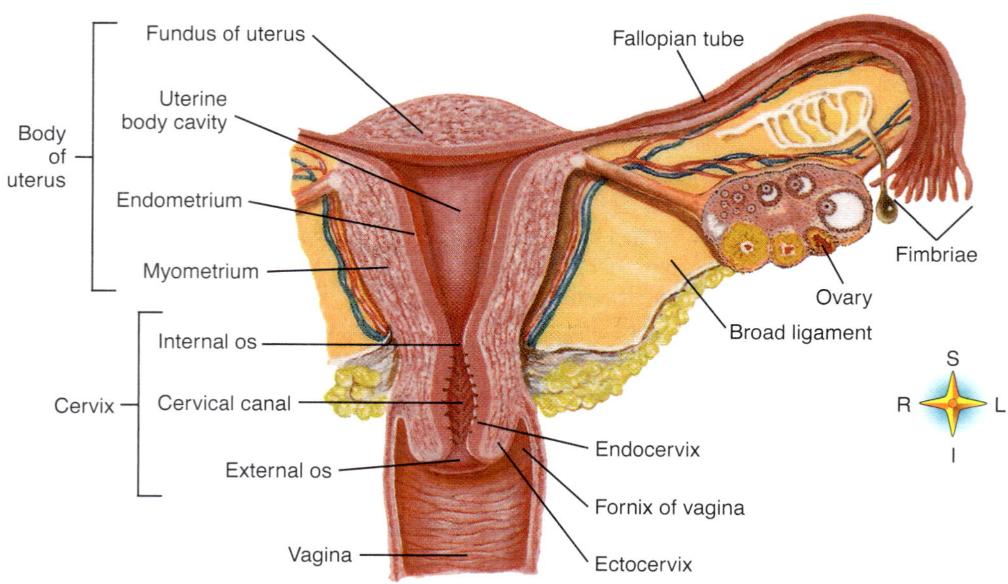

Fig. 23.1 The female reproductive system. (Modified from Thibodeau GA, Patton KT: *Anatomy and physiology*, ed 5, St. Louis, 2003, Mosby.)

BREAST EXAMINATION

The provider may begin the gynecologic examination with a clinical breast examination. The American College of Obstetricians and Gynecologists (ACOG) guidelines recommend a clinical breast examination every 1 to 3 years for women between the ages of 25 and 39. The ACOG further recommends a clinical breast examination every year for women 40 years of age and older. The medical assistant is responsible for assisting the patient into the supine position for the clinical breast examination. The provider inspects the breasts and nipples for swelling, dimpling, puckering, redness of the skin, and change in skin texture. The nipples are checked for abnormalities such as bleeding and discharge. The breasts and axillary lymph nodes are palpated for lumps, hard knots, and thickening.

In the past, a monthly breast self-examination (BSE) was recommended for women at average risk for breast cancer. A BSE is a detailed method of examining the breasts once a month following a specific pattern. Studies show that regular BSE does not help reduce deaths from breast cancer. Because of this, most major medical organizations now recommend *breast self-awareness* rather than a monthly BSE. Breast self-awareness means that a woman become familiar with how her breasts normally look and feel. If a lump or other change is discovered, the woman should schedule an appointment with her provider as soon as possible. Breast cancer is often found by a woman herself. (Refer to the Patient Coaching box: *Breast Self-Awareness*).

Breast Cancer Screening

Screening mammography is a radiographic examination of the breasts for the early detection of breast disease, particularly breast cancer. (Refer to Chapter 28 for a detailed discussion of mammography.) Breast cancer that is found early is more likely to be smaller and less likely to have spread outside the breast making it easier to treat successfully. Major medical organizations (e.g., ACS, ACOG) publish breast cancer screening recommendations for women at average risk for breast cancer. A woman at *average risk* does not have a personal history of breast cancer, a strong family history of breast cancer, a genetic mutation known to increase risk of breast cancer (e.g., *BRCA* gene mutation), and has not had chest radiation therapy before the age of 30. The breast cancer screening recommendations vary between medical organizations. The recommendations of the American Cancer Society (ACS) are outlined in Box 23.1. The decision of when to begin screening is one that a woman should make with her health care provider.

BOX 23.1 ACS Breast Cancer Screening Recommendations for Women at Average Breast Cancer Risk

- Women between 40 and 44 should have the option to start annual breast cancer screening with mammograms if they wish to do so.
- Women 45 to 54 should get mammograms every year.
- Women 55 and older should switch to a mammogram every other year, or they can choose to continue yearly mammograms.
- Screening should continue as long as a woman is in good health and is expected to live 10 more years or longer.
- All women should be familiar with how their breasts normally look and feel and report any changes to a health care provider right away.

ACS, American Cancer Society.

HIGHLIGHT on Breast Cancer

Breast cancer is one of the most common types of cancer among American women except for skin cancers. The American Cancer Society estimates that one of every eight women in the United States develops breast cancer at some point in her lifetime. Every year, about 300,000 new cases of breast cancer are diagnosed in women and about 2400 cases are diagnosed in men. Approximately 44,000 women and 500 men die each year from the disease.

Survival Rate

The 5-year survival rate for breast cancer that has spread to a distant site in the body (metastasized) is only 30%. The 5-year survival rate for small, localized tumors is 94%. If the cancer has only spread to lymph nodes in the region of the breast, the 5-year survival rate is 86%. These encouraging statistics are the result of advances in the early detection of breast cancer and better treatment, including improved surgical procedures, radiation therapy, chemotherapy, hormonal therapy, and biologic therapy.

Risk Factors

Breast cancer results from the abnormal growth of cells in breast tissue. It occurs more often in the left breast than in the right, and more often in the upper outer quadrant of the breast. The cause of abnormal growths in the breasts is unknown; therefore, every woman should consider herself at risk for breast cancer. Certain factors seem to place a woman at higher than normal risk for breast cancer, however, including the following:

- **Sex.** Women are much more likely than men to develop breast cancer.
- **Age.** The risk of breast cancer increases as women get older. Most women diagnosed with breast cancer are older than age 50.
- **Personal history.** Women with cancer in one breast have a greater chance of developing a new cancer in the other breast or in another part of the same breast.
- **Family history.** A woman's risk of developing breast cancer increases if her mother, sister, or daughter had breast cancer, especially at a young age.
- **Dense breast tissue.** Women with dense breast tissue (meaning they have more glandular tissue than fat tissue as seen on a mammogram) have a higher risk of developing breast cancer.
- **Breast biopsy.** Women who have had a breast biopsy that indicated certain types of benign breast disease (characterized by atypical hyperplasia) have an increased risk of developing breast cancer.
- **Breast cancer genes.** A woman who has inherited mutations in breast cancer genes (mutations of the *BRCA1* and

Continued

HIGHLIGHT on Breast Cancer—cont'd

BRCA2 genes) from either parent is more likely to develop breast cancer.

- **Reproductive history.** Women who began menstruating at an early age (younger than age 12) or who went through menopause at a late age (after age 55) have a slightly increased risk of breast cancer.
- **Childbearing.** Women who have never had a child or women who had their first child late (after age 30) have a slightly increased risk of developing breast cancer.
- **Hormone replacement therapy (HRT).** Studies indicate that the long-term use of estrogen and progesterone combination hormone replacement therapy for relief of menopausal symptoms increases the risk of breast cancer.
- **Radiation treatment.** Women who have had radiation of the chest before age 30 as treatment for another type of cancer (e.g., Hodgkin's disease) have a significantly increased risk of developing breast cancer.
- **Race.** Women of European ancestry are diagnosed more frequently than women of Hispanic, Asian, or African American origin.
- **Lifestyle factors.** Studies suggest that the use of alcohol (more than two drinks per day) increases the risk of breast cancer. Obesity, especially for women after menopause, also may increase the risk of breast cancer.

Warning Signs

The warning signs of possible breast cancer include a lump, hard knot, or thickening in the breast or armpit; a change in breast color or texture; dimpling or puckering; nipple discharge; changes in the size or shape of the breast; and an enlargement of the lymph nodes.

Diagnosis

A biopsy is the only conclusive method of determining whether a breast lump or suspicious area seen on a mammogram is benign or malignant. A biopsy involves the surgical removal and analysis of all or part of the lump. Biopsy methods include fine needle aspiration biopsy (collection of a sample of fluid from the lump), core needle biopsy (removal of a core of tissue from the lump), and surgical excisional biopsy (removal of all or part of the lump). The provider may recommend one or more of these procedures to evaluate a lump or other change in the breast.

Approximately 80% of breast lumps are benign. A lump or suspicious area is often the result of a benign breast condition, such as normal hormonal changes, fibrocystic breast disease, or a fibroadenoma. ■

Putting It All Into Practice

My name is Yin-Ling, and I am a Registered Medical Assistant. I work with 10 physicians in a large clinic. My primary job responsibilities include taking patient histories, measuring vital signs, and assisting physicians with patient examinations and procedures.

One experience that has probably affected me more than any other occurred while I was working in obstetrics and gynecology. A full-term prenatal patient came in for a routine weekly appointment late one afternoon. By this stage of the pregnancy, you have seen the patients often enough to develop a more personal relationship. I was taking her vital signs and asking the routine questions when she said, "I haven't felt the baby move for 2 days." This immediately sent up a red flag, but I was careful to hide my concern until I was out of her room. The physician was unable to pick up any fetal heart tones, so she immediately did an ultrasound. It showed that the fetus had died. The patient was alone and extremely upset. I stayed with her until her family arrived.

Although little medical treatment was given during this time, I do believe that my medical assisting training and experience made a difference in my knowing what to do and say to help comfort the patient during this difficult time. ■

PATIENT COACHING Breast Self-Awareness

Answer questions patients have about breast self-awareness.

What is breast self-awareness?

The purpose of breast self-awareness is to notice when there are changes in how your breasts look or feel. The best way to do this is to first become as familiar as possible with how your breasts normally look and feel. By examining your breasts, you will learn what is normal for you, and it will be easier to notice changes.

What is considered normal?

Breast tissue normally feels a little lumpy and uneven. The left and right breasts may not be the same size; most women's breasts are slightly different in size. Many women have a normal thickening or ridge of firm tissue under the lower curve of the breast where it attaches to the chest wall. Throughout your life, changes can also occur in the size, shape, and feel of your breasts because of aging, weight changes, the menstrual cycle, pregnancy, breastfeeding, and use of birth control pills or other hormones.

What symptoms should be reported to the provider?

Early breast cancer does not usually cause pain. When breast cancer first develops, there may be no symptoms at all. As the cancer grows, it can cause changes that should be reported to the provider. Contact your provider immediately if any of the following breast cancer warning symptoms occur:

- Any new lump or hard knot in the breast or underarm area
- Thickening or swelling of part of the breast
- Irritation or dimpling of the skin of the breast or nipple
- Redness or flaky skin in the nipple area or the breast
- Pulling in of the nipple or pain in the nipple area
- A discharge or bleeding from the nipple
- Any change in the size or shape of the breast
- Pain in any area of the breast

What Would You Do? What Would You *Not* Do?

Case Study 1

Carol Wooster, 47 years old, has come to the office for a gynecologic examination. She has not had a gynecologic examination in 10 years and has never had a screening mammogram. Mrs. Wooster is concerned because she found some unusual changes in her breasts. Her right breast is slightly larger than her left breast, her left nipple is pulled in, and she found some freckles on her right breast. Mrs. Wooster explains that she has not had a gynecologic examination in such a long time because her periods have been normal and regular. Mrs. Wooster is afraid that the physician will be annoyed with her for not having had the examination sooner. ■

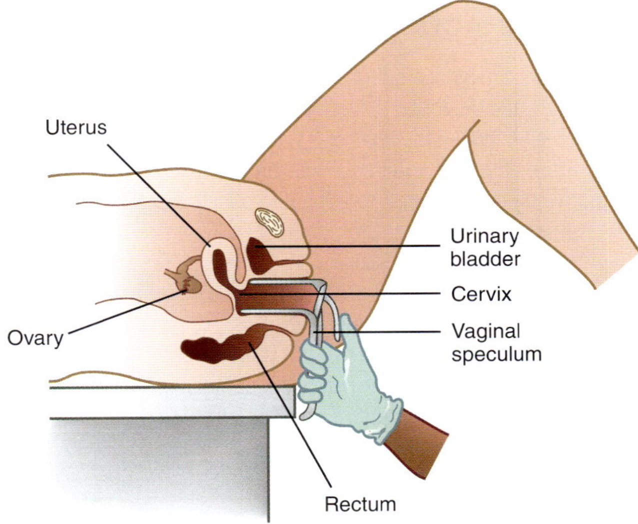

Fig. 23.2 Insertion of the vaginal speculum for visualization of the vagina and cervix.

PELVIC EXAMINATION

The purpose of the pelvic examination is to assess the size, shape, and location of the reproductive organs and to detect the presence of disease. The pelvic examination consists of the following components:

- Inspection of the external genitalia, vagina, and cervix
- Collection of a specimen for cervical cancer screening
- Bimanual pelvic examination
- Rectal–vaginal examination

For the pelvic examination, the patient is positioned in the lithotomy position. The patient lies on the table on her back, with her feet in the stirrups and her buttocks at the bottom edge of the table. The stirrups should be level with the examining table and pulled out approximately 1 foot from the edge of the table. The patient's knees should be bent and relaxed, and her thighs should be rotated outward as far as is comfortable. This position helps relax the vulva and perineum and facilitates insertion of the vaginal speculum. The patient should be properly draped to reduce exposure and to provide warmth. The lithotomy position is difficult to maintain, and the patient should not be placed in this position until the provider is ready to begin the examination.

The medical assistant can help the patient relax during the examination by telling her to breathe deeply, slowly, and evenly through the mouth. If the patient is relaxed, it is easier for the provider to insert the vaginal speculum and to perform the bimanual pelvic examination; it also is more comfortable for the patient. Procedure 23.1 outlines the medical assistant's role in assisting the provider with a gynecologic examination.

Inspection of External Genitalia, Vagina, and Cervix

The provider begins the pelvic examination with inspection of the external genitalia. The vulva is inspected for swelling, ulceration, and redness The **vulva** is the region of the external female genital organs.

Next, the provider inserts a *vaginal speculum* into the vagina. The function of a vaginal speculum is to hold the walls of the vagina apart to allow visual inspection of the vagina and cervix (Fig.23.2). Vaginal specula are available in two forms – plastic and metal. *Plastic specula* are used most often for the pelvic examination; they are disposable and are designed to be used only once and then discarded. A plastic speculum permits a light source to be directly attached to it to facilitate visualization of the vagina and cervix. *Metal specula* are reusable and must be sanitized and sterilized after each use.

Vaginal specula come in three sizes – small, medium, and large. The provider determines the size required based on the physical and sexual maturity of the patient.

The provider inspects the vagina and cervix for color, lacerations, ulcerations, redness, nodules, and discharge. If an abnormal discharge is present, the provider obtains a specimen for laboratory evaluation. Examples of pathologic conditions that may produce a discharge include vaginal infections such as *bacterial vaginosis (BV)*, *vulvovaginal candidiasis (VVC)*, *trichomoniasis*, *chlamydia*, and *gonorrhea*, which are discussed in detail later.

Cervical Cancer Screening

Cervical cancer screening is used for the early detection of cancer of the cervix. Almost all cervical cancers are caused by the human papillomavirus (HPV). HPV is a common virus that can be transmitted from one individual to another during sexual intercourse. There are many types of HPV, but most of these do not pose a health risk. Certain types of HPV are called *high-risk* because they can cause abnormal changes to the cervical cells (known as **dysplasia**) that can lead to cervical cancer over time. Although infection with a high-risk HPV is the most important risk factor for the development of cervical cancer, there are other factors that place a woman at higher risk for cervical cancer. These include:

- Cigarette smoking
- Weakened immune system due to human immunodeficiency virus (HIV) infection, organ transplantation, chemotherapy, or long-term steroid use
- Having given birth to three or more children

BOX 23.2 ACOG Cervical Cancer Screening Recommendations

- Cervical cancer screening should start at age 21. Women under age 21 should not be screened.
- Women between the ages of 21 and 29 should have a Pap test performed every 3 years. HPV testing alone can be considered for women who are 25 to 29, but Pap tests are preferred.
- Women between the ages of 30 and 65 have the following three options for screening:
  - Have a Pap test plus an HPV test (known as *co-testing*) performed every 5 years.
  - Have a Pap test alone every 3 years.
  - Have a primary high-risk HPV (primary hrHPV) test every 5 years. (A *primary hrHPV test* is an HPV test that is done by itself for screening. The FDA has approved certain tests to be primary hrHPV tests.)
- Women who are at high risk for cervical cancer or who have had abnormal Pap test results should be screened more often.
- Women over the age of 65 do not need screening if they have no history of cervical changes and either three negative Pap test results in a row, two negative HPV tests in a row, or two negative co-test results in a row within the past 10 years. The most recent test should have been performed within the past 3 or 5 years, depending on the type of test.
- A woman who has had her uterus and cervix removed (total hysterectomy) for reasons not related to cervical cancer and who has no history of cervical cancer or serious pre-cancer should not be screened.
- Women who have been vaccinated against HPV should still follow these guidelines for their age group.

ACOG, American College of Obstetricians and Gynecologists.

- Use of oral contraceptives for more than 5 years
- Diethylstilbestrol (DES) exposure before birth

Nearly all cancers of the cervix can be cured if detected early enough. The American College of Obstetricians and Gynecologists (ACOG) publishes recommendations for cervical cancer screening which are outlined in Box 23.2. Cervical cancer screening includes two types of tests, the Pap test and the HPV test, which are described in more detail as follows.

Pap Test

The Pap test is a simple and painless procedure named after its developer, Dr. George Papanicolaou (1883–1962). To perform the procedure, a sampling of cells is collected from the cervix and sent to an outside laboratory. The laboratory performs a **cytology** on the cells, which involves the examination of the cervical cells under the microscope for the presence of abnormal cells.

The primary purpose of the Pap test is to detect abnormal cervical cells (dysplasia) that may develop into cervical cancer if not treated. It usually takes years or even decades for abnormal cervical cells to develop into cancer. The Pap test can also determine the presence of noncancerous conditions such as infection and inflammation. The Pap test detects the presence of cancer cells, however in regularly screened individuals, most abnormal cells are discovered before they become cancerous. In some cases, the Pap test can detect cancer of the endometrium; however, it is less reliable in doing so.

Human Papillomavirus Test

The HPV test is a DNA test that detects the genetic material of high-risk types of HPV that have infected the cervical cells. Approximately 70% of all cervical cancers are caused by HPV types 16 and 18. The HPV test can be performed on the same liquid-based cytology specimen that is collected for a Pap test. Essentially, the Pap test looks for the presence of abnormal cells of the cervix while the HPV test looks for high-risk HPVs that may cause the cervical cells to become abnormal. Performing an HPV test is not necessary under the age of 30 (unless it is needed following an abnormal Pap test result). This is because cervical HPV infections in younger women usually go away on their own without causing problems.

Patient Instructions

The medical assistant should provide the patient with patient preparation instructions for Pap testing which helps to ensure accurate test results. No special preparation is needed before having an HPV test.

It is recommended that the Pap specimen not be collected during the patient's menstrual period. The patient should be instructed to schedule cervical cancer screening approximately 10 to 20 days after the first day of her last menstrual period. The patient should be told not to douche or insert tampons, vaginal medications, lubricants, or contraceptive spermicides into the vagina for 2 days before having cervical cancer screening. Douching and tampon insertion reduce the number of cervical cells available for analysis, and vaginal medications, lubricants, and spermicides change the pH of the vagina, making the specimen nonrepresentative or invalid. The patient also should be told to abstain from sexual intercourse for 2 days before undergoing a Pap test. Recent sexual intercourse can produce inflammatory changes that can interfere with visualization of abnormal cells that may be present.

Pap Specimen Collection Techniques

With a vaginal speculum in place, the provider collects a sampling of epithelial cells from the cervix for evaluation by the laboratory. A scraping of cells must be collected from both the ectocervix and the endocervix (refer to Fig. 23.1).

The **ectocervix** is the outermost layer of the cervix that projects into the vagina and consists of a thin, flat layer of cells, approximately 10 layers thick, known as *stratified squamous epithelial cells*. The **endocervix** is the inner part of the cervix that forms a narrow canal that connects the vagina to the uterus; it is lined with a mucous membrane made up of *simple columnar epithelial cells* that produce mucus. A scraping of epithelial cells may also be collected from the vagina; however, this is not usually done unless the provider has observed a lesion on the vaginal wall, or the maturation index is to be determined. The collection devices and techniques used by the provider to obtain the epithelial cells are described next.

Vaginal Specimen

If a vaginal specimen is needed, it is collected first, before the ectocervical and endocervical specimens are obtained. The rounded end of a plastic cytospatula is used to collect the specimen. If a routine vaginal specimen is being obtained, it is collected from the vaginal pool in the posterior fornix of the vagina, which is located just below the cervix (Fig. 23.3A). If the provider is collecting a specimen from a lesion on the vaginal wall, a scraping of cells is taken from the area of the lesion. To obtain a specimen for determination of the maturation index (discussed later), the provider obtains the vaginal specimen from the upper one-third of the lateral vaginal wall.

Ectocervical Specimen

The provider collects the ectocervical specimen by placing the S-shaped end of a plastic cytospatula just inside the cervical canal at the external os. The **external os** is the opening of the cervical canal of the uterus into the vagina. The provider next rotates the blade of the cytospatula 360 degrees over the surface of the ectocervix at the squamocolumnar junction, where cervical cancer is most often found (Fig. 23.3B).

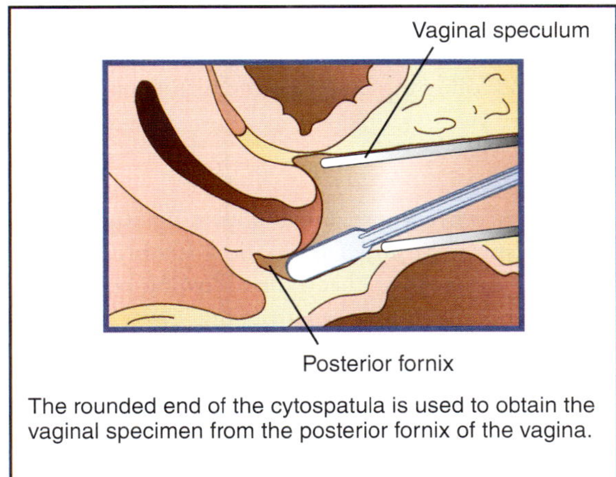

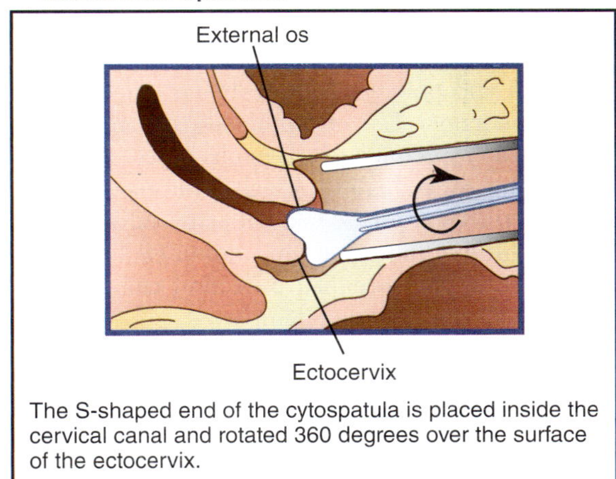

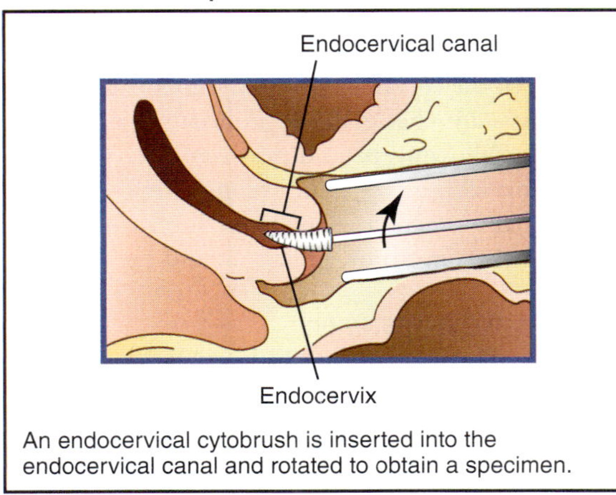

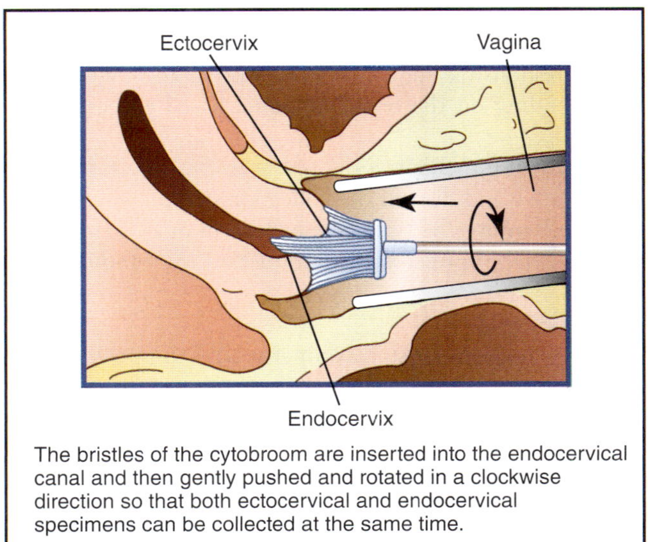

Fig. 23.3 Obtaining the Pap specimen. (A) Vaginal specimen. (B) Ectocervical specimen. (C) Endocervical specimen. (D) Cervical and endocervical combined specimen

Endocervical Specimen

The provider collects the endocervical specimen by inserting a cytobrush into the endocervical canal and rotating the cytobrush (Fig. 23.3C). The cytobrush is made up of soft bristles designed to be inserted into the canal without causing damage to it.

Ectocervical and Endocervical Combined Specimen

A scraping of cells from the ectocervix and endocervix can be collected at the same time using a flexible plastic collection device known as a *cytobroom*. The provider inserts the central bristles of the cytobroom into the endocervical canal deep enough to allow the shorter bristles to contact the outside of the cervix fully. The cytobroom is gently pushed and rotated in a clockwise direction to collect an ectocervical and endocervical combined specimen (Fig. 23.3D).

Preparation of the Pap Specimen

The most commonly used method to prepare a Pap specimen for evaluation is the liquid-based method; brand names of liquid-based systems include *ThinPrep* and *SurePath*. Following collection, the specimen is placed in a plastic collection vial containing a liquid preservative. The preservative maintains the specimen and prevents it from drying out during transport to the laboratory. Use of the liquid-based method provides a high-quality specimen which results in fewer slides that are unsatisfactory for evaluation. A high-quality specimen also reduces the occurrence of false-negative test results.

The specimen for a liquid-based preparation is obtained using one or more of the specimen collection techniques previously described; the technique employed is based on provider preference. A plastic cytospatula (S-shaped end) may be used to collect the ectocervical specimen and a cytobrush may be used to collect an endoectocervical specimen. Alternatively, a cytobroom can be used to collect an ectocervical and endocervical combined specimen. If a vaginal specimen is needed, it is collected first using the rounded end of a cytospatula.

Once the specimen has been collected, the medical assistant is responsible for performing one of the following steps depending on the brand of liquid-based preparation being used:

ThinPrep: Rinse the collection device in the vial of liquid preservative and discard the collection device.

SurePath: Remove the tip of the collection device, deposit it in the vial of preservative, and discard the handle.

Cytology Request

A cytology request must accompany all Pap specimens. Fig. 23.4 is an example of a cytology request form. The medical assistant is responsible for completing the request, which includes the following categories.

General Information

General information includes the provider's name, address, and phone number and the patient's name, address, identification number, date of birth, and date of last menstrual period (LMP). Insurance information also is required in this section for third-party billing.

Date and Time of Collection

The date and time of collection indicate to the laboratory the number of days that have passed since the collection, providing the laboratory with information regarding the freshness of the specimen.

Test(s) Requested

The test(s) desired by the provider are indicated by selecting the appropriate box adjacent to the test(s).

Source of the Specimen

The purpose of this category is to identify the origin of the specimen because it is impossible for the laboratory to obtain this information by looking at the specimen. The medical assistant selects one or more of the following boxes on the form: ectocervical, endocervical, or vaginal.

Collection Technique

The collection device or devices used to obtain the specimen must be indicated. The medical assistant selects one or more of the following boxes on the form: spatula, brush, or broom.

Patient History

Information on the present and past health status of the patient is specified under the patient history category. The medical assistant must check the following boxes that apply to the patient: pregnant, lactating, oral contraceptives, postmenopausal, hormone replacement therapy, postmenopausal (PMP) bleeding, postpartum, intrauterine device (IUD), postcoital bleeding, DES (diethylstilbestrol) exposure, and previous abnormal Pap test. This information assists the laboratory in evaluating the specimen.

Previous Treatment

Any previous treatment for a precancerous or cancerous condition of the cervix is indicated under this category. The medical assistant checks the appropriate box on the form if any of the following procedures have been performed on the patient: colposcopy and biopsy, cryotherapy, LEEP (loop electrocautery excision procedure), laser treatment, conization, hysterectomy, radiation, and chemotherapy.

Evaluation of the Specimen

Following collection, the liquid-based cytology specimen is transported to an outside laboratory for further processing and evaluation. Before a Pap evaluation can be performed, the specimen must undergo a processing procedure. The specimen is placed in an automated slide preparation processor which performs several important functions. First, it separates the cells from debris present in the specimen, and then it disperses a representative cell sample onto a slide in a thin, uniform layer. The slide is next immersed in a fixative to maintain the normal appearance of the cells.

GYN CYTOLOGY REQUISITION

THOMAS WOODSIDE, MD
501 MAIN ST
ST. LOUIS, MO 63146
(314) 555–0093

PATIENT INFO

Patient's Name (Last)	(First)	(MI)	Date of Birth MO | DAY | YR	Collection Time : AM PM	Collection Date MO | DAY | YR	Patient's ID #

Patient's Address | Phone

City | State | ZIP

RESP. PARTY

Name of Responsible Party (if different from patient)

Address of Responsible Party | APT #

City | State | ZIP

INSURANCE

Patient's Relationship to Responsible Party ☐ 1. Self ☐ 2. Spouse ☐ 3. Child ☐ 4. Other

Insurance Company Name	Plan	Carrier Code
Subscriber/Member #	Location	Group #

Insurance Address | Physician's Provider #

City | State | ZIP

Employer's Name or Number | Insured SSN

Diagnosis/Signs/Symptoms in ICD-9 Format (Highest Specificity)

REQUIRED

ICD-9 codes are the internationally accepted method of describing the clinical picture of the patient. All diagnoses should be provided by the ordering physician or his or her authorized designee. The following is a partial list of common diagnoses in ICD-9 format. Most third party payers require an ICD-9 code to indicate the medical necessity of the test(s) and or profile(s) ordered. For a complete list of all ICD-9 codes, please refer to a current ICD-9 manual.

Code	Diagnosis	Code	Diagnosis	Code	Diagnosis
V76.2	Routine Cervical Pap Smear	616.0	Cervicitis	626.8	Abnormal Bleeding
V15.89	High Risk Cervical Screening	616.10	Vaginitis	627.1	Postmenopausal Bleeding
V22.2	Pregnancy	617.0	Endometriosis, Uterus	627.3	Atrophic Vaginitis
079.4	Human Papillomavirus	622.1	Dysplasia, Cervix	795.0	Abnormal Cervical Pap Smear
180.0	Malignant Neoplasm, Cervix	623.0	Dysplasia, Vagina		

COLLECTION METHOD

Liquid-Based Prep
192055 ☐ ThinPrep Pap Test
192039 ☐ ThinPrep Pap Test w/reflex to HPV Hybrid Capture when ASC-US or SIL
192047 ☐ ThinPrep Pap Test w/reflex to high-risk only HPV Hybrid Capture when ASC-US

Pap Smear
009100 ☐ 1 Slide **009191** ☐ 2 Slides

Pap Smear and Maturation Index
009209 ☐ 1 Slide **190074** ☐ 2 Slides

SOURCE OF SPECIMEN

☐ **Ectocervical**
☐ **Endocervical**
☐ **Vaginal**

Date LMP

____/____/____
Mo **Day** **Year**

COLLECTION TECHNIQUE

☐ **Spatula**
☐ **Brush**
☐ **Broom**
☐ **Other** ____________

PATIENT HISTORY

☐ **Pregnant**
☐ **Lactating**
☐ **Oral Contraceptives**
☐ **Postmenopausal**
☐ **Hormone Replacement Therapy**
☐ **PMP Bleeding**
☐ **Postpartum**
☐ **IUD**
☐ **Postcoital Bleeding**
☐ **DES Exposure**
☐ **Previous Abnormal Pap Test**
☐ **Other** ____________

PREVIOUS TREATMENT | **Date/Results**

☐ **None**
☐ **Colposcopy and Bx** ____________
☐ **Cryosurgery** ____________
☐ **LEEP** ____________
☐ **Laser Vaporization** ____________
☐ **Conization** ____________
☐ **Hysterectomy** ____________
☐ **Radiation** ____________
☐ **Chemotherapy** ____________

Fig. 23.4 Cytology request form.

Before the Pap slide can be evaluated, it must be stained by a laboratory technician. The purpose of staining is to allow better viewing of the epithelial cells of the cervix. The slide is studied under a microscope for evidence of abnormalities by a specially trained technician, known as a *cytotechnologist*. When an abnormality is detected, it is reviewed by a *cytopathologist* (a provider specializing in pathology), who makes a final evaluation.

A more recent development in the evaluation of Pap slides is the use of automated cytology computer-imaging devices. An abnormal slide may contain only a few abnormal cells among thousands of normal cells. Because of this, these abnormal cells may be missed during the evaluation by the cytotechnologist. A cytology computer-imaging device is able to examine every cell on the slide and select and display cells that appear "most abnormal." The cytotechnologist can evaluate these cells further under a microscope. In this way, the cytotechnologist can focus their expertise and decision-making on preselected areas of the slide.

Maturation Index

The maturation index must be performed on a sampling of cells taken from the upper third of the lateral vaginal wall. The *maturation index* refers to the percentage of parabasal, intermediate, and superficial cells present in the specimen. The maturation index provides an endocrine evaluation of the patient, which can assist the provider in evaluating the cause of infertility, menopausal or postmenopausal bleeding, or amenorrhea and can help assess the results of treatment with hormones. Numerous factors affect the results of the maturation index; it is important to indicate on the cytology request the presence of abnormal bleeding; hormone treatment; or treatment with digitalis, corticosteroids, or thyroid medication.

Cytology Report

The Bethesda System (TBS) is the standard for reporting the results of a Pap test on the cytology report (Fig. 23.5). The National Cancer Institute in Bethesda, Maryland, developed this system. It provides a detailed cytologic description of the results. TBS is an effective means of communicating the results of the Pap test to the provider.

GYN CYTOLOGY REPORT

RIVERVIEW MEDICAL LABORATORY
DEPARTMENT OF PATHOLOGY
2501 GRANT AVENUE
ST. LOUIS, MO 63146
(314) 555–3443

PATIENT: **Heather Jones**
PATIENT NO: **45876**
DOB: **10/20/65**
SUBMITTING: **T. Woodside, MD**

Date of Specimen: 7/01/XX
Date Received: 7/02/XX
Date Reported: 7/06/XX
Performed By: Richard McVay, Cytotechnologist **Checked By:** Melissa Wagner, Pathologist

SPECIMEN TYPE
☒ ThinPrep ☐ Conventional Pap Smear

SPECIMEN ADEQUACY
☒ **Satisfactory for Evaluation**
☐ **Unsatisfactory for Evaluation**

GENERAL CATEGORIZATION
☐ **Negative for Intraepithelial Lesion or Malignancy (*see Interpretation/Result*)**
☒ **Epithelial Cell Abnormality (*see Interpretation/Result*)**
☐ **Other (*see Interpretation/Result*)**

INTERPRETATION/RESULT

A. BENIGN CELLULAR CHANGES
☐ Infection:
- ☐ Trichomonas vaginalis
- ☐ Fungal organisms morphologically compatible w/ Candida species
- ☐ Cellular changes associated with herpes simplex virus
- ☐ Bacterial infection morphologically compatible with gardnerella
- ☐ Cytoplasmic inclusions suggestive of chlamydia

☐ Reactive changes
- ☐ Without inflammation
- ☐ With inflammation
- ☐ Atrophy with inflammation (atrophic vaginitis)
- ☐ Radiation effect
- ☐ Repair
- ☐ Hyperkeratosis
- ☐ Parakeratosis

B. EPITHELIAL CELL ABNORMALITIES
☒ Squamous Cell
- ☒ Atypical Squamous Cells of Undetermined Significance (ASC-US)
- ☐ Atypical Squamous Cells of Higher Risk (ASC-H)
- ☐ Low-Grade Squamous Intraepithelial Lesion (LSIL)
- ☐ High-Grade Squamous Intraepithelial Lesion (HSIL)
- ☐ Squamous Cell Carcinoma

☐ Glandular Cell
- ☐ Atypical Glandular Cells of Undetermined Significance (AGUS)
- ☐ Adenocarcinoma

Fig. 23.5 Cytology report form (The Bethesda System).

TBS separates the cytology report into the following categories:

1. **Specimen Adequacy.** This category refers to the quality of the specimen collected by the provider. The specimen is described using one of the following classifications:
   - **Satisfactory for Evaluation.** This indicates that the specimen was of sufficient sampling and quality for a comprehensive assessment of the cells.
   - **Unsatisfactory for Evaluation.** This indicates that the overall sampling or quality of the specimen was inadequate. A reason is given for the inability to evaluate the specimen, such as too few cells were collected, or the presence of blood or inflammation is obscuring the cells.
2. **General Categorization.** This category provides the medical office with a quick review of the report. The following classifications are used to categorize the specimen:

   Negative for Intraepithelial Lesion or Malignancy. This indicates that the epithelial cells were normal and that there were no precancerous or cancerous findings. This classification also is assigned to a specimen that exhibits certain benign (noncancerous) changes. Benign changes can be caused by vaginal infections, such as bacterial vaginosis, chlamydia, trichomoniasis, candidiasis, and herpes. Benign changes also can be caused by inflammation resulting from the normal cell repair process, radiation, and chemotherapy. Any benign findings of importance (e.g., vaginal infections) are described in detail in the Interpretation/Result section of the cytology report.

   Epithelial Cell Abnormality. This classification indicates abnormal cell changes. The abnormality is described in detail in the Interpretation/Result section of the report.

   Other. This classification is used to indicate that no abnormality was found in the cells, but the findings indicate some increased risk. The presence of normal-appearing endometrial cells in a postmenopausal woman may indicate an abnormality of the endometrium. These findings are described in detail in the Interpretation/Result section of the report.
3. **Interpretation/Result.** This part of the report provides the provider with a detailed description of findings. This includes any significant benign changes (e.g., vaginal infections) and any abnormal changes in the epithelial cells. Table 23.1 lists and describes the findings most frequently reported.
4. **Automated Review.** This category indicates whether the specimen was evaluated using an automated computer-imaging device. The name of the device and the results are specified in this section.
5. **Ancillary Testing.** This category is used if an additional test method is used to evaluate the specimen. If abnormal cells are detected on the Pap slide, a human papillomavirus (HPV) test may be performed. The name of the test method and the results would be reported under this category.

Abnormal Pap Test Results

Abnormal Pap test results can be caused by infection and inflammation, precancerous lesions, and cancerous lesions. Although an abnormal Pap result is found in every 1 in 10 tests, most abnormal results are not due to cancer but rather are caused by infection or inflammation.

The Pap test is a screening test, therefore an abnormal test result requires further evaluation before a final diagnosis can be made. The type of test or procedure performed depends on the age of the patient and the Pap test result category (see Table 23.1). For example, a 21-year old patient with a result of ASC-US (atypical squamous cells of undetermined significance) may require a repeat Pap test in 12 months. On the other hand, a 35-year old patient with

Table 23.1 Pap Test Results

Test Result	Interpretation
Normal: Negative for intraepithelial lesion or malignancy	Epithelial cells were normal, and there were no precancerous or cancerous findings.
ASC-US: Atypical squamous cells of undetermined significance	Cells are only slightly abnormal. Nature and cause of abnormality cannot be determined. These slightly altered cells usually return to normal on their own, resulting in negative results on subsequent Pap tests.
ASC-H: Atypical squamous cells of higher risk	Minor abnormal changes in cells with unknown causes, but at risk of progressing to high-grade lesion (HSIL). Further testing is required to determine whether this is a minor condition or one that may progress to HSIL.
LSIL: Low-grade squamous intraepithelial lesion	Abnormal cells that show definite minor changes but are unlikely to progress to cancer (general term for this is *mild dysplasia*). LSIL may be caused by HPV infection, but of a type that is not likely to lead to cervical cancer.
HSIL: High-grade squamous intraepithelial lesion	Abnormal cell changes that have a higher likelihood of progressing to cancer. Although not cancerous yet, abnormal cells may become cancerous if treatment is not obtained (general term for this is *moderate-to-severe dysplasia*). HSIL is often caused by HPV infection of a type associated with cervical cancer.
Carcinoma	Usually means patient has cervical cancer. Most women with cervical cancer also test positive for HPV infection.

HPV, Human papillomavirus.

a result of HSIL (high-grade squamous intraepithelial lesion) may require colposcopy and biopsy or a LEEP (loop electrosurgical excision procedure). Procedures that are commonly performed following an abnormal Pap test result are outlined in Table 23.2.

Bimanual Pelvic Examination

After obtaining the smear for the Pap test, the provider withdraws the speculum and performs a bimanual pelvic examination. The provider inserts the index and middle fingers of a lubricated gloved hand into the vagina. The fingers of the other hand are placed on the woman's lower abdomen. Between the two hands, the provider can palpate the size, shape, and position of the uterus and ovaries and can detect tenderness or lumps (Fig. 23.6).

Rectal–Vaginal Examination

The last part of the pelvic examination is a rectal–vaginal examination. The provider inserts one gloved finger into the vagina and another gloved finger into the rectum to obtain information about the tone and alignment of the pelvic organs and the adjacent region (ovaries, fallopian tubes, and ligaments of the uterus). The presence of hemorrhoids, fistulas, and fissures also can be noted. During this examination, the provider may want to obtain a fecal specimen from the rectum to test for occult blood in the stool (e.g., Hemoccult). This is typically performed on women beginning at 40 years of age. The medical assistant is responsible for assisting with the collection and testing of the specimen for occult blood. This procedure (fecal occult blood testing) is presented in detail in Chapter 28.

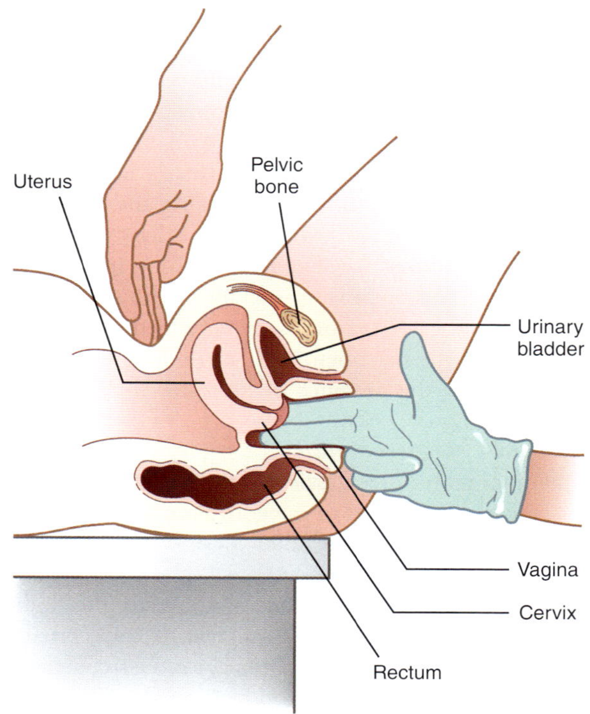

Fig. 23.6 The bimanual pelvic examination.

Table 23.2 Procedures Performed Following Abnormal Pap Test Results

Procedure	Description
Colposcopy (Refer to Ch. 25: Minor Office Surgery)	Colposcopy is performed to examine the vagina and cervix using a magnifying device (colposcope) to detect areas of abnormal tissue growth that may not be visible with the naked eye.
Cervical biopsy (Refer to Ch. 25: Minor Office Surgery)	A cervical biopsy is performed in combination with colposcopy to remove a cervical tissue specimen for examination by a pathologist to detect the presence of cervical dysplasia or cancer of the cervix.
LEEP (Loop electrosurgical excision procedure)	LEEP uses an electrical current which is passed through a thin wire loop which functions as a scalpel to remove abnormal cells from the cervix. The tissue is examined by a pathologist to detect the presence of cervical dysplasia or cancer of the cervix.
Cervical cryotherapy (Refer to Ch. 25: Minor Office Surgery)	Cryotherapy involves the application of extreme cold to destroy abnormal cervical cells that show changes that may lead to cancer. It is performed only after a colposcopy confirms the presence of cervical dysplasia.
Laser Treatment	Laser therapy involves the use of heat from a laser beam to destroy abnormal cervical cells.
Conization	Conization involves the removal of a cone-shaped section of the cervix containing abnormal cells using a scalpel, a laser, or the LEEP technique.

GYNECOLOGIC INFECTIONS

Gynecologic infections are commonly seen in the medical office and can be classified into the following categories: *vaginal infections* and *sexually transmitted infections (STIs).* Vaginal infections are caused by the overgrowth of an organism normally present in the vagina, while STIs are caused by the transmission of a pathogen through sexual contact with an infected partner. In most areas, vaginal infections are much more common than STIs.

The medical assistant is responsible for assembling the appropriate supplies for the collection of a suspected pathogen. The medical assistant must label the specimen with the patient's name and date of birth, the date, and the source of the specimen. A laboratory request form must be completed to accompany the specimen. The request form indicates the source of the specimen, the provider's clinical diagnosis, and the laboratory test requested. The provider's clinical assessment of the patient's signs and symptoms, along with the results of the laboratory evaluation of the specimen, are used to diagnose the presence of a gynecologic infection.

Medical assistants should protect themselves from infection with a pathogen while assisting with the collection of the specimen by practicing good techniques of medical asepsis. A thorough discussion of common vaginal infections and STIs is presented next.

VAGINAL INFECTIONS

The vagina provides a warm, moist environment, which tends to encourage the growth of various organisms that can result in a vaginal infection, or *vaginitis.* If an unusual vaginal discharge is present, suggesting a vaginal infection, a specimen is obtained to identify the invading organism. A specimen of the vaginal discharge is collected at the medical office and is evaluated there or placed in an appropriate specimen container that is picked up by a laboratory courier and transported to an outside medical laboratory for evaluation. The patient should be instructed not to douche or use a feminine hygiene product before coming to the medical office because the provider may not be able to observe the discharge or to obtain a specimen for analysis.

The most common vaginal infections include bacterial vaginosis, vulvovaginal candidiasis, and trichomoniasis, which are discussed in more detail as follows.

Bacterial Vaginosis

Description

Bacterial vaginosis (BV) is the most common cause of abnormal vaginal discharge in women of childbearing age (14 to 49). In the United States, as many as 30% of women of childbearing age are infected with BV. In the past, BV has been known by different names such as *Gardnerella vaginitis* and *nonspecific vaginitis.*

Many women with BV have no symptoms and are not aware of having the condition. When symptoms are present, they commonly include an abnormal amount of a thin, grayish-white vaginal discharge which has a foul-smelling or "fishy" odor. Any woman can develop BV, but some behaviors or activities have been found to increase the risk of developing this condition. They include vaginal douching, new or multiple sexual partners, IUD, recent antibiotic use, and cigarette smoking.

If left untreated, BV can lead to significant health complications. Having BV increases the risk of infection by a number of STIs such as chlamydia, gonorrhea, genital herpes and HIV. BV also increases the risk of pelvic inflammatory disease (PID), pregnancy complications, and post-surgical complications following gynecologic procedures such as a hysterectomy.

Diagnosis and Treatment

A nucleic acid hybridization test (NAT) known as a *DNA-probe test* is used to detect bacterial vaginosis. The brand name of this test is Affirm VP III (Becton Dickinson, San Jose, CA). The probe test uses DNA technology to detect the presence of bacterial vaginosis. The DNA-probe test can also simultaneously determine the presence of vulvovaginal candidiasis and trichomoniasis. The provider collects a vaginal specimen using sterile swab. After collection, the specimen is placed in a tube containing a transport medium to preserve the specimen until it reaches the laboratory.

Several antibiotics are effective in the treatment of bacterial vaginosis. These include metronidazole (Flagyl) taken either orally or as a vaginal gel (Metrogel). A vaginal clindamycin cream (Cleocin) is also effective in treating BV. Tinidazole (Tindamax) can be used to treat BV and tends to have fewer side effects than the other antibiotics. Once the natural balance of the vaginal flora has been disrupted, the body sometimes has difficulty in getting back to normal. Because of this, BV has a tendency to recur following treatment, requiring a second round of antibiotic therapy.

Vulvovaginal Candidiasis

Description

Candida albicans is a yeastlike fungus normally found in the intestinal tract and is a frequent contaminant of the vagina; however, it usually does not produce symptoms indicating a vaginal infection. Under a microscope *C. albicans* appears as yeast buds, spores, or hyphae (fungus) filaments (Fig. 23.7). Conditions such as pregnancy, diabetes mellitus, a weakened immune system, and prolonged antibiotic therapy may cause changes in the vagina that may precipitate vulvovaginal candidiasis (VVC), commonly referred to as a "yeast infection." The vaginal changes result in the overgrowth of *C. albicans* in the vagina. Symptoms of VVC include white patches on the mucous membrane of the vagina; a thick, odorless, cottage cheese–like discharge; vulval irritation; and dysuria. The discharge is extremely irritating and usually results in burning and intense itching of the vulva and vagina.

Diagnosis and Treatment

The recommended testing method for VVC is the DNA-probe test (Affirm VP III).

The provider collects a vaginal specimen using sterile swab. After collection, the specimen is placed in a tube

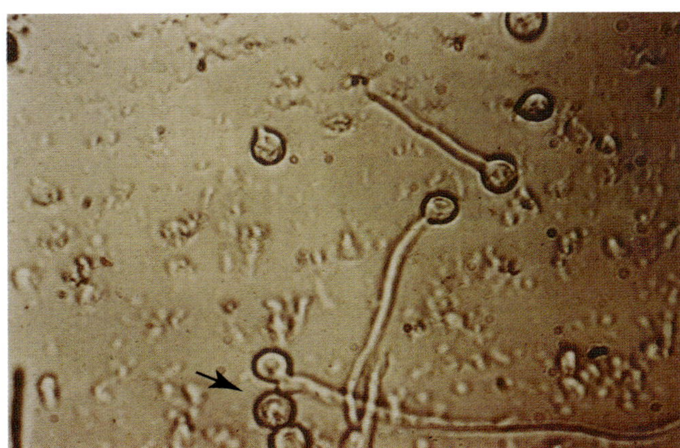

Fig. 23.7 *Candida albicans* (arrow) under a microscope. (Modified from Mahon C, Manuselis G: *Textbook of diagnostic microbiology*, ed 5, St. Louis, 2015, Saunders.)

containing a transport medium to preserve the specimen until it reaches the laboratory.

VVC is treated with the application of vaginal ointments or suppositories, such as miconazole (Monistat), clotrimazole (Gyne-Lotrimin), and nystatin (Mycostatin), or the oral administration of fluconazole (Diflucan). VVC has a tendency to recur; the patient should be instructed to contact the medical office if symptoms of the yeast infection reappear.

Trichomoniasis

Description

Trichomonas vaginalis, the causative agent of trichomoniasis (trich), is a one-celled pear-shaped protozoan with flagella, which allows for the motility of the organism (Fig. 23.8). Because trichomoniasis is spread through sexual intercourse, it is also classified as an STI. It is included in this section because the symptoms are similar to those of a vaginal infection. Women between the ages of 40 to 49 years are more likely than adolescents or young adults to be infected with trichomoniasis.

Women infected with trichomoniasis may not have any symptoms. When symptoms do occur they include a profuse, frothy vaginal discharge that is usually yellowish green and has an unpleasant odor; itching and irritation of the vulva and vagina; dyspareunia; and dysuria. The cervix may exhibit small red spots, a condition known as "strawberry cervix."

Diagnosis and Treatment

The recommended testing method for the diagnosis of trichomoniasis is the DNA-probe test (Affirm VP III). The provider collects a vaginal specimen using sterile swab. After collection, the specimen is placed in a tube containing a transport medium to preserve the specimen until it reaches the laboratory.

Trichomoniasis is treated with the oral administration of metronidazole (Flagyl) or tinidazole (Tindamax). The woman and her sexual partner must be treated at the same time to prevent reinfection because her partner may harbor the organism without displaying noticeable symptoms.

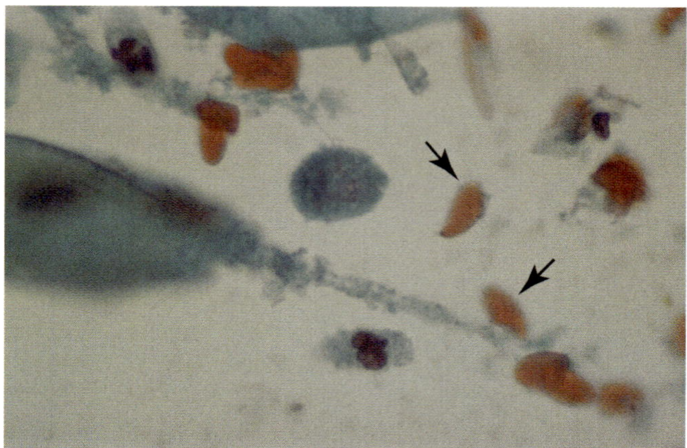

Fig. 23.8 *Trichomonas vaginalis* (arrows) under a microscope. (Modified from Mahon C, Manuselis G: *Textbook of diagnostic microbiology,* ed 3, St Louis, 2007, Saunders.)

SEXUALLY TRANSMITTED INFECTIONS

Sexually transmitted infections (STIs) are infections that are commonly spread through sexual contact with an infected individual and are among the most common infectious disease in the United States. (Refer to *Highlight on Sexually Transmitted Infections.*) Most STIs initially do not cause symptoms. This results in a greater risk of transmitting the infection to others. Because of this, the CDC has set forth screening recommendations for the detection of STIs in asymptomatic individuals. These recommendations are discussed in this section.

More than twenty STIs have been identified and are most often caused by bacteria and viruses. The most common STIs are chlamydia, gonorrhea, genital herpes, and human papillomavirus (HPV) which are discussed in this section. Other STIs include hepatitis B, syphilis, and human immunodeficiency virus (HIV), which are discussed in other chapters within this text. Of these, chlamydia, gonorrhea, and syphilis are curable with antibiotics, while genital herpes, HPV, hepatitis B, and HIV are treatable but not curable.

Chlamydia

Description

Chlamydia is caused by the bacterium *Chlamydia trachomatis.* It is a gram-negative intracellular bacterium that grows and multiplies in the cytoplasm of the host cell. Chlamydia is the most frequently reported and fastest spreading sexually transmitted disease in the United States, particularly among adolescent girls and young women. Because of this, the CDC recommends annual routine screening for chlamydia of all sexually active females 25 years of age or younger. The CDC also recommends annual screen for women older than 25 with risk factors such as new or multiple sex partners, or a sex partner who has an STI.

Most women with chlamydia have no symptoms and are not aware of having the condition. Because of this, many women do not seek medical care until serious complications have occurred. After infection, chlamydia first attacks the cervix, resulting in cervicitis. If symptoms do occur, they may include one or more of the following: dysuria, itching and irritation of the genital area, and a yellowish, odorless vaginal discharge. These symptoms usually appear 1 to 3 weeks after the patient has been infected.

If not treated, chlamydia can spread further into the female reproductive tract and cause *pelvic inflammatory disease* (PID). The symptoms of PID include lower abdominal pain, fever, nausea and vomiting, dyspareunia, vaginal discharge, and bleeding between periods. Complications of PID are serious and include chronic pelvic pain, scarring of the fallopian tubes, ectopic pregnancy, and infertility.

Symptoms of a chlamydial infection in men include mild dysuria and a thin, watery discharge from the penis. Men are more likely to have symptoms than women; however, the symptoms may appear only early in the day and be so mild that they are ignored. If the infection is not treated, it can cause *epididymitis,* a painful condition of the testicles that could result in infertility.

Diagnosis and Treatment

The recommended test method for chlamydia is a nucleic acid amplification (NAA) test. NAA testing became available within the last decade and is considered the most sensitive and promising test for the identification of chlamydia (and gonorrhea). NAA tests are able to detect the presence of the genetic material (DNA) of chlamydia bacteria.

The following types of specimens can be used with a NAA test:

- Endocervical specimen
- Vaginal specimen (provider-collected or patient-collected)
- Urethral specimen (male)

After collection, the specimen is placed in a tube containing a transport medium to preserve the specimen until it reaches the laboratory. See Box 23.3: *Chlamydia and*

BOX 23.3 Chlamydia and Gonorrhea Specimen Collection

NAA Test

The procedure for collecting an endocervical and urethral specimen for a NAA test is outlined below. Chlamydia and gonorrhea tests can be performed on the same specimen.

1. The medical assistant assembles supplies needed to collect the specimen, including a vaginal speculum, clean disposable gloves, and the specimen collection kit. The proper specimen collection kit should be selected based on whether the patient is a female or male. The medical assistant should check the expiration date on the collection kit to make sure it has not expired. The collection kit includes cotton-tipped swabs and a tube of transport medium.
2. The transport tube must be labeled with the following information: patient's name, date of birth, and identification number, date and time of collection, and provider's name and telephone number.

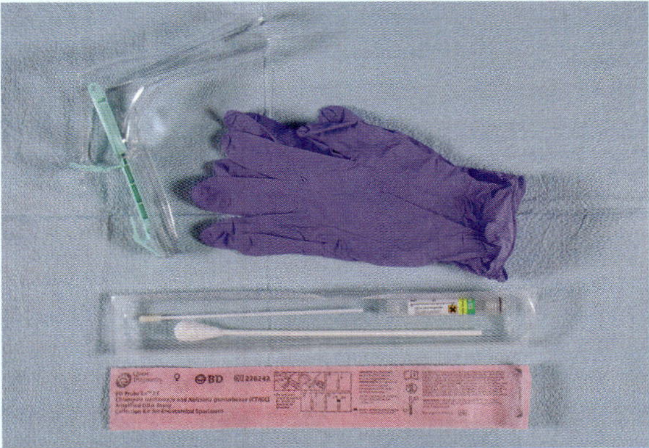

DNA probe setup (female patient).

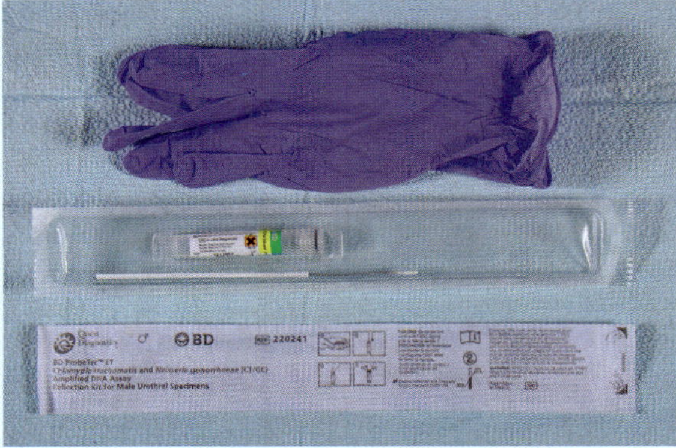

DNA probe setup (male patient).

3. The provider collects the specimen as follows:
   - **Female Patient:** The provider inserts a vaginal speculum into the vagina. Using a cotton-tipped swab, the provider first removes excess mucus or discharge from the cervix, and discards the swab. Next, the provider collects the specimen by inserting another cotton-tipped swab into the endocervical canal and rotating it for 15 to 30 seconds. This ensures a good sampling of the specimen.
   - **Male Patient:** The patient must not urinate for 1 hour before the collection to prevent any urethral discharge from being washed away. The provider inserts a small-tipped cotton swab 2 to 4 cm into the penis. The swab is gently rotated for 2 to 3 seconds to dislodge cells and to ensure contact with all urethral surfaces.
4. The provider carefully withdraws the swab.
5. The medical assistant should ensure that the transport medium is at the bottom of the tube. The medical assistant unscrews the cap and holds the tube for the provider.
6. The provider inserts the swab into the transport tube and breaks off the shaft of the swab at the score line and discards the top of the shaft.

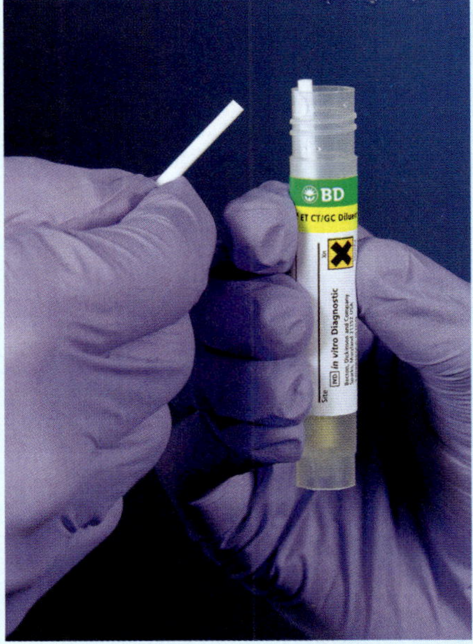

Breaking off shaft of swab.

7. The medical assistant places the cap on the tube and twists it until it clicks into place. The tube is placed in a biohazard specimen transport bag along with the laboratory requisition for pickup by the laboratory.

Gonorrhea Specimen Collection for instructions on how to assist with the collection of an endocervical and urethral specimen. NAA testing can also be performed on a liquid-based cytology specimen for a Pap test.

Women who do not need a pelvic exam as part of their clinical evaluation can be screened for chlamydia and gonorrhea by providing a *patient-collected* vaginal specimen. Many women prefer this method of collection over a provider-collected specimen. Studies show that the results from a patient-collected specimen are just as accurate as a provider-collected specimen. Refer to Box 23.4 which outlines the procedure for instructing a patient in obtaining a patient-collected vaginal specimen.

Many NAA tests on the market can also use a *first-catch* urine specimen to perform the test. A first-catch urine specimen involves the collection of urine that has remained

BOX 23.4 Patient-Collected Vaginal Specimen

Patient-collected specimens for chlamydia and gonorrhea are becoming more commonplace, especially among younger individuals. The specimen can be collected in the privacy of a rest room at the medical office. The medical assistant should provide the patient with an instruction sheet for the collection of the specimen and go over the instructions with the patient and offer to answer any questions.

The medical assistant should perform the following:

1. Sanitize the hands.
2. Obtain a NAA collection kit and check the expiration date. The kit includes a NAA transport tube and a sterile collection swab.
3. Open the collection kit package and label the transport tube with the patient's name, the date, the type of specimen (vaginal) and your initials.
4. Greet the patient and introduce yourself. Identify the patient and explain the procedure.
5. Escort the patient to the rest room and place the transport tube on a flat surface.
6. Partially open the swab package to expose the shaft of the swab and place the package on a flat surface within easy reach of the patient.

The medical assistant should instruct the patient in the collection of the specimen as follows:

7. Thoroughly wash your hands and dry them. Do not cleanse or wipe the genital area.
8. Remove all clothing from the waist down. Comfortably position yourself to maintain balance in a sitting or standing position by sitting on the toilet or standing with the legs spread apart.
9. Carefully remove the sterile swab from the package with your dominant hand taking care not to touch the tip, drop it, or lay it down. If the swab is contaminated request a new collection kit.
10. Hold the collection swab by placing your thumb and forefinger in the middle of the shaft covering the black score line.
11. Expose the vaginal opening by spreading apart the folds of skin around the vaginal opening (labia) with your nondominant hand.

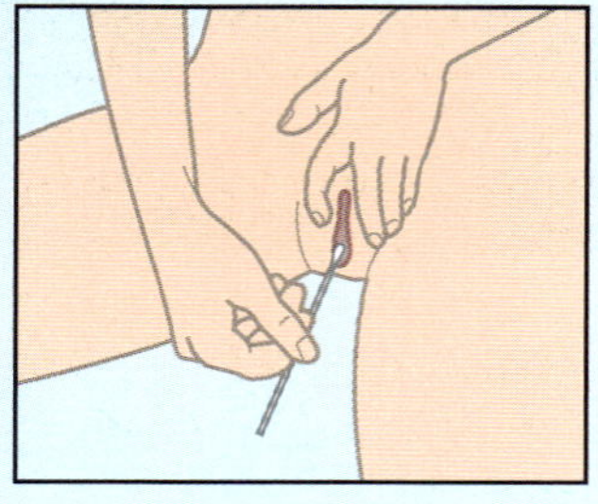

12. Carefully insert the soft tip of the swab into your vagina about 2 inches past the opening of the vagina (approximately the length of your little finger.
13. Gently rotate the swab for 10 to 30 seconds making sure the swab touches the walls of the vagina.

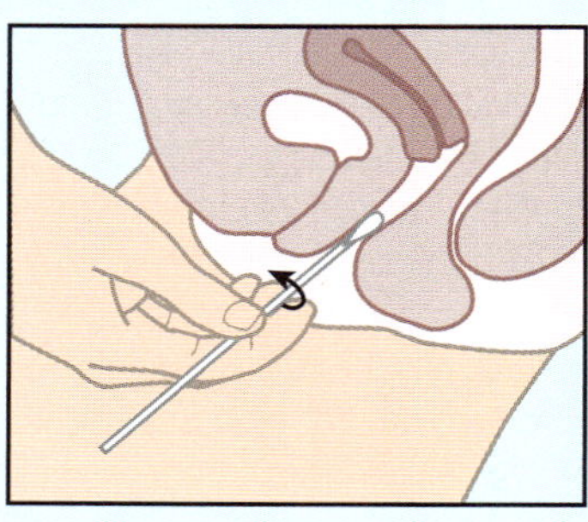

14. Withdraw the swab without touching the skin outside the vagina. Contamination of the swab may lead to inaccurate test results.
15. While still holding the swab in your dominant hand, carefully unscrew the cap from the transport tube.

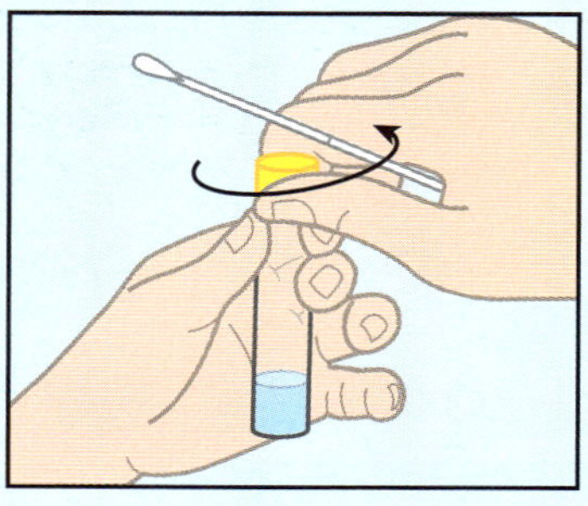

16. Immediately lower the swab in the transport tube until the visible black score-line on the shaft is lined up with the rim of the tube. Be careful not to touch the swab to any surface prior to placing it in the tube. The tip of the swab will be just above the liquid in the tube.

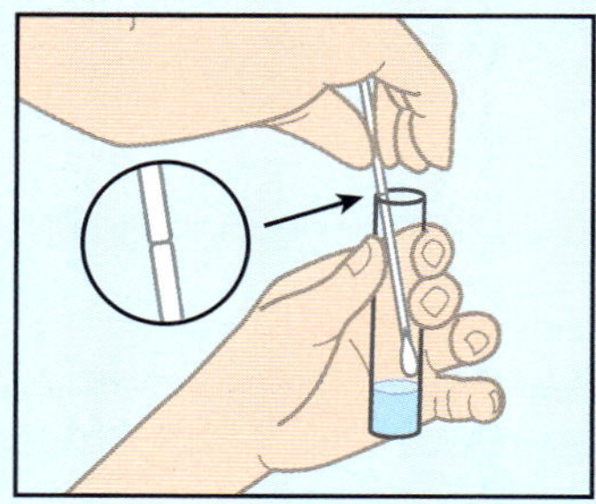

BOX 23.4 Patient-Collected Vaginal Specimen—cont'd

17. Carefully break the swab shaft at the black score-line by leaning the shaft against the tube rim and applying gentle pressure. Be careful not to spill the liquid. Dispose of the broken-off end of the shaft in the biohazard waste container provided.

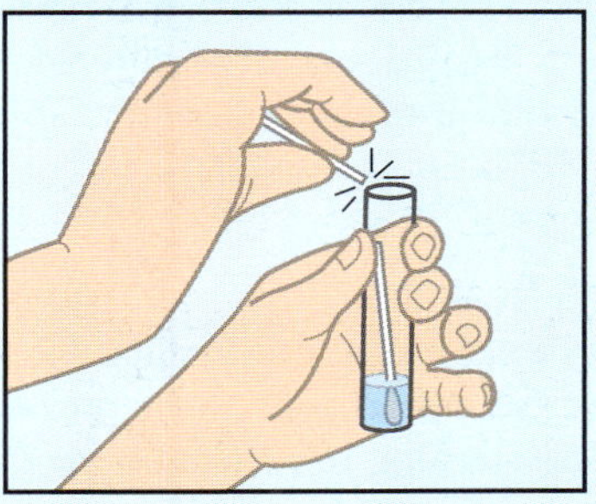

18. Tightly screw the cap onto the transport tube.
19. Thoroughly wash your hands.
20. Return the transport tube to the medical assistant.

The medical assistant should perform the following:

21. Apply gloves before accepting the transport tube from the patient.
22. Place the NAA transport tube in a biohazard specimen transport bag and seal the bag. Insert the laboratory requisition into the outside pocket of the bag.
23. Remove gloves and sanitize the hands.
24. Place the specimen bag in the appropriate location for pickup by the laboratory.

in the bladder for one hour. A first-catch urine specimen is the preferred specimen to test for chlamydia in a male. The procedure for obtaining a first-catch urine specimen is presented in Chapter 30 (Urinalysis).

When diagnosed early, chlamydia can be treated successfully with antibiotics. The antibiotics most often used are azithromycin (Zithromax) and doxycycline taken orally. The patient's partner(s) also should be tested for chlamydia so that if treatment is needed, it can be administered as soon as possible.

Gonorrhea

Description

Gonorrhea is caused by the bacterium *Neisseria gonorrhoeae*, which is a gram-negative diplococcus. Gonorrhea is an infection of the genitourinary tract that is transmitted through sexual intercourse. Chlamydia often occurs in association with gonorrhea; approximately 42% of women and 20% of men infected with gonorrhea also have chlamydia. The CDC recommends annual routine screening for gonorrhea of all sexually active females 25 years of age or younger. The CDC also recommends annual screen for women older than 25 with risk factors such as new or multiple sex partners, or a sex partner who has an STI.

Women who have contracted gonorrhea may have no symptoms or may exhibit dysuria and an increased vaginal discharge that is yellow in color. The symptoms of gonorrhea (if they occur) appear 2 to 10 days after infection and may be so mild that they are ignored. As the disease progresses, it can spread farther into the reproductive tract, resulting in PID. As mentioned previously, PID can lead to serious complications such as infertility.

Men who have contracted gonorrhea tend to exhibit more symptoms than women, including dysuria and a whitish discharge from the penis, which may progress to a thick and creamy discharge. The burning and pain experienced during urination are often severe, which usually prompts an infected man to seek early treatment. If not treated, gonorrhea may cause epididymitis, which could lead to infertility.

Diagnosis and Treatment

The recommended method for diagnosing gonorrhea is a NAA test which detects the presence of the genetic material (DNA) of gonorrhea bacteria. The type of specimens that can be used for the NAA gonorrhea test are the same as those previously described for the NAA test for chlamydia.

The CDC recommends the administration of ceftriaxone (Rocephin) by injection for the treatment of gonorrhea. The patient's partner(s) also should be tested for gonorrhea so that if treatment is needed, it can be administered as soon as possible.

Genital Herpes

Description

Genital herpes is one of the most common sexually transmitted infections in the United States. Approximately 50 million individuals in the United States are infected with genital herpes which translates to about one in six adults. Genital herpes occurs most often in individuals aged 14 to 49 and is more common in women than in men because it is more easily transmitted from men to women than from women to men during sexual intercourse.

Genital herpes is caused by the herpes simplex virus (HSV). There are two types of HSV; these include herpes simplex virus type 1 (HSV-1) and herpes simplex virus type 2 (HSV-2). The most common cause of genital herpes is HSV-2. HSV-1 is more often the cause of cold sores, however HSV-1 can be transmitted to the genital area during oral sex resulting in genital herpes.

Most individuals infected with HSV do not have symptoms or only have very mild symptoms which go unnoticed or are mistaken for another condition. Because of this, most individuals with genital herpes are not aware of having this condition. If symptoms do occur, they typically include small fluid-filled blisters on or around the genitals, anus, or lips.

These blisters break open resulting in painful sores or ulcers. The ulcers eventually scab over and heal within 2 to 4 weeks following an initial herpes infection. Systemic symptoms that may occur, especially during the first outbreak, include fever, muscle aches, swollen lymph nodes and headaches. There is no cure for herpes; once an individual is infected with HSV, the virus stays in the body for life causing recurrent outbreaks. Recurrent outbreaks are generally shorter in duration and less severe than the initial outbreak of genital herpes. Outbreaks are usually most frequent in the first year following infection and usually decrease in number over time.

Diagnosis and Treatment

The recommended test method for diagnosing genital herpes is a NAA test which detects the genetic material (DNA) of the herpes virus. Antiviral medications can be taken during an outbreak to shorten the length and severity of an outbreak. These antiviral medications include acyclovir, valacyclovir, and famciclovir. Taking a daily dose of an antiviral medication (known as *suppressive therapy*), can help to prevent or decrease the number of outbreaks and reduce the likelihood of transmitting the virus to a partner.

Human Papillomavirus Infection

Description

HPV infection is the most common STI in the United States. More than 79 million Americans are currently infected with HPV and approximately 14 million individuals become newly infected each year. There are 100 different types of HPV; approximately 40 of these types can affect the genitals and are transmitted through skin-to-skin contact during vaginal, anal, or oral sex. Genital HPV infections are so common that nearly all sexually active individuals will contract at least one type of HPV infection in their lifetime. Individuals who are not sexually active almost never develop HPV infections.

Most individuals with genital HPV infections do not exhibit symptoms and, therefore, do not know that they are infected. Because of this, they may unknowingly transmit the HPV infection to a partner. Most sexually transmitted HPV infections (90%) are cleared from the body by the immune system within 1 to 2 years following infection and the patient does not experience any health problems. In some instances, HPV infections persist and eventually cause genital warts or precancerous lesions.

Sexually transmitted HPVs are divided into the following two categories:

- *Low-Risk HPVs:* A low-risk HPV has a low-risk of causing cancer. Infection with a low-risk HPV can result in the development of genital warts. Genital warts rarely cause discomfort and pain and usually appear as flat lesions, cauliflower-like bumps, or tiny stem-like protrusions. Genital warts can affect the vulva, vagina, cervix and anus in women and the penis, scrotum, and anus in men. The diagnosis of genital warts is usually made through visual inspection. Treatment of genital warts may include topical medications, cryosurgery, electrocautery, laser treatments, or surgical excision.
- *High-Risk HPVs:* A high-risk HPV has a high risk of causing cancer. Infection with persistent high-risk HPVs cause abnormal cellular changes which may lead to precancerous lesions. These precancerous lesions may eventually result in cancer of the cervix, vulva, vagina, penis, anus, mouth, or pharynx. It usually takes years or even decades for cancer to develop following infection with a high-risk HPV.

Diagnosis and Treatment

The only HPV-related cancer for which routine screening is recommended is cervical cancer. As previously discussed, cervical cancer screening tests include the Pap test and the HPV test. The Pap test detects the presence of abnormal cervical cells that may develop into cancer if not treated while the HPV test detects the presence of high-risk HPV infections of the cervix which may cause the cervical cells to become abnormal. The ACOG guidelines (presented in Box 23.2) recommend that women ages 21 to 29 have a Pap test every 3 years. Women between the ages of 30 and 65 should have a Pap test combined with an HPV test every 5 years. This is known as *co-testing.* As alternatives, a woman in this age group can have a Pap test every 3 years or a primary HPV test every 5 years.

There are no screening tests available to detect high-risk HPV infections or abnormal cellular changes that may lead to HPV-related cancer of the vulva, vagina, penis, anus, mouth, or pharynx. The diagnosis of these conditions is usually made through visual inspection which is then confirmed through a biopsy.

There is currently no treatment available which will eliminate HPV from the body. There are treatments, however, for the health problems that may result from persistent HPV infections such as HPV-related cancers and genital warts. Although there is no cure for HPV infections, a vaccine is available to prevent sexually transmitted HPV infections that may lead to HPV-related cancers and genital warts. The HPV vaccine (Gardasil 9) does not protect against sexually transmitted HPV infections already contracted by an individual, therefore the HPV vaccine should be administered before an individual becomes sexually active (refer to Patient Coaching: HPV Vaccine).

PRENATAL CARE

Obstetrics is the branch of medicine that deals with the supervision of women's health during pregnancy, childbirth, and the puerperium. The **puerperium** is the period of time (usually 4 to 6 weeks following delivery) in which the body systems are returning to normal. **Prenatal** care refers to the care of a pregnant woman before delivery of the infant. Prenatal care consists of a series of scheduled medical office visits for promotion of the health of the mother and

PATIENT COACHING HPV Vaccine

Answer questions that patients have regarding the HPV vaccine.

What HPV vaccine is approved for use in the United States?

The HPV vaccine approved by the FDA for use in the United States is Guardasil 9 (Merck).

Guardasil 9 protects against infection with 9 types of HPV that are most likely to result in genital warts and HPV-related cancers. The vaccine is administered intramuscularly into the deltoid site or the vastus lateralis site located on the anterolateral thigh. Guardasil 9 does not protect against all the HPV types that may lead to cervical cancer, therefore it is important for women to continue routine cervical cancer screening.

What protection is provided by the HPV vaccine?

The HPV vaccine prevents HPV infections associated with the following HPV-related conditions:

Female:

- Cervical, vulvar, and vaginal cancer
- Anal cancer
- Certain head and neck cancers
- Genital warts

Male:

- Anal cancer
- Certain head and neck cancers
- Genital warts

Who should get the HPV vaccine?

The CDC recommends routine vaccination of both females and males starting at 11 or 12 years of age, but it can be administered as early as 9 years of age through 45 years of age.

What is the immunization schedule for the HPV vaccine?

- *Ages 9 to 14:* Pre-adolescents and adolescents between the ages of 9 and 14 years of age should receive the HPV vaccine as a two-dose series with the second dose being administered 6 to 12 months following the first dose. The vaccine can also be given as a three-dose series with the second dose administered 2 months after the first dose, and the third dose administered 6 months after the first dose (0, 2, 6).
- *Ages 15 to 45:* Individuals between the ages of 15 and 45 years of age should receive the HPV vaccine as a three-dose series as described above (0, 2, 6).

What are the side effects of the vaccine?

Many individuals who receive the HPV vaccine have no side effects at all or have very mild side effects. If side effects occur, they commonly include pain, redness and swelling at the injection site, fever, and headache. ■

HIGHLIGHT on Sexually Transmitted Infections

Sexually transmitted infections (STIs) are among the most common infectious diseases in the United States today. The CDC estimates that there are 20 million new infections each year in the United States. If this trend continues, over half of the population in the United States will contract an STI at some point in their lifetime. STIs are most prevalent among teenagers and young adults; more than half of all new STI cases are contracted by individuals 15 to 24 years old.

Transmission

STIs are spread most often by sexual contact with the penis, vagina, mouth, or anus of an infected person. They are less commonly spread by skin-to-skin contact and through the use of contaminated needles among drug users.

Symptoms

An STI sometimes causes no symptoms at all, particularly in women. If symptoms do occur, they include one or more of the following: an unusual discharge from the penis or vagina; itching, redness, or soreness of the genitals; sores or blisters on or around the genitals, anus, or both; and pain or burning during urination. With or without symptoms, an STI can be spread to someone else. If symptoms develop, they may be so mild that they go unnoticed, or they may be confused with symptoms of other diseases. Because of this, STIs may go undetected and untreated. If not treated, many STIs result in serious complications, such as infertility. In addition, some STIs can be passed from an infected mother to her infant before or during birth. An individual diagnosed with an STI should inform their sex partner immediately so that the partner can be also be treated. This reduces the risk that the sex partner will develop serious complications from the STI.

Treatment

When diagnosed early, most STIs can be treated effectively, and many can be cured. Antibiotics can cure STIs caused by bacteria, which include chlamydia, gonorrhea, and syphilis. Antiviral medications have been developed to control the symptoms of certain STIs caused by viruses (e.g. genital herpes, HIV), however these medications cannot eliminate the virus from the body. Currently, a preventive vaccine is available for hepatitis B and HPV.

Risk Factors

Sexually active individuals who are at increased risk for contracting an STI should have regular health checkups to be tested for STIs. Factors that increase the risk of contracting an STI include the following:

- Unprotected sex
- Multiple sexual partners
- Having a history of one or more STIs
- Alcohol use
- Illicit drug use
- Injecting drugs
- Being under 25 years of age
- Living in a community with a high prevalence of STIs

Continued

HIGHLIGHT on Sexually Transmitted Infections—cont'd

Individuals at increased risk should learn to recognize the symptoms of STIs and check themselves for signs of STI infection once a month. If an individual thinks they have an STI, a provider should be consulted as soon as possible. If an individual has been treated for an STI and still has symptoms, they should return to the provider for further evaluation. It is possible to have more than one STI at a time and to become reinfected with the same STI.

Prevention and Control Measures

All STIs can be prevented. The best way to prevent STIs is to practice abstinence or to have a mutually monogamous sexual relationship with an uninfected partner. If an individual's lifestyle does not follow one of these patterns, the following can be done to reduce the risk of contracting an STI:

- Get vaccinated for hepatitis B and HPV.
- Before having a sexual relationship, partners should discuss their sexual histories with each other and get tested for STIs.
- Use a condom during sexual intercourse. If the condom is not used correctly, however, an individual still could contract an STI. Make sure to use a water-based lubricant with condoms to keep the condom from breaking.
- Limit the number of sexual partners. The risk of an STI increases with each new partner, particularly if it is unknown how many previous partners that person has had.
- Do not have sex with anyone who exhibits the symptoms of an STI.
- Obtain annual STI testing if you have risk factors for contracting an STI.
- If you have an STI, take all prescribed medication and abstain from intercourse until a provider has determined that you are no longer contagious.

What Would You Do? What Would You *Not* Do?

Case Study 2

Brooke Madison comes to the office. She is 16 years old, and her father is a lawyer and her mother is a chemical engineer. Her boyfriend was diagnosed 2 days ago with chlamydia. Brooke was hesitant to come in because she does not have any symptoms and her boyfriend always uses a condom. She is worried about her parents finding out that she is sexually active and what they will think if she has an STI. Brooke also is afraid and extremely embarrassed about what will be "done to her" to determine whether she has chlamydia. She has never had a gyn exam and is visibly nervous and upset about it. She tells Yin-Ling that she is thinking of leaving the office and not seeing the provider at all. (*Note:* All 50 states now allow minors to give consent to STI testing and treatment.) ■

fetus through prevention of disease and early detection, diagnosis, and treatment of problems common to pregnancy (e.g., anemia, urinary tract infection, and preeclampsia). Early detection of medical problems helps prevent serious complications in the mother and the fetus.

Memories *from* Practicum

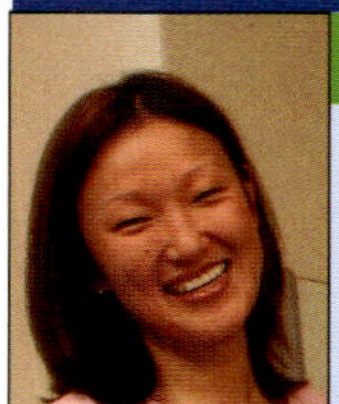

Yin-Ling: During my practicum, I was assigned to an OB/GYN clinic. They had an ultrasound technician working there who ran all the scans on prenatal patients. The ultrasound scans I observed always looked like a big blob to me—I could never see anything.

One day, a patient that the ultrasound technician knew really well came into the office. The patient agreed to let me come in for her ultrasound. It was her first time getting an ultrasound. When the technician put the ultrasound probe on her abdomen, we could see the outline of the whole baby. You could even see a tiny arm and fingers, and it looked like the baby was waving. The look of joy and amazement on the mom's face was unforgettable. After that, I knew I was in the right profession. ■

OBSTETRIC TERMINOLOGY

The medical assistant should know the common terms related to obstetrics, as follows:

Braxton Hicks contractions Intermittent and irregular painless uterine contractions that occur throughout pregnancy. They occur more frequently toward the end of pregnancy and are sometimes mistaken for true labor pains.

Dilation (of the cervix) Stretching of the external os (of the cervix) from an opening of a few millimeters to an opening large enough to allow the passage of an infant (approximately 10 cm).

Effacement Thinning and shortening of the cervical canal from its normal length of 1 to 2 cm to a structure with paper-thin edges in which there is no canal at all. Effacement occurs late in pregnancy, during labor, or both. The purpose of effacement, along with dilation, is to permit the passage of the infant into the birth canal.

Embryo The child in utero from the time of conception through the first 8 weeks of development (i.e., the first 2 months of development).

Engagement The entrance of the fetal head or the presenting part into the pelvic inlet.

Fetus The child in utero, from the third month after conception to birth; during the first 2 months of development, it is called an *embryo*.

Fundus The dome-shaped upper portion of the uterus between the fallopian tubes.

Gestation The period of intrauterine development from conception to birth; the period of pregnancy. The average pregnancy lasts about 280 days, or 40 weeks, from the date of conception to childbirth.

Gestational age The age of the fetus between conception and birth.

Infant A child from birth to 12 months old.

Multigravida A woman who has been pregnant more than once.

Multipara A woman who has completed two or more pregnancies to the age of viability regardless of whether they ended in live infants or stillbirths.

Nullipara A woman who has not carried a pregnancy to the point of fetal viability (20 weeks of gestation).

Position The relation of the presenting part of the fetus to the maternal pelvis.

Postpartum Occurring after childbirth.

Preeclampsia A major complication of pregnancy, the cause of which is unknown, characterized by increasing hypertension, albuminuria, and edema. If the condition is neglected or is not treated properly, preeclampsia may develop into eclampsia, which could cause maternal convulsions and coma. Preeclampsia generally occurs between the 20th week of pregnancy and the end of the first week postpartum.

Presentation Indication of the part of the fetus that is closest to the cervix and is delivered first. A cephalic presentation is a delivery in which the fetal head is presenting against the cervix. A breech presentation is a delivery in which the buttocks or feet are presented instead of the head.

Primigravida A woman who is pregnant for the first time.

Primipara A woman who has carried a pregnancy to fetal viability (20 weeks of gestation) for the first time regardless of whether the infant was stillborn or alive at birth.

Puerperium The period of time (usually 4 to 6 weeks) after delivery in which the uterus and the body systems are returning to normal.

Quickening The first movements of the fetus in utero as felt by the mother, which usually occurs between 16 and 20 weeks of gestation and is felt consistently thereafter.

Toxemia A condition that can occur in pregnant women that includes preeclampsia and eclampsia. If preeclampsia goes undiagnosed or is not satisfactorily controlled, it could develop into eclampsia, which is characterized by convulsions and coma.

Trimester Three months, or one third, of the gestational period. The 9 months of pregnancy are divided into three trimesters, each consisting of 3 months. From conception to 3 months is the first trimester, from 4 to 6 months is the second trimester, and from 7 to 9 months is the third trimester.

PRENATAL VISITS

Medical office visits for prenatal and postpartum care of the pregnant woman can be grouped into three major categories as follows:

1. First prenatal visit
2. Return prenatal visits
3. Six weeks postpartum visit

First Prenatal Visit

The first prenatal visit generally occurs after the woman has missed her second menstrual period; if problems exist, the woman is seen after missing her first menstrual period. Regardless of whether or not the patient is happy and excited about the pregnancy, the first visit is often a stressful experience for the patient. The medical assistant plays an important role in relaxing the patient and relieving her anxiety.

The first prenatal visit requires more time than subsequent prenatal visits; sufficient time should be scheduled to allow a complete and accurate initial assessment of the pregnant woman. The components of the first prenatal visit vary depending on the medical office, but they generally include the following:

- Completion of a prenatal record form
- Initial prenatal examination, consisting of a complete physical examination. Of particular importance are breast, abdominal, and pelvic examinations
- Prenatal patient education
- Laboratory tests

Prenatal Record

The prenatal record provides information regarding the past and present health of the patient and serves as a database and flow sheet for subsequent prenatal visits. The prenatal record is essential in helping identify high-risk patients. The medical assistant is usually responsible for collecting a portion of the information required for the prenatal record. Many types of prenatal record forms are available (Fig. 23.9). The specific form used in the medical office is based on the provider's preference and the method used for conducting the prenatal examination.

Obtaining and documenting information in the prenatal record from one visit to the next provides an opportunity for the medical assistant to develop a rapport with the patient. It is also an excellent time to relay information to her regarding various aspects of the prenatal and postnatal periods, such as an explanation of the changes occurring in her body, the signs and symptoms of labor, nutrition of the infant (breastfeeding and bottle feeding), and care of the newborn infant. The prenatal record form should be completed in a quiet setting that is free from distractions. This gives the patient the confidence to discuss areas of concern openly, which helps ensure a complete and accurate prenatal history.

During the first prenatal visit, the medical assistant should relay their name and position to the patient to help build a supportive relationship with her and to allow her to ask for the medical assistant by name when contacting the medical office. The prenatal record is similar to and contains much of the same information as the health history described in Chapter 20. Particular attention is given to factors that may influence the course of pregnancy, as described in the following paragraphs.

Past Medical History

The past medical history focuses on conditions that could affect the health of the mother and fetus, such as diabetes, hypertension, heart disease, autoimmune disorders, kidney disease, liver disease, varicosities or phlebitis, alcohol and tobacco intake, drug addiction, Rh sensitization, pulmonary disease (e.g., tuberculosis, asthma), bleeding tendencies, surgeries, anesthetic complications, previous abnormal Pap tests, infertility problems, sexually transmitted infections, and drug allergies. In addition, the medical assistant solicits information from the patient regarding immunizations and childhood diseases to provide the provider with the information needed to assess her antibody protection against such diseases.

Rubella, if contracted during pregnancy, can be dangerous to the developing fetus; the earlier in pregnancy the infection occurs, the greater is the chance of birth defects. The infant may be born with heart defects, cataracts, intellectual disabilities, and deafness. Patients who do not have antibody protection against rubella are given a rubella immunization within 6 weeks of delivery. Fortunately, rubella has become quite rare in the United States due to the routine rubella vaccination of children. The rubella vaccination cannot be given to a pregnant woman because it may be harmful to the fetus. These patients should be told to avoid exposure to children with rubella during their pregnancy.

PRENATAL HEALTH HISTORY

PATIENT INFORMATION

Date: ______ EDD: ______ Referred By: ______

Name: ______ (LAST, FIRST, MIDDLE) Phone (home): ______

Phone (work): ______

Address: ______ Emergency Contact: ______

______ (CITY, STATE, ZIP) Phone: ______

Date of Birth: ___/___/___ Age: ___ Marital Status: ______

Occupation: ______

Education: ☐ High School ☐ College ☐ Post-graduate

PAST MEDICAL HISTORY

	O Neg + Pos	DETAIL POSITIVE REMARKS INCLUDE DATE AND TREATMENT
1. DIABETES		
2. HYPERTENSION		
3. HEART DISEASE		
4. AUTOIMMUNE DISORDER		
5. KIDNEY DISEASE/UTI		
6. NEUROLOGIC/EPILEPSY		
7. PSYCHIATRIC		
8. HEPATITIS/LIVER DISEASE		
9. VARICOSITIES/PHLEBITIS		
10. THYROID DYSFUNCTION		
11. TRAUMA/DOMESTIC VIOLENCE		
12. BLOOD TRANSFUSION		

	AMT/DAY PREPREG.	AMT/DAY PREG.	# YEARS USE
13. TOBACCO			
14. ALCOHOL			
15. STREET DRUGS			

	O Neg + Pos	DETAIL POSITIVE REMARKS INCLUDE DATE AND TREATMENT
16. D (Rh) SENSITIZED		
17. PULMONARY (TB, ASTHMA)		
18. RHEUMATIC FEVER		
19. BLEEDING TENDENCY		
20. GYN SURGERY		
21. OPERATIONS/HOSPITALIZATIONS (YEAR AND REASON)		
22. ANESTHETIC COMPLICATIONS		
23. HISTORY OF ABNORMAL PAP		
24. UTERINE ANOMALY/DES		
25. INFERTILITY		
26. SEXUALLY TRANSMITTED DISEASE		
27. OTHER		

IMMUNIZATIONS:

Mark an X next to those you have had.

☐ Influenza ☐ Chickenpox
☐ Hepatitis B ☐ Pneumococcal
☐ Hib ☐ Tuberculin Test
☐ Polio ☐ Tetanus Booster
☐ MMR

ALLERGIES:

List all allergies (foods, drugs, environment). ☐ None

______

MENSTRUAL HISTORY

Menarche: Age of Onset ______

Frequency: Q ______ Days

Duration: ______ Days

Amount of Flow: ☐ Small ☐ Moderate ☐ Large

GYN Disorders (List): ______

On contraceptive at conception? ☐ Yes ☐ No

Fig. 23.9 Example of a prenatal record form.

OBSTETRIC HISTORY

G ________ (Total Pregnancies) T ________ (Term) P ________ (Preterm) A ________ (Abortions) L ________ (Living Children)

PREVIOUS PREGNANCIES:

DATE MONTH/ YEAR	WEEKS GEST.	LENGTH OF LABOR	BIRTH WEIGHT	SEX M/F	TYPE DELIVERY	ANES.	MATERNAL COMPLICATIONS	INFANT COMPLICATIONS

PRESENT PREGNANCY HISTORY

NAUSEA			ABDOMINAL PAIN		
VOMITING			URINARY COMPLAINTS		
FATIGUE			VAGINAL BLEEDING		
BREAST CHANGES			VAGINAL DISCHARGE		
INDIGESTION			PRURITIS		
CONSTIPATION			ACCIDENTS		
PERSISTENT HEADACHES			SURGERY		
DIZZINESS			X-RAYS		
VISUAL DISTURBANCE			RUBELLA EXPOSURE		
EDEMA (SPECIFY AREA)			OTHER VIRAL INFECTIONS		

LMP ______/______/______ (Mo Day Year) **Amount of Flow:** ☐ **Small** ☐ **Moderate** ☐ **Large**

CURRENT MEDICATIONS: (Include prescription, OTC, herbal, and vitamins). ☐ **None**

Medication **Frequency**

____

____

____

INITIAL PHYSICAL EXAMINATION

DATE ____/____/____

1. HEENT	☐ NORMAL	☐ ABNORMAL	12. VULVA	☐ NORMAL	☐ CONDYLOMA	☐ LESIONS
2. FUNDI	☐ NORMAL	☐ ABNORMAL	13. VAGINA	☐ NORMAL	☐ INFLAMMATION	☐ DISCHARGE
3. TEETH	☐ NORMAL	☐ ABNORMAL	14. CERVIX	☐ NORMAL	☐ INFLAMMATION	☐ LESIONS
4. THYROID	☐ NORMAL	☐ ABNORMAL	15. UTERUS SIZE	______ WEEKS		☐ FIBROIDS
5. BREASTS	☐ NORMAL	☐ ABNORMAL	16. ADNEXA	☐ NORMAL	☐ MASS	
6. LUNGS	☐ NORMAL	☐ ABNORMAL	17. RECTUM	☐ NORMAL	☐ ABNORMAL	
7. HEART	☐ NORMAL	☐ ABNORMAL	18. DIAGONAL CONJUGATE	☐ REACHED	☐ NO	______ CM
8. ABDOMEN	☐ NORMAL	☐ ABNORMAL	19. SPINES	☐ AVERAGE	☐ PROMINENT	☐ BLUNT
9. EXTREMITIES	☐ NORMAL	☐ ABNORMAL	20. SACRUM	☐ CONCAVE	☐ STRAIGHT	☐ ANTERIOR
10. SKIN	☐ NORMAL	☐ ABNORMAL	21. SUBPUBIC ARCH	☐ NORMAL	☐ WIDE	☐ NARROW
11. LYMPH NODES	☐ NORMAL	☐ ABNORMAL	22. GYNECOID PELVIC TYPE	☐ YES	☐ NO	

COMMENTS (Number and explain abnormals): ____

____

____

______________________ **EXAM BY** ______________________

Fig. 23.9, cont'd

Continued

PATIENT'S NAME ________________________________

INTERVAL PRENATAL HISTORY

Date 20___	Weeks Gestation	Height of Fundus (cm)	Weight	B/P	Urine Glucose	Urine Protein	FHT	Vaginal Examination	Presentation	Edema	Discharge	Bleeding	Contractions	Fetal Activity	NST	Next Appt.	Initials

PLANS/EDUCATION (COUNSELED ☑)

- ☐ ANESTHESIA PLANS ________
- ☐ TOXOPLASMOSIS PRECAUTIONS (CATS/RAW MEAT) ________
- ☐ CHILDBIRTH CLASSES ________
- ☐ PHYSICAL/SEXUAL ACTIVITY ________
- ☐ LABOR SIGNS ________
- ☐ NUTRITION COUNSELING ________
- ☐ BREAST OR BOTTLE FEEDING ________
- ☐ NEWBORN CAR SEAT ________
- ☐ POSTPARTUM BIRTH CONTROL ________
- ☐ ENVIRONMENTAL/WORK HAZARDS ________
- ☐ TUBAL STERILIZATION ________
- ☐ VBAC COUNSELING ________
- ☐ CIRCUMCISION ________
- ☐ TRAVEL ________
- ☐ LIFESTYLE, TOBACCO, ALCOHOL ________

REQUESTS ________

TUBAL STERILIZATION CONSENT SIGNED **DATE** ___/___/___ **INITIALS** ________

Fig. 23.9, cont'd

LABORATORY		PATIENT'S NAME ______		
INITIAL LABS	**DATE**	**RESULTS**	**REVIEWED**	**COMMENTS**
BLOOD TYPE	/ /	A B AB O		
Rh FACTOR	/ /	☐ Pos ☐ Neg		
Rh ANTIBODY SCREEN	/ /	☐ Pos ☐ Neg		
HCT/HGB	/ /	____% ____ g/dL		
RUBELLA ANTIBODY TITER	/ /	Immune Nonimmune		
VDRL	/ /	☐ NR ☐ R		
HBsAg (HEPATITIS B)	/ /	☐ Pos ☐ Neg		
HIV	/ /	☐ Pos ☐ Neg ☐ Declined		
URINE CULTURE/SCREEN	/ /			
PAP TEST	/ /	☐ Normal ☐ Abnormal		
CHLAMYDIA (DNA PROBE)	/ /	☐ Pos ☐ Neg		
GONORRHEA (DNA PROBE)	/ /	☐ Pos ☐ Neg		
7–20 WEEK LABS (WHEN INDICATED/ELECTED)	**DATE**	**RESULTS**	**REVIEWED**	**COMMENTS**
ULTRASOUND #1 (7–12 WEEKS)	/ /	EDD:		
ULTRASOUND #2 (18–20 WEEKS)	/ /	EFW:		
TRIPLE SCREEN (15–20 WEEKS)	/ /			
CVS	/ /			
AMNIOCENTESIS	/ /			
24–28 WEEK LABS (WHEN INDICATED)	**DATE**	**RESULTS**	**REVIEWED**	**COMMENTS**
HCT/HGB	/ /	____ % ____ g/dL		
GCT (24–28 WKS)	/ /	1 Hour ______		
GTT (IF SCREEN ABNORMAL)	/ /	____ FBS ____ 1 Hour ____ 2 Hour ____ 3 Hour		
D (Rh) ANTIBODY SCREEN	/ /			
D IMMUNE GLOBULIN (RhIG) GIVEN (28 WKS)	/ /	SIGNATURE		
32–36 WEEK LABS	**DATE**	**RESULTS**	**REVIEWED**	**COMMENTS**
HCT/HGB (32 WKS)	/ /	____ % ____ g/dL		
ULTRASOUND #3 (34 WKS)	/ /	EFW:		
GROUP B STREP (35–37 WKS)	/ /	☐ Pos ☐ Neg		
ADDITIONAL LAB TESTS	**DATE**	**RESULTS**	**REVIEWED**	**COMMENTS**
	/ /			
	/ /			
	/ /			
	/ /			
	/ /			

Fig. 23.9, cont'd

Menstrual History

A menstrual history is obtained from the patient. It includes the date of onset of menstruation, the menstrual interval cycle, the duration of the mentrual period and amount of flow (documented as small, moderate, or large), and any gynecologic disorders. The form also includes a space for the patient to indicate whether or not she was using a method of contraception when she became pregnant.

Obstetric History

A thorough obstetric history is a component of the prenatal record and provides the opportunity to obtain information from the patient related to previous pregnancies.

If a woman is a **multigravida** (having been pregnant more than once), information about each pregnancy is obtained, including the date of delivery, gestation in weeks, length of labor in hours, birth weight and sex of the newborn, type of delivery (vaginal or cesarean section), type of anesthesia, and any maternal or infant complications. The obstetric history assists in identifying areas that may need to be investigated further or monitored during the prenatal period. Women with previous complications, such as premature labor, gestational diabetes, or postpartum hemorrhaging, are at risk for having these problems again.

Present Pregnancy History

The present pregnancy history establishes a baseline for the present health status of the prenatal patient. In addition, the patient is queried regarding any warning signs that may be present and that may place the mother or fetus in jeopardy, such as persistent headaches, visual disturbances, abdominal pain, vaginal bleeding, or discharge. The patient also is asked whether she has experienced any of the early signs of pregnancy, such as nausea, vomiting, fatigue, spotting, and swollen/tender breasts.

All prescribed or over-the-counter medications (including vitamin supplements and herbal products) the patient is taking must be documented. Certain medications cross the placental barrier and could be harmful to the developing fetus. The patient should be instructed not to take any medications without first checking with the provider.

In the space provided under the present pregnancy history, the medical assistant needs to document the date of the first day of the patient's last menstrual period (LMP). The LMP is used to calculate the due date or **expected date of delivery (EDD)**.

Gestation calculators are commercially available that can be used to determine the EDD by lining up an arrow and the date of the LMP, using a movable inner cardboard wheel (Fig. 23.10). There are also many online gestation calculators available as well as a variety of gestation calculator applications designed for mobile devices. In addition, electronic health record software automatically calculates the EDD after the LMP has been entered into the computer. If the patient is unsure of the date of her LMP, the provider estimates the length of gestation by other methods, such as fundal height measurement and sonography.

Interval Prenatal History

The interval prenatal history also is included in the prenatal record form; its purpose is to update the record. During every return visit, essential data, including weight, blood pressure, urine testing results, fundal height measurement, and fetal heart rate, are collected and documented in this section. A general inquiry is made regarding the occurrence of additional signs of pregnancy, such as fetal movement or Braxton Hicks contractions, and how the patient is feeling and any concerns or symptoms since the last prenatal visit.

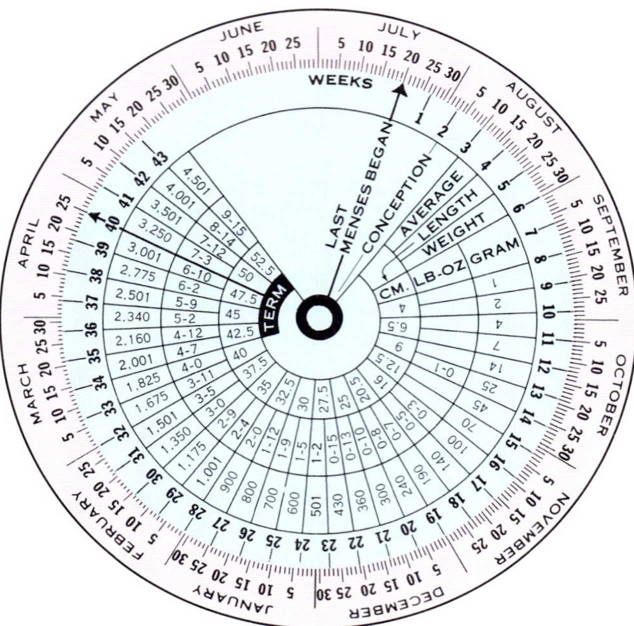

Fig. 23.10 Gestation calculator. The last menstrual period is July 20, and the expected date of delivery is April 25.

This information is documented in the prenatal record and assists the medical staff in planning, implementing, and evaluating individual needs. Particular attention is focused on risk factors, such as hypertension, thrombophlebitis, and uterine bleeding, which could influence the course of the pregnancy.

Initial Prenatal Examination

Purpose

The initial prenatal examination is of particular importance because it results in confirmation of the pregnancy and establishes a baseline for the woman's state of health. It includes a thorough gynecologic examination (breast and pelvic examinations), the measurement of vital signs, and a general physical examination of the other body systems, although the latter may be performed during a subsequent prenatal visit, depending on the medical office routine.

Women often have little or no medical supervision during their childbearing years; the physical examination is of particular importance in establishing a baseline for the woman's general state of health and in identifying high-risk prenatal patients. Conditions such as obesity, hypertension, severe varicosities, and uterine size inappropriate for the due date can be diagnosed by the provider, and necessary treatment or monitoring can be instituted to help prevent complications.

Preparation of the Patient

When the patient arrives at the medical office and the prenatal record form has been completed, the medical assistant is responsible for taking and documenting the patient's vital signs, height, and weight to provide a database for subsequent prenatal visits. The patient is asked to disrobe completely and put on an examining gown with the opening in front. The medical assistant must give complete and thorough instructions so the patient knows exactly what is expected. The patient should be asked whether she needs to empty her bladder because an empty bladder facilitates the examination and is more comfortable for her. If the office policy is such that a specimen is needed for urine testing at the initial prenatal visit, the patient will be required to void.

Special precautions should be taken in assisting the prenatal patient. The medical assistant should support the patient as she gets onto and off the scale and examining table to ensure her safety and comfort. This is especially important as the pregnancy progresses and the patient becomes more awkward and off balance.

The medical assistant is responsible for setting up the tray required for the examination. The setup includes the equipment and supplies required for the procedures to be performed. During the prenatal examination, the medical assistant is responsible for positioning the patient as required for each aspect of the examination and assisting the provider as necessary.

Patient Education

At the conclusion of the initial prenatal examination and after the patient is dressed, the provider counsels the patient on health promotion and disease prevention. Topics that are often discussed include nutrition, weight gain, rest, sleep, employment, exercise, travel, sexual intercourse, dental care, smoking, alcohol, and drugs. Many offices have a prenatal guidebook designed especially for this purpose that is given to each patient to use as a reference. Some offices also use educational videos that the patient views during return prenatal visits. The provider also prescribes a daily vitamin supplement to be taken during the prenatal period to ensure that the mother and fetus obtain an adequate supply of vitamins and minerals.

When the provider is finished talking with the patient, the medical assistant is responsible for scheduling the next prenatal visit and for ensuring that the patient understands the instructions for maintaining health and preventing disease during the pregnancy. The medical assistant should tell the patient to report the occurrence of any warning signs during the pregnancy (see Box 23.5: *Warning Signs During Pregnancy*) and not to take any medications without first checking with the provider. The patient also should be encouraged to contact the medical office should any questions or problems arise.

BOX 23.5 Warning Signs During Pregnancy

Signs of Infection

- Fever
- Vaginal discharge
- Dysuria
- Increased frequency of urination
- Marked decrease in urinary output

Signs of Spontaneous Abortion

- Vaginal bleeding
- Persistent low back pain
- Abdominal pain and cramping

Signs of Preeclampsia

- Severe, persistent headache
- Dizziness
- Blurred vision
- Sudden swelling of hands, feet, or face
- Sudden rapid weight gain
- Abdominal pain

Signs of Placental or Fetal Problems

- Vaginal spotting or bleeding
- Abdominal pain and cramping
- Back pain
- Noticeable decrease in fetal activity
- No fetal movement

Signs of Preterm Labor

- Regular or frequent contractions (more than four to six per hour)
- Recurring low, dull backache
- Menstrual-like cramping
- Unusual pressure in the pelvis, low back, abdomen, or thighs

Laboratory Tests

The provider orders many laboratory tests to assist in the assessment of the patient's state of health and to detect problems that may put the pregnancy at risk. Several tests, such as the Pap test and the chlamydia and gonorrhea tests, require the provider to collect the specimens at the medical office and have them transported by laboratory courier to an outside laboratory for evaluation. The specimen required for the prenatal blood tests (known as a prenatal profile) must be obtained through a venipuncture to provide a sufficient quantity of blood for the number of tests ordered. The blood specimen is collected at the medical office or at an outside laboratory.

It is important to have these initial tests completed as soon as possible to provide the provider with the test results by the time of the next scheduled prenatal visit. Based on the results of the prenatal examination and the laboratory tests, the provider may order additional tests to assess the patient's condition. Certain tests and procedures, such as the glucose challenge test (GCT) and the group B streptococcus (GBS) test, are scheduled later in the pregnancy. The prenatal laboratory tests that are usually performed on a pregnant woman are described next.

Urine Tests

Urinalysis

A complete urinalysis, including physical, chemical, and microscopic analyses of the urine, is performed; a clean-catch midstream urine specimen is generally required for the test. If bacteria are found in the urine specimen, the provider usually requests a urine culture and sensitivity test to determine the possible presence of a urinary tract infection. A pregnancy test also may be performed on the urine specimen, if ordered by the provider.

Swab Tests

Pap Test

The primary purpose of the Pap test is to detect abnormal cervical cells that may develop into cancer if not treated. It can also determine the presence of noncancerous conditions such as inflammation and infection. This test also can be used for hormonal assessment (maturation index) and to assist in the detection of vaginal infections.

Chlamydia and Gonorrhea

Specimens are taken from the vagina or endocervical canal and sent to the laboratory to rule out chlamydia and gonorrhea. A patient who is diagnosed with chlamydia or gonorrhea requires immediate treatment with an appropriate antibiotic to prevent problems for herself and her child.

If a chlamydial or gonorrheal infection is present at the time of delivery, the bacteria causing these conditions could infect the infant's eyes during passage through the birth canal. This may result in a type of conjunctivitis known as *ophthalmia neonatorum*, which, if not treated, could lead to blindness. For this reason, most states require that pregnant women be tested for chlamydia and gonorrhea, and that the eyes of newborns be treated with an antibiotic ointment immediately after birth to kill any harmful bacteria that may be present.

Vaginal Infections

If an excessively irritating vaginal discharge is present, the provider obtains a specimen to rule out bacterial infections including bacterial vaginosis, trichomoniasis and vulvovaginal candidiasis (VVC). If a vaginal infection is diagnosed, the prenatal patient will be treated with the appropriate medication. Bacterial vaginosis and trichomoniasis increase the risk of premature birth and low birth weight. It is important to control VVC before delivery to prevent the development of *thrush*, a yeastlike infection of the infant's mucous membranes of the mouth or throat.

Group B Streptococcus

Group B streptococcus (GBS) is a common bacterium often found in the vagina and rectum of healthy women. Normally, one in four pregnant women carries GBS. GBS is not harmful to a pregnant woman, but it can cause life-threatening infections in the newborn. While passing through the birth canal, a newborn can become infected with the bacteria carried by the mother. When infected, the infant may develop an infection of the blood (septicemia), pneumonia, or meningitis.

To prevent GBS infection of the newborn, a pregnant woman is tested for the bacteria between 35 and 37 weeks of gestation. Using two swabs, the provider collects specimens from the vagina and the rectum. The specimen swabs are placed in a transport tube and sent to the laboratory to be cultured for GBS. If GBS is found, intravenous antibiotics are administered to the woman every 4 hours during labor until delivery. In most cases, this antibiotic administration prevents the newborn from becoming infected with GBS. In situations in which the newborn does become infected with GBS, antibiotics are administered immediately, and the infant is closely monitored.

What Would You Do? What Would You *Not* Do?

Case Study 3

Johanna Kruger is 24 years old and pregnant with her first child. She is at the office for her first prenatal visit. She is quite upset. One of her neighbors had minimal prenatal care and just had a baby, and the baby died 24 hours later from a group B strep infection. Johanna is afraid that the same thing will happen to her baby. She wants to be tested for GBS as soon as possible. She has some antibiotics at home and is thinking of taking them. Johanna is worried because she has been experiencing some problems with her pregnancy. She feels nauseous all day, her breasts are swollen and tender, and yesterday she had some spotting. Johanna is hesitant to tell all of this to the physician because he might think she worries too much. ■

Blood Tests

Complete Blood Count

The complete blood count (CBC) is a basic screening test used to assist in assessing the patient's state of health. It includes a hemoglobin, hematocrit, white blood cell count, red blood cell count, differential white blood cell count, platelet count, and red blood cell indices. Of particular importance with respect to the prenatal patient are the hemoglobin and hematocrit evaluations, which are described here.

Hemoglobin and Hematocrit

Low hemoglobin and hematocrit values are seen in cases of anemia. Prenatal patients have a tendency to develop anemia because there is an increased demand for and correlating increased production of red blood cells during pregnancy; the provider carefully reviews the results of these tests. If the hemoglobin or hematocrit value is low, further hematologic evaluation is usually required. If necessary, therapy is instituted, which usually consists of an iron supplement and nutritional counseling. The hemoglobin and hematocrit values are checked again at approximately 32 weeks of gestation as a precaution against anemia before delivery.

Rh Factor and ABO Blood Type

Tests are performed to anticipate ABO blood type and Rh factor incompatibilities. If the patient is Rh-negative, the possibility of an Rh incompatibility exists. This situation warrants the performance of an Rh antibody titer test and repeat antibody titers throughout the pregnancy to determine whether the mother's antibody level is increasing. An increased Rh antibody level could be dangerous to the developing fetus. It can result in severe anemia, jaundice, brain damage, heart failure, and sometimes death of the fetus.

Glucose Challenge Test

A glucose challenge test is performed between 24 and 28 weeks of gestation to screen for gestational diabetes mellitus (GDM). This test works by assessing the body's response to a measured glucose solution. The patient does not need to fast for this test, and no preparation is required other than arriving at the laboratory at the scheduled time. To perform the glucose challenge test, the patient is asked to drink 50 g of a glucose solution, and her glucose level is measured 1 hour later. A woman with a glucose level of less than 140 mg/dL does not have GDM and requires no further testing. If the glucose level is greater than 140 mg/dL, the test is abnormal. Not all women with elevated results have diabetes, however, and further testing using the 3-hour oral glucose tolerance test (OGTT) must be performed before a final diagnosis can be made. (*Note:* Refer to Chapter 33 for information on the OGTT.)

Syphilis Test

The microorganism that causes syphilis, *Treponema pallidum*, is able to cross the placental barrier and infect the fetus; this could result in intrauterine death or could cause the fetus to be born with congenital syphilis. Infants with congenital syphilis are often born with deformities and may

HIGHLIGHT on Gestational Diabetes Mellitus

Definition of Gestational Diabetes Mellitus

Gestational diabetes mellitus (GDM) is a condition in which a pregnant woman who has never had diabetes mellitus develops an elevated glucose level (hyperglycemia). Every year, approximately 6% to 9% of pregnant women in the United States are diagnosed with GDM. Because most women with GDM have no symptoms, the American Diabetes Association recommends that all pregnant women be screened for GDM during the second trimester of the pregnancy.

Cause of Gestational Diabetes Mellitus

GDM develops from a physical interaction between the mother and the fetus. The placenta of the fetus produces hormones to preserve the pregnancy. These hormones are excreted into the mother's circulatory system in increasing amounts during the second trimester of pregnancy. These hormones counteract the effect of the mother's insulin, which results in a condition known as *insulin resistance.* In most cases, the mother's pancreas responds to insulin resistance by producing additional insulin to keep the blood glucose at a normal level. Some women are unable to produce enough extra insulin, however, which causes an elevation of their blood glucose level and results in GDM.

Problems for the Child

If GDM is not treated or if it is poorly controlled, problems can occur in the unborn child. The extra glucose crosses the placenta and enters the fetus' circulatory system. To decrease the elevated glucose level, the fetus' pancreas produces large amounts of insulin. The increased insulin converts the extra glucose into fat, resulting in the development of a large infant with a condition known as *macrosomia.* Infants with macrosomia may be too large to be born vaginally and may require a cesarean birth. Although the infant does not have diabetes, he or she is at risk for developing type 2 diabetes later in life. Other problems that can occur at birth include hypoglycemia, breathing difficulties, and jaundice.

Problems for the Mother

Problems that a mother with GDM can develop include an increased incidence of preeclampsia, infection, postpartum bleeding, and injury to the birth canal if the infant is delivered vaginally. Another problem is the development of polyhydramnios (excess amount of amniotic fluid), which causes the uterus to stretch and take up more space in the abdominal cavity. This can result in breathing difficulties for the mother during the pregnancy. GDM almost always resolves after delivery. This is because when the placenta is removed, the hormones causing the problem also are removed. The mother's insulin can work normally without resistance. Some women go on to develop type 2 diabetes later in life, however.

Risk Factors for Gestational Diabetes Mellitus

Certain factors put some women at greater risk for developing GDM. These women are usually screened earlier and more often for GDM during the pregnancy. Risk factors for GDM include the following:

- Obesity
- Family history of diabetes mellitus
- Previous birth of an infant weighing more than 9 lb
- Previous birth of an infant who was stillborn or had a birth defect
- Previous GDM diagnosis
- Age older than 25 years
- Polyhydramnios
- Belonging to an ethnic group known to have higher rates of GDM (Hispanic, African American, Native American, Asian, Pacific Islander)

Treatment

If a woman is diagnosed with GDM, the treatment is focused on keeping her glucose at a safe level. This includes special meal plans, exercise, daily blood glucose testing, and insulin injections, if needed. If the blood glucose is controlled during pregnancy, most women with GDM are able to prevent maternal or fetal complications. ■

become blind, deaf, paralyzed, and develop intellectual disabilities. The tests most commonly employed to screen for the presence of syphilis are the Venereal Disease Research Laboratory (VDRL) test and the rapid plasma reagin (RPR) test. The test results are reported as nonreactive, weakly reactive, or reactive. Because these tests are screening tests, a weakly reactive or reactive test result warrants more specific testing to arrive at a diagnosis for syphilis. Examples of these tests are the fluorescent treponemal antibody absorption (FTA-ABS) test and the *Treponema pallidum* particle agglutination assay (TPPA) test.

A prenatal test for syphilis is mandated by most states and should be performed early in the pregnancy, before fetal damage occurs. A patient who has contracted syphilis requires treatment with an appropriate antibiotic.

Rubella Antibody Titer

The rubella antibody titer assesses the level of antibody against rubella (German measles) in the patient's blood and is used to determine whether the woman is immune to rubella. If the mother contracts rubella during pregnancy, serious congenital abnormalities can occur in the fetus. Patients who lack immunity should be immunized against rubella within 6 weeks of delivery.

Rh Antibody Titer (on Rh-Negative Blood Specimens)

An Rh antibody titer detects the quantity of circulating Rh antibodies against red blood cells. These antibodies can occur in a pregnant woman who is Rh-negative and is carrying an Rh-positive fetus; an Rh antibody titer is performed on all Rh-negative blood specimens. Repeat antibody titer levels also are performed during the pregnancy to determine whether the woman's antibody level is increasing. As was previously indicated, an increased Rh antibody level could be dangerous to the developing fetus. As a preventive measure, Rh-negative women with the potential of having an Rh-positive infant and who test negative for Rh antibodies are given two injections of Rh immune globulin (RhoGAM).

The Rh immune globulin prevents the formation of Rh antibodies in the mother, which avoids Rh incompatibility complications during the next pregnancy. The first injection is given at 28 weeks of gestation, and the second injection is administered within 72 hours of delivery.

Hepatitis B and Human Immunodeficiency Virus

The Centers for Disease Control and Prevention (CDC) recommends that pregnant women have a hepatitis B test. Women who have positive test results have an increased risk of spontaneous **abortion** or preterm labor. In addition, the mother may transmit hepatitis B to the infant, particularly during delivery or in the first few days of life. This risk can be greatly reduced by administering hepatitis B immune globulin (HBIG) and the hepatitis B vaccine within 12 hours of birth to the newborns of women who have tested positive for hepatitis B.

Infants born to women who are human immunodeficiency virus (HIV) positive are at risk of developing the disease. If antiretroviral drugs are taken during pregnancy and the infant is delivered by cesarean section, the chance of transmitting HIV to the infant is reduced significantly. Because of this, the CDC recommends that testing for HIV be included in the routine panel of prenatal screening tests for all pregnant women, and that separate written consent is not required. The CDC further recommends that the patient should be notified that HIV testing will be performed unless the patient declines the test. The CDC recommends that repeat HIV screening be performed in the third trimester in geographic areas that have elevated rates of HIV infection among pregnant women.

Return Prenatal Visits

Return prenatal visits provide the opportunity for a continuous assessment of the health of the mother and the fetus. During each visit, essential data are collected and documented in the prenatal record, resulting in an updated record at each visit, as is discussed in this section. If signs or symptoms of a pathologic condition are present, the provider performs select aspects of the physical examination as necessary to diagnose and treat the condition. In addition, diagnostic and laboratory tests may be ordered to assist in diagnosis and treatment. The usual schedule of visits for prenatal care is listed below. A patient who exhibits complications is seen more frequently for closer monitoring.

- 0 to 28 weeks of gestation: Every 4 weeks
- 29 to 35 weeks: Every 2 weeks
- 36 weeks until delivery: Every week

The return prenatal visit also provides the opportunity for the provider and the medical assistant to lend support to the mother, to provide her with ongoing prenatal education to reduce apprehension and anxiety, and to ensure that the mother is well informed and prepared during her pregnancy, childbirth, and the postpartum period. The medical assistant plays an important role in prenatal education and should take the necessary time with each patient to provide appropriate information and to allow the patient to ask questions. outlines the medical assistant's role in the return prenatal visit.

The patient is asked to provide a urine specimen during each return prenatal visit. The medical assistant is responsible for testing the specimen for glucose and protein using a reagent strip and for documenting results in the prenatal record. A positive reaction to glucose may indicate the development of gestational diabetes mellitus or a prediabetic condition, and a positive reaction to protein may indicate a urinary tract infection or preeclampsia. Further testing usually is needed to arrive at a final diagnosis and to institute treatment. Hypertension is the most common medical disorder of pregnancy. Because of this, the medical assistant must make sure to obtain an accurate blood pressure measurement at each prenatal visit.

During the return visit, the provider performs one or more of the following procedures, depending on the stage of the pregnancy: (1) palpation of the woman's abdomen to measure fundal height, (2) measurement of the fetal heart rate, and (3) a vaginal examination. These procedures are discussed in detail next.

Fundal Height Measurement

The pregnant uterus rises gradually into the abdominal cavity, and the fundus is palpable between 8 and 13 weeks of gestation. The first fundal height measurement, which is usually performed during the first prenatal visit, is used as a guideline for all subsequent measurements. The provider measures the fundal height by placing one end of a flexible, nonstretchable centimeter tape measure on the superior aspect of the symphysis pubis and measuring to the crest or top of the uterine fundus (Fig. 23.11). The measurement is documented on a flow chart in the patient's prenatal record. By 20 weeks, the fundus reaches the lower border of the umbilicus, and between 36 and 37 weeks, it reaches the tip of the sternum. During the first and second trimesters, measuring the fundal height provides a rough estimate of

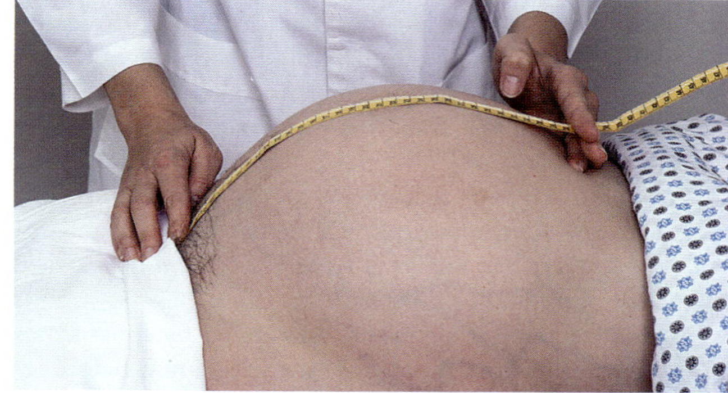

Fig. 23.11 Measurement of fundal height. The provider places one end of a centimeter tape measure on the superior aspect of the symphysis pubis and measures to the top of the uterine fundus. (From Ball JW, Dains JE, et al. *Seidel's Guide to Physical Examination: An Interprofessional Approach.* Elsevier; 2022.)

the duration of the pregnancy (Fig. 23.12). Because fetal weights vary considerably during the third trimester, it is difficult to use fundal height measurements as an estimate of the duration of the pregnancy in the last trimester.

In addition to assessing the duration of the pregnancy, the fundal height measurements permit variations from normal to become apparent and are used to assess whether fetal growth is progressing normally. Growth that is too rapid or too slow must be evaluated further by the provider as a possible indication of high-risk conditions, such as multiple pregnancies, polyhydramnios, ovarian tumor, intrauterine growth retardation, intrauterine death, or an error in estimating the fetal progress.

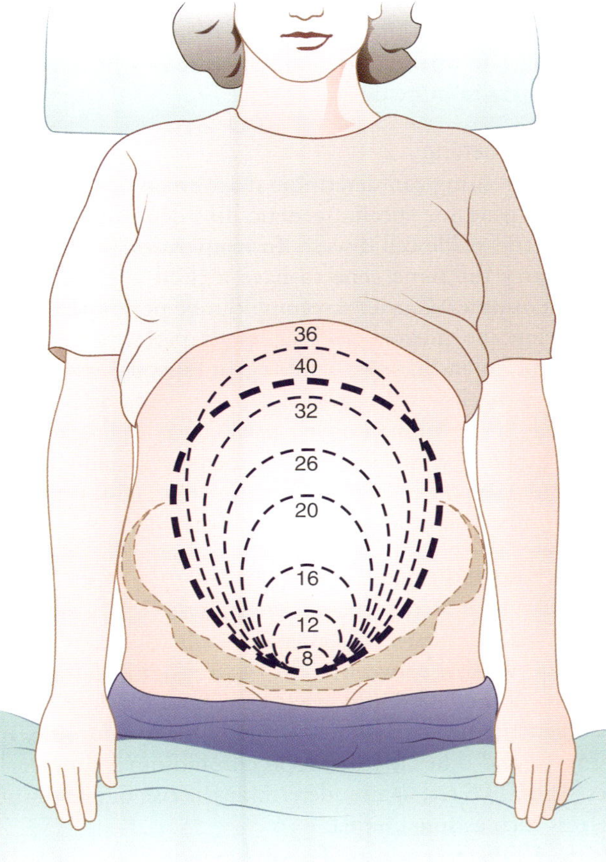

Fig. 23.12 Fundal height showing gestational age in weeks.

Fetal Heart Tones

Fetal heart tones refer to the heartbeat of the fetus as heard through the mother's abdominal wall and the **fetal heart rate** is the number of times per minute that the fetal heart beats. The normal range for the fetal heart rate is between 120 and 160 beats per minute with a regular rhythm. A very slow or rapid fetal heart rate usually indicates fetal distress. The fetal heart tones can be heard with a Doppler fetal pulse detector between 10 and 12 weeks of gestation. The Doppler fetal pulse detector converts ultrasonic waves into audible sounds of the fetal pulse.

The Doppler device consists of a main control unit and a probe (Fig. 23.13A). The probe head contains a transducer and electronic components, which generate the sound waves. The probe head is delicate and must be handled carefully, making sure not to drop or knock the head to prevent damaging it.

Because air is a poor conductor of sound, an ultrasound coupling gel must first be spread on the mother's abdomen in the area to be examined. The gel is usually applied by the medical assistant, and its purpose is to increase conductivity of the sound waves between the abdomen and the transducer.

The provider places the head of the probe into the gel on the mother's abdomen and slowly moves it until the fetal heart tones are located. The Doppler device amplifies the fetal heart tones, and they are broadcast through a built-in loudspeaker in the main unit. A volume control provides adjustment of the sound level as required. (Fetal heart tones sound like the hoofbeats of a galloping horse, and when the

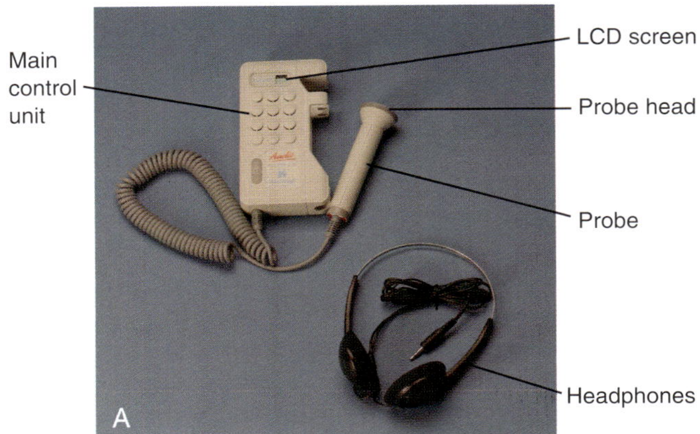

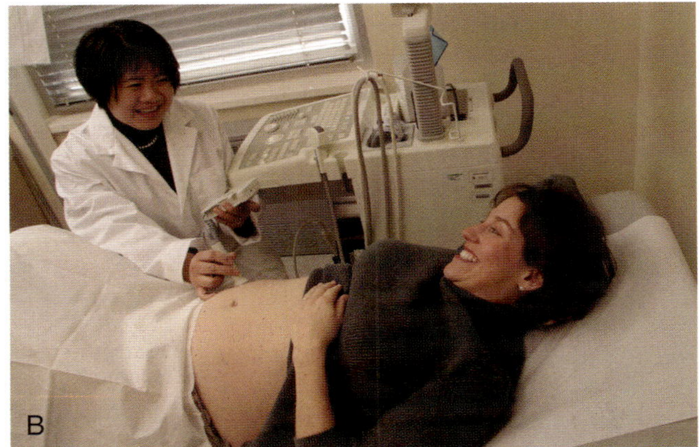

Fig. 23.13 (A) Parts of a Doppler device. (B) The probe of the Doppler device is moved across the abdomen to detect the fetal pulse.

probe is over the placenta, a windlike sound is heard.) The Doppler device also may have an LCD screen, which provides a digital display of the fetal heart rate. Headphones come with the Doppler device to allow private listening. The loudspeaker is muted when the headphones are connected (Fig. 23.13B).

After the procedure, the medical assistant should remove excess gel from the mother's abdomen with a paper towel. The probe head is cleaned using a damp cloth or a paper towel. The Doppler device should be properly stored in its carrying case to prevent it from becoming damaged.

Vaginal Examination

In the absence of vaginal bleeding, vaginal examinations may be performed at any time during the pregnancy; however, in a normal pregnancy, there is usually no need to perform a vaginal examination until the patient nears term. The vaginal examination is usually begun approximately 2 to 3 weeks from the EDD and is performed to confirm the presenting part and to determine the degree, if any, of cervical dilation and effacement. The purpose of dilation and effacement is to permit the passage of the infant from the uterus into the birth canal (Fig. 23.14).

What Would You Do? What Would You *Not* Do?

Case Study 4

Wynita Lopez is at the office with her husband following a prenatal visit. She is 36 years old and 14 weeks pregnant. It took Wynita a long time – almost 8 years – to get pregnant. She is excited and happy about being pregnant but, at the same time, upset and confused. Her test results on her first trimester prenatal screening test came back indicating an increased risk for Down syndrome. Wynita and her husband understand that the only way to know for sure is to have an amniocentesis. Wynita does not know what to do and cannot stop crying. She is afraid of having an amniocentesis because of the slight risk of miscarriage. Wynita and her husband are unsure what their decision would be if the baby did have Down syndrome. Her husband is visibly distressed and wants Wynita to be the one to decide whether or not to have an amniocentesis. Right now Wynita wants as much information as she can get about all of this before she makes a decision. ■

Special Tests and Procedures

The pregnancy can be evaluated with one or more of the following special tests and procedures: carrier screening, first trimester prenatal screening test, non-invasive prenatal test, multiple marker test, obstetric ultrasound scan, amniocentesis, and fetal heart rate monitoring. These are not considered routine tests and procedures; however, they involve a slight risk or no risk at all to the mother or the fetus. It is important for the medical assistant to have a general knowledge of these tests and procedures which are described next in more detail.

Carrier Screening

Carrier screening can determine if a woman or her partner carries a gene for specific genetic disorders such as cystic fibrosis and sickle cell disease. In many cases, both parents must carry the same gene to have a child affected with a genetic disorder. Carrier screening can be performed before or during the pregnancy. The test is performed using a blood specimen or tissue sample that is swabbed from inside the cheek. The provider often recommends carrier screening if the woman or her partner has a genetic disorder, has a child with a genetic disorder, has a family history of a genetic disorder, or belongs to an ethnic group that has an increased risk of a specific genetic disorder.

First Trimester Prenatal Screening Test

The first trimester prenatal screening (FTPS) test, also known as *Ultrascreen*, is a prenatal evaluation available to pregnant women between 11 to 14 weeks of gestation. The purpose of the FTPS is to assess the patient's risk of certain fetal genetic disorders which include Down syndrome, trisomy 18 and other less common chromosomal abnormalities. The FTPS test cannot determine the risk of neural tube defects such as spina bifida.

The FTPS test consists of a combination of the following two tests: (a) a blood test to measure a protein (pregnancy-associated protein A) and a hormone (human chorionic gonadotropin) present in the blood of a pregnant woman; and (b) an ultrasound to measure the fluid accumulation behind the neck of the fetus known as *nuchal translucency*. The FTPS is a screening test. Abnormal test results always necessitate further testing to determine whether a fetal abnormality actually exists, such as amniocentesis.

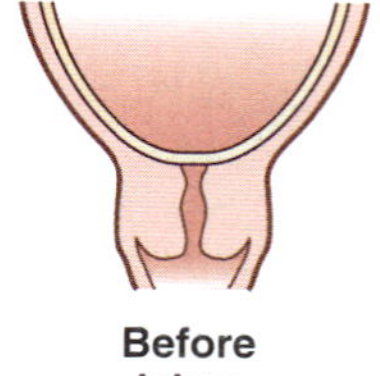

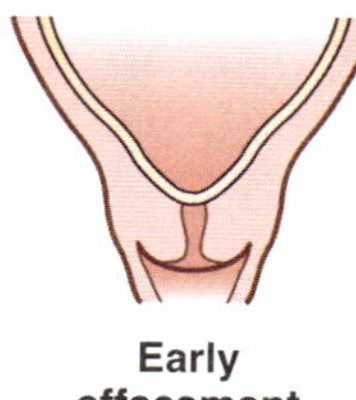

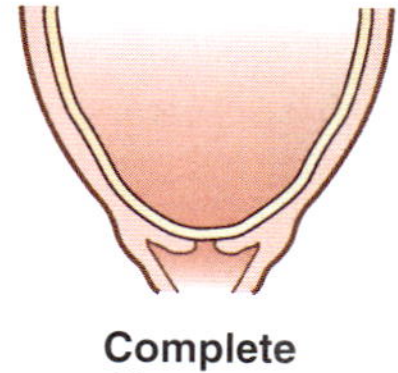

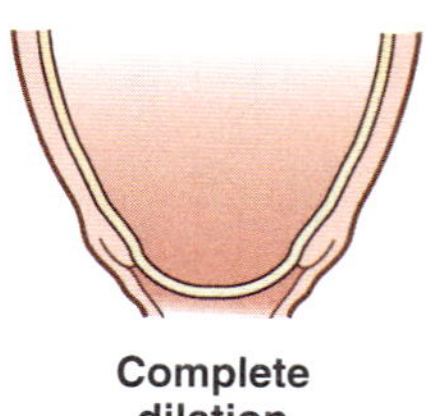

Fig. 23.14 Effacement and dilation occur to permit the passage of the infant into the birth canal. The cervical canal shortens from its normal length of 1 to 2 cm to a structure with paper thin edges in which there is no canal at all. The cervix dilates from an opening a few millimeters wide to an opening large enough to allow the passage of the infant (approximately 10 cm).

Non-Invasive Prenatal Test

The non-invasive prenatal test (NIPT), also known as *cell-free DNA test*, is a laboratory test used to assess whether a patient is at increased risk of having a fetus affected by certain genetic disorders. During pregnancy some of the DNA from the baby crosses into the mother's bloodstream. This DNA carries the baby's genetic information. This fetal DNA is tested to check for certain genetic disorders which include Down syndrome, trisomy 13, trisomy 18, and problems with the number of sex chromosomes. This test can also determine the gender of the baby. This NIPT can be performed as early as 9 to 10 weeks of gestation and up until delivery. The NIPT is a screening test. Abnormal test results always necessitate further testing, such as amniocentesis, to determine whether a fetal abnormality actually exists.

Multiple Marker Test

The multiple marker (quad screen) test is a laboratory test available to pregnant women between 15 and 20 weeks of gestation. Its purpose is to screen for the presence of certain fetal abnormalities, which include neural tube defects, Down syndrome, trisomy 18, and ventral wall defect. Because the multiple marker test has a high incidence of false-positive test results, it is not a mandatory prenatal test; however, the ACOG believes that this test should be offered to all pregnant women regardless of maternal age. The multiple marker test is a screening test. Abnormal test results always require further testing, such as amniocentesis, to determine whether a fetal abnormality actually exists.

Obstetric Ultrasound Scan

An obstetric ultrasound scan is a diagnostic imaging technique, similar to sonar, used to view the fetus in utero. It allows continuous viewing of the fetus and shows fetal movement. An ultrasound technologist usually performs the procedure. The primary purpose of an ultrasound scan is to evaluate the health of the fetus and to determine gestational age. This is accomplished by viewing the image of the fetus and by taking various measurements of the image, such as crown–rump length; biparietal diameter, which is a side-to-side measurement of the fetal head; femur length; and abdominal circumference. (Refer to Box 23.6 for various ultrasound images.)

Obstetric ultrasound scanning uses high-frequency sound waves that are directed into the uterus through a transducer. When the sound waves reach the uterus, they "bounce" back to the transducer, similar to an echo. These reflected sound waves are converted into an image, or *sonogram* (Fig. 23.15), which is displayed on a monitor screen. The monitor is positioned so the mother can view the image on the screen. There are two methods for performing an ultrasound scan: the transabdominal method and the endovaginal method.

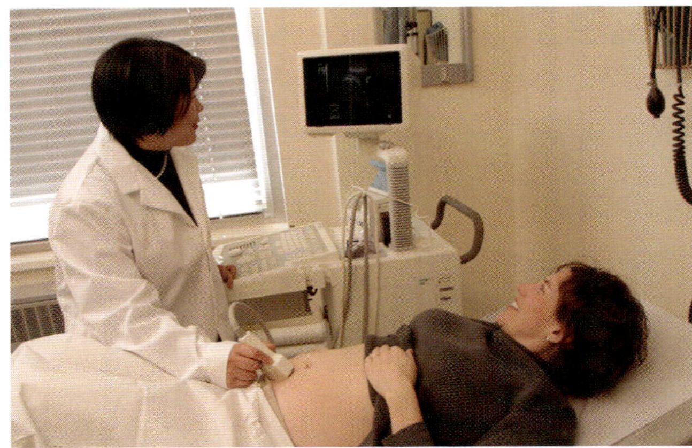

Fig. 23.15 Obstetric ultrasound scan.

Although an obstetric ultrasound scan can be performed at any time during the pregnancy, it is often performed at between 7 and 12 weeks of gestation and again at between 18 and 20 weeks. A third scan is sometimes done around 34 weeks of gestation. Box 23.6 outlines this schedule and what can be assessed at these times.

Transabdominal Ultrasound Scan

Transabdominal ultrasound is the scanning method performed most often. The patient must have a full bladder for this examination. This is accomplished by instructing the patient to consume 32 oz of fluid approximately 1 hour before the procedure. A full bladder acts as an "acoustic window" through which the sound waves can travel to provide a clear visualization of the uterus. In addition, a full bladder holds the uterus stable and pushes away any bowel that might interfere with the image. The patient lies on an examining table in a supine position and is draped with the abdomen exposed. A coupling agent, in the form of a liquid gel, is applied to the patient's abdomen to increase the transmission of the sound waves. An abdominal probe (containing a transducer) is placed into the gel, and the probe is moved slowly over the patient's abdomen; the image of the fetus is displayed on the screen of the monitor.

Three-dimensional and four-dimensional (3-D and 4-D) ultrasound are types of transabdominal ultrasound. A 3-D ultrasound exam takes thousands of images at once. These images are formatted into a 3-D image which looks more lifelike (refer to Box 23.6). A 4-D image is similar to a 3-D image, but it also shows movement, such as the baby kicking or the opening and closing of the eyes of the baby.

Endovaginal Ultrasound Scan

In the early stages of the pregnancy (up to 12 weeks), endovaginal scanning is preferred over transabdominal scanning. The patient must have an empty bladder for this scan, which makes the examination more comfortable. The patient is placed in the lithotomy position, and a vaginal probe is placed in the patient's vagina. The image of the embryo is displayed on the screen of the monitor. An endovaginal ultrasound scan provides clearer visualization of the uterus at the beginning of the pregnancy because the probe is situated in the vagina, which places it closer to the uterus.

BOX 23.6 Purpose of Obstetric Ultrasound Scanning

1. Between 7 and 12 Weeks

- To confirm pregnancy by detecting fetal heart motion
- To determine gestational age by taking measurements of the embryo and embryonic sac
- To measure nuchal translucency
- To detect an ectopic pregnancy

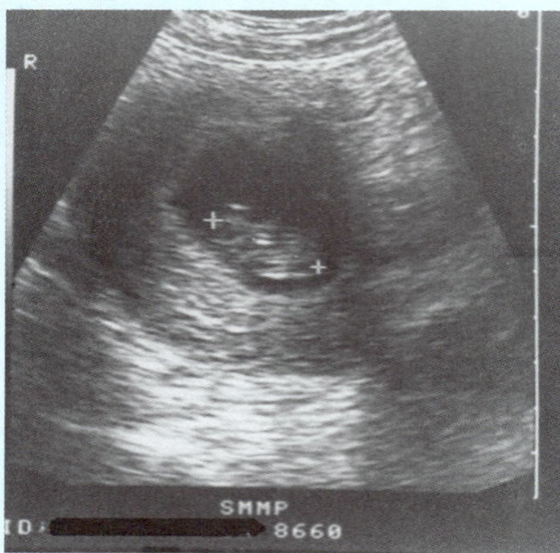

Embryo at approximately 9 weeks of gestation. (From Greer I, Cameron I, Kitchner H, et al: *Mosby's color atlas and text of obstetrics and gynecology*, St. Louis, 2001, Mosby.)

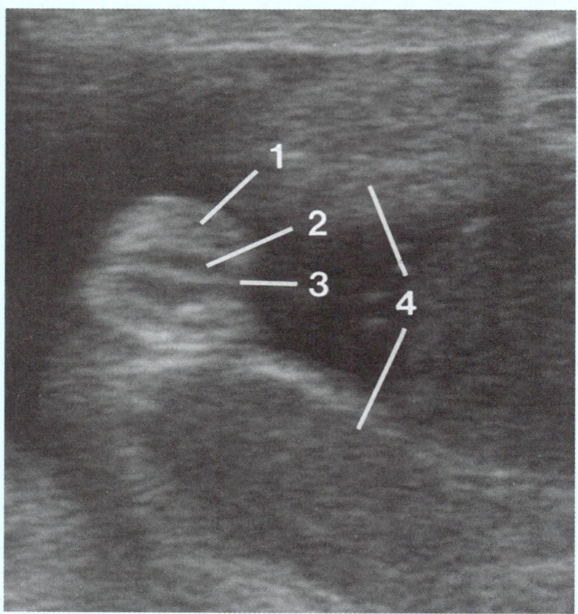

External female genitalia. *1*, major labium; *2*, minor labium; *3*, vaginal cleft; *4*, thighs. (From Callen P: *Ultrasonography in obstetrics and gynecology*, ed 4, Philadelphia, 2000, Saunders.)

2. Between 18 and 20 Weeks

- To determine fetal growth, size, and weight by taking measurements of the fetus
- To detect the presence of multiple fetuses
- To examine the brain, spinal cord, heart, lungs, gastrointestinal tract, reproductive organs, kidneys, bladder, bowel, and extremities of the fetus
- To detect congenital abnormalities
- To determine the location of the placenta
- To determine the cause of bleeding or spotting
- To determine if the fetus is male or female.

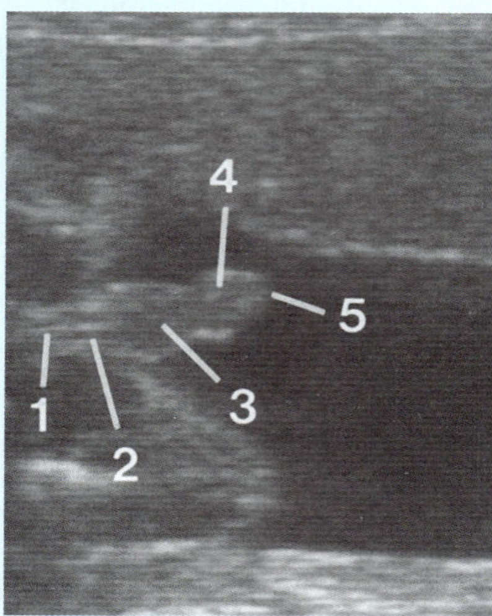

Erect fetal penis. *1*, urethra; *2*, corpus cavernosum; *3*, shaft; *4*, glans; *5*, foreskin. (From Callen P: *Ultrasonography in obstetrics and gynecology*, ed 4, Philadelphia, 2000, Saunders.)

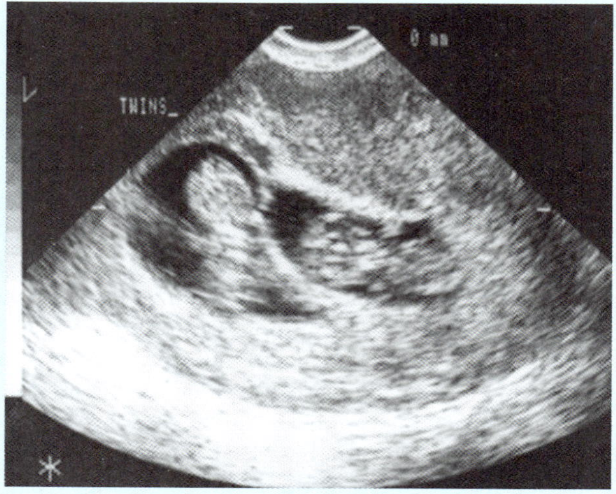

Sonogram of twins. (From Greer I, Cameron IT, Kitchener HC, Prentice, A: *Mosby's color atlas and text of obstetrics and gynecology*, St. Louis, 2001, Mosby.)

3. At 34 Weeks

- To evaluate fetal growth, size, and weight by taking measurements of the fetus
- To verify the location of the placenta
- To confirm fetal presentation in uncertain cases

4. Other Purposes

- To diagnose uterine and pelvic abnormalities during pregnancy
- To view the fetus, placenta, and amniotic fluid during tests such as amniocentesis and chorionic villus sampling
- To confirm intrauterine death

BOX 23.6 Purpose of Obstetric Ultrasound Scanning—cont'd

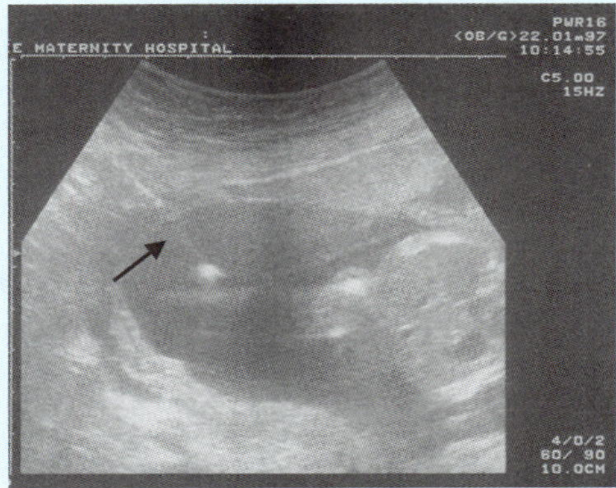

Amniocentesis being performed under ultrasound guidance. (From Greer I, Cameron I, Kitchner H, et al: *Mosby's color atlas and text of obstetrics and gynecology*, St. Louis, 2001, Mosby.)

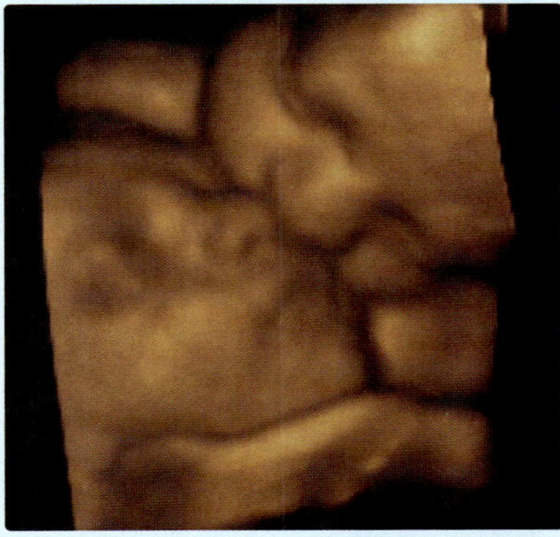

Three-dimensional ultrasound examination. (From Andonotopo W, Zumendi GA, Salihagic-Kadic A, KurjakA: *YMOB*, St. Louis, 2007, Mosby.)

Amniocentesis

Amniocentesis is a diagnostic procedure that can be performed between 15 and 18 weeks of gestation. Amniocentesis aids in prenatal diagnosis of certain genetically transmitted errors of metabolism, congenital abnormalities, and chromosomal disorders such as Down syndrome. It also is used to detect fetal jeopardy or distress and, later in the pregnancy, to assess fetal lung maturity. Amniocentesis also can determine whether the fetus is a boy or a girl.

To perform the procedure, the provider inserts a long, thin needle through the mother's abdomen and into the amniotic sac surrounding the fetus (Fig. 23.16 and Box 23.6). An obstetric ultrasound scan is always performed in conjunction with amniocentesis so that the provider can view the position of the fetus, placenta, and amniotic fluid. This allows the provider to know the exact place to insert the needle. The provider withdraws a sample (about 1 tablespoon) of fluid, which contains fetal cells. The fluid is sent to a laboratory for study. It usually takes 1 to 3 weeks to evaluate the amniotic fluid and report the results.

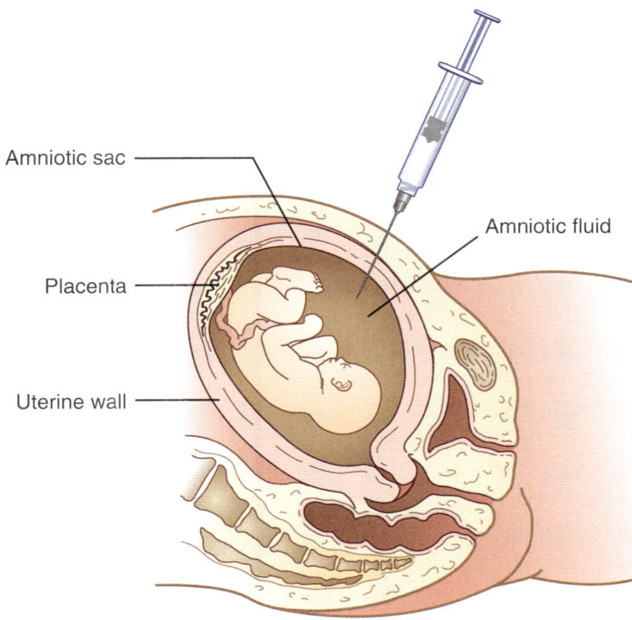

Fig. 23.16 Amniocentesis.

Although the complication rate for an amniocentesis is extremely low, the procedure is not risk free. There is a slight risk of bleeding, leakage of fluid, and infection of the amniotic fluid. There also is a slight possibility (less than 1%) of miscarriage. Because of these risks, amniocentesis is offered only to women whose pregnancies are at risk for fetal abnormalities. This includes women who are 35 years old or older, women who have a child with a genetic or neural tube defect, women who have abnormal multiple marker test results, women who have or whose partner has a chromosomal abnormality, and women who are or whose partner is a carrier for a metabolic disease.

Fetal Heart Rate Monitoring

Fetal heart rate (FHR) monitoring is performed later in the pregnancy to obtain information on the physical condition of the fetus. Specific conditions that may warrant this procedure are fetal growth that is not progressing well, decreased amniotic fluid, decreased fetal activity, elevation of the mother's blood pressure, gestational diabetes, and an overdue infant.

To perform the procedure, an electronic microphone is strapped to the mother's abdomen to amplify the fetal heartbeat. A gel is usually applied under the microphone to make the sounds clearer. The fetal heartbeat is heard and displayed on a screen and printed on special paper. There are two kinds of fetal heart rate monitoring procedures: the nonstress test and the contraction stress test.

Nonstress Test (NST): The NST monitors changes in the fetal heart rate in response to the fetus' spontaneous movements. The mother is instructed to press a button when she feels the fetus move. In a normal test, the fetus' heart rate increases when the fetus moves. To prepare for the NST, the mother must be instructed to eat a light meal within 2 hours of the procedure to stimulate fetal movement.

Contraction Stress Test (CST): If the results of the NST are abnormal, a CST may be performed. This test is similar to the NST except that mild contractions of the uterus are stimulated for a short period of time. The CST is used to evaluate the response of the fetus' heart rate to the contractions to determine whether the fetus would be able to withstand the stress of repeated contractions during labor. If the results of the test are abnormal, further evaluation is required to evaluate the well-being of the fetus and to determine how and when delivery of the fetus should be carried out.

MEDICAL ASSISTING RESPONSIBILITIES

The medical assistant has many important responsibilities during the return prenatal examination, which are outlined in Procedure 23.1. The medical assistant is responsible for assembling the equipment and supplies required for the examination, for obtaining information to update the prenatal record, for preparing the patient for the examination, and for assisting the provider during the examination. The provider depends on the medical assistant to have the urine test results and certain measurements, such as blood pressure and weight, completed and documented in advance to allow the provider the opportunity to review these measurements before examining the patient.

What Would You Do? What Would You *Not* Do? RESPONSES

Case Study 1

Page 497

What Did Yin-Ling Do?

- ❑ Reassured Mrs. Wooster that the physician is there to help her and emphasized that he will be pleased that she has come to the office for a gynecological examination.
- ❑ Commended Mrs. Wooster for paying attention to changes in her breasts.
- ❑ Told Mrs. Wooster that some breast changes are normal and others are not normal, and the only way to know for sure is to be seen by the physician.
- ❑ Told Mrs. Wooster that it is important to have a periodic gynecologic examination and recommended screening mammograms even if her periods are normal. Explained to her that some conditions can be present without symptoms. Gave Mrs. Wooster a patient information brochure on gynecologic examinations and mammography.
- ❑ Took plenty of time with Mrs. Wooster so that she would feel comfortable coming back again in the future for a gynecologic examination.

What Did Yin-Ling* Not *Do?

- ❑ Did not criticize Mrs. Wooster for never having a mammogram and waiting so long to schedule a gynecologic examination.

Case Study 2

Page 512

What Did Yin-Ling Do?

- ❑ Stressed to Brooke how important it is that she be seen by the physician. Explained that she could be infected with chlamydia and not know it because chlamydia often has no symptoms, especially in women.
- ❑ Explained to Brooke that state law allows her to give consent to be tested and treated for a sexually transmitted infection without permission from her parents. Told her the law was created to encourage minors to seek treatment for sexually transmitted infections.
- ❑ Commended Brooke on practicing safe sex. Relayed to her that if a condom is not used correctly, or if it tears, she might not be protected from getting a sexually transmitted infection. That is another reason she should be tested.
- ❑ Calmly explained to Brooke what occurs during the examination. Relayed techniques that Brooke could use to relax during the procedure.

What Did Yin-Ling* Not *Do?

- ❑ Did not tell Brooke everything would be all right and that she probably does not have chlamydia.
- ❑ Did not try to prevent Brooke from leaving if she still insists on doing so.

Case Study 3

Page 520

What Did Yin-Ling Do?

- ❑ Tried to calm Johanna by telling her that it is normal for her to be worried and concerned. Explained that the purpose of her prenatal visits is so that the physician can keep a close watch on her and detect any problems that might occur.
- ❑ Reassured Johanna that she does not need to be afraid to tell the physician any of her concerns because he is there to help her and her baby.
- ❑ Told Johanna that it is important not to take any medications during her pregnancy without first checking with the physician because some medications could be harmful to her baby.
- ❑ Told Johanna that her problems and concerns would be relayed to the physician and that he would want to talk to her about them. Explained that the physician also would talk with her about being tested for group B streptococcus.

What Would You Do? What Would You *Not* Do? RESPONSES—cont'd

What Did Yin-Ling* Not *Do?

- Did not tell Johanna that it was all right to take the antibiotics.
- Did not tell Johanna that her neighbor should have gotten better prenatal care.

Case Study 4

Page 524

What Did Yin-Ling Do?

- Escorted Mr. and Mrs. Lopez to a private room in the office. Tried to relax them and told them that whatever they choose to do will be the right decision for them.
- Gave Mrs. Lopez the information she requested that was available at the office and provided her with a list of resources approved by the physician that she could contact for further information.
- Asked Mr. and Mrs. Lopez whether they had any more questions they wanted to ask the physician.
- Made the physician aware of the anxiety that Mr. and Mrs. Lopez are experiencing.

What Did Yin-Ling* Not *Do?

- Did not give Mr. and Mrs. Lopez advice on what they should do.

TERMINOLOGY REVIEW

Medical Term	Word Parts	Definition
Abortion		The termination of the pregnancy before the fetus reaches the age of viability (20 weeks).
Amenorrhea	*a-:* without *men/o:* menstruation- *orrhea:* flow, excessive discharge	The absence or cessation of the menstrual period. Amenorrhea occurs normally before puberty, during pregnancy, and after menopause.
Braxton Hicks contractions		Intermittent and irregular painless uterine contractions that occur throughout pregnancy. They occur more frequently toward the end of pregnancy and are sometimes mistaken for true labor pains.
Cervix		The lower narrow end of the uterus that opens into the vagina.
Colposcopy	*colp/o:* vagina- *scopy:* visual examination	Examination of the cervix using a colposcope (a lighted instrument with a magnifying lens).
Cytology	*cyt/o:* cell- *ology:* study of	The science that deals with the study of cells, including their origin, structure, function, and pathology.
Dilation (of the cervix)		The stretching of the external os from an opening a few millimeters wide to an opening large enough to allow the passage of an infant (approximately 10 cm).
Dysmenorrhea	*dys-:* difficult, painful, abnormal *men/o:* menstruation *-orrhea:* flow, excessive discharge	Pain associated with the menstrual period.
Dyspareunia	*dys-:* difficult, painful, abnormal	Pain in the vagina or pelvis experienced by a woman during sexual intercourse.
Dysplasia	*dys-:* difficult, painful, abnormal *plasia:* a growth	The growth of abnormal cells. Dysplasia is a precancerous condition that may or may not develop into cancer.
Ectocervix	*ecto-:* outside, outer	The outermost layer of the cervix that projects into the vagina.
Effacement		The thinning and shortening of the cervical canal from its normal length of 1 to 2 cm to a structure with paper-thin edges in which there is no canal at all. Effacement occurs late in pregnancy, during labor, or both. The purpose of effacement along with dilation is to permit the passage of the infant into the birth canal.
Embryo		The child in utero from the time of conception through the first 8 weeks of development.
Endocervix	*endo-:* within	The inner part of the cervix that forms a narrow canal that connects the vagina to the uterus.

Continued

TERMINOLOGY REVIEW—cont'd

Medical Term	Word Parts	Definition
Engagement		The entrance of the fetal head or the presenting part into the pelvic inlet.
Expected date of delivery (EDD)		Projected birth date of the infant.
External os		The opening of the cervical canal of the uterus into the vagina.
Fetal heart rate		The number of times per minute the fetal heart beats.
Fetal heart tones		The sounds of the heartbeat of the fetus heard through the mother's abdominal wall.
Fetus		The child in utero from the third month after conception to birth; during the first 2 months of development, it is called an *embryo.*
Fundus		The dome-shaped upper portion of the uterus between the fallopian tubes.
Gestation		The period of intrauterine development from conception to birth; the period of pregnancy. The average pregnancy lasts about 280 days, or 40 weeks, from the date of conception to childbirth.
Gestational age		The age of the fetus between conception and birth.
Gynecology	*gynec/o:* woman *-ology:* study of	The branch of medicine that deals with health maintenance and diseases of the female reproductive system.
Infant		A child from birth to 12 months of age.
Menopause	*men/o:* menstruation	The permanent cessation of menstruation, which usually occurs between the ages of 45 and 55.
Menorrhagia	*men/o:* menstruation *-orrhagia:* rapid flow of blood	Excessive bleeding during a menstrual period, in the number of days or the amount of blood or both. Also called *dysfunctional uterine bleeding* (DUB).
Metrorrhagia	*metr/o:* uterus *-orrhagia:* rapid flow of blood	Bleeding between menstrual periods.
Multigravida	*multi-:* many *gravid/o:* pregnancy	A woman who has been pregnant more than once.
Multipara	*multi-:* many *par/o:* bear, give birth to	A woman who has completed two or more pregnancies to the age of fetal viability regardless of whether they ended in live infants or stillbirths.
Nullipara	*nulli-:* none *par/o:* bear, give birth to	A woman who has not carried a pregnancy to the point of fetal viability (20 weeks of gestation).
Obstetrics		The branch of medicine concerned with the care of the woman during pregnancy, childbirth, and the puerperium.
Perimenopause	*peri-:* surrounding *men/o:* menstruation	Before the onset of menopause, the phase during which the woman with regular periods changes to irregular cycles and increased periods of amenorrhea.
Perineum		The external region between the vaginal orifice and the anus in a female and between the scrotum and the anus in a male.
Position		The relation of the presenting part of the fetus to the maternal pelvis.
Postpartum	*post-:* after *par/o:* bear, give birth to	Occurring after childbirth.
Preeclampsia		A major complication of pregnancy, the cause of which is unknown, characterized by increasing hypertension, albuminuria, and edema. If this condition is neglected or is not treated properly, it may develop into eclampsia, which could cause maternal convulsions and coma. Preeclampsia generally occurs between the 20th week of pregnancy and the end of the first week postpartum.
Prenatal	*pre-:* in front of, before *nat/o:* birth *-al:* pertaining to	Before birth.
Presentation		Indication of the part of the fetus that is closest to the cervix and is delivered first. A cephalic presentation is a delivery in which the fetal head is presenting against the cervix. A breech presentation is a delivery in which the buttocks or feet are presented instead of the head.
Primigravida	*prim/i:* first *gravid/o:* pregnancy	A woman who is pregnant for the first time.

TERMINOLOGY REVIEW—cont'd

Medical Term	Word Parts	Definition
Primipara	*prim/i:* first *par/o:* bear, give birth to	A woman who has carried a pregnancy to fetal viability (20 weeks of gestation) for the first time regardless of whether the infant was stillborn or alive at birth.
Puerperium		The period of time, usually 4 to 6 weeks after delivery, in which the uterus and the body systems are returning to normal.
Quickening		The first movements of the fetus in utero as felt by the mother, which usually occur between 16 and 20 weeks of gestation and are felt consistently thereafter.
Risk factor		Anything that increases an individual's chance of developing a disease. Some risk factors (e.g., smoking) can be avoided, but others cannot (e.g., age and family history).
Toxemia		A condition that can occur in pregnant women that includes preeclampsia nd eclampsia. If preeclampsia goes undiagnosed or is not satisfactorily controlled, it could develop into eclampsia, characterized by convulsions and coma.
Trimester	*tri-:* three	Three months, or one third, of the gestational period of pregnancy.
Vulva		The region of the external female genital organs.

PROCEDURE 23.1 Assisting with a Gynecologic Examination

Outcome
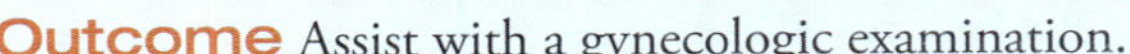
Assist with a gynecologic examination.

The following procedure describes the medical assistant's role in assisting with a gynecologic examination consisting of breast and pelvic examinations, including a liquid-based Pap test and a fecal occult blood test.

Equipment/Supplies

- Disposable gloves
- Examining gown and drape
- Disposable vaginal speculum
- Collection vial (ThinPrep, SurePath)
- Plastic cytospatula and cytobrush or cytobroom
- Water-based lubricant
- Gauze pads
- Fecal occult blood test
- Tissues
- Cytology request form
- Biohazard specimen transport bag

1. **Procedural Step.** Sanitize your hands.
2. **Procedural Step.** Assemble the equipment. Complete as much of the cytology request form as possible. Some information on the form, such as the last menstrual period (LMP), requires input from the patient and must be completed later.

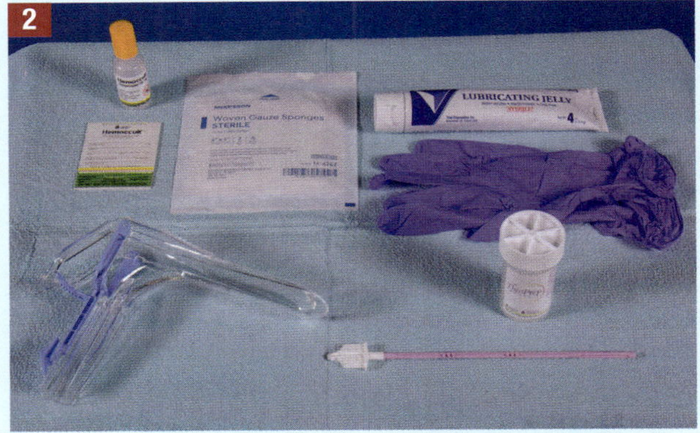

Assemble the equipment

Continued

PROCEDURE 23.1 Assisting with a Gynecologic Examination—cont'd

3. **Procedural Step.** Check the expiration date on the specimen vial. Label the vial with the date and the patient's name, date of birth, and identification number. The identification number is located on the cytology request form.
   Principle. If the vial is outdated, it should be discarded because it may lead to inaccurate test results.
4. **Procedural Step.** Greet the patient and introduce yourself.
5. **Procedural Step.** Escort the patient to the examining room and ask her to be seated. Identify the patient. Seat yourself so that you are facing the patient. Ask the patient whether she has any problems or concerns, and document this information in the patient's medical record. Ask the patient the necessary questions to complete the rest of the cytology request form.
6. **Procedural Step.** Measure the patient's vital signs, height, and weight, and document the results in the patient's medical record.
7. **Procedural Step.** Instruct and prepare the patient for the examination as follows:
   a. Ask the patient whether she needs to empty the bladder before the examination. If a urine specimen is needed, instruct the patient in the proper collection of the specimen.
   b. Provide the patient with a patient gown. Instruct the patient to remove all clothing and to put on the patient gown with the opening in front. If the patient is wearing socks, tell her she can keep them on. Offer assistance if you sense the patient may have trouble undressing.

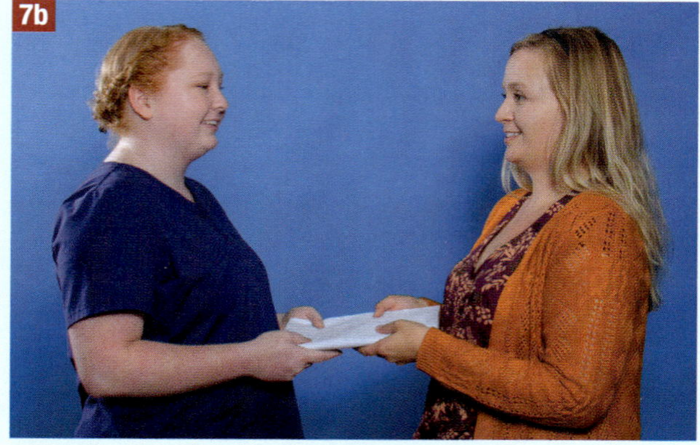

7b

Instruct and prepare the patient for the examination.

   c. Tell the patient to have a seat on the examining table after she has put on the examining gown.
   d. Leave the room to give the patient privacy.

   Principle. An empty bladder makes the examination easier and is more comfortable for the patient. Wearing socks helps keep the patient's feet warm during the examination.
8. **Procedural Step.** Check to make sure the patient is ready to be seen by the provider. Before entering the room, always knock lightly on the door to let the patient know you are getting ready to enter the room. Inform the provider that the patient is ready. This may be done using a color-coded flagging system mounted on the wall next to the examining room.
9. **Procedural Step.** Assist the patient into a supine position if a clinical breast exam is being performed. Properly drape the patient for the breast examination.
10. **Procedural Step.** Assist the patient into the lithotomy position for the pelvic examination.
11. **Procedural Step.** Prepare the vaginal speculum by thinly lubricating the blades of the speculum with a water-based lubricant. Never apply lubricant to the tip of the speculum.
    Principle. Lubricating the vaginal speculum facilitates its insertion into the vagina.
12. **Procedural Step.** Prepare the light for the provider as follows:
    a. *Overhead examination lamp:* Adjust and focus the light for the provider.
    b. *Speculum-illumination system:* Snap the light source device into the light holder on the vaginal speculum and turn it on. The lighting system produces a beam of light that shines through the blades of the speculum for visualization of the vagina and cervix.
    Principle. Visualization of the vagina and cervix requires direct light.
13. **Procedural Step.** Hand the vaginal speculum to the provider. Reassure the patient, and help her relax the abdominal muscles during the examination by telling her to breathe deeply, slowly, and evenly through the mouth.
    Principle. If the patient is relaxed, the examination proceeds more smoothly and is more comfortable for her.
14. **Procedural Step.** Apply gloves, and assist with the collection of the Pap specimen.
15. **Procedural Step.** Collect a specimen for ThinPrep using the cytospatula and cytobrush method:
    (1) Remove the cap from the ThinPrep vial, and hold it so that the provider can insert the cytospatula into the vial.
    (2) Rinse the plastic cytospatula in the liquid preservative by vigorously swirling it around in the solution 10 times.

PROCEDURE 23.1 Assisting with a Gynecologic Examination—cont'd

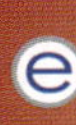

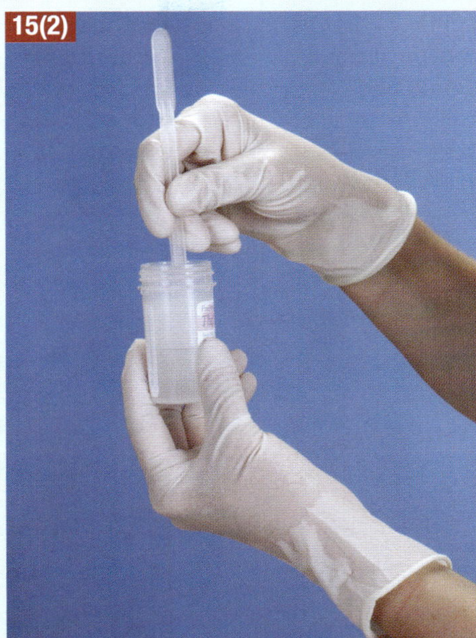

Vigorously swirl the cytospatula in the preservative.

(3) Discard the cytospatula in a biohazard waste container.
(4) Hold the vial so that the provider can insert the cytobrush into the vial.
(5) Rinse the cytobrush in the liquid preservative by vigorously rotating it in the solution 10 times while pushing the cytobrush against the vial wall. Swirl the cytobrush in the solution to further release cellular material.

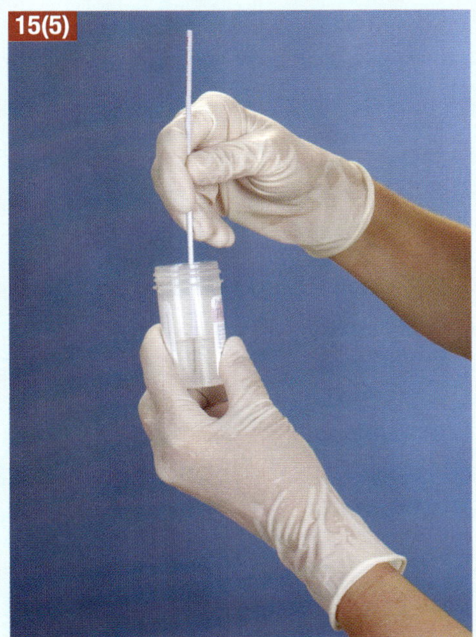

Rotate the cytobrush in the preservative.

(6) Discard the cytobrush in a biohazard waste container. Securely tighten the cap so that the torque line on the cap passes the torque line on the vial.

16. **Procedural Step.** Collect a specimen for ThinPrep using the cytobroom method.
(1) Remove the cap from the ThinPrep vial and hold it so that the provider can insert the cytobroom into the vial.
(2) Rinse the cytobroom in the liquid preservative by pushing the cytobroom vigorously into the bottom of the vial 10 times. This motion forces the cytobroom bristles apart, releasing cervical cells into the solution. Swirl the cytobroom vigorously in the liquid preservative to further release cellular material.

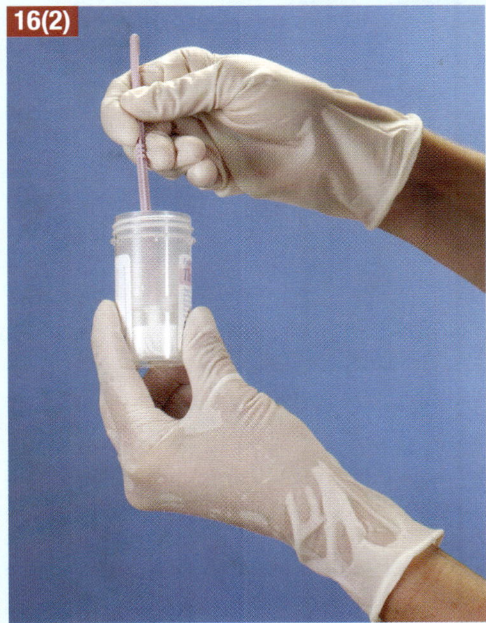

Push the cytobroom vigorously into the bottom of the vial.

(3) Discard the cytobroom in a biohazard waste container. Tighten the cap so that the torque line on the cap passes the torque line on the vial.

17. **Procedural Step.** Collect a specimen for SurePath.
(1) Remove the cap from the SurePath vial, and hold it so that the provider can insert the collection device into the vial.
(2) Break off (cytospatula and cytobrush method) or disconnect the tip (cytobroom method) of the collection device from the handle.
(3) Discard the handle of the collection device in a waste container.
(4) Repeat the above steps until the provider has collected all of the specimens needed for the Pap test.
(5) Securely tighten the cap on the vial.

Continued

PROCEDURE 23.1 Assisting with a Gynecologic Examination—cont'd

18. Procedural Step. Turn off the examining lamp or disconnect the light source from the vaginal speculum. Discard the disposable vaginal speculum in a biohazard waste container. Apply lubricant to a gauze square. Hold it out so that the provider can apply lubricant to their gloves to perform the bimanual and rectal–vaginal examinations. Assist with the collection of the fecal specimen for the fecal occult blood test.

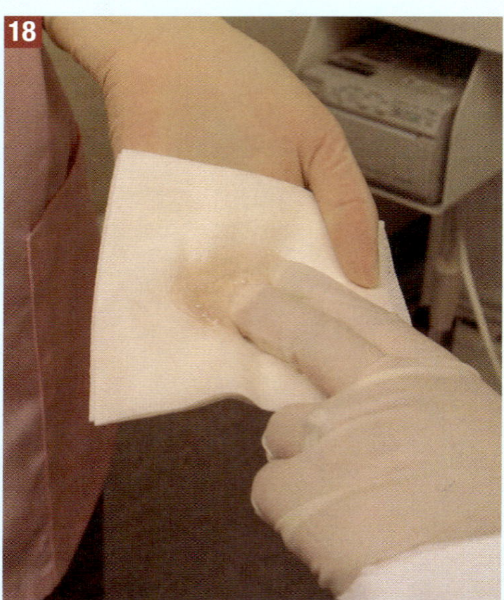

18 Hold the gauze with the lubricant for the provider.

Principle. Applying lubricant to a gauze square (rather than directly to the provider's gloved fingers) prevents the opening of the tube of lubricant from touching the provider's gloves and contaminating the contents of the tube.

19. Procedural Step. After the examination, assist the patient into a sitting position, and allow her the opportunity to rest for a moment. Offer the patient tissues to remove excess lubricant from the perineum. Assist the patient off the examining table.

Principle. Some patients (especially the elderly) become dizzy after lying on the examining table and should be allowed to rest after sitting up.

20. Procedural Step. Instruct the patient to get dressed. Tell the patient how and when she will be notified of the Pap test results.

21. Procedural Step. Test the fecal occult blood specimen, and document the results in the patient's medical record.

22. Procedural Step. Prepare the Pap specimen for transport to the laboratory. Place the vial in a biohazard specimen transport bag and seal the bag. Insert the cytology requisition into the outside pocket of the bag and tuck the top of the requisition under the flap. Place the bag in the appropriate location for pickup by the laboratory.

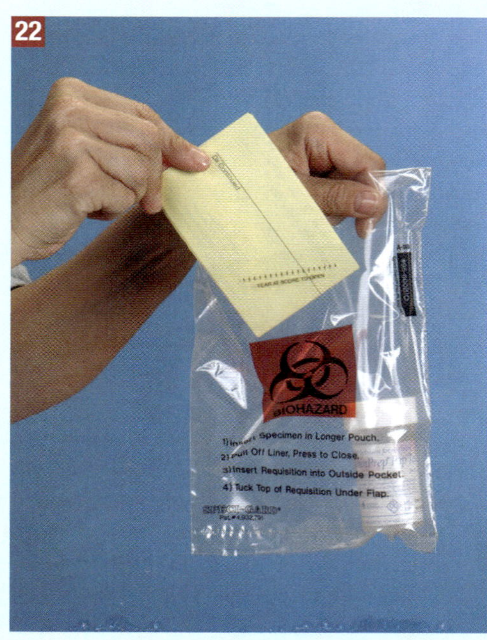

22 Insert the laboratory request into the outside pocket.

23. Procedural Step. Document the transport of the specimen to an outside laboratory in the patient's medical record.

23

DOCUMENTATION EXAMPLE

Date	
9/7/XX	10:00 a.m. Hemoccult: negative.
	ThinPrep Pap specimen to Medical Center
	Laboratory for cytology. ______________
	______________ Y. Wu, RMA

24. Procedural Step. Clean the examining room.

PROCEDURE 23.2 Assisting with a Return Prenatal Examination

Outcome Assist with a return prenatal examination.

Equipment/Supplies

- Urine specimen container
- Centimeter tape measure
- Doppler fetal pulse detector
- Ultrasound coupling gel
- Paper towel
- Disposable vaginal speculum
- Disposable gloves
- Water-based lubricant
- Gauze pads
- Examining gown and drape

1. **Procedural Step.** Sanitize your hands.
2. **Procedural Step.** Set up the tray for the prenatal examination. The equipment and supplies depend on the procedures to be included in the examination, which may include one or more of the following:
   a. Fundal height measurement
   b. Measurement of fetal heart tones
   c. Examination of the legs, feet, and face for edema and development of varicosities
   d. Taking a specimen for the diagnosis of a vaginal infection
   e. Vaginal examination

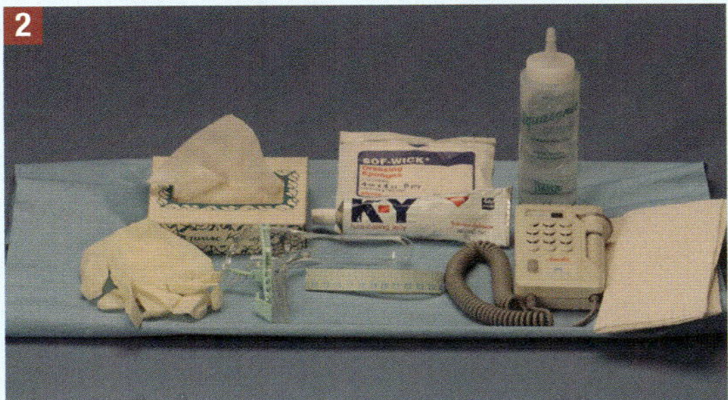

Set up the prenatal tray.

3. **Procedural Step.** Greet the patient and introduce yourself. Identify the patient and explain the procedure. Provide the patient with a urine specimen container, and ask her to obtain a urine specimen.
   Principle. A urine specimen is needed to test for glucose and protein at each prenatal visit. In addition, an empty bladder makes the examination easier and is more comfortable for the patient.
4. **Procedural Step.** Escort the patient to the examining room, and ask her to be seated. Seat yourself so that you are facing the patient. Ask the patient whether she has experienced any problems since the last prenatal visit, and document information in the appropriate section in her prenatal record.
   Principle. The provider investigates any unusual or abnormal signs or symptoms relayed by the patient.
5. **Procedural Step.** Measure the patient's blood pressure, and document the results in the prenatal record. If the blood pressure is elevated, allow the patient to relax, and then measure the blood pressure again.
   Principle. Taking the blood pressure again gives you the opportunity to determine whether the elevation was due to emotional excitement.

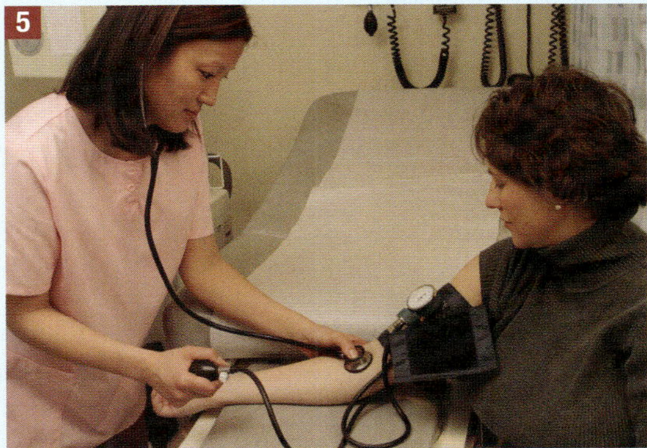

Measure the patient's blood pressure.

6. **Procedural Step.** Weigh the patient, and document the results in the prenatal record.
   Principle. Maternal weight gain or loss assists in assessing fetal development, as well as the mother's nutrition and state of health.

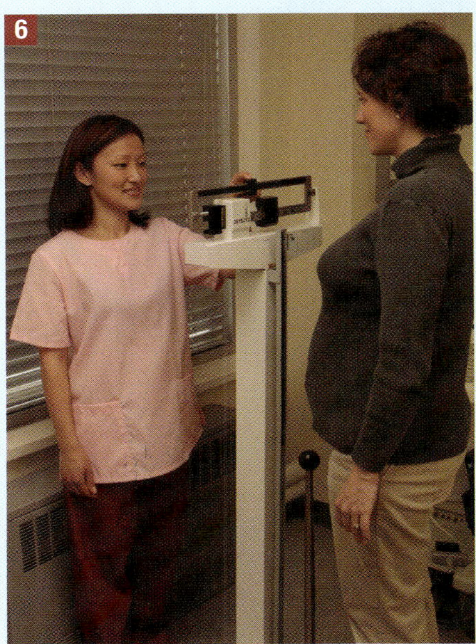

Weigh the patient.

Continued

PROCEDURE 23.2 Assisting with a Return Prenatal Examination—cont'd

7. **Procedural Step.** Instruct and prepare the patient for the examination. Have her remove or pull up her outer clothing to expose the abdominal area. If the provider will be performing a vaginal examination, the patient also must remove her panties; otherwise, she may leave them on. Tell the patient to have a seat on the examining table when she is finished getting ready for the examination. Leave the room to give the patient privacy.
8. **Procedural Step.** Using a reagent strip, test the urine specimen for glucose and protein, and document the results in the prenatal record. *Note:* The urine specimen may be tested at any time before the provider examines the patient; however, a convenient time to test the specimen is while the patient is disrobing.
   Principle. The prenatal patient's urine must be tested at every visit to assist in early detection and prevention of disease.
9. **Procedural Step.** Check to make sure the patient is ready to be seen by the provider. Before entering a patient's room, always knock lightly on the door to let the patient know you are getting ready to enter the room. Inform the provider. This may be done using a color-coded flagging system mounted on the wall next to the examining room.
10. **Procedural Step.** Assist the patient into a supine position, and properly drape her. Provide support and reassurance to the patient to help her relax during the examination.
    Principle. The patient should be properly draped so that she is warm and comfortable.
11. **Procedural Step.** Assist the provider as required for the prenatal examination, as follows:
    a. *Fundal height measurement:* Hand the provider the tape measure for determination of the fundal measurement.
    b. *Fetal heart tones:* Apply a liberal amount of coupling gel to the patient's abdomen. Turn on the Doppler fetal pulse detector and hand it to the provider. When the provider is finished, remove excess gel from the patient with a paper towel. Clean the probe head of the Doppler device with a damp cloth or a paper towel. Place the probe head back in its holder.

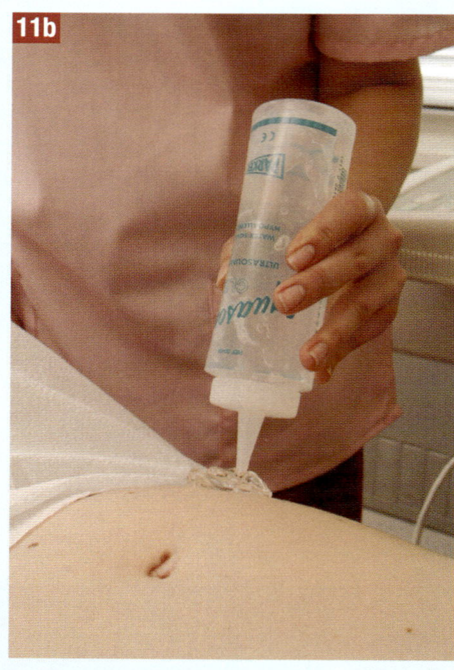

Apply a liberal amount of coupling gel.

    c. *Vaginal specimen:* Assist the patient into the lithotomy position if a specimen is to be taken for the detection of a vaginal infection. Assist with collection of the specimen as required.
    d. *Vaginal examination:* Assist the patient into the lithotomy position if a vaginal examination is to be performed.
12. **Procedural Step.** After the examination, assist the patient into a sitting position, and allow her the opportunity to rest for a moment. If a vaginal examination was performed, offer the patient tissues to remove excess lubricating jelly from the perineum. Assist her off the examining table to prevent falls. Instruct the patient to get dressed. Leave the room to provide the patient with privacy.

PROCEDURE 23.2 Assisting with a Return Prenatal Examination—cont'd

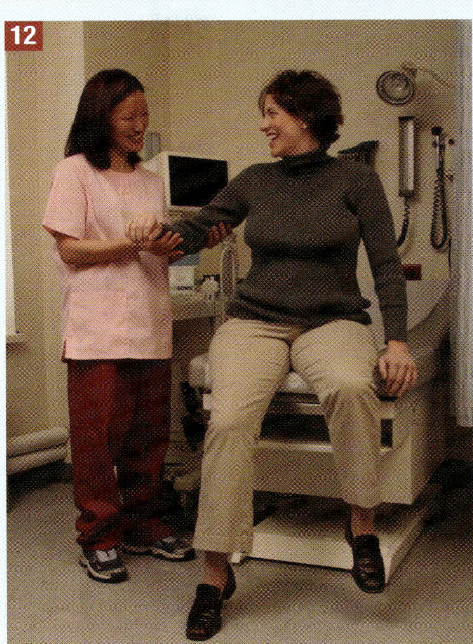

Assist the patient off the examining table.

Principle. The patient may become dizzy after being on the examining table and should be allowed to rest before getting off the table. The medical assistant must provide for the safety of the prenatal patient while she is getting off the examining table.

13. **Procedural Step.** Provide the prenatal patient with educational materials and further explanation of the provider's instructions as required to meet individual patient needs. Escort the patient to the reception area.
14. **Procedural Step.** Clean the examining room in preparation for the next patient, and, if necessary, prepare specimens for transport to an outside medical laboratory.

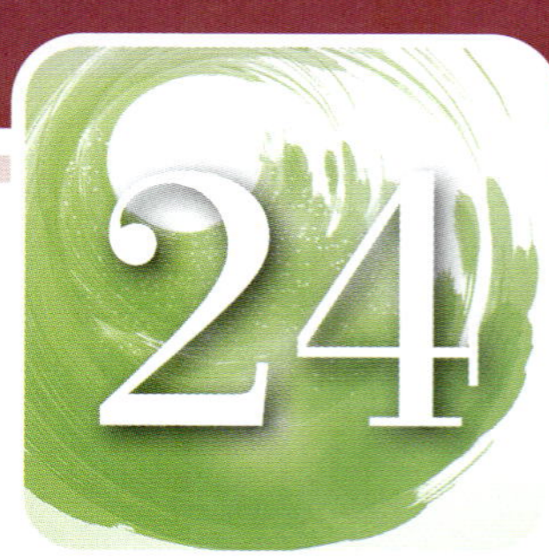

24 The Pediatric Examination

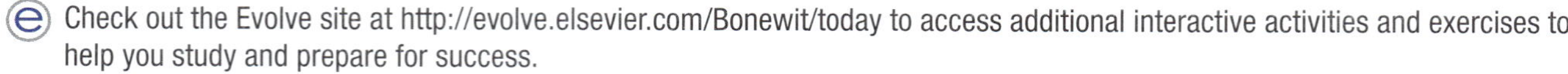

Check out the Evolve site at http://evolve.elsevier.com/Bonewit/today to access additional interactive activities and exercises to help you study and prepare for success.

LEARNING OBJECTIVES	PROCEDURES
Pediatric Office Visits	
1. List the components of the well-child visit. 2. State the usual schedule for well-child visits. 3. Explain the purpose of the sick-child visit. 4. List the procedures performed by the medical assistant during pediatric office visits. 5. Explain why it is important to develop a rapport with the pediatric patient.	Carry an infant using the following positions: • Cradle • Upright
Growth Measurements	
6. State the importance of measuring the child's weight, height (or length), and head circumference during each office visit. 7. State the functions served by a growth chart.	Measure the weight and length of an infant. Measure the head and chest circumference of an infant.
Pediatric Blood Pressure Measurement	
8. State the importance of measuring a child's blood pressure. 9. List the three factors that determine whether a child has hypertension.	Measure the blood pressure of a child. Plot pediatric growth values on a growth chart.
Collection of a Urine Specimen	
10. List the reasons for collecting a urine specimen from a child.	Collect a urine specimen using a pediatric urine collector.
Pediatric Injections	
11. State the range for the gauge and length of needles used for intramuscular and subcutaneous pediatric injections. 12. Explain the use of each of the following pediatric injection sites: vastus lateralis and deltoid.	Locate the following pediatric intramuscular injection sites: • Vastus lateralis • Deltoid Administer an intramuscular injection to an infant. Administer a subcutaneous injection to an infant.
Immunizations	
13. Describe the schedule for immunization of children and adolescents recommended by the Centers for Disease Control. 14. State the information that must be provided to parents as required by the National Childhood Vaccine Injury Act. 15. List the information that must be documented in the medical record after administering a vaccine.	Read and interpret a vaccine information statement. Document information on an immunization administration record.
Newborn Screening Test	
16. Explain the purpose of a newborn screening test. 17. List the symptoms of phenylketonuria. 18. State what occurs if phenylketonuria is left untreated.	Collect a specimen for a newborn screening test.

CHAPTER OUTLINE

KEY TERMS

adolescent
immunity (ih-MYOO-nih-tee)
immunization (IM-yoo-nih-ZAY-shun)
infant
length
pediatrician (PEE-dee-uh-TRIH-shun)
pediatrics (pee-dee-AT-riks)
preschool (PREE-skool) child
school-age child
toddler (TOD-ler)
toxoid (TOKS-oid)
vaccine (vak-SEEN)
vertex (VER-teks)

INTRODUCTION TO THE PEDIATRIC EXAMINATION

Pediatrics is the branch of medicine that deals with the care and development of children and the diagnosis and treatment of diseases in children. A **pediatrician** is a physician who specializes in pediatrics. Many physicians in general practice accept pediatric patients. It is essential that the medical assistant develop the skills needed to assist the physician in the care and treatment of children.

PEDIATRIC OFFICE VISITS

There are two broad categories of pediatric patient office visits. The first is the *well-child visit* (also termed *health maintenance visit*), in which the provider progressively evaluates the growth and development of the child. A patient history update and physical examination are performed during each well-child visit and are directed toward discovering any abnormal conditions commonly associated with the stage of development reached by the child. Table 24.1 provides an outline of normal development during infancy. The child also receives necessary immunizations during these visits.

The interval between well-child visits depends on the medical office, but it frequently follows this schedule after birth: 3 to 5 days, 1 month, 2 months, 4 months, 6 months, 9 months, 12 months, 15 months, 18 months, 24 months, 2½ years, 3 years, 4 years, and once a year thereafter.

The second category of pediatric patient office visits is the *sick-child visit.* The child is exhibiting the signs and symptoms of disease, and the provider evaluates the patient's condition to arrive at a diagnosis and to prescribe treatment.

During well-child and sick-child visits, the medical assistant performs many of the same procedures that have been presented in previous and subsequent chapters (e.g., measurement of temperature, pulse, respiration, and blood pressure; measurement of weight and height; measurement of visual and hearing acuity; assisting with the physical examination; administration of medication; collection of specimens). This chapter discusses procedures specifically related to the pediatric patient and variations in procedures previously presented.

What Would You Do? What Would You *Not* Do?

Case Study 1

My-Lai Chang comes into the office with Christopher Chang, her 1-month-old son. Christopher is here for his 1-month well-child visit. Mrs. Chang is distraught and says that Christopher has episodes of nonstop crying every day that last 2 to 3 hours at a time. She is breast feeding Christopher and says that the crying is worse after he nurses. Although Mrs. Chang realizes that Christopher has colic, she feels guilty because it seems "her milk" is making it worse. She also is having problems with sore nipples and engorgement. She really wanted to breast feed Christopher, but she is thinking of stopping because it just seems too hard to do. Christopher measures in the 50th percentile for weight and length. Mrs. Chang is worried that he is not growing and thinks she may not be producing enough milk. ■

Table 24.1 Milestones of Gross and Fine Motor Development in Infancy

Average Age (mo)	Gross Motor	Fine Motor
1	Turns head from side to side	Grasping reflex present
2	Holds head at 45-degree angle when prone	Holds rattle briefly
3	Begins rolling over	Grasps rattle or dangling objects
4	Slight head lag when pulled to sitting position	Brings objects to mouth
5	No head wobble when held in sitting position	Transfers objects from hand to hand
6	Sits without support	Manipulates and examines large objects with hands
7	Stands while holding on	Reaches for, grabs, and retains object
8	Pulls self to stand	Grasps objects with thumb and finger
9	Crawls backward	Begins to show hand preference
10	Creeps on hands and knees	Hits cup with spoon
11	Walks using furniture for support	Picks up small objects with thumb and forefinger (pincer grasp)
12	Stands alone easily	Puts three or more objects into container
12–16	Walks alone easily	Turns two or three pages in large cardboard book

From Leahy JM, Kizilay PE: *Foundations of nursing practice*, Philadelphia, 1998, Saunders.

DEVELOPING A RAPPORT

The medical assistant must establish a rapport with the pediatric patient. If the medical assistant gains the child's trust and confidence, the child is likely to cooperate during an examination or procedure. Interacting with children requires special techniques. The techniques employed depend on the age of the child. **Infants** (birth to 12 months old) respond best to a calm environment and physical contact with a parent or caregiver to comfort them during the visit. **Toddlers** (1 to 3 years old) and **preschool children** (3 to 6 years old) often respond well to making a game of the procedure. Explaining the purpose of an instrument (e.g., the stethoscope) to a **school-age child** (6 to 12 years old) and allowing them to hold the instrument or even to help during the procedure may overcome fears in that age group (Fig. 24.1) **Adolescents** (12 to 18 years old) respond best by discussing the risks of a procedure and allowing them to have input in the decision-making process.

The medical assistant should always explain the procedure to children who are able to understand. Each child must be approached at their level of understanding. To do this, the medical assistant should know what to expect from a child at a particular age, in terms of motor and social development. Each child has their own individual rate of development; the descriptions of normal development

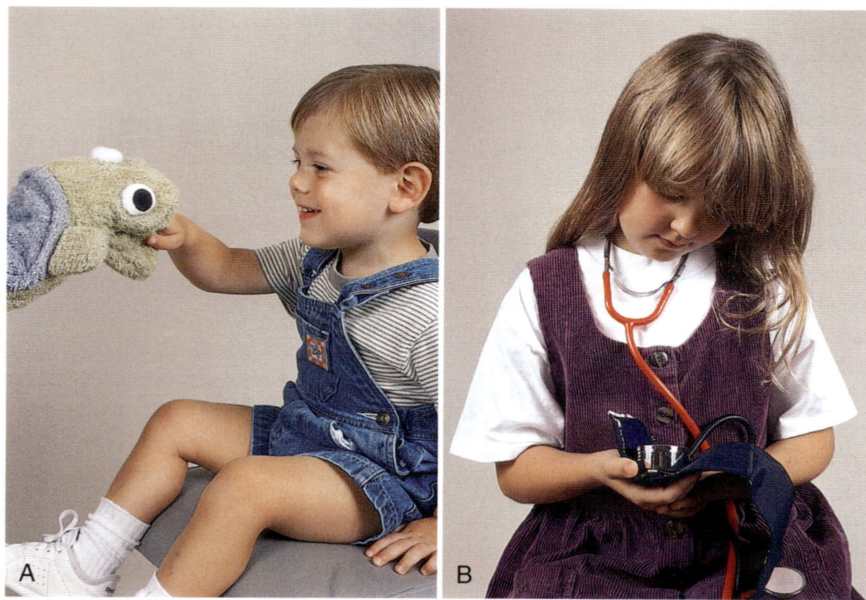

Fig. 24.1 The medical assistant should develop a rapport with children to gain their trust and cooperation. Making a game of the procedure (A) and explaining the purpose of the stethoscope and allowing the child to hold it (B) help the child overcome fears.

Table 24.2 Techniques for Interaction with Children

Technique	Infant (Birth to 1 yr)	Toddler (1–3 yr)	Preschool (3–6 yr)	School Age (6–12 yr)	Adolescent (12–18 yr)
Avoid sudden motion and loud or abrupt noises	•		•		
Limit number of strangers in room	•				
Use distractions, bright objects, rattles, and talking to gain cooperation	•				
Physically restrain child if necessary to ensure safety	•	•	•		
Allow physical contact with parent during procedure	•	•	•		
Encourage parent to comfort child after procedure	•	•	•		
Use play to explain procedure (e.g., dolls, puppets)		•	•		
Perform procedures quickly, if possible		•	•		
Use concrete terms, rather than abstract terms		•	•		
Avoid words that have more than one meaning (e.g., shot)		•	•		
Give child permission to cry, yell, or otherwise express pain verbally		•	•		
Praise child for cooperative behavior		•	•	•	
Allow child to handle equipment, if possible			•	•	
Make sure child understands body part to be involved			•	•	
Try to describe how procedure will feel			•	•	
Tell child about any discomfort that may be felt, but don't dwell on it			•	•	
Stress benefits of anything child may find pleasurable afterward (e.g., stickers, feeling better)			•	•	
Give child choices when possible (e.g., arm to use)			•	•	
Suggest ways to maintain control (e.g., counting, deep breathing, relaxation)			•	•	
Use drawing and diagrams to illustrate parts of body that will be involved			•	•	
Encourage participation such as holding instrument during procedure			•	•	
Include child in decision-making process				•	•
Discuss risks of procedure					•
Provide information about appearance changes that might result					•
Give child educational brochures or have them view videos about procedure					•
Ask parent to step out if child does not want parent in examining room					•

based on age are meant to serve as a guide only and may have to be modified to meet individual needs. In addition, it is normal for an ill child to regress to an earlier level of behavior. Table 24.2 outlines techniques that can be used with various age groups to gain their cooperation during an examination or procedure.

CARRYING THE INFANT

The medical assistant needs to lift and carry the infant to perform various procedures, such as measurement of length and weight. The infant should be lifted and carried in a manner that is safe and comfortable. Proper positions include the cradle and upright positions.

CRADLE POSITION

To place an infant in a cradle position, the medical assistant slides one hand and forearm under the infant's back and grasps the infant's arm from behind. The thumb and fingers should encircle the infant's forearm. The infant's head, shoulders, and back are supported by the medical assistant's forearm. Next, the medical assistant slips the other hand and forearm up and under the infant's buttocks. The infant is cradled in the arm with their body resting against the medical assistant's chest (Fig. 24.2).

UPRIGHT POSITION

To place an infant in an upright position, the medical assistant slips one hand and forearm under the infant's head

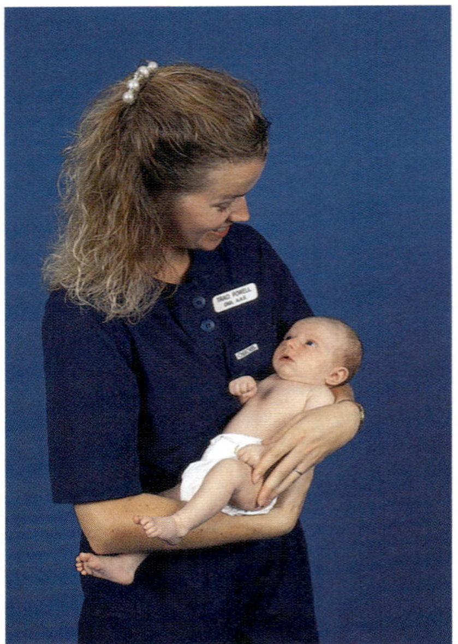

Fig. 24.2 Traci holds the infant in the cradle position.

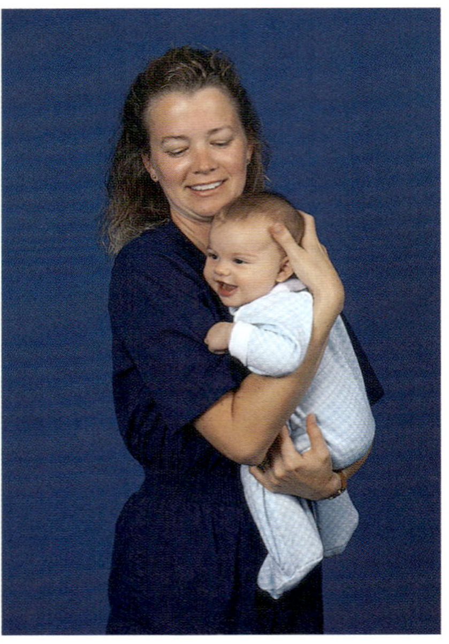

Fig. 24.3 Traci holds the infant in the upright position.

and shoulders. The fingers should be spread apart to support the infant's head and neck. The other hand and forearm are slipped under the infant's buttocks to help support the infant's weight. The infant should be allowed to rest against the medical assistant's chest with the cheek resting on the medical assistant's shoulder (Fig. 24.3).

GROWTH MEASUREMENTS

One of the best methods to evaluate the progress of children is to measure their growth. The weight, height (or length), and head circumference (up to age 3 years) of a child should be measured during each office visit and plotted on a growth chart.

WEIGHT

A child's weight is often used to determine nutritional needs and the proper dosage of medication to administer to the child. The medical assistant should exercise care in measuring weight. Infants are weighed in a recumbent position, as outlined in Procedure 24.1. Older children are weighed in a standing position, as presented in Chapter 20.

LENGTH AND HEIGHT

Another measure of a child's growth is length, or height (stature). Length is measured in children younger than 24 months. The recumbent **length** is a measurement from the **vertex** (top) of the head to the heel of a child in a supine position, as outlined in Procedure 24.1. Two people are often needed to determine the length of an infant accurately. A parent or caregiver's help can be requested; the medical assistant must provide thorough instructions on what is to be done. Older children have their height measured in a standing position (Fig. 24.4), as presented in Chapter 20.

Putting It All Into Practice

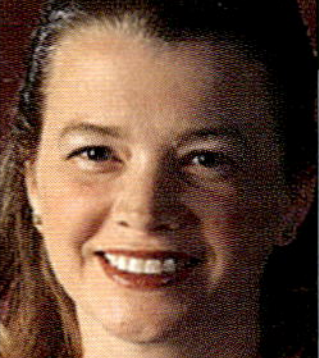

My name is Traci, and I am a Certified Medical Assistant. I work in the pediatrics department of a large multispecialty clinic. My job responsibilities are mostly clinical; however, I do assist in the front office when needed. I love working with the children and have enjoyed watching them grow over the years.

A co-worker and I recently organized a local AAMA (American Association of Medical Assistants) chapter. Our chapter provides AAMA continuing education units (CEUs). Our members attend state and national conventions every year, and they hold state and national leadership positions. It is my goal to see the medical assisting profession continue to grow and advance in the health care field.

It is interesting how your education, training, and experience all come together, especially in a crisis. Early one morning when I arrived at work, a mother rushed in with a small child who was approximately 2 years old. The child was dusky in color, panicky, and having trouble breathing. Apparently the child had gotten into some dry beans the previous night and had inhaled one into her lung. The physicians were not in the building yet, and this child was in respiratory distress. We immediately called a Code Blue, put her on oxygen, and made arrangements for an ambulance to take her to Children's Hospital, where a surgeon was waiting. All went well, and she is a healthy little girl today.

Looking back, I am grateful for a good, solid medical assisting education; a PALS (Pediatric Advance Life Support) certification; and experience in working with children so that I was able to help that child through a life-threatening experience. I firmly believe that no matter how long a person has been in the medical field or what their profession is, continuing education is essential to stay current in the ever-changing health care field. ■

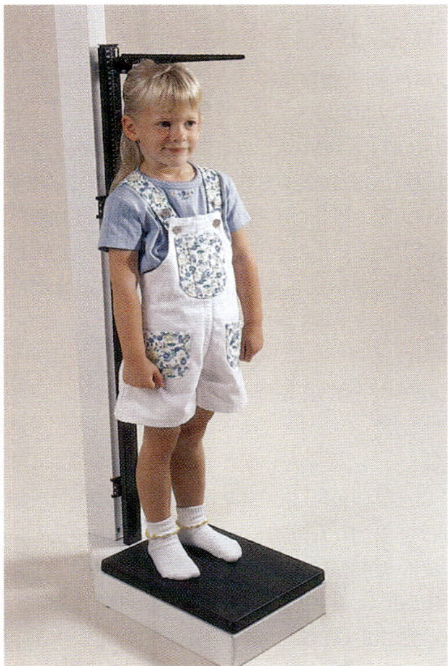

Fig. 24.4 Measuring the height of a child.

HEAD AND CHEST CIRCUMFERENCE

Infancy is a period of rapid brain growth. Because of this, the head circumference is an important measurement. Head circumference is usually measured in centimeters and is performed during well-child visits. The head circumference for a newborn ranges from 32 to 38 cm (12½ to 15 inches). A 10-cm (4-inch) increase in head circumference occurs within the first year of life.

The head circumference of children younger than 3 years should be routinely measured and plotted on a head circumference growth chart. Measurement of head circumference is an important screening measure for microencephaly and macroencephaly.

At birth a newborn's head circumference is about 2 cm larger than their chest circumference. The chest grows at a faster rate than the cranium, and between 6 months and 2 years of age the measurements are about the same. After age 2 years, the chest circumference is greater than the head circumference. The measurement of the chest circumference is valuable in a comparison with the head circumference, but not by itself. The chest circumference is not typically measured on a routine basis; this measurement is done only when a heart or lung abnormality is suspected. Procedure 24.2 outlines the procedure for measuring the head and chest circumference of an infant.

GROWTH CHARTS

Growth charts should be part of every child's permanent record. The National Center for Health Statistics developed growth charts to assist providers in determining whether the growth of a child is normal. The charts can be used to identify children with growth or nutritional abnormalities. In offices with an electronic medical record, the growth percentiles are automatically calculated and plotted on a growth chart when the child's growth measurements are entered into the computer. This "electronic" growth chart is maintained in the child's electronic medical record and can be printed out if needed. In some offices, the medical assistant may be responsible for manually plotting the child's measurements on a preprinted growth chart (Procedure 24.3).

Growth charts provide a means of comparing a child's weight and length (or height) with those of other children of the same age. For example, the medical assistant calculates the growth percentile of an 18-month-old boy and finds that he is in the 25th percentile for weight and the 80th percentile for length. This means that 75% of 18-month-old boys weigh more than he does, and 25% weigh less than he does. It also means that 20% of 18-month-old boys are taller, and 80% are shorter. Although comparing a child with other children of the same age is one use of growth charts (particularly by parents), it is not the most important use.

The primary use of growth charts is to look at the child's growth pattern. If a child has always hovered around a certain percentile in height and weight, there is no need for concern. If a child is in the 20th percentile for weight but has always been in this percentile, she is likely growing normally. It would be more of a concern if the child had been in the 75th percentile for weight and dropped to the 40th percentile. The provider investigates any significant change or rapid increase or decrease in a child's growth pattern.

HIGHLIGHT on Childhood Obesity

Statistics

An epidemic of childhood obesity is occurring in the United States and has become a serious public health problem. Childhood obesity occurs when a child consumes more calories than the body can burn. Approximately 20% of American children between the ages of 2 years and 19 years are obese. A child is considered overweight if their weight falls in the 85th to 95th percentile for age, sex, and height on the National Center for Health Statistics growth charts. When a child's weight exceeds the 95th percentile for age, sex, and height, the child is considered obese.

Causes

The primary causes of childhood obesity are overeating and inadequate exercise. Other causes include the following:

- Family history of obesity
- Illnesses (e.g., endocrine or neurological problems)
- Certain medications (e.g., steroids, certain psychiatric medications)
- Stressful life events (e.g., divorce, moves, deaths, abuse)
- Family and peer problems
- Low self-esteem
- Depression or other emotional problems

Continued

HIGHLIGHT on Childhood Obesity—cont'd

Related Problems

Problems associated with childhood obesity include high blood pressure, elevated blood cholesterol levels, type 2 diabetes, orthopedic problems caused by increased stress on weight-bearing joints, skin disorders (e.g., dermatitis), sleep apnea, low self-esteem, social isolation, and feelings of rejection and depression. Some authorities believe that the social and psychological problems are the most significant consequences of childhood obesity.

Prevention

The risk of obesity tends to be greater among children who have obese parents. After age 3, the likelihood that obesity will persist into adulthood increases as an obese child gets older. When an obese child reaches age 6, the probability is more than 50% that obesity will persist into adulthood. Among obese adolescents, 70% to 80% remain obese as adults.

It is much easier to prevent childhood obesity than to treat it after it has occurred. Authorities believe that the primary focus should be on educating parents about the problems associated with childhood obesity and helping them employ preventive measures. Preventing obesity in childhood is critical because habits formed during childhood frequently carry into adulthood. Guidelines for preventing childhood obesity include the following:

- Provide a healthy diet with a focus on fruits and vegetables.
- Avoid oversized portions.
- Encourage physical activity.
- Promote healthy snacks.
- Do not use food for reward, comfort, or bribes.
- Limit television, video games, and computer time.
- Limit the amount of "junk" food kept in the home.
- Do not make the child eat when he or she is not hungry.
- Do not offer dessert as a reward for finishing a meal.
- Encourage the child to drink water instead of sweet beverages.
- Do not frequently eat at fast-food restaurants.

Treatment

The treatment of childhood obesity is difficult, and the success rate is not particularly high. Children seem to be most successful at losing weight and keeping it off when the entire family is involved. Parents should eat healthy meals and snacks with their children. The most successful diets are those that use ordinary foods in controlled portions, rather than diets that require the avoidance of specific foods. Parents also should spend time being active with their children. Activities should stress self-improvement rather than competition. ■

PEDIATRIC BLOOD PRESSURE MEASUREMENT

The American Academy of Pediatrics recommends that all children 3 years and older have their blood pressure measured annually. Measuring pediatric blood pressure helps to identify children at risk for developing hypertension as adults. High blood pressure in children can be caused by kidney disease and to a lesser degree by heart disease. When the condition is treated, the blood pressure usually returns to normal. Overweight children usually have higher blood pressure than children of normal weight. Losing weight through a prescribed diet and regular physical activity often reduces blood pressure in these children.

SPECIAL GUIDELINES FOR CHILDREN

The procedure for measuring blood pressure in children is the same as that for adults and is presented in Chapter 19. Some special pediatric guidelines must be taken into consideration.

CORRECT CUFF SIZE

The most important criterion in obtaining an accurate pediatric blood pressure measurement is in the selection of the correct cuff size. If the cuff is too small, the reading may be falsely high. If the cuff is too large, the reading may be falsely low. Blood pressure cuffs come in a variety of sizes and are measured in centimeters. The size of a cuff refers to its inner inflatable bladder, rather than its fabric cover. Table 24.3 lists the range of cuff sizes commercially available. The name of the cuff (e.g., child, adult) does not imply that it is appropriate for that age. An 8-year-old obese child may need an adult-sized cuff.

The correct cuff size can be determined based on the circumference of the upper mid-arm which is located midway between the acromion process (shoulder) and the olecranon process (elbow). The circumference of the upper mid-arm must be measured with a flexible centimeter tape measure wrapped around the arm (Fig. 24.5). To select the correct cuff size, the measurement is then compared to Table 24.3 which outlines the cuff sizes and the mid-arm circumference range of each. If the correct cuff size has been selected, the bladder of the cuff should encircle 80% to 100% of the circumference of the upper mid-arm (Fig. 24.5). The correct cuff size can also

Table 24.3 Acceptable Bladder Dimensions for Arms of Different Sizes

Cuff	Bladder Length (cm)	Upper Mid-Arm Circumference Range (cm)
Newborn	6	Less than 6 cm
Infant	15	6–15 cm
Child	21	16–21 cm
Small adult	24	22–26 cm
Adult	30	27–34 cm
Large adult	38	35–44 cm
Adult thigh	42	45–52 cm

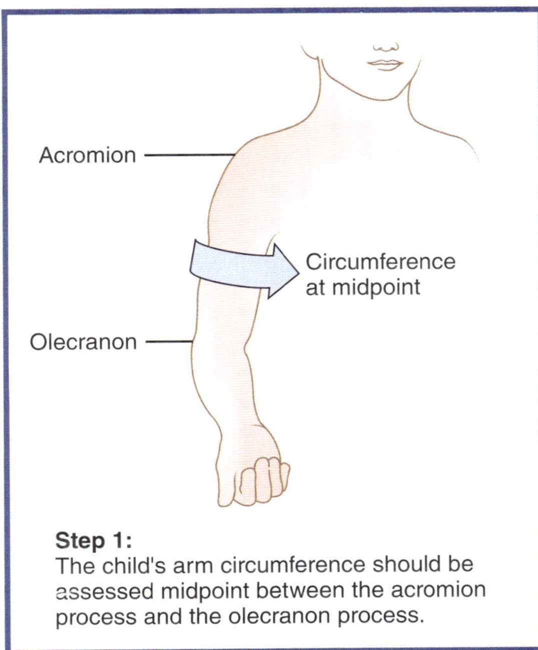

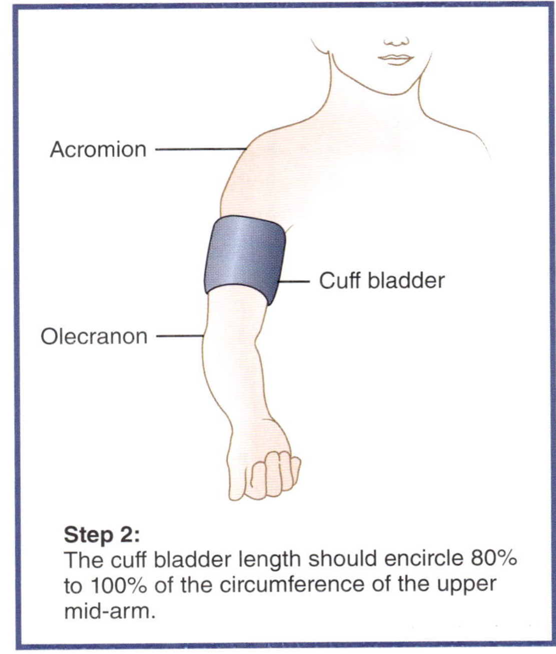

Fig. 24.5 Determination of proper blood pressure cuff size.

be determined using a cuff marked with range and index lines which is described in Chapter 19.

COOPERATION OF THE CHILD

Another important factor to consider when taking pediatric blood pressure is preparing the child for the procedure. It is important to gain the child's cooperation and to ensure that the child is relaxed. Apprehension can cause the blood pressure to be falsely high. To reduce a child's anxiety level, carefully explain the procedure to the child, and, if appropriate, allow them to handle the equipment before measurement of the blood pressure. The blood pressure should be measured after the child has been sitting quietly for 3 to 5 minutes (Fig. 24.6).

What Would You Do? What Would You *Not* Do?

Case Study 2

Wanda Tilley comes to the office with her 10-year-old daughter, Courtney. Courtney has a skin condition on her legs that needs to be evaluated by the physician. Courtney has been obese since she was 4 years old. Mrs. Tilley also is obese and is not too concerned about Courtney's weight. She says that Courtney must have inherited her "fat gene," and there's not much that can be done about it. Courtney's favorite activities are playing video games and reading. Courtney would like to join the community swim team, but she's too embarrassed for anyone to see her in a swim suit. Courtney says the other kids are always making fun of her at school. She says that they call her "two-ton Tilley" and "double-roll," and they don't want to sit with her at lunch. Courtney wants her mom to home-school her because she's getting to the point where she can't take it anymore. She doesn't want the doctor to examine her because she thinks he will scold her for being so fat. ■

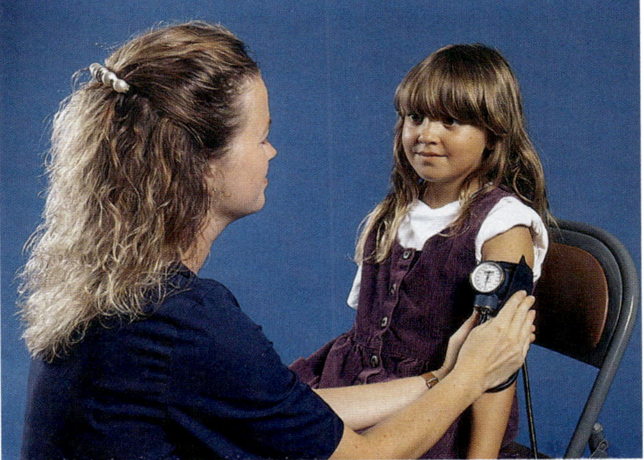

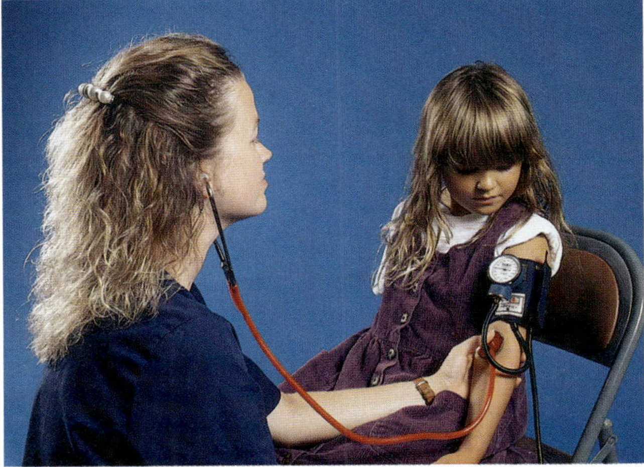

Fig. 24.6 Traci measures the blood pressure of a pediatric patient.

BLOOD PRESSURE CLASSIFICATIONS

Blood pressure varies depending on the age, height, and sex of the child. The National High Blood Pressure Education Program (NHBPEP) prepared a set of tables that providers use to determine whether a child's blood pressure is higher than the average among children of the same age, height, and sex. If a child has a blood pressure that is higher than 90% to 95% of most other children of the same age, height, and sex, the child may have high blood pressure.

The NHBPEP tables (one for boys and one for girls) allow precise classification of blood pressure according to body size, which avoids misclassifying children at the extreme ends of normal growth. A very tall child would not be mistakenly diagnosed as having hypertension, and hypertension would not be missed in a very short child. The NHBPEP tables used by providers to assist in the diagnosis of hypertension in children can be found at the National Heart, Lung, and Blood Institute website.

Blood pressure varies throughout the day in children as a result of normal fluctuations in physical activity and emotional stress. A single blood pressure reading taken on one occasion does not characterize the child's blood pressure accurately. If a child's blood pressure is elevated, an average of two or more blood pressure readings taken on two or more separate office visits must be taken before the provider can make a diagnosis of hypertension.

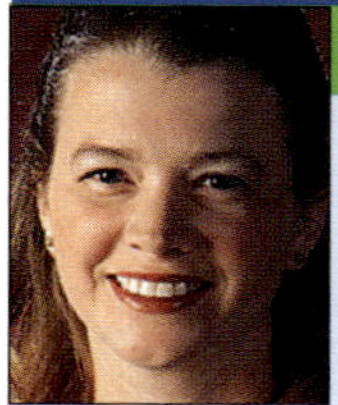

Memories *from* Practicum

Traci: I still remember how difficult it was at times as a student. I had been out of high school for more than a year, so I had to get back into the routine of studying. I worried about whether I would do well, whether I would be able to find a good job, and whether I would like medical assisting. Adding to these concerns was the financial burden of putting myself through two years of school. I took advantage of grants and student loans. Throughout the last 6 months of my education, I also worked full-time as an aide on the midnight shift at a nursing home while attending school full-time during the day. As if that were not enough, my first child was well on her way into this world as I was finishing up the last quarter of my degree. There were so many times that I was tired, frustrated, and broke, but I kept pushing myself to do my best because I knew this was going to be my lifetime career, and I wanted to excel in my profession. My determination paid off. Today I have a great medical assisting position that I love, with a medical clinic that is one of the best employers in the area. ■

COLLECTION OF A URINE SPECIMEN

A urinalysis may be performed on a pediatric patient for the following reasons: to screen for the presence of disease as part of a general physical examination, to assist in the diagnosis of a pathologic condition (e.g., urinary tract infection), or to evaluate the effectiveness of therapy. The collection of a urine specimen from a child who exhibits bladder control is performed using the technique outlined in Chapter 30. Collecting a urine specimen from an infant or young child who cannot urinate voluntarily involves the use of a pediatric urine collector. Pediatric urine collectors are designed to be used with both female and male children. The urine collector consists of a clear plastic disposable bag containing a hypoallergenic pressure-sensitive adhesive around the opening of the bag. The adhesive firmly attaches the urine collector to the skin surrounding the genitalia. Procedure 24.4 outlines the procedure for applying a pediatric urine collector.

PEDIATRIC INJECTIONS

Administering an injection to a child is an important responsibility. The experience a child has with early injections influences the child's attitude toward later ones. If the child is old enough to understand, the procedure should be explained. The medical assistant should be honest and should attempt to gain the child's trust and cooperation. The child should be told the truth about the injection—that it will hurt, but only for a short time. It also is advisable to explain to the child that the medicine is being given to help them. Another person (e.g., parent, caregiver, health care worker) should be present to assist. The assistant can help position the child and can divert or restrain the child if necessary. If the child struggles and fights excessively, the medical assistant should delay the injection and consult the provider. After the injection has been administered, the child's parent or caregiver should hold the child, provide comfort, and show approval so that the child associates something other than pain with this procedure.

The administration of injections is presented in Chapter 26. Before undertaking the study of pediatric injections, the medical assistant should review this chapter thoroughly, concentrating on the locations of injection sites and the procedures for preparing and administering injections. The same basic technique is used to administer an injection to an adult and a child. Variations in procedure are explained in the following section.

INTRAMUSCULAR INJECTIONS

An intramuscular injection is administered directly into muscle tissue. The gauge of the needle used for an intramuscular injection varies depending on the consistency of the medication to be administered; thick or oily preparations require a larger needle lumen than thin aqueous preparations. The size of the needle used depends on the size of the child. The needle must be long enough to reach the largest part of the muscle, but not so long as to reach the underlying bone. A needle length ranging from ⅝ inch to 1 inch is typically used to administer an intramuscular injection to a child, and in general the gauge of the needle ranges from 22 to 25, depending on the viscosity (thickness) of the medication.

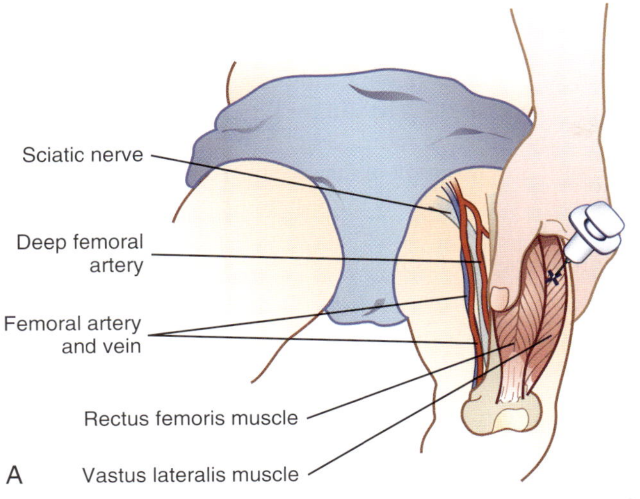

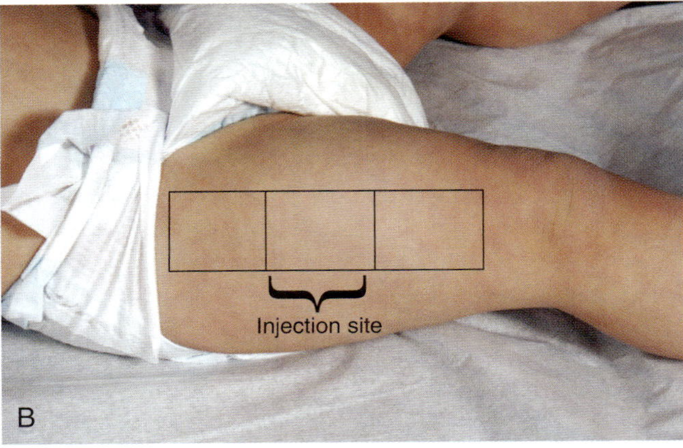

Fig. 24.7 (A) Vastus lateralis intramuscular injection site. (B) Location of the vastus lateralis injection site in an infant. Divide the mid-anterior thigh into thirds. The injection is administered into the middle third of the thigh. (A, Courtesy of Wyeth Laboratories, Philadelphia, PA.)

INTRAMUSCULAR INJECTION SITES

The specific site for injection of the medication depends on the age of the child which is indicated in the package insert accompanying the medication. The two most commonly used pediatric injection sites are the vastus lateralis site and the deltoid site. The dorsogluteal site is not recommended for infants and children. This is because an injection into this site may come dangerously close to the sciatic nerve; an injection into the sciatic nerves results in pain, numbness and weakness of the leg and foot.

Vastus Lateralis Site

The vastus lateralis site is recommended for infants and young children under the age of 3 years. The vastus lateralis muscle is located on the anterolateral thigh, away from major nerves and blood vessels, and it is large enough to accommodate the injected medication (Fig. 24.7A). To locate the vastus lateralis site in an infant or young child, divide the anterolateral thigh into thirds. The injection is administered into the middle third of the thigh (Fig. 24.7B).

The length of the needle used depends on the overall size of the thigh. The needle should be long enough to penetrate the muscle belly for proper absorption to occur. A 1-inch needle is typically used for a normal-sized infant or child; however, the length of the needle may need to be decreased (e.g., ⅝ inch) for a newborn or preterm infant and increased (e.g., 1¼ inches) for an obese child. For administration of the injection, the infant or toddler should be held on the lap of the assistant (parent, caregiver, or health care worker) in a "cuddle" or semi-recumbent position. The child may also be placed in a supine position for administration of the injection. The site should be clearly visible and the assistant should restrain the child to prevent as much movement as possible. The medical assistant should grasp the anterolateral thigh to compress the muscle tissue and to stabilize the extremity (Fig. 24.8A). The injection is administered at a 90-degree angle as illustrated in Fig. 24.8B, by following the procedure outlined in Chapter 26.

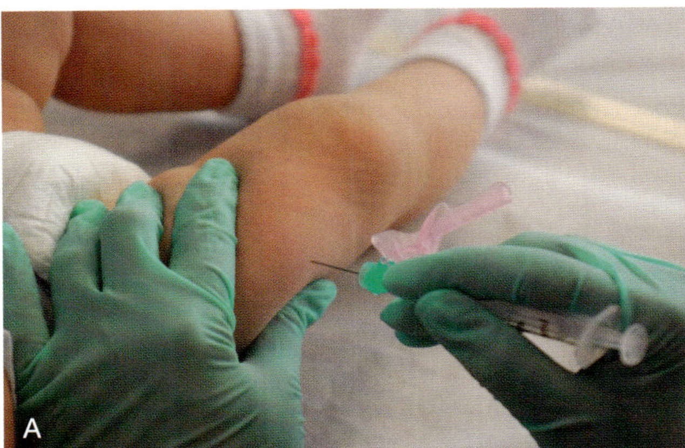

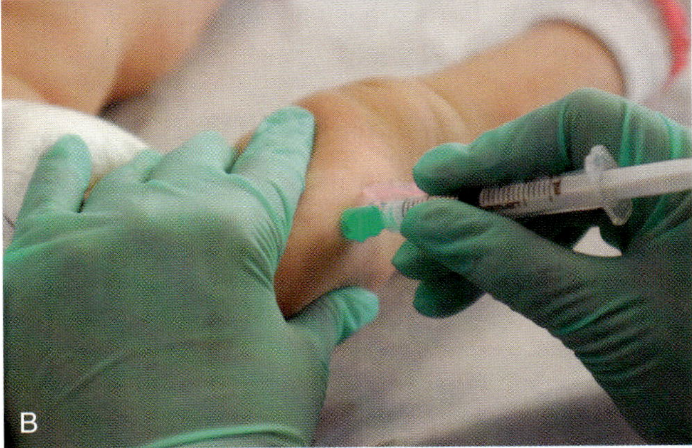

Fig. 24.8 (A) Compression of the vastus lateralis muscle. (B) Intramuscular injection into the vastus lateralis injection site.

Deltoid Site

The deltoid muscle is shallow and can accommodate only a small amount of medication (0.5 to 1 mL). In addition,

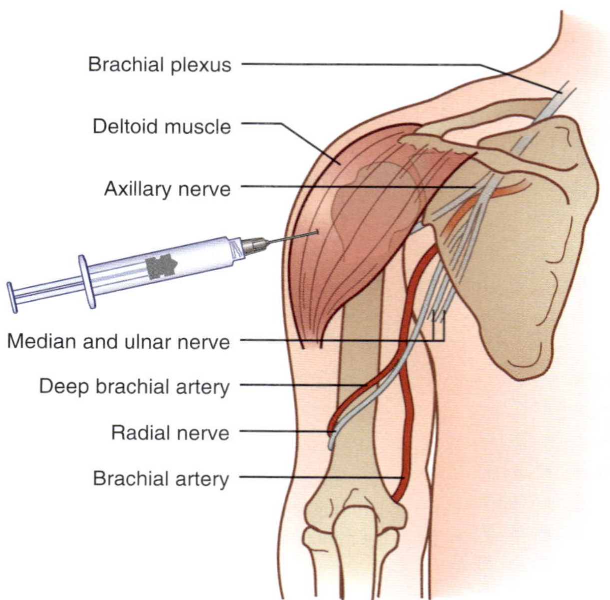

Fig. 24.9 Deltoid intramuscular injection site. (Courtesy of Wyeth Laboratories, Philadelphia, PA.)

repeated injections at this site are painful. Because the deltoid muscle is so small in an infant, the deltoid site should not be used to administer an injection until a child is 3 years of age when the muscle mass is more developed. The length of the needle should be adjusted according to the amount of subcutaneous tissue over the injection site. For example, a ⅝-inch needle is often used for a normal-sized 4-year-old, but a 1-inch needle may be required for an obese child of the same age. For administration of the injection, the deltoid muscle mass should be grasped at the injection site and compressed between the thumb and fingers. The needle should be inserted pointing slightly upward toward the shoulder (Fig. 24.9).

SUBCUTANEOUS INJECTIONS

A subcutaneous injection is made into the subcutaneous tissue, which consists of adipose (fat) tissue located just under the skin. The length of the needle used to administer a pediatric subcutaneous injection ranges from ½ inch to ⅝ inch, and the gauge of the needle ranges from 23 to 25.

Subcutaneous (fatty) tissue is located all over the body; however, certain sites are more commonly used because they are located where bones and blood vessels are not near the surface of the skin. The recommended subcutaneous site for an infant younger than 12 months of age is the fatty tissue of the anterolateral thigh. For a child 12 months of age or older, the recommended subcutaneous site is the lateral part of the upper arm or the anterolateral thigh.

For administration of the injection, the area surrounding the injection site should be grasped and held in a cushion fashion and the needle should be inserted at a 45-degree angle. This ensures that the subcutaneous tissue and not muscle tissue is entered. The designated pediatric subcutaneous injection sites do not contain any large blood vessels. Because of this, the CDC recommends that aspiration of the syringe is not necessary before administration of a vaccine through the subcutaneous route. Studies show that not aspirating before administration of the vaccine reduces pain at the injection site. It is extremely important, however, that the medical assistant always review and follow the medication administration policies set forth at their medical office.

IMMUNIZATIONS

Immunity is the resistance of the body to pathogenic microorganisms and their toxins. Immunization is the process of making an individual immune (resistant to a disease) through the administration of a vaccine. A **vaccine** is a suspension of weakened microorganisms, killed microorganisms, or toxoids administered to an individual to prevent an infectious disease by stimulating the production of antibodies in that individual. A **toxoid** is a toxin (a poisonous substance produced by a bacterium) that has been treated by heat or chemicals to destroy its harmful properties. Vaccines build the body's defenses and protect an individual from attack by certain infectious diseases.

Vaccines should be administered to infants and children during well-child visits according to an immunization schedule. The Centers for Disease Control (CDC) recommends that the schedule outlined in Fig. 24.10 be followed. This schedule is intended as a guide to be used with any modifications needed to meet the requirements of an individual or group.

The medical assistant should be familiar with each vaccine that is administered, including its use, common side effects, route of administration, dose, and method of storage. The drug manufacturer includes a package insert with each vaccine that contains this information. Drug references, such as the *Prescriber's Digital Reference* (available online), also can be used to locate information on vaccines. Vaccines administered to children and adolescents, along with brand names, abbreviations, and route of administration are listed in Table 24.4. Certain vaccines can be administered together in the same injection. A combined vaccine is just as effective as the individual vaccine and results in fewer injections for the child or adolescent. For example, diphtheria, tetanus, and pertussis (DTaP), hepatitis B, and polio (DTaP-HepB-IPV) vaccines can be combined together in the same injection. Table 24.5 provides a list of combined vaccines administered to children and adolescents, along with brand names and the routes of administration.

Parents should be provided with an immunization record card (Fig. 24.11) at their infant's first well-child visit. They should be instructed to bring this card to every visit so that their child's immunizations can be recorded. Parents should be informed of the possible normal side effects of each vaccine and given instructions on how to respond if they occur.

Recommended Child and Adolescent Immunization Schedule for Ages 18 Years or Younger, United States, 2024

These recommendations must be read with the notes that follow. For those who fall behind or start late, provide catch-up vaccination at the earliest opportunity as indicated by the green bars.
To determine minimum intervals between doses, see the catch-up schedule (Table 2).

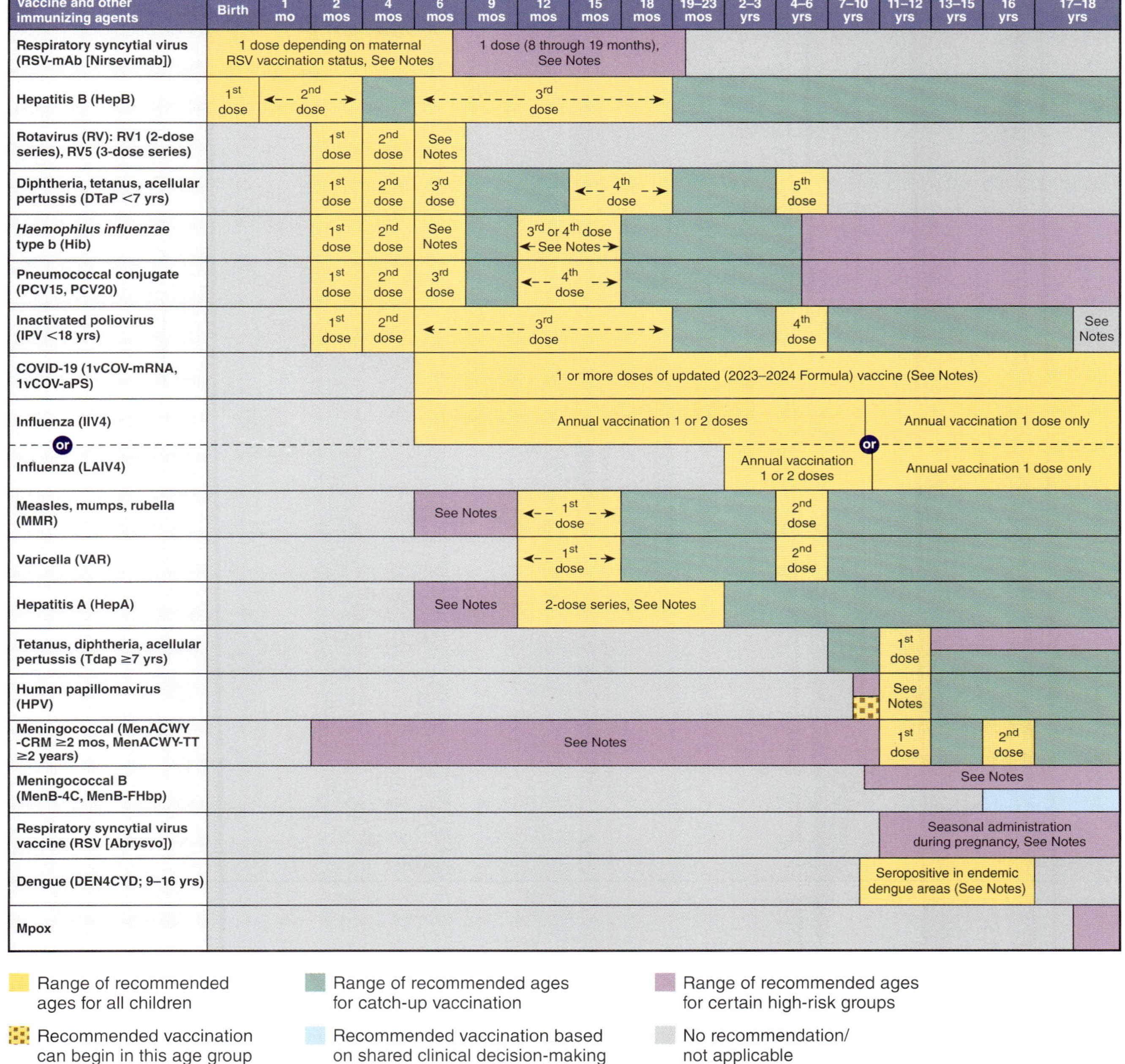

Fig. 24.10 Immunization schedule. (From Department of Health and Human Services, Centers for Disease Control and Prevention, United States, 2015.)

NATIONAL CHILDHOOD VACCINE INJURY ACT

The National Childhood Vaccine Injury Act (NCVIA) requires that parents be provided with information about the benefits and risks of childhood immunizations. To help medical offices comply with these regulations, the Centers for Disease Control and Prevention developed a set of vaccine information statements (VISs). Using lay terminology, a VIS provides a description of the vaccine and the benefits and risks of the vaccine. It also includes potential side effects and adverse reactions, information on reporting

Table 24.4 Child and Adolescent Vaccines

Vaccine	Abbreviation	Brand Name(s)	Route of Administration
COVID-19	1vCOV-mRNA 2vCOV-mRNA 1vCOV-aPS	Comirnaty Spikevax Pfizer-BioNTech Moderna Novavax	IM
Dengue vaccine	DEN4CYD	Dengvaxia	SC
Diphtheria, tetanus, and acellular pertussis vaccine	DTaP	Daptacel Infanrix	IM
Haemophilus influenzae type b vaccine	Hib	ActHIB Hiberix PedvaxHIB	IM
Hepatitis A vaccine	HepA	Havrix Vaqta	IM
Hepatitis B vaccine	HepB	Engerix-B Recombivax HB	IM
Human papillomavirus vaccine	HPV	Gardasil 9	IM
Influenza vaccine (inactivated)	IIV4	Afluria Fluarix FluLaval Flucelvax Fluzone	IM
Influenza vaccine (live, attenuated)	LAIV4	FluMist	IN
Measles, mumps, and rubella vaccine	MMR	M-M-R II Priorix	SC
Meningococcal serogroups A,C,W,Y vaccine	MenACWY-D	Menactra	IM
Meningococcal serogroup B vaccine	MenB-4C	Bexsero	IM
Pneumococcal conjugate vaccine	PCV13 PCV15	Prevnar Vaxneuvance	IM
Pneumococcal polysaccharide vaccine	PPSV23	Pneumovax 23	IM or SC
Poliovirus vaccine (inactivated)	IPV	IPOL	IM or SC
Rotavirus vaccine	RV1 RV5	Rotarix RotaTeq	PO
Tetanus and diphtheria vaccine	Td	Tenivac TDvax	IM
Varicella vaccine	VAR	Varivax	SC

ID, intradermal; *IM*, intramuscular; *IN*, intranasal; *PO*, oral; *SC*, subcutaneous.

Table 24.5 Child and Adolescent Combination Vaccines

Combined Vaccines	Brand Name	Route of Administration
DTaP-HepB-IPV	Pediarix	IM
DTaP-IPV-Hib	Pentacel	IM
DTaP-IPV	Kinrix Quadracel	IM
DTaP-IPV-Hib-HepB	Vaxelis	IM
MMRV	ProQuad	SC

DTaP, Diphtheria, tetanus, and pertussis; *HepB*, hepatitis B; *Hib*, *Haemophilus influenzae* type b; *IPV*, inactivated polio vaccine; *MMRV*, measles, mumps, rubella, varicella; *IM*, intramuscular; *SC*, subcutaneous.

adverse reactions, information on the National Vaccine Injury Compensation Program, and how to obtain more information about the vaccine. See Fig. 24.12 for a DTaP VIS.

The NCVIA requires that the appropriate and most current VIS be given to the child's parent or (or legal representative) each and every time before the child receives a dose of any vaccine listed in Table 24.4. The medical assistant must give the parent or representative enough time to read the VIS and an opportunity to ask questions before the vaccine is administered. In addition, the medical assistant must document the following information in the patient's medical record: the name and edition date of each VIS

IMMUNIZATION RECORD					
Name					
Birthdate					
Immunization	DATE	DATE	DATE	DATE	DATE
Hep B (Hepatitis B)					
DTaP (Diphtheria, Tetanus, and Pertussis)					
Hib (*Haemophilus influenzae* Type b)					
IPV (Inactivated Polio Vaccine)					
PCV (Pneumococcal Conjugate Vaccine)					
RV (Rotavirus vaccine)					
MMR (Measles, Mumps, Rubella)					
Varicella (Chickenpox)					
Hep A (Hepatitis A)					
MCV4 (Meningococcal Vaccine)					
HPV (Human Papillomavirus)					
Influenza					
Tuberculin (Mantoux) RESULT					
Tetanus Booster					
Other					

Fig. 24.11 Immunization record card.

VACCINE INFORMATION STATEMENT

DTaP (Diphtheria, Tetanus, Pertussis) Vaccine: *What You Need to Know*

Many vaccine information statements are available in Spanish and other languages. See www.immunize.org/vis

Hojas de información sobre vacunas están disponibles en español y en muchos otros idiomas. Visite www.immunize.org/vis

1. Why get vaccinated?

DTaP vaccine can prevent **diphtheria**, **tetanus**, and **pertussis**.

Diphtheria and pertussis spread from person to person. Tetanus enters the body through cuts or wounds.

- **DIPHTHERIA (D)** can lead to difficulty breathing, heart failure, paralysis, or death.
- **TETANUS (T)** causes painful stiffening of the muscles. Tetanus can lead to serious health problems, including being unable to open the mouth, having trouble swallowing and breathing, or death.
- **PERTUSSIS (aP)**, also known as "whooping cough," can cause uncontrollable, violent coughing that makes it hard to breathe, eat, or drink. Pertussis can be extremely serious especially in babies and young children, causing pneumonia, convulsions, brain damage, or death. In teens and adults, it can cause weight loss, loss of bladder control, passing out, and rib fractures from severe coughing.

2. DTaP vaccine

DTaP is only for children younger than 7 years old. Different vaccines against tetanus, diphtheria, and pertussis (Tdap and Td) are available for older children, adolescents, and adults.

It is recommended that children receive 5 doses of DTaP, usually at the following ages:

- 2 months
- 4 months
- 6 months
- 15–18 months
- 4–6 years

DTaP may be given as a stand-alone vaccine, or as part of a combination vaccine (a type of vaccine that combines more than one vaccine together into one shot).

DTaP may be given at the same time as other vaccines.

3. Talk with your health care provider

Tell your vaccination provider if the person getting the vaccine:

- Has had an **allergic reaction after a previous dose of any vaccine that protects against tetanus, diphtheria, or pertussis**, or has any **severe, life-threatening allergies**
- Has had **a coma, decreased level of consciousness, or prolonged seizures within 7 days after a previous dose of any pertussis vaccine (DTP or DTaP)**
- Has **seizures or another nervous system problem**
- Has ever had **Guillain-Barré Syndrome** (also called "GBS")
- Has had **severe pain or swelling after a previous dose of any vaccine that protects against tetanus or diphtheria**

In some cases, your child's health care provider may decide to postpone DTaP vaccination until a future visit.

Children with minor illnesses, such as a cold, may be vaccinated. Children who are moderately or severely ill should usually wait until they recover before getting DTaP vaccine.

Your child's health care provider can give you more information.

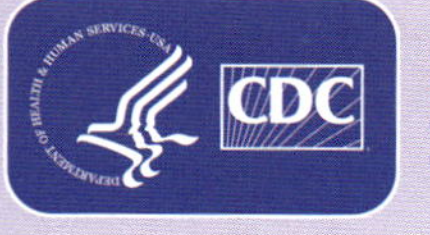

U.S. Department of Health and Human Services
Centers for Disease Control and Prevention

Fig. 24.12 Vaccine information statement for diphtheria, tetanus, and pertussis (DTaP). (Courtesy of Centers for Disease Control and Prevention, Atlanta, GA.)

4. Risks of a vaccine reaction

- Soreness or swelling where the shot was given, fever, fussiness, feeling tired, loss of appetite, and vomiting sometimes happen after DTaP vaccination.
- More serious reactions, such as seizures, non-stop crying for 3 hours or more, or high fever (over 105°F) after DTaP vaccination happen much less often. Rarely, vaccination is followed by swelling of the entire arm or leg, especially in older children when they receive their fourth or fifth dose.

As with any medicine, there is a very remote chance of a vaccine causing a severe allergic reaction, other serious injury, or death.

5. What if there is a serious problem?

An allergic reaction could occur after the vaccinated person leaves the clinic. If you see signs of a severe allergic reaction (hives, swelling of the face and throat, difficulty breathing, a fast heartbeat, dizziness, or weakness), call **9-1-1** and get the person to the nearest hospital.

For other signs that concern you, call your health care provider.

Adverse reactions should be reported to the Vaccine Adverse Event Reporting System (VAERS). Your health care provider will usually file this report, or you can do it yourself. Visit the VAERS website at **www.vaers.hhs.gov** or call **1-800-822-7967**. *VAERS is only for reporting reactions, and VAERS staff members do not give medical advice.*

6. The National Vaccine Injury Compensation Program

The National Vaccine Injury Compensation Program (VICP) is a federal program that was created to compensate people who may have been injured by certain vaccines. Claims regarding alleged injury or death due to vaccination have a time limit for filing, which may be as short as two years. Visit the VICP website at **www.hrsa.gov/vaccinecompensation** or call **1-800-338-2382** to learn about the program and about filing a claim.

7. How can I learn more?

- Ask your health care provider.
- Call your local or state health department.
- Visit the website of the Food and Drug Administration (FDA) for vaccine package inserts and additional information at **www.fda.gov/vaccines-blood-biologics/vaccines**.
- Contact the Centers for Disease Control and Prevention (CDC):
  - Call **1-800-232-4636** (**1-800-CDC-INFO**) or
  - Visit CDC's website at **www.cdc.gov/vaccines**.

Vaccine Information Statement
DTaP (Diphtheria, Tetanus, Pertussis) Vaccine

42 U.S.C. § 300aa-26
8/6/2021

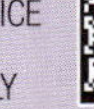

Fig. 24.12, cont'd

provided, and the date the VIS was given to the parent or representative. The edition date of the VIS is located at the bottom right corner of the VIS. Following the administration of the vaccine, the NCVIA requires the following information be documented in the patient's medical record: the date of administration, the manufacturer and lot number of the vaccine, the signature and title of the health care provider who administered the vaccine, and the name and address of the medical office where it was administered. Fig. 24.13 shows an example of an immunization administrative record that is included in a patient's medical record.

IMMUNIZATION ADMINISTRATION RECORD

Name ______________________________
(first) (MI) (last)

DOB ______________________________

Physician ______________________________

Address ______________________________

____

SITE ABBREVIATIONS:

- **RVL:** Right vastus lateralis
- **LVL:** Left vastus lateralis
- **RD:** Right deltoid
- **LD:** Left deltoid
- **PO:** By mouth
- **IN:** Intranasal

Vaccine	Type of Vaccine[1] (generic abbreviation)	Date Given (mo/day/yr)	Dose	Site	Vaccine		Vaccine Information Statement		Signature and Title of Vaccinator
					Lot #	Mfr.	Date on VIS	Date Given	
Hepatitis B[2] (e.g., HepB, Hib-HepB, DTaP-HepB-IPV) Give IM.									
Diphtheria, Tetanus, Pertussis[2] (e.g., DTaP, DTaP-Hib, DTaP-HepB-IPV, DT, DTaP-Hib-IPV, Tdap, DTaP-IPV, Td) Give IM.									
***Haemophilus influenzae* type b[2]** (e.g., Hib, Hib-HepB, DTaP-Hib-IPV, DTaP-Hib) Give IM.									
Polio[2] (e.g., IPV, DTaP-HepB-IPV, DTaP-Hib-IPV, DTaP-IPV) Give IPV SC or IM. Give all others IM.									
Pneumococcal (e.g., PCV, conjugate; PPV, polysaccharide) Give PCV IM. Give PPV SC or IM.									
Rotavirus Give oral.									
Measles, Mumps, Rubella[5] (e.g., MMR, MMRV) Give SC.									
Varicella[5] (e.g., Var, MMRV) Give SC.									
Hepatitis A Give IM									
Meningococcal (e.g., MCV4, MPSV4) Give MCV4 IM and MPSV4 SC.									
Human papillomavirus (e.g., HPV) Give IM									
Influenza[5] (e.g., TIV, inactivated; LAIV, live attenuated) Give TIV IM. Give LAIV IN.									
Other									

1. Record the generic abbreviation for the type of vaccine given (e.g., DTaP-Hib, PCV), *not* the trade name.
2. For combination vaccines, fill in a row for each separate antigen in the combination.

Fig. 24.13 Immunization administration record included in a patient's medical record. (Modified from Immunization Action Coalition, St Paul, MN.)

What Would You Do? What Would You *Not* Do?

Case Study 3

Stacy Jones, a legal secretary, brings her 5-year-old son, Matthew, in for a kindergarten physical. Stacy has read the vaccine information statements for the DTaP, IPV, varicella, and MMR vaccines that Matthew will be getting at this visit and has some questions. She wants to know why polio is not given orally anymore. She also wants to know why children are immunized against chickenpox because it is such a harmless disease. She is annoyed because she thinks that children are receiving too many unnecessary vaccines these days. Matthew is extremely afraid of "shots" and says that no one with a needle is getting anywhere near him. Stacy is protective of Matthew and knows that he will be hard to handle. She wants to know whether this set of vaccines could just be skipped. She says that most of these diseases do not even exist anymore and that she noticed, from reading the vaccine sheets, that there are a lot of possible side effects. ■

NEWBORN SCREENING TEST

PURPOSE OF THE TEST

A newborn screening test is performed on an infant to screen for the presence of certain metabolic and endocrine diseases. The diseases that are screened for vary by state but typically include phenylketonuria (PKU), biotinidase deficiency, congenital adrenal hyperplasia, maple sugar urine disease, congenital hypothyroidism, galactosemia, homocystinuria, and sickle cell anemia. The most important of these is PKU, which is discussed in greater detail in the following paragraphs.

PHENYLKETONURIA (PKU)

PKU is a congenital hereditary disease caused by a lack of the enzyme *phenylalanine hydroxylase.* This enzyme is needed to convert phenylalanine, an amino acid, into tyrosine, which is an amino acid needed for normal metabolic functioning. Without this enzyme, phenylalanine accumulates in the blood and, if the accumulation is left untreated, causes mental retardation and other abnormalities, such as tremors and poor muscle coordination. In most cases, on early detection a special low-phenylalanine diet and close periodic monitoring can prevent adverse effects. Normal development usually occurs if treatment is started before the child reaches 3 to 4 weeks of age. To promote the best development of cognitive abilities, most authorities recommend lifelong dietary restriction of phenylalanine. Although PKU is not a common condition (affecting 1 in every 12,000 births), early diagnosis and treatment lead to a better prognosis.

Phenylalanine can be detected in the blood of an affected infant only after the infant has been receiving breast or formula milk. Infants taking formula can be tested earlier than breast-fed infants because formula contains phenylalanine, whereas the "first breast milk," or colostrum, does not. The test results of breast-fed infants are usually invalid until the mother begins producing milk.

NEWBORN SCREENING REQUIREMENTS

All states require by law that infants undergo newborn screening. The best time to perform the test is between 1 and 7 days after birth. In most states the newborn screening test is performed before the infant leaves the hospital. If the test has abnormal or invalid results, the infant needs to be retested. Most repeat tests are required because of invalid test results caused by the collection of an inadequate amount of the blood specimen. Newborn screening retesting is usually performed at a hospital laboratory but may sometimes be performed in the medical office.

The newborn screening test card (Fig. 24.14) includes an information section that must be completed before the

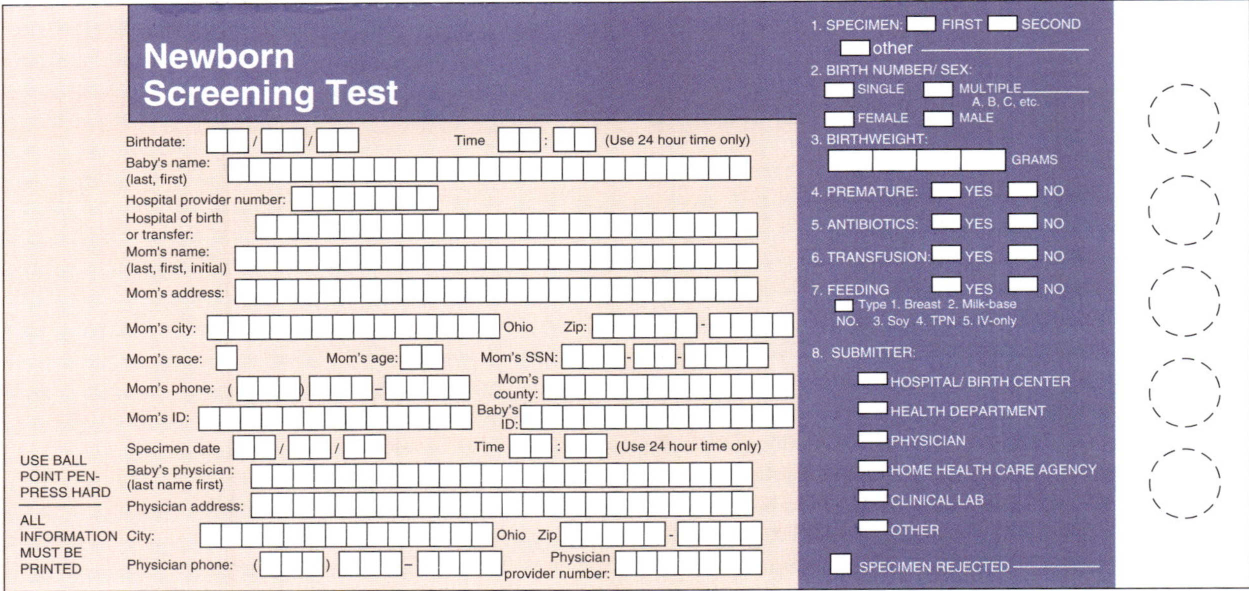

Newborn Screening Test

Birthdate: __/__/__ Time __:__ (Use 24 hour time only)
Baby's name: (last, first)
Hospital provider number:
Hospital of birth or transfer:
Mom's name: (last, first, initial)
Mom's address:
Mom's city: Ohio Zip: -
Mom's race: Mom's age: Mom's SSN: - -
Mom's phone: ( ) -
Mom's county:
Mom's ID:
Baby's ID:
Specimen date __/__/__ Time __:__ (Use 24 hour time only)
Baby's physician: (last name first)
Physician address:
City: Ohio Zip -
Physician phone: ( ) -
Physician provider number:

USE BALL POINT PEN-PRESS HARD
ALL INFORMATION MUST BE PRINTED

1. SPECIMEN: FIRST SECOND other
2. BIRTH NUMBER/ SEX: SINGLE MULTIPLE A, B, C, etc. FEMALE MALE
3. BIRTHWEIGHT: GRAMS
4. PREMATURE: YES NO
5. ANTIBIOTICS: YES NO
6. TRANSFUSION: YES NO
7. FEEDING YES NO Type 1. Breast 2. Milk-base NO. 3. Soy 4. TPN 5. IV-only
8. SUBMITTER: HOSPITAL/ BIRTH CENTER; HEALTH DEPARTMENT; PHYSICIAN; HOME HEALTH CARE AGENCY; CLINICAL LAB; OTHER

SPECIMEN REJECTED

Fig. 24.14 Newborn screening test card.

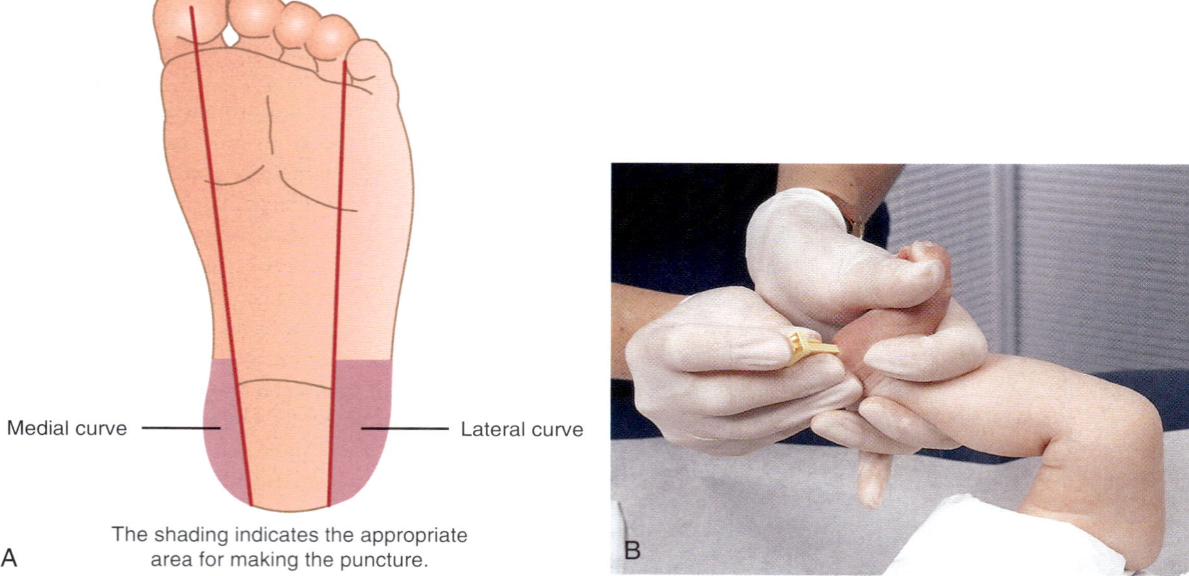

Fig. 24.15 (A) Heel puncture sites for a pediatric patient. (B) Puncture of the medial posterior curve of the plantar surface of an infant's heel.

test is performed. The newborn screening test is performed on capillary blood obtained from the fleshy part of the lateral or medial posterior curve of the plantar surface of the infant's heel (Fig. 24.15). The blood specimen is placed on a special filter paper attached to the newborn screening test card (Fig, 24.16) and is mailed to an outside laboratory for analysis. The results are ready in a few days. If one of the newborn screening test results is positive, further testing is performed.

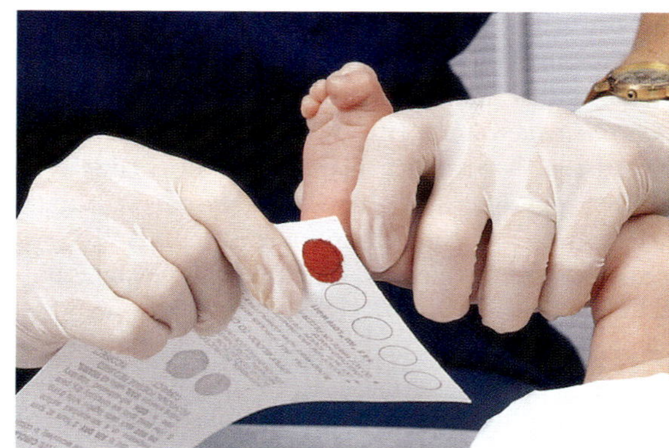

Fig. 24.16 Applying a drop of blood to the first circle on the filter paper of the newborn screening test card.

PATIENT COACHING Childhood Immunizations

- Encourage parents to have their children immunized.
- Emphasize to parents the importance of maintaining an immunization record card that documents all of their child's immunizations.
- Provide parents with educational materials on the importance of immunizations.
- Answer questions patients have about childhood immunizations.

What is immunity?

Immunity is the resistance of the body to microorganisms that cause disease. When an individual is infected with a pathogenic microorganism such as a virus or bacteria, the body responds by producing disease-fighting substances known as *antibodies*. Antibodies usually remain in the body even after the individual has recovered from the disease. This protects the individual from getting that disease again.

How do vaccines prevent disease?

The pathogens that cause disease or their toxins are weakened or killed and made into vaccines. These vaccines are administered to an individual, usually through injection. The body reacts to these vaccines the same way that it responds to the disease itself—by producing antibodies which fight disease. These antibodies last for a long time, often for life, to defend the body against disease.

What childhood diseases can be prevented through immunization?

The reduction of childhood disease by immunization during the past 50 years has been dramatic. Eighteen diseases can be prevented by routine immunization of children: hepatitis B, diphtheria, tetanus, pertussis (whooping cough), *Haemophilus influenzae* type b infections, polio, measles, mumps, rubella (German measles),

PATIENT COACHING Childhood Immunizations—cont'd

chickenpox (varicella), pneumococcal disease, respiratory syncytial virus (RSV) respiratory infections , COVID-19, human papillomavirus (HPV) infection, meningococcal disease, hepatitis A, rotavirus, and influenza (flu). Except for tetanus, all these diseases are contagious. They can be spread from child to child and from one community to another. When children are not protected against them, serious outbreaks of disease can still occur.

Haven't most of these diseases been eliminated in the United States?

Although most of the vaccine-preventable diseases have been reduced to very low levels in the United States, this is not true worldwide. Some of these diseases are quite prevalent in other countries. An infected traveler can bring these diseases into the United States without knowing it. If Americans were not immunized, these diseases could quickly spread throughout the population and cause an epidemic. Only when a disease has been eradicated worldwide is it safe to stop immunizing for that particular disease.

Do vaccines have side effects?

Vaccines are among the safest and most reliable medications available. Minor side effects may occur, however, after administration of a vaccine. They do not last long and may include a slight fever and irritability; redness, swelling, and soreness at the injection site; and a mild rash. Rarely, the effects can be more serious; if any unusual symptoms occur after a vaccine is administered, it is important to contact the provider immediately. Overall, the benefits of vaccines to prevent childhood diseases are greater than the possible risks for almost all children.

Are immunizations required by law?

Every state has laws requiring immunization against some or all of these diseases before children enter school. Children who get their immunizations benefit from the protection these immunizations provide. Immunizations also contribute to the well-being of everyone by reducing the chance for disease to spread. School immunization requirements for each state can be found on the CDC (Centers for Disease Control) website.

What Would You Do? What Would You *Not* Do? RESPONSES

Case Study 1

Page 539

What Did Traci Do?

- ❑ Listened patiently to Mrs. Chang and allowed her to vent her frustrations.
- ❑ Reassured Mrs. Chang that her milk is very nutritious for Christopher. Gave her a brochure on breast feeding that included information on what to do for sore nipples and engorgement.
- ❑ Gave Mrs. Chang the names and phone numbers of community resources for nursing mothers.
- ❑ Told Mrs. Chang that Christopher's weight and length do not fall in the underweight category on his growth chart. Showed her Christopher's growth chart so that she could see that Christopher is progressing normally.

What Did Traci Not Do?

- ❑ Did not tell Mrs. Chang to cheer up because the colic would eventually go away on its own.
- ❑ Did not give a personal opinion on whether Mrs. Chang should breast feed or bottle feed her infant.

Case Study 2

Page 545

What Did Traci Do?

- ❑ Explained to Mrs. Tilley that childhood obesity has increased dramatically in the United States and has become a serious health concern.
- ❑ Told Mrs. Tilley that she could have a big impact on Courtney's life by preparing healthy meals and eating them with her and by becoming involved in activities with Courtney, such as taking walks.
- ❑ Spent some time talking with Courtney about her interests and complimented Courtney on her achievements.
- ❑ Encouraged Courtney to join the swim team. Told her that lots of people do not like to be seen in a swim suit and encouraged her not to let that stand in her way of doing something she wants to do.
- ❑ Reassured Courtney that the doctor wants to help her and that he would never say anything bad about her weight.

What Did Traci Not Do?

- ❑ Did not agree with Mrs. Tilley that there is nothing that can be done about Courtney's weight problem.
- ❑ Did not tell Courtney that she needs to lose weight or she might develop serious health problems such as diabetes.

Case Study 3

Page 555

What Did Traci Do?

- ❑ Explained to Stacy that it is rare, but sometimes a child develops polio from getting the oral polio vaccine. Told her that this does not occur with the injectable polio vaccine.
- ❑ Explained to Stacy that chickenpox is usually a mild disease, but it can be serious, especially in young infants and adults.

Continued

What Would You Do? What Would You *Not* Do? RESPONSES—cont'd

- ❑ Explained to Stacy that most side effects from vaccines are mild and that complications from the diseases far outweigh the possible side effects.
- ❑ Told Stacy that these diseases have been reduced to very low levels in the United States, but they still occur in other countries. Explained that infected travelers can bring these diseases to the United States and infect individuals who are not immunized.
- ❑ Reminded Stacy that these vaccines are required for Matthew to start kindergarten.
- ❑ Talked with Matthew on his level about why he needs to be immunized.
- ❑ Told Matthew that they would play a game so that it wouldn't hurt as much. Taught him to hold up his finger and pretend that it was a birthday candle; when the injection was given, told him to keep blowing out the candle until he was told to stop.
- ❑ Told Matthew that he could choose a prize from the treasure chest after he had his immunizations.

What Did Traci Not Do?

- ❑ Did not ignore or minimize Stacy's concerns.
- ❑ Did not tell Stacy it would be all right to skip Matthew's immunizations.
- ❑ Did not refer to the immunizations as "shots" when talking with Matthew.
- ❑ Did not tell Matthew that it would not hurt when he gets his immunizations.

TERMINOLOGY REVIEW

Key Term	Word Parts	Definition
Adolescent		An individual from 12 to 18 years old.
Immunity		The resistance of the body to pathogenic microorganisms and their toxins.
Immunization (active, artificial)		The process of making an individual immune through the administration of a vaccine.
Infant		A child from birth to 12 months old.
Length (recumbent)		The measurement from the vertex of the head to the heel of the foot of an individual in a supine position.
Pediatrician	*pedi/a:* child	A physician who specializes in the care and development of children and the diagnosis and treatment of children's diseases.
Pediatrics	*pedi/a:* child	The branch of medicine that deals with the care and development of children and the diagnosis and treatment of children's diseases.
Preschool child	*pre-:* in front of; before	A child from 3 to 6 years old.
School-age child		A child from 6 to 12 years old.
Toddler		A child from 1 to 3 years old.
Toxoid		A toxic substance produced by a bacterium that has been treated by heat or chemicals to destroy its harmful properties. It is administered to an individual in a vaccine to prevent an infectious disease by stimulating the production of antibodies in that individual.
Vaccine		A suspension of weakened microorganisms, killed microorganisms, or toxoids administered to an individual to prevent an infectious disease by stimulating the production of antibodies in that individual.
Vertex		The top of the head.

PROCEDURE 24.1 Measuring the Weight and Length of an Infant

Outcome Measure the weight and length of an infant.

Equipment/Supplies

- Pediatric balance scale (table model)

1. **Procedural Step.** Sanitize your hands.
2. **Procedural Step.** Greet the infant's parent and introduce yourself. Identify the infant and explain the procedure to the parent. The weight of the infant is usually measured first. Depending on the medical office policy, ask the parent to perform one of the following:
   a. Remove the infant's clothing and put a dry diaper on the infant.
   b. Remove the infant's clothing, including the diaper.

   Principle. The infant should not be weighed with a wet diaper because it could increase the infant's weight considerably. Also, growth charts for infants and young children base their percentiles on the weight of the child without clothing.
3. **Procedural Step.** Unlock the pediatric scale, and place a clean paper protector on it. Check the balance scale for accuracy, making sure to compensate for the weight of the paper.

   Principle. The paper protector prevents cross-contamination and reduces the spread of disease from one patient to another.
4. **Procedural Step.** Gently place the infant on their back on the table of the scale. Place one hand slightly above the infant as a safety precaution.
5. **Procedural Step.** Balance the scale as follows:
   a. Move the lower weight to the notched groove that does not cause the indicator point to drop to the bottom of the calibration area. Ensure that the lower weight is seated firmly in its groove.
   b. Slowly slide the upper weight along its calibration bar by tapping it gently until the indicator point comes to rest at the center of the balance area.

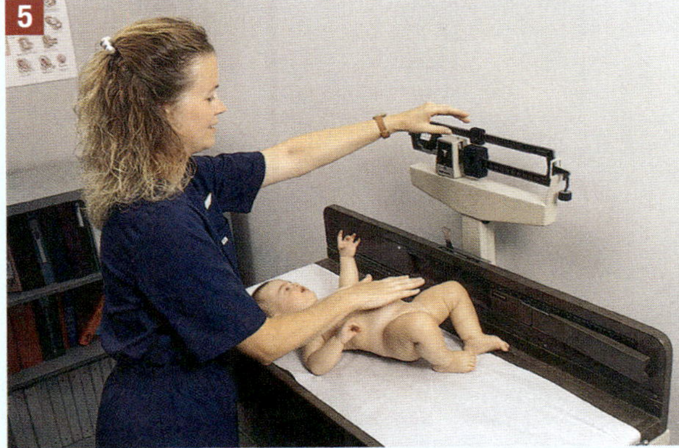

Balance the scale.

   Principle. Not seating the lower weight firmly in its groove results in an inaccurate reading.
6. **Procedural Step.** Read the results while the infant is lying still. Jot down this value or make a mental note of it. (*Note:* The result on the pictured scale is 15 lb, 2 oz.)

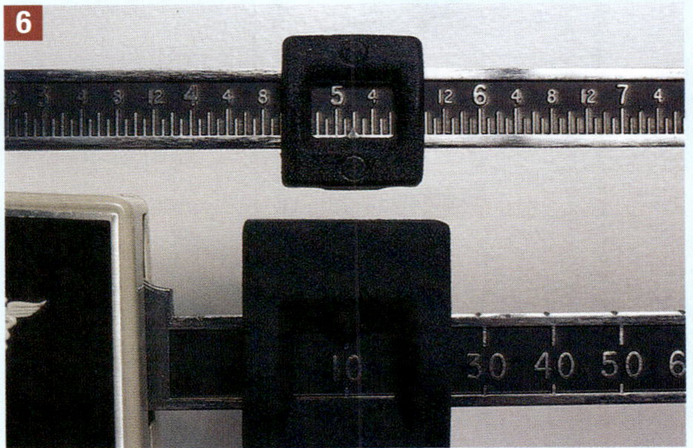

Read the results in pounds and ounces.

7. **Procedural Step.** Return the balance to its resting position, and lock the scale.
8. **Procedural Step.** Place the vertex (top) of the infant's head against the headboard at the zero mark. Ask the parent to hold the infant's head in this position.

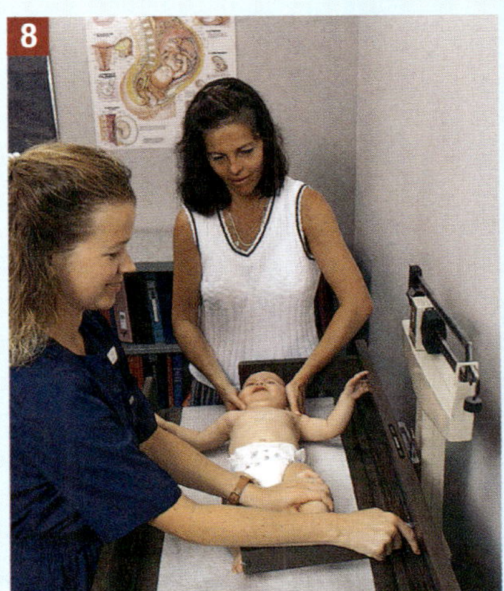

Properly position the infant.

9. **Procedural Step.** Straighten the infant's knees, and place the soles of their feet firmly against the upright footboard (to create a right-angle).

Continued

PROCEDURE 24.1

PROCEDURE 24.1 Measuring the Weight and Length of an Infant—cont'd

10. **Procedural Step.** Read the infant's length in inches to the nearest ⅛ inch from the measure. Jot down this value or make a mental note of it. (*Note:* The result on this scale is 25½ inches.)

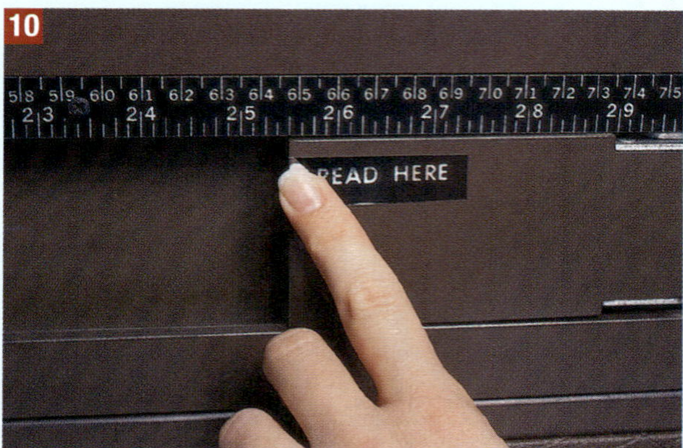

Read the length in inches.

11. **Procedural Step.** Gently remove the infant from the table, and hand them to the parent. Return the headboard and footboard to their resting positions.
12. **Procedural Step.** Sanitize your hands.
13. **Procedural Step.** Document the results in the patient's medical record.
    a. *Electronic medical record:* Document the infant's weight and length measurements using the appropriate radio buttons, drop-down menus, and free text fields. The electronic medical record will automatically calculate the child's growth percentiles and plot them on a growth chart once you enter the infant's weight and length measurements into the computer.
    b. *Paper-based patient record:* Document the date and time and the infant's weight and length measurements.

13b DOCUMENTATION EXAMPLE

Date	
8/10/XX	9:30 a.m. Wt. 15 lb 2 oz. Length 25 1/2 in.——
	———————— T. Powell, CMA (AAMA)

PROCEDURE 24.2 Measuring Head and Chest Circumference of an Infant

Outcome Measure the head and chest circumference of an infant.

Equipment/Supplies

- Flexible nonstretch centimeter tape measure

Measurement of Head Circumference

1. **Procedural Step.** Sanitize your hands and assemble the equipment.
2. **Procedural Step.** Greet the infant's parent and introduce yourself. Identify the infant and explain the procedure to the parent.
3. **Procedural Step.** Position the infant. The infant should be placed on their back on the examining table. An alternative position is to have the parent hold the infant.
4. **Procedural Step.** Position the centimeter tape measure around the infant's head at the greatest circumference. This is usually accomplished by placing the tape measure slightly above the eyebrows and pinna of the ears and around the occipital prominence at the back of the skull.

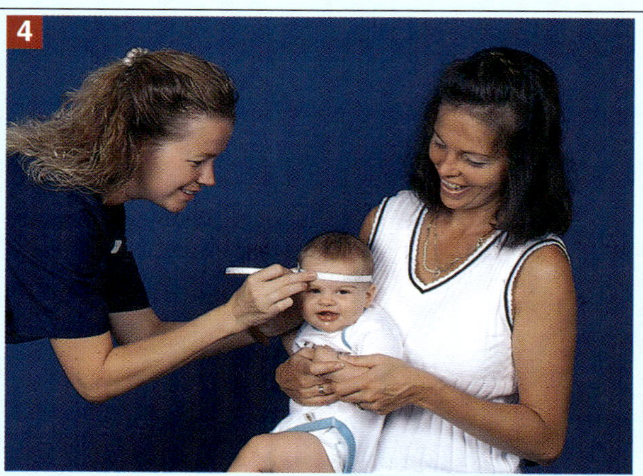

Position the tape measure around the infant's head.

PROCEDURE 24.2

PROCEDURE 24.2 Measuring Head and Chest Circumference of an Infant—cont'd

5. **Procedural Step.** Read the results in centimeters to the nearest 0.5 cm. Jot down this value or make a mental note of it. Sanitize your hands.
6. **Procedural Step.** Document the results in the patient's medical record.
   a. *Electronic medical record:* Document the infant's head circumference measurement using the appropriate radio buttons, drop-down menus, and free text fields. The electronic medical record will automatically calculate the child's head circumference percentile and plot it on a growth chart once you enter the infant's head circumference measurement into the computer.
   b. *Paper-based patient record:* Document the date and time and the infant's head circumference measurement in centimeters.

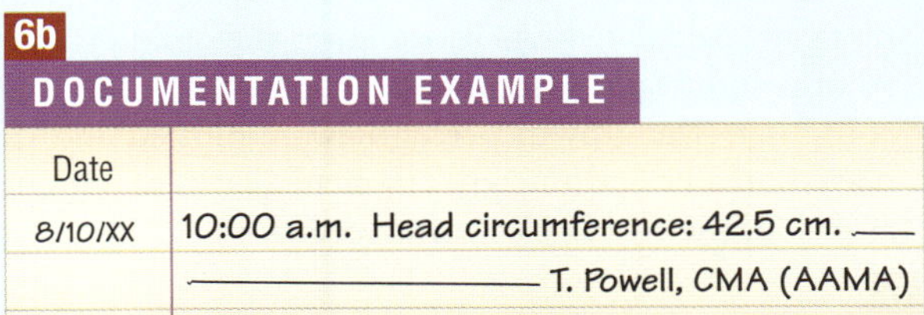

6b

DOCUMENTATION EXAMPLE

Date	
8/10/XX	10:00 a.m. Head circumference: 42.5 cm. ___
	________________ T. Powell, CMA (AAMA)

Measurement of Chest Circumference

1. **Procedural Step.** Sanitize your hands and assemble the equipment.
2. **Procedural Step.** Greet the infant's parent and introduce yourself. Identify the infant and explain the procedure to the parent.
3. **Procedural Step.** Position the infant on their back on the examining table.
4. **Procedural Step.** Encircle the centimeter tape measure around the infant's chest at the nipple line. It should be snug, but not so tight that it leaves a mark.

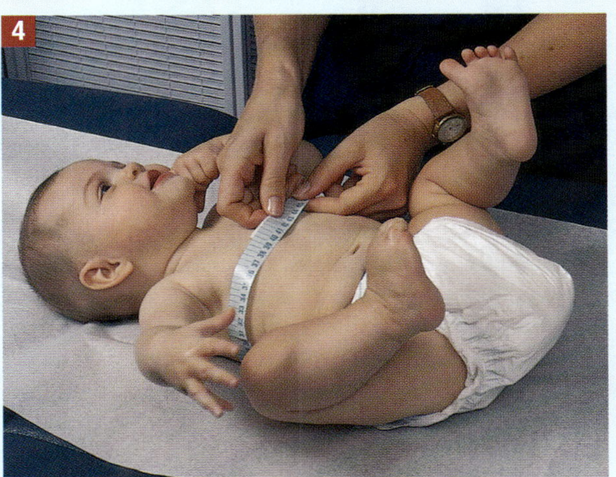

Encircle the tape around the infant's chest.

5. **Procedural Step.** Read the results in centimeters to the nearest 0.5 cm. Jot down this value or make a mental note of it. Sanitize your hands.
6. **Procedural Step.** Document the results in the patient's medical record.
   a. *Electronic medical record:* Document the infant's chest circumference measurement using the appropriate radio buttons, drop-down menus, and free text fields.
   b. *Paper-based patient record:* Document the date and time and the infant's chest circumference measurement in centimeters.

6b

DOCUMENTATION EXAMPLE

Date	
8/15/XX	10:00 a.m. Chest circumference: 42 cm. ___
	________________ T. Powell, CMA (AAMA)

PROCEDURE 24.3 Calculating Growth Percentiles

Outcome Plot a pediatric growth value on a growth chart.

Equipment/Supplies

- Pediatric growth chart

1. **Procedural Step.** Select the proper growth chart.
2. **Procedural Step.** Locate the child's age in the horizontal column at the bottom of the chart.
3. **Procedural Step.** Locate the growth value in the vertical column under the appropriate category (weight, length or stature, and head circumference).
4. **Procedural Step.** Draw an imaginary vertical line from the child's age mark and an imaginary horizontal line from the child's growth mark. Find the site at which the two lines intersect on the graph and place a dot on this site.

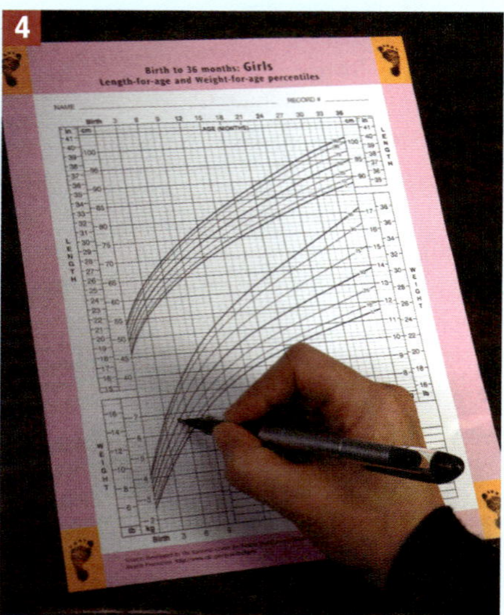

5. **Procedural Step.** To determine the percentile in which the child falls, follow the curved percentile line upward to read the value located on the right side of the chart. Interpolation is needed if the value does not fall exactly on a percentile line. (*Interpolation* means that you must estimate a percentile that falls between a larger and a smaller known percentile.)
6. **Procedural Step.** Document the results in the patient's medical record. Include the date and time and each growth percentile. In a medical office that uses an electronic medical record, the growth percentiles are automatically calculated when you enter the child's weight, length, and head circumference measurements into the computer. The growth percentiles are plotted and displayed on an electronic growth chart that is maintained as part of the child's electronic record.

6

DOCUMENTATION EXAMPLE

Date	
10/22/XX	10:30 a.m. Weight: 55%. Length: 70%. ———
	Head Circum: 67% —— T. Powell, CMA (AAMA)

PROCEDURE 24.3 Calculating Growth Percentiles—cont'd

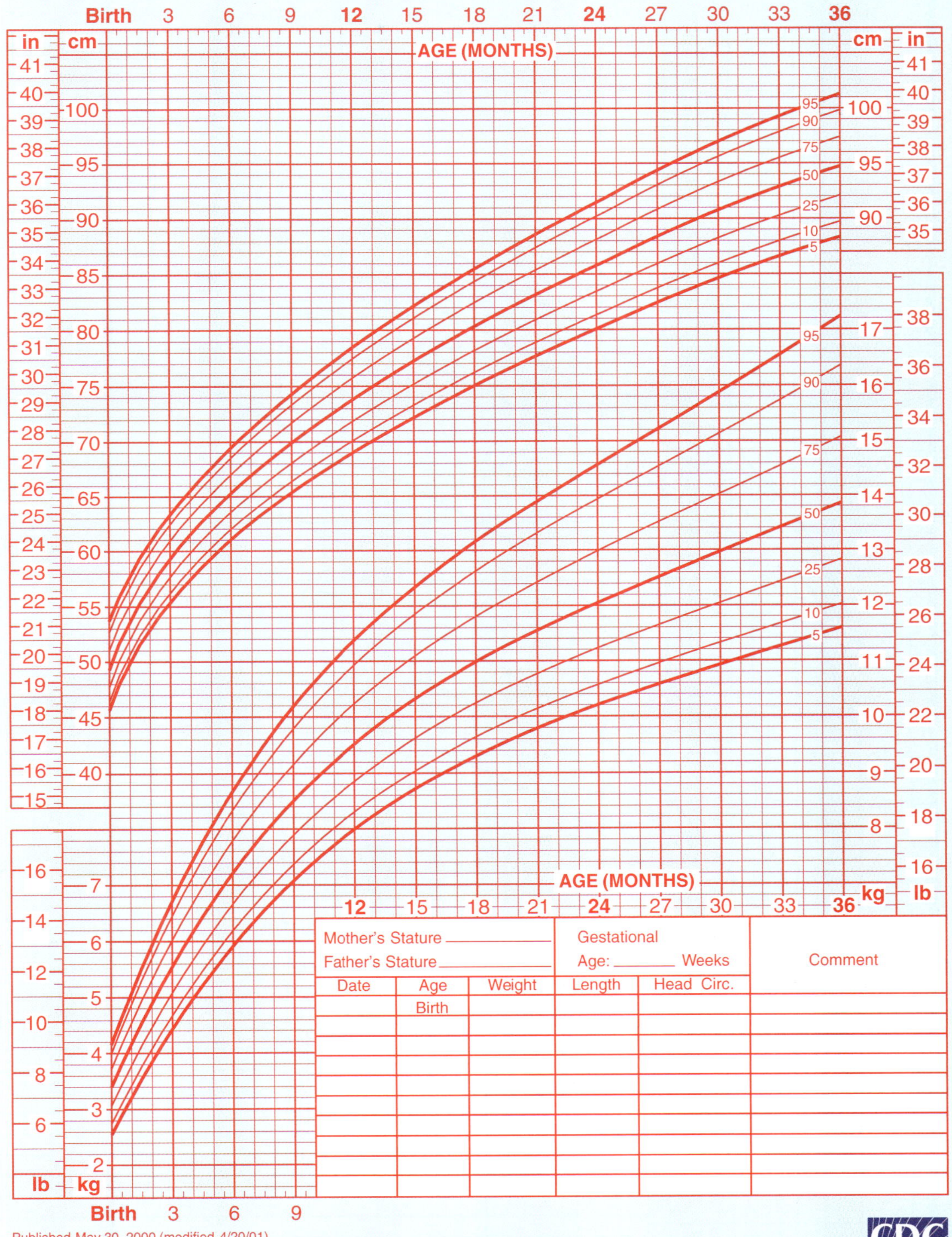

Birth to 36 months: Girls
Length-for-age and Weight-for-age percentiles

NAME ______________________

RECORD# ______________

Birth 3 6 9 12 15 18 21 24 27 30 33 36

AGE (MONTHS)

LENGTH: in 15–41; cm 40–100 (left scale); cm 90–100, in 35–41 (right scale)

Length percentiles: 95, 90, 75, 50, 25, 10, 5

WEIGHT: kg 8–17, lb 16–38 (right scale)

Weight percentiles: 95, 90, 75, 50, 25, 10, 5

WEIGHT: lb 6–16, kg 2–7 (left scale)

AGE (MONTHS)

12 15 18 21 24 27 30 33 36 kg lb

Mother's Stature ______ Father's Stature ______			Gestational Age: ______ Weeks		Comment
Date	Age	Weight	Length	Head Circ.	
	Birth				

Birth 3 6 9

Published May 30, 2000 (modified 4/20/01).
SOURCE: Developed by the National Center for Health Statistics in collaboration with the National Center for Chronic Disease Prevention and Health Promotion (2000).
http://www.cdc.gov/growthcharts

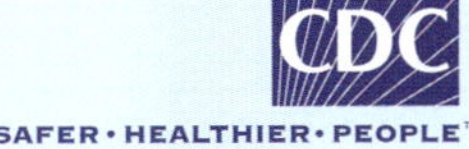

Continued

PROCEDURE 24.3 Calculating Growth Percentiles—cont'd

Birth to 36 months: Boys
Length-for-age and Weight-for-age percentiles

NAME ______________________

RECORD# ______________

Birth 3 6 9 12 15 18 21 24 27 30 33 36

AGE (MONTHS)

LENGTH (in / cm) — percentiles 95, 90, 75, 50, 25, 10, 5

WEIGHT (lb / kg) — percentiles 95, 90, 75, 50, 25, 10, 5

Mother's Stature ______________ Gestational

Father's Stature ______________ Age: ________ Weeks

Date	Age	Weight	Length	Head Circ.	Comment
	Birth				

Published May 30, 2000 (modified 4/20/01).
SOURCE: Developed by the National Center for Health Statistics in collaboration with the National Center for Chronic Disease Prevention and Health Promotion (2000).
http://www.cdc.gov/growthcharts

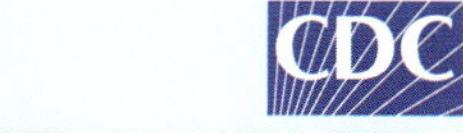

SAFER • HEALTHIER • PEOPLE™

PROCEDURE 24.4 Applying a Pediatric Urine Collector

Outcome Apply a pediatric urine collector.

Equipment/Supplies

- Disposable gloves
- Personal antiseptic wipes
- Pediatric urine collector bag
- Urine specimen container and label
- Regular waste container

1. **Procedural Step.** Sanitize your hands.
2. **Procedural Step.** Assemble the equipment.
3. **Procedural Step.** Greet the child's parent and introduce yourself. Identify the child and explain the procedure to the parent.
4. **Procedural Step.** Apply gloves. Position the child. The child should be placed on their back with the legs spread apart. The medical assistant may need another individual to hold the child's legs apart.
   Principle. This position facilitates cleansing of the genitalia and permits proper application of the urine collector bag.
5. **Procedural Step.** Cleanse the child's genitalia.
   a. *Female:* Using a front-to-back motion (pubis to anus), cleanse each side of the meatus with a separate wipe. With a third wipe, cleanse directly down the middle (directly over the urinary meatus). Discard each wipe after cleansing. Allow the area to dry completely.
   b. *Male:* If the child is not circumcised, retract the foreskin of the penis. Cleanse the area around the meatus and the urethral opening (meatal orifice) in a manner similar to that used to cleanse the female patient. Use a separate wipe for each swipe. Cleanse the scrotum last, using a fresh wipe. Discard each wipe after cleansing. Allow the area to dry completely.
   Principle. The urinary meatus and surrounding area must be cleansed to prevent contaminants, such as baby powder, fecal material, and microorganisms, from entering the urine specimen, which could affect the test results. A front-to-back motion must be used to prevent drawing microorganisms from the anal area into the area being cleansed. The area must be completely dry to ensure an airtight adhesion of the collection bag to prevent leakage of urine.
6. **Procedural Step.** Remove the paper backing from the urine collector bag. This exposes the hypoallergenic adhesive surface around the opening of the bag.

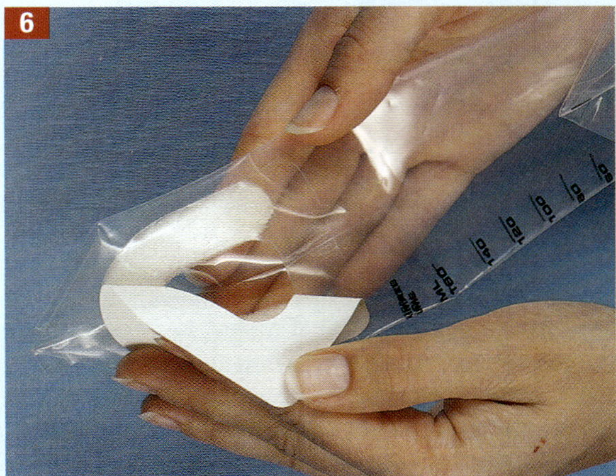

Remove paper backing from the urine collector bag.

7. **Procedural Step.** Firmly attach the bag in the following manner:
   a. *Female:* Stretch the perineum taut, and firmly place the bottom of the adhesive surface on the infant's perineum. Starting at the perineum and working upward, firmly press the adhesive surface to the skin surrounding the external genitalia, ensuring there is no puckering. The opening of the bag should be directly over the urinary meatus. The excess of the bag should be positioned toward the child's feet.

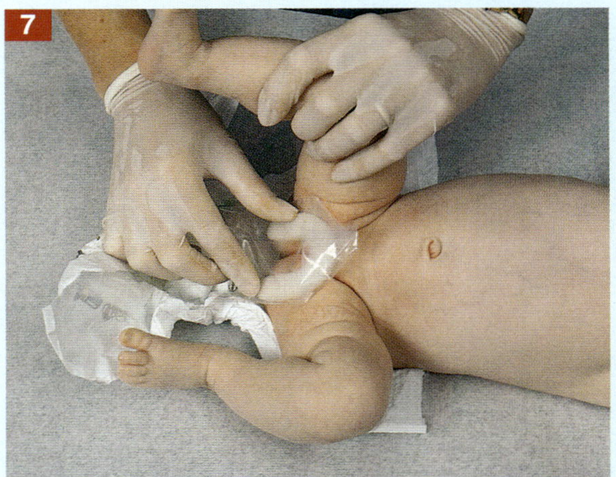

Firmly press the adhesive surface to the skin surrounding the external genitalia.

PROCEDURE 24.4

Continued

PROCEDURE 24.4 Applying a Pediatric Urine Collector—cont'd

7a

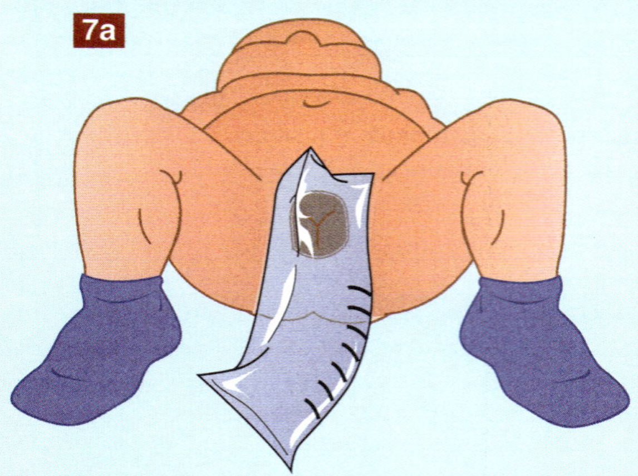

Female: The opening of the bag should be directly over the urinary meatus.

b. *Male:* Position the bag so that the child's penis and scrotum are projected through the opening of the bag. Starting at the perineum and working upward, firmly press the adhesive surface to the skin surrounding the penis and scrotum, ensuring there is no puckering. The excess of the bag should be positioned toward the child's feet.

7b

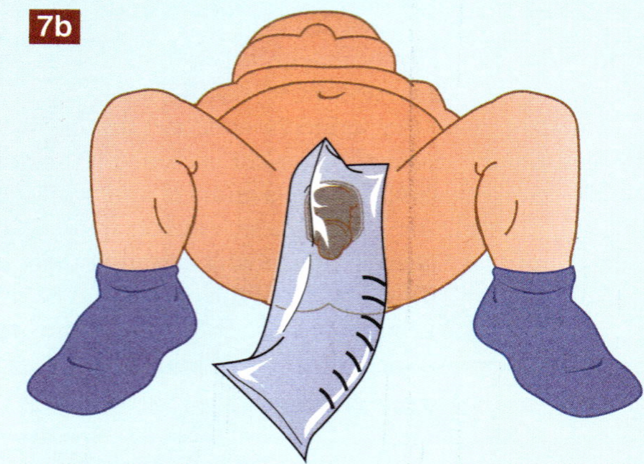

Male: The penis and scrotum are projected through the opening of the bag.

Principle. The adhesive surface of the bag must be attached securely with no puckering to prevent leakage.

8. **Procedural Step.** Loosely diaper the child. Check the urine collector bag every 15 minutes until a urine specimen is obtained.
   Principle. The diaper helps hold the urine collector bag in place. The bag must be checked frequently. Once the infant has urinated, moisture from the urine may cause the adhesive surface to become loose and leak, especially with an active infant.
9. **Procedural Step.** When the child has voided, gently remove the urine collector bag by holding the bottom of the adhesive surface against the infant's skin and carefully peeling the bag off from the top to the bottom.
   Principle. The bag must be removed gently because pulling the adhesive away too quickly may cause discomfort and irritation of the child's skin.
10. **Procedural Step.** Cleanse the genital area with a personal antiseptic wipe. Rediaper the child.
11. **Procedural Step.** Transfer the urine specimen into a urine specimen container, and tightly apply the lid. Label the container with the child's name and date of birth, the date, the time of collection, and the type of specimen (i.e., urine). Dispose of the collector bag in a regular waste container. (*Note:* The urine collector bag can be used as a urine container to transport the specimen to the laboratory. This is accomplished by folding the adhesive sponge ring in half along its vertical axis and pressing the adhesive surfaces firmly together to ensure a tight seal.)
12. **Procedural Step.** Based on the medical office routine, test the urine specimen or prepare it for transfer to an outside laboratory; be sure to include a completed laboratory request form. If the specimen cannot be tested or transferred immediately, preserve it by placing it in the refrigerator.
    Principle. Changes occur in a urine specimen that is left sitting out at room temperature, which can lead to inaccurate test results.
13. **Procedural Step.** Remove the gloves, and sanitize your hands.
14. **Procedural Step.** Document the procedure in the patient's medical record.
    a. *Electronic medical record:* Document the type of specimen (i.e., urine) and the testing that was completed, using the appropriate radio buttons, drop-down menus, and free text fields. If the specimen is to be transported to an outside laboratory, document this information, including the laboratory tests ordered.
    b. *Paper-based patient record:* Document the date, the time of collection, and the type of specimen (i.e., urine). If the specimen is to be transported to an outside laboratory, indicate this information, including the laboratory tests ordered.

14b

DOCUMENTATION EXAMPLE

Date	
8/12/XX	10:15 a.m. Urine specimen collected for
	culture. Picked up by Medical Center Lab on
	8/12/XX. ———— T. Powell, CMA (AAMA)

Minor Office Surgery

Check out the Evolve site at http://evolve.elsevier.com/Bonewit/today to access additional interactive activities and exercises to help you study and prepare for success.

LEARNING OBJECTIVES/ PROCEDURES

Surgical Asepsis

1. State the characteristics of a minor surgical procedure.
2. Identify procedures that require the use of surgical asepsis.
3. Describe the medical assistant's responsibilities during a minor surgical procedure.
4. List the guidelines to follow to maintain surgical asepsis during a sterile procedure.
5. Identify surgical instruments commonly used in the medical office and explain the use and care of each instrument.

Apply and remove surgical gloves.
Open a sterile package.
Add an item to a sterile field.
Pour a sterile solution.

Wound Healing

6. Explain the differences between a closed and an open wound and give examples.
7. List and explain the three phases of the healing process.
8. List and describe the different types of wound exudates.
9. List the functions of a dressing.

Change a sterile dressing.

Methods of Wound Closure

10. Explain the method used to measure the diameter of suturing material.
11. Describe the two types of sutures (absorbable and nonabsorbable) and give examples of their uses.
12. Categorize suturing needles according to type of point and shape.
13. State the advantages and wound care instructions for each of the following wound closure methods: sutures, surgical skin staples, topical tissue adhesives, and skin closure tape.

Set up a tray for suture insertion.
Remove sutures.
Remove surgical staples.
Assist the provider with the application of a topical tissue adhesive.
Apply and remove skin closure tape.

Minor Office Surgical Procedures

14. Explain the purpose of and procedure for each of the following minor surgical operations: sebaceous cyst removal, incision and drainage of a localized infection, mole removal, needle biopsy, ingrown toenail removal, colposcopy, cervical punch biopsy, and cryosurgery.
15. Explain the principles underlying each step in the minor office surgery procedures.

Assist the provider with minor office surgery.

Bandaging

16. State the functions of a bandage, and list the guidelines for applying a bandage.
17. Identify the common types of bandages used in the medical office.

Apply each of the following bandage turns:

- Circular
- Spiral
- Spiral-reverse
- Figure-eight
- Recurrent

CHAPTER OUTLINE

KEY TERMS

abrasion (ah-BRAY-shun)
abscess (AB-sess)
absorbable sutures (ab-SOR-ba-bul SOO-chur)
approximation (ah-PROKS-ih-MAY-shun)
bandage
biopsy (BYE-op-see)
colposcope (KOL-poh-skope)
colposcopy (kol-POS-koh-pee)
contaminate (kon-TAM-in-ate)
contusion (kon-TOO-shun)
cryosurgery (KRY-oh-SURJ-er-ee)
exudate (EKS-oo-date)
fibroblast (FYE-broh-blast)
forceps (FORE-seps)
furuncle (FYOOR-un-kul)
hemostasis (hee-moe-STAY-sis)
incision (in-SIH-shun)
infection (in-FEK-shun)
infiltration (in-fill-TRAY-shun)
inflammation (in-flah-MAY-shun)
laceration (lass-ur-AY-shun)
ligate (LIH-gate)
local anesthetic (LOE-kul an-es-STET-ik)
needle biopsy (NEE-dul BYE-op-see)
nonabsorbable suture (non-ab-SOR-ba-bul SOO-chur)
postoperative (post-OP-er-uh-tiv)
preoperative (pree-OP-er-uh-tiv)
puncture (PUNK-shur)
scalpel (SKAL-pul)
scissors
sebaceous cyst (suh-BAY-shus SIST)
sterile (STARE-ul)
surgery
surgical asepsis (SUR-jih-kul ay-SEP-sis)
sutures (SOO-churz)
swaged (SWAYJD) needle
wound

INTRODUCTION TO MINOR OFFICE SURGERY

The term **surgery** is defined as the branch of medicine that deals with operative and manual procedures for correction of deformities and defects, repair of injuries, and diagnosis and treatment of certain diseases. *Minor office surgery* (also known as *minor surgery*) refers to a surgical procedure that is restricted to the management of minor conditions and injuries that does not require the use of general anesthesia. Minor surgical procedures have the following characteristics:

- Are performed in an ambulatory health care facility, such as a medical office or clinic
- Can be performed in a short period of time, usually in less than 1 hour
- Require a local anesthetic, a topical anesthetic, or no anesthetic
- Can be performed safely with a minimum of discomfort to the patient
- Do not, under normal circumstances, pose a major risk to life or to the function of an organ or body parts

Various types of minor surgical procedures are performed in the medical office, such as insertion of sutures, sebaceous cyst removal, incision and drainage of infections, mole removal, needle biopsies, cervical biopsies, and ingrown toenail removal. The provider explains the nature of the surgical procedure and any risks to the patient and offers to answer questions. The medical assistant is responsible for **preoperative** (before a surgical operation) instructions such as explaining the patient preparation required for the procedure) and obtaining the patient's signature on a written consent to treatment form, which grants the provider permission to perform the surgery (Fig. 25.1).

Additional responsibilities of the medical assistant include preparing the treatment room, preparing the patient, preparing the minor surgery tray, assisting the provider during the procedure, administering **postoperative** (after a surgical operation) care to the patient, and cleaning the treatment room after the procedure.

The treatment room must be spotlessly clean, and the medical assistant should ensure that the provider has adequate lighting for the procedure. The patient is positioned and draped according to the procedure to be performed. The skin is prepared as specified by the provider. Hair

(Attach label or complete blanks)

First name: ____________ Last name: ____________

Date of Birth: ______ Month ______ Day ______ Year

Account Number: ______________________

Procedure Consent Form

I, ______________________________, hereby consent to have

Dr. ____________ perform ______________________.

I have been fully informed of the following by my physician:

1. The nature of my condition.
2. The nature and purpose of the procedure.
3. An explanation of risks involved with the procedure.
4. Alternative treatments or procedures available.
5. The likely results of the procedure.
6. The risks involved with declining or delaying the procedure.

My physician has offered to answer all questions concerning the proposed procedure.

I am aware that the practice of medicine and surgery is not an exact science, and I acknowledge that no guarantees have been made to me about the results of the procedure.

Patient ______________________ Date ____________

(or guardian and relationship)

Witnessed ______________________ Date ____________

Fig. 25.1 Consent to treatment form.

around the operative site is a contaminant and may need to be removed by shaving. The skin is cleansed, and an appropriate antiseptic is applied to the area to reduce the number of microorganisms present.

The medical assistant is responsible for preparing the minor surgery tray. The specific instruments and supplies included in each setup vary, depending on the type of surgery to be performed and the provider's preference. The medical assistant must become familiar with the instruments and supplies required for each surgical procedure performed in the medical office.

During the minor surgery, the medical assistant is present to assist the provider as needed and to lend support to the patient. The medical assistant should become completely familiar with the assisting techniques (e.g., swabbing blood from the operative site) required for each surgical procedure performed in the medical office and should learn to anticipate the provider's needs to help the procedure go quickly and smoothly.

After the minor surgery, the medical assistant should remain with the patient as a safety precaution to prevent accidental falls and other injuries and to make sure the patient understands the postoperative instructions. The medical assistant removes and properly cares for all used instruments and supplies and cleans the treatment room in preparation for the next patient.

SURGICAL ASEPSIS

The term **sterile** is defined as free from all living microorganisms and bacterial spores. **Surgical asepsis** refers to practices that keep objects and areas sterile. Surgical asepsis protects the patient from pathogenic microorganisms that may enter the body and cause disease. It is always employed under the following circumstances: when caring for broken skin, such as open wounds and suture punctures; when a skin surface is being penetrated, as by a surgical incision for a mole removal or the administration of an injection (the needle must remain sterile); and when a body cavity is entered that is normally sterile, such as during the insertion of a urinary catheter. Sterility of instruments and supplies is achieved through the use of disposable sterile items or by sterilizing reusable articles.

A sterile object that touches any unsterile object is automatically considered contaminated and must not be used. The term **contaminate** refers to the situation in which a sterile object or surface becomes uinsterile. If the medical assistant is in doubt or has a question concerning the sterility of an article, they should consider it contaminated and replace it with a sterile article.

Sterility of the hands cannot be attained. Sanitizing the hands renders them medically aseptic and must be performed before and after every surgical procedure using proper technique (see Chapter 17). To prevent contamination of sterile articles, surgical (sterile) gloves must be worn while picking up or transferring articles during a sterile procedure. Procedure 25.1 describes the procedure for applying and removing surgical gloves.

INSTRUMENTS USED IN MINOR OFFICE SURGERY

A variety of surgical instruments are used for minor office surgery. Most surgical instruments are made of stainless steel and have either a bright, highly polished finish or a dull finish. The medical assistant should become familiar with the name, use, and proper care of all instruments used in the medical office. Surgical instruments are named according to one or more of the following: (1) function (e.g., splinter forceps); (2) design (e.g., mosquito hemostatic forceps); and (3) the individual who developed the instrument (e.g., Kelly hemostatic forceps). The parts of an instrument are illustrated in Fig. 25.2; some common instruments are described here and are illustrated in Fig. 25.3.

SCALPELS

A **scalpel** is a small, straight surgical knife consisting of a handle and a thin, sharp steel blade. A scalpel is used to make surgical incisions and can divide tissue with the least possible trauma to surrounding structures. Both disposable and reusable scalpels are available. A disposable scalpel consists of a nonslip plastic handle and a permanently attached steel blade that is individually packaged to maintain sterility. Scalpels that are reusable consist of a reusable stainless steel handle to which a disposable steel blade is attached. The blade comes individually packaged in a moisture-proof sterile package.

SCISSORS

Scissors are cutting instruments that have ring handles and straight (str) or curved (cvd) blades. Both blade tips may be sharp (s/s), both may be blunt (b/b), or one tip may be blunt and the other sharp (b/s). The two parts of a pair of scissors come together at a hinge joint known as a *box lock* (see Fig. 25.2). The type of scissors employed depends on

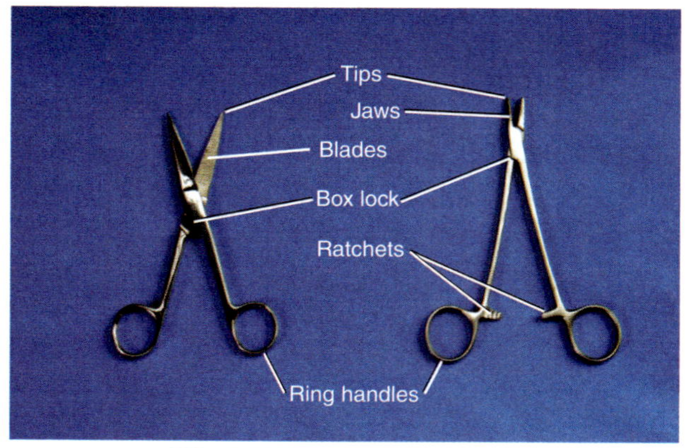

Fig. 25.2 Parts of an instrument.

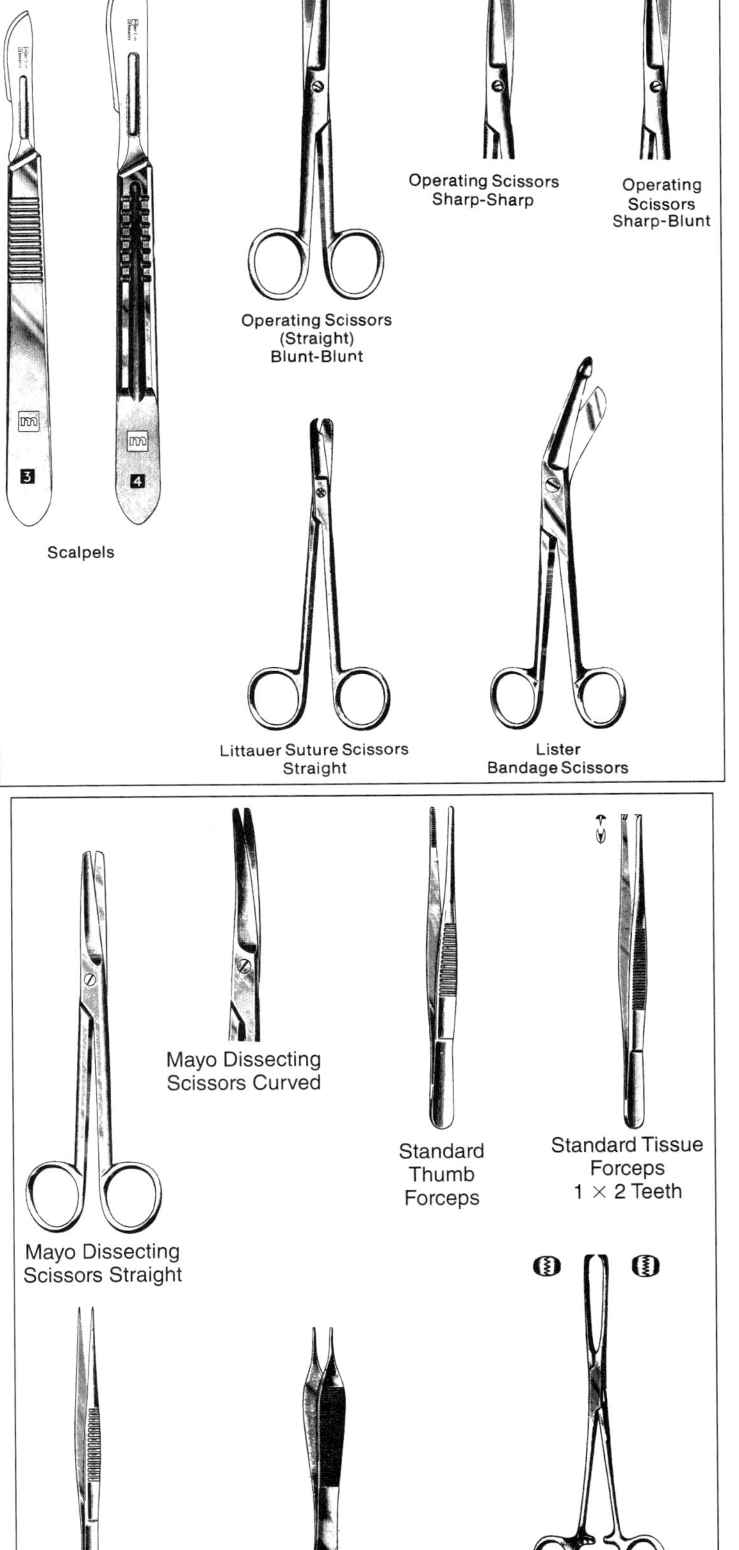

Fig. 25.3 Instruments used in minor office surgery. (Courtesy of Elmed, Addison, IL.)

Continued

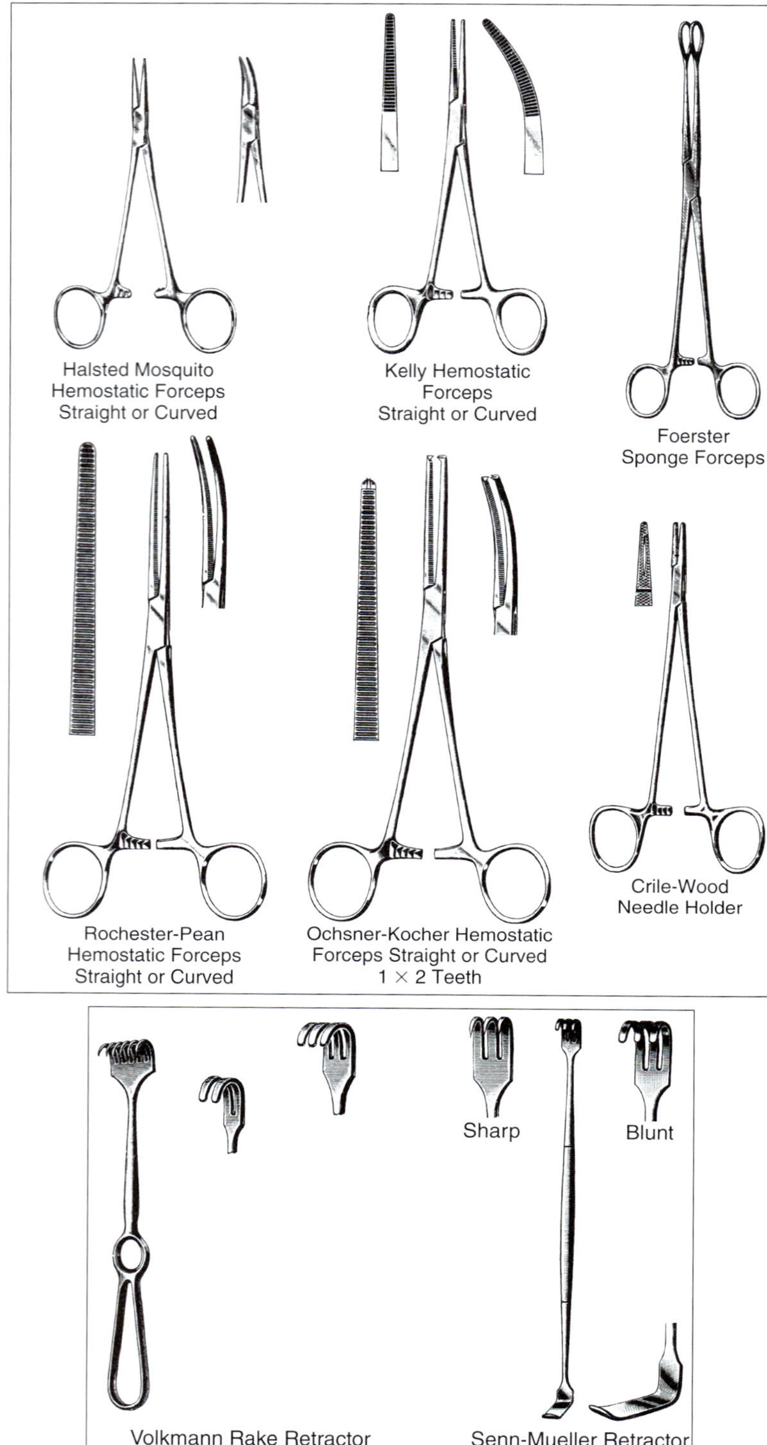

Fig. 25.3, cont'd

the intended use. The various types of scissors are listed and described next.

- *Operating scissors* have straight delicate blades with sharp cutting edges and are used to cut through tissue. They are available with sharp/sharp, blunt/blunt, or blunt/sharp blade tips.
- *Suture scissors* are used to remove sutures. The hook on the tip aids in getting under a suture, and the blunt end prevents puncturing of the tissues.
- *Bandage scissors* are inserted beneath a dressing or bandage to cut it for removal. The flat blunt prow can be inserted beneath a dressing without puncturing the skin.

- *Dissecting scissors* have thick beveled blades with a fine cutting edge used to divide or separate tissue rather than cut it. Dissecting scissors are available with straight or curved blades. Both blade tips of dissecting scissors are blunt.

FORCEPS

Forceps are instruments for grasping, squeezing, or holding tissue or an item such as sterile gauze. Some forceps have two prongs and a spring handle (e.g., thumb, tissue, splinter, dressing forceps) that provides the proper tension for grasping an object such as tissue, a foreign object, or sterile gauze. Some forceps have *serrations* (e.g., thumb and hemostatic forceps), which are sawlike teeth that grasp tissue and prevent it from slipping out of the jaws of the instrument. As is shown in Fig. 25.3, some varieties have toothed clasps on the handle, known as *ratchets* (see Fig. 25.2), to hold the jaws of the instrument securely together and lock them in place (e.g., Allis tissue forceps, hemostatic forceps). The ratchets are designed to allow locked closure of the jaws at two or more positions. The various types of forceps are listed and described next.

- *Thumb forceps* have serrated jaws and are used to pick up tissue or to hold tissue between adjacent surfaces.
- *Tissue forceps* have teeth, which are used to grasp tissue and prevent it from slipping. Tissue forceps are identified by the number of apposing teeth on each jaw (e.g., 1 × 2, 2 × 3, 3 × 4). Tissue forceps are sometimes referred to as "rat-toothed" forceps because the pointed projections resemble the teeth of a rat. The teeth should approximate tightly when the instrument is closed.
- *Splinter forceps* have sharp points that are useful in removing foreign objects, such as splinters, from the tissues.
- *Dressing forceps* are used in the application and removal of dressings. They are also used to hold or grasp sterile gauze or sutures during a surgical procedure. Dressing forceps have blunt ends that contain coarse cross-striations used for grasping.
- *Hemostatic forceps* have serrated jaws, ratchets, ring handles, and a box lock and are available with straight or curved blades. Hemostats are used to clamp off blood vessels and to establish **hemostasis** (arrest of bleeding) until the vessels can be closed with sutures. The serrations on a hemostat prevent the blood vessel from slipping out of the jaws of the instrument. The ratchets keep the jaws of the hemostat tightly shut and locked in place when it is closed. The ring handles allow for a secure grasp of the hemostat and also are used to select the desired ratchet position. The serrated jaws should mesh together smoothly when the hemostat is closed; if they spring back open, the instrument is in need of repair. *Mosquito hemostatic forceps* have small, fine jaws and are smaller and more delicate than standard Kelly hemostatic forceps. Mosquito hemostatic forceps are used to hold delicate tissue or to clamp off smaller blood vessels, whereas standard hemostatic forceps are used to grasp and compress larger blood vessels.
- *Sponge forceps* have ring handles, ratchets, a box lock, and oval serrated jaws for holding sponges. A *sponge* is a porous, absorbent pad, such as a 4-inch gauze pad, used to absorb fluids, apply medication, or cleanse an area.

MISCELLANEOUS INSTRUMENTS

Various miscellaneous instruments used in the medical office are listed and described next.

- *Needle holders* have serrated jaws, ring handles, ratchets, and a box lock. A needle holder is used to firmly grasp, hold, and manipulate a suture needle during suture insertion. The serrated jaws of a needle holder are designed to hold the suture needle securely without damaging it. A needle holder is sometimes referred to as a "needle driver" because it functions to drive a suture needle through the skin during wound closure.
- *Retractors* are used to hold tissues aside to improve the exposure of the operative area.

CARE OF SURGICAL INSTRUMENTS

Surgical instruments are expensive, are delicate yet durable, and last for many years if handled and maintained properly. The care an instrument receives depends to a large degree on the parts making up the instrument (e.g., blades, jaws, serations, ratchets, ring handles, box lock). The medical assistant works with instruments while setting up a sterile tray, performing certain procedures such as suture removal and sterile dressing change, and cleaning up after minor office surgery and during the sanitization and sterilization process. During each of these procedures, guidelines must be followed to prolong the life span of each instrument and to ensure its proper functioning:

1. Always handle instruments carefully. Dropping an instrument on the floor or throwing an instrument into a basin could damage it.
2. Do not pile instruments in a heap because they become entangled and might be damaged when separated.
3. Keep sharp instruments separate from the rest of the instruments to prevent damaging or dulling the cutting edge. Also, keep delicate instruments, such as lensed instruments, separate to protect them from damage.
4. To prolong the proper functioning of the ratchet, keep instruments with a ratchet in an open position when not in use.
5. Rinse blood and body secretions off an instrument as soon as possible to prevent them from drying and hardening on the instrument.
6. When performing procedures that require surgical instruments, always use the instrument for the purpose for which it was designed. Substituting one type of instrument for another could damage it.
7. Sanitize and sterilize instruments using proper technique.

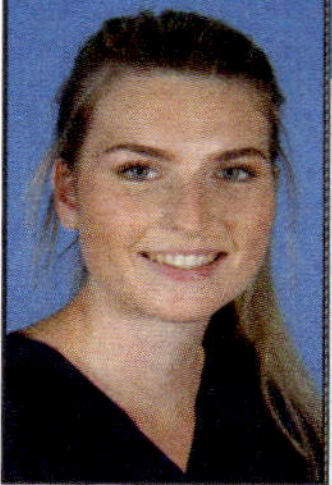

Putting It All Into Practice

My name is Heather, and I have worked as the office manager of an internal medicine office for the past 7 years. My job includes front and back office duties, including scheduling appointments, transcription, patient calls, patient workups, injections, electrocardiograms, and venipuncture. The most interesting part of my job is dealing with the many different personalities of the patients I come in contact with daily.

A patient who had not been to the clinic for a while came in one day. His graduation from college had been delayed because he had developed a pilonidal cyst that needed to be surgically removed. At onset, these cysts can be very painful and usually require daily cleaning and packing. From my experience with pilonidal cyst care, I knew that 1 to 2 months of treatment are usually required before full recovery is achieved.

The physician and I prepared for the initial treatment and noticed that the surgical site was very large and deep. We knew this treatment would take much longer than usual. Treatment was provided daily for 3 months. Subsequent treatments continued every other day for 2 months. Through our continuous contact, we became good friends with the patient.

Our patient graduated at the end of the spring quarter and moved out of state. He stays in contact with us and is still undergoing treatment. He made a difference in our lives because he always maintained a positive attitude and was very pleasant, making our job easier. We made a difference in his life through the good health care we provided and our continuing friendship. ■

COMMERCIALLY PREPARED STERILE PACKAGES

Commercially prepared disposable packages are used frequently and may contain one particular article (e.g., sterile dressing) or a complete sterile setup (e.g., one for the removal of sutures). The directions for opening the package are stated on the outside of the package; they should be followed carefully to prevent contamination of the sterile contents. Procedure 25.2 describes opening a sterile package.

One type of commercially prepared package is the peel-apart package (commonly referred to as a *peel-pack*). This type of sterile package has an edge with two flaps that can be pulled apart in the following manner: Grasp each unsterile flap between your bent index finger and extended thumb, and, rolling your hands outward, pull the package apart (Fig. 25.4A). The inside of the wrapper and the contents are sterile, and to prevent contamination, they must not be touched with the bare hands. The medical assistant can place the contents of the peel-pack directly on the sterile field by stepping back slightly from the field and gently ejecting or "flipping" the contents onto the center of the sterile field (Fig. 25.4B). Stepping back prevents the unsterile outer wrapper and the medical assistant's hands from crossing over the sterile field, which would result in contamination.

The contents of the package also can be removed with a sterile gloved hand. This technique is useful during minor office surgery, when the provider needs additional supplies, such as gauze pads and sutures. The medical assistant opens the sterile package, and the provider removes the sterile contents from the package using a gloved hand (Fig. 25.4C). The inside of the package can be used as a sterile field by opening the peel-apart package completely and laying it flat on a clean dry surface (Fig. 25.4D).

Once a sterile package has been opened and set up, the medical assistant may need to pour a sterile solution, such as an antiseptic, into a container located on the field. To do so, the steps of surgical asepsis outlined in Procedure 25.3 should be followed.

WOUNDS

A **wound** is a break in the continuity of an external or internal surface caused by physical means. Wounds can be accidental or intentional (as when the provider makes an incision during a surgical operation). There are two basic types of wounds: closed and open.

A *closed wound* involves an injury to the underlying tissues of the body without a break in the skin surface or mucous membrane; an example is a contusion, or bruise. A **contusion** results when the tissues under the skin are injured and is often caused by a blunt object. Blood vessels rupture, allowing blood to seep into the tissues, which results in a bluish discoloration of the skin. After several days, the color of the contusion turns greenish yellow as a result of oxidation of blood pigments. Bruising commonly occurs with injuries such as fractures, sprains, strains, and black eyes. *Open wounds* involve a break in the skin surface or mucous membrane that exposes the underlying tissues; examples include incisions, lacerations, punctures, and abrasions. Fig. 25.5 illustrates specific wounds.

- An **incision** is a clean, smooth cut caused by a sharp instrument, such as a knife, razor, or piece of glass. Deep incisions are accompanied by profuse bleeding; in addition, damage to muscles, tendons, and nerves may occur.
- A **laceration** is a wound in which the tissues are torn apart (rather than cut) leaving ragged and irregular edges. Lacerations are caused by dull knives, large objects that have been driven into the skin, and heavy machinery. Deep lacerations result in profuse bleeding, and a scar often results from the jagged tearing of the tissues.
- A **puncture** is a wound made by a sharp-pointed object piercing the skin layers—for example, a nail, splinter, needle, wire, knife, bullet, or animal bite. A puncture wound has a very small external skin opening, and for

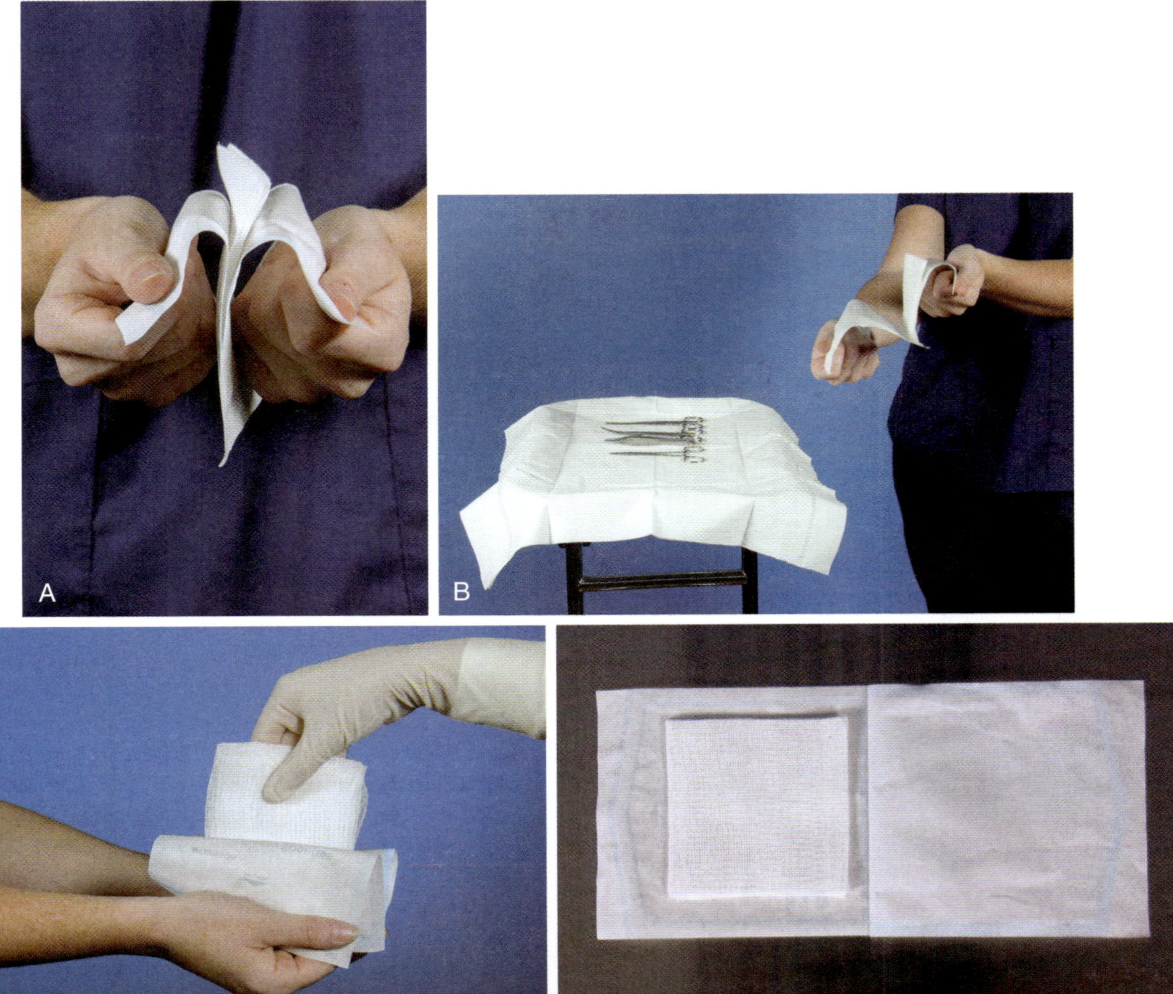

Fig. 25.4 Methods for removing the sterile contents of a peel-apart package so that sterility is maintained. (A) Grasp each flap between a bent index finger and an extended thumb, and roll hands outward to pull apart. (B) Step back and eject the contents onto the field. (C) The medical assistant opens the pack, and the provider removes the sterile contents with a gloved hand. (D) The inside of the peel-apart package can be used as a sterile field.

this reason bleeding is usually minor. A tetanus booster may be administered with this type of wound because the tetanus bacteria grow best in a warm anaerobic environment, such as the one in a puncture.

- An **abrasion** or scrape is a wound in which the outer layers of the skin are scraped or rubbed off, resulting in oozing of blood from ruptured capillaries. Abrasions are often caused by falling on gravel and floors (floor burn). These falls can result in skinned knees and elbows.

WOUND HEALING

The skin is a protective barrier for the body and is considered its first line of defense. When the surface of the skin has been broken, it is easy for microorganisms to enter and cause **infection.** The body has a natural healing process that works to destroy invading microorganisms and to restore the structure and function of damaged tissues, as is described next.

Phases of Wound Healing

Wound healing occurs in three phases, which are described here and illustrated in Fig. 25.6.

Phase 1

Phase 1, also called the *inflammatory phase*, begins as soon as the body is injured. This phase lasts approximately 3 to 4 days. During this phase, a fibrin network forms, resulting in a blood clot that "plugs" up the opening of the wound and stops the flow of blood. The blood clot eventually becomes the scab. The inflammatory process also occurs during this phase. **Inflammation** is the protective response of the body to trauma, such as cuts and abrasions, and to the

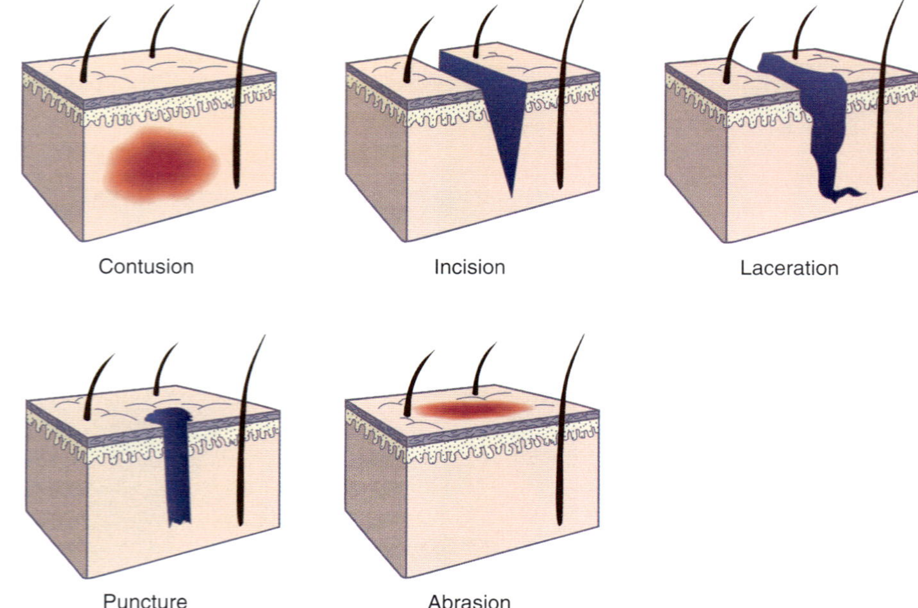

Fig. 25.5 Types of wounds.

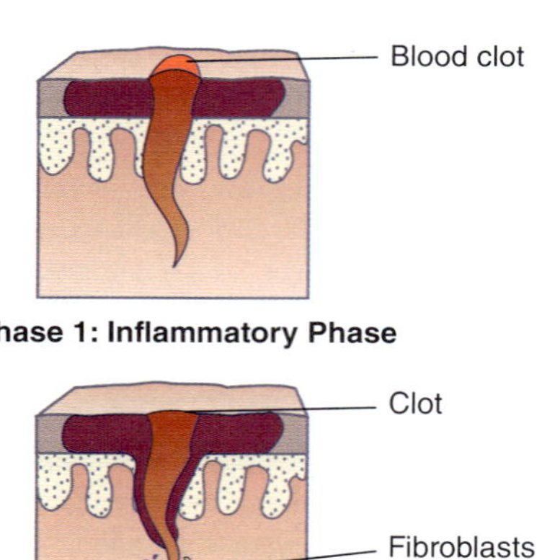

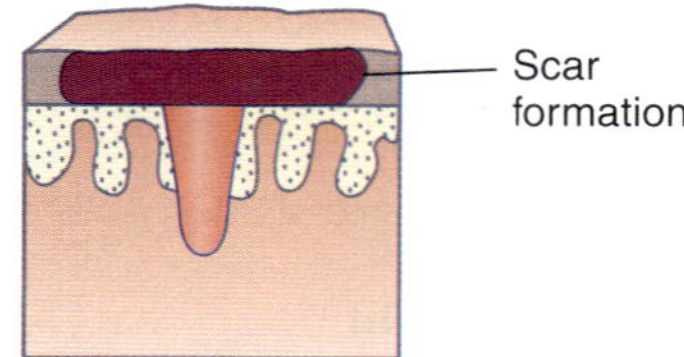

Fig. 25.6 Phases of wound healing.

entrance of foreign matter into the body, such as microorganisms. During inflammation, the blood supply to the wound increases, which brings white blood cells and nutrients to the site to assist in the healing process. The four local signs of inflammation are redness, swelling, pain, and warmth. The purpose of inflammation is to destroy invading pathogens and to remove damaged tissue debris from the area so that proper healing can occur.

Phase 2

Phase 2 is also called the *proliferative phase* and typically lasts 4 to 20 days. During this phase, the wound is rebuilt with new connective tissue known as *granulation tissue.* The function of granulation tissue is to fill in the wound and protect the surface of the wound. Granulation tissue consists primarily of collagen and microscopic blood vessels and is formed in the following sequence. **Fibroblasts** (immature cells from which connective tissue develops) migrate to the wound and begin to synthesize collagen. Collagen is a white protein that provides strength to the wound. As the amount of collagen increases, the wound becomes stronger, and the chance that the wound will open decreases. There also is a growth of new capillaries to provide an abundant blood supply to the granulation tissue. The presence of granulation tissue is part of the natural healing process and its presence indicates that wound healing is progressing normally. Granulation tissue exhibits the following characteristics:

- Translucent red or dark pink in color
- Soft and moist to the touch
- Bumpy or granular in appearance
- Painless

Phase 3

Phase 3, also known as the *maturation phase*, begins as soon as granulation tissue forms and can last for 2 years. During this phase, collagen continues to be synthesized, and the granulation tissue eventually hardens to white scar tissue. Scar tissue is not true skin and does not contain nerves or have a blood supply.

The medical assistant should always inspect the wound when providing wound care. The wound should be observed for signs of inflammation and the amount of healing that has occurred. This information should be documented in the patient's record.

Wound Drainage

The medical term for drainage is **exudate** which is produced as a normal part of the healing process. An exudate consists of material such as fluid and cells that have escaped from blood vessels during the inflammatory process and is deposited in tissue or on tissue surfaces. The function of an exudate is to flush foreign debris and dead tissue from the wound and to provide a moist environment to assist in wound healing. When providing wound care, the medical assistant should always inspect the wound for drainage and document this information in the patient's medical record. There are three major types of exudates: serous, sanguineous, and purulent.

- *Serous exudate.* A serous exudate consists chiefly of serum, which is the clear portion of the blood. Serous drainage is clear and watery. An example of a serous exudate is the fluid in a blister from a burn.
- *Sanguineous exudate.* A sanguineous exudate is red and consists of red blood cells. This type of drainage results when capillaries are damaged, allowing the escape of red blood cells, and is frequently seen in open wounds. A bright-red sanguineous exudate indicates fresh bleeding, and a dark exudate indicates older bleeding.
- *Purulent exudate.* A purulent exudate contains pus, which consists of leukocytes, dead liquefied tissue debris, and dead and living bacteria. Purulent drainage is usually thick and has an unpleasant odor. It is white in color but may acquire tinges of pink, green, or yellow depending on the type of infecting organism. The process of pus formation is *suppuration.*

In addition to the exudates just described, mixed types of exudates are often observed in a wound. A *serosanguineous exudate* consists of clear serous fluid and blood and is commonly seen in surgical incisions. A *purosanguineous exudate* consists of pus and blood and is often seen in a new wound that is infected.

STERILE DRESSING CHANGE

Surgical asepsis must be maintained when one is caring for and applying a dry sterile dressing (abbreviated as *DSD*) to an open wound. The medical assistant must take care to prevent infection in clean wounds and to decrease infection in wounds already infected. The function of a sterile dressing is to protect the wound from contamination and trauma, to absorb drainage, and to restrict motion, which may interfere with proper wound healing. The size, type, and amount of dressing material used during a sterile dressing change depend on the size and location of the wound and the amount of drainage.

Sterile folded *gauze pads* are used in the medical office for a sterile dressing change. This type of dressing absorbs drainage, but the gauze has a tendency to stick to the wound when the drainage dries. Gauze pads come in a variety of sizes, including 4 × 4, 3 × 3, and 2 × 2; the 4 × 4 size is used most frequently.

Nonadherent pads also are used as a sterile dressing; they have one surface impregnated with agents that prevent the dressing from sticking to the wound. One brand of this type of material is Telfa pads. The nonadherent side, which is shiny, is placed next to the wound. Telfa dressings are often used to cover burned skin. Procedure 25.4 presents the procedure for changing a sterile dressing.

METHODS OF WOUND CLOSURE

Wound closure may be required to close a surgical incision or to repair an accidental wound. It is typically required when tissue has been damaged to the extent that it cannot heal naturally on its own.

The most common methods of wound closure include sutures, surgical staples, topical skin adhesives (surgical glue), and skin closure tape. The goal of wound closure is to bring together the edges of the wound and holds them in place until enough healing has taken place so that the wound can withstand ordinary stress. The actual process of bringing together the edges of the wound is known as **approximation.** Wound closure also protects the wound from further contamination and minimizes the amount of scar formation. The method of wound closure chosen by the provider depends on the characteristics of the wound and the location of the wound. These four methods are described next along with the advantages and disadvantages of each.

SUTURES

Sutures are commonly used to close a wound. Suturing is a method of wound closure used to sew skin and other body tissues together to close a surgical incision or to close a wound caused by an injury. A **local anesthetic** is necessary to numb the area before the sutures are inserted. The suture is applied using a surgical needle and suturing material and secured with a surgical knot. Sutures minimize the risk of bleeding and infection that accompany surgical incisions and skin injuries. Closing a wound with sutures is one of the oldest known medical procedures. The ancient Egyptians are believed to have been the first to close wounds with a needle and thread nearly 4000 years ago.

Types of Sutures

Sutures are available in two types: absorbable and nonabsorbable. **Absorbable sutures** are made of a material that is gradually digested and absorbed by the body in a relatively short period of time. The amount of time can range from 7 days to several months, depending on the type of tissue being sutured and the size and type of absorbable suture being used.

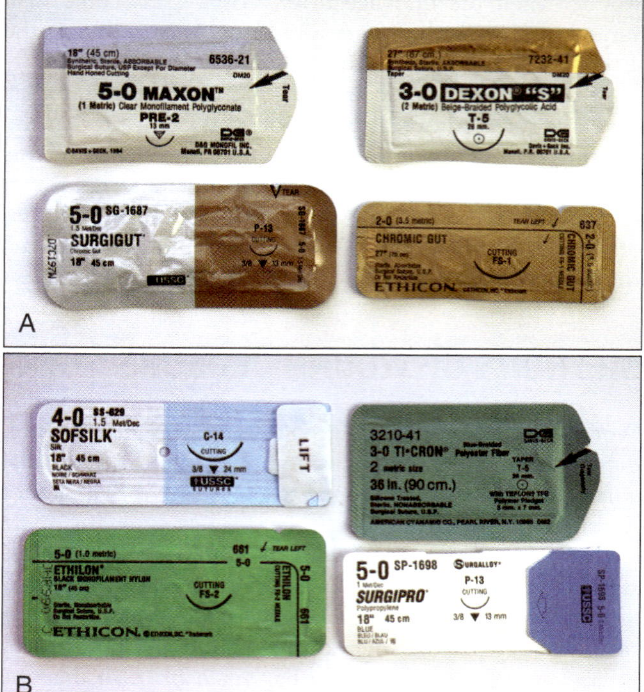

Fig. 25.7 Swaged suture packets. (A) Absorbable sutures. (B) Nonabsorbable sutures.

Absorbable sutures consist of surgical gut (Surgigut) or synthetic materials, such as polyglycolic acid (Dexon), polyglactin 910 (Vicryl), polydioxanone (PDS II), polyglyconate (Maxon), and poliglecaprone (Monocryl), lactomer (Polysorb), and Caprosyn (Fig. 25.7A). Surgical gut is made from sheep or cow intestine. This type of suturing material is gradually digested by tissue enzymes and is absorbed by the body's tissues 7 to 21 days after insertion, depending on the kind of surgical gut employed. *Plain surgical gut* has a rapid absorption time, whereas *chromic surgical gut* is treated to slow down its rate of absorption in the tissues. Absorbable sutures frequently are used to suture subcutaneous tissue, fascia, intestines, bladder, and peritoneum and to **ligate,** or tie off, vessels. Because suturing of this type of tissue is typically done during surgery performed by the provider in the hospital with the patient under a general anesthetic, the medical office may not stock absorbable suture material.

Nonabsorbable sutures (Fig. 25.7B) are not absorbed by the body and may remain permanently in the body tissues and become encapsulated by fibrous tissue or may be removed (e.g., skin sutures). Nonabsorbable sutures are used to suture skin; this type of suture is used frequently in the medical office. Nonabsorbable sutures are made from materials that are not affected by tissue enzymes. These materials include silk (Sofsilk), nylon (Ethilon), polyester (Ti-Cron, Surgidac), polypropylene (Prolene, Surgipro), polybutester (Novafil and Vascufil), and stainless steel wire.

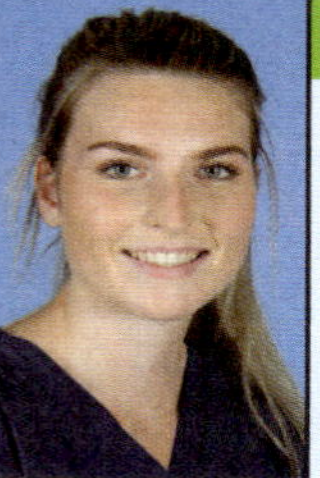

Memories *from* Practicum

Heather: I remember observing my first minor office surgery during my practicum. It was a sebaceous cyst removal. The cyst was located on the calf of the patient's left leg. I helped in setting up the surgical tray and prepared and draped the site. I tried to explain to the patient what was going to occur to prepare her for the procedure. I think the patient was calmer than I was. The physician entered the room with a medical assistant on hand. Although I was in the room primarily to observe, I helped the physician with his surgical gloves and in numbing the site. I watched the physician make the incision and remove a large cyst.

Everything was going smoothly until the physician started to suture the wound. I felt like someone had turned the heat up really high; the room seemed to get really hot. I started to feel dizzy. I smiled at the physician and excused myself. He just smiled back at me, and I left the room. I went outside the room and caught my breath. I regained my composure and reentered the room. The physician was still suturing the wound. As I watched him insert the needle through the skin and pull the suture tight, it really got to me. I smiled and told the physician that I would wait outside until they were done. After the provider left the room, I went back to help clean up. I felt so stupid. Later that day, the physician looked at me and said, "Got a little warm in there, didn't it?" He just laughed and said that what I did was normal and not to worry about it. He made me feel better about myself. After that incident, I went in alone and helped him with cyst removals, and it didn't bother me at all. ■

Suture Size and Packaging

Sutures are measured by their gauge, which refers to the diameter of the suturing material. The sizes range from numbers below 0 (pronounced "aught") to numbers above 0. The diameter of the suture material increases with each number above 0 and decreases with each number below 0. If the size of a particular suture material ranges from 7-0 to 5, available sizes include 7-0, 6-0, 5-0, 4-0, 3-0, 2-0, 0, 1, 2, 3, 4, and 5. Size 7-0 sutures are very fine sutures, and size 5 sutures are very heavy sutures. Size 2-0 (00) sutures have a smaller diameter than size 0 sutures.

Nonabsorbable sutures with a smaller gauge (5-0 to 6-0) are used for suturing incisions in delicate tissue, such as the face and neck, whereas nonabsorbable heavy sutures are used for firmer tissue, such as the chest and abdomen. Finer sutures leave less scar formation and are used when cosmetic results are desired.

Sutures come in a box of individually packaged sutures (Fig. 25.8A). The box of sutures is stamped with an expiration date that must be checked each time a suture package is removed from the box. Each individual suture package consists of an outer peel-apart envelope and a sterile inner packet (Fig. 25.8B).

Suture packages are labeled with the following information:

- Type of suture material (e.g., surgical silk)
- Size of the suturing material (e.g., 4-0)

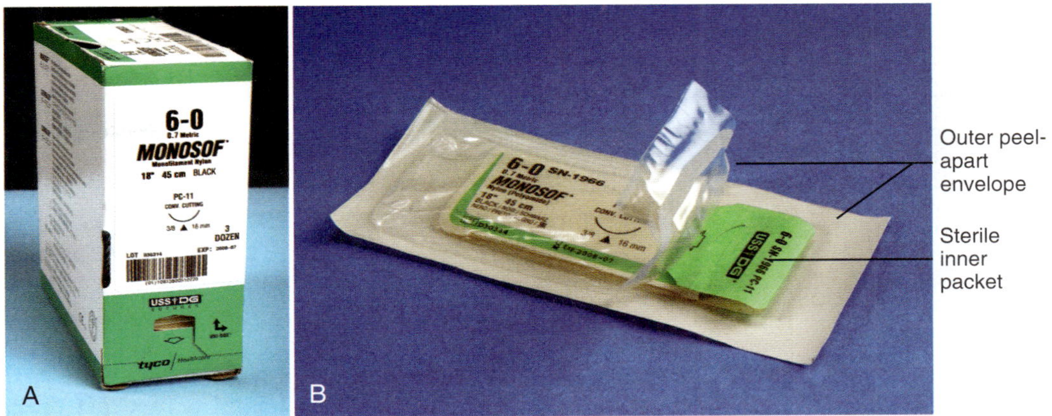

Fig. 25.8 (A) Sutures come in a box of individually packaged sutures. (B) Each individual suture package consists of an outer peel-apart envelope and a sterile inner packet.

- Length of the suturing material (e.g., 18 inches)
- Date of manufacture
- Expiration date of the suture

The type and size of material used are based on the nature and location of the tissue being sutured and the provider's preference. To repair a laceration of the arm, the provider might use a 4-0 surgical silk suture. The provider informs the medical assistant of the type and size of sutures needed.

Suture Needles

Needles used for suturing are made from stainless steel alloys and are categorized according to their type of point and their shape. A needle with a sharp point is a *cutting needle*, and one with a round point is a *noncutting needle*. Cutting needles (Fig. 25.9A) are used for firm tissues such as skin; the sharp point helps push the needle through the tissue. Noncutting or blunt needles are used to penetrate tissues that offer a small amount of resistance, such as the fascia, intestine, liver, spleen, kidneys, subcutaneous tissue, and muscle.

A suture needle may be curved or straight (see Fig. 25.9A). *Curved needles* come in various sizes and curves and are the most commonly used suture needles. Curved needles permit the provider to dip in and out of the tissue. A needle holder must be used with a curved needle. A *straight needle* is used when the tissue can be displaced sufficiently to permit the needle to be manually pushed and pulled through the tissue. Straight needles do not require the use of a needle holder.

Some needles have an eye through which the suture material is inserted; however, most needles are **swaged needles** (Fig. 25.9B). *Swaged* means that the suture and needle are one continuous unit; the needle is permanently attached to the end of the suture. Swaged needles are used frequently because they offer several advantages over eyed needles. One advantage is that the suture material does not slip off the needle, as might occur with suture material threaded through the eye of a needle. Another advantage is that tissue trauma is reduced because a swaged needle has only a single strand of suture that must be pulled through the tissue compared with a double strand in an eyed needle. The swaged needle can be pulled

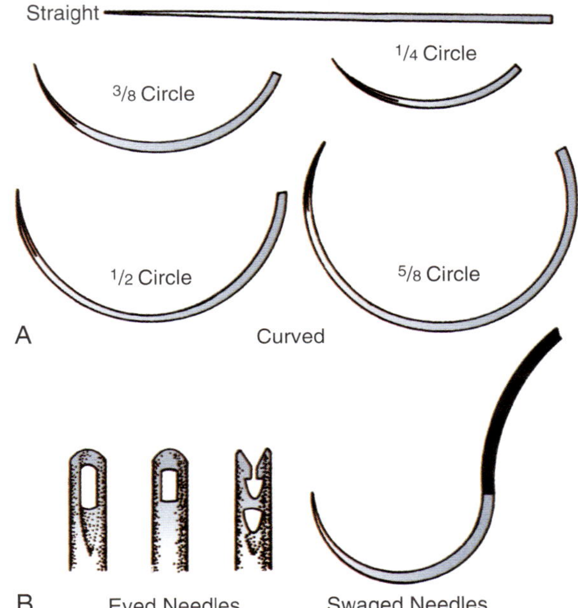

Fig. 25.9 Common suture needles. (A) Needles with a cutting point. (B) Eyed needles and a swaged needle. (B, Modified from Nealon TF Jr: *Fundamental skills in surgery*, ed 4, Philadelphia, 1994, Saunders.)

through the tissue with less resulting trauma. Swaged suture packets are labeled to specify the type, size and length of suture material, the type of needle point (cutting or noncutting), and the needle shape (curved or straight) (see Fig. 25.7).

Insertion of Sutures

The medical assistant may be responsible for preparing the suture tray and for assisting the provider during the insertion of the sutures. The provider designates the size and type of suture material and needle required. Because sutures, needles, and suture-needle combinations (swaged needles) are contained in peel-apart packages, they can be added to the sterile field by flipping them onto the sterile field or by placing them there with a sterile gloved hand (Fig. 25.10).

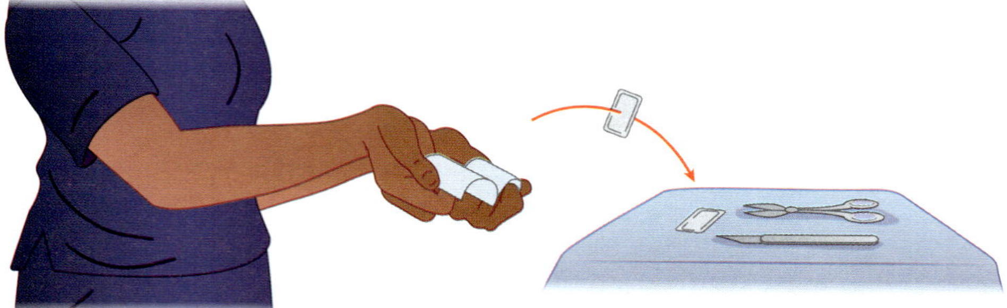

Flipping sutures onto the sterile field.

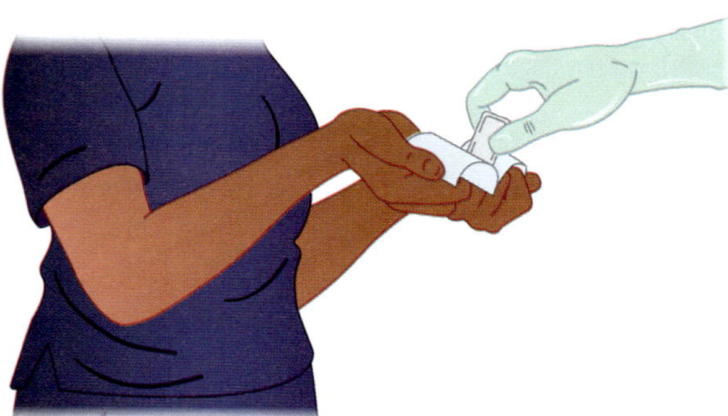

The physician removing the sutures with a sterile gloved hand.

Fig. 25.10 Adding sutures to a sterile field.

Suture Insertion Setup

The items required for a suture insertion setup are listed next.

Items Placed to the Side of the Sterile Field

- Clean disposable gloves
- Antiseptic solution
- Surgical scrub brush
- Antiseptic swabs
- Surgical gloves
- Local anesthetic
- Antiseptic wipe to cleanse the vial
- Tetanus toxoid with needle and syringe

Items Included on the Sterile Field

- Fenestrated drape
- Syringe and needle for drawing up the local anesthetic
- Hemostatic forceps
- Thumb forceps
- Tissue forceps
- Dissecting scissors
- Operating scissors
- Needle holder
- Suture
- Sterile 4 × 4 gauze

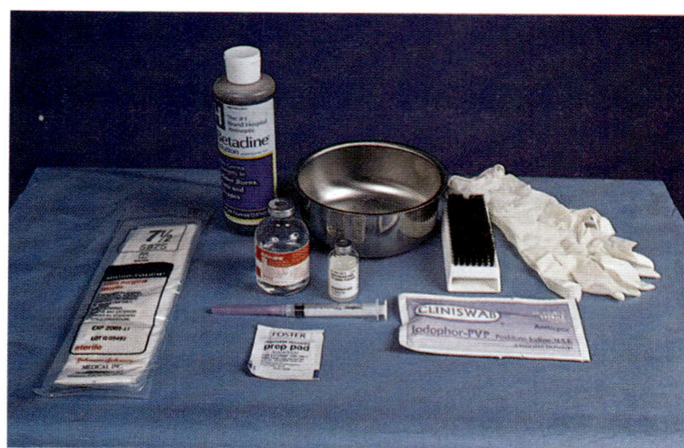

Suture insertion side table.

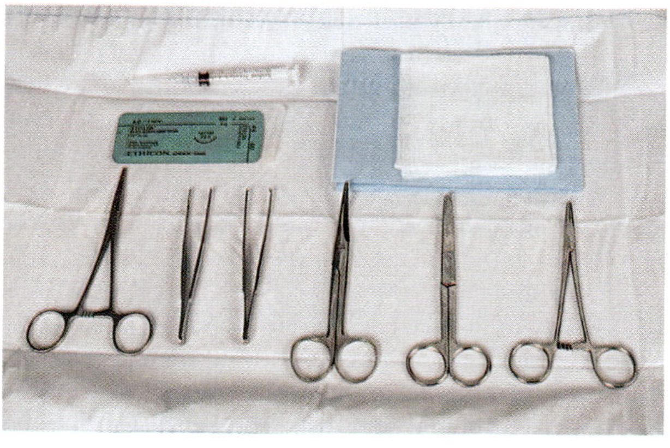

Suture insertion sterile field.

Procedure: Suture Insertion

Sutures are inserted as follows:
1. A local anesthetic is used to numb the area.
2. The provider inserts sutures to close a surgical incision or to repair an accidental wound.
3. A sterile dressing may be applied to the operative site.

Postoperative Instructions: Suture Insertion

Postoperative instructions include the following:
1. Keep the dressing clean and dry.
2. Contact the medical office if any signs of infection occur at the incision site, including excessive redness, swelling, discharge, or an increase in pain.
3. Notify the medical office if the sutures become loose or break.

Provide the patient with written instructions on wound care to refer to at home (Table 25.1) and instruct the patient when to return for removal of the sutures.

Suture Removal

When the wound has healed such that it no longer needs the support of nonabsorbable suture material, the sutures must be removed. The length of time the sutures remain in place depends on their location and the amount of healing that must occur. Some areas of the body, such as the head and neck, have a good blood supply; the sutures do not need to remain there as long as they do in other areas because this area heals more rapidly.

Sutures must always be left in place long enough for proper healing to occur. The provider determines the length of time, but in general, skin sutures inserted in the face and neck are removed in 3 to 5 days, and sutures inserted in other areas, such as the skin of the chest, arms, legs, hands, and feet, are removed in 7 to 14 days.

What Would You Do? What Would You *Not* Do?

Case Study 1

Kerry Ventura brings her 6-year-old son Cory to the medical office. Cory got a new bike for his birthday and just learned how to ride it without training wheels. While going around a corner, he lost his balance and fell and cut his left knee. The incision is almost 2 inches long. Cory is going to need sutures to approximate the wound. Mrs. Ventura is very upset and blames herself. She says that she should have been watching him more closely. Mrs. Ventura wants to know why Steri-Strips can't be used to close the incision. She says that it would be a lot less painful for Cory than having stitches. When asked to sign the consent to treatment form for Cory, Mrs. Ventura says she does not want to sign the form until her husband is back from his weeklong business trip to Japan and has a chance to assess the situation. ■

Table 25.1 Wound Care Instructions

General Wound Care Instructions

Explain the following to the patient regarding wounds:
- The type of wound that the patient has: incision, laceration, puncture, or abrasion.
- If a tetanus toxoid has been administered, explain the purpose of this immunization: to protect against tetanus (lockjaw).

Instruct the patient how to care for the wound, as follows:
- Keep the dressing clean and dry especially for the first 24 to 48 hours.
- Some swelling, redness, and pain are common with all wounds and will go away as the wound heals.
- Apply an ice bag for swelling (if prescribed by the provider).
- Report immediately any signs that the wound is infected. These signs include the following:
  a. Fever
  b. Persistent or increased pain, swelling, drainage, or foul odor
  c. Red streaks radiating away from the wound
  d. Increased redness or warmth
- Avoid any activities that may put strain on the wound. This could cause the wound to re-open.
- Return as instructed by the provider.

Give the patient written instructions on wound care to refer to at home.

Sutures and Staples

Instruct the patient how to take care of sutures or staples (in addition to general wound care instructions).
- The purpose of suturing or stapling the wound: to close the skin and protect against further contamination, to facilitate healing, and to leave a smaller scar.
- Do not take a tub bath or swim until the sutures or staples have been removed.
- After showering, gently pad the area dry with a soft towel.
- Do not pick at your sutures or staples.
- Notify the medical office if the sutures become loose or break.
- Return as instructed by the provider for removal of the sutures or staples.

Skin Closure Tape and Tissue Adhesives

Instruct the patient how to take care of skin closure tape and tissue adhesives (in addition to general wound care instructions).
- The purpose of applying skin closure tape or tissue adhesives: to close the skin and protect against further contamination, to facilitate healing, and to leave a smaller scar.
- Do not take a tub bath or swim.
- After showering, gently pad the area dry.
- Do not scratch, pick at or rub the tape or adhesive film.
- Do not apply any topical ointments or creams to the wound.
- Notify the medical office if the wound re-opens.

SURGICAL SKIN STAPLES

Surgical skin staples are often used to close wounds. Stapling is the fastest method of closure of long skin incisions. In addition, trauma to the tissue is reduced because the tissue does not have to be handled much when the staples are inserted. Surgical staples are stainless steel and are inserted into the skin using a special skin stapler. Skin staplers are available as reusable or disposable devices. The skin stapler holds a cartridge that contains a prescribed number and size of staples (Fig. 25.11).

The provider first administers a local anesthetic and then inserts the staples by gently approximating the tissues

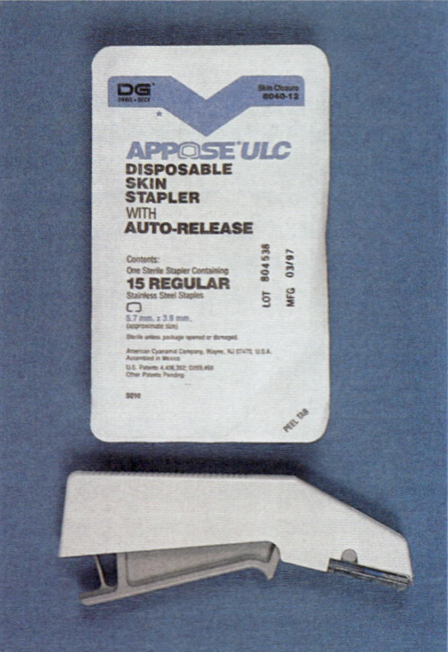

Fig. 25.11 Disposable skin stapler.

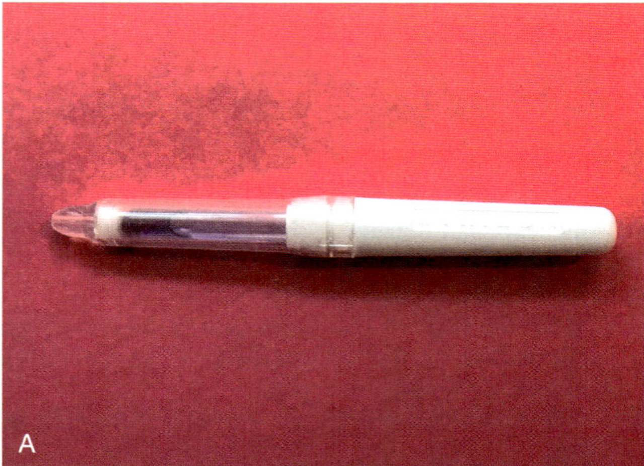

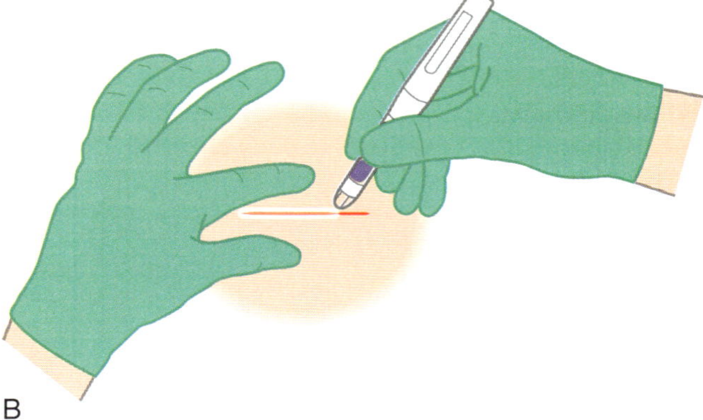

Fig. 25.12 Topical tissue adhesive.

with tissue forceps. The skin stapler is held over the site, and the staple is inserted into the skin. The medical assistant should provide the patient with instructions for caring for the wound (see Table 25.1). Skin stapling produces excellent cosmetic results, and the staples are easy to remove with a specially designed staple remover.

The medical assistant is frequently responsible for removing sutures and staples. This procedure should be done only after the provider has given a written or verbal order to the medical assistant. Procedure 25.5 presents the method used to remove sutures and skin staples.

TOPICAL TISSUE ADHESIVES

Topical tissue adhesives (also known as surgical glue) are the newest method of skin closure. In 1998, the Food and Drug Administration (FDA) approved the use of 2-octyl cyanoacrylate which is marketed as Dermabond (Ethicon, Somerville, NJ) and is available in a pre-filled single-use applicator.

Tissue adhesives work by forming a strong transparent flexible bond across the top of the skin that binds the skin edges together. Before applying a tissue adhesive, it is important to make sure the wound is clean and dry. The provider applies the tissue adhesive by approximating the edges of the wound with surgical gloves or forceps. The tissue adhesive is then applied as a liquid to the outer surface of the skin (Fig. 25.12). The liquid quickly dries into a film that holds the edges of the wound together. The film lasts for 5 to 10 days and then naturally falls off on its own. The medical assistant should provide the patient with instructions for caring for the wound (see Table 25.1).

Tissue adhesives are best suited to close small superficial lacerations or surgical incisions of the face, torso, and limbs. They cannot be used on wounds of the mucous membranes such as the lips or oral cavity. They also cannot be used on areas that harbor moisture (e.g., palms of the hands, soles of the feet, axillae) and hairy areas of the body (e.g., scalp) and areas that are subjected to too much tension or flexion (e.g., joints). The advantages of tissue adhesives are that they eliminate the need for sutures and a local anesthetic, they are easy to apply, they form a water-resistant protective covering over the wound, and they result in less scarring than sutures.

SKIN CLOSURE TAPE

Skin closure tape may be used for wound repair to approximate the edges of a laceration or incision. Skin closures consist of sterile, hypoallergenic adhesive tape that is commercially available in a variety of widths and lengths and is strong enough to approximate a wound until healing occurs. Brand names for skin closure tape are Steri-Strip (3M Corporation, St. Paul, MN) and Proxi-Strip (Ethicon, Bridgewater, NJ) (Fig. 25.13).

Skin closure tape may be used when not much tension exists on the skin edges. The strips of tape are applied transversely

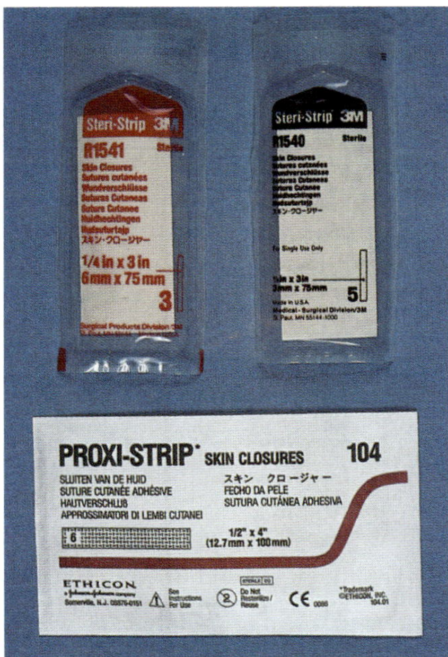

Fig. 25.13 Skin closure tape in different sizes.

across the line of incision to approximate the skin edges. The advantages of skin closure tape are that they eliminate the need for sutures and a local anesthetic, they are easy to apply and remove, they have a lower incidence of wound infection compared with sutures, and they result in less scarring than sutures. The disadvantage of this method is that there is less precision in bringing the wound edges together compared with suturing the wound. In addition, skin closure tape cannot be used on certain areas of the body where the tape has difficulty adhering to the skin. This includes areas that harbor moisture (e.g., palms of the hands, soles of the feet, axillae) and hairy areas of the body (e.g., scalp, a man's chest).

The medical assistant frequently is responsible for applying skin closure tape (Procedure 25.6) and for providing the patient with instructions for caring for the wound (see Table 25.1). Approximately 5 to 10 days after application, the skin closures usually loosen and fall off on their own. If they require removal by the medical assistant, the method presented at the end of Procedure 25.6 should be followed.

ASSISTING WITH MINOR OFFICE SURGERY

TRAY SETUP

Assisting with minor office surgery requires a thorough knowledge of the instruments and supplies for each tray setup and the type of assistance required by the provider during the surgery. The medical assistant must be able to work quickly and efficiently and to anticipate the provider's needs.

The instruments and supplies for the surgery must be set on a sterile field. Many offices maintain a written reference source such as a file on the office computer or index cards indicating the appropriate instruments and supplies for each minor office surgery tray setup. The reference source may also include information regarding the type of skin preparation, the position of the patient, the provider's glove size, the type of suture material, preoperative instructions, and postoperative instructions. The medical assistant should use the reference source as a guide to ensure that all required articles are placed on the sterile field. The medical assistant may set up the sterile tray before or after preparing the patient's skin. The sterile tray setup must not become contaminated. If the medical assistant must turn away from the sterile tray or leave the room after setting up, a sterile towel must be placed over the tray to maintain sterility.

Methods Used to Set up a Sterile Tray

There are two common methods used to set up a sterile tray described as follows.

Prepackaged Sterile Setup

A common method used to set up a sterile tray is to use prepackaged sterile setups wrapped in disposable sterilization paper that are prepared by the medical office through autoclave sterilization (see Procedure 25.2). These setups are labeled according to use (e.g., suture pack, cyst removal pack) and contain most of the instruments and supplies required for the minor office surgery indicated on the label. The medical assistant opens the wrapped package on a small, flat, metal tray (Mayo tray) with a moveable stand (Mayo stand). The inside of the wrapped package is sterile and serves as the sterile field. Several additional articles not contained in the prepackaged setup (e.g., an antiseptic, sterile 4 × 4 gauze pads, disposable syringes and needles, sutures) may need to be added to the sterile field when the package is opened. Items in peel-apart packages are added by flipping them onto the sterile field or by placing them on the field using a sterile gloved hand. If an antiseptic solution is poured into a basin on the sterile field, this is performed according to Procedure 25.3.

Transferring Items onto a Sterile Field

Another method used to set up a sterile tray is to place all necessary articles on the sterile field by flipping them onto the sterile field from peel-apart packages. With this method, the sterile field is prepared by placing a sterile towel over a portable instrument tray. The sterile towel must be handled by the corners so as not to contaminate it. It must not be fanned through the air, but instead must be laid down gently and slowly to prevent airborne contamination.

Specific guidelines must be observed during a sterile procedure to maintain the sterile field on the instrument tray. See the accompanying box, *Guidelines for Maintaining a Sterile Field.*

Guidelines for Maintaining a Sterile Field

1. Set up the sterile tray as close as possible to the time of use. Sterile items can become contaminated by prolonged exposure to airborne particles.
2. Take precautions to prevent sterile packages from becoming wet. Wet packages draw microorganisms into the package resulting in contamination of the sterile package. If a sterile package that has been prepared at the medical office becomes wet, it must be rewrapped and resterilized; if a disposable sterile package becomes wet, it must be discarded.
3. All items used in a sterile field must be sterile. A sterile item becomes contaminated if it is touched by a non-sterile item.
4. A 1-inch border around the sterile field is considered contaminated or unsterile because this area may have become contaminated while the sterile field was being set up.
5. Always face the sterile field. A sterile field must always be kept in sight to be considered sterile. If you must turn your back to it or leave the room, a sterile towel must be placed over the sterile field.
6. Hold all sterile items above waist level. Items held below waist level are considered non-sterile. Sterile items should be held in front of you and should not touch your uniform.
7. To avoid contamination, place all sterile items in the center, not around the edges, of the sterile field.
8. Do not talk, laugh, cough, or sneeze over a sterile field. Moisture droplets from the nose, mouth, and lungs are carried outward by the air and contaminate the sterile field.
9. Do not reach over a sterile field. Dead skin cells, dust, or lint from your clothing may fall onto the sterile field contaminating it.
10. Do not pass soiled dressings over the sterile field.
11. Always acknowledge if you have contaminated the sterile field so that proper steps can be taken to regain sterility.
12. If there is any doubt about the sterility of an item, it is considered contaminated and should not be used.

Side Table

Some articles required for minor office surgery are not placed on the sterile field but are set on an adjacent table or counter. These articles, such as a surgical scrub brush, are not sterile and must not be placed on the sterile field. The local anesthetic, which is a sterile solution, is in a vial that is not sterile and must *not* be placed on the sterile field. The provider needs to apply gloves to perform the surgery. Although the gloves are sterile, the outside wrapper is not; the package of gloves must not be placed on the sterile field. In addition, it is easier for the provider to apply gloves from a side table or counter. To facilitate application of the gloves, the medical assistant opens the outside wrapper for the provider.

SKIN PREPARATION

The patient's skin must be prepared before the minor office surgery because the skin contains an abundance of microorganisms. If these microorganisms were to enter the body through the operative site, a wound infection could develop. It is impossible to sterilize skin because chemical agents required to kill all living microorganisms are too strong to be placed on the skin surfaces. The operative site and an area surrounding it must be cleaned and prepared in such a way as to remove as many microorganisms as possible to reduce the risk of surgical wound contamination.

Shaving the Site

Hair supports the growth of microorganisms, and the provider may want the medical assistant to shave the skin at and around the operative site. Shave preparation trays are commercially available and include several gauze sponges, a measured amount of antiseptic soap, a container for soapy water, and a disposable safety razor. The skin should be pulled taut as it is shaved, and the medical assistant must be careful to prevent nicks. When all the hair has been removed, the shaved area should be rinsed and dried thoroughly.

Cleansing the Site

The operative site must be cleaned with an antiseptic solution such as povidone-iodine (Betadine Surgical Scrub) or chlorhexidine gluconate (Hibiclens) (Fig. 25.14). The medical assistant should scrub the operative area with a surgical scrub brush using a firm circular motion, moving from the inside outward. The area is rinsed using gauze pads saturated with water and is blotted dry with sterile gauze.

Antiseptic Application

When the patient's skin has been shaved (if required) and cleansed, an antiseptic is applied to the operative area, followed by the application of a sterile drape. The antiseptic decreases the number of microorganisms on the patient's skin; a common antiseptic is Betadine. A disposable sterile *fenestrated drape* (Fig. 25.15) is the type of drape most commonly used. It has an opening that is placed directly

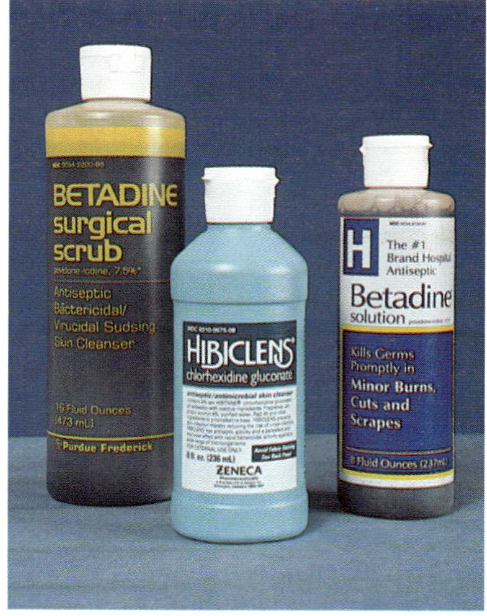

Fig. 25.14 Cleansing solutions.

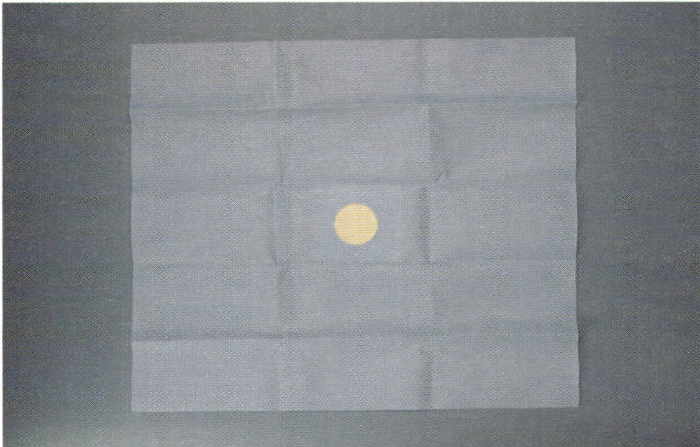

Fig. 25.15 Fenestrated drape.

over the operative site. A fenestrated drape covers a wide area of skin around the operative area, leaving only the operative site exposed. This provides a sterile area around the operative site and decreases contamination of the patient's surgical wound.

LOCAL ANESTHETIC

Minor office surgeries often require the use of a local anesthetic; the local anesthetic most frequently used in the medical office is lidocaine hydrochloride (Xylocaine). The provider injects the local anesthetic into the tissue surrounding the operative site, a process termed **infiltration,** to produce a loss of sensation in that area and prevent the patient from feeling pain during the surgery. When first injected into the tissues, lidocaine causes the patient to experience a brief burning or stinging sensation at the injection site. The local anesthetic begins working in 5 to 15 minutes and has a duration of action of 1 to 3 hours, depending on the type of anesthetic.

Some providers prefer to use a local anesthetic containing *epinephrine.* Epinephrine is a vasoconstrictor that prolongs the local effect of the anesthetic and decreases the rate of systemic absorption of the local anesthetic. It accomplishes this by constricting blood vessels at the operative site. The provider informs the medical assistant of the type, strength, and amount of local anesthetic needed for the minor office surgery. Xylocaine is available in 0.5%, 1%, 1.5%, and 2% solutions. The provider may order 1 mL of Xylocaine 2% with epinephrine to suture a laceration of the forearm.

Preparing the Anesthetic

The local anesthetic is drawn up into the syringe from a vial according to the procedure presented in Chapter 26. The vial must first be cleansed using an antiseptic wipe. The correct amount of anesthetic solution is withdrawn into the syringe. This may be performed by the medical assistant or the provider. The medical assistant withdraws the anesthetic into the syringe and hands it to the provider, who has not yet applied surgical gloves. The provider injects the anesthetic into the patient's tissues and then applies surgical gloves to begin the surgery.

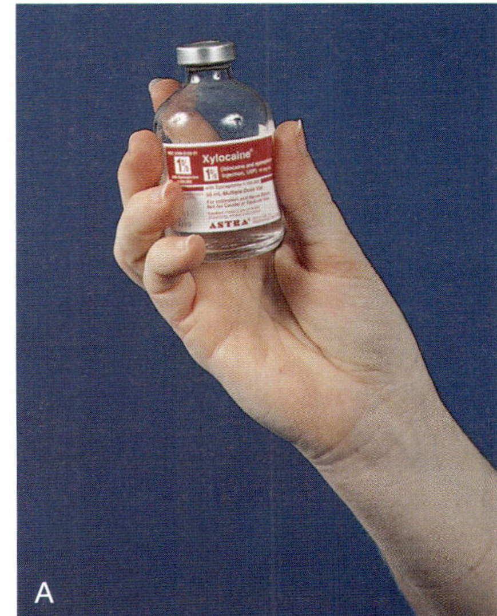

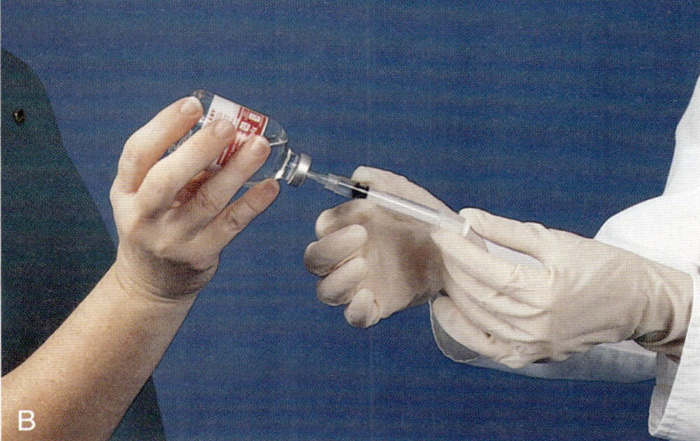

Fig. 25.16 Drawing up the local anesthetic. (A) Heather holds up the vial so that the provider can verify the name and strength of the local anesthetic. (B) Heather holds the vial securely while the provider withdraws the medication.

The provider may prefer to draw the anesthetic solution into the syringe after they have applied surgical gloves. The medical assistant should first show the label of the vial to the provider and should then hold the vial securely while the provider withdraws the medication (Fig. 25.16). The medical assistant must hold the vial because the outside of the vial is medically aseptic and cannot be touched by the provider's sterile gloved hand.

If the medical assistant prepares the anesthetic injection, the needle and syringe are not placed on the sterile field, but are assembled off to the side. If the provider withdraws the anesthetic, the needle and syringe are placed on the sterile field.

ASSISTING THE PROVIDER

The type of assistance required by the provider during minor office surgery is based on the type of surgery and the provider's preference. Some providers want the medical

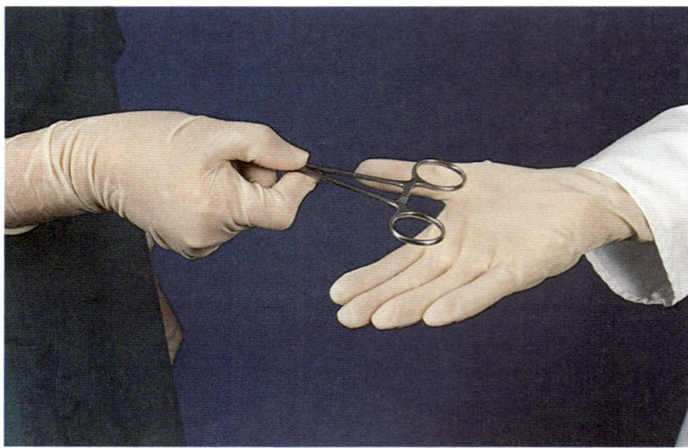
Fig. 25.17 Heather hands a hemostat to the provider in its functional position.

assistant to apply surgical gloves and assist directly by handing instruments and supplies from the sterile field. An instrument should be handed to the provider in a firm, confident manner so that the instrument does not slip out of the provider's hand and drop on the floor. The instrument should be placed in the provider's hand in its functional position—that is, the position in which it is to be used (Fig. 25. 17). If the instrument is handed correctly, the provider should not have to reposition the instrument to use it.

The medical assistant is responsible for adding any instruments or supplies to the sterile field that the provider requires after the surgery has begun, such as another hemostat, additional 4 × 4 gauze pads, and sutures. This is usually accomplished by using peel-apart packages and either flipping the contents onto the sterile field or holding the package open and allowing the provider to remove the contents with a gloved hand. In assisting with minor office surgery, it is essential to know all steps in the procedure so that the provider's needs can be anticipated and the surgery proceeds smoothly and efficiently.

The provider may obtain a tissue specimen that is sent to the laboratory for histologic examination. The specimen must be placed in an appropriate-sized container with a preservative. The medical assistant is responsible for labeling the specimen container. An unlabeled specimen is a cause for rejection of the specimen by an outside laboratory. Two *unique identifiers* should be used to label the specimen. A unique identifier is information that clearly identifies a specific patient, such as the patient's name and date of birth. A specimen can be labeled by attaching a computerized bar code label to the specimen. A specimen can also be labeled by hand-writing the information on the label, which should include the patient's name and date of birth, the date and time of collection, the medical assistant's initials, and any other information required by the laboratory, such as the source of the specimen. The information should be printed legibly, and the medical assistant should be certain that the information is accurate to avoid a mix-up of specimens. The medical assistant also must complete a laboratory requisition to accompany the specimen; this is known as a *biopsy requisition* (Fig. 25.18).

DIAGNOSTIC PATHOLOGY ASSOCIATES, INC

HISTOPATHOLOGY/CYTOPATHOLOGY REQUISITION

BILL TO: ☐ ACCOUNT ☐ PATIENT ☐ MEDICARE ☐ MEDICAID ☐ BLUE SHIELD ☐ OTHER	PATIENT NAME (LAST, FIRST, MIDDLE INITIAL)	PATIENT ID	ROOM NO.

SEX	BIRTHDATE / /	DATE COLLECTED	TIME COLLECTED A.M. P.M.	REQUESTING PHYSICIAN	SPECIAL INSTRUCTIONS

RESPONSIBLE PARTY NAME	RESPONSIBLE PARTY ADDRESS	CITY, STATE, ZIP

PHONE	MEDICAID ID NUMBER	MEDICARE HIC NUMBER	INSURANCE COMPANY NAME

INSURANCE COMPANY ADDRESS	GROUP NUMBER	CONTRACT NUMBER	COVERAGE CODE	PATIENT/INSURED RELATIONSHIP ☐ SELF ☐ SPOUSE ☐ DEPEND.

PATIENT AUTHORIZATION: I AUTHORIZE THE RELEASE OF ANY MEDICAL INFORMATION NECESSARY TO PROCESS A CLAIM, I PERMIT A COPY OF THIS AUTHORIZATION TO BE USED IN PLACE OF THE ORIGINAL AND REQUEST PAYMENT OF ANY MEDICAL INSURANCE BENEFITS EITHER TO ME OR TO THE PARTY WHO ACCEPTS ASSIGNMENT.	SIGNED X__________	DATE ________

TISSUE EXAM: ☐ GROSS & MICROSCOPIC ☐ GROSS ONLY **SPECIMEN TYPE:** ☐ BIOPSY ☐ SCRAPING ☐ BRUSHING ☐ WASHING ☐ FLUIDS ☐ FINE NEEDLE ☐ OTHER ________	**SOURCE OF SPECIMEN:** ☐ PHONE REPORT (NEXT WORKING DAY) COPIES TO:________	CLINICAL DIAGNOSIS: PATIENT HISTORY:

Fig. 25.18 Biopsy requisition. (Courtesy of Diagnostic Pathology Associates, Columbus, OH.)

When the minor office surgery is completed, the provider may want the medical assistant to place a DSD over the surgical wound to protect it from contamination or injury or to absorb drainage. The medical assistant also is responsible for assisting the patient and cleaning the examining room.

Procedure 25.7 describes the medical assistant's responsibilities while assisting with minor office surgery. Specific instruments and supplies required for the minor office surgery depend on the type of surgery being performed and the provider's preference. Knowing the name and function of the surgical instruments shown in Fig. 25.3 enables the medical assistant to set up for each type of minor surgery performed in the medical office. If the medical office uses prepackaged sterile setups, the medical assistant should have already assembled the instruments and supplies in the package during the sanitization and sterilization process; however, the instruments and supplies should be checked after the pack is opened to ensure that all the sterile articles are included.

What Would You Do? What Would You *Not* Do?

Case Study 2

Abbey Mendy is having a sebaceous cyst removed from her neck. She wants to know why the antiseptic applied to her neck is orange and whether it is going to permanently stain her skin. During the procedure, Abbey reaches her hand up to adjust her hair and accidentally touches the physician's gloved hand. After the procedure, a sterile dressing is applied to her neck, and she is given an appointment to return to have her sutures removed. Abbey becomes alarmed when she is told that the cyst will be sent to the laboratory for a biopsy. She wants to know if the physician is not telling her everything, and is concerned that she might have cancer. Abbey asks if her neighbor can take out her sutures. She says that he has worked as a veterinary assistant for the past 8 years and has lots of experience in removing stitches. ■

HIGHLIGHT on the History of Surgery

Primitive Surgery

Surgery evolved from very primitive beginnings. The first record of a surgical operation dates back to 350,000 BCE. Primitive humans believed that headaches were caused by demons that had gained entrance to the head and were unable to get out. To release the demons, a hole was chiseled through the patient's skull with a sharp flint. Early operating instruments consisted of sharpened flints and crude hammers. Sharpened animal teeth were used for bloodletting and drainage of abscesses. Ancient records show that suturing materials consisted of dried gut, dried tendon, strips of hide, horsehair, and fibers from tree bark. To help form a clot, bleeding wounds were covered with materials such as rabbit fur, shredded tree bark, egg yolk, and cobwebs.

Early 1800s

In the early 1800s, surgical instruments were still almost nonexistent. Kitchen knives and penknives doubled as scalpels, and table forks were used as retractors. Providers would use household pincushions to hold their suturing needles. The same sponges were used for every patient to wipe away blood and other secretions. Because of these conditions, the most trivial operations were likely to be followed by infection, and death occurred in half of all surgical operations. Joseph Lister, an English surgeon, was one of the first individuals to advocate the use of antiseptics during surgery. Lister insisted on the use of antiseptics on the hands of his surgical team, instruments, wounds, and dressings. Many surgeons ridiculed Lister's ideas, but in 1879 his antiseptic principles were, at long last, formally adopted by the medical profession. Today, Lister is known as the father of modern surgery.

Mid-1800s

Anesthetic agents, such as ether and chloroform, were discovered in the mid-1800s. Before this time, various methods were used to subdue and restrain patients during surgery, such as having the patient consume alcohol before the operation and strapping the patient to the operating table. With the advent of anesthetics, new surgical procedures never before considered possible came into existence. This resulted in new demands for surgical instruments and the necessity for smaller and more delicate instruments.

Late 1800s and Early 1900s

The late 1800s and early 1900s saw dramatic advances in surgical operations and techniques. The most notable include the invention of the steam sterilizer, which permitted sterilization of surgical instruments and supplies; the use of surgical gowns, caps, masks, and gloves during surgery; the monitoring of the condition of patients under anesthesia; the development of stainless steel, which provided a superior material for manufacturing surgical instruments; and the establishment of standards for manufacturing and packaging sutures. Other discoveries important to surgery during this time included the discovery of x-rays by Wilhelm Röntgen; the discovery of penicillin by Alexander Fleming; the discovery by William Halsted that cocaine could be used as a local anesthetic; and the development of endoscopic instruments, such as the laryngoscope, bronchoscope, and sigmoidoscope, for viewing internal structures of the body.

Breakthroughs in surgical technology established through the ages laid the foundation for present-day complex surgical procedures, such as laser surgery, open heart surgery, microsurgery, robotic surgery, and telesurgery. It is incredible to think that it all started with a sharpened flint! ■

MINOR OFFICE SURGICAL PROCEDURES

The most common surgical procedures performed in the medical office are presented on the following pages. A discussion of the procedure and the items required for each tray setup are included. The medical assistant should take into account, however, that the instruments and supplies may vary slightly from those listed here, based on the provider's preference.

SEBACEOUS CYST REMOVAL

A **sebaceous cyst** (also known as an *epidermal cyst*) is a thin, closed sac or capsule located just under the surface of the skin. A sebaceous cyst forms when the outlet of a sebaceous (oil) gland becomes obstructed. The cyst contains *sebum,* which is made up of secretions from the sebaceous gland. The built-up secretion of sebum causes swelling, and the lining of the cyst consists of the stretched sebaceous gland. A sebaceous cyst is usually white or yellow in appearance and varies in size from less than ¼ inch (6 mm) in diameter to nearly 2 inches (5 cm) in diameter. It is usually a movable, dome-shaped mass with a smooth surface that is filled with a thick, fatty-white, cheesy material that has a foul odor. This type of cyst can occur anywhere on the body except on the palms of the hands and the soles of the feet—these areas do not contain sebaceous glands. Sebaceous cysts tend to occur most frequently on the scalp, face (Fig. 25.19), ears, neck, back, and genital area.

A sebaceous cyst is usually slow-growing, painless, and nontender and may disappear on its own. A sebaceous cyst usually does not require surgical removal unless it becomes infected. An infected cyst is painful, tender, red, and swollen and may have a grayish-white, foul-smelling discharge. Because it is difficult to remove an infected sebaceous cyst, the provider usually drains the cyst and allows it to heal and then performs the cyst excision at a later time. Other reasons for removing a sebaceous cyst include cosmetic concerns and the need to reduce discomfort from a cyst that is located in a body area that is easily irritated, such as the armpit.

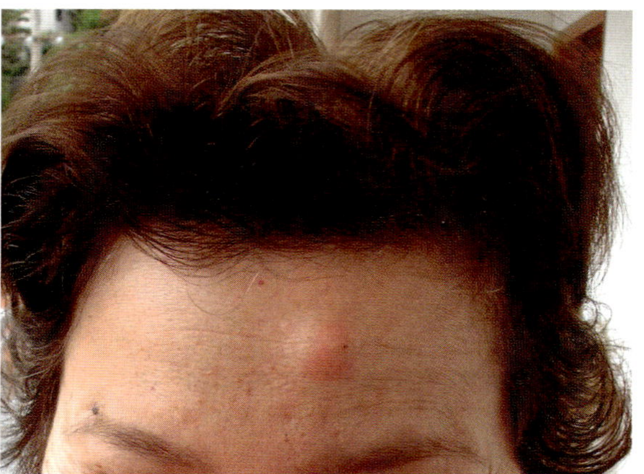

Fig. 25.19 Sebaceous cyst. (From Scully C: *Medical problems in dentistry*, ed 6, Norwalk, 2010, Churchill Livingstone.)

Surgical excision of a sebaceous cyst is a simple procedure that involves complete removal of the sac wall and its contents. Most sebaceous cysts are benign and are not usually biopsied unless they have an unusual appearance that may indicate a more serious problem. The side tray setup includes the items needed for a tissue biopsy (specimen container and laboratory request form); however, these items would not be placed on the tray if the provider determines that a biopsy of the sebaceous cyst is not warranted.

Procedure: Sebaceous Cyst Removal

A sebaceous cyst is removed as follows:

1. A local anesthetic is used to numb the area.
2. The provider makes an incision using either a single cut down the center or an oval cut on both sides of the cyst. The provider then removes the cyst and sutures the surgical incision (Fig. 25.20).
3. If the cyst is to be biopsied, it is placed in a specimen container with a preservative and sent to the laboratory for examination by a pathologist.
4. A sterile dressing is applied to the operative site.

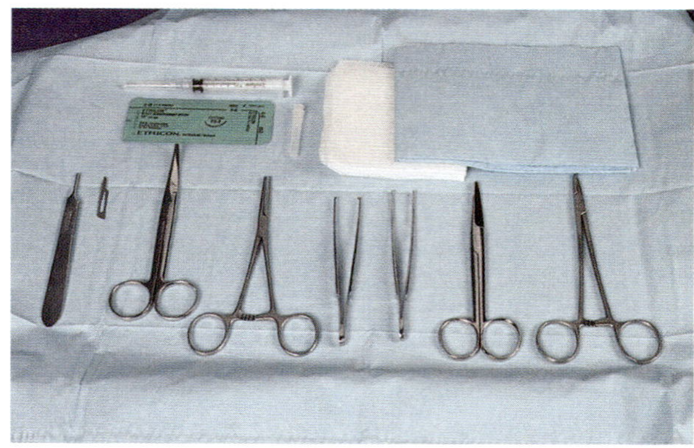

Sebaceous cyst removal sterile field.

Postoperative Instructions: Sebaceous Cyst Removal

Postoperative instructions include the following:

1. Keep the dressing clean and dry.
2. Report any signs that the wound is infected, which include fever, increased pain, swelling, redness, warmth, and discharge.
3. Notify the medical office if the sutures become loose or break.

Provide the patient with written instructions on wound care to refer to at home (see Table 25.1).

SURGICAL INCISION AND DRAINAGE OF LOCALIZED INFECTIONS

An **abscess** is a collection of pus in a cavity surrounded by inflamed tissue (Fig. 25.21A). It is caused by a pathogen

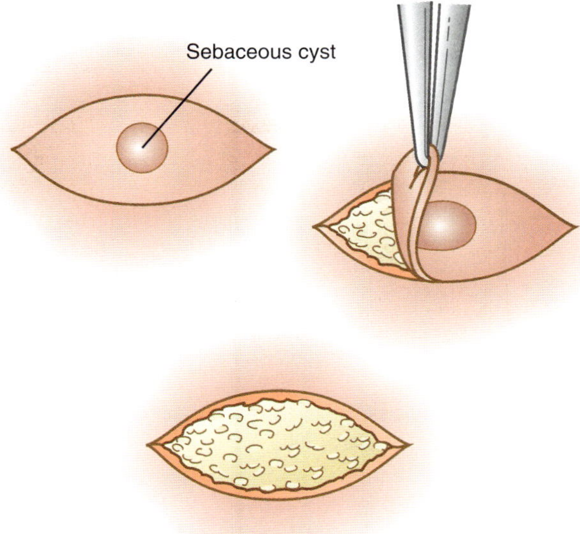

Fig. 25.20 Sebaceous cyst removal. The provider makes an incision, removes the cyst, and sutures the surgical incision. (From Nealon TF Jr: *Fundamental skills in surgery*, ed 4, Philadelphia, 1994, Saunders.)

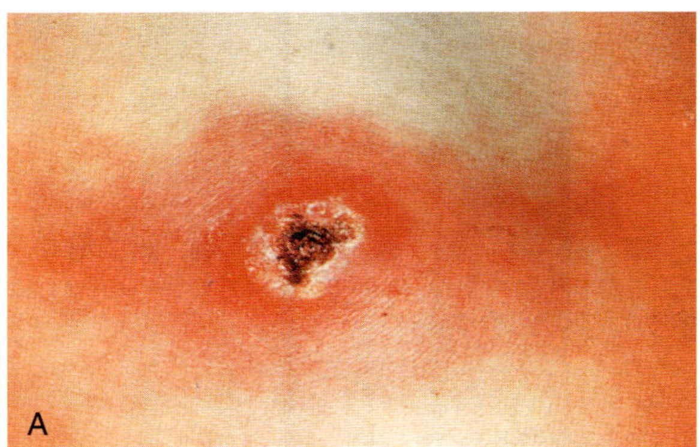

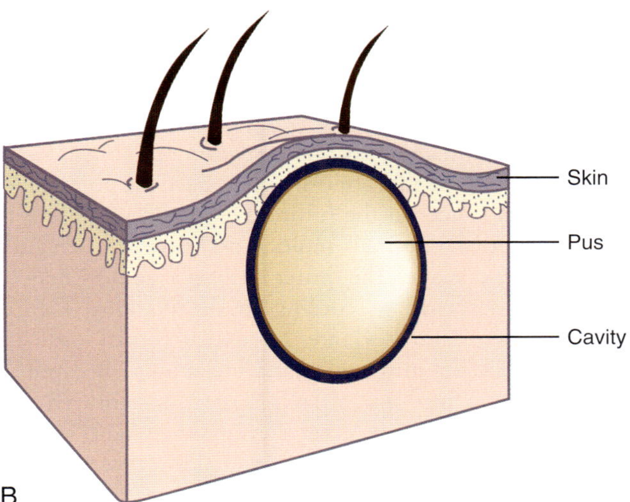

Fig. 25.21 (A) *Staphylococcus* skin abscess. (B) An abscess is a collection of pus in a cavity surrounded by inflamed tissue. (A, From Braverman IM: *Skin signs of systemic disease*, ed 3, Philadelphia, 1998, Saunders. B, From Nealon TF Jr: *Fundamental skills in surgery*, ed 4, Philadelphia, 1994, Saunders.)

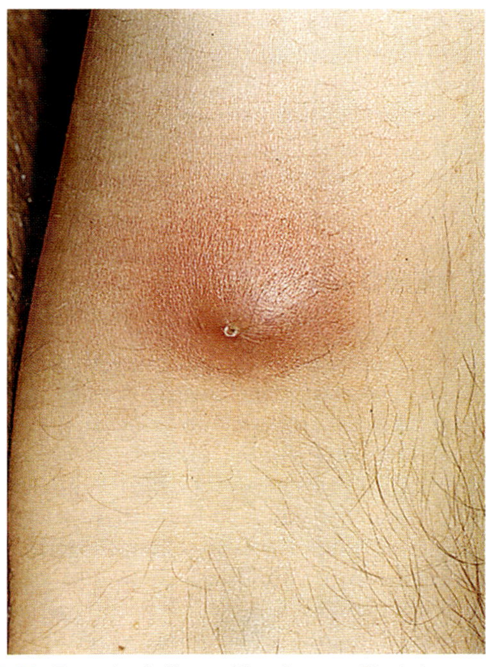

Fig. 25.22 Furuncle (boil) resulting from a *Staphylococcus aureus* infection. (From LaFleur Books M: *Exploring medical language: a student-directed approach*, ed 9, St. Louis, 2014, Mosby.)

that invades the tissues, usually via a break in the skin. An abscess serves as a defense mechanism of the body to keep an infection localized by walling off the microorganisms, preventing them from spreading through the body (Fig. 25.21B). A **furuncle,** also known as a *boil*, is a localized staphylococcal infection that originates deep within a hair follicle (Fig. 25.22). Furuncles produce pain and itching. The skin initially becomes red and then turns white and necrotic over the top of the furuncle. Erythema and induration usually surround it.

Procedure: Incision and Drainage

Localized infections, such as abscesses, furuncles, and infected sebaceous cysts, that do not rupture and drain naturally, may need to be incised and drained by the provider as follows:

1. A local anesthetic is typically used for the procedure.
2. A scalpel is used to make the incision. The provider then allows the pus to drain out and uses gauze to absorb pus and blood. Either gauze packing or a rubber Penrose drain is inserted into the wound to keep the edges of the tissues apart; this facilitates drainage of the exudate. The exudate contains pathogenic microorganisms; the medical assistant should be careful to avoid contact with the exudate while assisting with the minor surgery.
3. A sterile dressing of several thicknesses is applied over the operative site to absorb the drainage.

Postoperative Instructions: Incision and Drainage

Postoperative instructions include the following:

1. Keep the dressing clean and dry.

2. Report any signs that the wound is infected, which include fever, increased pain, swelling, redness, warmth, and discharge.

Provide the patient with written instructions on wound care to refer to at home (see Table 25.1) and instruct the patient when to return for removal of the gauze packing or Penrose drain.

MOLE REMOVAL

A mole (also known as a *nevus*) is a small growth on the human skin. An individual may be born with moles, which are known as *congenital nevi,* but may develop moles over time, known as *acquired nevi.* According to the American Academy of Dermatology, the majority of moles appear during the first 20 years of an individual's life. Moles can occur anywhere on the skin, and between 10 and 40 moles on the body is considered normal. Large numbers of moles can be concentrated on the back, chest, and arms. Most moles are benign and exhibit the following characteristics:

- Usually range in color from brown to nearly black but can be a pinkish flesh color to dark blue or even black. Dark-colored moles consist of a cluster of melanocytes. Melanocytes produce the pigment *melanin,* which is responsible for the dark color of these moles.
- Shape is usually round or oval and may be smooth or rough.
- Size is usually smaller than a pencil eraser but can range from barely visible to quite a large area.
- May form a raised area on the skin or may be flat.
- May sometimes have hairs growing out of them.

The most common types of moles are skin tags, flat moles, and raised moles. *Skin tags* or *acrochordon* are small, painless, benign growths that project from the skin from a small narrow stalk known as a *peduncle.* They are flesh colored or slightly darker, often appear in groups, and range from 1 mm to 5 mm in size (Fig. 25.23). Skin tags occur most often during and after middle age in adults who are overweight or have diabetes. Skin tags are most frequently found in body areas where the skin creases, such as the eyelids, neck, armpits, upper chest, and groin. Occasionally a skin tag becomes irritated as a result of shaving or rubbing from clothing or jewelry.

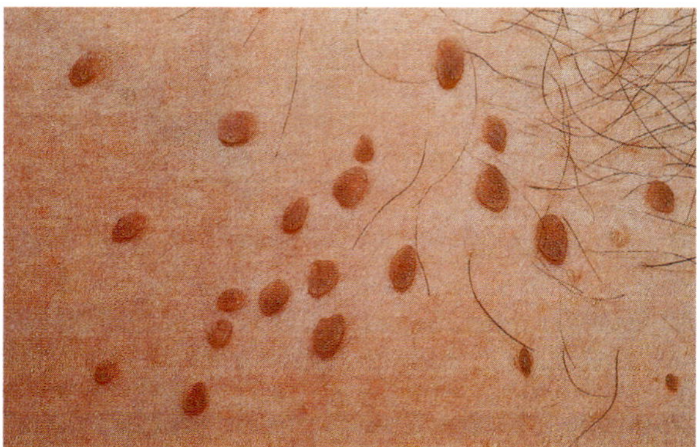

Fig. 25.23 Skin tags. (From White GM, Cox NH: *Diseases of the skin: a color atlas and text*, ed 2, St. Louis, 2006, Mosby.)

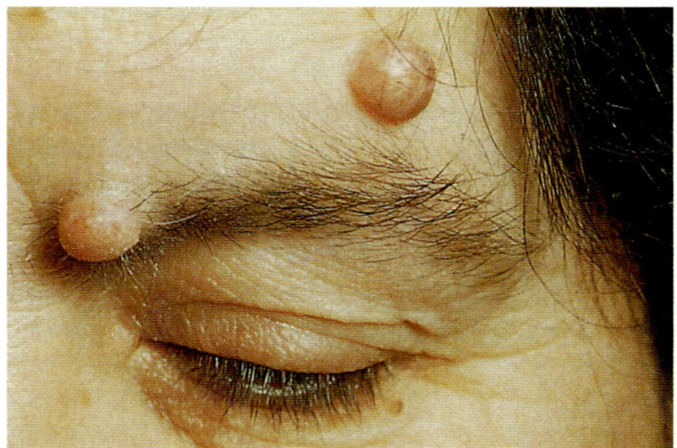

Fig. 25.24 Raised moles. (From Forbes CD: *Color atlas and text of clinical medicine*, ed 3, St. Louis, 2003, Mosby.)

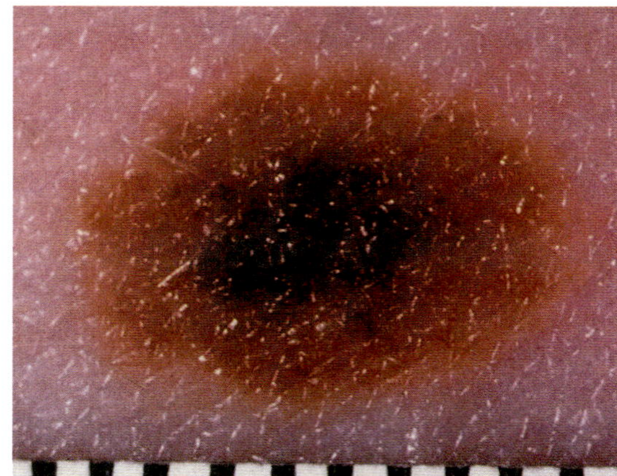

Fig. 25.25 Dysplastic nevi. (From Goldman L: *Cecil medicine*, ed 24, Philadelphia, 2012, Saunders.)

A *flat mole* is any dark spot or irregularity in the skin. A *raised mole*, as the name implies, extends above the skin. It can be a variety of colors and runs deeper than flat moles (Fig. 25.24).

Although most moles are benign, some moles may be precancerous and are known as *dysplastic nevi* (Fig. 25.25). *Precancerous* means that abnormal cells have the potential to develop into cancer in the future. Dysplastic nevi are usually larger than normal moles and have an irregular coloration and shape. The center of dysplastic nevi may be raised and darkened. According to the National Cancer Institute, dysplastic nevi are more likely than ordinary moles to develop into malignant melanoma. Because of this, dysplastic nevi are often biopsied or removed and biopsied to determine whether they are malignant.

Melanoma is a very serious type of skin cancer that can sometimes develop within a mole. Melanoma is most apt to be found on the upper backs of men and on the lower legs of women. Studies show that excessive sun exposure, especially severe blistering sunburns early in life, increases the risk of developing certain melanomas. If discovered early, it may be possible to completely remove the melanoma and

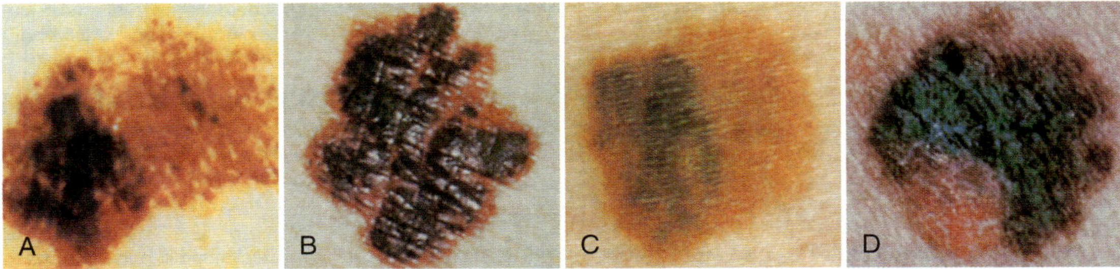

Fig. 25.26 The *ABCDs* of melanoma. A: Asymmetry (one half unlike the other half). B: Border (edges of mole are notched, uneven, or blurred). C: Color varied from one area to another; shades of tan, brown, and black, and sometimes white, red, or blue. D: Diameter larger than ¼ inch or 6 mm (diameter of a pencil eraser). (From Cooper K, Gosnell K: *Adult health nursing*, ed 7, St. Louis, 2015, Mosby.)

reduce the spread of skin cancer. Left untreated, melanoma can be fatal.

Any moles exhibiting the following characteristics common to melanoma (Fig. 25.26) should be evaluated by a provider:

- Asymmetric: one half of the mole is different from the other half.
- Irregular border: the edges of the mole are notched, uneven, or blurred rather than round or distinct.
- Color varies from one area of the mole to another: various shades of tan, brown, and black (and sometimes white, red, or blue) are present.
- Diameter is larger than ¼ inch (6 mm), which is about the diameter of a pencil eraser.
- Other signs: the mole is painful or tender, itches, bleeds, oozes, or has a scaly appearance.

Moles are removed for a variety of reasons, which include cosmetic issues (i.e., to improve an individual's appearance) and reduction of irritation and discomfort from a mole that is rubbing against clothing or that is in the way when shaving. A more serious reason for removing a mole is that the mole is suspected of being precancerous (dysplastic nevus) or cancerous (melanoma). Several methods may be used for mole removal. The most common methods include shave excision, surgical excision, and laser surgery. The method used depends on the type of mole being removed, including its size, shape, color, and location. In some cases a biopsy of the mole is performed before the mole is removed to determine whether the mole is benign or malignant.

Procedure: Mole Shave Excision

A shave excision is most commonly used to remove protruding moles. It can also be used to remove skin tags. This procedure is not used to remove dysplastic nevi because it might leave mole cells beneath the surface of the skin, which could cause the mole to grow back again. Sutures are not usually required for a shave excision. After the numbing effect of the anesthetic wears off, the area will be tender and sore. As healing occurs, a scab forms, which usually falls off within 1 to 2 weeks, leaving a red mark. As healing progresses, a flat, white mark usually remains in the place of the mole, which is approximately the same size as the mole. Over time, it fades to a barely visible scar. A mole is removed using the shave excision procedure as follows:

1. The provider numbs the area with a local anesthetic.
2. The provider uses a sharp razor or scalpel to shave off the protruding part of the mole until the area is flush with the level of the surrounding skin.
3. The provider may use electrosurgery to destroy the tissue below the surface of the mole and to control bleeding.
4. A topical antibiotic is applied to the area.
5. A sterile dressing is applied to the operative site.
6. The mole shavings may be placed in a specimen container with a preservative and sent to the laboratory for examination by a pathologist.

Procedure: Surgical Mole Excision

The surgical excision procedure is often used when the provider suspects that a mole is precancerous or cancerous. A scalpel is used to remove the entire mole, as well as a border of surrounding skin and tissue underlying the mole, to remove all the mole cells. A scar commonly forms after this procedure; however, it usually fades over time. A mole is removed using the surgical excision procedure as follows:

1. The provider numbs the area with a local anesthetic.
2. The provider uses a scalpel to cut an oval border surrounding the mole and removes the mole with tissue forceps.
3. The provider may use an electrocautery instrument to control bleeding.
4. The provider inserts sutures to close the surgical incision.
5. A sterile dressing is applied to the operative site.
6. The mole is placed in a specimen container with a preservative and is sent to the laboratory for examination by a pathologist.

Postoperative Instructions: Shave Excision and Surgical Excision

Postoperative instructions for both a shave excision and a surgical excision of a mole include the following:

1. Keep the dressing clean and dry.
2. Report any signs that the wound is infected, which include fever, increased pain, swelling, redness, warmth, and discharge.

3. If sutures have been inserted, notify the medical office if they become loose or break.
4. To reduce scarring, protect the area from the ultraviolet (UV) rays of the sun by staying out of the sun or using a good sunscreen with a sun protection factor (SPF) of 15 or higher.

Provide the patient with written instructions on wound care to refer to at home (see Table 25.1).

LASER MOLE SURGERY

Laser surgery is used to remove small or flat moles that are brown or black in color and noncancerous. This procedure involves the use of a laser beam of light, which evaporates the mole tissue. The laser beam also seals off blood vessels, which avoids the need for sutures. Because the laser light cannot penetrate deeply enough, this method usually is not used on raised moles, deep moles, large moles, or dysplastic nevi.

Removing a mole with a laser reduces the amount of tissue destruction in the surrounding tissue, which minimizes scarring. This procedure does not require a local anesthetic. No pain is involved during the procedure; the patient feels only a mild tingling when the laser pulses. A scab forms, which usually falls off within 1 to 2 weeks. Once the scab falls off, the area is usually reddish, and it may take several weeks before normal skin color returns. Repeated treatments (one to three) may be required before the mole is completely removed.

The medical assistant should instruct the patient to keep the area clean and dry. The patient should also protect the area from the UV rays of the sun by staying out of the sun or by using a good sunscreen with an SPF of 15 or higher.

NEEDLE BIOPSY

A **biopsy** is the removal and examination of tissue from the living body. The tissue usually is examined under a microscope. Biopsies are most often performed to determine whether a tumor is malignant or benign; however, a biopsy also may be used as a diagnostic aid for other conditions, such as infections. A **needle biopsy** is a type of biopsy in which tissue from deep within the body is obtained by the insertion of a biopsy needle through the skin. The advantage of a needle biopsy is that a sample of tissue can be obtained that might otherwise require a major surgical operation.

Procedure: Needle Biopsy

1. The procedure is performed with the patient under a local anesthetic, and because an incision is not required, the patient does not have to undergo the discomfort and inconvenience of an operative recovery.
2. The tissue specimen is placed in a container with a preservative and is sent to the laboratory for examination by a pathologist.
3. A small dressing, placed over the needle puncture site, is usually sufficient to protect the operative site and promote healing.
4. After the procedure, the patient should be observed for any evidence of complications related to the procedure.

Postoperative Instructions: Needle Biopsy

1. A bruise typically occurs at the biopsy site and will gradually disappear within several weeks.
2. Keep the dressing clean and dry.
3. Rest and avoid strenuous activity and heavy lifting for 2 days after the procedure.
4. Report any signs that the wound is infected, which include fever, increased pain, swelling, redness, warmth, and discharge.

INGROWN TOENAIL REMOVAL

An ingrown toenail occurs when the edge of the toenail grows deeply into the nail groove and penetrates the surrounding skin, resulting in pain, swelling, and and discomfort (Fig. 25.27A). An ingrown nail can occur in both the nails of the hands and those of the feet; however, it is more apt to occur in the toenails. An ingrown toenail can be caused by external pressure to the toe (such as from tight shoes, or trauma to the toe), improper nail trimming, or a nail infection. The protruding nail acts as a foreign body, usually resulting in secondary infection and inflammation. In mild cases, this condition is treated by inserting a small piece of cotton packing under the toenail to raise the nail edge away from the tissue of the nail groove (Fig. 25.27B). In severe and recurring cases, part of the nail must be surgically removed (Fig. 25.27C and D). Severe cases cause pain, swelling, redness, and drainage (Fig. 25.28). The toenail removal procedure relieves pain by decreasing nail pressure on the soft tissues.

Procedure: Ingrown Toenail

An ingrown toenail is removed as follows:

1. Before the surgical procedure is performed, the affected foot must be soaked in tepid water containing an antibacterial

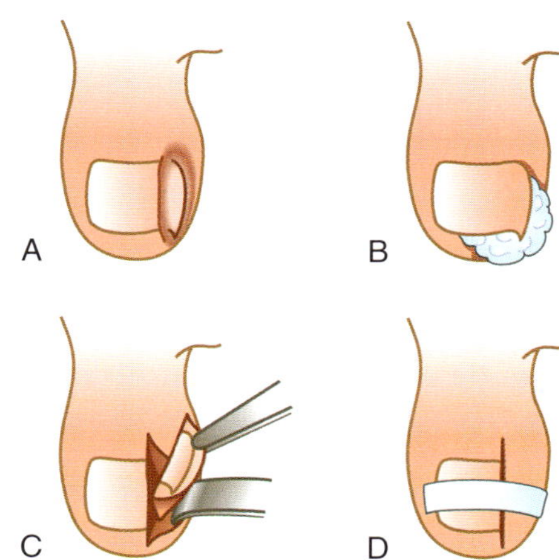

Fig. 25.27 Ingrown toenail. (A) The edge of the toenail grows deeply into the nail groove. (B) In mild cases, treatment consists of inserting a small piece of cotton packing under the toenail. (C) In severe and recurring cases, a wedge of the nail is surgically removed. (D) A strip of surgical tape is applied over the area. (From Nealon TF Jr: *Fundamental skills in surgery*, ed 4, Philadelphia, 1994, Saunders.)

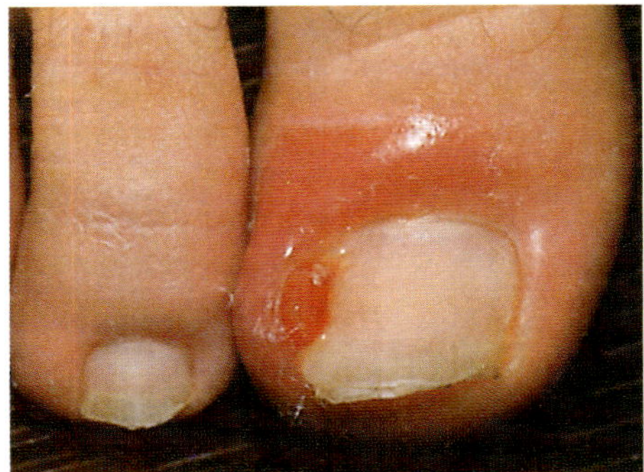

Fig. 25.28 Ingrown toenail. (From Seidel HM: *Mosby's guide to physical examination*, ed 6, St. Louis, 2006, Mosby.)

skin solution for 10 to 15 minutes to soften the nail plate and decrease the possibility of bacterial infection.

2. The patient is placed in a reclining position with the foot adequately supported, and the toe is shaved to remove hair, which would act as a contaminant.
3. An antiseptic is applied to the affected toe, which is then numbed using a local anesthetic.
4. Using surgical toenail scissors, the provider surgically removes a wedge of the nail (see Fig. 25.27C).
5. An antibiotic ointment is applied to the area.
6. A sterile gauze dressing or a strip of surgical tape is applied over the area to protect the operative site and to promote healing (see Fig. 25.27D).

Postoperative Instructions: Ingrown Toenail

Postoperative instructions include the following:

1. Elevate the foot for 24 hours following the procedure.
2. Keep the area clean and dry.
3. Cleanse the toe daily with warm water and gently dry the area.
4. Apply an antibiotic ointment daily until the wound has completely healed.
5. Wear loose-fitting shoes for 2 weeks after the procedure.
6. Avoid strenuous exercise for 2 weeks after the procedure.
7. Contact the medical office if any signs of infection occur, which include increasing pain, redness, swelling, and drainage from the toe.

Provide the patient with written instructions on wound care to refer to at home (see Table 25.1) and instruct the patient on the importance of wearing properly fitting shoes and on the proper procedure for nail trimming. The nail should be cut straight across with the corners of the nail protruding from the end of the toe.

COLPOSCOPY

Colposcopy is the visual examination of the vagina and cervix by means of a lighted instrument with a binocular magnifying lens, known as a **colposcope** (Fig. 25.29). The purpose of colposcopy is to examine the vagina and cervix to detect areas of abnormal tissue growth that may not be visible with the naked eye (Fig. 25.30). Colposcopy is performed after abnormal Pap test results and to evaluate a vaginal or cervical lesion observed during a pelvic examination. The primary goal of colposcopy is to prevent cervical cancer by detecting precancerous lesions early and treating them.

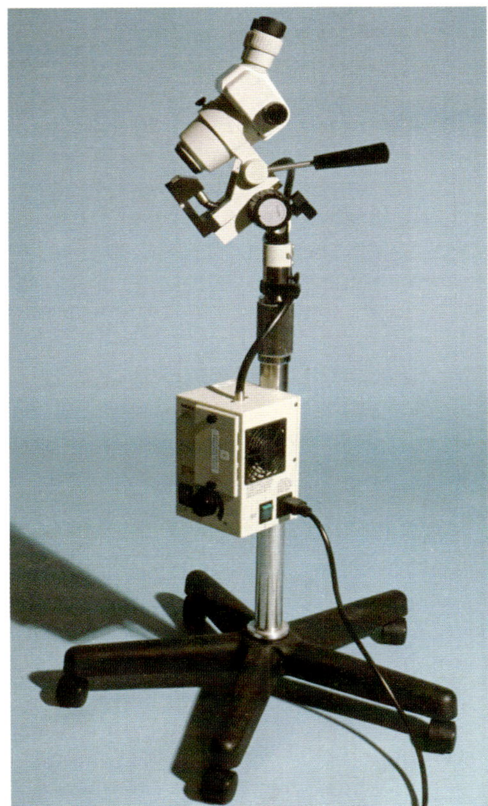

Fig. 25.29 A colposcope. (From Apgar BS, Brotzman GL, Spitzer M: *Colposcopy: principles and practice—an integrated textbook and atlas*, Philadelphia, 2002, Saunders.)

Blood cells make it more difficult for the provider to observe the cervix; therefore, a colposcopy is usually performed 1 week after the end of the menstrual period. To prepare for the procedure, the patient should be told not to douche; use tampons, vaginal medications, or spermicides; or have intercourse for 24 hours before the examination. The lens of the colposcope is positioned approximately 12 inches (30 cm) from the opening of the vagina. The lens magnifies tissue, facilitating the inspection of cervical cells and the obtaining of a biopsy specimen. For a routine colposcopic examination, a magnification ranging from 6× to 15× is typically used. The colposcope may be placed on an adjustable stand or attached to the side of the examining table and swung out before use.

Procedure: Colposcopy

Colposcopy is performed as follows:

1. The patient is assisted into a lithotomy position and is prepared as for a pelvic examination.
2. The provider inserts a vaginal speculum into the vagina.
3. A long, cotton-tipped applicator moistened with saline is used to wipe the cervix to remove the mucous film that

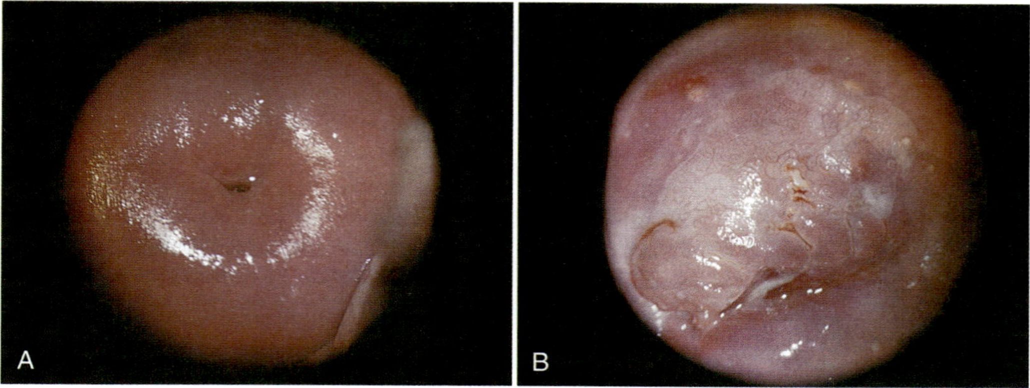

Fig. 25.30 (A) Normal cervix. (B) Abnormal cervix. (From Damjanov I: *Pathology for the health-related professions*, ed 4, St. Louis, 2012, Saunders.)

normally covers it. The saline also provides better visualization of the cervical epithelium because dry cervical epithelium is not transparent and does not allow satisfactory viewing of the vascular pattern of the cervix.

4. The colposcope is focused on the cervix, and the provider inspects the saline-moistened cervix.
5. The cervix is swabbed with acetic acid, using a long, cotton-tipped applicator. The acetic acid dissolves cervical mucus and other secretions. It also causes abnormal tissue to turn white, which allows easier visualization of abnormal areas of the cervix.
6. The cervical epithelium also may be stained with Lugol iodine solution using a long, cotton-tipped applicator. This provides another means to identify unhealthy epithelium. The healthy epithelium of the cervix contains glycogen, which is able to absorb the iodine, causing the epithelium to stain a dark brown color. Conversely, abnormal epithelium, such as would constitute a malignancy, does not contain glycogen and is unable to absorb the iodine.
7. If an abnormal area is observed, the provider obtains a cervical biopsy specimen using punch biopsy forceps, which is described next.

CERVICAL PUNCH BIOPSY

A cervical biopsy is performed in combination with colposcopy to remove a cervical tissue specimen for examination by a pathologist. The purpose of the biopsy is to detect the presence of cervical dysplasia or cancer of the cervix. *Cervical dysplasia* is an abnormal growth of cells on the surface of the cervix that are precancerous. Cervical dysplasia can range from mild to moderate to severe. A cervical punch biopsy can also be used to diagnose polyps on the cervix and genital warts. Genital warts may indicate infection with human papillomavirus (HPV), which is a risk factor for developing cervical cancer. Performing a cervical punch biopsy helps the provider determine the type of abnormal tissue present on the cervix so that the provider can determine the best form of treatment for the patient's condition.

Cervical biopsies are most frequently performed after abnormal Pap test results. Although an abnormal Pap test result is a cause for concern, the majority of abnormal Pap test results are not caused by cervical cancer, but rather by a vaginal infection. To prevent inaccurate test results, the cervical biopsy is usually performed 1 week after the end of the menstrual period, when the cervix is the least vascular. To prepare for the procedure, the patient should be told not to douche; use tampons, vaginal medications, or spermicides; or have intercourse for 24 hours before the procedure to prevent inaccurate test results.

What Would You Do? | What Would You *Not* Do?

Case Study 3

Sadira Wisal has been referred to the office by her family physician for a colposcopy. Her last Pap test results came back as abnormal, and a repeat Pap test 3 months later also had abnormal results. While having her vital signs taken, Sadira bursts into tears. She tearfully explains that she's afraid that she has cancer, and that no one at her family physician's office told her what to expect from this procedure. Sadira does not understand why she has to have this procedure, and does not know what will be done during the procedure. She says that she feels stupid, but she does not even know what a cervix is. Sadira also worries that the procedure will affect her ability to have children. ■

Procedure: Cervical Punch Biopsy

A cervical punch biopsy is performed as follows:

1. The patient is positioned and draped in a lithotomy position. An anesthetic is not needed because the cervix has few pain receptors. The patient may experience no discomfort during the procedure or a certain amount of discomfort ranging from mild to moderate in intensity. Some patients experience mild cramping and pinching when the specimen is being removed from the cervix.
2. The provider inserts a vaginal speculum into the vagina for proper visualization of the cervix.
3. The cervix is wiped with saline and then swabbed with ascetic acid.

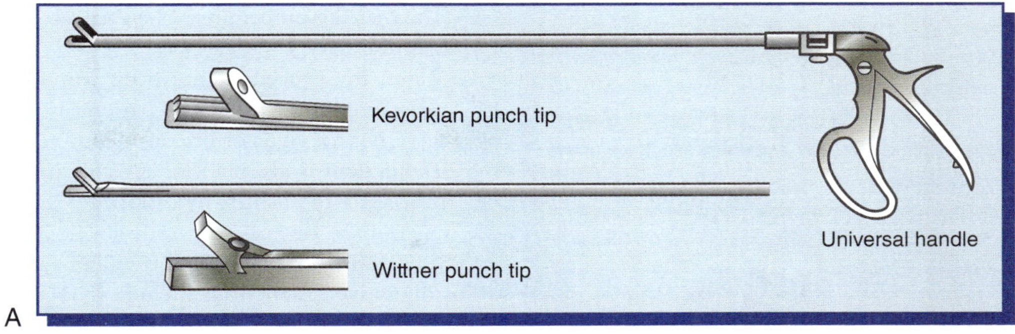

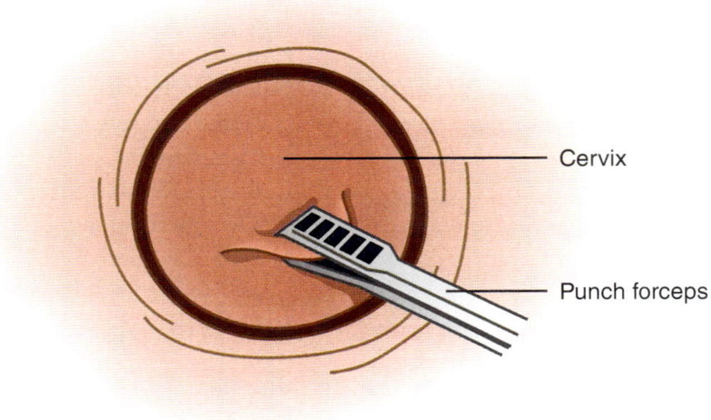

Fig. 25.31 Cervical punch biopsy. (A) Cervical biopsy punch forceps. (B) Obtaining a tissue specimen from the cervix using cervical biopsy punch forceps. (Courtesy of Elmed, Addison, IL.)

4. To assist in obtaining the specimen, the provider may stain the cervix with Lugol iodine solution.
5. The colposcope is focused on the cervix, and the provider inspects the cervix.
6. Using cervical biopsy punch forceps, the provider obtains several tissue specimens (Fig. 25.31A) from the abnormal cervical epithelium (Fig. 25.31B). The patient may feel a pinching sensation and mild cramps each time a specimen is removed from the cervix.
7. The specimen is placed in a container with a preservative and is sent to the laboratory for examination by a pathologist.
8. If bleeding occurs, the provider controls it with gauze packing, a hemostatic solution (e.g., Monsel solution), or electrocautery.
9. The patient is given a sanitary pad at the office after the procedure to absorb any discharge.

Postoperative Instructions: Cervical Punch Biopsy

Postoperative instructions include the following:

1. A minimal amount of cramping and bleeding may follow the procedure and last up to 1 week. Contact the medical office if the bleeding lasts longer than 2 weeks.
2. A thick, dark-colored vaginal discharge may occur after the procedure (if Monsel solution was used to control bleeding) and may last for several days.
3. Do not douche, use tampons, or have intercourse for 1 week after the procedure to allow proper healing of the cervix to take place.
4. Contact the medical office if any of the following occurs: bleeding that is heavier than normal menstrual bleeding, a foul-smelling vaginal discharge, fever, or lower abdominal pain.

Provide the patient with written instructions to refer to at home. An appointment is scheduled approximately 1 week after the procedure to make sure that healing is taking place and to discuss the biopsy results.

CRYOSURGERY

Cervical Cryosurgery

Cervical **cryosurgery,** also known as *cryotherapy,* uses freezing temperatures to treat certain gynecologic conditions. Cryosurgery is most often performed as a treatment for cervical dysplasia to destroy abnormal cervical cells that show changes that may lead to cancer. Cryosurgery is done only after a colposcopy confirms the presence of cervical dysplasia. Cryosurgery is also used for the treatment of chronic cervicitis, which is inflammation of the cervix.

Cervical cryosurgery can be performed without an anesthetic, although occasionally a mild analgesic is necessary immediately afterward. The cryosurgery unit consists of a

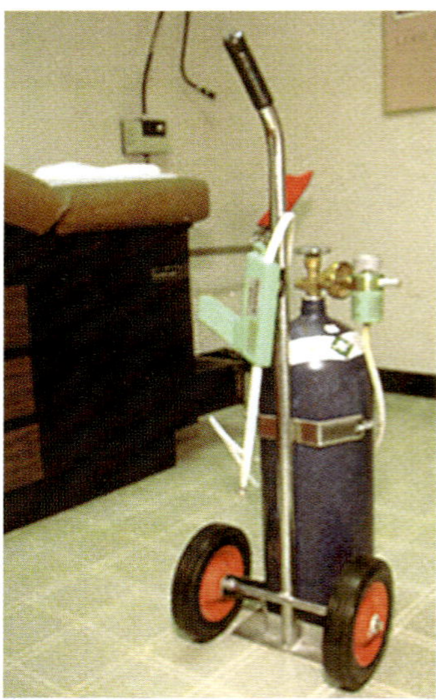

Fig. 25.32 Cryosurgery unit. (From Zakus S: *Clinical skills for medical assistants*, ed 4, Philadelphia, 2001, Saunders.)

long metal cryoprobe attached to a cooling-agent tank (Fig. 25.32). The principal cooling agents are liquid nitrogen and compressed nitrogen gas. The cryoprobe is inserted into the vagina and placed firmly in contact with the abnormal area. The cooling agent flows through the cryoprobe, freezing the cervical tissue to -20°C. This causes the abnormal cells to die and slough off so that the cervical covering can eventually be replaced with new, healthy epithelial tissue. Regeneration of cervical tissue occurs within approximately 4 to 6 weeks after the procedure. After cryosurgery, the patient will be required to have a Pap test every 3 to 6 months for a period of time determined by the provider.

Procedure: Cervical Cryosurgery

Cryosurgery is performed as follows:

1. The patient is draped and assisted into the lithotomy position.
2. The provider inserts a vaginal speculum for proper visualization of the cervix.
3. The cervix is swabbed with an acid-saline solution to remove mucus and other contaminants.
4. The metal cryoprobe is inserted into the vagina and placed firmly in contact with the affected area, and the cryosurgery unit is turned on.
5. The cooling agent flows through the cryoprobe and causes the metal probe to freeze and destroy superficial abnormal cervical tissue. The provider allows the cryoprobe to come in contact with the cervical area for approximately 3 minutes. During the procedure, the patient may experience some pain resembling menstrual cramping.
6. The cryoprobe is removed for 3 to 5 minutes to permit the cervical tissue to return to its normal temperature. The freezing procedure is then repeated for an additional 3 minutes.
7. When the procedure has been completed, the medical assistant should assist the patient as necessary and observe her for signs of discomfort or vertigo.
8. The patient is given a sanitary pad at the office after the procedure to absorb any discharge.

Postoperative Instructions: Cervical Cryosurgery

Postoperative instructions include the following:

1. Normal activities can be resumed the day after the cryosurgery.
2. On the first postoperative day, a clear, watery vaginal discharge occurs, which lasts for 2 to 4 weeks. The discharge is caused by the shedding of the dead cervical tissue and gradually diminishes as the healing progresses.
3. Use sanitary pads (rather than tampons) to absorb the watery discharge.
4. Do not douche, use tampons, or have intercourse for 2 to 3 weeks after the procedure to allow proper healing of the cervix to take place.
5. Contact the medical office if any of the following occurs: bleeding that is heavier than normal menstrual bleeding, a foul-smelling vaginal discharge, fever, or lower abdominal pain.

Provide the patient with written instructions to refer to at home. The patient must schedule a return visit 6 weeks after the procedure to ensure that proper healing has occurred.

Skin Lesions

In the medical office, cryosurgery also may be used to remove benign skin lesions, such as common warts and skin tags. Only a small amount of cooling agent is required for skin lesions, so the cryosurgery unit is considerably smaller than the one described for cervical cryosurgery. Most providers use liquid nitrogen contained in a small, pressurized, stainless steel canister with an attached probe. The provider applies the liquid nitrogen to the skin lesion until it turns white, which indicates that freezing of the tissue has occurred. During the procedure, the patient feels a slight burning or stinging sensation as the cooling agent is applied. After cryosurgery, a blister develops and dries to a scab in 1 week to 10 days and eventually sloughs off. The patient should be told to keep the area clean and dry until the scab has sloughed off. In some cases the treatment may not result in complete destruction of the lesion; two or more treatments may be required to remove the lesion.

BANDAGING

A **bandage** is a strip of woven material used to wrap or cover a part of the body. The function of a bandage may be to protect, support, or immobolize an injured part of the body, apply pressure to control bleeding, and to hold a dressing in place and protect it from external contamination.

GUIDELINES FOR APPLICATION

The bandage should be applied so that it feels comfortable to the patient, and it must be fastened securely with metal clips or adhesive tape. Guidelines for applying a bandage are as follows:

1. Observe the principles of medical asepsis during the application of a bandage.
2. Ensure that the area to which a bandage is applied is clean and dry.
3. Do not apply a bandage directly over an open wound. To prevent contamination of the wound, first apply a sterile dressing and then the bandage. The bandage should extend at least 2 inches (5 cm) beyond the edge of the dressing.
4. To prevent irritation, do not allow the skin surfaces of two body parts (e.g., two fingers) to touch. In addition, the patient's perspiration provides a moist environment that encourages the growth of microorganisms. A piece of gauze should be inserted between the two body parts.
5. Ensure that joints and prominent parts of bones are padded to prevent the bandage from rubbing the skin and causing irritation.
6. Bandage the body part in its normal position with joints slightly flexed to avoid muscle strain.
7. Apply the bandage from the distal to the proximal part of the body to aid the venous return of blood to the heart.
8. As you apply the bandage, ask the patient whether it feels comfortable. The bandage should fit snugly enough that it does not fall off, but not so tightly that it impedes circulation.
9. If possible, leave the fingers or toes exposed when bandaging an extremity. This provides the opportunity to check them for signs of impairment in circulation. Signs exhibited by the fingers or toes of a bandaged extremity indicating that the bandage is too tight include coldness, pallor, numbness, cyanosis of the nail beds, swelling, pain, and tingling sensations. If any of these signs occurs, loosen the bandage immediately.
10. If a bandage roll is dropped during the procedure, obtain a new bandage and begin again.

TYPES OF BANDAGES

Three basic types of bandages are used in the medical office. A *roller bandage* is a long strip of soft material wound on itself to form a roll. It ranges from ½ inch to 6 inches (1.3 to 15.2 cm) wide and from 2 to 5 yards (1.83 to 4.57 m) long. The width used depends on the part being bandaged. Roller bandages usually are made of sterilized gauze. Gauze is porous and lightweight, molds easily to a body part, and is relatively inexpensive and easily disposed of. Because it is made of loosely woven cotton, however, it may slip and fray easily. *Kling gauze* is a special type of gauze that stretches; this allows it to cling, and as a result it molds and conforms better to the body part than does regular gauze.

Elastic bandages are made of woven cotton that contains elastic fibers. One brand name of elastic bandages is the Ace bandage. Although elastic bandages are expensive, they can be washed and used again. The medical assistant must be extremely careful when applying an elastic bandage because it is easy to apply it too tightly and impede circulation. Elastic adhesive bandages also may be used; these have an adhesive backing to provide a secure fit.

BANDAGE TURNS

Five basic bandage turns are used, alone or in combination. The type of turn used depends on which body part is to be bandaged and whether the bandage is used for support or immobilization or for holding a dressing in place.

The *circular turn* is applied to a part of uniform width, such as toes, fingers, or the head. Each turn completely overlaps the previous turn. Two circular turns are used to anchor a bandage at the beginning and end of a spiral, spiral-reverse, figure-eight, or recurrent turn (Fig. 25.33).

The *spiral turn* is applied to a part of uniform circumference, such as the fingers, arms, legs, chest, or abdomen. Each spiral turn is carried upward at a slight angle and should overlap the previous turn by one-half to two-thirds the width of the bandage (Fig. 25.34).

The *spiral-reverse turn* is useful for bandaging a part that varies in width, such as the forearm or lower leg. Reversing each spiral turn allows for a smoother fit and prevents gaping caused by variation in the contour of the limb. The thumb is used to make the reverse halfway through each spiral turn. The bandage is directed downward over the thumb towards the lower edge of the previous turn. Each turn should overlap the previous one by two-thirds the width of the bandage. The reverse turn is used as often as necessary to provide a uniform fit (Fig. 25.35).

In general, the *figure-eight turn* is used to hold a dressing in place or to support and immobilize an injured joint, such as the ankle, knee, elbow, or wrist. The figure-eight turn consists of slanting turns that alternately ascend and descend around the part and cross over one another in the middle, resembling the figure eight. Each turn overlaps the previous one by two-thirds the width of the bandage (Fig. 25.36).

The *recurrent turn* is a series of back-and-forth turns used to bandage the tips of fingers or toes, the stump of an amputated extremity, or the head. The bandage is anchored by using two circular turns and is passed back and forth over the tip of the part to be bandaged, first on one side and then on the other side of the first center turn. Each turn should overlap the previous turn by two-thirds the width of the bandage (Fig. 25.37).

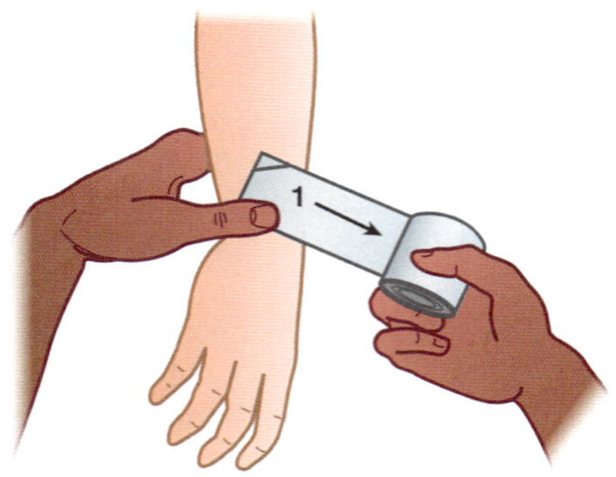

1. Place the end of the roller bandage on a slant.

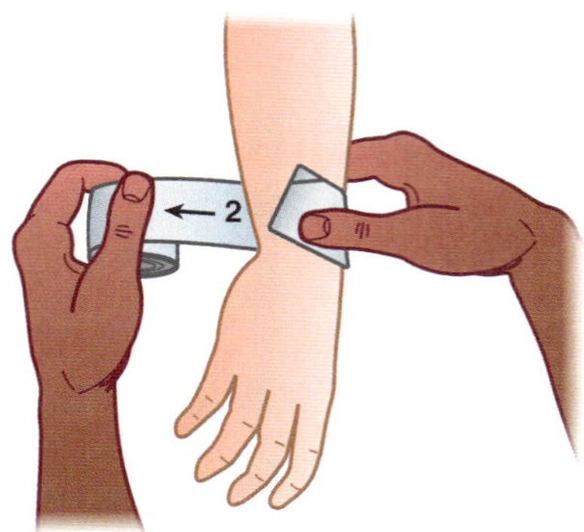

2. Encircle the part while allowing the corner of the bandage to extend.

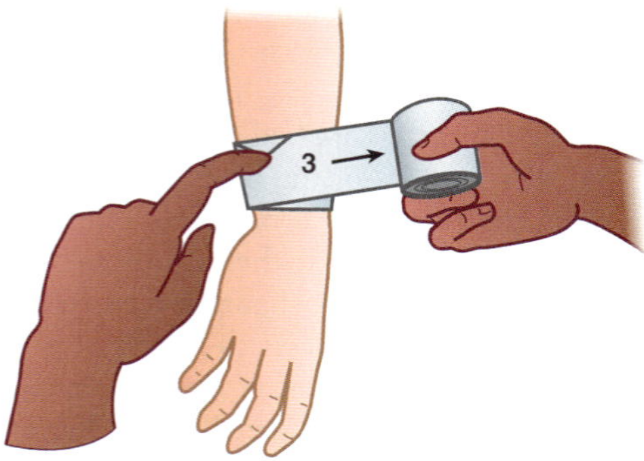

3. Turn down the corner of the bandage.

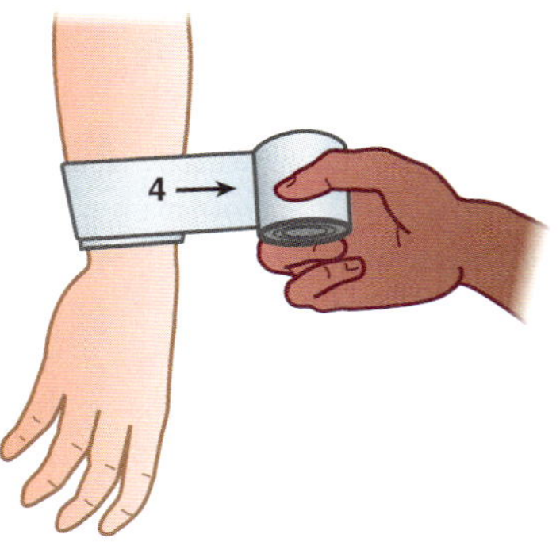

4. Make another circular turn around the part.

Fig. 25.33 Anchoring a bandage.

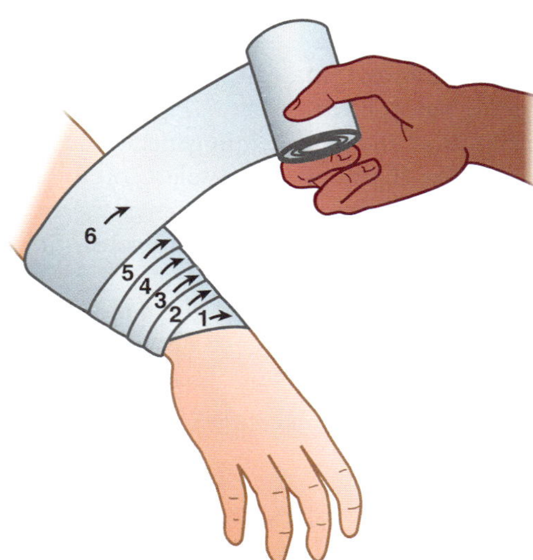

Fig. 25.34 Spiral turn.

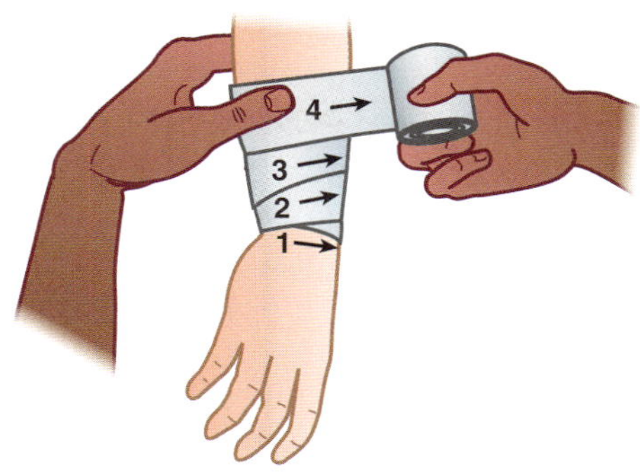

1. Encircle the lower arm while keeping the bandage at a slant.

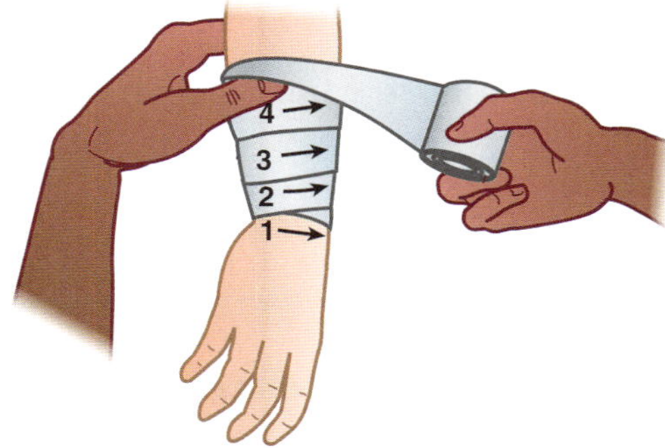

2. Direct the bandage downward over the thumb towards the lower edge of the previous turn.

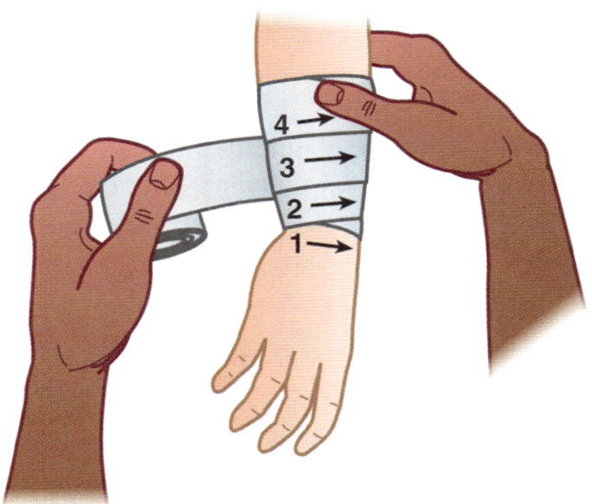

3. Keep the bandage parallel to the lower edge of the previous turn.

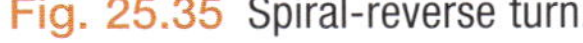

Fig. 25.35 Spiral-reverse turn.

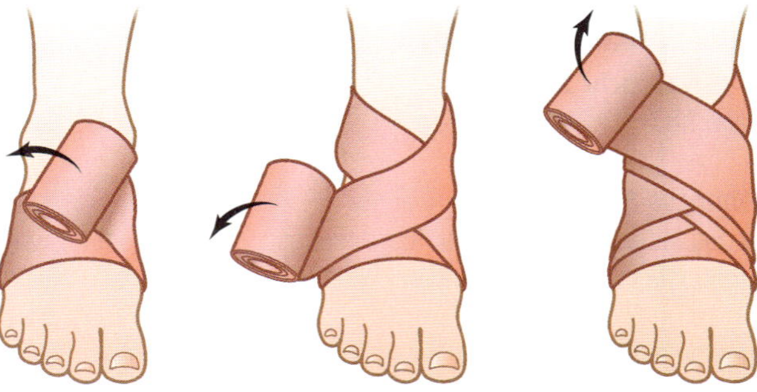

Fig. 25.36 Figure-eight turn. (From Leake MJ: *A manual of simple nursing procedures*, Philadelphia, 1971, Saunders.)

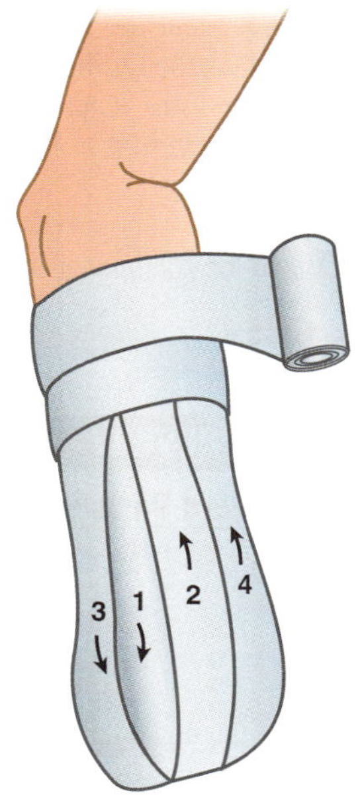

Fig. 25.37 Recurrent turn.

What Would You Do? What Would You *Not* Do? RESPONSES

Case Study 1

Page 581

What Did Heather Do?

- ❑ Tried to calm and reassure Mrs. Ventura. Told her that children at this age are prone to accidents and that she should not blame herself.
- ❑ Told Mrs. Ventura that Cory's wound could not be held together effectively with Steri-Strips. Explained that sutures would help the wound heal better.
- ❑ Told Mrs. Ventura that the doctor could not suture the wound unless she signs the consent form. Explained that Cory's wound should be sutured as soon as possible to prevent infection and to minimize scarring.
- ❑ Asked Mrs. Ventura if she would like to talk with the doctor again before signing the form.

What Did Heather Not Do?

- ❑ Did not prepare Cory for the suture insertion procedure until Mrs. Ventura signed the consent to treatment form.

Continued

What Would You Do? What Would You *Not* Do? RESPONSES—cont'd

Case Study 2
Page 587

What Did Heather Do?
- ❑ Explained to Abbey that the antiseptic contains iodine, which appears orange when it is applied to the skin. Assured her that the iodine would not stain her skin permanently and that it would wear off in a few days.
- ❑ Calmly and discreetly opened a new pair of surgical gloves so that the physician could reapply surgical gloves. Reminded Abbey not to move during the procedure.
- ❑ Told Abbey that most tissues removed from patients are routinely sent to the laboratory for a biopsy. Reassured her that the doctor has told her everything he knows about her condition.
- ❑ Made it clear to Abbey that her neighbor is not permitted to remove her sutures. Stressed to her that the doctor needs to check her incision before the sutures are removed to ensure that proper healing has occurred.

What Did Heather Not Do?
- ❑ Did not scold Abbey for contaminating the physician's sterile gloved hand.

Case Study 3
Page 594

What Did Heather Do?
- ❑ Listened empathetically to Sadira, and tried to calm and reassure her.
- ❑ Spent some time going over the colposcopy procedure and what to expect.
- ❑ Answered as many of Sadira's questions as possible. Reassured her that a lot of people do not know what a cervix is and that she is asking some very good questions.
- ❑ Asked the physician to spend some time talking with Sadira before the procedure to answer questions that Heather is not qualified to answer.
- ❑ Ensured that Sadira understood all of the information about the procedure before asking her to sign the consent to treatment form.

What Did Heather Not Do?
- ❑ Did not tell Sadira that her family physician should have explained the procedure to her.
- ❑ Did not tell Sadira that she does not have cancer.

TERMINOLOGY REVIEW

Key Term	Word Parts	Definition
Abrasion		A wound in which the outer layers of the skin are damaged; a scrape.
Abscess		A collection of pus in a cavity surrounded by inflamed tissue.
Absorbable suture		Suture material that is gradually digested and absorbed by the body.
Approximation		The process of bringing two parts, such as tissue, together through the use of sutures or other means.
Bandage		A strip of woven material used to wrap or cover a part of the body.
Biopsy	*bi/o:* life *-opsy:* to view	The surgical removal and examination of tissue from the living body. Biopsies are typically performed to determine whether a tumor is benign or malignant.
Colposcope	*colp/o:* vagina *-scope:* instrument used for visual examination	A lighted instrument with a binocular magnifying lens used to examine the vagina and cervix.
Colposcopy	*colp/o:* vagina *-scopy:* visual examination	The visual examination of the vagina and cervix using a colposcope.
Contaminate		As it relates to surgical asepsis, to cause a sterile object or surface to become unsterile.
Contusion		An injury to the tissues under the skin that causes blood vessels to rupture, allowing blood to seep into the tissues; a bruise.
Cryosurgery	*cry/o:* cold	The therapeutic use of freezing temperatures to destroy abnormal tissue.
Exudate		A discharge produced by the body's tissues.
Fibroblast	*fibr/o:* fibrous tissue *-blast:* developing cell	An immature cell from which connective tissue can develop.
Forceps		A two-pronged instrument for grasping and squeezing.
Furuncle		A localized staphylococcal infection that originates deep within a hair follicle. Also known as a *boil.*
Hemostasis	*hem/o:* blood *-stasis:* control, stop	The arrest of bleeding by natural or artificial means.
Incision		A clean cut caused by a cutting instrument.

TERMINOLOGY REVIEW—cont'd

Key Term	Word Parts	Definition
Infection		The condition in which the body, or part of it, is invaded by a pathogen.
Infiltration		The process by which a substance passes into and is deposited within the substance of a cell, tissue, or organ.
Inflammation		A protective response of the body to trauma and the entrance of foreign matter. The purpose of inflammation is to destroy invading pathogens and to remove damaged tissue debris from the area so that proper healing can occur.
Laceration		A wound in which the tissues are torn apart, leaving ragged and irregular edges.
Ligate		To tie off and close a structure such as a severed blood vessel.
Local anesthetic		A drug that produces a loss of feeling and an inability to perceive pain in only a specific part of the body.
Needle biopsy	*bi/o:* life *-opsy:* to view	A type of biopsy in which tissue from deep within the body is obtained by the insertion of a biopsy needle through the skin.
Nonabsorbable suture		Suture material that is not absorbed by the body and either remains permanently in the body tissue and becomes encapsulated by fibrous tissue or is removed.
Postoperative	*post-:* after	After a surgical operation.
Preoperative	*pre-:* before	Before a surgical operation.
Puncture		A wound made by a sharp-pointed object piercing the skin.
Scalpel		A surgical knife used to divide tissues.
Scissors		A cutting instrument.
Sebaceous cyst		A thin, closed sac or capsule that contains fatty secretions from a sebaceous gland.
Sterile		Free of all living microorganisms and bacterial spores.
Surgery		The branch of medicine that deals with operative and manual procedures for correction of deformities and defects, repair of injuries, and diagnosis and treatment of certain diseases.
Surgical asepsis	*a:* without or absence of *-sepsis:* infection	Practices that keep objects and areas sterile or free from microorganisms.
Sutures		Material used to approximate tissues with surgical stitches.
Swaged needle		A needle with suturing material permanently attached to its end.
Wound		A break in the continuity of an external or internal surface caused by physical means.

PROCEDURE 25.1 Applying and Removing Surgical Gloves

Outcome Apply and remove surgical gloves.

The medical assistant must wear surgical gloves to perform a sterile procedure, such as a dressing change, or to assist the provider during minor office surgery. The medical assistant must learn to put on the gloves using the principles of surgical asepsis so as not to contaminate them.

Gloves must be removed in a manner that protects the medical assistant from contaminating the clean hands with pathogens that might be on the outside of the gloves. This is accomplished by not allowing the bare hands to come in contact with the outside of the gloves.

Equipment/Supplies

- Surgical gloves in correct size

Continued

PROCEDURE 25.1 Applying and Removing Surgical Gloves—cont'd

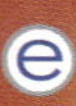

A. Applying Surgical Gloves

1. **Procedural Step.** Remove all rings and put them in a safe place. Wash your hands with an antimicrobial soap.
   Principle. Rings may cause the gloves to tear. The warm, moist environment inside gloves provides ideal growing conditions for the multiplication of transient microorganisms on the hands. Washing the hands with an antimicrobial removes these microorganisms and also deposits an antibacterial film on your hands to discourage the growth of bacteria. This prevents the transmission of pathogens.
2. **Procedural Step.** Choose appropriate-sized gloves; they should not be too small or too large. The gloves should fit snugly but not be too tight. (Refer to Chapter 17, Box 17.2: *Determination of Glove Size*).
   Principle. If your gloves are too small, they may rip as you apply them or become uncomfortable to wear. If they are too large, you may find it difficult to perform your tasks.
3. **Procedural Step.** Place the glove package on a clean flat surface. Open the glove package without touching the inside of the wrapper. The tops of the gloves are turned down to form a cuff.
   Principle. The hands are not sterile, and the inside of the wrapper is sterile.
4. **Procedural Step.** Pick up the first glove on the inside of the cuff with the fingers of the opposite hand, being sure not to touch the outside of the glove with your ungloved hand.
   Principle. After applying the gloves, the inside of the cuff lies next to your skin and does not remain sterile; therefore it is permissible to pick up the glove by the cuff. The outside of the glove is sterile, and touching it would contaminate it. If a glove becomes contaminated, you must obtain a new pair of gloves and repeat the procedure.

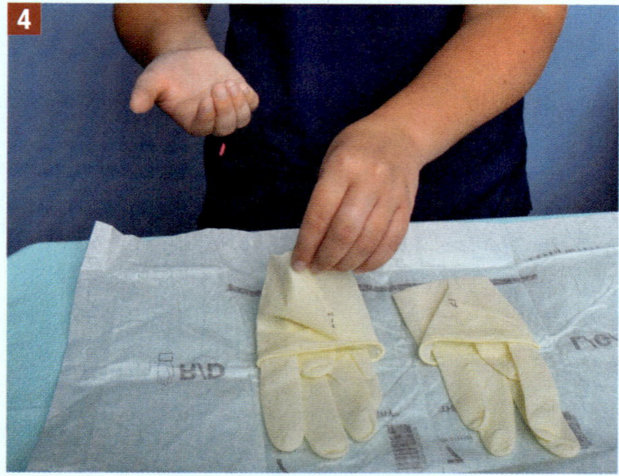

Pick up the first glove on the inside of the cuff.

5. **Procedural Step.** Step back and pull the glove on. Allow the cuff to remain turned back on itself.
   Principle. Stepping back prevents your unsterile hand from passing over the glove still in the glove package, which would contaminate it.
6. **Procedural Step.** Pick up the second glove by slipping your sterile gloved fingers under its cuff.
   Principle. The underside of the cuff is sterile and may be touched by the sterile gloved hand.

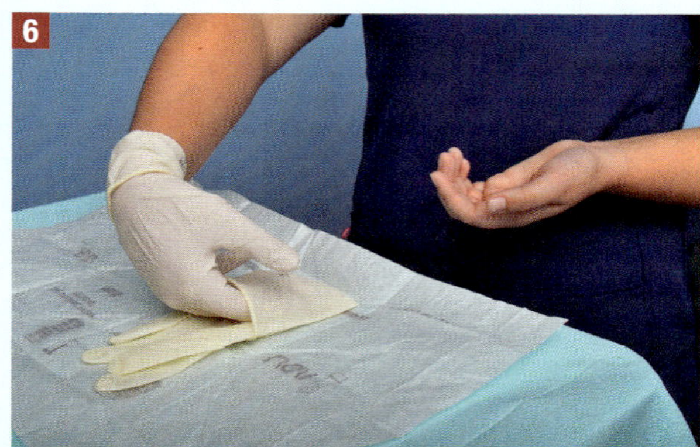

Pick up the second glove.

7. **Procedural Step.** Pull the glove onto your hand and turn back the cuff.
8. **Procedural Step.** Turn back the cuff of the first glove by reaching under the cuff with the other gloved hand. Do not allow your sterile gloved hand to come in contact with the inside of the cuff. Adjust the gloves to a comfortable position. Inspect the gloves for tears.
   Principle. The area under the folded cuff is sterile and may be touched by the sterile gloved hand. The inside of the cuff has previously been touched by your clean hands and is not sterile. If a tear is present, a new pair of gloves must be applied.

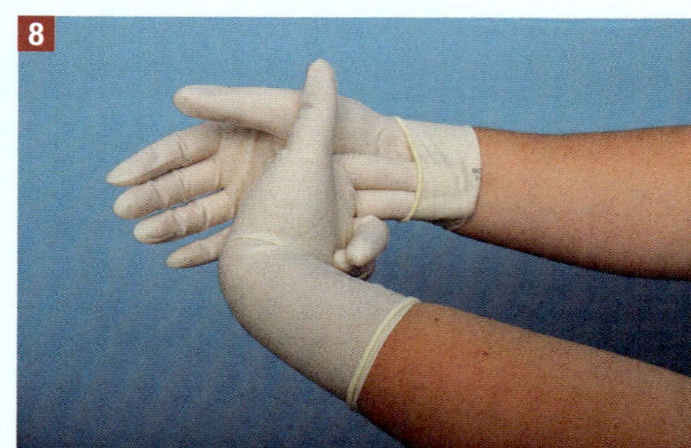

Turn back the cuff.

PROCEDURE 25.1 Applying and Removing Surgical Gloves—cont'd

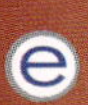

B. Removing Surgical Gloves

1. **Procedural Step.** With your gloved left hand, grasp the outside of the right glove 1 to 2 inches from the top. (*Note:* It does not matter which glove is removed first—you may start with the left glove if you prefer.)

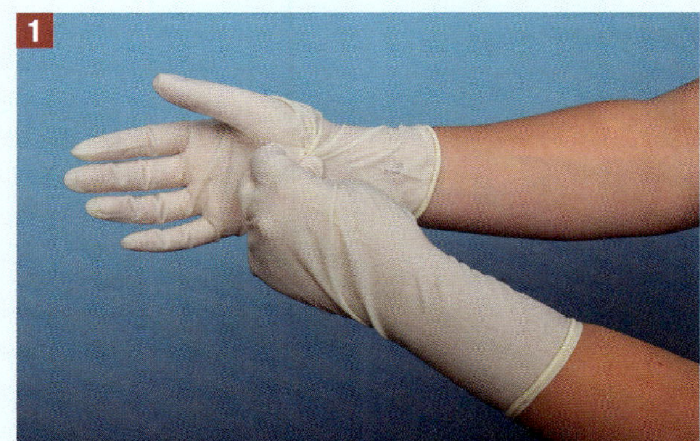

Grasp the outside of the glove.

2. **Procedural Step.** Slowly pull the right glove off the hand. It turns inside out as it is removed from your hand.

3. **Procedural Step.** Pull the right glove free, and scrunch it into a ball with your gloved left hand.

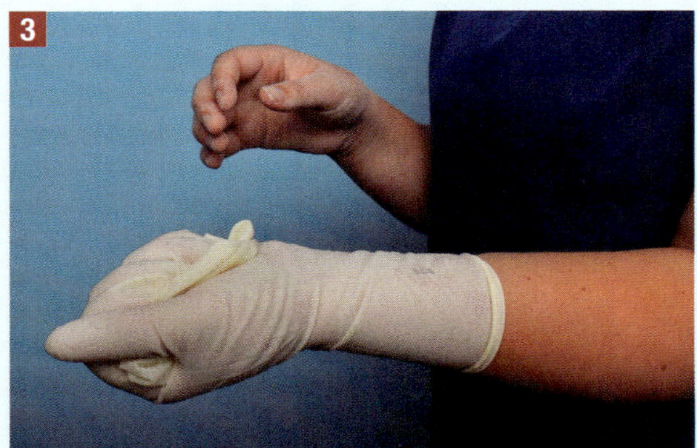

Scrunch the glove into a ball.

4. **Procedural Step.** Place the index and middle fingers of the right hand on the inside of the left glove. Do not allow your clean hand to touch the outside of the glove.

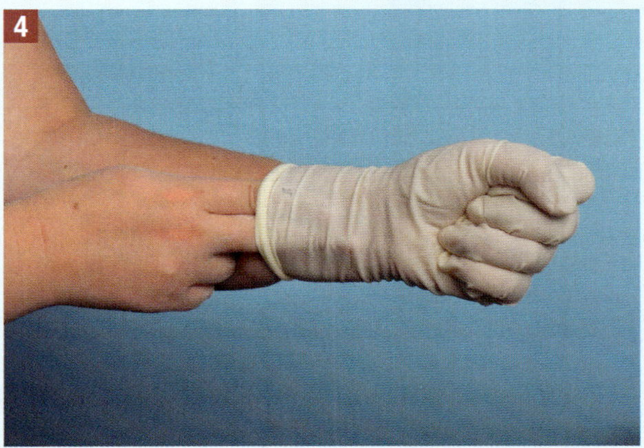

Place the fingers on the inside of the glove.

5. **Procedural Step.** Pull the second glove off the left hand. It turns inside out as it is removed from your hand, enclosing the balled-up right glove. Discard both gloves in an appropriate waste container. If your gloves are visibly contaminated with blood or other potentially infectious materials, discard them in a biohazard waste container; otherwise, they can be discarded in a regular waste container.

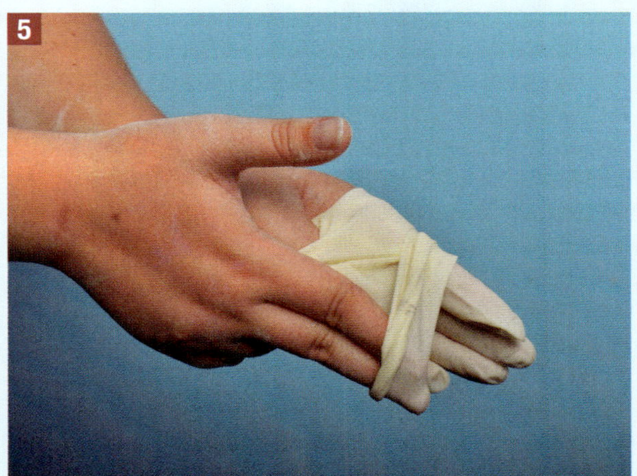

Pull the glove off the hand.

6. **Procedural Step.** Sanitize your hands thoroughly to remove any microorganisms that may have come in contact with your hands.

PROCEDURE 25.2 Opening a Sterile Package

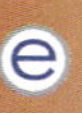

Outcome Open a sterile package. The sterile package may be in the form of a pack that has been assembled and sterilized at the medical office or a commercially prepared disposable; in both cases, the inside of the sterile wrapper serves as the sterile field.

Equipment/Supplies

- Sterile package

1. **Procedural Step.** Sanitize your hands.
2. **Procedural Step.** Assemble the equipment.
3. **Procedural Step.** Check the pack to make sure it is not wet, torn, or opened. These factors cause contamination of the sterile contents and the pack must not be used. If autoclave tape has been used to close the pack, check to make sure the tape has changed color.
   Principle. Autoclave tape indicates that the pack has been through the sterilization process, but it does not verify that the contents of the pack are sterile.

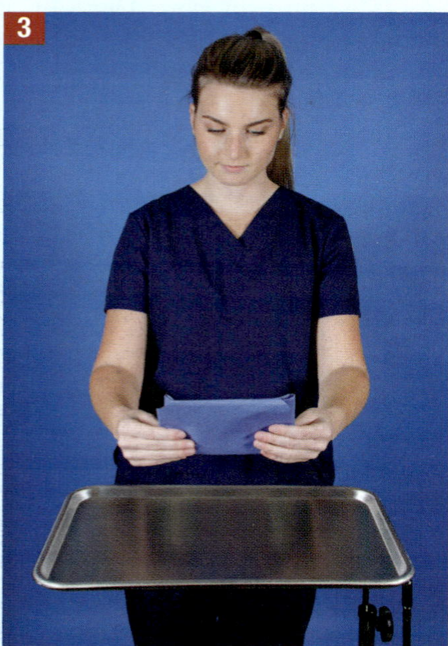

Check the sterilization indicator.

4. **Procedural Step.** Place the wrapped package on the table so that the top flap of the wrapper opens away from you. Always face the sterile field, and do not talk, laugh, cough, or sneeze over the field. These actions contaminate the sterile field.
5. **Procedural Step.** Loosen and remove the fastener on the wrapped package, and discard it in a waste container.
6. **Procedural Step.** Open the first flap away from the body. Handle only the outside of the wrapper.
   Principle. The medical assistant should open the sterile package so as not to reach over the sterile contents. Otherwise, dust or lint from unsterile clothing may fall on the contents of the package and cause contamination.

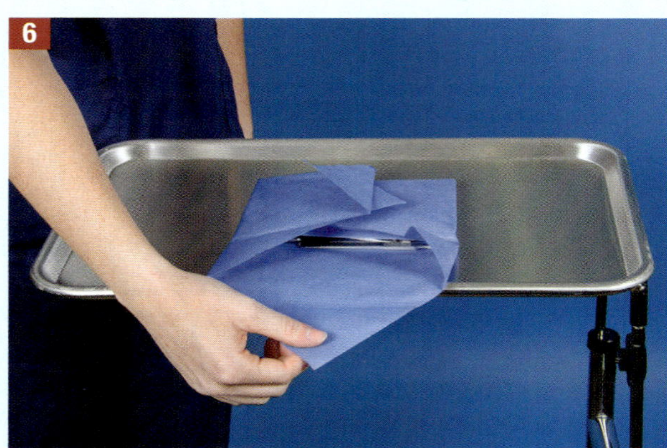

Open the first flap away from the body.

7. **Procedural Step.** Without crossing over the sterile field, open the left and right flaps.

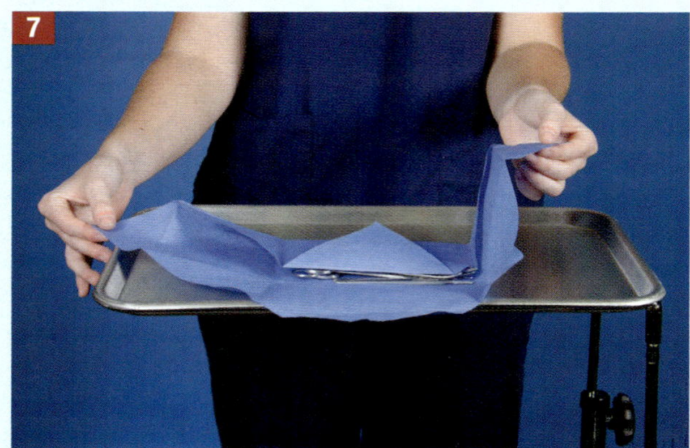

Open the left and right flaps.

8. **Procedural Step.** Open the flap closest to the body by lifting it toward you. Touch only the outside of the wrapper.

PROCEDURE 25.2 Opening a Sterile Package—cont'd

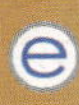
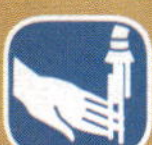

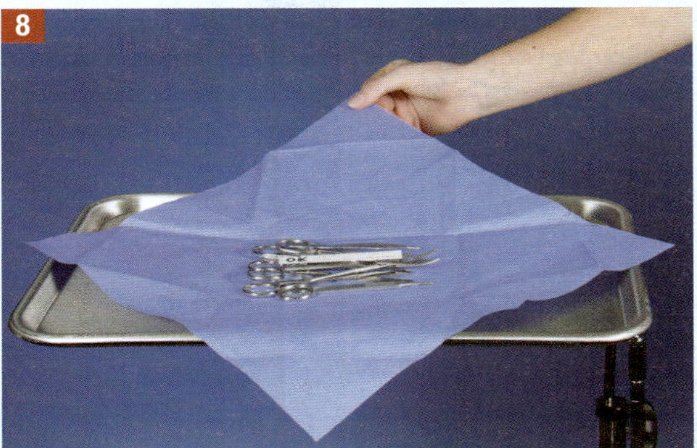

Open the flap closest to the body.

9. **Procedural Step.** Adjust the sterile wrapper by the corners as needed to make sure it lies in proper position on the tray or table.

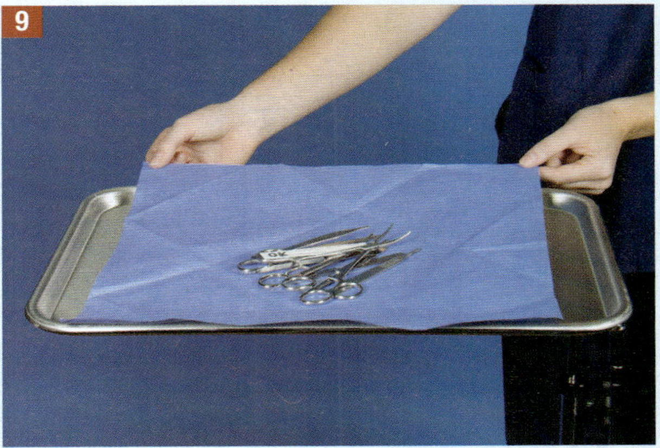

Adjust the sterile wrapper by the corners.

10. **Procedural Step.** Check the sterilization indicator on the inside of the pack to make sure it has changed appropriately. This indicates that the contents of the pack are sterile.

PROCEDURE 25.3 Pouring a Sterile Solution

Outcome Pour a sterile solution.

Equipment/Supplies

- Sterile solution
- Sterile container
- Sterile towel

1. **Procedural Step.** Read the label of the solution to ensure that you have the correct solution.
2. **Procedural Step.** Check the expiration date on the solution. Do not use an outdated solution.
   Principle. Outdated solutions may produce undesirable effects and should be discarded.
3. **Procedural Step.** Check the solution label a second time to make sure you have the correct solution.
4. **Procedural Step.** Place the palm of your hand over the label. Remove the cap by touching only the outside, and place the cap on a flat surface with the open end up. Do not place the cap on the sterile field, as the outside of the cap is contaminated.
   Principle. Palming the label prevents the solution from dripping on the label and obscuring it. Handling the cap by the outside prevents contamination of the inside. Placing the cap with the open end up prevents contamination of the inside of the cap by an unsterile surface.
5. **Procedural Step.** Rinse the lip of the bottle (if it has been previously used) by pouring a small amount of solution into a separate container.
   Principle. Rinsing the lip washes away any microorganisms that may be on it.
6. **Procedural Step.** Pour the proper amount of solution into the sterile container at a height of approximately 6 inches. Do not allow the neck of the bottle to come in contact with the sterile container, and be careful not to splash solution onto the sterile field.
   Principle. Pouring from a height of approximately 6 inches reduces splashing and prevents contamination of the sterile container with the outside of the (unsterile) bottle.

Continued

PROCEDURE 25.3 Pouring a Sterile Solution—cont'd

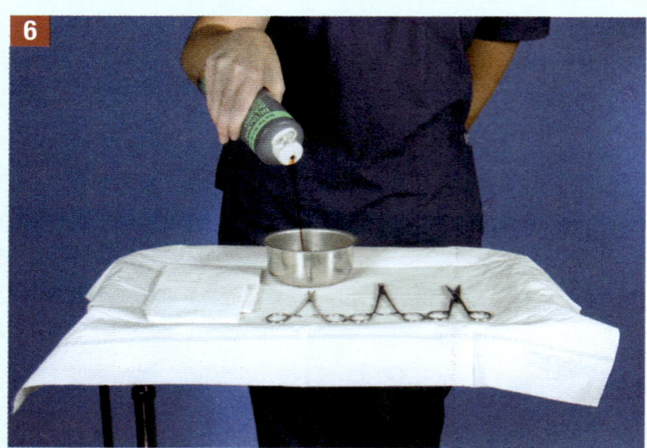

Pour the proper amount of solution.

7. **Procedural Step.** Replace the cap on the container without contaminating it. Check the label a third time to ensure that you have poured the correct solution.

PROCEDURE 25.4 Changing a Sterile Dressing

Outcome Change a sterile dressing.

Equipment/Supplies

- Mayo stand
- Biohazard waste container

Side Table

- Clean disposable gloves
- Antiseptic swabs
- Surgical gloves
- Plastic waste bag
- Surgical tape
- Scissors

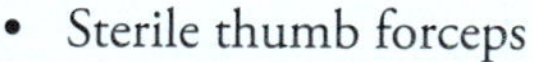

Sterile Field

- Sterile dressing
- Sterile thumb forceps

1. **Procedural Step.** Wash your hands with an antimicrobial soap.
2. **Procedural Step.** Assemble the equipment. Set up the nonsterile items on a side table or counter. Position the waterproof waste bag in a location convenient for disposal of contaminated items.

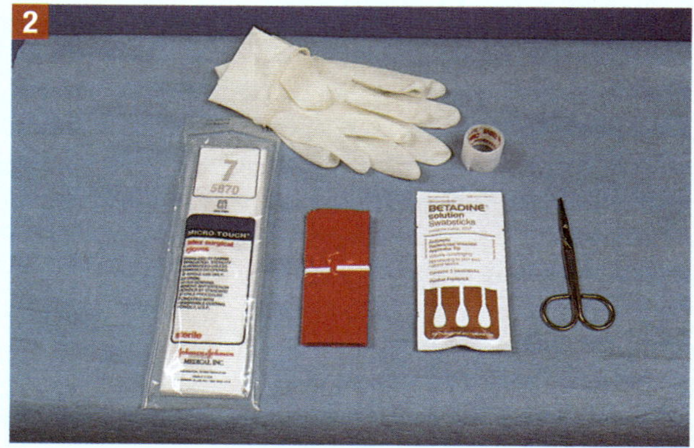

Prepare the side table.

PROCEDURE 25.4 Changing a Sterile Dressing—cont'd

3. **Procedural Step.** Greet the patient and introduce yourself. Identify the patient by full name and date of birth and explain the procedure. Instruct the patient not to move during the procedure. Adjust the light so that it is focused on the dressing.
4. **Procedural Step.** Apply clean gloves. Loosen the tape on the dressing, and pull it toward the wound. Carefully and gently remove the soiled dressing by pulling it upward. Do not touch the inside of the dressing that was next to the open wound. If the dressing is stuck to the wound, it can be loosened by moistening it with a normal saline solution. Place the soiled dressing in the waste bag without allowing the dressing to touch the outside of the bag.
   Principle. Gentle dressing removal avoids unnecessary stress on the wound. Touching the inside of the dressing can transfer an infected discharge to your gloves.

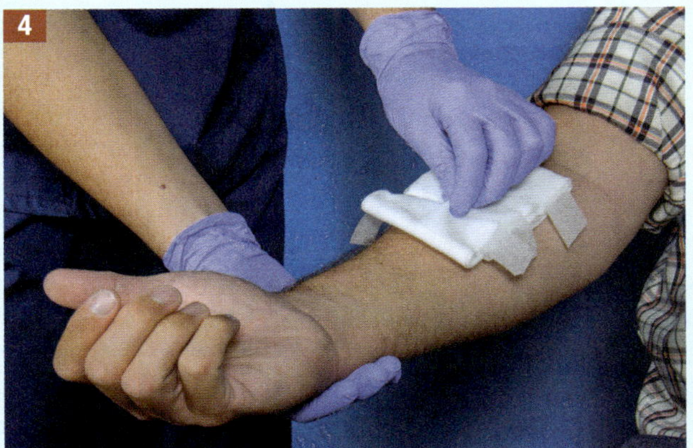

Remove the soiled dressing.

5. **Procedural Step.** Inspect the wound, and observe for the following: amount of healing; presence of inflammation; and presence of drainage, including the amount (scant, moderate, or profuse) and type of drainage.
   Principle. Drainage is classified as serous (containing serum), sanguineous (red and composed of blood), serosanguineous (containing serum and blood), or purulent (containing pus and appearing white with tinges of yellow, pink, or green, depending on the type of infecting microorganism). Purulent drainage is usually thick and has an unpleasant odor.
6. **Procedural Step.** Open the pouch containing the sterile antiseptic swabs, and place it in a convenient location or hold it in your nondominant hand.
7. **Procedural Step.** Using the antiseptic swabs, apply the antiseptic to the wound. Apply the antiseptic from the top to the bottom of the wound, working from the center to the outside of the wound. Use a new swab for each motion. Discard each contaminated swab in the waste bag after use.
   Principle. The purpose of the antiseptic is to decrease the number of microorganisms in the wound.

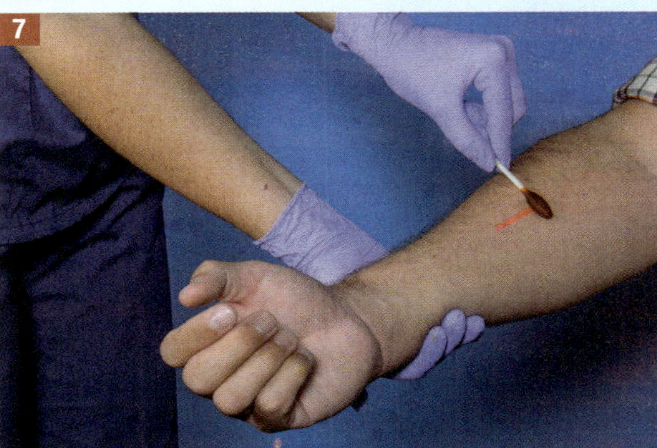

Apply an antiseptic to the wound.

8. **Procedural Step.** Remove the clean disposable gloves, and discard them in the waste bag without contaminating yourself. Sanitize your hands and prepare the sterile field using surgical asepsis. Items are either placed onto a sterile field or are contained in a prepackaged setup. Instruct the patient not to talk, laugh, sneeze, or cough over the sterile field.
   Principle. Microorganisms are carried in water vapor from the mouth, nose, and lungs and can be transferred onto the sterile field.
9. **Procedural Step.** Open a package of surgical gloves and apply them.
10. **Procedural Step.** Pick up the sterile dressing with your gloved hand or sterile forceps. Place the sterile dressing over the wound by lightly dropping it in place. Do not move the dressing once you have dropped it into place. Discard the gloves or forceps in the waste bag.
    Principle. Dropping the dressing over the wound and not moving it prevent the transfer of microorganisms from the skin to the center of the wound.

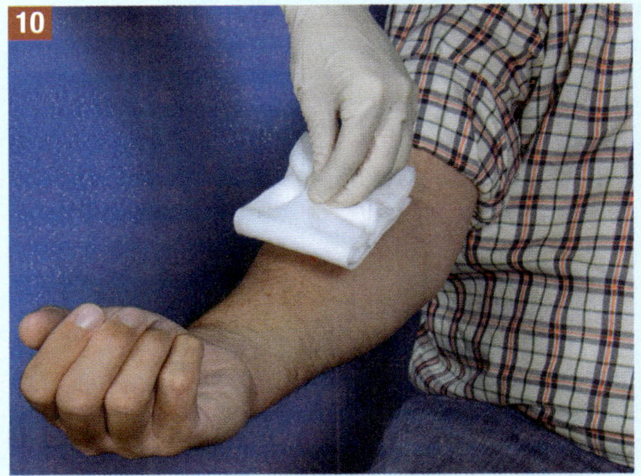

Place the dressing over the wound.

PROCEDURE 25.4

Continued

PROCEDURE 25.4 Changing a Sterile Dressing—cont'd

11. **Procedural Step.** Apply hypoallergenic adhesive tape to hold the dressing in place. The tape must be long enough to adhere to the skin, but not so long that it loosens when the patient moves. The strips of tape should be evenly spaced, with strips at each end of the dressing.

12. **Procedural Step.** Instruct the patient in wound care as follows:
    a. Provide the patient with written wound care instructions (refer to Table 25.1).
    b. Explain the wound care instructions and ask the patient whether they have any questions. Tell the patient to keep the dressing clean and dry and to contact the office if signs of infection occur, such as excessive swelling, pain, or discharge.
    c. Ask the patient to sign the instruction sheet on the appropriate line.
    d. Witness the patient's signature by signing your name in the appropriate space on the form. Include today's date.
    e. Before the patient leaves the medical office, make a copy of the instruction sheet. Give a signed copy of the wound care instructions to the patient.
    f. File the instruction sheet:

    Electronic health record: Scan the instruction sheet into the patient's electronic record.

    Paper-based patient record: File the original instruction sheet in the patient's medical record.

    Principle. The filed copy protects the provider legally in the event that the patient fails to follow the instructions and causes further harm or damage to the wound.

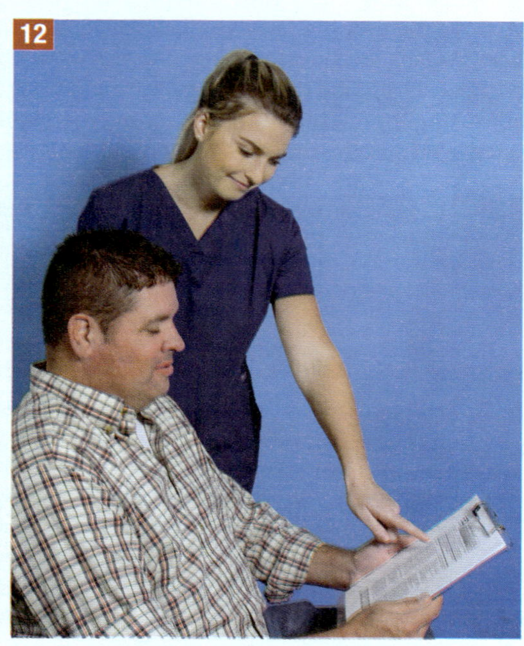

Instruct the patient in wound care.

13. **Procedural Step.** Return the equipment. Tightly secure the bag containing the soiled dressing and contaminated articles and dispose of it in a biohazard waste container.

    Principle. Contaminated items must be disposed of properly to prevent the spread of infection.

14. **Procedural Step.** Sanitize your hands.

15. **Procedural Step.** Document the procedure in the patient's medical record.
    a. *Electronic health record:* Document the location of the dressing, condition of the wound, type and amount of drainage, care of the wound, and any problems the patient has experienced with the wound using the appropriate radio buttons, drop-down menus, and free text fields. Also, document the instructions given to the patient on wound care.
    b. *Paper-based patient record*: Document the date and time, location of the dressing, condition of the wound, type and amount of drainage, care of the wound, and any problems the patient experienced with the wound. Also document the instructions given to the patient on wound care.

15b

DOCUMENTATION EXAMPLE

Date	
9/20/XX	10:30 a.m. Dressing changed (R) ant forearm.
	Scant amt of serous drainage noted. Sl
	redness around incision line. Sutures intact
	and suture line in good approximation. Incision
	cleaned c̄ Betadine and DSD applied. No
	complaints of pain or discomfort. Explained
	wound care. Written instructions provided.
	Signed copy filed in chart. To return in 2 days
	for suture removal. ————————
	———————— H. Hopstetter, CMA (AAMA)

PROCEDURE 25.5 Removing Sutures and Staples

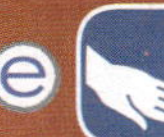

Outcome Remove sutures and staples.

Equipment/Supplies

- Antiseptic swabs
- Clean disposable gloves
- Sterile 4 × 4 gauze
- Surgical tape
- Mayo stand
- Biohazard waste container

For Suture Removal

- Suture removal kit, which includes the following:
  - Suture scissors
  - Thumb forceps
  - Sterile 4 × 4 gauze

For Staple Removal

- Staple removal kit, which includes the following:
  - Staple remover
  - Sterile 4 × 4 gauze

1. **Procedural Step.** Wash your hands with an antimicrobial soap. Assemble the equipment.
   Principle. Washing the hands with an antimicrobial soap removes microorganisms from the hands and also deposits an antimicrobial film on your hands to discourage the growth of bacteria.

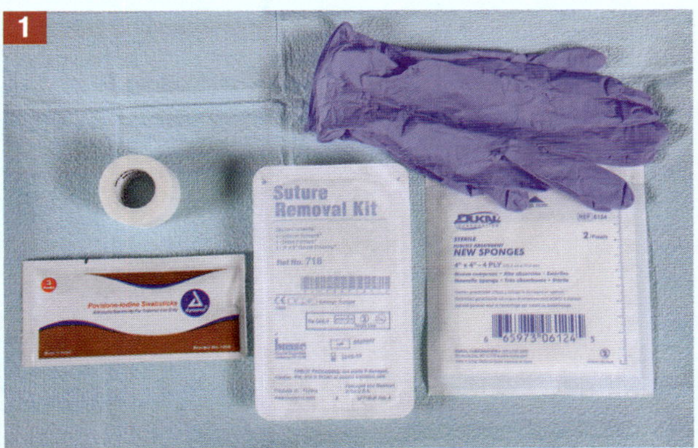

Suture removal setup.

2. **Procedural Step.** Greet the patient and introduce yourself. Identify the patient by full name and date of birth and explain the procedure.
3. **Procedural Step.** Position the patient as required to provide good access to the site. Adjust the light so that it is focused on the wound. Verify that the sutures (or staples) are intact and that the incision line is approximated and not gaping. Check that the incision line is not infected. If the incision line is not approximated, or if redness, swelling, or a discharge is present, do not remove the sutures; notify the provider.
   Principle. The sutures (or staples) should not be removed unless the incision line is approximated and free from infection.
4. **Procedural Step.** Open the suture or staple removal kit, keeping the contents of the kit sterile. Most kits are opened by peeling back a top cover, which exposes a plastic tray that holds the necessary instruments and supplies.

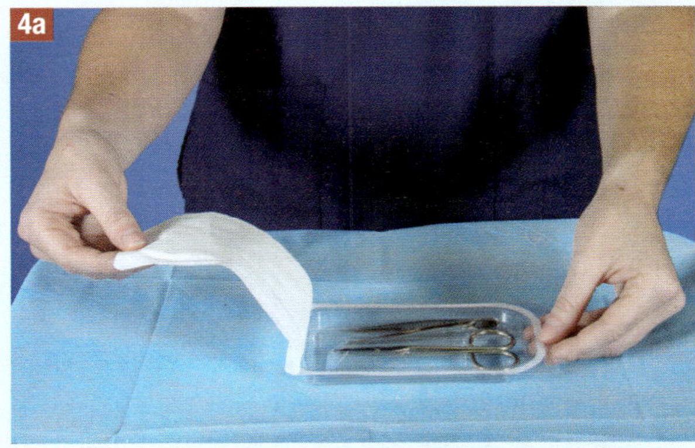
Open the suture removal kit.

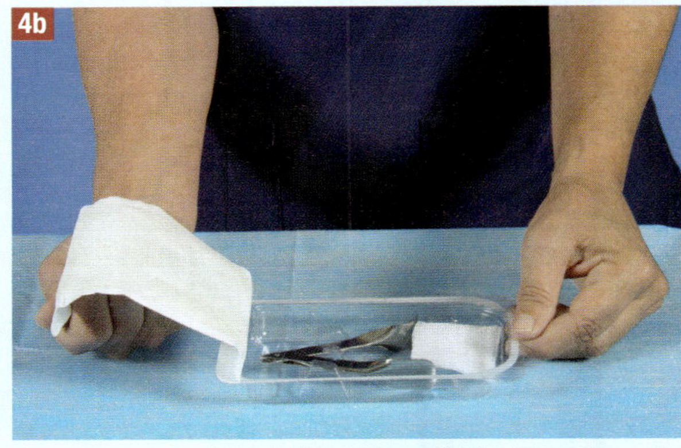
Open the staple removal kit.

Continued

PROCEDURE 25.5 Removing Sutures and Staples—cont'd

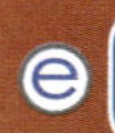   

5. **Procedural Step.** Apply clean gloves. Cleanse the incision line with an antiseptic swab to destroy microorganisms and to remove any dried exudate encrusted around the sutures or staples. Clean the wound from the top to the bottom, working from the center to the outside of the wound. Use a new swab for each cleansing motion. Allow the skin to dry.
   Principle. Dried exudate must be removed to allow unimpeded removal of the sutures or staples.
6. **Procedural Step.** Remove the sutures or staples. Tell the patient that they will feel a pulling or tugging sensation as each suture (or staple) is removed, but that it will not be painful. Count the number of sutures or staples removed. Check the patient's medical record to make sure the same number is removed as was inserted by the provider.
7. To remove sutures:
   a. Using the sterile thumb forceps provided in the kit, pick up the knot of the first suture.
   b. Place the curved tip of the suture scissors under the suture. Using the sterile suture scissors, cut the suture below the knot on the side of the suture closest to the skin. Cut the suture as close to the skin as possible.

7b

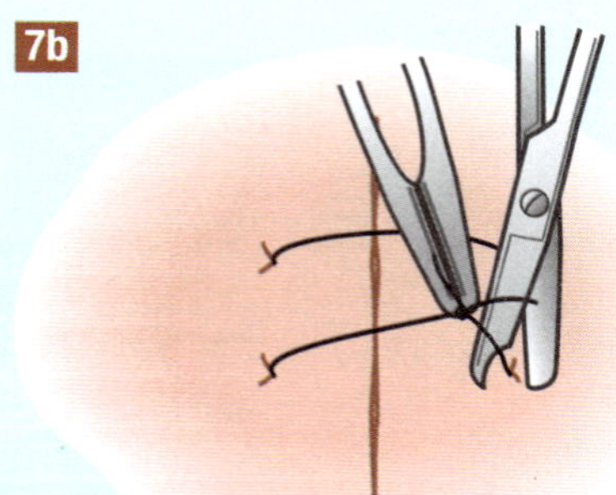

Cut the suture below the knot in the side closest to the skin. (Modified from Nealon TF, Jr.: *Fundamental skills in surgery*, ed 4, Philadelphia, 1994, Saunders.)

   c. Using a smooth, continuous motion, gently pull the suture out of the skin. Remove the suture without allowing any portion that was previously outside to be pulled back through the tissue lying beneath the incision line. Place the suture on the 4 × 4 gauze included in the suture kit.

7c

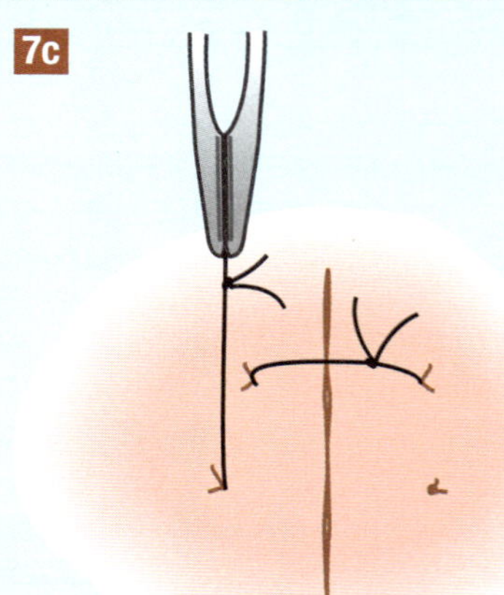

Gently pull the suture out. (Modified from Nealon TF, Jr.: *Fundamental skills in surgery*, ed 4, Philadelphia, 1994, Saunders.)

   d. Continue in this manner until all the sutures have been removed.
   Principle. To prevent infection, the suture must be removed without pulling any portion that has been outside the skin back through the tissue lying beneath the incision line.
8. To remove staples:
   a. Gently place the bottom jaws of the staple remover under the staple to be removed.

8a

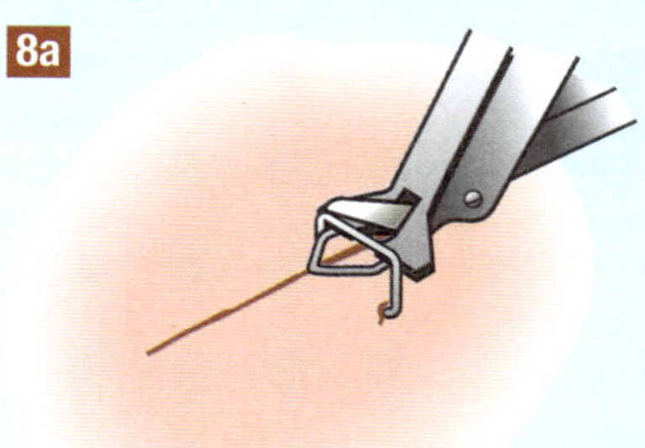

Place the bottom jaws of the staple remover under the staple. (© Ethicon, Inc. 2022. Reproduced with permission.)

   b. Firmly squeeze the staple handles until they are fully closed.

PROCEDURE 25.5 Removing Sutures and Staples—cont'd

8b

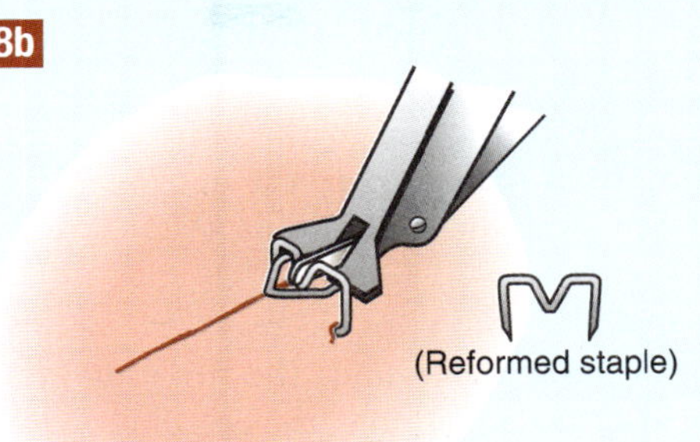

Firmly squeeze the staple handles until they are fully closed. (© Ethicon, Inc. 2022. Reproduced with permission.)

c. Carefully lift the staple remover upward to remove the staple from the incision line. Place the staple on the 4 × 4 gauze included in the staple kit.

d. Continue in this manner until all the staples have been removed.

9. **Procedural Step.** Cleanse the site with an antiseptic swab. Some providers want the medical assistant to apply skin closure tape after removing the sutures or staples to provide additional support to the wound as it continues to heal.

10. **Procedural Step.** Apply a dry sterile dressing if indicated by the provider.

11. **Procedural Step.** Dispose of the sutures (or staples) and the gauze in a biohazard waste container.

12. **Procedural Step.** Remove the gloves and sanitize your hands. Provide the patient with instructions on dressing care.

13. **Procedural Step.** Document the procedure in the patient's medical record.

a. *Electronic health record:* Document the status of the sutures (or staples) and incision line, the number of sutures (or staples) removed, the location of the site, the care of the wound (e.g., application of an antiseptic or dressing), and the patient's reaction using the appropriate radio buttons, drop-down menus, and free text fields.

b. *Paper-based patient record:* Document the date and time, the status of the sutures (or staples) and incision line, the number of sutures (or staples) removed, the location of the site, care of the wound (e.g., application of an antiseptic or dressing), and the patient's reaction. Document any instructions given to the patient.

13b

DOCUMENTATION EXAMPLE

Date	
9/20/XX	10:30 a.m. Sutures intact and incision line in
	good approximation. No signs of infection.
	Sutures x6 removed from Ⓡ ant forearm.
	Incision line cleaned c̄ Betadine and DSD
	applied. Instructions provided on dressing
	care. ———— H. Hopstetter, CMA (AAMA)

PROCEDURE 25.6 Applying and Removing Skin Closure Tape

Outcome Apply and remove skin closure tape.

Equipment/Supplies

- Clean disposable gloves
- Surgical gloves
- Antiseptic solution
- Surgical scrub brush
- Antiseptic swabs
- Tincture of benzoin
- Sterile cotton-tipped applicator
- Adhesive skin closure strips
- Sterile 4 × 4 gauze pads
- Surgical tape
- Biohazard waster container

Continued

PROCEDURE 25.6 Applying and Removing Skin Closure Tape—cont'd

Application of Skin Closure Tape

1. **Procedural Step.** Wash your hands with an antimicrobial soap and assemble the equipment. Check the expiration date on the skin closure tape.

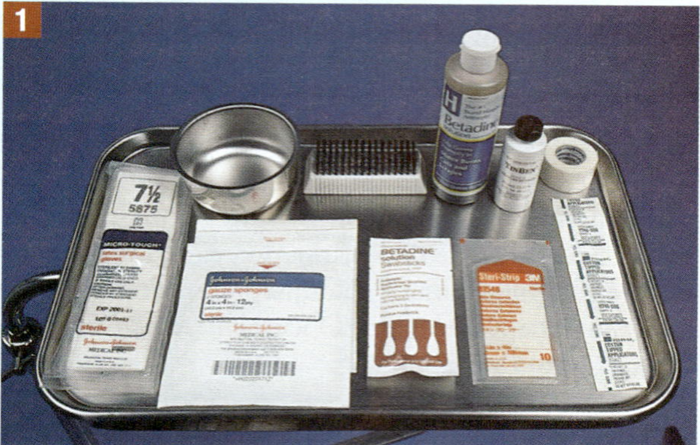

Assemble the equipment.

2. **Procedural Step.** Greet the patient and introduce yourself.
3. **Procedural Step.** Identify the patient by full name and date of birth and explain the procedure.
4. **Procedural Step.** Position the patient as required for application of the strips. Adjust the light so that it is focused on the wound. Apply clean gloves. Inspect the wound for signs of redness, swelling, and drainage. (*Note:* Document this information in the patient's record after completing the procedure.)
5. **Procedural Step.** Gently scrub the wound using an antiseptic solution (e.g., Betadine solution) and a sterile gauze pad or a surgical scrub brush. Clean at least 3 inches around the wound, removing all debris, skin oil, and exudates. Allow the skin to dry or pat dry with gauze pads. (*Note:* Change gloves as needed to maintain cleanliness.)

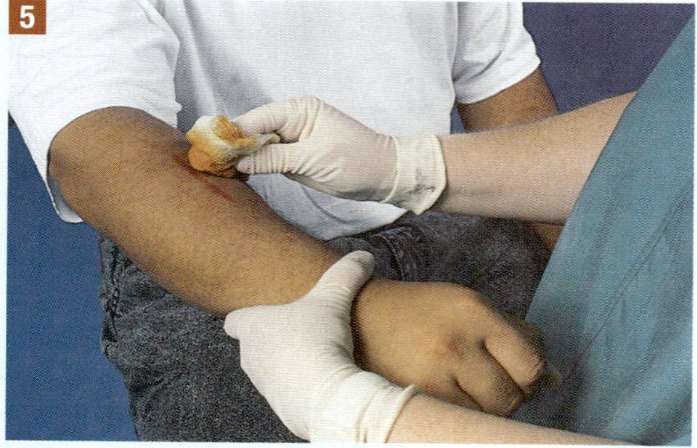

Clean the wound.

6. **Procedural Step.** Apply an antiseptic to the site using antiseptic swabs such as Betadine swabs. Apply the antiseptic from the top to the bottom of the wound, working from the center to the outside of the wound. Use a new swab for each motion. Allow the skin to dry completely.
   Principle. The antiseptic decreases the number of microorganisms in the wound. The skin must be completely dry to ensure adhesion of the skin closures to the skin.

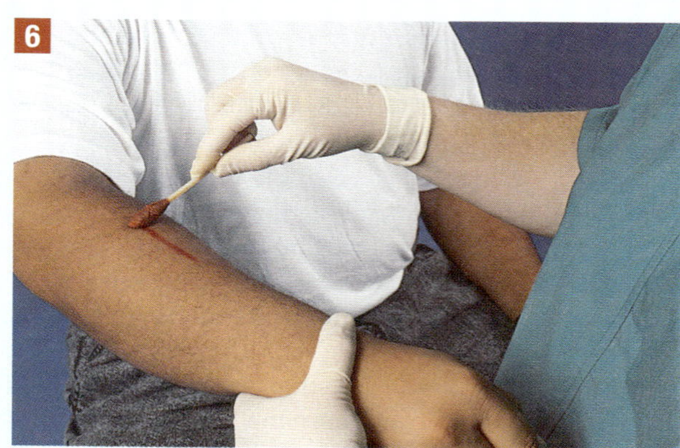

Apply an antiseptic to the wound.

7. **Procedural Step.** If dictated by the medical office policy, apply a thin coat of tincture of benzoin to the skin parallel to each side of the wound with a sterile cotton-tipped applicator. Do not allow the tincture of benzoin to touch the wound. Allow the skin to dry. Remove the gloves, and wash your hands with an antimicrobial soap.
   Principle. Tincture of benzoin facilitates adhesion of the strips to the skin.

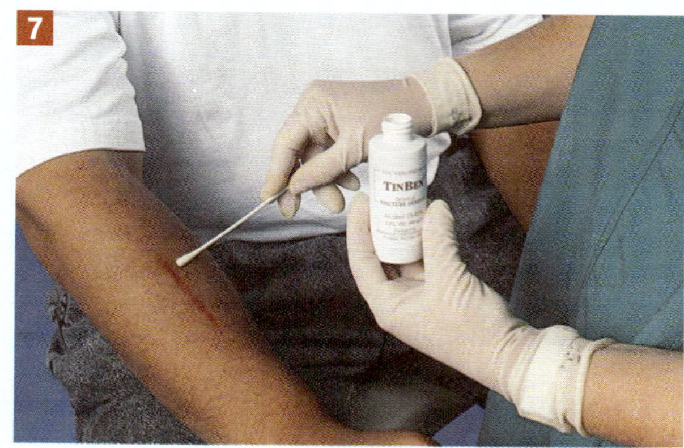

Apply tincture of benzoin.

PROCEDURE 25.6 Applying and Removing Skin Closure Tape—cont'd

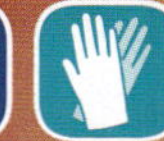

8. **Procedural Step.** Open the plastic peel-apart package of strips using surgical asepsis as follows:
   a. Grasp each flap of the package between the thumbs and bent index fingers. Pull the package apart.
   b. Peel back the package until it is completely open.
   c. Lay the opened package flat on a clean dry surface. The inside of the package serves as the sterile field.

9. **Procedural Step.** Apply surgical gloves. Fold the card of strips along its perforated tab, and tear off the tab, which exposes the ends of the tape strips, making them easier to grasp. Peel a strip of tape off the card at a 45-degree angle to the card.

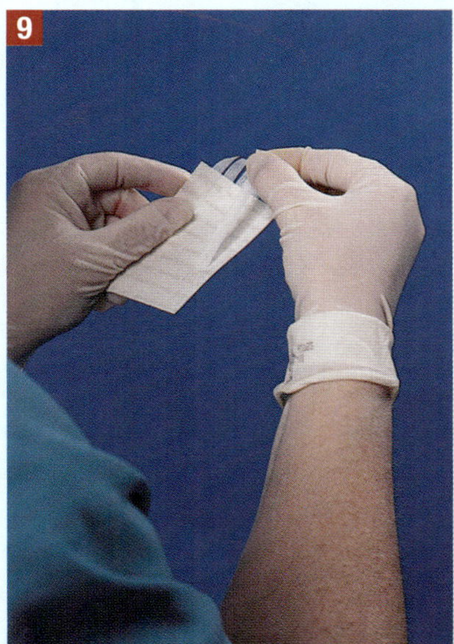

Peel a strip of tape off the card.

10. **Procedural Step.** Check that the skin surface is dry. Position the first strip over the center of the wound as follows:
   a. Secure one end of the strip of tape to the skin on one side of the wound by pressing down firmly on the tape.
   b. Use your gloved hand to assist in bringing the edges of the wound together as closely as possible.
   c. Apply the second half of the strip transversely across the line of the incision making sure the edges of the wound are approximated exactly.
   d. Secure the strip on the skin on the other side of the wound by pressing down firmly on the tape.

   Principle. Approximating the wound exactly facilitates good healing and minimizes scar formation.

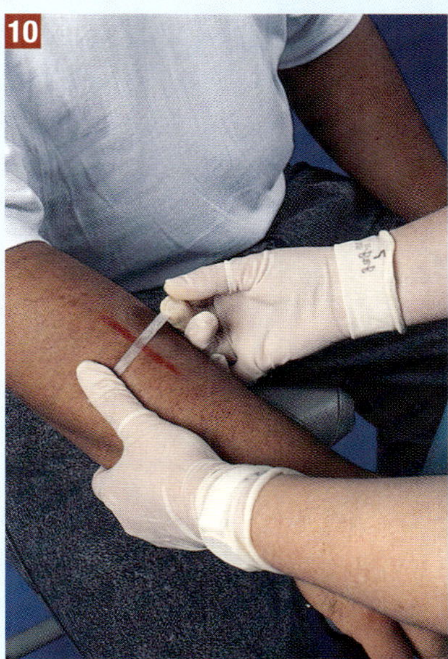

Apply the second half of the strip transversely across the incision.

11. **Procedural Step.** Apply the second strip perpendicular to the wound on one side of the center strip. The space between the strips should be approximately ⅛ inch. Apply a third strip on the other side of the center strip at a ⅛-inch interval. Continue applying the strips at ⅛-inch intervals until the edges of the wound are approximated. If at any time the skin surfaces become moist with perspiration, blood, or serum, wipe the area dry with a sterile gauze pad before applying the next strip.

   Principle. Applying the strips of tape in this manner facilitates good approximation of the wound. Spacing the strips at ⅛-inch intervals allows proper drainage of the wound.

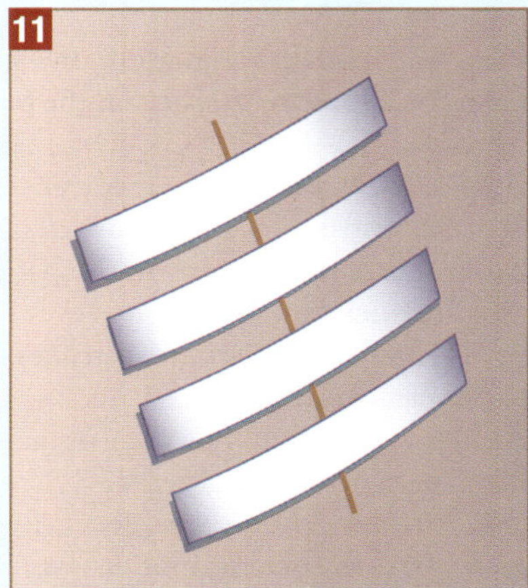

Apply the strips until the edges of the wound are approximated.

Continued

PROCEDURE 25.6 Applying and Removing Skin Closure Tape—cont'd

12. Procedural Step. Apply two closures approximately ½ inch from the ends of the strips and parallel to the wound (ladder fashion).

Principle. Applying a strip along each edge redistributes the tension and assists in holding the strips firmly in place.

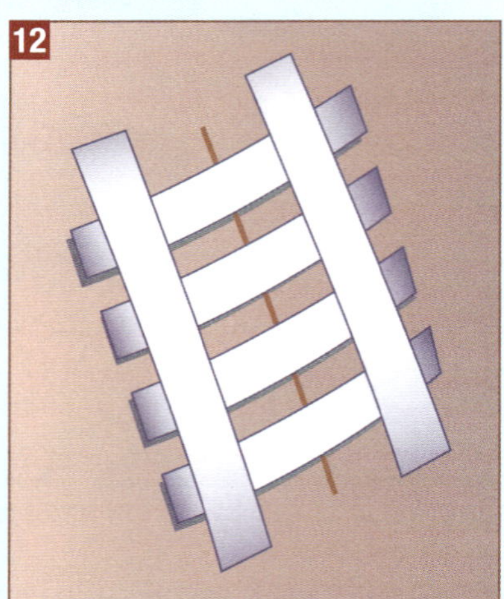

Apply a strip along each edge.

13. Procedural Step. Apply a dry sterile dressing over the strips if indicated by the provider (see Procedure 25.4).

14. Procedural Step. Remove the gloves, and sanitize your hands.

15. Procedural Step. Instruct the patient in wound care as follows:

a. Provide the patient with written wound care instructions (see Table 25.1).
b. Explain the wound care instructions and ask the patient whether they have any questions.
c. Ask the patient to sign the instruction sheet on the appropriate line.
d. Witness the patient's signature by signing your name in the appropriate space on the form. Include today's date.
e. Before the patient leaves the medical office, make a copy of the instruction sheet. Give a signed copy of the wound care instructions to the patient.
f. File the instruction sheet.

Electronic health record: Scan the instruction sheet into the patient's electronic record.

Paper-based patient record: File the original instruction sheet in the patient's medical record.

Principle. An instruction sheet signed by the patient provides legal documentation that wound care instructions were provided to the patient in the event that the patient fails to follow the instructions and causes further harm or damage to the wound.

16. Procedural Step. Document the procedure in the patient's medical record.

a. *Electronic health record:* Document the appearance of the wound, wound preparation, the number of strips applied, the location of the wound, the care of the wound, and the patient's reaction using the appropriate radio buttons, drop-down menus, and free text fields. Also, document verbal and written instructions given to the patient concerning wound care.
b. *Paper-based patient record:* Document the date and time, the appearance of the wound, the wound preparation, the number of strips applied, the location of the wound, the care of the wound, and the patient's reaction. Document verbal and written instructions given to the patient concerning wound care.

16b DOCUMENTATION EXAMPLE

Date	
9/20/XX	10:30 a.m. Incision approx. 5 cm long located
	on Ⓡ post forearm. Redness noted on edge
	of wound. Sl amt of serous drainage noted.
	Wound scrubbed c̄ Betadine sol and Betadine
	antiseptic applied. Applied Steri-Strips x4.
	Incision in good approximation. Applied DSD.
	Explained wound care. Written instructions
	provided. Signed copy filed in chart. To return
	in 5 days for removal of strips. ________
	________ H. Hopstetter, CMA (AAMA)

Removal of Skin Closure Tape

Skin closure tapes usually loosen and fall off on their own approximately 5 to 10 days after application. If they require removal, the procedure outlined here should be followed by the medical assistant.

1. Procedural Step. Sanitize your hands. Greet the patient and introduce yourself. Identify the patient by full name and date of birth and explain the procedure.

2. Procedural Step. Position the patient as required. Adjust the light so that it is focused on the wound. Check that the skin closures are intact and that the incision line is approximated and not gaping. Check that the incision line is not infected. If the incision line is not approximated, or if redness, swelling, or a discharge is present, do not remove the skin closures; notify the provider.

PROCEDURE 25.6 Applying and Removing Skin Closure Tape—cont'd

3. **Procedural Step.** Position a 4 × 4 gauze pad in a convenient location. Apply clean gloves.
4. **Procedural Step.** Remove the skin closures as follows:
   a. Gently grasp one end of a strip of tape with the dominant hand.
   b. Stabilize the skin with one finger of the nondominant hand.
   c. Slowly loosen and peel off one-half of the strip of tape from the outside to the wound margin, keeping the peeled-off section of the strip close to the skin surface and pulled back over itself. As you remove the strip from the skin, continue moving the finger as necessary to support the newly exposed skin. Always pull the strip toward the wound. Never pull the strip away from the wound because tension on the wound site could disrupt the healing process.
   d. Remove the other half of the strip of tape from the outside to the wound margin in the manner just described.
   e. When both halves of the strip are completely loosened, gently lift the strip up and away from the wound surface. Place the strip on a 4 × 4 gauze pad.
   f. Continue in this manner until all the skin closures have been removed.
5. **Procedural Step.** Cleanse the site with an antiseptic swab. Apply a dry sterile dressing if indicated by the provider (see Procedure 25.4).
6. **Procedural Step.** Dispose of the strips and gauze in a biohazard waste container. Remove the gloves, and sanitize your hands.
7. **Procedural Step.** Document the procedure in the patient's medical record.
   a. *Electronic health record:* Document the status of the skin closures, the number of skin closures removed, the location of the site, the care of the wound, and the patient's reaction, using the appropriate radio buttons, drop-down menus, and free text fields. Also, document any instructions given to the patient.
   b. *Paper-based patient record:* Document the date and time, the status of the skin closures, the number of skin closures removed, the location of the site, the care of the wound, and the patient's reaction. Document any instructions given to the patient.

7b

DOCUMENTATION EXAMPLE

Date	
9/25/XX	10:30 a.m. Skin closures intact and in good
	approximation. No signs of infection. Strips
	x 4 removed from Ⓡ post forearm. Incision
	line cleaned c̄ Betadine and DSD applied.
	Instructions provided on dressing care.
	———————— H. Hopstetter, CMA (AAMA)

PROCEDURE 25.7 Assisting with Minor Office Surgery

Outcome Set up a surgical tray, and assist with minor office surgery.

Equipment/Supplies

- Mayo stand
- Instruments and supplies for the type of surgery to be performed
- Biohazard waste container

Preparing the Tray

1. **Procedural Step.** Determine the type of minor office surgery to be performed. The provider instructs the medical assistant as to the type of surgery and provides any additional information needed to set up for the surgery, such as the type of local anesthetic and sutures to be used. If the medical office maintains a minor office surgery filing system, pull the file card that indicates the instruments and supplies required for the type of surgery to be performed.
2. **Procedural Step.** Prepare the examining room. Make sure the room is clean and well lighted.
3. **Procedural Step.** Sanitize your hands.

Continued

PROCEDURE 25.7 Assisting with Minor Office Surgery—cont'd

PROCEDURE 25.7

4. **Procedural Step.** Set up nonsterile articles on a side table or counter. If a specimen container is included in the setup, perform one of the following (based on the medical office policy):
   a. Attach a computer-generated bar code label to the specimen container *or*
   b. Clearly label the tubes and containers with the patient's name and date of birth, the date, your initials, and any other information required by the laboratory, such as the source of the specimen.

   Principle. Articles that are not sterile cannot be placed on the sterile field because they would contaminate it. Two unique identifiers should be used when labeling the specimen (e.g., patient's name and date of birth).
5. **Procedural Step.** Wash your hands with an antimicrobial soap and set up the minor office surgery tray on a clean, dry, flat surface, using the principles of surgical asepsis. The sterile tray can be set up as follows:

   Prepackaged setup
   a. Select the appropriate package from the supply shelf, and place it on a Mayo tray or other flat surface.
   b. Open the sterile pack using the inside of the wrapper as the sterile field. Check the sterilization indicator to make sure the contents of the pack are sterile.

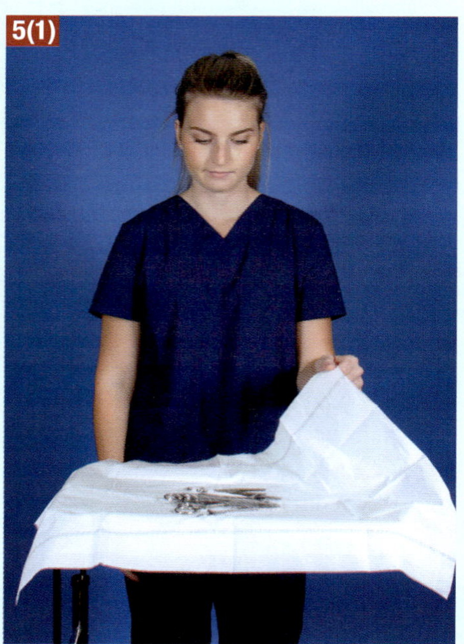

Open the sterile pack using the inside of the wrapper as the sterile field.

   c. Add other articles to the sterile field that are needed for the surgery but not contained in the sterile package, such as 4 × 4 gauze, sutures, and a fenestrated drape. If sutures are required for the setup, make sure to check the expiration date of the sutures.

   Transferring articles to a sterile field
   a. Pick up the folded sterile towel by two corner ends and allow it to unfold; make sure it does not touch an unsterile surface.
   b. Lay the sterile towel down gently and slowly over the Mayo tray, making sure it does not brush against an unsterile surface such as your uniform. Do not allow your arms to pass over the towel as you lay it down because this would result in contamination of the sterile field.

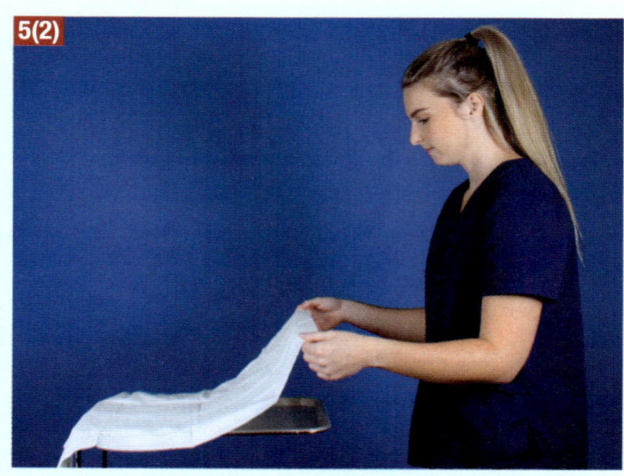

Lay the sterile towel down gently and slowly.

   c. Transfer instruments and supplies to the sterile field from wrapped or peel-apart packages.

   Principle. The principles of surgical asepsis must be followed to prevent contamination of the sterile field.
6. **Procedural Step.** Apply a sterile glove, and arrange the articles neatly on the sterile field. Do not allow one article to lie on top of another. Check that all the instruments and supplies required for the surgery are available on the sterile field.

   Principle. Instruments and supplies can be located quickly and efficiently on a neat and orderly sterile field. Surgical gloves must be used to prevent contamination of the sterile articles.

PROCEDURE 25.7 Assisting with Minor Office Surgery—cont'd

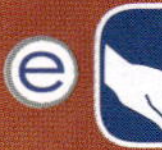   

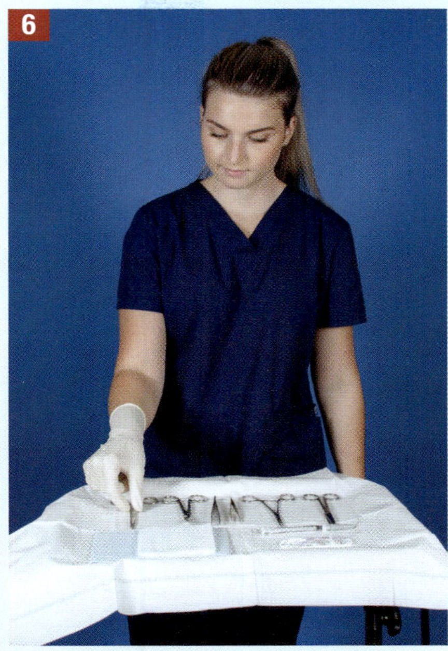

Arrange the articles neatly on the sterile field.

7. Procedural Step. Cover the tray setup with a sterile towel by picking up the towel by two corner ends and placing it gently and slowly over the setup. Do not allow your arms to pass over the sterile field as you lay it down.

Principle. The towel prevents the sterile tray from becoming contaminated. The towel must be picked up by the corner ends to prevent contaminating it and should be moved slowly and not fanned through the air to prevent airborne contamination. Passing the arms over the sterile field results in contamination of the field.

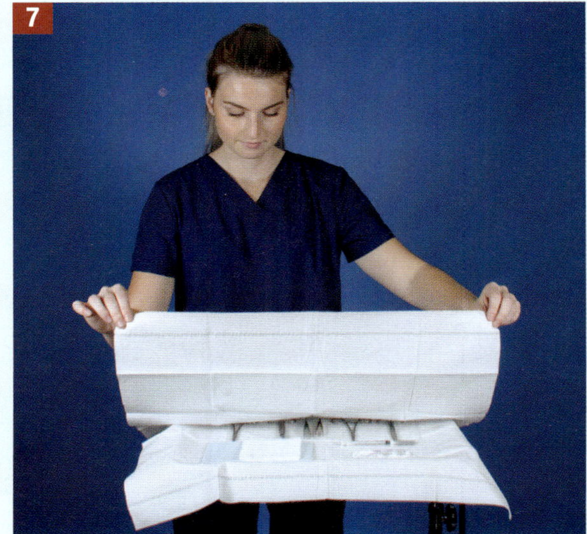

Cover the tray setup with a sterile towel.

Preparing the Patient

8. Procedural Step. Greet the patient and introduce yourself. Identify the patient by full name and date of birth. Explain the procedure, and prepare the patient for the minor office surgery as follows:

a. Try to allay the patient's fear or anxiety.
b. Ask the patient whether they need to void before the surgery.
c. Provide instructions to the patient about any clothing that must be removed and putting on an examination gown, if required. Enough clothing must be removed to expose the operative area completely and to avoid getting the antiseptic or blood on the patient's clothing.
d. Instruct the patient not to move during the procedure and not to talk, laugh, sneeze, or cough over the sterile field.

Principle. Minor office surgery is often a frightening experience for the patient, and reassurance should be offered to reduce apprehension. The amount of clothing that must be removed depends on the type of minor office surgery being performed. By moving, the patient may accidentally contaminate the sterile field or touch the operative site. Microorganisms are carried in water vapor from the mouth, nose, and lungs and can be transferred onto the sterile field.

9. Procedural Step. Position the patient. The position is determined by the type of minor office surgery to be performed. The patient is positioned in such a way as to provide the best possible exposure and accessibility to the operative site. *Note:* If a difficult position must be maintained, such as the knee–chest position, the patient should not be positioned until the provider is ready to begin the minor office surgery.

10. Procedural Step. Adjust the light so that it is focused on the operative site.

11. Procedural Step. Prepare the patient's skin by performing the following:

a. Apply clean disposable gloves.
b. If hair is present, the skin at and around the operative site may need to be shaved. The skin should be pulled taut as it is shaved. The area is rinsed and dried thoroughly.
c. Cleanse the patient's skin with an antiseptic solution and a surgical scrub brush using a firm, circular motion and moving from the inside outward. Do not return to an area just cleansed. The area is rinsed using gauze pads saturated with water and blotted dry with a sterile gauze pad.

Continued

PROCEDURE 25.7 Assisting with Minor Office Surgery—cont'd

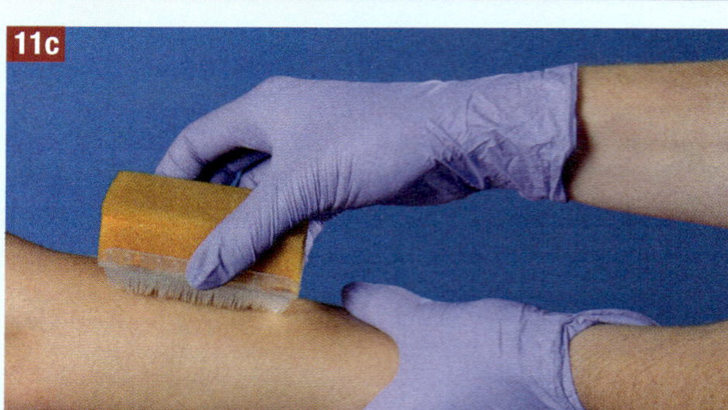

11c

Cleanse the patient's skin with an antiseptic solution.

d. Apply an antiseptic to the site using antiseptic swabs such as Betadine. Allow the skin to dry. Alternatively, the provider may place a fenestrated drape over the operative site and then apply the antiseptic.

e. Remove the gloves, and sanitize your hands.

12. **Procedural Step.** Verify that everything is prepared for the minor office surgery, and inform the provider that the patient is ready.

Assisting the Provider

13. **Procedural Step.** Assist the provider as required during the minor office surgery, following the principles of surgical asepsis. The provider drapes the patient, injects the local anesthetic, and performs the surgery. The responsibilities of the medical assistant may include the following:

a. Uncover the sterile tray setup by picking up the sterile towel covering it. The towel should be picked up by two corner ends and removed slowly and gently without allowing the arms to pass over the sterile field.

b. Open the outer glove wrapper for the provider to facilitate the application of surgical gloves.

c. Withdraw the local anesthetic into a syringe and hand it to the provider, or hold the vial while the provider withdraws the local anesthetic. If lidocaine (Xylocaine) is used, the provider or medical assistant should inform the patient to expect a brief burning or stinging sensation as it is injected into the tissues.

d. Adjust the light as needed by the provider for good visualization of the operative site.

e. Restrain patients such as children.

f. Relax and reassure the patient during the minor office surgery.

g. Hand instruments and supplies to the provider. (Surgical gloves are required.)

h. Keep the sterile field neat and orderly. (Surgical gloves are required.)

i. Hold a basin in which the provider can deposit soiled instruments and supplies, such as hemostats and gauze sponges. (Clean gloves are required.)

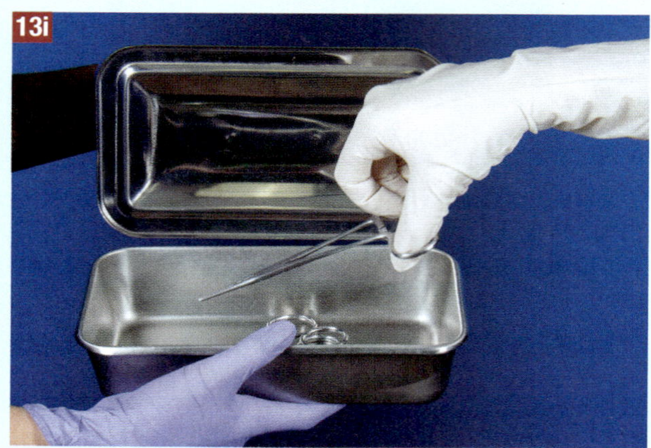

13i

Hold a basin for the provider to deposit soiled instruments.

j. Retract tissue from an area to allow the provider the best access to and visibility of the operative site. (Surgical gloves are required.)

k. Sponge blood from the operative site. (Surgical gloves are required.)

l. Add instruments and supplies to the sterile field as required by the provider.

m. Hold the specimen container to accept a tissue specimen received from the provider. (Clean gloves are required.) Do not touch the inside of the container because it is sterile. After the provider inserts the specimen, replace the container lid and close it tightly.

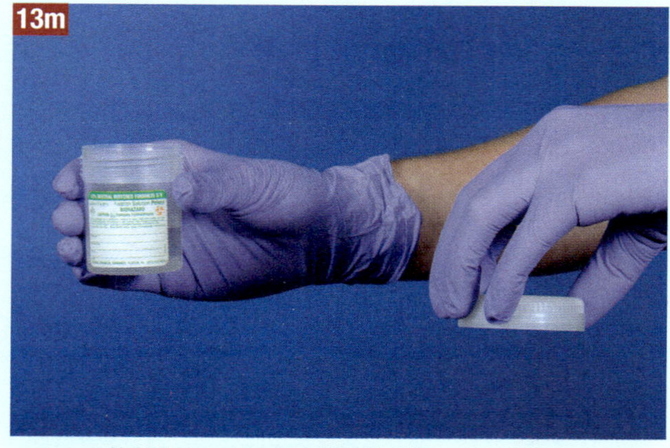

13m

Hold the container to accept a tissue specimen.

PROCEDURE 25.7 Assisting with Minor Office Surgery—cont'd

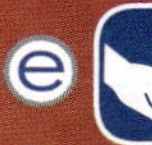

n. After the provider has inserted a suture, cut the ends of the suture material approximately ⅛ inch above the knot of the suture. (Surgical gloves are required.)

14. Procedural Step. Apply a sterile dressing to the surgical wound, if ordered by the provider (see Procedure 25-4).

Principle. The sterile dressing protects the wound from contamination and injury and absorbs drainage.

15. Procedural Step. After the surgery, perform the following:

a. Stay with the patient as a safety precaution and to assist and instruct the patient.

b. Ensure that postoperative instructions regarding any type of medical care to be administered at home are understood. If the patient has a wound or if sutures have been inserted, they should be told to keep the area clean and dry and to report any signs of infection, such as excessive redness, swelling, discharge, or increased pain. Provide the patient with written wound care instructions (see Table 25.1). Ask the patient if they have any questions. Have the patient sign the instruction sheet. Witness the patient's signature. Before the patient leaves the office, make a copy of the instruction sheet. Give a copy to the patient.

c. File the instruction sheet.

Electronic health record: Scan the instruction sheet into the patient's electronic record.

Paper-based patient record: File the original instruction sheet in the patient's medical record.

d. Relay information regarding the return visit for postoperative care, such as the removal of sutures or a dressing change.

e. Help the patient off the table to prevent falls.

f. Instruct the patient to get dressed, offering assistance if needed.

g. Any instructions or information given must be documented in the patient's medical record.

Principle. The patient (especially an elderly one) may become dizzy after the minor office surgery and may fall when getting off the examining table. The filed copy protects the provider legally, in the event that the patient fails to follow instructions and causes harm or damage to the operative site.

16. Procedural Step. If a specimen was collected, it must be transferred to the laboratory in a tightly closed, properly labeled specimen container. Prepare the specimen for transport. Complete a biopsy request form to accompany the specimen. Place the specimen container in a biohazard specimen bag and seal it. Insert the biopsy request in the outer pocket of the bag and tuck the requisition under the flap. Place the bag in the appropriate location for pickup by the laboratory.

17. Procedural Step. Document specimen transport information in the patient's medical record.

a. *Electronic health record:* Document the date the specimen was picked up or sent to the laboratory, as well as the name of the laboratory, using the appropriate radio buttons, drop-down menus, and free text fields.

b. *Paper-based patient record:* Document the date the specimen was picked up or sent to the laboratory and the name of the laboratory.

17b

DOCUMENTATION EXAMPLE

Date	
9/25/XX	2:00 p.m. Applied DSD to Ⓡ post forearm.
	Instructed patient on suture care. Written
	instructions provided. Signed copy filed in
	chart. To return in 5 days for removal of
	sutures. Sebaceous cyst specimen sent to
	Medical Center Laboratory for biopsy on
	9/25/XX. —— H. Hopstetter, CMA (AAMA)

Principle. Documenting information regarding transport of the specimen documents that the specimen was sent to the laboratory.

18. Procedural Step. Clean the examining room. Handle the instruments carefully so as not to damage them. Be especially careful with sharp instruments to prevent cutting yourself. Blood and body secretions should be rinsed off the instruments immediately to prevent them from drying and hardening. The instruments must be sanitized and sterilized when it is convenient to do so; follow the procedures presented in Chapter 18. Discard disposable articles contaminated with blood or other potentially infectious materials in a biohazard waste container.

Principle. Surgical instruments are expensive and must be handled carefully to prolong their life span. Hardened blood and secretions on an instrument are difficult to remove. Disposable articles must be discarded in an appropriate manner to prevent the spread of infection.

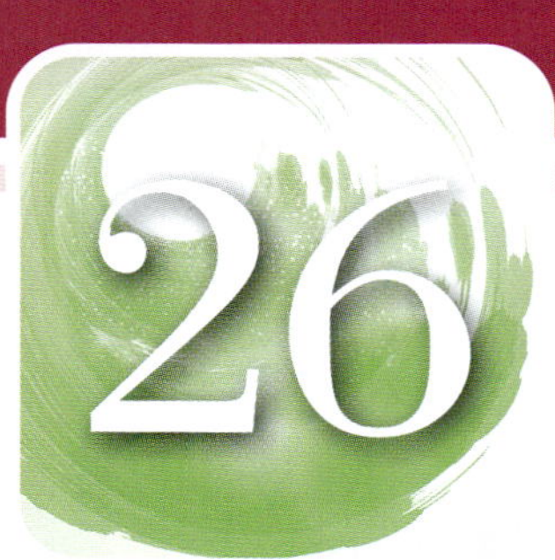

Administration of Medication

Check out the Evolve site at http://evolve.elsevier.com/Bonewit/today to access additional interactive activities and exercises to help you study and prepare for success.

LEARNING OBJECTIVES

Introduction to the Administration of Medication

1. Explain the difference between administering, prescribing, and dispensing medication.
2. State the common routes for administering medication.
3. List and describe the categories of information included in a drug package insert.
4. Describe the Food and Drug Administration's responsibilities with respect to drugs.
5. List and define the four names of drugs.
6. Classify drugs according to form.
7. Classify drugs according to the action they have on the body.
8. List the guidelines for writing metric notations.
9. List and describe the five schedules for controlled drugs.
10. List and explain the parts of a prescription.
11. Describe the functions performed by an electronic health record (EHR) prescription program.
12. Explain the purpose of a medication record.
13. List and describe the factors that affect the action of drugs in the body.
14. List and describe the possible adverse effects of medication.
15. List the guidelines for preparing and administering medication.

PROCEDURES

- Interpret a drug package insert.
- Calculate drug dosage.
- Complete a prescription using a paper form and an EHR prescription program.
- Complete a medication record form.

Oral Administration

17. Explain why the oral route is most frequently used to administer medication.
18. State where the absorption of most oral medications occurs.

PROCEDURES

- Prepare and administer oral medications.

Parenteral Administration

19. State the advantages and disadvantages of the parenteral route of administration.
20. Identify the parts of a needle and syringe and explain their functions.
21. State the ranges of gauge and length of needles for each of the following injections: intradermal, subcutaneous, and intramuscular.
22. State the purpose of safety-engineered syringes.
23. Describe the dispensing units available for injectable medications.
24. State which tissue layers of the body are used for intradermal, subcutaneous, and intramuscular injections.
25. List the medications commonly administered through each of the following routes: intradermal, subcutaneous, and intramuscular.
26. Explain the reason for administering medication with the Z-track method.

PROCEDURES

- Withdraw medication from a vial.
- Withdraw medication from an ampule.
- Reconstitute a powdered drug for parenteral administration.
- Locate appropriate subcutaneous injection sites.
- Administer a subcutaneous injection.
- Locate each of the following intramuscular injection sites: deltoid, vastus lateralis, ventrogluteal, and dorsogluteal.
- Administer an intramuscular injection.
- Administer an injection using the Z-track method.
- Administer an intradermal injection.

LEARNING OBJECTIVES

Tuberculin Testing

27. Explain the difference between active and latent tuberculosis.
28. Explain the purpose of tuberculin testing.
29. Identify the categories of individuals who should have a tuberculin test.
30. Explain the significance of a positive reaction to a tuberculin test.
31. List the diagnostic procedures that might be performed following a positive tuberculin test.
32. State the guidelines that should be followed when administering and reading a Mantoux tuberculin skin test.
33. State the advantages and disadvantages of the tuberculosis blood test.

Allergy Testing

34. Define an allergy, and name common allergens.
35. Explain what occurs during an allergic reaction.
36. List the guidelines for direct skin allergy testing.
37. State the purpose of each of the following types of allergy tests: patch testing, skin-prick testing, intradermal skin testing, and in vitro blood testing.

PROCEDURES

Administer a Mantoux tuberculin skin test, and read the test results.
Complete a tuberculosis test record card.

Perform allergy skin testing.

CHAPTER OUTLINE

KEY TERMS

adverse reaction (AD-vers ree-AK-shun)
allergen (AL-er-jen)
allergy (AL-er-jee)
ampule (AM-pyool)
anaphylactic reaction (an-uh-ful-AK-tik ree-AK-shun)
controlled drug
conversion (kon-VER-shun)
cubic centimeter (KYOO-bik SEN-tih-mee-ter)
DEA number
dose
drug
gauge (GAYJ)
induration (in-dur-AY-shun)
inscription (in-SKRIP-shun)
intradermal injection (in-tra-DER-mal in-JEK-shun)
intramuscular (in-tra-MUS-kyoo-lar) injection
oral (OR-ul) administration
parenteral (par-EN-ter-al)
pharmacology (far-ma-KOL-oh-jee)
prescription
signatura (sig-na-CHUR-ah)
subcutaneous (sub-kyoo-TAY-nee-us) injection
subscription (sub-SKRIP-shun)
superscription (soo-per-SKRIP-shun)
vial (VIE-ul)
wheal (WEE-ul)

INTRODUCTION TO THE ADMINISTRATION OF MEDICATION

Pharmacology is the study of drugs and includes the preparation, use, and action of drugs in the body. A **drug** is a chemical that is used for the treatment, prevention, or diagnosis of disease. Most drugs are produced synthetically, but they also can be obtained from other sources, such as animals, plants, and minerals.

ADMINISTERING, PRESCRIBING, AND DISPENSING MEDICATION

Medication may be administered, prescribed, or dispensed in the medical office. Medication that is *administered* is actually given to a patient at the office. Medication is *prescribed* when a provider authorizes the dispensing of a drug by a pharmacist. *Dispensed* medication is given to a patient at the office to be taken at home; for example, the provider gives a patient drug samples to take home.

LEGAL ASPECTS

An important responsibility of the medical assistant is the administration of medication. The medical assistant should administer medication only under the direction of the provider. In all states, it is unlawful to administer medication in the medical office without the consent of the provider.

ROUTES OF ADMINISTRATION

Common routes of administration of medication are oral, sublingual, inhalation, buccal, rectal, vaginal, topical, intradermal, subcutaneous (subcut), intramuscular (IM), and intravenous (IV). The route of administration depends on the type of drug being given, the dosage form, the intended action, and the rapidity of response desired. The route by which medication is most commonly administered in the medical office is the parenteral route. **Parenteral** refers to sites outside the gastrointestinal tract; this term is most commonly used to refer to the administration of medication by injection.

DRUG REFERENCES

The medical assistant is obligated to become familiar with the drugs that are most frequently used in their office. It is essential to know their indications, contraindications, adverse reactions, routes of administration, dosage, and storage. With each drug (including drug samples and injectable medications), the manufacturer includes a *package insert* (PI), which contains important information regarding the drug. The information included in a package insert is divided into categories which are listed and described in Fig. 26.1. Drug information is also available in drug reference books and on the Internet on certain recognized websites such as the *Prescriber's Digital Reference* (*pdr.net*).

FOOD AND DRUG ADMINISTRATION

The U.S. Food and Drug Administration (FDA) is a federal agency in the Department of Health and Human Services. The FDA is responsible for determining whether new food products, drugs, vaccines, medical devices, cosmetics, and other products are safe before they are released for human use.

The FDA determines the safety and effectiveness of prescription and nonprescription (over-the-counter [OTC]) drugs. Pharmaceutical manufacturers are required to submit new drug applications to the FDA for review and approval before products can be released for human use.

The FDA is also responsible for determining whether a medication will be available with or without a prescription. Medications that require a prescription have been determined by the FDA to be safe and effective when used under the guidance of a provider.

Nonprescription medications are drugs that the FDA determines to be safe and effective for use without provider supervision. Nonprescription medications have a low incidence of adverse reactions when the consumer follows the

DRUG PACKAGE INSERT

The categories of information included in a drug package insert are listed and described as follows:

DESCRIPTION: This category consists of a general description of the drug and includes the following information: brand name (with pronunciation), generic name, drug category, dosage form (e.g., tablets, capsules), route of administration, chemical name and structural formula, and the inactive ingredients contained in the drug. This category also indicates if the product requires a prescription (Rx) or if it is available over-the-counter (OTC). The symbol C and a Roman numeral appearing next to the drug indicates that it is a scheduled drug and that a prescription written for this drug requires the physician's DEA number.

CLINICAL PHARMACOLOGY: This category describes how the drug functions in the body to produce its therapeutic effect. Also included is an analysis of the absorption, distribution, metabolism, and excretion of the drug after it enters the body.

INDICATIONS AND USAGE: This category presents a list of the conditions that the drug has been formally approved to treat by the U.S. Food and Drug Administration (FDA).

CONTRAINDICATIONS: This category includes situations in which the drug should not be used because the risk of using the drug in these situations outweighs any possible benefit. Contraindications include administration of the drug to patients known to have a hypersensitivity (allergy) to it and use of the drug in patients who have a substantial risk of being harmed by it because of their particular age, sex, concurrent use of another drug, disease state, or condition (e.g., pregnancy).

WARNINGS: This category describes serious adverse reactions and potential safety hazards that may occasionally occur with the use of the drug and what should be done if they occur.

PRECAUTIONS: This category includes information regarding any special care that needs to be taken by the physician for the safe and effective use of the drug. Information typically presented in this category includes:

- **General Precautions:** Lists any disease states or situations that may require special consideration when the drug is being taken.
- **Information for Patients:** Includes information that should be relayed to the patient to ensure safe and effective use of the drug.
- **Laboratory Tests:** Indicates the laboratory tests that may be helpful in following the patient's response to the drug or in identifying possible adverse reactions to the drug.
- **Drug Interactions:** Lists any known interactions of this drug with other drugs that can affect the proper functioning of the drug.
- **Laboratory Test Interactions:** Includes any laboratory tests that may be affected when taking the medication.
- **Pregnancy:** Indicates the pregnancy category of the drug.

ADVERSE REACTIONS: This category describes the unintended and undesirable effects that may occur with the use of the drug. Some adverse reactions are harmless and therefore often tolerated by the patient in order to obtain the therapeutic effect of the drug. Other adverse reactions may be harmful to the patient and warrant discontinuing the medication.

OVERDOSAGE: This category describes symptoms associated with an overdosage of the drug, as well as the complications that can occur and the treatment to institute for an overdosage.

DOSAGE AND ADMINISTRATION: This category lists the recommended adult dosage, the usual dosage range of the drug, and the route of administration (e.g., by mouth, sublingual, IM). Also included is information about the intervals recommended between doses, the usual duration of treatment, and any modification of dosage needed for special groups such as children, the elderly, and patients with renal or hepatic disease.

HOW SUPPLIED: This category indicates the dosage forms that are available (e.g., 20-mg tablets), the units in which the dosage form is available (e.g., bottles of 100; 5-ml multiple-dose vial), information to help identify the dosage form (shape and color), and the handling and storage conditions for the drug.

Fig. 26.1 Information included in a drug package insert.

directions and warnings on the label. Examples of nonprescription medications include mild pain relievers; cough, cold, and allergy medications; antacids; topical antibiotics and antifungals; antidiarrheals; and laxatives.

DRUG NOMENCLATURE

Each drug has four names: chemical, generic, official, and brand (also known as *trade*) names.

1. *Chemical name.* The chemical name provides a precise description of the drug's chemical composition; pharmaceutical manufacturers and pharmacists are most concerned with the chemical makeup of a drug.
2. *Generic name.* After a drug has received official approval from the FDA, a generic name is assigned to it by the United States Adopted Names (USAN) Council. The responsibility of the USAN Council is to select a simple, short, informative, and unique generic name for each new drug developed by a pharmaceutical manufacturer.
3. *Official name.* The official name is the name under which the drug is listed in official publications, such as the *United States Pharmacopeia* (USP) and the *National Formulary* (NF). Official publications set specific standards to regulate the strength, purity, packaging, safety, labeling, and dosage form of each drug. The generic name is frequently used for the official name.
4. *Brand name.* The brand name is the common or trade name under which a pharmaceutical manufacturer markets a drug. Because a drug may be manufactured by more than one pharmaceutical company, it may have several brand names (but only one generic name). Brand names are usually less complicated and easier to remember than

generic names. The generic name of a common analgesic is acetaminophen; brand names for this drug include Tylenol, FeverAll, Tylophen, and Cetafen.

The medical assistant should be familiar with the generic and brand names of medications commonly prescribed and administered in the medical office.

What Would You Do? What Would You *Not* Do?

Case Study 1

Carol Okasinski, 56 years old, is a new patient who just moved to the community. Mrs. Okasinski is obese and has hypertension, type 2 diabetes, osteoarthritis in her hands and knees, and problems with depression. While completing her health history form, she says she cannot fill in the names of her medications.. She is on a lot of medications prescribed by her previous physician. She says she could not get the childproof pill containers open because of the arthritis in her hands, so she had her husband throw away the childproof containers and transfer each medication into an easy-to-open plastic container. She knows when to take her medications, but she does not know the names of them or why she is taking them. She has brought in a bag with all her medications in their plastic containers. ■

CLASSIFICATION OF DRUGS BASED ON FORM

Drugs are available in two basic forms: liquid and solid. A medication may be available in both these forms (liquid and solid), which permits it to be administered to different types of patients. The liquid form of an antibiotic is administered to young children, and the solid form (e.g., tablets) of the same medication is administered to older children and adults. The following list includes the common categories of drugs based on form.

LIQUID FORMS

Elixir A drug that is dissolved in a solution of alcohol and water. Elixirs are sweetened and flavored and are taken orally. *Example:* Dimetapp elixir.

Emulsion A mixture of fats or oils in water. *Example:* Durezol ophthalmic emulsion.

Liniment A drug combined with oil, soap, alcohol, or water. Liniments are applied externally, using friction, to produce a feeling of heat or warmth. *Example:* Heet liniment.

Lotion An aqueous preparation that contains suspended ingredients. Lotions are used to treat external skin conditions. They work to soothe, protect, and moisten the skin and to destroy harmful bacteria. *Example:* Caladryl lotion.

Solution A liquid preparation that contains one or more completely dissolved substances. The dissolved substance is known as the *solute*, and the liquid in which it is dissolved is known as the *solvent*. Most drugs administered parenterally (by injection) consist of solutions. *Example:* Depo-Provera injectable solution.

Spirit A drug combined with an alcoholic solution that is volatile (a substance that is volatile evaporates readily). *Example:* Aromatic spirit of ammonia.

Spray A fine stream of medicated vapor, usually used to treat nose and throat conditions. *Example:* Dristan nasal spray.

Suspension A drug that contains solid insoluble drug particles in a liquid; the medication must be shaken before administration. *Example:* Amoxicillin oral suspension.

Suspension aerosol A pressurized form in which solid aerosol or liquid drug particles are suspended in a gas to be dispensed in a cloud or mist. *Example:* Proventil inhalation aerosol.

Syrup A drug dissolved in a solution of sugar, water, and sometimes a flavoring to disguise an unpleasant taste. *Example:* Robitussin cough syrup.

Tincture A drug dissolved in a solution of alcohol or alcohol and water. *Example:* Tincture of iodine.

SOLID FORMS

Tablet A powdered drug that has been pressed into a disc. Some tablets are scored—that is, they are marked with an indentation so that they can be broken into halves or quarters for proper dosage. *Example:* Tylenol tablets.

Chewable tablet A powdered drug that has been flavored and pressed into a disc. Chewable tablets are often used for antacids, antiflatulents, and children's medications. *Example:* Pepto-Bismol chewable tablets.

Sublingual tablet A powdered drug that has been pressed into a disc and is designed to dissolve under the tongue, which permits its rapid absorption into the bloodstream. *Example:* Nitroglycerin sublingual tablets (Nitrostat).

Enteric-coated tablet A tablet coated with a substance that prevents it from dissolving until it reaches the intestines. The coating protects the drug from being destroyed by gastric juices and also prevents the drug from irritating the stomach lining. To prevent the active ingredients from being released prematurely in the stomach, enteric-coated tablets must not be crushed or chewed. *Example:* Ecotrin enteric-coated aspirin.

Capsule A drug contained in a gelatin capsule that is water-soluble and functions to prevent the patient from tasting the drug. *Example:* Benadryl capsules.

Sustained-release capsule A capsule that contains granules that dissolve at different rates to provide a gradual and continuous release of medication. This reduces the number of doses that must be administered. (Sustained-release medication also comes in other forms, such as tablets and caplets.) *Example:* Sudafed 12-hour sustained-release capsules.

Caplet A drug contained in an oblong tablet with a smooth coating to make swallowing easier. *Example:* Advil caplets.

Lozenge A drug contained in a candy-like base. Lozenges are circular and are designed to dissolve on the tongue. *Example:* Chloraseptic throat lozenges.

Cream A drug combined in a base that is usually nongreasy, resulting in a semisolid . Creams are applied externally to the skin. *Example:* Hydrocortisone topical cream.

Ointment A drug with an oil base, resulting in a semisolid preparation. Ointments are applied externally to the skin and are usually greasy. *Example:* Cortisporin topical ointment.

Suppository A drug mixed with a firm base, such as cocoa butter, that is designed to melt at body temperature. A suppository is shaped into a cylinder or a cone for easy insertion into a body cavity, such as the rectum or vagina. *Example:* Preparation H suppositories.

Transdermal patch A patch with an adhesive backing, which contains a drug, that is applied to the skin. The drug enters the circulation after being absorbed through the skin. *Example:* Nitroglycerin patches (Nitro-Dur).

CLASSIFICATION OF DRUGS BASED ON ACTION

Drugs also can be classified according to the action they have on the body. The medical assistant should know in which category a particular drug belongs and its primary uses and major therapeutic effects. Table 26.1 contains classifications based on action and examples of drugs that are commonly administered and prescribed in the medical office.

Text continued on p. 636

Table 26.1 Classification of Drugs Based on Action

		COMMONLY PRESCRIBED DRUGS	
Drug Category	**Primary Use and Major Therapeutic Effects**	**Generic**	**Brand**
Analgesics (opioid)	*Indications for use:* Used to manage moderate to severe pain *Desired effects:* Work by altering perception of and response to painful stimuli *Side effects:* Sedation, pruritis, dizziness, nausea, vomiting, constipation, physical dependence, tolerance, respiratory depression	codeine/acetaminophen (APAP) fentanyl hydrocodone/APAP meperidine morphine oxycodone xycodone/APAP propoxyphene propoxyphene N/APAP tramadol	▶ Tylenol w/ Codeine (III) ▶ Duragesic Skin Patch ▶ Vicodin (III) Demerol (II) MS Contin (II) ▶ OxyContin (II) ▶ Percocet (II) Darvon (IV) ▶ Darvocet-N (IV) ▶ Ultram
Analgesics (barbiturate)	*Indications for use:* Used to manage moderate to severe pain of tension headaches *Desired effects:* Work by relieving pain and relaxing muscle contractions *Side effects:* Drowsiness, lightheadedness, dizziness, sedation, shortness of breath, naurea, vomiting, abdominal pain, intoxicated feeling	butalbital/APAP/ caffeine butalbital/ASA/ caffeine	▶ Fioricet (III) Fiorinal (III)
Analgesics/ antipyretics	*Indications for use:* Used to manage mild to moderate pain and to reduce fever *Desired effects:* Work by relieving pain and reducing fever *Side effects:* Nausea, dyspepsia, ulceration or bleeding, diarrhea, headache, dizziness	Acetaminophen aspirin	▶ Tylenol* ▶ Bayer* ▶ Ecotrin* ▶ Bufferin
Analgesics/ antipyretics		**Nonsteroidal antiinflammatory drugs (NSAIDs)** diclofenac ibuprofen naproxen	 ▶ Cataflam ▶ Advil* ▶ Motrin* Aleve*
Anesthetics (local)	*Indications for use:* Used to produce local anesthesia through loss of feeling to a body part *Desired effects:* Work by preventing initiation and conduction of normal nerve impulses in body part *Side effects:* Mild bruising, swelling, or itching at the injection site	lidocaine dibucaine	▶ Xylocaine Nupercainal ointment*
Antacids	*Indications for use:* Used to treat heartburn, hyperacidity, indigestion, and gastroesophageal reflux disease and to promote healing of ulcers *Desired effects:* Work by neutralizing gastric acid to relieve gastric pain and irritation *Side effects:* Nausea, constipation, diarrhea, headache, hyperacidity	aluminum hydroxide/ magnesium hydroxide calcium carbonate sodium bicarbonate/ASA	Maalox* Mylanta* Tums* Alka-Seltzer*

Continued

Table 26.1 Classification of Drugs Based on Action—cont'd

Drug Category	Primary Use and Major Therapeutic Effects	COMMONLY PRESCRIBED DRUGS Generic	Brand
Anthelmintics	*Indications for use:* Used to treat worm infections (pinworms, roundworms, hookworms) *Desired effects:* Work by destroying worms *Side effects:* Abdominal pain, diarrhea, headache, dizziness	mebendazole	Vermox
Anti-Alzheimer agents	*Indications for use:* Used to treat mild to moderate dementia associated with Alzheimer disease *Desired effects:* Work by elevating acetylcholine concentration in the cerebral cortex *Side effects:* Headache, fatigue, dizziness, nausea, vomiting, diarrhea, loss of appetite, joint pain, insomnia	donepezil memantine	► Aricept Namenda
Antianemics	**Iron Supplements** *Indications for use:* Used to prevent or cure iron-deficiency anemia *Desired effects:* Work by increasing amount of iron in body *Side effects:* Upset stomach, cramps, constipation, diarrhea, nausea, vomiting	ferrous sulfate iron dextran	► Feosol* DexFerrum INFeD
	Vitamin B_{12} *Indications for use:* Used to treat pernicious anemia *Desired effects:* Work by increasing amount of vitamin B_{12} in body *Side effects:* Headache, dizziness, weakness, nausea, upset stomach, diarrhea, numbness or tingling, pain, swelling and redness at injection site, joint pain	cyanocobalamin	Cobex injection Cyanoject injection
	Folic Acid Supplements *Indications for use:* Used to promote normal fetal development *Desired effects:* Work by stimulating production of red blood cells, white blood cells, and platelets *Side effects:* Allergic reaction	folic acid	Folvite
Antianginals	*Indications for use:* Used to relieve or prevent angina attacks *Desired effects:* Work by increasing blood supply to myocardial tissue *Side effects:* Headache, dizziness, lightheadedness, fainting, fatigue	**Nitrates** isosorbide mononitrate nitroglycerin **Beta-Blockers** atenolol propranolol metoprolol **Calcium Channel Blockers** amlodipine diltiazem nifedipine	 ► Imdur Nitrostat Sublingual Tenormin Inderal ► Toprol-XL ► Norvasc ► Cardizem Adalat Procardia XL
Antianxiety agents	*Indications for use:* Used to treat anxiety *Desired effects:* Work at many levels in central nervous system to produce anxiolytic (anxiety-relieving) effect *Side effects:* Drowsiness, lack of energy, clumsiness, slurred speech, confusion, disorientation, depression, dizziness, impaired thinking, memory loss	alprazolam chlordiazepoxide diazepam lorazepam	► Xanax (IV) Librium (IV) ► Valium (IV) ► Ativan (IV)
Anticholinergics	*Indications for use:* Used preoperatively to decrease oral and respiratory secretions *Desired effects:* Work by blocking effects of acetylcholine in autonomic nervous system *Side effects:* Dry mouth and eyes, decreased sweating, blurred vision, constipation, flushing of the face, urinary retention	atropine tiotropium	Atro-Pen ► Spiriva

Table 26.1 Classification of Drugs Based on Action—cont'd

Drug Category	Primary Use and Major Therapeutic Effects	COMMONLY PRESCRIBED DRUGS	
		Generic	Brand
Anticoagulants	*Indications for use:* Used to prevent and treat venous thrombosis, pulmonary embolism, and myocardial infarction by preventing clot extension and formation *Desired effects:* Work by delaying or preventing blood coagulation *Side effects*: Hemorrhaging, hematuria, bruising, bleeding gums, nosebleeds, bloody or black stools, menorrhagia	heparin sodium	► heparin
		enoxaparin	► Lovenox
		warfarin	► Coumadin
		clopidogrel	Plavix
		rivaroxaban	► Xarelto
		apixaban	► Eliquis
		dabigatran	► Pradaxa
		dabigantran	► Fragmin
Anticonvulsants	*Indications for use:* Used to prevent or relieve seizures *Desired effects:* Work by decreasing incidence and severity of seizures *Side effects*: Constipation, nausea, vomiting, dizziness, drowsiness	clonazepam	► Klonopin (IV)
		divalproex	► Depakote
		gabapentin	► Neurontin
		lamotrigine	► Lamictal
		phenytoin	► Dilantin
		pregabalin	► Lyrica
		levetiracetam	► Keppra
Antidepressants	*Indications for use:* Used to prevent, cure, or alleviate depression and to treat anxiety disorders (panic attacks) and obsessive–convulsive disorder *Desired effects:* Work by inhibiting reuptake of neurotransmitters in the central nervous system *Side effects*: Nausea, increased appetite, weight gain, loss of sexual desire, fatigue, drowsiness	**Selective Serotonin Reuptake Inhibitors (SSRIs)**	
		citalopram	► Celexa
		escitalopram	► Lexapro
		fluoxetine	► Prozac
		fluvoxamine	Luvox
		paroxetine	► Paxil
		sertraline	► Zoloft
		Serotonin-Norepinephrine Reuptake Inhibitors (SNRIs)	
		desvenlafaxine	► Pristiq
		duloxetine	► Cymbalta
		venlafaxine	► Effexor XR
		levomilnacipran	► Fetzima
		tricyclic nortriptyline	► Pamelor
		imipramine	► Tofranil
		amitriptyline	► Elavil
			► Vanatrip
		Miscellaneous	
		bupropion	Wellbutrin SR
		mirtazapine	Remeron
		trazodone	► Desyrel
	Non-Insulin Medications		
Antidiabetics	*Indications for use:* Used to manage non–insulin-dependent type 2 diabetes mellitus *Desired effects:* Work by lowering blood glucose levels by stimulating release of insulin from pancreas and increasing sensitivity to insulin *Side effects*: Headache, stomach upset, loss of appetite, nausea, diarrhea, vomiting, hypoglycemia	glimepiride	► Amaryl
		glipizide	► Glucotrol XL
		glyburide	► Micronase
		metformin	► DiaBeta
		sitagliptin	► Glucophage
		semaglutide (injectable)	► Januvia
		dulaglutide (injectable)	► Ozempic
			► Trulicity

Continued

Table 26.1 Classification of Drugs Based on Action—cont'd

Drug Category	Primary Use and Major Therapeutic Effects	COMMONLY PRESCRIBED DRUGS	
		Generic	**Brand**
	Insulins		
Antidiabetics	*Indications for use:* Used to manage diabetes mellitus *Desired effects:* Work by reducing blood glucose levels *Side effects*: Hypoglycemia, headache, weight gain, pain, redness and irritation at the injection site	regular insulin insulin glargine insulin lispro insulin aspart insulin detemir insulin isophane canagliflozin liraglutide	Humulin R* Novolin R* ► Lantus ► Humalog ► Novolog ► Levemir ► Humulin ► Invokana ► Saxenda ► Victoza
Antidiarrheals	*Indications for use:* Used to control and relieve diarrhea *Desired effects:* Work by inhibiting peristalsis, reducing fecal volume, and preventing loss of fluids and electrolytes *Side effects*: Abdominal pain, constipation, dizziness, dry mouth, drowsiness	bismuth subsalicylate diphenoxylate/atropine kaolin/pectin loperamide	Pepto-Bismol* Lomotil (V) Kaopectate* Imodium*
Antidysrhythmics	*Indications for use:* Used to control or prevent cardiac dysrhythmias *Desired effects:* Work by decreasing myocardial excitability and slowing conduction velocity *Side effects*: Dry mouth and throat, dizziness, diarrhea, loss of appetite, lightheadedness, blurred vision	Metoprolol procainamide propranolol	► Lopressor ► Toprol-XL Pronestyl Inderal
Antiemetics	*Indications for use:* Used to prevent or relieve nausea and vomiting *Desired effects:* Work by depressing chemoreceptor trigger zone in central nervous system to inhibit nausea and vomiting *Side effects*: Dry mouth, drowsiness, dysuria, dizziness, blurred vision	Granisetron ondansetron prochlorperazine promethazine meclizine	► Kytril ► Sancuso ► Zofran Compazine Phenergan Bonine*
Antiflatulents	*Indications for use:* Used to relieve discomfort of excess gas and bloating in gastrointestinal tract *Desired effects:* Work by causing coalescence of gas bubbles in intestinal tract *Side effects*: Nausea, constipation, hypersensitivity reaction	simethicone	Gas-X* Mylanta Gas*
Antifungals	*Indications for use:* Used to treat fungal infections *Desired effects:* Work by killing or inhibiting growth of susceptible fungi *Side effects*: Mild stomach pain, headache, dizziness, unusual or unpleasant taste in the mouth	amphotericin B clotrimazole fluconazole ketoconazole miconazole nystatin terbinafine	Fungizone ► Lotrisone ► Diflucan ► Nizoral Topical Monistat* Mycostatin* Lamisil
Antigout agents	*Indications for use:* Used to prevent attacks of gout *Desired effects:* Work by inhibiting production of uric acid *Side effects*: Skin rash, diarrhea, nausea, itching, drowsiness	Allopurinol colchicine	► Zyloprim ► Colcrys ► Mitigare
Antihistamines	*Indications for use:* Used to relieve symptoms associated with allergies (increased sneezing, rhinorrhea, itchy eyes, nose, and throat) *Desired effects:* Work by blocking the effect of histamine at histamine receptor sites *Side Effects*: Dry mouth, drowsiness, dizziness, nausea, vomiting, blurred vision, urinary retention	cetirizine chlorpheniramine hydrocodone desloratadine diphenhydramine fexofenadine/ pseudoephedrine loratadine promethazine	Zyrtec* ► Tussionex (II) ► Pennkinetic(II) Clarinex ► Benadryl* Allegra Claritin* Phenergan

Table 26.1 Classification of Drugs Based on Action—cont'd

		COMMONLY PRESCRIBED DRUGS	
Drug Category	**Primary Use and Major Therapeutic Effects**	**Generic**	**Brand**
Antihypertensives	*Indications for use:* Used to manage hypertension	**ACE Inhibitors**	
	Desired effects: Work by causing systemic vasodilation to reduce blood pressure	perindopril	► Aceon
	Side effects: Constipation, dehydration, dizziness, lightheadedness, drowsiness	captopril	Capoten
		enalapril	► Vasotec
		lisinopril	► Epaned
		quinapril	► Prinivil
		ramipril	Accupril
			► Altace
			► Tritace
		Peripherally Acting Adrenergic Blockers	
		clonidine	Catapres
		doxazosin	► Cardura
		prazosin	Minipress
		Angiotensin II Receptor Antagonists	
		candesartan	Atacand
		irbesartan	Aprovel
		losartan	► Cozaar
		olmesartan	Olmetec
		Beta-Blockers	
		atenolol	► Tenormin
		carvedilol	► Coreg
		metoprolol	► Lopressor
		bisoprolol	► Toprol-XL
		propranolol	► Zebeta
			Inderal
		Calcium Channel Blockers	
		amlodipine	► Norvasc
		diltiazem	Cardizem
		nifedipine	Adalat
		Vasodilators	
		hydralazine	► Apresoline
Antiimpotence agents	*Indications for use:* Used to treat erectile dysfunction	sildenafil	► Viagra
	Desired effects: Work by promoting increased blood flow to penis	tadalafil	► Cialis
	Side effects: Headache, flushing, indigestion, stuffy or runny nose, temporary vision changes		
Antiinfectives	*Indications for use:* Used to treat infections	**Penicillins**	
	Desired effects: Work by killing or inhibiting growth of bacteria	amoxicillin	Amoxil
	Side effects: Vomiting, diarrhea, allergic reaction, abdominal cramps, vaginal itching or discharge, white patches on the tongue	amoxicillin/clavulanate	Trimox
		ampicillin	► Augmentin
		benzathine penicillin G	Omnipen
		penicillin VK	Bicillin L-A
			► Pen-V
			► PC Penn VK
		Macrolides	
		Azithromycin	► Zithromax (Z-Pak)
		clarithromycin	► Biaxin
		erythromycin	► Ery-Tab
			► E-mycin
		Cephalosporins	
		cefdinir	► Omnicef
		ceftriaxone	Rocephin
		cefuroxime	► Ceftin
		cephalexin	► Keflex

Continued

Table 26.1 Classification of Drugs Based on Action—cont'd

Drug Category	Primary Use and Major Therapeutic Effects	COMMONLY PRESCRIBED DRUGS	
		Generic	**Brand**
		Fluoroquinolones ciprofloxacin levofloxacin moxifloxacin	 ► Cipro ► Proquin ► Levaquin ► Avelox
		Tetracyclines doxycycline tetracycline	 ► Adoxa ► Vibramycin ► Ala-Tet ► Broadspec ► Sumycin
		Aminoglycosides gentamicin kanamycin	 Garamycin Kantrex
		Sulfonamides sulfamethoxazole trimethoprim/sulfamethoxazole	 Gantanol Bactrim
		Miscellaneous clindamycin chloramphenicol nitrofurantoin	 ► Cleocin Chloromycetin ► Macrobid Macrodantin
Antiinflammatories	*Indications for use:* Used to relieve signs and symptoms of osteoarthritis and rheumatoid arthritis in adults *Desired effects:* Work by decreasing pain and inflammation *Side effects:* Vomiting, nausea, constipation, reduced appetite, headache, dizziness, rash, drowsiness	aspirin ibuprofen meloxicam nabumetone naproxen cyclosporin	Bayer* Ecotrin* Advil* Motrin* ► Mobic ► Relafen Aleve* ► Sandimmune ► Neoral
Antimanics	*Indications for use:* Used to treat bipolar affective disorders *Desired effects:* Work by altering cation transport in nerves and muscles *Side effects:* Restlessness, mild tremor of hands, mild thirst, loss of appetite, stomach pain, flatulence, indigestion, weight gain or loss	lithium	Eskalith Eskalith CR
Antimigraine agents	*Indications for use:* Used in acute treatment of migraine attacks *Desired effects:* Work by causing vasoconstriction in large intracranial arteries *Side effects:* Dizziness, flushing, nausea, vomiting, sore throat, tingling sensation, abdominal pain	sumatriptan topiramate eletriptan zolmitriptan	► Imitrex ► Topamax ► Relpax ► Zomig
Antineoplastics	*Indications for use:* Used to treat tumors *Desired effects:* Work by preventing development, growth, or proliferation of malignant cells *Side effects:* Nausea, vomiting, loss of appetite, diarrhea, hair loss, bone marrow depression	cyclophosphamide methotrexate pemetrexed bevacizumab	Cytoxan ► Otrexup ► Alimta ► Avastin
Anti-Parkinson agents	*Indications for use:* Used to treat symptoms of Parkinson disease *Desired effects:* Work by restoring balance between acetylcholine and dopamine in central nervous system *Side effects:* Nausea, vomiting, sleepiness, dizziness, headache, low blood pressure	carbidopa/levodopa benztropine	► Sinemet ► Stalevo ► Dopar ► Inbrija ► Larodopa ► Congentin

Table 26.1 Classification of Drugs Based on Action—cont'd

Drug Category	Primary Use and Major Therapeutic Effects	COMMONLY PRESCRIBED DRUGS	
		Generic	Brand
Antiprotozoals	*Indications for use:* Used to treat protozoal infections *Desired effects:* Work by destroying protozoa *Side effects*: Diarrhea, nausea, vomiting, stomach pain	metronidazole	► Flagyl
Antipsychotics	*Indications for use:* Used to treat psychotic disorders *Desired effects:* Work by blocking dopamine and serotonin receptors in central nervous system *Side effects*: Drowsiness, rapid heartbeat, dizziness, weight gain	haloperidol olanzapine risperidone clozapine quetiapine	Haldol ► Zyprexa ► Risperdal ► Clozaril ► Seroquel
Antiretrovirals	*Indications for use:* Used to manage human immunodeficiency virus (HIV) infections and to reduce maternal-fetal transmission of HIV *Desired effects:* Work by inhibiting replication of retroviruses *Side effects*: Nausea, diarrhea, loss of appetite, headache, fatigue, peripheral neuropathy, lipodystrophy	raltegravir tenofovir zidovudine	► Isentress ► Atripla Retrovir
Antispasmodics	*Indications for use:* Used to control hypermotility in irritable bowel syndrome, spastic colitis, spastic bladder, and pylorospasm *Desired effects:* Work by preventing or relieving spasms of gastrointestinal or genitourinary tract *Side effects*: Flatulence, bloating, dizziness, heartburn, dry mouth, constipation	dicyclomine hyoscyamine	► Bentyl Levsin
Antituberculars	*Indications for use:* Used to treat tuberculosis *Desired effects:* Work by killing or inhibiting growth of mycobacteria *Side effects*: Diarrhea, stomach pain, nausea, vomiting, loss of appetite, unusual tiredness or weakness	isoniazid rifampin	INH Rifadin
Antitussives	*Indications for use:* Used in prevention or relief of coughs caused by minor viral upper respiratory infections or inhaled irritants *Desired effects:* Work by suppressing cough reflex by direct effect on cough center in central nervous system *Side effects*: Irritability, dizziness, drowsiness, nausea, vomiting	benzonatate chlorpheniramine/ hydrocodone dextromethorphan guaifenesin/codeine	Tessalon ► Tussionex (II) ► PennKinetic (II) Robitussin DM* Robitussin A-C (V)
Antiulcer agents	*Indications for use:* Used to manage ulcers, gastroesophageal reflux disease, heartburn, indigestion, and gastric hyperacidity *Desired effects:* Work by decreasing the amount of acid produced by the stomach. *Side effects*: Headache, mild diarrhea, nausea, stomach pain, flatulence, constipation, dry mouth	**Proton Pump Inhibitors** esomerazole lansoprazole omeprazole pantoprazole rabeprazole **H_2-Receptor Antagonists** cimetidine famotidine ranitidine	 ► Nexium ► Prevacid ► Prilosec* ► Protonix ► AcipHex Tagamet* ► Pepcid AC* ► Zantac*
Antivirals	*Indications for use:* Used to manage viral infections *Desired effects:* Work by inhibiting viral replication *Side effects*: Nausea, vomiting, dizziness, diarrhea, headache, insomnia	acyclovir famciclovir valacyclovir oseltamivir	► Zovirax Famvir ► Valcyte ► Valtrex ► Tamiflu
Bone resorption inhibitors	*Indications for use:* Used to treat and prevent osteoporosis *Desired effects:* Work by inhibiting reabsorption of bone *Side effects*: Nausea, vomiting, stomach pain, diarrhea, headache, dizziness, pain in the extremities, loss of voice	alendronate ibandronate raloxifene zoledronic acid risedronate	► Fosamax ► Boniva ► Evista ► Reclast ► Zometa ► Actonel

Continued

Table 26.1 Classification of Drugs Based on Action—cont'd

Drug Category	Primary Use and Major Therapeutic Effects	COMMONLY PRESCRIBED DRUGS Generic	Brand
Bronchodilators	*Indications for use:* Used to manage reversible airway obstruction caused by asthma or chronic obstructive pulmonary disease *Desired effects:* Work by relaxing smooth muscle of respiratory tract resulting in bronchodilation *Side effects*: Dry mouth, constipation, diarrhea, headache, heart palpitations, dizziness, trembling, nervousness, muscle aches or cramps	albuterol budesonide/formoterol fluticasone montelukast salmeterol theophylline ipratropium/albuterol	► Proventil ► ProAir HFA ► Symbicort ► Advair Diskus ► Singulair Serevent Bronkodyl ► Combivent ► Respimat
Cardiac glycosides	*Indications for use:* Used to treat congestive heart failure and cardiac arrhythmias *Desired effects:* Work by increasing strength and force of myocardial contractions and slowing heart rate *Side effects*: Cardiac arrhythmias, nausea, vomiting, diarrhea, loss of appetite, dizziness, weakness headache, blurred vision, depression	digitoxin digoxin	Crystodigin ► Digitek Lanoxicaps ► Lanoxin
Central nervous system stimulants	*Indications for use:* Used to treat narcolepsy and manage attention-deficit/hyperactivity disorder *Desired effects:* Work by increasing level of catecholamines in central nervous system *Side effects*: Loss of appetite, increased anxiety level, weight loss, dizziness, headache, irritability, facial tics, restlessness, panic attacks insomnia, tachycardia	atomoxetine dextroamphetamine dextroamphetamine saccharate and sulfate lisdexamfetamine methylphenidate	► Strattera Dexedrine (II) ► Adderall (II) ► Vyvanse (II) ► Ritalin (II) ► Concerta
Contraceptives (hormonal)	*Indications for use:* Used to prevent pregnancy and to regulate menstrual cycle *Desired effects:* Work by inhibiting ovulation *Side effects*: Headache, dizziness, lightheadedness, stomach upset, bloating, nausea, weight gain, metrorrhagia, breast tenderness, mood changes	**Oral Contraceptives** ethinyl estradiol/ drospirenone ethinyl estradiol ethinyl estradiol/ norethindrone ethinyl estradiol/ norgestimate	 ► Yaz Yasmin Brevicon Modicon ► Loestrin Fe Sprintec
		Injectable Contraceptives Medroxyprogesterone	 ► Depo-Provera
		Vaginal Ring Contraceptives ethinyl estradiol/etonogestrel	 NuvaRing
Corticosteroids	**Systemic Corticosteroids** *Indications for use:* Used to treat inflammation, allergies, asthma, and autoimmune disorders and as replacement therapy in adrenal insufficiency *Desired effects:* Work by suppressing inflammation and modifying normal immune response *Side effects*: Increased appetite, weight gain, sudden mood swings, easy bruising, muscle weakness, blurred vision, increased growth of body hair, swollen face	cortisone hydrocortisone prednisolone methylprednisolone prednisone triamcinolone	Cortone ► Ala-Cort ► Flo-Pred Medrol Depo-Medrol ► Deltasone ► Rayos ► Aristocort
	Nasal Corticosteroids *Indications for use:* Used to treat chronic nasal inflammatory conditions (e.g., allergic rhinitis) *Desired effects:* Work by suppressing inflammation and reducing hypersecretions of respiratory tract *Side effects*: Nosebleed, sinus pain, sore throat, burning, dryness or irritation inside the nose	fluticasone mometasone triamcinolone	► Flonase Nasonex Nasacort

Table 26.1 Classification of Drugs Based on Action—cont'd

Drug Category	Primary Use and Major Therapeutic Effects	COMMONLY PRESCRIBED DRUGS Generic	Brand
Decongestants	*Indications for use:* Used to decrease nasal congestion *Desired effects:* Work by producing vasoconstriction in respiratory tract mucosa *Side effects:* Irritation of the lining of the nose, headache, nausea, dry mouth, nervousness, insomnia, dizziness	oxymetazoline phenylephrine pseudoephedrine	Afrin* Dristan* Neo-Synephrine* Sudafed*
Disease-Modifying Antirheumatic Drugs (DMARD)	*Indications for use:* Used in the treatment of severe inflammatory arthritis and management of connective tissue diseases *Desired effects*: Work by reducing the immune system's response to attacking its healthy tissue *Side effects:* Loss of appetite, nausea, diarrhea, abdominal pain, liver problems, increased risk of infections	Methotrexate Etanercept adalimumab	Oxtrexup Enbrel Humira
Diuretics	*Indications for use:* Used to manage hypertension, edema in congestive heart failure, and renal disease *Desired effects:* Work by removing excess fluid from the body by increasing urine output *Side effects*: Dry mouth, increased thirst, weakness, lethargy, drowsiness, muscle pain or cramps, confusion, oliguria, headache, dizziness	**Loop Diuretics** bumetanide furosemide **Thiazide Diuretics** chlorthalidone hydrochlorothiazide **Potassium-Sparing Diuretics** spironolactone triamterene	 Bumex ► Lasix Hygroton ► Microzide ► Hyzaar ► Aldactone ► Dyrenium
Electrolyte replacements	*Indications for use:* Used to treat or prevent electrolyte depletion *Desired effects:* Work by replacing electrolytes in body *Side effects*: Nausea, vomiting, diarrhea, flatulence, high blood pressure, arrhythmias	**Potassium Supplements** potassium chloride	 K-Dur Klor-Con
Emetics	*Indications for use:* Used to treat poisoning *Desired effects:* Work by inducing vomiting *Side effects*: Diarrhea, lethargy, stomach cramps, prolonged vomiting	syrup of ipecac	
Expectorants	*Indications for use:* Used to manage coughs by expelling mucus *Desired effects:* Work by decreasing viscosity of bronchial secretions to promote clearance of mucus from respiratory tract *Side effects*: Nausea, vomiting, stomach upset, dizziness, headache, drowsiness, diarrhea, constipation	guaifenesin	Robitussin* Mucinex* Naldecon*
Hormone replacements	*Indications for use:* Used to treat moderate to severe vasomotor symptoms of menopause *Desired effects:* Work by restoring hormonal balance *Side effects*: Headache, nausea, vaginal discharge, fluid retention, weight gain, breast tenderness	conjugated estrogens conjugated estrogen/ progesterone estradiol estradiol/norethindrone	► Premarin Prempro Estrace Activella

Continued

Table 26.1 Classification of Drugs Based on Action—cont'd

Drug Category	Primary Use and Major Therapeutic Effects	COMMONLY PRESCRIBED DRUGS	
		Generic	**Brand**
Immunizations	*Indications for use:* Used to prevent (vaccine-preventable) diseases *Desired effects:* Work by stimulating body to produce antibodies *Side effects*: Pain, redness, tenderness and swelling at the injection site, fatigue, headache, nausea, dizziness, fever	diphtheria, tetanus toxoids, and acellular pertussis vaccine *Haemophilus* b conjugate vaccine hepatitis A vaccine hepatitis B vaccine human papillomavirus vaccine inactivated polio vaccine influenza virus vaccine types A and B measles, mumps, and rubella vaccine meningococcal conjugate vaccine pneumococcal conjugate vaccine rotavirus rubella vaccine varicella vaccine	Acel-Imune Certiva Daptacel Infanrix Tripedia ActHIB HibTITER Havrix Vaqta Engerix-B Recombivax HB Gardasil IPOL Afluria FluShield Fluzone FluMist M-M-R II Menactra Prevnar Pneumovax II Rotarix RotaShield Meruvax II Varivax
Immunosuppressants	*Indications for use:* Used to treat severe rheumatoid arthritis and to prevent and treat rejection of transplanted organs *Desired effects:* Work by inhibiting body's normal immune response *Side effects*: Abdominal discomfort, swollen and painful gums, acne, increased hair growth, headache, diarrhea, nausea, flushing, cramps	cyclosporine azathioprine prednisone	Sandimmune Neoral Imuran Deltasone
Laxatives	*Indications for use:* Used to relieve constipation *Desired effects:* Work by promoting defecation of normal, soft stool *Side effects*: Bloating, cramping, flatulence, diarrhea, nausea, dehydration	bisacodyl magnesium hydroxide polyethylene senna lactulose psyllium	Dulcolax* Milk of Magnesia* Miralax* ► Ex-Lax ► Senalax ► Constulose Metamucil*
Lipid-lowering agents	*Indications for use:* Used to lower cholesterol to reduce risk of myocardial infarction and stroke *Desired effects:* Work by inhibiting enzyme needed to synthesize cholesterol in body *Side effects*: Headache, diarrhea, constipation, muscle aches and weakness, nausea, vomiting, stomach upset, bloating, cramping	atorvastatin ezetimibe fenofibrate gemfibrozil lovastatin pravastatin rosuvastatin simvastatin	► Lipitor ► Zetia ► Tricor ► Lopid ► Mevacor ► Pravachol ► Crestor ► Zocor
Muscle relaxants (skeletal)	*Indications for use:* Used to treat acute painful musculoskeletal conditions *Desired effects:* Work by relaxing skeletal muscles *Side effects*: Headache, drowsiness, dizziness, dry mouth, nausea, blurred vision, stomach upset	baclofen cyclobenzaprine methocarbamol tizanidine	► Lioresal ► Flexeril ► Robaxin ► Zanaflex

Table 26.1 Classification of Drugs Based on Action—cont'd

Drug Category	Primary Use and Major Therapeutic Effects	COMMONLY PRESCRIBED DRUGS	
		Generic	Brand
Ophthalmic antiinfectives	*Indications for use:* Used to treat eye infections *Desired effects:* Work by destroying bacteria *Side effects*: Temporary blurred vision, tearing, eye redness, eye discomfort, allergic reaction	dexamethasone/tobramycin polymyxin/bacitracin polymyxin/neomycin polymyxin/trimethoprim tobramycin	TobraDex Polysporin Neosporin Polytrim Tobrex
Otic preparations	*Indications for use:* Used to treat ear conditions		
	Analgesics *Desired effects:* Work by relieving ear pain *Side effects*: Allergic reaction	Benzocaine	Auralgan
	Antiinfectives *Desired effects:* Work by treating otitis externa *Side effects:* Temporary stinging or burning in the ear, allergic reaction	neomycin/polymyxin/hydrocortisone ofloxacin	Cortisporin Otic Floxin Otic
	Cerumenolytics *Desired effects:* Work by softening cerumen *Side effects*: Temporary decrease in hearing and feeling of fullness in the ear	carbamide peroxide	Debrox*
Platelet inhibitors	*Indications for use:* Used to reduce incidence of myocardial infarction and stroke *Desired effects:* Work by interfering with ability of platelets to adhere to each other *Side effects*: Itching, eczema, rash, head or joint pain, bruising, diarrhea, stomach upset	clopidogrel salicylates	► Plavix Aspirin*
Sedatives and hypnotics	*Indications for use:* Used for short-term treatment of insomnia *Desired effects:* Work by promoting sleep by central nervous system depression *Side effects*: Burning or tingling in the extremities, change in appetite, constipation, diarrhea, dizziness, daytime drowsiness, loss of coordination, headache, mental slowing, stomach pain, unusual dreams	flurazepam hydroxyzine eszopiclone phenobarbital temazepam zaleplon zolpidem	Dalmane (IV) Atarax Vistaril ► Lunesta (IV) Luminal (IV) ► Restoril (IV) ► Sonata ► Ambien (IV)
Smoking deterrents	*Indications for use:* Used to manage nicotine withdrawal to cease cigarette smoking *Desired effects:* Work by providing nicotine during controlled withdrawal from cigarette smoking *Side effects*: Dry mouth, nausea, stomach pain, headache, dizziness, vision changes, sore throat, muscle pain	bupropion nicotine varenicline	Zyban Nicorette Gum* Nicotrol Inhaler Nicoderm Patch* Commit Lozenges* Chantix
Thrombolytic agents	*Indications for use:* Used for acute management of coronary thrombosis (myocardial infarction) *Desired effects:* Work by dissolving existing clots *Side effects*: Bleeding, arrhythmias, dizziness, headache, shortness of breath, allergic reaction	alteplase anistreplase reteplase streptokinase	Activase Eminase Retavase Streptase
	Thyroid Hormones	levothyroxine	► Synthroid
Thyroid preparations	*Indications for use:* Used as replacement or substitute therapy for diminished or absent thyroid functioning of many causes *Desired effects:* Work by increasing basal metabolic rate *Side effects*: Hair loss, fast or irregular heart rate, hot flashes, irritability, sweating, mood changes, insomnia, vomiting, diarrhea, appetite changes, weight changes		

Continued

Table 26.1 Classification of Drugs Based on Action—cont'd

Drug Category	Primary Use and Major Therapeutic Effects	COMMONLY PRESCRIBED DRUGS	
		Generic	Brand
	Antithyroid Agents	methimazole	Tapazole
	Indications for use: Used to treat hyperthyroidism *Desired effects:* Work by inhibiting thyroid hormone synthesis, reducing basal metabolic rate *Side effects*: Headache, drowsiness, dizziness, nausea, vomiting, stomach upset, itching, muscle, joint or nerve pain, hair loss		
Urinary tract antispasmodics	*Indications for use:* Used to treat overactive bladder function *Desired effects:* Work by inhibiting bladder contractions *Side effects*: Dry mouth, dry eyes, blurred vision, dizziness, drowsiness, constipation, diarrhea, stomach pain or upset, joint pain, headache	oxybutynin tolterodine	Ditropan ► Detrol
Vasopressors	*Indications for use:* Used to treat severe allergic reactions and cardiac arrest *Desired effects:* Work by increasing blood pressure and cardiac output and by dilating bronchi *Side effects*: Sweating, nausea, vomiting, pale skin, feeling short of breath, dizziness, weakness or tremors, headache, feeling nervous or anxious	epinephrine	Adrenalin EpiPen
Weight control agents	*Indications for use:* Used to manage obesity		
	Appetite Suppressants *Desired effects:* Work by suppressing appetite center in central nervous system *Side effects*: Nausea, vomiting, diarrhea, upset stomach, headache, blurred vision, nervousness, insomnia, dizziness, fatigue, dry mouth	diethylpropion phentermine sibutramine orlistat	Tenuate (IV) Fastin (IV) Meridia (IV) Xenical
	Lipase Inhibitors *Desired effects:* Work by inhibiting action of lipase to decrease absorption of dietary fats *Side effects*: Oily or fatty stools, orange or brown colored oil in stool, flatulence with an oily discharge, loose stools, increased number of bowel movements, stomach pain, nausea, vomiting		Alli*

►Top-200 most prescribed drugs.
(II), Schedule II drug; *(III)*, Schedule III drug; *(IV)*, Schedule IV drug.
*Available OTC (over the counter).

SYSTEMS OF MEASUREMENT FOR MEDICATION

Two systems of measurement are used in the United States for prescribing, administering, and dispensing medication: the metric system and the household system. The metric system is the most common system used to measure medication because it provides a more exact measurement and is easier to use. The household system is not as accurate as the metric system for the measurement of medication and usually is used only when a patient takes liquid medication at home.

Systems of measurement have units of weight, volume, and length. *Weight* refers to the heaviness of an item, and *volume* refers to the amount of space occupied by a substance. *Length* is a unit of linear measurement of the distance from one point to another. Although length is not used to administer medication, it is used in other aspects of the medical office. The head circumference of infants is measured in centimeters (cm), a metric unit of linear measurement.

To prepare and administer medication properly and to avoid medication errors, the medical assistant must have a thorough knowledge of the specific units of measurement for these two systems and must be able to convert within each system and from one system to another. A basic discussion of the metric and household systems is presented next. A more thorough study of these systems, including conversion of units and dose calculation, is included in Chapter 26 of the Study Guide.

METRIC SYSTEM

The metric system was developed in France in the latter part of the 18th century in an effort to simplify measurement. Most European countries are required by law to use this system for the measurement of weight, volume, and length. Overall, the metric system is used for most scientific and medical measurements. Pharmaceutical companies use the metric system to measure and label medications.

The metric system employs a uniform decimal scale based on units of 10, making it very flexible and logical. The basic metric units of measurement are the gram, liter, and meter. The *gram* is a unit of weight used to measure solids, the *liter* is a unit of volume used to measure liquids, and the *meter* is a linear unit used to measure length or distance. The metric units used most often in the administration of medication in the medical office are the milligram, gram, milliliter, and cubic centimeter. Because a **cubic centimeter** (cc) is the amount of space occupied by 1 milliliter (mL), these two units can be used interchangeably (i.e., 1 mL = 1 cc).

Prefixes added to the words *gram, liter*, and *meter* designate smaller or larger units of measurement in the metric system. The same prefixes are used with all three units. For example, *milli-* is used as follows: *milli*gram, *milli*liter, and *milli*meter. A prefix changes the value of the basic unit of measurement by the same amount. The prefix *milli-* describes a unit that is 1⁄1000 of the basic unit: 1 gram is equal to 1000 milligrams, 1 liter is equal to 1000 milliliters, and 1 meter is equal to 1000 millimeters. Box 26.1 *Metric Notation Guidelines* lists the metric units of measurement and equivalent values in different units. Specific guidelines are used in the medical notation of metric units and doses, which also are presented in the box. To read prescriptions and medication orders, to document medication administration, and, most important, to avoid medication errors, the medical assistant must be familiar with and be able to follow these guidelines.

HOUSEHOLD SYSTEM

The household system is more complicated and less accurate for administering liquid medication than the metric system. Nevertheless, most individuals are familiar with this system because of its frequent use in the United States. This system of measurement may be the only one the patient can understand and safely use to take liquid medication at home. Most patients are more comfortable measuring medication in teaspoons than in milliliters. In addition, the patient is more likely to have household measuring devices on hand than to have metric measuring devices. If a precise measurement is needed, however, the metric system must be used, and the medical assistant should instruct the patient in the use of the metric measuring device.

BOX 26.1 Metric Notation Guidelines

Follow these guidelines when using the metric notation of measurement and dosage.

1. The units of metric measurement are written using the following abbreviations.

   Weight

   microgram: mcg
   milligram: mg
   gram: g
   kilogram: kg

   Volume

   milliliter: mL
   liter: L

2. Do not use a period with the abbreviations for metric units because the period might be mistaken for another letter or symbol.

   Correct: mg
   mL
   Incorrect: mg.
   mL.

3. Place the numeral that expresses the quantity of the dose in front of the abbreviation. To make it easier to read, leave a (single) space between the quantity and the abbreviation.

   Correct: 5 mL
   Incorrect: mL 5
   5 mL

4. Write a fraction of a dose as a decimal rather than a fraction.

   Correct: 0.5 g
   Incorrect: ½ g

5. If the dose is a fraction of a unit, place a zero before the decimal point as a means of focusing on the fractional dose. This reduces the possibility of misreading the dose as a whole number.

   Correct: 0.5 g (this reduces the possibility of not seeing the decimal point and reading the dose as 5 grams)
   Incorrect: .5 g

6. Do not place a decimal point and a zero after a whole number. The decimal point may be overlooked, resulting in a 10-fold overdose error.

   Correct: 1 mL (this reduces the possibility of not seeing the decimal point and reading the dose as 10 mL)
   Incorrect: 1.0 mL

Metric System: Conversion of Equivalent Values

Weight

1000 micrograms = 1 milligram
1000 milligrams = 1 gram
1000 grams = 1 kilogram

Volume

1000 milliliters = 1 liter
1000 liters = 1 kiloliter
1 milliliter = 1 cubic centimeter

Table 26.2 Household System: Conversion of Common Values

Abbreviations	
drop	gtt
teaspoon	tsp
tablespoon	T
ounce	oz
cup	c
Volume	
60 gtt =	1 tsp
3 tsp =	1 T
6 tsp =	1 oz
2 T =	1 oz
6 oz =	1 teacup
8 oz =	1 glass

Table 26.3 Equivalences in Household and Metric Units (Volume)

Household	Metric
1 gtt	= 0.06 mL
15 gtts	= 1 mL (1 cc)
1 tsp	= 5 (4) mL*
1 T	= 15 mL
2 T	= 30 mL
1 oz	= 30 mL
1 teacup	= 180 mL
1 glass	= 240 mL

*The American standard teaspoon is accepted as 5 mL; however, 4 mL can be used as the equivalent to provide a more accurate conversion.

Volume is the only household unit of measurement used to administer medication. The basic unit of liquid volume in the household system is the *drop (gtt)*, which is approximately equal to 0.6 mL in the metric system. These two units cannot be considered exact equivalents because the size of the drop varies based on temperature, the viscosity of the liquid, and the size of the dropper. The remaining units, in order of increasing volume, are *teaspoon*, *tablespoon*, *ounce (fluid ounce)*, *cup*, and *glass*. Table 26.2 lists the units of liquid volume measurement in the household system and equivalent values in different units.

CONVERTING UNITS OF MEASUREMENT

Changing from one unit of measurement to another is known as **conversion.** Conversion is required when medication is ordered in a unit of measurement that differs from the medication's label. The dose quantity must be mathematically translated or converted to the unit of measurement of the medication on hand. If the provider orders 5 grams of an oral solid medication, and the medication label expresses the drug strength in milligrams, the medical assistant would need to convert the grams into milligrams to know how much medication to administer. Converting units of measurement can be classified into the following categories: (1) conversion of units within a measurement system, and (2) conversion of units from one measurement system to another.

Converting units within a measurement system allows a quantity to be expressed in two different but equal units of measurement within *one* system. An example of converting units of weight within the metric system is as follows: 1 gram is equal to 1000 milligrams. Converting from one measurement system to another allows a quantity written in one measurement system to be expressed in an equivalent unit of measurement in *another* system. An example of a conversion from the metric system to the household system is as follows: 5 milliliters (metric system) is equivalent to 1 teaspoon (household system).

Conversion requires the use of a conversion table to indicate the equivalent values of various units of measurement. Conversion tables of equivalent values are included in this chapter:

- Metric conversion—Box 26.1: *Metric Notation Guidelines*
- Household conversion—Table 26.2: *Household System*

Tables used to convert from one system to another consist of approximate rather than exact equivalents, and a 10% error usually occurs in making these conversions. Conversion tables used to convert from the household system to the metric system are presented in Table 26.3.

The medical assistant must be careful to avoid errors in interpolation when using conversion tables. The numbers on conversion tables are small and close together; it is easy to misread the chart from one column to the other. To reduce this possibility, a straightedge, such as a ruler, should be used when reading a conversion table.

CONTROLLED DRUGS

As a result of federal and state legislation, restrictions are placed on drugs that have potential for abuse that can lead to physical or psychological dependence. These drugs are known as **controlled drugs.** They are classified into five categories, called *schedules*, which are based on their accepted medical use and potential for abuse and dependence. Table 26.4 lists and describes each schedule and provides examples of drugs included in each schedule.

To administer, prescribe, or dispense controlled drugs, a provider must register with the Drug Enforcement Administration (DEA). The provider is assigned a registration number known as the **DEA number.** Each time a prescription for a controlled drug is authorized, the provider must include their DEA number on the prescription. The provider must renew their DEA number every 3 years.

Table 26.4 Classification of Controlled Drugs

Classification	Description and Prescription Regulations	EXAMPLES Generic	Brand
Schedule I	High potential for abuse Currently no accepted medical use in treatment in the United States There is a lack of accepted safety for use of the drug under medical supervision Use may lead to severe physical or psychological dependence May be used for research with appropriate limitations Not available for prescribing	GHB Heroin LSD MDMA ("ecstasy") Mescaline methaqualone (Quaalude) psilocybin	
Schedule II	High potential for abuse Currently accepted medical use in treatment in the United States or a currently accepted medical use with severe restrictions Abuse may lead to severe psychological or physical dependence No refills allowed Manufacturer's label marked C-II	**Analgesics**	
		cocaine	
		codeine	
		fentanyl	Duragesic
		hydrocodone combined with nonopioid analgesic	Vicodin, Lortab, Lorcet, Tussionex, Vicoprofen
		hydromorphone	Dilaudid
		meperidine	Demerol
		methadone	Dolophine
		morphine	MS Cotin
		oxycodone	OxyContin
		oxycodone/acetaminophen (APAP)	Percocet
		oxycodone/aspirin (ASA)	Percodan
		Central Nervous System Stimulants	
		dextroamphetamine	Adderall
		lisdexamfetamine	Vyvanse
		methylphenidate	Ritalin, Concerta
		methamphetamine	Desoxyn
		Sedatives/Hypnotics	
		amobarbital	Amytal
		glutethimide	Doriden
		pentobarbital	Nembutal
		secobarbital	Seconal
Schedule III	Less potential for abuse than drugs in Schedules I and II Currently accepted medical use in treatment in the United States Abuse may lead to moderate or low physical dependence or high psychological dependence If authorized by provider, prescription can be refilled up to five times within 6 months from issue date Manufacturer's label marked C-III	**Anabolic Steroids**	
		oxandrolone	Anavar
		oxymetholone	Anapolon
		Analgesics	
		buprenorphine	Suboxone Buprenex
		butalbital compound	Fioricet, Fiorinal
		codeine combined with nonopioid analgesic	Tylenol w/ Codeine, Empirin w/ Codeine
		Central Nervous System Stimulant	
		benzphetamine	Didrex
		Male Hormone	
		testosterone	Depotest, Delatestryl
		Sedative/Hypnotic	
		butabarbital	Butisol

Continued

Table 26.4 Classification of Controlled Drugs—cont'd

Classification	Description and Prescription Regulations	EXAMPLES Generic	Brand
Schedule IV	Lower potential for abuse than drugs in Schedule III Currently accepted medical use in treatment in the United States Abuse may lead to limited physical or psychological dependence If authorized by provider, prescription can be refilled up to five times within 6 months of issue date Manufacturer's label marked C-IV	**Analgesics**	
		butorphanol	Stadol
		pentazocine	Talwin
		propoxyphene	Darvon Darvocet-N
		Antianxiety Agents	
		alprazolam	Xanax
		chlordiazepoxide	Librium
		diazepam	Valium
		halazepam	Paxipam
		lorazepam	Ativan
		meprobamate	Equanil
		oxazepam	Serax
		Anticonvulsant	
		clonazepam	Klonopin
		Central Nervous System Stimulants	
		modafinil	Provigil
		pemoline	Cylert
		Sedatives/Hypnotics	
		chloral hydrate	Noctec
		eszopiclone	Lunesta
		ethchlorvynol	Placidyl
		flurazepam	Dalmane
		midazolam	Versed
		phenobarbital	Luminal
		temazepam	Restoril
		triazolam	Halcion
		zaleplon	Sonata
		zolpidem	Ambien
		Weight Control Agents	
		diethylpropion	Tenuate
		phentermine	Fastin
		sibutramine	Meridia
Schedule V	Low potential for abuse Accepted medical use in United States Abuse may lead to limited physical or psychological dependence Prescribing policies determined by state and local regulations. In most states: • Number of refills determined by provider • Prescription expires 1 year from the date it was filled. • Manufacturer's label marked C-V	Cough suppressants with small amounts of codeine	Robitussin A-C Cheracol syrup
		Antidiarrheals containing paregoric	Parepectolin Kapectolin PG
		diphenoxylate/atropine	Lomotil

PRESCRIPTION

A **prescription** is an order from a licensed provider (e.g., physician, physician's assistant, nurse practitioner) authorizing the dispensing of a drug by a pharmacist. Prescriptions can be authorized in different forms, including handwritten and computer-generated printed prescriptions, or they can be sent electronically, telephoned, or faxed, to a pharmacy. Over the past decade, there has been a substantial increase in the electronic prescribing of medication, known as *e-prescribing*, which is discussed in more detail later in this section.

Abbreviations and symbols are usually used to write a prescription. They also are used to document medication information in the patient's medical record. Common abbreviations used in the medical office for writing prescriptions are included in Table 26.5.

If the provider handwrites prescriptions on a prescription form, the medical assistant should ensure that all prescription pads are kept in a safe place and out of reach of individuals who may want to obtain drugs illegally. The stock supply of prescription pads should be locked in a drawer.

PARTS OF A PRESCRIPTION

A prescription consists of directions to the pharmacist for filling the prescription and instructions to the patient for taking the medication (Fig. 26.2). A prescription must include the following specific information:

- *Prescription Date.* A pharmacist cannot fill a prescription unless the date the prescription was issued is indicated on the prescription. The reason for this is that a prescription expires after a certain length of time. In most states, a prescription for a drug (with the exception of controlled drugs) expires 1 year from the date it was filled. After this time, any refills left on the prescription

Table 26.5 Common Abbreviations and Symbols Used in Medication Documentation

Abbreviation or Symbol	Meaning	Abbreviation or Symbol	Meaning
$\overline{aa}$	of each	OTC	over the counter
ac	before meals	oz	ounce
ad lib	as desired	$\bar{p}$	after
aq	water	pc	after meals
admin	administer, administration	Pt or pt	patient
AM or a.m.	morning	per	by
APAP	acetaminophen	PM or p.m.	evening
ASA	aspirin	po or PO	by mouth
bid	twice a day	prn	as needed
$\bar{c}$	with	qAM	every morning
cap(s)	capsule(s)	qh	every hour
DAW	dispense as written	q(2, 3, 4)h	every (2, 3, 4) hours
dil	dilute	qid	four times a day
g	gram	qs	of sufficient quantity
gtt(s)	drop(s)	Rx	prescription
h or hr	hour	$\bar{s}$	without
ID	intradermal	subcut	subcutaneous
IM	intramuscular	SL	sublingual
IV	intravenous	sol	solution
kg	kilogram	STAT	immediately
L	liter	T	tablespoon
liq	liquid	tab(s)	tablet(s)
mcg	microgram	tid	three times a day
med(s)	medication(s)	tsp	teaspoon
mg	milligram	#	number
min	minute	×	times
mL	milliliter		no, none
NPO	nothing by mouth		

Larry Douglas, M.D.
11 West Union Street
Athens, OH 45701

Phone 740-555-8993 FAX 740-555-7222

Patient Name Holly Roberts DOB 10/1/XX
Address 72 Hill St., Athens, OH 45701 Age 24
Date 07/12/XX

℞ } Superscription

Inscription { Amoxil 250 mg capsule

Subscription { Disp: #30 (thirty) capsules

Signatura { Sig: Take 1 capsule orally 3 times a day for 10 days

☐ Dispense as Written

Refill (NR) 1 2 3 4 5

Signature Larry Douglas, M.D.
DEA #

Fig. 26.2 Example of a handwritten prescription.

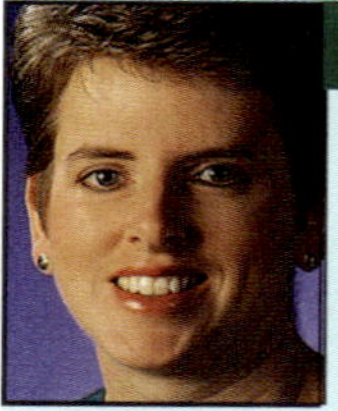

Putting It All into Practice

My name is Theresa, and I work for four physicians in a family practice medical office. I have worked there ever since I graduated from college with an associate's degree in medical assisting. One experience that I will never forget taught our entire office staff a valuable lesson. It involved a woman who came to our office because she had lacerated her wrist while using a butcher knife. After the wound was sutured, I gave her a tetanus injection because she was past due for one. Shortly thereafter, she became very nauseated and dizzy, and I had her lie down on the examining table. She asked me to get her a cold drink of water, and I left the room to do so. Apparently, while I was gone, she must have tried to sit up or turn over because she rolled off the table and struck the back of her head on the floor. She sustained a laceration to her scalp, which also had to be sutured. Owing to her persistent symptoms of severe nausea, vomiting, and headache, it was decided that she should be admitted to the hospital for neurologic observation and x-ray studies.

The vital lesson that this experience taught everyone in our office was that you must never leave a patient alone, not even for a minute to get something, if there is the slightest indication that he or she is not feeling perfectly fine. Another staff member should be called to obtain whatever is needed. From that point on, this has been our office policy and procedure. ■

cannot be filled and a new prescription must be issued by the provider.

- *Provider's name, address, telephone number, and fax number.* This information is preprinted on prescription forms that are handwritten and automatically printed on forms that are computer generated. This information identifies the provider issuing the prescription and provides the necessary information should the pharmacist have a question and need to contact the medical office.
- *Patient's name and address.* This information is important for insurance billing and for properly dispensing the medication.
- *Patient's date of birth and age.* It is important to include the patient's age on the prescription so that the pharmacist can double-check the provider's order to ensure the proper dose is being dispensed based on the patient's age. The most common errors in dosage occur among children and the elderly, who may not require the standard dose of a drug because patients in these age groups metabolize drugs differently. Knowing the patient's age also allows the pharmacist to double-check that the drug is age appropriate for the patient. For example, ciprofloxacin (e.g., Cipro) should not be taken by children and adolescents because this antibiotic can damage cartilage in individuals younger than 18 years.
- *Superscription.* The **superscription** consists of the abbreviation *Rx.* This abbreviation comes from the Latin word *recipe* and means "take."

- *Inscription.* The **inscription** identifies the name of the drug, the dose (e.g., Amoxil 250 mg), and the form in which the drug should be dispensed (e.g., capsule, tablet). Most drugs are available in various strengths; therefore, it is important that the correct dosage strength be prescribed. For example, Amoxil comes in the following strengths: 125 mg, 250 mg, and 500 mg.
- *Subscription.* The **subscription** designates the quantity of the drug to be dispensed. To prevent a prescription from being altered illegally, it is recommended that numbers as well as letters be used to indicate the quantity to be dispensed (e.g., #30 [thirty]).
- *Signatura.* The **signatura** (abbreviated *Sig.*) comes from the Latin term *signa,* which means "write" or "label." The signatura indicates the information to be included on the medication label. It consists of directions to the patient for taking the medication including how much of the drug to take (e.g., 1 capsule), the route of administration (orally), and how often and for how long to take the medication (e.g. 3 times a day for 10 days). The name of the medication is also included on the medication label so that the patient can identify the medication.
- *Refill.* This part of the prescription indicates the number of times the prescription may be refilled. If the medication cannot be refilled, this is indicated on the prescription form based on the setup of the form.
- *Provider's signature.* A prescription cannot be filled unless it is signed by the provider.
- *DEA number.* The number assigned to the provider by the Drug Enforcement Administration must appear on the prescription for a controlled drug. See Table 26.4 for examples of controlled drugs.

GENERIC PRESCRIBING

Generic prescribing means that the provider writes the prescription using the generic rather than the brand name of the drug. Because many pharmaceutical manufacturers may produce the same generic drug and sell it under different brand names, price competition often results. If the provider prescribes a drug using its generic name, the pharmacist is permitted to fill it with the drug that offers the best savings to the patient. In addition, most states allow the pharmacist the option of filling the prescription with a chemically equivalent generic drug, even if the drug has been prescribed by brand name. If the provider wants the prescription to be filled with a specific brand of drug, instructions must be indicated on the prescription form, such as "Dispense as Written (DAW)," or words of a similar meaning (see Fig. 26.2).

COMPLETING A PRESCRIPTION FORM

The provider is responsible for having accurate and pertinent information on the prescription form. If the provider so delegates, a prescription form can be completed by the medical assistant and signed by the provider. The provider must review the prescription thoroughly before signing it to ensure all of the information is correct. If the medical assistant is delegated this responsibility, they must carefully follow the important guidelines presented in Box 26.2.

BOX 26.2 Guidelines for Completing a Prescription Form

Using a Prescription Form

- Work in a quiet, well-lit area that is free of distractions.
- Use an indelible black ink pen to write on the form.
- Print all information on the form.
- Ensure that all information is spelled correctly.
- Review the metric notation guidelines presented in Box 26.1: *Metric Notation Guidelines.* (Most prescriptions are written in metric units.)
- Always ask the provider if you have questions about the prescription.
- Complete all of the required information on the form; it includes the following:
  1. Patient's name, address, date of birth, and age
     - Clearly print all of this information on the form. Never leave the address, date of birth, and age categories blank.
  2. Date
     - Indicate today's date on the prescription form.
  3. Name of the medication
     - The provider may prescribe the medication using either the generic or the brand name.
     - Make sure to spell the name of the drug correctly. If you are unsure, use a drug reference to find the correct spelling of a drug.
  4. Medication dosage
     - Never leave a decimal point "naked." If the dosage is a fraction of a unit, a zero must be placed before the decimal point as a means of focusing on the fractional dose. This reduces the possibility of misreading the dose as a whole number. *Example:* 0.5 mL (not .5 mL).
     - Never place a decimal point and a zero after a whole number because the decimal point may be overlooked, resulting in a 10-fold overdose error. *Example:* 5 mg (not 5.0 mg).
  5. Medication form
     - Indicate the medication form following the medication name and dosage. Examples of forms of medication include tablets, capsules, and ointment.
  6. Quantity to dispense
     - Use numbers and letters to indicate the quantity to be dispensed. *Example:* Disp: #30 (thirty).
     - Ensure that the quantity is correct. The number of prescribed pills should match the duration of treatment. *Example:* If the patient has been prescribed 3 tablets a day for 7 days, the quantity should be written as follows: Disp: #21 (twenty-one).

Continued

BOX 26.2 Guidelines for Completing a Prescription Form—cont'd

7. Directions for taking the medication
   - Clearly indicate the directions for taking the medication. Many authorities recommend writing the directions without abbreviations. *Example:* Sig: Take 1 capsule orally 3 times a day for 10 days.
8. Refills
   - Never leave this category blank.
   - If there are no refills, indicate this clearly on the form. The method for doing this is based on the setup of the preprinted form.
     Example: Refill:(NR)1 2 3 4 5
     (on this form, the information is circled)
     Example: Refill: Ø
     (on this form, the information is written in)
9. Dispense as written
   - If the provider does not allow a substitution (e.g., generic equivalent) for this medication, check this category.
10. DEA number
    - If the prescription is for a controlled drug, clearly indicate the provider's DEA number on the form.
11. Group practice
    - If there is more than one provider in the practice, circle (or check) the name of the provider prescribing the medication. This avoids confusion if the pharmacist cannot read the provider's signature.
      Example:
      James Ortman, MD, (Mark Rothstein, MD), Richard Bontrager, MD
    - Give the prescription to the provider to review and sign.
    - Document the prescription information in the patient's medication record. Give the prescription to the patient. Provide the patient with guidelines for taking the medication (see the *Patient Coaching* box on prescription medications).
    - Ask the patient whether they have any questions about the medication.

Using an EHR Prescription Program

1. Access the patient's electronic health record.
2. Access the prescription screen and verify the auto-filled information (i.e., date, patient name, date of birth, address, and age).
3. Select the correct medication from the drop-down menu.
4. The program will display a list of available dosage strengths (e.g., 250 mg, 500 mg) and dosage forms for that medication (e.g., tablets, oral suspension). Select the dosage strength and dosage form ordered by the provider using drop-down lists or check-boxes.
5. Select the dosage frequency and the route of administration using drop-down lists, check-boxes, or fill-in boxes.
6. Enter the correct information in the Refills field. This field should not be left blank; there should be either a number indicated or "no refills."
7. If the provider has indicated that there should be no substitution for this medication, the "Dispense as Written" radio button should be selected.
8. Forward the prescription to the provider for review and their electronic signature.
9. Send the prescription electronically to the pharmacy (or print a copy and have the provider review and sign it and then give it to the patient).
10. The prescription program automatically saves the prescription information in the patient's electronic medication record.

PATIENT COACHING Prescription Medications

To avoid adverse reactions, teach patients the proper guidelines for taking prescription medication. These guidelines are as follows:

- Know the names of all your prescription and nonprescription medications. Know the generic and brand names of each of your medications. Nonprescription drugs are known as over-the-counter (OTC) drugs; they are drugs that can be purchased without a prescription. Vitamin supplements and herbal products are considered OTC drugs.
- Know why you are taking each medication. It is important to know the desired therapeutic outcome, dose, frequency and time of administration, and common side effects of each medication, and guidelines ("do's and don'ts") to follow when taking the medication. Never take your medication in the dark or without your reading glasses (if needed for close vision).
- Take your medication exactly as prescribed, at the right times, and in the right amounts. The medication may not work properly if it is not taken as directed. If the dose is too small, the drug may not produce its intended therapeutic effect; exceeding the recommended dose could result in a toxic effect. Make sure you know what to do if you are late in taking a dose or miss a dose of your medication. It is also important to know if any other medication or food interferes with your medication and should be avoided.
- Inform the provider if new symptoms or adverse effects develop when you are taking the medication. The provider may need to change your dose or prescribe a different medication. There are usually alternative medications that the provider can prescribe to treat your condition.
- Take the medication for the prescribed duration of time, even after you begin to feel better. If you do not complete the entire course of drug therapy, your condition may recur. Not taking all of a prescribed antibiotic may cause an infection to return, and it may be worse than the first infection.
- Tell the provider if you decide not to take your medication. Otherwise, the provider may think your medication is not working. Not taking a medication prescribed by the provider could be serious because this may allow your condition to worsen.
- Do not take additional medications, including OTC medications, without checking with the provider. All drugs, including OTC medications, are designed to have an effect on the body.

PATIENT COACHING Prescription Medications—cont'd

Vitamin supplements and herbal products are considered OTC drugs. Some combinations of drugs cause serious reactions. In some cases, one drug cancels the effects of another and prevents it from working.

- Never take a medication that was prescribed for someone else. Providers prescribe medication based on an individual's age, weight, sex, and condition. Taking a medication prescribed for someone else can have serious results.
- Keep all medications in their original containers to avoid taking the wrong medication by mistake. Store your medications in their original containers from the pharmacy. Basic information about your medication is on the original container. Medications that are not clearly marked may be taken inadvertently by the wrong person.
- Store your medications in a safe place, away from the reach of children. If you have young children, make sure your medication is dispensed in containers with child-resistant safety closures. After taking your medication, make sure that the cap of the container is closed tightly. Accidental drug poisoning in children is a common and preventable problem. Also, do not take your medication in front of young children because they may want to mimic your behavior.
- Store medications in a cool, dry place or as stated on the label. Do not store capsules or tablets in the bathroom or kitchen because heat or moisture may cause the medication to break down.
- Properly discard unused portions of prescription medications and outdated OTC medications. Unused or expired medication should be disposed of as soon as possible to reduce the chance that individuals may accidentally take or misuse the medication. Because unwanted medications may pose a risk to human health and the environment, they should be disposed of properly. If a drug take-back program (described below) is not available, unused or expired medication should not be flushed down the toilet or drain unless the drug label or accompanying product package insert specifically instructs you to do so.

Disposal of Unwanted Medication

Medication can be safely disposed in the following ways:

1. **Drug Take-Back Programs**
   a. *Collection Events:* Federal, state, or local law enforcement may periodically host a community drug take-back day where residents drop off unwanted medication at a designated location during a specific time period.
   b. *On-Site Collection Receptacle:* Drug collection receptacles permanently located in specific locations such as pharmacies, health departments, and law enforcement locations allow individuals to safely dispose of unwanted medication.
   c. *Mail-Back Program:* Some pharmacies may offer mail-back envelopes to assist consumers in safely disposing of unwanted medication. The consumer places the medication in a specially-designed envelope which is shipped directly to a destruction facility.
2. **Household disposal:** If a take-back program is not available in the community, the following steps should be followed to dispose of unwanted medication:
   a. Remove the medication from its original container.
   b. Mix the medication with an undesirable substance, such as kitty litter or coffee grounds.
   c. Place the mixture in a disposable container such as a sealable plastic bag or an empty plastic container with a lid and discard it in the household trash.
   d. Remove personal information (including the prescription number) from an empty prescription medication container before discarding the container in the trash to protect the privacy of your personal health information. This can be accomplished by covering the information with a permanent marker or scratching it off. ■

ELECTRONIC PRESCRIBING

Electronic health record (EHR) software includes a prescription program for the electronic prescribing (*e-prescribing*) of medication. Electronic prescribing reduces medication errors, and the amount of time needed to prescribe and refill medication. The program allows the provider to issue a prescription with an electronic signature and then transmit it electronically to the patient's pharmacy. Many states now require the electronic prescribing of controlled drugs which increases security by sending the prescription information directly and securely to the pharmacy. The prescription program can also generate and print out a prescription, which is then signed by the provider and given to the patient (Fig. 26.3). Both of these features eliminate the need for the pharmacist to decipher the provider's handwriting.

To use a prescription program, the provider first selects the medication. The program then displays a list of available dosage strengths (e.g., 150 mg, 300 mg) and dosage forms (e.g., tablets, capsules, oral suspension) for that medication. The provider indicates the dosage strength and dosage form desired and enters the information into the computer. Next, the provider selects additional information related to the prescription, including dosage frequency, route of administration, and number of refills using fill-in boxes, drop-down lists, and check-boxes. The program automatically checks the prescription against any drug allergies the patient may have. It also checks for potential interactions with other medications being taken by the patient. The prescription program usually has the capability to compare the prescription against the *formulary* or list of drugs covered by the patient's insurance plan. If the prescription is not in the patient's formulary, the provider is advised of alternative drugs that are covered by the patient's insurance plan.

Once the provider has entered the prescription into the computer, the prescription information is automatically saved in the patient's electronic medication record. The prescription program also has the capability to quickly refill a prescription and produce a printout list of medications being taken by the patient. The patient can use this list to keep track of the medication they are taking (Fig. 26.4).

PRESCRIPTION: (Give to the pharmacist)	PRESCRIPTION: (Give to the pharmacist)
Huntington Clinic 701 Concord Ave Lexington, KY 48710 614-871-0033	Huntington Clinic 701 Concord Ave Lexington, KY 48710 614-871-0033
Doctor: John Blauser, MD	Doctor: John Blauser, MD
For: Danielle Travis Age: 28 DOB: 08/08/XX	For: Danielle Travis Age: 28 DOB: 08/08/XX
Date: 10/27/20XX	Date: 10/27/20XX
Address: 101 Coventry Lane Lexington, KY 48710	Address: 101 Coventry Lane Lexington, KY 48710
Rx: Amoxil (Generic - amoxicillin) (Dose/unit - 250 mg) (Form - Caps) (Disp - #30)(thirty) (Frequency - One three times daily for 10 days) (Route - By mouth) (Refills-0).	Rx: Tylenol-3 (Generic - Acetaminophen/Codeine) (Dose/unit - 1 to 2) (Form - Tabs) (Disp - #15)(fifteen) (Frequency - Every 4 hours as needed for moderate to severe pain) (Route - By mouth) (Refills-0).
Dr: *John Blauser, MD*	Dr: *John Blauser, MD*

Fig. 26.3 Example of a computer-generated prescription.

Huntington Clinic
701 Concord Ave
Lexington, KY 48710
614-871-0033

Patient: Clare Andrews
352 Pinewood Dr.
Lexington, KY 48710

Age/DOB: 12/25/xx
EMRN: 7016780

Medication List

Medication	Refills	Start
Abilify 15 mg tablet TAKE 1 TABLET DAILY	0	24Sep20XX
Acetaminophen-Codeine #3 300-30 mg tablet TAKE 1 TABLET EVERY 6 TO 8 HOURS AS NEEDED FOR PAIN	0	23Sep20XX
Clonazepam 1 mg tablet TAKE 1 TABLET EVERY 8 HOURS PRN	0	24Sep20XX
Etodolac CR 500 mg tablet extended release 24 hour 1-2 TABLETS PO ONCE DAILY WITH FOOD	0	21Sep20XX
Fish Oil 1000 mg capsule TAKE 1 CAPSULE DAILY	11	7Apr20XX
Flovent HFA 44 mcg/act aerosol INHALE 2 PUFFS TWICE DAILY	3	6Jan20XX
Fluticasone Propionate 50 mcg/act suspension USE 2 SPRAYS IN EACH NOSTRIL ONCE DAILY	3	9Sep20XX
Lamictal 200 mg tablet TAKE 2 TABLETS DAILY	0	24Sep20XX
Omeprazole 20 mg capsule delayed release TAKE 1 TABLET DAILY	11	24Sep20XX
Pamine 2.5 mg tablet TAKE 1 TABLET 3 TIMES DAILY	0	6Jan20XX
Proventil HFA 108 (90 base) mcg/act aerosol solution INHALE 1-2 PUFFS EVERY 4-6 HOURS AS NEEDED AND AS DIRECTED	3	21Jul20XX
Tramadol HCl 50 mg tablet TAKE 1 TABLET EVERY 6 HOURS	0	29Apr20XX
Voltaren 1% gel APPLY 2 GRAMS TOPICALLY 4 TIMES DAILY	6	24Sep20XX
WelChol 625 mg tablet TAKE 3 TABLETS TWICE DAILY WITH MEALS	11	29Apr20XX

Fig. 26.4 Example of a computer-generated patient medication list.

MEDICATION RECORD

Patient: John Walsh
Birthdate: 6/10/XX
ALLERGY: Ø

DATE	MEDICATION AND DOSAGE	FREQUENCY	RX	OTC	REFILLS	STOP
2/18/XX	Cipro 250 mg	ī q 12 h po x 10 days	X			2/28/XX
6/10/XX	Prevacid 15 mg	ī daily po	X			7/10/XX
6/10/XX	Lipitor 10 mg	ī daily po	X		1/6/XX	
6/10/XX	Prozac 20 mg	ī daily po	X		1/6/XX	
12/3/XX	Tobrex Ophthalmic Solution	ī drop q3h Ⓡ eye	X			12/10/XX
2/5/XX	Echinacea	ī daily po		X		
3/15/XX	Nitrostat 0.4 mg	ī prn pain SL Rep q 5 min prn pain, not to exceed 3 tabs	X			
3/15/XX	Inderal 40 mg	ī bid po	X			
3/15/XX	St. Joseph's ASA Enteric Coated 81 mg	ī daily po		X		

Fig. 26.5 Example of a medication record using a preprinted form.

MEDICATION RECORD

A medication record (Fig. 26.5) includes detailed information about each medication so that the provider can tell at a glance what medications and how much the patient is taking. Both prescription medications and OTC medications, including vitamin supplements and herbal products, must be documented in the medication record.

The medication record is part of the patient's medical record. The medical assistant is often responsible for documenting medication information in the medication record. Care must be taken to ensure the information is correct and clearly stated.

In a paper-based patient record (PPR), the medical office may use a preprinted form to document the medication that a patient is taking. With an EHR, the medical assistant enters this information into a digital form on the screen of the monitor using free text entry, drop-down lists, and check-boxes.

A medication record typically includes the following information:

- Patient's name and date of birth
- Any drug allergies
- Date the medication was prescribed (for prescription medications) or date the patient started taking the medication (for OTC medications)
- Name and dose of the medication
- Frequency of administration of the medication
- Route of administration
- Prescription or OTC medication category
- Refills (prescription medication only)
- Date the patient stopped taking the medication

What Would You Do? What Would You *Not* Do?

Case Study 2

Linda Cardwell calls the medical office. Her daughter Rachel, 9 years old, was seen in the office 10 days ago. Rachel was diagnosed with strep throat, and the provider ordered Amoxil 250 mg capsule 3 times a day by mouth for 7 days. Mrs. Cardwell says that after 3 days of taking the medication Rachel was much better, so she stopped giving her the Amoxil because it was causing her to have diarrhea. Mrs. Cardwell says that her 12-year-old son started feeling achy all over and she gave him the Amoxil for 2 days, and it seemed to help. She also says that her husband started complaining of sinus problems, so she also gave him the Amoxil for 2 days. Mrs. Cardwell says that now Rachel's throat is hurting again, and she has a fever. She wants to know whether Rachel has developed another case of strep throat. Mrs. Cardwell says she does not know what to do because she does not have any Amoxil left to give Rachel. ■

FACTORS AFFECTING DRUG ACTION

THERAPEUTIC EFFECT

Each drug has an intended therapeutic effect—the reason the patient takes the medication. Certain factors affect the therapeutic action of drugs in the body, causing patients to respond differently to the same drug. Because of this, the drug therapy may need to be adjusted to meet these variations, which include the following.

Age

Children and the elderly tend to respond more strongly to drugs than young and middle-aged adults. The provider may calculate smaller doses for very young and geriatric patients.

Route of Administration

Medications administered by different routes are absorbed at different rates. Drugs administered orally are absorbed slowly because they must be digested first. Parenterally administered drugs are absorbed more quickly than orally administered drugs because they are injected directly into the body.

Size

A patient's body size has an effect on drug action. A thin individual may require a smaller quantity of a drug, and an obese individual may require more.

Time of Administration

A drug administered by the oral route is absorbed more rapidly when the stomach is empty than when it contains food. A drug may not produce the desired effect or may be absorbed too slowly if it is taken when food is present. Some drugs irritate the stomach's lining, however, and must be taken with food. The drug package insert or a drug reference should always be consulted to determine when a drug should be taken.

Tolerance

A patient taking a certain drug over a period of time may develop a tolerance to it. This means that the same dose of a drug no longer produces the desired effect after prolonged administration. The provider should be notified to determine whether a change of drug or dosage is needed.

UNDESIRABLE EFFECTS OF DRUGS

A drug may cause undesirable effects, which may occur immediately or may be delayed hours or even days after administration of the medication.

Adverse Reactions

Most drugs produce unintended and undesirable effects known as **adverse reactions.** Adverse reactions are secondary effects that occur along with the therapeutic effect of the drug. Some adverse reactions, referred to as *side effects*, are harmless and are often tolerated by the patient to obtain the therapeutic effect of the drug. Most patients are willing to tolerate the dry mouth and drowsiness that may accompany an antihistamine to obtain its therapeutic effect. Other adverse reactions, such as a decrease in blood pressure or an allergic reaction, can be harmful to the patient and warrant discontinuing the medication.

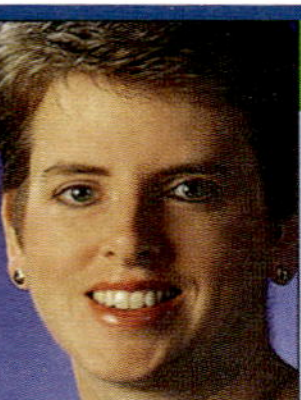

Memories *from* Practicum

Theresa: I can clearly remember the first time I gave an injection at my practicum site. I was worried that I would forget how to give an injection and look bad in front of my practicum supervisor and the patient. What made things worse is that the patient was a woman with very thin arms. I was giving her a flu shot, and I was so scared that the needle would hit her bone even though I was only using a 1-inch needle. When I walked into the room, my supervisor told the woman that I was a student and asked her if it was all right if I gave her the flu injection. The woman laughed and said, "Well, I guess so." That made me feel even more nervous. The patient then asked if it was my first shot. I told her "yes" and she said, "Just don't hurt me." When it came time to give the injection, everything that I had ever learned about injections came back to me. I gave the injection, and the woman told me I did a good job and that she didn't even feel it. That made me feel so good! My supervisor said, "If you can give a shot to her, you can give a shot to anyone." Every injection after that was a "piece of cake." I've learned just to take a deep breath before each difficult situation encountered in the office, and everything will work out. ■

Drug Interactions

When certain medications are used at the same time, drug interactions may produce undesirable effects. The medical assistant should inquire about other medications the patient is taking and document this information in the patient's medical record for review by the provider.

Allergic Drug Reaction

The patient may exhibit an allergic reaction to a drug. The reaction is usually mild and takes the form of a rash, rhinitis, or pruritus. Occasionally, a patient has a severe allergic reaction that occurs suddenly and immediately. This is known as an **anaphylactic reaction.**

An anaphylactic reaction is the least common but the most serious type of allergic reaction as it can be life-threatening. The early symptoms of an anaphylactic reaction begin with sneezing, urticaria (hives), itching, erythema, angioedema, and disorientation. *Erythema* is reddening of the skin caused by dilation of superficial blood vessels in the skin. *Angioedema* is a localized urticaria of the deeper tissues of the body. If not treated, the symptoms of an anaphylactic reaction quickly increase in severity and progress to dyspnea, cyanosis, and shock. Blood pressure decreases, and the pulse becomes weak and thready. Convulsions, loss of consciousness, and death may occur if treatment is not initiated soon enough.

To prevent an anaphylactic reaction to a drug or to reduce its danger, the medical assistant should stay with the patient after the administration of medication. The medical assistant should be especially alert for signs of an anaphylactic reaction after administering allergy skin tests or a penicillin or allergy injection. If a reaction occurs, the provider should be notified immediately so that treatment can be initiated as soon as possible. Treatment for an anaphylactic reaction consists of one or more injections of epinephrine; the number of injections depends on the severity of the reaction. Epinephrine goes to work immediately to reverse the life-threatening symptoms of an anaphylactic reaction. When the patient's condition has been stabilized, they are usually given an injection of an antihistamine. The antihistamine takes longer to begin working but helps alleviate urticaria, itching, angioedema, and erythema. The medical assistant must ensure that an ample supply of epinephrine is on hand at all times. Many offices maintain emergency crash carts for this purpose.

Idiosyncratic Reaction

An idiosyncratic reaction is an abnormal or peculiar response to a drug that is unexplained and unpredictable. Elderly patients are most prone to idiosyncratic reactions to drugs and should be monitored closely when they are taking a new medication.

PREPARATION AND ADMINISTRATION OF MEDICATION

To prevent medication errors, the medical assistant should follow these guidelines when preparing and administering any drug:

1. Work in a quiet, well-lit atmosphere that is free of distractions.
2. Always ask if you have a question about the medication order.
3. Know the drug to be given.
4. Select the proper drug. Check the label of the medication three times—as it is taken from its storage location, before preparing the medication, and after preparing the medication. Do not use a drug if the label is missing or is difficult to read.
5. Do not use a drug if the color has changed, if a precipitate has formed, or if it has an unusual odor.
6. Check the expiration date before preparing the drug for administration.
7. Prepare the proper dose of the drug. The term **dose** refers to the quantity of a drug to be administered at one time. Each medication has a dose range, or range of quantities of the drug that can produce therapeutic effects. It is important to administer the exact dose of the drug. A dose that is too small would not produce a therapeutic effect, and a dose that is too large could be harmful or even fatal to the patient.
8. Correctly identify the patient so that the drug is administered to the intended patient. When medication is administered, the patient should be identified by their full name and date of birth.
9. Before administering the medication, check the patient's records or question the patient to ensure that they are not allergic to the medication.
10. If you are giving an injection, determine the appropriate route and site at which to administer the injection; the route and site are dictated by the type of injection being given. An allergy injection is given by the subcutaneous route, and an antibiotic injection is given by the intramuscular route. The site must be free from abrasions, lesions, bruises, and edema.
11. Use the proper technique to administer the medication.
12. Stay with the patient after administering the medication.
13. Document information properly in the patient's medical record immediately after administering the drug. If using a PPR, include the date and time, the name of the medication, the manufacturer and lot number (if required), the dose given, the route of administration, the site of administration, and any unusual observations or patient reactions. Sign the recording with your name and credentials. If you administer a medication that contains a fraction of a unit, place a 0 before the decimal point (e.g., 0.5 mg, not .5 mg) so that the dose is not misread as 5 mg. A decimal point and a zero should never be placed after a whole number. The decimal point may be overlooked and misread, resulting in a 10-fold overdose error (e.g., 20 mg, not 20.0 mg). If using an EHR, document the name of medication, the manufacturer and lot number (if required), the dose given, the route of administration, and any unusual observations or patient reactions using the appropriate radio buttons, drop-down menus, and free text fields.
14. Always follow the seven "rights" of preparing and administering medication in the medical office:
    - Right patient
    - Right medication
    - Right dose
    - Right route
    - Right time
    - Right technique
    - Right documentation

ORAL ADMINISTRATION

The oral route is the most convenient and most used method for administering medication. **Oral administration** means that the drug is given by mouth in either a solid form (e.g., tablet, capsule) or a liquid form (e.g., suspension, syrup). Absorption of most oral medications occurs in the small intestine, although some may be absorbed in the mouth and stomach.

Many patients find it easier to swallow a tablet or a capsule with a glass of water. Water should not be offered after the patient has received a cough syrup, however, because the water would dilute the medication's beneficial effects. Unless the patient has a malabsorption problem or is unable to swallow the medication, the oral route is considered the safest and most desirable route for administering medication. Procedure 26.1 outlines the procedure for the administration of oral medications.

PARENTERAL ADMINISTRATION

The parenteral route of drug administration has several advantages. Medications given subcutaneously, intramuscularly, and intravenously are absorbed more rapidly and completely than medications given orally. In some cases, the parenteral route is the only way a drug can be given (e.g., insulin, most immunizations). If the patient is unconscious or has a gastric disturbance, such as nausea or vomiting, the parenteral route may be used to administer medication. Medical assistants are usually responsible for administering subcutaneous, intramuscular, and intradermal injections in the medical office. Intravenous medications are sometimes administered in the medical office but must be administered by health care workers thoroughly trained in IV medication administration.

The parenteral route also has disadvantages, such as pain and the possibility of infection as a result of breaking the skin. The medical assistant can minimize pain by inserting and withdrawing the needle quickly and smoothly and by withdrawing the needle at the same angle as for insertion. If injections are given repeatedly (e.g., allergy injections), the sites should be rotated to prevent the overuse of one site, which may cause irritation and tissue damage. Rotating sites also allows for better absorption of the drug.

When documenting the administration of a parenteral medication in the patient's medical record, the medical assistant must include the site of injection (e.g., right upper lateral arm, left ventrogluteal). This information provides a reference point should a problem arise with the injection site and allows a skin test site to be located if test results need to be read at a later date. It also assists in proper site rotation for patients who receive repeated injections to avoid overuse of a site.

Medical asepsis must be used when parenteral medications are administered. In addition, the needle and the inside of the syringe must remain sterile. These practices reduce the danger of microorganisms entering the patient's body during the administration of medication. The medical assistant must follow the OSHA standard when administering medication as a means of protecting themselves from bloodborne pathogens (see Chapter 17). Procedure 26.2 describes how to prepare an injection.

PARTS OF A NEEDLE AND SYRINGE

Needle

The needle for administering an injectable medication consists of several parts (Fig. 26.6). The *hub* of the needle fits onto the top of the syringe. The *shaft* of the needle is inserted into the body tissue. The opening in the shaft of the needle, known as the *lumen*, is continuous with the needle hub. Medication flows from the syringe and through the lumen of the needle. The *point* of the needle is located at the end of the needle shaft. The point is sharp so that it can penetrate body tissues easily. The top of the needle is slanted and is called the *bevel*. The bevel is designed to make a narrow, slitlike opening in the skin. This narrow opening closes quickly when the needle is removed to prevent leakage of medication, and it heals quickly.

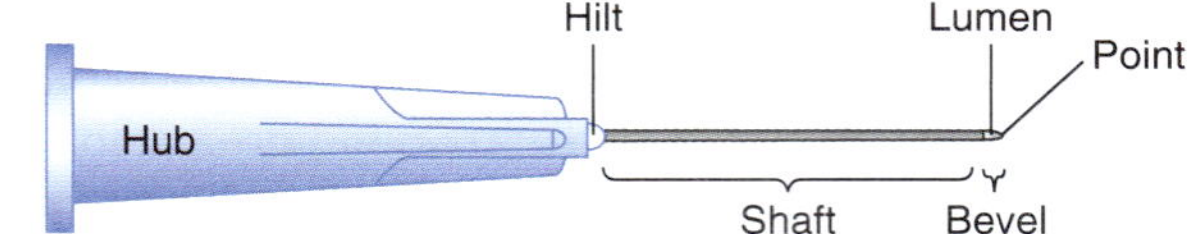

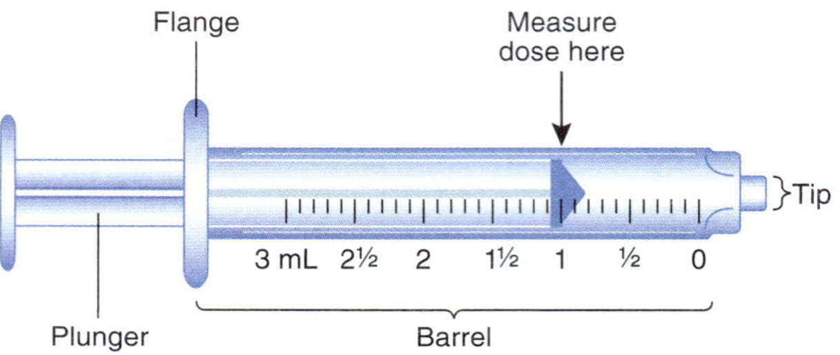

Fig. 26.6 Diagram of a needle and a 3-mL syringe, with parts identified.

The length of the needle ranges between ⅜ inch and 3 inches; the length used is based on the route of administration of the medication. For example, the needle used to administer an intramuscular injection must be longer than the one used for a subcutaneous injection so that the needle can penetrate deeply enough to reach muscle tissue. The length of the needle required also depends on the size of the patient. Administering an intramuscular injection to an obese adult requires a longer needle to reach muscle tissue than would be required for a normal-size adult. Administering an intramuscular injection to a thin patient requires a shorter needle to avoid inserting a needle too deeply and possibly penetrating the bone. Refer to Fig. 26.7 for examples of various needle lengths.

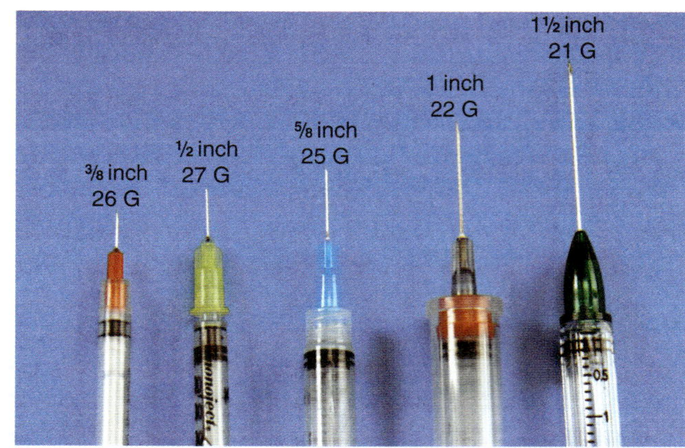

Fig. 26.7 Needle lengths and gauges.

Each needle has a certain gauge (G); needle gauges for administering medication range between 18 G and 27 G. The **gauge** of a needle refers to the diameter of the lumen of the needles; as the size of the gauge increases, the diameter of the lumen decreases (see Fig. 26.7). A needle with a gauge of 23 has a smaller lumen diameter than a needle with a gauge of 21. The gauge of the needle selected depends on the viscosity (thickness) of the medication being administered. Aqueous medications are thin and can be administered with a smaller lumen (higher gauge) needle. Thick or oily medications must be given with a large lumen (lower gauge) needle because they are too thick to pass through a smaller one. A needle with a larger lumen makes a larger needle track in the tissues. To reduce pain and tissue damage, a needle lumen with the smallest diameter appropriate for the solution and route of administration is always chosen.

Syringe

The syringe is used to draw up the medication and push it out through the needle into the patient's tissues. It is made of plastic and must be disposed of after one use. The syringe with an attached needle is packaged in a cellophane wrapper or a rigid plastic container. Information regarding the syringe's capacity and the needle's length and gauge is printed on the wrapper of the syringe and needle (Fig. 26.8). Syringes and needles also are available in separate packages. In this case, the medical assistant must attach a needle to the syringe before withdrawing medication into the syringe.

The parts of a syringe are the tip, barrel, flange, and plunger (see Fig. 26.6). The *tip* is the end of the syringe to which the needle hub attaches. The *barrel* of the syringe

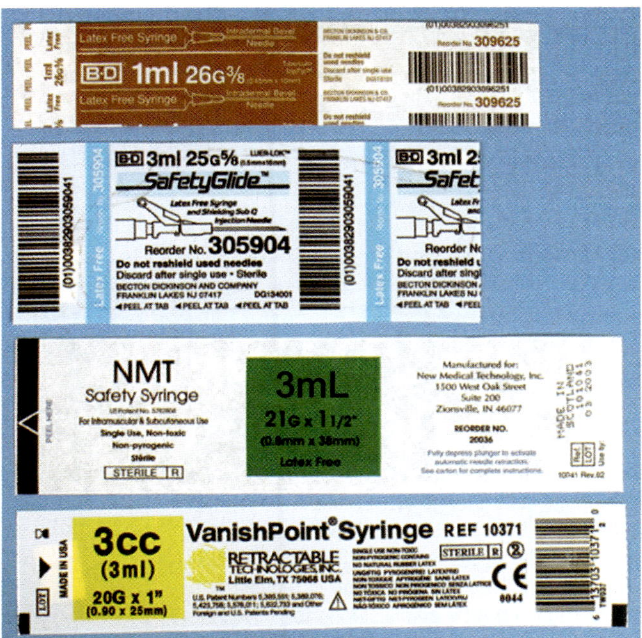

Fig. 26.8 Examples of syringe and needle packages labeled according to contents.

holds the medication and contains calibrated markings to measure the proper amount of medication. Syringes are usually calibrated in milliliters (mL), which is the unit of measurement used most often to administer parenteral medication. The medical assistant should become familiar with reading the graduated scales on syringes. At the end of the barrel is a rim known as the *flange*, which helps in injecting the medication. The flange also prevents the syringe from rolling when it is placed on a flat surface. The *plunger* is a movable cylinder with a seal tip that slides back and forth in the barrel. It is used to draw medication into the syringe when an injection is prepared and to push medication out of the syringe when an injection is administered. The medication should be measured at the widest part of the plunger seal closest to the needle (see Fig. 26.6).

Various types of syringes are available to administer injections. The choice is based on the type of injection being administered (e.g., tuberculin skin test [TST], insulin injection, antibiotic injection) and the amount of medication being administered. The types of syringes used most often in the medical office include hypodermic, insulin, and tuberculin (Fig. 26.9).

Hypodermic syringes are available in 2-, 2.5-, 3-, and 5-mL sizes and are calibrated in milliliters (or cubic centimeters). They are commonly used to administer intramuscular injections.

The *insulin syringe* is designed especially for the administration of an insulin injection, and the barrel is calibrated in units. The most common type is the U-100 syringe, which is calibrated into 100 units in increments of 2.

Tuberculin syringes are employed to administer a small dose of medication, such as when administering a TST. The tuberculin syringe has a capacity of 1 mL, and the calibrations are divided into tenths (0.10) and hundredths (0.01) of a milliliter.

Syringes also are available with capacities of 10, 20, 30, 50, and 60 mL; however, they are not used for administering medication, but rather for medical treatments, such as irrigating wounds and draining fluid from cysts.

SAFETY-ENGINEERED SYRINGES

OSHA stipulates requirements to reduce needlestick and other sharps injuries among health care workers. As discussed in Chapter 17, employers are required to evaluate and implement commercially available safer medical devices that reduce occupational exposure to the lowest extent feasible.

Safer medical devices include safety-engineered syringes. *Safety-engineered syringes* incorporate a built-in safety feature to reduce the risk of a needlestick injury. The three types of safety-engineered syringes most commonly used include the pivoting-shield syringe, the hinged-shield syringe, and the retractable needle syringe. Fig. 26.10 illustrates three types of safety-engineered syringes and the procedures for activating them.

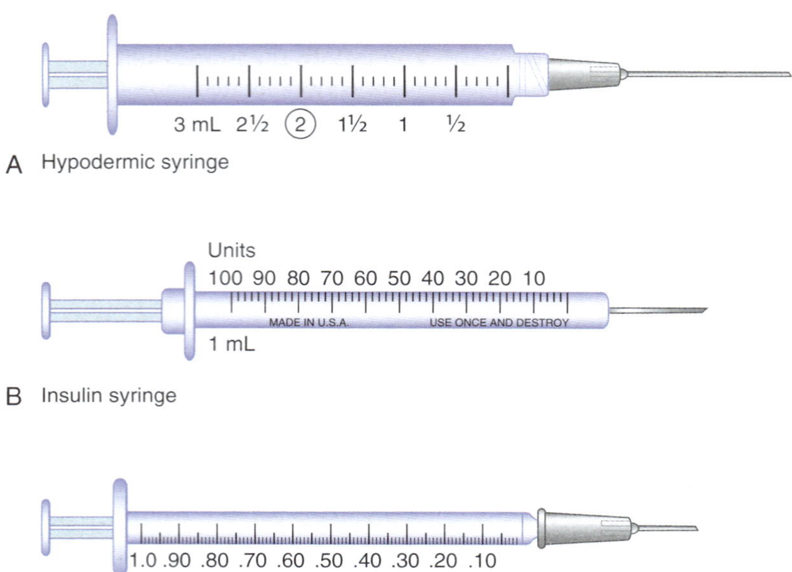

Fig. 26.9 Various syringes used to administer injections. (A) Hypodermic. (B) Insulin (U-100). (C) Tuberculin.

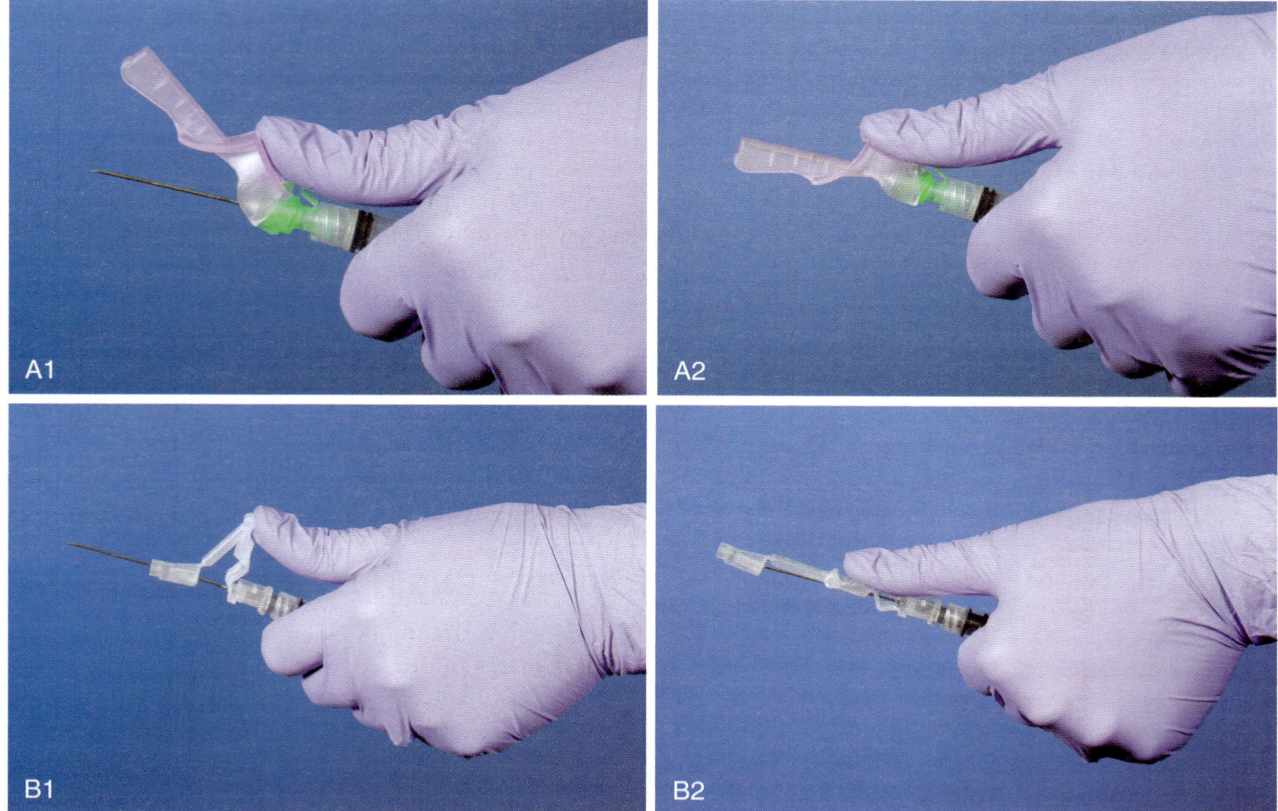

Fig. 26.10 Activation of safety-engineered syringes. (A) Pivoting-shield syringe (BD Eclipse Syringe). (1) After administering the injection, hold the syringe and needle away from yourself and others. Center the thumb (or forefinger) on the textured finger pad of the shield. (2) Push the shield forward until you hear a click and then visually confirm that the shield has fully encased the needle. Discard the syringe in a biohazard sharps container. (B) Hinged-shield syringe (BD Safety Glide Syringe). (1) After administering the injection, hold the syringe and needle away from yourself and others. Push the lever arm forward. (2) Continue pushing until the lever arm is fully extended and the needle tip is completely covered. Visually confirm that the needle tip is covered. Discard the syringe in a biohazard sharps container.

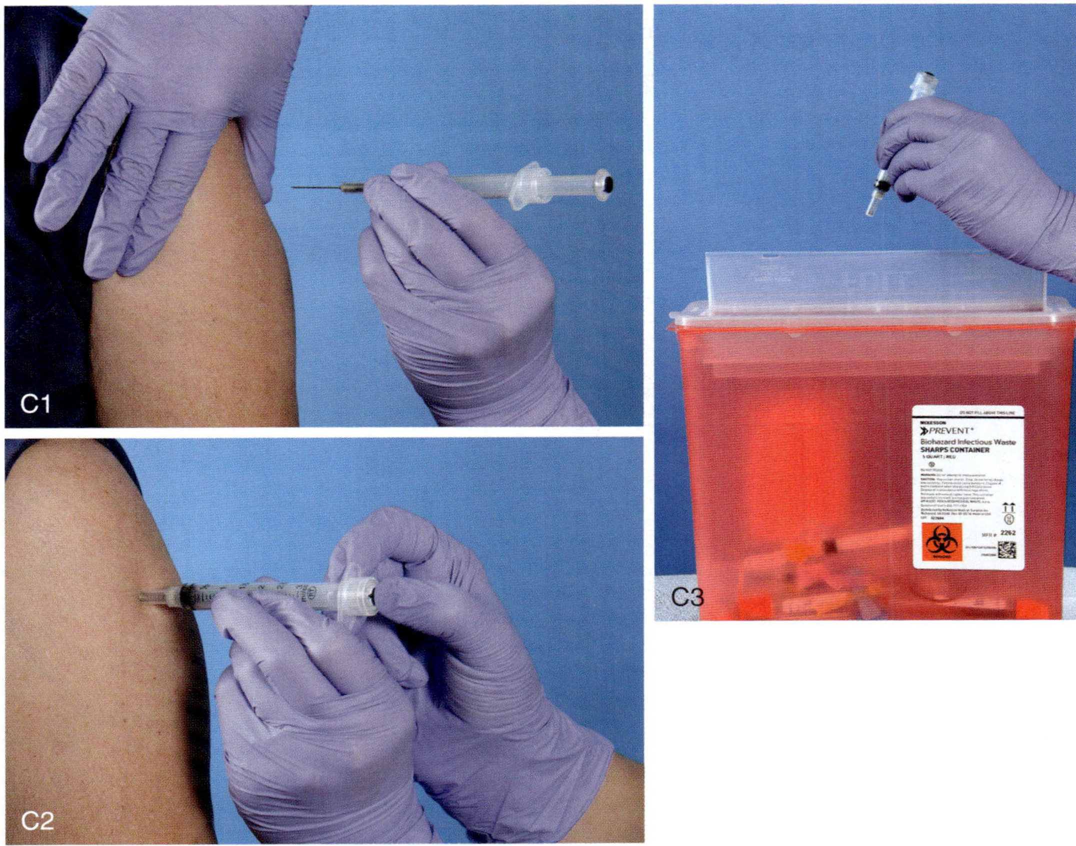

Fig. 26.10, cont'd (C) Retractable needle (Vanish Point Syringe). (1) Administer the injection by following the proper technique. (2) After administering the medication, continue depressing the plunger with the thumb. Use firm pressure past the point of initial resistance. This action delivers the full dose of medication to the patient and activates the needle retraction device, causing the needle to retract automatically from the patient's skin and into the barrel of the syringe. (3) Discard the syringe in a biohazard sharps container.

PREPARATION OF PARENTERAL MEDICATION

Medication used for injections is available in various types of dispensing units—vials, ampules, and prefilled syringes and cartridges.

Vials

A **vial** is a closed glass or plastic container with a rubber stopper; a soft metal or plastic cap protects the rubber stopper and must be removed the first time the medication is used. An injectable medication may be available in a single-dose vial, a multiple-dose vial, or both (Fig. 26.11). A vial is labeled with specific information as illustrated in Fig. 26.12.

Before the medication can be withdrawn, some vials require mixing (e.g., reconstituting a powdered drug, mixing a vial that separates on standing). Vials that require mixing should be rolled between the hands rather than shaken because shaking would cause the medication to foam, creating air bubbles that may enter the syringe when the medication is withdrawn.

To remove medication from a vial, an amount of air exactly equal to the amount of liquid to be removed is injected

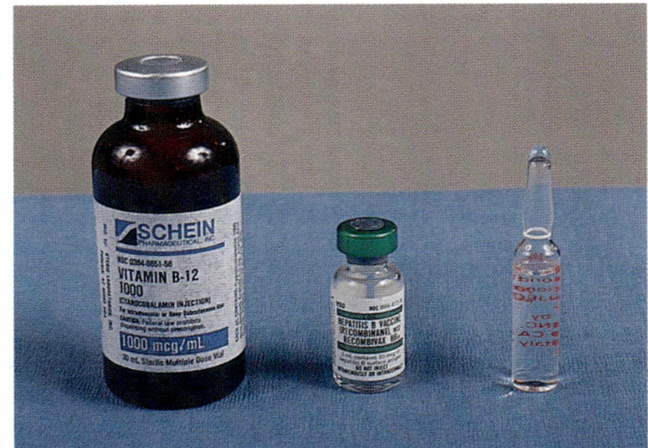

Fig. 26.11 The multiple-dose vial (left) and the single-dose vial (middle) consist of a closed glass container with a rubber stopper. The ampule (right) consists of a small, sealed glass container that holds a single dose of medication.

into the vial. The air should be inserted above the fluid level to avoid creating bubbles in the medication. If air is not injected first, a partial vacuum is created, and it is difficult to remove the medication. During the withdrawal of medication,

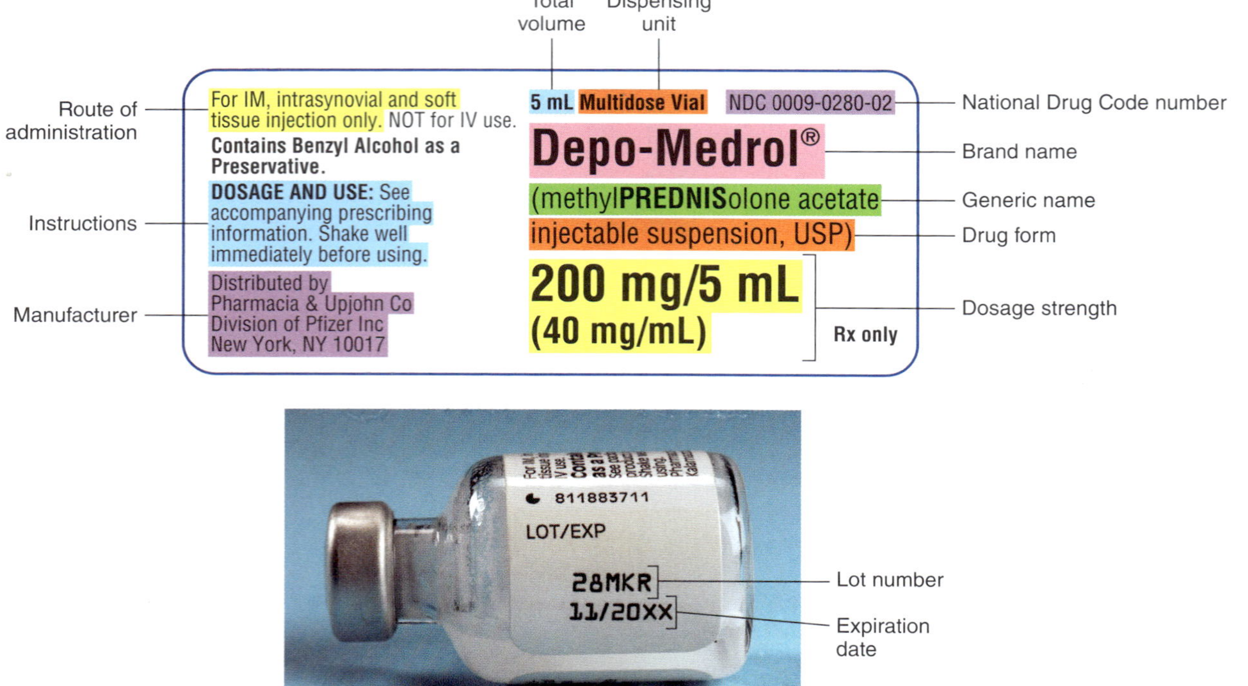

Fig. 26.12 Information included on the label of a medication vial.

the needle opening should be inserted below the fluid level to prevent the entrance of air bubbles into the syringe. Air bubbles can be removed by tapping the barrel of the syringe with the fingertips. If the bubbles are allowed to remain, they take up space that the medication should occupy, which would prevent the patient from receiving the full dose of medication.

Ampules

An **ampule** is a small, sealed glass container that holds a single dose of medication (see Fig. 26.11). An ampule has a constriction in the stem, known as the *neck*, which helps in opening it. Before opening, the medical assistant must ensure that there is no medication in the stem by tapping it lightly. A colored ring around the neck indicates where the ampule is prescored for easy opening. The ampule is opened by holding it firmly with gauze and breaking off the stem with a strong steady pressure.

A hazard with medication in ampules is the possibility of small glass particles getting into the ampule as the stem is broken off. When the medication is withdrawn into the syringe, the glass particles also might be withdrawn. To prevent this problem, a needle with a filter should be used that filters out small glass particles (Fig. 26.13).

The needle opening is inserted into the base of the ampule below the fluid level to withdraw medication. To prevent contamination, the needle should not be permitted to touch the outside of the ampule. Air should never be injected into the ampule because it could force out some of the medication.

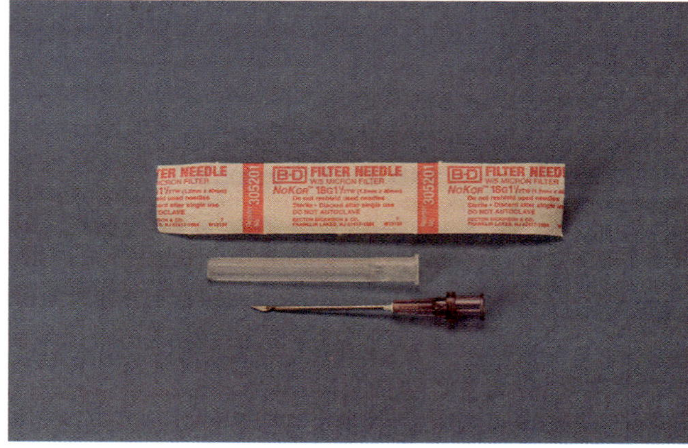

Fig. 26.13 Filter needle used to withdraw medication from an ampule.

Prefilled Syringes and Cartridges

Some medications are available in prefilled disposable syringes which contain a single dose of medication (Fig. 26.14A). Using this type of dispensing unit does not require drawing up the medication which helps reduce dosage errors and the time required to prepare the injection. The name of the drug,

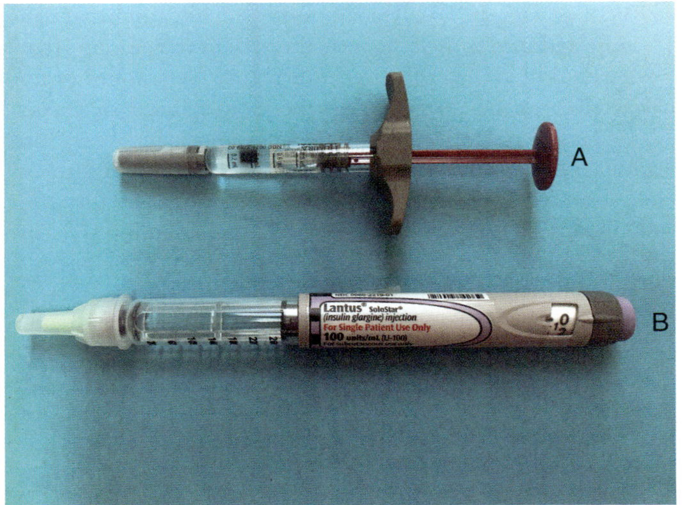

Fig. 26.14 (A) Prefilled disposable syringe. (B) Prefilled cartridge.

the dose, and the expiration date are printed on the syringe. Examples of medications that are available in a prefilled syringe include vaccines (e.g., influenza vaccine, COVID-19 vaccine) and injectable medications for rheumatoid arthritis (e.g., Humira).

Prefilled cartridges are also available for administering medication. The most common use of this type of dispensing unit are insulin pens (Fig. 26.14B). Insulin pens contain a prefilled insulin cartridge and are prescribed to insulin-dependent diabetic patients for administering insulin at home. Additional information on insulin pens is presented in Chapter 33: *Blood Chemistry and Immunologic Testing*.

STORAGE

The medical assistant should always read the drug package insert to determine the proper method for storing each parenteral medication because improper storage may alter the effectiveness of the medication.

RECONSTITUTION OF POWDERED DRUGS

Some parenteral medications are stable for only a short time in liquid form; these medications are prepared and stored in powdered form and require the addition of a liquid before administration. The process of adding a liquid to a powdered drug is known as *reconstitution.* The liquid used to reconstitute a powdered drug is known as the *diluent* and usually consists of sterile water or normal saline. The powdered drug is contained in a single-dose or multiple-dose vial and is accompanied by specific instructions for reconstitution. An example of a parenteral medication that requires reconstitution is the measles, mumps, and rubella (MMR) immunization (Fig. 26.15). The procedure for reconstituting powdered drugs is outlined in Procedure 26.3.

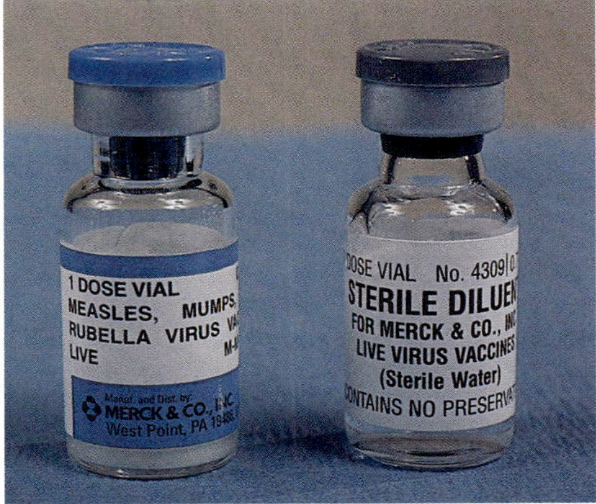

Fig. 26.15 The measles, mumps, and rubella (MMR) vaccine is a parenteral medication that requires reconstitution before administration. The vial on the left contains the medication in powdered form, and the vial on the right contains the sterile diluent.

TYPES OF INJECTIONS

In the medical office, medication is often administered through a subcutaneous injection, intramuscular injection and intradermal injection. Each of these are described as follows.

SUBCUTANEOUS INJECTION

A **subcutaneous injection** is made into the subcutaneous tissue, which consists of adipose (fat) tissue and is located just under the skin (Fig. 26.16). Subcutaneous tissue is located all over the body; however, certain sites are more commonly used because they are located where bones and

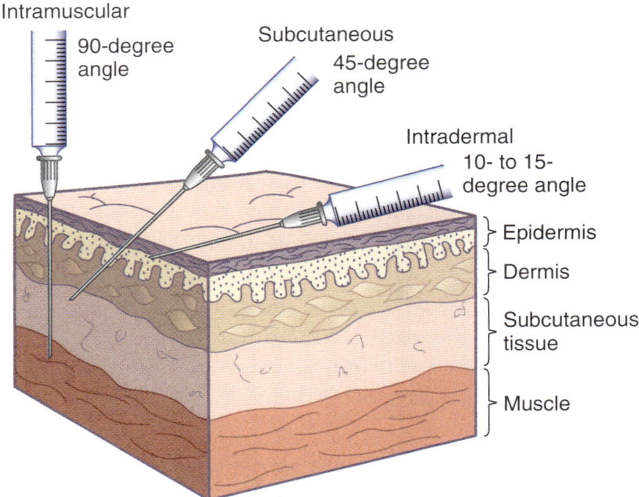

Fig. 26.16 Angle of insertion for intradermal, subcutaneous, and intramuscular injections.

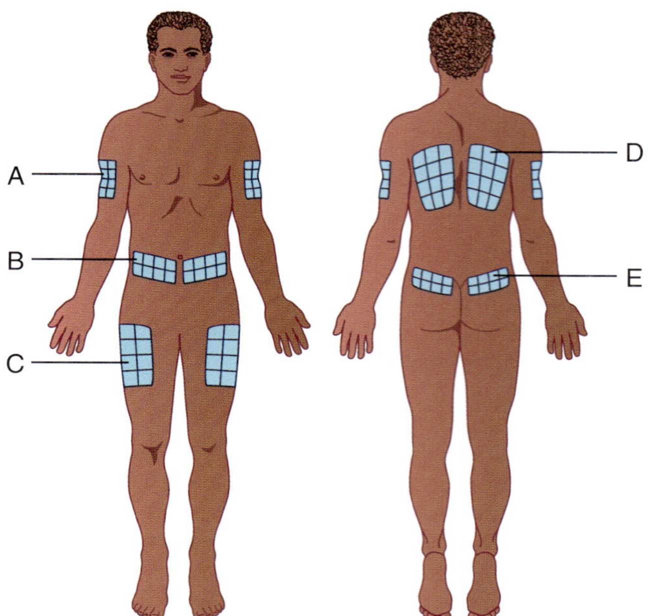

Fig. 26.17 Common sites for subcutaneous injections. (A) Upper lateral arm. (B) Lower abdomen. (C) Anterior thigh. (D) Upper back. (E) Flank region.

blood vessels are not near the surface of the skin. These sites include the upper lateral part of the arms, the anterior thigh, the upper back, and the lower abdomen (Fig. 26.17). Absorption of medication from a subcutaneous injection occurs mainly through capillaries, resulting in a slower absorption rate than with intramuscular injections. To ensure proper absorption, tissue that is grossly adipose, hardened, inflamed, or edematous should not be used as an injection site.

The needle length varies from ½ to ⅝ inch, and the gauge ranges from 23G to 25G. Elderly and dehydrated patients tend to have less subcutaneous tissue, and obese patients have more. The length of the needle should be adjusted accordingly to ensure the medication is administered into the subcutaneous tissue and not into muscle tissue.

Subcutaneous tissue is sensitive to irritating solutions and large volumes of medications; therefore, drugs given subcutaneously must be isotonic, nonirritating, nonviscous, and water-soluble. The amount of medication injected through the subcutaneous route should not exceed 1 mL. More than this amount results in pressure on sensory nerve endings, causing discomfort and pain.

Medications commonly administered through the subcutaneous route include epinephrine, insulin, and allergy injections. Patients who receive allergy injections must wait in the medical office for 15 to 20 minutes after the injection to be observed for an allergic reaction. Procedure 26.4 outlines the administration of a subcutaneous injection.

INTRAMUSCULAR INJECTION

Intramuscular injections are made into the muscular layer of the body, which lies below the skin and subcutaneous layers (see Fig. 26.16). The amount of medication that can be injected into muscle tissue is more than the amount that can be injected into subcutaneous tissue. An amount of up to 3 mL can be injected into the ventrogluteal or vastus lateralis muscles of an adult, although older and very thin adults are able to tolerate only 2 mL or less in these sites.

Absorption is more rapid by this route than by the subcutaneous route because there are more blood vessels in muscle tissue. Medication that is irritating to subcutaneous tissue is often given intramuscularly because there are fewer nerve endings in deep muscle tissue. Most parenteral medications administered in the medical office are given through the intramuscular route; examples include antibiotics, injectable contraceptives, vitamin B_{12}, corticosteroids, and most immunizations.

The needle for an adult must be long enough to reach muscle tissue and varies in length from 1 to 3 inches. A 1½-inch needle is typically used for an average-sized adult, whereas a 1-inch needle is often used for a thin adult or a child, and a needle length of 2 to 3 inches may be needed for an obese adult. The gauge of the needle used ranges from 18G to 23G, depending on the viscosity of the medication. Procedure 26.5 outlines the technique for the administration of an intramuscular injection.

Intramuscular Injection Sites

The sites chosen for intramuscular injections are away from large nerves and blood vessels. The medical assistant should practice locating these sites to become familiar with them. The area should always be fully exposed to permit clear visualization of the injection site.

Deltoid Site

The deltoid site can be used to administer an injection to an adult and children that are 3 years of age and older. This site is easily accessible and can be used when the patient is sitting or lying down. In most individuals the deltoid site is small and large amounts of medication (no more than 1 mL) and repeated injections should not be given in this area. This is the most common site used to administer vaccines (e.g., influenza vaccine).

When using the deltoid site, the medical assistant should make sure the entire arm is exposed by having the patient's sleeve completely pulled up or by removing the sleeve from the arm if it cannot be pulled up. A tight sleeve constricts the arm and causes unnecessary bleeding from the puncture site. In an adult, the deltoid site is located by palpating the lower edge of the acromion process and going two finger widths down from the acromion process. This forms the base of an inverted triangle with the midpoint of the triangle on the lateral side of the arm in line with the axilla. The injection is administered into the center of the triangle (Fig. 26.18A).

Vastus Lateralis Site

The vastus lateralis site is used because it is not near major nerves and blood vessels and is a relatively thick muscle.

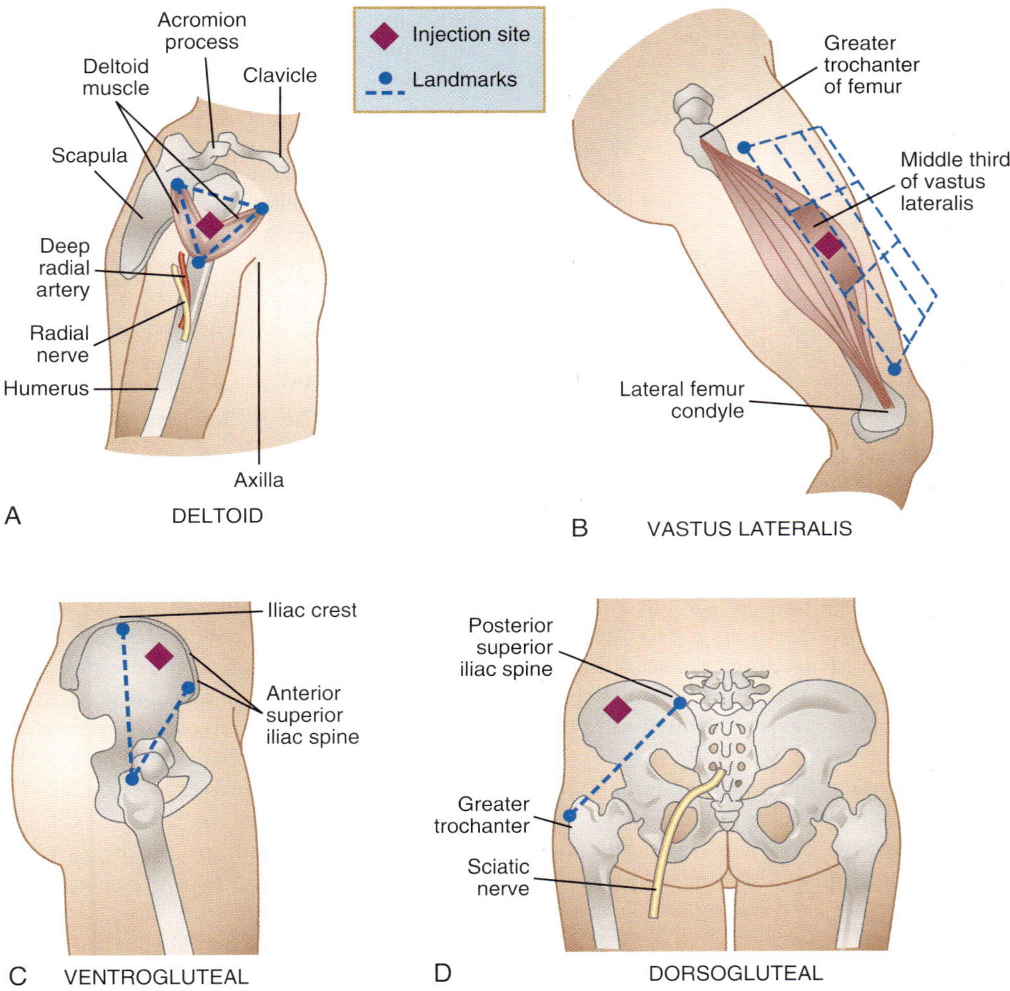

Fig. 26.18 Sites of intramuscular injections. (A) Deltoid muscle. (B) Vastus lateralis. (C) Ventrogluteal muscle. (D) Dorsogluteal muscle (From Leahy JM, Kizilay PE: *Foundations of nursing practice: a nursing process approach*, Philadelphia, 1988, Saunders.)

This site can be used for both children and adults and is particularly desirable for infants and children younger than 3 years of age. The area is bounded by the midanterior thigh on the front of the leg and the midlateral thigh on the side. In an adult, the proximal boundary is a handbreadth below the greater trochanter, and the distal boundary is a handbreadth above the knee. It is easier to give an injection in the vastus lateralis if the patient is lying down, but a sitting position also can be used.

The vastus lateralis site is located by dividing the front thigh into thirds both vertically and horizontally to make 9 squares. The injection is administered to the outer middle square (Fig. 26.18B).

Ventrogluteal Site

The ventrogluteal site can be used to administer an injection to both children and adults. It is considered an ideal intramuscular injection site because the subcutaneous layer over this site is relatively thin and the muscle layer is thick, allowing it to absorb a large amount of medication. It is also located away from major nerves and blood vessels.

To locate the ventrogluteal site, the patient is placed on their side with the injection site facing upwards. If the injection is being made into the patient's right side, the palm of the left hand is placed over the greater trochanter with the fingers pointing toward the patient's head and the thumb pointing towards the front of the leg. The index finger is then placed on the anterior superior iliac spine. The middle finger is spread posteriorly as far as possible away from the index finger towards the iliac crest to form a "V". (The hand position is reversed if the injection is being made into the patient's left side.) The injection is administered into the center of the "V" at the level of the knuckles between the index and middle fingers (Figs. 26.18C, 26.19).

Dorsogluteal Site

The dorsogluteal site has been used for many years by health care workers to administer intramuscular injections because

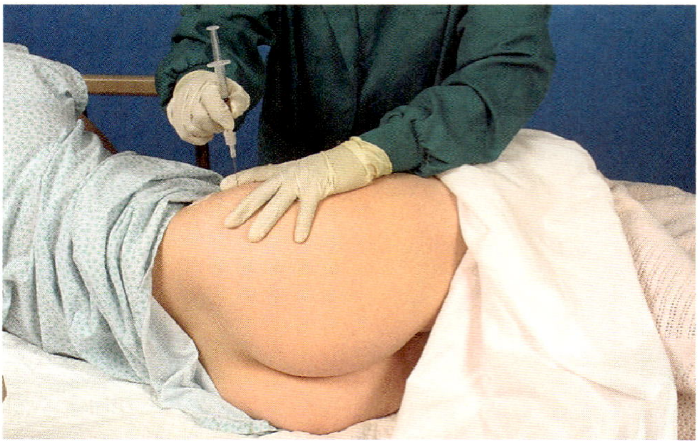

Fig. 26.19 Ventrogluteal intramuscular injection. This site is located away from major nerves and blood vessels. (From Perry AG, Potter PA, Elkin MK: *Nursing interventions and clinical skills*, ed 5, St. Louis, 2012, Mosby.)

it is a large muscle and can absorb a large amount of medication. Many researchers, however, no longer recommend the dorsogluteal site because of its close proximity to the sciatic nerve and the superior gluteal artery. Despite these recommendations, health care workers continue to use this site in adults.

To locate this site, the patient lies on the abdomen with the toes pointed inward, which aids in relaxation of the gluteal muscles. The medication is injected into the upper outer quadrant of the gluteal area. This site is located by palpating the greater trochanter and the posterior superior iliac spine. An imaginary line is then drawn between these two points, and the injection is administered above and outside of this area (Fig. 26.18D). The dorsogluteal site can also be located by dividing the buttocks into quadrants. The site is located in the upper outer quadrant approximately 2 to 3 inches below the iliac crest. The medical assistant must be *extremely* careful to maintain the proper boundary lines to avoid injection into the sciatic nerve or superior gluteal artery. Damage to the sciatic nerve can result in pain, numbness, and temporary or permanent leg paralysis.

Z-Track Method

Medications that are irritating to subcutaneous and skin tissue or that discolor the skin must be given intramuscularly using the Z-track method; one medication that is administered by this method is iron dextran (Imferon). The ventrogluteal and vastus lateralis sites can be used as areas to administer a Z-track injection.

The Z-track method is similar to the intramuscular injection procedure except that the skin and subcutaneous tissue at the injection site are pulled to the side before the needle is inserted. This causes a zigzag path through the tissues when the needle is removed and the skin is released. The zigzag path prevents the medication from reaching the subcutaneous layer or skin surface by sealing off the needle track (Fig. 26.20). The procedure for administering medication using the Z-track method is outlined in Procedure 26.6.

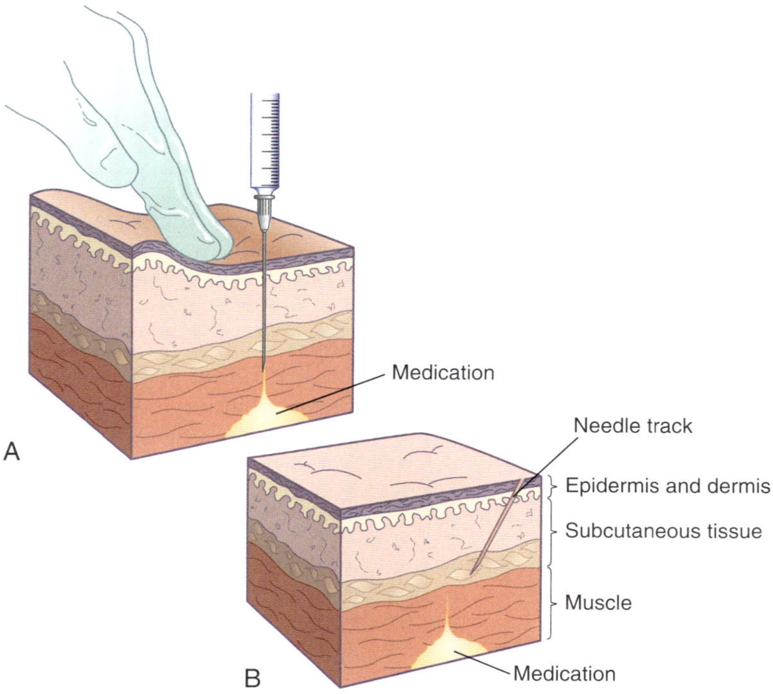

Fig. 26.20 Z-track intramuscular injection method. (A) The skin and subcutaneous tissue are pulled to the side before the needle is inserted. (B) This causes a zigzag path through the tissue when the skin is released, which seals off the needle track.

What Would You Do? What Would You *Not* Do?

Case Study 3

Danielle Roush, 16 years old, has come to the office with her mother. Danielle is complaining of a painful sore throat, fever, and severe aching in both of her ears. The physician diagnoses her with strep throat and otitis media and prescribes a parenteral antibiotic to be given deep IM in the ventrogluteal site. Danielle says that she's a basketball player and on the varsity team at her high school. She says that she is always too embarrassed to change or take a shower in front of the other girls because she's so skinny. Danielle would like to have the injection in her arm because it would be too embarrassing to have it in her hip. ■

INTRADERMAL INJECTION

An **intradermal injection** is given into the dermal layer of the skin, at an angle almost parallel to the skin (see Fig. 26.16). Absorption is slow; only a small amount of medication may be injected (0.01 to 0.2 mL). The sites most often used for an intradermal injection are areas where the skin is thin, such as the anterior forearm and the middle of the back. The upper arm also is used to administer an intradermal injection.

The needle used is short, usually ⅜ to ⅝ inch long, and the lumen has a small diameter, usually 25G to 27G. A tuberculin syringe is often used for administering the injection. The capacity of the syringe is small (1 mL), and the calibrations are divided into tenths and hundredths of a milliliter. The fine calibrations allow a very small amount of medication to be administered, which is required with an intradermal injection. Procedure 26.7 outlines the technique for the administration of an intradermal injection.

The most frequent use of intradermal injections is to administer a skin test, such as an allergy test or a tuberculin skin test. The medication for the appropriate test is placed into the skin layers, and a small, raised area known as a **wheal** is produced at the injection site, owing to distention of the skin (Fig. 26.21). At a time dictated by the type of test being administered, the results are read and interpreted. Most allergy tests can be read and interpreted at the medical office a short time (usually 15 to 20 minutes) after administration of the test, whereas tuberculin testing requires 48 hours before the results can be read.

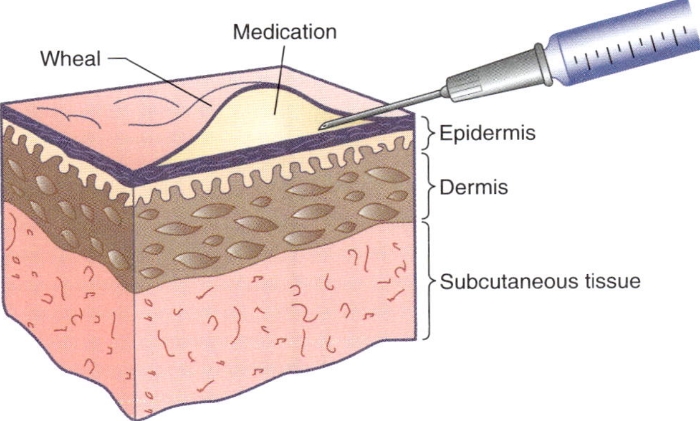

Fig. 26.21 Intradermal injections are used to administer skin tests. Enough medication must be deposited in the skin layers to form a wheal.

The skin testing medication interacts with the body tissues; if no reaction occurs, the wheal disappears within a short time, and the only visible sign left is the puncture site. If a reaction to the skin test occurs, induration results, indicating a positive reaction. Erythema also may be present at the test site; however, for most skin tests the extent of induration is the only criterion used to assess a positive reaction.

TUBERCULIN TESTING

TUBERCULOSIS

Tuberculosis (TB) is an infectious bacterial disease that can occur in almost any part of the body but usually attacks the lungs. Tuberculosis affecting the lungs is known as *pulmonary tuberculosis*, whereas tuberculosis occurring in other parts of the body is known as *extrapulmonary tuberculosis* and is most apt to occur in the brain, spine, kidneys, bones, and joints. The name of the bacterium that causes tuberculosis is *Mycobacterium tuberculosis*, which is a rod-shaped bacterium. Shortly (within weeks) after infection, a small percentage of individuals infected with TB bacteria develop active pulmonary tuberculosis.

Active Tuberculosis

Active tuberculosis develops when TB bacteria are able to overcome the body's defense system which occurs in 10% of infected individuals. Active tuberculosis is most apt to occur in young children and individuals with a weakened immune system. The TB bacteria then begin to multiply and attack the body, resulting in the destruction of tissue. Symptoms of active pulmonary tuberculosis include a chronic cough lasting 3 weeks or longer that produces a mucopurulent sputum, occasional hemoptysis (coughing up blood), and chest pain. Systemic symptoms include fatigue, loss of appetite, weakness, unexplained weight loss, chills, low-grade fever, and sweating at night. If active tuberculosis is left untreated, it can result in serious complications such as permanent lung damage and even death.

Latent Tuberculosis

Most people (90%) infected with the TB bacterium do not develop the active disease because their body defenses protect them. Body defenses may be able to destroy the TB bacteria immediately after they enter the body and completely clear them from the body. If this is not possible, the TB bacteria are engulfed by white blood cells known as macrophages. The body then builds a fibrous wall of tissue around these macrophages (infected with TB bacteria) to encapsulate them. Some of the TB bacteria may remain alive inside the capsule in a dormant or inactive state. During this time, the individual experiences no symptoms and cannot spread the disease to others. Individuals are said to have a latent tuberculosis infection (LTBI), and the only sign indicating that they have been infected with tuberculosis is a positive reaction to a TB test.

Individuals with latent tuberculosis may go on to develop active tuberculosis. This occurs in approximately 10% of individuals with LTBI. About half of these individuals develop active tuberculosis within 2 years after the initial infection, and the other half develop tuberculosis many years, even decades, after having become infected. The TB bacteria break out of the capsule and cause the symptoms of active tuberculosis (described previously). The development of LTBI into active tuberculosis is most apt to occur when the body's immune system is weakened, such as during a serious illness, or in patients who have an immune disorder such as human immunodeficiency virus (HIV) infection. The difference between active tuberculosis and latent tuberculosis is outlined in Table 26.6.

PURPOSE OF TUBERCULIN TESTING

The purpose of tuberculin testing is to identify individuals who are infected with *M. tuberculosis*. Early identification of individuals with active infectious tuberculosis leads to early treatment and prevents the spread of tuberculosis.

A tuberculin test is recommended for individuals who are at higher risk for tuberculosis exposure or infection, or at higher risk for progressing from latent tuberculosis to active tuberculosis. Examples include individuals who have close day-to-day contact with someone with active tuberculosis, individuals who have immigrated from a country with a high incidence of TB, and individuals who work or reside in facilities or institutions with people who are at high risk for TB (e.g., hospitals and other health care facilities, correctional facilities, and nursing homes). Tuberculin testing may also be required as a prerequisite for employment, college entrance, entrance into the military service, and so on. A positive reaction to a tuberculin test occurs 2 to 10 weeks after an individual is infected with tuberculosis. Because of this, a patient recently infected with TB bacteria may show a false-negative test result and should be retested 10 weeks later.

There are two main types of tuberculin tests. They include the tuberculin skin test (TST) and the tuberculin blood test, which are described in more detail in this section.

MANTOUX TUBERCULIN SKIN TEST

The Mantoux test is most commonly used for tuberculin skin testing and is named after Charles Mantoux, the French physician who developed the test. The Mantoux TST is administered through an intradermal injection using a tuberculin syringe with a capacity of 1.0 mL and a short (⅜ to ½ inch) needle with a gauge of 26 to 27. The substance used for the test is tuberculin, which consists of a purified protein derivative (PPD) extracted from a culture of *M. tuberculosis* (the causative agent of tuberculosis), to test for sensitivity to the TB organism. The tuberculin PPD solution contains no live tuberculosis organisms and is completely harmless, making it safe to administer to people of all ages.

The standard injected dose is 0.1 mL of tuberculin PPD solution containing 5 TU (tuberculin units). Brand names for Mantoux tests include TUBERSOL (Sanofi Pasteur Ltd) and Aplisol (JHP Pharmaceuticals, LLC). Once opened, a vial of tuberculin PPD solution expires after 30 days and must be discarded. This is because oxidation and degradation of tuberculin reduce its potency, which can lead to inaccurate test results. The medical assistant should write the expiration date on the vial on opening. Before withdrawing tuberculin from the vial, the medical assistant should check both the manufacturer's expiration date and the 30-day expiration date marked by the medical assistant on the vial.

It is important to properly store the tuberculin PPD solution because it can be adversely affected by exposure to light and heat. The vial should be stored in the dark as much as possible; exposure to bright light should be avoided because this can diminish the potency of the PPD solution. A vial that has been exposed to light for an extended period of time should be discarded. The vial must be stored in the refrigerator at a temperature between 35°F to 46°F (2°C to 8°C). The vial should be returned to its refrigerated storage area as soon as possible after the proper dose has been drawn up into a syringe.

Table 26.6 Differences Between Active and Latent Tuberculosis (TB)

Characteristics	Active TB	Latent TB
Symptoms	Patient usually feels sick and has symptoms of TB such as cough, fever, and weight loss	Patient feels fine and has no symptoms
TB bacterial status	Active TB bacteria are present in the body	TB bacteria are present in the body that are alive but inactive
TB test results	Patient usually has a positive TST or QFT-G blood test result.	Patient usually has a positive TST or QFT-G blood test result.
Diagnostic tests	Patient may have an abnormal chest radiograph and a positive sputum test result.	Patient has a normal chest radiograph and a negative sputum test result
Ability to infect others	Patient is infectious and may spread the disease to others	Patient is not infectious and cannot spread the TB to others
Treatment	Patient needs treatment for active TB	Provider may consider treatment for latent TB to prevent active TB disease

QFT-G, QuantiFERON-TB Gold; *TST*, tuberculin skin testing.

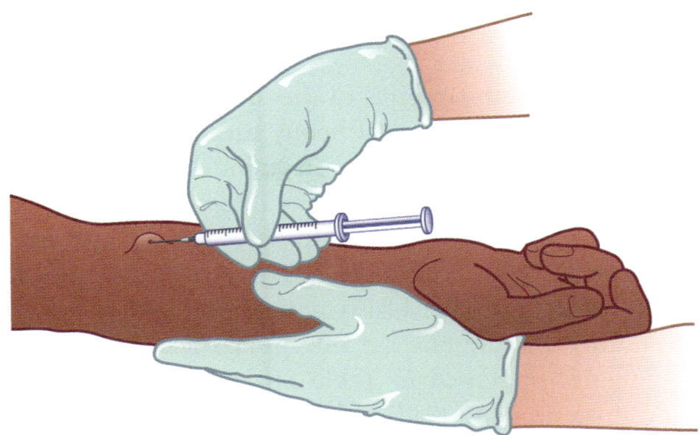

Fig. 26.22 Intradermal skin testing. Intradermal skin testing involves the injection of a small amount of allergen extract into the superficial skin layers through the intradermal route of administration.

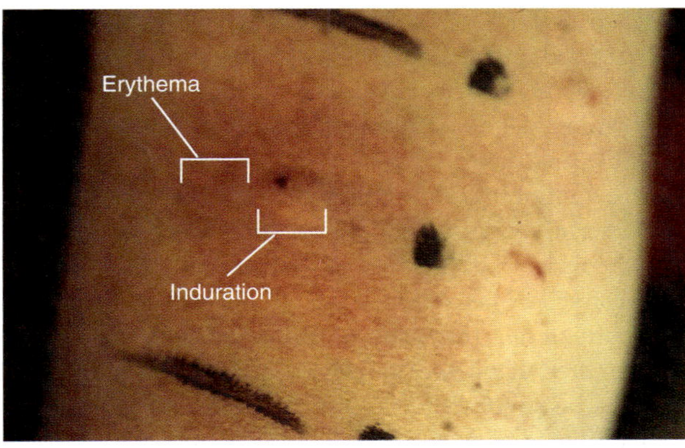

Fig. 26.23 Positive tuberculin skin test showing induration and erythema. Induration is the only criterion used to determine a positive reaction. (From Abbas AK, Lichtman AH, Pillai S: *Basic immunology functions and disorders of the immune system*, ed 4, Philadelphia, 2014, Saunders.)

It is important that the medical assistant draw up the proper amount of tuberculin PPD solution. Injecting too much of the solution might elicit a reaction not caused by a tuberculous infection and injecting too little of the solution results in insufficient solution being injected into the skin to elicit a reaction. This will invalidate the test because if no reaction occurs, it cannot be accepted as a negative reaction.

The medical assistant must make sure to inject the tuberculin solution into the superficial skin layers to form a tense, pale, raised area known as a **wheal** (Fig. 26.22). If the injection is made into the subcutaneous layer, a wheal will not form and the test will yield a false-negative result, whereas a too-shallow injection may cause leakage of the tuberculin solution onto the skin. In either case, the medical assistant must repeat the TST at a site at least 2 inches (5 cm) away.

The medical assistant should not apply pressure to the site after injecting the tuberculin PPD solution because the solution is not intended to be absorbed into the tissues. In addition, applying pressure may cause leakage of the solution through the needle puncture site. The wheal will disappear on its own within a few minutes and should not be covered with an adhesive bandage.

TUBERCULIN SKIN TEST REACTIONS

When PPD solution is introduced into the skin of an individual with an active or latent case of tuberculosis, it causes localized thickening of the skin, resulting in induration. **Induration**, which indicates a positive reaction, is an abnormally raised hardened area with clearly defined margins caused by an accumulation of small, sensitized lymphocytes (a type of white blood cell) that occurs in the area in which the tuberculin was injected into the skin (Fig. 26.23). TST reactions are based on the amount of induration present and are interpreted according to the manufacturer's instructions that accompany the test.

A positive reaction to a TST indicates the presence of a tuberculous infection; however, it does not differentiate between active and latent forms of the infection. Therefore, a positive reaction warrants additional diagnostic procedures before the provider can make a final diagnosis. Other procedures used to detect an active tuberculous infection include chest x-ray and microbiologic examination and culture of the patient's sputum for TB bacteria.

Guidelines for Administering a Mantoux Tuberculin Skin Test

1. Use the anterior forearm, approximately 4 inches (10 cm) below the bend in the elbow, as the site of administration of the test. Avoid the following areas because they make the test harder to perform and interfere with good visualization and palpation of test reactions:
   - Hairy areas of the skin
   - Areas with visible veins
   - Scar tissue
   - Red or swollen areas
   - Bruised areas
   - Areas with lesions, dermatitis, or other skin irritations
   - Muscle ridges
2. Cleanse the skin thoroughly with an antiseptic wipe and allow it to dry completely before administering the test.
3. Be sure to inject the PPD tuberculin solution slowly into the superficial layers of the skin. If the injection is performed correctly, a wheal should appear that is approximately 6 to 10 mm (⅜ inch) in diameter. If blood appears at the puncture site once the TST has been administered, this is not significant and will not interfere with the test. The blood can be removed by gently blotting the area with a gauze pad, making sure not to apply pressure.
4. Once the TST has been administered, the results must be read within 48 to 72 hours.

Guidelines for Reading Mantoux Tuberculin Skin Test Results

1. The TST results must be read in good lighting within 48 to 72 hours.
2. Use both inspection and palpation to read the TST results. Induration may not always be visible and therefore must be assessed through palpation.
3. If induration is present, rub your fingertip lightly from the area of normal skin (without induration) to the indurated

area to assess its size. The diameter of induration must be assessed and measured transversely to the long axis of the forearm (left to right, not up and down). Measure the widest diameter of induration in millimeters using a flexible millimeter ruler.

4. The extent of induration present is the only criterion used to determine a positive TST reaction (see Fig. 26.23). If erythema is present without induration, the results are interpreted as negative.
5. Document all reactions in millimeters to the nearest millimeter. If no induration is present, the TST results should be documented as 0 mm. Results should never be documented as positive or negative.
6. The interpretation of the TST test results depends on the following:
   a. Measurement (in mm) of the induration
   b. The individual's risk of being infected with tuberculosis (e.g., close contact with an individual with active TB increases the risk of being infected)
   c. The individual's risk of progression to disease if infected (e.g., HIV-infected individuals are more apt to progress from LTBI to active TB)
7. Mantoux TST results are interpreted according to the guidelines presented in Table 26.7. The procedure for administering and reading a Mantoux TST is presented in Procedure 26.7.

Table 26.7 Interpretation of the Tuberculin Mantoux Skin Test*

Interpretation of the Mantoux skin test results is based on the individual's risk of being infected with tuberculosis (TB) and the risk of progression to disease if infected. Individuals with impaired immunity are more likely to have a weaker response to a tuberculin skin test. Because of this, there are three cutoff points for identifying a positive reaction to a Mantoux test.

Positive Reaction

An induration of 5 mm or more is classified as positive in individuals with the following high-risk factors for developing TB:

1. Individuals infected with HIV
2. Individuals who have had recent close contact with individuals who have active TB
3. Individuals who have fibrotic changes on a chest radiograph consistent with previously healed TB
4. Individuals who have had organ transplants
5. Individuals on immunosuppressive drug therapy (e.g., prolonged high-dose corticosteroid therapy, TNF-alpha–antagonist drug therapy [Remicade, Enbrel, Humira])

Negative Reaction

An induration of 4 mm or less

Positive Reaction

An induration of 10 mm or more is classified as positive in individuals who do not meet the aforementioned criteria but who have other risk factors for TB, including the following:

1. Individuals who inject illegal drugs
2. Individuals with the following conditions that weaken the immune system: diabetes mellitus; chronic renal failure; body weight that is 10% or more below ideal body weight; silicosis; gastrectomy; jejunoileal bypass; certain hematologic disorders such as leukemias and lymphomas; carcinoma of the head, neck, or lungs
3. Residents and employees of the following high-risk congregate settings: hospitals and other health care facilities, correctional facilities, nursing homes, homeless shelters, drug rehabilitation centers, residential facilities for patients with AIDS
4. Recent immigrants from countries with a high incidence of TB (countries in Asia, Africa, the Caribbean, Latin America, and Eastern Europe and Russia)
5. Children younger than 4 years
6. Infants, children, and adolescents exposed to adults at high risk for developing TB
7. Mycobacteriology laboratory personnel

Negative Reaction

An induration of 9 mm or less

Positive Reaction

An induration of 15 mm or more is classified as positive in individuals at low risk for developing TB, including individuals with no known risk factors for TB

Negative Reaction

An induration of 14 mm or less

AIDS, Acquired immunodeficiency syndrome; *HIV*, human immunodeficiency virus; *TNF*, tumor necrosis factor.
*The cutoff point may sometimes vary from state to state from those presented in this table.

TUBERCULOSIS BLOOD TEST

Interferon gamma release assays (IGRAs) are blood tests used to identify individuals who are infected with *M. tuberculosis* (the causative agent of tuberculosis). Currently, there are two IGRAs approved for use by the FDA; these include the QuantiFERON-TB Gold In-Tube test (QFT-GIT) manufactured by Cellestis, Inc. and the T-SPOT TB test (T-SPOT) manufactured by Oxford Immunotec, Ltd.. As with the TST, IGRAs cannot differentiate between active and latent forms of the infection. Therefore, a positive result warrants additional diagnostic procedures, such as a chest radiograph and microbiologic examination and culture of the patient's sputum, before the provider can make a diagnosis.

If the blood specimen for the IGRA test is drawn in the medical office, it is important for the medical assistant to carefully follow the test manufacturer's instructions for the collection of the specimen to ensure accurate test results. Following collection, the blood specimen for an IGRA must be stored at room temperature and transported to the laboratory within a specified time period for processing. The blood specimen for a QFT-GIT test must be transported within 14 hours following collection while the blood specimen for a T-SPOT must be transported within 8 hours following collection.

When an individual is infected with *M. tuberculosis* certain lymphocytes in their blood become sensitized and release a substance known as interferon gamma (IFN-gamma). IGRA tests are able to detect the presence of INF-gamma in a patient infected with *M. tuberculosis.* The patient is likely to be infected with *Mycobacterium* if they register an IFN-gamma level above the positive cutoff value. On the other hand, if the patient is not infected with *M. tuberculosis,* his or her blood will not contain sensitized lymphocytes and there will not be a release of IFN-gamma. In this case, the test result is documented as negative, indicating that the patient is unlikely to be infected with *M. tuberculosis.*

IGRA test results are interpreted as follows:

Positive: Individuals who test positive are likely to be infected with *M. tuberculosis* and should be evaluated further for latent TB or active TB.

Negative: Healthy adults who test negative are unlikely to have an *M. tuberculosis* infection and usually do not require further evaluation.

Indeterminate/borderline: An indeterminate/borderline result indicates that the *M. tuberculosis* infection status cannot be determined because of factors that invalidate the test results. These factors include the following: improper technique used in the collection, handling, and storage of the blood specimen; a delay in transporting the specimen to the laboratory; and the inability of the patient's blood to respond to the test because of a severely weakened immune system, such as in a patient undergoing chemotherapy. If a test result is indeterminate/borderline, the IGRA test should be repeated using a fresh blood specimen.

IGRA tests offer several advantages over the Mantoux TST, which include the following:

1. The patient needs to visit the office only one time to have their blood drawn. This alleviates the problem that sometimes occurs with patients undergoing a TST, in which a patient does not return for the second visit to have the results read.
2. The results are available within 24 hours compared with the 48 to 72 hours required for a TST.
3. IGRA tests provide an objective evaluation, whereas the TST is a subjective evaluation. If the TST test is not measured correctly, inaccurate test results may occur.
4. IGRA tests provide a positive or negative test result, and risk factors do not have to be taken into consideration when positive reactions are interpreted, as is required with the TST.
5. An individual who has been vaccinated for tuberculosis with the bacillus Calmette-Guérin (BCG) vaccine does not show a false-negative result with IGRA tests, as can occur with a TST.

IGRA tests have some disadvantages which are outlined as follows:

1. The patient's blood specimen must be delivered within a specified time period following collection. This is because the lymphocytes in the blood specimen begin to die after this time period has elapsed.
2. Errors in the collection, handling, or storage of the specimen can affect the accuracy of IGRA tests.
3. The cost of an IGRA test is significantly higher than that of a TST.

ALLERGY TESTING

ALLERGY

An **allergy** is an abnormal hypersensitivity of the immune system of the body to a substance that is ordinarily harmless; this substance is known as an **allergen.** Allergens enter the body by being inhaled, by being swallowed, by being injected, or by coming into contact with the skin. Almost any substance in the environment can be an allergen. Some common allergens are plant pollens, mold, house dust, animal dander, latex, dyes, soaps, detergents, cosmetics, certain foods and medications, and venom from insect stings. (Refer to *Highlight on Allergens* for detailed information on certain allergens).

The exact cause of allergies is not fully understood. In many cases, the tendency to develop allergies seems to be inherited because children of allergic parents tend to exhibit more allergic symptoms than children of nonallergic parents. Although allergies can develop at any age, children are more apt to develop allergies than are older individuals.

ALLERGIC REACTION

The immune system of an individual with allergies interprets certain allergens (e.g., pollen, mold, house dust) as invaders. The first time the allergen enters the body of an allergic individual it stimulates the body to produce antibodies to that allergen. These antibodies are usually of a type known as *immunoglobulin E (IgE) antibodies.* After the initial sensitization, allergic antibodies combine with the allergen in the body, resulting in an allergen-antibody reaction. When such a reaction occurs, histamine is released in significant amounts, causing allergic symptoms (e.g., sneezing, watery eyes, runny nose). Allergen-antibody reactions may involve any system of the body; however, they most frequently affect the respiratory and integumentary systems. Allergic symptoms can range from mild to very severe, as is the case with the potentially fatal anaphylactic reaction.

Depending on the allergen and the body system affected, allergies appear in different forms in an individual and commonly include hay fever (allergy to mold and pollen), allergic rhinitis (runny and inflamed nose), asthma, urticaria, contact dermatitis, eczema, and food allergies. Symptoms exhibited by an allergic individual depend on an individual's form of allergy. Table 26.8 lists and describes the common clinical forms of allergies including the signs and symptoms of each.

Table 26.8 Clinical Forms of Allergies

Hay fever (seasonal allergic rhinitis)	Caused by allergy to mold or the pollen of trees, grasses, or weeds. The term *hay fever* is misleading because hay fever is not caused by hay, and it does not result in fever. English physicians first used the term *hay fever* in the early 1800s when treating patients with allergies to grass pollens. Symptoms of hay fever and the common cold are almost identical: episodes of sneezing, itching, and watery eyes; runny and stuffy nose; and burning sensation of the palate and throat. Hay fever is seasonal, occurring when there is pollen in the air. Depending on geographic location, hay fever may occur in spring, summer, or fall, and last until first frost.
Perennial allergic rhinitis	Inflammation of mucous membranes of the nose caused by allergies. Symptoms include nasal congestion, sneezing, and runny nose. With perennial rhinitis, the nasal mucosa is inflamed year-round. This type of allergic rhinitis is commonly caused by allergens that are always present in the environment, such as house dust and animal dander.
Allergic asthma	Condition characterized by coughing, chest tightness, shortness of breath, and wheezing. During an asthma attack, the bronchiole tubes constrict and become clogged with mucus, which accounts for many of the symptoms of allergic asthma. Asthma can occur at any age but is more common in children and young adults and, if not treated, can lead to serious complications such as permanent lung damage. It is frequently, but not always, associated with a family history of allergy. Any common allergen, such as house dust, pollens, mold, or animal dander, may trigger an allergic asthma attack.
Urticaria	Urticaria, or hives, is an outbreak on the skin of welts of varying sizes that are redder or paler than surrounding skin and are accompanied by intense itching. When swellings are large and invade deeper tissues, the condition is known as *angio-edema.* Hives may develop on the face or lips or even internally. Allergies to food or drugs (especially penicillin and aspirin) and insect bites often cause hives, but they also may result from underlying disease or occur after exercise. In many cases the exact causes of urticaria cannot be determined. 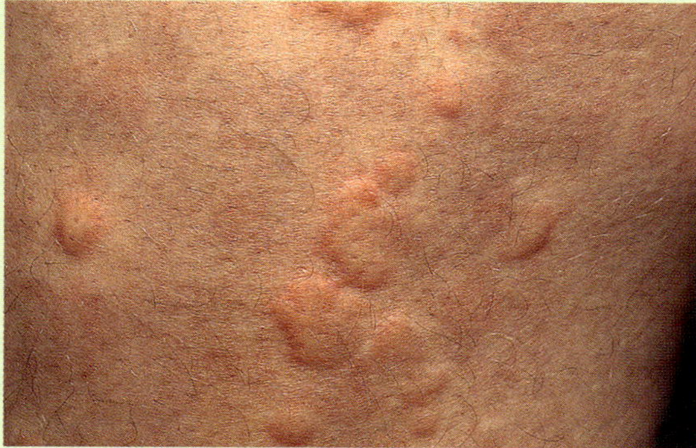
Contact dermatitis	Rash caused by direct contact of the skin with an allergen, such as cosmetics, perfumes, deodorants, latex, plastics, certain plants, and clothing treated with certain preservatives or dyes. Symptoms include swelling, blistering, oozing, and scaling. Rash usually occurs only on the areas of the body that have been in contact with the allergen. The most common causes of contact dermatitis are poison ivy, poison oak, and sumac. 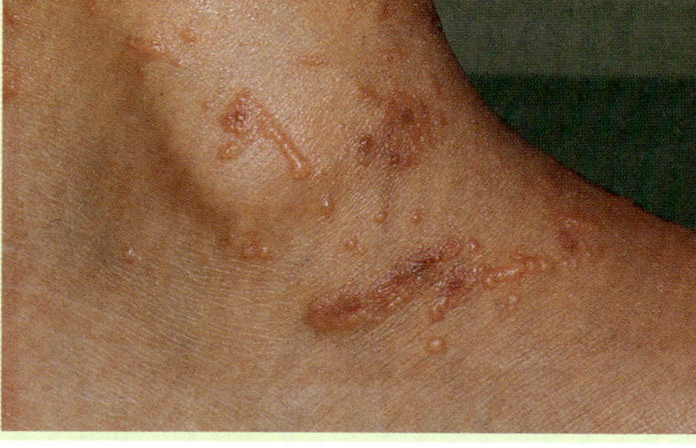

Table 26.8 Clinical Forms of Allergies—cont'd

Eczema	Noncontagious rash accompanied by redness, itching, vesicles, oozing, crusting, and scaling. Eczema is a common allergic reaction in children, but it also may occur in adults, usually in a more severe form. A rash commonly appears on the face, neck, and folds of the elbows and knees. Eczema frequently is associated with allergies, and substances to which a person is allergic may aggravate it. Foods may be important factors, particularly milk, fish, or eggs. Allergens that are inhaled, such as dust and pollen, rarely cause eczema. 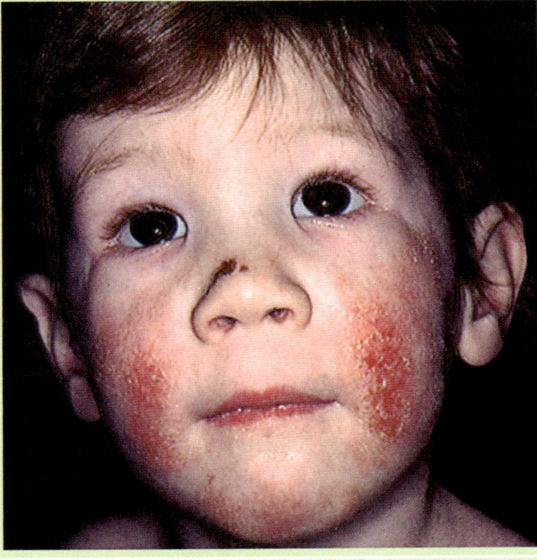
Food allergy	An immune system reaction that occurs soon after eating a food to which an individual is allergic. The most common symptoms that occur when a patient has a food allergy are urticaria (hives), asthma symptoms (such as wheezing and shortness of breath), gastrointestinal symptoms (such as nausea, vomiting, diarrhea, abdominal pain), and swelling of the lips, face, tongue, or throat. The most common foods that cause allergies are milk, soy, eggs, peanuts, tree nuts (e.g., walnuts), fish, shellfish, and wheat. The primary treatment for a food allergy involves avoidance of the food. If the individual has a severe allergy to a food, such as peanuts, consuming the food can cause an anaphylactic reaction, which can be life-threatening. Treatment involves the immediate injection of epinephrine.

DIAGNOSIS AND TREATMENT

The best way to prevent allergic symptoms is to identify and avoid the offending allergen or allergens. The first and most important step in this process is the completion of a careful and detailed medical history by the provider. Of particular importance to the diagnosis of an allergy are the patient's home and work environments, diet, and living habits. The provider also performs a thorough physical examination to detect conditions resulting from allergies, such as nasal polyps, wheezing, skin rashes, and urticaria.

When the medical history and physical examination have been completed, the provider may order diagnostic tests. Allergy testing is performed to confirm information obtained through the medical history and physical examination. The allergy tests ordered most often are direct skin testing and in vitro blood testing, which are described in greater detail in the following section. The general treatment of allergies includes avoiding the allergen(s) (if possible); alleviating the symptoms through drug therapy such as antihistamines, decongestants, bronchodilators, and inhaled steroids; and decreasing the sensitivity of the body to the allergen by the administration of allergy injections, or desensitization injections (known as *immunotherapy*).

TYPES OF ALLERGY TESTS

The purpose of allergy testing is to determine the specific substances or allergens that are causing the patient's allergic symptoms. The two main categories of allergy tests are direct skin tests and the in vitro blood test. The medical assistant is often responsible for performing direct skin testing in the medical office. The in vitro blood test is performed on a blood specimen by an outside laboratory. The medical assistant may be responsible for performing a venipuncture to obtain the blood specimen.

Direct Skin Testing

Direct skin testing involves applying extracts of common allergens to the skin and observing the body's reaction to them. The extract is applied either topically to the skin (patch testing) or into the superficial skin layers (skin-prick testing and intradermal testing). The advantage of direct skin testing is that test results are obtained immediately.

This in vivo administration of allergens has the potential, however, to cause adverse reactions, the least common but most serious being an anaphylactic reaction. The medical assistant should have a thorough knowledge of the signs of an anaphylactic reaction and should alert the provider immediately if the patient begins to exhibit them.

Regardless of the specific type of direct skin test used (patch, skin-prick, or intradermal), some general guidelines should be followed:

1. Instruct the patient to discontinue the use of antihistamines for 3 days before the skin testing. Antihistamines block the response of histamine, which may suppress skin testing reactions and lead to false-negative test results. Certain medications decrease the immune response of the body to skin testing, which could cause a false-negative test result. These medications include tricyclic antidepressants, corticosteroids, theophylline, beta-blockers, angiotensin-converting enzyme (ACE) inhibitors, and nifedipine. If the patient is taking any of these medications, the provider must determine if it is possible to take the patient off of the medication. If it is not feasible, the provider may order in vitro allergy blood testing, which is not affected by medication.
2. Verify that the area of application is free from hair, scar tissue, and dermatitis to permit good visualization and palpation of test reactions. Recommended sites include the anterior forearm, the upper arm, and the middle of the back. The back is usually used for patch and skin-prick testing, and the upper arm and forearm are typically used for intradermal skin testing.
3. Cleanse the area of application thoroughly with an antiseptic wipe, and allow it to dry completely.
4. Wear gloves when the allergy testing involves puncture of the skin, which includes skin-prick testing and intradermal skin testing. Gloves protect the medical assistant from exposure to bloodborne pathogens, as required by the OSHA standard.
5. Space the allergen extracts at least 1 inch apart to provide enough surface area for a sizable reaction. If not enough surface area is available, large adjacent reactions may run together, making it difficult to read test results.
6. Label the test sites so that the application site of each allergen extract can be identified later when reading results.
7. Closely observe the patient after the procedure for a systemic reaction to the skin testing. The patient should remain at the office for at least 30 minutes after the procedure for observation.
8. Make the patient aware that the skin testing may cause a mild allergic reaction, such as a runny nose, sneezing, and mild wheezing 8 to 24 hours after skin-prick and intradermal skin testing. Instruct the patient to contact the provider immediately if a more severe reaction than this occurs, such as difficulty in breathing, dizziness, or swelling of the face, lips, or mouth.

Quality Control

Positive and negative controls should be performed with each skin testing procedure to ensure reliable and valid test results. Controls are performed at the same time and in the same way that the allergy skin testing is performed.

Negative Control

To perform a negative skin test control, a substance that should not cause a reaction in a normal person is inserted into the patient's superficial skin layers. The negative control usually consists of normal saline. Some patients have a condition known as *dermographism*, which causes them to have a reaction just from the irritating effect of a needle pricking their skin. Running a negative control ensures that positive skin test reactions are truly positive and are not the result of another factor, such as dermographism.

Positive Control

For a positive control, a substance that should cause a reaction in a nonallergenic patient is inserted into the patient's superficial skin layers. The substance used for the positive control is histamine. The positive control should produce a reaction that consists of at least 3 mm of induration surrounded by erythema. Patients who are taking an antihistamine or who have a depressed immune system because of a disease or immunosuppressive medication may have a false-negative reaction to a skin test. Running a positive control ensures that negative skin test reactions are truly negative and are not just the result of another factor, as in a patient who has taken an antihistamine.

HIGHLIGHT on Allergens

House Dust

There are many components in house dust to which an individual may be allergic; the most significant of these is the house dust mite. Dust mites thrive in warm humid conditions and feed on scales shed from human skin; they are often found in mattresses, carpets, stuffed animals, and upholstered furniture. An individual who is allergic to house dust reacts to the waste products of these dust mites.

There is no shortage of food for the dust mite because one person sheds up to 1 gram of scales per day, which is enough to feed thousands of mites for months. *Dermatophagoides pteronyssinus* and *Dermatophagoides farinae* are the most common house dust mites and are present in varying numbers in virtually every home. Mites occur in greatest numbers in bedding, particularly in mattresses; there may be 1000 mites in each gram of dust from a mattress. Sufferers often notice that symptoms become much worse

HIGHLIGHT on Allergens—cont'd

when the bedding is disturbed and allergenic material becomes airborne. Practices that eliminate dust also reduce the number of dust mites in a household.

Insect Stings

It is estimated that between 5% and 7.5% of Americans are allergic to the venom from insect stings. Approximately 50 people in the United States die each year from a severe allergic reaction to insect venom. The incidence of deaths is low because most people know they need to obtain medical attention immediately if an allergic reaction begins.

Almost all insects whose venom can cause allergic reactions belong to the order Hymenoptera, which includes honeybees and bumblebees, wasps, yellow jackets, and hornets. When a honeybee stings, its stinger remains embedded in the victim's skin, causing the bee to die as it tries to tear itself away. Wasps, yellow jackets, and hornets are more aggressive than bees and can sting repeatedly. Hornets are the most aggressive of the group and may sting even when not provoked. Yellow jackets are close behind in aggressiveness, but wasps usually sting only if someone interferes with them near their nest.

If an insect sting does not cause an allergic reaction within 30 minutes, chances are excellent that no problem will occur. A normal reaction to an insect sting includes localized pain, redness, swelling, and itching lasting 1 to 2 days. Any generalized reaction not arising directly from the area of the sting is almost certain to be an anaphylactic reaction, which begins with such symptoms as sneezing, urticaria, itching, angioedema, erythema, and disorientation and progresses to difficulty in breathing, cyanosis, shock, convulsions, loss of consciousness, and death. Medical care should be sought immediately because most fatalities occur within 2 hours after the sting. Because time is a factor, individuals who are known to have a severe allergy to insect stings are provided with an anaphylactic emergency treatment kit that contains epinephrine in a prefilled syringe and oral antihistamines. They can carry the kit with them so that treatment for a severe allergic reaction can be started as soon as possible.

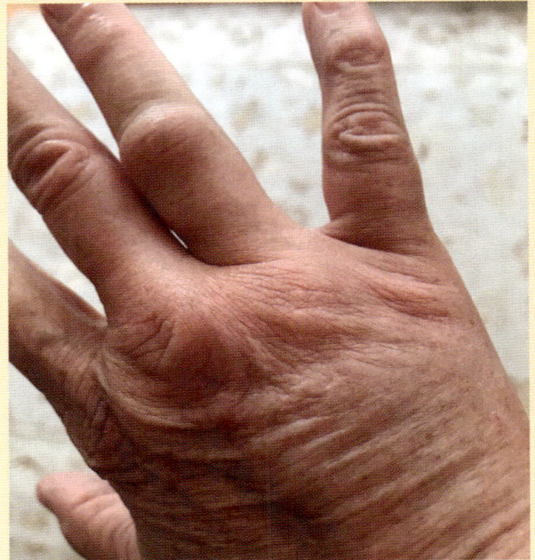

Localized reaction to a wasp sting.

Penicillin

Penicillin is a common cause of allergic drug reactions. Approximately 2% of the American population are allergic to penicillin. The reaction may be mild and completely overlooked or confused with the symptoms of the disease being treated with penicillin, or it can be more serious and take the form of severe dermatitis or an anaphylactic reaction. Death as a result of a severe anaphylactic reaction is rare, occurring in only 0.01% of patients being treated with penicillin.

Penicillin was discovered in 1929 by Sir Alexander Fleming, but it was not used as a therapeutic drug until 1940. By 1944, it was evident that some of the side effects of penicillin were allergic reactions; the first documented death as a result of an anaphylactic reaction to penicillin occurred in 1945.

Oral administration of penicillin is safer than a penicillin injection because it has a lower frequency of severe allergic reactions. There have been only six reported deaths from oral administration of penicillin.

Approximately 95% of serious reactions occur within 1 hour after a penicillin injection. The best preventive measure is to keep the patient under direct observation for at least 30 minutes after administration of the injection. ■

Types of Direct Skin Tests

Patch Testing

Patch testing is primarily used to identify allergens that cause contact dermatitis. Patch testing involves the topical application of each allergen to the skin, using a "patch." A patch consists of a small piece of gauze or filter paper impregnated with the allergen, which is applied to the skin and taped in place with hypoallergenic tape (Fig. 26.24). Allergens commonly applied include plants, topical drugs, latex, resins, metals, cosmetics, dyes, and chemicals. The patient should be instructed to leave the patches in place, keep them dry, and return to the medical office in 48 hours to have the results read. When the patient returns to the

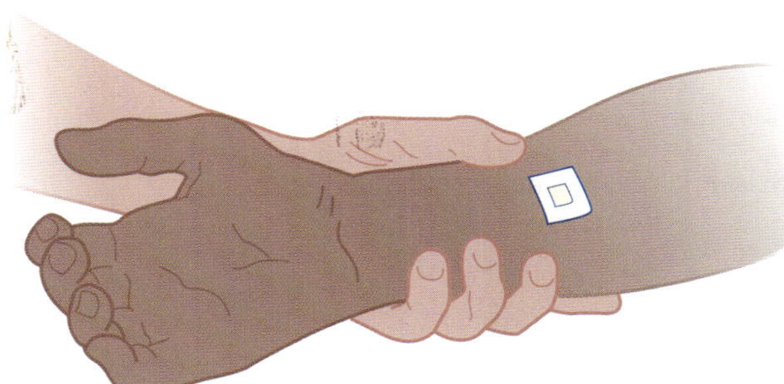

Fig. 26.24 Patch testing. A patch consists of a small piece of gauze or filter paper impregnated with the allergen, which is applied to the skin and taped in place.

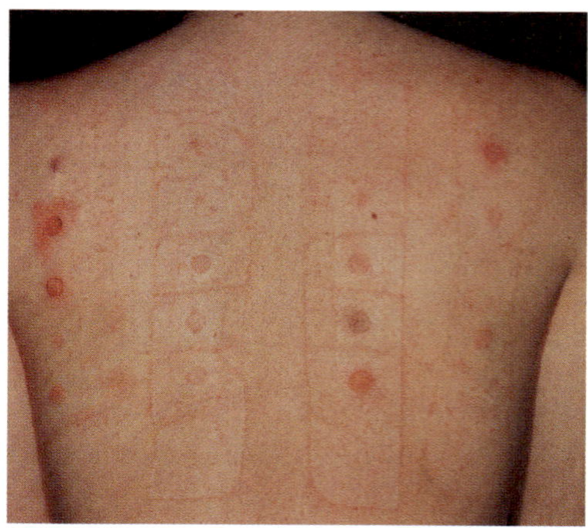

Fig. 26.25 Patch test showing positive results.(From Shiland BJ: *Mastering healthcare terminology*, ed 4, St. Louis, 2013, Mosby.)

office, the patches are carefully removed, and the results are read 20 minutes later. The delayed reading time allows lessening of redness that may occur from the tape removal.

Test results are documented as positive or negative. Positive reactions cause a small area of contact dermatitis characterized by itching, erythema, induration, and vesiculation (Fig. 26.25). In strongly positive responses, the reaction may extend beyond the margins of the patch. Positive results are graded further on a quantitative 1+ to 3+ scoring system according to the type of reaction (Table 26.9).

Skin-Prick Testing

Skin-prick testing usually is performed to diagnose allergies to common allergens, particularly those that are inhaled, such as house dust, pollens, and molds. It is also used to test for food allergies; the most common foods that cause allergies are milk, soy, eggs, peanuts, tree nuts (e.g., walnuts), fish, shellfish, and wheat.

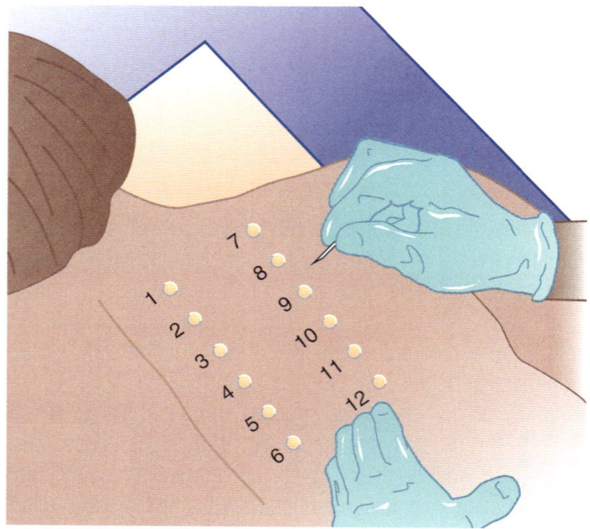

Fig. 26.26 Skin-prick testing. Skin-prick testing involves the application of numerous allergen extracts to the skin, followed by the pricking of each with a sterile needle.

Skin-prick testing involves the application of numerous allergen extracts to the skin, followed by the pricking of each with a sterile needle or another sharp instrument (Fig. 26.26). The number of allergen extracts applied during one office visit usually ranges between 20 and 30. Pricking the skin deposits the allergens in the outer layers of the skin to allow each to react with the body tissues.

The following guidelines should be followed for skin-prick testing: The extracts should be placed on the skin in rows in a specific pattern. This, along with labeling the test sites with a felt-tipped pen, tracks the location of each extract. Only a single drop of extract should be placed on the skin; more than this amount may cause the extracts to diffuse and run together. A sterile needle should be passed through the drop, and the point should lightly lift the top layer of skin without causing bleeding. It is important to wipe the needle dry with a sterile swab between pricks to prevent one extract from mixing with the next, leading to inaccurate test results.

The maximum reaction is usually seen in 15 to 20 minutes. During this time, the test sites should be left uncovered, and the patient should be instructed not to touch them. These areas should not be wiped because this removes the allergen extract, resulting in false-negative results. The results are read (after 15 to 20 minutes) using a millimeter ruler.

An area of induration surrounded by redness and itching characterizes a positive reaction. Positive results are documented by measuring the size of the induration in millimeters and converting it to a numeric scale based on the extent of the induration (see Table 26.8). Any redness should be ignored. See Fig. 26.27 for an illustration of skin test results. If a negative or only a mild reaction occurs and the

Table 26.9 Guidelines for Documenting Direct Skin Test Results

Patch Test	
–	No reaction
+1	Presence of erythema and edema, possibly papules
+2	Presence of erythema, edema, and vesicles, possibly papules
+3	Erythema, vesicles, and severe edema
Skin-Prick Testing and Intradermal Testing	
–	No reaction
±1	Induration 1 mm or less
+1	Induration greater than 1 mm and up to 5 mm in diameter
+2	Induration greater than 5 mm and up to 10 mm in diameter
+3	Induration greater than 10 mm and up to 15 mm in diameter
+4	Induration greater than 15 mm in diameter

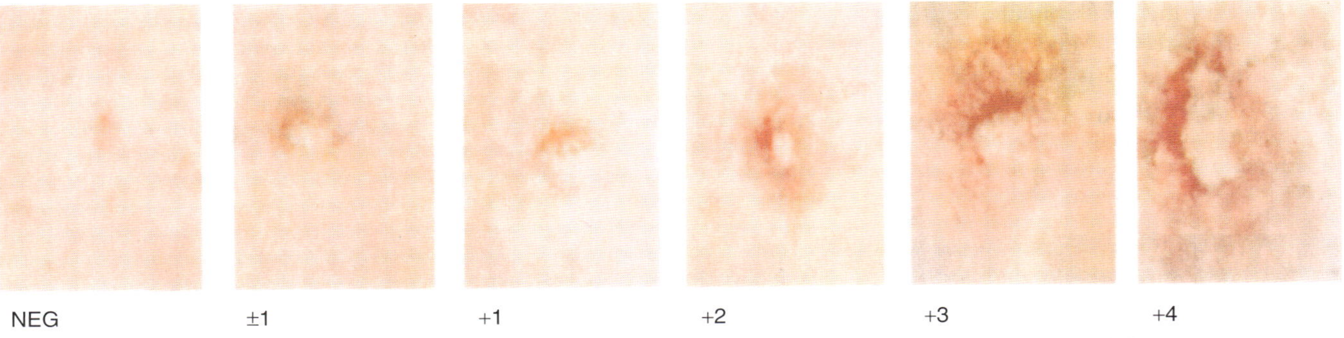

Fig. 26.27 Skin-prick and intradermal skin test results. (Copyright and courtesy Hollister-Stier, Spokane, WA.)

provider still suspects the presence of an allergy, the provider may order intradermal skin testing.

Intradermal Skin Testing

Intradermal skin testing is similar to skin-prick testing but is more sensitive. The number of skin tests performed during one office visit ranges from 5 to 30. Because there is a greater chance of adverse allergic reactions to intradermal skin testing, the provider often starts with skin-prick testing in individuals who are suspected of being highly allergic as determined by the medical history and results of the physical examination.

Intradermal skin testing involves the injection of a small amount (0.02 mL to 0.05 mL) of allergen extract into the superficial skin layers through the intradermal route of administration. A tuberculin syringe is used to administer the test, and the allergen extract is injected until a wheal forms (see Procedure 26.7). After 15 to 20 minutes, the test sites are observed for reactions. Positive reactions are characterized by an area of induration surrounded by redness and itching (Fig. 26.28). As with skin-prick testing, positive results are documented by measuring the size of the induration in millimeters and converting it to a numeric scale based on the amount of induration present (see Table 26.9).

In Vitro Allergy Blood Testing

An in vitro allergy blood test measures the amount of IgE antibodies in the blood that respond to common allergens. Examples of in vitro blood tests include enzyme-linked immunosorbent assay (ELISA), the radioallergosorbent test (RAST), and ImmunoCAP. For an in vitro allergy blood test, a sample of the patient's blood is sent to an outside laboratory, where it is exposed to allergens suspected of causing an allergic reaction in that patient. A detection device is used to measure the level of IgE antibodies that respond to each allergen being tested, and the results are reported as a numeric value. An elevated level of IgE antibodies responding to an allergen indicates the patient is allergic to that allergen.

Advantages of the in vitro blood test over direct skin testing are as follows. The results are not affected by

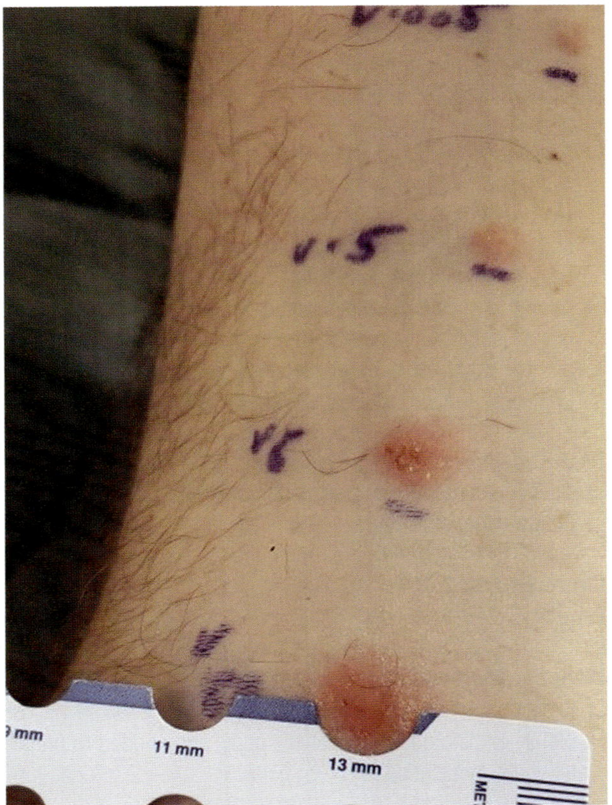

Fig. 26.28 Intradermal skin testing results. Positive results are characterized by an area of induration surrounded by redness. (From Kwah J, Banerji A. Delayed intradermal skin testing to diagnose culprits drugs in drug reaction with eosinophilia and systemic symptoms (DRESS). *Journal of Allergy and Clinical Immunology: In Practice*, 2023, vol 11, issue 5, pp 1572–3.)

medication (e.g., antihistamines); there is no danger of adverse allergic reactions because the test is performed in vitro, meaning outside the body; and in vitro blood testing can be performed on patients who have skin eruptions and are unable to undergo direct skin testing because of the lack of an intact skin surface area. In vitro blood testing is expensive, however, and does not provide immediate test results, which are available with direct skin testing. Blood testing is often used to test for allergies when it is not possible to perform skin testing. These situations include the following:

1. The provider does not want the patient to be taken off of a medication that interferes with skin test results.
2. The provider suspects that skin testing could result in an anaphylactic reaction in that patient.
3. The patient has a severe skin condition such as widespread dermatitis.
4. The skin testing may be difficult to perform, as in a child younger than 4 years.

What Would You Do? What Would You *Not* Do? RESPONSES

Case Study 1
Page 624

What Did Theresa Do?

- ❑ Asked Mrs. Okasinski what pharmacy she uses. Called the pharmacy and asked them to send an electronic copy of Mrs. Okasinski's medications to the medical office. Used the information to identify Mrs. Okasinski's medications.
- ❑ Documented the medications in her medical record for the physician to review.
- ❑ Explained to Mrs. Okasinski that when she has her prescriptions filled, she should request non-childproof containers so that she will be able to use the original containers, which have the name and prescription information on them. This will make it easier to tell her medications apart.
- ❑ After the physician was finished with Mrs. Okasinski, printed out a list of all the medications she would be taking based on the physician's orders. Reviewed each medication with Mrs. Okasinski, and told her to keep the list as a reference.

What Did Theresa Not Do?

- ❑ Did not criticize Mrs. Okasinski for taking her medications out of their original containers.

Case Study 2
Page 647

What Did Theresa Do?

- ❑ Explained to Mrs. Cardwell that for the infection to be completely eliminated from Rachel's body, she needed to be given all of the medication.
- ❑ Stressed to Mrs. Cardwell that medication prescribed to one person should never be given to someone else because it might cause them to have a bad reaction.
- ❑ Explained to Mrs. Cardwell that if side effects of medication ever occur, it is important to call the medical office for information on what to do.
- ❑ Told Mrs. Cardwell that Rachel needs to be seen by the doctor again, and scheduled an appointment for her. Asked if any other family members needed an appointment with the doctor.

What Did Theresa Not Do?

- ❑ Did not scold Mrs. Cardwell for giving Rachel's antibiotic to the other family members.

Case Study 3
Page 659

What Did Theresa Do?

- ❑ Explained to Danielle that if the injection were given in her arm, it would not be absorbed very well and she might not get better.
- ❑ Explained to Danielle that injections are given to patients every day in the hip at the office and that Danielle does not need to be embarrassed.
- ❑ Told Danielle that she would be draped extra well and that it would only take a minute to give the injection.

What Did Theresa Not Do?

- ❑ Did not disregard Danielle's concerns.
- ❑ Did not give the injection in the deltoid.

TERMINOLOGY REVIEW

Key Term	Word Parts	Definition
Adverse reaction		An unintended and undesirable effect produced by a drug.
Allergen		A substance that is capable of causing an allergic reaction.
Allergy		An abnormal hypersensitivity of the body to a substance that is ordinarily harmless.
Ampule		A small sealed glass container that holds a single dose of medication.
Anaphylactic reaction		A serious allergic reaction that can be life-threatening and requires immediate treatment.
Controlled drug		A drug that has restrictions placed on it by the government because of its potential for abuse and dependence.
Conversion		Changing from one system of measurement to another.
Cubic centimeter		The amount of space occupied by 1 milliliter (1 mL = 1 cc).

TERMINOLOGY REVIEW—cont'd

Key Term	Word Parts	Definition
DEA number		A registration number assigned to providers by the Drug Enforcement Administration for prescribing or dispensing controlled drugs.
Dose		The quantity of a drug to be administered at one time.
Drug		A chemical used for the treatment, prevention, or diagnosis of disease.
Gauge		The diameter of the lumen of a needle used to administer medication.
Induration		An abnormally raised, hardened area of the skin with clearly defined margins.
Inscription		The part of a prescription that indicates the name of the drug and the drug dosage.
Intradermal injection	*intra-:* within *derm/o:* skin *-al:* pertaining to	Introduction of medication into the dermal layer of the skin.
Intramuscular injection	*intra-:* within *muscul/o:* muscle *-ar:* pertaining to	Introduction of medication into the muscular layer of the body.
Oral administration		Administration of medication by mouth.
Parenteral		Administration of medication by injection.
Pharmacology	*pharmac/o:* drugs *-ology:* study of	The study of drugs.
Prescription		An order from a licensed provider authorizing the dispensing of a drug by a pharmacist.
Signatura		The part of a prescription that indicates the information to print on the medication label.
Subcutaneous injection	*sub-:* under, below *cutane/o:* skin *-ous:* pertaining to	Introduction of medication beneath the skin, into the subcutaneous or fatty layer of the body.
Subscription	*sub-:* under, below	The part of the prescription that gives directions to the pharmacist and usually designates the number of doses to be dispensed.
Superscription	*super-:* over, above	The part of a prescription consisting of the abbreviation *Rx* (from the Latin word *recipe*, meaning "take").
Vial		A closed glass container with a rubber stopper that holds medication.
Wheal		A tense, pale, raised area of the skin.

PROCEDURE 26.1

PROCEDURE 26.1 Administering Oral Medication

Outcome Administer oral solid and liquid medications.

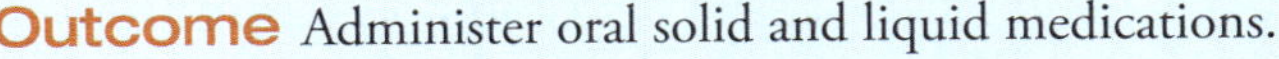

Equipment/Supplies

- Medication ordered by the provider
- Medication order
- Medicine cup
- Medication tray

1. **Procedural Step.** Sanitize your hands.
2. **Procedural Step.** Assemble the equipment.
3. **Procedural Step.** Work in a quiet, well-lit atmosphere.
   Principle. Good lighting aids the medical assistant in reading the medication label.
4. **Procedural Step.** Select the correct medication from the shelf. Compare the medication with the provider's instructions and medication order. Check the drug label three times—while removing the medication from storage, while preparing the medication, and after preparing the medication. Check the expiration date.

Continued

PROCEDURE 26.1 Administering Oral Medication—cont'd

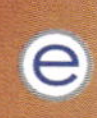

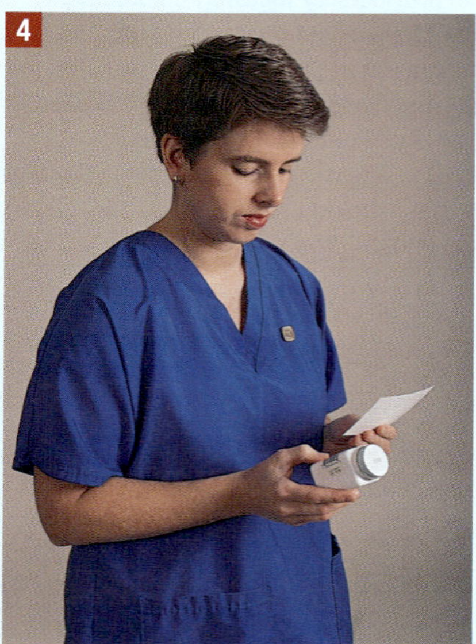
Compare the medication with the provider's instructions.

Principle. If the medication is outdated, consult the provider because it may produce undesirable effects for which the medical assistant could be held responsible. To prevent a drug error, the medication should be carefully compared with the provider's instructions.

5. **Procedural Step.** Calculate the correct dose to be given, if necessary.
6. **Procedural Step.** Remove the bottle cap, touching the outside of the lid only.
   Principle. Touching the inside of the lid contaminates it.
7. **Procedural Step.** Check the drug label again, and pour the medication.
   a. *Solid medications:* Pour the correct number of capsules or tablets into the bottle cap. Transfer the medication to a medicine cup, being careful not to touch the inside of the cup.

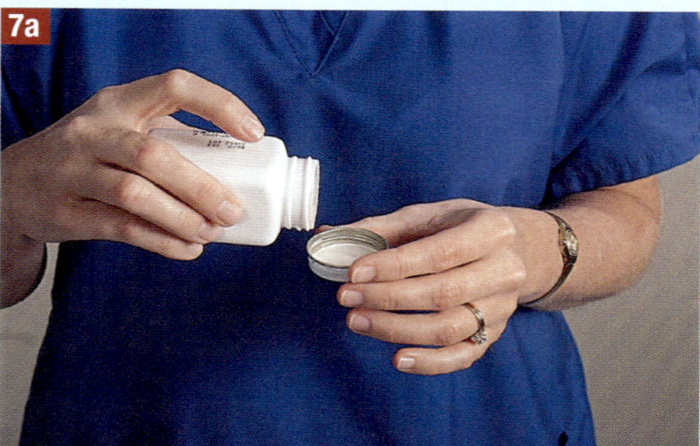
Pour the correct number of capsules or tablets into the bottle cap.

Principle. Pouring the medication into the lid prevents contamination of the medication and lid.

   b. *Liquid medications:* Place the lid of the bottle on a flat surface with the open end facing up. Palm the surface of the label.

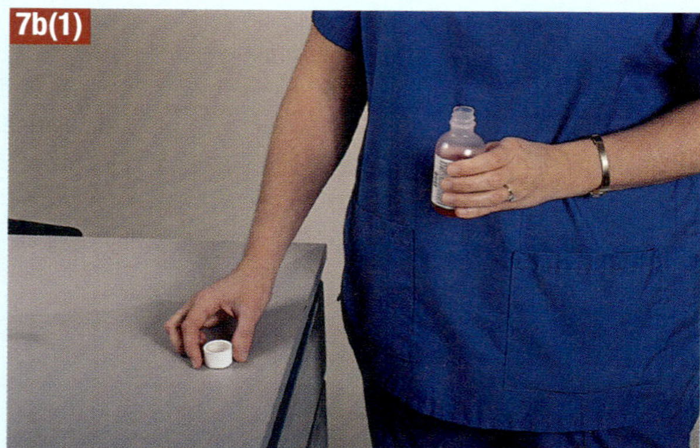
Place the lid of the bottle on a flat surface with the open end facing up.

With the opposite hand, place the thumbnail at the proper calibration on the medicine cup, and hold the cup at eye level. Pour the medication, and read the dose at the lowest level of the meniscus. (The meniscus is the curved surface of the liquid in a container. When a liquid is poured into a medicine cup, capillary action causes the liquid in contact with the cup to be drawn upward, resulting in a curved surface in the middle.)

PROCEDURE 26.1 Administering Oral Medication—cont'd

7b(2)

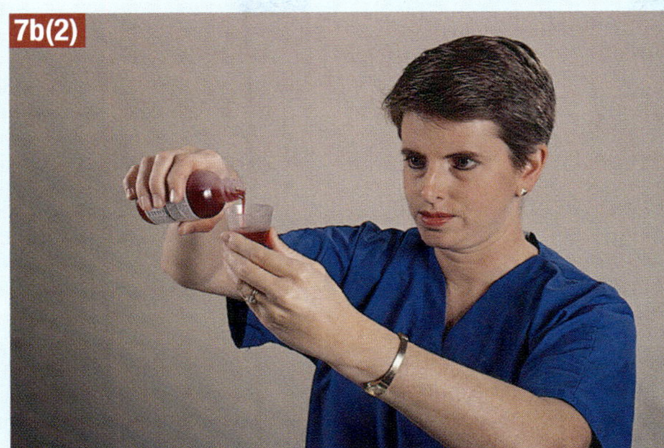

Hold the cup at eye level and pour the medication.

Principle. Placing the bottle cap with the open end up prevents contamination of the inside of the cap. Palming the medication label prevents the medication from dripping on the label and obscuring it.

8. **Procedural Step.** Replace the bottle cap, and check the drug label a third time to ensure it is the correct medication. Return the medication to its storage location.
9. **Procedural Step.** Greet the patient and introduce yourself. Identify the patient by full name and date of birth and explain the procedure. Explain the purpose of administering the medication.
   Principle. It is crucial that no error be made in patient identity.
10. **Procedural Step.** Hand the medicine cup containing the medication to the patient, along with a glass of water. (If the medication is a cough syrup, do not offer water.)
    Principle. Water helps the patient swallow the medication.
11. **Procedural Step.** Remain with the patient until the medication is swallowed. If the patient experiences any unusual reaction, notify the provider.
12. **Procedural Step.** Sanitize your hands.
13. **Procedural Step.** Document the procedure in the patient's medical record.
    a. *Electronic health record:* Document the name of the medication, the dose given, the route of administration, and any significant observations or patient reactions, using the appropriate radio buttons, drop-down menus, and free text fields.
    b. *Paper-based patient record:* Document the date and time, the name of the medication, the dose given, the route of administration, and any significant observations or patient reactions. The Latin abbreviation *po*, which means "by mouth," can be used to indicate the route of administration.

13b

DOCUMENTATION EXAMPLE

Date	
2/12/XX	9:30 a.m. Acetaminophen, 650 mg, po.
	———————— T. Cline, CMA (AAMA)

PROCEDURE 26.2 Preparing an Injection

Outcome Prepare an injection from an ampule and a vial.

Equipment/Supplies

- Medication ordered by the provider
- Medication order
- Appropriate needle and syringe
- Antiseptic wipe
- Medication tray
- Sharps container

1. **Procedural Step.** Sanitize your hands.
2. **Procedural Step.** Assemble the equipment.
3. **Procedural Step.** Work in a quiet and well-lit atmosphere.
   Principle. Good lighting aids the medical assistant in reading the medication label.
4. **Procedural Step.** Select the proper medication. Check the expiration date. Compare the medication with the provider's instructions. Check the drug label three times—while removing the medication from storage, before withdrawing the medication into the syringe, and after preparing the medication.

Continued

PROCEDURE 26.2 Preparing an Injection—cont'd

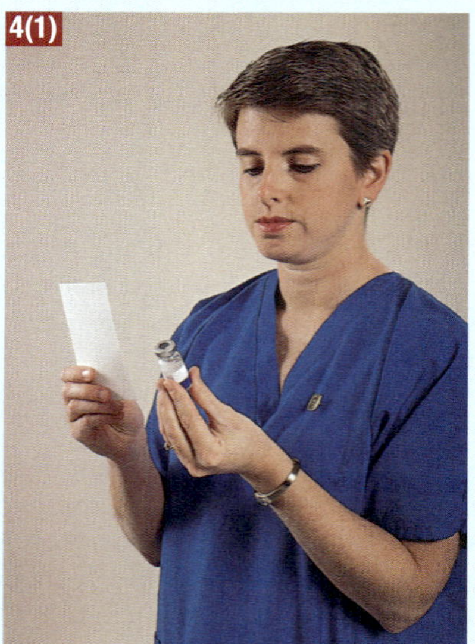

Compare the medication with the provider's instructions.

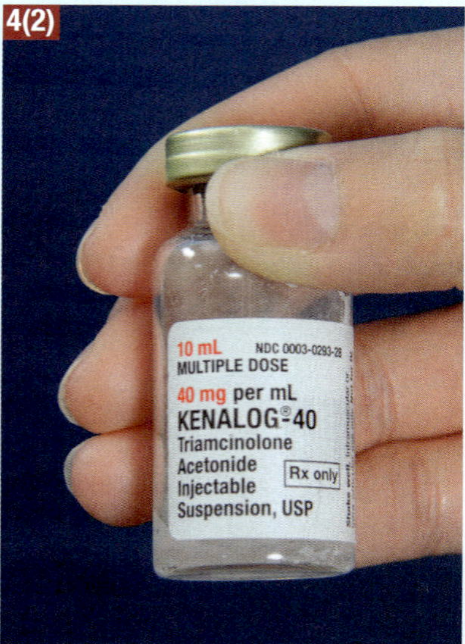

Check the drug label three times.

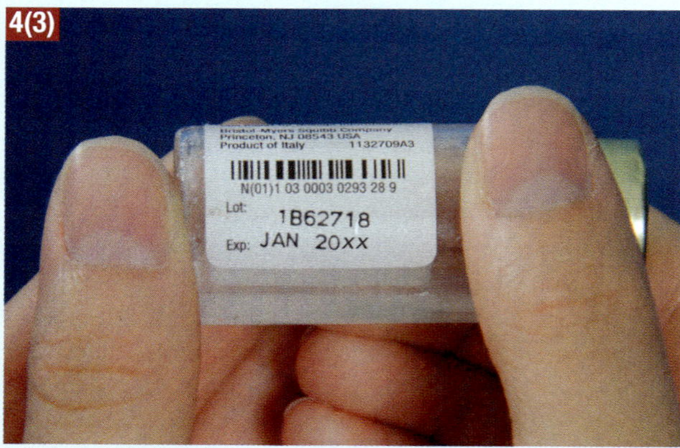

Check the expiration date.

Principle. The medication should be carefully identified to prevent administration of the wrong medication. Outdated medication should not be used because it could produce undesirable effects.

5. Procedural Step. Calculate the correct dose to be given, if necessary. If you have any questions regarding the administration of the medication, check the package insert accompanying the drug.

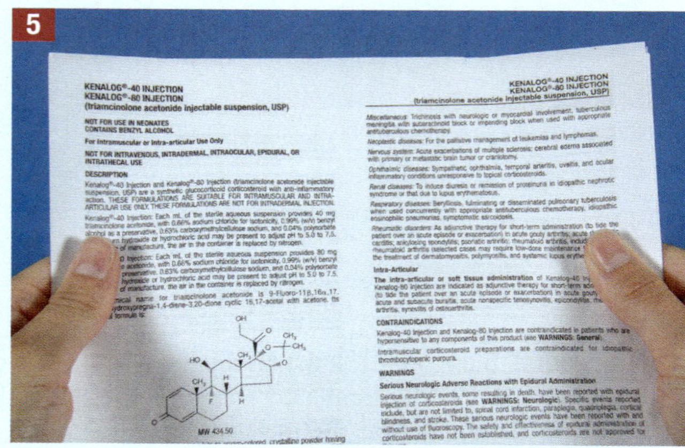

Check the package insert.

6. Procedural Step. Open the syringe and the needle package. If necessary, assemble the needle and syringe.
Principle. Disposable needles and syringes may come already assembled together in a package or in separate packages that require assembly of the needle and syringe.

7. Procedural Step. Check to ensure that the needle is attached firmly to the syringe by loosening the guard on the needle, grasping the needle at the hub, and tightening it. Break the seal on the syringe by moving the plunger back and forth several times.

8. Procedural Step. Check the drug label again to ensure it is the correct medication. If required, mix the medication by rolling the vial between your hands to obtain a uniform suspension of the medication.

9. Procedural Step. Withdraw the medication from the dispensing unit.

10. Procedural Step. Withdraw the medication from a vial.

a. Procedural Step. Remove the soft metal or plastic cap protecting the rubber stopper of an unused vial to expose the rubber stopper. Open the antiseptic; wipe and cleanse the rubber stopper and allow it to dry.

PROCEDURE 26.2 Preparing an Injection—cont'd

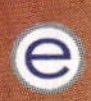

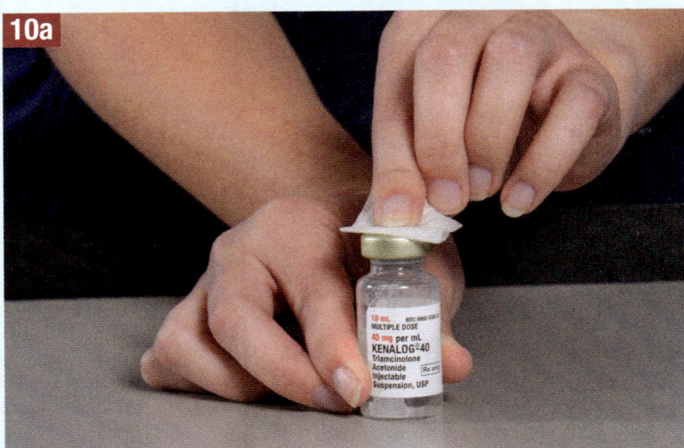

Cleanse the rubber stopper.

Principle. Cleansing the top of the vial removes dust and bacteria. The alcohol must be allowed to dry to prevent it from adhering to the needle and mixing with the medication.

b. Procedural Step. Place the vial in an upright position on a flat surface. Remove the needle guard. Pull back on the plunger to draw an amount of air into the syringe equal to the amount of medication to be withdrawn from the vial.

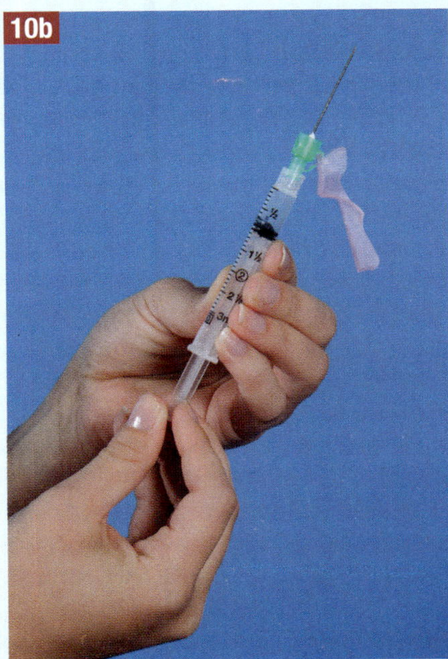

Draw the air into the syringe.

Principle. Air must be injected into the vial first to prevent the formation of a partial vacuum in the vial, which would make it difficult to remove medication.

c. Procedural Step. With the vial on a flat surface, use moderate pressure on the barrel of the syringe to insert the needle through the center of the rubber stopper at a 90-degree angle. Continue to apply pressure until the needle reaches the empty space between the stopper and fluid level. Be careful not to bend the needle. Push down on the plunger to inject the air into the vial, keeping the needle opening above the fluid level. (*Note:* If you are using a retractable safety syringe, do not push too hard on the plunger to avoid activating the retracting mechanism prematurely.)

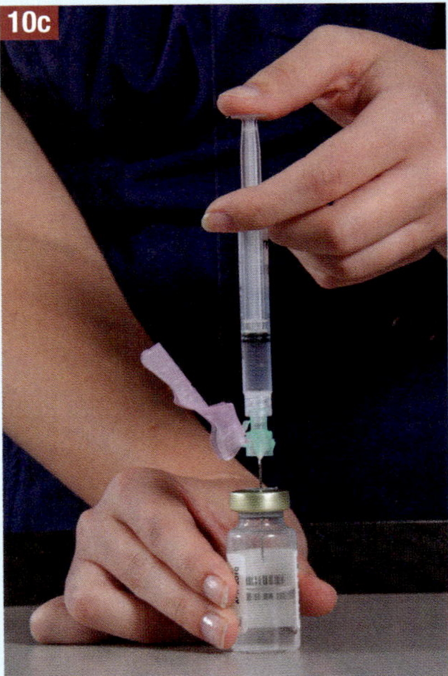

Inject air into the vial.

Principle. The center of the rubber stopper is thinner and easier to penetrate. The air must be inserted above the fluid level to avoid creating air bubbles in the medication.

d. Procedural Step. Invert the vial while holding onto the syringe and plunger. Hold the syringe at eye level, and withdraw the proper amount of medication. The medication should be measured at the widest part of the plunger seal closest to the needle. Make sure to keep the needle opening below the fluid level.

Continued

PROCEDURE 26.2 Preparing an Injection—cont'd

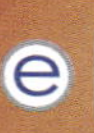

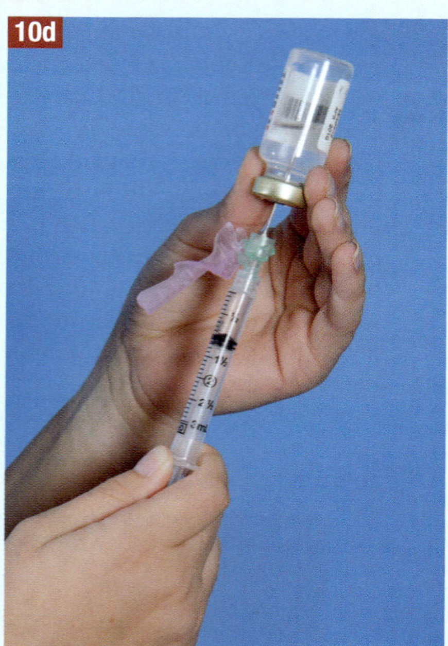

Withdraw the proper amount of medication.

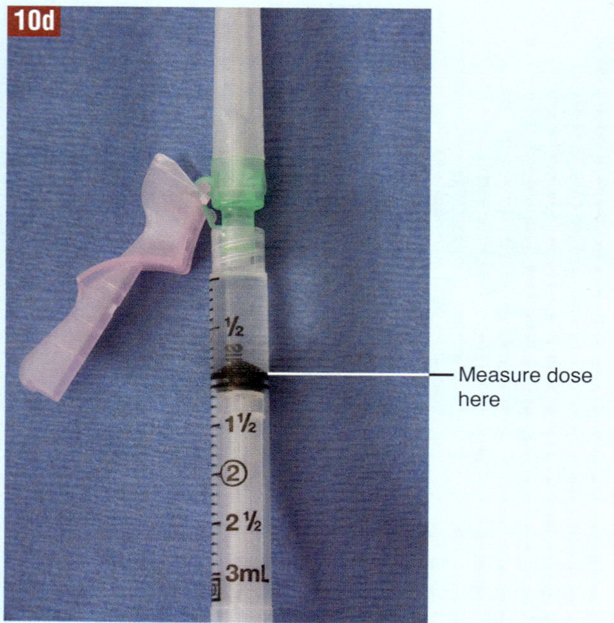

Measure the medication at the widest part of the plunger seal closest to the needle.

Principle. The needle opening must be below the fluid level to prevent the entrance of air bubbles into the syringe.

e. **Procedural Step.** Remove any air bubbles in the syringe by holding the syringe in a vertical position and tapping the barrel carefully with the fingertips until they disappear.

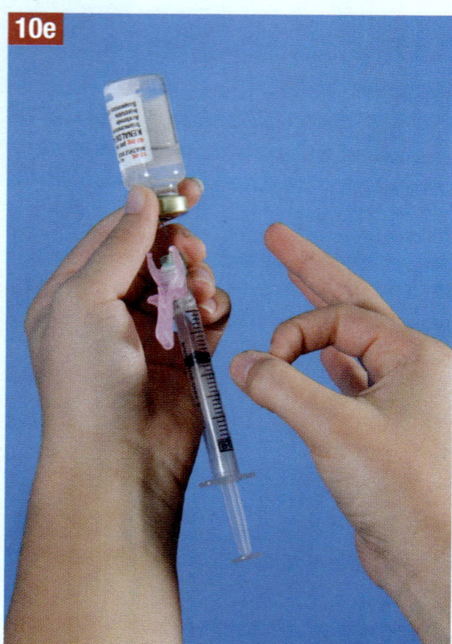

Tap the barrel with the fingertips to remove air bubbles.

Principle. Tapping the barrel too forcefully could cause the needle to bend. Air bubbles take up space the medication should occupy, preventing the patient from getting the proper dose of medication.

f. **Procedural Step.** Remove any air remaining at the top of the syringe by slowly pushing the plunger forward and allowing the air to flow back into the vial.

g. **Procedural Step.** Holding the syringe at eye level, check again to make sure you have drawn up the proper amount of medication. Carefully remove the needle from the rubber stopper, and replace the needle guard. (*Note:* After drawing up the medication, some facilities require that the needle used to draw up the medication be removed from the syringe and replaced with a new sterile needle. This is because the point of the needle may not be as sharp after it has been inserted into rubber stopper of the medication vial. The medical assistant should follow the policy set forth by his or her medical office.)
Principle. The needle must remain sterile. The needle guard prevents the needle from becoming contaminated.

h. **Procedural Step.** Check the drug label for the third time, and return the medication to its proper storage location.

11. **Procedural Step.** Withdraw medication from an ampule.
    a. **Procedural Step.** Remove the needle (and needle guard) from the syringe, and attach a filter needle (and needle guard).

PROCEDURE 26.2 Preparing an Injection—cont'd

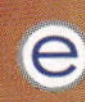

b. **Procedural Step.** Open the antiseptic wipe, and cleanse the neck of the ampule.
Principle. Cleansing the neck of the ampule removes dust and bacteria.

c. **Procedural Step.** Tap the stem of the ampule lightly to remove any medication in the neck of the ampule.

d. **Procedural Step.** Check the medication label a second time and place a piece of gauze around the neck of the ampule. Hold the base of the ampule between the first two fingers and the thumb of one hand. Hold the neck of the vial between the first two fingers and the thumb of the other hand. Apply a strong steady pressure with the thumbs, and break off the stem by snapping it quickly and firmly away from the body. Discard the stem and gauze in a biohazard sharps container.

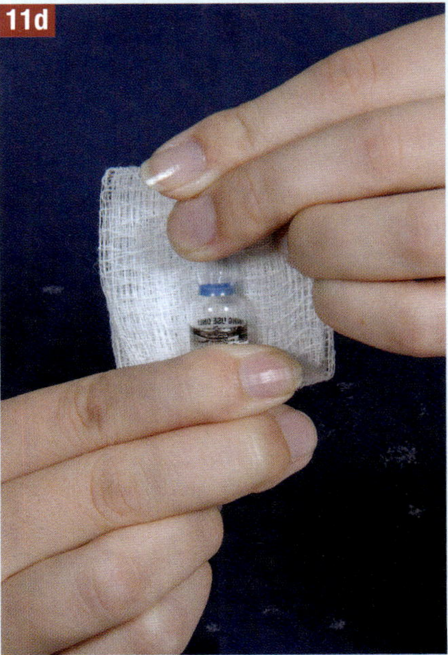

Snap the stem away from the body.

e. **Procedural Step.** Place the ampule on a flat surface. Remove the needle guard. Insert the filter needle opening below the fluid level.
Principle. The filter needle prevents glass particles from being withdrawn into the syringe.

f. **Procedural Step.** Withdraw the proper amount of medication by pulling back on the plunger. The medication should be measured at the widest part of the plunger seal closest to the needle. Make sure to keep the needle opening below the fluid level to prevent the entrance of air bubbles into the syringe. Tilt the ampule as needed to keep the needle opening immersed in the fluid. *Note:* There is another method that can be used to remove medication from an ampule. Choose the method that is easiest for you. To perform this method, invert the ampule, making sure to keep the needle opening below the fluid level. Withdraw the proper amount of medication by pulling back on the plunger. Move the needle downward as necessary to keep the needle opening immersed in the fluid.

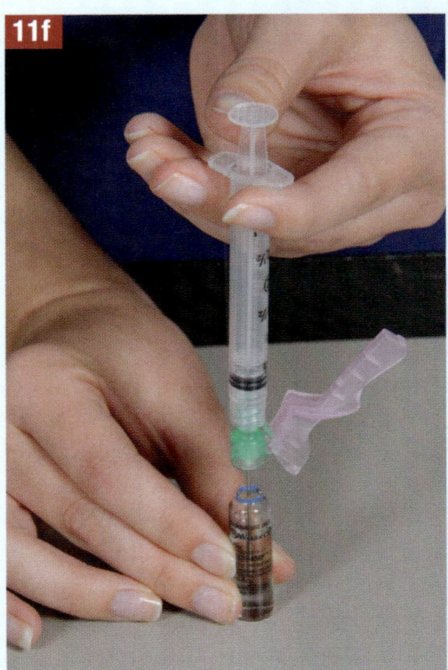

Withdraw the medication.

Principle. Air bubbles take up space the medication should occupy, resulting in an inaccurate measurement of medication.

Continued

PROCEDURE 26.2 Preparing an Injection—cont'd

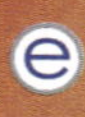

g. **Procedural Step.** Remove the needle from the ampule, and replace the needle guard. Check the drug label for the third time, and dispose of the glass ampule in a biohazard sharps container.
h. **Procedural Step.** Remove the filter needle (and guard) from the syringe, and discard it in a biohazard sharps container. Reapply the needle (and guard) for administering the medication.
i. **Procedural Step.** If air bubbles are in the syringe, remove the needle guard, hold the syringe in a vertical position, and tap the barrel with the fingertips until the bubbles disappear. Remove the air at the top of the syringe by slowly pushing the plunger forward. If the syringe contains excess fluid, hold the syringe vertically over a sink with the needle tip up and slanted toward the sink. Slowly eject the excess fluid into the sink. Holding the syringe at eye level, check again to make sure you have drawn up the proper amount of medication. Replace the needle guard.

PROCEDURE 26.3 Reconstituting Powdered Drugs

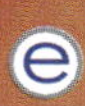

Outcome Reconstitute a powdered drug for parenteral administration.

Equipment/Supplies

- Medication ordered by the provider
- Medication order
- Appropriate needle and syringe
- Antiseptic wipe
- Medication tray

1. **Procedural Step.** Follow steps 1 through 8 of Procedure 26.2.
2. **Procedural Step.** From the vial of the powdered drug, withdraw an amount of air equal to the amount of liquid to be injected into the vial.
   Principle. Removing air from the powdered drug vial allows room for injection of the diluent.
3. **Procedural Step.** Inject the air removed from the powdered drug vial into the vial of diluent.
   Principle. Air must be injected into the vial to prevent formation of a partial vacuum in the vial, which would make it difficult to remove the diluent.
4. **Procedural Step.** Invert the diluent vial, and withdraw the proper amount of liquid into the syringe. Remove air bubbles from the syringe. Holding the syringe at eye level, check again to make sure you have drawn up the proper amount of diluent. Carefully remove the needle from the vial.
5. **Procedural Step.** Insert the needle into the powdered drug vial, and inject the diluent into the vial. Remove the needle from the vial, and replace the needle guard.

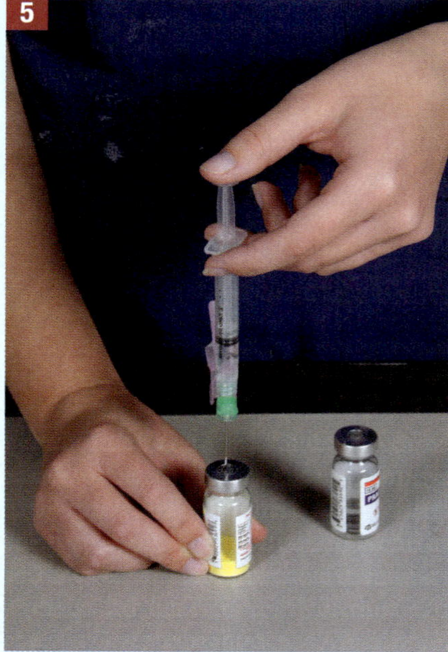

Inject the diluent into the vial.

PROCEDURE 26.3 Reconstituting Powdered Drugs—cont'd

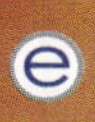

6. Procedural Step. Roll the vial between the hands to mix the powdered drug and liquid (unless indicated otherwise by the drug package insert).

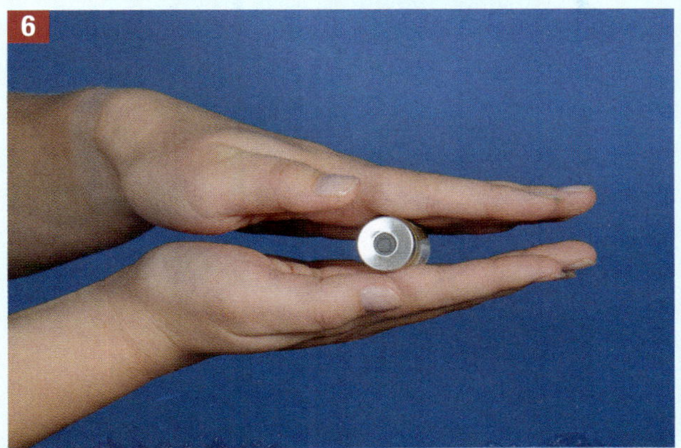

Roll the vial between the hands.

Principle. Shaking the vial may cause air bubbles to form.

7. **Procedural Step.** Label multiple-dose vials with the date of preparation and your initials.
8. **Procedural Step.** Prepare the mediation and administer the injection.
9. **Procedural Step.** Store multiple-dose vials as indicated by the manufacturer's instructions. Because reconstituted drugs are stable for a short time, carefully check the date of preparation on the multiple-dose vial before administering the medication again.

PROCEDURE 26.4 Administering a Subcutaneous Injection

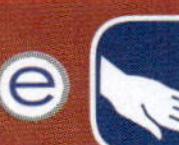
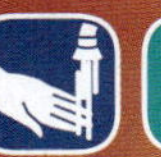

Outcome Administer a subcutaneous injection.

Equipment/Supplies

- Medication ordered by the provider
- Medication order
- Appropriate needle and syringe
- Antiseptic wipe
- Sterile 2 × 2 gauze pad
- Disposable gloves
- Biohazard sharps container

1. **Procedural Step.** Sanitize your hands and prepare the injection (see Procedure 26.2).
2. **Procedural Step.** Greet the patient and introduce yourself. Identify the patient by full name and date of birth. Explain the procedure and the purpose of the injection.
   Principle. It is crucial that no error be made in patient identity. An apprehensive patient may need reassurance.
3. **Procedural Step.** Select an appropriate injection site. The upper arm, thigh, back, and abdomen are recommended sites for a subcutaneous injection. See Fig. 26.17.
   Principle. The entire area should be exposed to ensure a safe and comfortable injection.
4. **Procedural Step.** Prepare the injection site. Cleanse the area with an antiseptic wipe. Using a circular motion, start with the injection site and move outward. Do not touch the site after cleansing it.

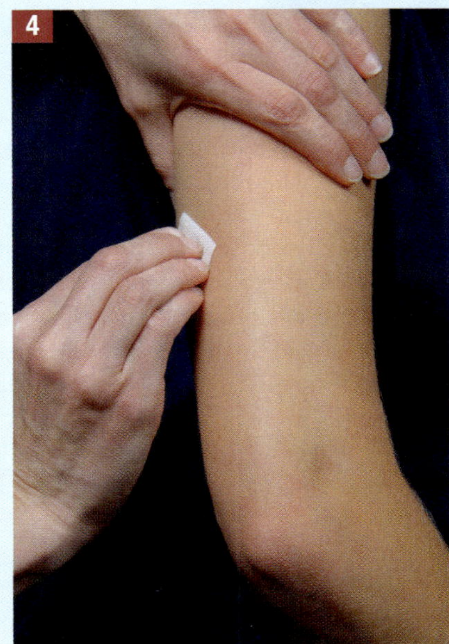

Cleanse the area with an antiseptic wipe.

Continued

PROCEDURE 26.4 Administering a Subcutaneous Injection—cont'd

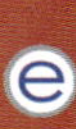

Principle. Using a circular motion carries contaminants away from the injection site. Touching the site after cleansing contaminates it, and the cleansing process needs to be repeated.

5. **Procedural Step.** Allow the area to dry completely.
Principle. If the area is not permitted to dry, the antiseptic may enter the tissues when the skin is pierced, resulting in irritation and patient discomfort.

6. **Procedural Step.** Apply gloves, and remove the needle guard. Position your nondominant hand on the area surrounding the injection site. The skin may be held taut, or the area surrounding the injection site may be grasped and held in a cushion fashion.

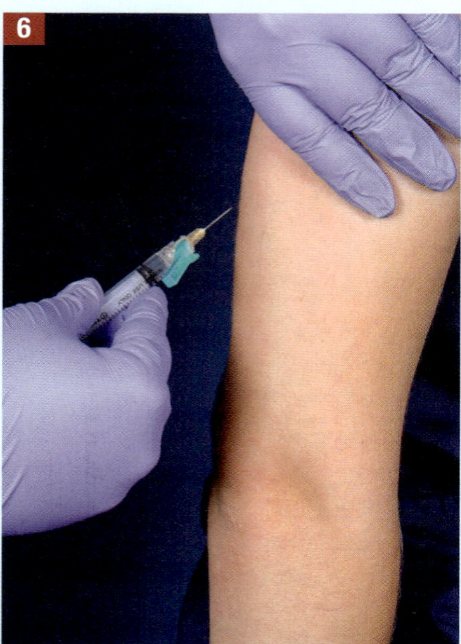

Grasp the area surrounding the injection site.

Principle. Gloves provide a barrier against bloodborne pathogens. In normal adults the needle enters the subcutaneous tissue when the skin is held taut. Grasping the area around the injection site is recommended for a thin or dehydrated patient. This ensures that the subcutaneous tissue, and not muscle tissue, is entered.

7. **Procedural Step.** Hold the barrel of the syringe between your thumb and index finger. Insert the needle quickly and smoothly at a 45-degree or 90-degree angle, depending on the length of the needle. With a ½-inch needle, a 90-degree angle should be used; with a ⅝-inch needle, a 45-degree angle should be used. Insert the needle to the hub.

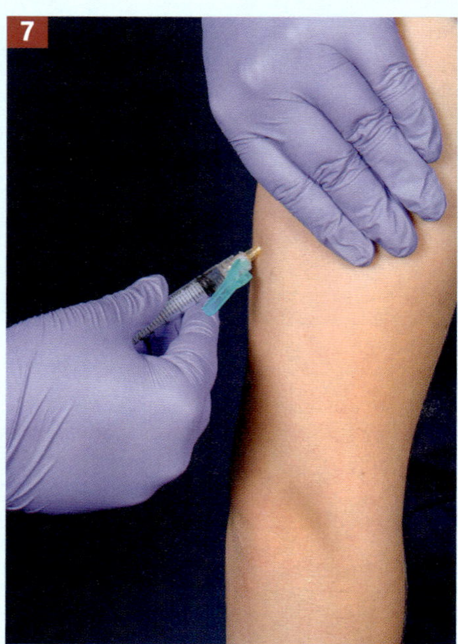

Insert the needle at a 45-degree angle.

Principle. Inserting the needle quickly and smoothly minimizes tissue trauma and pain. Needle length determines the angle of insertion to ensure placement of the medication in subcutaneous tissue.

8. **Procedural Step.** Remove your hand from the skin.
Principle. Medication injected into compressed tissue causes pressure against nerve fibers and is uncomfortable for the patient.

9. **Procedural Step.** Inject the medication slowly and steadily by depressing the plunger while holding the syringe steady. If you are using a retractable safety syringe, activate it at this time by following the steps outlined in Fig. 26.10C, and continue to Step 12.

PROCEDURE 26.4 Administering a Subcutaneous Injection—cont'd

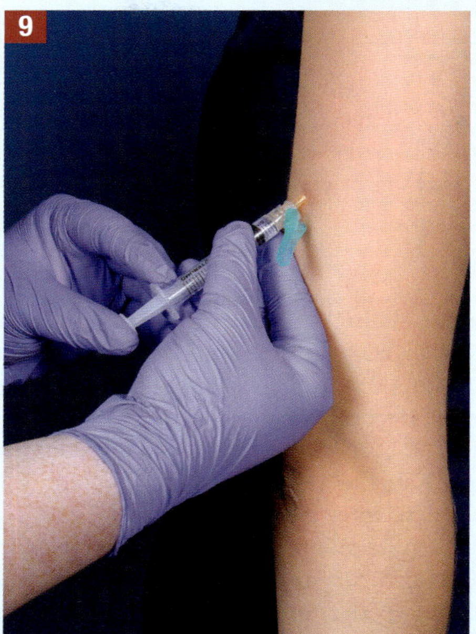
9

Inject the medication slowly and steadily.

(*Note:* Unless otherwise required by the package insert accompanying the medication to be administered or by your medical office policy, aspiration of the syringe for blood is not necessary because there are no large blood vessels located in subcutaneous tissue).

Principle. Rapid injection creates pressure and destroys tissue, both of which are uncomfortable for the patient. Moving the syringe after the needle has entered the tissue causes patient discomfort.

10. **Procedural Step.** Place a gauze pad gently over the injection site and quickly remove the needle, keeping it at the same angle as for insertion.

    Principle. Withdrawing the needle quickly and at the same angle as for insertion reduces patient discomfort. The gauze pad placed over the injection site helps prevent tissue movement as the needle is withdrawn, reducing patient discomfort.

11. **Procedural Step.** Apply gentle pressure to the injection site with a gauze pad. If you are using a safety syringe with a pivoting-shield or hinged-shield, activate the safety feature at this time by following the steps outlined in Fig. 26.10.

    Principle. Gentle pressure helps distribute the medication so that it is completely absorbed. Avoid vigorous massaging because this could damage underlying tissue.

12. **Procedural Step.** Properly dispose of the needle and syringe in a biohazard sharps container.

    Principle. Proper disposal is required by the OSHA standard to prevent accidental needlestick injuries.

13. **Procedural Step.** Remove gloves, and sanitize your hands.
14. **Procedural Step.** Document the procedure in the patient's medical record.
    a. *Electronic health record:* Document the name of the medication, the manufacturer and lot number (if required), the dose given, the route of administration, the injection site used, and any significant observations or patient reactions, using the appropriate radio buttons, drop-down menus, and free text fields.
    b. *Paper-based patient record:* Document the date and time, the name of the medication, the manufacturer and lot number (if required), the dose given, the route of administration, the injection site used, and any significant observations or patient reactions.

14b

DOCUMENTATION EXAMPLE

Date	
2/17/XX	3:30 p.m. Ragweed allergy inj, 0.20 mL, subcut, Ⓡ
	upper arm. Arm checked 15 min. after admin. No
	reaction noted. ______T. Cline, CMA (AAMA)

Principle. The lot number indicates the batch in which the medication was made. Should a problem arise with that batch, the drug can be recalled, and the individuals who received it can be identified.

15. **Procedural Step.** Stay with the patient to ensure that they are not experiencing any unusual reactions. (*Note:* If an allergy injection has been given, the patient should remain at the medical office for 15 to 20 minutes to ensure that an allergic reaction does not occur.) Check the patient's arm after the waiting period, and observe for induration and redness. If the patient experiences such a reaction, notify the provider immediately. Document the inspection of the injection site in the patient's medical record.

PROCEDURE 26.5 Administering an Intramuscular Injection

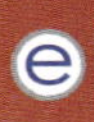

Outcome Administer an intramuscular injection

Equipment/Supplies

- Medication ordered by the provider
- Medication order
- Appropriate needle and syringe
- Antiseptic wipe
- Sterile 2 × 2 gauze pad
- Disposable gloves
- Biohazard sharps container

1. **Procedural Step.** Sanitize your hands and prepare the injection (see Procedure 26.2).
2. **Procedural Step.** Greet the patient and introduce yourself. Identify the patient by their full name and date of birth. Explain the procedure and purpose of the injection.
   Principle. Make sure that you administer the medication to the right patient. Explain the purpose of the injection. Assistance may be needed for restraining infants and children.
3. **Procedural Step.** Select an appropriate intramuscular (IM) injection site. See Fig. 26.18 for the recommended intramuscular injection sites. Remove the patient's clothing as necessary to ensure the entire area is exposed.
   Principle. The medical assistant should develop skill and accuracy in locating the proper sites.
4. **Procedural Step.** Prepare the injection site. Cleanse the area with an antiseptic wipe. Using a circular motion, start with the injection site and move outward. Do not touch the site after cleansing it.

4

Cleanse the site with an antiseptic wipe.

   Principle. Using a circular motion carries contaminants away from the injection site. Touching the site after cleansing contaminates it, and the cleansing process needs to be repeated.
5. **Procedural Step.** Allow the area to dry completely.
   Principle. If the area is not permitted to dry, the antiseptic may enter the tissues when the skin is pierced, resulting in irritation and patient discomfort.
6. **Procedural Step.** Apply gloves, and remove the needle guard. Using the thumb and first two fingers of the nondominant hand, stretch the skin taut over the injection site.
   Principle. Gloves provide a barrier against bloodborne pathogens. Stretching the skin taut permits easier insertion of the needle and helps ensure that the needle enters muscle tissue.
7. **Procedural Step.** Hold the barrel of the syringe like a dart, and insert the needle quickly and smoothly at a 90-degree angle to the patient's skin with a firm motion. Insert the needle to the hub.

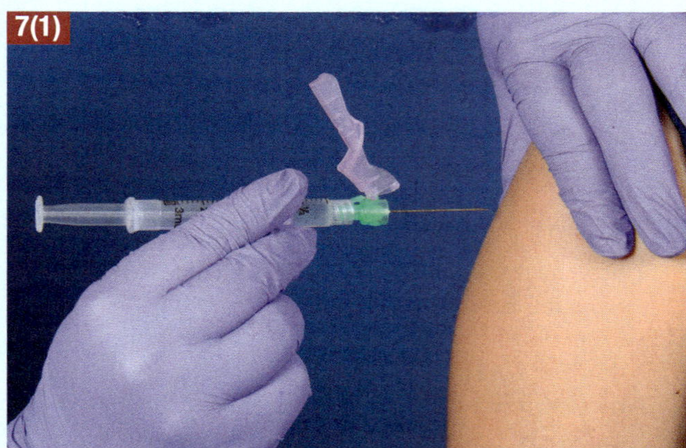

Insert the needle at a 90-degree angle (deltoid site).

PROCEDURE 26.5 Administering an Intramuscular Injection—cont'd

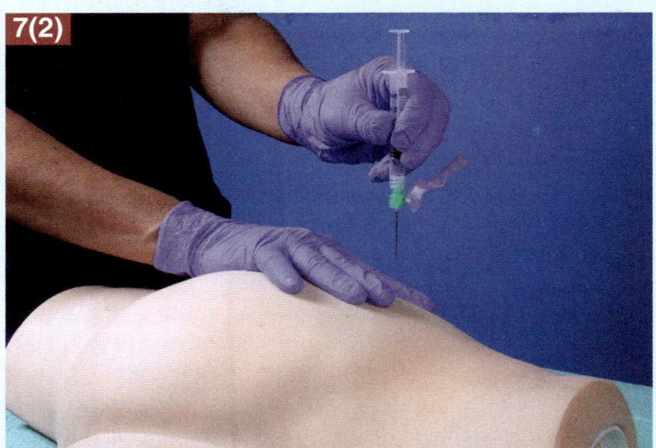

Insert the needle at a 90-degree angle (ventrogluteal site).

Principle. The needle is inserted at a 90-degree angle and to the hub to ensure that it reaches muscle tissue. Inserting the needle quickly and smoothly minimizes tissue trauma and pain.

8. Procedural Step. Hold the syringe steady, and pull back gently on the plunger for 5 to 10 seconds to determine whether the needle is in a blood vessel. If blood appears, withdraw the needle, prepare a new injection, and begin again. (Note: Some IM injections (e.g., vaccines) do not require aspiration. The medical assistant should review the drug package insert and follow the aspiration recommendations stated by the manufacturer).

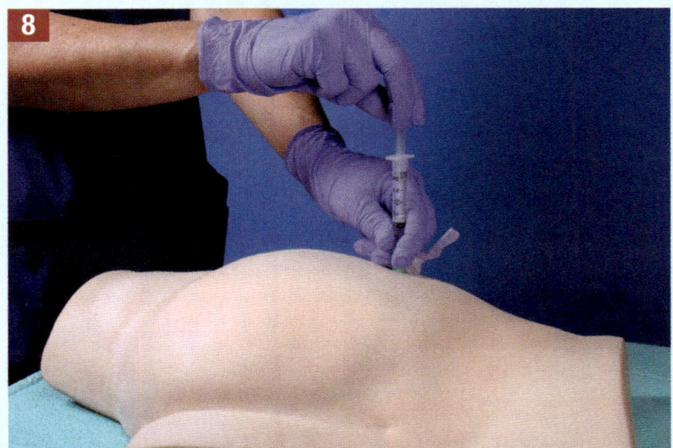

Aspirate to determine if the needle is in a blood vessel.

Principle. Moving the syringe after the needle has penetrated the tissue causes patient discomfort. If the needle is in a small blood vessel, it takes 5 to 10 seconds for the blood to appear in the syringe. If drugs intended for intramuscular administration are injected into a blood vessel, the result is faster absorption of the medication. This may produce undesirable results.

9. Procedural Step. Inject the medication slowly and steadily by depressing the plunger. If you are using a retractable safety syringe, activate it at this time while following the steps outlined in Fig. 26.10C, and continue to Step 11.

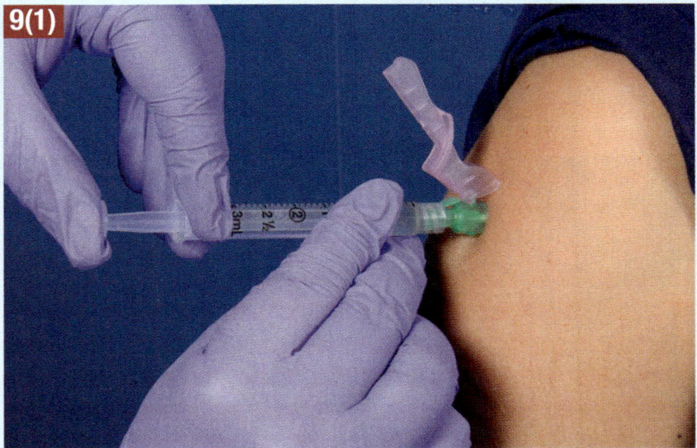

Inject the medication slowly and steadily into the deltoid site.

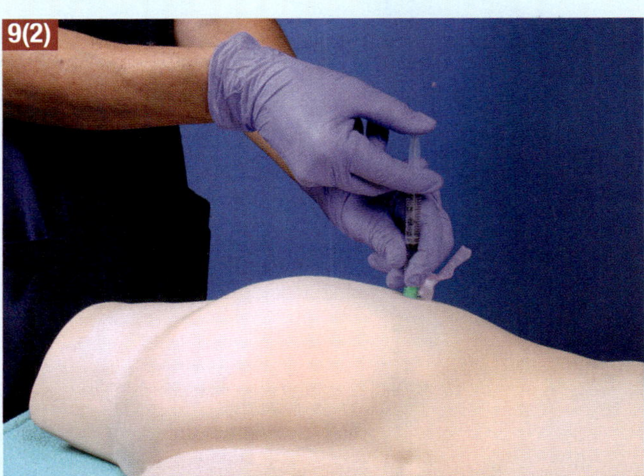

Inject the medication slowly and steadily into the ventrogluteal site.

Principle. Rapid injection creates pressure and destroys tissue, causing discomfort for the patient. Inject the medication slowly and steadily.

Continued

PROCEDURE 26.5 Administering an Intramuscular Injection—cont'd 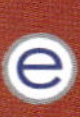   

10. Procedural Step. Place a gauze pad gently over the injection site and remove the needle quickly, keeping it at the same angle as for insertion.

Principle. Withdrawing the needle quickly and at the same angle as for insertion reduces patient discomfort. Placing a gauze pad over the injection site helps prevent tissue movement as the needle is withdrawn, also reducing patient discomfort. Using a gauze pad prevents a stinging sensation from the alcohol.

11. Procedural Step. Apply gentle pressure to the injection site with a gauze pad. If you are using a safety syringe with a pivoting-shield or a hinged-shield, activate the safety feature at this time by following the steps outlined in Fig. 26.10.

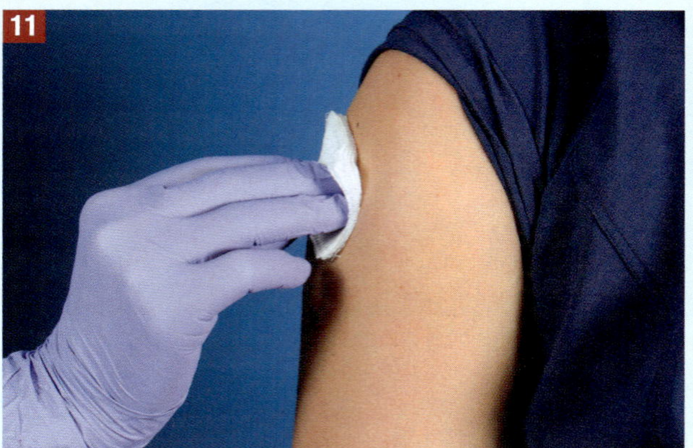

Apply gentle pressure to the injection site.

Principle. Gentle pressure helps distribute the medication so that it is absorbed by the muscle tissue. Avoid vigorous massaging because this could damage underlying tissues.

12. Procedural Step. Properly dispose of the needle and syringe in a biohazard sharps container.

Principle. Proper disposal is required by the OSHA standard to prevent accidental needlestick injuries.

13. Procedural Step. Remove the gloves, and sanitize your hands.

14. Procedural Step. Document the procedure in the patient's medical record.

a. *Electronic health record:* Document the name of the medication, the manufacturer and lot number, the dose given, the route of administration, the injection site used, and any significant observations or patient reactions, using the appropriate radio buttons, drop-down menus, and free text fields.

b. *Paper-based patient record:* Document the date and time, the name of the medication, the manufacturer and lot number, the dose given, the route of administration, the injection site used, and any significant observations or patient reactions.

14b

DOCUMENTATION EXAMPLE

Date	
2/20/XX	9:30 a.m. Rocephin (Hoffmann-LaRoche, Lot #: U6261).
	Admin 1 gram, IM, (L) deltoid. Tolerated injection
	well. ———————— T. Cline, CMA (AAMA)

Principle. The lot number indicates the batch in which the medication was made. Should a problem arise with that batch, the drug can be recalled, and individuals who received it can be identified.

15. Procedural Step. Stay with the patient to ensure they are not experiencing any unusual reactions. If the patient experiences an unusual reaction, notify the provider immediately.

PROCEDURE 26.6 Z-Track Intramuscular Injection Technique

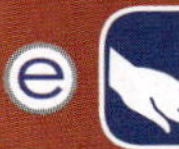

Outcome Administer an intramuscular injection using the Z-track method.

Equipment/Supplies

- Medication ordered by the provider
- Medication order
- Appropriate needle and syringe
- Antiseptic wipe
- Disposable gloves
- Biohazard sharps container

1. **Procedural Step.** Follow steps 1 through 5 of Procedure 26.5.
2. **Procedural Step.** Apply gloves, and remove the needle guard. With the nondominant hand, pull the skin away laterally from the injection site approximately 1 to 1½ inches.
3. **Procedural Step.** Insert the needle quickly and smoothly at a 90-degree angle.
4. **Procedural Step.** If required, aspirate for 5 to 10 seconds to determine whether the needle is in a blood vessel. If blood appears, withdraw the needle and discard the needle and syringe. Prepare another injection and begin again.
5. **Procedural Step.** Inject the medication slowly and steadily.
6. **Procedural Step.** After injecting the medication, wait 10 seconds before withdrawing the needle to allow initial absorption of the medication.
7. **Procedural Step.** Withdraw the needle quickly, keeping it at the same angle as for insertion.
8. **Procedural Step.** Release the traction on the skin to seal off the needle track; doing so prevents the medication from reaching the subcutaneous tissue and skin surface.
9. **Procedural Step.** Do not apply pressure to the site because this could cause the medication to seep out.
10. **Procedural Step.** If you are using a safety syringe with a shield, activate the safety feature at this time by following the steps outlined in Fig. 26.10.
11. **Procedural Step.** Properly dispose of the needle and syringe in a biohazard sharps container.
12. **Procedural Step.** Remove your gloves, and sanitize your hands.
13. **Procedural Step.** Document the procedure in the patient's medical record.
    a. *Electronic health record:* Document the name of the medication, the manufacturer and lot number, the dose given, the route of administration, the injection site used, and any significant observations or patient reactions using the appropriate radio buttons, drop-down menus, and free text fields.
    b. *Paper-based patient record:* Document the date and time, the name of the medication, the manufacturer and lot number, the dose given, the route of administration, the injection site used, and any significant observations or patient reactions.

13b

DOCUMENTATION EXAMPLE

Date	
2/20/XX	10:30 a.m. Iron dextran (Watson Pharmaceuticals,
	Lot #: 1445). Admin 100 mg, IM, Z-track into (R)
	ventrogluteal. No complaints of discomfort.———
	——————————— T. Cline, CMA (AAMA)

14. **Procedural Step.** Stay with the patient to ensure they are not experiencing any unusual reactions. If the patient experiences an unusual reaction, notify the provider immediately.

PROCEDURE 26.7A Administering an Intradermal Injection

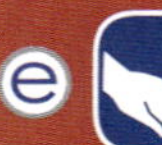  

Outcome Administer an intradermal injection and read the test results.

Equipment/Supplies

- Skin test solution ordered by the provider
- Medication order
- Appropriate needle and syringe
- Antiseptic wipe
- Sterile 2 × 2 gauze pad
- Disposable gloves
- Millimeter ruler
- Tuberculosis (TB) skin test record card
- Biohazard sharps container

1. **Procedural Step.** Sanitize your hands and prepare the injection (see Procedure 26.2).
2. **Procedural Step.** Greet the patient and introduce yourself. Identify the patient by full name and date of birth. Explain the procedure and purpose of the injection.
   Principle. It is crucial that no error be made in patient identity. Explain the purpose of the injection to reassure an apprehensive patient.
3. **Procedural Step.** Select an appropriate injection site. The anterior forearm and the middle of the back are recommended sites for an intradermal injection. If using the anterior forearm, position the arm on a firm surface with the palm facing upward.
   Principle. The entire area should be exposed to ensure a safe and comfortable injection.
4. **Procedural Step.** Prepare the injection site. Cleanse the area with an antiseptic wipe. Using a circular motion, start with the injection site and move outward. Do not touch the site after cleansing it.
   Principle. Using a circular motion will carry material away from the injection site. Touching the site after cleansing will contaminate it, and the cleansing process will need to be repeated.
5. **Procedural Step.** Allow the area to dry completely.
   Principle. If the area is not permitted to dry, the antiseptic may enter the tissue when the skin is pierced, resulting in irritation and patient discomfort. In addition, the antiseptic may cause a reaction that could be mistaken for a positive test response.
6. **Procedural Step.** Apply gloves, and remove the needle guard. With the nondominant hand, stretch the skin taut at the proposed site of administration. Insert the needle at a 10- to 15-degree angle (almost parallel to the skin), with the bevel upward. The needle should be inserted about ⅛ inch until the bevel of the needle just penetrates the skin. Slight resistance may be felt as the needle is inserted. No aspiration is needed.

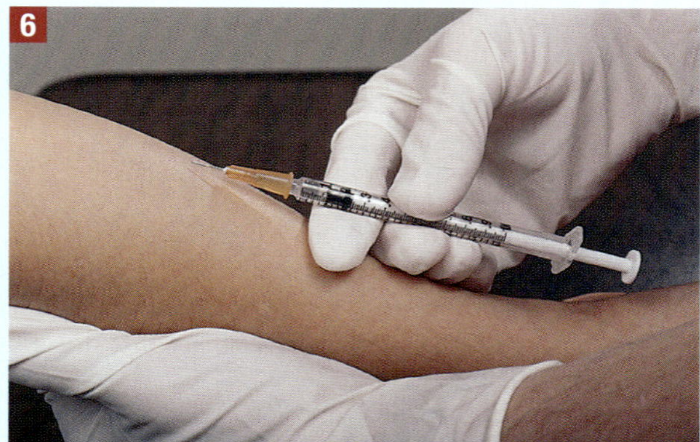

Insert the needle at a 10- to 15-degree angle with the bevel upward.

   Principle. Gloves provide a barrier against bloodborne pathogens. Stretching the patient's skin taut will permit easier insertion of the needle. The needle should be inserted at an angle almost parallel to the skin, to ensure penetration within the dermal layer of the skin. The needle must be inserted with the bevel facing up to allow proper wheal formation. If the needle is inserted with the bevel facing down, the skin test solution will be absorbed into the underlying subcutaneous tissue, and a wheal will not form.
7. **Procedural Step.** Release the stretched skin. Hold the syringe steady, and inject the skin test solution slowly and steadily by depressing the plunger until a firm, tense, pale wheal forms (approximately 6 to 10 mm in diameter). Expect to feel a certain amount of resistance as you inject the solution; this helps in indicating that the needle is properly located in the superficial skin layers rather than in the deeper subcutaneous tissue. If a wheal does not form, the test must be repeated at another site that is at least 2 inches (5 cm) from the first site. If you are using a retractable safety syringe, activate it at this time by following the steps outlined in Fig. 26.10C, and continue to Step 9.

PROCEDURE 26.7A Administering an Intradermal Injection—cont'd

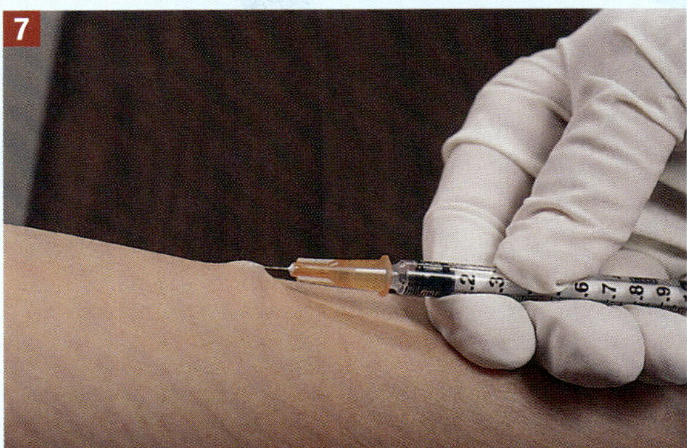
7

Inject the medication to form a wheal.

Principle. Moving the syringe once the needle has entered the skin causes patient discomfort. Test results are considered reliable only if a wheal forms.

8. **Procedural Step.** Place a gauze pad gently over the injection site and remove the needle quickly and at the same angle as for insertion.
   Principle. Withdrawing the needle quickly and at the angle of insertion reduces patient discomfort. The gauze pad placed over the injection site helps prevent tissue movement as the needle is withdrawn, also reducing patient discomfort.
9. **Procedural Step.** Do not apply pressure to the injection site. If blood appears at the injection site, blot the site lightly with a gauze pad. If you are using a safety syringe with a pivoting-shield or hinged-shield, activate the safety feature at this time by following the steps outlined in Fig. 26.10.
   Principle. Applying pressure may cause leakage of the testing solution through the needle puncture site, resulting in inaccurate test results.
10. **Procedural Step.** Properly dispose of the needle and syringe in a biohazard sharps container.
    Principle. Proper disposal of the needle and syringe is required by the OSHA standard to prevent accidental needlestick injuries.
11. **Procedural Step.** Remove gloves and sanitize your hands.
12. **Procedural Step.** Stay with the patient to make sure that they are not experiencing any unusual reactions. The medical assistant should be especially careful and alert for any sign of a patient reaction when administering allergy skin tests. If the patient experiences an unusual reaction, notify the provider immediately.
13. **Procedural Step.** Perform one of the following, based on the type of skin test being administered.
14. **Procedural Step.** Read the allergy skin test results.
    a. Read the test results within 20 to 30 minutes, using inspection and palpation at the site of the injection to assess the presence of and to determine the amount of induration. Interpret the skin test results according to the information outlined in Table 26.9.
    b. Document the procedure in the patient's medical record.
       (1) *Electronic health record:* Document the injection site, the names of the skin tests, the skin test results, and any significant observations or patient reactions using the appropriate radio buttons, drop-down menus, and free text fields.
       (2) *Paper-based patient record:* Document the date and time, the injection site used, the names of the skin tests, the skin test results, and any significant observations or patient reactions.

14b(2)

DOCUMENTATION EXAMPLE

Date	
2/15/XX	Allergy skin tests, ID, (R) ant forearm.
	Results: House dust +2
	Cat dander +4
	Dog dander –
	Ragweed +4
	Mixed fungi +3
	———————— T. Cline, CMA (AAMA)

15. **Procedural Step.** Provide patient instruction for the Mantoux tuberculin skin test.
    a. Inform the patient of the date and time to return to the medical office to have the results read. Results must be read within 48 to 72 hours after the test has been administered. Stress the importance of returning to the office to have the results read, even if the test site does not exhibit a reaction. Failure to return warrants having to repeat the test.
    b. Document the procedure in the patient's medical record.
       (1) *Electronic health record:* Document the name of the tuberculin purified protein derivative (PPD) solution, the dose given, the manufacturer and lot number, the route of administration, the injection site used, and any significant observations or patient reactions, using the appropriate radio buttons, drop-down menus, and free text fields.

Continued

PROCEDURE 26.7A Administering an Intradermal Injection—cont'd

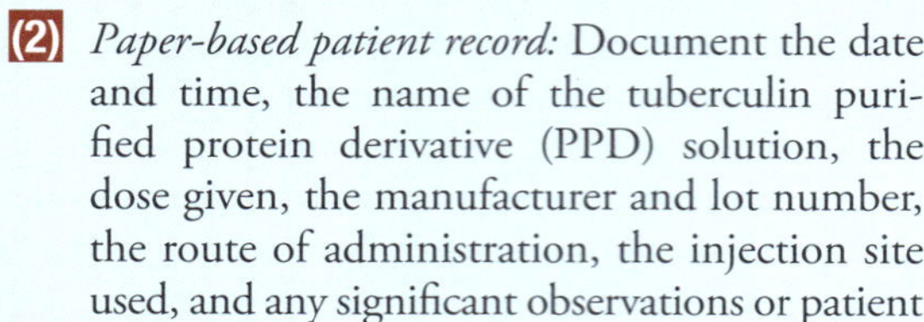

(2) *Paper-based patient record:* Document the date and time, the name of the tuberculin purified protein derivative (PPD) solution, the dose given, the manufacturer and lot number, the route of administration, the injection site used, and any significant observations or patient reactions.

15b(2)

DOCUMENTATION EXAMPLE

Date	
2/15/XX	10:00 a.m. Tubersol Mantoux test 5 TU,
	0.10 mL, ID. (Connaught Laboratories,
	Lot #: C0832AA). Admin (R) ant forearm.
	Pt to return on 2/17/XX to have results
	read. ——————— T. Cline, CMA (AAMA)

Principle. The lot number indicates the batch in which the tuberculin solution was made. Should a problem arise with that batch, the tuberculin solution can be recalled and the individuals who received it can be identified.

c. Instruct the patient in the care of the test site as follows:
   - Continue your normal daily personal hygiene activities.
   - Do not cover the test site with an adhesive bandage.
   - Avoid the use of ointments, lotions, and sunscreens.
   - Mild itching, swelling, or irritation may normally occur at the test site.
   - Do not touch, scratch, press on, or rub the test site. This could alter the test results. If the test site itches, apply a cold compress to the area.
   - Pat the arm dry after washing it. Do not rub it dry.

PROCEDURE 26.7B Read a Tuberculin Skin Test Result

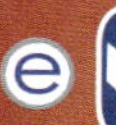  

Equipment/Supplies

- Millimeter ruler
- Disposable gloves
- Tuberculin test record card

1. **Procedural Step.** Greet the patient and introduce yourself. Identify the patient by full name and date of birth and explain the procedure.
2. **Procedural Step.** Work in a quiet well-lit atmosphere. Check the patient's medical record to determine which arm was used to administer the test.
3. **Procedural Step.** Sanitize your hands and apply gloves.
4. **Procedural Step.** Position the patient's arm on a firm surface with the arm flexed at the elbow.
5. **Procedural Step.** Locate the application site. The result should be read transversely to the long axis of the forearm, meaning "across" the forearm.
6. **Procedural Step.** Gently rub your fingertip over the test site and lightly palpate for the presence of induration. If induration is present, the area should be lightly rubbed from the area of normal skin (without induration) to the indurated area to assess the size of the area of induration. If the margins of induration are irregular, assess the widest diameter of induration across the forearm.

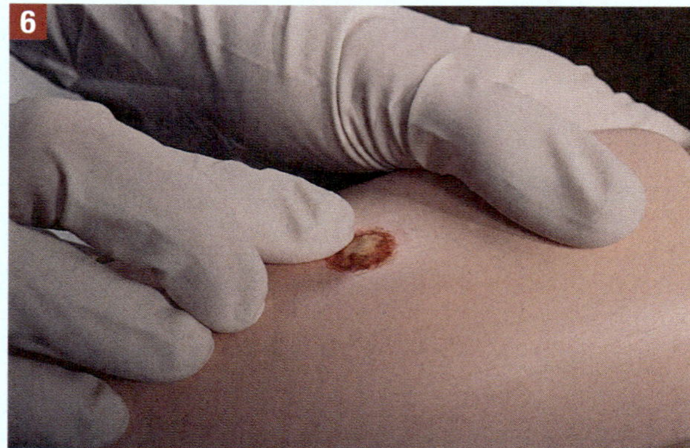

Lightly palpate for induration.

PROCEDURE 26.7B Read a Tuberculin Skin Test Result—cont'd

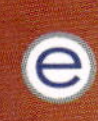  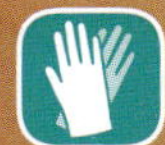

Principle. Induration is the only criterion used in determining a positive reaction. If erythema is present without induration, the results are interpreted as negative.

7. Procedural Step. Measure the diameter of the induration with a flexible millimeter ruler (supplied by the manufacturer).

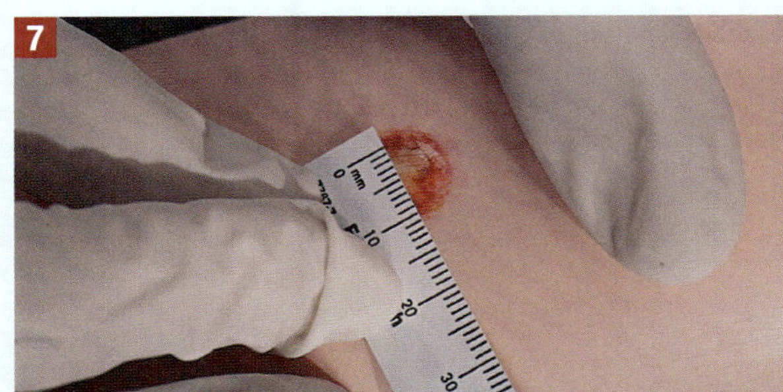

Measure the induration.

8. Procedural Step. Remove gloves and sanitize your hands.

9. Procedural Step. Document the results in the patient's medical record.

a. *Electronic health record:* Document the name of the test (Mantoux TST) and the test results (documented in millimeters) using the appropriate radio buttons, drop-down menus, and free text fields. If no induration is present, 0 mm should be documented. The results of the Mantoux TST are interpreted according to the guidelines outlined in Table 26.7.

b. *Paper-based patient record:* Document the date and time, the name of the test, and the test results (documented in millimeters). If no induration is present, 0 mm should be documented. The results of the Mantoux TST are interpreted according to the guidelines outlined in Table 26.7.

9b

DOCUMENTATION EXAMPLE

Date	
2/17/XX	3:00 p.m. Tubersol Mantoux test: 9mm.
	Pt provided c̄ TB record card. Scheduled
	for TB retesting on 2/28/XX. ————
	———— T. Cline, CMA (AAMA)

10. Procedural Step. Complete a tuberculin test record card and give it to the patient.

Principle. The record card provides the patient with a permanent record of the test results.

10

TUBERCULOSIS TEST RECORD

Name	Date Admin: 2/15/XX
Carrie Fee	Date Read: 2/17/XX
MANTOUX TEST	**RESULT**
Tubersol, 5 TU	9 mm

Logan Family Practice
401 St. George St.
St. Augustine, FL 32084
(904) 555-3933

Performed by T. Cline, CMA (AAMA)

PROCEDURE 26.7B

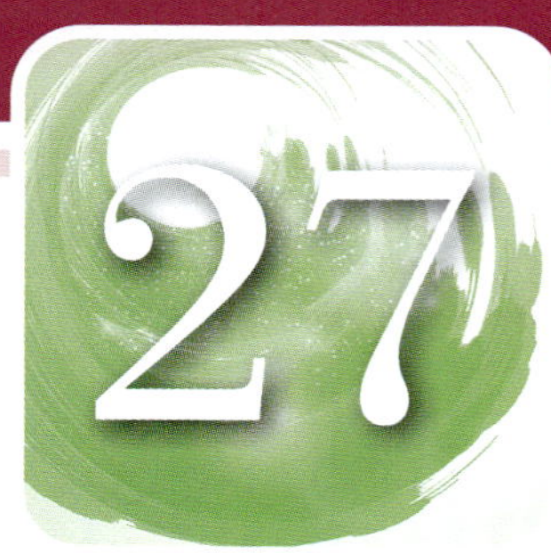

27 Cardiopulmonary Procedures

Check out the Evolve site at http://evolve.elsevier.com/Bonewit/today to access additional interactive activities and exercises to help you study and prepare for success.

LEARNING OBJECTIVES

Electrocardiography

1. State the purpose of electrocardiography.
2. Identify each of the following components of the ECG cycle:
   - P wave
   - QRS complex
   - T wave
   - P–R segment
   - ST segment
   - P–R interval
   - Q–T interval
   - Baseline following the T wave
3. State the purpose of the standardization mark.
4. State the functions of the electrodes, amplifier, and output device.
5. List the 12 leads that are included in an ECG.
6. Describe the function served by each of the following:
   - Three-channel recording capability
   - Interpretive electrocardiography
   - Electronic medical record connectivity
   - Teletransmission
7. Identify each of the following types of artifacts, and state its causes:
   - Muscle
   - Wandering baseline
   - 60-cycle interference
   - Interrupted baseline

Holter Monitor Electrocardiography

8. List the reasons for applying a Holter monitor.

Cardiac Dysrhythmias

9. Identify the different types of cardiac dysrhythmias.

Pulmonary Function Testing

10. Identify the different pulmonary function tests.
11. List indications for performing spirometry testing.
12. Describe patient preparation for spirometry.
13. Explain the purpose of post-bronchodilator spirometry.
14. Identify the symptoms of an asthma attack.
15. List examples of asthma triggers.
16. Explain the difference between long-term control and quick-relief asthma medications.
17. Describe the purpose of a peak flow meter.
18. State the purpose of a peak flow chart.
19. Identify the information included in an asthma action plan.

PROCEDURES

Record a 12-lead, three-channel ECG.

Measure a patient's peak expiratory flow rate.

Home Oxygen Therapy

20. Explain why the body needs oxygen.
21. Describe what occurs when the body cannot maintain an adequate blood oxygen level.
22. Identify the conditions that may require home oxygen therapy.
23. List and describe the three common types of oxygen delivery systems along with the advantages and disadvantages of each.
24. List and describe the two types of devices used to administer home oxygen therapy.
25. State the usage and safety guidelines that should be followed by a patient on home oxygen therapy.

CHAPTER OUTLINE

KEY TERMS

artifact (AR-tih-fakt)
atherosclerosis (ath-roe-skler-OH-sus)
baseline
cardiac cycle
dysrhythmia (dis-RITH-mee-ah)
ECG cycle
electrocardiogram (ee-LEK-troe-KAR-dee-oh-gram) (ECG)
electrocardiograph (ee-LEK-troe-KAR-dee-oh-graf)
electrode (ee-LEK-trode)
electrolyte (ee-LEK-troe-lite)
flow rate
hypoxemia
hypoxia
interval (IN-ter-val)
ischemia (is-KEEM-ee-ah)
normal sinus rhythm
oxygen therapy
peak expiratory flow rate
segment
spirometer (spih-ROM-ih-ter)
spirometry (spih-ROM-ih-tree)
wheezing

INTRODUCTION TO ELECTROCARDIOGRAPHY

The **electrocardiograph** is an instrument used to record the electrical activity of the heart. The **electrocardiogram** (ECG) is the graphic representation of this activity. The ECG exhibits the amount of electrical activity produced by the heart and the time required for the impulse to travel through the heart.

Cardiovascular disorders can cause abnormal changes to occur on the ECG. Because of this, electrocardiography is used for the following purposes:

- To evaluate the following symptoms: chest pain, shortness of breath, dizziness, or heart palpitations
- To detect an abnormality in the heart's rate or rhythm (**dysrhythmia**)
- To detect the presence of impaired blood flow to the heart muscle, known as myocardial ischemia. The term **ischemia** refers to a deficiency of blood in a body part, usually caused by a blocked artery
- To help diagnose damage to the heart caused by a myocardial infarction
- To determine the presence of hypertrophy (enlargement) of the heart
- To detect inflammation of the heart muscle (myocarditis) or the lining of the heart (pericarditis)
- To assess the effect on the heart of digitalis and other cardiac drugs
- To determine the presence of electrolyte disturbances
- To assess the progress of rheumatic fever
- To detect congenital heart defects
- Performed before surgery to assess cardiac risk during surgery
- As part of a complete physical examination

A 12-lead resting ECG cannot detect all cardiovascular disorders, nor can it always detect impending heart disease such as a myocardial infarction. An ECG is taken with the patient in a resting state and records only about 10 seconds of the heart's electrical activity. If a patient has a dysrhythmia that occurs intermittently, the abnormal heartbeat may not occur during this brief time period. A patient who experiences angina pectoris does not typically have symptoms while in a resting state, and an ECG run on such a patient may appear normal. Because of this, an ECG must be used in combination with the patient's symptoms, health history, physical examination, and other diagnostic and laboratory tests to obtain a complete assessment of cardiac functioning.

The medical assistant is frequently responsible for recording ECGs in the medical office. The medical assistant must acquire knowledge, and skill must be acquired in the following aspects of electrocardiography: preparation of the patient, operation of the electrocardiograph, identification and elimination of artifacts, and care and maintenance of the electrocardiograph.

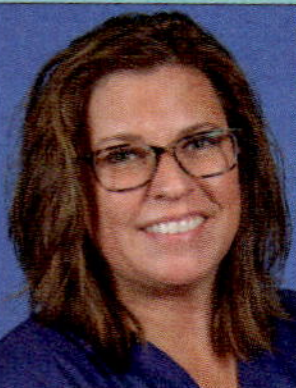

Putting It All Into Practice

My name is Anitra, and I work in the medical laboratory of an internal medicine office. I also run electrocardiograms, apply and remove Holter monitors, perform pulmonary function tests, and assist with cardiac stress testing.

One of my most rewarding experiences was when a young woman came into the office with severe chest pain. I immediately helped her back to an examining room. I ran an electrocardiogram, as ordered by the physician. After the physician read the electrocardiogram, he indicated the results did not look good and that the patient would have to be transported to the hospital. I went into the patient's room to comfort her. She asked me if she was going to have to go to the hospital. I replied, "Possibly." She immediately said, "I don't want to go!" Then I began to explain to her how important it was to have more tests to make sure she would be all right. She finally agreed to go. After being taken to the hospital by an ambulance, she was later transferred to another hospital for the insertion of a stent. A few weeks passed, and she came into the office. She hugged me and thanked me for possibly saving her life. It felt so good that I could help make a difference in a patient's life. ■

CARDIAC CYCLE

The **cardiac cycle** represents one complete heartbeat. It consists of the contraction of the atria, the contraction of the ventricles, and the relaxation of the entire heart (as described previously in Chapter 12: *Circulatory System*). The electrocardiograph records the electrical activity that causes these events in the cardiac cycle. The **ECG cycle** is the graphic representation of the cardiac cycle (Fig. 27.1).

Waves

The normal ECG cycle consists of a P wave; the Q, R, and S waves (known as the *QRS complex*); and a T wave. The ECG cycle is recorded from left to right, beginning with the P wave.

P wave The P wave represents the electrical activity associated with the contraction of the atria, or *atrial depolarization.*

QRS complex The QRS complex represents the electrical activity associated with the contraction of the ventricles, or *ventricular depolarization*, and consists of the Q wave, the R wave, and the S wave. The ventricles are larger than the atria and therefore require a stronger electrical stimulus to depolarize the ventricles. That is why the R wave is taller than the P wave on the ECG graph cycle.

T wave The T wave represents the electrical recovery of the ventricles, or *ventricular repolarization.* The muscle cells are recovering in preparation for another impulse. (*Note:* Electrical recovery, known as *atrial repolarization*, follows the P wave. This repolarization occurs at the same time as ventricular depolarization [QRS complex]. Because of this, atrial repolarization is masked or hidden

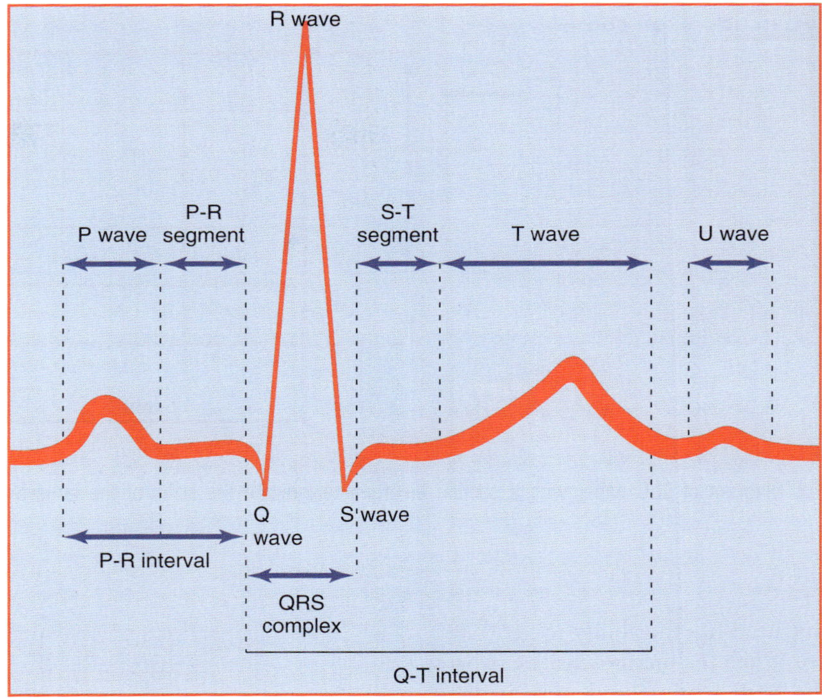

Fig. 27.1 ECG cycle.

by the QRS complex and does not appear as a separate wave on the ECG cycle.)

U wave Occasionally a U wave follows a T wave. It is a small round wave that is associated with repolarization of the Purkinje fibers in the papillary muscle of the heart.

Baseline, Segments, and Intervals

The flat, horizontal line that separates the various waves is known as the **baseline**. Following the U wave, the heart is at rest or *polarized.* Because no electrical activity is occurring in the heart during this time, the electrocardiograph does not have anything to record, which is why the baseline is flat.

The waves deflect either upward (positive deflection) or downward (negative deflection) from the baseline. The ECG cycle between the P wave and the T wave is divided into segments and intervals for the purpose of interpretation and analysis of the ECG by the provider. A **segment** is the portion of the ECG between two waves, and an **interval** is the length of one or more waves and a segment.

Segments

PR segment The PR segment represents the time interval from the end of the atrial depolarization to the beginning of the ventricular depolarization. It is the time needed for the impulse to be delayed at the AV node and then travel through the bundle of His and Purkinje fibers to the ventricles.

ST segment The ST segment represents the time interval from the end of the ventricular depolarization to the beginning of repolarization of the ventricles.

Intervals

PR interval The PR interval represents the time interval from the beginning of the atrial depolarization to the beginning of the ventricular depolarization.

QT interval The QT interval is the time interval from the beginning of the ventricular depolarization to the end of repolarization of the ventricles.

Baseline The baseline after the T wave (or U wave, if present) represents the period when the entire heart returns to its resting, or polarized, state.

ELECTROCARDIOGRAPH PAPER

Electrocardiograph paper is divided into two sets of squares for the accurate and convenient manual measurement of the waves, intervals, and segments (Fig. 27.2). Each small square is 1 mm high and 1 mm wide. Each large square (made up of 25 small squares) is 5 mm high and 5 mm wide. By manually measuring the various waves, intervals, and segments of the ECG graph cycle with ECG calipers or an ECG ruler, the provider is able to determine whether the electrical activity of the heart falls within normal limits. Heart disease can trigger abnormal changes in the ECG cycle, causing the results to fall outside of normal limits. For example, myocardial ischemia (often caused by coronary artery disease) can cause a depressed ST segment and an inverted T wave. A myocardial infarction can cause a larger than normal Q wave and an elevated ST segment.

Electrocardiograph paper contains a thermosensitive coating. A black or red graph is printed on top of this coating. The electrocardiograph uses a thermal print head to produce

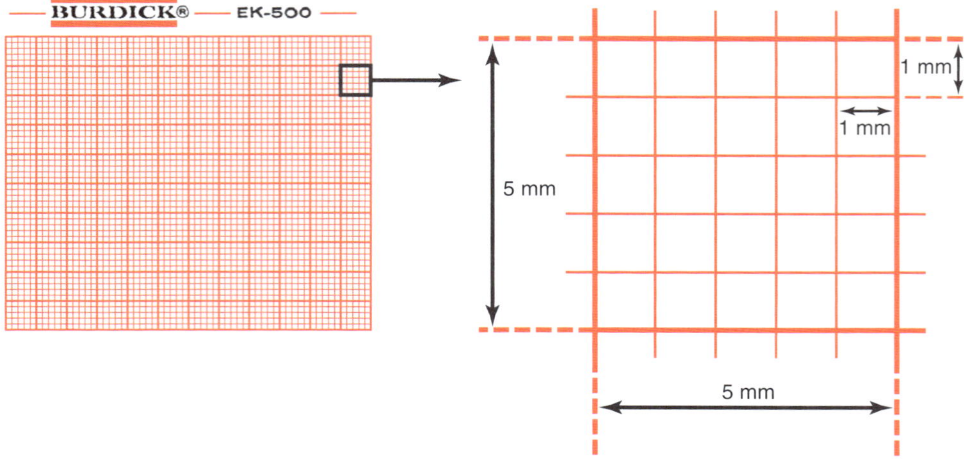

Fig. 27.2 Diagram of ECG paper with a section enlarged to indicate the sizes of the large and small squares.

the ECG tracing. The print head has the ability to generate heat in a prescribed pattern. When the thermosensitive paper comes in contact with the heated print head, the coating turns black in the areas where it is heated, producing the ECG tracing. In addition to being heat sensitive, ECG paper is pressure sensitive and should be handled carefully to avoid making impressions that would interfere with proper reading of the ECG.

STANDARDIZATION OF THE ELECTROCARDIOGRAPH

The electrocardiograph must be standardized, or calibrated, when an ECG is recorded. This is a quality control measure that ensures an accurate and reliable recording. It also means that an ECG run on one electrocardiograph compares in accuracy with a recording run on another machine. An ECG run on a properly calibrated electrocardiograph results in an accurate and reliable representation of the electrical activity of the patient's heart.

By international agreement, 1 millivolt (mV) of electricity should cause the stylus to move 10 mm high (10 small squares). During the recording, the machine allows 1 mV to enter the electrocardiograph, which should result in an upward deflection of 10 mm. The marking that occurs on the ECG paper is known as a *standardization mark* (Fig. 27.3). In other words, if the electrocardiograph is properly standardized, the standardization mark will be 10 mm high. The width of the mark made by the machine is approximately 2 mm (two small squares). The electrocardiograph automatically records standardization marks on the ECG; a standardization mark is recorded at the beginning and end of each of the ECG strips (see Fig. 27.8, presented later). If the standardization mark is more or less than 10 mm high, the electrocardiograph must be adjusted; otherwise, the ECG recording may not be accurate. The manufacturer's operating manual must be consulted for proper adjustment information.

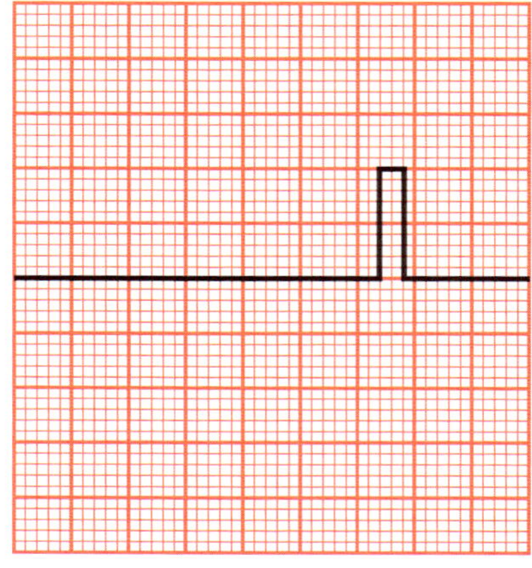

Normal Standard
Standardization mark is
10 mm high

Fig. 27.3 Standardization mark.

ELECTROCARDIOGRAPH LEADS

The standard ECG consists of 12 leads. A *lead* is a tracing of the electrical activity of the heart between two electrodes. Each lead provides an electrical "photograph" of the heart's activity from a different angle. Together, the 12 leads, or "photographs," facilitate a thorough interpretation of the heart's activity.

Ten lead wires are attached to the patient and are used to take the 12 electrical "photographs" of the heart. There are four limb lead wires: the right arm lead wire (RA), the left arm lead wire (LA), the right leg lead wire (RL), and the left leg lead wire (LL). The right leg lead wire is known as the *ground.* It is not used for the actual recording, but serves as an electrical reference point. There are six chest lead wires; each is abbreviated with a "V" and includes V_1, V_2, V_3, V_4, V_5, and V_6.

Electrodes

The electrical impulses given off by the heart are picked up by **electrodes** placed on the skin and conducted into the electrocardiograph through lead wires. Electrodes are composed of a substance that is a good conductor of electricity. The electrical impulses given off by the heart are very small (0.0001 to 0.003 volt). To produce a readable ECG, they must be made larger, or amplified, by a device known as an *amplifier*, located within the electrocardiograph. The amplified voltages are then relayed to an *output device*. The output device graphically records the ECG cycles on electrocardiograph paper using a thermal print head or electronically sends the recording to a computer where it is displayed on the screen of the computer (Fig. 27.4).

Disposable electrodes are used to record a resting 12-lead ECG. The electrode contains a thin layer of a metallic substance; this metallic substance is a good conductor of electricity. The electrode is square in shape and has a tab extending from one end (Fig. 27.5A). The tab allows for the firm attachment of an alligator clip (Fig. 27.5B). The back of the electrode contains an electrolyte gel combined with an adhesive (Fig. 27.5C). An **electrolyte** is a substance that facilitates the transmission of the heart's electrical impulses. Skin is a poor conductor of electricity; therefore, an electrolyte must be used when recording an ECG. The adhesive allows for firm adherence of the electrode to the patient's skin. There is no adhesive on the tab of the electrode, to allow for attachment of the alligator clip. The electrode is applied to the skin and held in place with its adhesive backing; it is thrown away after use.

Disposable 12-lead electrodes come on a card containing 10 electrodes (Fig. 27.5D). A foil-lined pouch is used to hold 10 cards of electrodes (or 100 electrodes per pouch). The foil-lined pouch preserves moisture to prevent the electrolyte from drying out. Each elexctrode pouch (and the box containing the pouches) is stamped with an expiration date. The medical assistant must always check the expiration date of the electrodes before applying them. The electrolyte gel on outdated electrodes may be dried out; a dried out electrolyte is unable to transmit a good electrical impulses from the heart.

Electrodes are sensitive to environmental conditions and must be stored properly to prevent electrolyte drying. They should be stored in a cool area (less than 75°F or 24°C) away from sources of heat. When an electrode pouch is opened, the medical assistant should seal the pouch by folding over the end of it and then place the pouch (containing

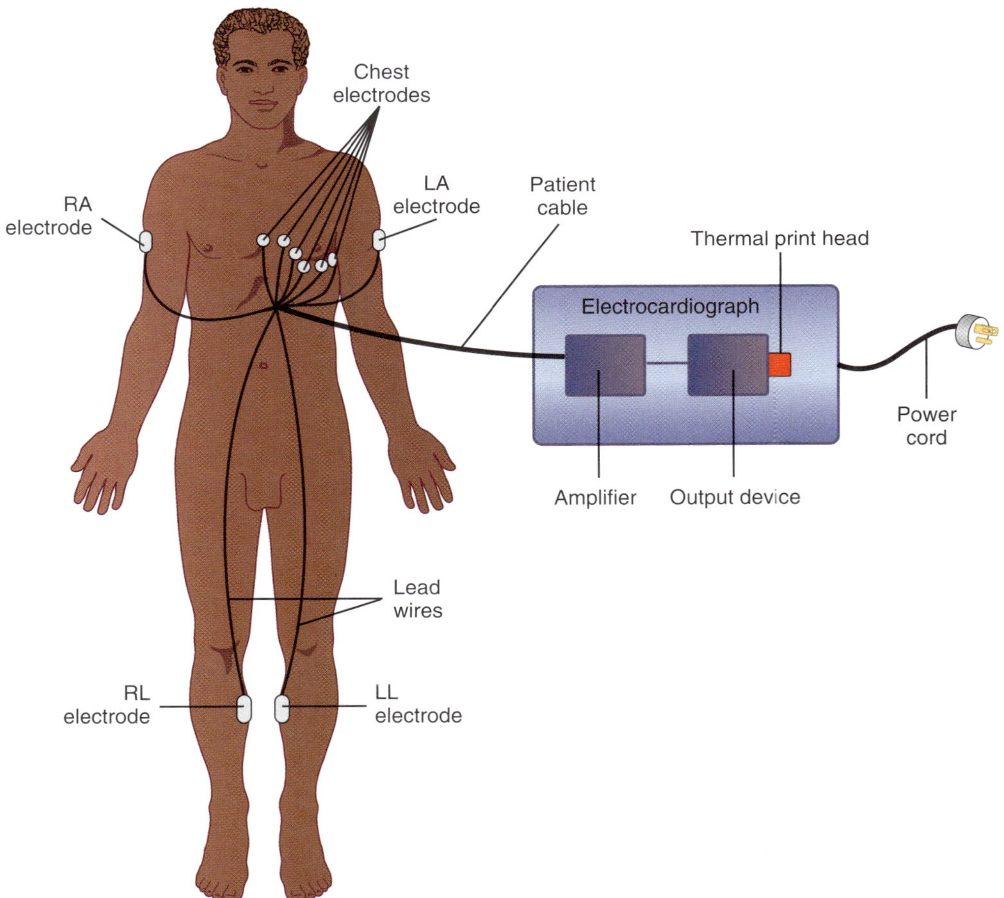

Fig. 27.4 Diagram of the basic components of the electrocardiograph. The limb electrodes are attached to the fleshy parts of the limbs, and the lead wires are arranged to follow body contour. The patient cable is not dangling, and the power cord points away from the electrocardiograph.

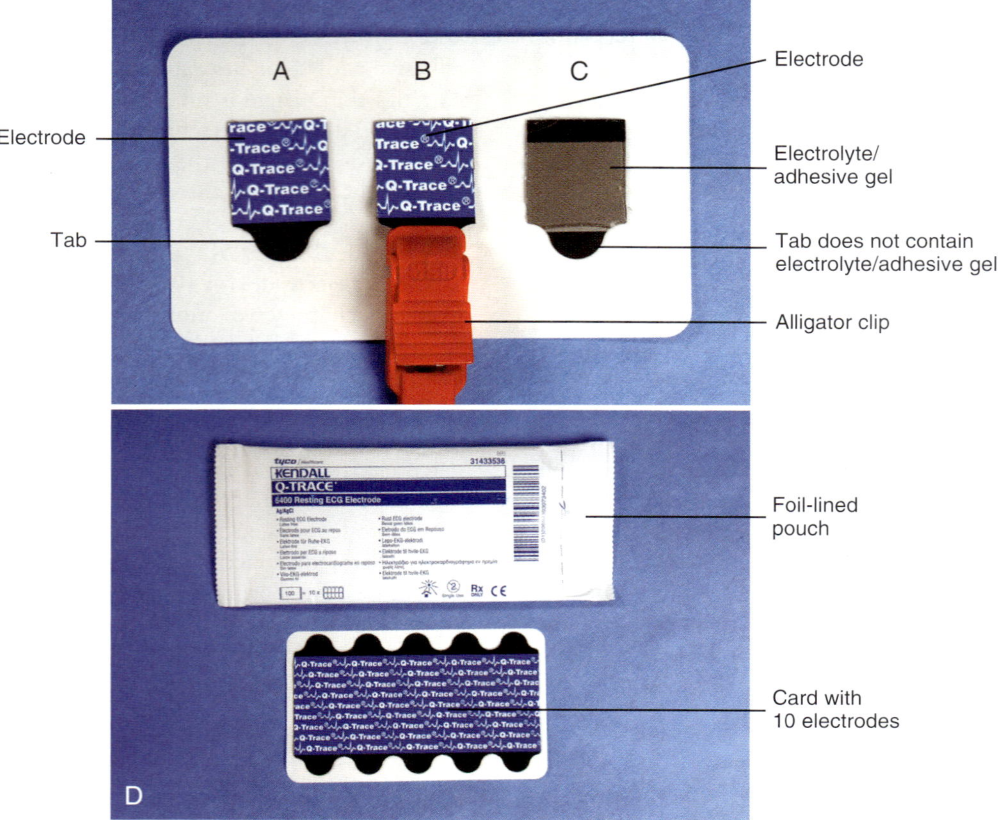

Fig. 27.5 Resting 12-lead ECG electrodes. (A) Disposable resting 12-lead electrode. (B) The tab allows for attachment of the alligator clip. (C) The back of the electrode contains an electrolyte gel combined with an adhesive. (D) Disposable 12-lead electrodes are packaged in a foil-lined pouch and come on a card that contains 10 electrodes.

the remaining electrode cards) in a zipper-lock plastic bag to preserve moisture.

Bipolar Leads

The first three leads of the 12-lead ECG are the bipolar leads; they are leads I, II, and III. The bipolar leads use two of the limb electrodes to record the heart's electrical activity. Lead I records the electric current traveling between the right arm and the left arm electrodes, lead II records the electric current traveling between the right arm and the left leg electrodes, and lead III records the electric current traveling between the left arm and the left leg electrodes (Fig. 27.6).

Lead II shows the heart's rhythm more clearly than the other leads. Because of this, the provider often requests a *rhythm strip*, which is a longer recording (approximately 12 inches) of lead II (see Fig. 27.8, presented later).

Augmented Leads

The next three leads are the augmented leads: aVR (augmented voltage—right arm), aVL (augmented voltage—left arm), and aVF (augmented voltage—left leg or foot). Lead aVR records the electric current traveling between the right arm electrode and a central point between the left arm and left leg electrodes. Lead aVL records the electric current traveling between the left arm electrode and a central point between the right arm and left leg electrodes. Lead aVF records the electric current traveling between the left leg electrode and a central point between the right and left arm electrodes. Leads I, II, III, aVR, aVL, and aVF provide an electrical "photograph" of the heart's activity from side to side and from the top to the bottom of the heart (see Fig. 27.6).

Chest Leads

The last six leads are the chest, or precordial, leads (V_1, V_2, V_3, V_4, V_5, and V_6). These leads record the heart's voltage from front to back. The electric current traveling through the heart is recorded from a central point "inside" the heart to a point on the chest wall where the electrode is placed. These points correspond to the chest electrode placement sites. Fig. 27.7 shows the proper location of the electrodes for the six chest leads. To ensure an accurate and reliable recording, the medical assistant must be able to locate these electrode placement sites accurately (by palpating the patient's chest). For example, if V_1 and V_2

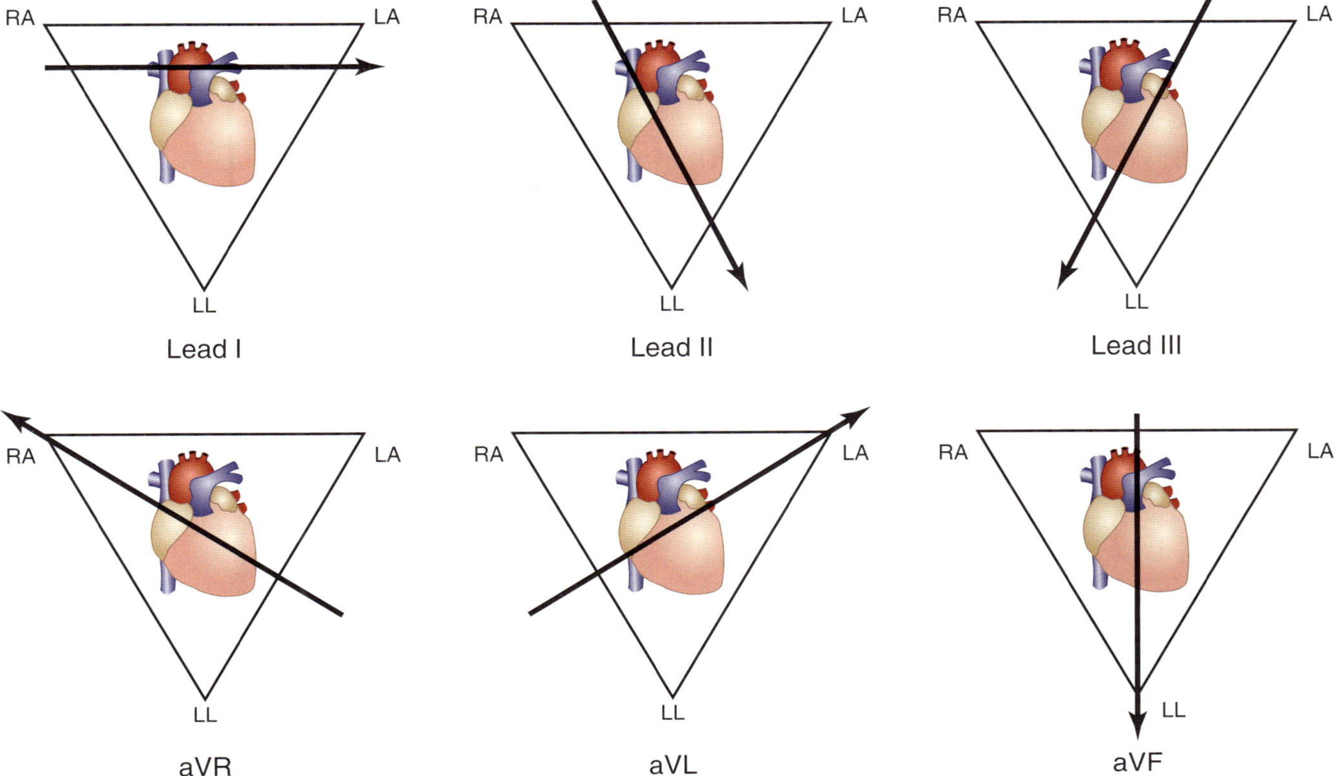

Fig. 27.6 Diagram of the heart's voltage for leads I, II, III, aVR, aVL, and aVF. *LA*, Left arm electrode; *RA*, right arm electrode; *LL*, left leg electrode.

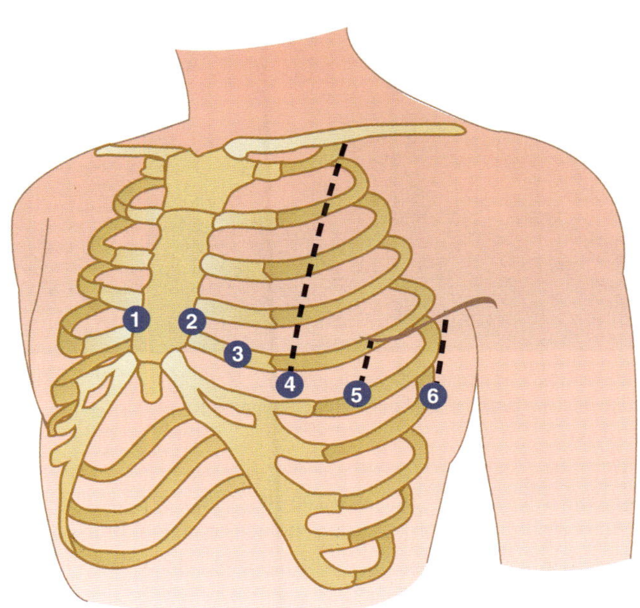

Fig. 27.7 Recommended positions for ECG chest electrodes: V_1, fourth intercostal space at right margin of sternum; V_2, fourth intercostal space at left margin of sternum; V_3, midway between positions 2 and 4; V_4, fifth intercostal space at junction of left midclavicular line; V_5, at horizontal level of position 4 at left anterior axillary line; V_6, at horizontal level of position 4 at left midaxillary line.

are placed in the third intercostal space (instead of the fourth intercostal space), changes can occur to the P and T waves, which can falsely indicate heart disease. When first learning to locate the electrode sites for each chest lead, it helps to mark their locations on the patient's chest with a felt-tipped pen.

What Would You Do? What Would You *Not* Do?

Case Study 1

Camilla Rossi is 22 years old and works at a Waffle House during the day and goes to business school at night. She comes to the office because she has been experiencing some heart problems. Over the past month, she has had three episodes of tachycardia, palpitations, difficulty in breathing, and profuse sweating. She is really scared that she has heart disease because her grandfather just died from a heart attack. The physician orders an ECG, but Camilla is reluctant to have the procedure. She is embarrassed about having to disrobe from the waist up, and she is worried that all the wires coming out of the machine will shock her. She says that she does not have health insurance, and she does not know how she would pay for the test. She wants to know whether there is a less expensive way to find out what is wrong with her. ■

HIGHLIGHT on Cardiac Stress Testing

Description

A cardiac stress test (also known as an *exercise tolerance test* or *exercise electrocardiogram* [ECG]) is a diagnostic procedure used to evaluate the cardiovascular health of individuals with known heart disease and individuals at high risk for developing heart disease, particularly coronary artery disease (CAD). Cardiac stress testing is usually performed in a hospital under the direction of a cardiologist and a cardiac technician so that emergency equipment and trained personnel are available to deal with any unusual situations that might arise. (*Note:* A *nuclear cardiac stress test* is a type of stress test that employs the use of a radioactive material injected through an intravenous line and is described in Chapter 28.)

Purpose

The purpose of cardiac stress testing is as follows:

1. To evaluate symptoms of ischemic heart disease that cannot be assessed by a resting ECG. Ischemic heart disease occurs as a result of an inadequate blood supply to the myocardium, which is most commonly caused by atherosclerosis. **Atherosclerosis** is a condition in which fibrous plaques of fatty deposits and cholesterol build up on the inner walls of arteries. This causes narrowing and partial blockage of the lumen of these arteries, along with hardening of the arterial wall. Atherosclerosis in the coronary arteries is called *coronary artery disease.* During rest, the myocardium supplied by the partially blocked artery may receive an adequate blood supply. If the individual exercises, however, the artery may not be able to supply enough blood to the myocardium, resulting in myocardial ischemia. Myocardial ischemia can cause chest discomfort and certain abnormal changes on the ECG.
2. To assist in evaluating symptoms indicating the presence of cardiac dysrhythmias.
3. To assess the effectiveness of cardiac drug therapy.
4. To follow the course of rehabilitation after a myocardial infarction or a cardiac surgical procedure, such as a coronary bypass operation or a coronary stent placement.
5. To determine an individual's fitness level for a strenuous exercise program, such as jogging.

Patient Preparation

Patient preparation for a cardiac stress test includes the following:

1. Refrain from smoking for 4 hours before the test.
2. Avoid strenuous physical activities for 8 to 12 hours before the test.
3. Do not consume alcohol or food and beverages containing caffeine for 12 hours before the test. These substances may interfere with obtaining accurate results.
4. Do not eat or drink anything except water for 4 hours before the test. This reduces the likelihood of nausea that may accompany strenuous activity after a meal.
5. Certain cardiac medications may need to be discontinued 1 to 2 days before the test; the provider makes this determination.
6. Wear loose, comfortable clothing and sports shoes suitable for exercising.

How the Test Works

- Cardiac stress testing involves the continuous electrocardiographic monitoring of an individual during physical exercise. During exercise, the body's need for oxygen places added demands or "stress" on the heart, making it work harder. A cardiac stress test evaluates the response of the heart to maximum or near-maximum exertion.
- A resting 12-lead ECG is usually performed before a cardiac stress test, and the results of the resting ECG are compared with the results of the cardiac stress test.
- The stress test is accomplished by having the patient use a treadmill while connected to an electrocardiograph machine through lead wires and electrodes (see illustration).
- The intensity of the physical exertion starts with a slow warm-up walk on the treadmill. The speed and incline of the treadmill are gradually increased every 3 minutes until the patient's target heart rate is reached. During this time the ECG is continuously displayed on a computer screen. The patient's blood pressure, heart rate, and physical symptoms are also monitored during the test.
- If the signs and symptoms of myocardial ischemia appear, the test is stopped. These symptoms include severe dyspnea, chest discomfort or pain, pallor, weakness, and dizziness. The test is also stopped if the ECG shows abnormal changes, if a serious, irregular heartbeat occurs, or if there is an abnormal change in blood pressure.
- Once the exercising is complete, the patient's blood pressure, heart rate, and ECG are monitored until they return to normal.

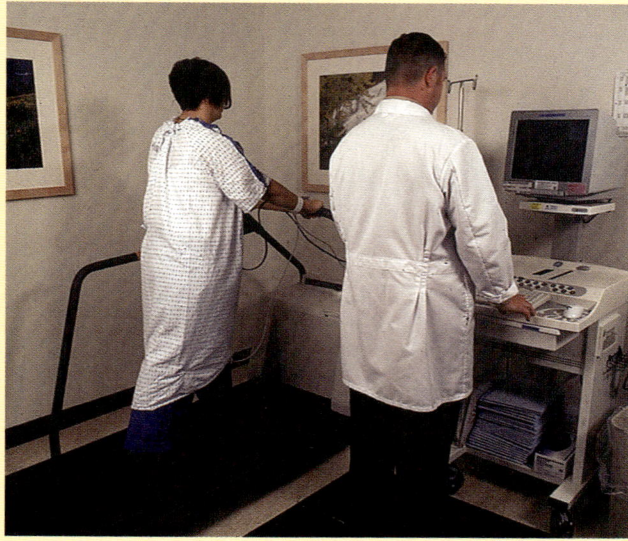

Cardiac treadmill stress test. (From deWit SC: *Medical-surgical nursing: concepts and practice*, St. Louis, 2008, Saunders.)

Interpretation of Results

The patient's response to the cardiac stress test is used to determine normal or abnormal results. A normal response is a gradual increase in the patient's blood pressure as physical exertion increases, whereas an abnormal response is a sudden increase or decrease in the patient's blood pressure. The ECG of a normal individual undergoing exercise exhibits a shortened PR interval and a compressed QRS complex. An abnormal tracing indicative of myocardial ischemia results in a depressed ST segment and an inverted T wave. An abnormal cardiac stress test result usually warrants further testing, such as coronary angiography, to assess the extent and severity of the heart disease. ■

PATIENT PREPARATION

Minimal preparation is required for an ECG. The medical assistant should instruct the patient in the following guidelines, which facilitate placement of the electrodes and ensure good adhesion of the electrodes to the patient's skin.

1. Do not apply body lotion, oil, or powder on the day of the procedure. This may make it more difficult to apply the electrodes.
2. Wear comfortable clothing and a shirt or blouse that can be removed easily.
3. Avoid wearing tights since the electrodes need to be placed on the lower legs.

MAINTENANCE OF THE ELECTROCARDIOGRAPH

Electrocardiographs require periodic maintenance. The casing of the electrocardiograph should be cleaned frequently with a soft cloth, slightly dampened with a mild detergent, to remove dust and dirt. Commercial solvents and abrasives should not be used because they can damage the finish of the casing.

The patient cable, lead wires, and power cord should be cleaned periodically with a cloth moistened with a disinfectant cleaner. The cables should never be immersed in the cleaning solution because this could damage them. Inspect the cables frequently for cracks or fraying, and replace them if needed. Check the metal tip of each lead wire for adhesive/electrolyte gel residue, which can interfere with the transmission of good electrical impulses from the heart. Remove any residue with an alcohol wipe using pressure and friction.

The reusable alligator clips should be cleaned thoroughly with an alcohol wipe after patient use. Check the alligator clips periodically to make sure they fit snugly on the metal tip of each lead wire.

ELECTROCARDIOGRAPHIC CAPABILITIES

Electrocardiographs have a variety of capabilities that permit specific recording and transmittal options.

Three-Channel Recording Capability

Most medical offices use a three-channel electrocardiograph. An electrocardiograph with a three-channel recording capability can record the electrical activity of the heart through three leads simultaneously. This is in contrast to a single-channel electrocardiograph, which records only one lead at a time. The advantage of a three-channel electrocardiograph is that an ECG can be produced in less time than would be required if each lead were recorded separately.

The leads that are recorded simultaneously are leads I, II, and III; followed by aVR, aVL, and aVF; followed by V_1, V_2, and V_3; followed by V_4, V_5, and V_6. Each lead is automatically labeled by the electrocardiograph with its appropriate abbreviation. Fig. 27.8 is an example of a three-channel ECG

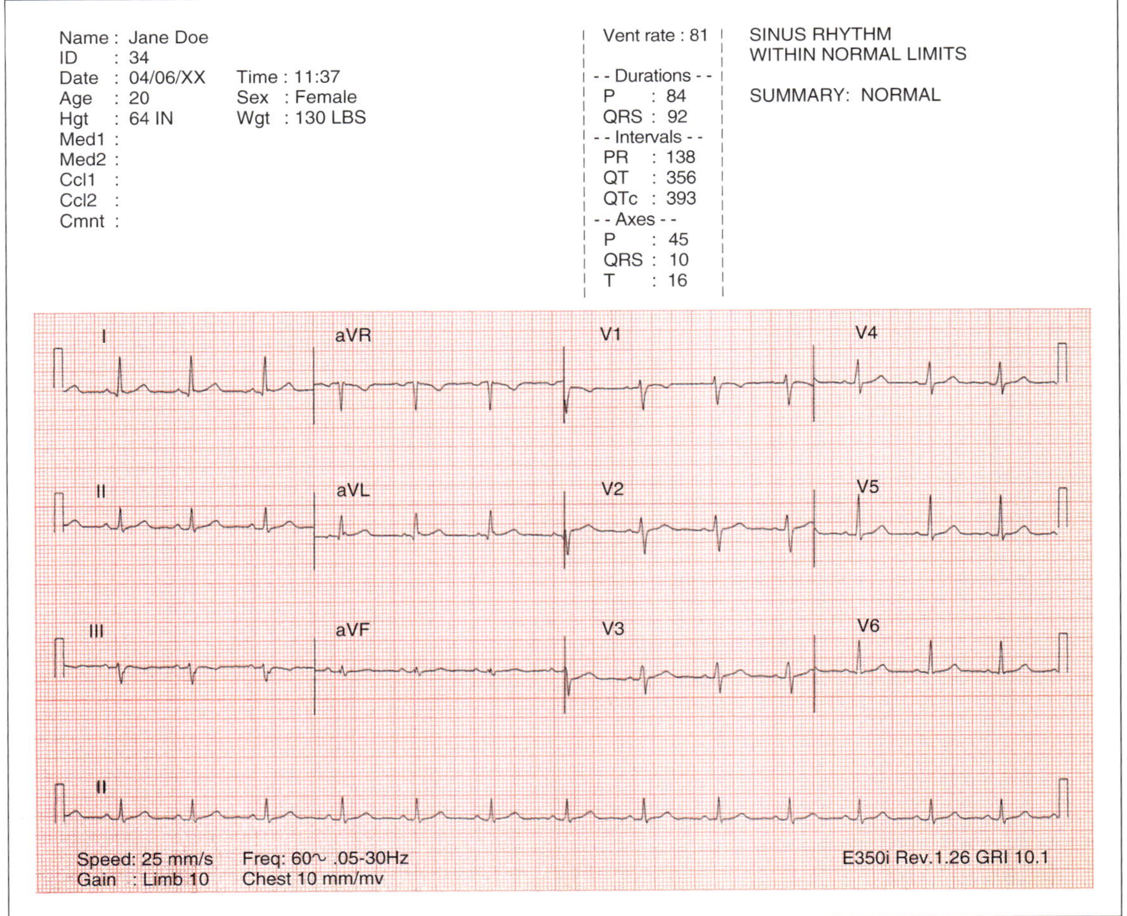

Fig. 27.8 A three-channel ECG with a rhythm strip.

recording that also includes a rhythm strip. Procedure 27.1 describes how to run a 12-lead three-channel ECG.

Interpretive Electrocardiograph

An electrocardiograph with interpretive capabilities has a software program that analyzes the recording as it is being run. Interpretive electrocardiographs provide immediate information on the heart's activity, leading to earlier diagnosis and treatment. Patient data are used in the interpretation of the ECG and must be entered into the electrocardiograph using a keyboard before running the recording. The data generally required are the patient's age, sex, height, weight, and medications, which are presented at the top of the recording. The computer analysis of the ECG is also printed at the top of the recording, along with the reason for each interpretation (Figs. 27.8 and 27.9). The results are reviewed and interpreted further by the provider before a diagnosis is made and treatment is initiated.

Electronic Health Record Connectivity

Electronic health record (EHR) connectivity allows the electrocardiograph to be linked with a computer system. The electrical activity of the heart is converted into a digital format which is sent electronically to a computer where it is displayed on the screen of the computer. If needed, a copy of the ECG report can be printed out on a regular sheet of paper. The ECG report is reviewed and interpreted by the provider and then stored electronically in the patient's EHR.

Teletransmission

An ECG that has been recorded in a digital format can be transmitted electronically to an ECG data interpretation site. The recording is interpreted by a cardiologist (often along with a computer analysis) at the interpretation site, and the ECG recording and its interpretation is electronically transmitted to the sending office the same day.

ARTIFACTS

The medical assistant is responsible for producing a clear and concise ECG recording that can be read and interpreted by both a computer and the provider. Structures sometimes appear in the recording that are not natural and

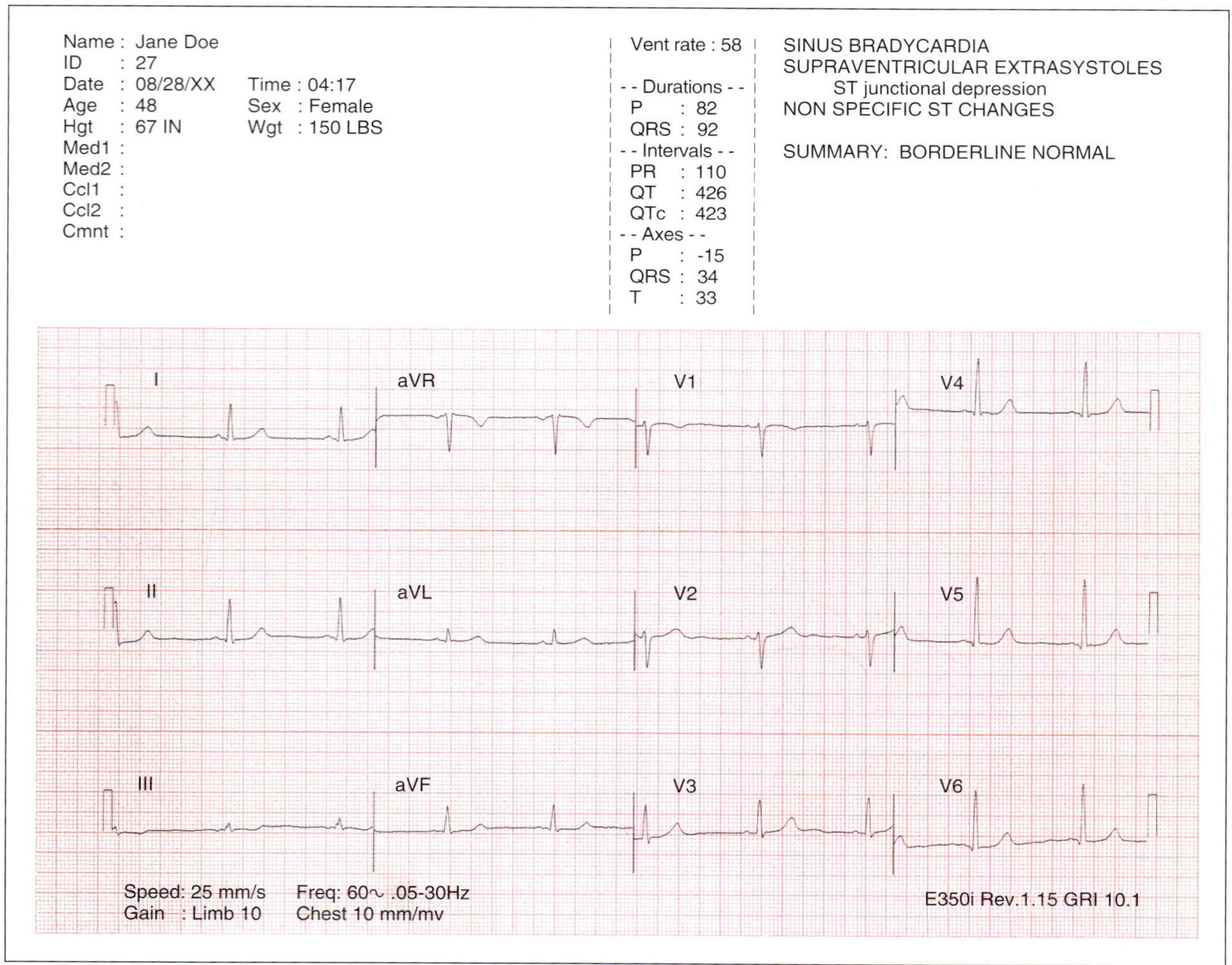

Fig. 27.9 An ECG recording that has been analyzed by an interpretive electrocardiograph. The computer analysis is printed at the top of the recording, along with the reason for each interpretation.

interfere with the normal appearance of the ECG cycles. They are known as **artifacts** and represent additional electrical activity that is picked up by the electrocardiograph. The presence of artifacts affects the quality of the recording, making it difficult to manually measure the ECG cycles. Artifacts can also sometimes cause a false-positive result on an ECG that is analyzed by a computer. The medical assistant should be able to identify artifacts and eliminate them. There are several types of artifacts; the most common are muscle, wandering baseline, and 60-cycle interference.

If the medical assistant is unable to correct an artifact, it is possible that the electrocardiograph is broken. If an electrocardiograph service technician needs to be contacted, the medical assistant should have the following information available to aid the technician in locating the problem:

1. What already has been done to locate and correct the problem
2. Leads in which the artifact occurs
3. A sample of the artifact recorded by the electrocardiograph

Muscle Artifact

A muscle artifact (Fig. 27.10A) can be identified by its fuzzy, irregular baseline. There are two types of muscle artifacts: those caused by involuntary muscle movement (somatic tremor) and those caused by voluntary muscle movement. The cause of muscle artifacts and the action to take to eliminate them is presented below:

1. *An apprehensive patient.* To reduce the patient's apprehension and relax muscles, explain the procedure and reassure the patient that having an ECG recorded is a painless procedure.
2. *Patient discomfort.* Ensure that the table is wide enough to support the patient's arms and legs adequately. The patient can be made more comfortable by placing a pillow under their head. Check that the room temperature is comfortable for the patient. A temperature that is warm enough for the medical assistant may be too cold for the patient who has removed clothing. This could result in shivering, which also would produce a muscle artifact on the ECG.
3. *Patient movement.* The patient must be instructed to lie still and not talk during the recording.
4. *A physical condition.* Several nervous system disorders, such as Parkinson disease, prevent relaxation, and the patient trembles continually. For these individuals, it is difficult to obtain an ECG that is free of artifacts. The artifacts can be reduced, however, by asking the patient to place their hands under the buttocks with the palms facing downward.

Wandering Baseline Artifact

A wandering baseline artifact appears as a slow wavy baseline on the ECG (Fig. 27.10B). The cause of wandering baseline artifacts and the action to take to eliminate them is presented below:

1. *Loose electrodes.* The medical assistant should ensure that the electrodes are attached firmly to the patient's skin. A loose electrode results in poor transmission of the electrical impulse from the patient's skin to the electrode. If an electrode pulls loose, it can be reattached with hypoallergenic tape or replaced with a new electrode. The alligator clips should be attached firmly to the tabs of the electrodes. To prevent pulling of the lead wires on the electrodes, the patient cable should be well supported on the table or the patient's abdomen and should not be allowed to dangle. Pulling on the electrodes can cause the electrodes to pull away from the patient's skin.
2. *Dried-out electrolyte.* If the electrolyte gel on an electrode is dried out, the medical assistant must replace it with a new electrode. Always check the expiration date stamped on the electrode pouch (or box) to make sure the electrodes are within their expiration date.
3. *Body creams, oils, or lotions on the skin in the area where the electrode is applied.* Creams, oils, or lotions prevent good adhesion of the electrodes to the patient's skin. The medical assistant should remove these substances by rubbing with alcohol, using friction.
4. *Excessive movement of the chest wall during respiration.* The medical assistant should encourage the patient to relax and breathe more calmly, using the diaphragm rather than expanding the chest.

60-Cycle Interference Artifact

A 60-cycle interference artifact (also known as an *AC artifact*) is caused by electrical interference. Electric current can "leak" or spread out from the power used by electrical appliances in the room in which the ECG is being run. This current may be picked up by the patient and carried into the electrocardiograph, where it would show up on the ECG recording as a 60-cycle interference artifact. This type of artifact appears as small, straight, spiked lines that are consistent in nature (Fig. 27.10C), causing the baseline to be thick and unreadable. The cause of 60-cycle interference artifacts and the action to take to eliminate them is presented below:

1. *Lead wires not following body contour.* Dangling lead wires can pick up electric current. Arrange the wires to follow body contour and to lie flat.
2. *Other electrical equipment in the room.* Lamps, autoclaves, electrically powered examining tables, or other electrical equipment that is plugged in may be leaking electric current. Unplug all nearby electrical equipment. (*Note:* Jewelry and watches do not interfere with the recording; therefore it is not necessary for the patient to remove these items unless they interfere with proper placement of the electrodes.)
3. *Wiring in the walls, ceilings, or floors.* Try moving the patient table away from the walls.
4. *Improper grounding of the electrocardiograph.* The machine is automatically grounded when it is plugged in. Check the three-pronged plug of the electrocardiograph to make sure the prongs are not loose or damaged. Ensure that the plug fits securely in the wall outlet. The right leg electrode is not used for recording the leads, but it picks up electric

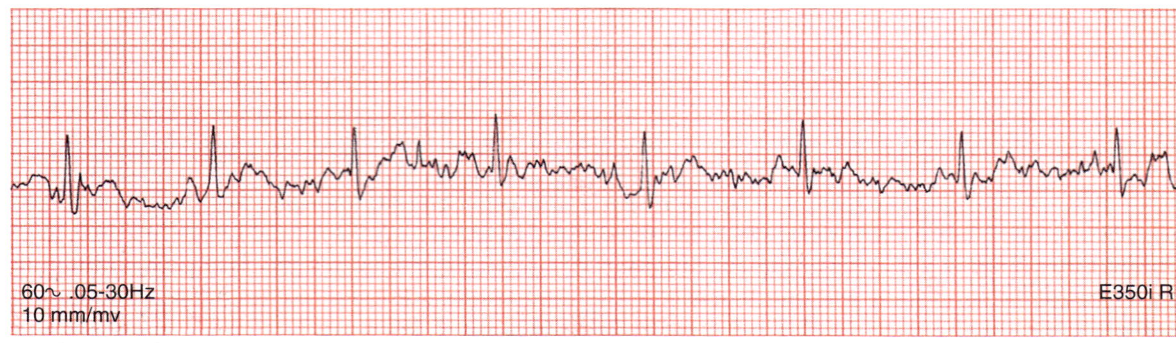

A
Muscle artifact

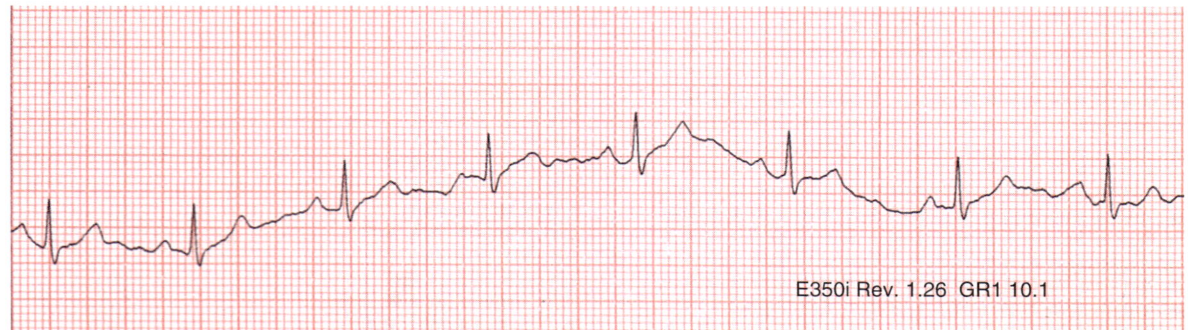

B
Wandering baseline

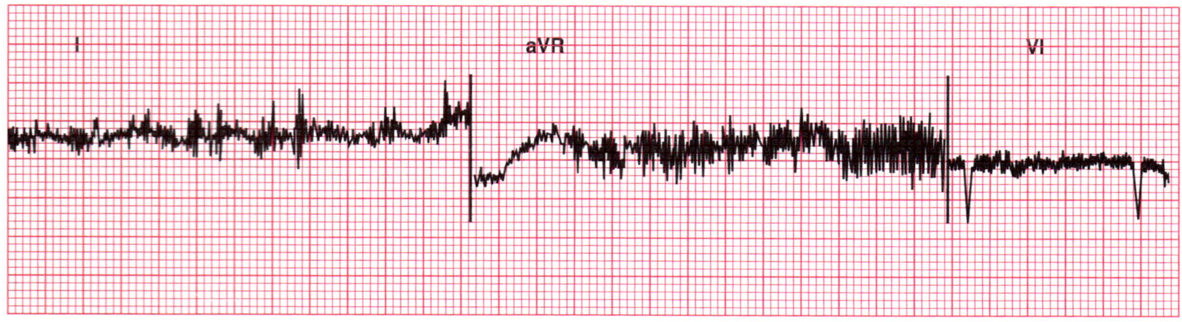

C
60-cycle interference

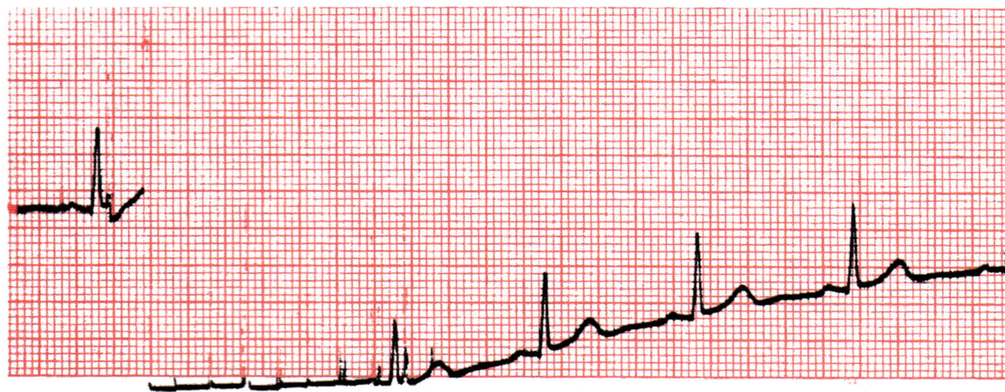

D
Interrupted baseline

Fig. 27.10 (A–D) Examples of ECG artifacts. (D from Long BW: *Radiography essentials for limited practice*, ed 3, St. Louis, 2010, Saunders.)

current that has "leaked" onto the patient and carries it into the electrocardiograph. The electric current is carried away by the machine's grounding system.

Interrupted Baseline Artifact

Occasionally, an interrupted baseline artifact (Fig. 27.10D) occurs that may be caused by the metal tip of a lead wire becoming detached or by a frayed or broken patient cable. If the latter is the case, a new patient cable should be ordered from the manufacturer.

HOLTER MONITOR ELECTROCARDIOGRAPHY

A Holter monitor is also known as an *ambulatory electrocardiographic monitor* (AEM). A Holter monitor is a portable ambulatory monitoring system for the continuous recording of the electrical activity of the heart for 24 hours or longer (Fig. 27.11). The monitor is named for Dr. Norman Holter, an American biophysicist who invented this cardiac monitoring device. The original Holter monitor consisted of a large pack of equipment worn on the patient's back.

The purpose of a Holter monitor is to detect cardiac abnormalities that occur while the patient is engaged in their normal daily routine. Because of this, the Holter system is designed so that the patient is able to maintain their usual daily activities with minimal inconvenience while being monitored.

A Holter monitor is similar to a resting 12-lead ECG in that the electrical impulses given off by the heart are picked up by electrodes and transmitted through lead wires to a recording device (Fig. 27.12). It is different from a resting 12-lead ECG in that only about 10 seconds of the heart's activity are recorded with a 12-lead ECG, whereas a Holter monitor records the heartbeat continuously for an extended period of time. This allows the Holter monitor to pick up cardiac abnormalities that do not occur during the brief recording period of a resting 12-lead ECG.

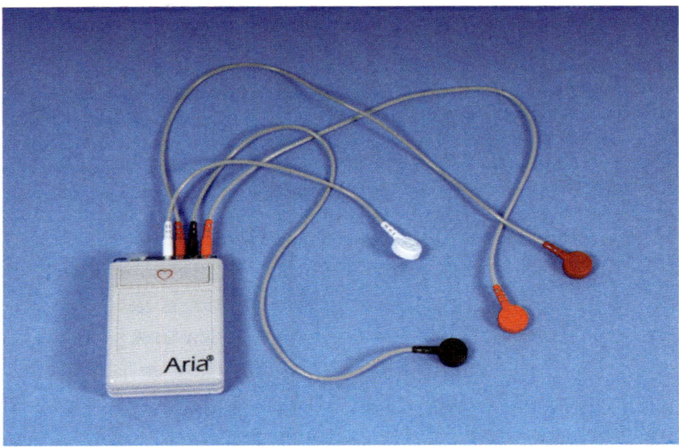

Fig. 27.11 Digital Holter monitor.

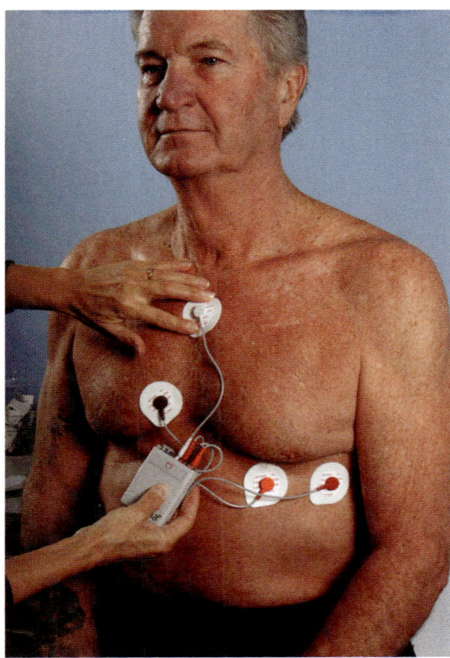

Fig. 27.12 Digital Holter monitor. Electrical impulses given off by the heart are picked up by electrodes placed on the patient's chest.

Purpose

Holter monitor electrocardiography is an important noninvasive procedure used to diagnose cardiac rate, rhythm, and conduction abnormalities. Specifically, it is most frequently used for the following purposes:

- To assess the rate and rhythm of the heart during daily activities.
- To evaluate patients with unexplained chest pain, dizziness, or syncope (fainting).
- To discover intermittent cardiac dysrhythmias not picked up on a routine resting 12-lead ECG. A resting ECG records only 40 to 50 heartbeats, whereas a Holter monitor records approximately 100,000 heartbeats in a 24-hour period.
- To detect myocardial ischemia.
- To assess the effectiveness of antidysrhythmic medications (e.g., digitalis, antianginal medications).
- To assess the effectiveness of a pacemaker.

Digital Holter Monitor

A digital Holter monitor is lightweight and battery powered, and uses a memory card to document the heart's activity (see Fig. 27.11). The monitor can be clipped onto a belt around the patient's waist. It can also be held in a protective pouch, which is hung around the patient's neck with a strap known as a *lanyard* (Fig. 27.13). Digital monitors can continuously record the electrical activity of the heart for 24 hours, 48 hours, or 72 hours. Most providers order a 24-hour recording, but they may occasionally order a 48- or 72-hour recording when the heart's activity needs to be recorded for a longer period of time. Throughout the monitoring period, the system continuously

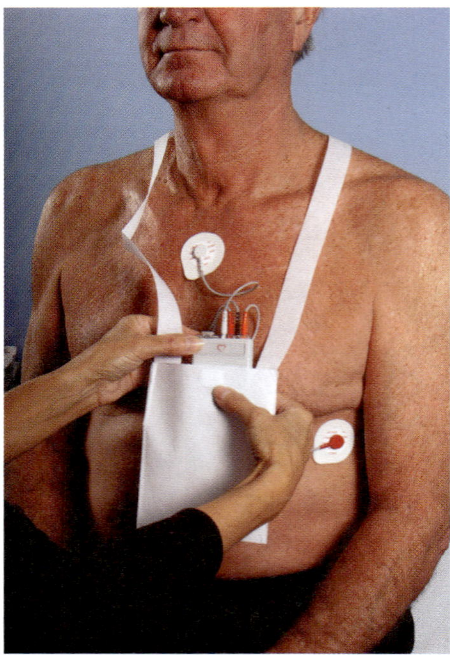

Fig. 27.13 The digital Holter monitor is placed in a pouch hung around the patient's neck by a strap.

records the electrical activity of the heart and stores it on the memory card. The monitor may have a small LCD screen that displays the date and time along with the remaining recording time. The Holter monitor automatically stops recording after the monitoring period has been completed.

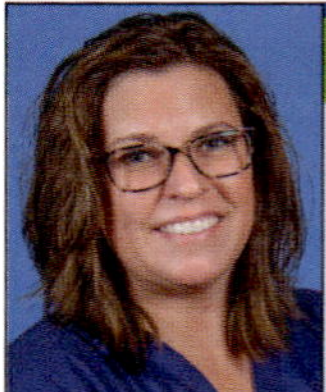

Memories *From* Practicum

Anitra: During my practicum, I was at an office where electrocardiograms were one of the many procedures performed. For my first electrocardiogram, the patient was a man who had a lot of hair on his chest, and I would need to shave the electrode placement sites on his chest. I was very nervous, but the procedure went well. When the electrocardiogram was run, he told me that I did a wonderful job and that it did not hurt at all to have his chest shaved. I realized then that it was not so bad after all. That patient made me feel so good about what I do and helped me feel confident in the procedures I had ahead of me. ■

Evaluating Results

At the end of the monitoring period, the Holter monitor system is removed from the patient. The information on the memory card is then uploaded to a computer. Specialized ECG software performs calculations on the data and prepares an ECG summary report of the monitoring period, which is then displayed on the screen of the computer.

The computer-generated ECG report summarizes information about the patient's heart rate and rhythm and any abnormalities that occurred during the monitoring period. The summary report also includes selected samples of the patient's cardiac activity, and any abnormal cardiac activity exhibited by the patient (e.g., cardiac dysrhythmias). The results of the ECG summary report are reviewed and interpreted further by the provider. The ECG summary report can be stored electronically in the patient's EHR (electronic health record) or printed out and stored in a PPR (paper-based patient record).

CARDIAC DYSRHYTHMIAS

The normal ECG graph cycle consists of a P wave, a QRS complex, and a T wave, which repeat in a regular pattern (see Fig. 27.1). The term **normal sinus rhythm** refers to an ECG that is within normal limits. This means that the waves, intervals, segments, and cardiac rate fall within the normal range. The normal heart rate ranges from 60 to 100 beats per minute. A rate slower than 60 beats per minute is *sinus bradycardia,* and a rate faster than 100 beats per minute is *sinus tachycardia.*

Cardiac **dysrhythmia** is the term used to describe abnormal electrical activity in the heart causing an irregular heartbeat. Cardiac dysrhythmias can be classified into one of the following categories: (1) extra beats, (2) an abnormal rhythm, or (3) an abnormal heart rate. Most cardiac dysrhythmias are harmless; however, some can be serious or even life-threatening. Cardiac dysrhythmias include: premature atrial contraction (PAC), paroxysmal supraventricular tachycardia (PVST), atrial flutter (AFL), atrial fibrillation (A-fib), premature ventricular contraction (PVC), ventricular tachycardia (V-tach), and ventricular fibrillation (V-fib).

PULMONARY FUNCTION TESTS

The purpose of a pulmonary function test (PFT) is to assess lung functioning which assists in the detection and evaluation of pulmonary disease. Pulmonary function tests performed in the medical office include spirometry, peak flow measurement, and pulse oximetry. Other types of pulmonary function tests include lung volumes, diffusion capacity, arterial blood gas studies, and cardiopulmonary exercise tests. Spirometry and peak flow measurement are described in the next section and pulse oximetry is presented in Chapter 19: Vital Signs.

SPIROMETRY

Spirometry is a simple, noninvasive screening test that is often performed in the medical office. A computerized electronic instrument known as a **spirometer** is used to conduct the test (Fig. 27.14). A spirometer measures how much air is exhaled by the lungs and how fast it is exhaled. The spirometry report is printed out as a table and graph. Spirometry is considered a screening test, and abnormal test results require that the patient undergo additional pulmonary

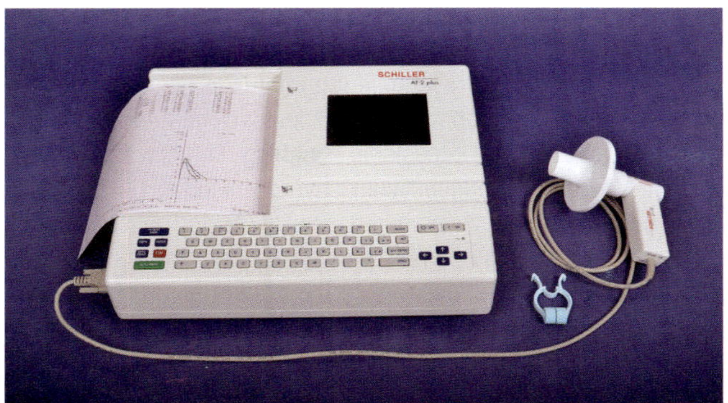

Fig. 27.14 Spirometer (From Pepper J, Niedzwiecki B, Shearer M, Welch Haynes K. *Kinn's the clinical medical assistant: an applied learning approach*, ed 15, St. Louis, 2023, Elsevier.)

function tests and possibly a computed tomography (CT) scan before a diagnosis can be made. Indications for performing spirometry include the following:

1. Patients who exhibit symptoms of lung dysfunction such as dyspnea
2. Individuals at high risk for lung disease because of smoking or exposure to environmental pollutants such as coal dust, asbestos, and exhaust fumes
3. Patients with lung disease, such as asthma, chronic bronchitis, and emphysema
4. Patients who are to undergo surgery (to assess probable lung performance during an operation)
5. Patients who need to be evaluated for lung disability or impairment for a compensation program (e.g., coal miners)

What Would You Do? What Would You *Not* Do?

Case Study 2

Joel Matthews, 48 years old, is at the office for a checkup. Joel had a mild heart attack 2 years ago. Since then, he has made significant changes to his lifestyle. He's become a vegetarian and practices yoga every morning before going to work. After he gets home, he jogs 10 miles. He also lifts weights every other day and takes herbal vitamin supplements. Since his heart attack, he has lost 40 pounds and says that he has never felt better. The only thing he cannot seem to do is give up smoking. He started smoking when he was 17 years old and has cut back from 2 packs to 1 pack a day. He keeps trying to stop but says that he has been smoking so long that it might not be possible. Besides, with all the other healthy stuff he is doing, he thinks it probably cancels out the bad effect of the cigarettes. Joel is very concerned that if he does stop smoking, he will gain back all of the weight that it took him so long to lose. ■

Patient Preparation

Patient preparation is essential to obtain accurate test results. To prepare for the test, the patient should be instructed to do the following:

1. Do not eat a heavy meal for 8 hours before the test. (The patient must exert the diaphragm muscles, and a full stomach may interfere with this action.)
2. Stop smoking at least 8 hours before the test.
3. Do not take bronchodilators for 4 hours before the test.
4. Do not engage in strenuous activity for 4 hours before the test.
5. Wear loose, nonrestrictive clothing to keep the chest area as free as possible, which makes it easier to perform the breathing maneuver.

POST-BRONCHODILATOR SPIROMETRY

If the results of the spirometry test indicate a possible obstruction, the provider usually orders a post-bronchodilator spirometry test. This test is performed by having the patient inhale a bronchodilator and running a spirometry test approximately 10 to 15 minutes later. The purpose of this test is to inform the provider as to how treatment would work in patients whose airways are obstructed.

HIGHLIGHT on Smoking and Chronic Obstructive Pulmonary Disease (COPD)

Chronic Obstructive Pulmonary Disease Defined

COPD is a chronic airway obstruction that results from emphysema or chronic bronchitis or a combination of these conditions. COPD is a chronic, debilitating, irreversible, and sometimes fatal disease.

More than 16 million Americans have been diagnosed with COPD; however, it is estimated that an additional 8 million Americans have the disease and remain undiagnosed. Smoking tobacco is the primary cause of COPD. In the United States, approximately 85% to 90% of deaths from COPD are caused by smoking. According to the American Lung Association, COPD is the fourth leading cause of death in the United States, behind heart disease, cancer, and stroke. COPD claims the lives of more than 140,000 Americans each year.

Emphysema

Emphysema is most often seen in older individuals with a long history of smoking. Emphysema due to smoking is caused by

Continued

HIGHLIGHT on Smoking and Chronic Obstructive Pulmonary Disease (COPD)—cont'd

irreversible damage to the alveoli in the lungs from toxins present in cigarette smoke (see illustration). As alveoli continue to be damaged, the lungs are able to transfer less and less oxygen to the bloodstream. In addition, air becomes trapped in the damaged alveoli, making it difficult to remove during exhalation. Because of this, the primary symptom of emphysema is shortness of breath. Other symptoms include chronic cough, tiredness, and limited exercise tolerance. More than 3 million people in the United States currently have been diagnosed with emphysema. The reason is not yet understood, but only 15% to 20% of long-term smokers develop emphysema.

Chronic Bronchitis

Chronic bronchitis is an inflammation of the lining of the bronchiole tubes that causes swelling and excess production of mucus. Swelling and excess mucus narrow the bronchiole tubes and restrict airflow into and out of the lungs. Symptoms include chronic cough, shortness of breath, and coughing up of mucus. To be classified as chronic bronchitis, the symptoms must last 3 or more months out of the year for at least 2 years. As the disease progresses, the lips and skin may exhibit cyanosis resulting from lack of oxygen in the blood. Chronic bronchitis is most often caused by long-term irritation of the bronchial tubes as a result of cigarette smoking; other causes include air pollution and exposure to dust or toxic gases in the workplace (e.g., coal mines). Chronic bronchitis often precedes or accompanies emphysema. It is estimated that 10 million Americans have chronic bronchitis. This condition affects individuals of all ages but has a higher incidence in individuals older than 45 years. Women are more than twice as likely to be diagnosed with chronic bronchitis as men.

Symptoms of Chronic Obstructive Pulmonary Disease

Damage to the lungs caused by COPD occurs gradually over many years. In fact, more than 90% of patients who have COPD are over the age of 45 at the time of their diagnosis. Because there are no early symptoms, many people do not know they have COPD. By the time an individual experiences symptoms, it is usually a sign that irreversible lung damage has already occurred. The first symptoms of COPD include mild shortness of breath on exertion and occasional coughing. The disease slowly becomes more pronounced with severe episodes of dyspnea and coughing after even modest activity. As the disease progresses, the heart also can be affected and shortness of breath is present all the time, even while the patient is sitting quietly. At this point the individual's quality of life is greatly diminished. When the lungs and the heart are no longer able to deliver oxygen to the body's tissues, death occurs.

Treatment for Chronic Obstructive Pulmonary Disease

The best treatment for COPD caused by smoking is for the patient to stop smoking. Continued smoking makes the COPD worse; quitting smoking slows the disease process. There are programs, support groups, nicotine replacement aids (e.g., nicotine patch, gum, lozenges, inhalers, nasal sprays), and prescription medications (e.g., Chantix, Zyban) to help individuals quit smoking. Other forms of treatment depend on the patient's condition and degree of lung impairment and may include the following:

1. Bronchodilators to relax and widen the bronchial tubes to increase airflow. They may be inhaled as aerosol sprays or taken orally.
2. Expectorants to thin the mucus so that it is easier to expel.
3. Antibiotics to treat infections that could interfere further with breathing and lung function.
4. Corticosteroids to reduce inflammation in the airways.
5. Breathing exercises to strengthen the muscles used to breathe.
6. Maintenance of overall good health habits, which include proper nutrition, adequate sleep, and regular exercise.
7. Oxygen therapy for patients with low blood oxygen to help with shortness of breath, allowing them to be more active.
8. Special measures including avoiding extremes of temperature (heat and cold), getting an annual influenza immunization, avoiding individuals with respiratory infection, and reducing exposure to air pollution.
9. Lung transplantation surgery is being performed on some patients who are in the later stages of COPD.

PEAK FLOW MEASUREMENT

Peak flow measurement using a peak flow meter is performed in the medical office and by the patient at home to determine how well a patient's asthma is being controlled. An overview of asthma followed by the procedure for using a peak flow meter is presented next.

ASTHMA

Asthma is a chronic inflammatory lung disease that affects the airways of the lungs. Asthma is characterized by recurrent episodes of coughing, chest tightness, shortness of breath, and wheezing known as an *asthma attack* or *flare-up*. **Wheezing** is a continuous, high-pitched, whistling, musical sound heard particularly during exhalation and sometimes during inhalation.

Asthma can develop at any age but is more common in children and young adults. In the United States, there are approximately 26 million individuals with asthma; of these, 6 million are children. Each year, more than 4000 deaths result from asthma.

The exact cause of asthma is not known. It is thought to be caused by a combination of factors, including genetics, certain childhood respiratory infections, and contact with allergens or exposure to certain viral infections in infancy or early childhood.

Asthma Triggers

In a normal individual, the airways to the lungs are fully open, allowing air to move easily into and out of the lungs. In a patient with asthma, the airways are always inflamed and hypersensitive to certain stimuli that do not affect the airways of normal individuals. These stimuli are known as *asthma triggers* because they can "trigger" an asthma attack. Asthma triggers vary from one patient to another and may also vary from one season to the next. Examples of common allergens that may trigger an asthma attack include dust mites, pollens, molds, animal dander, and cockroaches. Asthma attacks can also be triggered by environmental irritants, activities, or events, including air pollutants, tobacco smoke, chemical fumes (e.g., perfume, paint, and gasoline), vigorous physical exercise, upper respiratory viral infections, exposure to cold, and emotional stress. It is sometimes difficult to determine what specific triggers cause a patient's asthma attacks.

Asthma Attack

When the inflamed airways of a patient with asthma are stimulated by a trigger, the inflamed airways become even more inflamed causing a series of reactions to occur. The bronchial tubes begin to constrict and swell, causing the patient to experience the symptoms of an asthma flare-up. Sometimes the symptoms are mild and go away, either on their own or with treatment with medication. At other times, the symptoms become worse, leading to a severe asthma attack. During a severe attack the bronchial tubes continue to constrict and swell and become clogged with mucus (Fig. 27.15). This results in less air moving into and out of the lungs, which leads to a decrease in the amount of oxygen available to the body. The narrowed bronchial tubes and decreased oxygen supply cause the patient to experience coughing, chest tightness, shortness of breath, and wheezing, making it hard to breathe. A severe asthma attack that does not improve with medication therapy can become a life-threatening emergency.

Depending on the patient, asthma attacks vary in frequency and severity and may come on suddenly or gradually. An asthma attack may last for only 10 to 15 minutes or it may last for hours or even days.

Diagnosis and Treatment

The provider diagnoses asthma through a careful and detailed medical history. Of particular importance to the diagnosis of asthma are the patient's symptoms, family history of asthma, home and work environment, and living habits. The provider also performs a thorough physical examination to detect symptoms resulting from asthma, such as wheezing. When the medical history and physical examination have been completed, the provider usually orders laboratory and diagnostic tests, which may include pulmonary function tests (e.g., spirometry), allergy testing, and arterial blood gas studies.

Although asthma is a chronic disease with no cure, most patients with asthma are able to lead a normal life through proper management and treatment. It is important to treat symptoms when they first begin to occur to prevent them from getting worse and causing a severe asthma attack, which may require emergency treatment. The general treatment of asthma includes identifying and avoiding asthma triggers (if possible) and preventing and alleviating asthma symptoms through medication therapy. Two general categories of medication are prescribed for asthma: long-term–control medication and quick-relief medication.

- **Long-term–control medication** helps relieve bronchial inflammation and prevents symptoms from occurring. Control medication helps the patient have fewer and milder asthma attacks and is typically taken every day. Corticosteroids are an example of a control medication; brand names include Flovent, Pulmicort, Asmanex, Qvar, and AeroBid. Other examples of long-term–control medication include Singulair and Advair.
- **Quick-relief medication** (also called *rescue medication*) opens the airways quickly by dilating the bronchial tubes. It is taken when the patient is experiencing symptoms to prevent or control an asthma attack. Fast-acting bronchodilators are an example of quick-relief medication; brand names include Proventil, Ventolin, and Xopenex.

Many asthma medications are delivered through an *inhaler* (Fig. 27.16), which allows the medication to go directly to the lungs. Quick-relief medications can be used in a breathing machine known as a *nebulizer* to treat an asthma attack at home. A nebulizer converts liquid quick-relief

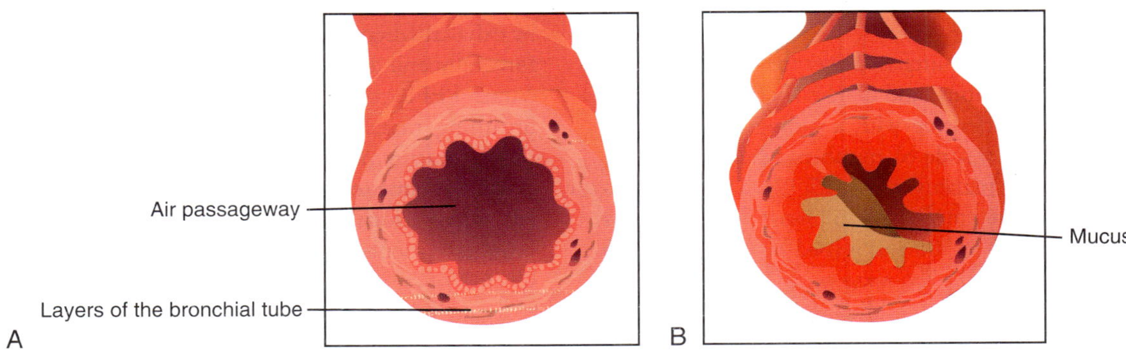

Fig. 27.15 (A) Normal bronchial tube. (B) Bronchial tube during an asthma attack.

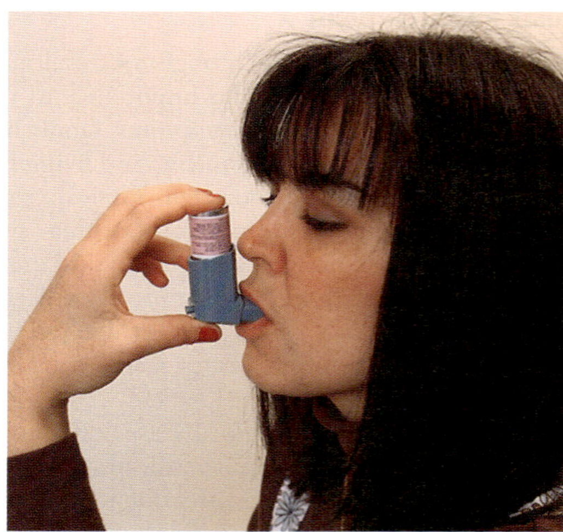

Fig. 27.16 An inhaler is often used to deliver asthma medication to the bronchial tubes of the lungs. (From Potter PA: *Basic nursing: essentials for practice*, ed 7, St. Louis, 2011, Mosby.)

medication into a mist that can be easily inhaled through a mouthpiece or mask. A nebulizer can deliver a larger dose of medication at a faster rate than an inhaler. Other asthma medications are administered orally; however, they take longer to work because they first have to travel through the digestive and circulatory systems before reaching the lungs.

PEAK FLOW METER

A peak flow meter is a portable, handheld device used to measure airflow out of the lungs. It is recommended that a peak flow meter be used on a regular schedule by patients with moderate to severe asthma to determine how well their asthma is being controlled. The measurements obtained from a peak flow meter are not as accurate as those obtained by spirometry; however, a peak flow meter can be used easily by a patient at home. The provider determines each patient's schedule of use based on the severity and frequency of asthma symptoms. Most providers recommend that the patient use a peak flow meter at least once a day, preferably in the morning before taking asthma medication. A peak flow measurement should also be obtained when the patient is having symptoms. If the patient has a more severe form of asthma, the provider may want the patient to use a peak flow meter twice a day—in the morning and in the evening.

Peak flow meters can be purchased over the counter and are available in two types: manual and digital. *A manual peak flow meter* consists of a plastic tube with a sliding indicator that manually moves along a scale of numbers when the patient performs the breathing maneuver (Fig. 27.17). They are available in two ranges: a low range and a full range. The *low-range meter* has a range from 0 to 300 and is used by young children and some older patients. The *full-range meter* has a range from 0 to 800 and is used by older children, teenagers, and adults (Fig. 27.18). An adult has much larger bronchial tubes than

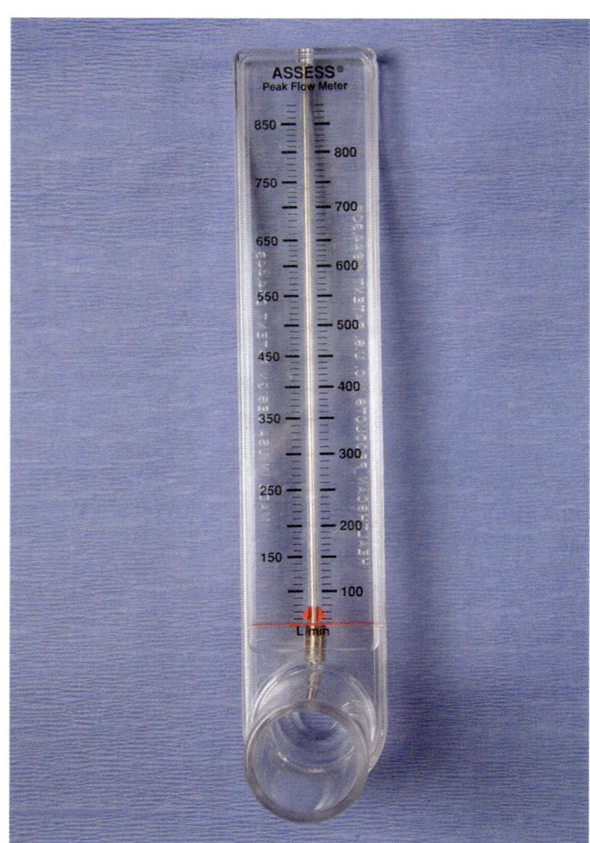

Fig. 27.17 Manual peak flow meter.

a child and needs the wider range. A *digital peak flow meter* automatically measures the breathing maneuver and displays the measurement digitally on a screen (Fig. 27.19).

Several different brands of peak flow meter are available, and peak flow measurements may vary among brands. Because of this, a patient who purchases more than one meter should always use the same brand to attain consistency among measurements.

PEAK EXPIRATORY FLOW RATE

The peak flow measurement obtained from a breathing maneuver performed by the patient is known as the **peak expiratory flow rate** (PEFR). The PEFR is the maximum volume of air measured in liters per minute (L/min) that can be exhaled when the patient blows into a peak flow meter as forcefully and as rapidly as possible. To obtain the most accurate PEFR, the patient should perform three acceptable breathing maneuvers and then record the highest of the three measurements. The three measurements should be about the same to show that an acceptable breathing maneuver was performed each time. Peak flow measurements provide patients with important information such as the severity of an asthma attack and when to take medication.

Peak flow measurements may show changes before the patient feels them. A patient's PEFR may drop hours or

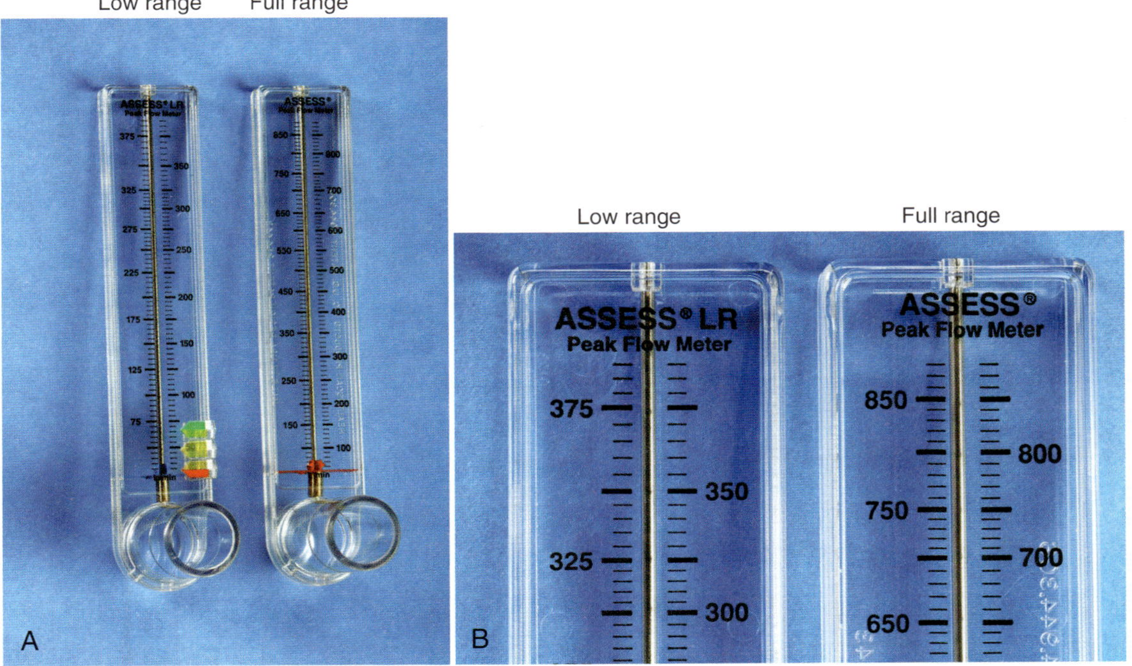

Fig. 27.18 Comparison of a low-range (A, B: left) and full-range (A, B: right) peak flow meter.

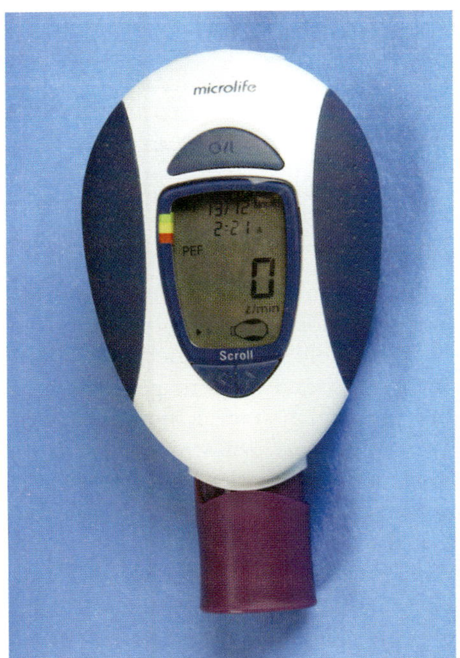

Fig. 27.19 Digital peak flow meter.

even days before any asthma symptoms occur. For example, the patient may feel fine, but when a peak flow measurement is taken, the reading is slightly decreased. By taking medication before symptoms occur, it may be possible to stop the attack quickly to avoid a severe asthma attack.

Peak Flow Chart

Peak flow measurements may be recorded on a peak flow chart (Fig. 27.20), which allows the patient and the provider to track changes in the patient's lung function over a period of time. A peak flow chart consists of graph paper with a range of peak flow numbers (usually from 50 to 800 L/min) listed in a vertical column on the left side of the graph paper. The patient indicates the date and time at the top of the chart. After obtaining a peak flow measurement, the patient places a dot across from the peak flow number in the appropriate column. A sample peak flow chart usually accompanies a peak flow meter and can be photocopied for ongoing use or downloaded from the internet.

Peak flow charts allow providers and patients to monitor changes in the patient's airflow over time to determine how well the patient's asthma is being controlled. They also help the provider determine if a patient's daily medications need to be adjusted or changed. If the patient is doing well as indicated by high peak flow measurements, the provider may be able to lower the dosage of the patient's medication or discontinue certain medications altogether.

The medical assistant is often responsible for instructing a newly diagnosed asthma patient in the procedure for using a peak flow meter and recording results on a peak flow chart. In addition, the medical assistant may be responsible for obtaining the PEFR of a patient with asthma at the

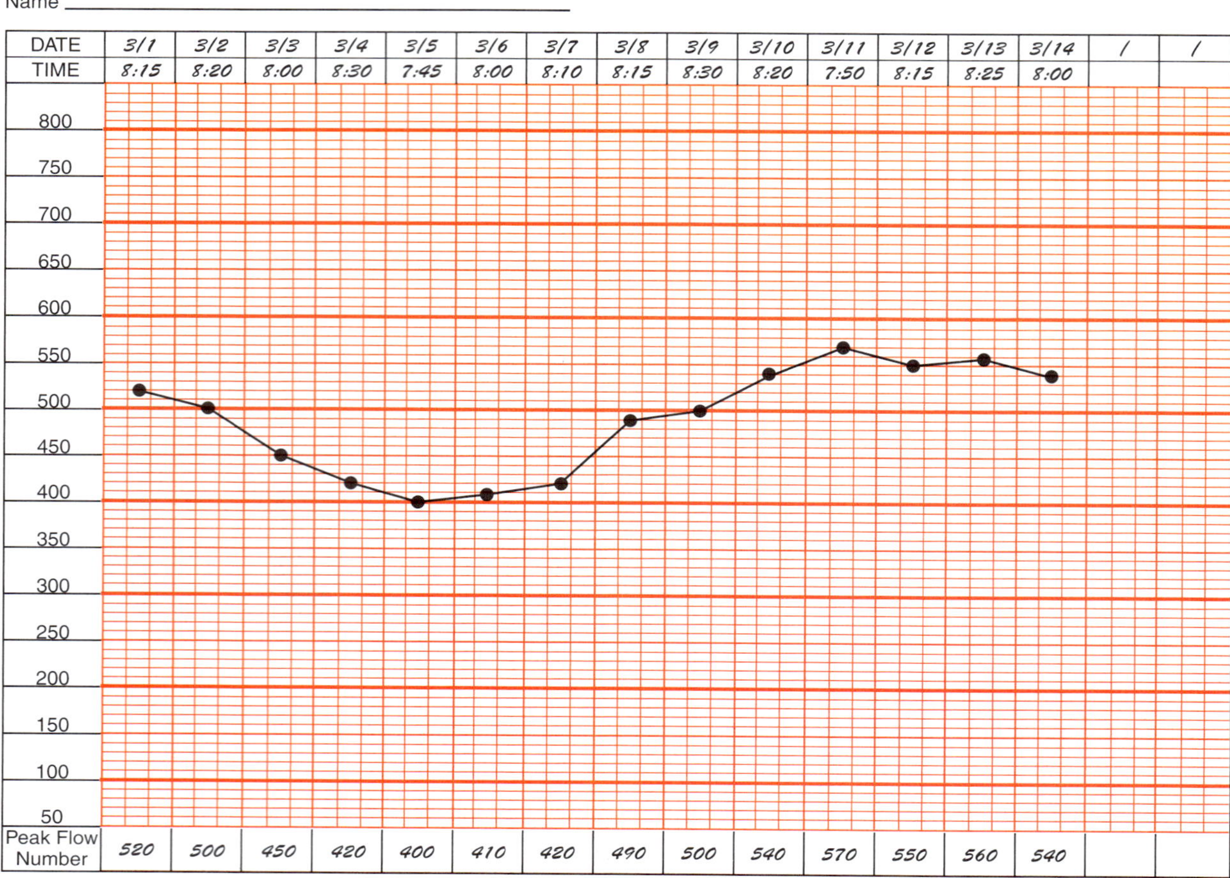

Fig. 27.20 An example of a peak flow chart.

medical office. The procedure for measuring PEFR is outlined in Procedure 27.2.

ASTHMA ACTION PLAN

An *asthma action plan* (AAP) is a written individualized management plan developed jointly by the provider and the patient. The goal of an AAP is to provide the patient with guidelines to follow for the control and treatment of their asthma which usually leads to fewer asthma attacks. An example of an individualized Asthma Action Plan developed by the American Lung Association is presented in Fig. 27.21.

An AAP typically includes the following information:

- A list of possible asthma triggers that should be avoided
- Instructions for taking asthma medications
- Guidelines for determining the severity of an asthma attack based on symptoms and peak flow measurements
- Recommendations on what to do during an asthma attack
- Instructions on when to call a doctor and/or obtain emergency care
- Emergency telephone numbers

Asthma Zones

An AAP is divided into three asthma zones that can be compared to the colors on a traffic light (green, yellow, and red). The threshold level for each zone is based on the patient's symptoms and percentage determinations of the patient's personal best peak flow measurement (see Fig. 27.21). The *personal best measurement* is the highest peak flow measurement a patient can achieve over a period of 2 to 3weeks when under good asthma control. The patient must obtain a peak flow measurement (i.e., the highest of three acceptable measurements) twice a day; in the morning upon awakening and in the late afternoon or early evening. The highest measurement (personal best) during this time period is then used to determine the threshold level for each of the patient's three asthma zones. As an example, the threshold level for the green zone is 80% to 100% of the patient's personal best measurement. Therefore, if a patient's personal best is 500 L/min, the threshold level for their green zone would be between 400 L/min (*80% of 500 L/min*) and 500 L/min (*100% of 500 L/min*).

Provider: ______________________ Clinic: ______________________

American Lung Association.

My Asthma **Action Plan**

Name: ______________________ DOB:____ /____ /______

Severity Classification: ☐ Intermittent ☐ Mild Persistent ☐ Moderate Persistent ☐ Severe Persistent

Asthma Triggers (list): ______________________

Peak Flow Meter Personal Best: __________

Green Zone: Doing Well

Symptoms: Breathing is good – No cough or wheeze – Can work and play – Sleeps well at night

Peak Flow Meter __________ (more than 80% of personal best)

Flu Vaccine—Date received: _______ Next flu vaccine due: ________ COVID19 vaccine—Date received:_______

Control Medicine(s)	Medicine	How much to take	When and how often to take it
	______________	______________	______________
	______________	______________	______________

Physical Activity ☐ Use Albuterol/Levalbuterol _____ puffs, 15 minutes before activity

☐ with all activity ☐ when you feel you need it

Yellow Zone: Caution

Symptoms: Some problems breathing – Cough, wheeze, or tight chest – Problems working or playing – Wake at night

Peak Flow Meter _______ to _______ (between 50% and 79% of personal best)

Quick-relief Medicine(s) ☐ Albuterol/Levalbuterol _____ puffs, every 20 minutes for up to 4 hours as needed

Control Medicine(s) ☐ Continue Green Zone medicines

☐ Add ______________________ ☐ Change to ______________________

You should feel better within 20-60 minutes of the quick-relief treatment. If you are getting worse or are in the Yellow Zone for more than 24 hours, THEN follow the instructions in the RED ZONE and call the doctor right away!

Red Zone: Get Help Now!

Symptoms: Lots of problems breathing – Cannot work or play – Getting worse instead of better – Medicine is not helping

Peak Flow Meter __________ (less than 50% of personal best)

Take Quick-relief Medicine NOW! ☐ Albuterol/Levalbuterol _____ puffs, ______________ (how frequently)

Call 911 immediately if the following danger signs are present:

- Trouble walking/talking due to shortness of breath
- Lips or fingernails are blue
- Still in the Red Zone after 15 minutes

Emergency Contact Name ______________________ Phone (______)______ - ________

Date: _____ /_____ /_______

1-800-LUNGUSA | Lung.org

ALA Asthma AP V4 3 1 2023

Fig. 27.21 Asthma Action Plan. (American Lung Association, 2021).

What Would You Do? What Would You *Not* Do?

Case Study 3

Deisha Williams comes to the medical office for a check-up appointment for her 12-year-old son, Damonte. Damonte developed asthma at age 6 and has recently taken an interest in learning more about his condition. He wants to know if asthma triggers are the same for everyone with asthma. He also wants to know what causes him to have trouble breathing during a severe asthma attack. The physician recommends that Damonte obtain a peak flow measurement every day. Damonte says his asthma hasn't been a problem lately and wants to know if he could perform the peak flow procedure twice a week instead of every day. ■

HOME OXYGEN THERAPY

Oxygen is a colorless, odorless, and tasteless gas that is vital to the human body. Oxygen is transported by the blood to various tissues of the body. When it reaches the tissues, oxygen is taken into the cells, where it combines with glucose to produce energy. Energy is necessary to the body for carrying out all metabolic processes that sustain life such as breathing and beating of the heart.

When the lungs cannot deliver enough oxygen to the body, there is a reduction in the amount of oxygen in the blood, resulting in hypoxemia. **Hypoxemia** is defined as a decrease in the oxygen saturation of the blood. Hypoxemia, in turn, leads to **hypoxia,** which is a reduction in the oxygen supply to the tissues of the body. Failure to maintain an adequate blood oxygen level can result in progressive deterioration of the patient, beginning with the death of cells and, if prolonged, continuing to organ failure and eventually body system failure and death.

There are certain conditions, such as severe chronic obstructive pulmonary disease (COPD), that reduce the amount of oxygen in the body, resulting in hypoxemia. In these cases, the provider may write a prescription for home oxygen therapy. **Oxygen therapy** is the administration of supplemental oxygen at concentrations greater than room air to treat or prevent hypoxemia. Oxygen therapy increases the oxygen supply to the lungs, which in turn raises blood oxygen to normal levels and increases the availability of oxygen to the tissues. Oxygen therapy helps to alleviate the effects of low oxygen levels such as shortness of breath and fatigue and helps the patient have a better quality of life and live longer.

Home oxygen therapy is most commonly prescribed for patients with severe COPD caused by smoking. Other common causes of hypoxemia that may require home oxygen therapy include asthma, occupational lung disease, lung cancer, cystic fibrosis, and congestive heart failure.

OXYGEN PRESCRIPTION

The provider determines a patient's need for oxygen therapy through clinical observation of the patient and by measuring the oxygen level of the patient's blood. Clinical signs of hypoxemia include cyanosis, dyspnea, tachypnea, tachycardia, and anxiety. The oxygen level of the blood is typically measured by arterial blood gas (ABG) analysis and through pulse oximetry. A normal individual should have an ABG analysis of 75 to 100 mmHg and a pulse oximetry reading above 94%. An ABG analysis less than or equal to 55 mgHg and a pulse oximetry reading of 88% or less warrants the use of supplemental oxygen. The goal of oxygen therapy is to maintain a blood oxygen level of 65 mmHg (as measured through ABG analysis) and 90% to 93% (as measured through pulse oximetry).

Once the need for supplemental oxygen has been determined, the provider must write a prescription for oxygen therapy that is filled by a home medical supply company. The prescription must include the amount and duration of supplemental oxygen needed by the patient, which are based on the severity of the patient's condition. In addition, the prescription includes the recommended oxygen delivery system and the oxygen administration device, which are described in the next section.

The amount of supplemental oxygen prescribed for a patient is known as the **flow rate**, which is measured in liters per minute (L/min). For example, if a patient has been prescribed 2 L/min, each minute, 2 liters of oxygen will flow from the patient's oxygen delivery system into tubing, and then into the patient's upper airway. As previously described, the flow rate prescribed by the provider is targeted at raising the patient's ABG analysis to 65 mmHg and the pulse oximetry measurement to 90% to 93%. Most people with COPD start out with a flow rate of 1 to 2 liters per minute. As their COPD worsens over time, the flow rate might increase to 3 to 6 L/min.

The duration of oxygen therapy refers to the number of hours per day oxygen therapy is administered and, depending on the patient's lung function, can vary from a few hours a day up to 15 or more hours per day. Some patients need oxygen only when sleeping or exercising, whereas other patients with more severe hypoxemia may require continuous oxygen therapy. *Continuous oxygen therapy* refers to the use of oxygen for more than 15 hours a day.

Once oxygen therapy is initiated, periodic assessment of the patient's blood oxygen level is required. This assessment is necessary to make sure that the patient still requires oxygen therapy, and that the amount and duration of oxygen are adequate to meet the patient's oxygen needs.

OXYGEN DELIVERY SYSTEMS

There are three common delivery systems for providing supplemental oxygen to a patient: compressed oxygen gas, liquid oxygen, and an oxygen concentrator. The type of delivery system prescribed by the provider is based on the patient's condition, the patient's personal preference, the ease of equipment use, and cost. Each of these delivery systems can be used alone or in combination with another system to meet the oxygen needs of the patient. These systems are described in greater detail in the next section.

Compressed Oxygen Gas

Compressed oxygen gas is oxygen gas compressed under high pressure and then stored in a container referred to as a *cylinder* or *tank*. Compressed oxygen cylinders vary in size from very large stationary cylinders to small portable cylinders that can be carried around (Fig. 27.22A). The patient uses a large cylinder of compressed oxygen at home. When the patient goes outside of the home, they use a small cylinder that has been placed in a carrying device such as a shoulder bag.

The cylinder is equipped with a regulator and a flow meter that control the flow rate of the oxygen (Fig. 27.22B). The flow of oxygen out of the cylinder is constant. To conserve oxygen and avoid waste, an oxygen-conserving device may be attached to the system. An oxygen-conserving device releases the oxygen gas only when the patient inhales and cuts off the release of oxygen when the patient exhales. Advantages and disadvantages of compressed oxygen gas include the following:

Advantage:

- Compressed oxygen gas is less expensive than liquid oxygen.

Disadvantages:

- The oxygen cylinders must be refilled frequently.
- A compressed oxygen gas cylinder cannot be taken on a commercial airliner.

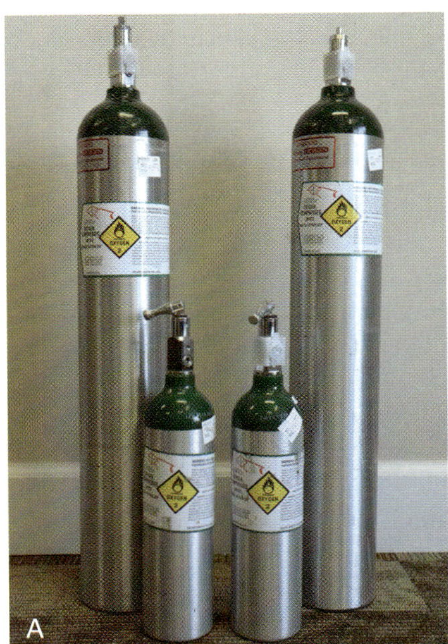

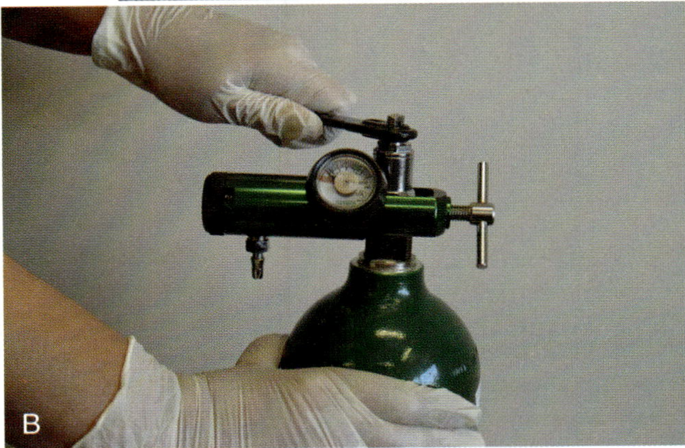

Fig. 27.22 (A) Compressed oxygen cylinders. (B) Oxygen cylinder with regulator and flow meter attached. (Courtesy of Family Oxygen and Medical Equipment, Athens, OH.)

Liquid Oxygen

When oxygen gas is subjected to an extremely cold temperature, it changes from a gas to a very cold liquid. The liquid oxygen is stored in an insulated tank with a lining similar to a Thermos. Oxygen in a liquid form takes up much less space than compressed oxygen gas—for example, 1 liter of liquid oxygen is equal to 860 liters of compressed oxygen gas. Because of this, a container of liquid oxygen lasts four times longer than compressed oxygen gas of the same weight.

A liquid oxygen system consists of a large stationary tank that serves as the primary reservoir of oxygen. A small portable tank weighing between 5 and 13 pounds is filled from the large primary tank for use outside the home (Fig. 27.23). The portable tank can be hung over the shoulder or pulled on a roller cart. When liquid oxygen is released from its tank, it changes into a gas and the patient breathes it in, similar to breathing in compressed oxygen gas. Advantages and disadvantages of liquid oxygen include the following:

Advantage:

- Because it takes up less space and is easier to transport than compressed oxygen gas, liquid oxygen is often preferred by individuals who want to maintain an active life.

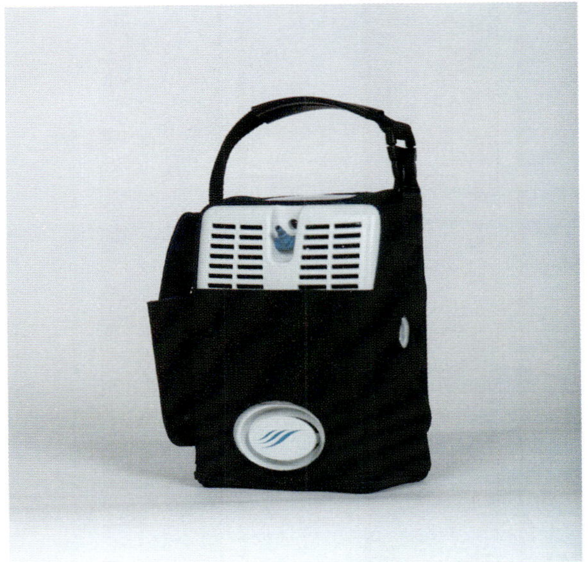

Fig. 27.23 Liquid oxygen portable tank. (From Perry AG: *Clinical nursing skills and techniques*, ed 8, St. Louis, 2014, Saunders.)

Disadvantages:

- Liquid oxygen is more expensive than compressed oxygen gas.
- The contents of a liquid oxygen tank evaporate, making it necessary to have the tank refilled often.
- A liquid oxygen portable tank cannot be taken on a commercial airliner.

Oxygen Concentrator

An oxygen concentrator is an electrically powered device that weighs about 35 pounds and is about the size of a large suitcase (Fig. 27.24A). It works by separating oxygen out of the air, concentrating it, and then storing it for use by the patient. The oxygen concentrator is equipped with a built-in flow meter, which allows the prescribed flow rate to be set.

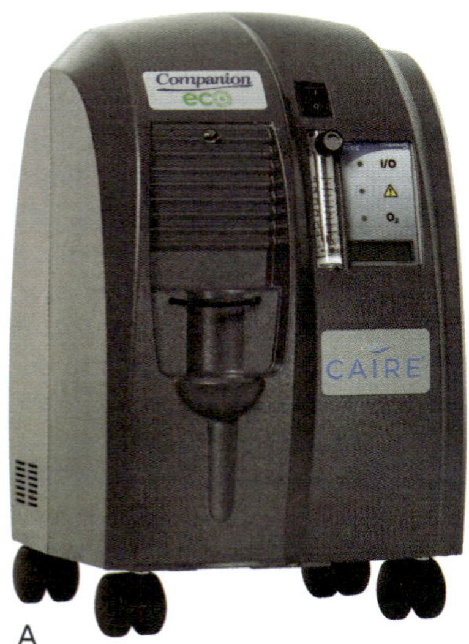

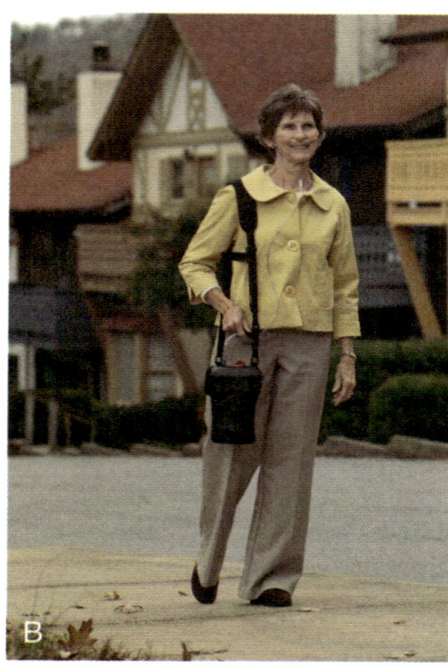

Fig. 27.24 (A) Oxygen concentrator. (B) Portable oxygen concentrator. (A and B, Courtesy CAIRE Inc.)

Small, portable, battery-powered oxygen concentrator systems weighing about 10 pounds have been developed (Fig. 27.24B). They can provide a patient with oxygen for about 8 hours when used at a flow rate of 2 L/min. For many patients, portable oxygen concentrators have replaced liquid oxygen or compressed gas cylinders for mobility. Advantages and disadvantages of oxygen concentrators include the following:

Advantages:

- Oxygen concentrators do not need to be resupplied with oxygen from a home medical supply company.
- Oxygen concentrators are less expensive and safer than oxygen cylinders.
- Portable oxygen concentrators that are battery powered offer the patient even greater freedom and mobility than other oxygen delivery systems.
- Some portable oxygen concentrators have been approved by the Federal Aviation Administration (FAA) for use on commercial airlines.

Disadvantage:

- Because oxygen concentrators use electricity, if the power goes out the patient must have a compressed oxygen gas cylinder for use as a backup.

OXYGEN ADMINISTRATION DEVICES

A device must be used to administer the oxygen to the upper airway of the patient from the delivery system. The device used depends on the expected duration of therapy and the personal preference and needs of the patient. The most commonly used devices to administer home oxygen therapy are a nasal cannula and a face mask, which are described in greater detail here.

Nasal Cannula

A nasal cannula is the most frequently used device for administering home oxygen therapy. A nasal cannula consists of soft plastic tubing with a two-pronged device that is inserted into the patient's nose (Fig. 27.25A). The tubing of the prongs loops over the patient's ears and is secured under the chin (Fig. 27.25B). The tubing connects to the delivery system (i.e., compressed oxygen cylinder, liquid oxygen, or oxygen concentrator). The primary advantage of a nasal cannula is that it does not interfere with the patient's ability to talk, eat, or drink.

The concentration of oxygen inhaled by the patient depends on the flow rate prescribed by the provider. A nasal cannula can deliver oxygen at a flow rate between 0.25 and 6 L/min. If the flow rate is greater than 4 L/min, it can dry out the patient's nasal passages. To prevent this from occurring, a humidifier should be used to provide moisture for a flow rate above 4 L/min.

The cannula should be washed once or twice a week using liquid soap and water, rinsed thoroughly, and allowed to air-dry. The cannula should be replaced with a new cannula every 2 to 4 weeks.

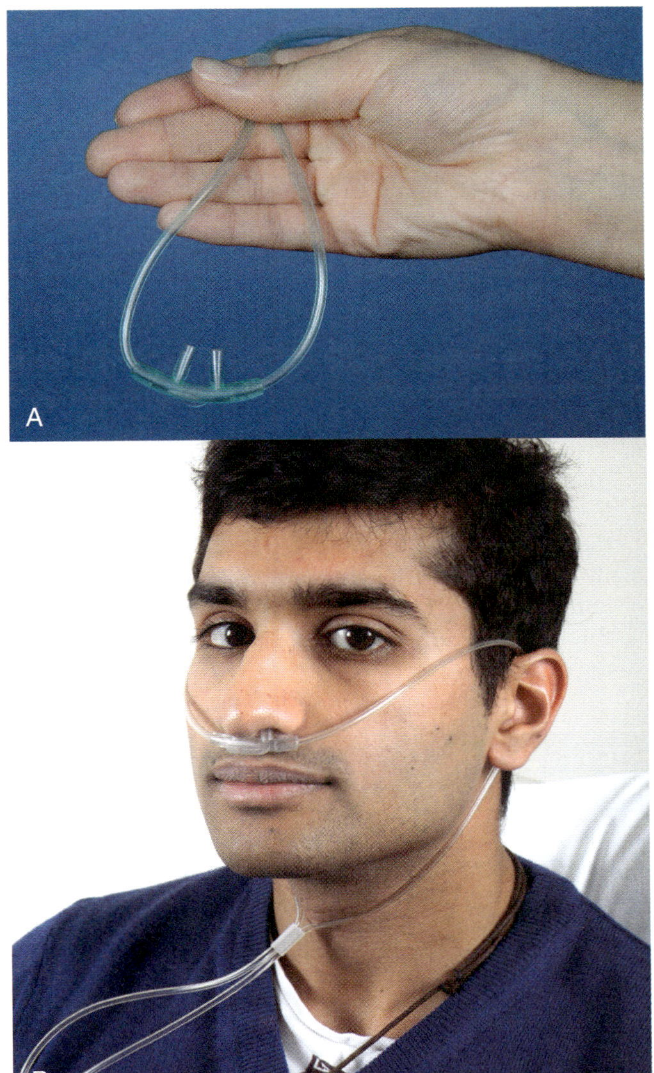

Fig. 27.25 (A) Nasal cannula showing prongs. (B) The tubing of the prongs loops over the patient's ears and is secured under the chin. (B, From *The unofficial guide to practical skills*, ed 2, 2024, Elsevier Ltd.)

Face Mask

A face mask consists of plastic and fits over the patient's nose and mouth. A face mask strap is then tightened around the patient's head to ensure a secure fit (Fig. 27.26). Oxygen tubing is used to connect the face mask to the oxygen delivery system. A face mask is not used as frequently as a nasal cannula to administer oxygen because it is bulky and must be removed for eating or drinking and to communicate effectively.

A face mask is often used for patients who need a high flow rate of oxygen. It can deliver oxygen to the patient at a flow rate between 5 and 15 L/min. Wearing a nasal cannula for an extended period of time can irritate the nose. Because of this, the patient might prefer to wear a nasal cannula during the day and a face mask at night to reduce the irritation that may occur from a nasal cannula.

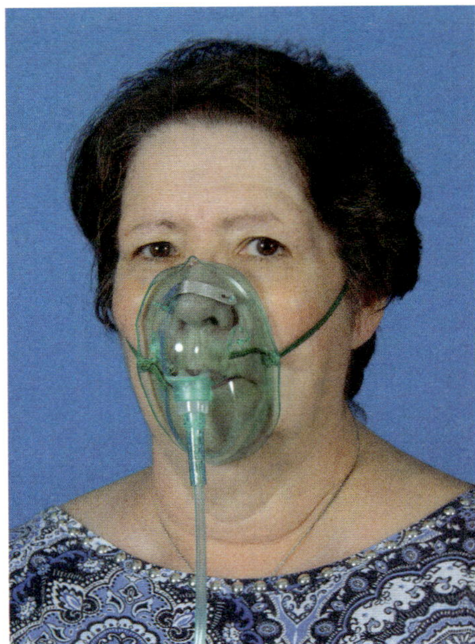

Fig. 27.26 Face mask.

The patient who has nasal congestion from a cold will also prefer a face mask.

The face mask should be washed once or twice a week using liquid soap and water, then rinsed thoroughly and dried. The face mask should be replaced with a new one every 2 to 4 weeks, or sooner if it becomes cracked or discolored.

OXYGEN GUIDELINES

The home medical supply company that provides the patient with the oxygen equipment gives the patient specific instructions on safe use, care, and maintenance of the equipment. Listed below are general usage and safety guidelines that the patient should follow.

Usage

1. Contact the provider if any of the symptoms of a low blood oxygen level occur, which include frequent headaches, anxiety, cyanosis of the lips or fingernails, drowsiness, confusion, restlessness, and slow, shallow, difficult, or irregular breathing.
2. Keep the oxygen delivery system clean and free from dust.
3. Do not change the oxygen flow rate unless directed to do so by the provider.
4. Do not use alcohol or take any other sedating drugs, as these substances will slow the breathing rate.
5. Order more oxygen from a home medical company in a timely manner.
6. To prevent the cheeks or skin behind the ears from becoming irritated from the tubing, tuck some gauze under the tubing. If you have persistent redness under your nose, contact the provider.

7. Oxygen therapy dries out the inside of the patient's nose and mouth. Use water-based lubricants (e.g., K-Y Jelly) on the lips or nostrils to relieve the drying effect. Do not use oil-based products such as petroleum jelly.
8. Do not use more than 40 to 50 feet of tubing with the oxygen delivery system to avoid bending or twisting of tubing to ensure unobstructed oxygen flow.
9. People are not allowed to bring compressed oxygen cylinders or liquid oxygen tanks on board an airplane. Many airlines will provide oxygen if notified 48 to 72 hours in advance.

Safety

Oxygen is a safe gas as long as it is used properly. Oxygen itself is not flammable, nor will it explode; however, it greatly increases the combustion rate of a fire. If something catches fire, oxygen will make the flame hotter and cause it to burn faster and more vigorously. The result is that a fire involving oxygen can appear explosive-like.

1. Store oxygen in a clean, dry, well-ventilated room. If kept in a closed area such as a closet, the small amount of oxygen gas that is continually vented from these units can accumulate in a confined space and become a fire hazard.
2. Compressed oxygen cylinders and liquid oxygen tanks must remain upright at all times. Secure oxygen cylinders and tanks to a fixed object, or place in a stand.
3. Never smoke while using oxygen. Do not allow smoking in the room where the oxygen is kept. Post "No Smoking: Oxygen in Use" signs where oxygen is kept.
4. Keep the oxygen supply at least 6 to 8 feet away from open flames such as gas stoves, lighted fireplaces, and candles.
5. Keep the oxygen supply at least 6 to 8 feet away from intense heat such as radiators, furnaces, and space heaters.
6. Keep the oxygen supply away from flammable products such as cleaning fluid, paint thinner, and aerosol sprays.
7. Do not lubricate oxygen equipment with oil or grease, as these substances are flammable.
8. Be sure to have functioning smoke detectors in the home.
9. Buy a fire extinguisher, and be familiar with how to use it.

What Would You Do? What Would You *Not* Do? RESPONSES

Case Study 1

Page 697

What Did Anitra Do?

- ❑ Tried to reduce Camilla's fears by talking with her calmly and quietly.
- ❑ Explained to Camilla that an ECG is the best screening test available to check for heart problems.
- ❑ Reassured Camilla that she would be draped during the procedure and that she would be exposed as little as possible.
- ❑ Told Camilla that the wires may look a little scary, but there is no chance of being shocked by them. Explained that she will not feel anything when the test is being run.
- ❑ Told Camilla that she could talk with the billing clerk about setting up a payment plan for the test. Provided her with information about community resources that might help her pay for the test.

What Did Anitra Not Do?

- ❑ Did not tell Camilla that she was too young to have heart problems.
- ❑ Did not tell Camilla that she needed to be more mature about being tested.

Case Study 2

Page 705

What Did Anitra Do?

- ❑ Commended Joel for his weight loss and lifestyle changes.
- ❑ Shared a positive story with Joel about a patient who stopped smoking and did not gain weight.
- ❑ Asked Joel whether he would like any of the latest information on smoking cessation.

What Did Anitra Not Do?

- ❑ Did not agree that Joel's lifestyle changes would counteract the bad effects of smoking.
- ❑ Did not lecture Joel on the dangers of smoking, because if he has been smoking since age 17 and has been trying to quit, he already knows what they are.

Case Study 3

Page 712

What Did Anitra Do?

- ❑ Complimented Damonte on wanting to take more of an interest in his asthma condition.
- ❑ Told Damonte that asthma triggers vary from one asthmatic patient to another.
- ❑ Explained to Damonte that during a severe asthma attack, his airways get smaller and become clogged with mucus. This causes less oxygen to be able to enter his lungs making it harder for him to breathe.
- ❑ Told Damonte that his peak flow measurements are used to know how well his asthma is being controlled and for making decisions on his asthma medications, so it is important to get a peak flow measurement every day. Also explained to Damonte that he may feel fine but his peak flow measurements may be decreasing. If this happens, he can start taking his medication to possibly stop the asthma attack.

What Did Anitra Not Do?

- Did not scold Damonte for wanting to take a shortcut with his peak flow measurements.

TERMINOLOGY REVIEW

Key Term	Word Parts	Definition
Artifact		Additional electrical activity picked up by the electrocardiograph that interferes with the normal appearance of the ECG cycles.
Atherosclerosis	*ather/o:* yellowish, fatty plaque *-sclerosis:* hardening of	Buildup of fibrous plaques of fatty deposits and cholesterol on the inner walls of an artery that causes narrowing, obstruction, and hardening of the artery.
Baseline		The flat horizontal line that separates the various waves of the ECG cycle.
Cardiac cycle	*cardi/o:* heart	One complete heartbeat.
Dysrhythmia	*dys-:* difficult, painful, abnormal *rhythm*: rhythm *-ia:* condition of diseased or abnormal state	An irregular heart rate or rhythm; also termed *arrhythmia.*
ECG cycle		The graphic representation of the cardiac cycle.
Electrocardiogram (ECG)	*electr/o:* electrical, electrical activity *cardi/o:* heart *-gram:* record of	The graphic representation of the electrical activity of the heart.
Electrocardiograph	*electr/o:* electrical, electrical activity *cardi/o:* heart *-graph:* instrument used to record	The instrument used to record the electrical activity of the heart.
Electrode	*electr/o:* electrical, electrical activity	A device placed on the skin that picks up electrical impulses given off by the heart.
Electrolyte	*electr/o:* electrical, electrical activity	A substance that facilitates transmission of the heart's electrical impulses.
Flow rate		The number of liters of oxygen per minute that come out of an oxygen delivery system.
Hypoxemia	*hypo-:* below, deficient *ox/i:* oxygen *-emia:* blood condition	A decrease in the oxygen saturation of the blood.
Hypoxia	*hypo-:* below, deficient *ox/i:* oxygen *-ia:* condition of diseased or abnormal state	A reduction in the oxygen supply to the tissues of the body.
Interval		The length of one or more waves and a segment.
Ischemia	*isch/o:* deficiency, blockage *-emia:* blood condition	Deficiency of blood in a body part.
Normal sinus rhythm		Refers to an ECG that is within normal limits.
Oxygen therapy		The administration of supplemental oxygen at concentrations greater than room air to treat or prevent hypoxemia.
Peak expiratory flow rate		The maximum volume of air that can be exhaled when the patient blows into a peak flow meter as forcefully and as rapidly as possible.
Segment		The portion of the ECG between two waves.
Spirometer	*spir/o:* breathe, breathing *-meter:* instrument used to measure	An instrument that measures how much air is exhaled by the lungs and how fast it is exhaled.
Spirometry	*spir/o:* breathe, breathing *-metry:* measurement	Measurement of an individual's breathing capacity by means of a spirometer.
Wheezing		A continuous, high-pitched whistling musical sound heard particularly during exhalation and sometimes during inhalation.

PROCEDURE 27.1 Recording a 12-Lead Electrocardiogram

Outcome Record a 12-lead electrocardiogram (ECG).

Equipment/Supplies

- Three-channel electrocardiograph
- Disposable electrodes
- ECG paper

1. **Procedural Step.** Work in a quiet, relaxing atmosphere away from sources of electrical interference.
2. **Procedural Step.** Sanitize your hands, and assemble the equipment. Check the expiration date of the electrodes.
   Principle. The electrolyte gel on outdated electrodes may be dried out, which can cause artifacts on the ECG.
3. **Procedural Step.** Greet the patient and introduce yourself. Identify the patient by full name and date of birth. Help the patient relax by explaining the procedure. Tell the patient that having an ECG recording is painless. Explain that they must lie still, breathe normally, and not talk while the ECG is being recorded so that an accurate ECG can be obtained.
   Principle. Explaining the procedure helps reassure apprehensive patients. The patient should be mentally and physically relaxed for an accurate ECG recording; an apprehensive or moving patient produces muscle artifacts. Heavy breathing or sighing can cause a wandering baseline artifact.
4. **Procedural Step.** Prepare the patient. Ask them to remove clothing from the waist up. The lower legs also must be uncovered. Provide a female patient with a gown, and instruct her to put it on with the opening in front. Assist the patient into a supine position on the table. The table should support the arms and legs adequately so that they do not dangle. Properly drape the patient to prevent exposure and to provide warmth. A pillow can be used to support the patient's head.
   Principle. The chest, upper arms, and lower legs must be uncovered to allow proper placement of the electrodes. The patient should be kept warm, and the arms and legs should not be allowed to dangle; otherwise, muscle artifacts could result.
5. **Procedural Step.** Position the electrocardiograph so that the power cord points away from the patient and does not pass under the table. It is usually easier for the medical assistant to work on the left side of the patient.
   Principle. Proper positioning of the electrocardiograph reduces 60-cycle interference artifacts.
6. **Procedural Step.** Prepare the patient's skin for application of the disposable electrodes. If the patient has sweaty or oily skin or has used lotion, rub the area to which the electrode will be applied with alcohol, and allow it to dry. If the patient's chest is hairy, dry shave it at each electrode site before applying the electrode.
   Principle. The patient's skin must be dry and free of oil and body hair so that the adhesive backing of the electrodes sticks to the patient's skin and stays on during the procedure.
7. **Procedural Step.** Remove a card containing 10 electrodes from its foil-lined pouch and reseal the pouch. Apply the limb electrodes. Firmly apply the adhesive backing of the electrodes to the fleshy part of each of the four limbs (upper arms and lower legs). The electrode tabs should point toward the center of the body. The tabs of the arm electrodes should point downward, and the tabs of the leg electrodes should point upward. The adhesive backing of the electrode allows it to adhere firmly to the patient's skin.

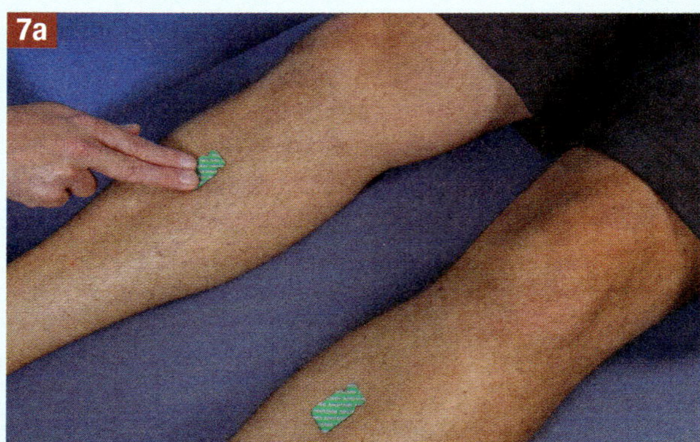

Apply the leg electrodes.

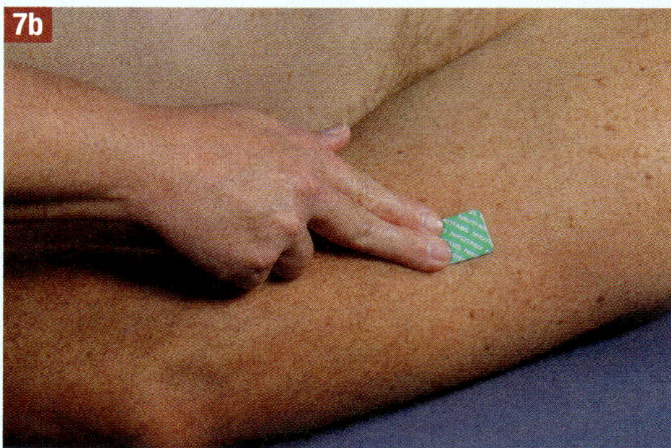

Apply the arm electrodes.

Principle. The pouch should be resealed to preserve moisture and prevent the electrolyte on the remaining electrodes from drying out. The electrodes must be

PROCEDURE 27.1 Recording a 12-Lead Electrocardiogram—cont'd

firmly attached to permit good transmission of the electrical impulse from the patient's skin to the electrode. Loose electrodes can cause artifacts to occur on the recording, making it difficult to analyze the recording. The tabs of the electrodes should be positioned toward the center of the body to provide a more stable connection when the lead wire is attached to the electrode and to prevent the lead wires from pulling onto the electrodes and causing artifacts.

8. **Procedural Step.** Apply the chest electrodes. Properly locate each electrode placement site using palpation, and apply the electrode with the tab pointing downward. Continue until all six of the chest electrodes have been applied.
   Principle. Positioning the tabs of the electrodes downward prevents the lead wires from pulling and causing artifacts.

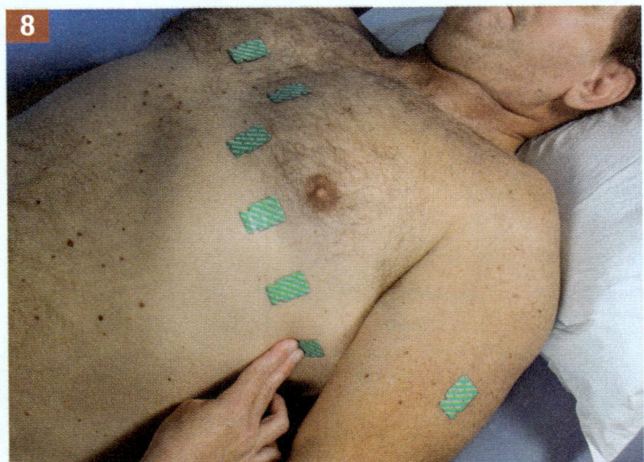

Apply the chest electrodes.

9. **Procedural Step.** Connect the lead wires to the electrodes. This is accomplished by inserting an alligator clip onto the metal tip of each lead wire. Next, firmly attach an alligator clip to the tab of each electrode. The ends of the lead wires are usually color coded (e.g., red for the arms and green for the legs) and identified with abbreviations to help the medical assistant connect the proper lead to each electrode. Arrange the lead wires to follow body contour.
   Principle. The lead wires must be attached correctly to ensure an accurate and reliable ECG. Arranging the lead wires to follow body contour reduces the possibility of 60-cycle interference artifacts.

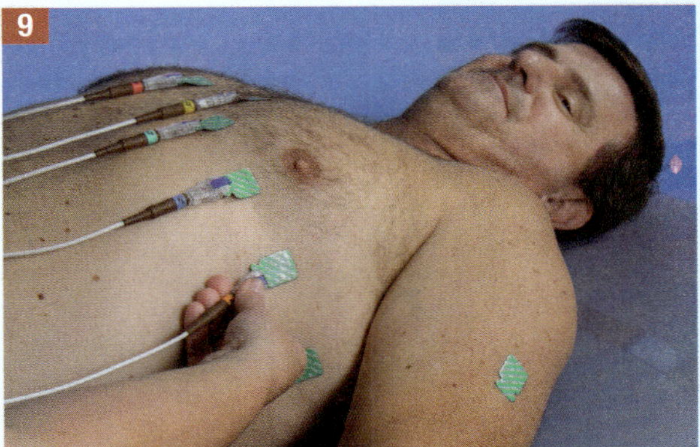

Connect the lead wires to the electrodes.

10. **Procedural Step.** Plug the patient cable into the electrocardiograph. The cable should be supported on the table or on the patient's abdomen to prevent pulling of the lead wires on the electrodes.
    Principle. Pulling of the lead wires on the electrodes can cause the electrodes to pull away from the skin, resulting in artifacts.
11. **Procedural Step.** Turn on the electrocardiograph. Enter patient data using the soft-touch keypad. Always use your fingertips to enter the data. Pencils and other sharp objects can damage the keyboard. As the data are entered, they are displayed on the liquid crystal diode (LCD) screen. Patient data to be entered typically include the patient's name, a patient identification number, age, sex, height, weight, and medications.

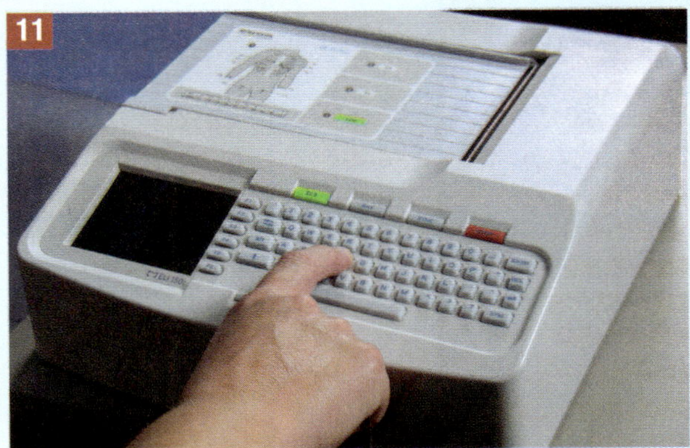

Enter patient data.

12. **Procedural Step.** Remind the patient to lie still, breathe normally, and not talk. Press the AUTO (automatic) button, and run the recording. The electrocardiograph automatically inserts a standardization mark at the beginning of each ECG strip, followed by the recording of the 12-lead ECG in a three-channel format. Another standardization mark is inserted at the end of each ECG strip.

Continued

PROCEDURE 27.1

PROCEDURE 27.1 Recording a 12-Lead Electrocardiogram—cont'd

(*Note:* With most three-channel electrocardiographs, the machine checks for a clear electrical impulse from the heart after the AUTO button is pressed. If the electrical impulse is "noisy," this may indicate that an electrode does not have a good connection with the patient's skin. The machine usually indicates which electrode is causing the problem [e.g., "V_6 noisy"]. Apply firm pressure to the electrode causing the problem. If this does not correct the problem, replace the electrode with a new one and/or place a piece of nonallergenic tape over the electrode.)

13. Procedural Step. After the ECG has been recorded:

a. Check the printout to ensure that the standardization mark is 10 mm high. If it is more or less than 10 mm, adjust the standardization mark according to the manufacturer's instructions, and run another ECG.

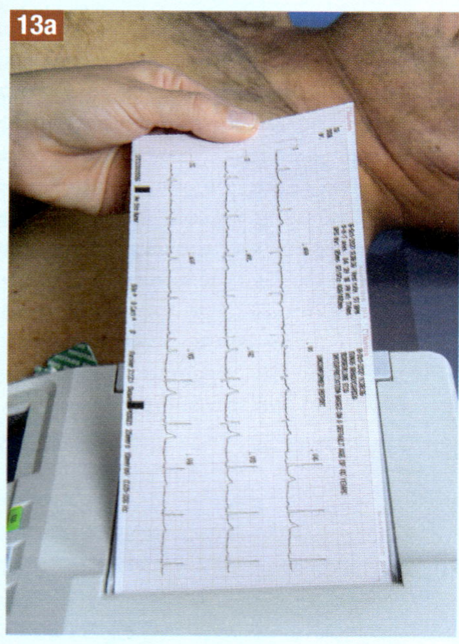

13a Check the standardization mark.

b. Check the direction of the R wave in lead I. If your patient's limb leads are attached correctly, the R wave on lead I should have a positive deflection. If it has a negative deflection, the limb leads are not attached correctly. Reattach the limb leads properly and run another recording.

c. Observe the recording for artifacts. If an artifact is present, determine the cause of the artifact, correct the problem, and run another ECG.

14. Procedural Step. Inform the patient that you are finished and they can now talk or move. Turn the machine off. Disconnect the lead wires. Remove and discard the electrodes.

15. Procedural Step. Assist the patient in stepping down from the table.

16. Procedural Step. Sanitize your hands.

17. Procedural Step. Document the procedure in the patient's medical record.

a. *Electronic medical record:* Document the procedure performed (12-lead ECG) using the appropriate radio buttons, drop-down menus, and free text fields.

b. *Paper-based patient record:* Document the date and time and the name of the procedure.

17b

DOCUMENTATION EXAMPLE

Date	
6/12/XX	10:30 a.m. Completed a 12-lead ECG.
	Recording to physician for review. ———
	——————— A. Martin, CMA (AAMA)

18. Procedural Step. Return all equipment to its proper storage place.

PROCEDURE 27.2 Measuring Peak Expiratory Flow Rate

Outcome Measure a patient's peak expiratory flow rate.

Equipment/Supplies

- Peak flow meter
- Disposable mouthpiece
- Waste container

1. **Procedural Step.** Sanitize the hands. Assemble and prepare the equipment. Move the sliding indicator on the peak flow meter to the bottom of the numbered scale. Apply a disposable mouthpiece to the mouthpiece holder.
Principle. Not placing the marker at the bottom of the numbered scale leads to inaccurate test results. The disposable mouthpiece prevents the spread of microorganisms from one patient to another.

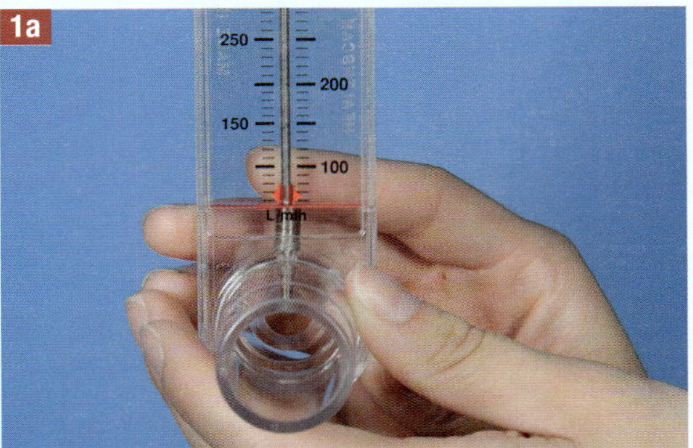

Move indicator to bottom of scale.

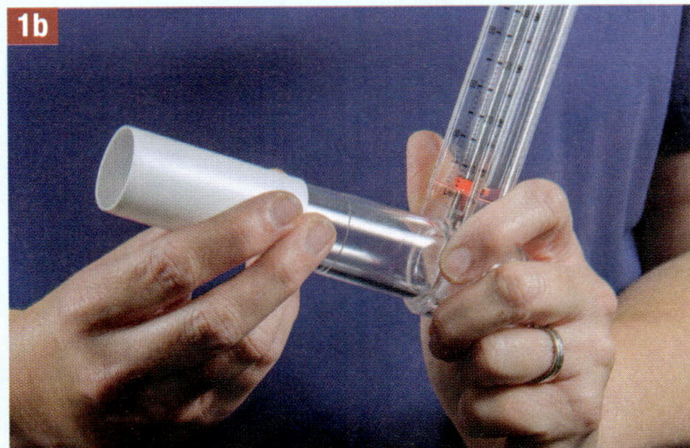

Apply a disposable mouthpiece.

2. **Procedural Step.** Greet the patient and introduce yourself. Identify the patient and explain the procedure. Tell the patient that they will be performing a breathing maneuver several times to see how well their lungs are functioning.
3. **Procedural Step.** Prepare the patient. Have the patient remove any heavy or constricting clothing, such as a jacket or a sweater. Also, ask the patient to loosen tight clothing, such as a necktie or a tight collar. If the patient is chewing gum, ask them to discard it in a waste container.
Principle. Heavy outer clothing, tight clothing, or gum may make it difficult for the patient to perform the breathing maneuver.
4. **Procedural Step.** Instruct the patient in the breathing maneuver. The following procedure should be described and demonstrated to the patient:
   a. Relax and take the deepest breath possible until your lungs are completely filled with air.

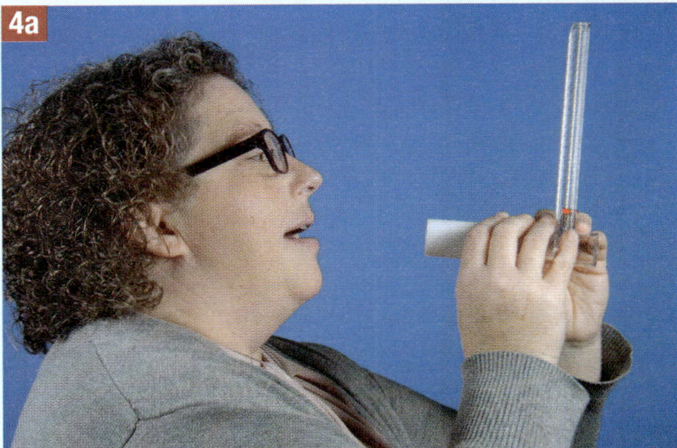

The patient takes a deep breath.

   b. Place the mouthpiece in your mouth, and seal your lips tightly around it.
   c. Blow out as hard and fast as you can until your lungs are completely empty. Try to move the marker as high as you can on the numbered scale. Do not block the opening of the mouthpiece with your tongue.

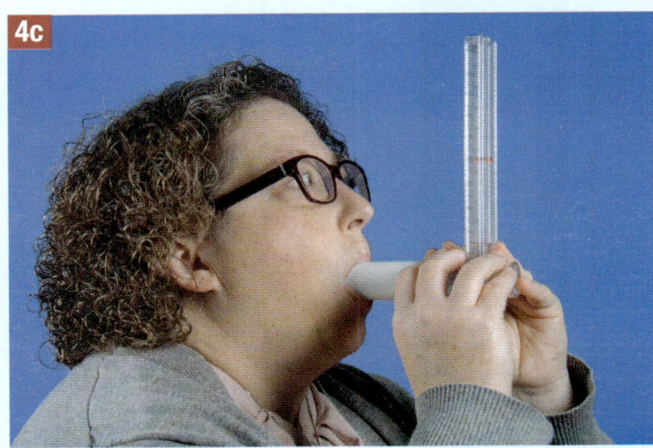

The patient blows out hard and fast.

   d. Remove the mouthpiece from your mouth.

Continued

PROCEDURE 27.2 Measuring Peak Expiratory Flow Rate—cont'd

Principle. The lips must be tightly sealed around the mouthpiece so that all of the air leaving the mouth enters the mouthpiece. The force of the air coming out of the patient's lungs causes the marker to move upward on the scale. The reading depends on how hard the patient blows out the air in their lungs.

5. **Procedural Step.** Tell the patient you will repeat the instructions during the test. Encourage the patient to remain calm during the procedure.
   Principle. Fear or anxiety can make the results less reliable.
6. **Procedural Step.** Place a new disposable mouthpiece on the peak flow meter, and slide the marker to the bottom of the numbered scale. Hand the peak flow meter to the patient.
7. **Procedural Step.** Instruct the patient to stand up straight and look straight ahead.
8. **Procedural Step.** Begin the test. Actively coach the patient as follows:
   a. "Now relax and take in a big breath—in—in—in—"
   b. "Put the mouthpiece in your mouth and blow hard."
   c. "Take out the mouthpiece and rest for a while. You did a great job."
9. **Procedural Step.** Note the number at which the indicator stopped on the scale of the peak flow meter. Jot down the number on a piece of paper. The peak flow measurement on the meter illustrated is 400 L/min.

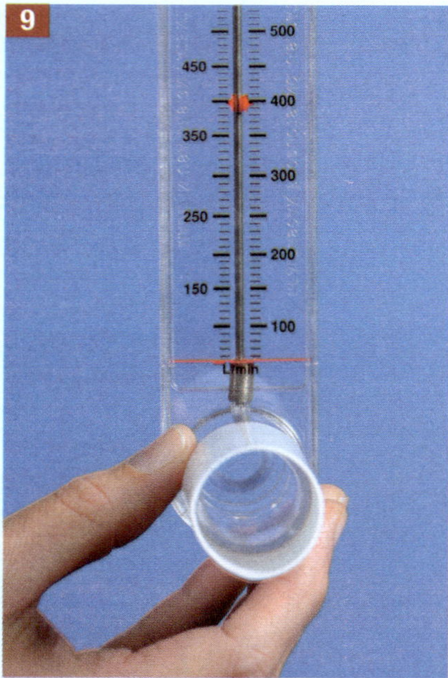

Note where the indicator stopped on the scale.

10. **Procedural Step.** If the patient coughs or does not perform the breathing maneuver correctly, do not write down the number. Inform the patient of what modifications are needed for the next effort.
11. **Procedural Step.** Continue until three acceptable breathing maneuvers have been obtained. Make sure to slide the marker to the bottom of the scale before each measurement.
    Principle. Three acceptable efforts must be obtained to ensure valid test results. If the patient performs the breathing maneuver correctly, the measurements from the three tests should be about the same.
12. **Procedural Step.** Take the peak flow meter from the patient, and remove the mouthpiece from the mouthpiece holder. Dispose of the mouthpiece in a regular waste container.
13. **Procedural Step.** Sanitize your hands. Note the highest of the three peak flow measurements. (Do not calculate an average.)
14. **Procedural Step.** Document the procedure in the patient's medical record.
    a. *Electronic medical record:* Document the name of the procedure and the highest of the three acceptable peak flow measurements using the appropriate radio buttons, drop-down menus, and free text fields.
    b. *Paper-based patient record:* Document the date, the time, the name of the procedure, and the highest of the three acceptable peak flow measurements.

14b DOCUMENTATION EXAMPLE

Date	
6/21/XX	10:30 a.m. PEFR: 400 L/min. Pt stated she
	was tired following the test. ———
	——— A. Martin, CMA (AAMA)

15. **Procedural Step.** Clean the peak flow meter by washing it in warm soapy water, rinsing it thoroughly, and allowing it to dry completely.

Specialty Tests and Procedures

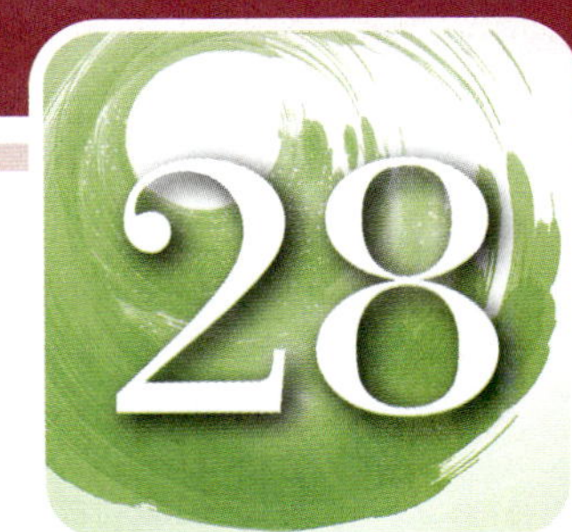

Check out the Evolve site at http://evolve.elsevier.com/Bonewit/today to access additional interactive activities and exercises to help you study and prepare for success.

LEARNING OBJECTIVES	PROCEDURES
Stool-Based Colorectal Screening Tests	
1. List the symptoms of colorectal cancer.	
2. Identify the recommended colorectal cancer screening guidelines.	
3. Identify three types of stool-based colorectal screening tests.	
4. Explain the recommended follow-up for a positive stool-based colorectal screening test.	
5. State the purpose of a guaiac fecal occult blood test (gFOBT).	
6. Identify the patient preparation required for a gFOBT.	Instruct a patient in the preparation requirements and the collection procedure for a gFOBT.
7. Describe the quality control measures that should be employed with a gFOBT.	Develop and interpret the results of a gFOBT.
8. State the purpose of a fecal immunochemical test (FIT).	
9. Identify the two types of tests included in the FIT-DNA (fecal immunochemical and DNA) test.	
10. Describe the meaning of a positive FIT-DNA test.	
Sigmoidoscopy	
11. Explain the purpose of sigmoidoscopy.	Instruct a patient in the preparation required for a sigmoidoscopy. Assist the provider with a sigmoidoscopy.
12. Explain the importance of proper bowel preparation prior to a sigmoidoscopy.	
13. Explain the purpose of a digital rectal examination (DRE) prior to a sigmoidoscopy.	
Colonoscopy	
14. Explain the purpose of a colonoscopy.	Instruct a patient in the preparation required for a colonoscopy.
15. List the conditions that can be detected and assessed during a colonoscopy.	
16. Describe the procedure for a colonoscopy.	
Prostate Cancer Screening Tests and Procedures	
17. List the symptoms of prostate cancer.	
18. Explain how the digital rectal examination (DRE) is used to screen for prostate cancer screening.	Assist the provider with a digital rectal examination.
19. Explain the purpose of the prostate-specific antigen (PSA) test.	Instruct a patient in the preparation for a PSA test.
Testicular Cancer Screening Procedure	
20. State the risk factors for testicular cancer.	Teach a patient how to perform a testicular self-examination.
21. Identify the testicular self-examination schedule.	

LEARNING OBJECTIVES

Radiology

22. State the function of radiographs in medicine.
23. Explain the importance of proper patient preparation for a radiographic examination.
24. Explain the difference between film-based radiography and digital radiography.
25. State the advantages of digital radiography.
26. Explain the function of a contrast medium.
27. Describe the purpose of a fluoroscope.
28. Explain the purpose of each of the following types of radiographic examinations:
    - Mammography
    - Bone density scan
    - Upper gastrointestinal radiography
    - Lower gastrointestinal radiography
    - Intravenous pyelography

Diagnostic Imaging

29. Explain the purpose of each of the following diagnostic imaging procedures:
    - Ultrasonography
    - Computed tomography
    - Magnetic resonance imaging
    - Nuclear medicine imaging
30. Explain how nuclear medicine is used to produce an image of a body part.
31. State the purpose of a bone scan.
32. State the purpose of a nuclear cardiac stress test.
33. Describe a PET scan.

PROCEDURES

Instruct a patient in the guidelines for the following radiographic examinations:
- Mammography
- Upper gastrointestinal examination
- Lower gastrointestinal examination
- Intravenous pyelography

Instruct a patient in the guidelines for the following diagnostic imaging procedures:
- Ultrasonography
- Computed tomography
- Magnetic resonance imaging

Nuclear medicine imaging

CHAPTER OUTLINE

KEY TERMS

biopsy (BIE-op-see)
colonoscope (KOL-un-oh-skope)
colonoscopy (KOL-un-OS-koe-pee)
contrast medium
echocardiogram (EK-oh-KAR-dee-oh-gram)
endoscope (EN-doe-skope)
enema (EN-em-ah)
fluoroscope (FLOOR-oh-skope)
fluoroscopy (floor-OS-koe-pee)
insufflate (IN-suf-flate)
occult (ah-KULT) blood
polyp
radiograph (RAY-dee-oh-graf)
radiography (ray-dee-OG-rah-fee)
radiologist (ray-dee-AH-lah-jist)
radiology (ray-dee-AH-lah-jee)
radiolucent (ray-dee-oh-LOO-sent)
radiopaque (ray-dee-oh-PAYK)
screening
sigmoidoscope (sig-MOYD-oh-skope)
sigmoidoscopy (sig-moyd-OS-koe-pee)
sonogram (SON-oh-gram)
ultrasonography (ul-trah-son-AH-grah-fee)

INTRODUCTION TO COLORECTAL TESTS AND PROCEDURES

Colorectal tests and procedures are often performed for the early detection of colorectal cancer and precancerous polyps. Other, less serious conditions can also be detected through these tests and procedures including hemorrhoids, anal fissures, diverticulitis, peptic ulcers, ulcerative colitis, gastroesophageal reflux disease (GERD), and Crohn's disease. The most commonly used tests and procedures include stool-based colorectal screening tests, sigmoidoscopy, and colonoscopy.

The medical assistant is often responsible for coaching the patient on any advance preparation required for these tests and procedures. The medical assistant should make sure the patient thoroughly understands the instructions. If the patient does not prepare properly, inaccurate results may occur. To completely understand colorectal tests and procedures, the medical assistant should be familiar with the structure of the large intestine. Refer to Chapter 14: *Digestive System* to review the structure of the large intestine.

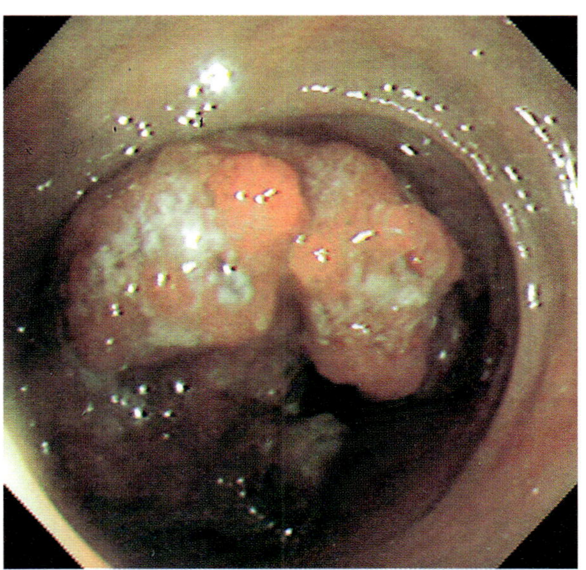

Fig. 28.1 Colon cancer. (From Forbes CD: *Color atlas and text of clinical medicine*, ed 3, Philadelphia, 2003, Mosby.)

COLORECTAL CANCER

Colorectal cancer (CRC) is used to describe both cancer of the colon (Fig. 28.1) and cancer of the rectum. While colorectal cancer may occur in young adults, the majority of cases (90%) occur in individuals older than 50 years of age. Colorectal cancer is the third most common type of cancer in the United States and the second leading cause of cancer-related deaths for both men and women. According to the American Cancer Society, every year more than 150,000 people are diagnosed with colorectal cancer, and approximately 50,000 of these individuals die from this disease.

Colorectal cancer usually starts from small precancerous polyps in the colon or rectum. A colorectal **polyp** is an abnormal growth that protrudes from the mucous membrane of the large intestine (Fig. 28.2). Most cases of colorectal cancer arise from a type of polyp known as an *adenomatous polyp* that gradually increases in size and becomes malignant and spreads to other parts of the body over a long period of time (typically 10 to 15 years). Adenomatous polyps usually cause no symptoms and there is no way to prevent them. However, detecting polyps

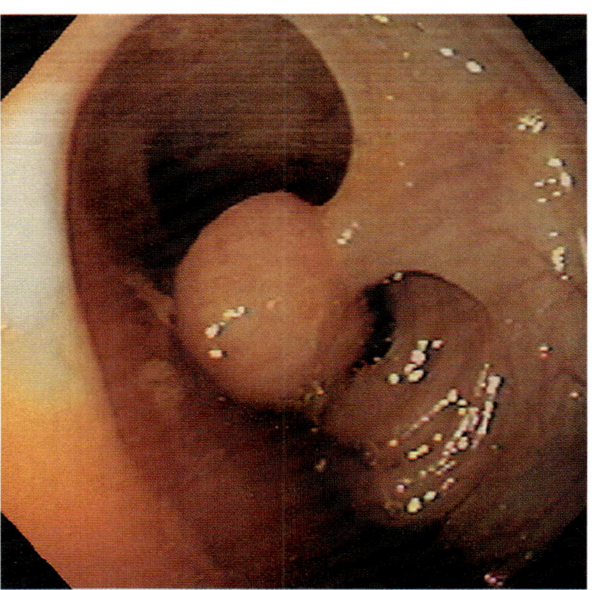

Fig. 28.2 Colon polyp. (From Lewis S: *Medical-surgical nursing*, ed 9, St. Louis, 2014, Mosby.)

early through colorectal cancer screening allows them to be removed before they can develop into cancer and spread to other parts of the body. Once a polyp is removed, it is examined by a pathologist to determine if it is benign or malignant which then dictates whether further treatment is necessary.

Symptoms

No symptoms or very few symptoms occur during the early stages of colorectal cancer. If colorectal cancer is detected and treated while the patient is still asymptomatic, the patient has a 90% chance of 5-year survival. By comparison, the 5-year survival rate for patients in whom colorectal cancer is diagnosed after symptoms appear is only 40% and the 5-year survival rate when the cancer has spread to distant organs (metastasized) such as the liver or lungs is only 11%.

Symptoms that occur when colorectal cancer is more developed include the following:

- Bleeding from the rectum
- Blood in or on the stool
- A change in the shape of the stool (e.g., stools that are narrower than usual)
- A change in bowel habits (e.g., diarrhea, constipation)
- General abdominal discomfort (e.g., aches, pains, cramps that don't go away)
- Unexplained weight loss
- Constant fatigue

Risk Factors for Colorectal Cancer

The exact cause of colorectal cancer is not known, but certain factors increase the risk of developing this disease. A *risk factor* is anything that increases an individual's chance of developing a disease such as cancer. Although colorectal cancer risk factors often influence the development of cancer, most do not directly cause it. For example, some people with several colorectal risk factors never develop cancer, while others with no known risk factors do. Some colorectal risk factors can be changed (e.g., smoking, diet, and physical activity) while others cannot be changed (e.g., age and family history). The risk factors for colorectal cancer are outlined in Box 28.1.

BOX 28.1 Colorectal Cancer Risk Factors

The following factors may increase the risk of developing colorectal cancer:

- ***Gender.*** Men have a slightly higher risk of developing colorectal cancer than women.
- ***Personal history of adenomatous polyps.*** Individuals with adenomatous polyps have an increased risk of developing colorectal cancer. Approximately 10% of adenomatous polyps become cancerous if not removed. Adenomatous polyps that become cancerous are known as adenocarcinomas.
- ***Personal or family history of colorectal cancer.*** Individuals who have been diagnosed previously with colorectal cancer are at higher risk for developing it in other parts of the colon and rectum, even if it was completely removed. Individuals with colorectal cancer in a first-degree relative (e.g., parent, sibling) are also at increased risk for developing the disease.
- ***Personal history of inflammatory bowel disease.*** Individuals with inflammatory bowel disease of long duration such as ulcerative colitis and Crohn's disease are at increased risk for colorectal cancer.
- ***Personal or family history of an inherited genetic syndrome.*** Approximately 5% to 10% of individuals who develop colorectal cancer have an inherited genetic colorectal cancer syndrome. These syndromes occur when a genetic mutation associated with colon or rectal cancer is passed down through a family's genes. The most common of these syndromes include familial adenomatous polyposis (FAP) and hereditary nonpolyposis colon cancer (Lynch syndrome).
- ***Racial and ethnic background.*** African Americans have the highest incidence of colorectal cancer and mortality rates of all racial groups in the United States. The reasons for this are not fully understood.
- ***Other factors*** that have been associated with a higher incidence of colorectal cancer include:
  - Type 2 diabetes
  - Smoking
  - Moderate to heavy alcohol consumption
  - Physical inactivity and obesity
  - Diet high in fat, red meat (e.g., beef, pork, lamb) and processed meats (e.g., hot dogs, bacon, cold cuts)
  - Low intake of fresh fruits and vegetables

COLORECTAL CANCER SCREENING GUIDELINES

Screening refers to the process of testing to detect disease in an individual who is not yet experiencing symptoms. For certain types of cancer (e.g., colorectal cancer and breast cancer), screening allows the cancer to be discovered early, when it is more treatable, which increases the patient's survival rate.

For the early prevention and detection of colorectal cancer, the American Cancer Society (ACS) recommends that all adults ages 45 to 75 years who are at average risk be screened for colorectal cancer. Previous to this, the ACS stipulated 50 as the age to begin screening. In recent years, however, there has been an increase in colorectal cancer among younger adults resulting in the recommendation to begin screening at 45 years of age. Individuals are considered to be at *average risk* for colorectal cancer if they do not have any of the following: personal or family history of colorectal cancer, adenomatous polyps, or an inherited genetic syndrome; inflammatory bowel disease of long duration; personal history of getting radiation to the abdomen or pelvic area to treat a prior cancer. Individuals with these conditions have an increased risk for developing colorectal cancer and should be screened at an earlier age and with greater frequency following the recommendations of their providers.

BOX 28.2 American Cancer Society Colorectal Cancer Screening Guidelines

Individuals Between the Ages of 45 and 75 at Average Risk for Colorectal Cancer

Stool-Based Colorectal Screening Tests

- Guaiac fecal occult blood test: every year*
- Fecal immunochemical test: every year*
- FIT-DNA test: every 3 years*

Visualization Examination Procedures

- Colonoscopy: every 10 years
- CT colonography (virtual colonoscopy): every 5 years*
- Flexible sigmoidoscopy: every 5 years*

Individuals Between the Ages of 76 and 85

The decision to be screened should be based on an individual's preferences, life expectancy, overall health, and prior screening history.

Individuals Over the Age of 85

No longer need to be screened.

*Colonoscopy should be performed if the results are positive

There are many colorectal cancer screening options available; therefore individuals should talk with their healthcare providers to determine which option is best for them. Colorectal cancer screening guidelines and options are outlined in Box 28.2.

STOOL-BASED COLORECTAL SCREENING TESTS

Stool-based tests are used to screen for the possible presence of colorectal cancer and polyps. They require that a patient collect a stool specimen at home and return it to the medical office or an outside laboratory for testing. The medical assistant is often responsible for providing the patient with instructions on any patient preparation required, collection of the stool specimen, and the proper care and storage of the specimen. Some patients initially may be reluctant to comply with the patient preparation and specimen collection requirements. The medical assistant can help by explaining the purpose of the test to patients to help them understand the benefits to be derived from the test.

Most stool-based colorectal screening tests work by detecting the presence of blood in the stool. During the early asymptomatic stages, almost all cancers and large polyps of the colon and rectum bleed a small amount on an intermittent basis. This is because the blood vessels in cancer or polyps are often fragile and easily damaged by the passage of stool. The damaged vessels usually bleed into the colon or rectum, but only rarely is there enough bleeding for it to be seen by the unaided eye. This hidden, or nonvisible, blood is termed **occult blood**, and its presence can be detected with a stool-based test.

The patient should be instructed *not* to collect a stool specimen when any of the following conditions are present: diarrhea, blood in the urine or stool, bleeding cuts or wounds on the hands, rectal bleeding, and menstruation. These conditions may cause blood to appear in the stool resulting in a false-positive test result.

A positive test result for a stool-based colorectal screening test does not mean the patient has colorectal cancer. It only indicates the presence of blood in the stool; the source and cause of the bleeding must still be determined. This means that further diagnostic procedures must be performed before the provider can make a diagnosis. These procedures may include colonoscopy, CT colonography, and sigmoidoscopy. A negative result does not guarantee the absence of cancer and the patient should continue to follow the colorectal cancer screening guidelines outlined in Box 28.2.

Types of Tests

There are three types of stool-based colorectal screening tests commonly used to screen for colorectal cancer, which include the following:

- Guaiac fecal occult blood test (gFOBT)
- Fecal Immunochemical Test (FIT
- Fecal Immunochemical-DNA Test (FIT-DNA Test)

Guaiac Fecal Occult Blood Test

The guaiac fecal occult blood test (gFOBT) is a CLIA-waived test that uses guaiac to screen for occult blood in the stool. Guaiac is a chemical that changes to a blue color if blood is present. Brand names for the gFOBT (Fig. 28.3) include Hemoccult (Beckman Coulter, Inc.) and ColoScreen (Helena Laboratories). The gFOBT is designed to detect the presence of occult blood in three stool specimens collected on three different days. The purpose of using three specimens is to allow detection of blood from colorectal lesions that exhibit

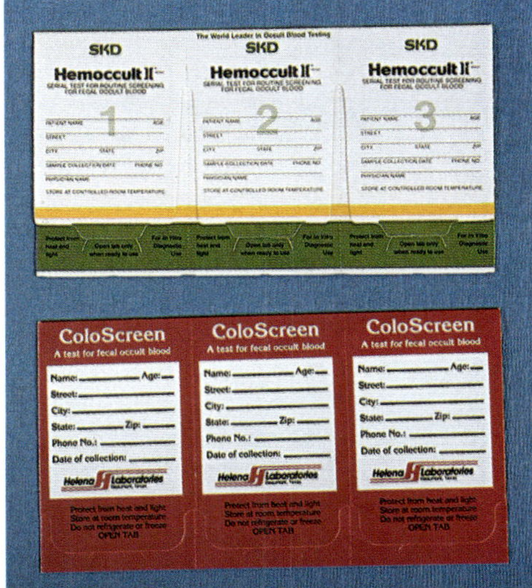

Fig. 28.3 Examples of fecal occult blood testing kits. Hemoccult (top) and ColoScreen (bottom).

intermittent bleeding. The gFOBT is an inexpensive test that is easy to perform; however, care must be taken to prevent false-positive and false-negative test results.

Patient Instructions

Patient instructions for a gFOBT play an important role in ensuring accurate test results. The patient must follow a special diet, beginning 3 days before the test, and must continue the diet until all three specimens have been collected. The patient is placed on a high-fiber diet that is free of red meat. Red meat contains animal blood, which could lead to a false-positive test result. A high-fiber diet is used because it encourages bleeding from colorectal lesions that may bleed only occasionally. In addition, fiber adds bulk to the stool, which promotes bowel elimination and ensures adequate specimen collection.

Certain medications irritate the gastrointestinal tract, which can result in a small amount of bleeding that could cause a false-positive result on a gFOBT. Medications that should be avoided before testing include ibuprofen, naproxen, and more than one adult aspirin per day. In addition, vitamin C (greater than 250 mg per day) from supplements and citrus fruits and juices can cause a false-negative test result. An iron supplement will not affect the test results. Table 28.1 lists patient instructions for a gFOBT.

Quality Control

Quality control methods must be employed with a gFOBT to ensure reliable and valid results. It is important to properly store the testing kit containing the gFOBT cardboard collection slides and developing solution. Adverse storage conditions can result in deterioration of the developing solution and the active reagents impregnated on the filter paper of the slides, leading to inaccurate test results. The testing kit must be stored at a room temperature which is between 59°F and 86°F (15°C and 30°C). The contents of the kit must be protected from heat, sunlight, and strong fluorescent light. In addition, the testing kit should not be stored in close proximity to volatile chemicals such as ammonia, bleach, bromine, iodine, and disinfectant cleaners. If stored properly, the slides and developing solution will remain effective until the expiration date that is stamped on the side of the testing kit box, each slide itself, and the container of developing solution.

A quality control procedure must be performed *after* the patient's test has been developed, read, and interpreted. This ensures that the test results are accurate and valid. The Hemoccult test includes an on-slide performance monitor that consists of a positive and negative monitor area. Failure of the expected control results to occur indicates an error, and the test results are not considered valid; possible causes include the use of an outdated test or developing solution; an error in technique; and subjection of the test to heat, sunlight, strong fluorescent light, or volatile chemicals. Procedure 28.1 outlines the procedure for coaching a patient in the collection of a specimen for a Hemoccult test. Procedure 28.2 describes the development and interpretation of a Hemoccult test.

Table 28.1 Patient Instructions for the gFOBT

Diet	**For 3 days before and during the collection period:**
Meats	• Eat no red or rare meat (beef and lamb) or liver. • Small amounts of well-cooked pork, poultry, and fish are permitted.
Fruits and Vegetables	• Eat moderate amounts of raw and cooked fruits and vegetables. • Do not consume melons, horseradish, turnips, broccoli, cauliflower, and radishes.
High-Fiber Foods	• Eat moderate amounts of whole-wheat bread, bran cereal, and popcorn. Foods high in fiber provide roughage to promote bowel elimination and encourage bleeding from "silent" lesions that bleed only occasionally.
Vitamins	• Do not take vitamin C in excess of 250 mg from supplements or citrus fruits and juices. • An iron supplement will not affect the test results.
Medications	**For 7 days before and during the collection period:** Avoid nonsteroidal antiinflammatory drugs (NSAIDs) and more than one adult aspirin a day. • Examples of NSAIDs include ibuprofen (Advil, Motrin) and naproxen (Aleve). • Acetaminophen (Tylenol) can be taken as needed.
Special Guidelines	• Do not consume any of the food items listed previously if you know, from past experience, that they cause you severe gastrointestinal discomfort or serious diarrhea. • The provider may stipulate additional medication restrictions. • Do not initiate the test during a menstrual period or in the first 3 days after a menstrual period. • Do not conduct the test when blood is visible in the stool or urine, such as from bleeding from hemorrhoids or a urinary tract infection. These conditions result in false-positive test results. • Store the slides with the flaps in a closed position at room temperature, and protect them from heat, sunlight, and fluorescent light. • Store the slides away from volatile chemicals such as ammonia, bleach, and other household cleaners.

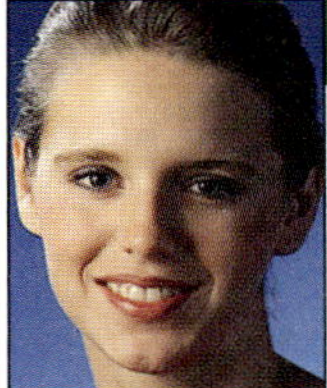

Putting It All Into Practice

My name is Megan, and I work in a large clinic that includes the specialties of family practice, gastroenterology, immunology, and dermatology. I am the clinical supervisor and oversee all of the clinical medical assistants as well as our "in-house" laboratory. I work closely with all physicians to meet the growing needs of the clinic.

Working with a gastroenterologist has been interesting and educational. When preparing patients for a sigmoidoscopy, you must help them feel relaxed. This is an embarrassing situation for patients, so you need to them feel as comfortable as possible and maintain their privacy and modesty. During the procedure, I talk to patients about the weather, their pets, and other interests to make them feel more relaxed and comfortable. This can help take their minds off of the procedure.

One day I was assisting with a sigmoidoscopy, and a few minutes into the procedure the look on the physician's face told me something was wrong. When the examination was finished, the physician and I left the room and went back to his office. He informed me that what he saw on his examination was rectal cancer in an advanced stage, and at this stage, not much could be done for the patient. The worst thing a physician has to do is give unpleasant news to a patient and see the look on the patient's face. Going into the room of a patient who has just received life-threatening information is something you don't forget. All you can do is be sympathetic and understanding and be a good listener. You have to be strong and not show your emotions even though your heart is breaking for the patient and their family. Always let patients know you are there for them.

Being with a patient who receives bad news about their health can make you think about your own life, and how it affects not only you, but also your family and friends. I often think of how I would feel about receiving such news. I try to put myself in the patient's place and to be sincere and understanding and willing to lend an ear. ■

Fecal Immunochemical Test

The fecal immunochemical test (FIT) is a CLIA-waived fecal occult blood test that uses antibodies to detect human hemoglobin which is a component of red blood cells. Examples of brand names for this test (Fig. 28.4) are QuickVue iFOB (Quidel Inc., San Diego, CA) and Hemoccult ICT (Beckman-Coulter/HemoCue, Brea, CA). The stool specimen for a FIT is collected by the patient at home and then returned to the medical office for processing and interpretation. The method used to collect and process the stool specimen and interpret the test results varies based on the brand of test used. Because of this, it is important for the medical assistant to become completely familiar with the FIT test brand used in their office by reading the product instructions that accompanies the testing kit. The medical assistant is responsible for providing the patient with instructions for collection of the specimen and the proper care and storage of the specimen until it is returned to the medical office.

What Would You Do? What Would You *Not* Do?

Case Study 1

Beatrice Bernard is 52 years old and has come to the office for a physical examination. The physician wants Mrs. Bernard to collect a stool specimen for a Hemoccult test. After being told the purpose of the test, how to prepare for it and collect the stool specimen, Mrs. Bernard expresses some concerns. She does not like the idea of collecting a stool specimen because it does not seem sanitary to her. She also thinks it will hard for her to follow the diet and medication modifications. She says she has red meat for dinner at least four times a week, and she does not understand why she has to eliminate it for 3 days. She says she takes a baby aspirin every day for "heart health" and would prefer not to stop taking it. Mrs. Bernard says that she has always taken very good care of herself, and she has never had any problems with her colon. She also says there is no history of colorectal cancer in her family. Mrs. Bernard is too embarrassed to talk about this topic with the physician. She says she may just throw the test away when she gets home. ■

Although the FIT is more expensive than the gFOBT, it is more sensitive to the presence of lower gastrointestinal (GI) bleeding than is the gFOBT test. It is also not affected by drugs or food and therefore does not require any medication or dietary modifications. In addition, FIT has fewer false-positive test results than the gFOBT. When a FIT test is positive, the patient must undergo further testing such as a colonoscopy.

Fecal Immunochemical-DNA Test

A FIT-DNA test is the newest type of stool-based colorectal screening test. It is approved by the FDA for use in the United States only under the brand name of Cologuard (Exact Sciences Corp., Madison, WI). The Cologuard test is much more expensive than other stool-based colorectal screening tests, however most insurance companies will

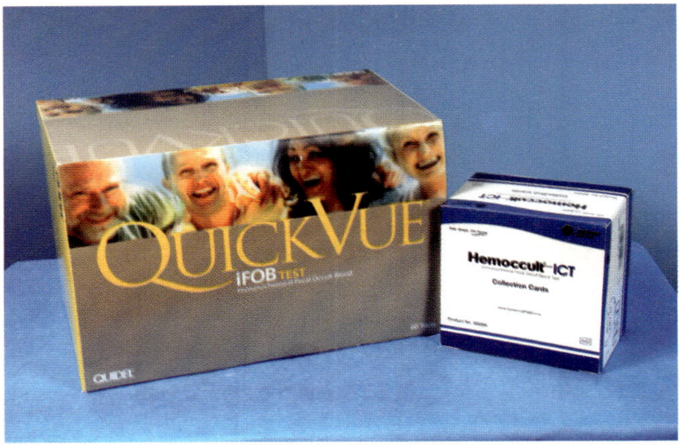

Fig. 28.4 FIT tests: QuickVue iFOB (left) and Hemoccult ICT (right).

cover the cost of it. Cologuard is a combination of two tests: a FIT test and a DNA test. As previously discussed, the FIT test detects the presence of human hemoglobin in the stool. The DNA test detects altered DNA in the stool shed from cells that may be associated with colorectal cancer or precancerous polyps. Studies show that Cologuard detects 92% of colorectal cancers and 42% of precancerous polyps.

The Cologuard test must be prescribed by a healthcare provider. A Cologuard collection kit is shipped directly to the patient from a Cologuard laboratory. The kit includes step-by-step instructions for the proper collection and processing of the stool specimen. No special patient preparation (e.g., dietary or medication modifications) are required for the test; however, certain guidelines must be followed, which are outlined in Fig. 28.5. The general procedure for the collection and processing of the stool specimen by the patient for the Cologuard test is presented in Box 28.3.

The laboratory tests the specimen and sends the test results to the patient's provider. A positive test result indicates the presence of altered DNA and/or human hemoglobin in the stool sample; however, it does not confirm the presence of colorectal cancer or precancerous polyps. It is therefore recommended that patients with positive test results undergo a colonoscopy. A negative result does not guarantee the

Cologuard Patient Guidelines

The following guidelines should be followed when using a Cologuard kit:

1. Check the expiration date on the collection kit to make sure it has not expired. If the kit has expired, request a new collection kit.
2. Store the collection kit at room temperature which is between 59°F and 86°F (15°C and 30°C) and keep it away from direct sunlight.
3. Do not collect a stool specimen when any of the following are present:
   - Diarrhea
   - Blood in the urine or stool
   - Bleeding cuts or wounds on the hands
   - Rectal bleeding
   - Menstrual period
4. Avoid getting urine or toilet paper into the collection container.
5. Do not let the liquid preservative touch your skin or eyes. If this occurs, flush the area with water.
6. To ensure the integrity of the stool specimen, it must be received by the laboratory within 72 h (3 days) of collection. This means that the specimen must be mailed back within 24 h following collection to ensure enough delivery time.

Fig. 28.5 Cologuard Patient Guidelines.

BOX 28.3 Cologuard Procedure

1. Collect an entire bowel movement in the large container (included in the kit).
2. Remove the grooved probe from the collection tube (included in the kit).
3. Obtain a small stool sample from the bowel movement in the large container by scraping the surface of the stool with the probe making sure to cover the grooves at the end of the probe.

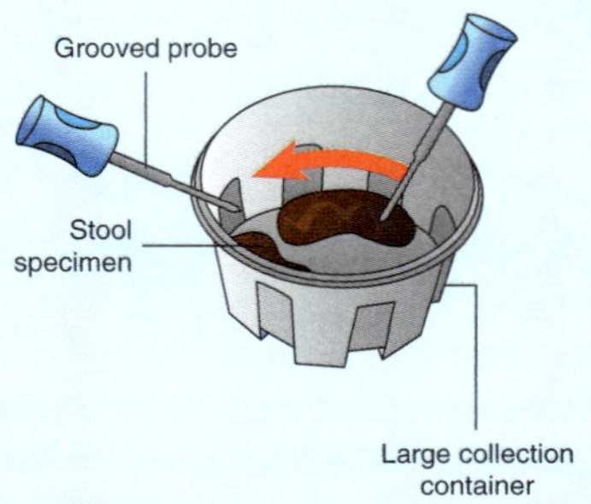

4. Place the probe containing the stool in the collection tube and seal it tightly with the screw cap.

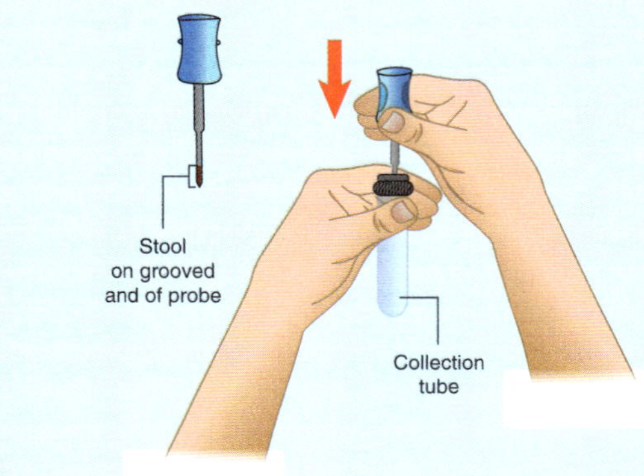

5. Immediately pour the preservative over the stool specimen in the large container and seal it tightly with the screw-on lid.

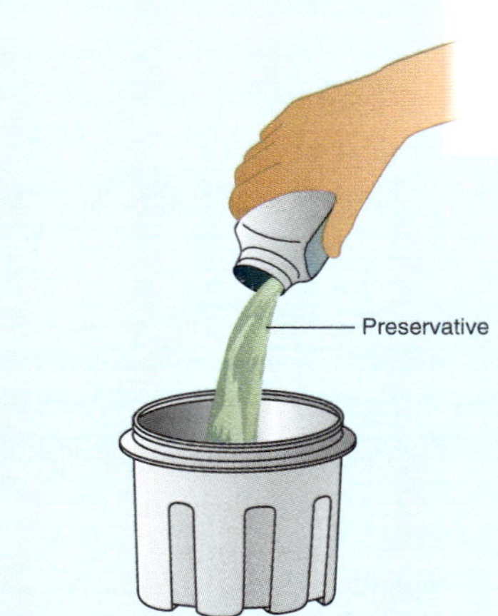

6. Label the collection container and tube.
7. Place the large container and the tube in the shipping box and mail it back to the Cologuard laboratory within 24 hours.

absence of cancer or precancerous polyps and the patient should continue following the colorectal cancer screening guidelines outlined in Box 28.2.

DIAGNOSTIC COLORECTAL PROCEDURES

Flexible Sigmoidoscopy

Sigmoidoscopy is the visual examination of the mucosa of the rectum and sigmoid colon (lower third of the colon) using a flexible fiberoptic **sigmoidoscope** (Fig. 28.6). The sigmoidoscope consists of a control head and a long flexible insertion tube attached to a light source (Fig. 28.7). The insertion tube is ½ inch (1.3 cm) in diameter and 24 inches (60 cm) long. The sigmoidoscope has a tiny video camera attached to the distal end of the flexible insertion tube. The camera magnifies and transmits images of the sigmoid colon to a video screen for viewing by the provider.

Before a patient undergoes a sigmoidoscopy, the provider explains the nature of the procedure and any risks to the patient and offers to answer questions. The medical assistant is responsible for obtaining the patient's signature on a written consent form, which grants the provider permission to perform the procedure.

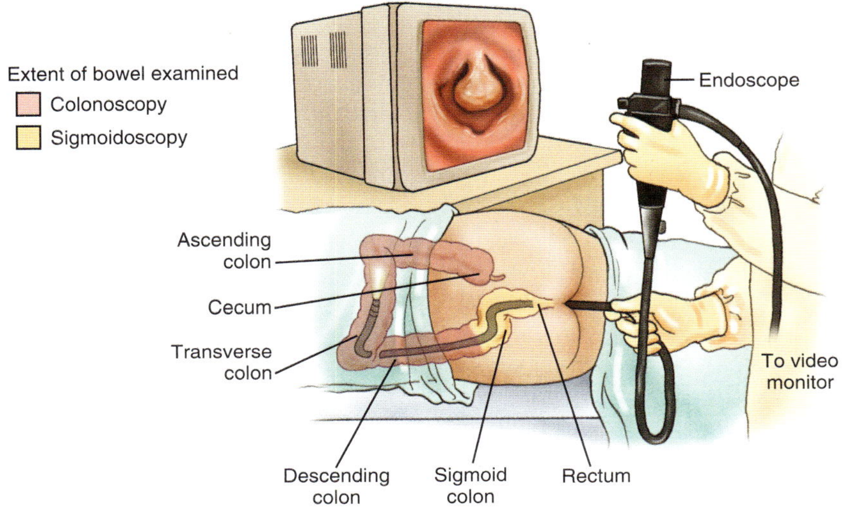

Fig. 28.6 Sigmoidoscopy and colonoscopy. (From Lafleur Brooks M: *Exploring medical language: a student-directed approach*, ed 9, St. Louis, 2014, Mosby.)

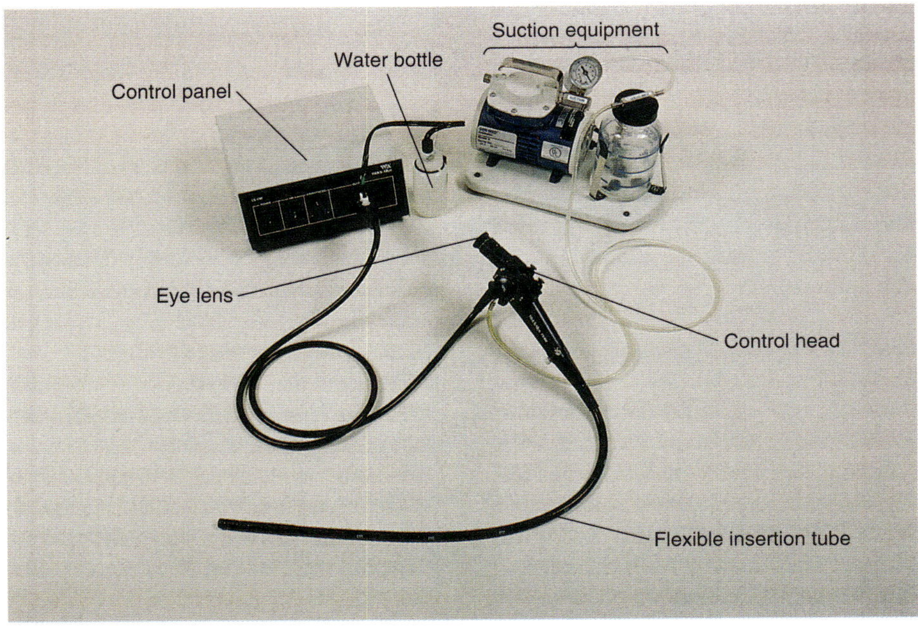

Fig. 28.7 Flexible fiberoptic sigmoidoscope.

Purpose

Sigmoidoscopy may be performed following a positive stool-based colorectal screening test to determine the source and cause of the bleeding. It is also performed to evaluate patient symptoms related to the lower colon such as lower abdominal pain, diarrhea, or constipation. Conditions of the lower colon that can be detected and assessed during a sigmoidoscopy include lesions (benign or malignant tumors), polyps, hemorrhoids, fissures, infection, and inflammation. It is especially valuable as a diagnostic procedure for detecting inflammatory bowel disease such as ulcerative colitis and Crohn's disease.

A sigmoidoscopy has certain limitations. Because a sigmoidoscopy reaches only the lower third of the colon, the provider may not be able to determine the cause of the patient's symptoms or fecal occult bleeding. In this situation, the provider may order a colonoscopy to be performed at a later date. If the sigmoidoscopy detects the presence of a precancerous polyp or colorectal cancer, a colonoscopy must be performed to detect additional polyps or cancer that may be present in the rest of the colon.

Patient Preparation for Flexible Sigmoidoscopy

The patient is required to prepare the colon before the sigmoidoscopy. The lower third of the colon must be flushed out completely, so that it is empty and free of fecal material; this is known as a *partial bowel prep* because only a portion of the colon needs to be prepared. Bowel preparation is one of the most important parts of sigmoidoscopy. Fecal material can interfere with good visualization of the wall of the sigmoid colon, making it difficult for the provider to detect abnormalities.

The medical assistant is responsible for providing the patient with instructions on preparing the colon. The medical assistant should encourage the patient to follow the instructions exactly. If the patient does not prepare properly, the sigmoidoscopy is usually canceled and must be rescheduled, which requires the patient to go through the bowel preparation procedure again. The patient preparation instructions may vary slightly from one facility to another. General patient preparation recommendations for a sigmoidoscopy are outlined in Table 28.2.

Procedure

When the sigmoidoscopy is performed, the patient is placed on their left side in a modified left lateral recumbent position. A digital rectal examination (DRE) of the anal canal and rectum is performed before a sigmoidoscopy. Using a well-lubricated, gloved index finger, the provider palpates the rectum for the presence of tenderness, hemorrhoids, polyps, and tumors. Any palpable abnormality is viewed directly when the endoscope is inserted. An **endoscope** is an instrument (e.g., sigmoidoscope and colonoscope) that consists of a tube and an optical system used for direct visual inspection of organs or cavities. The digital examination also helps relax the sphincter muscles of the anus and prepares the patient for the insertion of the endoscope.

The distal end of the sigmoidoscope is lubricated and inserted into the anus and rectum and then slowly advanced into the colon until it reaches the sigmoid colon. A small amount of air is usually blown, or **insufflated**, into the colon through tubing attached to the air control valve located on the head of the sigmoidoscope. The function of the air is to distend (expand) the lumen of the colon for better visualization. In addition, suction equipment can be used to remove secretions, such as mucus, blood, and liquid feces, which interfere with proper visualization of the intestinal mucosa. The provider then slowly withdraws the sigmoidoscope while carefully observing the mucosa of the sigmoid colon for abnormalities.

If an abnormal lesion is discovered during the examination, the provider will perform a biopsy using a long thin instrument passed through the lumen of the endoscope to obtain a specimen (Fig. 28.8). A **biopsy** is the surgical removal and examination of tissue from the body to determine

Table 28.2 Patient Preparation for Sigmoidoscopy

Beginning 7 days before the procedure	• Discontinue taking iron, aspirin, and aspirin products. Iron can alter the color of the wall of the colon. Aspirin may cause bleeding if a polyp is removed from the colon.
Beginning 5 days before the procedure	• Discontinue taking nonsteroidal antiinflammatory drugs such as ibuprofen and naproxen to minimize the risk of bleeding if a polyp is removed.
The day before the procedure	• Do not consume any solid food (until completion of the procedure). • Drink only clear liquids (water, apple juice, sport drinks [e.g., Gatorade], soft drinks, clear broth). • Do not drink alcohol. • Consume only gelatin (Jell-O) or Popsicles (except purple or red, which could be mistaken for blood in the colon). • Coffee or tea is permitted with no milk or cream.
The evening before the procedure	• Drink a laxative solution (such as magnesium citrate) as directed by your provider. • Continue drinking plenty of clear liquids to stay hydrated.
The day of the procedure	• Continue drinking clear liquids until 4 hours before the procedure. • Two hours before the examination: Use an OTC enema kit to cleanse out the lower colon following the package instructions. • One hour before the procedure: Perform another enema.

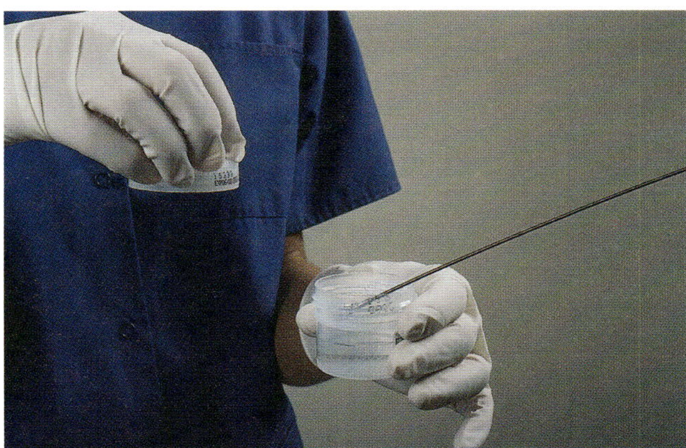

Fig. 28.8 Collection of a specimen during a sigmoidoscopy.

whether a lesion is benign or malignant. If a polyp is discovered, the provider may remove it (polypectomy) and/or perform a biopsy. Removal of a precancerous polyp prevents it from developing into colon cancer.

The medical assistant must prepare the patient for the procedure and assist the provider during the sigmoidoscopy. These responsibilities include the following:

1. Determine whether the patient has prepared properly for the sigmoidoscopy.
2. Ask the patient to void before the procedure.
3. Position and drape the patient in a modified left lateral recumbent position.
4. Reassure the patient and help the patient to relax.
5. Lubricate the provider's gloved index finger for the digital rectal examination.
6. Lubricate the distal end of the sigmoidoscope before the provider inserts it (Fig. 28.9).

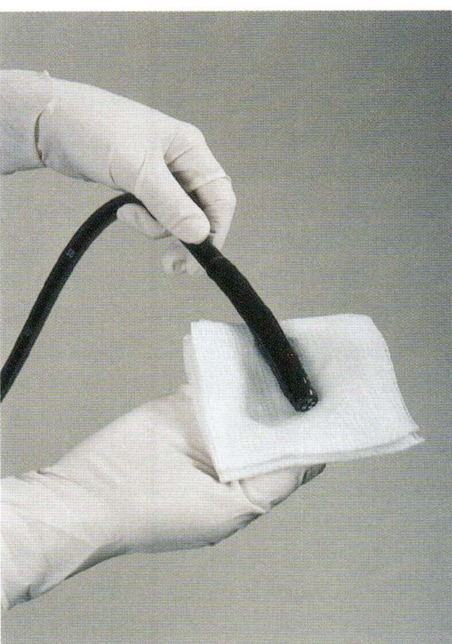

Fig. 28.9 The distal end of the sigmoidoscope must be lubricated before insertion.

7. Assist with suction equipment.
8. Hold the specimen container to accept a specimen (if required).
9. Assist the patient after the examination.
10. Prepare the specimen for transport to the laboratory.
11. Clean the examining room.
12. Sanitize and disinfect the sigmoidoscope.

Colonoscopy

A **colonoscopy** is the visual examination of the mucosa of the rectum and the entire length of the colon (sigmoid colon, descending colon, transverse colon, and ascending colon) using a flexible fiberoptic **colonoscope**. The colonoscope has a tiny video camera attached to the distal end of the flexible insertion tube. The camera magnifies and transmits images of the colon to a video screen for viewing by the provider (see Fig. 28.6).

Before a patient undergoes a colonoscopy, the provider explains the nature of the procedure and any risks to the patient and offers to answer questions. The medical assistant may be responsible for obtaining the patient's signature on a written consent form, which grants the provider permission to perform the procedure.

Purpose

Colonoscopy is often performed following a positive stool-based colorectal screening test to determine the source and cause of the bleeding. It is also performed to evaluate patient symptoms related to the colon, such as lower abdominal pain, rectal bleeding, chronic constipation, and chronic diarrhea. Colonoscopy is considered the "gold standard" for assessing abnormalities of the colon. Conditions that can be detected and assessed during a colonoscopy include the following:

- Lesions of the colon or rectum (e.g., benign or malignant growths)
- Colorectal polyps
- Hemorrhoids
- Fissures
- Infection and inflammation

Colonoscopy is particularly valuable for the detection of symptomatic and asymptomatic colorectal cancer. Early detection of colorectal cancer leads to early diagnosis and treatment, which increases the chance of survival for patients with this disease.

Patient Preparation for Colonoscopy

A colonoscopy is usually performed in a hospital on an outpatient basis or in a large medical clinic. The rectum and the entire colon must be flushed out completely so that it is empty and free of fecal material; this is known as a *full bowel prep*. This is one of the most important parts of the colonoscopy. Fecal material can interfere with good visualization of the wall of the colon, making it difficult for the provider to detect abnormalities.

The medical assistant may be responsible for providing the patient with instructions on preparing the colon, which includes a strong laxative and a liquid diet. The patient should be encouraged to follow the instructions exactly. If the patient does not prepare properly, the colonoscopy is usually canceled and must be rescheduled, which requires the patient to go through the bowel preparation procedure again. The patient preparation instructions may vary from one facility to another. General patient preparation recommendations for a colonoscopy are outlined in Table 28.3, along with patient instructions following the procedure.

Procedure

A sedative is administered intravenously before the colonoscopy. The sedative causes the patient to become relaxed, sleepy, and less aware of what is taking place. Some patients do not remember the procedure at all afterward.

The procedure itself is similar to a sigmoidoscopy. The patient is placed on their left side in a modified left lateral recumbent position. The provider performs a digital rectal examination before inserting the colonoscope. The colonoscope is advanced all the way through the entire colon (approximately 4 to 5 feet) until it reaches the cecum. The provider then slowly withdraws the colonoscope while carefully observing the mucosa of the colon for abnormalities.

If an abnormal lesion is discovered during the examination, the provider will perform a biopsy using a long thin instrument passed through the lumen of the endoscope to obtain a specimen. If a polyp is discovered, the provider may remove it and/or perform a biopsy. Removal of a precancerous polyp prevents it from developing into colon cancer in the future.

MALE REPRODUCTIVE TESTS AND PROCEDURES

Important tests and procedures related to male reproductive health include prostate cancer screening tests and testicular self-examination, which assist in the early detection of prostate and testicular cancers.

Table 28.3 Patient Preparation for Colonoscopy

Beginning 7 days before the procedure	• Discontinue taking iron, aspirin, and aspirin products.
Beginning 5 days before the procedure	• Discontinue taking nonsteroidal antiinflammatory drugs such as ibuprofen and naproxen to minimize the risk of bleeding if a polyp is removed.
Beginning 3 days before the procedure	• Eat only low fiber foods which can be cleared easily from the colon. • High fiber foods that should be avoided include: seeds, nuts, popcorn, raw vegetables, and fruits with skin, dried beans, and whole grains. These foods are not easily removed from the colon and may interfere with proper visualization of the colon.
Beginning 1 day before the procedure	• Do not consume any solid food (until completion of the procedure). • Drink only clear liquids (water, apple juice, sport drinks [e.g., Gatorade], soft drinks, clear broth). • Do not drink alcohol. • Consume only gelatin (Jell-O) or Popsicles (except purple or red, which could be mistaken for blood in the colon). • Coffee or tea is permitted with no milk or cream.
Begin bowel preparation 1 day before the procedure	• Drink a laxative solution as directed by your provider; examples include GoLytely, NuLytely, MoviPrep, Visicol, and Suprep. • It is best to drink the solution quickly rather than slowly sipping it. • You may experience nausea and a bloated feeling. This is temporary and will disappear once you start having bowel movements. • Liquid stools will usually start within a few hours after you begin drinking the solution. You will have the urge to have a bowel movement about 10 to 15 times. • If you have prepared properly, your stool will be a clear or yellow liquid. • Continue drinking plenty of clear liquids to stay hydrated.
The day of the procedure	• You may be asked to drink another laxative solution the morning of the procedure. • Continue drinking clear liquids until 4 hours before the procedure.
Following the procedure	• Arrange to have someone drive you home following the procedure. You will be sedated during the procedure and cannot drive yourself. • It takes about an hour to recover from the sedative. • You may experience some bloating, abdominal cramping, and flatulence for several hours following the procedure. • If you had a polyp removed or a biopsy taken, it is normal to experience traces of blood in the stool for 1 to 2 days. • Contact your provider if you experience significant rectal bleeding, abdominal pain, fever, faintness, dizziness, shortness of breath, or heart palpitations.

PROSTATE CANCER

The prostate is a small gland that surrounds the urethra and is located just below the bladder and in front of the rectum (Fig. 28.10). It is approximately the size and shape of a large walnut and its function is to secrete fluid that transports sperm.

According to the American Cancer Society, prostate cancer is the most common type of cancer in American males and is the second most common cause of cancer deaths in men, with lung cancer being the most common. Every year, nearly 300,000 men are diagnosed with prostate cancer, and more than 35,000 men die each year from this disease. The incidence of prostate cancer increases with age; approximately 60% of cases are diagnosed in men over the age of 65. Prostate cancer is found more often in African American men and men with a family history of prostate cancer.

In the early stages, prostate cancer often causes no symptoms. Symptoms that occur when the cancer is more developed include the following:

- Frequent urination, especially at night
- Difficulty in starting or holding back urination
- Weak or interrupted urinary flow
- Painful or burning urination
- Difficulty in having an erection
- Blood in the urine or semen
- Pain or stiffness in the lower back, hips, pelvis, or thighs

PROSTATE CANCER SCREENING

The purpose of prostate cancer screening is to detect prostate cancer at an early stage when it is more treatable. The primary screening tests for prostate cancer are the digital rectal examination (DRE) and the prostate-specific antigen (PSA) test.

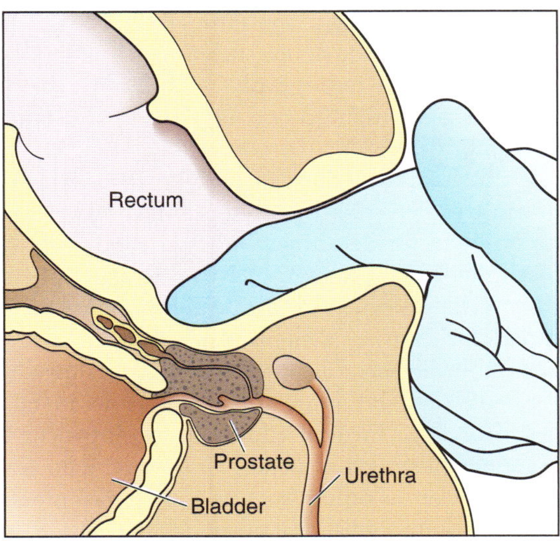

Fig. 28.10 Digital rectal examination.

Digital Rectal Examination

The digital rectal examination (DRE) is a quick and simple procedure that causes only momentary discomfort. During the examination, the provider inserts a lubricated gloved finger into the patient's rectum. Because the prostate gland is located in front of the rectum, the provider is able to palpate the surface of the prostate through the rectal wall (see Fig. 28.10). The provider palpates the prostate to determine whether it is enlarged or has an abnormal consistency. Normally, the prostate gland should feel soft, whereas malignant tissue is firm and hard. The sensitivity of the DRE is limited, however, because the provider can palpate only the posterior and lateral aspects of the prostate gland.

Prostate-Specific Antigen Test

The prostate-specific antigen (PSA) test is a screening test primarily used to screen for the presence of prostate cancer in healthy men without symptoms. PSA is a protein produced by cells in the prostate gland (both normal cells and cancer cells) and is mostly found in semen, but a small amount is also found in blood.

The PSA test measures the amount of PSA in the blood measured in units called nanograms per milliliter (ng/mL). When there is a problem with the prostate gland, such as prostate cancer, more PSA is released into the blood. The possibility of having prostate cancer goes up as the PSA level goes up, however there is no set cut-off value that indicates whether or not a man might have prostate cancer. Most men without prostate cancer have a PSA level below 4 ng/mL. A PSA level of 4 to 10 ng/mL is considered borderline high and the chance of having prostate cancer is 25%. Men with a PSA level above 10 ng/mL have a 50% chance of having prostate cancer. The higher the PSA level, the more likely that cancer is present. Other conditions that can cause an elevated PSA level include benign prostatic hyperplasia (BPH) and prostatitis.

The PSA level may normally increase after vigorous physical exercise (e.g., jogging and biking) therefore the patient should be instructed to engage only in normal activity for 2 days before having blood drawn for a PSA test. The patient also should be instructed not have sexual intercourse for 2 days before the test because ejaculation can cause a significant increase in the PSA level.

If the DRE is abnormal and/or the PSA test is elevated, further testing may be performed to determine if prostate cancer is present. To make this assessment, one or more of the following tests may be performed: transrectal ultrasound (TRUS), biopsy of the prostate gland, magnetic resonance imaging (MRI), bone scan, and computed tomography (CT) scan.

Prostate Screening Guidelines

The DRE and PSA screening tests for prostate cancer have certain limitations. Abnormal results from these tests do not necessarily indicate that cancer is present. Furthermore, normal results from these tests do not mean that cancer is *not* present. An abnormal DRE and/or an elevated PSA test may lead to further testing and the detection of cancer in an individual, which can pose a dilemma. Most types of prostate cancer grow very slowly and do not result in death. In fact, many men with this disease live long and healthy lives without ever knowing they have prostate cancer. Fast-growing prostate cancer is less common, but more serious and is often life-threatening. The follow-up tests used to diagnose the presence of prostate cancer can be invasive, stressful, and expensive and lead to a diagnosis of a type of cancer that would never have caused a man any harm. Treatment of a man with prostate cancer can have major side effects such as erectile dysfunction, urinary incontinence, and problems with bowel function.

The American Cancer Society (ACS) believes that available evidence does not currently support routine testing for prostate cancer. The ACS recommends that health care providers discuss the potential benefit and harm of prostate cancer screening and treatment with men older than 50 years of age. Following this discussion, the PSA test and the DRE should be offered annually to men 50 years and older who are at average risk for prostate cancer and have at least a 10-year life expectancy. Those men who indicate a preference for testing should be tested. The ACS recommendation provides men with knowledge of the advantages and disadvantages of early detection and treatment of prostate cancer, which then allows them to share in the decision of whether or not to be tested.

What Would You Do? What Would You *Not* Do?

Case Study 2

Peter Bota, a 62-year-old retired male, came to the medical office one week ago for a physical examination. The physician performed a DRE but did not palpate anything abnormal. At that visit, Mr. Bota's blood was drawn for a PSA test, and the results came back as borderline high (8 ng/mL). Mr. Bota was informed of the test results, and has returned to the office and is waiting to talk with the provider about the results and possible follow-up testing. Mr. Bota is extremely worried that he has cancer and wants to know the symptoms of prostate cancer. He also wants to know whether he did anything to cause prostate cancer. He says he does not smoke, drinks very little, and walks his dog twice a day for exercise. ■

TESTICULAR SELF-EXAMINATION

The purpose of testicular self-examination (TSE) is early detection of testicular cancer. Although testicular cancer can develop at any age, it is most common in males 15 to 34 years old. If detected early, it has a very high cure rate. Most cases of testicular cancer are detected by men themselves, either by accident or when performing a TSE. Certain risk factors increase a man's chance of getting testicular cancer, including the following:

- History of cryptorchidism (undescended testicles)
- Family history of testicular cancer
- Cancer of the other testicle
- White race (testicular cancer is five times more common in White men than in African American men)

TSE should be performed monthly, starting at 15 years of age. A good idea is for the patient to choose an easy-to-remember date each month, such as the first day of the month. The best time to perform the examination is after taking a warm bath or shower. Heat allows the scrotal skin to relax and become soft, making it easier to palpate the underlying testicular tissues.

The most common sign of testicular cancer is a small, hard, painless lump (about the size of a pea) located on the front or side of the testicle. Any abnormality of the testicles should be reported to the provider immediately. It does not mean that the patient has cancer, however; the provider must make that determination. Fig. 28.11 outlines the procedure for a TSE.

INTRODUCTION TO RADIOLOGY

Radiology is the branch of medicine that uses radiation and other imaging techniques to diagnose and treat disease; examples include x-rays, ultrasound, computed tomography (CT), magnetic resonance imaging (MRI), and nuclear medicine imaging. A **radiologist** is a physician who specializes in the diagnosis and treatment of disease using radiation and other imaging techniques.

Wilhelm Konrad Röentgen, a German physicist, discovered x-rays on November 8, 1895, while working with a cathode ray tube. He noticed that these rays could pass through solid materials, such as paper, wood, and human skin. Because he did not know what they were, he named them *x-rays.* The rays have since been renamed *roentgen rays* after their discoverer; however, they are better known as "x-rays."

X-rays are high-energy electromagnetic waves that are invisible and have a short wavelength that enables them to penetrate solid materials in varying degrees. **Radiography** is the taking of permanent images of internal body organs and structures by passing x-rays through the body to act on a radiosensitive receptor device such as a digital detector or radiographic film. A **radiograph** is the term used for the permanent image produced by x-rays acting on a radiosensitive receptor device.

X-rays are used to visualize internal organs and structures which assist in detecting the presence of disease. They are especially useful for detecting abnormal conditions associated with the skeletal system, such as fractures. X-rays also are used in the treatment of disease conditions, such as for the radiation therapy of malignant neoplasms.

An orthopedic medical office may have its own radiographic equipment, but more often radiographs are taken in a hospital or large medical clinic on an outpatient basis. Some radiographs, such as a chest x-ray, require no advance preparation, whereas others, such as a lower gastrointestinal (GI) study, require a great deal of special preparation. Medical assistants are usually responsible for patient instruction in

TESTICULAR SELF-EXAMINATION

1
Take a warm bath or shower.

2
Stand in front of a mirror. Look for any swelling of the skin of the scrotum.

3
Place the index and middle fingers of both hands on the underside of one testicle and the thumbs on top of the testicle.

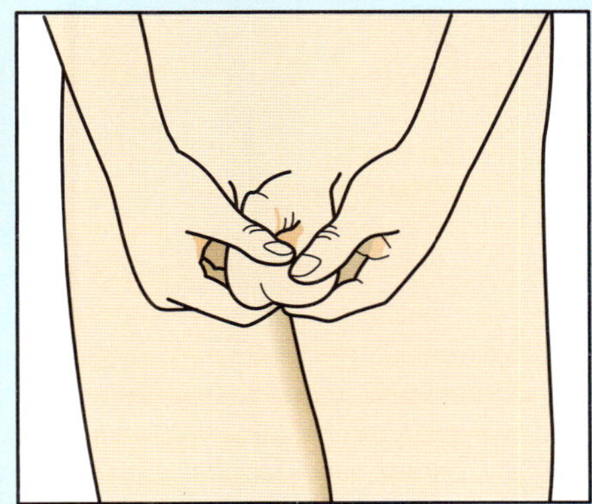

4
Apply a small amount of pressure and gently roll the testicle between the thumb and fingers of both hands, feeling for lumps, swelling, or any change in the size, shape, or consistency of the testicle. A normal testicle should feel smooth, egg-shaped and rather firm. It is also normal for one testicle to be larger or hang lower than the other testicle.

5
Find the epididymis so that you do not confuse it with a lump. The epididymis is a soft tubular cord, located behind the testicle, that functions in storing and carrying sperm.
(Note: Tenderness in the area of the epididymis is considered normal.)

6
Repeat the examination outlined above on the other testicle.

7
Report any of the following abnormalities to the provider: any unusual lump, a feeling of heaviness in the scrotum, a dull ache in the lower abdomen or groin, enlargement of one of the testicles, tenderness or pain in a testicle, or any change in the way the testicle feels.

Fig. 28.11 Testicular self-examination.

the type of preparation necessary for a particular radiographic examination and for ensuring that the patient understands the importance of the preparation. If the patient does not prepare properly, the radiograph may be of poor quality, and the procedure may need to be rescheduled. This section introduces the study of radiographs, with a focus on the patient preparation necessary for common radiographs.

FILM-BASED RADIOGRAPHY

X-rays can be taken using the conventional film-based method or digitally using a computer and digital detectors. With film-based radiography, radiographic film is loaded into a device known as an *x-ray cassette*. The cassette is placed behind the part being examined, and a shadow or image of the internal body structure photographed is produced on the film. After the x-ray has been taken, the film must be processed in order to develop the image on the film. A radiologic technician takes the cassette into a darkroom and develops the image using an x-ray processor. The image on the film is then reviewed by a radiologist on a high-intensity light box.

DIGITAL RADIOGRAPHY

Advances in digital imaging technology have made inroads into the field of radiology. The result is the transformation of film-based radiography into a system of computer-displayed and stored digital images. To assist in understanding digital radiography, this transformation can be compared with the replacement of film cameras with digital cameras.

With digital radiography, permanent images of internal body organs and structures are obtained by passing x-rays through the body to act on a digital detector. A *digital detector* converts x-rays into electronic signals which are sent to a computer to produce a digital image. The radiologist then reviews the digital image on a high-resolution computer monitor. Digital radiography allows images to be taken and viewed immediately and also allows them to be sent electronically to a network of computers.

Important benefits of digital radiography include a shorter radiation exposure time, higher-quality images and the ability to manipulate the images (e.g., enhance and enlarge the image) and the ability to transfer the images electronically. The medical assistant is responsible for using the medical office computer to access, display (Fig. 28.12), and permanently save digital radiographs.

CONTRAST MEDIA

Radiography relies on differences in density between various body structures to produce shadows of varying intensity on the radiograph. There is a difference in density between bone and soft tissue and organs; bone is denser than soft

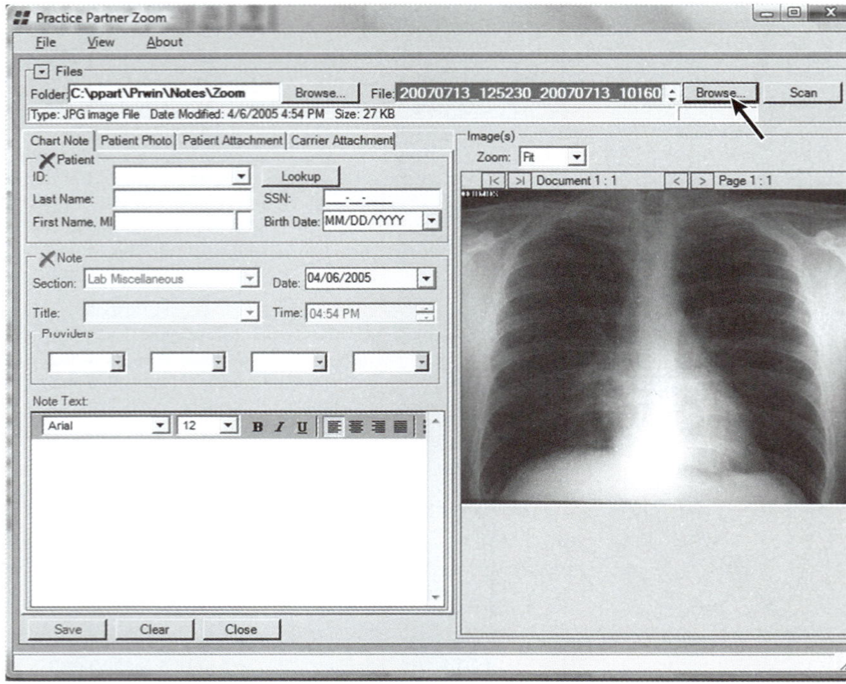

Fig. 28.12 Digital image of a chest x-ray. (Screenshot used by permission of MCKESSON Corporation. All rights reserved. © MCKESSON Corporation, 2011. From Buck CJ: *Electronic health record booster kit for the medical office*, St. Louis, 2009, Saunders.)

tissue and organs. Bone absorbs more x-rays and does not allow them to reach the radiosensitive receptor device. This leaves that part of the radiograph unexposed and causes white images to appear on the radiograph. If the x-rays penetrate structures that have a low density (soft tissue and organs), a black area appears on the radiograph. For example, the lungs are filled with air giving them a low density; therefore, x-rays are able to penetrate them easily. As a result, the lungs appear black on the radiograph while the ribs absorb the x-rays and appear as white images on the radiograph (Fig. 28.13). A structure such as the lungs that permits the passage of x-rays is termed **radiolucent**. Other examples of radiolucent structures include the stomach, intestines, and urinary bladder. A structure such as bone that obstructs the passage of x-rays and causes a (white) image to be cast on the radiograph is termed **radiopaque**.

In many cases, the natural densities of two adjacent structures are similar. In this instance, a **contrast medium** must be used to make a particular structure, such as an organ, visible on the radiograph. Contrast media are typically radiopaque chemical compounds that cause a body structure to absorb more radiation resulting in a contrast in density between the body structure and the surrounding area. The structure becomes visible and appears white on the radiograph. Substances used as contrast media must be able to be ingested or injected into the body without causing harm to the patient. Contrast media are administered to the patient through various routes. Some are administered orally; others are injected into a vein or are delivered through an intravenous (IV) line or an enema.

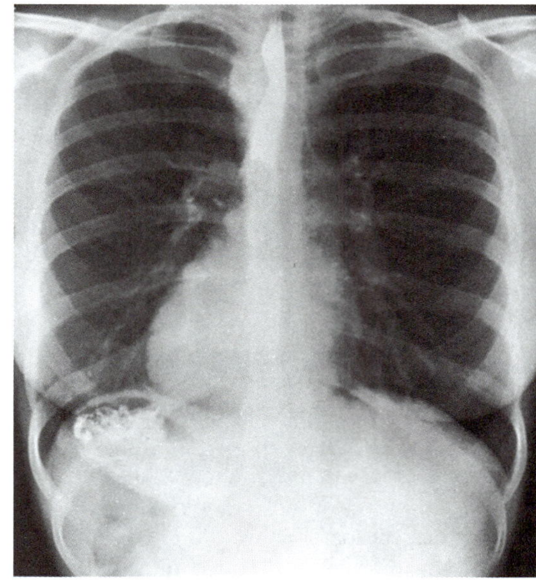

Fig. 28.13 Chest radiograph. The lungs are radiolucent and the rib bones are radiopaque. (From Meschan I: *Synopsis of radiologic anatomy with computed tomography*, Philadelphia, 1980, Saunders.)

Barium sulfate and inorganic iodine compounds are commonly used radiopaque contrast media. Barium sulfate is a chalky compound that is water insoluble and does not allow penetration by x-rays. It is frequently used for examination of the GI tract because barium is not absorbed into the body through the GI tract and does not alter its normal function. Iodine salts are radiopaque and are combined with other compounds for radiographic examination of structures such as the urinary tract and blood vessels. Iodine sometimes produces an allergic reaction, and before administration, patients should be asked whether they have an allergy to iodine. Patients with known allergies may be given an iodine sensitivity test as a precautionary measure.

What Would You Do? What Would You *Not* Do?

Case Study 3

Jose Ramirez is a 10-year-old boy with episodes of unexplained abdominal pain and vomiting during the past 6 months. The medical office has scheduled an upper GI radiographic study at the local hospital. Mrs. Ramirez wants to know how best to prepare Jose for the procedure, so that he will not be so afraid of the x-ray room and equipment. She asks what she can do so that he will drink the barium solution. She says he will not drink milk, and if the barium tastes anything like milk, it will be hard to get him to drink the barium. Mrs. Ramirez wants to know whether Jose can hold his favorite toy (a metal truck) during the procedure to comfort him. She also wants to know whether the barium solution has any side effects. ■

FLUOROSCOPY

A **fluoroscope** is an instrument used to view internal organs and structures of the body directly in real time on a display screen. The procedure for viewing internal organs and structures directly in real time is known as **fluoroscopy**. A radiopaque contrast medium is often used with fluoroscopy to outline various parts of the body. The patient is positioned between the radiographic tube and a fluorescent screen composed of cesium iodide crystals. When the x-rays pass through the body and strike the crystals, visible light is emitted so that the radiologist can view the action of body structures (e.g., stomach and intestines) on the screen of a monitor. During fluoroscopy, the radiologist can take radiographs that permit the study of the structures in detail and serve as a permanent record.

POSITIONING THE PATIENT

The position of the patient is determined by the purpose of the examination and the area examined. The patient is typically placed in several different positions so that different views can be obtained to provide a complete three-dimensional picture of the part examined. Articles such as jewelry and hairpins must be removed so the image on the radiograph is not obscured. To prevent blurring of the image on the radiograph, patients must maintain the position in which they are placed and not move during the radiographic examination. Blurring prevents good visualization of the part and may warrant retaking of the radiograph.

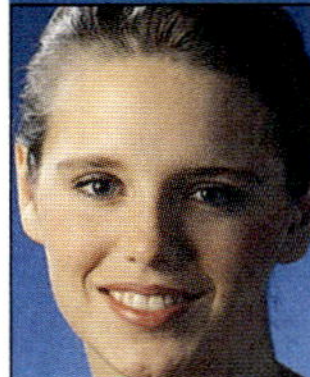

Memories *from* Practicum

Megan: My first practicum was terrifying at first, but at the same time I was overwhelmed with excitement. I remember worrying how I was going to remember all my clinical and administrative skills. I was worried that I would hurt someone or forget to do something important.

One day a patient came into our office upset and crying. The examination rooms were full, so I took her into our staff lounge. I sat her down, fixed her a cup of coffee, and asked her if I could help. She told me that her son had drowned 2 years ago on that day, her mother had cancer, and her husband had passed away 8 months previously. I listened to everything she had to say, and I comforted her until the physician was ready to see her. She walked over to me, hugged me, and said my smile and people skills were the best treatment for her depression that she had ever had. Her telling me that made me feel good about my career choice, and it made me realize how fulfilling it was. It did not take me long to realize that all the hands-on skills that I had learned in the classroom were not forgotten. I also realized that a smile and listening to people are just as important as my skills. ■

RADIOGRAPHIC EXAMINATIONS

The medical assistant should understand the purpose of commonly performed radiographic examinations and should be able to instruct a patient on the proper preparation for each (Fig. 28.14). Frequently performed radiographic examinations and the advance preparation necessary for each are described in this section.

Mammography

Mammography is a radiographic examination of the breasts used to detect many forms of breast disease, such as benign

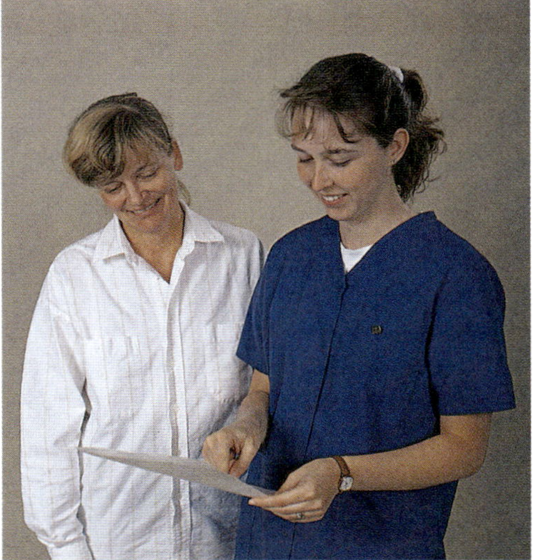

Fig. 28.14 A patient is instructed in the proper preparation for a radiographic examination.

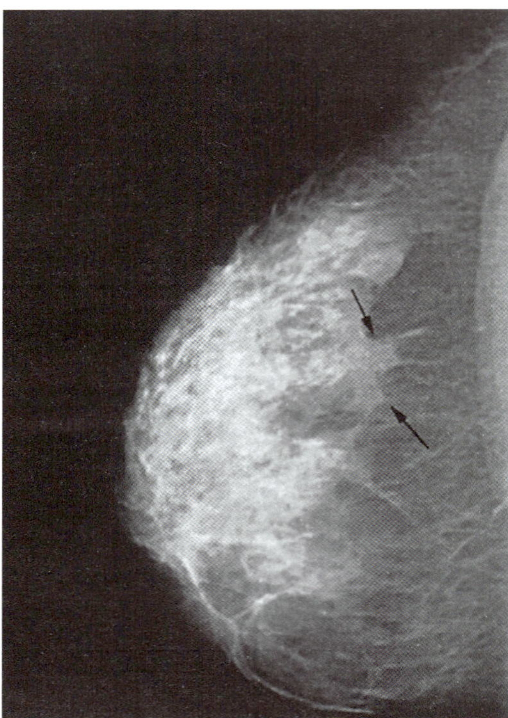

Fig. 28.15 Mammogram. Arrows indicate suspicious areas of increased density that needs further evaluation. (From Prue L: *Atlas of mammographic positioning*, Philadelphia, 1994, Saunders.)

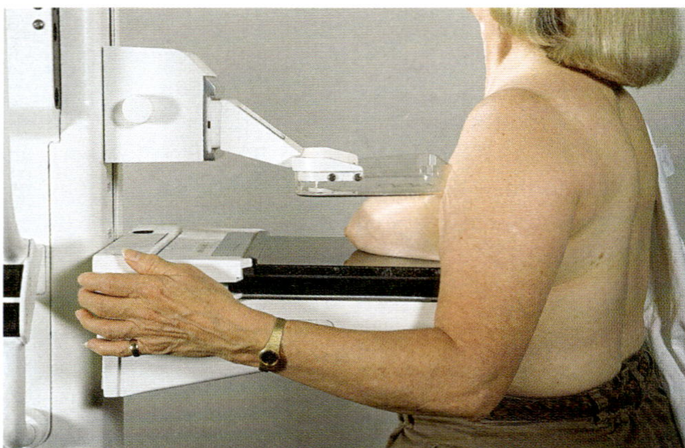

Fig. 28.16 Patient positioning for mammography. (From Ballinger PW, Frank ED, eds: *Merrill's atlas of radiographic positions and radiologic procedures*, vol 2, ed 12, St. Louis, 2012, Mosby.)

breast masses, breast calcifications, fibrocystic breast disease, and particularly breast cancer. It also is used to monitor the effects of surgery and radiation therapy on breast tumors.

Mammography uses low doses of x-rays that pass through the breast and act on a radiosensitive receptor device to create a permanent image of each breast (Fig. 28.15). On the mammogram, an abnormal area appears noticeably different from normal breast tissue. Mammography can be used to detect a breast tumor when the growth is less than 1 cm in diameter (about the size of a pea) and before it is clinically palpable. This permits a malignant tumor to be removed at an early stage which usually results in conservative treatment with less disfigurement and a high survival rate. With early diagnosis and treatment, breast cancer survival rates for women can reach as high as 94%.

Very little preparation is required for mammography. The patient should not wear any lotions, creams, powders, or deodorants on the breasts or under the arms because they may contain small amounts of metal that can be seen on the radiograph and may interfere with interpretation. For the mammogram, the patient must remove clothing from the waist up and put on an upper body wrap. The patient should be told that it is easier to wear pants or a skirt so that she only needs to remove clothing above the waist.

A radiology technician generally performs the mammogram which takes approximately 20 minutes. The patient's breast is positioned on the mammography platform, and pressure is applied for 10 to 15 seconds with a plastic compression paddle that flattens the breast (Fig. 28.16). Compression of the breast is necessary to obtain a clear radiograph and to lower the radiation dosage as much as possible. During the procedure, the patient must hold her breath and remain still momentarily because any type of motion, even breathing, can blur the image and make a repeat radiograph necessary. Two radiographs are taken of the breast—one from above and one from the side. The procedure is then repeated on the other breast.

A radiologist then checks the mammogram and occasionally orders additional images to obtain a more complete view of the breast tissue. The current mammogram is compared with the patient's previous mammograms. After the procedure, the radiologist studies the mammogram for any signs of breast cancer or other breast problems and sends a written report of the findings to the patient's provider.

Three-Dimensional Mammography

Three-dimensional (3D) mammography, also known as *digital breast tomosynthesis* (DBT), is a new technology designed to improve detection of breast cancer in its earliest stages. A 3D mammogram is similar to a conventional two-dimensional (2D) mammogram; the amount of compression of the breasts is the same and it takes the same amount of time. The procedure uses multiple low-dose x-ray images from different angles to create a mammogram that allows the radiologist to view the breast tissue in thin slices. This makes it easier for the radiologist to detect cancer since each breast can be observed one layer at a time. In fact, 3D mammography can detect up to 40% more invasive breast cancers than 2D mammography. In addition, there are fewer false-positive results as compared with 2D mammography which requires the patient to return for additional images and evaluation.

During 3D mammography, an x-ray arm moves in a small arc over the breast acquiring multiple images which are reconstructed by a computer into a 3D image. As previously discussed, conventional 2D mammography only obtains two images of each breast (one from above and one from the side). The radiation exposure for a 3D mammography is the same as that for 2D mammography.

PATIENT COACHING Mammography

Answer questions patients may have about mammography.

What is the purpose of mammography?

Mammography is a safe, low-dose radiographic examination used to screen for abnormal changes in the breasts. Mammography allows the provider to detect small lumps in the breast long before they can be felt. Although most breast lumps are not cancerous, breast cancer can be removed at an early stage when detected early, which usually results in treatment that is less deforming and has a much higher survival rate.

Who should have a mammogram?

The American Cancer Society recommendations for mammography for women of average breast cancer risk are as follows:

- Women between 40 and 44 should have the choice to start annual breast cancer screening with mammograms if they wish to do so.
- Women 45 to 54 should get mammograms every year.
- Women 55 and older should switch to a mammogram every other year, or they can choose to continue yearly mammograms.
- Screening should continue as long as a woman is in good health and is expected to live 10 more years or longer.
- All women should be familiar with how their breasts normally look and feel and report any changes to a health care provider right away.

Women at high risk for breast cancer such as a family or personal history of breast cancer or a known *BRCA1* or *BRCA2* gene mutation should follow the advice of their provider regarding mammography; age guidelines do not apply because these women undergo examination on a more frequent basis.

What occurs during the mammography procedure?

During mammography, the breast is positioned on a special platform table and is flattened with a compression paddle. Breast compression may be uncomfortable for some women. The discomfort can be reduced with avoidance of caffeine several days before the procedure and by scheduling the mammography the week after a menstrual period, when the breasts are less tender. Each breast is radiographed from above and from the side. A radiologist studies the resulting mammogram to detect any abnormalities. The results are reported to the provider.

- Encourage the patient to have a mammogram according to the schedule recommended by the American Cancer Society.
- Provide the patient with educational materials on mammography.

Bone Density Scan

A bone density scan is an enhanced form of x-ray technology that measures the bone mineral density of the human skeleton to detect bone loss. As individuals age, their bones may become less dense, causing them to become brittle and weak which may lead to a bone fracture. Factors that cause bones to lose density include osteoporosis, thyroid and parathyroid conditions, and certain medications (e.g., corticosteroids). Postmenopausal women are at particular risk for osteoporosis. *Osteoporosis* is a condition in which a gradual loss of calcium causes the bones to become thinner, more fragile, and more likely to break. It is recommended that women 65 years of age and older and men 70 years of age and older undergo a bone density scan.

Dual energy x-ray absorptiometry (DXA) scanning is the most widely used bone density testing method. DXA (pronounced "dexa") uses x-rays to determine the amount of bone in the human skeleton. During a DXA scan, bone density measurements are taken at different parts of the body. The bone density measurements indicate if the patient has lost bone density. They also assist in detecting the presence of osteoporosis and can be used to predict the patient's risk of bone fracture. Patients on medication therapy for osteoporosis (e.g., Fosamax, Boniva, and Actonel) undergo a DXA screen every 1 to 2 years to determine if the medication is working.

The patient should be instructed to abstain from taking a calcium supplement or medication containing calcium (e.g., Rolaids and Tums) for 24 hours prior to the scan. If the calcium is not completely dissolved, it may be interpreted by the DXA equipment as extra bone which results in inaccurate bone density measurements. For the examination, the patient is positioned on an x-ray table and instructed to remain as still as possible during the test. The radiologic technician then scans one or more areas of bone with the DXA equipment. Areas that are typically scanned include the lower spine and head of the femur because the bone in these areas is more likely to fracture from osteoporosis.

Test results are in the form of two scores (a T-score and a Z-score), which are sent to the patient's provider. These scores assist the provider in diagnosing and treating the patient. The *T- score* is derived by comparing the patient's measurements with those of healthy young normal adults with peak bone density of the same gender as the patient. A T-score of −1.0 or above indicates normal bone density. A T-score between −1.0 and −2.5 indicates low bone density or *osteopenia*. A T-score of −2.5 or below indicates the presence of osteoporosis. The T-score is used to estimate the patient's risk of developing a fracture. The *Z-score* is derived by comparing the patient's measurements with an established database of healthy individuals of the same age and gender as the patient. An unusually high or low Z-score may indicate the need for further testing.

Gastrointestinal Series

Upper Gastrointestinal Radiography

An upper GI study is an examination of the upper digestive tract using fluoroscopy and radiography. The examination is helpful in the diagnosis of disorders of the esophagus, stomach, and duodenum. These disorders include gastroesophageal reflux disease (GERD), hiatal hernias, ulcers, inflammation or blockages of the upper GI tract, and benign and malignant tumors. The procedure may be ordered when the patient complains of difficulty in swallowing, vomiting, abdominal pain, gastric reflux (burping up food), severe indigestion, and blood in the stool.

Proper patient preparation is important for this procedure. The patient's stomach must be empty at the beginning of the study, so food does not obscure the radiographic image. To prepare for the examination, the patient must eat a light evening meal and then not eat or drink anything, including water and medications, after midnight on the day before the examination. Food and fluid in the GI tract have a degree of density and could cause confusing shadows on the radiograph.

The upper GI tract varies little in density from the structures around it, and to make it show up on a radiograph, a contrast medium must be used. The patient drinks a suspension of barium mixed with water and flavoring, which resembles a milkshake and has a chalky taste. Before drinking the barium, the patient may be asked to drink a carbonated solution which puts air into the upper GI tract, causing it to expand. The combination of air and barium, known as a *double contrast study*, allows the radiologist to view the esophagus, stomach, and duodenum in greater detail.

As the patient swallows the barium mixture, the radiologist observes its passage down the esophagus and into the stomach and duodenum with fluoroscopy. The barium coats the lining of the upper GI tract, making it visible on the screen of the fluoroscope. Radiographs are taken periodically during the examination to allow a detailed study of the upper GI tract and to provide a permanent record. The patient's position is changed at various times so that the upper GI tract can be visualized from different profiles. After the procedure, the radiologist prepares a report of the findings, which is sent to the patient's provider.

The medical assistant should explain to the patient that the barium suspension will appear in the stool for 1 to 3 days following the procedure and will cause the stool to have a whitish color. The barium mixture may cause constipation and the need for a laxative. To help prevent constipation, the patient should be instructed to increase fiber and fluid intake for several days following the procedure.

Lower Gastrointestinal Radiography

A lower GI study is an examination of the lower GI tract using fluoroscopy and radiography. A lower GI examination involves filling the colon with a barium sulfate mixture with a catheter (tube) inserted into the rectum through the anus. Because of this, the procedure is sometimes called a *barium enema*. The examination is used to observe and obtain permanent pictures of the colon, sigmoid colon, and rectum (Fig. 28.17). A lower GI assists in diagnosis of disorders of the lower GI tract, such as polyps, cancerous tumors, diverticulosis, and the extent of inflammatory bowel disease (e.g., ulcerative colitis, Crohn disease). The procedures may be ordered when the patient complains of chronic diarrhea, blood in the stool, constipation, irritable bowel syndrome, unexplained weight lost, and change in bowel habits.

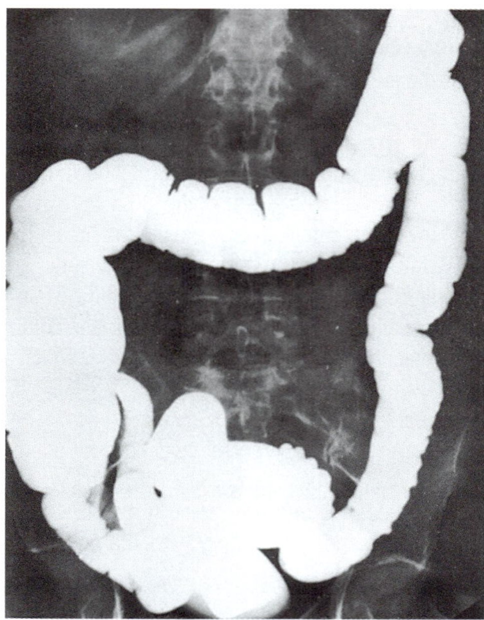

Fig. 28.17 Lower GI radiograph. Colon is distended with barium. (From Meschan I: *Synopsis of radiologic anatomy with computed tomography*, Philadelphia, 1980, Saunders.)

The colon must be thoroughly cleansed in advance to remove gas and fecal material. Gas has a certain degree of density and shows up as confusing shadows on the radiograph. If fecal material appears on the radiograph, the image of the colon is obscured. Instructions for cleansing the colon may vary from one medical office to another, but in general, the patient is instructed to consume only clear liquids the day before the examination, such as water, plain coffee and tea, clear broth, and strained fruit juice. A laxative should be taken on the day before the scheduled examination; an enema also may be necessary. An **enema** is an injection of fluid into the rectum to aid in the elimination of feces from the colon. The patient should not drink anything (except water) after midnight on the day before the examination. On the morning of the examination, the patient may be required to perform a warm water cleansing enema until the returns are clear.

The patient should report at the scheduled time and is instructed to relax on one side while the rectal catheter is inserted. As the barium enters the colon, the radiologist watches it on the fluoroscopic screen and periodically takes radiographs. The patient has a sensation of fullness and the urge to defecate as the barium enters the colon. The patient is moved into various positions to allow the barium to fill the colon completely and to obtain better visualization of the colon. The tip of the enema tube is specially designed to hold the barium in the lower GI tract. Once the examination is completed, most of the barium is emptied through the rectal catheter. The patient is then allowed to evacuate the remainder of the barium.

A *double-contrast study* of the lower GI tract is similar to a lower GI study; however (in addition to the barium), it also employs the use of air that is inserted into the colon through the same catheter as the barium. The air distends the wall of the colon and allows the radiologist to view the colon in greater detail, making it easier to detect polyps and small cancerous tumors. After the procedure, the radiologist prepares a report of the findings, which is sent to the patient's provider.

The medical assistant should explain to the patient that the barium suspension will appear in the stool for 1 to 2 days following the procedure and will cause the stool to have a whitish color. The barium mixture may cause constipation and the need for a laxative. To help prevent constipation, the patient should be instructed to increase fiber and fluid intake for several days following the procedure.

Intravenous Pyelography

An intravenous pyelogram (IVP) is a radiograph of the kidneys, ureters, and urinary bladder (Fig. 28.18). An IVP is used to assist in the diagnosis of kidney stones, kidney cysts, an enlarged prostate gland, blockage or narrowing of the urinary tract, and tumors of the urinary tract.

The patient should consume only clear liquids on the day before the examination. The evening before the examination, the patient must take a laxative to remove gas and fecal material from the intestines to permit proper visualization of the urinary tract. Starting at midnight the day before the examination, the patient should not eat, drink, smoke, or chew gum. Unless the patient is allergic to iodine, a contrast medium containing iodine is used and is administered intravenously to the patient. As the iodine enters the bloodstream, the patient may feel warm and flushed, have a mild itching sensation, and a metallic or salty taste in the mouth. This reaction is normal and lasts for only a few minutes. If the patient is allergic to iodine, a different type of contrast medium must be used. After the procedure, the radiologist prepares a report of the findings, which is sent to the patient's provider.

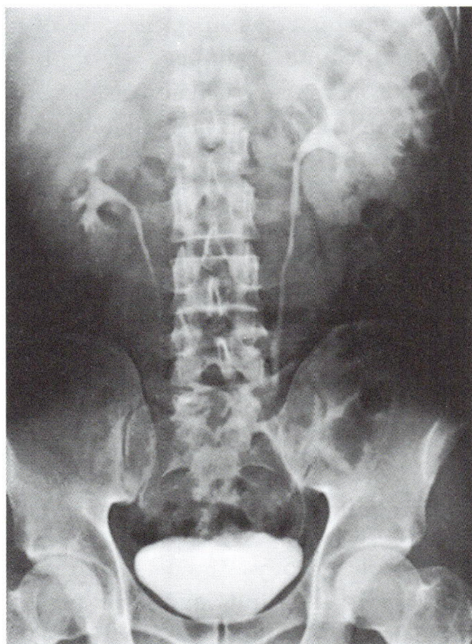

Fig. 28.18 Intravenous pyelogram. (From Meschan I: *Synopsis of radiologic anatomy with computed tomography*, Philadelphia, 1980, Saunders.)

Other Types of Radiographs

Other types of radiographs that the medical assistant may encounter include the following:

Angiocardiogram. Radiograph of the valves and blood vessels of the heart using a contrast medium and fluoroscopy to determine if there is a restriction in the blood flow going to the heart.

Bronchogram. Radiograph of the lungs using a contrast medium to assist in the diagnosis of lung cancer, tuberculosis, and pneumonia.

Cerebral angiogram. Radiograph of the major arteries of the brain using a contrast medium to detect blockages or other abnormalities in the blood vessels of the head and neck.

Chest radiograph. Radiograph of the chest to assist in diagnosing conditions affecting the chest, its contents, and nearby structures to detect conditions such as pneumonia, heart failure, and emphysema. (No contrast medium is required.)

Cholangiogram. Radiograph of the bile ducts after administration of a contrast medium to detect bile duct blockages.

Coronary angiogram. Radiograph of the coronary arteries using a contrast medium to detect a restriction in blood flow to the heart.

Cystogram. Radiograph of the urinary bladder using a contrast medium to assist in diagnosing problems of the urinary bladder.

Hysterosalpingogram. Radiograph of the uterus and fallopian tubes using a contrast medium to evaluate the shape of the uterus and determine if the fallopian tubes are patent (open and unobstructed).

Myelogram. Radiograph of the spinal canal using a contrast medium to detect conditions affecting the spinal cord and nerves within the spinal canal.

Retrograde pyelogram. Radiograph of the kidneys and urinary tract using a contrast medium injected directly into the ureter through a ureteral catheter. The dye flows to the kidneys through the ureters to detect abnormalities of the urinary tract.

INTRODUCTION TO DIAGNOSTIC IMAGING

Diagnostic imaging procedures allow for the visualization of internal body structures in great detail. The most common diagnostic imaging procedures are ultrasonography, computed tomography, magnetic resonance imaging, and nuclear medicine imaging. Diagnostic imaging procedures are usually performed in a hospital or a large clinic on an outpatient basis. The medical assistant may need to relay information to a patient scheduled for such a procedure, including what to expect during the procedure and any patient preparation that may be required. The medical assistant should have a basic knowledge of diagnostic imaging procedures and the preparation necessary for each.

ULTRASONOGRAPHY

Ultrasonography, also called ultrasound (US), is the oldest of the diagnostic imaging procedures. Ultrasound uses high-frequency sound waves for the study of soft tissue structures. Advances have been made in ultrasound technology. These include three-dimensional (3-D) ultrasound, in which sound waves are formatted into 3-D images (Fig. 28.19). Four-dimensional (4-D) ultrasound is another new technology that consists of 3-D ultrasound, but in motion.

Ultrasound is frequently used in the diagnosis of conditions of the abdominal and pelvic organs, particularly the breasts, gallbladder, liver, spleen, pancreas, kidneys, uterus, ovaries, and abdominal aorta. Some examples of conditions that can be detected using ultrasound include breast cysts, gallstones, kidney stones, uterine polyps, and abdominal aorta aneurysms. An ultrasound examination of the heart is known as an **echocardiogram** and is used to determine the size, shape, and position of the heart and the movement of the heart valves and chambers. Ultrasonography is also used for guiding a needle or other device during a minimally invasive procedure, such as amniocentesis, a needle biopsy, cortisone injection into a joint, and needle aspiration of fluid in a joint.

Ultrasonography offers many advantages as a diagnostic imaging procedure. It shows movement, allows continuous viewing of a structure, uses sound waves rather than radiation, and is less expensive than other imaging procedures. Ultrasound does have some minor limitations. Because sound waves are unable to penetrate bone and air or gas-filled cavities such as the lungs, stomach, and intestines, ultrasound cannot be used in the evaluation of these structures. In addition, ultrasound may be difficult to use with obese patients because adipose tissue can interfere with sound wave transmission.

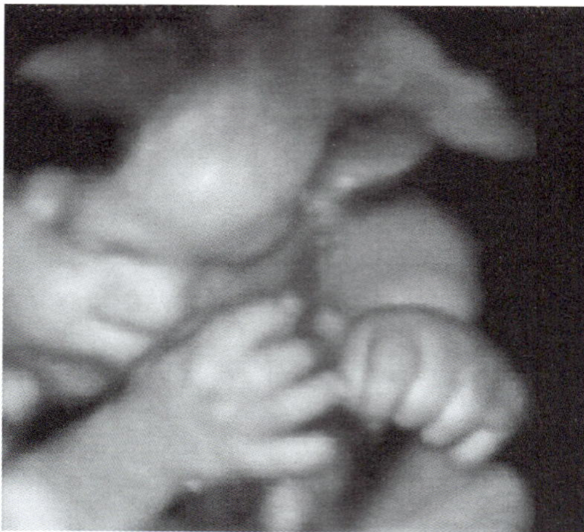

Fig. 28.19 3-D ultrasound of a third-trimester fetus. (From Leonard PC: *Building a medical vocabulary: with Spanish translations*, ed 8, St. Louis, 2011, Saunders.)

Before performing an ultrasound examination, a warm ultrasound gel must first be spread on the area to be examined. The purpose of the gel is to increase conductivity of the sound waves between the skin and the transducer. During the ultrasound examination, the ultrasound technician places a probe containing a transducer firmly on the patient's skin and moves it over the body areas to be examined. The transducer generates sound waves that are directed into the patient's tissues and reflected back to the transducer, similar to an echo. The transducer converts the waves into electrical signals. A computer then converts these signals into digital images. The size, shape, and consistency of the images are displayed on a video display screen; this image is known as a **sonogram** (Fig. 28.20). The patient is often permitted to view the sonogram on the screen of the monitor as the procedure is performed. The digital images can be permanently stored on a computerized storage medium. A radiologist reviews and interprets the images and prepares a report of the findings that is sent to the patient's provider.

Although ultrasound is commonly used for a wide variety of noninvasive imaging procedures, individuals are most familiar with its use in obstetrics. Obstetric ultrasound is most frequently used to confirm a pregnancy, determine the gestational age of a fetus and to confirm the due date; to detect congenital abnormalities, ectopic pregnancy, and multiple pregnancy; and to determine the fetus's position and size late in pregnancy. If the fetus is old enough and is positioned correctly, it is usually possible to determine its gender. Because the ultrasound machine is a compact unit, most obstetricians perform this procedure in their medical offices. Ultrasound is also used by gynecologists to evaluate and treat infertility problems.

Doppler ultrasound is a special application of ultrasound. It measures the direction and speed of blood as it flows through blood vessels, such as major arteries and veins in the abdomen, arms, legs, and neck. Doppler ultrasound images can assist the provider in diagnosing blood flow blockages, narrowing of blood vessels due to atherosclerosis, and congenital malformations.

Patient Guidelines

The medical assistant should tell the patient what to expect during an ultrasound examination and instruct the patient in the preparation required for the procedure, as follows:

1. Ultrasound is a safe and painless procedure that takes approximately 15 to 45 minutes to complete, depending on the body part examined.
2. The patient may need to prepare for the procedure, depending on the part of the body examined. An ultrasound of the gallbladder, liver, spleen, and pancreas necessitates that the patient fast for 8 to 12 hours. For an obstetric ultrasound, the patient needs to have a full bladder. The patient should be instructed to consume approximately 32 ounces (1 liter) of fluid about 1 hour before the procedure.

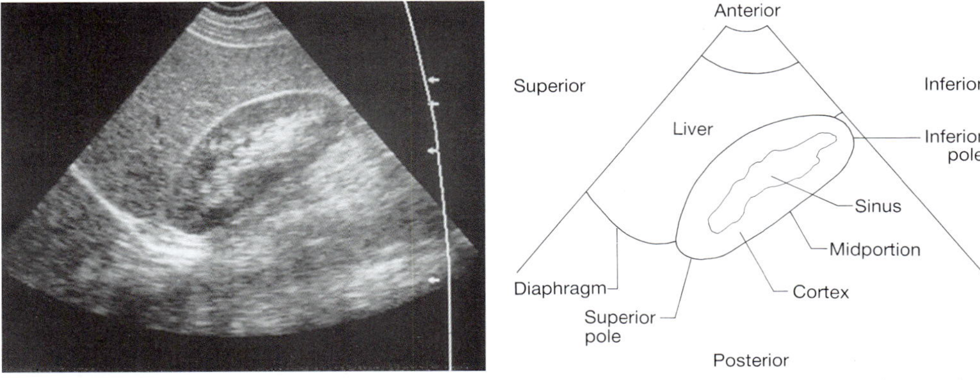

Fig. 28.20 Sonogram of the right kidney. (From Tempkin BB: *Ultrasound scanning: principles and protocols*, ed 3, St. Louis, 2009, Saunders.)

3. The patient must remain still when requested during the procedure because movement can interfere with accurate results. In addition, the patient may be asked to change positions so that the organs can be seen at different angles.

COMPUTED TOMOGRAPHY

Computed tomography (also known as a *CT scan*) is a diagnostic imaging procedure that uses x-ray technology to produce detailed images of the inside of the body. The CT machine, known as the *CT scanner*, takes a series of images of a body part, permitting the imaging of structures that cannot be visualized with conventional radiographic procedures. The series of images is processed with a computer to produce 3-D cross-sectional images of a body part similar to the slices of bread in a loaf (Fig. 28.21). Newer CT scanners take continuous pictures of a body part in a spiral fashion; a spiral CT scanner is faster and produces better quality images of areas inside the body as compared to a conventional scanner.

CT scans are used primarily to detect and evaluate tumors and other abnormalities and to monitor the effects of surgery, radiation therapy, or chemotherapy on tumors. CT is particularly well suited to quickly examine individuals who may have internal injuries and bleeding from automobile accidents or other types of trauma. CT scans are used to detect tumors or lesions within the abdomen. A CT scan of the heart may be ordered when various types of heart disease or abnormalities are suspected. CT is also used to image the head in order to locate injuries, tumors, or clots that may lead to a stroke, brain hemorrhage, and other conditions. It can image the lungs in order to reveal the presence of tumors, pulmonary embolisms (blood clots), excess fluid, and other conditions such as emphysema or pneumonia. A CT scan is often used to image complex bone fractures, severely eroded joints, or bone tumors since it usually produces more detail than would be possible with a conventional x-ray.

Some CT examinations require the use of a contrast medium. The contrast medium may be given by mouth, injected into a vein, or given by enema. The contrast medium allows for a sharper image of internal structures of the body.

A CT scan is conducted by a diagnostic imaging technician. The patient is positioned on a narrow motorized table (Fig. 28.22). From an adjoining room, the technician mechanically moves the table into the large doughnut-shaped CT scanner. The x-ray tube within the CT scanner rotates around the patient taking multiple images as the table is slowly moved through the scanner. The images are processed with a computer to produce 3-D cross-sectional digital images of a body part which are stored digitally on electronic media for evaluation by a radiologist. The radiologist reviews and interprets the images and prepares a report of the findings, which is sent to the patient's provider (Fig. 28.23).

Patient Guidelines

The medical assistant should tell the patient what to expect during the CT scan and should instruct the patient on the preparation required for the procedure, as follows:

1. If a contrast medium is to be used, the patient may need to fast for several hours before the procedure. It is important to ask the patient whether they are allergic to radiographic contrast media to avoid an adverse reaction.
2. Before the procedure, the patient must remove all radiopaque objects, such as dentures, eyeglasses, and jewelry, because they interfere with a clear image of the body part examined.
3. The technician will be in an adjacent room where the scanner controls are located. The patient is in constant sight of the technician and speakers inside the scanner enable communication with the technician.
4. The patient should lie motionless and breathe normally during the procedure. When a radiograph is being taken, the patient is usually asked to hold their breath to prevent blurring of the images. The patient hears slight buzzing, clicking and whirring sounds from the scanner as pictures are taken.
5. The entire procedure, which includes set-up, the scan itself, checking the images, and removing the IV (if needed), takes 15 to 45 minutes depending on what part of the body is being scanned.

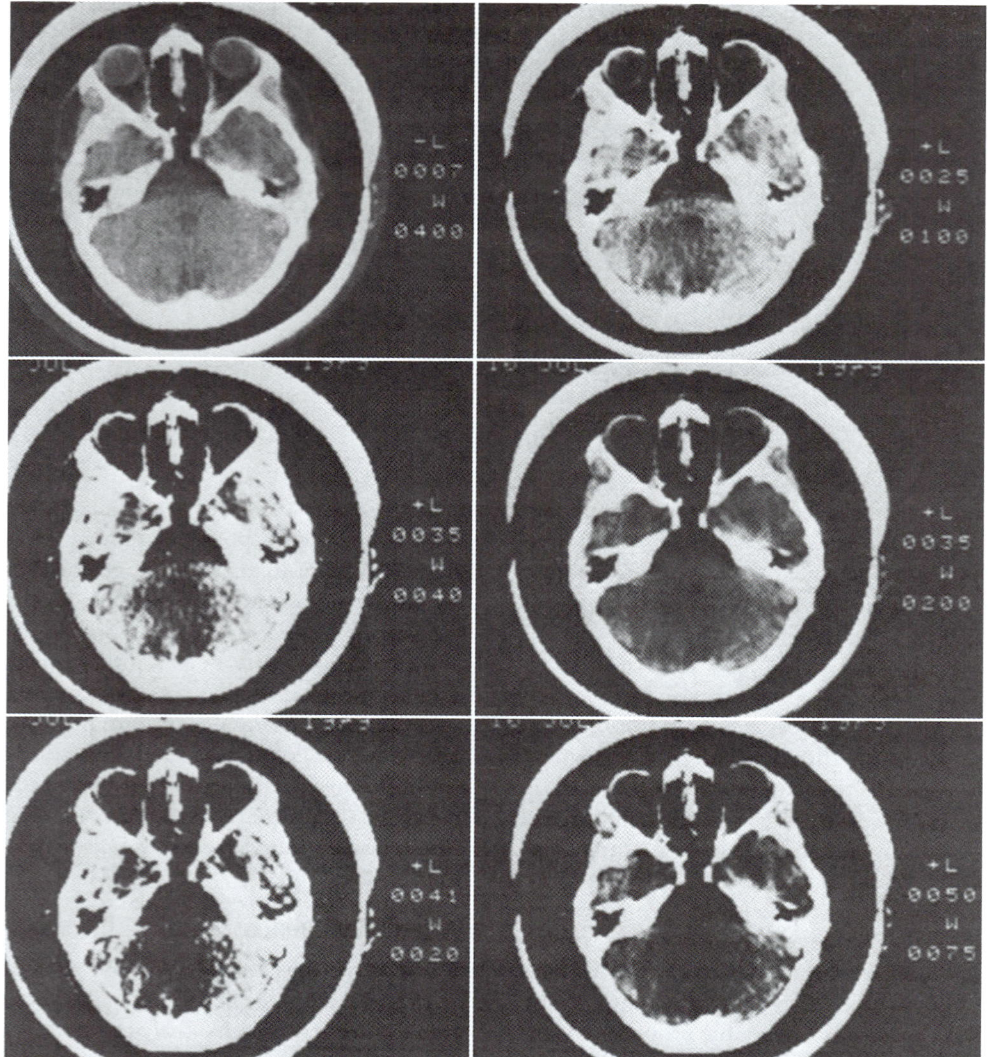

Fig. 28.21 CT cross-sectional images of the head. (From Snopek A: *Fundamentals of special radiographic procedures*, ed 5, Philadelphia, 2007, Saunders.)

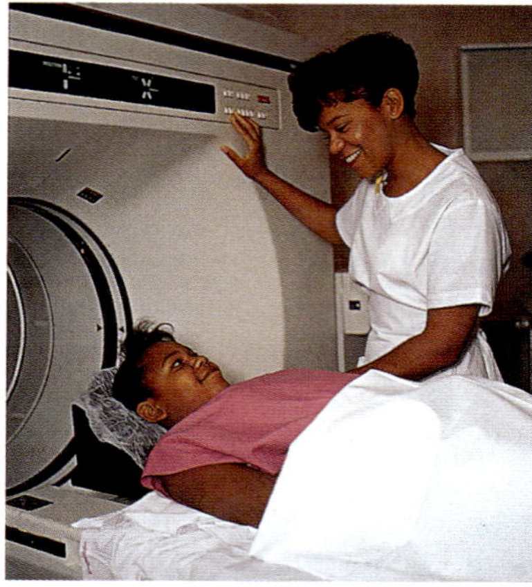

Fig. 28.22 Positioning a patient for a CT scan. (From Kowalczyk N, Donnett K: *Integrated patient care for the imaging professional*, St. Louis, 1996, Mosby.)

MAGNETIC RESONANCE IMAGING

Magnetic resonance imaging (MRI) is a diagnostic imaging procedure that uses a strong magnetic field, radio waves, and a computer to produce detailed 3D cross-sectional images of internal body structures. Because MRI does not involve radiation, the U.S. Food and Drug Administration has classified the MRI machine as a low-risk device.

MRI is used for imaging tissues of high fat and water content that cannot be seen with other radiologic techniques. MRI assists in the diagnosis of intracranial and spinal lesions and cardiovascular and soft tissue abnormalities, such as herniated discs, torn ligaments, and joint diseases. MRI allows the examiner to see through bone and view fluid-filled soft tissue in great detail. The brain, spinal cord and nerves, along with muscles, ligaments, and tendons, are seen much more clearly with MRI than with regular x-rays and CT.

CT Diagnostic Imaging Report

Patient: Regina Bach
Gender: F
DOB: 10/22/xx

Ordering Physician: Brian Mendelssohn
Exam Date: 7/28/xx
Radiologist Reviewer: Daniel Baldwin

Type of Exam: CT scan of the abdomen and pelvis with intravenous and oral contrast media.

Clinical History: This is a 66-year-old female with a history of breast cancer and new onset abdominal pain.

Comparison: Comparison is made to a CT scan of the abdomen and pelvis performed 10/1/xx.

Technique: 5 mm axial images from the lung bases through the pubic symphysis following the administration of intravenous and oral contrast media.

Findings:

- Lung bases: No pulmonary nodules or evidence of pneumonia.
- Cardiac: Base of heart is within normal limits. No pericardial effusion.
- Liver: Normal size and contour. There is a new 2 cm hypoattenuating focus in segment 8. Gallbladder is surgically absent.
- Spleen: No splenomegaly.
- Pancreas: No mass or ductal dilation.
- Kidneys and adrenals: No masses, stones or hydronephrosis. No adrenal nodules.
- Bladder: Within normal limits.
- Uterus and adnexa: The uterus and bilateral ovaries are within normal limits for age.
- Lymph nodes: No lymphadenopathy.
- Bones: No aggressive osseous lesions. Degenerative changes are present in the spine.

Impression:

1. No findings on the current CT to account for the patient's clinical complaint of abdominal pain.
2. There is a new 2 cm lesion in the liver which is indeterminate and cannot be definitely diagnosed by the study.

Recommendation:
Given the patient's personal history of breast cancer, an MRI of the liver is recommended to better characterize the indeterminate liver lesion to exclude the possibility of cancer metastases.

Fig. 28.23 CT diagnostic imaging report.

An MRI is conducted by a diagnostic imaging technician. The patient lies on a table that is moved to the inside of the cylindrical MRI machine while a diagnostic imaging technician in an adjoining room monitors the procedure (Fig. 28.24). Because of the closed space, some patients may have difficulty with claustrophobia. The provider may order a sedative for these patients. Open MRI machines are less confining than traditional MRI machines and are helpful for examining obese patients and patients with claustrophobia; however, they are a newer technology and may not be available at some facilities.

The 3-D cross-sectional images are electronically stored on a computer for evaluation by a radiologist. The radiologist reviews and interprets the images and prepares a report of the findings, which is sent to the patient's provider.

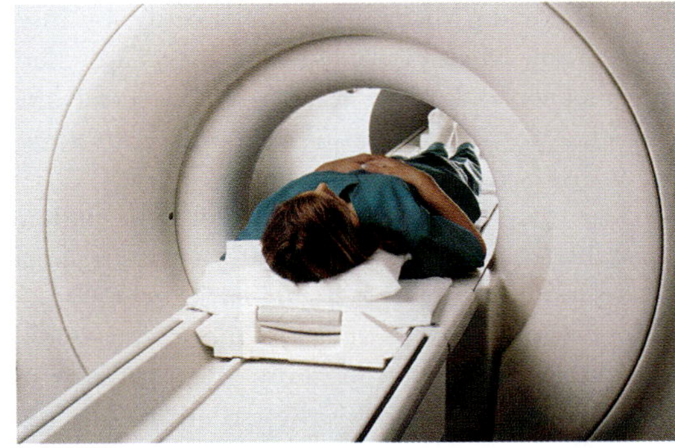

Fig. 28.24 Magnetic resonance imaging (MRI). The patient lies on a table inside the cylindrical MRI machine while an MRI technician in an adjoining room monitors the procedure. (From Ballinger PW, Frank ED, eds: *Merrill's atlas of radiographic positions and radiologic procedures*, vol 3, ed 12, St. Louis, 2012, Mosby.)

Patient Guidelines

The medical assistant should tell the patient what to expect during the MRI and instruct the patient in the preparation required for the procedure, as follows:

1. MRI is a safe and painless procedure which typically takes between 20 and 60 minutes depending on the size of the area being scanned and the number of images being taken.
2. A contrast medium may be used for the procedure. It improves the resolution of the image by increasing the brightness in various parts of the body.
3. No special preparation is necessary for the MRI examination. The patient may eat or drink before the examination and take any prescribed medication.

What Would You Do? What Would You *Not* Do?

Case Study 4

Michael Wendl is an 18-year-old high school varsity football player. For the past 3 months, he has had pain and swelling in his left shoulder. The provider schedules an MRI to assist in determining the cause of the problem. Michael has had several radiographs over the past 2 years and is worried about radiation exposure to his body. He wants to know how much radiation will be involved with the procedure. Michael has problems with claustrophobia and wants to know whether he can play a game on his cellphone during the procedure to distract him. He also wants to know whether he is allowed to eat anything before the procedure. ■

4. Because the procedure involves a strong magnet, the patient should remove any metal or magnetic-sensitive items, such as coins, cell phones, eyeglasses, hearing aids, dentures, watches, rings, and keys. Avoid wearing cosmetics, as certain types of cosmetic preparations contain small amounts of metal. Individuals with a pacemaker or cochlear implant may not be able to undergo an MRI.
5. The patient must remain completely still for 15- to 20-minute intervals during the procedure. The patient hears a metallic clacking sound like a muffled drumbeat during the procedure. Earplugs or headphones are available for use if the patient desires.

NUCLEAR MEDICINE IMAGING

Nuclear medicine imaging is an advanced diagnostic procedure in which a tiny amount of radioactive material (known as a *radiopharmaceutical*) is introduced into the patient using one of the following methods: intravenously, by ingestion, or by inhalation. Most radiopharmaceuticals are chemically bound to a complex known as a *tracer*. A tracer is designed to be attracted to specific areas of the body or, in some cases, to types of diseased tissue.

A nuclear imaging technician positions the patient on a scanning table that works in association with a specialized piece of equipment known as a *gamma camera*. The gamma camera is positioned above or below the scanning table and is able to detect the radiation being given off by the body part that has been targeted by the radiation. The resulting information is displayed as still images or functional animations of body parts and organs. Because it can show the actual function of organs, nuclear medicine imaging provides more detailed information for certain conditions than is provided by other diagnostic imaging examinations (e.g., CT scan, MRI).

The most common nuclear medicine imaging procedures include bone scans and nuclear cardiac stress tests, which are described in more detail in the next section. Other types of nuclear medicine imaging procedures that may be performed include gallbladder procedures, thyroid studies, brain scans, and lung scans.

Bone Scan

A bone scan is performed to detect bone fractures that are difficult to locate (e.g., stress fractures and hip fractures), osteomyelitis, arthritis, bone tumors, and metastatic bone cancer. When a bone scan is performed, the patient is intravenously injected with a radiopharmaceutical. The patient must then wait at the facility for a predetermined period of time, based on the area being examined. The purpose of the waiting period is to allow the radiopharmaceutical to be absorbed sufficiently so that an accurate diagnosis can be made. The gamma camera detects radiation given off by a bone abnormality and shows up as a "hot spot" on the nuclear images (Fig. 28.25). The radiologist reviews the nuclear images and prepares a bone scan report, which is sent to the patient's provider.

Nuclear Cardiac Stress Test

A nuclear cardiac stress test is a diagnostic procedure used to evaluate the cardiovascular health of individuals with known heart disease or individuals at high risk for developing heart disease, particularly coronary artery disease (CAD). Although a nuclear stress test is more time consuming and expensive to perform than a simple stress test (described in Chapter 27), it provides more accuracy in diagnosing CAD.

The radiopharmaceutical used for a nuclear stress test is administered intravenously and targets the heart. Nuclear images included in the stress test are taken by the gamma

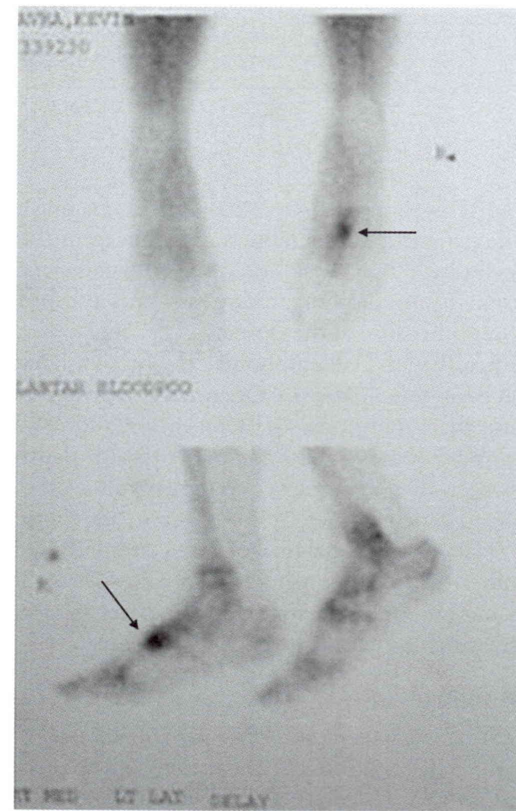

Fig. 28.25 Bone scans of the feet. *Arrows* show the hot spot that indicates a stress fracture. (From Donatelli RA: *Sports-specific rehabilitation*, St. Louis, 2007, Churchill Livingstone.)

camera during two phases: a *resting phase* and a *stress phase* (which is a functional study). The resting phase is performed with the heart at a normal rate, whereas the stress phase is performed immediately after the patient exercises at his or her maximal (target) heart rate. The two sets of nuclear images—the resting images and the images taken under cardiac stress—are then compared with each other. These images assist the radiologist in determining which parts of the heart are healthy and functioning normally. The images also identify areas of the heart that exhibit decreased blood flow during exercise, meaning that a portion of the heart muscle is not receiving enough oxygen. A decreased oxygen supply to a portion of the heart is known as cardiac ischemia and is typically due to the presence of coronary artery disease. The radiologist reviews and interprets the images and prepares a report of the findings which is sent to the patient's provider.

Positron Emission Tomography Scan

A positron emission tomography (PET) scan is a special type of nuclear imaging procedure. PET uses a special camera and computer to construct a 3-D image of the area being scanned. This procedure is particularly useful in diagnosing conditions of the brain and heart, such as brain cancer and heart disease.

What Would You Do? What Would You *Not* Do? RESPONSES

Case Study 1

Page 729

What Did Megan Do?

- ❑ Relayed to Mrs. Bernard that this is not the most fun test to perform, but that if colorectal cancer is detected early, the cure rate is very high.
- ❑ Explained to Mrs. Bernard that colorectal cancer increases after age 50, and that an individual can develop colorectal cancer without a family history of it.
- ❑ Told Mrs. Bernard that during the early stages of colorectal cancer no symptoms occur, so it is possible to feel fine but still have a problem.
- ❑ Explained to Mrs. Bernard in greater detail the reason for not eating red meat or taking aspirin during the testing period.
- ❑ Told Mrs. Bernard that disposable gloves could be given to her to wear when she collects the specimens.
- ❑ Explained to Mrs. Bernard that the physician talks with patients every day about these types of things, and it is important to talk with him about all aspects of her health so that she receives the best care possible.
- ❑ Told Mrs. Bernard that the office would call her in 3 days to see whether she has any questions or is having any problems with the test.

What Did Megan Not Do?

- ❑ Did not tell Mrs. Bernard that she is getting older and needs to be more concerned about performing health screening tests.

Case Study 2

Page 736

What Did Megan Do?

- ❑ Listened patiently and tried to reassure and calm Mr. Bota. Told him that physicians do not yet know what causes prostate cancer.
- ❑ Explained that the PSA test is a screening test and that he should not jump to conclusions about the results.
- ❑ Told Mr. Bota that the physician would talk with him about his test results in a short while.
- ❑ Commended Mr. Bota on his healthy lifestyle habits and encouraged him to continue with them.
- ❑ Gave Mr. Bota some brochures on male reproductive health to read while he waited to be seen by the physician.

What Did Megan Not Do?

- ❑ Did not tell Mr. Bota that there was nothing to worry about.

Case Study 3

Page 739

What Did Megan Do?

- ❑ Told Mrs. Ramirez that a role-playing game with Jose might help. Suggested that she play the "doctor" and pretend she is taking an x-ray of Jose.
- ❑ Told Mrs. Ramirez that the barium will have a flavoring in it but that it does taste chalky. Suggested that she explain to Jose why he needs to drink the barium—to help the doctor find what is wrong with him so that he will not get sick anymore.
- ❑ Told Mrs. Ramirez that Jose's metal truck would interfere with a good radiograph. Suggested that she bring the truck and tell Jose he can have it after the procedure.
- ❑ Explained that the barium might cause constipation and would cause Jose's next bowel movement to be white. Told her that she should encourage Jose to drink a lot of water after the procedure to help prevent constipation.

What Did Megan Not Do?

- ❑ Did not tell Mrs. Ramirez that the barium solution would taste good and that she should not have any trouble getting Jose to drink it.

Case Study 4

Page 748

What Did Megan Do?

- ❑ Explained to Michael that an MRI does not use radiation, so he would not be exposed to any radiation during the procedure.
- ❑ Told Michael that he would not be able to play a game on his cellphone during the procedure. Explained that the MRI works with a strong magnet that might damage his cellphone and also interfere with a good image of the shoulder. Told Michael that he would need to lie still during the procedure.
- ❑ Told Michael the physician would be informed of his problem with claustrophobia. Explained that the physician may want to give him something to help him relax during the procedure.
- ❑ Told Michael that it was fine to eat before the procedure.

What Did Megan Not Do?

- ❑ Did not overlook or minimize Michael's concern about claustrophobia.

TERMINOLOGY REVIEW

Medical Term	Word Parts	Definition
Biopsy	*bi/o-:* life *-opsy:* to view	The surgical removal and examination of tissue from the living body. Biopsies generally are performed to determine whether a tumor is benign or malignant.
Colonoscope	*colon/o-:* colon *-scope:* instrument used for visual examination	An endoscope that is specially designed for passage through the anus to permit visualization of the rectum and the entire length of the colon.
Colonoscopy	*colon/o-:* colon *-scopy:* visual examination	The visualization of the rectum and the entire colon using a colonoscope.
Contrast medium		A substance used to make a particular structure visible on a radiograph.
Echocardiogram	*ech/o-:* sound *cardi/o-:* heart *-gram:* record	An ultrasound examination of the heart.
Endoscope	*endo-:* within *-scope:* instrument used for visual examination	An instrument that consists of a tube and an optical system used for direct visual inspection of organs or cavities.
Enema		An injection of fluid into the rectum to aid in the elimination of feces from the colon.
Fluoroscope	*fluor/o-:* fluorescence *-scope:* instrument used for visual examination	An instrument used to view internal organs and structures directly in real time.
Fluoroscopy	*fluor/o-:* fluorescence *-scopy:* visual examination	An x-ray procedure for viewing internal organs and structures directly in real time.
Insufflate		To blow a powder, vapor, or gas (e.g., air) into a body cavity.
Occult blood		Blood in such a small amount that it is not detectable by the unaided eye.
Polyp (colorectal)		An abnormal noncancerous growth that protrudes from the mucous membrane of the large intestine.
Radiograph	*radi/o-:* radiation *-graph:* instrument used to record, x-ray film	The permanent image produced by x-rays acting on a radiosensitive receptor device such as a digital detector or radiographic film.
Radiography	*radi/o-:* radiation *-graphy:* process of recording, x-ray filming	The taking of permanent images (radiographs) of internal body organs and structures by passing x-rays through the body to act on a radiosensitive receptor device.
Radiologist	*radi/o-:* radiation *-ologist:* one who studies and practices (specialist)	A provider who specializes in the diagnosis and treatment of disease using radiation and other imaging techniques.
Radiology	*radi/o-:* radiation *-ology:* study of	The branch of medicine that uses radiation and other imaging techniques to diagnose and treat disease.
Radiolucent	*radi/o-:* radiation *-lucent:* transparent	Describing a structure that permits the passage of x-rays.
Radiopaque	*radi/o-:* radiation *-opaque:* opaque	Describing a structure that obstructs the passage of x-rays.
Screening		The process of testing to detect disease in an individual who is not yet experiencing symptoms.
Sigmoidoscope	*sigmoid/o-:* sigmoid (colon) *-scope:* instrument used for visual examination	An endoscope that is specially designed for passage through the anus to permit visualization of the rectum and sigmoid colon.
Sigmoidoscopy	*sigmoid/o-:* sigmoid (colon) *-scopy:* visual examination	The visual examination of the rectum and sigmoid colon using a sigmoidoscope.
Sonogram	*son/o-:* sound *-gram:* record	The image obtained with ultrasonography.
Ultrasonography	*ultra-:* beyond, excess *sono-:* sound *-graphy:* process of recording	The use of high-frequency sound waves to produce an image of an organ or tissue.

PROCEDURE 28.1 Patient Coaching: Collection of a Specimen for a Hemoccult Test

Outcome Coach a patient in specimen collection for a Hemoccult test.

Equipment/Supplies

- Hemoccult kit

1. Procedural Step. Obtain a Hemoccult kit and check the expiration date.

Principle. An outdated kit can lead to inaccurate test results.

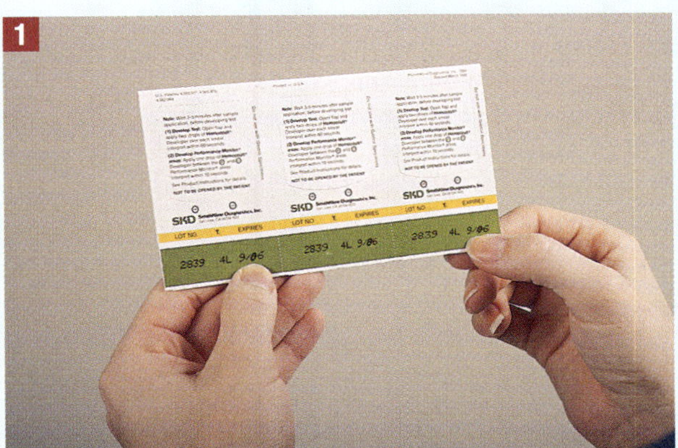

Check the expiration date.

2. Procedural Step. Greet the patient and introduce yourself. Identify the patient and explain the purpose of the Hemoccult test. Tell the patient that the stool specimens should not be collected during a menstrual period or when hemorrhoids are bleeding or a urinary tract infection is present.

Principle. Bleeding from other (identifiable) sources causes a false-positive test result.

3. Procedural Step. Provide patient instructions for the test following the guidelines in Table 28.1. Instruct the patient to begin the diet modifications 3 days before collecting the first stool specimen and to continue them throughout the collection period. Encourage the patient to adhere to the diet modifications.

Principle. The diet modifications may discourage patient compliance. The medical assistant should reinforce the importance of adhering to the diet requirements. Improper patient preparation can lead to inaccurate test results.

4. Procedural Step. Provide the patient with the Hemoccult kit. The kit consists of three identical cardboard slides attached to one another; each slide contains two squares, labeled "A" and "B." Three wooden applicator sticks and written instructions also are included in the testing kit.

Principle. Three slides are provided so that three stool specimens can be collected. The two squares in each slide (A and B) contain filter paper impregnated with guaiac, a chemical necessary for detection of blood in the stool.

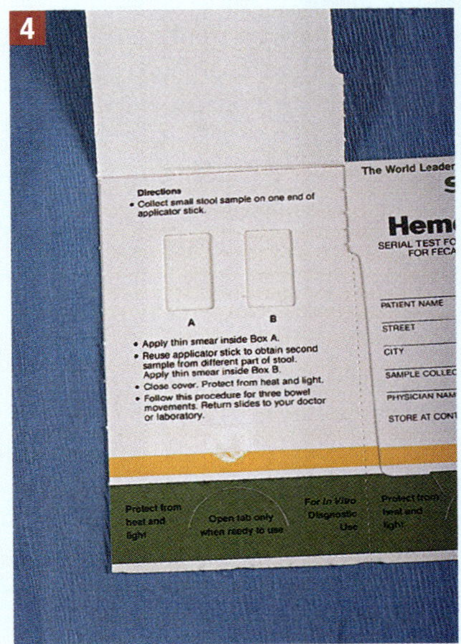

Each slide contains two squares labeled "A" and "B."

5. Procedural Step. Instruct the patient on completion of the information required on the front flap of each collection slide. This includes the patient's name, address, phone number, and age and the date of the specimen collection. A pen should be used to write this information.

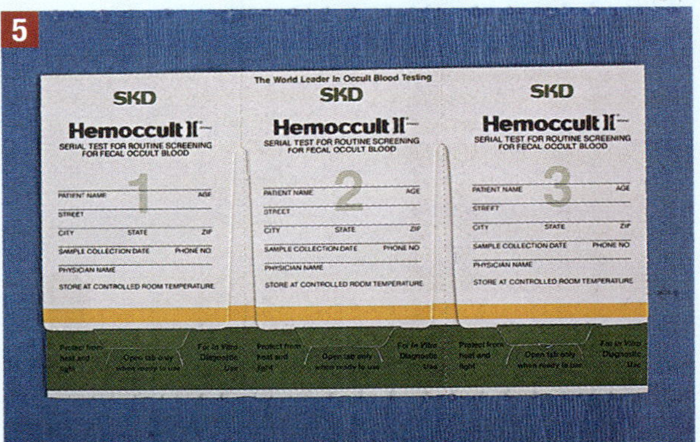

Instruct the patient on how to complete the information section on the slides.

Continued

PROCEDURE 28.1 Patient Coaching: Collection of a Specimen for a Hemoccult Test—cont'd

6. **Procedural Step.** Provide instructions on proper care and storage of the cardboard slides. Make it clear that the slides must be stored (with the flaps in a closed position) at room temperature and protected from heat, sunlight, strong fluorescent light, and volatile chemicals.
   Principle. Adverse storage conditions can result in deterioration of the active reagents impregnated on the filter paper of the slides, leading to inaccurate test results.
7. **Procedural Step.** Instruct the patient on the initiation of the test by telling them to begin the diet modifications and then to collect a stool specimen from the first bowel movement after the 3-day preparatory period.
8. **Procedural Step.** Instruct the patient on proper collection of the stool specimen:
   a. Right before a bowel movement, fill in the collection date on the front flap of the first cardboard slide.
   b. Use a clean, dry container to collect the stool specimen. The specimen must be collected before it comes in contact with toilet bowl water. Allow the stool to fall into the collection container.
   c. Use one of the wooden applicators to obtain a specimen from one part of the stool sample.
   d. Open the front flap of the first cardboard slide (located on the left in the series of three).
   e. Spread a very thin smear of the specimen over the filter paper in the square labeled "A."
   f. Using the same wooden applicator, obtain another specimen from a different area of the stool.
   g. Spread a thin smear of the specimen over the filter paper in the square labeled "B."

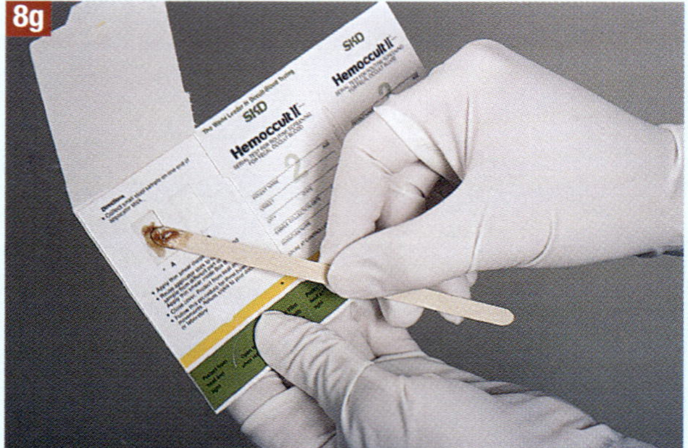

Spread a thin smear of the specimen over the filter paper.

   h. Close the front flap of the cardboard slide.
   i. Discard the wooden applicator in a waste container. Do not flush it down the toilet.
   j. Place the slides in a regular paper envelope to air-dry overnight.

   Principle. Two squares are included in each slide to allow specimen collection from different parts of the stool since occult blood is not always uniformly distributed throughout the stool. Thick specimens prevent adequate light penetration through the filter paper, making it difficult to interpret the test results.
9. **Procedural Step.** Instruct the patient to continue the collection period on 3 different days until all three specimens have been obtained as follows.
   a. Repeat Procedural Step 8 after the second bowel movement the next day. If you do not have a bowel movement on the next day, then collect the specimen on the following day. The specimens should be collected on 3 different days. Use the cardboard slide located in the middle of the series of three.
   b. Repeat Procedural Step 8 after the third bowel movement, using the cardboard slide located to the right in the series of three.
   c. Allow the completed slides to air-dry overnight in the paper envelope.
10. **Procedural Step.** Instruct the patient to place the cardboard slides in the envelope lined with foil, seal carefully, and return them as soon as possible to the medical office. Emphasize to the patient that only the foil-lined envelope can be used to mail the slides; a standard envelope cannot be used. Inform the patient that the slides must be returned to the medical office as soon as possible but no later than 10 days after the first specimen is collected.
    Principle. Standard paper envelopes are not approved by U.S. postal regulations for mailing fecal occult blood testing slides. Slides should not be developed after 10 days, as the test results may not be accurate.

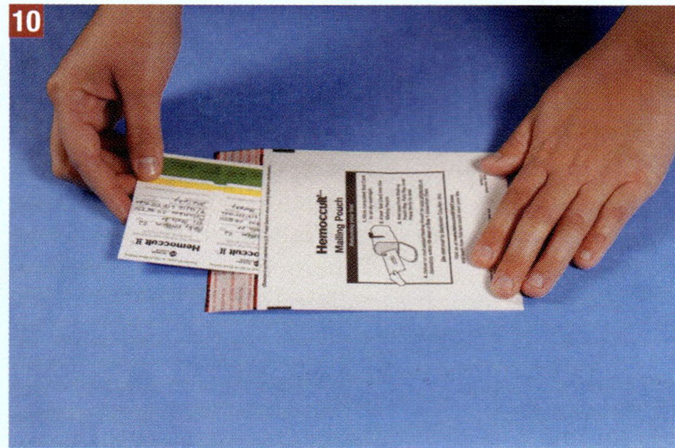

Place the cardboard slides in the envelope.

11. **Procedural Step.** Give the patient an opportunity to ask questions; ensure that the patient understands the instructions for patient preparation and collection of the stool specimen and for storage of the slides.

PROCEDURE 28.1 Patient Coaching: Collection of a Specimen for a Hemoccult Test—cont'd

Principle. Improper patient preparation and poor collection technique can lead to inaccurate test results.

12. Procedural Step. Document in the patient's medical record.

a. *Electronic medical record:* Document that the Hemoccult kit and instructions were given to the patient using the appropriate radio buttons, drop-down menus, and free text fields.

b. *Paper-based patient record:* Document the date and verification that the Hemoccult kit and instructions were given to the patient.

12b

DOCUMENTATION EXAMPLE

Date	
9/08/XX	9:00 a.m. Pt provided with a Hemoccult
	test and instructions for the procedure.
	———————— M. Baer, CMA (AAMA)

PROCEDURE 28.2 Developing a gFOBT

Outcome Develop a Hemoccult test.

Equipment/Supplies

- Disposable gloves
- Prepared cardboard slides
- Hemoccult developing solution
- Waste container

1. Procedural Step. Assemble the equipment. Check the expiration date on the developing solution bottle. The developing solution contains hydrogen peroxide and must be stored away from heat and light. It must be tightly capped when not in use.

Principle. Outdated solution should not be used because it can lead to inaccurate test results. The solution should be stored properly because it is flammable and evaporates easily.

2. Procedural Step. Sanitize your hands and apply gloves. Open the back flap of the cardboard slides. Apply 2 drops of the developing solution to the filter paper underlying the back of each smear.

Principle. The developing solution is absorbed through the filter paper and into the stool specimen. This solution could irritate the skin and eyes; if contact occurs, immediately rinse the area with water.

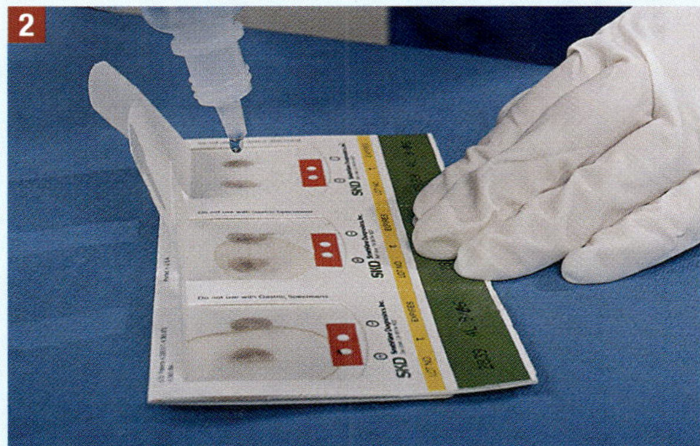

Apply 2 drops of developing solution.

3. Procedural Step. Read and interpret the results within 60 seconds. Fecal blood loss greater than 5 mL per day

Continued

PROCEDURE 28.2 Developing a gFOBT—cont'd

results in a positive reaction, which is indicated by any trace of blue on or at the edge of the fecal smear. If no detectable color change occurs, the result is considered negative.

Principle. In the presence of hydrogen peroxide, the heme compound in hemoglobin oxidizes the guaiac, causing it to turn blue within 60 seconds after the developer is added. The reading time is important because the color reaction may fade after 2 to 4 minutes.

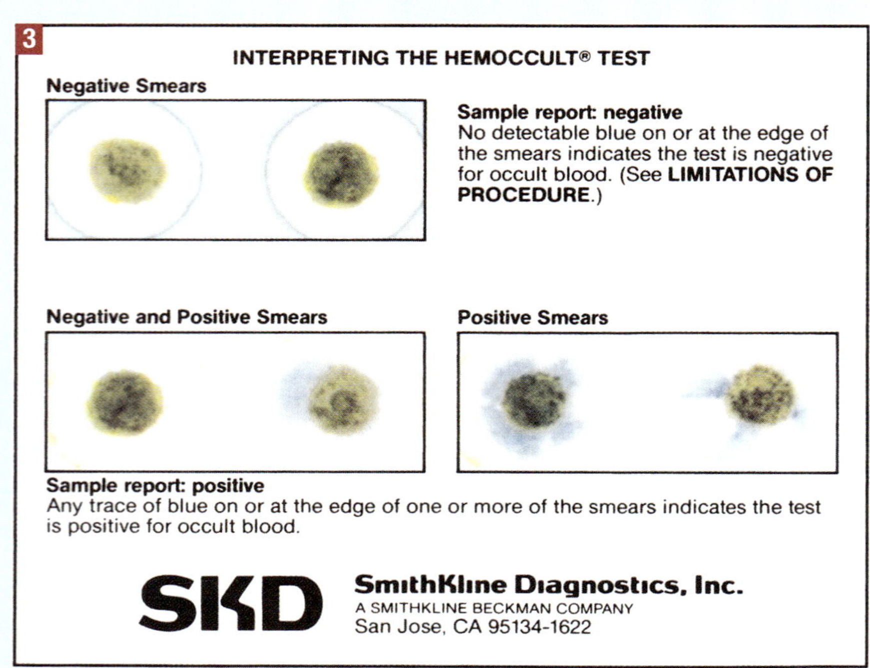
3

INTERPRETING THE HEMOCCULT® TEST

Negative Smears

Sample report: negative
No detectable blue on or at the edge of the smears indicates the test is negative for occult blood. (See **LIMITATIONS OF PROCEDURE.**)

Negative and Positive Smears

Positive Smears

Sample report: positive
Any trace of blue on or at the edge of one or more of the smears indicates the test is positive for occult blood.

SKD **SmithKline Diagnostics, Inc.**
A SMITHKLINE BECKMAN COMPANY
San Jose, CA 95134-1622

4. Pocedural Step. Perform the quality control procedure as follows:

a. Apply 1 drop of developing solution between the positive and negative control performance indicators on each of the three slides.

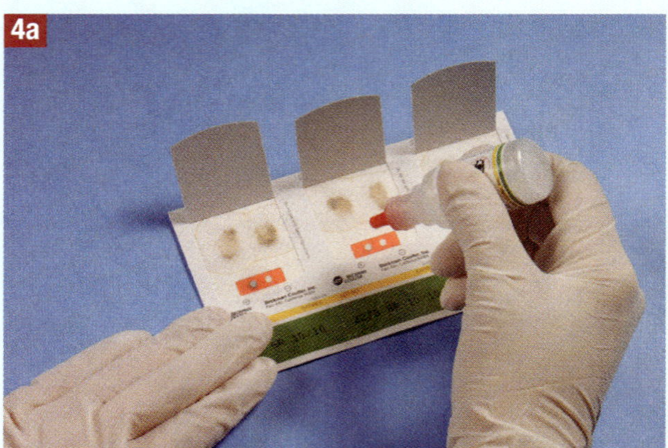

Apply 1 drop of developing solution to the control area.

b. Read the results within 10 seconds.

c. The positive area should turn blue and the negative area should show no color change. Failure of the expected control results to occur indicates an error and that the test results are invalid.

Principle. The quality control procedure must be performed after developing, reading, and interpreting the slides. Quality control procedures ensure the accuracy and reliability of the test results.

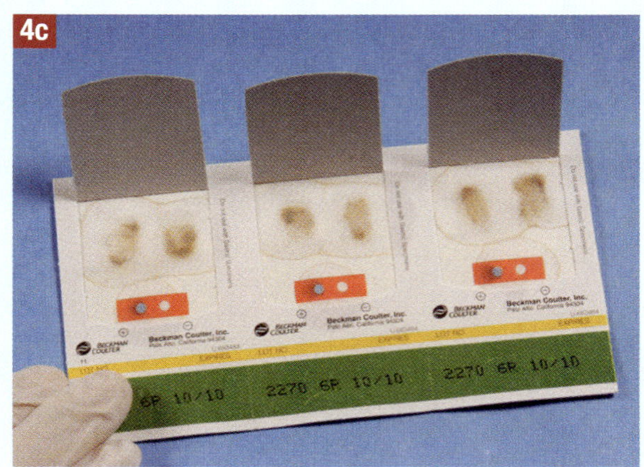

The positive area should turn blue, and the negative area should show no color change.

PROCEDURE 28.2 Developing a gFOBT—cont'd

5. **Procedural Step.** Properly dispose of the Hemoccult slides in a regular waste container.
   Principle. Fecal material is not considered regulated medical waste and can be discarded in a regular waste container.
6. **Procedural Step.** Remove gloves and sanitize your hands.
7. **Procedural Step.** Document the results in the patient's medical record.
   a. *Electronic medical record:* Document the brand name of the test (Hemoccult) and the test results for each slide (documented as positive or negative).
   b. *Paper-based patient record:* Document the date and time, the brand name of the test (Hemoccult), and the test results for each slide (documented as positive or negative).

7b

DOCUMENTATION EXAMPLE

Date	
9/14/XX	10:30 a.m. Hemoccult test:
	Slide 1: Negative
	Slide 2: Negative
	Slide 3: Negative
	——————— M. Baer, CMA (AAMA)

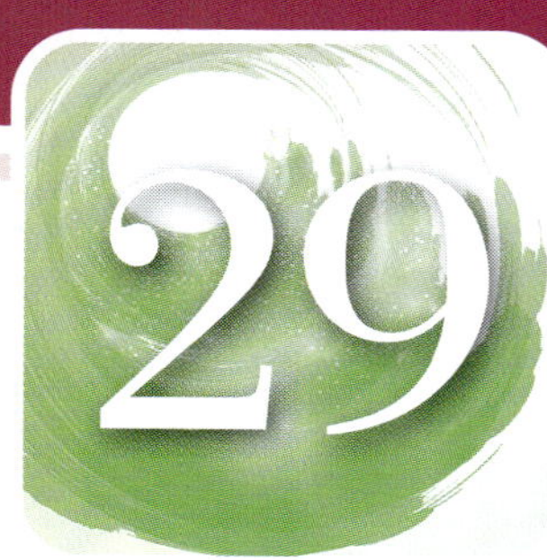

Introduction to the Clinical Laboratory

Check out the Evolve site at http://evolve.elsevier.com/Bonewit/today to access additional interactive activities and exercises to help you study and prepare for success.

LEARNING OBJECTIVES	PROCEDURES
Clinical Laboratory	
1. Identify the use of laboratory test results.	
2. Explain what occurs when the body is not in homeostasis.	
3. Explain the purpose of a physician's office laboratory (POL).	
4. List and describe the components of POL.	
5. Identify the purpose of an emergency eyewash station.	Operate an emergency eyewash station. Inspect an emergency eyewash station.
6. Describe an outside laboratory.	
7. List and describe the information included in a laboratory test directory.	Use a laboratory test directory.
Laboratory Tests	
8. Explain the purpose of laboratory testing.	
9. List examples of specimens collected for laboratory analysis.	
10. Identify the eight categories of laboratory tests based on function.	
11. Explain the meaning of a reference range.	
12. Explain the difference between a specific laboratory panel and a general laboratory panel.	
13. Explain the use of laboratory test results.	
Laboratory Forms	
14. Identify the purpose of a laboratory request.	Complete a laboratory request.
15. List and describe the information included on a laboratory request.	
16. Explain the difference between a preprinted and a computerized-generated laboratory request.	
17. Identify the purpose of a laboratory report.	Review a laboratory report.
18. List and describe the information included on a laboratory report.	
19. Identify methods for transmitting laboratory reports to the medical office.	
20. Describe ways in which laboratory test results can be accessed and manipulated by a computer.	
Patient Instructions	
21. Explain the purpose of patient preparation for a laboratory test.	Instruct a patient in the preparation necessary for a laboratory test that requires fasting.
22. Explain the purpose of fasting before a laboratory test.	
Specimen Collection for Transport to an Outside Laboratory	
23. Identify the guidelines to follow when collecting a specimen for transport to an outside laboratory.	Collect a specimen for transport to an outside laboratory.
24. Explain the procedure for proper identification of the patient.	
25. Describe two methods for labeling a specimen.	
26. Describe the guidelines to follow when handling and storing specimens for transport to an outside laboratory.	Handle and store a specimen for transport to an outside laboratory.

LEARNING OBJECTIVES	PROCEDURES
CLIA-Waived Laboratory Tests	
27. Describe the following CLIA test categories: waived, moderate complexity, and high complexity.	
28. List and describe the information included in a package insert that accompanies a CLIA-waived test kit.	
29. List the advantages of a CLIA-waived automated analyzer.	
30. Explain the purpose of quality control in the laboratory.	Perform quality control procedures on a quality control test system.
31. Describe the guidelines to follow for CLIA-waived tests.	Perform a CLIA-waived laboratory test.
32. Explain the difference between an internal control and an external control.	
33. Explain the difference between a qualitative and a quantitative test result.	
34. List the laboratory safety guidelines to follow to prevent accidents in the POL.	Practice laboratory safety.

CHAPTER OUTLINE

INTRODUCTION TO THE CLINICAL LABORATORY

Physician's Office Laboratory

Components of a POL

Maintenance of the POL

Outside Laboratory

Laboratory Test Directory

LABORATORY TESTS

Reference Range

Laboratory Panels

USE OF LABORATORY TEST RESULTS

LABORATORY DOCUMENTS

Laboratory Request

Parts of a Laboratory Request

Types of Laboratory Request

Laboratory Report

Parts of a Laboratory Report

Electronic Transmission of Laboratory Reports

Specimen Labels

Handwritten Label

Barcode Label

PATIENT INSTRUCTIONS

Patient Preparation

Fasting

Medication Restrictions

SPECIMEN COLLECTION FOR TRANSPORT TO AN OUTSIDE LABORATORY

Causes for Rejection of a Specimen

Guidelines for Specimen Collection and Handling

CLINICAL LABORATORY IMPROVEMENT AMENDMENTS

Categories of Tests

CLIA-Waived Tests

CLIA-Nonwaived Tests

CLIA-WAIVED TESTS IN THE POL

CLIA-Waived Test Systems

CLIA-Waived Test Kits

CLIA-Waived Automated Analyzers

POL LABORATORY TESTING

Quality Control

Storage of Test Components

Stability of Test Components

Calibration Procedure

Control Procedure

Collecting the Specimen

Testing the Specimen

Interpreting and Reading the Test Results

Documenting the Test Results

LABORATORY SAFETY

Specimen Collection and Testing

Hazardous Chemicals

KEY TERMS

analyte
calibration
CLIA-nonwaived test
CLIA-waived test
clinical diagnosis
clinical laboratory
control
critical value
fasting
homeostasis (hoe-mee-oh-STAY-sis)
laboratory panel
laboratory test
package insert
qualitative test
quality control
quantitative test
reagent (REE-ajent)
reference range
screening test
serum (SEER-um)
specimen (SPES-i-men)
test system
unique identifier

INTRODUCTION TO THE CLINICAL LABORATORY

A clinical laboratory is a facility in which laboratory tests are performed on biologic specimens to obtain valuable information regarding the health of a patient. Laboratory test results are used, along with the health history, physical examination, and diagnostic procedures, to obtain essential data needed by the provider for the diagnosis, treatment, and management of a patient's condition.

When the body is healthy, its systems function normally, and a state of equilibrium of the internal environment is said to exist; this is termed **homeostasis.** When the body is in a state of homeostasis, the physical and chemical characteristics of body substances are within an acceptable range.

When a pathologic condition exists, changes occur which alter the normal functioning of the body resulting in an imbalance; in other words, the body is no longer in homeostasis. These changes cause the patient to experience the symptoms of a particular pathologic condition. For example, iron-deficiency anemia may cause the patient to experience weakness, fatigue, dizziness, pallor, irritability, and shortness of breath. These changes may also cause an alteration in the characteristics of body substances leading to abnormal laboratory test results. Iron-deficiency anemia causes an alteration in normal red blood cell morphology and decreased hemoglobin, hematocrit, blood iron, and ferritin levels.

This chapter serves as an introduction to the clinical laboratory by providing an overview of clinical laboratory methods and techniques. It is important that the medical assistant have knowledge of the laboratory tests that are performed most often, including the purpose and normal range of these tests, any substances that might interfere with accurate test results, and factors that may cause abnormal test results.

PHYSICIAN'S OFFICE LABORATORY

A medical office may house its own laboratory for performing laboratory tests, known as a *physician's office laboratory (POL)*. There are several advantages to performing laboratory tests in a POL. The test results are available while patients are still at the medical office which may allow the provider to diagnose or monitor their conditions immediately. The provider is also able to initiate or adjust the course of treatment for patients before they leave the office, rather than delaying treatment until test results are received from the laboratory.

The laboratory tests performed in a POL are usually CLIA-waived tests. CLIA is an abbreviation for the *Clinical Laboratory Improvement Amendments* which consist of regulations that have been developed by the federal government to improve the quality of laboratory testing in the United States to ensure accurate and reliable test results.

A **CLIA-waived test** is a laboratory test that has been determined to be a simple procedure that is easy to perform and has a low risk of erroneous test results, such as urinalysis using a reagent strip (Fig. 29.1). CLIA-waived tests are exempt from most of the CLIA regulations. Medical assistants trained in the proper collection and testing procedures are qualified to perform CLIA-waived tests in the POL.

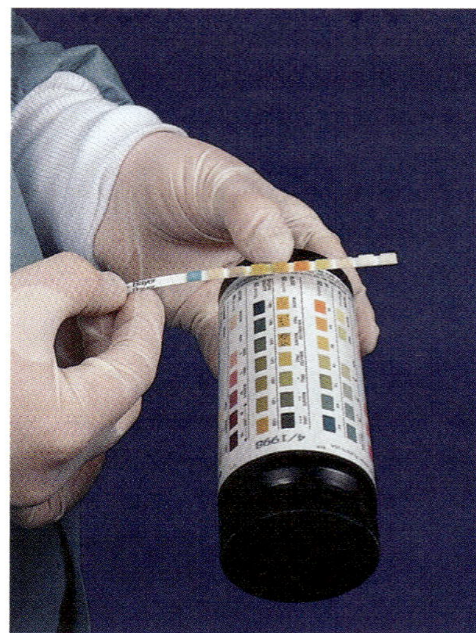

Fig. 29.1 Urinalysis using a reagent strip is a CLIA-waived test.

A **CLIA-nonwaived test** is a laboratory test that does not meet the criteria for waiver and is subject to the CLIA regulations. Nonwaived tests require a complex testing method and are usually performed in an outside laboratory by certified medical laboratory personnel. Additional information on CLIA is presented later in this chapter.

Components of a POL

The components of a POL should meet certain requirements to provide a safe and effective working environment as outlined below.

Physical Structure

The POL should be a separate room or work area in the medical office. Laboratory work counters should be large enough to provide ample space for testing specimens. Cabinets should be available for storing equipment and supplies. The medical assistant should check the supply inventory periodically and reorder as needed.

Room Temperature and Lighting

The temperature of the POL should be maintained at room temperature (RT), which is a temperature that falls between 59°F and 86°F (15°C and 30°C). This temperature range is conducive to storing test components requiring RT storage. Temperatures outside of this range may cause deterioration of the test components, such as controls and test reagents.

Temperature requirements are also important when using an automated analyzer. When a specimen is tested using an automated analyzer, a chemical reaction occurs between the specimen and the test reagents to produce the test results. With some analyzers, the chemical reaction can occur only at RT. If the temperature is outside of RT, the analyzer cannot perform the test, resulting in an error message appearing on the screen of the analyzer. The temperature of the POL should be checked daily to ensure that it is at RT.

Adequate lighting is essential for the proper collection, handling, and testing of specimens. Good lighting is also needed for the proper interpretation of test results that use color comparison to determine test results, such as urinalysis using a reagent strip.

Refrigerator

A medical refrigerator should be available in a POL for the storage of specimens and test components requiring refrigeration. The temperature of the refrigerator must be maintained between 36°F and 46°F (2°C and 8°C) to retard alterations in the physical and chemical composition of specimens and to prevent deterioration of test components. The temperature of the refrigerator should be checked at least once each day and documented in a refrigerator temperature log. As required by the OSHA Standard, food and beverages must not be stored in the medical refrigerator, and a biohazard warning label must be attached to the refrigerator to alert employees to the presence of potentially infectious materials.

Protective Equipment and Supplies

Laboratory testing involves the collection and handling of specimens that may contain pathogens. Protective equipment and supplies necessary to comply with the OSHA Standard should be readily accessible in the POL. This includes handwashing facilities, alcohol-based hand sanitizers, gloves, safety goggles and masks, laboratory coats, and safety-engineered syringes and needles. Biohazard sharps containers and bags must be available for disposal of medical waste, such as contaminated needles and syringes and used collection supplies.

Emergency Eyewash Station

An *emergency eyewash station* should be available in a POL in the event of an accidental exposure incident to the eyes. An emergency eyewash station (Fig. 29.2) is a device that is used to flush the eyes with tepid water when substances such as blood or hazardous chemicals enter the eye. *Tepid* water consists of water with a temperature between 60°F and 100°F (16°C and 38°C). An eyewash station flushes both eyes simultaneously with water at a velocity low enough not to injure the eyes of the user.

The eyewash station is activated by pressing a lever attached to the station; the lever must be clearly identified and operate with a single easy motion. Once activated, the nozzle covers pop off the nozzle heads and each of the nozzles begin discharging water. The eyes should be flushed for a full 15 minutes which is the minimum amount of time needed to clear the eyes of hazardous substances. Following activation, the eyewash station remains operational without requiring the user's hands for 15 minutes (or until it is manually turned off).

The eyewash station should be easily accessible and located within a 10 second walking distance (approximately 55 feet) of potential hazards. The first 10–15 seconds after exposure of the eye to a hazardous substance are critical, especially if it is a corrosive chemical. A delay in treatment could result in permanent damage to the eye.

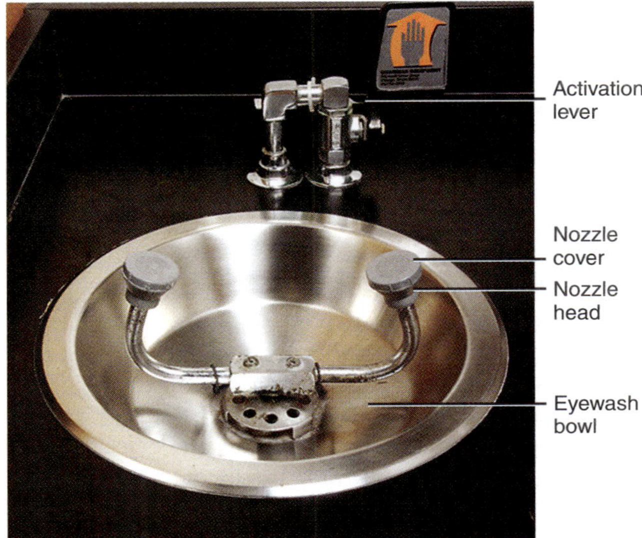

Fig. 29.2 Emergency eyewash station.

It is important that the medical assistant inspect and activate the eyewash station each week to ensure that it is operating properly and to flush out the water supply lines. A more detailed inspection should be performed on an annual basis by a qualified service technician. The procedure for operating an eyewash station and performing a weekly eyewash inspection is outlined Procedure 29.1.

Maintenance of the POL

The medical assistant is responsible for making sure the POL is clean and free of clutter. Biohazard sharps containers and bags should be replaced as needed and not be allowed to overfill. An approved disinfectant should be readily available for disinfecting laboratory work surfaces each day. The medical assistant should know how to care for each piece of laboratory equipment; this information is included in the operating manual that accompanies the equipment.

OUTSIDE LABORATORY

Outside laboratories use highly sophisticated automated analyzers for performing tests that provide the medical office with fast and reliable test results. Medical offices typically use a combination of a POL and an outside laboratory to fulfill their laboratory testing requirements.

Outside laboratories include hospital and privately-owned independent laboratories. Independent laboratories range from large, national corporations (e.g., *LabCorp* and *Quest Diagnostics*) to small, local independent laboratories. Because the medical assistant works closely with an outside laboratory, knowledge of the relationship between the medical office and an outside laboratory is important.

A specimen can be collected at the medical office and transported to an outside laboratory for testing or it can be collected (and tested) at the outside laboratory. If the specimen is collected at the medical office, the laboratory usually provides the medical office with the supplies necessary to collect and handle the specimen. The medical assistant is responsible for checking these supplies periodically and reordering them as needed.

Laboratory Test Directory

Most outside laboratories publish a *laboratory test directory* which serves as a valuable reference source for the medical office. It is usually in the form of an online directory to provide for quick and easy access of laboratory information. The directory includes a *test menu*, which consists of an alphabetic listing of all the tests performed by the outside laboratory. Information is provided for each test in the test menu and includes patient preparation requirements, specimen collection and processing requirements, and proper preparation and storage of the specimen for transport to the outside laboratory (Fig. 29.3). If the medical assistant has a question regarding any aspect of the procedure, the laboratory should be contacted before proceeding.

The following information is typically included in the laboratory test directory for each test performed by the laboratory:

- Name and CPT (Current Procedural Terminology) code of the test
- Synonyms for the test name
- Type and amount of specimen required
- Collection container(s) required
- Patient preparation
- Collection and processing requirements
- Specimen storage and transport requirements
- Specimen stability
- Causes for rejection of the specimen by the laboratory
- Reference range of the test
- Uses and limitations of the test
- Form requirements
- Methodology used to perform the test

LABORATORY TESTS

A **laboratory test** is defined as the clinical analysis and study of a body substance to obtain objective data for the diagnosis, treatment, and management of a patient's condition. Laboratory tests are performed on specimens collected from the body. A **specimen** is a small sample taken from the body to represent the nature of the whole. Most laboratory tests are performed on specimens that are easily obtained from the body, such as blood and urine. Other examples of specimens collected for laboratory analysis and study include stool, sputum, cervical and vaginal scrapings of cells, and secretions and discharges from various parts of the body. The medical assistant is usually responsible for the collection of most patient specimens. Certain specimens must be collected by the provider, such as a specimen for a Pap test, a sample of vaginal or urethral discharge, and a tissue specimen for biopsy. In these cases, the medical assistant assists with the collection.

Laboratory tests can be classified by function into categories. Use of these categories makes it easier to refer to laboratory tests. Table 29.1 lists and describes each of these categories and provides examples of tests in each category.

The number of laboratory tests ordered for a patient depends on the provider's clinical diagnosis. A **clinical diagnosis** is defined as a tentative diagnosis of a patient's condition obtained through the evaluation of the health history and the physical examination, without the benefit of laboratory tests or diagnostic procedures. A clinical diagnosis of strep throat usually requires only a strep (*Streptococcus*) test for confirmation. However, most diseases cause more than one alteration in the physical and chemical characteristics of body substances, and a series of laboratory tests is necessary to arrive at a diagnosis.

There are some pathologic conditions that do not require the use of laboratory test results to determine a diagnosis. In some cases, the information obtained from the patient's clinical signs and symptoms is sufficient enough for the diagnosis of a condition. In these instances, the provider is so certain of the diagnosis that treatment can be instituted without laboratory confirmation. For example, most providers diagnose otitis media (middle ear infection) with the information obtained from patient symptoms (earache, fever, and feeling of fullness in the ear) and from an otoscopic examination of the tympanic membrane (the tympanic membrane is red and bulging). Information obtained through these clinical signs and symptoms is sufficiently specific to otitis media to allow the provider to make a diagnosis and to prescribe treatment.

REFERENCE RANGE

A **reference range** is defined as a certain established and acceptable range with upper and lower limits within which the laboratory test results of a healthy individual are expected to fall. A range, rather than a single value, is necessary because of individual differences within a general population caused by factors such as age, sex, race, and geographic location. The reference range for each test varies slightly from one laboratory to another, depending on the test method, equipment, and chemical reagents used to perform the test. It is essential that test results be compared with the reference ranges supplied by the laboratory performing the test rather than with a laboratory reference source.

A test result falling outside of the reference range for a particular test may be seen with more than one pathologic condition. A decrease in the hemoglobin level may occur with iron-deficiency anemia, leukemia, cirrhosis, chronic kidney failure and certain autoimmune diseases. In this regard, the provider cannot rely solely on a low hemoglobin level to make a diagnosis, but must acquire data from additional sources such as the health history, physical examination, diagnostic imaging, and further laboratory testing.

LABORATORY TEST DIRECTORY Triglycerides	
CPT Code:	84478
Synonyms:	Trig, Tg
Type of Specimen:	Serum
Amount of Specimen:	2 mL
Collection Container:	SST (send entire tube)
Patient Preparation:	Fasting for 9–12 h prior to collection. No alcohol consumption for 24 h prior to collection.
Collection and Processing:	1. Collect and label specimen. 2. Gently invert tube 5 times immediately after collection. 3. Place specimen in a vertical position and allow to clot for a minimum of 30 min and a maximum of 2 h. 4. Centrifuge specimen for 10 min.
Storage and Transport:	Store at RT or refrigerate until pickup by lab courier.
Specimen Stability:	RT (59°F-86°F): 5 days Refrigerated (2°C–8°C): 7 days
Causes for Rejection:	Nonfasting specimen Specimen other than serum Improper labeling of specimen Improper storage temperature
Reference Range:	Desirable: Less than 150 mg/dL Borderline high: 150–199 mg/dL High: 200–499 mg/dL Very high: 500 mg/dL or greater
Uses:	Measurement of triglycerides levels assist with the diagnosis and treatment of diabetes mellitus, nephrosis, liver obstruction, and other diseases involving lipid metabolism. In conjunction with HDL cholesterol and total cholesterol, a triglycerides determination assists in the assessment of the risk for developing coronary artery disease. Elevated levels may occur with liver disease, nephritic syndrome, hypothyroidism, increased alcohol consumption, poorly controlled diabetes, and pancreatitis.
Limitations:	Pregnancy and women on estrogens may cause an increase in triglycerides level.
Forms:	Order electronically or print the lab request form and submit with specimen.
Methodology:	Quantitative enzymatic

Fig. 29.3 Laboratory Test Directory indicating triglycerides specimen requirements.

Table 29.1 Categories of Laboratory Tests[a]

Category	Description and Tests
Hematology	Hematology is the science of the study of blood and blood-forming tissues. Laboratory analysis in hematology involves the examination of blood for detection of abnormalities including blood cell counts, cellular morphology, clotting ability of blood, and identification of cell types. Tests include: White blood cell (WBC) count Red blood cell count (RBC) Differential white cell count (Diff) Hemoglobin (Hgb) Hematocrit (Hct) Platelet count Reticulocyte count Prothrombin time (PT) Sedimentation rate
Immunology and Blood Banking	Laboratory analysis in immunology and blood banking involves studying antigen–antibody reactions to assess the presence of a substance or to determine the presence of disease. Tests include: *Immunology* Allergy blood tests Antinuclear antibody (ANA) Antistreptolysin O (ASO) C-Reactive protein (CRP) COVID-19 test *H. pylori* test Hepatitis tests HIV tests Mononucleosis test Pregnancy test PSA test Rheumatoid factor (RF) Syphilis test (VDRL, RPR) TB blood test Thyroid fnction tests *Blood Banking* ABO blood typing Rh typing Rh antibody test
Clinical Chemistry	Laboratory analysis in clinical chemistry determines the amount of chemical substances present in blood, body fluids, excreta, and tissues. The largest area in clinical chemistry is blood chemistry. Tests include: Albumin ALP ALT AST Bilirubin Blood alcohol Blood lead BUN Calcium Carbon dioxide Chloride Cholesterol Cortisol Creatine kinase (CK) Creatinine Glucose Inorganic phosphorus LDH Potassium Protein (total) Sodium T_3 and T_4 Triglycerides Uric acid
Urinalysis	The physical, chemical, and microscopic analyses of urine to detect deviations from normal. A. *Tests included in physical analysis of urine:* Color Appearance Specific gravity B. *Tests included in chemical analysis of urine:* Glucose Bilirubin Blood Ketones Leukocytes Nitrite pH Protein Urobilinogen C. *A microscopic analysis of urine looks for the following structures:* Red blood cells White blood cells Bacteria Yeast Epithelial cells Casts Crystals

Table 29.1 Categories of Laboratory Tests[a]—cont'd

Category	Description and Tests	Category	Description and Tests
Microbiology	Microbiology is the scientific study of microorganisms and their activities. Laboratory analysis in microbiology involves identification of pathogens present in body specimens (e.g., urine, blood, throat, sputum, wound, urethra, vagina, cerebrospinal fluid). Tests include: Throat culture Urine culture Genital cultures Blood culture Stool culture Wound culture Sputum cultures Nasopharyngeal culture Eye and ear culture	**Cytology**	Laboratory analysis in cytology deals with detection of the presence of abnormal cells: Chromosome studies Pap test
Parasitology	Laboratory analysis in parasitology involves detection of disease-producing human parasites or eggs present in body specimens (e.g., stool, vagina, blood). Human diseases caused by parasites include the following: Amebiasis Ascariasis Hookworms Malaria Pinworms Scabies Tapeworms Toxoplasmosis Trichinosis Trichomoniasis	**Histology**	Histology is the microscopic study of the form and structure of various tissues making up living organisms. Laboratory analysis in histology involves the detection of diseased tissues. Tests include: Biopsy studies Tissue analyses

[a]Categories of laboratory tests are listed, including definitions of each and commonly performed tests or pathologic conditions in each category. Tests commonly known by their abbreviations are listed this way.
ALP, Alkaline phosphatase; *ALT*, alanine aminotransferase; *AST*, aspartate aminotransferase; *BUN*, blood urea nitrogen; *HIV*, human immunodeficiency virus; *LDL*, low-density lipoprotein; *PSA*, prostate-specific antigen; T_3, triiodothyronine; T_4, thyroxine; *TB*, tuberculosis.

LABORATORY PANELS

A **laboratory panel** (also known as a *laboratory profile*) consists of a combination of laboratory tests that have been determined to be the most sensitive and specific means of identifying a disease state or evaluating a particular organ or organ system. The panels performed by an outside laboratory and the tests included in each are listed in the laboratory test directory.

A laboratory panel may be *specific* in nature—that is, all tests included in the panel relate to a specific organ of the body or a particular disease state. A specific panel is usually ordered when the provider does not have a definite clinical diagnosis but has a good idea of the patient's condition or what organ or organs are involved in the patient's condition. The provider orders a panel of the condition or organ in question. An example of a panel used to identify a disease state is the *rheumatoid arthritis panel*, which assists in the diagnosis of rheumatoid arthritis. An example of a panel used to evaluate an organ is the *hepatic panel*, which is used to assess liver function and assist in the diagnosis of pathologic conditions that affect the liver.

A laboratory panel may be *general* in nature. A general metabolic panel contains a number of routine laboratory tests. It is used primarily for a routine health evaluation of a patient to screen for any changes in the body that may be present, even though there are no symptoms to indicate these changes have occurred. A general metabolic panel is also used when the patient's symptoms are so vague that the provider does not have enough concrete evidence to support a clinical diagnosis. An example of a general panel is a *comprehensive metabolic panel*; refer to Table 29.2 for a list of the tests included in this panel. The medical assistant should know the names of common laboratory panels and the tests included in each, which are listed in Table 29.2.

USE OF LABORATORY TEST RESULTS

The most frequent use of laboratory test results is to assist in the diagnosis of a patient's condition. Laboratory test

Table 29.2 Laboratory Panels

Laboratory Panel	Tests Included	Use
Comprehensive Metabolic Panel	Albumin ALP ALT AST Bilirubin (total) BUN Calcium Carbon dioxide Chloride Creatinine Glucose Potassium Total protein Sodium	General health screen that provides information on kidneys, liver, acid–base balance, blood glucose level, and blood proteins Evaluation of organ function and to check for conditions such as diabetes, liver disease, and kidney disease Routinely ordered as part of blood workup for physical or medical examination (particularly when patient's symptoms are vague) Abnormal test results are usually followed up with more specific tests before a diagnosis is made
Electrolyte Panel	Carbon dioxide Chloride Potassium Sodium	Screens for electrolyte or acid–base imbalance Monitors effect of treatment on disease or condition that causes electrolyte imbalance Evaluation of patients taking medication that can cause electrolyte imbalance
Hepatic Panel	Albumin ALP ALT AST Bilirubin (direct) Bilirubin (total) Total Protein	Detection of pathologic conditions affecting the liver Monitor liver function of an individual with liver disease or a condition known to affect the liver Monitor the effectiveness of treatment of the liver May be ordered when an individual has been exposed to hepatitis, has a family history of liver disease, has excessive alcohol consumption, or is taking medication that can result in liver damage
Hepatitis Panel	Hepatitis A antibody, IgM Hepatitis B core antibody, total Hepatitis B surface antigen Hepatitis C antibody	Detection of viral hepatitis.
Lipid Panel	Total cholesterol LDL cholesterol HDL cholesterol Triglycerides VLDL cholesterol (calculation) Total cholesterol/HDL ratio (calculation)	Determination of the risk of coronary artery disease
Prenatal Panel	ABO grouping and Rh typing CBC w/diff and w/plt Hepatitis B surface antigen Red blood cell (RBC) antibody screen Rubella antibody Syphilis serology (RPR)	Establish health status of prenatal patients early in the pregnancy Screening of prenatal patients for disease or potential problems
Renal Function Panel	Albumin BUN Calcium Carbon dioxide Chloride Creatinine Glucose Phosphorus Potassium Sodium	Detection of kidney problems Provides information on how well the kidneys are functioning to remove excess fluid and waste When a problem is detected, diagnostic imaging tests may be used for further evaluation and diagnosis

Table 29.2 Laboratory Panels—cont'd

Laboratory Panel	Tests Included	Use
Rheumatoid Arthritis Panel	Rheumatoid factor (RF) Cyclic citrullinated peptide (CCP) Antinuclear antibody (ANA) C-reactive protein (CRP) Erythrocyte sedimentation rate (ESR)	Assists in diagnosis of rheumatoid arthritis and helps distinguish it from other forms of arthritis and conditions with similar symptoms Evaluation of the severity of rheumatoid arthritis Monitors rheumatoid arthritis and its complications, and assesses response to treatment
Thyroid Panel	Thyroxine (T_4) Triiodothyronine (T_3) Uptake Thyroid stimulating hormone (TSH) Free thyroxine intake (FTI)	Evaluation of thyroid function Detection of disorders affecting the thyroid gland

ALP, Alkaline phosphatase; *ALT*, alanine aminotransferase; *AST*, aspartate aminotransferase; *BUN*, blood urea nitrogen; *CBC*, complete blood count; *HDL*, high-density lipoprotein; *IgM*, immunoglobulin M; *LDH*, lactate dehydrogenase; *VLDL*, very-low-density lipoprotein; *w/diff*, with differential; *w/plt*, with platelet count.

results also have other significant medical uses. A summary of the use of laboratory test results follows.

1. *To assist in the diagnosis of pathologic conditions.* Laboratory test results are most frequently used to assist in the diagnosis of pathologic conditions. Along with the health history and the physical examination, test results provide essential data needed by the provider to arrive at a diagnosis and prescribe treatment. After obtaining the health history and performing the physical examination, the provider may order laboratory tests for these reasons:
   - *To confirm a clinical diagnosis.* The patient's signs and symptoms may provide a strong clinical diagnosis of a particular condition, and the provider may use laboratory test results to confirm that diagnosis. For example, the patient may have the typical signs and symptoms of diabetes mellitus, which would give the provider a fairly certain clinical diagnosis. In this instance, a hemoglobin A1c test or an oral glucose tolerance test (OGTT) may be ordered to confirm the diagnosis and to institute therapy.
   - *To assist in the differential diagnosis of a patient's condition.* Two or more diseases may have similar signs and symptoms and the provider must use laboratory test results to assist in the differential diagnosis of the patient's condition. A diagnosis of strep throat must be made with a laboratory test to differentiate it from other pathologic conditions with similar signs and symptoms, such as pharyngitis and mononucleosis.
   - *To obtain information regarding a patient's condition* when not enough concrete evidence exists to support a clinical diagnosis. The patient sometimes may have vague signs and symptoms, and laboratory tests are ordered to obtain information on what may be causing the patient's problems. For example, the patient may have nonspecific abdominal pain, and the physical examination may not yield enough information to support a clinical diagnosis. In this case, the provider may order a laboratory panel to assist in pinpointing the cause of the patient's problems.
2. *To evaluate the patient's progress and to regulate treatment.* When a diagnosis has been made, laboratory testing may be performed to monitor the patient's progress and to regulate treatment. On the basis of the laboratory test results, the therapy may need to be adjusted or further treatment prescribed. A patient undergoing iron therapy for iron-deficiency anemia should have a CBC (complete blood count) performed every month to assess the response to treatment and to ensure that the condition is improving. A patient with diabetes who measures their blood glucose level each day to regulate insulin dosage is an example of using laboratory test results to regulate treatment.
3. *To establish a baseline level.* On the basis of such factors as age, sex, race, and geographic location, individuals have different normal levels within the established reference range for a particular test. In this respect, laboratory test results can establish each patient's baseline level with which future results can be compared. A patient who is going to receive warfarin (Coumadin) therapy should have a blood specimen drawn for a prothrombin time test before administration of this anticoagulant. The results serve as a baseline recording for that particular patient against which future prothrombin time test results can be compared.
4. *To prevent or reduce the severity of disease.* Laboratory test results can help to prevent or reduce the severity of disease through the early detection of abnormal findings. Certain conditions, such as anemia and diabetes, are relatively common disorders and sometimes may exist without symptoms, especially early in the development of the disease. Laboratory tests known as **screening tests** are performed on a routine basis on apparently healthy individuals to assist in the early detection of disease. Screening tests are relatively easy to perform and present a minimal hazard to the patient; the most commonly performed laboratory screening tests include urinalysis, CBC, and a comprehensive metabolic panel.
5. *To comply with state laws.* Another reason for a laboratory test is its requirement by state law. The statutes of most

states require a syphilis test be performed on pregnant women. The purpose of this test is to protect the mother and fetus from harm in the event of a positive test result.

LABORATORY DOCUMENTS

The most common laboratory documents include laboratory requests, laboratory reports, and specimen labels, which are described below.

LABORATORY REQUEST

A laboratory request serves as a means of communication between the medical office and the outside laboratory to designate the test(s) ordered by the provider. The request provides the outside laboratory with essential information necessary for accurate testing, reporting of results, and billing. It is required when the specimen is collected at the medical office and transported to an outside laboratory for testing or when the specimen is collected and tested at an outside laboratory.

Once completed, the laboratory request must be transmitted to the outside laboratory. The medical assistant should realize the significance of this simple but important step. Without the request the laboratory does not have the information it needs to carry out the provider's orders, causing delays in completing the tests and reporting results. The most common methods used to transmit laboratory requests to an outside laboratory include:

- Electronic transmission
- Faxed
- Hand-delivered (along with the specimen) by a laboratory courier
- Hand-delivered by a patient having a specimen collected and tested at an outside laboratory

Parts of a Laboratory Request

Specific information that is required on the laboratory request includes:

1. *Name and address of the laboratory.* The name and address of the laboratory performing the test must appear on the laboratory request.
2. *Medical office name, address, and account number.* This information must appear on the laboratory request to facilitate the reporting of test results to the provider.
3. *Name and signature of the ordering provider.* This information must be included on the request in order for the tests to be performed. In the case of an electronic laboratory request, the provider's signature is in the form of an electronic signature.
4. *Patient's name, address, and telephone number and ID number.* The patient's full legal name must be entered on the request in the following format: last name, first name and middle initial. The patient's name and address is needed for billing purposes and must include the city, state, and zip code.
5. *Patient's date of birth and sex.* The reference ranges for some tests vary depending on the patient's age and sex. The reference range for hemoglobin concentration varies according to sex (12–16 g/dL for a female; 14–18 g/dL for a male).
6. *Date and time of collection of the specimen.* The date and time of specimen collection must be documented on the request. The date of collection indicates to the laboratory the number of days that have passed since the collection, providing the laboratory with information regarding the freshness of the specimen. A time lapse that is too long between collection and testing of a specimen may affect the accuracy of some test results. The time of collection is significant with respect to certain laboratory tests. The reference range for serum cortisol varies depending on whether the specimen is collected in the morning or in the afternoon.
7. *Fasting or non-fasting.* The laboratory request must specify if the patient was in a fasting or nonfasting state when the specimen was collected. The composition of the blood is altered by the consumption of food and fluid which can affect the results of certain laboratory tests.
8. *Name of Responsible Party.* The responsible party is the individual assuming the financial responsibility for payment of the tests.
9. *Third-party billing information.* Third-party billing information must be indicated on the request to provide the necessary information to bill the patient's insurance company for the tests performed.
10. *Laboratory tests ordered.* The test(s) ordered by the provider must be indicated on the request. The laboratory test directory contains a complete listing of all the laboratory tests and panels performed by the laboratory.
11. *Source of the microbiologic specimen.* Microbiologic tests require that the source of the specimen (e.g., throat swab, wound swab, and vaginal swab) be documented on the laboratory request. This is done for identification of the origin of the specimen for the laboratory, because this information is not available by looking at the specimen. In many instances, the source dictates the test method used by the laboratory to evaluate the specimen for the presence of pathogens.
12. *Clinical diagnosis in ICD format.* ICD (International Classification of Disease) diagnosis codes must be used to indicate the patient's clinical diagnosis. This assists the laboratory in correlating clinical laboratory data with the needs of the provider. In some instances, further testing is performed by the laboratory if one test method proves inconclusive to confirm or reject the clinical diagnosis. Another function of the clinical diagnosis is to assure laboratory personnel that the test results are within the framework of the diagnosis. When the results of a test disagree with the clinical diagnosis, the laboratory may repeat the test on the same or another specimen. The clinical diagnosis also alerts laboratory personnel to the

possibility of the presence of a dangerous pathogen, such as the hepatitis virus. In addition, ICD codes are necessary for third-party billing by the laboratory. If the laboratory bills the patient's insurance company for the tests, the ICD codes for the clinical diagnosis must be indicated on the insurance form.

13. *Medications.* Certain medications may interfere with the accuracy and validity of test results and are specified in the laboratory test directory. The medical assistant should document any medications being taken by the patient that could affect the accuracy of the test results. For example, antibiotics being taken by a patient may cause a falsely-negative test result on a strep test.
14. *STAT.* The provider may want the laboratory test results reported as soon as possible. In this case STAT must be indicated on the laboratory request. Requests that are marked STAT are performed as soon as possible after receipt by the laboratory, and the results are telephoned, sent electronically, or faxed to the provider as soon as they are available. STAT testing is only available for a limited number of tests in the test menu and requires additional fees for the expedited service.

Types of Laboratory Requests

There are two types of laboratory requests, the preprinted request and the electronic request, which are described in more detail below.

Preprinted Laboratory Request

A preprinted laboratory request is completed by writing in the required information on a preprinted form (Fig. 29.4). The request form includes spaces for indicating patient demographic and insurance information and includes a list of the most frequently ordered laboratory tests. The tests ordered by the provider are indicated by marking a box adjacent to those tests (and their corresponding CPT codes). A space designated as "other tests" is provided on the request form for specifying the name and CPT code of a test that is desired but not listed on the preprinted request form.

Electronic Laboratory Request

An electronic laboratory request (e-request) is completed by entering the required information into a computer using drop-down lists, radio buttons, checkboxes, and fill-in boxes (Fig. 29.5). The patient's demographic and insurance information is automatically entered by the computer which eliminates errors in reentering this information. Once the request is completed, barcode specimen labels are automatically generated and printed out by the computer.

An electronic laboratory request can be transmitted electronically to the outside laboratory. In order for this to occur, the medical office computer system must be interfaced with the computer system in the outside laboratory. An electronic request can also be printed out by the computer and placed with the specimen for pickup by a laboratory courier.

What Would You Do? What Would You *Not* Do?

Case Study 1

Hans Volkman, age 28, is getting ready to leave the medical office after being seen by the physician. The physician gave him a laboratory request for a CBC and a lipid panel to take to the hospital laboratory. Hans notices that the clinical diagnosis on the form indicates iron-deficiency anemia and wants to know why the physician did not prescribe any medication for him if he thought he had anemia. Hans says that he told the physician he has never had a cholesterol test and asked the physician if he would order one for him. Hans says the physician must have forgotten because the test was not included on the request. Hans has been instructed to fast for the laboratory tests. He says that he stops every morning at the Coffee Cup restaurant and has coffee with cream and sugar, orange juice, and doughnuts. He would like to know whether he could just have the coffee with cream and sugar before the tests. Hans says he has a hard time functioning in the morning without coffee. ■

LABORATORY REPORT

The purpose of a laboratory report is to relay laboratory test results to the provider. The report is usually generated by a computer. It may consist of a preprinted form with the test results printed in the appropriate spaces on the form by a computer (as illustrated in Fig. 29.6), or the entire report may be electronically generated by the computer as illustrated in Fig. 29.7.

Most laboratory computer systems automatically flag abnormal results on the laboratory report as shown in Fig. 29.7. For example, an "H" next to a test result means the result is higher than the reference range and an "L" means it is lower than the reference range.

STAT test results and tests results with critical values are telephoned to the medical office as soon as possible, with the entire report transmitted immediately thereafter. A **critical value** is a laboratory test result that is dangerously abnormal and must be reported immediately to the ordering provider. Critical values are considered life-threatening and require immediate attention.

Laboratory reports can be transmitted to the medical office by one or more of the following methods: electronic transmission, faxed, mailed, or hand-delivered by a laboratory courier. Once received, the provider reviews each laboratory report and the data obtained are correlated with information obtained from the health history and physical examination. The provider indicates that he or she is finished with the report by signing the report.

The medical assistant may be responsible for reviewing laboratory reports as they are received. The medical assistant should compare the patient's test results with the reference ranges supplied by the laboratory and notify the provider of any abnormal test results.

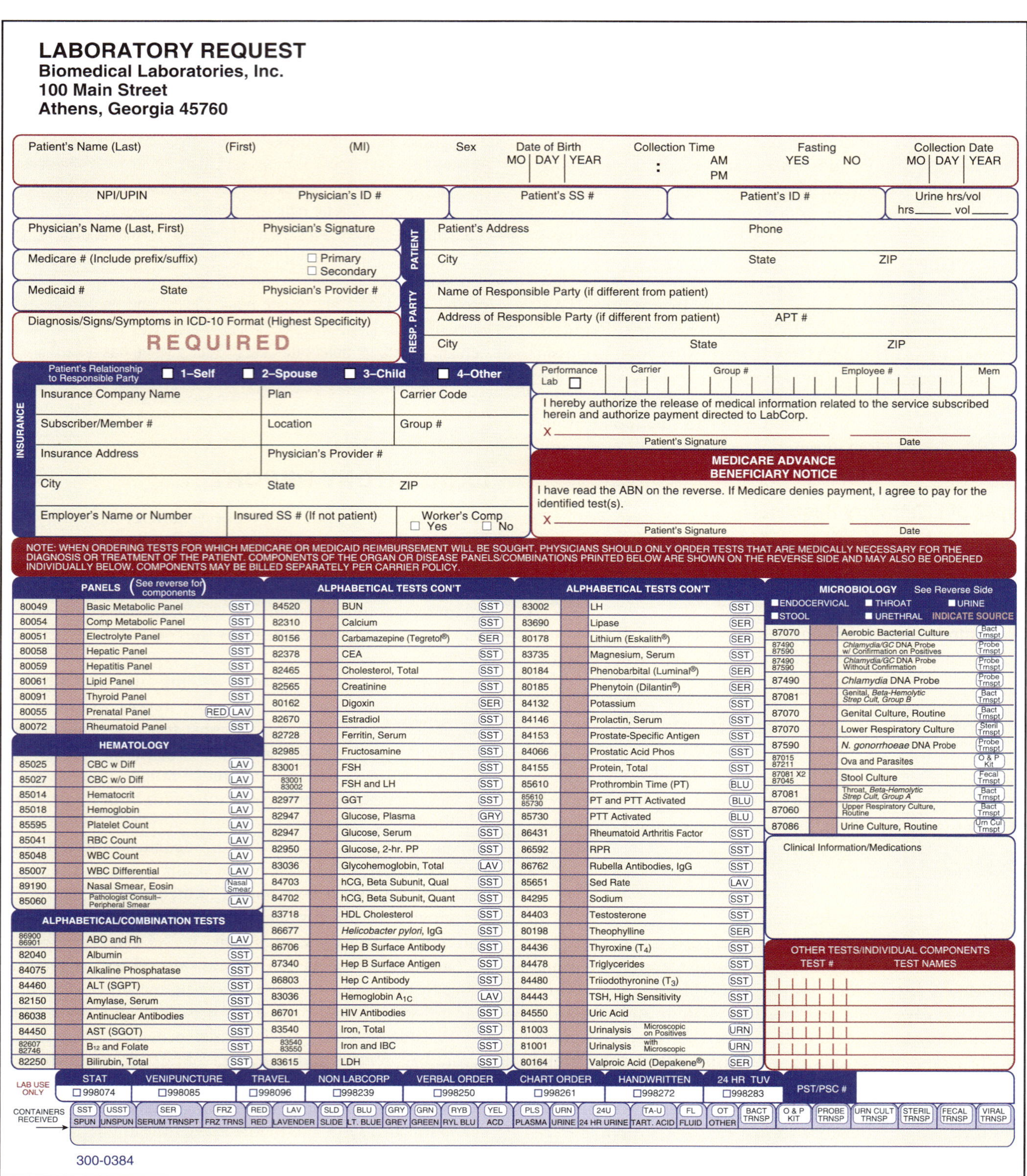

LABORATORY REQUEST
Biomedical Laboratories, Inc.
100 Main Street
Athens, Georgia 45760

Patient's Name (Last) (First) (MI) Sex | Date of Birth MO | DAY | YEAR | Collection Time : AM PM | Fasting YES NO | Collection Date MO | DAY | YEAR

NPI/UPIN | Physician's ID # | Patient's SS # | Patient's ID # | Urine hrs/vol hrs_____ vol_____

Physician's Name (Last, First) Physician's Signature

Medicare # (Include prefix/suffix) ☐ Primary ☐ Secondary

Medicaid # State Physician's Provider #

Diagnosis/Signs/Symptoms in ICD-10 Format (Highest Specificity)
REQUIRED

PATIENT: Patient's Address Phone
City State ZIP

RESP. PARTY: Name of Responsible Party (if different from patient)
Address of Responsible Party (if different from patient) APT #
City State ZIP

INSURANCE: Patient's Relationship to Responsible Party ■ 1–Self ■ 2–Spouse ■ 3–Child ■ 4–Other

Insurance Company Name | Plan | Carrier Code
Subscriber/Member # | Location | Group #
Insurance Address | Physician's Provider #
City | State | ZIP
Employer's Name or Number | Insured SS # (If not patient) | Worker's Comp ☐ Yes ☐ No

Performance Lab ☐ | Carrier | Group # | Employee # | Mem

I hereby authorize the release of medical information related to the service subscribed herein and authorize payment directed to LabCorp.
X________________ Patient's Signature ________ Date

MEDICARE ADVANCE BENEFICIARY NOTICE
I have read the ABN on the reverse. If Medicare denies payment, I agree to pay for the identified test(s).
X________________ Patient's Signature ________ Date

NOTE: WHEN ORDERING TESTS FOR WHICH MEDICARE OR MEDICAID REIMBURSEMENT WILL BE SOUGHT, PHYSICIANS SHOULD ONLY ORDER TESTS THAT ARE MEDICALLY NECESSARY FOR THE DIAGNOSIS OR TREATMENT OF THE PATIENT. COMPONENTS OF THE ORGAN OR DISEASE PANELS/COMBINATIONS PRINTED BELOW ARE SHOWN ON THE REVERSE SIDE AND MAY ALSO BE ORDERED INDIVIDUALLY BELOW. COMPONENTS MAY BE BILLED SEPARATELY PER CARRIER POLICY.

PANELS (See reverse for components)

Code	Test	Container
80049	Basic Metabolic Panel	SST
80054	Comp Metabolic Panel	SST
80051	Electrolyte Panel	SST
80058	Hepatic Panel	SST
80059	Hepatitis Panel	SST
80061	Lipid Panel	SST
80091	Thyroid Panel	SST
80055	Prenatal Panel	RED LAV
80072	Rheumatoid Panel	SST

HEMATOLOGY

Code	Test	Container
85025	CBC w Diff	LAV
85027	CBC w/o Diff	LAV
85014	Hematocrit	LAV
85018	Hemoglobin	LAV
85595	Platelet Count	LAV
85041	RBC Count	LAV
85048	WBC Count	LAV
85007	WBC Differential	LAV
89190	Nasal Smear, Eosin	Nasal Smear
85060	Pathologist Consult–Peripheral Smear	LAV

ALPHABETICAL/COMBINATION TESTS

Code	Test	Container
86900 86901	ABO and Rh	LAV
82040	Albumin	SST
84075	Alkaline Phosphatase	SST
84460	ALT (SGPT)	SST
82150	Amylase, Serum	SST
86038	Antinuclear Antibodies	SST
84450	AST (SGOT)	SST
82607 82746	B_{12} and Folate	SST
82250	Bilirubin, Total	SST

ALPHABETICAL TESTS CON'T

Code	Test	Container
84520	BUN	SST
82310	Calcium	SST
80156	Carbamazepine (Tegretol®)	SER
82378	CEA	SST
82465	Cholesterol, Total	SST
82565	Creatinine	SST
80162	Digoxin	SER
82670	Estradiol	SST
82728	Ferritin, Serum	SST
82985	Fructosamine	SST
83001	FSH	SST
83001 83002	FSH and LH	SST
82977	GGT	SST
82947	Glucose, Plasma	GRY
82947	Glucose, Serum	SST
82950	Glucose, 2-hr. PP	SST
83036	Glycohemoglobin, Total	LAV
84703	hCG, Beta Subunit, Qual	SST
84702	hCG, Beta Subunit, Quant	SST
83718	HDL Cholesterol	SST
86677	*Helicobacter pylori*, IgG	SST
86706	Hep B Surface Antibody	SST
87340	Hep B Surface Antigen	SST
86803	Hep C Antibody	SST
83036	Hemoglobin A_{1C}	LAV
86701	HIV Antibodies	SST
83540	Iron, Total	SST
83540 83550	Iron and IBC	SST
83615	LDH	SST

ALPHABETICAL TESTS CON'T

Code	Test	Container
83002	LH	SST
83690	Lipase	SER
80178	Lithium (Eskalith®)	SER
83735	Magnesium, Serum	SST
80184	Phenobarbital (Luminal®)	SER
80185	Phenytoin (Dilantin®)	SER
84132	Potassium	SST
84146	Prolactin, Serum	SST
84153	Prostate-Specific Antigen	SST
84066	Prostatic Acid Phos	SST
84155	Protein, Total	SST
85610	Prothrombin Time (PT)	BLU
85610 85730	PT and PTT Activated	BLU
85730	PTT Activated	BLU
86431	Rheumatoid Arthritis Factor	SST
86592	RPR	SST
86762	Rubella Antibodies, IgG	SST
85651	Sed Rate	LAV
84295	Sodium	SST
84403	Testosterone	SST
80198	Theophylline	SER
84436	Thyroxine (T_4)	SST
84478	Triglycerides	SST
84480	Triiodothyronine (T_3)	SST
84443	TSH, High Sensitivity	SST
84550	Uric Acid	SST
81003	Urinalysis Microscopic on Positives	URN
81001	Urinalysis with Microscopic	URN
80164	Valproic Acid (Depakene®)	SER

MICROBIOLOGY See Reverse Side

■ ENDOCERVICAL ■ THROAT ■ URINE ■ STOOL ■ URETHRAL INDICATE SOURCE

Code	Test	Container
87070	Aerobic Bacterial Culture	Bact Trnspt
87490 87590	*Chlamydia/GC* DNA Probe w/ Confirmation on Positives	Probe Trnspt
87490 87590	*Chlamydia/GC* DNA Probe Without Confirmation	Probe Trnspt
87490	*Chlamydia* DNA Probe	Probe Trnspt
87081	Genital, *Beta-Hemolytic Strep Cult, Group B*	Bact Trnspt
87070	Genital Culture, Routine	Bact Trnspt
87070	Lower Respiratory Culture	Steril Trnspt
87590	*N. gonorrhoeae* DNA Probe	Probe Trnspt
87015 87211	Ova and Parasites	O & P Kit
87081 X2 87045	Stool Culture	Fecal Trnspt
87081	Throat, *Beta-Hemolytic Strep Cult, Group A*	Bact Trnspt
87060	Upper Respiratory Culture, Routine	Bact Trnspt
87086	Urine Culture, Routine	Urn Cul Trnspt

Clinical Information/Medications

OTHER TESTS/INDIVIDUAL COMPONENTS
TEST # | TEST NAMES

LAB USE ONLY

STAT	VENIPUNCTURE	TRAVEL	NON LABCORP	VERBAL ORDER	CHART ORDER	HANDWRITTEN	24 HR TUV	PST/PSC #
☐998074	☐998085	☐998096	☐998239	☐998250	☐998261	☐998272	☐998283	

CONTAINERS RECEIVED →

SST	USST	SER	FRZ	RED	LAV	SLD	BLU	GRY	GRN	RYB	YEL	PLS	URN	24U	TA-U	FL	OT	BACT TRNSP	O & P KIT	PROBE TRNSP	URN CULT TRNSP	STERIL TRNSP	FECAL TRNSP	VIRAL TRNSP
SPUN	UNSPUN	SERUM TRNSPT	FRZ TRNS	RED	LAVENDER	SLIDE	LT. BLUE	GREY	GREEN	RYL BLU	ACD	PLASMA	URINE	24 HR URINE	TART. ACID	FLUID	OTHER							

300-0384

Fig. 29.4 Preprinted laboratory request form.

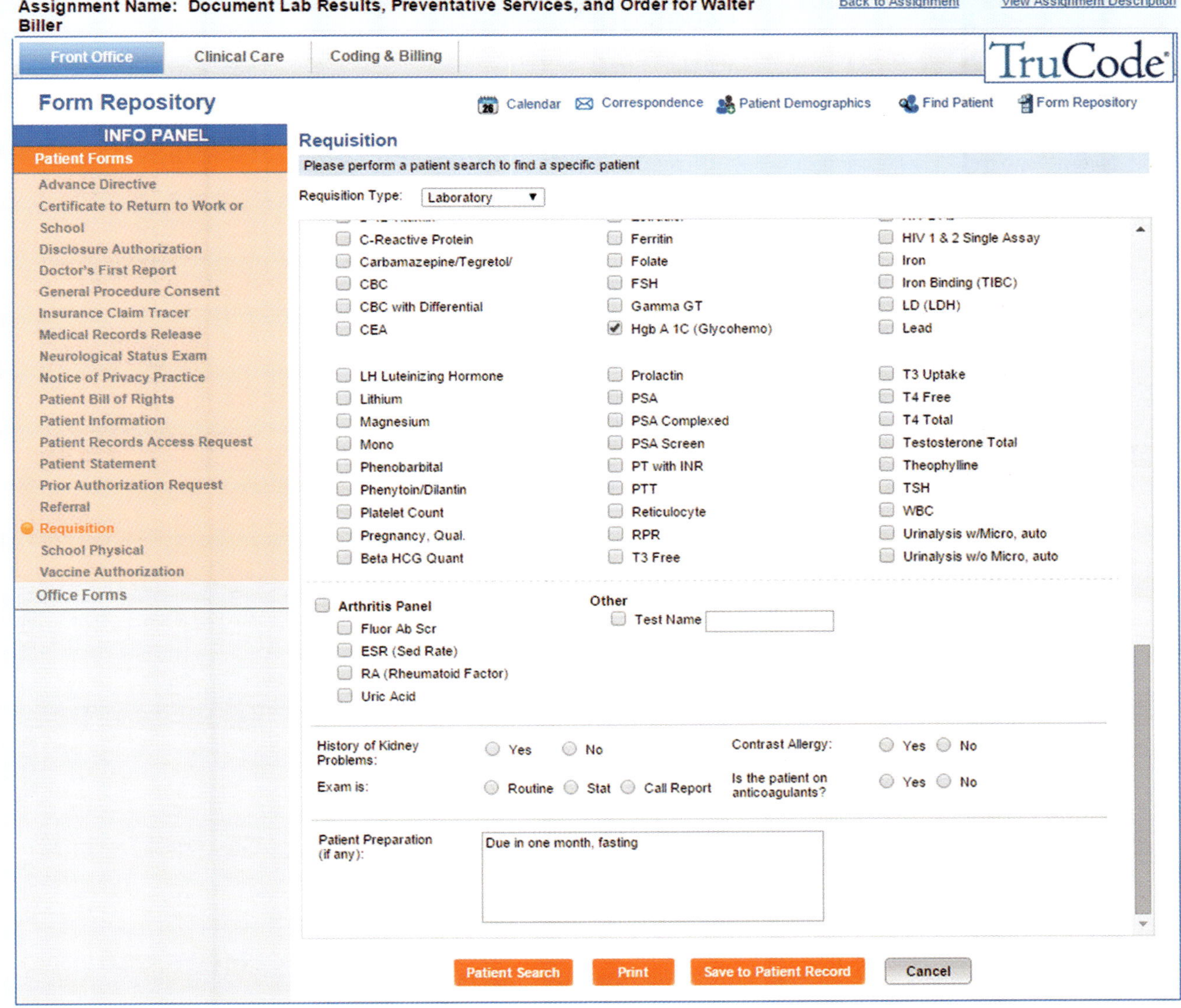

Fig. 29.5 Electronic laboratory request computer entry screen.

Parts of a Laboratory Report

A laboratory report includes the following information:

1. Name and address of the laboratory
2. Name and address of the medical office
3. Name of the provider ordering the test(s)
4. Patient's name, address, phone number, and laboratory identification number
5. Patient's date of birth, age, and sex
6. Laboratory specimen accession number
7. Date and time of specimen collection
8. Fasting or nonfasting specimen
9. Date and time the specimen was received by the laboratory
10. Date and time the results were reported by the laboratory
11. Name of the laboratory test(s) ordered
12. Test results
13. Reference range for each test performed
14. Identification of test results outside of the reference range

Electronic Transmission of Laboratory Reports

Computer-generated laboratory reports are often transmitted electronically from the laboratory computer system to the medical office computer system. The laboratory report is placed in the provider's "electronic review box" for review. After reviewing the report the provider signs it with an electronic signature. The report is then automatically filed in the patient's electronic health record (EHR).

Computer-generated laboratory reports stored in an EHR can be accessed by the computer and manipulated according to the needs of the provider. Examples include the following:

- Laboratory reports can be displayed in chronological order or reverse-chronological order.
- Current and previous results for a specific test (or tests) can be accessed by the computer and displayed in chronological order. This permits the provider to compare changes in test results over a period of time.

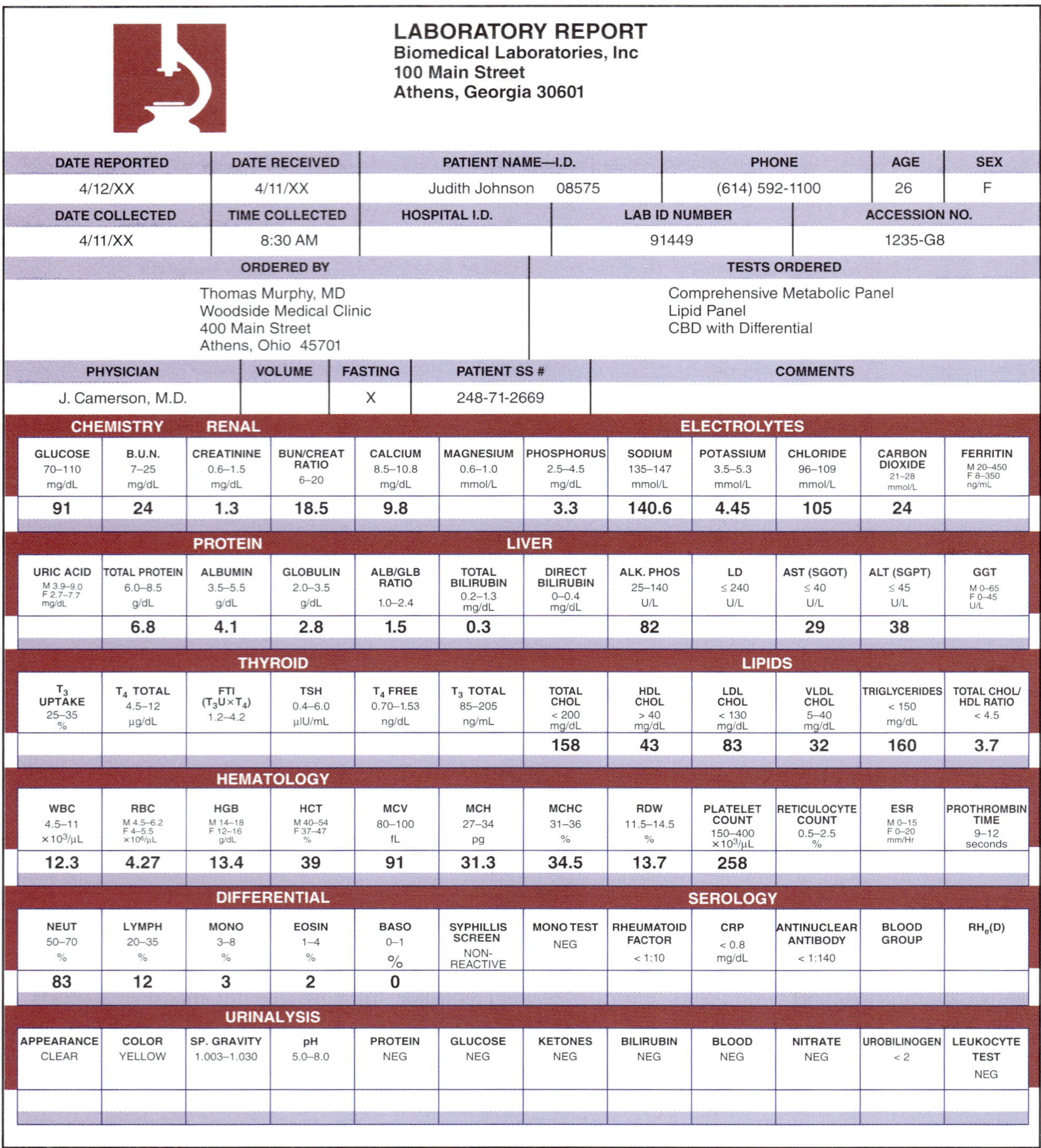

LABORATORY REPORT
Biomedical Laboratories, Inc
100 Main Street
Athens, Georgia 30601

DATE REPORTED	DATE RECEIVED	PATIENT NAME—I.D.	PHONE	AGE	SEX
4/12/XX	4/11/XX	Judith Johnson 08575	(614) 592-1100	26	F

DATE COLLECTED	TIME COLLECTED	HOSPITAL I.D.	LAB ID NUMBER	ACCESSION NO.
4/11/XX	8:30 AM		91449	1235-G8

ORDERED BY	TESTS ORDERED
Thomas Murphy, MD Woodside Medical Clinic 400 Main Street Athens, Ohio 45701	Comprehensive Metabolic Panel Lipid Panel CBD with Differential

PHYSICIAN	VOLUME	FASTING	PATIENT SS #	COMMENTS
J. Camerson, M.D.		X	248-71-2669	

CHEMISTRY / RENAL / ELECTROLYTES

GLUCOSE	B.U.N.	CREATININE	BUN/CREAT RATIO	CALCIUM	MAGNESIUM	PHOSPHORUS	SODIUM	POTASSIUM	CHLORIDE	CARBON DIOXIDE	FERRITIN
70–110 mg/dL	7–25 mg/dL	0.6–1.5 mg/dL	6–20	8.5–10.8 mg/dL	0.6–1.0 mmol/L	2.5–4.5 mg/dL	135–147 mmol/L	3.5–5.3 mmol/L	96–109 mmol/L	21–28 mmol/L	M 20–450 F 8–350 ng/mL
91	24	1.3	18.5	9.8		3.3	140.6	4.45	105	24	

PROTEIN / LIVER

URIC ACID	TOTAL PROTEIN	ALBUMIN	GLOBULIN	ALB/GLB RATIO	TOTAL BILIRUBIN	DIRECT BILIRUBIN	ALK. PHOS	LD	AST (SGOT)	ALT (SGPT)	GGT
M 3.9–9.0 F 2.7–7.7 mg/dL	6.0–8.5 g/dL	3.5–5.5 g/dL	2.0–3.5 g/dL	1.0–2.4	0.2–1.3 mg/dL	0–0.4 mg/dL	25–140 U/L	≤ 240 U/L	≤ 40 U/L	≤ 45 U/L	M 0–65 F 0–45 U/L
	6.8	4.1	2.8	1.5	0.3		82		29	38	

THYROID / LIPIDS

T_3 UPTAKE	T_4 TOTAL	FTI ($T_3U \times T_4$)	TSH	T_4 FREE	T_3 TOTAL	TOTAL CHOL	HDL CHOL	LDL CHOL	VLDL CHOL	TRIGLYCERIDES	TOTAL CHOL/ HDL RATIO
25–35 %	4.5–12 µg/dL	1.2–4.2	0.4–6.0 µIU/mL	0.70–1.53 ng/dL	85–205 ng/mL	< 200 mg/dL	> 40 mg/dL	< 130 mg/dL	5–40 mg/dL	< 150 mg/dL	< 4.5
						158	43	83	32	160	3.7

HEMATOLOGY

WBC	RBC	HGB	HCT	MCV	MCH	MCHC	RDW	PLATELET COUNT	RETICULOCYTE COUNT	ESR	PROTHROMBIN TIME
4.5–11 $\times 10^3/\mu L$	M 4.5–6.2 F 4–5.5 $\times 10^6/\mu L$	M 14–18 F 12–16 g/dL	M 40–54 F 37–47 %	80–100 fL	27–34 pg	31–36 %	11.5–14.5 %	150–400 $\times 10^3/\mu L$	0.5–2.5 %	M 0–15 F 0–20 mm/Hr	9–12 seconds
12.3	4.27	13.4	39	91	31.3	34.5	13.7	258			

DIFFERENTIAL / SEROLOGY

NEUT	LYMPH	MONO	EOSIN	BASO	SYPHILLIS SCREEN	MONO TEST	RHEUMATOID FACTOR	CRP	ANTINUCLEAR ANTIBODY	BLOOD GROUP	$RH_o(D)$
50–70 %	20–35 %	3–8 %	1–4 %	0–1 %	NON-REACTIVE	NEG	< 1:10	< 0.8 mg/dL	< 1:140		
83	12	3	2	0							

URINALYSIS

APPEARANCE	COLOR	SP. GRAVITY	pH	PROTEIN	GLUCOSE	KETONES	BILIRUBIN	BLOOD	NITRATE	UROBILINOGEN	LEUKOCYTE TEST
CLEAR	YELLOW	1.003–1.030	5.0–8.0	NEG	NEG	NEG	NEG	NEG	NEG	< 2	NEG

Fig. 29.6 Laboratory report form.

- Current and previous test results can be accessed by the computer and plotted graphically on a flowsheet in chronological order. This permits an abnormal trend to be visually identified, so that appropriate action can be taken. Fig. 29.8 illustrates a flow sheet of hemoglobin test results.

If the medical office is not networked through computers with an outside laboratory, the laboratory reports received by the office through other means (e.g., faxed) must be scanned into the computer. A scanned report has some limitations. The computer can display the report, but the data on the report cannot be accessed or manipulated by the computer. Because of this, laboratory data cannot be used for many of the functions previously described. For example, the data on scanned reports cannot be accessed and incorporated into a flowsheet for trend analysis.

Laboratory Report
Comprehensive Metabolic Panel

PATIENT		ORDERED BY	RESULTS PROVIDED BY
Colbert, Jason K. 2963 Flint Dr. S Clearwater, FL 33759 PH: 740-541-3575	ID #: 336879 DOB: 4/28/1970 AGE: 53 SEX: M	Thomas Murphy, MD Pinellas Medical Office 3477 Arrowhead Ave Clearwater, FL 33759	Medical Center Laboratory 33 West Main St Clearwater, FL 33759

SPECIMEN COLL. DATE	11/25/20XX	FASTING/NONFASTING	Fasting
SPECIMEN COLL. TIME	08:00 am	ACCESSION NUMBER	3380837
SPECIMEN RECEIVED DATE/TIME	11/25/20XX 05:30 pm	LAB ID NUMBER	773978
RESULTS REPORTED DATE/TIME	11/26/20XX 10:00 am	TEST(S) ORDERED	CPT: 80053 Comprehensive Metabolic Panel

TEST	RESULT	REFERENCE RANGE	UNITS	FLAG
Albumin	**3.1**	**3.5-5.2**	**g/dL**	**L**
Alanine Aminotransferase (ALT)	16	0-45	u/L	
Alkaline Phosphastase (ALP)	81	25-140	u/L	
Aspartate Aminotransferase (AST)	9	0-40	u/L	
Bilirubin, Total	0.6	0.3-1.2	mg/dL	
Urea Nitrogen (BUN)	**28**	**7-25**	**mg/dL**	**H**
Calcium	9.3	8.5-10.2	mg/dL	
Carbon Dioxide	29.6	21.0-32.0	mEq/L	
Chloride	102.9	98.0-107.0	mmol/L	
Creatinine	**1.35**	**0.60-1.10**	**mg/dL**	**H**
Glucose	90	70-99	mg/dL	
Potassium	4.12	3.50-5.10	mmol/L	
Protein, Total	6.6	6.4-8.3	g/dL	
Sodium	139.1	136.0-145.0	mmol/L	

Fig. 29.7 Computer-generated laboratory report.

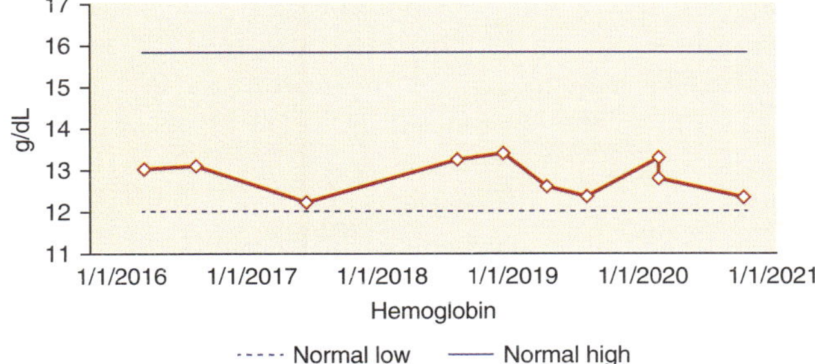

Fig. 29.8 Hemoglobin flowsheet generated by a computer.

SPECIMEN LABEL

Each specimen must be properly identified with a label before it is transported to an outside laboratory. Specimen labeling errors that are not discovered may cause misinterpretation of test results leading to an incorrect diagnosis and unnecessary treatment.

Two unique identifiers must be used to label each specimen. A **unique identifier** is information directly associated with an individual that reliably identifies the individual as the person for whom the service or treatment is intended. The most common identifiers used to label specimens are the patient's full legal name and date of birth. It is important to label the specimen container itself and not the lid of the container or the biohazard specimen bag used to transport the specimen.

Handwritten Label

A specimen can be labeled by handwriting the information on the label using a ball point pen (do not use a felt-tipped pen). The label information should include the patient's full legal name and date of birth, the date and time of collection, the initials of the individual collecting the specimen, and

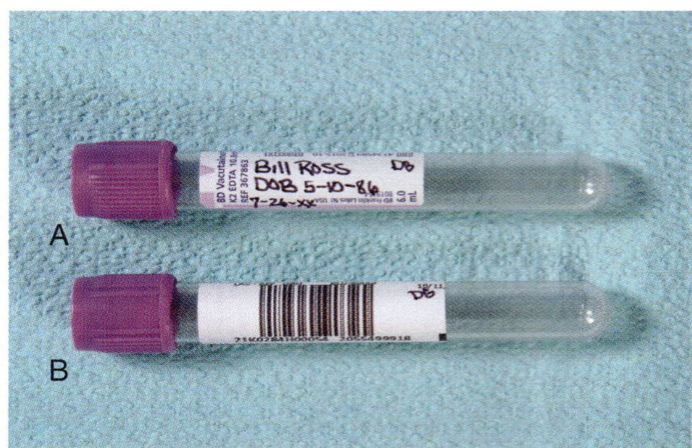

Fig. 29.9 **A**, Handwritten specimen label. **B**, Computer-generated barcode specimen label.

any other information required by the laboratory (e.g., the source of a microbiologic specimen). It is important to print legibly and to make certain that the information is accurate (Fig. 29.9A).

Barcode Label

As part of the electronic laboratory request process, the medical office computer also prints out custom barcode labels. The specimen is identified by properly attaching the adhesive barcode label to the specimen container (Fig. 29.9B). Laboratory analyzers incorporate a barcode reader that is able to read the information on the barcode necessary for testing the specimen and generating test results. To enable the barcode reader to read the label, it must be aligned in a straight (not diagonal) position on the specimen container with no wrinkles, folds, or tears. Barcode labels result in faster processing of the specimen once it arrives at the outside laboratory leading to a faster turnaround time for test results.

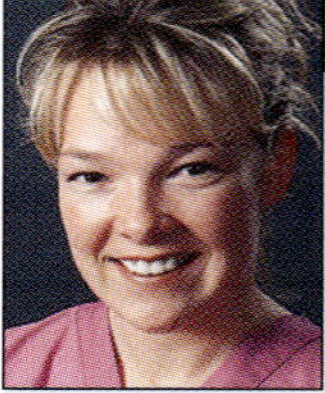

Putting It All Into Practice

My name is Korey, and I am employed by a group of physicians in a family practice medical office. Some of my duties include showing patients to examining rooms, taking vital signs, administering medication, and performing CLIA-waived laboratory tests. I have found that being a medical assistant has been challenging and rewarding, and I wish you the best of luck in reaching your goals.

When I first started working as a practicing medical assistant, I had a challenging venipuncture experience. The patient was a kind and personable 74-year-old man with hardening of the arteries. I tried to obtain the blood specimen from his arm but was not successful. The patient was calm and was not bothered at all by the unsuccessful stick. He said that it was hard to draw blood on him and to go ahead and try again. I decided to try taking the blood from a vein on the back of his hand with a butterfly setup. To my relief, I obtained the blood specimen. I think that I was more nervous about this experience than the patient was. It is important to remain calm on the outside around patients even if you are nervous on the inside. ■

PATIENT INSTRUCTIONS

The medical assistant is often responsible for providing instructions to a patient for a laboratory test ordered for that patient. The medical assistant should inform the patient of the name and purpose of the test, how to prepare for the test, and how and when to expect the test results. After the instructions have been explained, the medical assistant should verify that the patient understands them and offer to answer any questions. It also is advisable to provide the patient with a written information sheet (Fig. 29.10) to serve as a reference, should the patient forget some of the information after leaving the medical office.

Some laboratory tests require that the patient remain at the collection site for a specified period of time; an example of this is the OGTT, which requires several hours for the collection of multiple, timed specimens. The patient should be told in advance of the time requirement, so that any necessary arrangements can be made with an employer or child care provider.

There are some specimens that need to be collected at home by the patient. For example, if a first-voided morning urine specimen is necessary for a laboratory test, the medical assistant must provide the patient with the appropriate specimen container and instruct the patient in the proper collection, handling, and storage of the specimen until it reaches the medical office. It also is advisable to provide the patient with a written information sheet to serve as a reference, should the patient forget some of the information after leaving the medical office. The instructions should be available in the languages used in the community served by the medical office.

PATIENT PREPARATION

Advance patient preparation is necessary for some laboratory tests to obtain a high-quality specimen suitable for testing. Factors such as food and fluid consumption, medication, activity, alcohol consumption, and time of day may affect the results of certain tests. The medical assistant should make sure to explain the reason for the advance preparation, so the patient will be more likely to comply with the necessary preparation. A specimen obtained from a patient who has not prepared properly may invalidate the test results and necessitate calling the patient back to collect the specimen again.

The type of preparation necessary for a particular test depends on the test ordered. If an outside laboratory is performing the test, the patient preparation can be found in the laboratory test directory. If the test is performed in the POL, the medical assistant should consult the manufacturer's instructions that accompany the laboratory test to obtain this information. Advance patient preparation usually consists of fasting and medication restrictions, which are described next in more detail.

ORAL GLUCOSE TOLERANCE TEST
Patient Information Sheet

General information
Your provider has ordered an oral glucose tolerance test (OGTT) for you. The purpose of this test is to see how well your body processes glucose (sugar). Glucose is the primary source of energy for your body. The OGTT is primarily used for diagnosis of prediabetes and diabetes and to screen pregnant women for gestational diabetes.

Preparation for the Test
It is very important that you prepare properly to ensure accurate test results.
1. For 3 days prior to the test you should consume a high-carbohydrate diet consisting of at least 150 grams of carbohydrate each day. High carbohydrate foods include: bread, pasta, cereal, rice, potatoes, and crackers.
2. Do NOT drink or eat anything except water for 9 –12 h before the test.
3. Your test is performed in the morning because of the overnight fast.
4. Your provider will discuss what medication (if any) to discontinue before the test.
5. You will need to stay at the testing facility for the duration of the collection procedure which is approximately 2–3 h.
6. You may want to bring something to read or work on during your wait at the facility.

Collection Procedure
The collection procedure includes the following:
1. After arrival, a fasting blood specimen will be collected.
2. Following this, you will be given a very sweet glucose solution to drink. You must drink all of the glucose solution within a 5-min period of time. Some people experience a brief period of nausea after consuming the solution.
3. A blood specimen will be collected 60 min after drinking the glucose solution.
4. Another specimen will be collected 120 min (2 h) after drinking the glucose solution.
5. Another specimen may be collected 180 min (3 h) after drinking the glucose solution.

Testing Information
It is important to adhere to the following guidelines to ensure accurate test results.
1. Remain quietly seated during the testing period and do not leave the testing facility. Any form of exercise should be avoided because it can affect the test results.
2. Do not eat or drink anything except small sips of water during the collection procedure.
3. Do not smoke or chew gum during the collection procedure.
4. Following the procedure, you can eat and drink as usual and resume your normal activities.

Normal Side Effects
During the procedure, you may experience some normal side effects such as weakness, a feeling of faintness, or perspiration. They are caused by a decrease in your body's glucose level as insulin is secreted in response to the glucose solution.

Fig. 29.10 Patient information sheet for an oral glucose tolerance test.

Fasting

Some blood specimens require the patient to fast before collection. **Fasting** involves abstaining from food and fluids (except water) for a specified period of time before the collection of the specimen (usually 8–12 hours) to allow food and fluid from the previous meal to be completely digested and absorbed. Fasting specimens are usually collected in the morning which causes the least amount of inconvenience to the patient in terms of abstaining from food and fluid.

Fasting is an important component of certain laboratory tests. The composition of blood is altered by the consumption of food and fluid because digested food and fluid are absorbed into the circulatory system, changing the results of certain laboratory tests. Food intake causes fasting blood glucose (FBG) and triglycerides tests to yield falsely-high results. Any laboratory panel including the test (e.g., comprehensive metabolic panel) requires the patient to fast before the specimen is collected.

The medical assistant must give detailed instructions to the patient, ensuring that the patient understands that fasting includes abstaining from food and fluid for the specified period of time. The patient should be told, however, that it is permissible—in fact, advisable—to drink water because dehydration caused by water abstinence can alter certain test results.

Medication Restrictions

Medication may affect the physical and chemical characteristics of body substances and lead to inaccurate test results. The provider may want the patient to stop taking a medication that might interfere with the test results for a certain period of time before the collection of the specimen. The medical assistant should instruct the patient concerning the name of the medication to discontinue, the period of time to discontinue it, and the reason for discontinuing it.

What Would You Do? What Would You *Not* Do?

Case Study 2

Kathleen O'Leary will be coming to the medical office today for a follow-up appointment. She was seen last week complaining of fatigue, shortness of breath, weight loss, insomnia, and joint pain. The provider gives Kathleen a laboratory request to have her blood drawn and tested at an outside laboratory. The provider ordered a CBC with differential and a comprehensive metabolic panel. A review of Kathleen's EHR shows that she did not get her lab testing done. Kathleen is contacted by phone; she says she knows she should have gone to the laboratory to have her blood drawn, but she is afraid of needles and panics at the sight of blood. She says that the last time she had her blood drawn she started feeling warm and lightheaded and had to lie down and was embarrassed by that. Kathleen says she also is worried the laboratory results might show something is wrong with her. She is thinking of not coming for her appointment today with the hope that she starts feeling better on her own. ■

SPECIMEN COLLECTION FOR TRANSPORT TO AN OUTSIDE LABORATORY

There are a number of steps involved in the collection and handling of a specimen for transport to an outside laboratory. These steps include patient preparation, collecting and processing the specimen, and preparing and storing the specimen for transport to the laboratory. The most important goal of specimen collection is to provide the laboratory with a sample that is as biologically representative as possible of the body substance collected. If the specimen is collected or handled improperly, the integrity of the specimen may be adversely affected. This may cause inaccurate test results and interfere with the accurate diagnosis and treatment of the patient's condition.

Once the specimen arrives at the outside laboratory, it is assigned an accession number. The purpose of an accession number is to provide positive identification of each specimen within the laboratory and to allow easy access to laboratory records should a test result need to be located again. If the provider desires to have the laboratory test repeated, the accession number (printed on the laboratory report) must be entered on the laboratory request.

CAUSES FOR REJECTION OF A SPECIMEN

It may not be possible to test a specimen if the specimen requirements have not been met; in these cases, the outside laboratory rejects the specimen. Sometimes the situation can be rectified, such as when a laboratory request is missing and the medical office is able to quickly supply it to the laboratory. When the situation cannot be rectified, another specimen must be collected from the patient, such as when an insufficient amount of specimen was submitted. Causes of specimen rejection by an outside laboratory include the following:

- No label on the specimen container or incorrect information on the specimen label
- Specimen label information and information on the lab request do not match
- Specimen is received without a laboratory request
- Specimen is collected in the wrong container or in a container past its expiration date
- Insufficient type or amount of specimen is submitted for the test requested
- Hemolyzed serum or plasma specimen is submitted
- Leakage of the specimen container
- Damaged specimen container (broken, chipped, or cracked)
- Improper storage of the specimen
- Significant time delay between specimen collection and receipt of the specimen by the laboratory

GUIDELINES FOR SPECIMEN COLLECTION AND HANDLING

Specific guidelines must be followed when collecting a specimen for transport to an outside laboratory. The medical assistant is responsible for performing the following:

1. *Provide patient instructions.* Explain the patient instructions thoroughly (e.g.; patient preparation), and provide the patient with written instructions to take home as a reference. Notify the patient of the time to report to the medical office for the specimen collection.
2. *Review the collection and handling requirements.* Review the collection and handling requirements in the laboratory test directory for the test(s) ordered by the provider. A review of the requirements beforehand prevents errors in collection and handling of the specimen. Contact the outside laboratory if you have any questions regarding any aspect of collection procedure. Specimen requirements include the following:
   a. Collection materials required
   b. Type of specimen to be collected (e.g., whole blood, serum, urine)
   c. Amount of the specimen needed to perform the laboratory test
   d. Procedure to follow to collect the specimen
   e. Proper handling and storage of the specimen awaiting transport
3. *Identify the patient.* Identify the patient by asking the patient to state their full name and date of birth. Compare this information with the demographic data in the patient's medical record. The patient should *not* be asked whether he or she is a certain patient. For example, the patient should not be asked, "Are you Brad Thompson?" The patient may not hear this information correctly or may not be paying attention and may answer in the affirmative even if he is not that patient. Collecting a specimen

on the wrong patient by mistake may lead to an inaccurate diagnosis and the wrong treatment.

4. *Determine whether the patient has prepared properly.* If the patient was required to prepare for the test, determine whether this was performed properly. If the patient has not prepared properly, inform the provider. The provider may want the patient to prepare properly and return to the medical office. If the provider wants to go ahead with the collection, indicate this information on the laboratory request. For example, if the patient did not fast for a FBG, indicate "nonfasting specimen" on the laboratory request.
5. *Assemble the equipment and supplies.* Assemble the appropriate equipment and supplies specified in the laboratory test directory. Substituting collection containers may not yield the proper type of specimen required, which can affect the test results. Check each container before use to ensure it is not broken, chipped, cracked, or otherwise damaged. Damaged containers are unsuitable for specimen collection and should be discarded. Check the expiration date on the container (Fig. 29.11). Outdated specimen containers may affect the accuracy of the test results.
6. *Complete a laboratory request.* The request may be a preprinted request or an electronic request. The completed request provides the outside laboratory with the information necessary to test the specimen.
7. *Label the specimen container.* Properly label each specimen container to prevent a mix-up of specimens. At a minimum, the label should include the patient's full legal name, date of birth, and the date and time of collection of the specimen. (*Note:* The medical assistant should follow the medical office policy as to when the container should be labeled. Some offices prefer that the container be labeled *before* the specimen is collected; other offices want the container to be labeled *after* the specimen is collected.)
8. *Collect the specimen.* Proper collection of the specimen provides the outside laboratory with a biologically representative sample of the body substance collected. The specimen should be collected according to the following guidelines:
   a. Adhere to the OSHA Bloodborne Pathogens Standards (see Chapter 17) when collecting and handling the specimen to prevent an exposure incident (Fig. 29.12).
   b. Collect the specimen according to the requirements specified in the laboratory directory.
   c. Collect the proper type of specimen (e.g. whole blood, serum, plasma, and urine).
   d. Collect the proper amount of specimen. It is critical that an adequate amount of specimen be submitted for analysis. If the amount of the specimen is insufficient to perform the test(s), a report is sent to the medical office indicating QNS (quantity not sufficient). This situation warrants calling the patient back for the collection of another specimen.
   e. Securely tighten the lids on specimen containers to prevent leakage of the specimen during storage and transport.
   f. Properly discard used collection materials in a biohazard waste container.
9. *Process the specimen.* Process the specimen according to the requirements specified in the laboratory directory. For example, a serum specimen collected in a *serum separator tube (SST)* must be centrifuged to separate the serum from the cells with a gel barrier, as shown in Fig. 29.13. **Serum** is the clear, straw-colored part of the blood that remains after the solid elements and the clotting factor fibrinogen have been separated out of it.
10. *Prepare and store the specimen for transport.* It is important to store the specimen under environmental conditions that will not affect the integrity of the specimen and to transport the specimen to an outside laboratory in a timely manner as follows:
    a. Place the specimen in a biohazard specimen bag and seal the bag (Fig. 29.14). Biohazard bags prevent contamination of the specimen and protect healthcare workers and laboratory couriers from the possibility of an exposure incident.

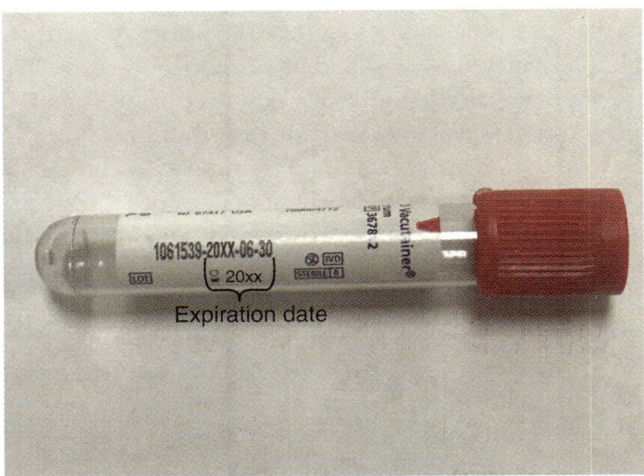

Fig. 29.11 Blood tube showing expiration date.

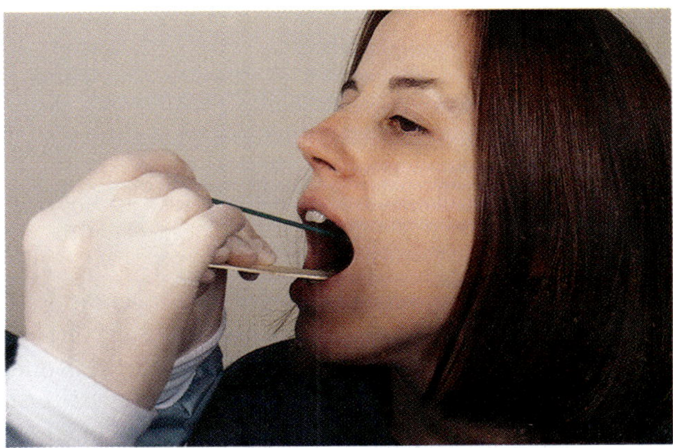
Fig. 29.12 The OSHA Standard must be followed during specimen collection.

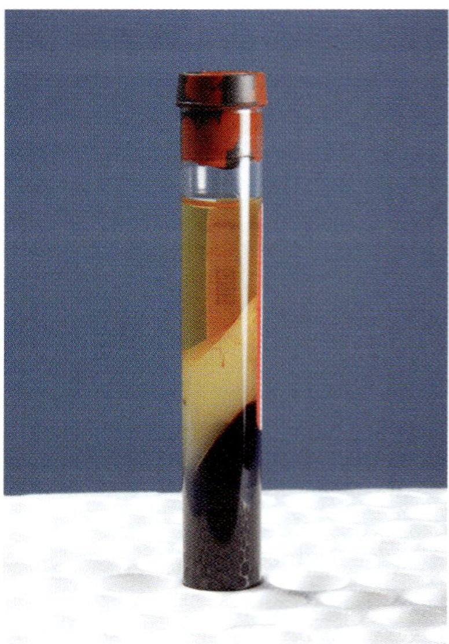

Fig. 29.13 Serum specimen in a serum separator tube (SST) that has been centrifuged.

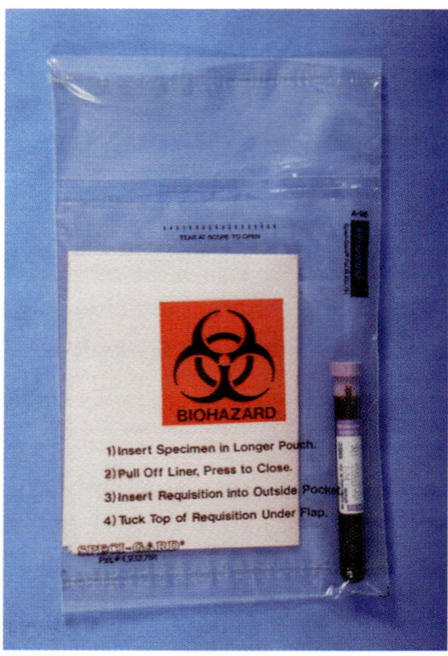

Fig. 29.14 Biohazard specimen bag.

b. Depending on the policy of the outside laboratory, transmit the laboratory request electronically and/or place the request in the outside pocket of the biohazard specimen bag.

c. Properly store specimens awaiting pickup following the storage requirements in the laboratory directory. Many specimens can be stored at RT while others may need to be refrigerated or frozen. Definitions of storage temperatures are outlined in Box 29.1. An outside laboratory may provide the medical office with a large lockable container, known as a *lockbox*, for storing specimens awaiting pickup. The laboratory provides instructions on the proper placement and storage of specimens in the lockbox.

BOX 29.1 Specimen Storage Temperatures

Storage Temperature	Temperature Range
Room temperature (RT)	59° F to 86° F (15° C to 30° C)
Refrigerated	36° F to 46° F (2° C to 8° C)
Frozen	-4° F or below (-20° C or below)

CLINICAL LABORATORY IMPROVEMENT AMENDMENTS

As previously discussed, the CLIA regulations were developed by the federal government to improve the quality of laboratory testing in the United States to ensure accurate and reliable test results. The CLIA regulations govern all facilities that perform laboratory tests for health assessment or for the diagnosis, prevention, or treatment of disease such as hospital and independent laboratories, medical offices, health departments, and nursing homes.

The Centers for Medicare and Medicaid Services (CMS) is a division of the Department of Health and Human Services (HHS). The CMS is responsible for regulating and operating the CLIA program. In addition to following CLIA regulations, a clinical laboratory must also be in compliance with all other federal, state, and local legislation such as the OSHA Standard.

CATEGORIES OF TESTS

CLIA establishes three categories of laboratory tests based on the complexity of the test method: basically, the more complex the test method, the more stringent the CLIA regulations. These three categories include waived tests, moderate complexity tests, and high complexity tests, which are described as follows.

CLIA-Waived Tests

A CLIA-waived test is a laboratory test that has been determined to be a simple procedure that is easy to perform and has a low risk of erroneous test results. Waived tests also include tests that have been approved for use by patients at home (e.g., urine pregnancy test). POLs that perform only waived tests must apply for a CLIA certificate of waiver (CW) from CMS which must be renewed every two years. POLs holding a CW are exempt from most of the CLIA regulations but are still expected to adhere to good laboratory practices. CLIA requires that the manufacturer's instructions that accompany the test system be followed *exactly* which includes the following:

- Proper storage of the test system
- Adherence to expiration dates
- Proper collection and handling of the specimen
- Performance of quality control procedures
- Proper testing of the specimen
- Correct interpretation of test results
- Accurate documentation of test results

CLIA-Nonwaived Tests

Laboratories performing nonwaived tests must be certified by CLIA and adhere to the CLIA regulations. These regulations include the following: proper educational and training qualifications for laboratory personnel; participation in a proficiency testing program; procedures to ensure proper test performance and accurate test results; an overall plan to monitor the quality of the laboratory's operation; and unannounced on-site inspections by CMS every 2 years. Nonwaived tests include moderate complexity and high complexity tests described as follows.

Moderate Complexity Tests

Moderate complexity tests account for 75% of the estimated 7 to 10 billion laboratory tests performed in the United States each year. Most of these tests are performed by hospital and independent laboratories on highly sophisticated clinical laboratory equipment. Moderate complexity tests include electrolyte profiles, chemistry profiles, CBC, drug screens, and automated immunoassays. Some medical office providers perform moderate complexity tests known as *provider-performed microscopy* (PPM) procedures, which involve the examination of a specimen under the microscope. An example of a PPM procedure is the microscopic analysis of urine sediment. PPM procedures are a subcategory of the moderate complexity test category and must be performed by an individual with the proper training and skill qualifications, such as a medical office provider. A CLIA certificate is required for PPM procedures and the CLIA regulations must be followed, however the POL is exempt from on-site inspections.

High Complexity Tests

High complexity tests are those that require the expertise of a clinical laboratory professional such as a pathologist. Examples include cytology (e.g. Pap test), immunohistochemistry, peripheral blood smears, flow cytometry, gel electrophoresis, and most molecular diagnostic tests.

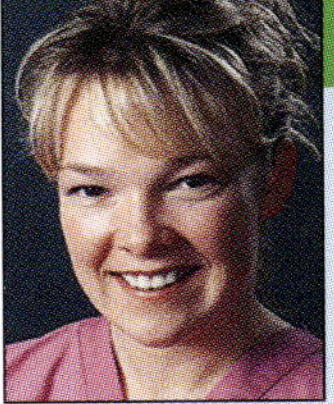

Memories *from* Practicum

Korey: One of my most difficult situations as a medical assisting student was taking the temperature of a patient who started to have a seizure. I was scared because I was only a student, and I had never been in a situation like that before. I knew I had to act immediately, and luckily one of the certified medical assistants (CMA [AAMA]) was nearby. We immediately put the patient on the floor and moved things away from him to keep him from hurting himself. We then notified the physician, who was with a patient in another examining room. The seizure lasted only about 4 minutes, and the patient was fine. The CMA (AAMA) told me that the patient had a history of seizures and that I did a good job of staying calm. That surely was a difficult but valuable learning experience for me. ■

CLIA-WAIVED TESTS IN THE POL

Approximately 1400 CLIA-waived tests are commercially available that test for 120 different analytes. An **analyte** is a body substance that is being identified or measured by a laboratory test, such as glucose, hemoglobin, and group A streptococci. The number of waived tests is expected to increase as new technology becomes available.

CLIA-waived tests that are performed most frequently in the POL include the following:

- **Urine and Fecal Tests**
  - Urinalysis test (using a reagent strip or a CLIA-waived urine chemistry analyzer)
  - CLIA-waived urine drug test
  - Urine pregnancy test with visual color comparisons
  - Fecal occult blood test
- **Hematology Tests**
  - Hemoglobin test (using a CLIA-waived analyzer)
  - Spun microhematocrit test
  - Prothrombin time test (using a CLIA-waived analyzer)
- **Blood Chemistry and Immunologic Tests**
  - Blood glucose test (using CLIA-waived analyzer)
  - Hemoglobin A1C test (using a CLIA-waived analyzer)
  - Cholesterol test (using a CLIA-waived analyzer)
  - Triglycerides test (using a CLIA-waived analyzer)
  - Rapid COVID test
  - Rapid HIV test
  - Rapid mononucleosis test
- **Microbiologic Tests**
  - Group A rapid *Streptococcus* test
  - Rapid influenza A and B test

CLIA-WAIVED TEST SYSTEMS

A **test system** is a setup that includes all of the equipment and supplies needed to perform laboratory tests such as blood analyzers, testing devices, test reagents, and controls. A **reagent** is a chemical that reacts with a specimen to allow the detection or measurement of an analyte. CLIA-waived test systems include CLIA-waived test kits and CLIA-waived automated analyzers described as follows:

CLIA-Waived Test Kits

A CLIA-waived test kit consists of a box packaged with the items needed to perform the test (Fig. 29.15). Each kit contains enough supplies to perform a specific number of tests as indicated on the package label. Examples of CLIA-waived test kits include:

- Hemoccult fecal occult blood test (SmithKline Diagnostics, Palo Alto, CA)
- QuickVue HCG urine pregnancy test (Quidel, San Diego, CA)
- QuickVue In-Line Strep A test (Quidel, San Diego, CA)

Each test kit includes a **package insert,** which is a printed document developed by the manufacturer of a laboratory test that provides detailed information on the use of the test

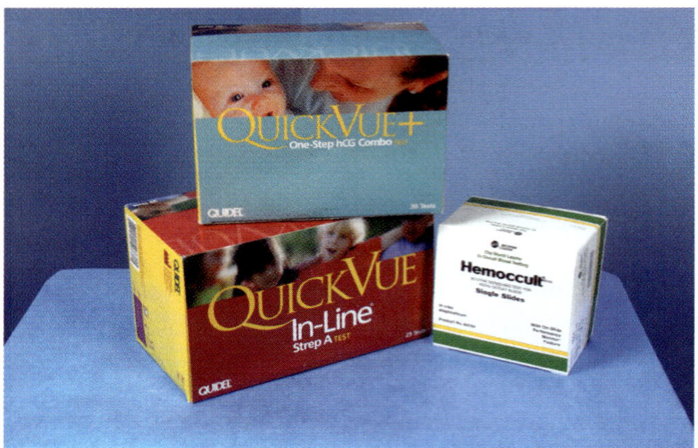

Fig. 29.15 CLIA-waived test kits.

and how to perform the test. The information included in a package insert is listed and described in Table 29.3. The medical assistant should carefully read the package insert and follow the instructions *exactly* to ensure accurate and reliable test results. The test kit often includes a *procedure reference card*, which is a condensed version of the steps in the testing procedure, and can be used as a quick reference guide when performing the test. Because the procedure reference card is a summary of the testing procedure, it should never be substituted for the package insert when first learning about the test.

Test kits often use a *unitized test device* to perform the test. A unitized test device is a self-contained device, such as a cassette, to which a specimen is added directly and in which all of the steps of the testing procedure occur (Fig. 29.16). A unitized device is used to perform one laboratory test (e.g., urine pregnancy test) and is discarded after testing.

Many of the test kits rely on a color change for interpretation of results. A color chart or diagram is provided with the kit for making a visual comparison and interpreting results. When the test results are documented, the brand name and lot number of the test kit should be indicated.

CLIA-Waived Automated Analyzers

CLIA-waived automated analyzers have been developed for performing laboratory tests in the POL; they are

Table 29.3 Information Included in the Package insert of a Test Kit

Section	Information Included
Intended Use	A description of the purpose of the test and the reason for performing the test
Summary and Explanation	Provides a brief overview of the condition being detected by the test, including the symptoms, prevalence, and complications of the condition
Principles of the Procedure	A detailed explanation of how the test works to detect the substance in the patient's specimen
Precautions and Warnings	Outlines precautions that must be taken when running the test to ensure accurate and reliable test results. Also includes guidelines for safe handling, use, and disposal of chemical reagents included in the test kit
Reagents and Materials Provided	A list of the collection devices, controls, reagents, and other supplies included in the test kit. Describes each component in detail, including the number of tests in the kit and the types and amounts of reagents and supplies
Materials Not Provided	A list of the materials needed to perform the test, but not included in the test kit
Storage and Stability	A description of the proper storage requirements of the test kit such as temperature range. Also identifies how long each testing component is stable for both unopened and opened components
Specimen Collection and Handling	Type of specimen required and procedures that must be followed when collecting, handling, and storing the specimen to ensure a high-quality and reliable specimen. Also includes safety precautions to take when handling the specimen
Test Procedure	Presents a step-by-step procedure that must be followed to test the specimen. Diagrams and illustrations of the procedural steps are often included in this section
Interpretation and Reading Results	Guidelines for reading and interpreting the test results. If a color change is involved in reading the results, a color comparison chart or color diagram is included with the test kit. Also explains the action to take if the test results are invalid
Quality Control	An explanation of the quality control procedures that must be performed to ensure accurate and reliable test results. Includes instructions for performing control procedures. Also includes information on how often and when controls should be run and the expected results. Describes what should be done if the controls do not produce expected results
Limitations of the Procedure	A test system works only within certain prescribed conditions and situations. Identifies conditions or situations that might prevent the test from performing correctly and influence the test results, such as medications or the presence of certain medical conditions. Also identifies any supplemental testing needed to confirm a waived test
Expected Values	Identifies the test result(s) that should be expected by the user
Performance Characteristics	Presents the results of research studies that have been conducted to evaluate test performance

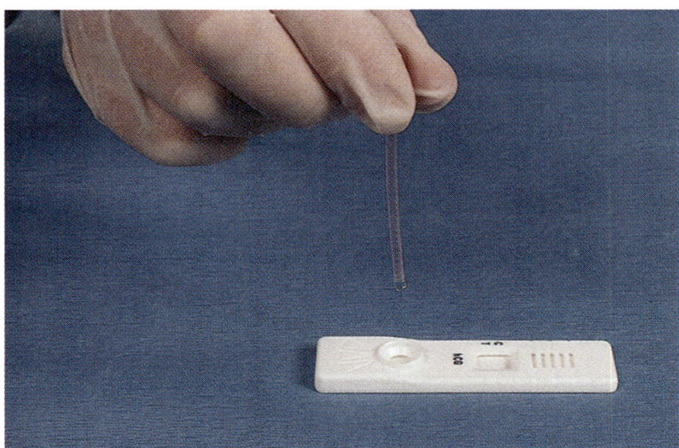

Fig. 29.16 Unitized test device.

continually increasing in number as new technology becomes available. These analyzers consist of compact or handheld devices that permit the processing of a specimen in a short time with accurate test results. Reagent strips or test cassettes are often used with CLIA-waived analyzers. Test results are obtained through a direct (digital display or printed) readout (Fig. 29.17).

The ease of operating automated analyzers should not lead to a false sense of security because they have limitations which must be recognized—the most critical one being the failure of the equipment. One of the most important aspects of use of an automated analyzer is the ability to recognize signs that indicate it is malfunctioning, because this can lead to inaccurate test results.

The manufacturer of each automated analyzer provides an operating manual that includes information needed to perform quality control procedures, collect and handle the specimen, and test the specimen. Medial assistants should be completely familiar with all aspects of automated analyzers used to perform laboratory tests in their POLs.

When a CLIA-waived automated analyzer is purchased, the test components (e.g., controls, test reagents) are usually purchased separately. The medical assistant is responsible for checking the supplies periodically and reordering them as needed. Each test component comes with a package insert, which indicates its use, and proper storage and stability requirements.

Some examples of brand names of CLIA-waived automated analyzers (Fig. 29.18) include:

- Cholestech LDX (Cholestech, Hayward, CA)
- STAT-Site Hemoglobin Meter (Stanbio Laboratory, Boerne, TX)
- CoaguChek system and Accu-Chek (Roche Diagnostics, Branchburg, NJ)
- A1C Now (Bayer Corporation, Morrisville, NJ)
- Clinitek urine analyzer (Siemens Corporation, New York, NY)

What Would You Do? What Would You *Not* Do?

Case Study 3

Zachary Tyler, 21 years of age, comes to the medical office complaining of fever, sore throat, painful swallowing, and red, swollen tonsils with white patches. The physician examines Zachary and orders a CLIA-waived rapid strep test to make a differential diagnosis of his condition. As Korey is preparing the supplies to collect a throat specimen, Zachary wants to know why the physician wasn't able to tell if he has strep throat from looking at his throat. He also says that he thought lab testing could only be done at a clinical laboratory by medical laboratory technologists. Zachary says that he has an overly sensitive gag reflex and wants to know if Korey could run the test using a blood sample. After Korey collects the throat specimen, Zachary says he forgot to tell the physician that he took an antibiotic this morning hoping it would help with his throat pain. The test results indicate that Zachary has group A strep and the physician electronically orders amoxicillin from Zachary's preferred pharmacy. When leaving the office, Zachary asks Korey for his antibiotic prescription. ■

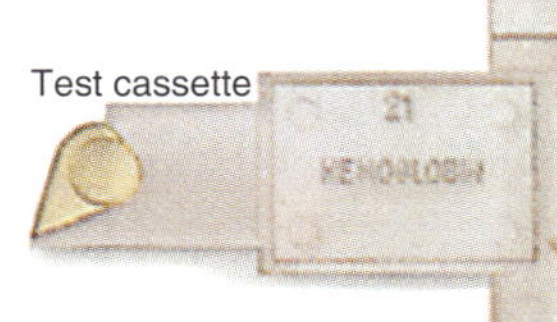

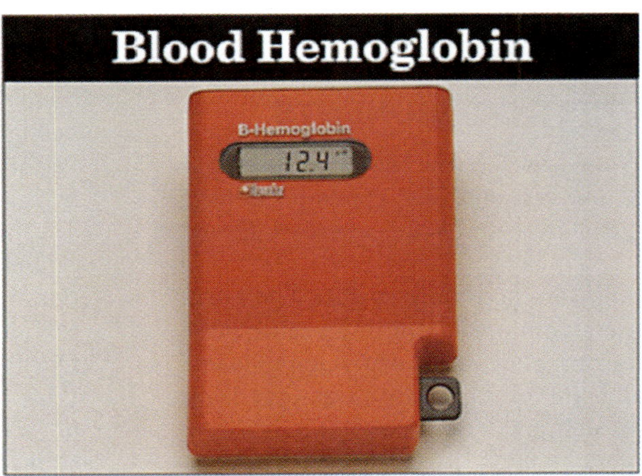

Fig. 29.17 Digital readout of test results on an automated analyzer. (Modified from Garrels M: *Laboratory and diagnostic testing in ambulatory care*, ed 4, St. Louis, 2019, Elsevier.)

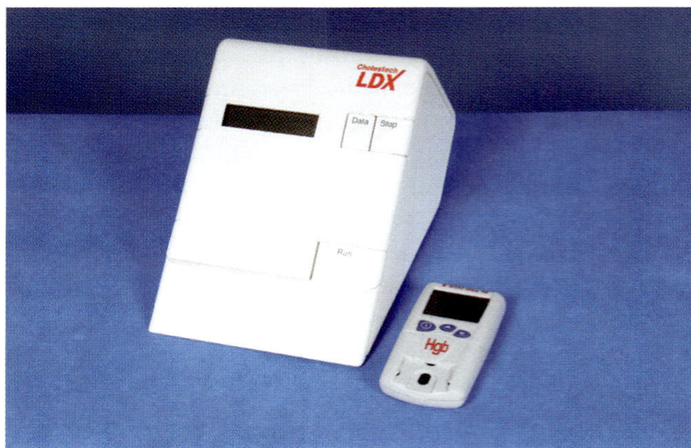

Fig. 29.18 CLIA-waived automated analyzers. Cholesterol analyzer (left) and hemoglobin analyzer (right).

POL LABORATORY TESTING

Testing a specimen in a POL involves a series of steps to determine the presence of a specific analyte in the specimen. The remainder of this chapter focuses on guidelines that should be followed when performing a CLIA-waived test in a POL.

QUALITY CONTROL

It is important to ensure that a laboratory test accurately measures what it is supposed to measure; this involves practicing and maintaining a quality control program. **Quality control** is defined as the application of methods and means throughout the entire test procedure to ensure that test results are reliable and accurate, and that errors are detected and eliminated. Quality control methods ensure reliable information that enables the provider to make an accurate diagnosis leading to the correct treatment. Quality control is an ongoing process that encompasses every aspect of test storage, patient preparation and specimen collection, handling, and testing.

STORAGE OF TEST COMPONENTS

Test components are used to perform laboratory tests and include controls and test reagents. Test components have specific storage requirements that must be carefully followed as outlined below.

1. Store the test components according to the information in the package insert. Improper storage can cause deterioration of the test components. Most test components need to be stored at RT in a cool, dry area away from sources of heat and sunlight as these conditions can alter their effectiveness.
2. Some test components may need to be stored in the refrigerator (e.g., controls and test reagents). Allow time for a refrigerated test component to reach RT before using it, which usually takes approximately 15–30 minutes.
3. If indicated, gently shake the control bottle to mix it.
4. Do not transfer test components from one test kit to another.
5. Make sure environmental conditions (e.g., RT) are appropriate for running the test as specified in the package insert.

STABILITY OF TEST COMPONENTS

Stability refers to the reliability of test components to perform as expected. Guidelines to ensure the stability of test components include the following:

1. Check the expiration date of each test component before using it. Do not use a test component if it is past its expiration date. Outdated components can lead to inaccurate test results.
2. An unopened control is stable until the manufacturer's expiration date stamped on the label is reached. Once opened, some controls are stable only for a certain period of time (e.g., 30 days). For these controls, the date the control is opened *and* the date it should be discarded (expiration date) must be written on the label of the control after it has been opened. An opened control is stable until it reaches the manufacturer's expiration date or the hand-written expiration, whichever comes first.
3. Discard outdated test components as soon as they reach their expiration dates.

CALIBRATION PROCEDURE

Calibration is a mechanism used to check the precision and accuracy of an automated analyzer to determine if it is providing accurate test results. A calibration check detects errors caused by an analyzer that is not working properly. Calibration is typically performed using a device known as a *calibration standard*. The calibration standard may come in the form of a calibration strip or cassette. The calibration standard is inserted into the analyzer (Fig. 29.19A), and the calibration results are displayed on the screen of the analyzer or printed out by the analyzer. The calibration results are then compared with the expected results provided in the package insert or shown on the calibration standard (Fig. 29.19B). Calibration guidelines include the following:

1. Perform the calibration check following the instructions in the operating manual accompanying the analyzer. The instructions include information on the type of calibration standard to use, how to perform the calibration procedure, and what action should be taken if the calibration procedure does not perform as expected.
2. Document calibration results in a quality control log. (This is a CLIA recommendation for waived tests and not a requirement.)
3. If the calibration procedure does not perform as expected, patient testing should not be conducted until the problem has been identified and resolved.

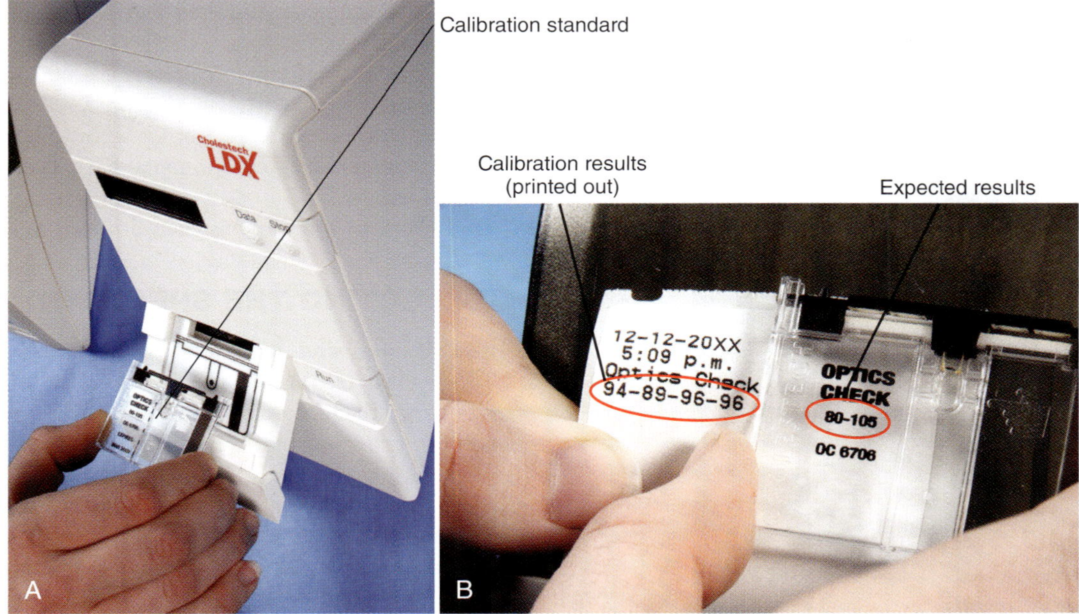

Fig. 29.19 **A**, Calibration of an analyzer using a calibration standard. **B**, Calibration results are compared with expected results shown on the calibration standard.

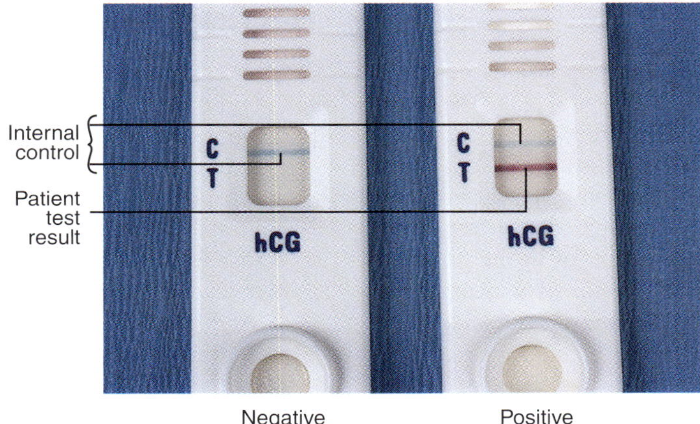

Fig. 29.20 Internal control. The blue line next to the letter C indicates that the internal control has performed as expected.

4. The frequency of performing the calibration procedure is indicated in the operating manual. At a minimum, a calibration check should be performed when using a new lot number of test reagents.

CONTROL PROCEDURE

A **control** is a solution used to monitor a test system to ensure reliable and accurate test results. Controls come with a package insert, which lists the expected ranges for control results. There are two categories of controls: external controls and internal controls.

Internal controls: An internal control is built into a test device (Fig. 29.20). It evaluates whether certain aspects of the testing procedure are working properly. An internal control is performed at the same time that the testing procedure is performed. It checks for one or more of the following: whether a sufficient amount of the specimen was added, whether a sufficient amount of test reagent was added, and whether the test reagent migrated through the test device properly. If the internal control does not perform as expected, the test result is invalid and the specimen must be retested. If the test result continues to be invalid, the manufacturer of the test system should be contacted.

External controls: External controls are used to determine if the test reagents are performing properly and to detect any errors in technique used to perform the test. External controls consist of commercially available solutions with known values. They may be included with the test system or may need to be purchased separately. In general, two levels of

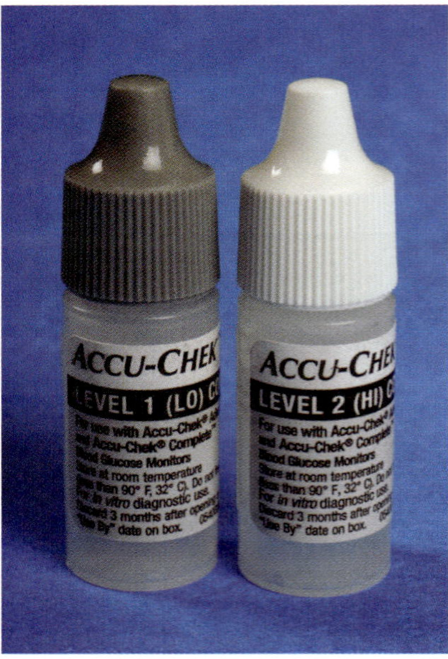

Fig. 29.21 External controls. Low or level 1 control (left) and high or level 2 control (right).

controls must be performed on a test system. A *low-level control* (also known as a *Level 1 control*) produces results that fall below the reference range for the test; a *high-level control* (also known as a *Level 2 control*) produces results that fall above the reference range for the test (Fig. 29.21). The control procedure is performed using the same procedure for performing the test on a patient. Instead of adding the patient specimen to the testing device, however, the control is added to it. Control results are compared with expected results provided on the control container or in the package insert accompanying the control. Failure of a control to produce expected results may be caused by outdated test components, improper storage of test components, improper environmental testing conditions and an error in the technique used to perform the control procedure.

External control guidelines include the following:

1. Perform the control check following the information in the package insert which includes instructions on how to perform the control procedure and what action should be taken if the control does not perform as expected.
2. Document control results in a quality control log (Fig. 29.22). (This is a CLIA recommendation for waived tests and not a requirement.)
3. If the control procedure does not perform as expected, patient testing should not be conducted until the problem is identified and resolved. If the problem cannot be resolved, the manufacturer of the test system should be contacted.
4. The frequency of performing the external control procedure is specified in the manufacturer's instructions accompanying the test system and usually includes:
   - When first receiving the test system
   - For periodic routine checking of analyzers, test strips and reagents
   - When a new lot number of test strips or reagents are used
   - When the test system does not seem to be working properly
   - When the test results do not seem to be accurate
   - When the test components have been improperly stored
   - When an analyzer has been dropped or damaged

COLLECTING THE SPECIMEN

The collection and handling requirements necessary for CLIA-waived testing are presented in the manufacturer's instructions that accompany the test system. General guidelines for collecting and handling specimens include the following:

1. Use the appropriate collection device to collect the specimen. Do not substitute other devices.
2. Follow the manufacturer's instructions *exactly* for collecting and handling the specimen.
3. If a specimen (e.g., urine) cannot be tested immediately, the specimen should be stored according to the information provided in the manufacturer's instructions.

TESTING THE SPECIMEN

Guidelines for performing a CLIA-waived laboratory test include the following:

1. If more than one patient is being tested at a time, label each test device with the patient's name to prevent mix-up of specimens.
2. Follow the procedure in the manufacturer's instructions *exactly* for testing the specimen. Specific requirements may include the following:
   - Adding the proper amounts of reagents
   - Adding reagents in the proper order
   - Adhering to proper time intervals for various steps in the procedure
   - Reading results within the proper time frame

INTERPRETING AND READING THE TEST RESULTS

A laboratory test can be either a qualitative test or a quantitative test. A **qualitative test** indicates whether or not a particular analyte is present in a specimen and also may provide an approximate indication of the amount of the analyte present. Most CLIA-waived test kits are qualitative tests. Qualitative tests are useful for screening purposes because they are easy to perform and can be used to screen large numbers of individuals—a procedure that otherwise might be too expensive and time-consuming.

Interpretation and reading of qualitative tests usually involve the use of a color comparison chart or a color diagram (Fig. 29.23). Qualitative test results are expressed in descriptive terms such as positive or negative; 1+, 2+, or 3+; reactive, weakly reactive, or nonreactive; and

ACCU-CHEK QUALITY CONTROL LOG
High/low Level Controls

Control Level	Lot Number	Expiration Date	Expected Range (mg/dL)
High Level Control	63330	11/29/XX	270 to 324
Low Level Control	42693	11/29/XX	18 to 64

Date	High Level Results (mg/dL)	Accept	Reject	Low Level Results (mg/dL)	Accept	Reject	Technician
2/9/XX	300	X		25	X		K. McGrew
2/10/XX	290	X		30	X		K. McGrew
2/11/XX	295	X		29	X		K. McGrew
2/12/XX	302	X		32	X		K. McGrew
2/13/XX	298	X		33	X		K. McGrew

Fig. 29.22 Quality control log.

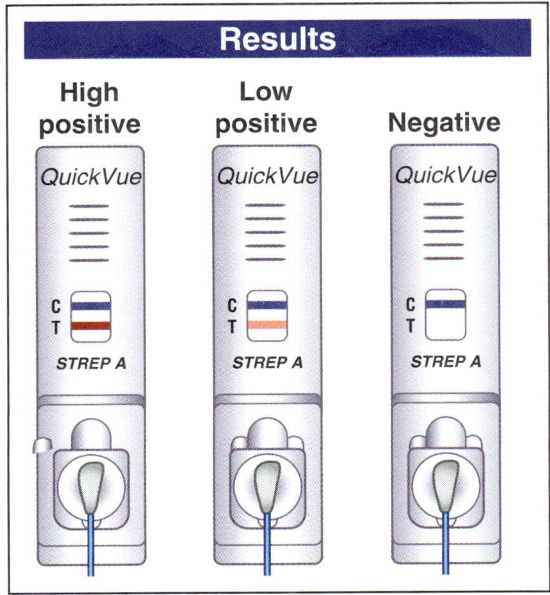

Fig. 29.23 Color diagram used to interpret test results.

invalid. An invalid test result means there was a problem with the collection or testing of the specimen such as an outdated test kit, improper storage of the kit, or an error in technique during the procedure. In this case, the problem must be identified and resolved before the specimen can be retested. If the problem cannot be resolved, the manufacturer of the test should be contacted.

A **quantitative test** measures the exact amount of an analyte present in a specimen with the test results expressed in measurable units (e.g., mg/dL). CLIA-waived automated analyzers provide quantitative test results and the results are printed out or displayed on the screen of the analyzer. No interpretation is required to read quantitative test results.

DOCUMENTING THE TEST RESULTS

Careful documentation is essential to avoid errors, which could affect the patient's diagnosis. Documentation of test results should include the following: the date and time, name of the test, and test results. Qualitative test results should be documented using words or abbreviations (e.g., positive, negative) and not symbols (e.g., +, −), because symbols can be accidentally changed or misinterpreted. Quantitative test results should be documented using the unit of measurement of the test system (e.g., mg/dL). The office may maintain a log of patient test results for each test performed in the POL The log includes the name and reference range of the test, the date the test was performed, the patient's name and identification number, the test results with abnormal values flagged, and the name of the individual performing the test (Fig. 29.24).

LABORATORY SAFETY

Laboratory safety is an important aspect of laboratory testing in the POL. Many of the laboratory tests performed in the POL involve the use of hazardous chemical reagents, the handling of specimens that may contain pathogens, and the use of laboratory equipment. Practicing good technique in testing specimens and recognizing potential hazards help to reduce accidents in the laboratory. Guidelines for laboratory safety in the POL are outlined here.

ACCU-CHEK GLUCOSE TEST
Patient Test Results Log

Test Name: *Fasting blood glucose*

Reference Range: *70 to 110 mg/dL*

Date	Patient Name	Patient ID	FBG Test Results (mg/dL)	Flag	Technician
2/11/XX	Edward Stanton	1341	98		K. McGrew
2/11/XX	Danella Baldwin	3744	74		K. McGrew
2/12/XX	Tristen Westfall	6497	115	H	K. McGrew
2/12/XX	Amy Longstreet	5310	78		K. McGrew
2/12/XX	Andrew Johnson	2333	85		K. McGrew
2/13/XX	Benjamin Harris	1466	65	L	K. McGrew
2/13/XX	Thomas Jeffers	5399	102		K. McGrew
2/14/XX	John Adams	2512	92		K. McGrew
2/15/XX	James Grant	1788	88		K. McGrew
2/15/XX	John Tyler	3903	120	H	K. McGrew
2/16/XX	Franklin Hoover	4559	102		K. McGrew

Fig. 29.24 Patient test results log.

SPECIMEN COLLECTION AND TESTING

Follow the OSHA Bloodborne Pathogens Standard during the collection, handling, and testing of specimens. In the event of an exposure incident, perform first aid measures immediately and then report the incident to the provider so that medical treatment and post-exposure prophylaxis (if needed) can be initiated.

1. Tie back or pin up long hair when working with specimens.
2. Cover any break in the skin, such as a cut or scratch, with a bandage.
3. Disinfect work counters before and after performing a laboratory test.
4. Wash hands immediately if any specimen is accidentally touched.
5. Avoid hand-to-mouth contact when working with specimens (e.g., eating, drinking, handling contact lenses, applying cosmetics).
6. Immediately clean up a specimen spilled on the work counter or floor and thoroughly disinfect the area with an approved disinfectant.
7. Ensure that all specimen containers are tightly capped to prevent leakage.
8. Do not store food or beverages in refrigerators, freezers, and cabinets where specimens and testing supplies are stored.
9. Properly handle all laboratory equipment and supplies as indicated in the manufacturer's instructions. For example, wait until a centrifuge comes to a complete stop before opening it.
10. Properly dispose of medical waste in biohazard containers such as contaminated needles and syringes, used collection devices, and infectious waste.

HAZARDOUS CHEMICALS

Review the safety data sheet (SDS) before using a laboratory chemical reagent to become familiar with its health hazards, and measures to take to prevent injury and illness when handling the chemical reagent. Measures include:

1. Ensure that all reagent containers are clearly and properly labeled.
2. If a label is loose, reattach it immediately.
3. Recap reagent containers immediately after use to prevent spills.

The first aid measures to be taken if exposed to a hazardous chemical should also be reviewed.

What Would You Do? What Would You *Not* Do? RESPONSES

Case Study 1

Page 767

What Did Korey Do?

- ❑ Told Hans that the term *clinical diagnosis* means what the physician "thinks" is wrong before the laboratory tests are performed.
- ❑ Explained that when the test results are returned, the physician would be able to make a diagnosis, and then he would determine what treatment is needed.
- ❑ Told Hans that a lipid panel includes several tests, and one of those tests is a cholesterol test. Explained that the tests in a lipid panel all help to determine whether someone is at risk for heart disease.
- ❑ Told Hans that he could not have any coffee with cream and sugar until after his blood was drawn because it would affect the test results. Told him that his test could be scheduled first thing in the morning if that would help.

What Did Korey Not Do?

- ❑ Did not tell Hans he could have a cup of coffee before his blood was drawn.
- ❑ Did not tell Hans that he should not be eating doughnuts if he is concerned about his heart.

Case Study 2

Page 774

What Did Korey Do?

- ❑ Stressed to Kathleen that if the laboratory test results are abnormal, it is better to know so that the physician can help make her better.
- ❑ Told Kathleen that many patients feel the same way about having blood drawn, so she is not alone. Relayed to her that her fear is normal, and she has no reason to be embarrassed.
- ❑ Told Kathleen that she should tell the laboratory about her last experience so they can make it easier for her. Explained that they would probably put her in a reclining position to draw her blood so that she would not get lightheaded.
- ❑ Gave Kathleen some suggestions on how to relax during the venipuncture. Told her to breathe deeply and to turn her head when the blood is drawn.
- ❑ Asked Kathleen whether she had any additional symptoms.
- ❑ Checked with the provider to see whether he wanted to keep her appointment for today or have her appointment rescheduled after the laboratory tests are completed.

What Did Korey Not Do?

- ❑ Did not ignore or minimize Kathleen's concerns and fears.
- ❑ Did not tell Kathleen that her test results would probably be fine.

Case Study 3

Page 779

What Did Korey Do?

- ❑ Explained to Zachary that the physician cannot tell if he has strep throat by looking at his throat because there are other conditions that resemble strep throat and the only way to know for sure is to run a lab test.
- ❑ Told Zachary that there are certain tests that the federal government allows medical offices to perform without having to follow strict regulations and the rapid strep test is one of those tests.

Continued

What Would You Do? What Would You *Not* Do? RESPONSES—cont'd

- ❑ Explained to Zachary that the manufacturer's instructions for the strep test require that the test be performed on a specimen swabbed from the throat and using a different specimen would invalidate the test results.
- ❑ Explained to Zachary that it is important to first check with the physician before taking a prescription medication.
- ❑ Informed the physician that Zachary took an antibiotic before coming to the medical office and documented this information in Zachary's medical record.
- ❑ Told Zachary that he doesn't need a paper prescription because the physician sent the prescription directly to his pharmacy using a computer.

What Did Korey Not Do?

- ❑ Did not scold Zachary for taking a "left-over" antibiotic that might possibly be outdated.
- ❑ Did not tell Zachary that he asks a lot of questions.

TERMINOLOGY REVIEW

Key Term	Definition
Analyte	A body substance that is being identified or measured by a laboratory test.
Calibration	A mechanism to check the precision and accuracy of an automated analyzer to determine if it is providing accurate test results. Calibration is typically performed using a calibration device, often called a standard.
CLIA-nonwaived test	A complex laboratory test that does not meet the criteria for waiver and is subject to the CLIA regulations.
CLIA-waived test	A laboratory test that meets the criteria for being a simple procedure that is easy to perform and has a low risk of erroneous test results.
Clinical diagnosis	A tentative diagnosis of a patient's condition obtained through an evaluation of the health history and the physical examination, without the benefit of laboratory or diagnostic tests.
Clinical laboratory	A facility in which tests are performed on biologic specimens to obtain information regarding the health of a patient.
Control	A solution that is used to monitor a test system to ensure reliable and accurate test results.
Critical value	A laboratory test result that is dangerously abnormal and is life-threating requiring immediate attention.
Fasting	Abstaining from food or fluids (except water) for a specified amount of time before the collection of a specimen.
Homeostasis	The state in which body systems are functioning normally and the internal environment of the body is in equilibrium; the body is in a healthy state.
Laboratory panel	A combination of laboratory tests that have been determined to be the most sensitive and specific means of identifying a disease state or evaluating a particular organ or organ system.
Laboratory test	The clinical analysis and study of a body substance to obtain objective data for the diagnosis, treatment, and management of a patient's condition.
Package insert (laboratory test)	A printed document developed by the manufacturer of a laboratory test that provides detailed information on the use of a test and how to perform the test.
Qualitative test	A test that indicates whether or not a particular analyte is present in a specimen and may also provide an approximate indication of the amount of the analyte present.
Quality control	The application of methods and means to ensure that test results are reliable and accurate and that errors are detected and eliminated.
Quantitative test	A test that indicates the exact amount of an analyte that is present in a specimen, with the results being reported in measurable units.
Reagent	A chemical that reacts with a specimen to allow the detection or measurement of an analyte.
Reference range	A certain established and acceptable range within which the laboratory test results of a healthy individual are expected to fall.
Screening test (laboratory)	A laboratory test performed routinely on apparently healthy individuals to assist in the early detection of disease.
Serum	The clear, straw-colored part of the blood that remains after the solid elements and the clotting factor fibrinogen have been separated out of it.
Specimen (body)	A small sample taken from the body to represent the nature of the whole.
Test system	A test system is a setup that includes all of the equipment and supplies needed to perform laboratory tests such as blood analyzers, testing devices, test reagents, and controls.
Unique identifier	Information directly associated with an individual that reliably identifies an individual as the person for whom a service or treatment is intended.

PROCEDURE 29.1 Operating an Emergency Eyewash Station

Outcome Operate and inspect an emergency eyewash station.

Equipment/Supplies

- Emergency eyewash station
- Disinfectant

Operate an Emergency Eyewash Station

1. **Procedural Step.** Immediately proceed to the emergency eyewash station after the eye(s) come in contact with a hazardous substance. Ask for assistance if needed.
2. **Procedural Step.** Activate the eyewash station using the activation lever. Once activated, the protective nozzle covers will automatically pop off the nozzle heads and water will begin to flow out of the nozzles. Once activated, the eyewash station remains operational for 15 minutes without requiring the use of the user's hands (or until it is manually turned off).
   Principle. The nozzle covers protect the nozzle heads from airborne contaminants.
3. **Procedural Step.** Hold both eyelids apart with your thumbs and forefingers to keep the eyes open.
   Principle. Most individuals respond to foreign substances in the eyes by closing their eyes tightly, therefore the eyes must be forcibly held open.

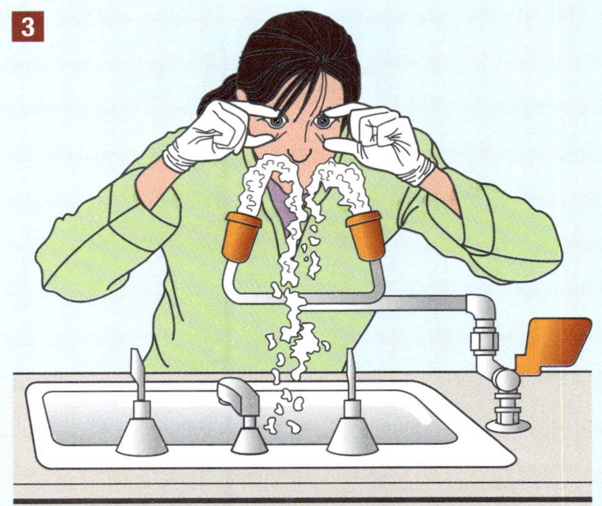

Hold both eyelids apart with your thumbs and forefingers.

4. **Procedural Step.** Lower your eyes into the stream of water coming from the nozzles and flush both eyes simultaneously.
5. **Procedural Step.** If necessary, gently remove contact lenses once the flushing process has begun. Flushing the eyes should not be delayed by removing the lenses before activating the eyewash station. In most cases, however, contact lenses are flushed out of the eyes by the water flow and do not need to be removed manually.
   Principle. Removing contact lenses prevents the hazardous substance from becoming trapped under the lens.
6. **Procedural Step.** Continue to hold the eyelids apart and gently roll your eyeballs from left to right and up and down.
   Principle. Rolling the eyeballs makes sure the water is reaching all areas of the eye.
7. **Procedural Step.** Continue flushing for a full 15 minutes. If the irritation persists, repeat the flushing procedure.
   Principle. Fifteen minutes is the minimum amount of time it takes to sufficiently clear the eyes of harmful substances. Not flushing the eyes for the full 15 minutes may result in permanent damage to the eyes.
8. **Procedural Step.** Return the activation lever to its resting position to turn off the flow of water.
9. **Procedural Step.** Seek medical attention immediately to determine if further treatment is required.
10. **Procedural Step.** A staff member should clean, disinfect, rinse, and completely dry the eyewash device.

Inspect and Activate an Emergency Eyewash Station

Inspect and activate the eyewash station each week to ensure that it is operating properly and to flush out the water supply lines.

1. **Procedural Step.** Make sure the access route to the eyewash station is well lit and free of obstructions.
2. **Procedural Step.** Make sure the eyewash station is well lit and the area around the eyewash station is free of clutter.
   Principle. This avoids unnecessary delay in activating the eyewash station.

Continued

PROCEDURE 29.1

PROCEDURE 29.1 Operating an Emergency Eyewash Station—cont'd

3. **Procedural Step.** Make sure the protective nozzle covers are in place and in good condition.
   Principle. The covers protect the nozzle heads from airborne contaminants.
4. **Procedural Step.** Make sure the eyewash bowl is clean and free of debris.
5. **Procedural Step.** Activate the eyewash device using the activation lever. The water flow from the nozzles should occur in one second or less following activation of the eyewash device.
6. **Procedural Step.** Make sure the protective nozzle covers come off automatically when the eyewash device is activated.
7. **Procedural Step.** Activate the eyewash station for at least 3 minutes.
   Principle. Activation of the eyewash station flushes out sediment, debris, or bacteria from the water supply lines.
8. **Procedural Step.** Make sure the water flows continuously (once activated) without the use of the hands.
9. **Procedural Step.** Make sure that the nozzle heads are not clogged, and that water flows equally from both nozzle heads.
10. **Procedural Step.** Return the activation lever to its resting position to turn off the flow of water.
11. **Procedural Step.** Clean, disinfect, rinse, and completely dry the eyewash device including the nozzle heads and protective covers.
12. **Procedural Step.** Replace the nozzle covers on the nozzle heads.
13. **Procedural Step.** Report any problems to the appropriate personnel.
14. **Procedural Step.** Document the inspection date and your initials on either an eyewash inspection log sheet or an eyewash inspection tag that is attached to the device.

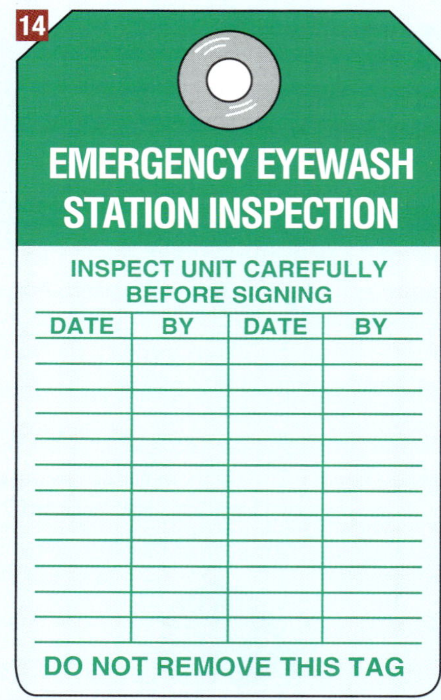

Emergency eyewash station inspection tag.

PROCEDURE 29.1

Urinalysis

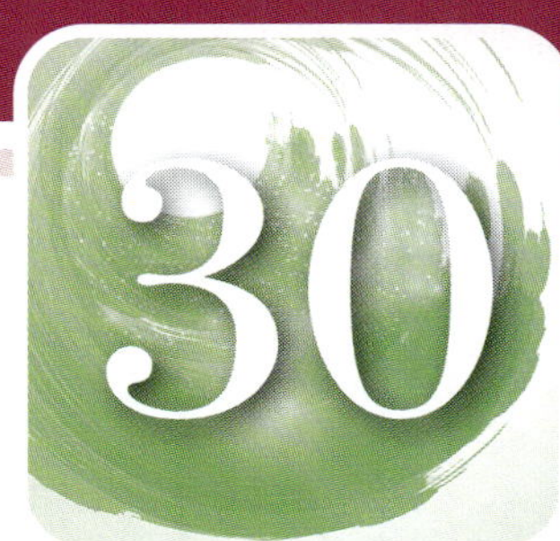

 Check out the Evolve site at http://evolve.elsevier.com/Bonewit/today to access additional interactive activities and exercises to help you study and prepare for success.

LEARNING OBJECTIVES/PROCEDURES

Urinary System

1. State the function of the urinary system.
2. Identify the structures making up the urinary system.
3. Identify the composition of urine.
4. List conditions that may cause polyuria and oliguria.
5. List and define the terms used to describe symptoms associated with the urinary system.

Collection of Urine

6. Explain why a first-voided morning specimen is often preferred for urinalysis.
7. Explain the purpose for collecting a clean-catch midstream specimen, a first-voided morning specimen and a first-catch specimen.
8. Explain the purpose for collecting a 24-hour urine specimen.
9. List changes that may occur if urine is allowed to remain standing for longer than 1 hour.

Procedures:
- Instruct a patient in the collection of a clean-catch midstream urine specimen.
- Instruct a patient in the collection of a 24-hour urine specimen.

Urinalysis

10. Identify the purpose of a urinalysis.
11. List factors that may cause urine to have an unusual color or become cloudy.
12. List and describe the various tests included in a physical and chemical examination of urine.
13. List the structures that may be found in a microscopic examination of urine.

Procedures:
- Assess the color and appearance of a urine specimen. Perform a chemical assessment of a urine specimen using a CLIA-waived reagent strip.
- Prepare a urine specimen for microscopic examination by the provider.

Urine Pregnancy Testing

14. Explain the basis for urine pregnancy tests.
15. List the guidelines that must be followed during a urine pregnancy test to ensure accurate test results.

Procedures:
- Perform a CLIA-waived urine pregnancy test.

CHAPTER OUTLINE

KEY TERMS

anuria (ah-NOOR-ee-ah)
bilirubinuria (bill-ih-roo-bin-YUR-ee-ah)
bladder catheterization
diuresis (di-ah-REE-sis)
dysuria (dis-YUR-ee-ah)
frequency
glycosuria (glie-koe-SOO-ree-ah)
hematuria (hem-ah-TOOR-ee-ah)
ketonuria (kee-toe-NOO-ree-ah)
ketosis (kee-TOE-sis)
micturition (mik-tur-ISH-un)
nephron (NEF-ron)
nocturia (nok-TOOR-ee-ah)
nocturnal enuresis (nok-TOOR-nal en-YUR-ee-sis)
oliguria (oh-lig-YUR-ee-ah)
pH (PEE-AYCH)
polyuria (pol-ee-YUR-ee-ah)
proteinuria (proe-teen-YUR-ee-ah)
pyuria (pi-YUR-ee-ah)
renal threshold (REE-nul THRESH-hold)
retention
specific gravity
supernatant (soo-per-NAY-tent)
suprapubic aspiration
urgency
urinalysis (yur-in-AL-ih-sis)
urinary incontinence

INTRODUCTION TO URINALYSIS

The urinary system consists of the kidneys, the ureters, the urinary bladder, and the urethra. The function of the urinary system is to regulate the fluid and electrolyte balance of the body and to remove waste products. A physiologic change in the body caused by disease may create a disturbance in one or more of the functions of the kidney. Detection of such a disturbance can be made with the examination of urine and other body fluids such as blood.

Urinalysis is the analysis of urine and is the laboratory test most commonly performed in the medical office because a urine specimen is readily obtainable and can be easily tested. Urinalysis consists of a physical, chemical, and microscopic examination of urine. Deviation from normal in any of the three areas assists the provider in the diagnosis and treatment of pathologic conditions, not only of the urinary system, but also of other body systems. Urinalysis may be performed as a screening measure for the early detection of disease or to assist in the diagnosis of a pathologic condition. It also may assist in the evaluation of effectiveness of therapy after treatment has been initiated for a pathologic condition. Before beginning a study of this chapter, it is important to thoroughly review the chapter on the anatomy and physiology of the urinary system presented in Chapter 15: Urinary System.

COMPOSITION OF URINE

Urine is composed of 95% water and 5% organic and inorganic waste products. Organic waste products consist of urea, uric acid, ammonia, and creatinine. Urea is present in the greatest amounts and is derived from the breakdown of proteins. Inorganic waste products include chloride, sodium, potassium, calcium, magnesium, phosphate, and sulfate.

A normal adult excretes approximately 750 to 2000 mL of urine per day. This amount varies according to the amount of fluid consumed and the amount of fluid lost through other means, such as perspiration, feces, and water vapor from the lungs. An excessive increase in urine output is known as **polyuria,** with the urine volume exceeding 2000 mL in 24 hours. Polyuria may be caused by the excessive intake of fluids or the intake of fluids that contain caffeine (e.g., coffee, tea, cola), which is a mild diuretic. Certain drugs, such as diuretics, and the pathologic conditions of diabetes mellitus, diabetes insipidus, and renal disease, also may result in polyuria. Decreased or scanty urine output is known as **oliguria.** In the case of oliguria, the urine volume is less than 400 mL in 24 hours. Oliguria may occur with decreased fluid intake, dehydration, profuse perspiration, vomiting, diarrhea, or kidney disease. The normal act of voiding urine is known as **micturition.**

TERMS RELATED TO THE URINARY SYSTEM

The medical assistant should have a thorough knowledge of the following terms used to describe symptoms associated with the urinary system:

Anuria Failure of the kidneys to produce urine
Diuresis Secretion and passage of large amounts of urine
Dysuria Difficult or painful urination
Frequency The condition of having to urinate often

Hematuria Blood present in the urine
Nocturia Excessive (voluntary) urination during the night
Nocturnal enuresis Inability of an individual to control urination at night during sleep (bedwetting)
Oliguria Decreased or scanty output of urine
Polyuria Increased output of urine
Pyuria Pus present in the urine
Retention The inability to empty the bladder. The urine is being produced normally but is not being voided
Urgency The immediate need to urinate
Urinary incontinence The inability to retain urine in the bladder

COLLECTION OF URINE

The advantages of urine testing are that urine is readily available and obtaining it does not require an invasive procedure or the use of special equipment. For accurate test results, the medical assistant must adhere to proper urine collection procedures to obtain the correct specimen for the type of test being performed.

GUIDELINES FOR URINE COLLECTION

The following guidelines should be followed in the collection of a urine specimen:

1. Make sure to obtain an adequate volume of urine as necessary for the type of test being performed (usually 30 to 50 mL of urine).
2. Each specimen must be labeled properly with the patient's full name and date of birth, the date and time of collection, and the type of specimen (i.e., urine).
3. Medications being taken by the patient that may affect the test results should be documented on the laboratory request and in the patient's medical record.
4. If possible, the collection of a urine specimen should be avoided in women during menstruation and for several days thereafter because the specimen may become contaminated with blood. This results in a false-positive test result for blood in the urine.
5. Take into consideration that voiding may be difficult for patients under stress and anxiety. In these instances, understanding and patience should be conveyed to the patient.
6. A urine specimen may be difficult to obtain from a child, even with the assistance of a parent. In this case, the provider should be informed because another collection method may be used, such as a urine collection bag, suprapubic aspiration, or catheterization of the patient.

COLLECTION METHODS

The type of test to be performed on the urine dictates the method used to collect the urine specimen. A first-voided morning specimen is recommended for pregnancy testing, and a clean-catch midstream specimen is necessary for identification of the presence of a urinary tract infection (UTI).

Most offices use disposable plastic urine specimen containers. These containers are available in different sizes and come with screw-on lids to prevent spillage and to reduce bacterial and other types of contamination.

What Would You Do? What Would You *Not* Do?

Case Study 1

Yusuke Urameshi is at the office with fever and chills, urinary frequency, and painful and difficult urination. The physician suspects that Mr. Urameshi has prostatitis and orders a clean-catch urine specimen for a complete urinalysis, including a microscopic examination of the urine sediment. Mr. Urameshi tries to collect the specimen but is able to collect only 5 mL of urine. He says that he is worried about what is wrong with him and he thinks his nervousness is making it hard to get a specimen. Mr. Urameshi says that it is probably just as well because he did not understand how to cleanse himself, and he is not sure that he did it correctly. ■

Random Specimen

Urine testing in the medical office is often performed on freshly voided, random specimens. The medical assistant instructs the patient to void into a clean, dry, wide-mouthed container, and the urine is tested immediately at the medical office.

First-Voided Morning Specimen

In many cases a first-voided morning specimen may be desired for testing because it contains the greatest concentration of dissolved substances, and a small amount of an abnormal substance that is present would be more easily detected. The patient should be instructed to collect the first specimen of the morning after rising and to preserve the specimen by refrigerating it until it is brought to the medical office. It is important to provide the patient with a specimen container to prevent the patient's use of a container from home that might harbor contaminants and affect the test results.

Clean-Catch Midstream Specimen

The urinary bladder and most of the urethra are normally free of microorganisms, whereas the distal urethra and the urinary meatus normally harbor microorganisms. If the urine is being cultured and examined for bacteria, a clean-catch midstream specimen is necessary to prevent contamination of the specimen with these normally present microorganisms. Only microorganisms that may be causing the patient's condition are desired in the urine specimen. A clean-catch midstream collection may be ordered for the detection of a UTI or for the evaluation of the effectiveness of drug therapy in a patient undergoing treatment for such an infection.

The purpose of a clean-catch midstream collection is to remove microorganisms from the urinary meatus and the distal urethra. This is accomplished by instructing the patient to thoroughly cleanse the area surrounding the meatus and to void a small amount of urine into the toilet, which flushes out microorganisms in the distal urethra. The urine specimen is collected in a sterile container using medically aseptic techniques. A properly collected specimen reduces the possibility of having to perform a bladder catheterization or a suprapubic aspiration of the bladder. **Bladder catheterization** involves the passing of a sterile tube (the catheter) through the urethra and into the bladder to remove urine. **Suprapubic aspiration** involves the passing of a sterile needle through the abdominal wall into the bladder to remove urine. Both of these procedures must be performed using sterile technique.

Guidelines

Guidelines that should be followed when collecting a clean-catch midstream specimen are as follows:

1. A clean-catch midstream specimen is collected by the patient at the medical office. The medical assistant must provide complete instructions for collection of this specimen. Failure to instruct the patient adequately may necessitate a return to the medical office for the collection of another specimen because of bacterial contamination. Patient instructions for obtaining a clean-catch midstream specimen are presented in Procedure 30.1.
2. If the specimen is to be tested at an outside laboratory, a laboratory request must be completed.
3. The container must be labeled with the patient's name and date of birth, the date, the time of collection, and the type of specimen (clean-catch midstream urine specimen).
4. For reliable test results, the specimen should be tested immediately and should not be allowed to stand. If this is not possible, the specimen should be refrigerated, or a preservative should be added to it.
5. The procedure should be documented in the patient's medical record. The information to be documented for a specimen tested at the medical office includes the date and time, the type of specimen collected, and the laboratory test results. If the specimen is being transported to an outside laboratory for testing, document the date and time of the specimen collection, the type of specimen collected, and the date the specimen was transported to the laboratory.

First-Catch Urine Specimen

A first-catch urine specimen can be used to test for the presence of chlamydia and gonorrhea using a nucleic acid amplification (NAA) test. (Refer to Chapter 23 for more information on chlamydia and gonorrhea and the NAA test.) To obtain a first-catch urine specimen, the patient should not urinate for at least one hour prior to the collection of the urine specimen. The patient should not cleanse the genital area before collecting the specimen as this results in the removal of pathogens from the area which could lead to false-negative test results. The patient should be instructed to collect only 15 to 30 mL (1 to 2 tablespoons) of the initial urine stream in the specimen container. If more than 30 mL of urine is collected, the patient must start the procedure over again. The first 15 to 30 mL of urine voided by the patient contains the greatest concentration of chlamydia and/or gonorrhea bacteria resulting in a greater likelihood that the NAA test will detect the presence of these pathogens. Collection of more than 30 mL of urine results in dilution of the specimen which may affect the accuracy of the test results.

Following collection of the specimen, the medical assistant is responsible for transferring 2 mL of the urine specimen to a transport tube using a disposable pipette. The specimen should then be placed in a biohazard specimen bag and stored in the refrigerator for pick-up by a courier from an outside laboratory.

Twenty-four–Hour Urine Specimen

A 24-hour urine specimen is used for the quantitative measurement of specific urinary components. Collecting urine over a 24-hour period provides greater accuracy in the measurement of urinary components than with a random specimen. This is because body metabolism, exercise, and hydration can affect the excretion rate of substances in the urine. Examples of substances measured in a 24-hour specimen include calcium, cortisol, lead, potassium, protein, and urea nitrogen. A 24-hour specimen is often used in the diagnosis of the cause of kidney stone formation and in the control and prevention of new stone formation. It may also be used to perform a creatinine clearance test, which provides information on kidney function.

A large wide-mouthed container (3000 mL) is used to store the urine collected over the 24-hour period. To prevent changes in the quality of the urine specimen, the specimen must be kept refrigerated or placed in an ice chest. Some containers also contain a chemical preservative (in the form of crystals, tablets, or a liquid) to assist in maintaining the quality of the specimen. Examples of urine preservatives include hydrochloric acid, boric acid, acetic acid, and toluene. A hazardous chemical warning label should be attached to a specimen container with a preservative, and the patient should be instructed not to discard or touch the preservative in the container.

The patient is provided with a smaller container to collect each urine specimen. A female patient may be given a urine "hat," which is placed under the seat of the commode, and a male patient is often provided with a collection cup. After collection, the urine is poured into the large specimen container. This method makes collection easier and safer for the patient. If the patient voids urine directly into a specimen container that holds a preservative, the preservative could splash onto the patient's skin, resulting in a chemical burn.

The medical assistant should provide the patient with verbal and written instructions for collection of the urine specimen. The patient should be advised to drink a normal amount of fluid during the collection period. The patient should be instructed to avoid alcohol intake for 24 hours before and during the collection period. The patient should stay at home during the collection period, so that the urine container does not have to be transported. The test should not be performed when the patient is menstruating. Because certain medications, such as thiazides, phosphorus-binding antacids, allopurinol, and vitamin C, can alter the test results, the provider usually requires the patient to discontinue any of these medications being taken by the patient for one week before the test. The procedure for instructing a patient in the collection of a 24-hour urine specimen is presented in Procedure 30.2.

URINALYSIS

Urinalysis is the analysis of urine and is the laboratory test most commonly performed in the medical office because a urine specimen is readily obtainable and can be easily tested. Urinalysis consists of a *physical*, *chemical*, and *microscopic examination* of urine. Deviation from normal in any of the three areas assists the provider in the diagnosis and treatment of pathologic conditions, not only of the urinary system, but also of other body systems. Urinalysis may be performed as a screening measure as part of a routine health examination or to assist in the diagnosis of a pathologic condition. It also may assist in the evaluation of effectiveness of therapy after treatment has been initiated for a pathologic condition.

Urinalysis should be performed on a fresh or preserved specimen. If a specimen cannot be examined within 1 hour of voiding, it should be preserved at once in the refrigerator in a closed container and later returned to room temperature and mixed before testing. Chemical additives can be used to preserve urine specimens but are typically only used with specimens that require prolonged storage.

If the urine is allowed to stand at room temperature for longer than 1 hour, the following changes may occur:

1. Bacteria in the environment that get into the specimen work on urea present in the urine, converting it to ammonia. Because ammonia is alkaline, acid urine becomes alkaline which increases the pH of the urine. An alkaline pH may result in a false-positive result on the protein test.
2. Bacteria multiply rapidly in the urine, resulting in a cloudy specimen and an increase in the nitrite.
3. If glucose is present in the specimen, it decreases in amount because microorganisms use the glucose as a source of food.
4. Any red or white blood cells present in the urine may break down.
5. Casts decompose after several hours.

PHYSICAL EXAMINATION OF URINE

The physical examination of urine includes a determination of the color, appearance, and specific gravity of the urine. The color and appearance of the urine specimen may be evaluated during the preparation of the urine for another test, such as the chemical testing of the urine. For an accurate evaluation of the color and appearance, the urine specimen must be collected in a clear plastic container.

Color

The normal color of urine ranges from almost colorless to dark yellow. Dilute urine tends to be a lighter yellow in color because it does not contain many dissolved substances. Concentrated urine contains more dissolved substances causing it to be a darker yellow. A first-voided morning specimen is usually the most concentrated because consumption of fluids is decreased during the night. Urine becomes more dilute as the day progresses as more fluids are consumed.

The color of the urine is the result of the presence of a yellow pigment known as *urochrome*, produced by the breakdown of hemoglobin. It is common for the color of urine to vary among different shades of yellow within the course of a day. Classifications that can be used to describe the color of urine include light yellow, yellow, dark yellow, amber, and dark amber (Fig. 30.1).

An abnormal urine color assists in determining additional tests that may be necessary. Abnormal colors may be caused by the presence of hemoglobin or blood (resulting in a red or reddish color), bile pigments (resulting in a yellow-brown or greenish color), and fat droplets or pus (resulting in a milky color). Some foods and medications also may cause the urine to change to an abnormal color. Phenazopyridine (Pyridium), a urinary tract analgesic, causes the urine to change to an orange-to-red color.

Appearance

Evaluation of the appearance of urine is usually performed at the same time as the color evaluation. Fresh urine is usually clear, or transparent, but becomes cloudy if left standing out too long. Cloudiness in a freshly voided specimen may be the result of the presence of bacteria, pus, blood, fat, yeast, sperm, mucous threads, or fecal contaminants. A microscopic examination of the urine sediment is usually performed on all cloudy specimens to determine the cause of the cloudiness. Cloudiness resulting from bacteria may be caused by a UTI.

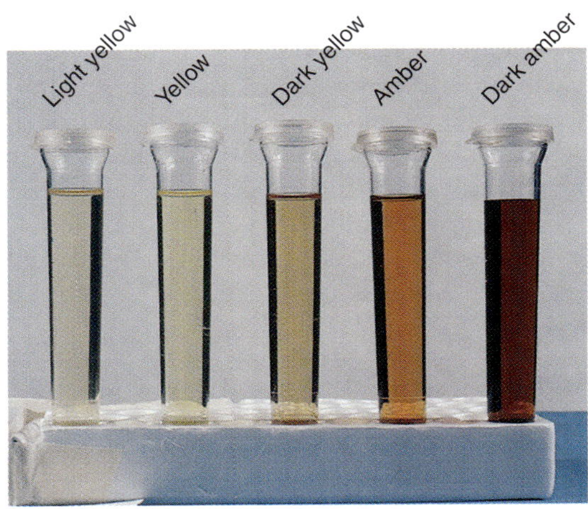

Fig. 30.1 Color of urine.

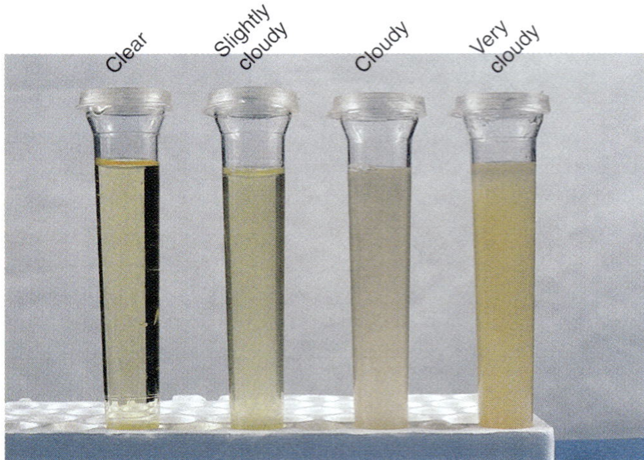

Fig. 30.2 Appearance of urine.

Classifications used to describe the appearance of urine include clear, slightly cloudy, cloudy, and very cloudy (Fig. 30.2). The medical assistant should develop skill in recognizing the varying degrees of urine clarity.

Odor

Freshly voided urine normally should have a slightly aromatic odor. Urine left standing out for a long time develops an ammonia odor from the breakdown of urea by bacteria in the specimen. The urine of a patient with diabetes mellitus may have a fruity odor from the presence of ketone. The urine of a patient with a UTI is usually foul smelling, and the odor becomes worse on standing. Certain foods, such as asparagus, can cause the urine to have a musty smell. Although urine may have many characteristic odors, as a rule the odor of urine is not typically used in the diagnosis of a patient's condition.

Specific Gravity

The **specific gravity** of urine measures the weight of the urine compared with the weight of an equal volume of distilled water. Specific gravity indicates the amount of dissolved substances present in the urine, providing information on the ability of the kidneys to dilute or concentrate the urine. Specific gravity is decreased in conditions in which the kidneys cannot concentrate the urine, such as chronic renal insufficiency, diabetes insipidus, and malignant hypertension. The specific gravity is increased in patients with adrenal insufficiency, congestive heart failure, hepatic disease, diabetes mellitus with glycosuria, and conditions that cause dehydration, such as fever, vomiting, and diarrhea.

The normal specific gravity of urine ranges from 1.005 to 1.030 but is usually between 1.010 and 1.025 (the specific gravity of distilled water is 1.000). Specific gravity varies greatly with fluid intake and the state of hydration of an individual. Dilute urine contains fewer dissolved substances and has a lower specific gravity. Concentrated urine has a higher specific gravity because of the increased amount of dissolved substances. In general, a urine specimen is more concentrated in the morning and becomes more dilute after fluid consumption.

In the medical office, specific gravity is most commonly measured using a reagent strip. This involves a color comparison determination with a reagent strip that includes a reagent pad for specific gravity. The reagent strip is dipped into the urine specimen, and the results are compared with a color chart (Procedure 30.3).

What Would You Do? What Would You *Not* Do?

Case Study 2

Nora Sheridan is at the clinic complaining of urinary frequency, urgency, dysuria, and blood in her urine. During the past 6 months, Nora has been having problems with UTIs. She wants to know why these infections continue to occur and whether she can do anything to prevent them. Nora says that she has a lot of deadlines at work and that it is difficult to find time to come to the medical office. She says that her drugstore sells urine testing strips. Nora wants to know whether she could get a container of the strips and test her urine at home when she is having problems. That way she could just contact the office when she has positive test results, and the physician could call in a prescription for an antibiotic for her. ■

Putting It All Into Practice

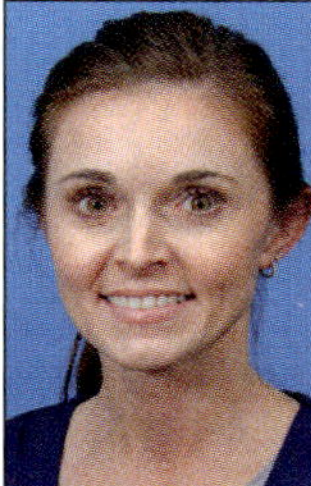

My name is Kayla, and I work for a urologist and his wife, who is a pediatrician. I work primarily in the urology practice and only occasionally in pediatrics. I am responsible for having the medical records ready when the patients are seen and for doing their urinalysis. Another one of my responsibilities is to assist with special procedures, such as catheter insertions, male and female dilations, ultrasound examinations of the bladder, and prostate examinations.

When I first started working in the urology office, I was trained to assist with transrectal ultrasounds of the prostate in case the ultrasound technician was sick. When she retired, I inherited the position. At first, I dreaded doing the procedures and would be so nervous that I would get the shakes and forget the order in which things were supposed to be done. My physician was understanding and would help by talking me through it. I think the reason I was so nervous was that sometimes patients have trouble and we have to administer oxygen and run intravenous lines. One time, a patient had a reaction to the sedative we gave before the procedure. Time, practice, and confidence in myself have improved my nerves, even with the occasional emergency situation. ■

HIGHLIGHT on Drug Testing in the Workplace

Statistics

Statistics suggest that the problem of drug abuse is growing in the workplace. The effects of on-the-job drug use extend into every segment of the population and touch every business and industry. The U.S. Department of Labor estimates that 65% of all work-related accidents can be traced to substance abuse. According to the National Council on Alcoholism and Drug Dependence (NCADD), drug abuse costs industry billions of dollars annually because of accidents, health insurance claims, high employee turnover, absenteeism, lost productivity, and workplace theft.

Drug-testing programs

Because of these economic and safety factors, businesses across the United States are adopting a less permissive attitude toward drug use and are requiring drug testing in the workplace. Approximately one-half of U.S. employers have implemented drug-testing programs in the workplace. These employers include utility companies, transportation operations, construction companies, sports associations, and governmental agencies. Currently, many companies test blue-collar and white-collar employees for drug use. Companies with drug-testing programs report a significant reduction in employee accidents, fewer sick days, and healthier employees.

A comprehensive drug-testing program includes the detection of drug use in the workplace, policies to discourage further abuse, and the referral of employees for treatment and rehabilitation. Drug testing may be performed for one or more of the following purposes: (1) preemployment drug screening; (2) random sample testing of the workforce to detect use of controlled substances by employees on the job; (3) testing for probable cause after unexplained behavior or an incident (e.g., an accident on the job).

Drug-testing methods

Drug testing can be performed on several different types of specimens, which include blood, urine, saliva, and hair. Blood testing is the best means for determining precise information concerning the amount of drug used and when the drug was taken. Blood tests are costly, however, and are time-consuming to perform. Urine drug testing offers the next best alternative; it is noninvasive and technically easier and less expensive to perform. Current urine screening tests target the most common drugs of abuse: amphetamines and methamphetamines, barbiturates, benzodiazepines, cocaine, fentanyl, marijuana, opioids, phencyclidine (PCP), and methadone. CLIA-waived urine drug-testing kits are available for testing the specimen in the medical office. These kits provide immediate results and take only a few minutes to perform. Alcohol may also be included in a drug-testing program, but it is usually detected through a breath test.

Chain of custody

The usual procedure for urine drug testing involves screening the specimen and confirming positive results with more specific urine tests. The specimen may be collected at the workplace, at the medical office, or at an outside laboratory. To help ensure reliable and valid drug-testing results, a security system or "chain of custody" must be followed in the collection and handling of the specimen. This includes ensuring the identification of the individual undergoing drug testing, taking precautions to avoid falsification of or tampering with specimens, proper collection and labeling of the urine specimen, sealing the specimen container after collection, and immediately sending the specimen to an outside laboratory for analysis or refrigerating it if there is a delay in transport.

Disadvantages

The main disadvantage of urine drug testing is that a positive test result indicates only the presence of a drug in the urine; it does not provide any information as to when the drug was taken. Drugs that are detected in the urine may or may not still be present in the blood, where they can affect an individual's behavior and impair performance. Because of this, a positive urine test result does not determine whether an individual is impaired by drugs. In addition, the initial urine screening tests are sometimes unreliable; unless positive results are confirmed with a more specific test, an individual may be unjustly accused of drug use. These factors and the violation of an individual's right to privacy are the main areas of dispute for individuals who oppose drug testing in the workplace.

Intervention

Companies with drug-testing programs have various options when results are positive, such as recommendations for drug treatment programs or disciplinary action. Many companies have established in-house employee assistance programs that include counseling and drug withdrawal therapy for employees who desire help. Most companies prefer to help current employees with rehabilitation instead of discharging them and hiring and training new employees. Studies show a 35% to 60% recovery rate for employees enrolled in drug treatment programs. ■

CHEMICAL EXAMINATION OF URINE

The chemical examination of urine is used to assist in the evaluation of kidney function, urinary tract infections, carbohydrate metabolism (diabetes mellitus), and liver function. Substances present in excessive (abnormal) amounts in the blood are usually removed by the urine. For example, glucose is normally present in the blood, but if it exceeds a certain level or threshold, the excess amount is excreted in the urine. Chemical testing of urine is an indirect means of detecting abnormal amounts of chemicals in the body, indicating a pathologic condition. The chemical examination of urine also can be used to detect the presence of substances that, in the absence of disease, do not normally appear in the urine, such as blood and nitrite.

Chemical tests that are routinely performed during a urinalysis include testing for pH, glucose, protein, and ketone. Other chemical tests that may be performed include

LABORATORY REPORT Complete Urinalysis				
Patient Colbert, Evelyn K. 2963 Flint Dr. S Clearwater, FL 33759 PH: 727-541-3575	ID #: 336879 DOB: 4/28/1990 Age: 34 Gender: F	**Ordered By** Thomas Murphy, MD Pinellas Medical Office 3477 Arrowhead Ave Clearwater, FL 33759		**Results Provided By** Medical Center Laboratory 33 West Main St Clearwater, FL 33759
Specimen Coll. Date	6/25/20XX	Fasting/Nonfasting		Nonfasting
Specimen Coll. Time	02:53 pm	Laboratory Accession Number		33804237
Specimen Received Date/Time	6/25/20XX 05:30 pm	Lab ID Number		373978
Results Reported Date/Time	6/26/20XX 10:00 am	Test(s) Ordered		CPT: 81001 Complete Urinalysis

Test	**Result**	**Reference Range**	**Units**	**Flag**
Physical Examination				
Color	Yellow	Yellow		
Appearance	**Cloudy**	**Clear**		**Abnormal**
Specific gravity	1.020	1.005-1.030		
Chemical Examination				
Glucose	Negative	Negative		
Bilirubin	Negative	Negative		
Ketone	Negative	Negative		
Blood	Negative	Negative		
pH	6.5	5-7.5		
Protein	Trace	Negative/Trace		
Urobilinogen	0.2	0.2-1.0	mg/dL	
Nitrite	**Positive**	**Negative**		**Abnormal**
Leukocytes	**2+**	**Negative**		**Abnormal**
Microscopic Examination				
WBC	**8-10**	**0-5**	**/HPF**	**Abnormal**
RBC	0-2	0-3	/HPF	
Epithelial Cells	0-8	0-10	/HPF	
Casts	None seen	None	/LPF	
Mucus Threads	Present	Not Established		
Bacteria	**Moderate**	**None Seen/ Few**	**/HPF**	**Abnormal**

Fig. 30.3 Urinalysis laboratory report.

testing for blood, bilirubin, urobilinogen, nitrite, and leukocytes. A computer-generated laboratory report for a complete urinalysis is illustrated in Fig. 30.3.

pH

The **pH** is the unit that indicates the acidity or alkalinity of a solution. The pH scale ranges from 0.0 to 14.0. The lower the number, the greater the acidity; the higher the number, the greater the alkalinity. A pH reading of 7.0 is neutral; a reading below 7.0 indicates acidity; a reading above 7.0 indicates alkalinity.

The kidneys help regulate the acid–base balance of the body. For an accurate pH reading of the urine, the measurement should be performed on freshly voided urine. If the urine is allowed to remain standing out too long, it becomes more alkaline as urea is converted to ammonia by bacterial action.

Although the pH of urine can normally range from 4.6 to 8.0, the pH of a freshly voided specimen of a patient on a normal diet is usually acidic and has a pH reading of about 6.0. An abnormally high pH reading on a fresh specimen (i.e., alkaline urine) may indicate a bacterial infection of the urinary tract.

Glucose

Normally, no glucose should be detectable in the urine. Glucose in the blood is filtered through the **nephrons** (functional units of the kidney) and is reabsorbed into the body. If the glucose concentration in the blood becomes too high, the kidneys are unable to reabsorb all of it back into the blood, the renal threshold is exceeded, and glucose is spilled into the urine—a condition known as **glycosuria.** (The **renal threshold** is the concentration at which a substance in the blood that is not normally excreted by the kidneys begins to appear in the urine.) The renal threshold for glucose is typically 160 to 180 mg/dL (100 mL of blood), but this number may vary among individuals. Diabetes mellitus is the most common cause of glycosuria. Some individuals have a low renal threshold, and glucose may appear in their urine after the consumption of a large quantity of foods containing sugar. This condition is known as *alimentary glycosuria.*

Protein

The presence of protein in the urine is known as **proteinuria.** Protein in the urine usually indicates a pathologic condition if found in several samples over a period of time. A temporary increase in urine protein may be caused by stress or strenuous exercise. Some of the conditions that may cause proteinuria include glomerular filtration problems, renal disease, and bacterial infection of the urinary tract. If proteinuria occurs, the provider usually requests an examination of the sediment to determine, through visual observation, what is causing protein to be in the urine.

Ketones

Ketones are the normal products of fat metabolism and can be used by muscle tissue as a source of energy. There are three types of ketone bodies: beta-hydroxybutyric acid, acetoacetic acid, and acetone. When more than normal amounts of fat are metabolized by the body, the muscles cannot handle all of the ketones that result. Large amounts of ketone accumulate in the tissues and body fluids; this condition is known as **ketosis.** The body rids itself of these excess ketones by excreting them in the urine. **Ketonuria** is the term that refers to the presence of ketone bodies in the urine. Conditions that can cause increased fat metabolism resulting in ketonuria include uncontrolled diabetes mellitus, starvation, and a diet composed almost entirely of fat.

Bilirubin

The average life span of a red blood cell is 120 days. When a red blood cell breaks down, one of the substances released from the breakdown of hemoglobin is a vivid yellow pigment known as *bilirubin.* Normally, bilirubin is transported to the liver by the blood and excreted into the bile, and it eventually leaves the body through the intestines in the feces giving the stool its brown color. If damaged, the liver is unable to remove bilibrubin from the blood. The bilirubin builds up in the blood and is excreted in the urine. Certain liver conditions and gallbladder problems, such as gallstones, hepatitis, and cirrhosis, may result in the presence of bilirubin in the urine, or **bilirubinuria.** The urine becomes yellow-brown or greenish, and a yellow foam appears when the urine is shaken.

Urobilinogen

Normally, bilirubin is excreted by the liver into the intestinal tract. Bacteria present in the intestines convert it to urobilinogen. Approximately 50% of the urobilinogen is reabsorbed into the body for reexcretion by the liver. Small amounts may appear in the urine, but most of the urobilinogen is excreted in the feces. An increase in the production of bilirubin increases the amount of urobilinogen excreted in the urine. Conditions such as excessive hemolysis of red blood cells, infectious hepatitis, cirrhosis, congestive heart failure, and infectious mononucleosis may increase the level of urobilinogen in the urine.

Blood

Blood is considered an abnormal constituent of urine, unless it is present as a contaminant during menstruation. The condition in which blood is found in the urine is termed *hematuria.* Hematuria may be the result of injury or disorders such as cystitis, tumors of the bladder, urethritis, kidney stones, and certain kidney disorders.

Nitrite

Nitrite in the urine indicates the presence of a pathogen in the (normally sterile) urinary tract, which results in a UTI. The pathogen possesses the ability to convert nitrate, which normally occurs in the urine, to nitrite, which is normally absent. The nitrite test must be performed with urine that has been in the bladder for at least 4 to 6 hours to ensure that bacteria have converted nitrate to nitrite. Therefore, use of a first-voided morning specimen is recommended. The test should *not* be performed on specimens that have been left standing out because a false-positive result may occur from bacterial contamination from the environment. The nitrite test is a screening test and is usually followed by a quantitative urine culture and identification of the invading pathogen.

Leukocytes

The presence of leukocytes in the urine is known as *leukocyturia* and accompanies inflammation of the kidneys and the lower urinary tract. Examples of specific conditions include acute and chronic pyelonephritis, cystitis, and urethritis. Urine reagent strips are available that contain a reagent pad that permits the chemical detection of intact and lysed leukocytes in the urine. The advantage of detecting lysed leukocytes is that these cells cannot be observed during a microscopic examination of urine sediment and would otherwise remain undetected. The recommended urine specimen, particularly for women, is a clean-catch midstream collection to prevent contamination of the specimen with leukocytes from vaginal secretions leading to a false-positive test result.

CLIA-Waived Reagent Strips

CLIA-waived reagent strips are frequently used in the medical office for the chemical testing of urine. Reagent strips consist of disposable plastic strips on which separate reagent pads are affixed for testing specific chemicals that may be present in the urine during pathologic conditions.

The number and type of reagent pads included on the reagent strip depend on the particular brand of reagent strips. Multistix 10 SG (Siemens Healthcare Diagnostics, Tarrytown, NY) is a CLIA-waived test that contains 10 reagent pads for testing pH, protein, glucose, ketone, bilirubin, blood, urobilinogen, nitrite, specific gravity, and leukocytes. The procedure for performing urinalysis using a Multistix 10 SG reagent strip is presented in (Procedure 30.3).

Test results are qualitative results, and a positive result may indicate the need for further testing. *Qualitative test results* indicate whether a substance is present in the urine and also may provide an approximate indication of the amount of the substance present. Interpretation of reagent strip results involves the use of a color comparison chart, with results documented in terms of positive or negative; 1+, 2+, or 3+; trace, and small, moderate, or large.

The chemical testing of urine using a reagent strip provides information that assists in the diagnosis of the following:

- Conditions affecting kidney function (e.g., kidney stones)
- Urinary tract infections
- Conditions affecting carbohydrate metabolism (e.g., diabetes mellitus)
- Conditions affecting liver function (e.g., hepatitis)

Test results also provide information related to the status of the patient's acid–base balance and urine concentration.

Guidelines

Testing urine with a reagent strip is a relatively easy procedure to perform. Specific guidelines must be followed, however, to ensure accurate test results.

1. *Type of specimen.* The best results are obtained with a freshly voided and thoroughly mixed urine specimen. If the medical assistant is unable to test the specimen within 1 hour of voiding, the specimen should be refrigerated immediately and then allowed to return to room temperature before testing.
2. *Type of collection.* Most reagent strips are designed to be used with a random specimen collection; however, clean-catch midstream and first-voided morning specimens are suggested for specific tests. The nitrite test results are optimized with a first-voided morning specimen, whereas a clean-catch midstream collection is recommended for the leukocyte test.
3. *Urine specimen container.* The specimen container used must be thoroughly clean and free from any detergent or disinfectant residue because cleansing agents contain oxidants that react with the chemicals on the reagent strip, leading to inaccurate test results. The container should be large enough to allow for complete immersion of all of the reagent pads on the strip.
4. *Time intervals.* Read the test results at the exact time intervals specified on the color chart. Do not read any test results after 2 minutes.
5. *Interpretation and reading of results.* Of particular importance is the comparison of the reagent strip with the color chart on the strip container. The reagent strip must be compared with the color chart in good lighting to obtain a good visual match to ensure accurate test results.
6. *Storage of reagent strips.* The reagents on the strips are sensitive to light, heat, and moisture, and the container of strips must be stored in a cool, dry area away from direct sunlight, with the cap tightly closed to maintain reactivity of the reagents. Most reagent strips are packaged in opaque containers to protect them from light. The container may include a desiccant that should not be removed because its purpose is to promote dryness by absorbing moisture. The container of reagent strips must be stored at a temperature between 59°F (15°C) and 86°F (30°C). The strips should not be stored in the refrigerator or freezer. The reagent strips must never be transferred from their original container to another because the other container may harbor traces of moisture, dirt, or chemicals that could affect the test results. A tan-to-brown discoloration or darkening of the reagent pads may indicate deterioration of the pads, in which case the strips should not be used because the test results would be inaccurate. A container of reagent strips past its expiration date should be discarded to prevent inaccurate test results.

Quality Control Test

A quality control procedure should be performed when testing urine with reagent strips. The quality control procedure ensures the reliability of test results by (1) determining whether the reagent strips are reacting properly, and (2) confirming that the testing procedure is being properly performed and accurately interpreted.

To check the reliability of Multistix reagent strips, a Chek-Stix control (Siemens Healthcare Diagnostics, Tarrytown, NY) should be used (Fig. 30.4). The control procedure must be performed according to the manufacturer's instructions outlined in the package insert. The values to be expected from the control procedure are also included in the package insert. The results of the control procedure should be documented in a quality control log. If the expected values are not obtained, the cause of the problem must be determined and corrected. Factors that can cause a

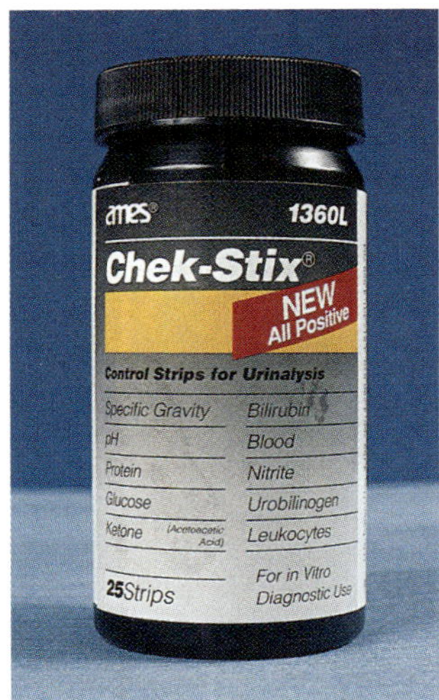

Fig. 30.4 Chek-Stix control.

problem include outdated reagent strips, improper storage of the reagent strips, and an error in testing technique. The quality control procedure should be performed when each new container of reagent strips is opened for the first time or when a question of reliability arises regarding the reagent strips.

Urine Analyzer

CLIA-waived urine analyzers are used to perform an automatic chemical examination of urine with reagent strips. They offer the advantage of the ability to perform the chemical analysis quickly and to interpret results automatically. These analyzers are used most often in medical offices that perform moderate-volume to large-volume urine testing.

The Clinitek Analyzer (Siemens Healthcare Diagnostics, Tarrytown, NY) is an example of a CLIA-waived urine analyzer that automatically reads Multistix SG and other (Siemens) urine reagent strips (Fig. 30.5A). The results are printed out, and abnormal results are flagged to call attention to them (Fig. 30.5B).

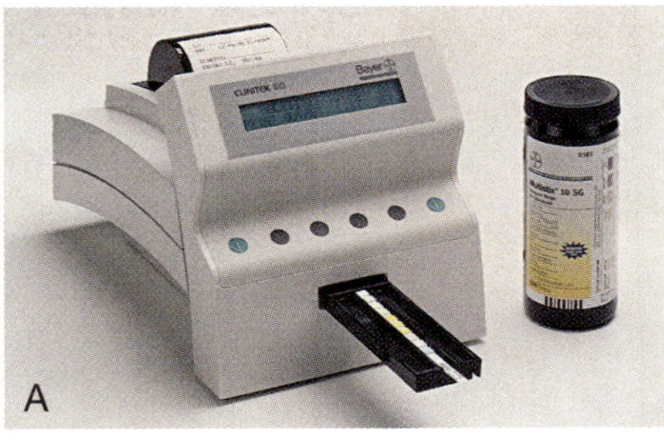

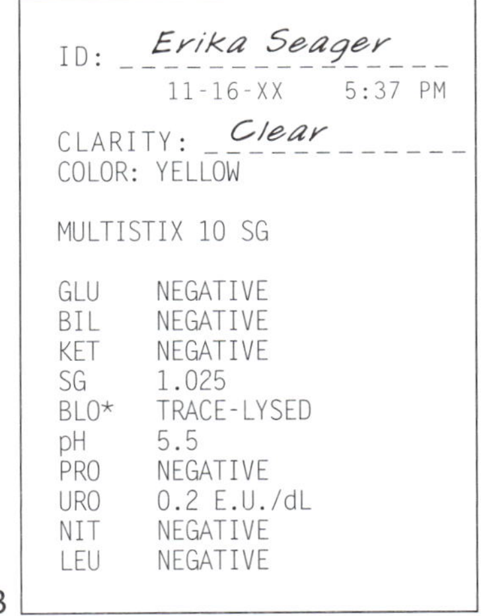
ID: Erika Seager
11-16-XX 5:37 PM
CLARITY: Clear
COLOR: YELLOW

MULTISTIX 10 SG

GLU	NEGATIVE
BIL	NEGATIVE
KET	NEGATIVE
SG	1.025
BLO*	TRACE-LYSED
pH	5.5
PRO	NEGATIVE
URO	0.2 E.U./dL
NIT	NEGATIVE
LEU	NEGATIVE

B

Fig. 30.5 (A) Clinitek urine analyzer. (B) Clinitek printout of test results.

MICROSCOPIC EXAMINATION OF URINE

As discussed in Chapter 29, some medical offices perform moderate complexity tests known as *provider-performed microscopy* (PPM) procedures, which involve the examination of a specimen under the microscope. The microscopic examination of urine sediment is a PPM procedure and must be performed by an individual with the proper training and skill qualifications, such as a medical office provider. A CLIA certificate for PPM procedures is required and the CLIA regulations must be followed, however a physician's office laboratory (POL) is exempt from on-site inspections for PPM procedures.

Urine sediment is the solid material contained in the urine. A microscopic examination of the urine sediment helps to clarify the results of the physical and chemical examination of urine. A first-voided morning specimen is preferred because it is more concentrated and contains more dissolved substances; small amounts of abnormal substances are more likely to be detected. A fresh urine specimen should be used to perform the examination because of the changes that occur in a specimen left standing out. These changes can affect the reliability of the test results. The medical assistant is responsible for preparing the urine specimen for microscopic examination by the provider, as presented in Procedure 30.4.

Red Blood Cells

Red blood cells appear as round, colorless, biconcave discs that are highly refractive (Table 30.1). The presence of 0 to 3 per high-power field (HPF) is considered normal. More than this number may indicate bleeding somewhere along the urinary tract. Table 30.1 lists the possible causes of an abnormal number of red blood cells in the urine. Concentrated urine causes the red blood cells to become shrunken or *crenated*, whereas dilute urine causes them to swell and become rounded, which may cause them to hemolyze. If the red blood cells have hemolyzed, they cannot be seen under the microscope. The presence of blood in the urine still can be identified, however, with a reagent strip, such as Multistix, which is designed to detect free hemoglobin.

Table 30.1 Structures in Urine Sediment

Structure	Possible Causes	Microscopic Appearance
Red blood cells	Inflammatory diseases Acute glomerulonephritis Pyelonephritis Hypertension Renal infarction Trauma Stones Tumor Bleeding diseases Use of anticoagulants	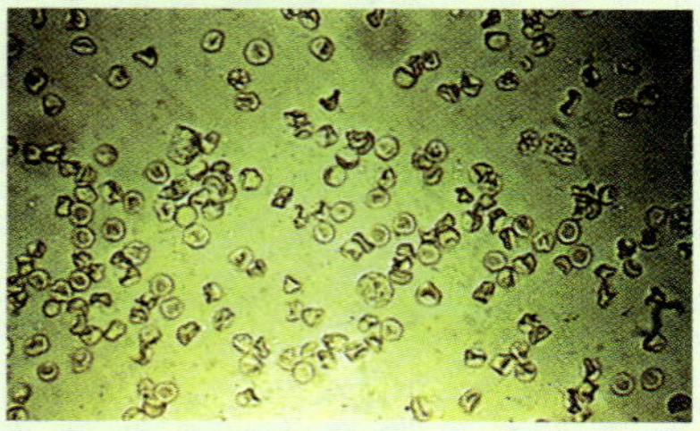 Red blood cells
White blood cells	Pyelonephritis Cystitis Urethritis Prostatitis Transplant rejection (manifested by lymphocytes in urine) Tissue injury accompanied by severe inflammation (manifested by monocytes in urine) Inflammation, immune mechanisms, and other host defense mechanisms (manifested by histiocytes in urine)	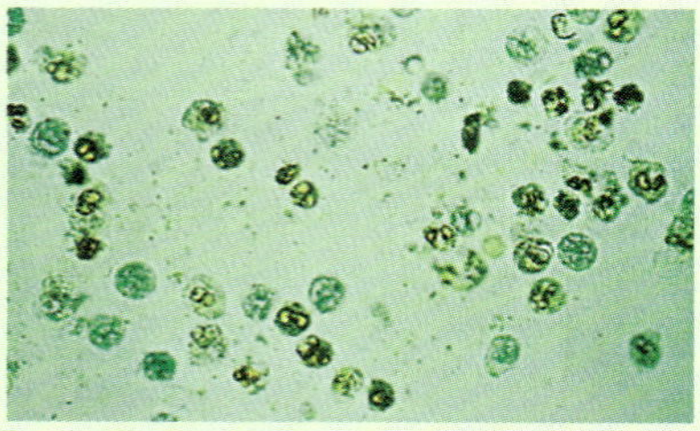 White blood cells
Squamous epithelial cells	Vaginal contamination	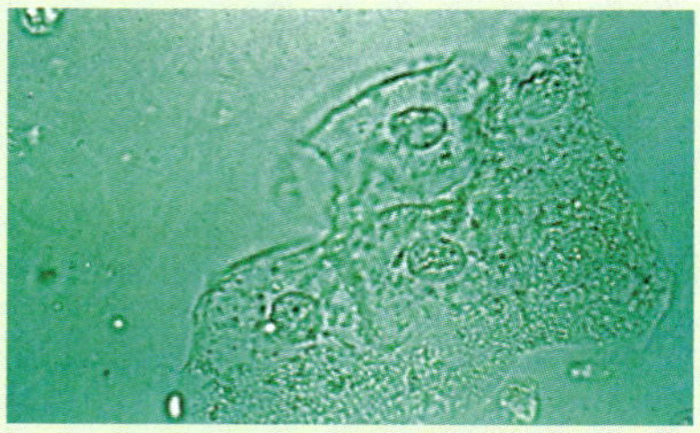 Squamous epithelial cells
Renal tubular epithelial cells	Acute tubular necrosis Glomerulonephritis Acute infection Renal toxicity Viral infection	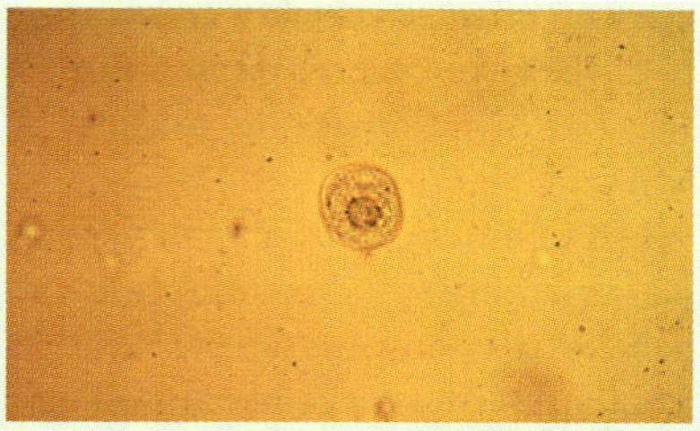 Renal tubular epithelial cells
Hyaline casts	Normal urine Strenuous exercise Acute glomerulonephritis Acute pyelonephritis Malignant hypertension Chronic renal disease	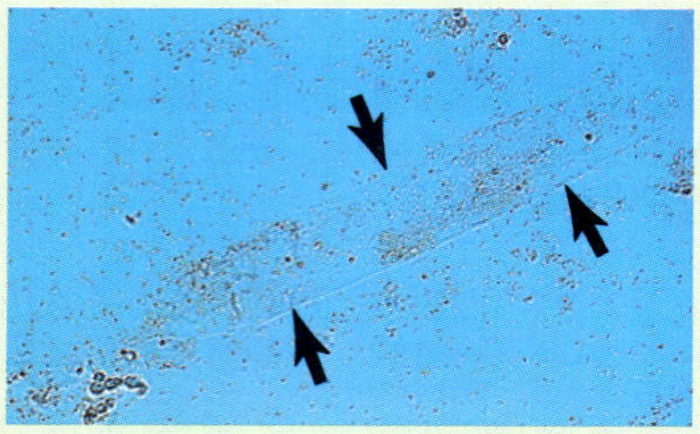 Hyaline cast*
Amorphous urate	Nonpathologic	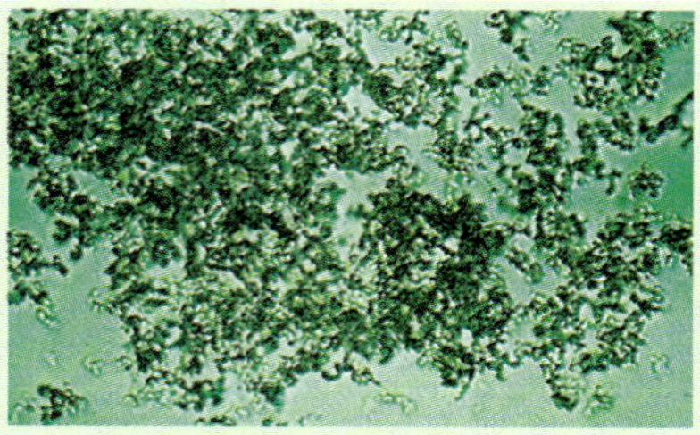 Amorphous urate crystals*

Table 30.1 Structures in Urine Sediment—cont'd

Structure	Possible Causes	Microscopic Appearance
Uric acid	Usually nonpathologic; in large numbers, may indicate gout	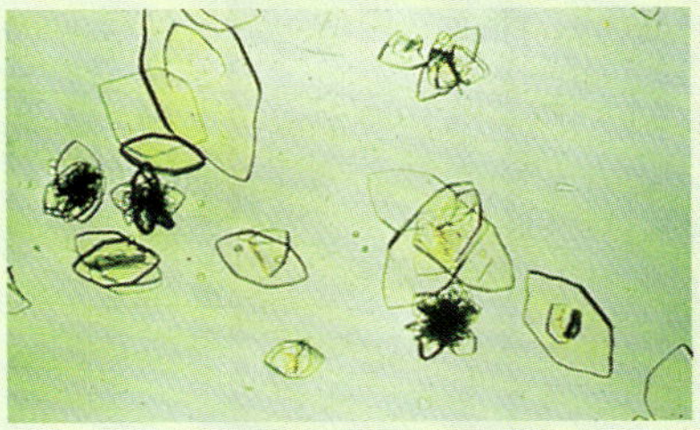 Uric acid crystals*
Calcium oxalate	Usually nonpathologic; may be associated with stone formation	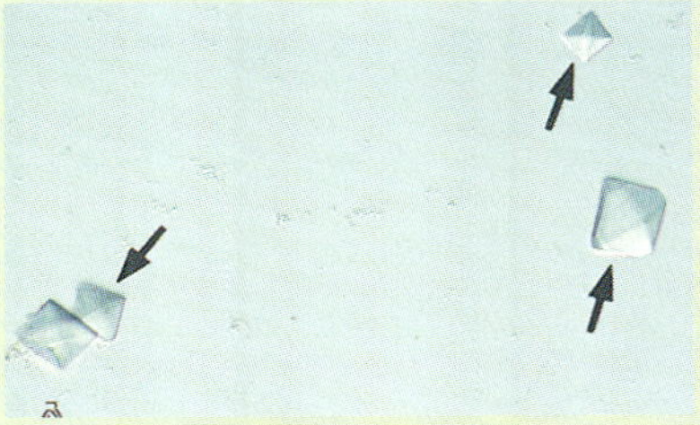 Calcium oxalate crystals†
Bacteria	More than 100,000 bacteria per mL indicates urinary tract infection 10,000–100,000 bacteria per mL indicates that tests should be repeated Less than 10,000 bacteria per mL may signify urine in which any bacteria are urethral organisms or the result of contamination Bacteria accompanied by white blood cells or white blood cell or mixed casts may indicate acute pyelonephritis	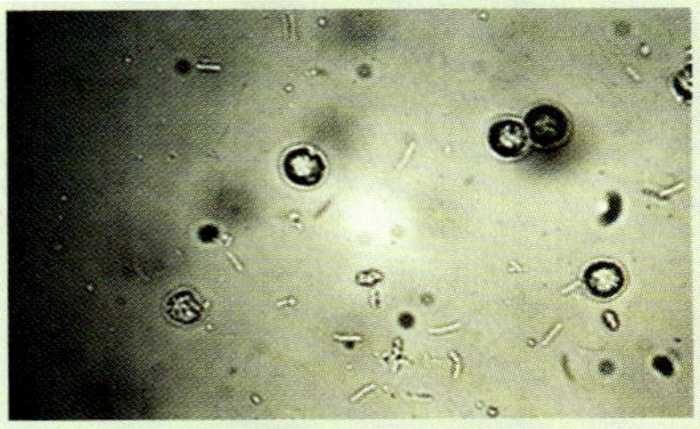 Bacteria (small rod structures)*
Yeast	May indicate contamination by yeasts from skin or hair May indicate diabetes mellitus or urinary tract infection *Candida albicans* may occur in patients with diabetes mellitus or in the contaminated urine of female patients with candidal vaginitis	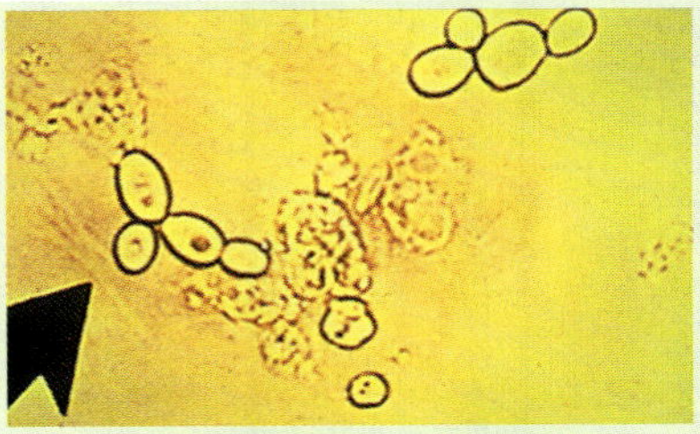 *C. albicans* (yeast)*
Parasites and parasitic ova	Usually indicate fecal or vaginal contamination and should be reported *Trichomonas* may be found in patients with urethritis and in contaminated urine of women with *Trichomonas* vaginitis Pinworm is a common contaminant and should be reported	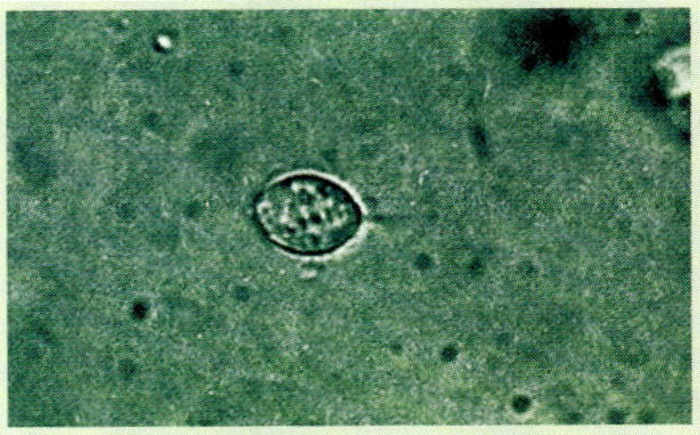 *Trichomonas* (parasite)*
Spermatozoa	Nonpathologic	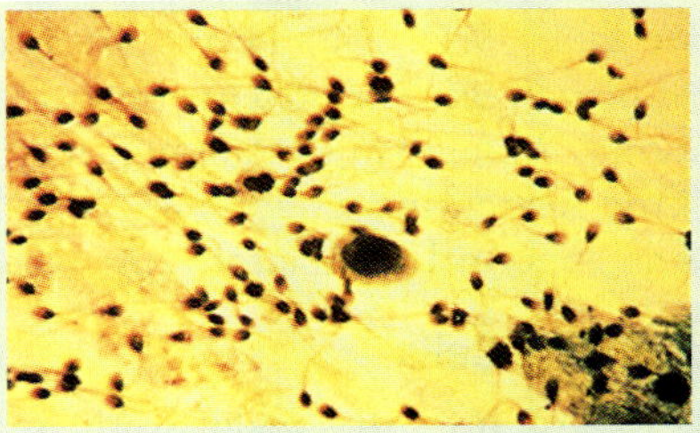 Spermatozoa*

Continued

Table 30.1 Structures in Urine Sediment—cont'd

Structure	Possible Causes	Microscopic Appearance
Urinary artifacts Hair (a) Pollen grains Bubbles Oil droplets Fibers (b) Powder (c) Dust Mucous threads (d) Glass particles	Nonpathologic May result from improper urine collection, improper slide preparation, or outside contamination	(a) Hair†
		(b) Fiber*
		(c) Powder*
		(d) Mucous threads‡

*Photomicrographs courtesy Bayer Corporation, Diagnostics Division, Elkhart, IN.
†Photomicrograph from Lehman CA: *Saunders manual of clinical laboratory science*, Philadelphia, 1998, Saunders.
‡Photomicrograph from Stepp CA, Woods M: *Laboratory procedures for medical office personnel*, Philadelphia, 1998, Saunders.
Text courtesy Boehringer Mannheim Diagnostics, Indianapolis, IN.

White Blood Cells

White blood cells are round and granular and have a nucleus (see Table 30.1). They are approximately 1.5 times as large as red blood cells. The presence of 0 to 5 per HPF is considered normal. More than this amount may indicate inflammation of the genitourinary tract. Table 30.1 lists the possible causes of an abnormal number of white blood cells in the urine.

Epithelial Cells

Most structures that make up the urinary system are composed of several layers of epithelial cells. The outer layer is constantly sloughed off and replaced by the cells underneath it. *Squamous epithelial cells* are large, clear, flat cells with an irregular shape. They contain a small nucleus and come from the urethra, bladder, and vagina. Squamous epithelial cells are normally present in small amounts in the urine. *Renal epithelial cells* are round and contain a large nucleus. They come from the deeper layers of the urinary tract, and their presence in the urine is considered abnormal. Table 30.1 lists the types of epithelial cells and possible causes of the presence of abnormal amounts in the urine.

Casts

Casts are cylindric structures formed in the lumen of the tubules that make up a nephron. Materials in the tubules harden, are flushed out, and appear in the urine in the form of casts. Various types of casts may be present in the urine. In general, their presence indicates a diseased condition.

Casts are named according to what they contain. *Hyaline casts* are pale, colorless cylinders with rounded edges that vary in size (see Table 30.1). *Granular casts* are hyaline casts that contain granules and are described as "coarsely granular" or "finely granular," depending on the size of the granules. *Fatty casts* are hyaline casts that contain fat droplets. *Waxy casts* are light yellow and have serrated edges; their name is derived from the fact that they appear to be made of wax. *Cellular casts* contain organized structures and are named according to what they contain. Examples include red blood cell casts, which are hyaline casts containing red blood cells; white blood cell casts, which are hyaline casts containing white blood cells; epithelial casts, which are hyaline casts containing epithelial cells; and bacterial casts, which are hyaline casts containing bacteria.

Crystals

A variety of crystals may be found in the urine. The type and number vary with the pH of the urine. Abnormal crystals include leucine, tyrosine, cystine, and cholesterol. Crystals that commonly appear in acid urine include amorphous urates, uric acid, and calcium oxalate (see Table 30.1). Crystals that commonly appear in alkaline urine include amorphous phosphate, triple phosphate, calcium phosphate, and ammonium urate crystals.

Miscellaneous Structures

Miscellaneous structures are illustrated in Table 30.1 and include the following:

Mucous threads are normally present in small amounts in the urine. They appear as long, wavy, threadlike structures with pointed ends.

Bacteria should not normally exist in the urinary tract. The presence of more than a few bacteria may indicate either contamination of the specimen during collection or a UTI. Bacteria are small structures that may be rod-shaped or round.

Yeast cells are smooth, refractile bodies with an oval shape. A distinguishing feature of yeast cells is small buds that project from the cells involved with reproduction. Yeast cells in the urine of female patients are usually a vaginal contaminant caused by the yeast *Candida albicans* and produce the vaginal infection known as *vulvovaginal candidiasis.* Yeast cells also may be present in the urine of patients with diabetes mellitus.

Parasites may be present in the urine sediment as a contaminant from fecal or vaginal material. *Trichomonas vaginalis* is a parasite that causes trichomoniasis vaginitis.

Spermatozoa may be present in the urine of a man or woman after intercourse. The spermatozoa have round heads and long, slender, hairlike tails.

Fig. 30.3 is an example of a laboratory report that includes a microscopic examination of urine.

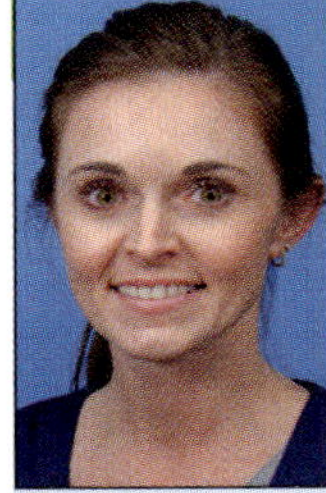

Memories *from* Practicum

Kayla: My main problem as a student on practicum was that I was a little shy. I learned that when your patient is relaxed, he or she is more likely to give you additional and important information about what is wrong. If your patient tenses up during a procedure, this can cause pain for the patient and make the procedure more difficult. When I started to make myself talk more to the patients and staff, things went more smoothly. ■

PATIENT COACHING Urinary Tract Infections (UTIs)

Answer questions that patients may have about UTIs.

What is a UTI?

Urinary tract infection (UTI) is a general term for the presence of bacteria in any portion of the urinary tract. UTIs, particularly those involving the bladder (cystitis) and urethra (urethritis), are common and treatable. A UTI is usually treated with an antibiotic. Use of all of the antibiotic for the total number of days prescribed is important, even if the symptoms disappear. If the medication is stopped too soon, the infection may recur and may be more difficult to treat than the original infection.

What are the symptoms of a UTI?

The symptoms of a simple UTI (cystitis) commonly include the frequent need to urinate, urgency (meaning the immediate need to urinate), a burning sensation during urination, and sometimes blood in the urine. Symptoms of a more complicated UTI involving the kidneys (pyelonephritis) include the aforementioned symptoms as well as lower abdominal discomfort, low back pain, fever, cloudy or foul-smelling urine, and blood in the urine.

Why do women have UTIs more frequently than men?

Women are more prone than men to the type of UTI called *cystitis* because the urethra of a woman is shorter than that of a man, which makes travel up the urethra and into the bladder easier for bacteria. The most common source of infection is bacteria (*Escherichia coli*). *E. coli* organisms are normally found in the large intestine but can travel from the anal area to the urinary bladder, often as the result of poor hygienic practices. Cystitis occurs if *E. coli* organisms are able to overcome the

Continued

PATIENT COACHING **Urinary Tract Infections (UTIs)—cont'd**

body's natural defenses when the bacteria reach the urinary bladder and set up an infection.

What can women do to prevent a UTI?

Women prone to development of UTIs should practice the following prevention measures:

- Practice good hygienic measures by always cleaning the genital area from front to back after a bowel movement.
- Avoid possible irritants, such as bubble baths, perfumed soaps, feminine hygiene sprays, and the use of strong powders and bleaches for washing underclothes.
- Avoid clothing that traps moisture and encourages the growth of microorganisms, such as tight, constricting clothing; nylon panties; and pantyhose.
- Avoid activities that can contribute to irritation of the urinary meatus, such as prolonged bicycling, motorcycling, horseback riding, and travel that involves prolonged sitting.
- Urinate as soon as possible when you feel the urge. Holding urine in the bladder gives the bacteria more time to grow, which can cause a more severe infection. The more often you urinate, the more quickly the bacteria are removed from the bladder.
- Seek prompt treatment if you experience any of the symptoms of a UTI.

Encourage the patient with a UTI to drink plenty of water to help flush the bacteria out of the urinary tract.

Emphasize to the patient the importance of taking all of the antibiotic for the duration of time prescribed.

Emphasize the importance of practicing preventive measures to prevent the occurrence of UTIs.

Provide the patient with educational materials on UTIs. ■

URINE PREGNANCY TESTING

The diagnosis of pregnancy can be accomplished in several ways. By the eighth week after conception, pregnancy can be confirmed with the medical history and physical examination. The provider may desire an earlier diagnosis, however, with a pregnancy test to initiate early prenatal care. A pregnancy test also may be necessary before certain medications are ordered or procedures are performed that may cause injury to a fetus.

HUMAN CHORIONIC GONADOTROPIN

Immunoassay tests are often used for pregnancy testing. These tests are performed on a concentrated urine specimen and rely on the presence of a hormone known as *human chorionic gonadotropin* (HCG) for a positive reaction.

HCG is produced by the developing fertilized egg, and small amounts of it are secreted into the urine and blood. Immediately after conception and implantation of the fertilized egg, the plasma level of HCG increases rapidly and can be used to detect pregnancy with a serum pregnancy test as early as 6 days before the first missed menstrual period. The highest plasma levels of HCG occur at about 8 weeks after conception. After this time, the production of HCG declines and remains at a lower level for the duration of the pregnancy. Within 72 hours of delivery, HCG disappears entirely from the plasma. As a result, pregnancy tests are more sensitive during the first trimester and may show a negative reaction when the level of HCG begins to decline during the second and third trimesters.

IMMUNOASSAY URINE PREGNANCY TEST

CLIA-waived immunoassay tests are used in the medical office for the detection of pregnancy. These tests are convenient to perform and provide immediate test results. Positive and negative reactions are evidenced by a specific visible reaction that is observed and interpreted by the individual performing the test.

Immunoassay urine pregnancy tests are commercially available in test kits that contain the required reagents and supplies to perform the test. Each kit can be used to perform a specific number of tests, ranging from 25 to 50. The instructions in the package insert accompanying the test kit should be followed *exactly* to prevent inaccurate test results. When performed correctly, most urine pregnancy tests are 99% accurate with low occurrences of false-positive test results.

Immunoassay pregnancy tests provide for the rapid, qualitative detection of HCG in a urine specimen; brand names include QuickVue HCG Urine Test (Quidel, San Diego, CA), OSOM HCG Urine Test (Genzyme Diagnostics, Cambridge, MA), and ICON HCG Pregnancy Test (Beckman Coulter, Brea, CA). Early prediction pregnancy tests may be able to detect pregnancy as early as 2 to 3 days before a first missed menstrual period. Urine pregnancy tests performed this early, however, may show a false-negative result and should be repeated later to confirm the results. Accurate results are much more probable if the urine is tested 1 week after a missed period.

Immunoassay tests take approximately 5 minutes to perform, and the test results are easily observed as a color change. Specific instructions for interpreting the test results are included in the package insert. The procedure for performing an immunoassay with the QuickVue HCG Urine Test (Quidel) is outlined in Procedure 30.5.

GUIDELINES FOR URINE PREGNANCY TESTING

Specific guidelines must be followed for urine pregnancy testing, to ensure accurate test results:

1. Use clean, preferably disposable, urine containers to collect the specimen. Traces of detergent in the specimen container may cause inaccurate test results.
2. The preferred specimen for a urine pregnancy test is a first-voided morning specimen because it contains the highest concentration of HCG; however, a random urine specimen can also be used. If the urine specimen cannot be tested immediately after voiding, it should be preserved in the refrigerator. A patient who collects the specimen at home should be given instructions on preserving the specimen.
3. The specific gravity of the urine specimen should be determined before the test is performed. A specific gravity of less than 1.007 is considered too dilute for pregnancy testing because it may lead to a false-negative test result.
4. The urine specimen should be at room temperature before the procedure is performed.
5. The urine pregnancy test kit should be stored according to the information in the package insert. Most test kits are stored at a room temperature between 59°F (15°C) and 86°F (30°C) and away from direct sunlight.
6. Test kits past their expiration dates should not be used.
7. If more than one patient is being tested at a time, label each test device with the patient's name to prevent a mix-up of specimens.
8. Most urine pregnancy test kits include a built-in internal control to evaluate whether certain aspects of the testing procedure are working properly. The internal control is performed at the same time that the testing procedure is performed. It determines whether a sufficient amount of the specimen was added to the test cassette and if the correct procedural technique was followed. If the internal control does not perform as expected, the test result is invalid and the specimen must be retested. It is recommended that the internal control results be documented in a quality control log for the first pregnancy test run each day.
9. It is recommended that a positive and a negative external control be performed with each new lot of test kits. External controls are used to determine if the test reagents are performing properly and to detect any errors in technique of the individual performing the test. External controls consist of commercially available solutions and may be included with the test system or may need to be purchased separately. The control procedure is performed using the same procedure for performing the test on a patient. Instead of adding the patient specimen to the test device, however, the control is added to it. The positive control should produce a positive result, and the negative control should produce a negative result. The results should be documented in a quality control log (Fig. 30.6). Failure of an external control to produce expected results may be caused by outdated controls or test reagents, improper storage of test components, improper environmental testing conditions and an error in the technique used to perform the procedure.
10. Conditions other than a normal pregnancy that can result in a positive result include ectopic pregnancy and molar pregnancy.

QUALITY CONTROL LOG

URINE PREGNANCY TEST

	Date	Name of test	Control lot #	Control expiration date	External positive control	External negative control	Technician
1	3/25 20XX	Quick Vue One Step HCG	140400	3/16/XX	+	–	L.Profit CMA (AAMA)
2	4/22 20XX	Quick Vue One Step HCG	140400	3/16/XX	+	–	L.Profit CMA (AAMA)
3	5/27 20XX	Quick Vue One Step HCG	140400	3/16/XX	+	–	L.Profit CMA (AAMA)
4							
5							
6							
7							
8							
9							
10							

Fig. 30.6 Quality control log for urine pregnancy testing.

What Would You Do? What Would You *Not* Do?

Case Study 3

Rita Lavelle is 8½ months pregnant and is at the clinic for a prenatal appointment. Lately, she has been having difficulty obtaining a urine specimen at the medical office because of her enlarged abdomen. At her last appointment, the office provided her with a urine specimen container so that she could obtain her specimen more easily at home. Rita brings in a first-voided urine specimen in a glass jar. She says her dog chewed up the specimen container from the office, so she used an empty peanut butter jar. The urine test results from her specimen show that her glucose level is normal, but her protein level is 4+. Until this time, her urine test results all have been normal. Rita is concerned about her baby. She says that she was cleaning her bathroom cabinet yesterday and came across a pregnancy test; just for the fun of it, she decided to run the test. The results were negative, and now she is worried that something is wrong. Rita says that she has not been sleeping as well at night and that she has noticed more Braxton–Hicks contractions, but the baby has been kicking and moving as usual. ■

SERUM PREGNANCY TEST

The radioimmunoassay (RIA) serum pregnancy test for HCG is a (nonwaived) quantitative test used to detect HCG in the serum of the blood. This test can detect pregnancy earlier and with greater accuracy than a urine pregnancy test. A serum pregnancy test can usually detect pregnancy at approximately the eighth day after fertilization, which is 6 days before the first missed menstrual period. This test uses a radioisotope technique and is capable of detecting minute amounts of HCG in the blood. This test is usually used to diagnose abnormalities, such as ectopic pregnancy; to follow the course of early pregnancy when abnormalities of embryonic development are suspected; and to provide an early diagnosis of pregnancy in individuals at high risk, such as patients with diabetes.

What Would You Do? What Would You *Not* Do? RESPONSES

Case Study 1

Page 791

What Did Kayla Do?

- ❑ Took some time to try to calm and relax Mr. Urameshi. Reassured him that the physician would do everything he could to make Mr. Urameshi better.
- ❑ Offered Mr. Urameshi something to drink and told him it might help him obtain a specimen.
- ❑ Went over the directions again with Mr. Urameshi.
- ❑ Asked Mr. Urameshi if he would try again to obtain a specimen.

What Did Kayla Not Do?

- ❑ Did not tell Mr. Urameshi that he was not trying hard enough.

Case Study 2

Page 794

What Did Kayla Do?

- ❑ Asked Nora whether she takes all of the antibiotic she is prescribed when she has a UTI.
- ❑ Explained to Nora in terms she can understand why women seem to be more prone to development of UTIs.
- ❑ Explained to Nora what she could do to help prevent UTIs. Gave her a patient education brochure on UTIs to take home.
- ❑ Told Nora that the physician is not legally or ethically permitted to call in a prescription for her without seeing her. Also explained that it is in the best interests of her health care to be seen by the physician.

What Did Kayla Not Do?

- ❑ Did not tell Nora that she could not test her urine at home.

Case Study 3

Page 806

What Did Kayla Do?

- ❑ Told Rita that some peanut butter residue might have been left in the jar she used and might have affected the test results. Asked her to try to collect another specimen at the office so that the urine could be tested again.
- ❑ Told Rita that if something happens to the specimen container again, she should come to the office and get another one.
- ❑ Told Rita that several things could have caused her pregnancy test result to be negative. Explained to her that the test could have been outdated or not stored properly. Also explained that as a pregnancy gets farther along, less of the hormone that causes the test to be positive is secreted, so negative test results at the end of a pregnancy are not unusual.
- ❑ Reassured Rita that many women have trouble sleeping during the last month of pregnancy and that it is normal to have more Braxton–Hicks contractions as she gets closer to delivery.
- ❑ Told Rita that she would inform the physician of her symptoms so that he could discuss them in more detail with her.

What Did Kayla Not Do?

- ❑ Did not criticize Rita for collecting her specimen in a peanut butter jar.
- ❑ Did not ignore or minimize Rita's concerns.

TERMINOLOGY REVIEW

Key Term	Word Parts	Definition
Anuria	*an-:* without, absence of *ur/o:* urine *-ia:* condition of disease or abnormal state	Failure of the kidneys to produce urine.
Bilirubinuria	*bilirubino/o:* bilirubin *ur/o-:* urine *-ia:* condition of disease or abnormal state	The presence of bilirubin in the urine.
Bladder catheterization		The passing of a sterile catheter through the urethra and into the bladder to remove urine.
Diuresis		Secretion and passage of large amounts of urine.
Dysuria	*dys-:* difficult, labored, painful *ur/o:* urine *-ia:* condition of disease or abnormal state	Difficult or painful urination.
Frequency		The condition of having to urinate often.
Glycosuria	*glyc/o:* sugar *ur/o:* urine *-ia:* condition of disease or abnormal state	The presence of glucose in the urine.
Hematuria	*hemato/o:* blood *ur/o:* urine *-ia:* condition of disease or abnormal state	Blood present in the urine.
Ketonuria	*keton/o:* ketone *ur/o:* urine *-ia:* condition of disease or abnormal state	The presence of ketone bodies in the urine.
Ketosis	*keton/o:* ketone *-osis:* abnormal condition	An accumulation of large amounts of ketone bodies in the tissues and body fluids.
Micturition		The act of voiding urine.
Nephron		The functional unit of the kidney that filters waste substances from the blood and dilutes them with water to produce urine.
Nocturia	*noct/i:* night *ur/o:* urine *-ia:* condition of disease or abnormal state	Excessive (voluntary) urination during the night.
Nocturnal enuresis		Inability of an individual to control urination at night during sleep (bedwetting).
Oliguria	*olig/o:* scanty, few *ur/o:* urine *-ia:* condition of disease or abnormal state	Decreased or scanty output of urine.
pH		The unit that describes the acidity or alkalinity of a solution.
Polyuria	*poly-:* many *ur/o:* urine *-ia:* condition of disease or abnormal state	Increased output of urine.
Proteinuria	*protein-:* protein *ur/o:* urine *-ia:* condition of disease or abnormal state	The presence of protein in the urine.
Pyuria	*py/o:* pus *ur/o:* urine *-ia:* condition of disease or abnormal state	The presence of pus in the urine.
Renal threshold		The concentration at which a substance in the blood that is not normally excreted by the kidneys begins to appear in the urine.
Retention		The inability to empty the bladder. The urine is being produced normally but is not being voided.

Continued

TERMINOLOGY REVIEW—cont'd

Key Term	Word Parts	Definition
Specific gravity (urine)		The weight of a substance compared with the weight of an equal volume of distilled water. In urinalysis, the *specific gravity* refers to the measurement of the amount of dissolved substances present in the urine compared with the same amount of distilled water.
Supernatant	*super:* over, above	The clear liquid that remains at the top after a precipitate has settled.
Suprapubic aspiration	*supra-:* above *pub/o:* pubis *-ic:* pertaining to	The passing of a sterile needle through the abdominal wall into the bladder to remove urine.
Urgency		The immediate need to urinate.
Urinalysis	*urin/o:* urine	The physical, chemical, and microscopic analyses of urine.
Urinary incontinence		The inability to retain urine in the bladder.

PROCEDURE 30.1 Collection of a Clean-Catch Midstream Urine Specimen

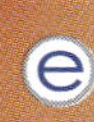

Outcome Instruct a patient in the collection of a clean-catch midstream urine specimen.

Equipment/Supplies

- Sterile specimen container and label
- Personal antiseptic towelettes
- Tissues

1. **Procedural Step.** Sanitize your hands. Greet the patient and introduce yourself. Identify the patient and explain the procedure.
2. **Procedural Step.** Assemble equipment. Label the specimen container with the patient's name and date of birth, the date, the type of specimen (clean-catch midstream), and your initials.

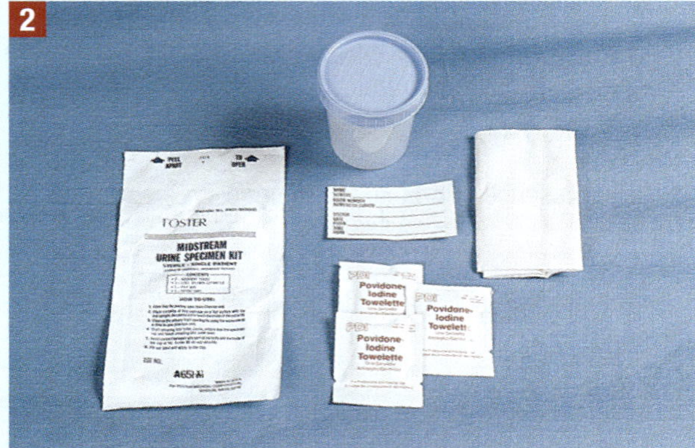

Assemble the equipment.

3. **Procedural Step.** Instruct a female patient on collection of the specimen as follows:
   a. Wash the hands, open the package of towelettes, and place them on their wrapper.
   b. Remove the lid from the specimen container and place it on a paper towel with the opening of the lid facing upward. Do not touch the inside of the lid or the inside of the specimen container.
   c. Pull undergarments down and sit on the toilet. Expose the urinary meatus by spreading apart the labia with one hand.
   d. Cleanse each side of the urinary meatus with an antiseptic towelette using a front-to-back motion (from pubis to anus). Use a separate antiseptic towelette for each side of the meatus. After use, discard each towelette in the toilet.

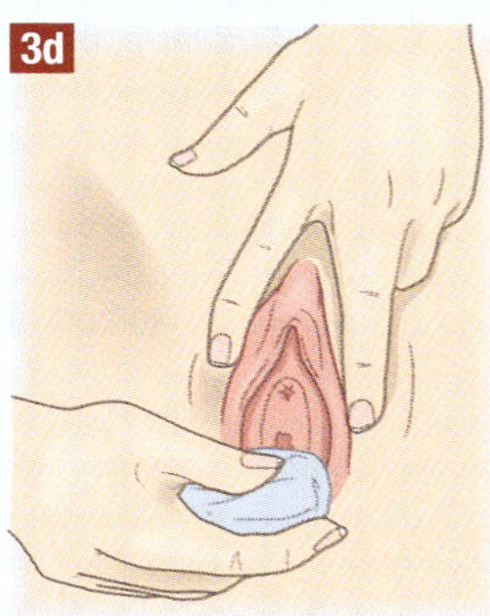

Cleanse the urinary meatus. (From Niedzwiecki B, Pepper J, Weaver P: *Kinn's the medical assistant*, ed 14, St. Louis, 2020, Elsevier.)

PROCEDURE 30.1 Collection of a Clean-Catch Midstream Urine Specimen—cont'd

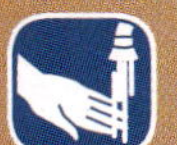

e. Cleanse directly across the meatus (front to back) with a third antiseptic towelette. Discard the towelette.

f. Continue to hold the labia apart and void a small amount of urine into the toilet.

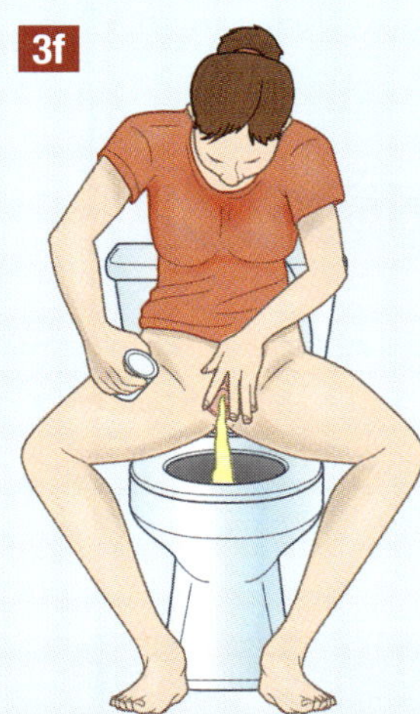

Void a small amount of urine into the toilet. (From Niedzwiecki B, Pepper J, Weaver P: *Kinn's the medical assistant*, ed 14, St. Louis, 2020, Elsevier.)

g. Without stopping the urine flow, collect the next amount of urine (midstream flow of urine) by voiding into the sterile container. Do not touch the inside of the sterile container. Fill the specimen container about half full with urine.

h. Void the last amount of urine into the toilet. This means that the first and last portions of the urine flow are not included in the specimen. Replace the lid of the specimen container.

i. Wipe the area dry with a tissue, and discard it in the toilet. Flush the toilet and wash the hands.

Principle. Cleansing removes microorganisms from the urinary meatus. A front-to-back motion must be used for cleansing to avoid drawing microorganisms from the anal region into the area that is being cleansed. Voiding a small amount flushes microorganisms out of the distal urethra. Touching the inside of the container contaminates it with microorganisms that normally reside on the skin.

4. Procedural Step. Instruct a male patient as follows:

a. Wash the hands, open the towelettes, remove the lid from the specimen container, and remove undergarments.

b. Stand in front of the toilet. Retract the foreskin of the penis (if uncircumcised).

c. Cleanse the area around the meatus (glans penis) and the urethral opening (meatal orifice) by wiping each side of the meatus with a separate antiseptic towelette.

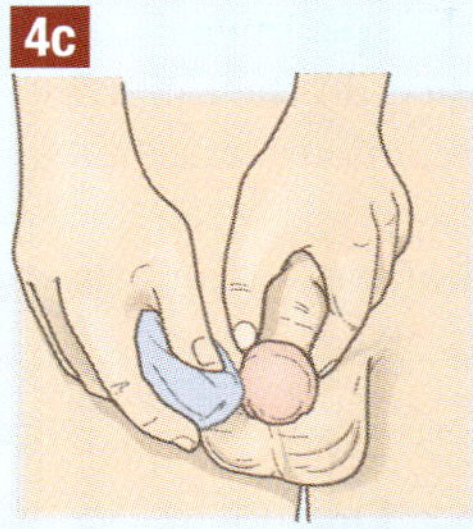

Cleanse the area around the meatus. (From Niedzwiecki B, Pepper J, Weaver P: *Kinn's the medical assistant*, ed 14, St. Louis, 2020, Elsevier.)

d. Cleanse directly across the meatus with a third antiseptic towelette. After use, discard each towelette in the toilet.

e. Void a small amount of urine into the toilet.

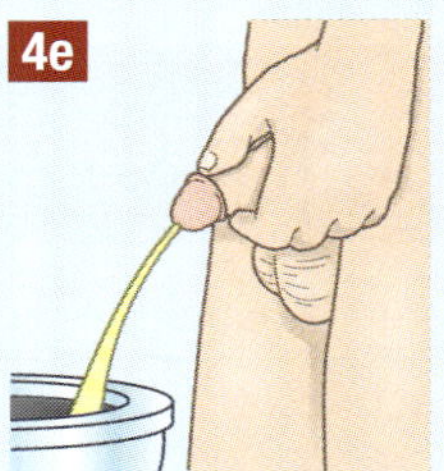

Void a small amount of urine into the toilet. (From Niedzwiecki B, Pepper J, Weaver P: *Kinn's the medical assistant*, ed 14, St. Louis, 2020, Elsevier.)

f. Collect the next amount of urine by voiding into the sterile container without touching the inside of the container with the hands or penis. Fill the container about half full with urine.

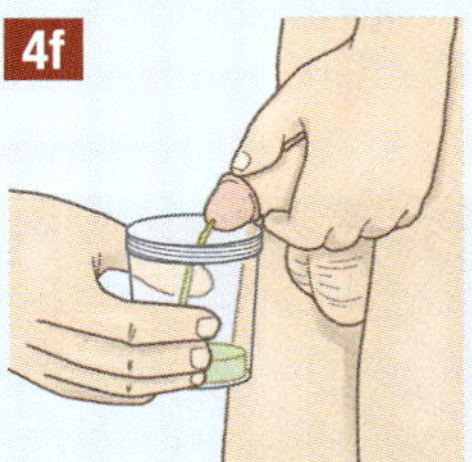

Void into the sterile container. (From Niedzwiecki B, Pepper J, Weaver P. *Kinn's the medical assistant*, ed 14, St. Louis, 2020, Elsevier.)

g. Void the last amount of urine into the toilet and replace the lid on the container.

Wipe the area dry with a tissue, and discard it in the toilet. Flush the toilet and wash the hands.

5. Procedural Step. Provide the patient with instructions about what to do with the specimen after it has been collected (e.g., placing it in a designated area, directly handing it to the medical assistant).

6. Procedural Step. Test the specimen at the office or prepare the specimen for transport to an outside laboratory

Continued

PROCEDURE 30.1 Collection of a Clean-Catch Midstream Urine Specimen—cont'd

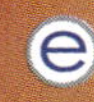

for testing. If the specimen is to be transported to an outside laboratory, do the following:

a. Place the specimen container in a biohazard specimen bag.
b. Place the laboratory request in the outside pocket of the specimen bag.
c. Properly preserve the specimen while awaiting pickup by a laboratory courier by placing it in a refrigerator.

7. Procedural Step. Document the procedure in the patient's medical record.

a. *Electronic health record:* Document the type of specimen collected (clean-catch specimen, midstream collection) and the test results or the date the specimen was transported to the laboratory using the appropriate radio buttons, drop-down menus, and free text fields.
b. *Paper-based patient record:* Document the date and time and the type of specimen collected (clean-catch midstream collection). Document either the test results or the date the specimen was transported to the laboratory. (Refer to the PPR documentation example.)

7b

DOCUMENTATION EXAMPLE

Date	
3/24/XX	10:15 a.m. Clean-catch midstream collected
	by pt. Sent to Medical Center Laboratory for
	C & S on 3/24/XX. ——K. Smith, CMA (AAMA)

PROCEDURE 30.2

PROCEDURE 30.2 Collection of a 24-Hour Urine Specimen

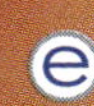

Outcome Instruct a patient in the collection of a clean-catch midstream urine specimen.

Equipment/Supplies

- Large urine collection container and label
- Collecting container
- Written instructions
- Laboratory requisition

1. Procedural Step. Sanitize your hands. Greet the patient and introduce yourself. Identify the patient, and explain the procedure.

2. Procedural Step. Assemble the equipment. Label the large specimen container with the patient's name and date of birth, the date, the type of specimen (24-hour urine specimen), and your initials.

2

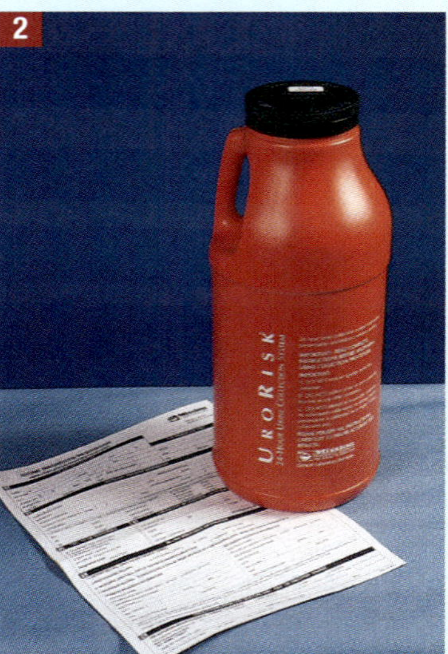

Assemble the equipment.

Instruct the patient on collection of the specimen as follows.

3. Procedural Step. When you get up in the morning, empty your bladder into the toilet just as you normally do. In other words, this urine is not to be saved. Make a note of what time it is, and write the date and start time in the appropriate space on the label of the container.

Principle. This urine was produced before the collection period began and should not be included in the collection.

4. Procedural Step. The next time you need to urinate, void in the collecting container and then pour the urine into the large wide-mouthed specimen container.

5. Procedural Step. Tightly screw the lid onto the 24-hour specimen container, and put the container in your refrigerator or into an ice chest.

6. Procedural Step. Repeat procedural steps 4 and 5 each time you urinate.

7. Procedural Step. Emphasize the importance of the following to the patient:

a. The urine must be stored only in the designated container.
b. Collect all of the urine during the 24-hour period, including urine that you void if you get up during

PROCEDURE 30.2 Collection of a 24-Hour Urine Specimen—cont'd

the night. The information this test provides would be inaccurate if any urine from the 24-hour period does not go into the container.

c. Urinate into the collection container before having a bowel movement to avoid losing urine you might pass during the bowel movement.

d. The collection must be started again from the beginning if any of the following occurs:
- You forget to collect the urine when you void.
- You spill some urine from the collection container.
- Your urine becomes contaminated with stool from a bowel movement.
- The child wets the bed (if the specimen is being obtained from a child).
- You go beyond the 24-hour collection period and collect too much urine.

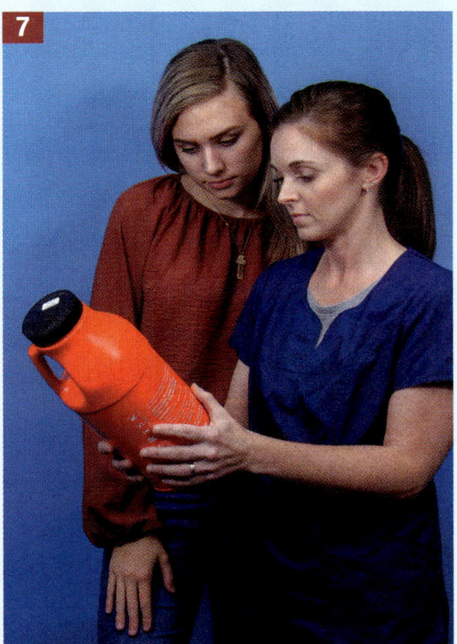

Explain the procedure.

8. Procedural Step. On the following morning, get up and void at the same time (exactly 24 hours after beginning the test). Void into the collection container for the last time and pour the urine into the large specimen container.

9. Procedural Step. Put the lid on the specimen container tightly, and write the date and time the test ended on the label in the appropriate space. Return the 24-hour specimen container to the office the same morning you complete the urine collection.

10. Procedural Step. Provide the patient with the 24-hour specimen container, a collection container, and written instructions. If the specimen container contains a chemical preservative, provide the patient with an MSDS (Material Safety Data Sheet) so that the patient has information regarding the chemical, its hazards, and measures to take to prevent injury and illness when handling the chemical. Document this information in the patient's medical record.

11. Procedural Step. When the patient returns the 24-hour urine specimen container, ask the patient if any difficulties were encountered in following the instructions. If any problems occurred that resulted in undercollection or overcollection of urine, the entire collection process must be repeated.

12. Procedural Step. Prepare the specimen for transport to the laboratory. Complete a laboratory request form.

13. Procedural Step. Document this information in the patient's medical record.

a. *Electronic health record:* Document the type of specimen collected (24-hour specimen) and information on sending the specimen to the laboratory using the appropriate radio buttons, drop-down menus, and free text fields.

b. *Paper-based patient record:* Document the date and time, the type of specimen collected (24-hour specimen), and information on sending the specimen to the laboratory (refer to the PPR documentation example).

13b

DOCUMENTATION EXAMPLE

Date	
3/26/XX	3:30 p.m. Container and verbal/written
	instructions provided on 24-hour specimen
	collection. ———— K. Smith, CMA (AAMA)
3/28/XX	10:00 a.m. 24-hour urine specimen sent to
	Medical Center Laboratory for kidney stone
	risk analysis. ———— K. Smith, CMA (AAMA)

PROCEDURE 30.3 Chemical Assessment of a Urine Specimen Using a Reagent Strip

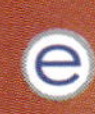

Outcome Perform a chemical assessment of a urine specimen using a reagent strip.

Equipment/Supplies

- Disposable gloves
- Container of Multistix 10 SG reagent strips
- Urine container
- Timer
- Laboratory report form

1. **Procedural Step.** Perform the quality control procedure if using a new container of reagent strips.
   Principle. Performing the quality control procedure ensures the reliability of test results.
2. **Procedural Step.** Obtain a freshly voided urine specimen from the patient in a clean, dry container. The specimen should be at room temperature and should be tested within 1 hour after voiding.
   Principle. The best results are obtained with a freshly voided specimen. The urine container should be clean because contaminants could affect the results. Uncentrifuged specimens ensure a homogeneous sample.
3. **Procedural Step.** Sanitize your hands.
4. **Procedural Step.** Assemble the equipment. Check the expiration date of the reagent strips.
   Principle. Outdated reagent strips may lead to inaccurate test results.
5. **Procedural Step.** Apply gloves. Thoroughly mix the urine specimen and remove the lid from the urine container. Set the container on a flat surface. Remove a reagent strip from its container, and recap the container immediately. It is important not to remove the strip from its container until just before testing. Do not touch the test reagent pads with your fingers.
   Principle. Removing the strip just before testing and recapping the container is necessary to prevent exposing the strips to environmental moisture, light, and heat, which cause altered reagent reactivity. Contamination of test pads by the hands may affect the accuracy of test results.
6. **Procedural Step.** Using the dominant hand, completely immerse the reagent strip in the urine specimen to moisten all the test pads. Remove the strip immediately. While removing, run the edge of the strip against the rim of the urine container to remove excess urine.
   Principle. The strip should be completely immersed to ensure that all test pads are moistened for accurate test results. Prolonged immersion of the reagent strip and failure to remove excess urine may cause the reagents to dissolve and leach onto adjacent test pads, affecting the accuracy of the test results.

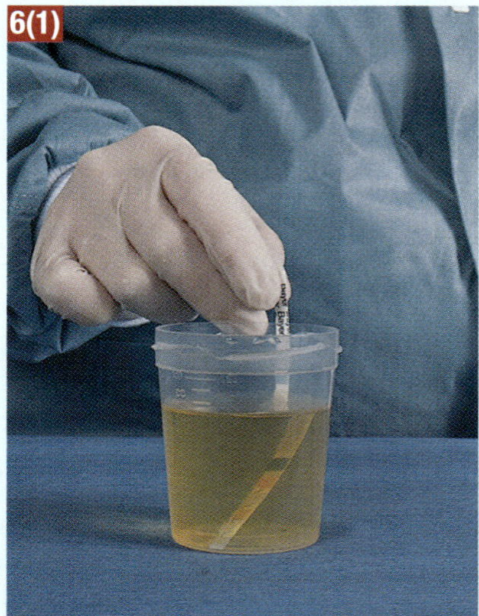

Completely immerse the reagent strip in the urine.

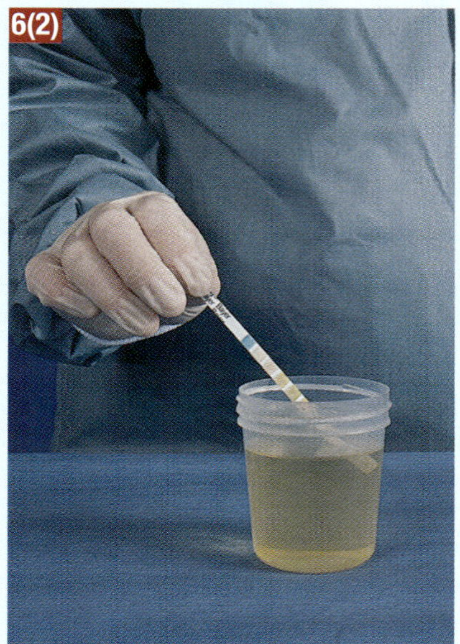

Run the edge of the strip against the urine container.

PROCEDURE 30.3 Chemical Assessment of a Urine Specimen Using a Reagent Strip—cont'd

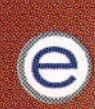

7. Procedural Step. With the nondominant hand, start the timer, pick up the reagent strip container, and rotate it to the color chart. Hold the reagent strip in a horizontal position and place it as close as possible to the corresponding color blocks on the color chart. Do not lay the strip directly on the color chart because this will result in soiling of the chart by the urine. In good lighting, compare each test pad to the corresponding row of color blocks on the container label. Read the results carefully and at the exact reading times, starting with the shortest time specified on the color chart (below). Do not read any test pad after 2 minutes have elapsed as the results will be inaccurate.

Glucose: 30 seconds	pH: 60 seconds
Bilirubin: 30 seconds	Protein: 60 seconds
Ketone: 40 seconds	Urobilinogen: 60 seconds
Specific gravity: 45 seconds	Nitrite: 60 seconds
Blood: 60 seconds	Leukocytes: 2 minutes

Principle. Holding the strip in a horizontal position avoids soiling your gloves with urine and prevents reagents from running over into adjacent test pads, causing inaccurate test results. The strip must be read at the proper time interval to avoid dissolving out reagents, leading to inaccurate test results.

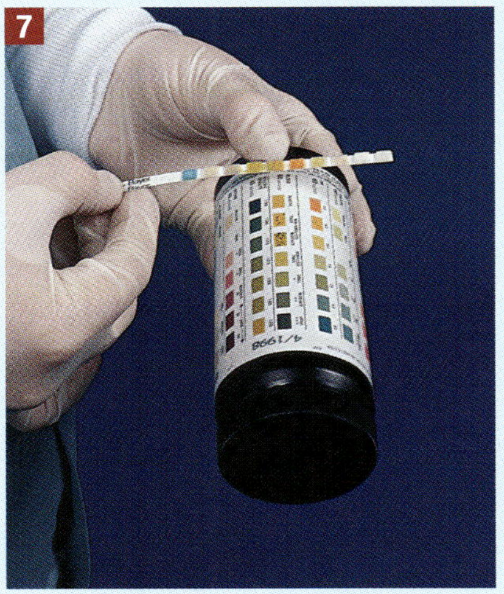

Hold the strip horizontally and read the results.

8. Procedural Step. Dispose of the strip in a regular waste container.

9. Procedural Step. Remove gloves, and sanitize your hands.

10. Procedural Step. Document the results in the patient's medical record. The results should be documented by following the interpretation guide provided above each color block on the color chart.

a. *Electronic health record:* Document the brand name of the test used (Multistix 10 SG) and the results using the appropriate radio buttons, drop-down menus, and free text fields.

b. *Paper-based patient record:* Most offices use a preprinted reporting form to make it easier to document results. The documentation should include the date and time, the brand name of the test used (Multistix 10 SG), and the results (refer to the PPR documentation example).

PROCEDURE 30.3

Continued

PROCEDURE 30.3 Chemical Assessment of a Urine Specimen Using a Reagent Strip—cont'd

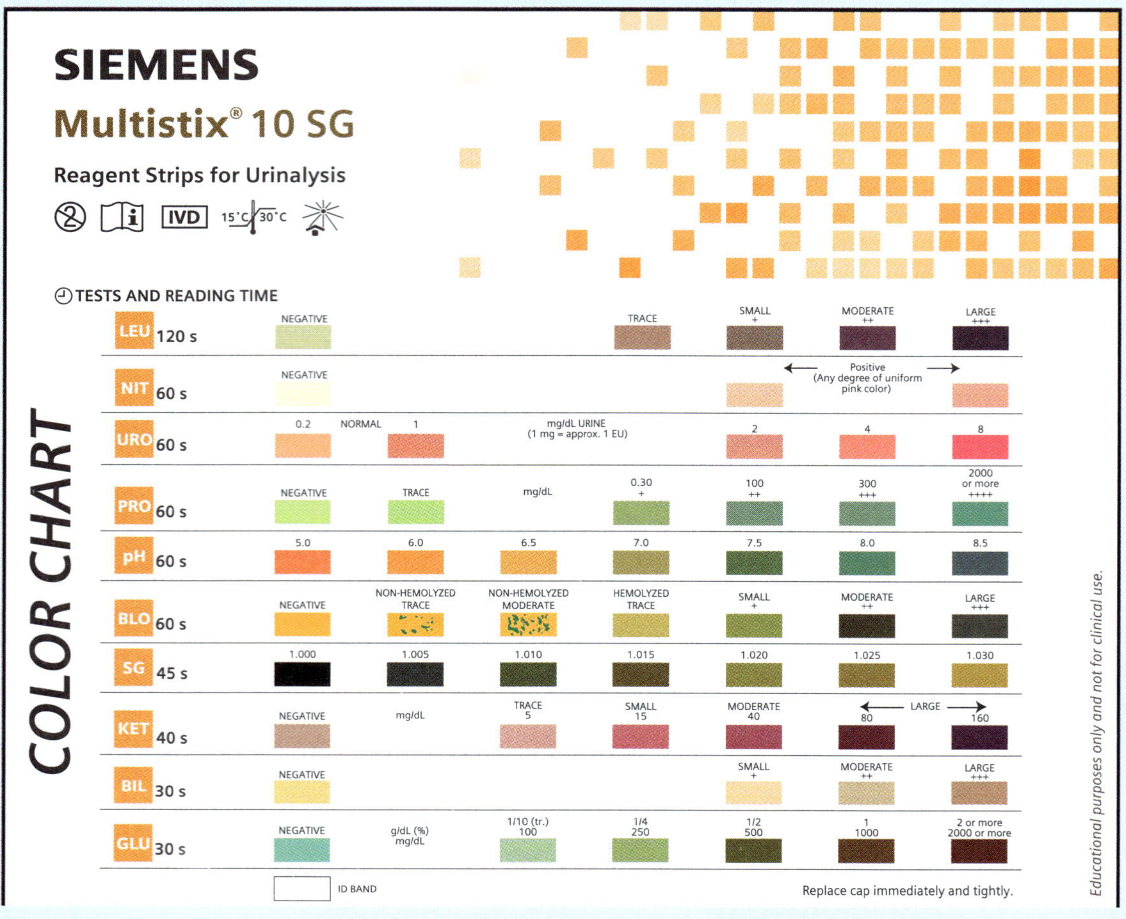

10b DOCUMENTATION EXAMPLE

Multistix® 10 SG Reagent Strips for Urinalysis

PATIENT Annette Ross

DATE 3/22/XX TIME 9:45 a.m.

LEUKOCYTES	NEGATIVE ☑		TRACE ☐	SMALL + ☐	MODERATE ++ ☐	LARGE +++ ☐	
NITRITE	NEGATIVE ☑		POSITIVE ☐	POSITIVE ☐	(Any degree of uniform pink color is found)		
UROBILINOGEN	NORMAL 0.2 ☑	NORMAL 1 ☐	mg/dL 2 ☐	4 ☐	8 ☐	(1mg = approx. 1 BU)	
PROTEIN	NEGATIVE ☐	TRACE ☑	mg/dL 30 + ☐	100 ++ ☐	300 +++ ☐	2000 OR MORE ☐	
pH	5.0 ☑	6.0 ☐	6.5 ☐	7.0 ☐	7.5 ☐	8.0 ☐	8.5 ☐
BLOOD	NEGATIVE ☑	NON-HEMOLYZED TRACE ☐	NON-HEMOLYZED MODERATE ☐	HEMOLYZED TRACE ☐	SMALL + ☐	MODERATE ++ ☐	LARGE +++ ☐
SPECIFIC GRAVITY	1.000 ☐	1.006 ☐	1.010 ☐	1.015 ☑	1.020 ☐	1.025 ☐	1.030 ☐
KETONE	NEGATIVE ☑	mg/dL	TRACE 5 ☐	SMALL 15 ☐	MODERATE 40 ☐	LARGE 80 ☐	LARGE 160 ☐
BILIRUBIN	NEGATIVE ☑		SMALL + ☐	MODERATE ++ ☐	LARGE +++ ☐		
GLUCOSE	NEGATIVE ☑	g/L (%) mg/dL	1/10 tr.) 100 ☐	1/6 250 ☐	1/2 500 ☐	1 1000 ☐	2 or more 2000 or more ☐

Multistix Color Chart. (Modified and printed by permission of Siemens Healthcare Diagnostics, Tarrytown, NY.)

PROCEDURE 30.4 Prepare a Urine Specimen for Microscopic Examination: Kova Method

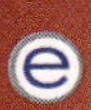

Outcome Prepare a urine specimen for microscopic examination by the provider.

Equipment/Supplies

- Disposable gloves
- Urine specimen (first-voided morning specimen)
- Kova (Biochemical Diagnostics, Inc., Edgewood, NY) urine centrifuge tube
- Kova cap
- Kova pipette
- Kova slide
- Kova stain
- Test tube rack
- Urine centrifuge
- Mechanical stage microscope

1. Procedural Step. Sanitize the hands, and assemble the equipment.

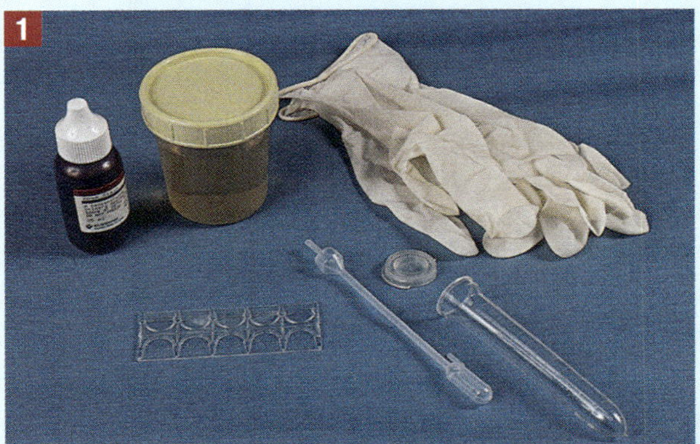
Assemble the equipment.

2. Procedural Step. Apply gloves. Mix the urine specimen with the Kova pipette.
Principle. The specimen must be well mixed to ensure accurate test results.

3. Procedural Step. Pour the urine specimen into the urine centrifuge tube. Fill it to the 12-mL graduation mark, and cap the tube.

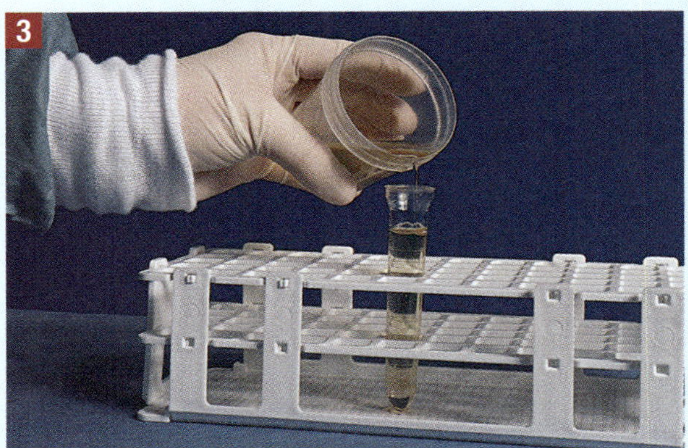
Pour the specimen into the urine tube.

4. Procedural Step. Centrifuge the tube for 5 minutes at approximately 1500 revolutions per minute (rpm).
Principle. Centrifuging the specimen causes the solid elements in the urine to settle to the bottom of the tube.

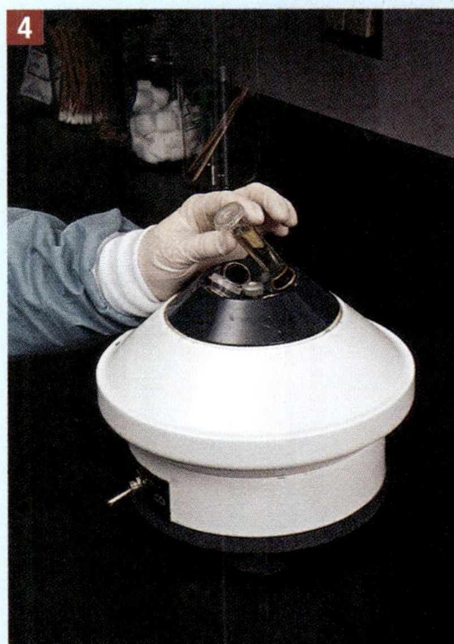
Centrifuge the specimen.

5. Procedural Step. Remove the urine tube from the centrifuge; do not disturb or dislodge the sediment.

6. Procedural Step. Remove the cap. Insert the Kova pipette into the urine tube, and push it to the bottom of the tube until it seats firmly. Ensure that the clip on the bulb is hooked over the outside edge of the tube.

Continued

PROCEDURE 30.4 Prepare a Urine Specimen for Microscopic Examination: Kova Method—cont'd

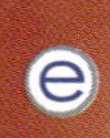

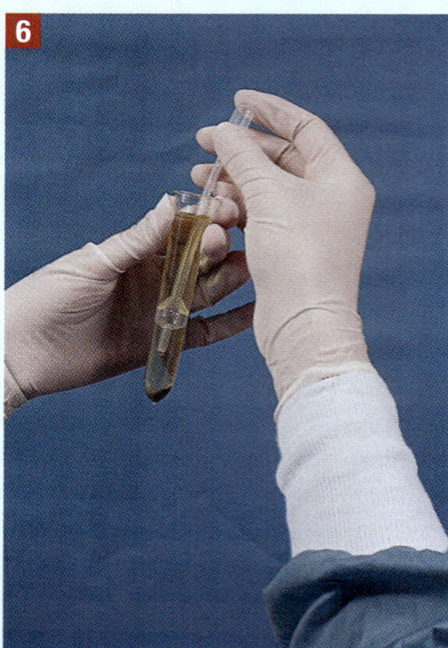
Insert the pipette until it seats firmly.

7. Procedural Step. Decant the specimen by inverting the tube and pouring off the **supernatant** fluid. Approximately 1 mL of sediment is retained in the bottom of the tube.

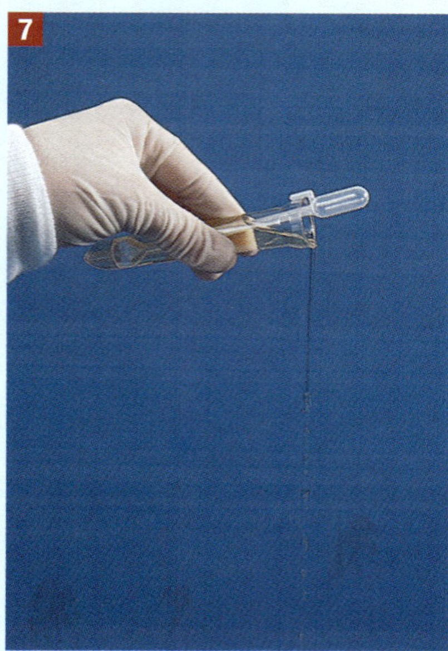
Pour off the supernatant fluid.

8. Procedural Step. Remove the pipette from the tube. Add 1 drop of Kova stain to the tube. Place the pipette back in the tube, and mix the sediment and stain together vigorously with the pipette. Ensure that the sediment and the stain are well mixed. Place the urine tube in a test tube rack.

Principle. Kova stain improves the detail of the sediment for better visualization of structures under the microscope.

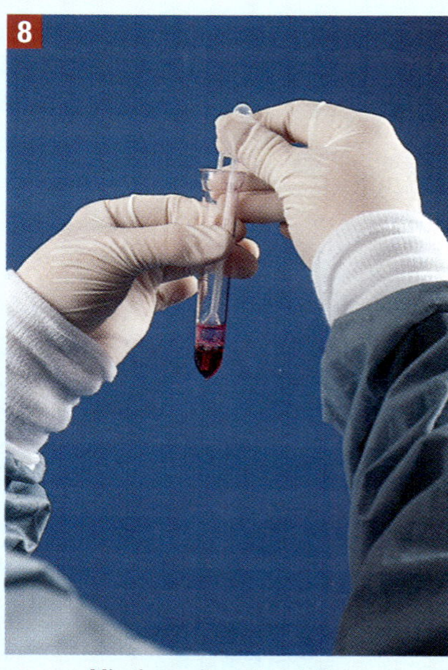
Mix the sediment and stain.

9. Procedural Step. Transfer a sample of the sediment to the Kova slide as follows:

a. Place the Kova slide on a flat surface with the open "envelope" areas facing upward.
b. Squeeze the bulb of the pipette to draw a sample of the sediment into the tip of the pipette.
c. Place the tip of the pipette so that it just touches the notched corner edge of the slide.
d. Gently squeeze the bulb to allow the specimen to fill the well. Do not overfill or underfill the well.
e. Place the pipette in the urine tube.

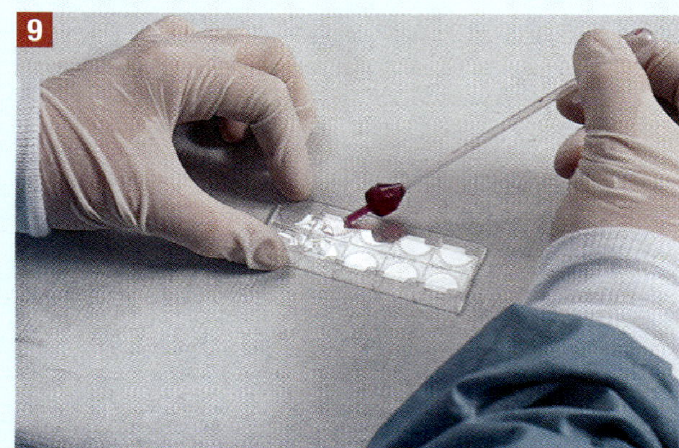
Fill the well with the specimen.

PROCEDURE 30.4 Prepare a Urine Specimen for Microscopic Examination: Kova Method—cont'd

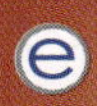

10. Procedural Step. Allow the specimen to sit for 1 minute to permit the sediment to settle in the well.

Principle. Allowing the sediment to settle prevents structures from moving when the slide is viewed under the microscope.

11. Procedural Step. Place the slide on the stage of the microscope. Focus the specimen for the provider under the microscope.

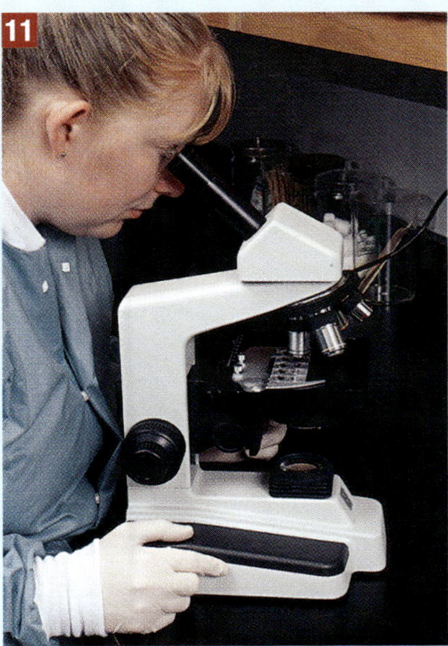

Focus the specimen for the provider.

12. Procedural Step. When the provider is finished examining the urine sediment and documenting results (refer to the laboratory report), remove the slide from the stage.

12

LAB REPORT

Date	Time	Name	
3/18/XX	10:00 a.m.	Tanya Howe	
	MICROSCOPIC		
	WBCs		20 /HPF
	RBCs		3 /HPF
	CASTS (Hyaline)		0 /LPF
	CASTS (Granular)		0 /LPF
	CASTS (Cellular)		0 /LPF
	CASTS (Waxy)		0 /LPF
	EPITHELIAL CELLS		0 /LPF
	BACTERIA		Freq
	MUCUS		Occ
	CRYSTALS		0 WBCs
			T. Bach, MD

13. Procedural Step. Dispose of the plastic slide and pipette in a regular waste container. Rinse the remaining urine down the sink. Cap the empty plastic urine tube and dispose of it in a regular waste container.

14. Procedural Step. Remove gloves and sanitize your hands.

PROCEDURE 30.5 Perform a CLIA-Waived Urine Pregnancy Test

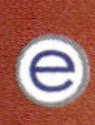

Outcome Perform a CLIA-waived urine pregnancy test.

Equipment/Supplies

- Disposable gloves
- Urine pregnancy test kit (QuickVue HCG Urine Test by Quidel)
- Urine specimen (first-voided morning specimen)

1. Procedural Step. Sanitize the hands, and assemble the equipment. Check the expiration date on the urine pregnancy test kit. It should not be used if the expiration date has passed. When a new test kit is opened (and thereafter on a monthly basis), external positive and negative controls should be performed according to the instructions in the package insert accompanying the controls. Document the control results in a quality control log. If the controls do not perform as expected, patient testing should not be conducted until the problem has been identified and resolved.

Principle. An expired pregnancy test may produce inaccurate test results. Running positive and negative external controls ensures that the test results are valid and reliable. Factors that can cause abnormal control results include outdated controls or test reagents, improper storage of test components, and an error in the technique used to perform the procedure.

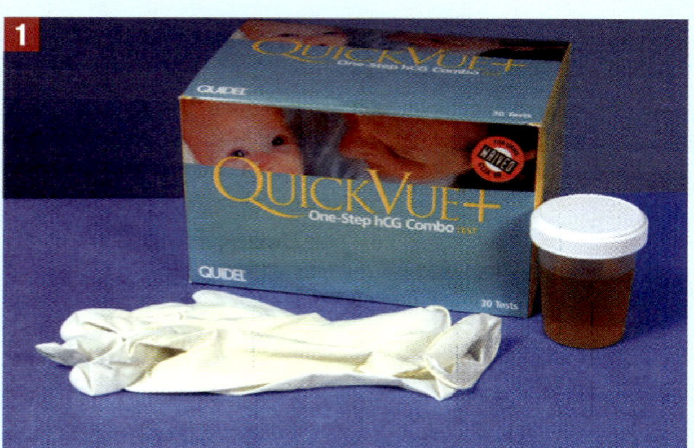

Assemble the equipment.

2. Procedural Step. Apply gloves. Rotate the urine specimen cup to mix the urine. Inspect the foil pouch containing the cassette. If it is torn or punctured, discard the test and obtain another one from the test kit. Remove the test cassette from its foil pouch, and place it on a clean, dry, level surface.

Principle. The foil pouch should not be opened until it is time to perform the test.

3. Procedural Step. Add 3 drops of urine to the round sample well on the test cassette with a disposable pipette supplied with the kit. The test cassette should not be handled or moved again until the test is ready for interpretation. Dispose of the pipette in a regular waste container.

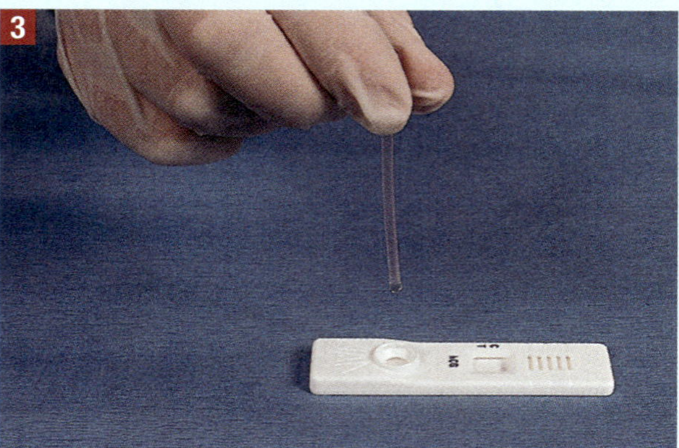

Add 3 drops of urine to the test well.

4. Procedural Step. Wait 3 minutes, and read the results by observing the test result window.

5. Procedural Step. Interpret the test results as follows:

Negative: The appearance of the blue internal control line next to the letter *C* only and no pink to purple test line next to the letter *T* in the test result window. In addition, the background of the test window should be clear and not interfere with the ability to read the test results. (*Note:* If the test result is negative and pregnancy is suspected, another specimen should be collected and tested 48 to 72 hours later.)

Positive: The appearance of any pink to purple line next to the letter *T* along with a blue internal control line next to the letter *C* in the test result window. In addition, the background of the test window should be clear and should not interfere with the ability to read test results.

Invalid result: If no blue internal control line appears within 3 minutes, or if the background of the test window interferes with reading the results, the test result is

PROCEDURE 30.5 Perform a CLIA-Waived Urine Pregnancy Test—cont'd

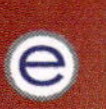  

invalid, and the specimen must be retested with a new cassette.

Principle. The blue control line is a positive internal control indicator designating that a sufficient urine sample was added to the cassette well and that the test is working properly. A background in the test window that is clear and does not interfere with reading the test results is a negative internal quality control indicator and also indicates that the test is working properly.

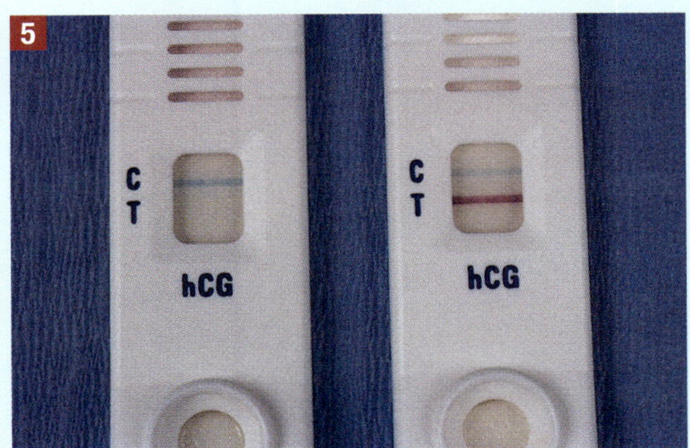

Negative Positive
Interpret the results.

6. **Procedural Step.** Dispose of the test cassette in a regular waste container. Remove gloves, and sanitize your hands.

7. **Procedural Step.** Document the results in the patient's medical record.
   a. *Electronic health record:* Document the date of the patient's last menstrual period (LMP), the name of the test, and the results documented as either positive or negative using the appropriate radio buttons, drop-down menus, and free text fields.
   b. *Paper-based patient record:* Document the date and time, the date of the patient's last menstrual period (LMP), the name of the test, and the results documented as either positive or negative (refer to the PPR documentation example).

7b DOCUMENTATION EXAMPLE

Date	
3/25/XX	10:30 a.m. LMP: 2/20/XX.
	QuickVue preg test: Positive. ________
	________ K. Smith, CMA (AAMA)

Phlebotomy

Check out the Evolve site at http://evolve.elsevier.com/Bonewit/today to access additional interactive activities and exercises to help you study and prepare for success.

LEARNING OBJECTIVES

Venipuncture

1. List and describe the guidelines that should be followed when performing a venipuncture.
2. Explain how each of the following blood specimens is obtained:
   - Clotted blood
   - Serum
   - Whole blood
   - Plasma
3. List the layers into which the blood separates when an anticoagulant is added to the specimen.
4. List the layers into which the blood separates when an anticoagulant is not added to the specimen.
5. List the OSHA safety precautions that must be followed during venipuncture.
6. State the additive content of each of the following evacuated blood collection tubes and list the types of blood specimens that can be obtained from each: red, lavender, gray, light blue, green, royal blue.
7. Identify and explain the order of draw for the Vacutainer and butterfly methods of venipuncture.
8. List and describe guidelines for use of blood collection tubes.
9. Identify problems that may occur during a venipuncture and how to prevent or respond to them.
10. List four ways to prevent a blood specimen from becoming hemolyzed.
11. Explain how a serum separator tube functions in the collection of a serum specimen.

Skin Puncture

12. Explain when a skin puncture is preferred over a venipuncture.
13. Identify skin puncture sites for adults and infants.
14. List and describe guidelines for performing a finger puncture.

PROCEDURES

Perform a venipuncture using the Vacutainer method.

Perform a venipuncture using the butterfly method.

Collect a capillary blood specimen using a disposable lancet.

CHAPTER OUTLINE

KEY TERMS

antecubital space (an-tih-KYOO-bih-tul SPAYS)
anticoagulant (an-tih-koe-AG-yoo-lent)
buffy coat
evacuated blood collection tube
hematoma (hee-mah-TOE-mah)
hemoconcentration (hee-moe-kon-sen-TRAY-shun)
hemolysis (hee-MOL-ih-sis)
osteochondritis (OS-tee-oh-kon-DRY-tis)
osteomyelitis (OS-tee-oh-mie-LIE-tis)
phlebotomist (fleh-BOT-oe-mist)
phlebotomy (fleh-BOT-oe-mee)
plasma
serum
venipuncture (VEN-ih-punk-chur)
venous reflux (VEEN-us REE-fluks)
venous stasis (VEEN-us STAE-sis)

INTRODUCTION TO PHLEBOTOMY

The purpose of phlebotomy is to collect a blood specimen for laboratory analysis. The word *phlebotomy* is derived from the Greek words for "vein" (*phlebos*) and "incision" (*otomy*) and literally means "making an incision into a vein." As used in the clinical laboratory sciences, **phlebotomy** is defined as the collection of blood. An individual who collects a blood sample is a **phlebotomist**. Phlebotomy encompasses three major areas of blood collection:

- *Arterial puncture* for the collection of an arterial blood specimen
- *Venipuncture* for the collection of a venous blood specimen
- *Skin puncture* for the collection of a capillary blood specimen

An arterial puncture is typically performed in a hospital setting to assess the oxygen level, carbon dioxide level, and acid–base balance of arterial blood; medical assistants do not perform arterial punctures. In the medical office, medical assistants perform venipunctures and skin punctures which are described in detail in this chapter.

Capillary blood specimens are tested in the medical office while venous blood specimens are usually transported to an outside laboratory for testing. Specimens for transport must be placed in a biohazard specimen bag to protect health care workers and laboratory couriers from an exposure incident (Fig. 31.1). A laboratory request must be completed for specimens being transported to an outside laboratory. The purpose of the request is to provide the outside laboratory with information necessary for accurate testing, reporting of results, and billing.

VENIPUNCTURE

Venipuncture means the puncturing of a vein for the removal of a venous blood specimen. Venipuncture is usually performed in the medical office using the following methods:

- Vacutainer method
- Butterfly method

The Vacutainer method is the fastest and most convenient method and is used most often. This method relies on the use of the Vacutainer blood collection system (Becton Dickinson, Franklin Lakes, NJ.) The Vacutainer setup consists of a blood collection needle, a collection tube holder, and an evacuated blood collection tube**.** An **evacuated blood collection tube** is a sterile plastic or glass blood collection tube with a color-coded closure that contains a vacuum. The butterfly method is used for difficult draws, such as when a vein is small or sclerosed (hardened).

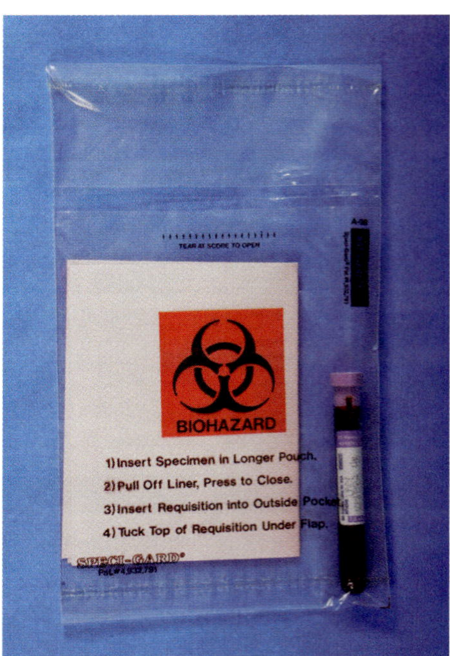

Fig. 31.1 Blood specimen in a biohazard specimen bag along with the laboratory request form.

The butterfly method also uses evacuated blood collection tubes and a collection tube holder; however, the collection needle is different than the one used with the Vacutainer method. This chapter presents the theory and procedure for both of these methods.

GENERAL GUIDELINES FOR VENIPUNCTURE

PATIENT PREPARATION

If advance preparation is required for a laboratory test, the patient should be given instructions an appropriate number of days before the specimen collection. Information on the preparation required is specified in the laboratory test directory provided by the outside laboratory. Although most tests require no preparation, some tests require fasting or the avoidance of certain medications. *Fasting* involves abstaining from food and fluids (except water) for a specified period of time before the collection of the specimen (usually 8 to 12 hours) to allow food and fluid from the previous meal to be completely digested and absorbed.

When a laboratory test requires advance preparation, the medical assistant must verify that the patient has prepared properly before performing the venipuncture. If the patient has not properly prepared, do not collect the specimen unless directed otherwise by the provider. If the venipuncture is to be rescheduled, carefully review the preparation requirements with the patient.

REVIEW COLLECTION AND HANDLING REQUIREMENTS

The medical assistant should carefully review the collection and handling requirements in the laboratory test directory for the test(s) ordered by the provider. These include the collection supplies necessary, the type of specimen to be collected, the amount of the specimen needed to perform the laboratory test, the procedure to follow to collect the specimen, and the proper handling and storage of the specimen awaiting transport to an outside laboratory.

A review of the requirements beforehand prevents errors in collection and handling of the specimen. The medical assistant should contact the outside laboratory if there are any questions regarding any aspect of collection procedure. Fig. 31.2 shows an example of the collection and handling requirements for a complete blood count (CBC) as it is presented in a laboratory test directory.

IDENTIFY THE PATIENT

The patient must be identified using two unique identifiers (e.g., full legal name and date of birth) before performing the venipuncture. Proper patient identification is essential to avoid collecting a specimen from the wrong patient by mistake which could lead to an inaccurate diagnosis and the wrong treatment. After greeting the patient, the medical assistant should ask the patient to state their full name and date of birth. This information should be compared with the demographic data indicated in the patient's medical record.

ASSEMBLE THE EQUIPMENT AND SUPPLIES

The medical assistant must make sure to use the appropriate blood collection tube for each test ordered by the provider as specified in the laboratory test directory. Substituting one collection tube for another will not yield the proper type of specimen required for the test, as shown by the following example. If a serum specimen is required (which requires a collection tube without an anticoagulant) and a tube containing an anticoagulant is used (instead of a tube without an anticoagulant), the blood separates into plasma and cells rather than serum and cells, and the wrong type of blood specimen is obtained. This is a cause for rejection of the specimen by the outside laboratory and necessitates collecting another specimen from the patient.

The medical assistant should check each blood collection tube before use to ensure that it is not broken, chipped, cracked, or otherwise damaged. Damaged collection tubes are unsuitable for specimen collection and should be discarded. Collection tubes have an expiration date (Fig. 31.3). The medical assistant should make sure to check the expiration date on the tube to avoid using an outdated collection tube which is a cause for rejection of the blood specimen by the outside laboratory.

LABORATORY TEST DIRECTORY CBC with Differential	
CPT Code:	85025
Tests Included:	WBC, RBC, Hemoglobin, Hematocrit, MCV, MCH, MCHC, RDW, Platelet Count, MPV and Differential (Absolute and Percent - Neutrophils, Lymphocytes, Monocytes, Eosinophils, and Basophils). If abnormal cells are noted on a manual review of the peripheral blood smear or if the automated differential information meets specific criteria, a full manual differential will be performed.
Alternative Names:	Complete blood count
Type of Specimen:	Whole blood
Amount of Specimen:	7 mL
Collection Container:	7-mL lavender-top tube
Patient Preparation:	None
Collection and Processing:	1. Red and SST tubes should be drawn before the lavender tube. 2. Completely fill tube to the exhaustion of the vacuum to ensure a proper blood-to-anticoagulant ratio. 3. Gently invert tube 8 to 10 times immediately after collection to mix the anticoagulant with the blood. 4. Traumatic draw can introduce thromboplastin and trap WBC and platelets. 5. Refrigeration can precipitate fibrin and trap WBC and platelets.
Storage and Transport:	Store at RT. Do not refrigerate.
Specimen Stability:	RT (15°-30° C): 48 hours
Causes for Rejection:	Hemolyzed or clotted specimen Underfilled tube Specimen collected in any tube other than an EDTA tube Improper labeling of specimen Improper storage temperature Specimen is more than 48 hours old
Reference Range:	Values given with laboratory report.
Use:	The CBC is used as a screening test to assess the overall health of an individual and to detect a wide range of hematologic conditions such as anemia, leukemia, infection, bleeding disorders, and inflammation. The CBC is also used to assist in managing medication and chemotherapeutic decisions.
Limitations:	A manual differential can identify cells that may be misidentified by an automated analyzer.
Forms:	Order electronically or print lab request and submit with specimen.
Methodology:	Automated cell counter and microscopy

Fig. 31.2 CBC collection and handling requirements from a laboratory directory.

Complete a Laboratory Request

The laboratory request may be a preprinted request form or a computer-generated electronic request. The completed request provides the outside laboratory with the information necessary to test the specimen.

Label the Blood Collection Tube(s)

The medical assistant must make sure to properly label each blood collection tube. At a minimum, the label should include the patient's full legal name, date of birth, and the date and time of collection of the specimen. (*Note:* The

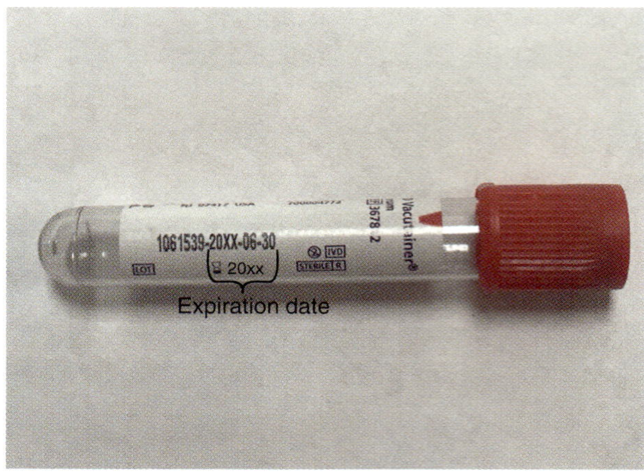

Fig. 31.3 Blood collection tube showing expiration date.

medical assistant should follow the medical office policy as to when the collection tube should be labeled. Some offices prefer that the tube be labeled *before* the specimen is collected; other offices want the tube to be labeled *after* the specimen is collected.

Barcode Label

A specimen can be labeled by attaching an adhesive barcode label to the blood collection tube (Fig. 31.4A). Barcode specimen labels are printed out once a laboratory request has been entered into the computer. The specimen label includes a barcode along with printed information (Fig. 31.5). A blood analyzer in an outside laboratory incorporates a barcode reader that is able to electronically read the information on a barcode necessary for testing the specimen and generating test results.

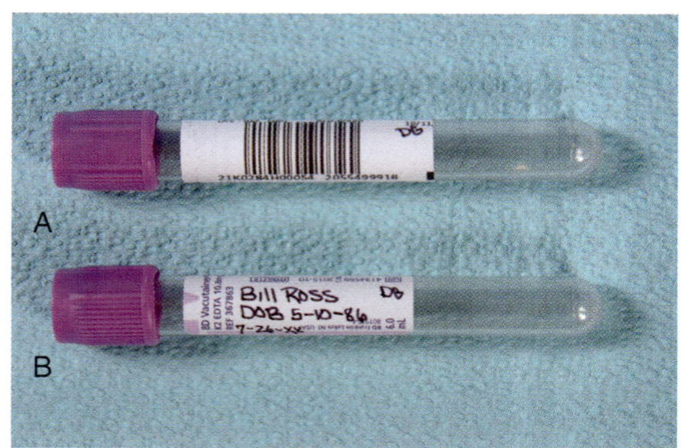

Fig. 31.4 (A) Barcode label. (B) Handwritten label.

It is important to attach the barcode label to the proper collection tube. Inspect the label for information indicating the color of the tube closure (e.g., LV for lavender) to which the label must be attached. For example, the barcode label illustrated in Fig. 31.5 must be placed on a lavender (LV) closure tube for a specimen that is being collected to perform a CBC.

The barcode label must be properly positioned on the collection tube. The label should be placed lengthwise on the tube with the patient's name towards the closure allowing the label to be read from left to right. The left side of the label should be aligned with the top of the manufacturer's label and no higher. To enable the barcode reader to read the barcode, the label must be placed in a straight (not diagonal) position on the collection tube with no wrinkles, folds, or tears. It is important not to write on the label as this may prevent the barcode reader from being able to electronically read the barcode.

Handwritten Label

A blood specimen can also be labeled by handwriting the required information on the label (patient's full legal name and date of birth, the date and time of collection, the medical assistant's initials, and any other information required by the laboratory) (see Fig. 31.4B). The information should be printed legibly with a pen, and the medical assistant should be certain that the information is accurate to avoid a mix-up of specimens.

REASSURE THE PATIENT

Venipuncture is often a frightening experience for the patient. For many patients, the anticipation of the procedure is worse than the actual drawing of the blood. The medical assistant should take time to explain the procedure to the

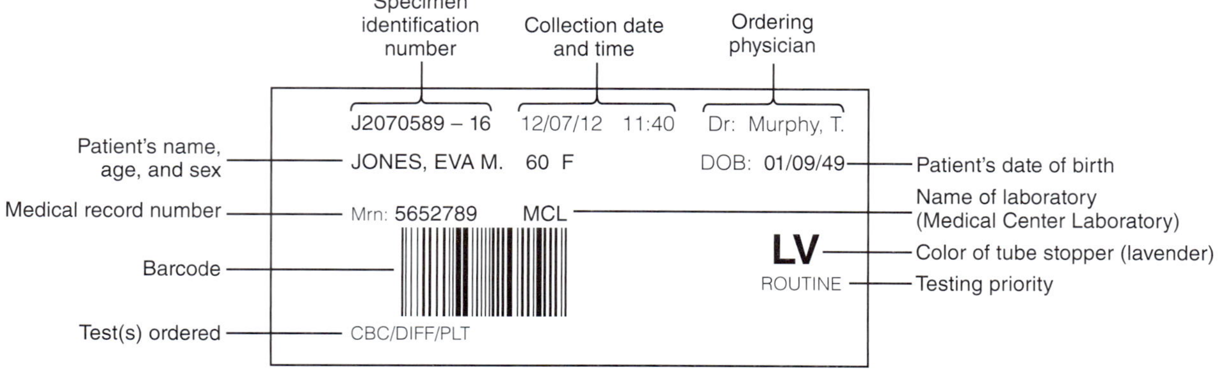

Fig. 31.5 Information included on a laboratory specimen barcode label.

patient in an unhurried and confident manner. This helps to alleviate the patient's fears, which relaxes the patient's veins. Relaxed veins make venipuncture easier to perform and result in less pain for the patient.

Instruct the patient to remain still during the procedure. Explain to the patient that a small amount of pain is associated with a venipuncture, but it is brief. Never tell the patient that the venipuncture will not hurt. Just before inserting the needle, tell the patient that they will "feel a small stick." This prevents startling the patient, which could cause the patient's arm to move resulting in movement of the needle in the vein. This causes pain for the patient and may also damage tissue at the venipuncture site.

PATIENT POSITION FOR VENIPUNCTURE

The patient position for venipuncture is especially important to the successful collection of a blood specimen. Proper positioning allows easy access to the vein and is more comfortable for the patient. The patient position depends on the vein to be used. The most common site for venipuncture is the **antecubital space** which is the surface of the arm in front of the elbow (Fig. 31.6). The information on positioning the patient presented next refers to the antecubital venipuncture site.

The patient should be seated comfortably in a phlebotomy chair. The arm should be extended downward to form a straight line from the shoulder to the wrist with the palm facing up; the arm should not bend at the elbow. The arm can be supported on the armrest by a rolled towel or by having the patient place the fist of the other hand under the elbow (see Fig. 31.6).

A venipuncture should never be performed with the patient sitting on a stool or standing. The patient may faint and injure themselves. If the patient appears nervous or has fainted in the past from a venipuncture, it is best to place the patient in a semi reclining position (semi-Fowler position) on the examining table.

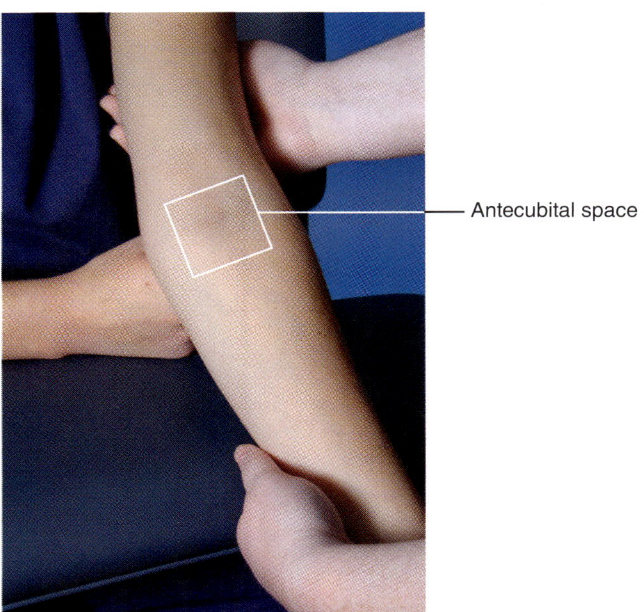

Fig. 31.6 Patient position for obtaining a blood specimen from the antecubital veins.

Although unusual, it is possible for blood to flow from the collection tube back into the patient's vein during the procedure. This condition is known as **venous reflux**. Venous reflux could cause the patient to have an adverse reaction to a tube additive, particularly if the additive in the tube is ethylenediaminetetraacetic acid (EDTA). Venous reflux can occur only if the contents of the collection tube are in contact with the tube stopper while the specimen is being drawn. Venous reflux is prevented by keeping the patient's arm in a downward position so that the collection tube remains below the venipuncture site and fills from the bottom up.

Putting It All Into Practice

My name is Dori, and I work in a very busy, fast-paced family practice office for two physicians. I love my job. The physicians are great, with very different styles; the pace is fast; and the time flies by. I am constantly challenged, learning new things, meeting and helping people, and being a part of a team that works well together.

While performing a venipuncture for a routine blood chemistry panel (a procedure I have performed many times), I accidentally stuck myself after collecting the specimen. I could see the blood inside my glove, and I could see the patient's blood clinging to the point of the needle—my heart sank. I activated the safety shield and placed the needle and holder in the sharps container and tried to keep my cool and not alarm the patient. I mentally assessed the patient. He was an older man from a rural community, but I know you cannot always judge a book by its cover.

I excused myself and immediately proceeded to wash my hands thoroughly with soap and water and rinse, rinse, rinse! I then notified the physician. The physician questioned the patient regarding operations he had had in the previous year. He had undergone bypass surgery and had received two units of blood. Although blood is effectively screened, I thought about that one-in-a-zillion chance that it could have been contaminated. Thankfully, I had received the hepatitis B immunization series, but there was still concern regarding hepatitis C and, of course, HIV.

The patient was gracious and complied with our request to be tested for hepatitis and HIV. The physician and I discussed the situation, and we determined the risk to be low, but he nonetheless offered me the option of getting the HIV postexposure prophylactic treatment. I decided not to get the treatment and proceeded to wait in agony for the patient's test results. The word *relief* hardly describes how I felt when the patient's laboratory results came back negative!

This incident confirmed the importance of getting the hepatitis B immunization and paying attention to good technique when performing procedures involving blood. ■

APPLICATION OF A TOURNIQUET

An important step in the venipuncture procedure is the application of the tourniquet. A tourniquet consists of a flat, soft band of rubber approximately 1 inch (2.5 cm) wide and 15 to 18 inches (38 to 45 cm) long. Most offices use latex-free tourniquets which consist of synthetic rubber. This protects both health care workers and patients with a hypersensitivity to latex.

The tourniquet makes the patient's veins stand out so that they are easier to palpate. The tourniquet acts as a "dam" that causes the venous blood to slow down and pool in the veins in front of the tourniquet. This pooling of blood makes the veins more prominent so that they are more visible and can be palpated.

When applying a tourniquet, it is important to obtain the correct tourniquet tension. The tourniquet should be applied with enough tension to slow the venous flow without affecting the arterial flow. A tourniquet that is too tight is uncomfortable for the patient; it also obstructs both the venous blood flow and arterial flow, which may result in a specimen that produces inaccurate test results. A tourniquet that is too loose fails to cause the veins to stand out enough to be palpated. A correctly applied tourniquet should fit snugly and not pinch the patient's skin.

Guidelines for Applying a Tourniquet

The following guidelines help to ensure successful application of the tourniquet:

1. Do not apply the tourniquet over sores or burned skin.
2. Hold each end of the tourniquet with one hand. Position the tourniquet 3 to 4 inches (7.5 to 10 cm) above the bend in the elbow. This allows adequate room for cleansing the site and performing the venipuncture without the tourniquet getting in the way. Make sure the tourniquet lies flat against the patient's skin and then pull the ends away from each other to create tension (see Fig. 31.7A).
3. Bring the ends of the tourniquet toward each other and cross one over the other at the point of your grasp, with enough tension that the tourniquet is snug but is not pinching the patient's skin or is otherwise painful to the patient (see Fig. 31.7B).
4. Tuck a portion of the top length into the bottom length, forming a loop between the tourniquet and the patient's arm. This allows for a one-handed release of the tourniquet when pulled on one end. Make sure the flaps are directed upward so that they do not dangle into the working area (see Fig. 31.7C).
5. Never leave the tourniquet on for longer than 1 minute because this would be uncomfortable for the patient. In addition, prolonged application of the tourniquet causes the venous blood to stagnate, or pool in one place too long—a condition known as **venous stasis**. When venous stasis occurs, the plasma portion of the blood filters into the tissues, causing hemoconcentration. **Hemoconcentration** is an increase in the concentration of nonfilterable blood components in the blood vessels, such as red blood cells, enzymes, iron, and calcium, as a result of a decrease in the fluid content of the blood. This can result in inaccurate results for a variety of laboratory tests.
6. Remove the tourniquet as soon as a good blood flow into the collection tube is established; however, this may not be practical when you are first learning the venipuncture procedure. Removing the tourniquet may cause the needle to move such that no more blood can be obtained, and the blood has to be redrawn. When first learning the venipuncture procedure, it is better to wait until just before the needle is removed to remove the tourniquet.

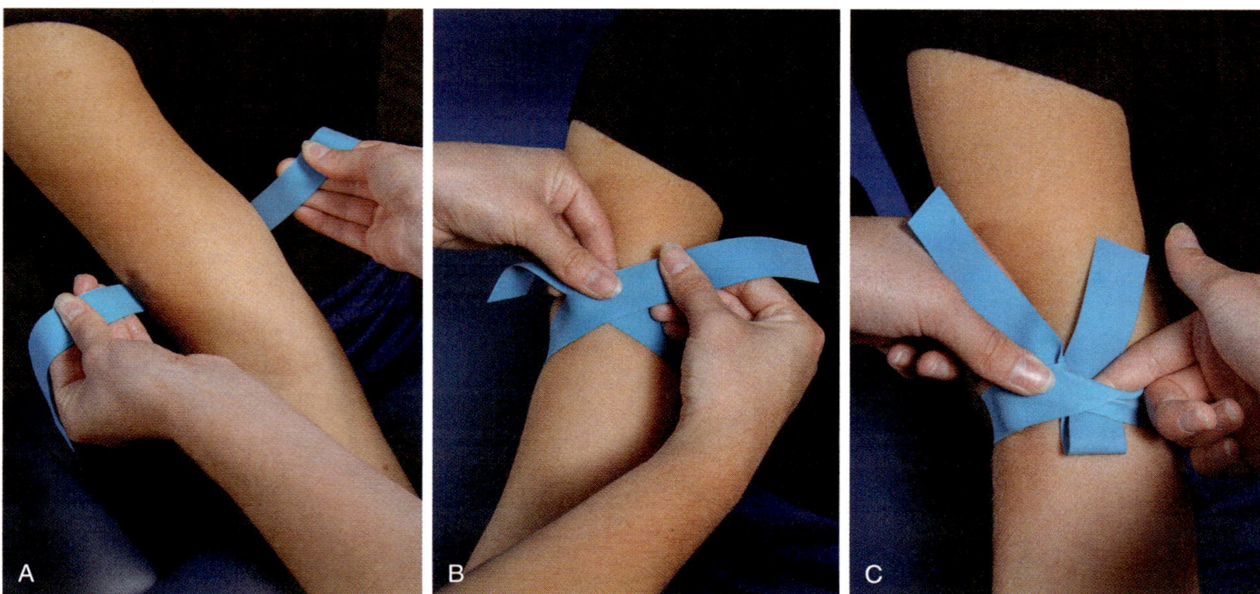

Fig. 31.7 Application of a latex-free tourniquet. (A) Create tension by pulling the ends of the tourniquet away from each other. (B) With tension, cross one flap over the other at the point of your grasp. (C) Form a loop by tucking a portion of the top length into the bottom length.

7. *Always* remove the tourniquet before removing the needle from the patient's arm. If the needle is removed first, the pressure of the tourniquet causes blood to be forced out of the puncture site and into the surrounding tissue, resulting in a hematoma. A **hematoma** is a swelling or mass of clotted blood within the tissues caused by a break in a blood vessel.

SITE SELECTION FOR VENIPUNCTURE

For most patients, the best site to use are the veins in the antecubital space (Fig. 31.8). If the patient has large, visible antecubital veins, drawing blood is easy. If the patient has small veins or veins that cannot be palpated, obtaining a blood specimen can be quite a challenge, even for the most experienced medical assistant.

The antecubital veins typically have a wide lumen and are close to the surface of the skin, which makes them easily accessible. In addition, these veins typically have thick walls, making them less likely to collapse. Using the antecubital space spares the patient unnecessary pain because the skin is less sensitive there than at other sites, such as the back of the hand. The medical assistant should not be misled by the presence in some patients of many small, very blue "spidery" veins that lie close to the surface of the skin. These veins are not suitable for performing a venipuncture. The antecubital veins lie beneath these veins.

The best vein to use in the antecubital space is the *median cubital* vein. The median cubital vein is a prominent vein in the middle of the antecubital space that does not roll (see Fig. 31.8). At times, however, the median cubital vein cannot be used—for example, when it lies deep in the tissues and cannot be palpated or is scarred from repeated venipunctures.

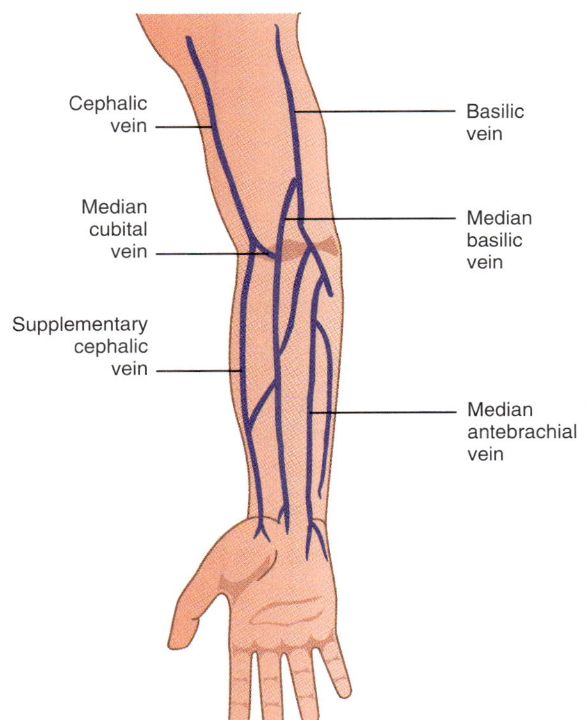

Fig. 31.8 Antecubital veins.

The *cephalic* and *basilic* veins are located on opposite sides of the antecubital space and provide an alternative site when the median cubital vein is unavailable. The cephalic vein is located on the thumb side of the antecubital space, and the basilic vein is located on the little finger side of the antecubital space. The disadvantage of these "side" veins is that they tend to roll or move away from the needle, escaping puncture. To prevent rolling, firm pressure should be applied below and to the side of the vein to stabilize it as the needle is inserted.

The brachial artery also is located in the antecubital space, but it lies deeper in the tissues. This is the artery that is used to measure blood pressure. Before performing a venipuncture, palpate for the presence of this artery. In contrast to a vein, an artery pulsates, is more elastic, and has a thicker wall than a vein. If the brachial artery is inadvertently punctured, the patient feels more than the usual amount of pain, and the blood is bright red and comes out in pulsing movements. If this situation occurs, the tourniquet should be removed and then the needle. Pressure with a gauze pad should be applied for 4 to 5 minutes.

Guidelines for Site Selection

Specific guidelines should be followed to facilitate the selection of a good vein:

1. *Ensure that the lighting is adequate.* Good lighting facilitates inspection of the veins.
2. *Ensure that the veins "stand out" as much as possible.* Before locating a venipuncture site, always apply the tourniquet. When the tourniquet is in place, ask the patient to clench their fist. This pushes blood from the lower arm into the veins making them more prominent and easier to palpate. You can ask the patient to clench and unclench the fist a few times; however, vigorous pumping should be avoided because it could lead to hemoconcentration, which could produce inaccurate test results.
3. *Examine the antecubital veins of both arms.* The best site to perform a venipuncture varies with each individual. The patient may have larger veins in one arm than in the other. It is advisable to ask the patient whether they have had a venipuncture before. Most adults have had previous venipunctures and know which of their veins are best to use and which should be avoided. Listen to and evaluate information offered by the patient.
4. *Use inspection and particularly palpation to select a vein.* A vein does not have to be seen to be a good selection. If you cannot see a vein, palpation alone can be used to locate it. A vein feels like an elastic tube that "gives" under the pressure of the fingertips.
5. *Always palpate for the median cubital vein (middle vein) first.* It usually is bigger, is anchored better, bruises less, and poses the smallest risk of injuring underlying structures (e.g., nerves and arteries) than the other veins. Because of this, if the patient's median cubital vein cannot be seen but still can be palpated, it should be used as the first choice when selecting a vein. If the median cubital vein is good in both arms, select the one that appears the

fullest. The cephalic vein located on the thumb side is the next best vein choice because it does not roll and bruise as easily as the basilic vein. The basilic vein, located on the little finger side of the antecubital space, is the least desirable venipuncture site in the antecubital space. Branches of the median nerve may lie close to this vein in some individuals. In addition, the basilic vein lies in close proximity to the brachial artery. Both of these conditions pose a risk of injury to underlying structures when blood is drawn from the basilic vein.

6. *Thoroughly assess the patient's veins.* To assess a vein as a possible site for venipuncture, place one or two fingertips (index and middle fingers) over it and press lightly, then release pressure. Do not use your thumb to palpate the vein because it is not as sensitive as the index finger. To be suitable for a venipuncture, the vein should feel round, firm, elastic, and engorged. When you depress and release an engorged vein, it should spring back in a rounded, filled state.
7. *Determine the size, depth, and direction of the vein.* When a suitable vein has been located, it should be palpated thoroughly and carefully to determine the direction of the vein and to estimate the size and depth of the vein. Palpate and trace the path of the vein several times by rolling your index finger back and forth over the vein to determine its size. Inspect and palpate the vein for problems. Some veins that appear suitable at first sight feel small, hard, bumpy, or flat when palpated.
8. *Map the location of the site.* After locating an acceptable vein, mentally "map" the location of the puncture site on the patient's arm with "skin marks." This technique is particularly helpful if the vein cannot be seen, but only palpated. The puncture site may be located on or next to a skin mark, such as a freckle, skin crease, or a pigmented area. Do not mark the site with a pen as this contaminates the site.
9. *Do not leave the tourniquet on for longer than 1 minute.* When first learning the venipuncture procedure, you may need to perform numerous assessments of the patient's arms to locate the best vein. After each assessment, remove the tourniquet for approximately 2 minutes to allow normal circulation of the blood to occur. This prevents patient discomfort and hemoconcentration, which can lead to inaccurate results for a variety of laboratory tests.
10. *If a suitable vein cannot be found*, the following techniques can be employed to make the veins more prominent:
    - Remove the tourniquet, and have the patient dangle the arm over the side of the chair for 1 to 2 minutes.
    - Tap the vein site sharply a few times with your index finger and second finger.
    - Gently massage the arm from the wrist to the elbow.
    - Apply a warm, moist washcloth to the area for 5 minutes.

Alternative Venipuncture Sites

If it is impossible to locate a suitable vein in the antecubital space, alternative sites are available, including the inner forearm, the wrist area above the thumb, and the back of the hand (Fig. 31.9). These alternative veins are smaller and have thinner walls than the antecubital veins and should be

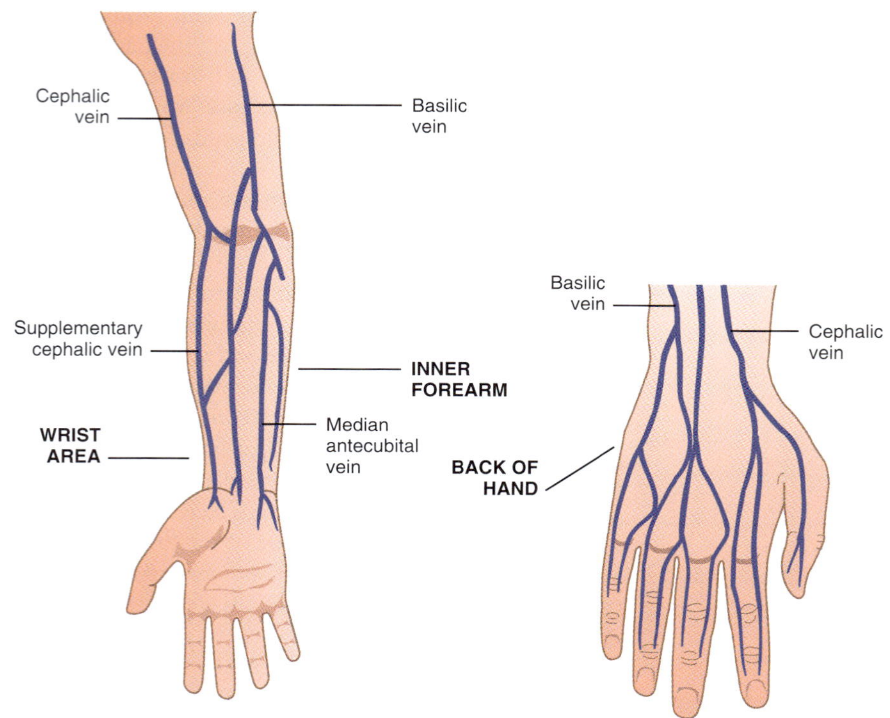

Fig. 31.9 Alternative venipuncture sites: the inner forearm, the wrist area above the thumb, and the back of the hand.

used for venipuncture only when all possibilities for obtaining the blood specimen at the antecubital site have been considered. If the medical assistant is able to palpate a small vein in the antecubital space, it may be possible to obtain blood there using the butterfly method of venipuncture.

The hand veins, in particular, should be used only as a last resort. The veins of the hand have a tendency to roll because they are not supported by much tissue and are close to the surface of the skin. This makes them more difficult to stick. In addition, an abundant supply of nerves is present in the hands, which makes this procedure more uncomfortable for the patient. Hand veins tend to have thin walls, which makes them more susceptible to collapsing, bruising, and phlebitis. In some patients, however, especially the obese and the elderly, the hand veins may be the only accessible site.

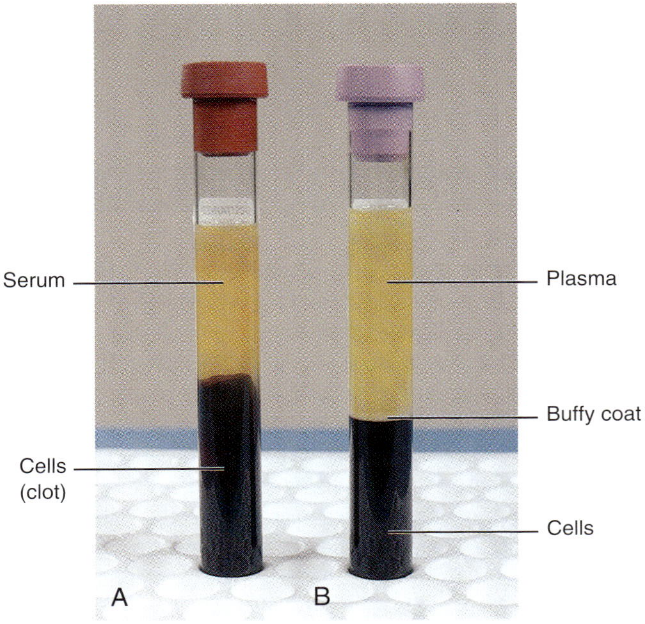

Fig. 31.10 Layers into which the blood separates when there is no anticoagulant (A) and when an anticoagulant is present (B).

TYPES OF BLOOD SPECIMENS

The type of blood specimen required depends on the type of test to be performed. Serum is required for most blood chemistry tests, whereas whole blood is required for a CBC. The various types of blood specimens that can be obtained through the venipuncture procedure are as follows:

1. *Clotted blood.* Clotted blood is obtained from a tube that does not contain an anticoagulant. A tube without an anticoagulant causes the blood cells to clot.
2. *Serum.* **Serum** is plasma from which the clotting factor fibrinogen has been removed. Serum is obtained from clotted blood by allowing the specimen to stand and then centrifuging it. Centrifuging a blood specimen that does not contain an anticoagulant causes the blood to separate into the following layers (Fig. 31.10A):
   - Top layer—serum
   - Bottom layer—clotted blood cells
3. *Whole blood.* Whole blood is obtained by using a tube that contains an **anticoagulant**. An anticoagulant is a substance that prevents the blood from clotting in the collection tube.
4. *Plasma.* **Plasma** is the liquid part of the blood consisting of a clear, straw-colored fluid that comprises approximately 55% of the blood volume. Plasma is obtained from whole blood that has been centrifuged. Centrifuging a blood specimen that contains an anticoagulant causes the blood to separate into the following layers (see Fig. 31.10B):
   - Top layer—plasma
   - Middle layer—**buffy coat** (contains white blood cells and platelets)
   - Bottom layer—red blood cells

OSHA SAFETY PRECAUTIONS

The OSHA Bloodborne Pathogens Standard presented in Chapter 17 must be carefully followed during the venipuncture procedure to avoid exposure to bloodborne pathogens. The following OSHA requirements apply specifically to the venipuncture procedure and the separation of serum from whole blood (see later):

1. Wear gloves when it is reasonably anticipated that you will have hand contact with blood.
2. Avoid hand-to-mouth contact, such as eating, drinking, handling contact lenses, and applying cosmetics while working with blood specimens.
3. Wear a face shield or mask in combination with an eye protection device whenever splashes, spray, splatter, or droplets of blood may be generated.
4. Perform all procedures involving blood in a manner so as to minimize splashing, spraying, splattering, and generating droplets of blood.
5. If your hands or other skin surfaces come in contact with blood, wash the area as soon as possible with soap and water.
6. If your mucous membranes (e.g., eyes, nose, and mouth) come in contact with blood, flush them with water as soon as possible.
7. Do not bend, break, or shear contaminated venipuncture needles.
8. Do not recap a contaminated venipuncture needle.
9. Locate the sharps container as close as possible to the area of use. Immediately after use, place the contaminated blood collection needle (and tube holder) in the biohazard sharps container.
10. Handle all laboratory equipment and supplies properly and with care as indicated by the manufacturer. For example, wait until the centrifuge comes to a complete stop before opening it.
11. Do not store food in refrigerators where testing supplies or specimens are stored.

12. Sanitize hands as soon as possible after removing gloves.
13. If you are exposed to blood, report the incident immediately to your provider-employer.

What Would You Do? What Would You *Not* Do?

Case Study 1

Camila Hernadez is 21 years old and comes to the office at 9:00 a.m. to have her blood drawn for a CBC and a thyroid panel. She has brought a friend along with her. Camila seems nervous, and her voice is shaking. She says this is the first venipuncture she has ever had. Camila asks whether her friend can stay with her to give her moral support while her blood is being drawn. Camila says that the blood has to be taken out of her left arm. She says she is right-handed and has a softball game this evening. When the veins of Camila's left arm are examined, a suitable vein cannot be located; however, she has a good median cubital vein in her right arm. Camila then wants to know whether the blood could be drawn from her left hand like they do on hospital television shows. ■

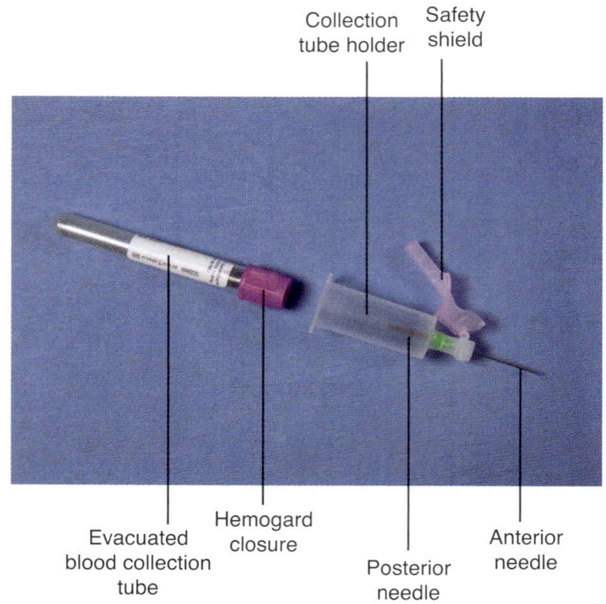

Fig. 31.11 Vacutainer system.

VACUTAINER METHOD OF VENIPUNCTURE

The Vacutainer method is frequently used to collect venous blood specimens. This method is considered ideal for collecting blood from normal healthy antecubital veins that are adequate in size to withstand the pressure of the vacuum in the collection tube. The Vacutainer system consists of a blood collection needle, a collection tube holder, and an evacuated blood collection tube (Fig. 31.11). Procedure 31.1 outlines the venipuncture Vacutainer method.

BLOOD COLLECTION NEEDLE

The safety-engineered needle used with the Vacutainer method consists of a double-pointed stainless-steel needle with a threaded hub near its center and a safety shield (Fig. 31.12). The needle is coated with silicon, enabling it to penetrate the skin smoothly. The threaded hub of the needle screws into a collection tube holder. Vacutainer blood collection needles are packaged in sealed twist-apart plastic containers.

The double-pointed needle consists of an anterior needle and a posterior needle. The *anterior needle* is longer and has a beveled point designed to facilitate entry into the skin and the vein. The *posterior needle* is shorter, and its purpose is to pierce the rubber stopper of the blood collection tube. The posterior needle has a rubber sleeve that functions as a valve which permits the collection of multiple blood specimens. Pushing the tube stopper of a collection tube onto the posterior needle compresses this rubber sleeve and exposes the opening of the needle, allowing blood to enter the tube. When a tube is removed, the sleeve slides back over the needle opening and stops the flow of blood.

Blood collection needles for the Vacutainer method are available in the following gauges: 21G and 22G. A 21-G needle is used most often for a routine venipuncture. A 22-G needle is recommended for children and adults

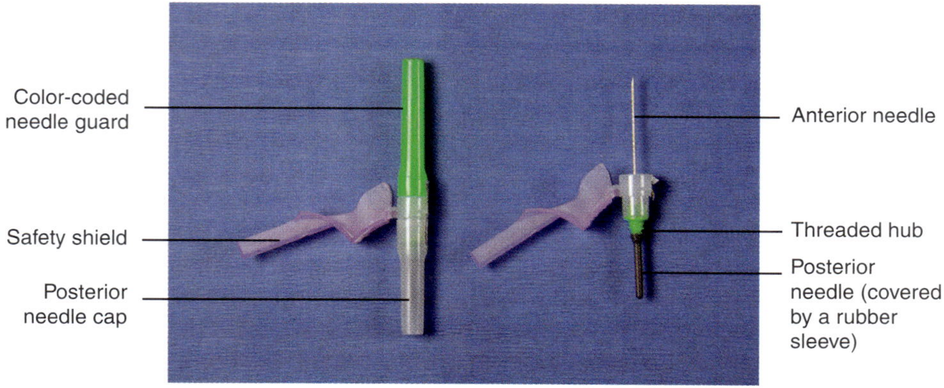

Fig. 31.12 Vacutainer blood collection needle with a safety shield.

with small veins. Manufacturers often color-code the needle guard by gauge for easier identification—for example, Becton Dickinson uses the following color-coding system: green for 21-G needles (see Fig. 31.12), and black for 22-G needles. Blood collection needles come in three lengths: 1 inch, 1¼ inch and 1½ inch. The length used is based on individual preference; most medical assistants prefer the 1- or 1½-inch needle for routine venipunctures; they are less intimidating to the patient and tend to offer greater control because they allow the medical assistant to rest the fourth and fifth fingers on the patient's arm for stability. A 1½-inch needle allows more room for stabilizing the vein.

OSHA stipulates requirements to reduce needlestick and other sharps injuries among health care workers. As discussed in Chapter 17, employers are required to evaluate and implement commercially available safer medical devices that reduce occupational exposure to the lowest extent feasible. Safer medical devices include safety-engineered blood collection needles which incorporate a built-in safety feature to reduce the risk of a needlestick injury. Fig. 31.13 illustrates a safety-engineered blood collection needle and the method for activating the safety shield.

COLLECTION TUBE HOLDER

The collection tube holder consists of a plastic cylinder with two openings. The small opening is used to secure the double-pointed needle, and the large opening is used to hold the blood collection tube. The large opening has a plastic extension known as the *flange.* The flange assists in the insertion and removal of collection tubes and prevents the tube holder from rolling when it is placed on a flat surface.

The tube holder has an indentation about ½ inch from the hub of the needle. This marks the point at which the posterior needle starts to enter the rubber stopper of the tube. If a tube stopper is inserted past this point before the vein is entered, the tube fills with air, which prevents blood from entering the tube.

EVACUATED BLOOD COLLECTION TUBES

Evacuated blood collection tubes consist of a sterile plastic or glass tube with either a *Hemogard closure* (Fig. 31.14) or a *conventional rubber stopper closure* (Fig. 31.15). A collection tube contains a vacuum that creates suction to pull the

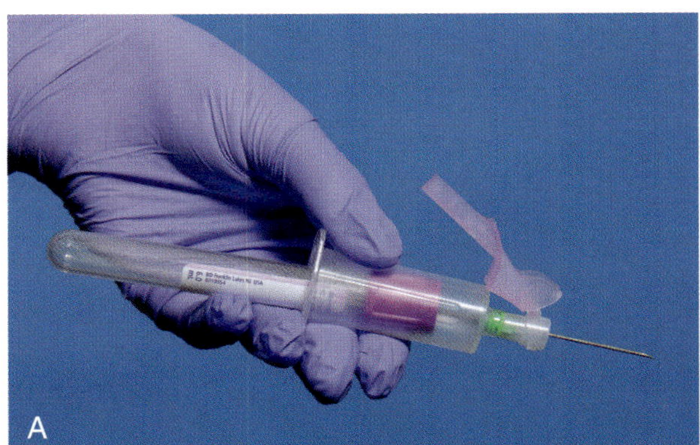

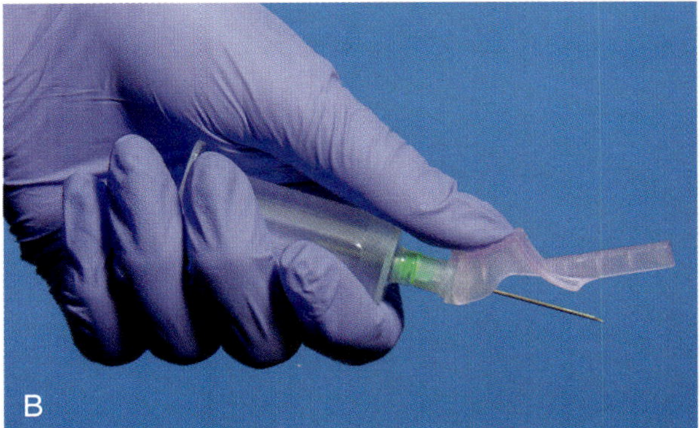

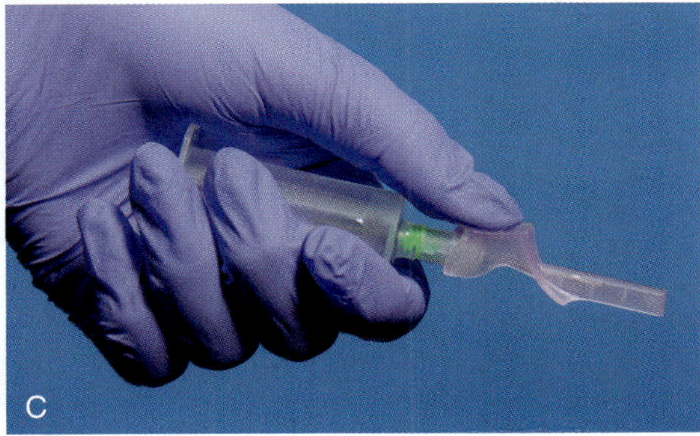

Fig. 31.13 Activation of the safety shield on a blood collection needle. (A) Perform the venipuncture with the safety shield straight back toward the holder. (B) After performing the venipuncture, place the thumb on the safety shield thumb pad and push the safety shield forward. (C) Continue pushing the safety shield forward with your thumb until an audible click is heard, which indicates the shield has locked into place. Discard the needle and holder in a biohazard sharps container.

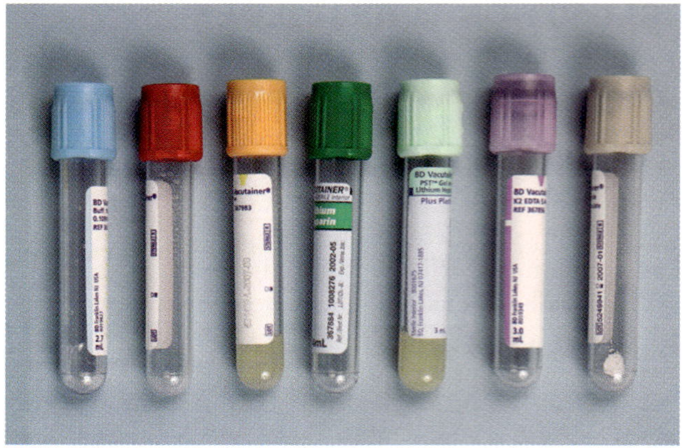

Fig. 31.14 Hemogard closure tubes. (From Garrels M: *Laboratory and diagnostic testing in ambulatory care*, ed 4, St. Louis, 2019, Elsevier. Photo by Zack Bent.)

blood specimen into the tube. The tube has a label affixed to it indicating the additive content, expiration date, and tube capacity. Evacuated blood collection tubes are available in varying capacities that range from 2 mL to 10 mL. The capacity of the tube used depends on the amount of the specimen required for the test.

A *Hemogard closure* consists of a special rubber stopper and a plastic safety-engineered closure that overhangs the outside of the tube. Together, these components act as a single unit to reduce the likelihood of coming in contact with the contents of the tube. After collecting a blood specimen, the medical assistant may need to gain access to the blood in the tube for further processing, such as when separating serum from whole blood. A conventional rubber stopper tube "pops" as the stopper is removed, which may result in splattering of blood. The design of the Hemogard closure works to prevent splattering of blood when the top is removed.

Additive Content of Blood Collection Tubes

Evacuated blood collection tubes use a color-coded system for ease in identifying the additive content of each tube (Table 31.1). A tube additive must not alter the blood components or affect the laboratory test to be performed. The medical assistant must determine the correct closure color to use for each test ordered by the provider as specified in the laboratory test directory. Substituting one type of collection tube for another may not yield the proper type of specimen required for the test. If a CBC has been ordered by the provider, a lavender-closure tube must be used, and a tube with a different closure color cannot be substituted for it.

The most frequently used blood collection tubes in the medical office are classified here according to the color of the closure and the additive content:

1. *Red.* A tube with a red closure does not contain an anticoagulant and is used to obtain clotted blood or serum. Clotted blood is used for blood banking. Serum is required for serologic tests and blood chemistry tests.
2. *Gold and marbled red/gray (often called a "tiger top" tube) closures.* These tubes are used to obtain serum. They do not contain an anticoagulant; however, they do contain an additive known as a *clot activator.* A clot activator consists of a substance that makes the red blood cells in the tube clot more quickly to yield serum. Tubes with a gold or marbled red/gray closure are known as serum separator tubes (SST) because they contain a gel that separates the cells from the serum when the tube is centrifuged. A tube with a clot activator must be inverted 5 times after the blood has been drawn to mix the clot activator with the blood specimen. The most common use of these tubes is to collect a specimen for blood chemistry testing.
3. *Lavender.* A tube with a lavender closure contains the anticoagulant EDTA and is used to obtain whole blood or plasma. The most common use of a lavender closure tube is to collect a blood specimen for a CBC.

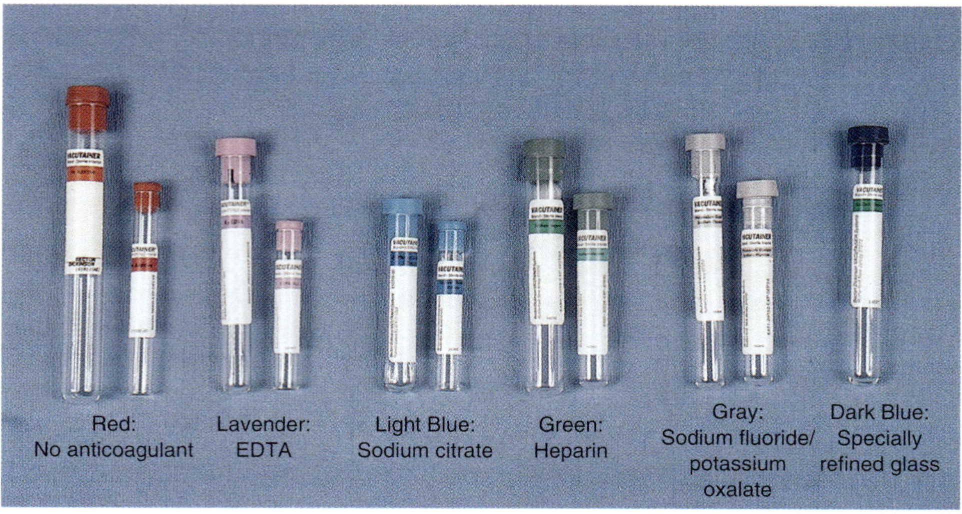

Fig. 31.15 Conventional rubber stopper closure tubes.

Table 31.1 Order of Draw forCollection of Multiple Evacuated Tubes

BD Hemogard Plastic Colors	Rubber Stopper Colors	Additive or Anticoagulant	Number of Inversions to Mix During Blood Draw	Laboratory Use
Yellow, Sterile	Yellow, Sterile	Sodium polyanetholsulfonate (SPS)	8–10	Blood cultures
Light blue	Light blue	Sodium citrate	3–4	Coagulation tests
Red	Red	Glass: no additive Plastic: clot activator	0 5	Chemistries Serology Blood bank
Gold	Marbled red and gray[a]	Serum separator Gel and clot activator	5	Most chemistry testing
Light green	Marbled green and gray[a]	Plasma separator gel and lithium heparin	8–10	Potassium determinations
Green	Green	Sodium heparin, or lithium heparin, or ammonium heparin	8–10	Blood gas determination and pH assays
Lavender	Lavender	EDTA	8–10	Whole blood hematology cell count, CBC
Gray	Gray	Sodium fluoride and potassium oxalate	8–10	Oral glucose tolerance test Blood alcohol test

[a]Note the mixing requirements.

CBC, Complete blood count; *EDTA,* ethylenediaminetetraacetic acid.

BD Hemogard plastic covers and rubber stopper colors from BD Diagnostics, Preanalytical Systems, 1 Becton Drive, Franklin Lakes, NJ, 07417, USA. www.bd.com/vacutainer. BD, BD Logo and all other trademarks are property of Becton, Dickinson, and Company. © 2014. Modified from Garrels M: *Laboratory and diagnostic testing in ambulatory care*, ed 3, St.Louis, 2014, Mosby.

4. *Light blue.* A tube with a light blue closure contains the anticoagulant sodium citrate and is used to obtain whole blood or plasma; the most common use is for coagulation tests, such as prothrombin time.
5. *Green.* A tube with a green closure contains the anticoagulant heparin and is used to collect a blood specimen to perform a blood gas determination or pH assay.
6. *Gray.* A tube with a gray closure contains sodium fluoride (a preservative) and potassium oxalate (an anticoagulant) and is used to obtain whole blood or plasma. The most common use of a gray closure tube is to collect a blood specimen to perform a blood alcohol test, drug test or an oral glucose tolerance test (OGTT).
7. *Royal blue.* A tube with a royal blue closure contains either EDTA or no additive at all. The tube is made of specially refined glass. A royal blue closure tube is used for the detection of trace elements, such as lead, zinc, arsenic, and copper, which are contracted through occupational or environmental exposure.

ORDER OF DRAW FOR MULTIPLE TUBES

When multiple tubes of blood need to be drawn, the order of draw presented in Table 31.1 is recommended by the *Clinical and Laboratory Standards Institute (CLSI).* Following the order of draw avoids cross-contamination of the specimen with additives found in different tubes.

A general overview of the order of draw is outlined below:

1. *Blood culture tube:* Yellow-closure glass tube that contains the anticoagulant sodium polyanethol sulfonate (SPS), which is used for blood cultures and other tests that require sterile specimens.
   Rationale: A blood culture tube is drawn first to prevent contamination of the specimen by other tubes which may lead to inaccurate test results.
2. *Coagulation tube:* Light blue-closure tube for coagulation tests.
   Rationale: To prevent additives from other tubes from getting into the tube.
   (*Note for Butterfly Setup:* The tubing of the butterfly setup contains 0.3 to 0.5 mL of air. If a light blue–closure tube is the first or only tube to be drawn, a 5-mL red-closure tube must be drawn first and discarded. This is because some of the tube's vacuum is exhausted by the air in the tubing (rather than blood), resulting in underfilling of the tube. If the light blue–closure tube is filled first, the underfilled tube results in an incorrect anticoagulant-to-blood ratio. An incorrect ratio when performing a coagulation test leads to inaccurate coagulation test results. It is also important to completely fill coagulation tubes to the exhaustion of the vacuum; failure to do so leads to erroneous coagulation test results.)
3. *Serum tubes:* Tubes with or without a clot activator, and tubes with or without a gel barrier (e.g., red-closure tube; marbled red/gray or gold-closure tubes).
   Rationale: To prevent contamination of serum tubes by tubes with an anticoagulant.
4. *Anticoagulant tubes* in this order of closure color: green, lavender, royal blue (tube that contains EDTA), and gray.
   Rationale: To prevent cross-contamination among different types of anticoagulants, which may lead to inaccurate test results.

What Would You Do? What Would You *Not* Do?

Case Study 2

Buzz Braydon had a heart attack 4 weeks ago and is taking the anticoagulant warfarin (Coumadin). He is at the office for a checkup and to have his prothrombin time tested. Blood is collected from a small vein in Buzz's left arm using the butterfly method. After the specimen has been collected, Buzz wants to know why a red-stoppered tube was used to draw blood from him and then thrown away. Buzz says that he is going on vacation in North Carolina for 2 weeks. He says that they explained to him at the hospital why he should have his blood tested every week, but he's not sure where to go to get his blood tested while he's on vacation. Buzz wants to know if, as long as he takes his medication exactly as he should, it would be all right to skip his weekly prothrombin test during that time. ■

BLOOD COLLECTION TUBE GUIDELINES

Certain guidelines should be followed when using evacuated blood collection tubes, as follows:

1. Select the proper blood collection tubes according to the type and amount of specimen required.
2. Check to ensure that the tube is not cracked. A cracked tube no longer has a vacuum.
3. Check the expiration date on each tube. Outdated tubes may no longer contain a vacuum, and as a result they would not be able to draw blood into the tube.
4. Make sure each tube is properly labeled. Proper labeling avoids mixing up specimens.
5. Before using tubes that contain powdered additives (e.g., gray-closure tube), gently tap the tube just below the stopper so that all of the additive is dislodged from the stopper. If an additive remains trapped in the stopper, erroneous test results may occur.
6. Take precautions to avoid premature loss of the tube's vacuum. Premature loss of vacuum can occur from the following:
   - Dropping the tube
   - Pushing the posterior needle through the tube closure before puncturing the vein
   - Partially pulling the needle out of the vein after penetrating the patient's vein
7. Use a continuous, steady motion to make the puncture. Performing the puncture with a slow, timid motion or a rapid, jabbing motion is painful for the patient. In addition, a rapid motion could cause the needle to go completely through the vein, resulting in failure to obtain blood and possibly a hematoma.

8. When multiple tubes are to be drawn, follow the proper *order of draw.* This prevents contamination of nonadditive tubes by additive tubes and cross-contamination among different types of additive tubes, which could lead to inaccurate test results.
9. Fill collection tubes until the vacuum is exhausted, as evidenced by cessation of blood flow into the tube. The tube is almost but not quite full when the vacuum is exhausted. If the collection tube is removed before the vacuum is exhausted, a rush of air enters the tube, damaging the red blood cells. A tube that contains an anticoagulant must be filled completely to ensure the proper ratio of anticoagulant to the blood specimen.
10. Remove the last tube from the tube holder before removing the needle from the patient's vein. This prevents blood from dripping out of the tip of the needle after it has been withdrawn from the patient's skin.
11. Mix tubes that contain a clot activator or an anticoagulant immediately after drawing by gently inverting them. Gentle inversion provides adequate mixing without causing **hemolysis**, or breakdown of blood cells. One inversion consists of one complete turn of the wrist (180 degrees) and then back again. Tubes with a clot activator should be inverted 5 times, and tubes with an anticoagulant (with the exception of sodium citrate tubes) should be inverted 8 to 10 times. Tubes containing sodium citrate (light-blue stopper) should be gently inverted 3 or 4 times (see Table 31.1). Inadequate mixing or not mixing tubes with an anticoagulant immediately after drawing the specimen may result in clotting of the blood, leading to inaccurate test results.
12. After the venipuncture, the top of a conventional rubber stopper tube may contain residual blood. Take precautions by following the OSHA Standard when handling these tubes.

BUTTERFLY METHOD OF VENIPUNCTURE

The butterfly method of venipuncture is also called the *winged infusion method.* This is because a winged infusion set is used to perform the procedure which consists of a blood collection needle, plastic wings and a length of tubing. The term *butterfly* is derived from the plastic "wings" located between the needle and the tubing of the winged infusion set (Fig. 31.16).

The gauge of the butterfly needle used to collect a blood specimen ranges from 21G to 23G, and the length of the needle ranges from ½ to ¾ inch. The needle is short and sharp, making it easier to stick difficult veins. For extremely small veins, a 23-G needle should be used to prevent rupture of the vein by a larger needle. In this case, it is preferable to use smaller-volume tubes (e.g., 2-mL collection tubes) because large collection tubes may put too much vacuum pressure on the vein, causing it to collapse. Manufacturers often color-code the wings of the infusion setup by gauge for easier identification—for example, Becton Dickinson uses the following color-coding system: green for 21-G needles and light blue for 23-G needles (see Fig. 31.16). Butterfly blood collection needles are available with a safety shield to reduce the risk of a needlestick injury by covering the contaminated needle after it has been withdrawn from the patient's vein. Fig. 31.17 illustrates a safety-engineered blood collection needle and the two techniques that can be used to activate the safety shield.

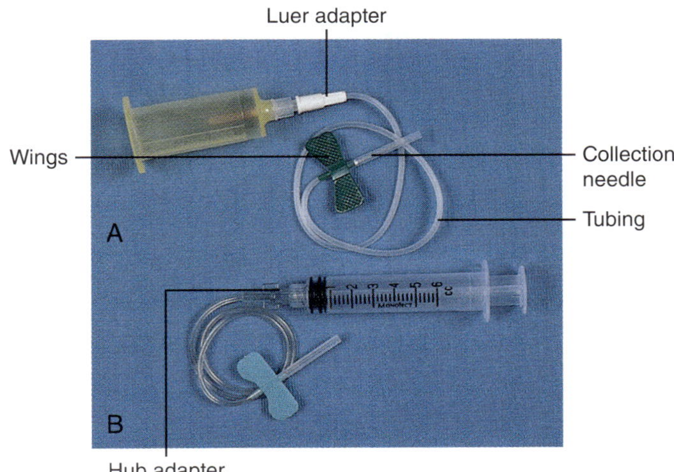

Fig. 31.16 Winged infusion set. (A) Luer adapter with collection tube. (B) Hub adapter with syringe.

The butterfly needle is attached to a 7- or 12-inch (18- or 30.5-cm) length of tubing and a *Luer adapter,* which is attached to a (posterior) needle with a rubber sleeve. A collection tube holder is screwed onto the Luer adapter, which allows it to be used with blood collection tubes (see Fig. 31.16A). Winged infusion sets also are available with a hub adapter that allows them to be used with a syringe (see Fig. 31.16B).

The butterfly method is used to collect blood from patients who are difficult to stick by conventional methods because it provides better control when making the puncture, and less pressure is exerted on the vein wall from the blood collection tube. The butterfly method is recommended for adults with small antecubital veins and children, who typically have small antecubital veins.

The butterfly method also is used when the antecubital veins are unavailable and veins in the forearm, wrist area, or back of the hand are used, as may occur with elderly and obese patients. These alternative veins are usually smaller and sometimes have a thin wall (e.g., hand veins), making them more likely to collapse with the Vacutainer method of venipuncture. With the Vacutainer method, the "sucking action" exerted on the vein when the pressure in the vacuum is released causes the vein to collapse, blocking the flow of blood into the tube. The butterfly method results in less pressure on the vein wall because the pressure exerted by the collection tube must travel through a length of

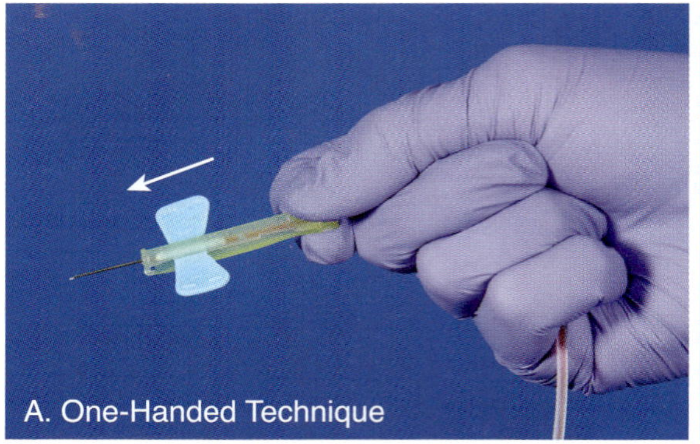

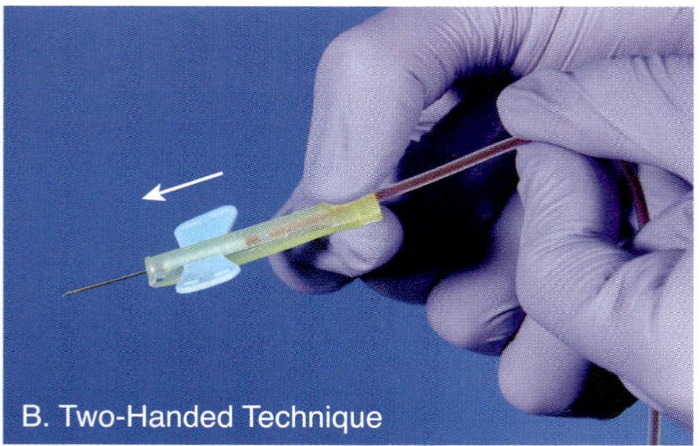

Fig. 31.17 Activation of the safety shield on a butterfly needle. (A) ***One-handed technique:*** 1, Grasp the yellow safety shield grip area with your thumb and index finger and at the same time grasp the tubing with your hand. 2, Push the safety shield forward with the thumb and index finger until a click is heard indicating the needle is completely retracted and the safety shield is locked into place. (B) ***Two-handed technique:*** 1, Grasp the yellow safety shield grip area with your thumb and index finger. With your opposite hand, grasp the tubing with the thumb and index finger. 2, Push the safety shield forward with the thumb and index finger until a click is heard indicating the needle is completely retracted and the safety shield is locked in placed.

tubing before reaching the vein. Because the pressure against the vein wall is minimized, the vein is less likely to collapse with the butterfly method. Procedure 31.2 describes the venipuncture procedure with the butterfly method.

GUIDELINES FOR THE BUTTERFLY METHOD

Certain guidelines should be followed when performing the butterfly method of venipuncture, as follows:

1. Position the patient according to the site selected for the venipuncture as follows:
   - *Antecubital, wrist, and forearm veins.* Position the arm in a straight line from the shoulder to the wrist as described for the Vacutainer method of venipuncture.
   - *Hand veins.* Position the patient's hand on the armrest, and ask the patient to make a loose fist or to grasp a rolled towel. This combination causes the hand veins to stand out so that accurate selection of a puncture site can be made. Locate a suitable vein between the knuckles and the wrist bones. Hand veins are usually visible and easy to locate.
2. Position the tourniquet according to the venipuncture site as follows: If the antecubital space is used, position the tourniquet 3 to 4 inches above the bend in the elbow. If the veins of the forearm or wrist are used, apply the tourniquet to the forearm, approximately 3 inches above the puncture site (Fig. 31.18A,B). For hand veins, position the tourniquet on the arm just above the wrist bone (Fig. 31.18C).

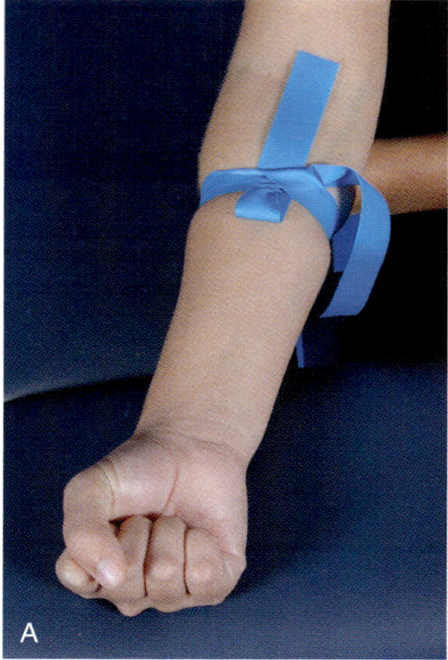

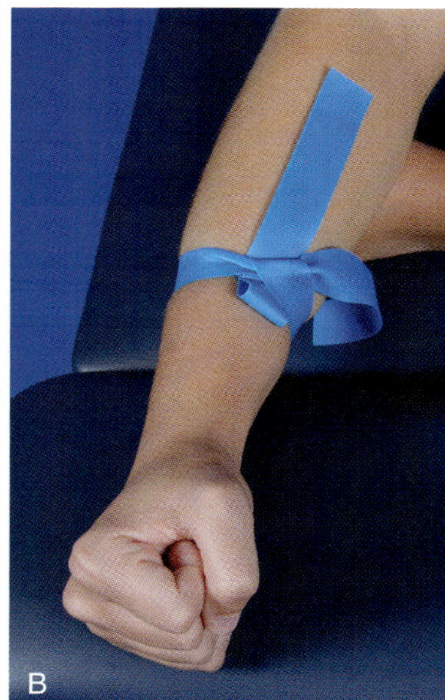

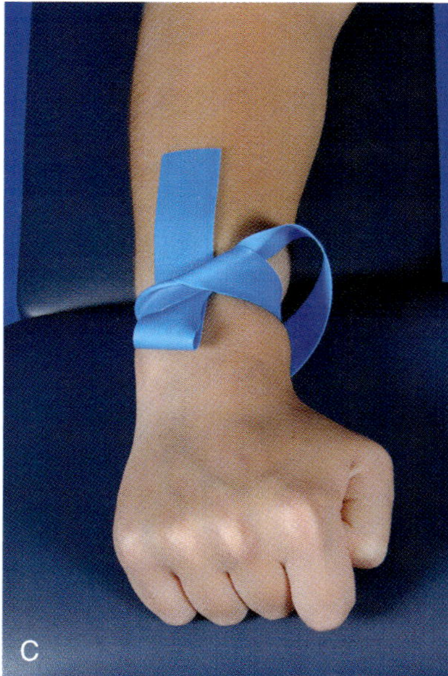

Fig. 31.18 Application of the tourniquet for alternative venipuncture sites. (A) Forearm site. (B) Wrist site. (C) Hand site.

3. Grasp the needle by compressing the plastic wings together. Insert the needle with the bevel facing up at a 15-degree angle to the skin. When the vein has been entered, decrease the angle to 5 degrees.
4. After decreasing the needle angle to 5 degrees, slowly thread the needle inside the vein an additional ¼ inch. This anchors or seats the needle in the center of the vein and allows the medical assistant to use both hands to change tubes.
5. To prevent venous reflux, keep the collection tube and holder (or syringe) in a downward position. This technique ensures that the blood fills from the bottom up and not near the rubber stopper.
6. When multiple blood collection tubes are to be drawn, follow the proper order of draw. Following the order of draw avoids cross-contamination of the specimen by additives found in different tubes.

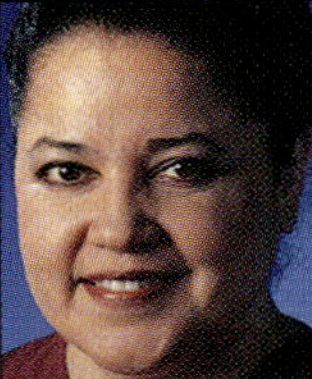

Memories *from* Practicum

Dori: One of the most terrifying things for me as a student was learning venipuncture. Even though I would practice during classroom laboratory hours and felt comfortable with it, it still scared me to know I would have to draw on a real person one day. When the day arrived to draw on my laboratory partner, I became sick to my stomach. In the end, we both got through it just fine and walked away without hurting each other. I spent days trying to prepare myself for that first experience, but after it was over, I felt more confident and relaxed that I could do this. At my practicum site, I was able to perform several venipunctures a day, which raised my confidence level. Today venipuncture is my favorite responsibility of all. I would draw blood all day if I could. I know I could even draw with my eyes closed, but never would, of course! ■

What Would You Do? What Would You *Not* Do?

Case Study 3

Porsha Coleman is at the office complaining of persistent headaches and abdominal pain over the past 3 months. The physician gives Mrs. Coleman a laboratory requisition to have her blood collected and tested at an outside laboratory. Mrs. Coleman says that her daughter who lives with her works as a phlebotomist at the local hospital. Mrs. Coleman wants to know whether her daughter can draw her blood at home and then drop it off at the laboratory. She says that the last time she had her blood drawn, they had to stick her two times and then she got a big bruise on her arm afterward. She says the laboratory technician kept digging around in her arm to find the vein and that it was quite painful. ■

PROBLEMS ENCOUNTERED WITH VENIPUNCTURE

Sometimes the medical assistant encounters problems when attempting to draw blood from a patient. The appropriate response depends on the type of problem.

FAILURE TO OBTAIN BLOOD

Periodically, even individuals highly skilled at performing venipuncture have difficulty obtaining blood. Although large and prominent veins make it easier to collect the blood specimen, conditions often exist that make the procedure more difficult.

It is often difficult to draw blood from obese patients who have small, superficial veins and whose veins suitable for venipuncture are buried in adipose tissue. Elderly patients with arteriosclerosis may have veins that are thick and hard, making them difficult to puncture. Other patients have veins that are small or have a thin wall, making the veins likely to collapse. After two unsuccessful attempts at venipuncture, the medical assistant should seek assistance in obtaining the blood specimen.

Another factor that results in failure to obtain blood is not using the correct angle of insertion of the needle into the vein. The needle should be positioned at a 15-degree angle to the arm. An angle of less than 15 degrees may cause the needle to enter above the vein, preventing puncture of the vein (Fig. 31.19B). Using an angle of more than 15 degrees may cause the needle to go through the vein (Fig. 31.19C). In these instances, most authorities recommend removing the needle rather than trying to probe the vein. Probing is often uncomfortable for the patient and can affect the integrity of the blood specimen, leading to inaccurate test results. Occasionally, a blood collection tube loses its vacuum because of a manufacturing defect or through improper handling of the tube. If suspected, this problem can be corrected by removing the defective tube and inserting another collection tube.

INAPPROPRIATE PUNCTURE SITES

If a patient complains of pain or soreness at a potential venipuncture site, this area should be avoided. In addition, any skin areas that are scarred, bruised, burned, or adjacent to areas of infection should not be used. A venipuncture should not be performed on an arm with edema. Swelling makes is more difficult to locate a vein and results in a longer time for healing of the puncture site to occur. Other sites to avoid include an arm that has a cast applied to it and an arm on the same side as a radical mastectomy.

SCARRED AND SCLEROSED VEINS

An individual who has had many venipunctures over a period of years often develops scar tissue in the wall of the vein. Elderly patients may have veins that have become thickened from arteriosclerosis. In both cases, the veins feel stiff and hard when palpated. A scarred or sclerosed vein is difficult to stick, and the blood return may be poor owing to a narrowed lumen; it is recommended that another vein be used for the venipuncture. If this is impossible, the needle should be inserted with careful pressure to avoid going completely through the vein.

ROLLING VEINS

The median cubital vein, located in the center of the antecubital space, is considered the best vein for a venipuncture.

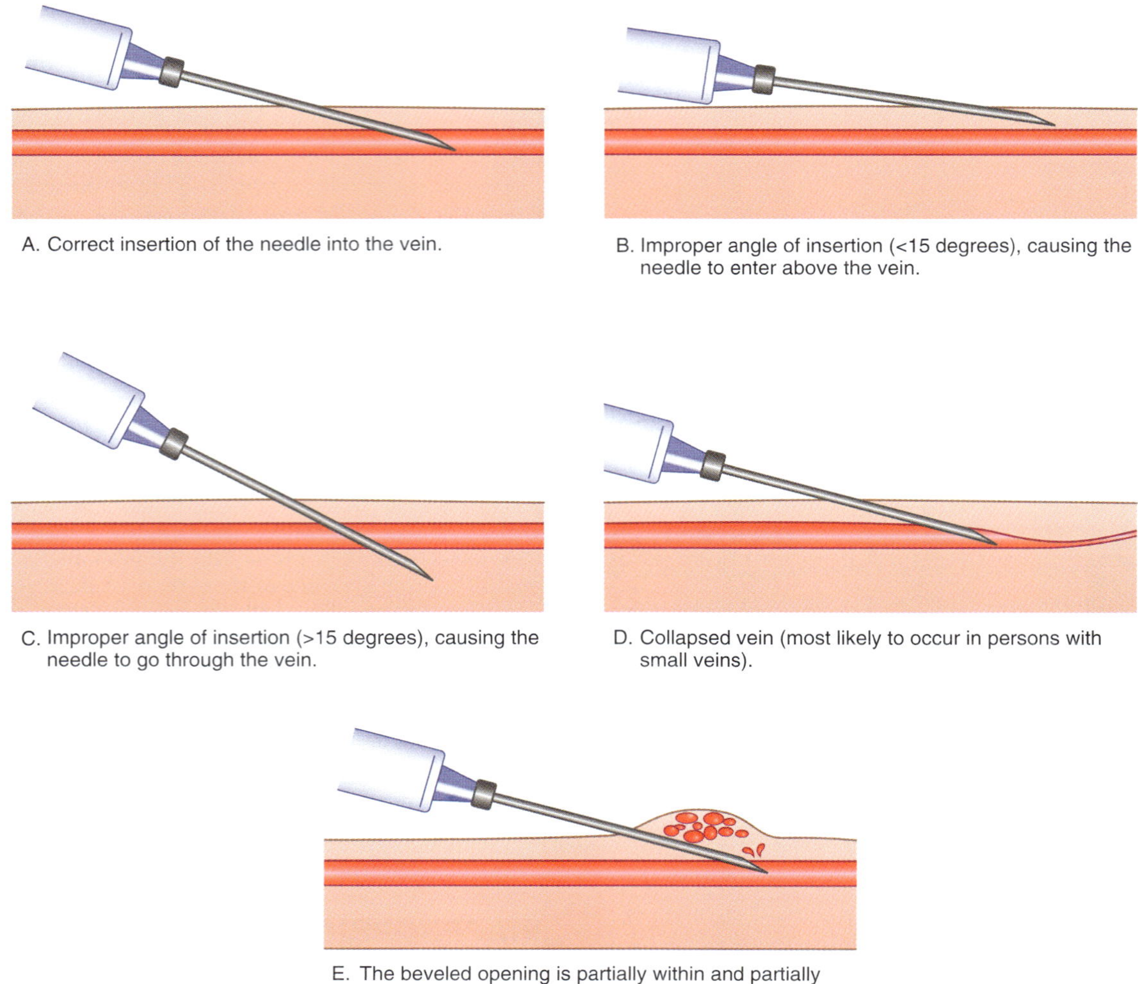

A. Correct insertion of the needle into the vein.

B. Improper angle of insertion (<15 degrees), causing the needle to enter above the vein.

C. Improper angle of insertion (>15 degrees), causing the needle to go through the vein.

D. Collapsed vein (most likely to occur in persons with small veins).

E. The beveled opening is partially within and partially outside of the vein, causing a hematoma.

Fig. 31.19 Problems encountered with venipuncture.

Sometimes it is impossible to use this vein, however, such as when it lies deep in the tissues and cannot be palpated or is scarred from repeated venipunctures. The veins on either side of the median cubital vein (cephalic vein or basilic vein) can be used, but they have a tendency to "roll," or move away from the needle, escaping puncture. To prevent rolling, firm pressure should be applied below and to the side of the vein to stabilize it as the needle is inserted.

COLLAPSING VEINS

Veins are most likely to collapse in individuals who have small veins or veins with thin walls. This is particularly true when the Vacutainer method is used. The "sucking action" exerted on the vein when the pressure in the vacuum is released causes the vein to collapse, blocking the flow of blood into the tube (see Fig. 31.19D). The typical result observed is that a small amount of blood enters the tube and then stops. Because better control and less pressure on the vein are possible, the butterfly method of venipuncture is recommended to obtain the specimen in patients with small veins.

PREMATURE NEEDLE WITHDRAWAL

Patient movement or improper venipuncture technique can cause the needle to come out of the vein prematurely. Because of the pressure exerted by the tourniquet, blood may be forced out of the puncture site, and immediate action is required to prevent a hematoma. The tourniquet should be removed at once, a gauze pad placed on the puncture site, and pressure applied until the bleeding has stopped.

HEMATOMA

When performing a venipuncture, a hematoma results if blood leaks from the puncture site of the vein and into the surrounding tissues. This can be caused by a needle that is inserted too far and goes through the vein, a bevel opening that is partially in the vein and partially out of the vein (see Fig. 31.19E), and insufficient pressure applied to the puncture site after removal of the needle. The first sign of a hematoma is a sudden swelling around the puncture site. If this occurs when the needle is in the patient's vein, first the tourniquet and then the needle should be removed immediately, and pressure should be applied to the puncture site until the bleeding stops.

HEMOLYSIS

The blood specimen should be handled carefully at all times. Blood cells are fragile, and rough handling may cause hemolysis, or breakdown of the blood cells. Hemolyzed blood specimens produce inaccurate test results. To prevent hemolysis, these guidelines should be followed:

1. Store the blood collection tubes at room temperature because chilled tubes can result in hemolysis.
2. Allow the alcohol to air-dry completely before performing the venipuncture. Alcohol entering a blood specimen can cause hemolysis.
3. Use an appropriate-gauge needle to collect the specimen. Using a needle with a small lumen (e.g., 25G) can cause the blood cells to rupture as they pass through the lumen of the needle.
4. Practice good technique in collecting the specimen; excessive trauma (e.g., probing) to the blood vessel can result in hemolysis.
5. Do not leave the tourniquet on for an extended period of time (more than 1 minute).
6. Always handle the collection tube carefully; do not shake it or handle it roughly.

FAINTING

Occasionally a patient experiences dizziness or fainting during or after a venipuncture. Should this occur, the most immediate concern is to protect the patient from injury—for example, by preventing the patient from falling. The patient should be placed in a position that promotes blood flow to the brain, and the provider should be notified for further treatment (see the box *Highlight on Vasovagal Syncope (Fainting)*).

HIGHLIGHT on Vasovagal Syncope (Fainting)

Most people experience no change in their sense of well-being when they have blood taken. A very small percentage of individuals experience a type of fainting, however, known as *vasovagal syncope.*

Cause and Symptoms

Vasovagal syncope is caused by unpleasant physical or emotional stimuli, such as pain, fright, and the sight of blood. A sudden pooling of blood occurs, which results in a sudden decrease in blood pressure. This momentarily deprives the brain of blood, causing a temporary loss of consciousness, usually lasting only 1 to 2 minutes. Vasovagal syncope usually occurs when an individual is in an upright position, as in standing or sitting. Before fainting, the patient usually experiences some warning signals, such as sudden lightheadedness, nausea, weakness, yawning, paleness, blurred vision, a feeling of warmth, and sweating followed by drooping eyelids; a weak, rapid pulse; and, finally, unconsciousness.

Treatment

A person who is about to faint should be placed in a position that facilitates blood flow to the brain and told to breathe deeply. The preferred position is lying down (supine) with the legs elevated and the collar and clothing loosened. This position may not always be possible, such as when a patient is seated and the venipuncture needle has already been inserted. In this case, the tourniquet and then the needle should be removed, and the patient's head should be lowered between the legs. An individual who has fainted should be protected from injury from falling and should be placed in a position that facilitates blood flow to the brain, as just described.

Prevention

Fainting during or after venipuncture is more likely in the following individuals: patients having a venipuncture for the first time, young patients, thin patients, patients with a low diastolic or high systolic blood pressure, patients with a history of fainting, nervous and apprehensive patients, and patients who are very quiet or very talkative. Fainting often can be prevented by identifying and closely observing individuals who are more likely to faint (as described). Talking to the patient often helps relax the patient and divert attention from the venipuncture procedure. If a patient has a history of fainting, they should be in a semi-reclining position for the venipuncture procedure because people rarely faint in this position. Other factors that contribute to fainting and that should be avoided include fatigue, lack of sleep, hunger, and environmental factors, such as a noisy, crowded, or overheated room. ■

OBTAINING A SERUM SPECIMEN

SERUM

Serum is plasma from which the clotting factor fibrinogen has been removed. Serum is normally clear in appearance and light yellow to yellow in color. Serum contains many dissolved substances, such as glucose, cholesterol, sodium, potassium, chloride, antibodies, hormones, and enzymes. As a result, many laboratory tests require a serum specimen to determine whether levels of these substances are within normal limits and to detect substances that should not normally be in the serum and that if present indicate a pathologic condition.

BLOOD COLLECTION TUBE SELECTION

A tube without an anticoagulant (e.g., SST or red-closure) must be used to collect the blood specimen, to allow the specimen to separate into serum and clotted blood cells. Because the amount of serum recovered is only a portion of the specimen, a blood specimen must be drawn that is 2.5 times the amount required for the test. If 2 mL of serum is required, a 5-mL tube of blood must be collected; if 3 mL of serum is required, an 8-mL tube of blood is collected; and if 4 mL of serum is required, a 10-mL tube of blood is collected.

PROCESSING THE SPECIMEN

After the blood specimen has been collected, the red-closure tube or SST must be allowed to stand upright at room temperature for 30 to 45 minutes before being centrifuged. This allows clot formation of the blood cells, which yields more serum from the specimen. If the specimen is centrifuged too soon after collection of the blood specimen, the clotting factors do not have an opportunity to settle down into the cell layer to form a blood clot. The result of this is the formation of a *fibrin clot* in the serum layer of the specimen. A fibrin clot is a spongy substance that occupies space, interfering with adequate serum collection from the specimen (Fig. 31.20). The blood specimen should not be allowed to stand for longer than 1 hour, however, because leaching of substances from the cell layer into the serum may occur. This leaching of substances changes the integrity of the serum, leading to inaccurate test results. After the specimen has been allowed to stand and the blood cells have clotted, the specimen is centrifuged for 10 minutes to separate the serum from the blood cells.

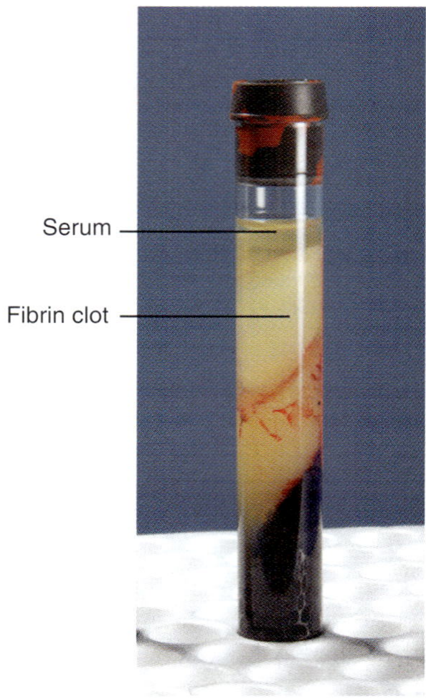

Fig. 31.20 A fibrin clot may interfere with adequate collection of serum.

SERUM SEPARATOR TUBES

A serum separator tube (SST), also known as a *gel barrier tube*, is a blood collection tube specially designed to facilitate the collection of a serum specimen. The SST is identified by a gold or marbled red/gray closure and is used for collection and separation of blood. The SST contains a thixotropic gel, which is in a solid state at the bottom of the unused tube (Fig. 31.21A).

The blood specimen is collected following the appropriate venipuncture method (Vacutainer or butterfly). The specimen must then be allowed to stand in an upright position for 30 to 45 minutes for proper clot formation of the blood cells and must be centrifuged as previously described. During centrifugation, the gel temporarily becomes fluid and moves to the dividing point between the serum and clotted cells, where it re-forms into a solid gel, serving as a physical barrier between the serum and the clot (Fig. 31.21B). It is important to centrifuge the specimen for the proper length of time (i.e., 10 minutes). Centrifuging the specimen for less than 10 minutes can result in an incomplete gel barrier between the serum and the clot.

The serum can be transported to an outside laboratory in the serum separator tube. The medical assistant must first inspect the tube carefully to ensure that the gel barrier is firmly attached to the glass wall. If a complete barrier has not formed, the serum specimen must be removed and placed in a transfer tube to prevent leaching of substances from the cell layer into the serum, affecting the accuracy of the test results.

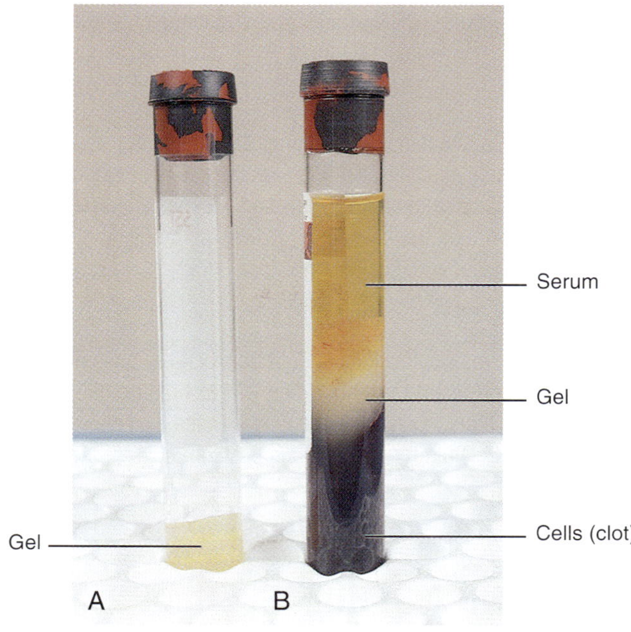

Fig. 31.21 Serum separator tubes. (A) An SST that contains a thixotropic gel in the bottom of the tube. (B) A tube that has been used to collect a blood specimen. During centrifugation, the gel temporarily becomes fluid and moves to the dividing point between the serum and blood cells in a fibrin clot.

RED-CLOSURE TUBES

If a red-closure tube has been used to collect the specimen, the serum must be removed from the clot to prevent leaching of substances from the cell layer into the serum which affects the accuracy of the test results. The serum is removed using a pipette and placed in a separate collection tube known as a transfer tube.

SKIN PUNCTURE

A skin puncture is used to obtain a capillary blood specimen and is also called a *capillary puncture.* Laboratory testing of a capillary blood specimen is usually performed in the medical office. Examples of such tests are hemoglobin, hematocrit, blood glucose, mononucleosis, and prothrombin time.

A skin puncture is performed when a test requires only a small blood specimen. Skin puncture is the method preferred for obtaining blood from infants and young children. Collecting blood from patients in this age group by venipuncture is often difficult and may damage veins and surrounding tissues.

PUNCTURE SITES

The puncture site varies depending on the age of the patient. The lateral part of the tip of the third or fourth finger is the preferred site for a skin puncture in an adult. In an infant (birth to 1 year old), the skin puncture should be performed on the lateral or medial plantar surface of the heel. A finger puncture should *never* be performed on infants. The amount of tissue between skin surface and bone is so small that an injury to the bone is likely. After a child has begun to walk, the skin puncture can be performed on the fingertip.

DISPOSABLE RETRACTABLE LANCET

According to OSHA, a skin puncture should be performed in the medical office using a disposable retractable lancet, which consists of a spring-loaded plastic holder with a metal blade inside the holder. The skin puncture must not penetrate deeper than 3.1 mm in adults (finger) and 2.0 mm in infants (plantar surface of the heel) and children. If the puncture is deeper than this, the bone may be penetrated, which could result in the painful and serious conditions of osteochondritis or osteomyelitis. **Osteochondritis** is inflammation of bone and cartilage, and **osteomyelitis** is inflammation of the bone or bone marrow caused by bacterial infection. To avoid these complications, lancet blades are available in different lengths to control the depth of puncture. The blade length selected depends on the size of the patient's fingers; for example, adults with thin fingers and children require a shorter blade to avoid penetration of the bone.

The gauge of the lancet blade used to perform the skin puncture is based on the amount of blood specimen required. The gauge refers to the diameter of the lancet blade; lancet blades are available in sizes ranging from 18G to 30G. As the size of the gauge increases, the diameter of the lancet blade decreases. For example, a blade with a gauge of 23 has a smaller diameter than a blade with a gauge of 19. A lancet blade with a large diameter (e.g., 19G) must be used to obtain enough blood to fill a microcollection device, whereas a lancet blade with a smaller diameter (e.g., 23G) should be used if only a drop of blood is needed.

The plastic holder of a disposable lancet may be color-coded by the manufacturer for ease in identifying the blade length of the lancet—for example, Surgilance Safety Lancet (Surgilance, Norcross, GA) (Fig. 31.22A). The plastic holder conceals the blade so the patient cannot see it during the puncture, as with the CoaguChek Lancet (Roche

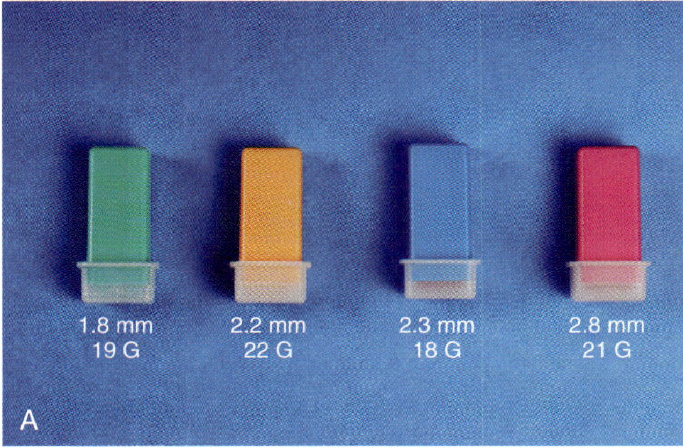

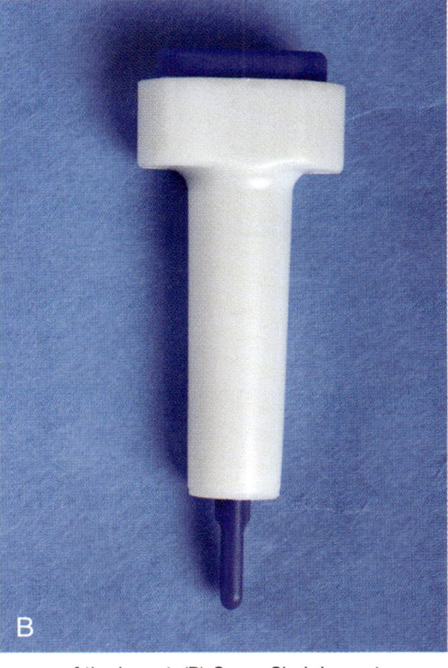

Fig. 31.22 (A) Surgilance color-coded lancets indicating length and gauge of the lancet. (B) CoaguChek Lancet.

Diagnostics, Branchburg, NJ) (Fig. 31.22B). Another example is the Quikheel Infant Lancet (Becton Dickinson), which is used for heel punctures in infants.

When performing a finger puncture, use the lateral part of the tip of the third or fourth finger (middle or ring finger) of the nondominant hand for the puncture site. The capillary beds in these fingers are large, and the skin is easy to penetrate. The puncture site should be free of lesions, scars, bruises, and edema. The index finger is not recommended as a puncture site. The index finger is more calloused, which makes it harder to penetrate than the other fingers. Also, the patient uses that finger more and would notice the pain longer. The little finger also should not be used as a puncture site. The amount of tissue between the skin surface and the bone is so small that using this finger as a puncture site could result in injury to the bone.

To perform the skin puncture, the retractable lancet is placed on the patient's skin and activated. Depending on the brand, this is accomplished by one of the following methods:

- Depressing an activation button located on the top of the lancet until an audible click is heard (e.g., Coagu-Chek Lancet)
- Pushing the lancet firmly onto the puncture site until an audible click is heard (e.g., Surgilance Safety Lancet)

When the lancet is activated, the spring forces the blade into the skin and retracts the blade into the holder. The concealed blade and automatic puncture tend to result in less patient apprehension. After the puncture, the entire lancet is discarded in a biohazard sharps container. Procedure 31.3 describes the skin puncture procedure for use of a disposable retractable lancet.

MICROCOLLECTION DEVICES

After the skin has been punctured, a capillary blood specimen must be collected. The blood specimen can be collected directly onto a reagent strip, such as occurs with blood glucose monitors. It also can be collected in a small container known as a *microcollection device*. The device depends on the laboratory equipment running the test. Common microcollection devices are capillary tubes and microcollection tubes.

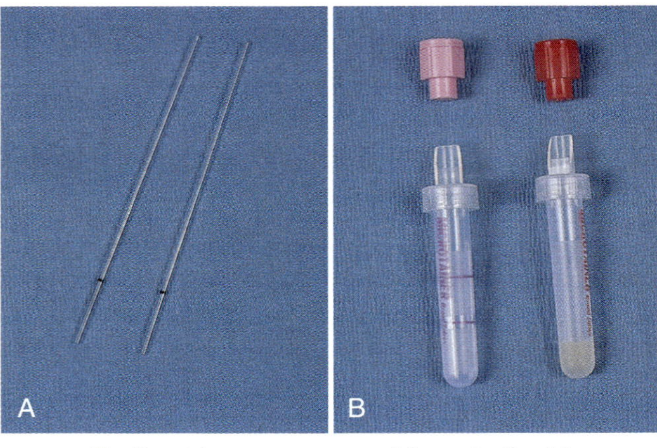

Capillary tubes Microcollection tubes

Fig. 31.23 Microcollection devices. (A) Microcollection tubes. (B) Capillary tubes.

Capillary tubes: A capillary tube consists of a disposable glass or plastic tube (Fig. 31.23A). Depending on the size of the tube, it can hold 5 to 75 μL of blood. In the medical office, a capillary tube is used to collect a blood specimen for a hematocrit determination. This procedure is presented in Chapter 32.

Microcollection tubes: A microcollection tube consists of a small plastic tube with a removable blood collector tip. The tip is designed to collect capillary blood from a skin puncture, which results in a relatively large blood specimen. After the specimen has been collected, the collector tip is removed, discarded, and replaced by a plastic plug. Microcollection tubes are available with or without an anticoagulant. The plugs are color-coded and correspond to the color-coded collection tube system used in venipuncture. One such device is the Microtainer (Becton Dickinson) (Fig. 31.23B).

What Would You Do? What Would You *Not* Do? RESPONSES

Case Study 1
Page 830

What Did Dori Do?

- ❑ Told Camila that it was fine to have her friend there while she gets her blood drawn.
- ❑ Told Camila that she could not have the blood drawn out of her left arm because a good vein could not be located in that arm.
- ❑ Told Camila that using the hand veins is always the last choice when drawing blood. Explained to Camila that there will just be a small stick and that it will heal quickly, and there should be no reason it would affect her softball game this evening.
- ❑ Tried to relax and reassure Camila before the venipuncture. Carefully explained the procedure to her because it was her first one.
- ❑ Because Camila is nervous, took precautions to prevent her from fainting by placing her in a semi-Fowler position on the examining table.
- ❑ Had Camila's friend stand near the head of the table to help calm her down.

What Did Dori Not Do?

- ❑ Did not try to draw Camila's blood from her left arm or hand.
- ❑ Did not ignore the fact that Camila was nervous about the venipuncture.

What Would You Do? What Would You *Not* Do? RESPONSES—cont'd

Case Study 2

Page 834

What Did Dori Do?

- ❑ Told Buzz that when a butterfly setup is used, the air in the tubing alters the test results. Explained that the red tube is used to get rid of the air, and because it is not needed for testing, it is thrown away.
- ❑ Stressed to Buzz how important it is to have his blood tested every week, which helps the physician determine if there is too much or too little Coumadin in his body. Explained to him again what might occur if his Coumadin were at the wrong level.
- ❑ Told Buzz that the office would help him locate a medical laboratory where he will be vacationing, so he can have his test done.
- ❑ Made sure that Buzz had a laboratory requisition so that he could have his test done while he was on vacation.

What Did Dori Not Do?

- ❑ Did not tell Buzz that it would be all right to skip his prothrombin test during his vacation.

Case Study 3

Page 837

What Did Dori Do?

- ❑ Told Mrs. Coleman that the laboratory can accept only specimens drawn at the laboratory or at the medical office.
- ❑ Told Mrs. Coleman that if it would make her feel more comfortable, the laboratory could drop off the blood-drawing supplies at the office, and her blood could be drawn tomorrow at the office.
- ❑ Informed the physician about Mrs. Coleman's experience at the laboratory.

What Did Dori Not Do?

- ❑ Did not tell Mrs. Coleman that probing a vein could cause the test results to be inaccurate.

TERMINOLOGY REVIEW

Key Term	Word Parts	Definition
Antecubital space	*ante-:* before	The surface of the arm in front of the elbow.
Anticoagulant	*anti-:* against	A substance that inhibits blood clotting.
Buffy coat		A thin, light-colored layer of white blood cells and platelets that lies between a top layer of plasma and a bottom layer of red blood cells when an anticoagulant has been added to a blood specimen.
Evacuated blood collection tube		A sterile glass or plastic blood collection tube with a color-coded closure that contains a vacuum.
Hematoma	*hemat/o:* blood *-oma:* tumor or swelling	A swelling or mass of clotted blood within the tissues caused by a break in a blood vessel.
Hemoconcentration	*hem/o:* blood	An increase in the concentration of the nonfilterable blood components in the blood vessels, such as red blood cells, enzymes, iron, and calcium, as a result of a decrease in the fluid content of the blood.
Hemolysis	*hem/o:* blood *-lysis:* breakdown	The breakdown of blood cells.
Osteochondritis	*oste/o:* bone *myel/o:* bone marrow *-itis:* inflammation	Inflammation of bone and cartilage.
Osteomyelitis	*oste/o:* bone *myel/o:* bone marrow *-itis:* inflammation	Inflammation of the bone or bone marrow as a result of bacterial infection.
Phlebotomist	*phleb/o:* vein *tomist:* specialist	A health care professional trained in the collection of blood specimens.
Phlebotomy	*phleb/o:* vein *-otomy:* incision	Incision of a vein for the removal of blood; the collection of blood.
Plasma		The liquid part of the blood consisting of a clear, straw-colored fluid that comprises approximately 55% of the blood volume.
Serum		Plasma from which the clotting factor fibrinogen has been removed.
Venipuncture	*ven/o:* vein	Puncturing of a vein.
Venous reflux	*ven/o:* vein *-ous:* pertaining to	The backflow of blood (from a blood collection tube) into the patient's vein.
Venous stasis	*ven/o:* vein *stasis:* control, stop	The temporary cessation or slowing of the venous blood flow.

PROCEDURE 31.1 Venipuncture—Vacutainer Method

Outcome Perform a venipuncture using the Vacutainer method.

Equipment/Supplies

- Disposable gloves
- Tourniquet
- Antiseptic wipe
- Blood collection needle with a safety shield
- Collection tube holder
- Blood collection tubes
- Sterile 2 × 2 gauze pad
- Adhesive bandage
- Biohazard sharps container
- Biohazard specimen bag

PROCEDURE 31.1

1. **Procedural Step.** Review the collection and handling requirements for the tests ordered by the provider in the laboratory test directory.
2. **Procedural Step.** Sanitize your hands. Greet the patient and introduce yourself. Identify the patient by asking the patient to state their full name and date of birth. Compare this information with the demographic data in the patient's medical record. Seat the patient comfortably in a phlebotomy chair.
   Principle. It is important to confirm that you have the correct patient to avoid collecting a specimen from the wrong patient.
3. **Procedural Step.** If the patient was required to prepare for the test (e.g., fasting, medication restriction), determine whether they have prepared properly. If the patient has not followed the patient preparation requirements, notify the provider for instructions on handling this situation.
   Principle. The patient must prepare properly so the medical assistant can obtain a high-quality specimen that will yield accurate test results.
4. **Procedural Step.** Assemble the equipment.
   a. Select the proper blood collection tubes for the tests ordered by the provider and check the expiration date on the tubes.
   b. Complete a laboratory request by writing in the information on a preprinted form or by entering the required information into a computer.
   c. Label each tube using one of the following methods: attaching a computer barcode label to each tube, or manually labeling each tube with the patient's name and date of birth, the date, and your initials. (*Note:* Follow the medical office policy as to when the tubes should be labeled. Some offices prefer that tubes be labeled *before* the specimen is drawn; other offices want the tubes to be labeled right *after* the specimen has been drawn.)

   Principle. Outdated tubes may no longer contain a vacuum, and as a result they may not be able to draw blood into the tube. Proper labeling of blood specimens avoids a mix-up of specimens.

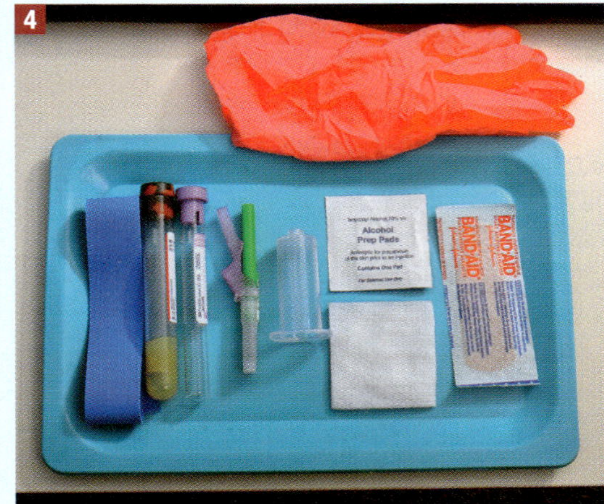

Assemble the equipment.

5. **Procedural Step.** Prepare the Vacutainer system. Remove the cap from the posterior needle using a twisting and pulling motion. Insert the posterior needle into the small opening on the collection tube holder. Screw the tube holder onto the Luer adapter, and tighten it securely.
   Principle. An unsecured needle can fall out of its tube holder.

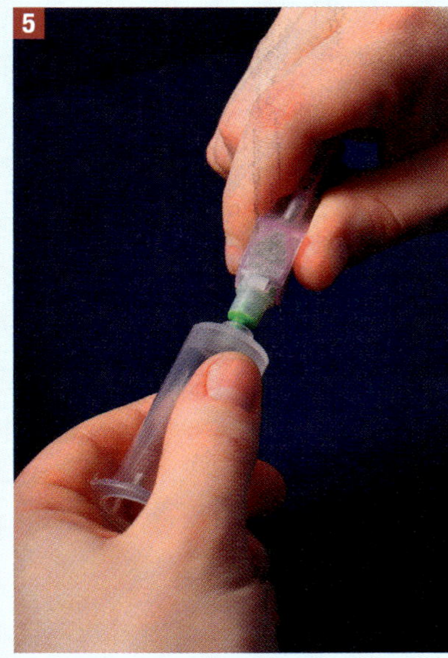

Insert the posterior needle into the collection tube holder.

PROCEDURE 31.1 Venipuncture—Vacutainer Method—cont'd

6. **Procedural Step.** Open the sterile gauze packet, and lay it flat to allow the gauze pad to rest on the inside of its wrapper. Position the blood collection tubes in the correct order of draw. If the collection tube contains a powdered additive, tap the tube just below the stopper to release any additive adhering to the stopper.
   Principle. If an additive remains trapped in the stopper, erroneous test results may occur.
7. **Procedural Step.** Place the first tube loosely in the collection tube holder.
8. **Procedural Step.** Explain the procedure to the patient, and reassure the patient. Perform a preliminary assessment of both arms to determine the best vein to use. It also is helpful to ask the patient which arm has been used in the past to obtain blood.
   Principle. Venipuncture is often a frightening experience for the patient, and reassurance should be offered to reduce apprehension.
9. **Procedural Step.** Apply the tourniquet. Position the tourniquet 3 to 4 inches above the bend in the elbow. The tourniquet should be snug but not tight. Ask the patient to clench the fist of the arm to which the tourniquet has been applied.
   Principle. The combined effect of the pressure of the tourniquet and the clenched fist should cause the antecubital veins to stand out so that accurate selection of a puncture site can be made. A tourniquet that is too tight is uncomfortable for the patient and may also result in a specimen that leads to inaccurate test results.

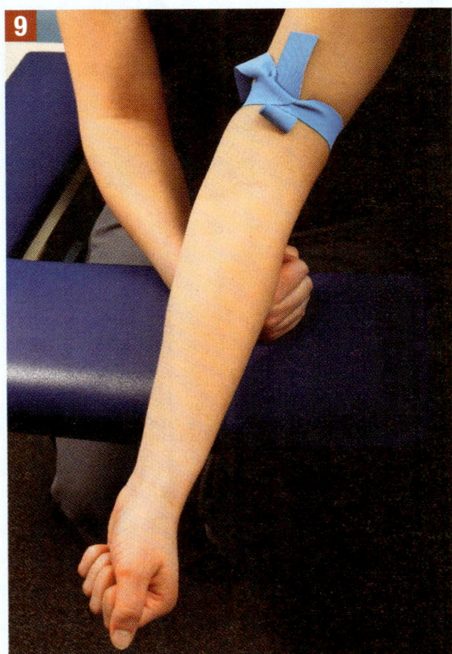

Apply the tourniquet.

10. **Procedural Step.** With a tourniquet in place, thoroughly assess the veins of first one arm and then the other to determine the best vein to use.
11. **Procedural Step.** Position the patient's arm. The arm with the vein selected for the venipuncture should be extended and placed in a straight line from the shoulder to the wrist with the antecubital veins facing anteriorly. The arm can be supported on the armrest by a rolled towel or by having the patient place the fist of the other hand under the elbow.
    Principle. This position allows easy access to the antecubital veins.
12. **Procedural Step.** Thoroughly palpate the selected vein. Gently palpate the vein with the fingertips to determine the direction of the vein and to estimate its size and depth. Never leave the tourniquet on an arm for longer than 1 minute at a time. (*Note:* If you need to perform several assessments to locate the best vein, the tourniquet must be removed and reapplied after a 2-minute waiting period.)
    Principle. Leaving the tourniquet on for longer than 1 minute is uncomfortable for the patient and may alter the test results.

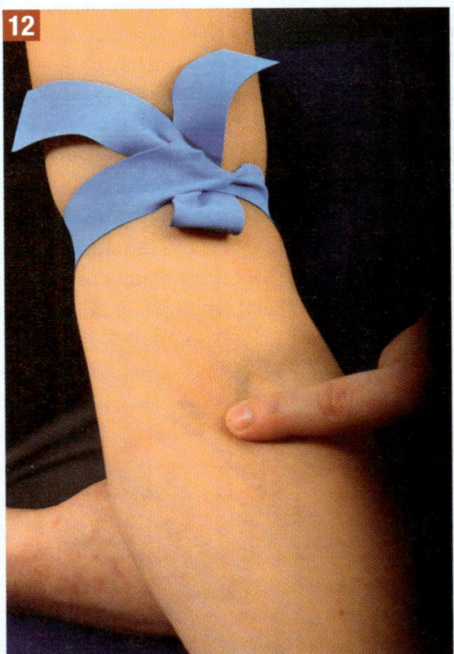

Palpate the vein.

13. **Procedural Step.** Remove the tourniquet (if more than 1 minute has elapsed) and cleanse the site with an antiseptic wipe. Cleansing should be done in a circular motion, starting from the inside and moving away from the puncture site. Allow the site to air-dry;

Continued

PROCEDURE 31.1 Venipuncture—Vacutainer Method—cont'd

after cleansing, *do not touch the area*, wipe the area with gauze, or fan the area with your hand. Place the remaining supplies within comfortable reach of your nondominant hand.

Principle. Using a circular motion helps carry foreign particles away from the puncture site. The site must be allowed to air-dry to allow the alcohol enough time to destroy microorganisms on the patient's skin. Residual alcohol entering the blood specimen can cause hemolysis, leading to inaccurate test results. In addition, residual alcohol causes the patient to experience a stinging sensation when the puncture is made. Touching or fanning the area causes contamination of the puncture site, and the cleansing process must be repeated. Items used during the procedure should be positioned so that you do not have to reach over the patient and possibly move the needle, resulting in pain, injury, or both.

14. Procedural Step. Reapply the tourniquet. Apply gloves. Gently position the pink safety shield straight back toward the holder (refer to Fig. 31.13A). Remove the needle guard from the needle using a twisting and pulling motion. Hold the Vacutainer system by placing the thumb of the dominant hand on top of the tube holder and the pads of the first three fingers underneath the holder and collection tube. The needle bevel is in the correct position (bevel facing up) when the pink safety shield is facing up. Position the collection tube so that the label is facing down.

Principle. Gloves provide a barrier against bloodborne pathogens. A bevel up position allows easier entry of the needle into the skin and the vein, resulting in less pain for the patient. With the label facing down, you are can observe the blood as it fills the tube, which allows you to know when the tube is full.

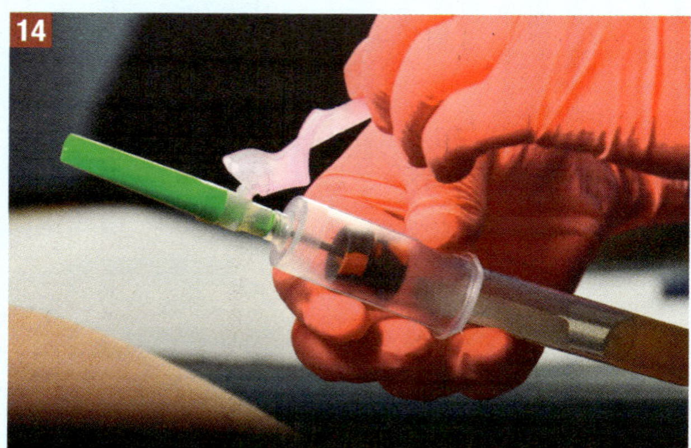

Position the safety shield straight back towards the holder.

15. Procedural Step. Anchor the vein. Grasp the patient's arm with the nondominant hand. Your thumb should be placed 1 to 2 inches below and to the side of the puncture site. Using your thumb, draw the skin taut over the vein in the direction of the patient's hand.

Principle. The thumb helps hold the skin taut for easier entry and helps stabilize the vein to be punctured. Placing the thumb to the side keeps it out of the way of the Vacutainer setup, so that you can maintain a 15-degree angle when entering the vein.

16. Procedural Step. Position the needle at a 15-degree angle to the arm. Rest the backs of the fingers on the patient's forearm. Ensure that the needle points in the same direction as the vein to be entered. The needle should be positioned so that it enters the vein approximately ⅛ inch below the place where the vein is to be entered.

Principle. An angle of less than 15 degrees may cause the needle to enter above the vein, preventing puncture of the vein. An angle of more than 15 degrees may cause the needle to go through the vein by puncturing the posterior wall. This could result in a hematoma.

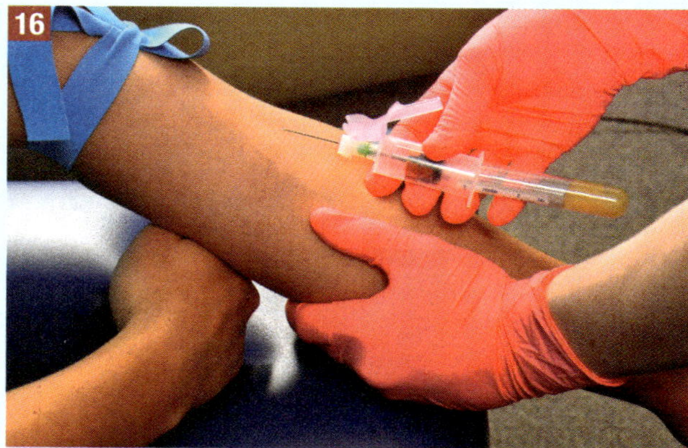

Position the needle.

17. Procedural Step. Tell the patient that they or she will "feel a small stick," and with one continuous steady motion, enter the skin and then the vein. You will feel a sensation of resistance followed by a "release" as the vein is entered. When the "release" is felt, you have entered the vein and should not advance the needle any farther.

Principle. Alerting the patient to the stick prevents startling the patient, which could cause the patient's arm to move. Movement of the needle in the vein causes pain for the patient, and it may damage tissue at the venipuncture site. Using one continuous steady motion helps to prevent tissue damage.

PROCEDURE 31.1 Venipuncture—Vacutainer Method—cont'd

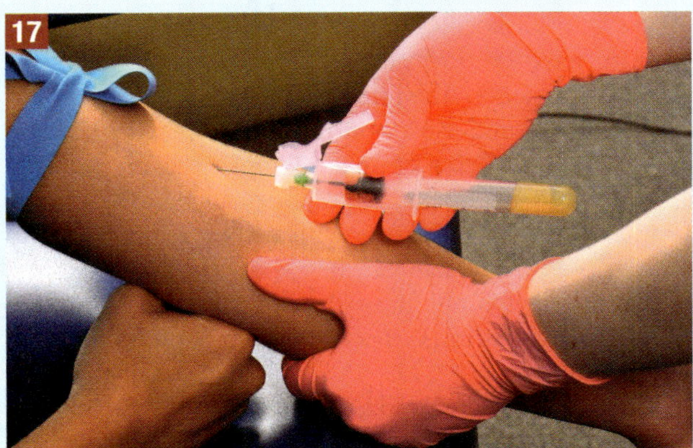
Make the puncture.

18. **Procedural Step.** Stabilize the Vacutainer setup by firmly grasping the holder between the thumb and the underlying fingers to prevent the needle from moving. Do *not* change hands during the procedure.
Principle. Stabilizing the holder helps prevent the needle from moving when a tube is inserted or removed. Changing hands may cause the needle to move, which is painful for the patient.
19. **Procedural Step.** With the nondominant hand, place the first two fingers on the underside of the flange on the tube holder, and with the thumb, slowly push the tube forward to the end of the holder. This allows the posterior needle to puncture the rubber stopper. Blood begins flowing into the tube if the (anterior) needle is in a vein.
Principle. Not using the flange may cause the needle to advance forward and go completely through the vein, resulting in failure to obtain blood; bleeding from the puncture site also occurs resulting in a hematoma.
20. **Procedural Step.** Allow the blood collection tube to fill to the exhaustion of the vacuum, as indicated by cessation of the blood flow into the tube. The suction of the collection tube automatically draws the blood into the tube.
Principle. If the collection tube is removed before the vacuum is exhausted, a rush of air enters the tube, damaging the red blood cells. Also, a tube containing an additive, such as an anticoagulant, must be filled completely to ensure accurate test results.
21. **Procedural Step.** Remove the tube from the holder by grasping the tube with the fingers, placing the thumb or index finger against the flange, and pulling the tube off the posterior needle. Do not change the position of the needle in the vein. If the tube contains a clot activator, gently invert the tube back and forth 5 times before laying it down. If the tube contains an anticoagulant, gently invert the tube 8 to 10 times.
Principle. The rubber sheath covers the point of the needle, stopping the flow of blood until the next tube is inserted. Not using the flange to remove the tube can cause the needle to come out of the vein prematurely, resulting in blood being forced out of the puncture site. A tube containing an anticoagulant must be inverted immediately to prevent the blood from clotting. Gentle inversion of a tube with a clot activator or an anticoagulant prevents hemolysis.

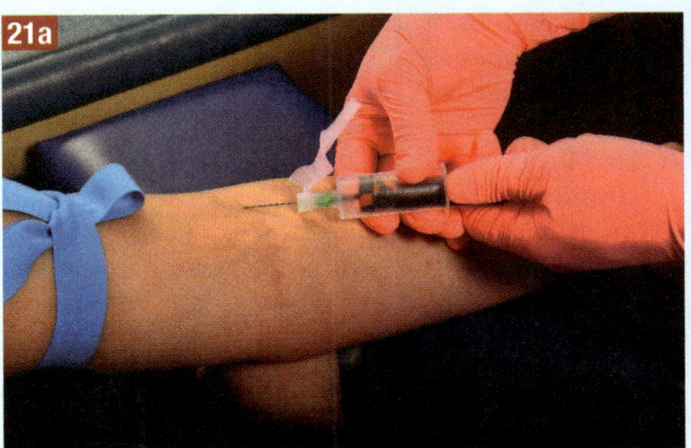
Remove the tube from the holder.

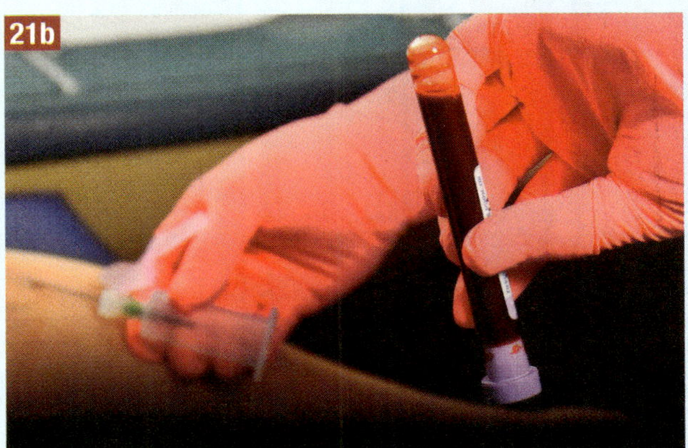
Invert the tube 8 to 10 times.

22. **Procedural Step.** Using the flange, carefully insert the next tube into the holder. Continue in this manner until the last tube has been filled.
23. **Procedural Step.** Remove the tension from the tourniquet (if it has not been previously released) by pulling upward on one of the flaps of the tourniquet. Ask the patient to unclench the fist.
Principle. The tourniquet tension must be removed before the needle. Otherwise, the pressure on the vein from the tourniquet could cause internal and external bleeding around the puncture site resulting in a hematoma.

Continued

PROCEDURE 31.1 Venipuncture—Vacutainer Method—cont'd

24. Procedural Step. Remove the last tube from the holder. Immediately invert the tube back and forth 5 times if it contains a clot activator and 8 to 10 times if it contains an anticoagulant.

Principle. Removing the last tube prevents blood from dripping out of the tip of the needle after it has been removed from the patient's arm.

25. Procedural Step. Place a sterile gauze pad slightly above the puncture site, and carefully withdraw the needle at the same angle as for penetration. Immediately move the gauze over the puncture site, and apply firm pressure. (Do not apply any pressure to the puncture site until the needle has been completely removed.) Activate the safety shield away from yourself and the patient and as illustrated in Fig. 31.13.

Principle. Placing the gauze pad above the puncture helps prevent tissue movement as the needle is withdrawn and reduces patient discomfort. Careful withdrawal prevents further tissue damage.

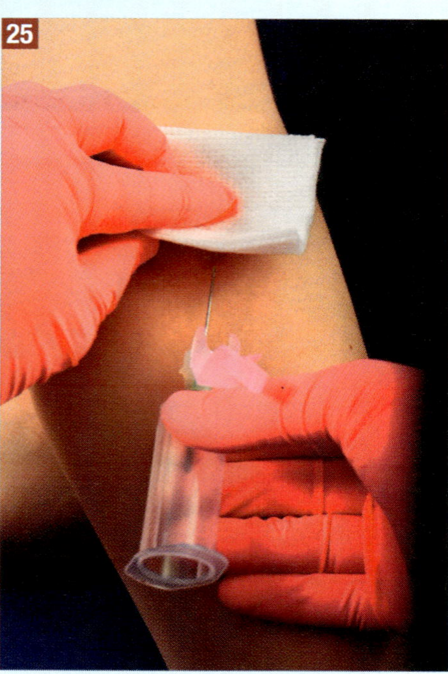

Withdraw the needle.

26. Procedural Step. Immediately discard the collection tube holder and attached needle as one unit in a biohazard sharps container. Do not remove the needle from the holder; the holder must be discarded and not reused.

Principle. Immediate disposal of the needle and holder unit is required by the OSHA Standard to prevent a needlestick injury; even though the safety shield encases the anterior needle, a needlestick injury can still occur from the posterior needle, which is covered only with a rubber sleeve. Tube holders are often contaminated with blood and must not be reused.

27. Procedural Step. Continue to apply pressure with the gauze pad. Cooperative patients can be asked to assist by applying pressure with the gauze pad for 1 to 2 minutes. The arm can be elevated to facilitate clot formation. Do not allow the patient to bend the arm at the elbow because this increases blood loss from the puncture site.

Principle. Applying pressure reduces the leakage of blood from the puncture site externally or internally. Internal leakage of blood into the tissues could result in a hematoma.

28. Procedural Step. Stay with the patient until the bleeding has stopped. Remove the gauze, and inspect the puncture site to ensure that the opening is sealed with a clot. Apply an adhesive bandage to the puncture site. As an alternative, the gauze pad can be folded into quarters and taped on the puncture site to be used as a pressure bandage. Instruct the patient not to pick up anything heavy for about an hour. (*Note:* If swelling or discoloration occurs, apply an ice pack to the site after bandaging it.)

Principle. Lifting a heavy object causes pressure on the puncture site, which could result in bleeding.

29. Procedural Step. Place the tubes in an upright position in a test tube rack. Remove the gloves, and sanitize your hands.

30. Procedural Step. Document the procedure in the patient's medical record.

a. *Electronic medical record:* Document which arm and vein were used, as well as any unusual patient reactions, using the appropriate radio buttons, drop-down menus, and free text fields.

b. *Paper-based patient record:* Document the date and time, which arm and vein were used, unusual patient reaction, and your initials (refer to the PPR documentation example).

31. Procedural Step. If needed, process the specimen by letting it stand for 30 to 45 minutes and then centrifuging it to separate serum from the cells. Prepare the specimen for transport to an outside laboratory as follows:

a. Place the specimen tube in a biohazard specimen bag.

b. Place the laboratory request in the outside pocket of the specimen bag (or transmit it electronically).

c. Properly handle and store the specimen while awaiting pickup by a laboratory courier.

PROCEDURE 31.1 Venipuncture—Vacutainer Method—cont'd

d. Document the date the specimen was transported to the laboratory in the patient's medical record.

Principle. The biohazard bag protects the laboratory courier from the possibility of an exposure incident. The outside laboratory must have the completed request form to know which laboratory tests have been ordered by the provider. The specimen must be handled and stored properly to maintain the in vivo characteristics of the specimen.

31d DOCUMENTATION EXAMPLE

Date	
4/5/XX	9:00 a.m. Venous blood specimen collected
	from (L) arm. Picked up by Medical Center
	Laboratory on 4/5/XX.
	D. Glover, CMA (AAMA)

PROCEDURE 31.2 Venipuncture—Butterfly Method

Outcome Perform a venipuncture using the butterfly method.

Equipment/Supplies

- Disposable gloves
- Tourniquet
- Antiseptic wipe
- Winged infusion set with a Luer adapter and safety shield
- Collection tube holder
- Blood collection tubes
- Sterile 2 × 2 gauze pad
- Adhesive bandage
- Biohazard sharps container
- Biohazard specimen bag

1. **Procedural Step.** Review the collection and handling requirements in the laboratory test directory for the tests ordered by the provider.
2. **Procedural Step.** Sanitize your hands. Greet the patient and introduce yourself. Identify the patient by asking the patient to state their full name and date of birth. Compare this information with the demographic data in the patient's medical record. Seat the patient comfortably in a phlebotomy chair.
3. **Procedural Step.** If the patient was required to prepare for the test (e.g., fasting, medication restriction), determine whether they have prepared properly. If the patient has not followed the patient preparation requirements, notify the provider for instructions on handling this situation.
4. **Procedural Step.** Assemble the equipment.
   a. Select the proper blood collection tubes for the tests ordered by the provider and check the expiration date on the tubes.
   b. Complete a laboratory request by writing in the information on a preprinted form or by entering the required information into a computer.
   c. Label each tube using one of the following methods: attaching a computer barcode label to each tube, or manually labeling each tube with the patient's name and date of birth, the date, and your initials. (*Note:* Follow the medical office policy as to when the tubes should be labeled. Some offices prefer that tubes be labeled *before* the specimen is drawn; other offices want the tubes to be labeled right *after* the specimen has been drawn.)

Principle. Outdated tubes may no longer contain a vacuum, and as a result they may not be able to draw blood into the tube. Proper labeling of blood specimens avoids the mix-up of specimens.

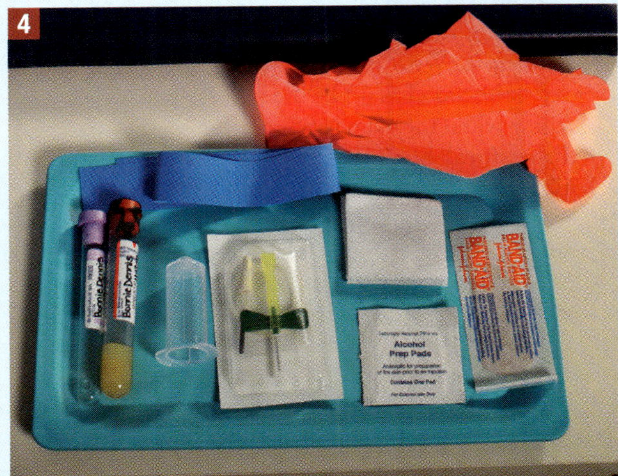

Assemble the equipment.

5. **Procedural Step.** Prepare the winged infusion set. Remove the winged infusion set from its package. Extend the tubing to its full length, and stretch it slightly to

Continued

PROCEDURE 31.2 Venipuncture—Butterfly Method—cont'd

prevent it from recoiling. Insert the posterior needle into the small opening on the collection tube holder. Screw the tube holder onto the Luer adapter, and tighten it securely.
Principle. Extending the tubing straightens it to permit a free flow of blood in the tubing. An unsecured needle can fall out of its tube holder.

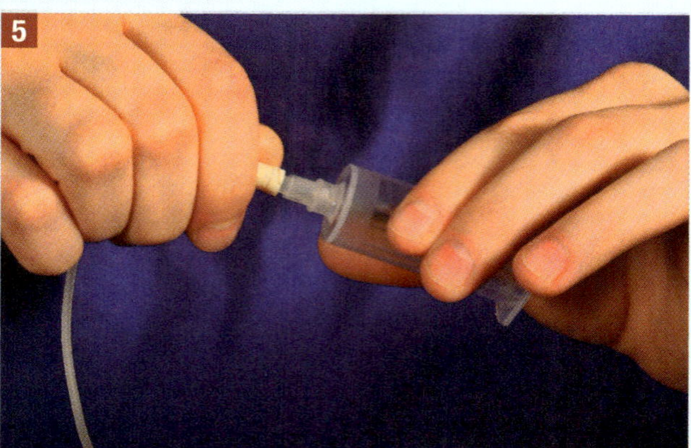

Screw the plastic tube holder onto the Luer adapter.

6. **Procedural Step.** Open the sterile gauze packet, and lay it flat to allow the gauze pad to rest on the inside of its wrapper. Position the blood collection tubes in the correct order of draw. If the collection tube contains a powdered additive, tap the tube just below the stopper to release any additive adhering to the stopper.
Principle. If an additive remains trapped in the stopper, erroneous test results may occur.
7. **Procedural Step.** Place the first tube loosely in the collection tube holder with the label facing down.
Principle. With the label facing down, you can observe the blood as it fills the tube, which allows you to know when the tube is full.
8. **Procedural Step.** Explain the procedure to the patient, and reassure the patient. Perform a preliminary assessment of both arms to determine the best vein to use. It also is helpful to ask the patient which arm has been used in the past to obtain blood.
Principle. Venipuncture is often a frightening experience for the patient, and reassurance should be offered to reduce apprehension.
9. **Procedural Step.** Apply the tourniquet. Position the tourniquet 3 to 4 inches above the bend in the elbow. The tourniquet should be snug but not tight. Ask the patient to clench the fist of the arm to which the tourniquet has been applied.
Principle. The combined effect of the pressure of the tourniquet and the clenched fist should cause the antecubital veins to stand out so that accurate selection of a puncture site can be made. A tourniquet that is too tight is uncomfortable for the patient and may also result in a specimen that leads to inaccurate test results.
10. **Procedural Step.** With a tourniquet in place, thoroughly assess the veins of first one arm and then the other to determine the best vein to use.
11. **Procedural Step.** Position the patient's arm. The arm with the vein selected for the venipuncture should be extended and placed in a straight line from the shoulder to the wrist with the antecubital veins facing anteriorly. The arm should be supported on the armrest by a rolled towel or by having the patient place the fist of the other hand under the elbow.
Principle. This position allows easy access to the antecubital veins.
12. **Procedural Step.** Thoroughly palpate the selected vein. Gently palpate the vein with the fingertips to determine the direction of the vein and to estimate its size and depth. Never leave the tourniquet on an arm for longer than 1 minute at a time. (*Note:* If you need to perform several assessments to locate the best vein, the tourniquet must be removed and reapplied after a 2-minute waiting period.)
Principle. Leaving the tourniquet on for longer than 1 minute is uncomfortable for the patient and may alter the test results.
13. **Procedural Step.** Remove the tourniquet (if more than 1 minute has elapsed) and cleanse the site with an antiseptic. Cleansing should be done in a circular motion, starting from the inside and moving away from the puncture site. Allow the site to air-dry; after cleansing, *do not touch the area*, wipe the area with gauze, or fan the area with your hand. Place your remaining supplies within comfortable reach.
Principle. Using a circular motion helps carry foreign particles away from the puncture site. The site must be allowed to air-dry to allow the alcohol enough time to destroy microorganisms on the patient's skin. Residual alcohol entering the blood specimen can cause hemolysis, leading to inaccurate test results. In addition, residual alcohol causes the patient to experience a stinging sensation when the puncture is made. Touching or fanning the area causes contamination of the puncture site, and the cleansing process must be repeated. Items used during the procedure should be positioned so that you do not have to reach over the patient and possibly move the needle, resulting in patient pain, injury, or both.
14. **Procedural Step.** Reapply the tourniquet. Apply gloves. With the dominant hand, grasp the winged infusion set by pressing the butterfly tips together. Remove the protective sheath from the needle of the

PROCEDURE 31.2

PROCEDURE 31.2 Venipuncture—Butterfly Method—cont'd

infusion set. The needle should be positioned with the bevel facing up.

Principle. Gloves provide a barrier against bloodborne pathogens. Positioning the needle with the bevel up allows easier entry into the skin and the vein, resulting in less pain for the patient.

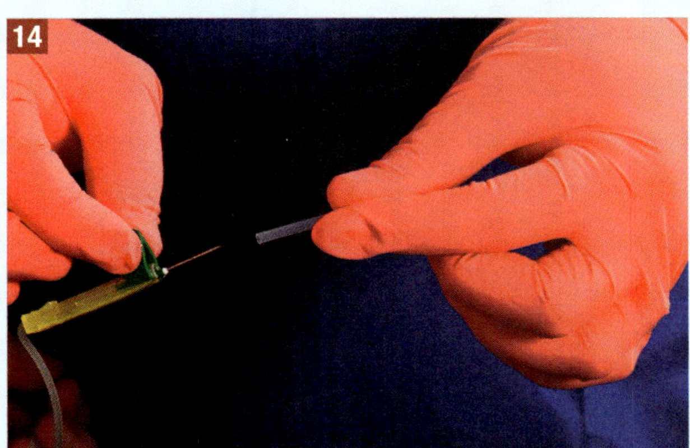

Remove the protective shield from the needle.

15. **Procedural Step.** Anchor the vein. Grasp the patient's arm with the nondominant hand. The thumb should be placed 1 to 2 inches below and to the side of the puncture site. Using the thumb, draw the skin taut over the vein in the direction of the patient's hand.

    Principle. The thumb helps hold the skin taut for easier entry and helps stabilize the vein to be punctured. Placing the thumb to the side keeps it out of the way of the winged infusion setup so that you can maintain a 15-degree angle when entering the vein.

16. **Procedural Step.** Position the needle at a 15-degree angle to the arm. Rest the backs of the fingertips on the patient's skin. Make sure the needle points in the same direction as the vein to be entered. The needle should be positioned so that it enters the vein approximately ⅛ inch below the place where the vein is to be entered.

    Principle. An angle of less than 15 degrees may cause the needle to enter above the vein, preventing puncture. An angle of more than 15 degrees may cause the needle to go through the vein by puncturing the posterior wall. This could result in a hematoma.

17. **Procedural Step.** Tell the patient that they will "feel a small stick," and with one continuous steady motion, enter the skin and then the vein. You will feel a sensation of resistance followed by a "release" as the vein is entered. After penetrating the vein, decrease the angle of the needle to 5 degrees. If the needle is in the vein, a flash of blood appears at the top of the tubing.

    Principle. Using one continuous motion reduces tissue damage.

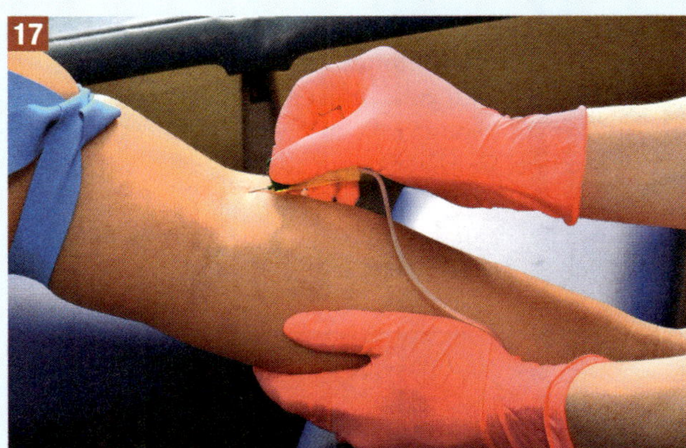

Make the puncture.

18. **Procedural Step.** Seat the needle by threading it forward an additional ¼ inch inside the center of the vein so that it does not twist out of the vein, even if you let go of it. Open the butterfly wings and securely rest the wings flat against the skin. Ensure that the needle does not move.

    Principle. Seating the needle anchors the needle in the center of the vein and allows the use of both hands for changing tubes. Moving the needle is painful for the patient.

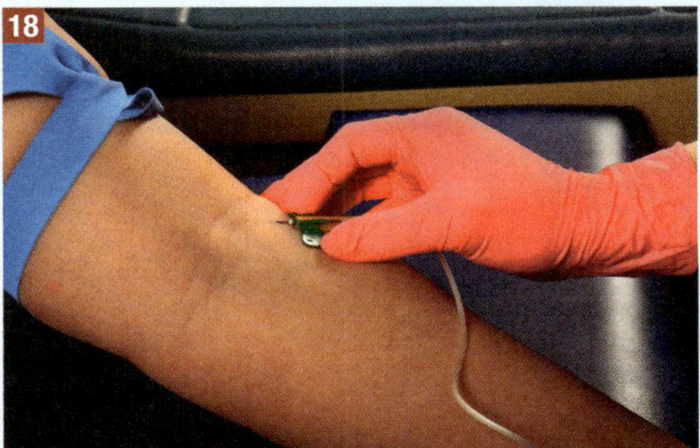

Rest the butterfly wings flat against the patient's skin.

19. **Procedural Step.** Keep the collection tube and holder in a downward position so that the tube fills from the bottom up and not near the rubber stopper. Slowly push the tube forward to the end of the holder. This allows the needle to puncture the rubber stopper.

Continued

PROCEDURE 31.2

PROCEDURE 31.2 Venipuncture—Butterfly Method—cont'd

Blood begins to flow into the tube. Allow the blood collection tube to fill to the exhaustion of the vacuum, as indicated by cessation of the blood flow into the tube. The suction of the collection tube automatically draws the blood into the tube.

Principle. The tube must fill from the bottom up to prevent venous reflux. If the collection tube is removed before the vacuum is exhausted, a rush of air enters the tube, damaging the red blood cells. Also, a tube containing an anticoagulant must be filled completely to ensure accurate test results.

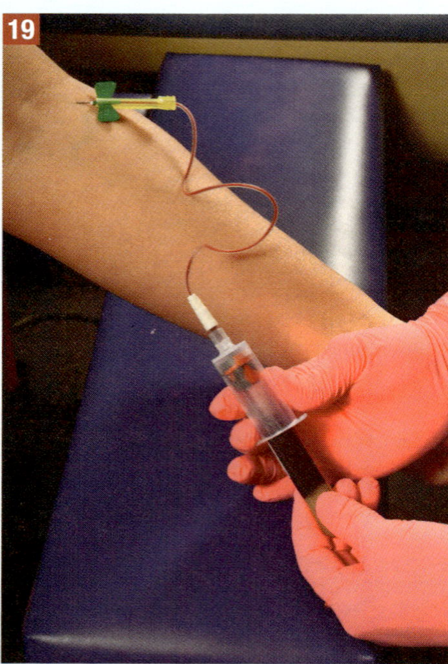

19 Fill the tube in a downward position.

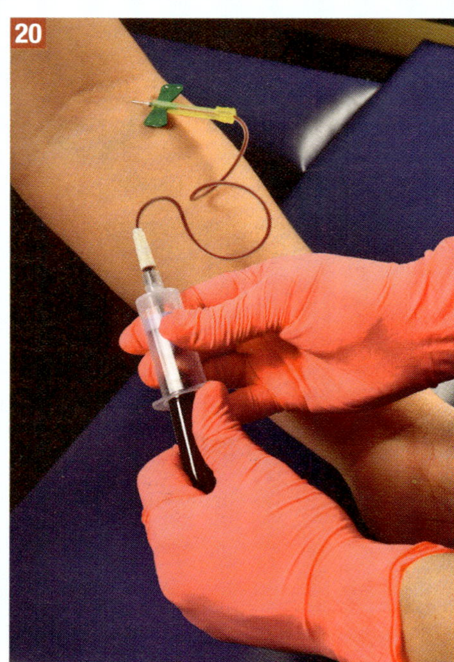

20 Remove the tube from the holder.

20. Procedural Step. Remove the tube from the tube holder. If the tube contains a clot activator, gently invert the tube back and forth 5 times before laying it down. If the tube contains an anticoagulant, gently invert the tube 8 to 10 times.

Principle. The rubber sheath covers the point of the needle, stopping the flow of blood until the next tube is inserted. You must invert a tube containing an anticoagulant before laying it down, to prevent the blood from clotting. Gentle inversion of a tube with a clot activator or an anticoagulant prevents hemolysis.

21. Procedural Step. Using the flange, carefully insert the next tube into the holder. Continue in this manner until the last tube has been filled.

22. Procedural Step. Remove the tension from the tourniquet (if it has not been previously released) by pulling upward on one of the flaps of the tourniquet. Ask the patient to unclench the fist.

Principle. The tourniquet tension must be removed before the needle. Otherwise, pressure on the vein from the tourniquet could cause internal and external bleeding around the puncture.

23. Procedural Step. Remove the last tube from the holder. Immediately invert the tube back and forth 5 times if it contains a clot activator and 8 to 10 times if it contains an anticoagulant.

Principle. Removing the last tube from the holder prevents blood from dripping out of the tip of the needle after it has been removed from the patient's arm.

24. Procedural Step. Place a sterile gauze pad slightly above the puncture site. Grasp the setup just below the wings, and slowly withdraw the needle at the same angle as for penetration. Immediately move the gauze over the puncture site, and apply firm pressure. (*Note:* Do not apply pressure to the puncture site until the

PROCEDURE 31.2 Venipuncture—Butterfly Method—cont'd

needle has been completely removed.) Cooperative patients can be asked to assist by applying pressure with the gauze pad. Activate the safety shield away from yourself and the patient and as illustrated in Fig. 31.17.

Principle. Placing the gauze pad above the puncture site helps prevent tissue movement as the needle is withdrawn and reduces patient discomfort. Careful withdrawal prevents further tissue damage.

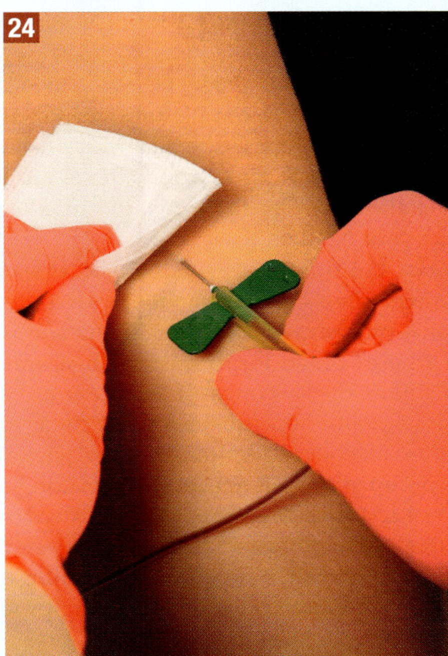

Release the tourniquet and remove the needle.

25. **Procedural Step.** Immediately discard the winged infusion set and attached tube holder. Holding onto the tube holder, first drop the needle into a biohazard sharps container, followed by the tubing and holder. Do not remove the tube holder from the setup; the tube holder must be discarded and not reused.

    Principle. Proper disposal is required by the OSHA Standard to prevent a needlestick injury; even though the safety shield has been activated to encase the butterfly needle, a needlestick injury can still result from the posterior needle, which is covered with only a rubber sleeve. Tube holders are often contaminated with blood and must not be reused.

26. **Procedural Step.** Continue to apply pressure with the gauze pad. The arm can be elevated to facilitate clot formation. Do not allow the patient to bend the arm at the elbow because this increases blood loss from the puncture site.

    Principle. Applying pressure reduces the leakage of blood from the puncture site externally or internally. Internal leakage into the tissues could result in a hematoma.

27. **Procedural Step.** Stay with the patient until the bleeding has stopped. Remove pressure, and inspect the puncture site to ensure that the opening is sealed with a clot. Apply an adhesive bandage to the puncture site. As an alternative, the gauze pad can be folded into quarters and taped onto the puncture site to be used as a pressure bandage. Instruct the patient not to pick up anything heavy for about an hour. (*Note:* If swelling or discoloration occurs, apply an ice pack to the site after bandaging it.)

    Principle. Lifting a heavy object causes pressure on the puncture site, which could result in bleeding.

28. **Procedural Step.** Place the tubes in an upright position in a test tube rack. Remove the gloves, and sanitize your hands.

29. **Procedural Step.** Document the procedure in the patient's medical record.
    a. *Electronic medical record:* Document which arm and vein were used and any unusual patient reactions using the appropriate radio buttons, drop-down menus, and free text fields.
    b. *Paper-based patient record:* Document the date and time, which arm and vein were used, unusual patient reactions, and your initials (refer to the PPR documentation example).

30. **Procedural Step.** If needed, process the specimen. Prepare the specimen for transport to an outside laboratory as follows:
    a. Place the specimen tube in a biohazard specimen bag.
    b. Place the laboratory request in the outside pocket of the specimen bag (or transmit it electronically).
    c. Properly handle and store the specimen while awaiting pickup by a laboratory courier.
    d. Document the date the specimen was transported to the laboratory in the patient's medical record.

    Principle. The biohazard bag protects the laboratory courier from the possibility of an exposure incident. The outside laboratory must have the completed request form to know which laboratory tests have been ordered by the provider. The specimen must be handled and stored properly to maintain the in vivo characteristics of the specimen.

30d

DOCUMENTATION EXAMPLE

Date	
4/10/XX	10:30 a.m. Venous blood specimen collected
	from (L) arm. Picked up by Medical Center
	Laboratory on 4/10/XX. ———
	——— D. Glover, CMA (AAMA)

PROCEDURE 31.3 Skin Puncture—Disposable Lancet

Outcome Obtain a capillary blood specimen.

Equipment/Supplies

- Disposable gloves
- Antiseptic wipe
- CoaguChek lancet
- Sterile 2 × 2 gauze pad
- Adhesive bandage
- Biohazard sharps container

1. **Procedural Step.** Sanitize your hands.
2. **Procedural Step.** Greet the patient and introduce yourself. Identify the patient by asking the patient to state their full name and date of birth. Compare this information with the demographic data in the patient's medical record. If the patient was required to prepare for the test (e.g., fasting, medication restriction), determine whether they have prepared properly. If the patient has not followed the patient preparation requirements, notify the provider for instructions on handling this situation.
3. **Procedural Step.** Assemble the equipment. Open the sterile gauze packet and lay it flat to allow the gauze pad to rest on the inside of its wrapper.

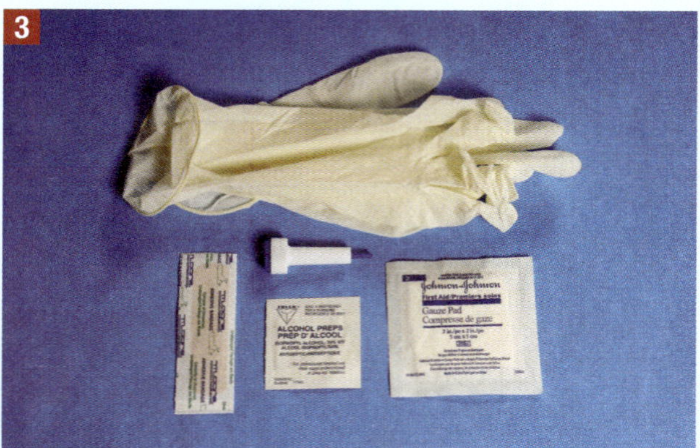

Assemble the equipment.

4. **Procedural Step.** Explain the procedure to the patient, and reassure the patient. Explain to the patient that the procedure should be relatively quick and only slightly uncomfortable.
   Principle. Reassurance should be offered to reduce apprehension.
5. **Procedural Step.** Seat the patient comfortably in a chair. The patient's arm should be firmly supported and extended with the palmar surface of the hand facing up.
6. **Procedural Step.** Select an appropriate puncture site. Use the lateral part of the tip of the third or fourth finger of the nondominant hand to make the puncture. If the patient's finger is cold, you can warm it by gently massaging the finger five or six times from base to tip, or by placing the hand in warm water for a few minutes.
   Principle. Warming the site increases the blood flow to the area and promotes bleeding from the puncture site.
7. **Procedural Step.** Cleanse the site with an antiseptic wipe. Allow the site to air-dry, and after cleansing it do not touch the area, wipe the area with gauze, or fan the area with your hand.
   Principle. The site must be allowed to air-dry to allow enough time for the alcohol to destroy microorganisms on the patient's skin. If the site is dry, a round drop of blood forms on the finger, making it easy to collect the specimen. If the site is not dry, the blood leaches out and runs down the finger, making it difficult to collect. Residual alcohol entering the blood specimen can cause hemolysis, leading to inaccurate test results. In addition, residual alcohol causes the patient to experience a stinging sensation when the puncture is made. Touching or fanning the area causes contamination, and the cleansing process has to be repeated.
8. **Procedural Step.** Apply gloves. Using a twisting motion, remove the plastic post from the lancet.
   Principle. Gloves provide a barrier precaution against bloodborne pathogens.
9. **Procedural Step.** Without touching the puncture site, firmly grasp the patient's finger in front of the most distal knuckle joint. Apply enough pressure to cause the fingertip to become hard and red. Position the blade of the lancet perpendicular to the lines of the fingerprint on the fleshy portion of the fingertip, slightly to the side of center. This facilitates the formation of a well-formed drop of blood that is easy to collect.
   Principle. The site must be grasped with enough pressure so that adequate penetration and depth of puncture can occur. Punctures that are not perpendicular cause the blood to run down the finger, making it difficult to collect. Puncturing the side or tip of the finger may cause the lancet to penetrate the bone.

PROCEDURE 31.3 Skin Puncture—Disposable Lancet—cont'd

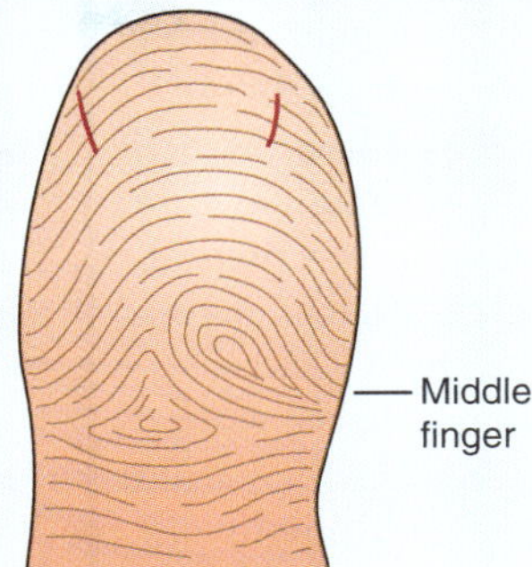

10. Procedural Step. Just before making the puncture, tell the patient that they will "feel a small stick." Firmly depress the activation button, without moving the lancet or finger, until an audible click is heard. Pressing the activation button causes the lancet to puncture the skin and then retract into its plastic casing. A well-made puncture results in a free-flowing wound that needs only slight pressure to make it bleed.
Principle. Alerting the patient to the stick prevents startling the patient, which could cause the patient to move. Moving the lancet or finger before the process is complete can result in an inadequate puncture and poor blood flow.

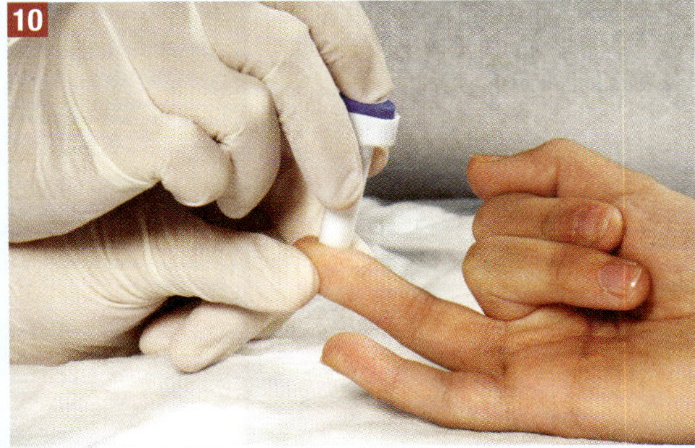

Make the puncture.

11. Procedural Step. Immediately dispose of the lancet in a biohazard sharps container.
Principle. Proper disposal of contaminated sharps is required by the OSHA Standard to prevent exposure to bloodborne pathogens.

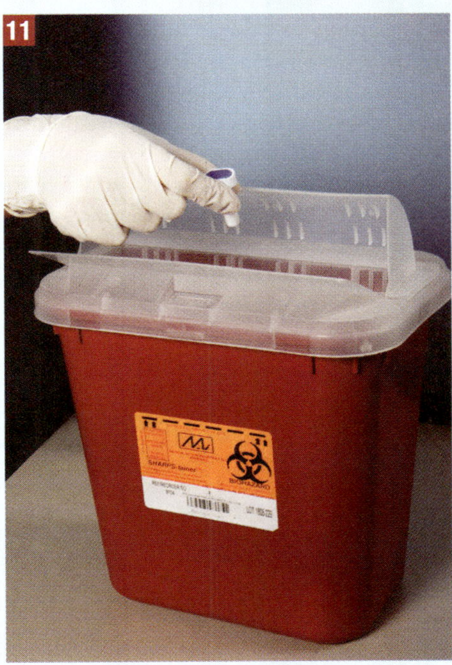

Discard the lancet.

12. Procedural Step. Wait a few seconds to allow blood flow to begin. Wipe away the first drop of blood with a gauze pad.
Principle. The first drop of blood is diluted with alcohol and tissue fluid and is not a suitable specimen.

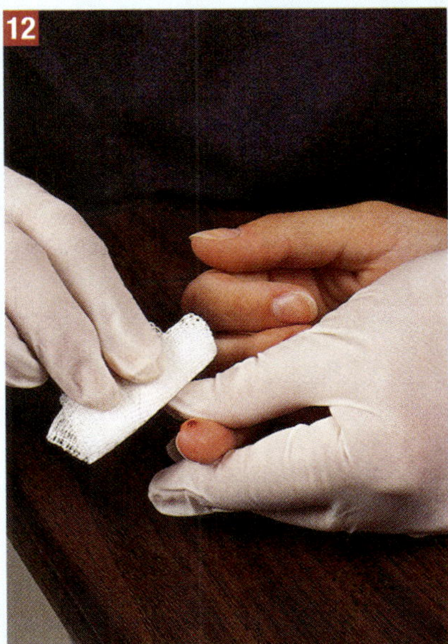

Wipe away the first drop of blood.

Continued

PROCEDURE 31.3 Skin Puncture—Disposable Lancet—cont'd

13. **Procedural Step.** Use the second drop of blood for the test. Allow a large well-rounded drop of blood to form by holding the hand in a downward position and applying gentle continuous pressure without squeezing the finger. You can massage the tissue surrounding the puncture firmly but gently to encourage blood flow.
Principle. Squeezing or massaging the site excessively causes dilution of the blood sample with tissue fluid, leading to inaccurate test results.

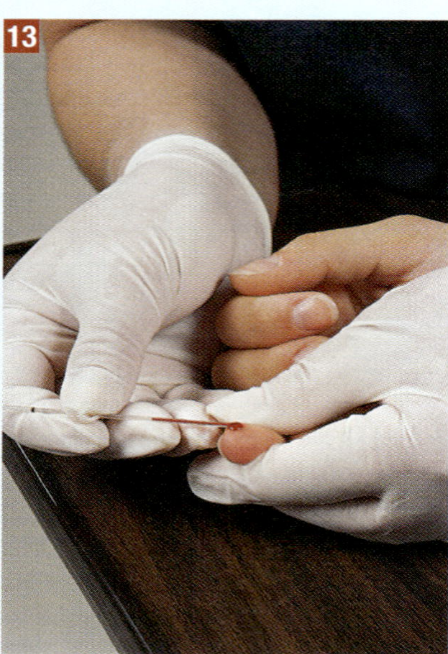

Collect the specimen.

14. **Procedural Step.** Collect the blood specimen on a test strip or in the appropriate microcollection device.
15. **Procedural Step.** Have the patient hold a gauze pad over the puncture and apply pressure until the bleeding stops. As a safety precaution, remain with the patient until the bleeding stops. If needed, apply an adhesive bandage. A bandage is not recommended for children younger than 2 years.
Principle. A bandage may irritate the skin of a young child, and the child might put the bandage in their mouth, aspirate it, and choke.
16. **Procedural Step.** Test the blood specimen by following the manufacturer's instructions that accompany the blood analyzer or test kit.
17. **Procedural Step.** Remove the gloves and sanitize your hands.

Hematology

 Check out the Evolve site at http://evolve.elsevier.com/Bonewit/today to access additional interactive activities and exercises to help you study and prepare for success.

LEARNING OBJECTIVES

Composition and Function of Blood

1. Identify the components of blood.
2. Describe the function of red blood cells.
3. Explain the purpose of the biconcave shape of an erythrocyte.
4. Describe the composition of hemoglobin and explain its function.
5. Explain the function of leukocytes.
6. Explain how leukocytes move from the circulatory system and into the tissues.
7. Explain the difference between granulocytes and agranulocytes.
8. List the five different types of white blood cells.
9. Identify the function of each of the five types of white blood cells.

Complete Blood Count

10. List the tests included in a complete blood count (CBC).
11. State the reference range for each test included in a CBC.
12. Identify conditions that can cause an increase or decrease in the hemoglobin level.
13. State the purpose of the hematocrit, and list the layers into which the blood separates after it has been centrifuged.
14. Identify conditions that cause an increase or decrease in the RBC count.
15. Identify conditions that cause an increase or decrease in the WBC count.
16. Explain how the RBC indices can help diagnose the various types of anemia.
17. Explain the purpose of a WBC differential count.
18. Explain the difference between an automated and manual WBC differential count.

Coagulation Tests

19. State the purpose of a platelet count.
20. Identify conditions that cause an increase or decrease in the platelet count.
21. State the purpose of the prothrombin time (PT) test.
22. Identify the symptoms of a bleeding disorder.
23. Identify the symptoms of a clotting disorder.
24. Explain why the sodium citrate tube for a PT test must be filled completely.
25. Explain what to do if a winged infusion set is used to collect a PT specimen.
26. Explain why a PT/INR test is performed on patients on long-term warfarin therapy.
27. Identify conditions for which warfarin therapy may be prescribed.
28. List the advantages of prothrombin time home testing.

PROCEDURES

Collect a specimen for a CBC for transport to an outside laboratory.

Perform a CLIA-waived hemoglobin test.

Perform a CLIA-waived hematocrit test.

Prepare a blood smear for transport to an outside laboratory.

Collect a specimen for a prothrombin time test for transport to an outside laboratory.

Perform a CLIA-waived prothrombin time test.

CHAPTER OUTLINE

KEY TERMS

ameboid movement (ah-MEE-boid-MOVE-ment)
anemia (ah-NEE-mee-ah)
anisocytosis
anticoagulant (an-tih-koe-AG-yoo-lent)
bilirubin (bill-ih-ROO-bin)
diapedesis (die-ah-pah-DEE-sis)
erythrocyte
hematology (hee-mah-TOL-oe-jee)
hematopoiesis
hemoglobin (HEE-moe-gloe-bin)
hemolysis (hee-MOL-oe-sis)
hypochromic (hahy-puh-KROH-mik)
leukocyte
leukocytosis (loo-koe-sie-TOE-sis)
leukopenia (loo-koe-PEE-nee-ah)
macrocytic (mak-ruh-SIT-ik)
microcytic (mahy-kruh-SIT-ik)
morphology
normochromic (NAWR-muh-kroh-mik)
normocytic (NAWR-muh-sahyt-ik)
oxyhemoglobin (ok-see-HEE-moe-gloe-bin)
phagocytosis (fay-goe-sie-TOE-sis)
polycythemia (pol-ee-sie-THEE-mee-ah)
thrombocyte
thrombocytopenia
thrombocytosis

INTRODUCTION TO HEMATOLOGY

Hematology is the study of blood, including the morphologic appearance and function of blood cells and diseases of the blood and blood-forming tissues. Laboratory analysis in hematology is concerned with the testing of a blood specimen for the purpose of detecting pathologic conditions. It includes performing blood cell counts, evaluating the clotting ability of the blood, and identifying blood cell types. These tests are valuable tools that allow the provider to determine whether each blood component falls within its reference range.

Examples of hematologic tests that are frequently ordered on patients include:

- Red blood cell count (RBC count)
- White blood cell count (WBC count)
- Hemoglobin (Hgb)
- Hematocrit (Hct)
- White blood cell differential count (differential)
- Platelet count (PLT count)
- Erythrocyte sedimentation rate (ESR)
- Prothrombin time (PT)

Several of these hematologic tests may be performed in the medical office using CLIA-waived analyzers. Each CLIA-waived analyzer is accompanied by a detailed operating manual that explains its operation, test parameters, care, and maintenance. CLIA-waived analyzers permit testing of the specimen in a short time with accurate and reliable test results. This allows the provider to evaluate the test results while the patient is still at the medical office without a delay in waiting for test results to be transmitted from an outside laboratory.

This chapter presents information on hematology, including the components and function of blood, with an emphasis on CLIA-waived testing in the medical office.

COMPOSITION AND FUNCTION OF BLOOD

The average adult body contains 10 to 12 pints (5 to 6 L) of blood which makes up about 8% of the total body weight. Blood consists of two parts—*plasma* and *formed elements* (Fig. 32.1). Women tend to have a lower blood volume than men.

Plasma, the liquid part of the blood, consists of a clear yellowish fluid that makes up approximately 55% of the total blood volume. Most of the plasma (90%) is made up of water and the remaining 10% consists of solutes such as proteins (albumin, globulins, and fibrinogen). Other solutes present in plasma include electrolytes, nutrients, and waste products. Plasma transports nutrients to the tissues of the body to nourish and sustain them. Plasma picks up wastes from the tissues which are then eliminated through the kidneys. Solutes also present in the plasma include regulatory substances such as antibodies, enzymes, and hormones. The plasma transports these substances throughout the body to help regulate normal body functioning.

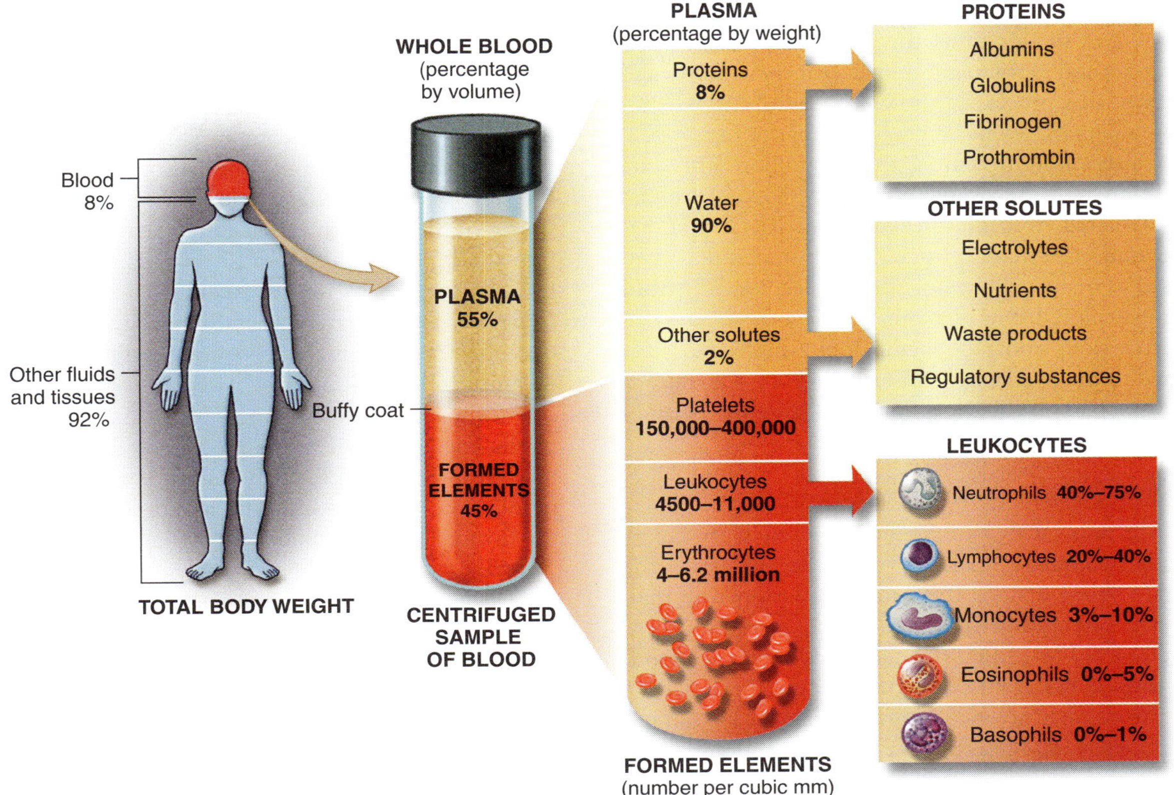

Fig. 32.1 Composition of Blood. (With permission from Huether S, McCance K: *Understanding pathophysiology*, ed 5, St. Louis, 2012, Mosby, : p. 479.)

The formed elements consist of three types of cells: erythrocytes, leukocytes, and thrombocytes. The formed elements make up approximately 45% of the total blood volume. The formed elements are produced in the red bone marrow and the process of blood cell formation is known as **hematopoiesis**. All blood cells are derived from *hematopoietic stem* cells which are able to differentiate into the various types of blood cells in the bone marrow. Hematopoietic stem cells are responsible for the constant renewal of blood cells in the body. Each day the bone marrow produces more than 300 billion new blood cells.

Red Blood Cells

Red blood cells (RBCs), or **erythrocytes**, are the most numerous blood cells in the circulating blood. An erythrocyte is approximately 7 to 8 micrometers in diameter. The primary function of red blood cells is to transport oxygen and carbon dioxide in the body (which is directly related to hemoglobin). The number of RBCs in a healthy adult ranges from 4 to 5.5 million per cubic millimeter of blood in a woman, and from 4.5 to 6.2 million per cubic millimeter of blood in a man.

In an adult, erythrocytes are produced in the red bone marrow of the ribs, sternum, skull, and pelvic bone and in the ends of the long bones of the limbs. The immature form of an erythrocyte contains a nucleus. As the cell develops and matures, however, it loses its nucleus and acquires the shape of a biconcave disc, thin in the middle and thicker around the rim. This shape gives the cell more room to carry hemoglobin and provides the erythrocyte with a greater surface area for the exchange of gases (oxygen and carbon dioxide) between the blood and tissues. The biconcave shape of the erythrocyte also provides it with flexibility to bend and squeeze through tiny capillaries.

A major portion of the erythrocyte consists of hemoglobin. **Hemoglobin** is a complex compound that carries the oxygen to the tissues and is responsible for the red color of the erythrocyte. The amount of hemoglobin in the blood averages 12 to 16 g/dL for a female and 14 to 18 g/dL for a male. A decrease in the number of erythrocytes or amount of hemoglobin in the blood is known as **anemia** and an increase in the number of erythrocytes or amount of hemoglobin is known as **polycythemia.**

A hemoglobin molecule consists of a globin, or protein, and an iron-containing pigment called *heme.* One hemoglobin molecule loosely combines with four oxygen molecules in the lungs to form a substance called **oxyhemoglobin.** Oxyhemoglobin is transported by the circulatory system and distributed to the tissues, where the oxygen is easily released from the hemoglobin. The blood then picks up carbon dioxide (a waste product) from the tissues and transports it back to the lungs to be expelled. When oxygen combines with hemoglobin, a bright red color results characteristic of arterial blood. Venous blood is darker red owing to its lower oxygen content.

The average life span of a red blood cell is 120 days. Toward the end of this time, the membrane of the RBC becomes more and more fragile and eventually ruptures and breaks down; this process is known as **hemolysis.** Hemolyzed RBCs are replaced by an equal number of new RBCs. Under typical conditions, more than 2 million RBCs are destroyed and replaced every second. Hemoglobin molecules are liberated from the breakdown of RBCs. The hemoglobin molecules release iron which is stored and then later reused to make new hemoglobin molecules. **Bilirubin** is an orange-colored bile pigment that is a by-product of heme destruction from the hemoglobin molecule. It is transported to the liver, where it is excreted as a waste product into the bile and then it eventually leaves the body in the stool.

White Blood Cells

White blood cells (WBCs), or **leukocytes**, are clear, colorless cells that contain a nucleus. They make up 1% of the total blood volume making them much less numerous than erythrocytes. The number of leukocytes in a healthy adult ranges from 4500 to 11,000 per cubic millimeter of blood. **Leukocytosis** is the condition of having an abnormal increase in the number of leukocytes (greater than 11,000 per cubic millimeter), and **leukopenia** is the condition of having an abnormal decrease in the number of leukocytes (less than 4500 per cubic millimeter).

The function of leukocytes is to defend the body against infection and foreign materials. The bone marrow stores an estimated 80% to 90% of the WBCs. When an infection or inflammatory response occurs, the bone marrow releases WBCs to fight the infection.

Pathogens can gain entrance into the body in a variety of ways (review the infection process cycle in Chapter 17). Leukocytes attempt to destroy invading pathogens and remove them from the body. In contrast to erythrocytes, leukocytes do their work in the tissues; they are transported to the site of infection by the circulatory system.

During inflammation, the capillaries in the infected area dilate, resulting in an increased blood supply. More oxygen, nutrients, and WBCs can be delivered to the infected area to aid in the healing process. The cells in the capillary walls spread apart, enlarging the pores between the cells. White blood cells squeeze through these pores by **ameboid movement** and move out into the tissues to fight the infection. This movement of the leukocytes through the pores of the capillaries and out into the tissues is known as **diapedesis.**

Types of White Blood Cells

There are five types of white blood cells, or leukocytes, each having a certain size, shape, appearance, and function. These include:

- Neutrophils
- Eosinophils
- Basophils
- Lymphocytes
- Monocytes

Leukocytes are classified into two major categories—granulocytes and agranulocytes. *Granulocytes* have a multilobed nucleus and contain distinct granules in the cytoplasm; they include the neutrophils, eosinophils, and basophils. The granules contain enzymes that damage and digest pathogens; these enzymes also trigger the inflammatory response. The *inflammatory response* is a protective response of the body to trauma and the entrance of pathogens into the body. The purpose of inflammation is to destroy invading pathogens and to remove damaged tissue debris from the area so that proper healing can occur. Symptoms of inflammation include pain, swelling, redness, and warmth at the infection site. *Agranulocytes* have a single round nucleus and contain few or no granules in the cytoplasm; they include the lymphocytes and monocytes. They play an important role in the immune system, such as the production of antibodies. The reference range for each of the five types of white blood cells is presented in Fig. 32.1.

Leukocytes (especially granulocytes) are phagocytic, and when they arrive at the site of infection, they begin the process of phagocytosis. **Phagocytosis** is the engulfing and destruction of foreign particles such as pathogens and damaged cells. In some conditions, pus forms in the infected area; pus contains dead leukocytes, dead bacteria, and dead tissue cells.

Each type of leukocyte has a specific function in defending the body against infection. Refer to Chapter 12: *Circulatory System* for detailed information on the different types of white blood cells and their function.

Platelets

Platelets, also known as **thrombocytes**, are tiny irregularly-shaped cell fragments. They lack a nucleus and are formed in the red bone marrow from giant cells known as *megakaryocytes*. The number of platelets in a healthy adult ranges from 150,000 to 400,000 per cubic millimeter of blood. An increase in the number of platelets is known as **thrombocytosis** and a decrease in the number of platelets in known as **thrombocytopenia**.

Platelets function by participating in the blood-clotting mechanism in the body. When the lining of a blood vessel breaks, platelets accumulate at the site of the injury and become sticky. This stickiness causes them to attach to one another as well as to the blood vessel wall. This results in a *platelet plug* that seals the opening in the blood vessel wall and stops the flow of blood. A fibrin network forms next which attaches to the platelet plug to hold it in place and to trap more platelets as well as red blood cells. This results in the platelet plug becoming harder and more durable. The platelet plug is now known as a *thrombus* or blood clot (Fig. 32.2). The blood clot eventually becomes the scab and remains in place until the wound heals.

Platelets survive in the circulatory system for approximately 8 to 10 days. The bone marrow must continuously produce new platelets that break down, are used up during the clotting process, or lost through bleeding.

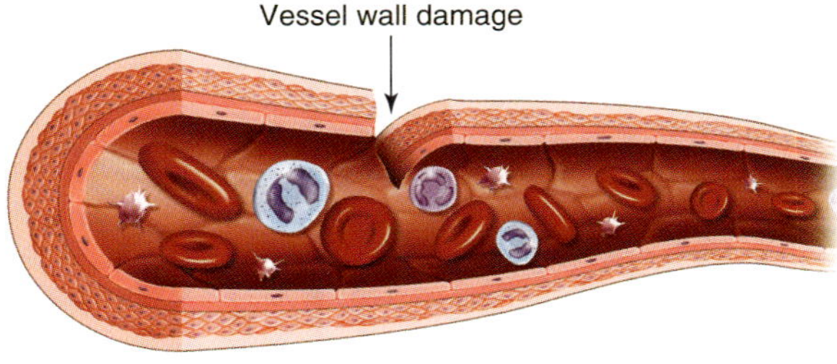

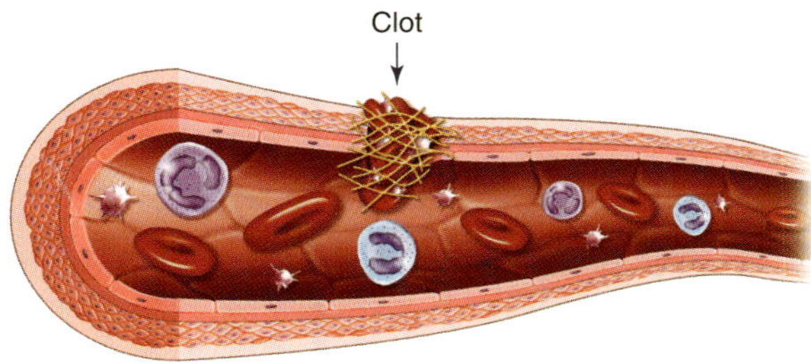

Fig. 32.2 Blood clotting. (From Yoost B, Crawford L: *Fundamentals of nursing: active learning for collaborative practice*, ed 2, St. Louis, 2020, Elsevier.)

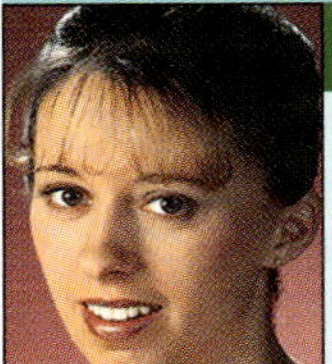

Putting It All Into Practice

My name is Latisha, and I work in a multiphysician office as a laboratory technician in our POL. I have worked in this office for 3 years and I really enjoy my job. My responsibilities mostly include venipuncture, preparing blood specimens for pickup by the lab courier, and performing CLIA-waived laboratory tests. One day, a frail older lady came in who had just been diagnosed with atrial fibrillation and was placed on Coumadin therapy. I needed to draw a blood specimen on her for a PT/INR test—a procedure I had done many times before. I looked up information on the test in the laboratory test directory. I next checked the veins in the lady's arms and couldn't find any veins that could be used. I knew that I would have to draw the blood from her hand and I really hated to do that to her because I know that a stick can hurt a lot more in the hand. I got out a blue-topped tube and the butterfly setup. I was just about ready to make the stick when I suddenly realized that I first needed to draw a red discard tube with a butterfly setup. I broke into a sweat thinking of what could have happened if I had forgotten the discard tube. I would have had to stick that sweet lady's hand again causing her more pain. To this day, I always read the information in the test directory more than one time. ■

COMPLETE BLOOD COUNT

The most frequently performed hematologic laboratory test is the complete blood count (CBC). Because a WBC differential count (differential) is often ordered with a CBC, it will also be discussed in this section. A CBC with differential includes a group of tests that determine the number of red blood cells, number and type of white blood cells, and the number of platelets in the circulatory system along with a determination of the hemoglobin and hematocrit levels and RBC indices.

A CBC is used as a screening test to assess the overall health of an individual and to diagnose a wide range of hematologic conditions such as anemia, leukemia, infection, bleeding disorders, and inflammation. The CBC is also used to monitor patients undergoing chemotherapy or radiation therapy for cancer because these treatments suppress the production of blood cells in the bone marrow. Test results from a CBC provide valuable information to assist the provider in making a diagnosis, evaluating the patient's progress, and regulating treatment. The tests included in a CBC and the reference range for each test is summarized in Table 32.1.

A CBC is usually performed by an outside laboratory since many of the tests included in a CBC are moderate complexity tests. Guidelines for collecting a specimen for a CBC to be transported to an outside laboratory are presented below.

There are two tests included in a CBC that can be performed using CLIA-waived analyzers: these tests include hemoglobin and hematocrit. These tests are presented first in this section followed by the moderate complexity tests included in a CBC (RBC count, WBC count, platelet count, WBC differential count, and the RBC indices).

SPECIMEN COLLECTION FOR A CBC

The medical assistant is often required to collect a blood specimen for a CBC for transport to an outside laboratory for testing. The guidelines listed below should be followed when collecting the specimen:

1. Collect the blood specimen in a lavender closure tube. A whole blood specimen is required for a CBC.
2. Completely fill the collection tube to the exhaustion of the vacuum to ensure a proper blood-to-anticoagulant ratio.
3. Gently invert the tube 8 to 10 times following collection to mix the anticoagulant with the blood. This prevents the formation of blood clots which can affect the accuracy of the test results.
4. Store the specimen at RT while awaiting pickup by a laboratory courier. The specimen is stable for 48 hours at RT. The specimen should not be refrigerated because refrigeration can precipitate the formation of a fibrin clot which traps WBCs and platelets affecting the accuracy of the test results.

After testing the specimen, the outside laboratory transmits the results to the medical office. An example of a computer-generated laboratory report indicating the results of a CBC is presented in Fig. 32.3.

HEMOGLOBIN

As previously discussed, hemoglobin (Hgb) is a major component of a red blood cell. It carries oxygen to the tissues of the body and is responsible for the red color of the erythrocyte. A hemoglobin determination is a measurement of the

Table 32.1 CBC Purpose and Reference Ranges

Complete Blood Count			
Test	**Purpose**	**Reference Range**	**Units**
RBC count	Measurement of the number of RBCs in the circulating blood	F: 4–5.5 M: 4.5-6.2	$\times 10^6/mm^3$
WBC count	Measurement of the number of WBCs in the circulating blood.	4.5–11.0	$\times 10^3/mm^3$
Hemoglobin	Measurement of the hemoglobin level to assess the oxygen-carrying capacity of the blood	F: 12–16 M: 14–18	g/dL
Hematocrit	To measure the percentage by volume of the packed RBCs in whole blood	F: 37–47 M: 40–54	%
Platelet count	Measurement of the number of platelets in the circulating blood to assess the clotting ability of the blood	150–400	$\times 10^3/mm^3$
Red Blood Cell Indices			
Test	**Purpose**	**Reference Range**	**Units**
MCV	Measurement of the average size of a RBC	80–100	f/L
MCH	Measurement of the average amount of hemoglobin in a RBC	27–31	pg
MCHC	Measurement of the average concentration of hemoglobin within a RBC	32–36	mg/dL
RDW	Measurement of any variation in size of the RBCs	11.5–14.5	%
WBC Differential Count			
Cell Type	**Function**	**Reference Range**	**Unit**
Neutrophils	Destruction of invaders through phagocytosis	40–75	%
Eosinophils	Destruction of parasitic worms Counteracts the effects of histamine in an allergic reaction	0–5	%
Basophils	Release of histamine and heparin	0–1	%
Lymphocytes	Production of antibodies to destroy foreign invaders	20–40	%
Monocytes	Clean up the infection site through phagocytosis	3–10	%

MCH, Mean corpuscular hemoglobin; *MCHC*, mean cell hemoglobin concentration; *MCV*, mean corpuscular volume; *RBC*, red blood cell; *RDW*, red cell distribution width; *WBC*, white blood cell.

hemoglobin level in the body to assess the oxygen-carrying capacity of the blood. A hemoglobin test is used to screen for anemia, determine its severity, and monitor the response to treatment. The reference range for hemoglobin for a healthy woman is 12 to 16 g/dL and the reference range for a healthy man is 14 to 18 g/dL.

A decreased hemoglobin level reduces the oxygen carrying capacity of the blood. This can occur with anemia (especially iron-deficiency anemia), hyperthyroidism, cirrhosis of the liver, severe hemorrhaging, hemolytic reactions, and certain systemic diseases, such as leukemia and Hodgkin disease. Increased levels of hemoglobin are present with chronic obstructive pulmonary disease, and congestive heart failure.

CLIA-WAIVED HEMOGLOBIN TEST

A CLIA-waived hemoglobin test is often performed in the medical office as a routine screening test on individuals who are at risk for developing iron-deficiency anemia, such as children younger than 2 years of age, adolescent girls, and pregnant women; all of whom have an increased demand for iron in the body. The hemoglobin test is a quantitative test that measures the specific amount of hemoglobin present in the body with the results being reported in grams per deciliter (g/dL).

There are several advantages of using a CLIA-waived hemoglobin analyzer. The analyzer only requires a capillary specimen collected through a finger or heel puncture to perform the test, rather than a venous blood specimen collected through venipuncture. The hemoglobin analyzer permits testing of the specimen in a short time with accurate and reliable results, allowing the provider to evaluate the patient while still at the medical office.

The manufacturer of the hemoglobin analyzer provides an operating manual that includes information needed to perform quality control procedures, collect the specimen, test the specimen, and properly store the test devices (e.g., microcuvettes or testing cards) and control reagents. It is important that the medical assistant become familiar with all aspects of the hemoglobin analyzer. Quality control procedures are of particular importance to ensure that the analyzer is functioning properly and that test results are reliable and

Laboratory Report
Complete Blood Count with Diff/Platelets

PATIENT		ORDERED BY	RESULTS PROVIDED BY
Yang, Hu 2963 Flint Dr. Clearwater, FL 33759 PH: 740-541-3575	ID #: 336879 DOB: 4/28/1970 AGE: 53 GENDER: M	Thomas Murphy, MD Pinellas Medical Office 3477 Arrowhead Ave Clearwater, FL 33759	Medical Center Laboratory 33 West Main St Clearwater, FL 33759
SPECIMEN COLL. DATE	11/25/20XX	FASTING/NONFASTING	Nonfasting
SPECIMEN COLL. TIME	02:53 pm	ACCESSION NUMBER	3380837
SPECIMEN RECEIVED DATE/TIME	11/25/20XX 05:30 pm	LAB ID NUMBER	773978
RESULTS REPORTED DATE/TIME	11/26/20XX 10:00 am	TEST(S) ORDERED	CPT: 85025 CBC with differential

TEST	RESULT	REFERENCE RANGE	UNITS	FLAG
RBC	**3.57**	**4.5-6.2**	**$\times 10^6/mm^3$**	**L**
WBC	4.6	4.5-11.0	$\times 10^3/mm^3$	
Hemoglobin	**12.2**	**14.0-18.0**	**g/dL**	**L**
Hematocrit	**35.6**	**40.0-54.0**	**%**	**L**
MCV	92	80-100	f/L	
MCH	31.4	27.0-31.0	pg	
MCHC	34	32.0-36.0	mg/dL	
RDW	**17.6**	**11.5-14.5**	**%**	**H**
Platelets	308	150-400	$\times 10^3/mm^3$	
Neutrophils	73	40-75	%	
Eosinophils	1	0%-5%	%	
Basophils	1	0%-1%	%	
Lymphoytes	14	20-40	%	
Monocytes	11	3-10	%	

Fig. 32.3 CBC laboratory report (computer-generated).

accurate. Examples of CLIA-waived hemoglobin analyzers include the HemoPoint H2 Meter (Stanbio Laboratory, Boerne, TX), Hemoglobin Hb 201+ Analyzer (HemoCue, Lake Forest, CA).

Procedure for the CLIA-Waived Hemoglobin Hb 201+ Analyzer

The medical assistant must follow the hemoglobin collection and testing procedure *exactly* as presented in the operating manual. An overview of the procedure for performing a CLIA-waived hemoglobin test using the Hemoglobin Hb 201+ Analyzer is outlined here:

1. Pull out the cuvette tray from the front of the analyzer.
2. Perform a finger puncture to obtain a capillary blood specimen and wipe away the first 2 or 3 drops of blood.
3. Touch the open end of the microcuvette to the drop of blood and fill the microcuvette in one continuous process (Fig. 32.4).
4. Wipe off excess blood from the outside of the microcuvette and place it in the cuvette holder on the analyzer (Fig. 32.5).
5. When three dashes appear on the LCD screen of the analyzer, push the tray back into the analyzer.
6. After a countdown, the hemoglobin test result is displayed on the LCD screen of the analyzer. The hemoglobin result for this test is 14.2 g/dL which is a normal result for both a male and a female (Fig. 32.6).
7. Document the results in the patient's medical record, including the date and time, the name of the test (hemoglobin), and the test result measured in g/dL.

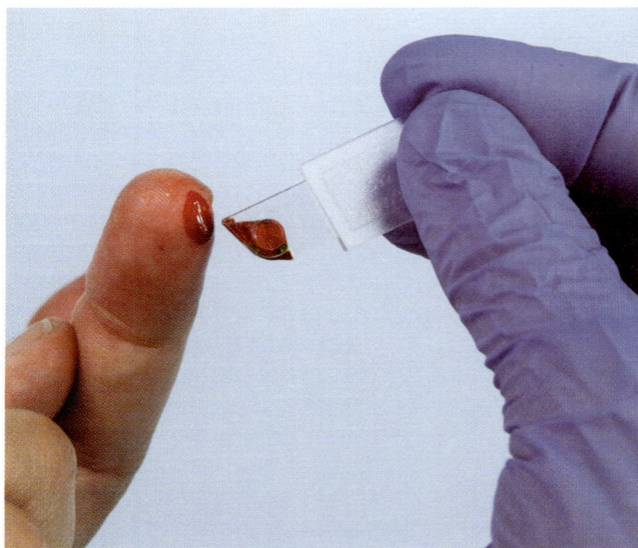

Fig. 32.4 The microcuvette is filled with blood. (From Garrels M: *Laboratory and diagnostic testing in ambulatory care*, ed 4, St. Louis, 2019, Elsevier.)

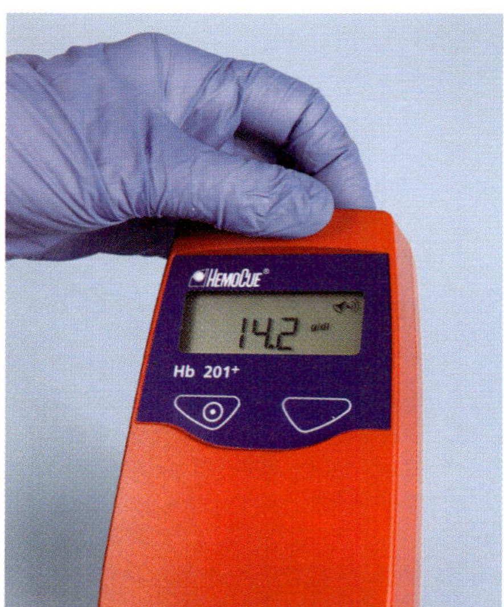

Fig. 32.6 Test results are displayed on the LCD screen. (From Garrels M: *Laboratory and diagnostic testing in ambulatory care*, ed 4, St Louis, 2019, Elsevier.)

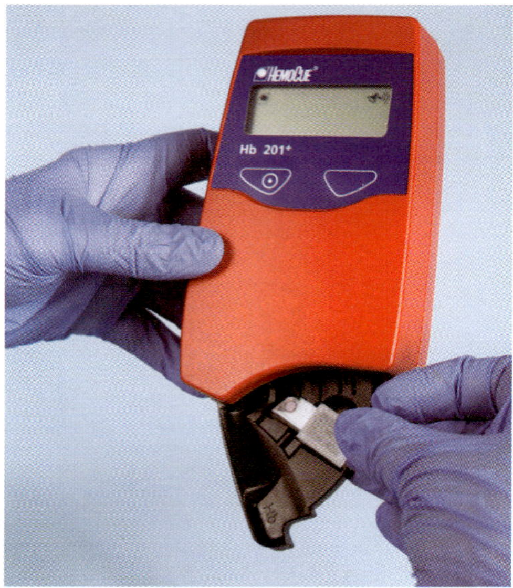

Fig. 32.5 Place the microcuvette in the cuvette holder. (From Garrels M: *Laboratory and diagnostic testing in ambulatory care*, ed 4, St. Louis, 2019, Elsevier.)

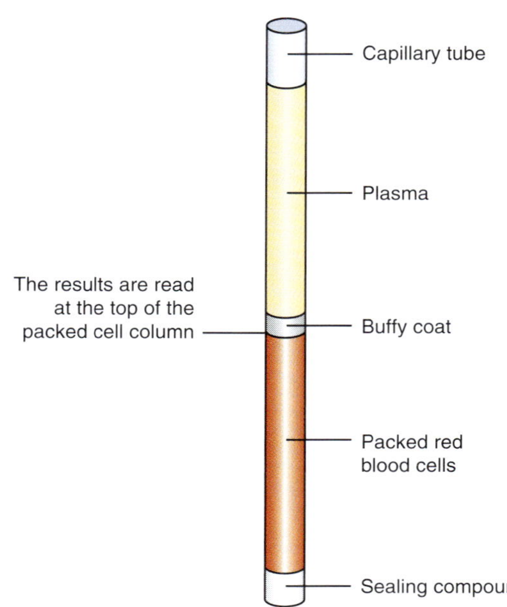

Fig. 32.7 Hematocrit test results. The blood cells are separated from the plasma by centrifuging an anticoagulated blood specimen, and the results are read at the top of the packed cell column.

HEMATOCRIT

The hematocrit (Hct) is a simple, reliable, and informative test that is frequently performed in the medical office. The word *hematocrit* means "to separate blood." The formed elements are separated from the plasma by centrifuging an anticoagulated blood specimen. The heavier RBCs become packed and settle to the bottom of a tube. The top layer contains the clear, straw-colored plasma. Between the plasma and the packed RBCs is a small, thin, yellowish-gray layer known as the *buffy coat,* which contains the platelets and WBCs (Fig. 32.7).

The purpose of the hematocrit is to measure the percentage by volume of packed RBCs in whole blood which is a determination of how much of the blood is made up of RBCs. The hematocrit is used as a screening measure for the early detection of anemia and is often included as part of a general health examination. The hematocrit reference range for a healthy woman is 37% to 47% and the reference range for a healthy man, 40% to 54%. A low hematocrit reading may indicate anemia, and a high reading may indicate polycythemia.

CLIA-WAIVED HEMATOCRIT TEST

The CLIA-waived *microhematocrit method* is used in the medical office to perform a hematocrit determination. Through capillary action, blood is drawn directly from a free-flowing skin puncture into a disposable capillary tube. After the specimen has been collected, one end of the capillary tube is sealed with a sealing compound and placed in a microhematocrit centrifuge. The centrifuge spins the blood at an extremely high speed for 3 to 5 minutes to pack the RBCs at the bottom of the tube. The results are read at the top of the packed red blood cell column. Procedure 32.1 describes how to perform a hematocrit test.

What Would You Do? What Would You *Not* Do?

Case Study 1

Theodore Pascal is at the office for a general health examination. The physician orders a CBC and CMP (comprehensive metabolic panel) on Theodore. Theodore says he has been feeling fine and wants to know why lab tests have been ordered for him. When Theodore realizes that the tests require a venipuncture, he says that he gets nervous about having blood drawn and wants to know if a finger stick could be done instead so it won't hurt so much. He also wants to know why two tubes of blood have to be drawn from him and why one tube of blood can't be used for the tests. ■

PATIENT COACHING Iron-Deficiency Anemia

Answer questions that patients have about iron-deficiency anemia.

What is anemia?

Anemia is a decrease in the number of RBCs or the amount of hemoglobin in the body. Hemoglobin, the part of the blood that gives RBCs their red color, carries oxygen to all the cells in the body. There are many types of anemia, of which iron-deficiency anemia is the most common. Other types of anemia include pernicious anemia, sickle cell anemia, hemolytic anemia, and aplastic anemia.

What causes iron-deficiency anemia?

In general, iron-deficiency anemia is caused by conditions that deplete the iron stored in the body; it can result from an increased need for iron by the body or an increased loss of iron from the body. Iron-deficiency anemia may occur in children younger than 2 years if their diet does not include enough iron to meet the demands of rapid growth. This is especially true in children whose main source of nutrition during these years is breast milk or bottle milk, because milk contains very little iron. Adolescent girls are prone to iron-deficiency anemia because of growth spurts during puberty and blood loss through menstruation. Pregnant women also are at increased risk because of the demands of the growing fetus. In adults, the most common cause of anemia is chronic blood loss, such as from a bleeding ulcer or bleeding hemorrhoids and heavy menstrual bleeding.

What can be done for individuals at risk for iron-deficiency anemia?

Individuals prone to developing iron-deficiency anemia are encouraged to increase foods in their diet that contain iron, such as beef, liver, spinach, eggs, and iron-fortified breads and cereals. As a preventive measure, the provider usually prescribes vitamin supplements containing iron for individuals who are at increased risk for developing iron-deficiency anemia, such as pregnant women, infants, and young children. Infant formulas and cereals that have been supplemented with iron are also available.

What are the symptoms of anemia?

All types of anemia have the same general symptoms. Often these symptoms do not develop right away; when they do develop, feeling tired and run down may be the only sign of anemia. Other symptoms that may occur, particularly as the anemia becomes worse, are paleness of the skin, fingernail beds, and mucous membranes; shortness of breath, especially during physical activity; dizziness; headache; irritability; and inability to concentrate. These symptoms result from the diminished ability of the blood to carry oxygen to the cells of the body. Blood tests are necessary to diagnose anemia and to determine the specific type of anemia present.

How is iron-deficiency anemia treated?

The most important part of treating anemia is to determine its cause, such as not enough iron consumed in the diet or chronic blood loss, and to correct that condition. The provider usually prescribes an iron supplement to replace the iron that has been depleted from the body. It is typically prescribed in oral form, but it is given through an injection if the patient cannot take iron by mouth because of the side effects. Iron may also be given through an injection if the iron content in the blood is so low that oral supplements would be too slow in increasing the iron level. An oral iron supplement causes the stool to turn a black, tarlike color. This is normal and should not be a cause for concern. Also, an effort should be made to consume foods high in iron content.

- For patients who have had a vitamin supplement prescribed to *prevent* iron-deficiency anemia, such as children younger than 2 years and pregnant women, emphasize to the patient (or parent) the importance of taking the vitamin supplement every day to prevent the development of iron-deficiency anemia.
- For patients who have had an iron supplement prescribed to *treat* iron-deficiency anemia, emphasize to the patient the importance of taking the iron supplement for the period of time prescribed by the provider, because replacement of iron takes time.
- Explain to patients that there are some side effects that may occur when taking oral iron which include stomach upset and pain, constipation or diarrhea, nausea, and vomiting. Explain that taking an iron supplements with food may reduce some of these side effects.
- Instruct patients to keep iron supplements out of the reach of children to prevent iron poisoning.
- Provide patients with written educational materials on iron-deficiency anemia.

RED BLOOD CELL COUNT

The red blood cell (RBC) count is a measurement of the number of RBCs in the circulating blood. The reference range for the RBC count in a healthy woman is 4 to 5.5 million RBCs per cubic millimeter of blood, expressed on laboratory reports as 4 to 5.5 ($\times 10^6/mm^3$). The reference range for a healthy man is 4.5 to 6.2 million RBCs per cubic millimeter of blood, expressed on a laboratory report as 4.5 to 6.2 ($\times 10^6/mm^3$). In the medical office, the RBC is performed using a nonwaived blood cell counter.

A decrease in the RBC count can be caused by blood loss, production of defective RBCs, decreased production of RBCs, and increased destruction of RBCs. An increase in the RBC count can be caused by the production of RBCs to compensate for chronically low oxygen levels in conditions such as lung or heart disease.

A RBC count is a moderate complexity test and is performed on an automated (nonwaived) blood cell counter. Blood cell counters are also able to perform a WBC count, platelet count, hemoglobin, hematocrit, and WBC differential count, as well as a calculation of the RBC indices. Examples of nonwaived blood cell counters include the QBC Autoread Plus (Druker Diagnostics), the Cell-Dyn (Abbott, Santa Clara, CA), and the Beckman Coulter Counter (Beckman Coulter, Brea, CA) (Fig. 32.8).

RED BLOOD CELL INDICES

The RBC indices help to determine the cause of anemia. They are measurements that are reported as part of the CBC. RBC indices provide information about the size and hemoglobin content of a patient's red blood cells. The RBC indices include the MCV (mean corpuscular volume), MCH (mean corpuscular hemoglobin), MCHC (mean cell hemoglobin concentration), and RDW (red cell distribution width). Most of the RBC indices are obtained from calculations performed on certain test results included in a CBC—specifically, the RBC count, hemoglobin, and hematocrit. The calculation is automatically performed by the automated blood cell analyzer that performs the CBC. Refer to Table 32.1 for the purpose and reference ranges of the red blood cell indices.

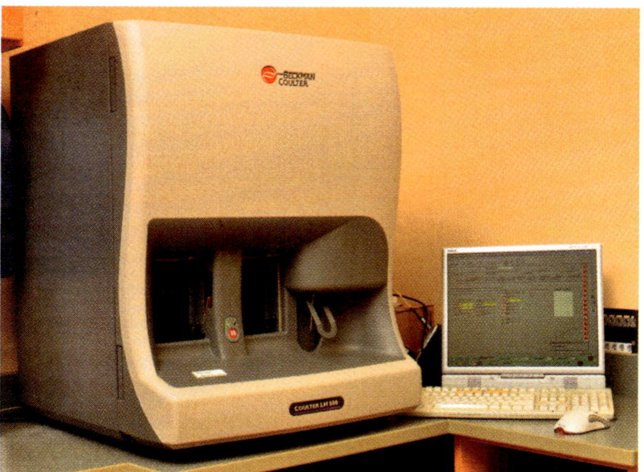

Fig. 32.8 Coulter blood cell counter. (Courtesy of Holzer Health Systems, Athens, OH.)

More than 400 types of anemia have been identified, but many of them are rare conditions. Each of the various forms of anemia (e.g., iron-deficiency anemia, pernicious anemia) may alter one or more of the RBC indices in a particular way. This information is used by the provider to assist in the diagnosis of the type of anemia a patient has and in determination of its cause.

MCV: MEAN CORPUSCULAR VOLUME

The MCV is a measurement of the average size of a single red blood cell. The MCV is the index used most often to assist in the diagnosis of a particular type of anemia. The MCV results are expressed in femtoliters (fL). The MCV reference range for a normal-sized red blood cell is 80 to 100 fL, and the cell is described as being **normocytic.**

An MCV result below 80 means that the patient's RBCs are smaller than normal and are described as being **microcytic.** The most common cause of microcytic anemia (low MCV) is a lack of iron in the diet, known as iron-deficiency anemia. Microcytic anemia may also be due to *thalassemia*, which is a hereditary type of anemia. An MCV result greater than 100 fL means that the cells are larger than normal, or **macrocytic.** The most common causes of macrocytic anemia (high MCV) are folic acid deficiency and a lack of vitamin B_{12} in the body, known as *pernicious anemia.*

MCH: MEAN CORPUSCULAR HEMOGLOBIN

The MCH measures the average amount of hemoglobin within a red blood cell. The results are expressed in picograms (pg). The reference range for an MCH is 27 to 31 pg. The cause of MCH values outside of the reference range are the same as those for MCV values outside of the reference range. For example, iron-deficiency anemia is associated with both a decreased MCV and a decreased MCH.

MCHC: MEAN CELL HEMOGLOBIN CONCENTRATION

The MCHC measures the average concentration of hemoglobin within red blood cells. The MCHC reference range for a red blood cell with a normal concentration of hemoglobin is 32% to 36%, and the cell is described as being **normochromic.** An example of a type of anemia that exhibits normochromia is pernicious anemia, which is caused by a lack of vitamin B_{12} in the body. An MCHC result below 32% means that the patient's red blood cells contain less than the normal concentration of hemoglobin or are **hypochromic,** a condition that occurs with iron-deficiency anemia and thalassemia. Because there is a physical limit to the amount of hemoglobin that can fit into an RBC, an

MCHC level above 36% does not occur (and therefore, RBCs cannot be *hyperchromic*).

RDW: RED CELL DISTRIBUTION WIDTH

The RDW measures any variation in the size of the red blood cells in a patient's specimen. Normally, all the red blood cells in a patient's specimen should be the same size, with very little variation. The RDW reference range is 11.5% to 14.5%. Certain anemias, such as iron-deficiency anemia, can change the size of some of the red blood cells, resulting in an increase in the RDW. **Anisocytosis** is the term used to describe a variation in the size of red blood cells.

WHITE BLOOD CELL COUNT

The white blood cell (WBC) count is used to assist in the diagnosis and management of pathologic conditions that affect the defense mechanism of the body that protects against infection and foreign materials. The WBC count is a measurement of the number of WBCs in the circulating blood. The reference range for a WBC count for a healthy adult is 4500 to 11,000 WBCs per cubic millimeter of blood, which is expressed as 4.5 to 11 ($\times 10^3/mm^3$) on laboratory reports. Conditions that result in an increase in leukocytes (leukocytosis) include acute infection such as appendicitis, chickenpox, diphtheria, infectious mononucleosis, meningitis, and rheumatic fever. Normal elevation of the white blood cell count can occur with pregnancy, strenuous exercise, stress, and treatment with corticosteroids. Conditions that result in a decrease in leukocytes (leukopenia), include viral infections, bone marrow damage, chemotherapy, and radiation therapy.

What Would You Do? What Would You *Not* Do?

Case Study 2

Paulina Torres brings in her 6-month-old son, Juan, for a well-child visit. Mrs. Torres has been breastfeeding Juan since he was born, and he is not yet on solid food. She says that Juan has been doing just fine, but he did not like his liquid vitamins, so she stopped giving them to him. Mrs. Torres says that she is eating a well-balanced diet and takes a multivitamin every day, so she didn't think it would be a problem. Juan's hemoglobin level is tested during the visit, and it is 9 g/dL. The physician prescribes ferrous sulfate drops for Juan. After the physician leaves the room, Mrs. Torres becomes quite upset. She says she does not understand why Juan's hemoglobin is low. She says that she thought that breast milk provided the best nutrition possible for infants. ■

WHITE BLOOD CELL DIFFERENTIAL COUNT

The purpose of the WBC differential count (differential) is to identify and count the five types of WBCs in a representative blood sample which include neutrophils, eosinophils, basophils, lymphocytes, and monocytes. The results are expressed as a percentage. The reference ranges for a differential count for an adult are presented in Table 32.1. The results of a differential count assist the provider in diagnosing conditions that affect one or more types of WBCs and in monitoring individuals undergoing treatment for these conditions.

The WBC differential count is a moderate complexity test that can be performed by an automated blood cell counter or manually through the examination of a blood smear. An automated differential count is faster and more convenient and permits the identification of many more WBCs than a manual differential count. A manual differential count, however, allows for closer inspection of abnormal WBCs.

AUTOMATED WBC DIFFERENTIAL COUNT

An automated WBC differential count involves the use of a sophisticated automated blood cell counter, such as the Sysmex XE2100 hematology analyzer (Sysmex Corporation, Kobe, Japan) or the Coulter cell counter (see Fig. 32.8). The specimen required is an EDTA–anticoagulated blood specimen obtained through venipuncture using a lavender-closure tube. The blood specimen is loaded into the automated analyzer which measures the various properties of WBCs (size, shape, and electrical properties) to determine which type of WBC it is. If abnormal features are present in the WBCs that the analyzer is unable to identify, the results are flagged and a manual differential count is performed by the outside laboratory. Between 10% and 25% of specimens are flagged by the analyzer for a manual review.

MANUAL WBC DIFFERENTIAL COUNT

If the provider orders a manual WBC differential count on a blood specimen, the medical assistant may need to prepare two blood smears using fresh whole blood for transport to an outside laboratory. The preparation of a blood smear is outlined in Procedure 32.2. Fresh whole blood is preferred for blood smears; however, a satisfactory smear can be made at the outside laboratory from an EDTA-anticoagulated blood specimen, provided that the smear is made within 24 hours after collection. Other anticoagulants should not be used because they could alter the morphology of the white blood cells. Blood cell **morphology** refers to the size, shape, and structure of a blood cell. After preparing the blood smear, the medical assistant must place the slides into a protective slide container for transport to an outside laboratory.

The blood smear is evaluated by a medical laboratory technologist at the outside laboratory. Because WBCs are clear and colorless, they must be stained with an appropriate dye (usually Wright's stain) before they can be identified. The nucleus, the cytoplasm, and any granules in the cytoplasm take on the characteristic colors of their cell type which aids in proper identification. A minimum of 100 WBCs are identified under a microscope based on the size,

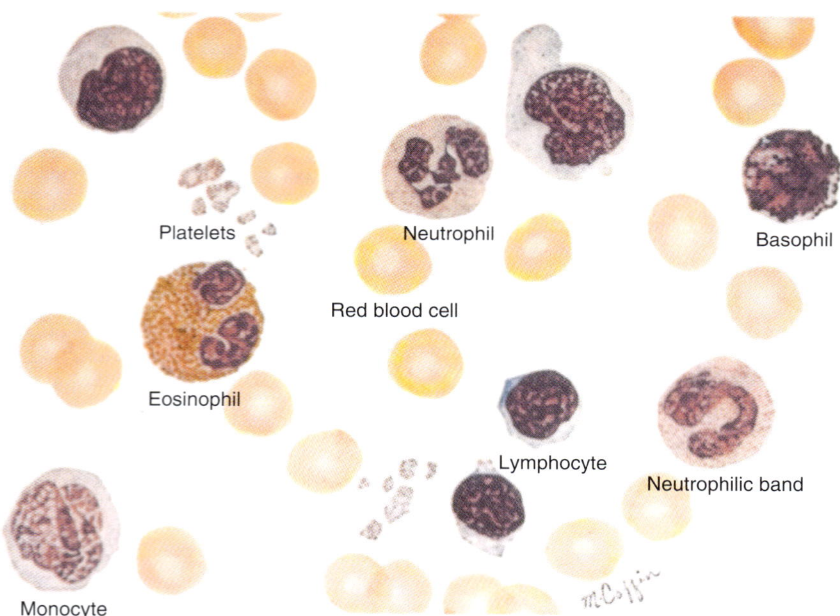

Fig. 32.9 Types of blood cells in a blood smear. (Modified from Custer RP: *An atlas of the blood and bone marrow*, ed 2, Philadelphia, 1974, WB Saunders.)

color, and structure of the nucleus and the color and texture of the cytoplasm. Each cell is assigned to its appropriate category: neutrophil, eosinophil, basophil, lymphocyte, or monocyte (Fig. 32.9). The number of each type of leukocyte is documented as a percentage and reflects the overall distribution of WBCs in the patient's bloodstream. During the manual evaluation of the blood smear, the laboratory technologist will also examine the morphology of RBCs and platelets including their size, shape, and structure. If immature or abnormal blood cells are observed on the slide, it is referred to a hematomorphologist and/or a pathologist for further evaluation and interpretation.

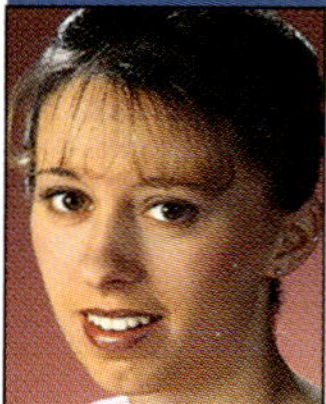

Memories *from* Practicum

Latisha: My practicum was at a cardiology office. A lot of venipunctures were performed at this office. Most of the blood specimens were picked up by Labcorp and taken to their laboratory for testing. I felt lucky I was able to get so much experience in drawing blood at this office. When I first started my practicum, the patients were apprehensive about someone new drawing their blood. This made me nervous because it seemed they were questioning my ability to perform the procedure. I explained to the patients that I had received the proper training for drawing blood and that I had successfully drawn blood on several of my classmates. Before drawing blood, I would go over the procedure many times in my head and I tried to be relaxed and confident performing the venipuncture. By doing this, I gained their trust and before long, they were requesting that I draw their blood. This taught me that if you believe in yourself and have confidence you can succeed at anything ■

What Would You Do? What Would You *Not* Do?

Case Study 3

Marjorie Merrick comes to the office for a follow-up visit to discuss her laboratory results with the physician. Marjorie is in perimenopause and has been having problems with heavy menstrual periods, bleeding between periods, hot flashes, insomnia, fatigue, and shortness of breath. Marjorie's laboratory tests indicate that she has iron-deficiency anemia. Because Marjorie's hemoglobin level is extremely low, the physician orders an injection of iron dextran, Z-track technique, and instructs Marjorie increase foods in her diet that contain iron. Marjorie says she has heard that an iron injection can stain the skin and wants to know whether that is true. She wants to know what foods contain iron. Marjorie says she has a friend who has received a vitamin B_{12} injection every 2 weeks. Marjorie wants to know whether she will have to do that, too. Marjorie signed up to donate blood this week at her church's Red Cross blood drive. She wants to know whether it is all right for her to donate. ■

COAGULATION TESTS

Most coagulation tests are moderate complexity tests and are performed at an outside laboratory. Examples of coagulation tests include: prothrombin time (PT), partial thromboplastin time (PTT), platelet count, fibrinogen level, factor V assay, and thrombin time. Commonly performed coagulation tests include the platelet count and the prothrombin time test, which are described in more detail below.

PLATELET COUNT

The platelet (PLT) count is included in a CBC; however, since it is a coagulation test, it is discussed in this section.

A PLT count is a moderate complexity test performed on an automated blood cell counter. The PLT count is a measurement of the number of platelets in the circulating blood. The reference range for a PLT count in a healthy adult is 150,000 to 400,000 platelets per cubic millimeter of blood, which is expressed as 150 to 400 ($\times 10^3/mm^3$) on a laboratory report.

The PLT count is used to assist in the diagnosis and management of conditions that affect the clotting mechanism of the body. A PLT count may be ordered when a patient has signs and symptoms associated with thrombocytopenia (decreased platelets) such as unexplained bruising, prolonged bleeding from a cut or wound, nosebleeds, heavy menstrual bleeding, small red spots on the skin known as *petechiae*, and small purplish spots on the skin known as *purpura* caused by bleeding under the skin. Conditions that can cause thrombocytopenia include iron-deficiency anemia, cancer, splenectomy, acute blood loss, and hemolytic anemia.

A PLT count may also be ordered when a patient has signs and symptoms associated with thrombocytosis (increased platelets) such as excessive clotting. Thrombocytosis is less common than thrombocytopenia and can be caused by the following conditions: viral infections (e.g., mononucleosis, hepatitis, HIV, and measles), leukemia, lymphoma, sepsis, cirrhosis, aplastic anemia, and autoimmune disorders.

PROTHROMBIN TIME TEST

Prothrombin is a protein produced by your liver. It is one of many factors in the blood that help it to clot appropriately. Vitamin K is needed for the production of prothrombin. A prothrombin time (PT) test measures the time it takes for the blood to form a clot. A PT test helps to detect bleeding and clotting disorders in patients exhibiting symptoms of these disorders. The reference range for a PT test for a healthy adult is 9 to 12 seconds.

If the PT result is more than 12 seconds, the blood is clotting slower than normal which could result in excessive bleeding. Symptoms of a bleeding disorder that may warrant a PT test include unexplained nosebleeds, excessive bleeding from the gums, easy bruising, heavy menstrual periods, and unexplained blood in the stool or urine. Conditions that can cause a prolonged prothrombin time include liver disease, vitamin K deficiency, or a deficiency of a clotting factor.

If the PT result is less than 9 seconds, the blood is clotting faster than normal which could result in excessive clot formation in arteries or veins. Symptoms of a clotting disorder that may warrant a PT test include swelling, redness, tenderness or warmth in a leg; redness or red streaks on the legs; shortness of breath, cough, and chest pain. The conditions causing these symptoms are those associated with the presence of a blood clot such as thrombophlebitis (usually in a leg) and a pulmonary embolism.

PT/INR TEST

A PT/INR (prothrombin time with INR) test is a combination of a PT test and a mathematical calculation performed on the PT test result to arrive at a standardized value known as an *INR (International Normalized Ratio)*.

The PT/INR test is most commonly used to monitor patients on long-term warfarin anticoagulant therapy to determine how well the warfarin is working to prevent blood clots. An **anticoagulant** inhibits the formation of blood clots by interfering with the blood clotting mechanism in the body. This causes the blood to take longer to clot. Warfarin works by reducing the available vitamin K in the liver responsible for producing some of the clotting factors, including prothrombin; brand names for warfarin include Coumadin and Jantoven.

PURPOSE OF THE PT/INR TEST

A PT/INR test is recommended for patients on long-term warfarin therapy. Patients on warfarin therapy have to have their blood tested every 2 to 4 weeks for as long as they are on warfarin, which may be for the rest of their lives. Reagents used to perform the test vary from one laboratory to another and sometimes even within the same laboratory over time. The INR is a calculation performed by the automated coagulation analyzer on the PT result that adjusts for changes in the reagents and allows results from different laboratories to be compared. The INR is expressed as a ratio and provides a good comparison of test results for patients on long-term warfarin therapy.

The INR is a standardized measurement of the rate at which the blood clots. It is expressed as a number, and because the value is a ratio, the result does not have a unit of measurement attached to it. A healthy individual with a normal clotting ability (and not on warfarin therapy) should have an INR result that falls between 0.9 and 1.2. Most laboratories report both the PT and INR values when a PT/INR test is performed.

A low INR means there is an increased risk of blood clot formation in an artery or vein. A high INR means that there is an increased risk of bleeding; the higher the number, the longer it takes for the blood to clot. For example, an individual with an INR of 3.0 (high INR) would have blood that takes longer to clot than an individual with an INR of 1.0 (normal INR). The risk of spontaneous bleeding begins to rise as the INR reaches a level of 4.0 or higher.

Long-Term Warfarin Therapy

Conditions for which long-term warfarin therapy is prescribed include the following:

- Patients who experience recurrent atrial fibrillation. *Arial fibrillation* is an irregular heartbeat, which can cause blood to pool in the atrium of the heart; the pooled blood may cause formation of a blood clot, which can travel to the brain, resulting in a stroke.
- Patients who have experienced a pulmonary embolism (PE) or thrombophlebitis (also known as *deep vein thrombosis* [DVT]) to prevent the formation of another clot.
- Patients who have had a heart valve replaced with a mechanical valve because of the increased risk that a

clot may form on the mechanical valve, causing heart blockage.

The goal of warfarin therapy is to increase the clotting time to a level that prevents the formation of blood clots in an individual with one of the conditions listed above, without causing excessive bleeding or bruising. The ideal INR range for a patient on warfarin therapy depends on the condition being treated. The ideal INR range for a patient on moderate-intensity warfarin therapy following a DVT or PE, or for a patient with recurring atrial fibrillation, is between 2.0 and 3.0. The ideal INR range for a patient with a mechanical valve replacement is between 2.5 and 3.5.

PT/INR TESTING SCHEDULE

To ensure that patients on long-term warfarin therapy remain within their ideal INR range, they must undergo periodic PT/INR testing. When patients are first placed on warfarin therapy, a PT/INR test is performed once or twice a week to assess their response to the warfarin. Based on the INR results, the dose of warfarin is adjusted so that the results become stable and consistently fall within their ideal INR range. Once the test results become stabilized, the patient should have a PT/INR test performed every 2 to 4 weeks.

PT/INR SPECIMEN COLLECTION FOR TRANSPORT

The medical assistant may be responsible for collecting the specimen for a PT/INR test for transport to an outside laboratory for testing. The PT/INR test requires only a small collection tube (usually 4 to 5 mL). The blood must be collected in a tube containing sodium citrate, which is a light-blue closure tube (Fig. 32.10). The sodium citrate prevents the specimen from clotting without affecting the test results.

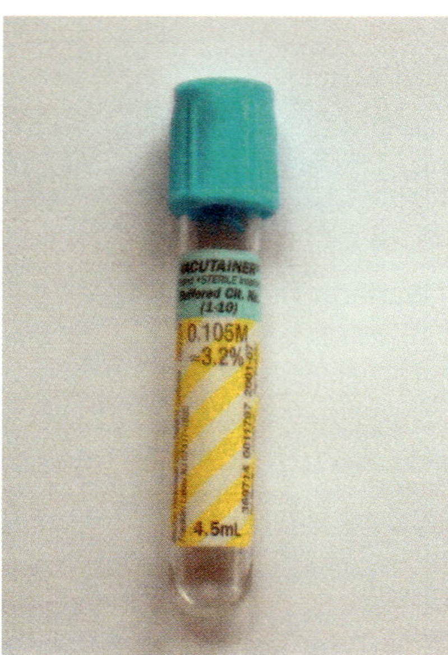

Fig. 32.10 Light-blue closure tube used to collect a specimen for a PT/INR test.

When collecting the specimen, it is very important to fill the light-blue closure tube to the exhaustion of the vacuum to provide for the correct anticoagulant-to-blood ratio. Failure to completely fill the tube is a cause for rejection of the specimen by the outside laboratory because it leads to inaccurate test results. Some light-blue tubes have a fill indicator, so that the medical assistant can verify visually that the tube is completely filled.

If the butterfly method is used to collect the specimen, a modification in the collection procedure is required under the following circumstances. If the light-blue closure tube is the first or only tube to be drawn, a 5-mL red closure tube must be drawn first and discarded. This must be done to remove the air in the butterfly tubing and replace it with blood. If the light-blue closure tube is filled without drawing a discard tube, some of the tube's vacuum is exhausted by the air in the butterfly tubing (rather than blood), resulting in underfilling of the tube. An underfilled tube results in an incorrect anticoagulant-to-blood ratio which is a cause for rejection of the specimen by the outside laboratory.

Once the tube has been drawn, it should be immediately and gently inverted three or four times to mix the anticoagulant with the blood to prevent the formation of clots. The tube should then be placed in a biohazard specimen bag for transport to an outside laboratory. A laboratory request form must be placed with the specimen or transmitted electronically to the laboratory. Information on the collection and handling of a specimen for a PT/INR test as presented in a laboratory test directory is outlined in Fig. 32.11.

CLIA-WAIVED PT/INR TEST

A PT/INR test can be performed in the medical office using a CLIA-waived automated coagulation analyzer. One of the advantages of CLIA-waived coagulation analyzers is that they only require a capillary specimen to perform the test. The manufacturer of each coagulation analyzer provides an operating manual that includes information needed to perform quality control procedures, collect and test the specimen, and properly store the test strips. It is important that the medical assistant become familiar with all aspects of the coagulation analyzer used to perform a PT/INR test. Quality control procedures are of particular importance to ensure that the analyzer is functioning properly and that the test results are reliable and accurate. Brand names of coagulation analyzers include HemoSense InRatio 2 (Hemosense Inc., San Diego, CA) and CoaguChek XS (Roche Diagnostics, Branchburg, NJ).

Procedure for the CLIA-Waived CoaguChek XS Test

The medical assistant must follow the PT/INR collection and testing procedure *exactly* as presented in the operating

Test Directory Prothrombin Time with INR	
CPT Code:	85610
Synonyms:	PT/INR, PT, Protime
Type of Specimen:	Whole blood or plasma
Amount of Specimen:	4.5 mL
Collection Container:	Light-blue top tube
Patient Preparation:	None
Collection and Processing:	1. Collect and label specimen. 2. With a winged-infusion setup, draw a 5 mL discard tube first to account for air in the tubing to prevent underfilling the tube. 3. Fill the light-blue top tube completely. 4. Gently invert tube 3-4 times immediately after collection.
Storage and Transport:	Store at RT
Specimen Stability:	RT 59°–86° F (15°–35° C): 24 hours If testing cannot be performed within 24 hours, centrifuge the specimen for 15 minutes and remove the plasma using a plastic pipet being careful not to disturb the buffy coat. Place the plasma in a labeled transfer tube freeze immediately at –20° C for pickup by a courier.
Causes for Rejection:	Specimen collected in any tube other than a sodium citrate tube Hemolyzed or clotted specimen. Underfilled tube (less than 90%) Collection tube past its expiration date Improper labeling of tube
Reference Range:	**INR:** *For patients with normal clotting ability:* 0.9-1.2 *For patients taking warfarin:* Moderate intensity warfarin therapy 2.0-3.0 Higher intensity warfarin therapy 2.5-3.5 **PT:** 9–12 seconds

Uses:
Detection of bleeding and clotting disorders.
Screening for congenital and acquired deficiencies of factors II, V, VII, X, and fibrinogen.
Therapeutic monitoring of warfarin (Coumadin®) anticoagulant therapy.

Limitations:	Consumption of food containing rich in Vitamin K can decrease the PT/INR Barbiturates, oral contraceptives, and HRT can decrease the PT/INR
Forms:	Order electronically or print the lab request form and submit with specimen.
Methodology:	Photo-optical clot detection analyzer.

Fig. 32.11 PT/INR test specimen requirements from a laboratory test directory.

manual. An overview of the procedure for performing a PR/INR test using the CLIA-waived CoaguChek XS is outlined here:

1. Perform a finger puncture to obtain a capillary blood specimen.
2. Apply the first drop of blood to the test strip (Fig. 32.12).
3. Read the results after a countdown period in which the analyzer determines the PT test results and then calculates the INR. The INR on this meter is 0.9 which is within the reference range for a healthy adult not on warfarin therapy (Fig. 32.13).
4. Document the results in the patient's medical record, including the date and time, the name of the test (PT/INR), and the INR ratio value.

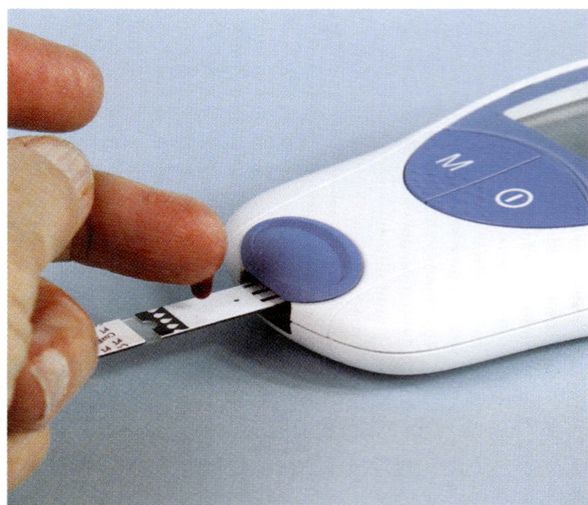

Fig. 32.12 A drop of blood is placed on the test strip. (From Garrels M: *Laboratory and diagnostic testing in ambulatory care*, ed 4, St.Louis, 2019, Elsevier.)

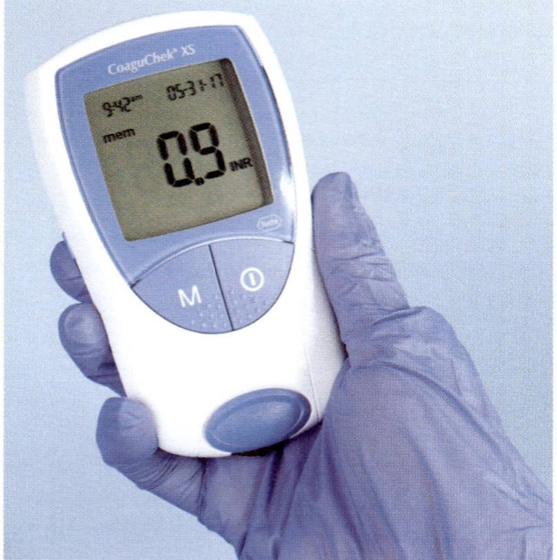

Fig. 32.13 Test results are displayed on the LCD screen. (From Garrels M: *Laboratory and diagnostic testing in ambulatory care*, ed 4, St. Louis, 2019, Elsevier.)

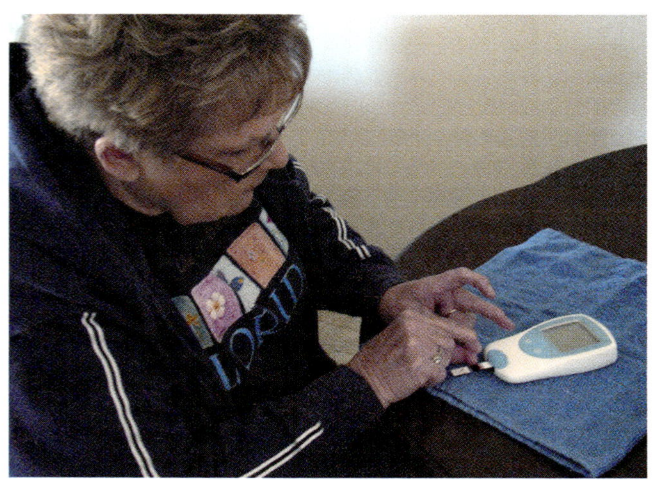

Fig. 32.14 PT/INR home testing.

HOME TESTING

Patients on long-term warfarin therapy are able to test their blood at home with a CLIA-waived coagulation analyzer (Fig. 32.14). Home PT/INR testing with a coagulation analyzer is covered by Medicare and most private insurance companies. Home testing provides patients with the convenience of not having to make periodic visits to a laboratory or medical office to have a PT/INR test performed. Patients can check their PT/INR when conditions occur that might indicate a problem, such as nosebleeds, bleeding gums, or unexplained bruising. In these situations, treatment can be instituted immediately to prevent the problem from getting worse.

Factors that can affect INR results and cause them to be outside of a patient's ideal range include the following: a change in diet; use of prescription or over-the-counter medications that interact with warfarin; vitamins and herbal preparations; a change in the level of exercise; illness; smoking; and alcohol consumption. It is important that the patient keep their provider informed of any factors that may alter the body's response to warfarin.

What Would You Do? What Would You *Not* Do? RESPONSES

Case Study 1
Page 865

What Did Latisha Do?

- ❑ Told Theodore that the tests are routine screening tests that are being run to make sure he is in good health.
- ❑ Told Theodore that it it not possible to obtain the specimen from his finger because it would not provide enough blood to perform the tests.
- ❑ Explained to Theodore that a small amount of pain is associated with a blood draw but it would be brief.
- ❑ Explained to Theodore that two different tests are being run on him and they each require a certain type of tube.
- ❑ Placed Theodore in a semi-reclining position for the venipuncture as a safety precaution.
- ❑ Helped Theodore to relax during the venipuncture by telling him to breathe deeply.
- ❑ Just before inserting the needle, told Theodore that he would feel a "small stick" to prevent startling him when the needle is inserted.

What Did Latisha Not Do?

- ❑ Did not tell Theodore that he is healthy and does not have anything wrong with him.
- ❑ Did not tell Theodore that he should try to be braver about having his blood drawn.
- ❑ Did not tell Theodore that the venipuncture would not hurt.

What Would You Do? What Would You *Not* Do? RESPONSES—cont'd

Case Study 2

Page 867

What Did Latisha Do?

- ❑ Commended Mrs. Torres on eating nutritiously.
- ❑ Told Mrs. Torres that breast milk does not contain very much iron. Explained that because of this, it is important to give Juan his liquid vitamins, which have iron in them.
- ❑ Reassured Mrs. Torres that breastfeeding does provide very good nutrition for Juan.
- ❑ Explained to Mrs. Torres that the iron supplement may cause Juan's stool to be a dark, tarlike color, and she should not be alarmed because this is normal.

What Did Latisha Not Do?

- ❑ Did not scold Mrs. Torres for not giving Juan his vitamins.
- ❑ Did not make Mrs. Torres feel like it was her fault that Juan's hemoglobin was low.

Case Study 3

Page 868

What Did Latisha Do?

- ❑ Explained to Marjorie that the iron injection can stain the skin but that it would be given in a special way to prevent that from happening.
- ❑ Told Marjorie that the following foods contain iron: beef, liver, spinach, eggs, and iron-fortified breads and cereals.
- ❑ Told Marjorie that she wouldn't be getting a vitamin B_{12} injection because vitamin B_{12} is not used to treat iron-deficiency anemia.
- ❑ Told Marjorie that the Red Cross requires that a blood donor's hemoglobin level be within the normal range to donate blood. Explained that she could not donate this time, but that when her hemoglobin is back to normal, she will be able to donate.
- ❑ Explained to Marjorie that the iron supplement may cause her stool to be a dark, tarlike color, and she should not be alarmed because this is normal.
- ❑ Gave Marjorie a patient education brochure on iron-deficiency anemia to take home with her.

What Did Latisha Not Do?

- ❑ Did not tell Marjorie that her hemoglobin level was really low and should be a cause for concern.
- ❑ Did not tell Marjorie that her friend has pernicious anemia because there is no way of knowing this.

TERMINOLOGY REVIEW

Medical Term	Word Parts	Definition
Ameboid movement		Movement used by leukocytes that permits them to propel themselves from the capillaries into the tissues.
Anemia	*an-:* without or absence of *-emia:* blood condition	A condition in which there is a decrease in the number of erythrocytes or the amount of hemoglobin in the blood.
Anisocytosis	*anis/o-:* unequal, dissimilar *cyt/o:* cell *-osis:* abnormal condition	A variation in the size of red blood cells.
Anticoagulant	*anti-:* against *-coagulant:* clotting	A substance that inhibits blood clotting.
Bilirubin	*bili-:* bile	An orange-colored bile pigment that is a by-product of heme destruction from the hemoglobin molecule.
Diapedesis	*dia-:* through	The ameboid movement of blood cells (especially leukocytes) through the wall of a capillary and out into the tissues.
Erythrocyte	*erythro-:* red *cyte:* cell	Red blood cell. RBCs are responsible for transporting oxygen and carbon dioxide in the body.
Hematology	*hemat/o-:* blood *-ology:* study of	The study of blood and blood-forming tissues.
Hematopoiesis	*hemat/o-:* blood *-poiesis*: formation of	The process of blood cell formation.
Hemoglobin	*hem/o-:* blood *-globin:* protein	The protein- and iron-containing pigment of erythrocytes that carries oxygen to the tissues of the body.
Hemolysis	*hem/o-:* blood *-lysis:* breakdown	The breakdown of erythrocytes with the release of hemoglobin into the plasma.
Hypochromic	*hypo-:* below, deficient *chrom/o:* color *-ic:* pertaining to	A red blood cell with a decreased concentration of hemoglobin.
Leukocyte	*leuk/o-:* white *cyt/o:* cell	White blood cell. WBCs functions in defending the body against infection and foreign materials.

Continued

TERMINOLOGY REVIEW—cont'd

Medical Term	Word Parts	Definition
Leukocytosis	*leuk/o-:* white *cyt/o:* cell *-osis:* abnormal condition (means increased when used with blood cell word parts)	An abnormal increase in the number of leukocytes (greater than 11,000 per cubic millimeter of blood).
Leukopenia	*leuk/o-:* white *-penia:* abnormal reduction in number	An abnormal decrease in the number of leukocytes (less than 4500 per cubic millimeter of blood).
Macrocytic	*macr/o-:* abnormally large *cyt/o:* cell *-ic:* pertaining to	An abnormally large red blood cell.
Microcytic	*micro-:* small *cyt/o:* cell *-ic:* pertaining to	An abnormally small red blood cell.
Morphology (blood cells)	*morpho-:* form and structure *-ology:* study of	The study of the size, shape, and structure of a blood cell.
Normochromic	*norm/o-:* normal *chrom/o:* color *-ic:* pertaining to	A red blood cell with a normal concentration of hemoglobin.
Normocytic	*norm/o:* normal *cyt/o:* cell *-ic:* pertaining to	A normal-sized red blood cell.
Oxyhemoglobin	*oxy/i-:* oxygen *hem/o:* blood *-globin:* protein	Hemoglobin that has combined with oxygen.
Phagocytosis	*phag/o-:* eat, swallow *cyt/o:* cell *-osis:* abnormal condition	The engulfing and destruction of foreign particles, such as pathogens and damaged cells, by certain cells in the body.
Polycythemia	*poly-:* many *cyt/o:* cell *hem/o:* blood *-ia:* condition of diseased or abnormal state	A disorder in which there is an increase in the number of red blood cells or the amount of hemoglobin.
Thrombocyte	*thrombo-:* clot *cyt/o:* cell	Platelets. Thrombocytes function by participating in the blood clotting mechanism of the body.
Thrombocytopenia	*thrombo-:* clot *cyt/o:* cell *-penia:* abnormal reduction in number	An abnormal decrease in the number of thrombocytes (less than 150,000 per cubic millimeter of blood).
Thrombocytosis	*thrombo-:* clot *cyt/o:* cell *-osis:* abnormal condition (means increased when used	An abnormal increase in the number of thrombocytes (greater than 400,000 per cubic millimeter of blood).

PROCEDURE 32.1 Perform a CLIA-Waived Hematocrit Test

Outcome Perform a hematocrit test.

Equipment/Supplies

- CLIA-waived microhematocrit centrifuge
- Disposable gloves
- Lancet
- Antiseptic wipe
- Gauze pads
- Capillary tubes
- Sealing compound
- Adhesive bandage
- Biohazard sharps container

1. **Procedural Step.** Sanitize your hands. Greet the patient and introduce yourself. Identify the patient by full name and date of birth, and explain the procedure.
2. **Procedural Step.** Assemble equipment. Open the gauze packet. Cleanse the puncture site with an antiseptic wipe, and allow it to air-dry. Apply gloves and perform a finger puncture, then dispose of the lancet in a biohazard sharps container.
   Principle. Personal protective equipment and proper disposal of the lancet are required by the OSHA standard to prevent exposure to bloodborne pathogens.
3. **Procedural Step.** Wipe away the first drop of blood with a gauze pad. Fill the first capillary tube by holding one end of it horizontally, but slightly downward, next to the free-flowing puncture. Keep the tip of the capillary tube in the blood, but do not allow it to press against the patient's skin. Calibrated tubes are filled to the calibration line; uncalibrated tubes are filled approximately three-quarters (within 10 to 20 mm of the end of the tube). The blood is drawn into the tube through capillary action. Fill a second tube using the method just described. Place a gauze pad over the puncture site and apply pressure.
   Principle. Not keeping the tip of the capillary tube in the blood can cause air bubbles in the stem of the tube, which leads to inaccurate test results. Allowing the capillary tube to press against the skin closes the opening of the capillary tubes and does not allow blood to enter. The type of tube (calibrated or uncalibrated) is based on the method used to read the test results. The hematocrit should be performed in duplicate to ensure accurate and reliable test results.

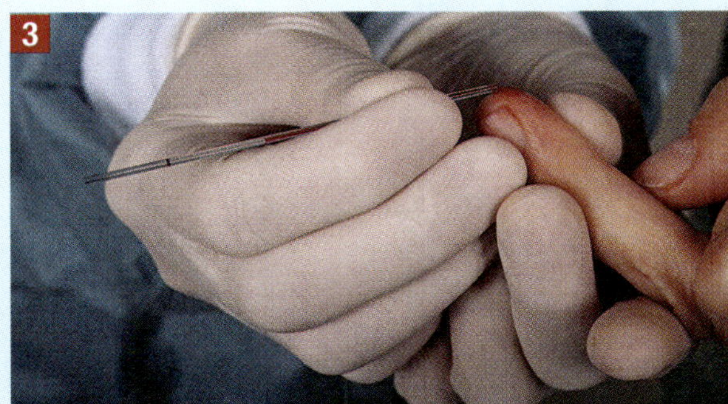

Fill the capillary tube.

4. **Procedural Step.** Push the dry end of the tube (end opposite the filling end that does not contain blood) down into the sealing compound. This seals the end of the capillary tube. The sealing compound can be used to hold the capillary tubes until they are ready to be placed in the microhematocrit centrifuge. To do this, place the sealing compound on a flat surface with the tubes in a vertical position. Before removing a capillary tube from the sealing compound, rotate the tube between the thumb and index finger to prevent the sealing compound from pulling out when the tube is lifted out of the sealing compound.
   Principle. Capillary tubes must be sealed properly to prevent leakage of the blood specimen during centrifugation.

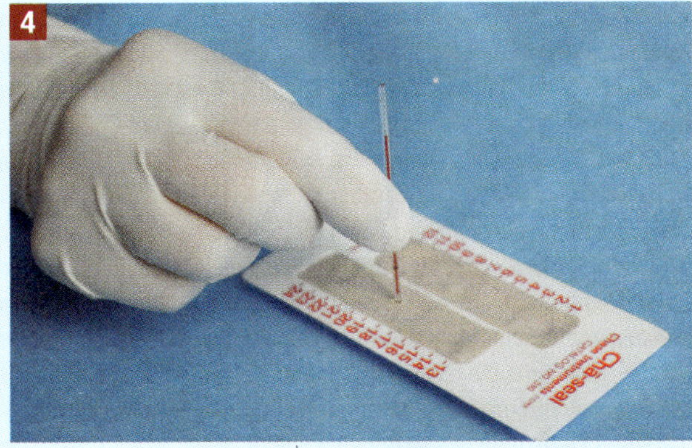

Seal the end of the tube.

Continued

PROCEDURE 32.1 Perform a CLIA-Waived Hematocrit Test—cont'd

5. **Procedural Step.** Check the patient's puncture site for bleeding and apply an adhesive bandage, if needed.
6. **Procedural Step.** Place the capillary tubes in the microhematocrit centrifuge with the sealed end facing out. Balance one tube with the other capillary tube placed on the opposite side of the centrifuge.
   Principle. Placing the sealed end toward the outside prevents the blood specimen from spinning out of the capillary tube when the centrifuge is in operation.

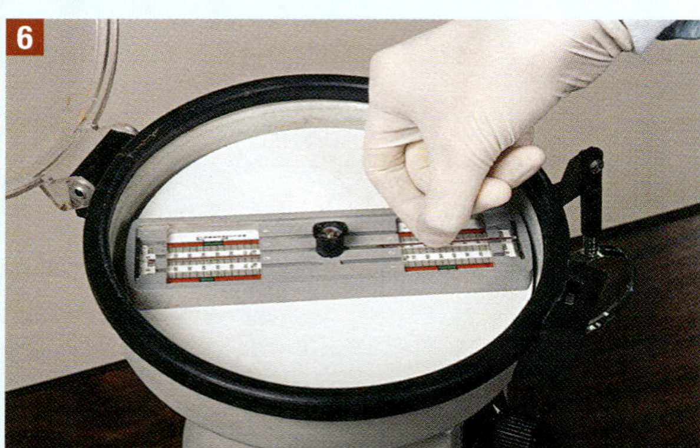

6

Place the tube in the centrifuge.

7. **Procedural Step.** Place the cover on the centrifuge, and lock it securely. Centrifuge the blood specimen for 3 to 5 minutes at a speed of 10,000 rpm.
   Principle. Centrifuging the blood specimen causes the red blood cells to become packed and to settle on the bottom of the tube.
8. **Procedural Step.** Allow the centrifuge to come to a complete stop. Read the results, as follows:
   Calibrated tube. If a capillary tube with a calibration line was used, read the results using the special graphic reading device that is part of the centrifuge. Adjust the capillary tube so that the bottom of the red blood cell column (just above the sealing compound) is placed on the 0 line. With a magnifying glass, read the results at the top of the packed red blood cell column, and you will see a percentage on the reading device.
   Uncalibrated tube. If an uncalibrated tube was used, you must use a microhematocrit reader card to determine the results; place the top of the plasma column on the 100% mark and the bottom of the cell column on the 0 line. Read the results on the scale, which corresponds to the top of the packed cell column.
   In both cases, the buffy coat should not be included in the reading. The answer represents the percentage of blood volume occupied by the RBCs. (The hematocrit test on this reading device is 38.)
   Principle. Stopping the centrifuge with your hands can injure you and can damage the machine.

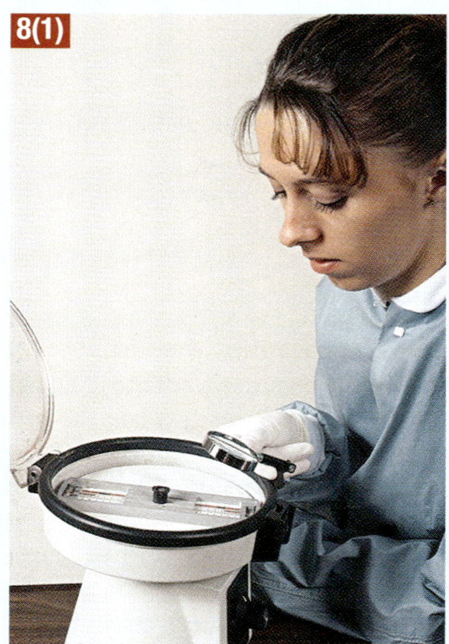

8(1)

Align the bottom of the red cell column with the 0 line.

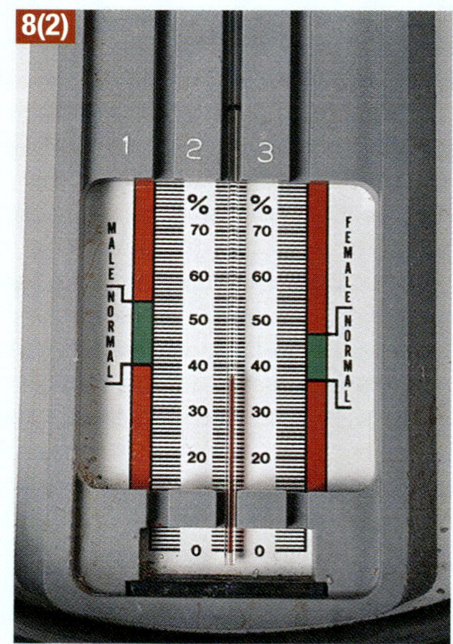

8(2)

Read the results.

9. **Procedural Step.** Read the second tube in the manner just described; the results of the tubes should agree within 4 percentage points. If not, the hematocrit procedure must be repeated. If they are within 4 percentage points, the two values are averaged to derive the test results.
10. **Procedural Step.** Properly dispose of the capillary tubes in a biohazard sharps container. Remove gloves and sanitize your hands.

PROCEDURE 32.1 Perform a CLIA-Waived Hematocrit Test—cont'd

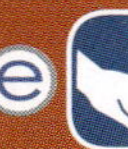  

11. Procedural Step. Document the results in the patient's medical record.

a. *Electronic medical record:* Document the hematocrit results using the appropriate radio buttons, drop-down menus, and free text fields.

b. *Paper-based patient record:* Document the date and time and the hematocrit results (refer to the PPR documentation example).

11b

DOCUMENTATION EXAMPLE

Date	
5/5/XX	11:15 a.m. Hct: 38%. ————
	———— L. Sharpe, CMA (AAMA)

12. Procedural Step. Return the equipment to its proper storage place. Store the sealing compound at room temperature. Exposing it to a temperature above 80° F adversely affects its consistency.

Reference range for hematocrit:

Female: 37% to 47%
Male: 40% to 54%

PROCEDURE 32.2 Preparation of a Blood Smear for a WBC Differential Count

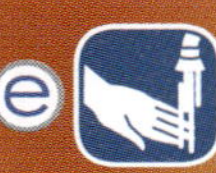 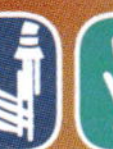  

Outcome Prepare a blood smear for a WBC Differential count.

Equipment/Supplies

- Disposable gloves
- Supplies to perform a finger puncture or venipuncture
- Slides with a frosted edge
- Slide container
- Biohazard specimen bag
- Laboratory request form
- Biohazard sharps container

1. Procedural Step. Sanitize your hands. Greet the patient and introduce yourself. Identify the patient by full name and date of birth, and explain the procedure.

2. Procedural Step. Assemble the equipment. Complete a laboratory request by writing in the information on a preprinted form or by entering the required information into a computer. Using a pencil, label two slides on the frosted edge with the patient's name and date of birth, and the date.

Principle. Laboratories request the preparation of two blood smears as a means of quality control.

3. Procedural Step. Open the gauze packet. Cleanse the puncture site with an antiseptic wipe. Perform a finger puncture, and wipe away the first drop of blood. Place a drop of blood from the patient's finger in the middle of each slide, approximately {1/4} inch from the slide's frosted edge, by touching the slide to the drop of blood. Do not allow the patient's finger to touch the slide.

Principle. If the patient's finger touches the slide, it will spread out the blood specimen, producing an uneven smear. In addition, moisture or oil from the patient's finger could interfere with the smear.

4. Procedural Step. Make the blood smear as follows:

a. Hold a second "spreader" slide between the thumb and index finger of the dominant hand. Position a nondominant finger (or fingers) at the end of the slide (end opposite the frosted edge). Position the spreader slide in front of the drop of blood and at a 30-degree angle to the first slide.

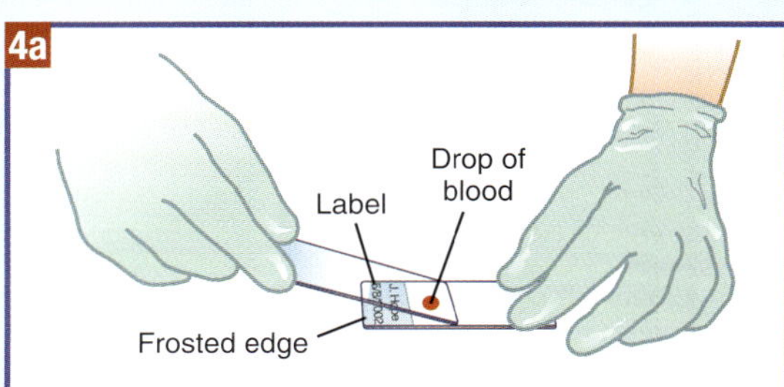

Hold the spreader slide in front of the drop of blood.

b. Move the spreader slide until it touches the drop of blood. The blood distributes itself along the edge of the spreader by capillary action.

Continued

PROCEDURE 32.2 Preparation of a Blood Smear for a WBC Differential Count—cont'd

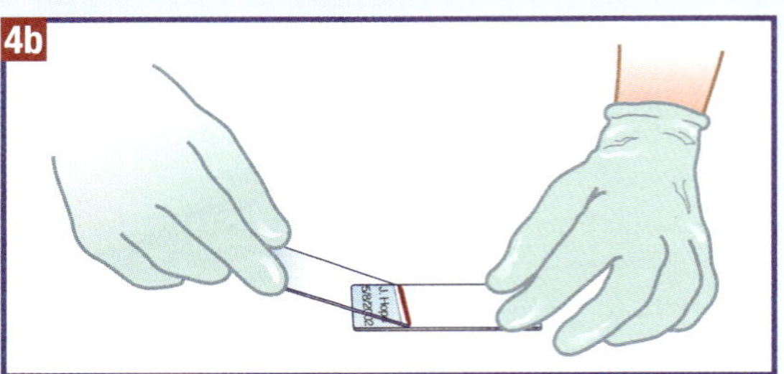

Move the spreader into the drop of blood.

c. Using a smooth, continuous motion with a light but firm pressure, spread the blood thinly and evenly across the surface of the first slide, ending the motion by lifting the spreader slide off the specimen in a smooth, low arc. The smear should be approximately 1½ inches long. The blood smear is thickest at the beginning and gradually thins to a very fine "feathered" edge which is only one cell layer thick.

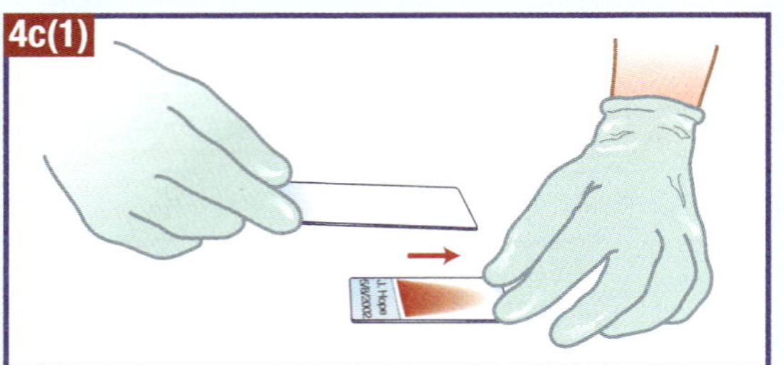

Spread the blood across the slide.

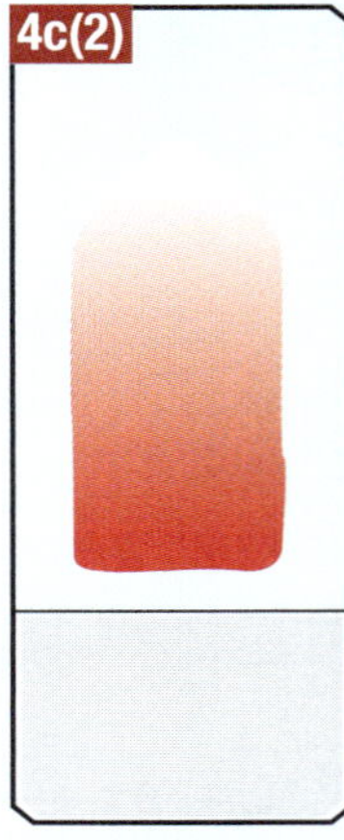

Properly prepared blood smear. (From Rodak BF: *Hematology: clinical principles and applications*, ed 4, St. Louis, 2012, Elsevier.)

Repeat the above procedure to prepare the second blood smear.

If the blood smear has been prepared correctly, it exhibits the following characteristics: (1) It is smooth and even with no ridges, holes, lines, streaks, or clumps; (2) it is not too thick or too thin; (3) a feathered edge is seen at the thin end of the smear; and (4) a margin is evident on all sides of the smear.

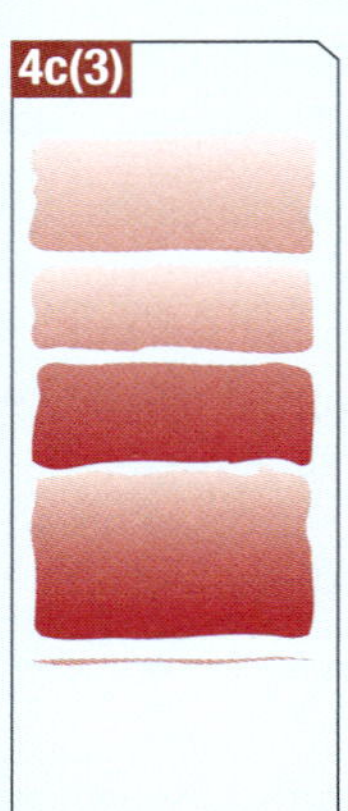

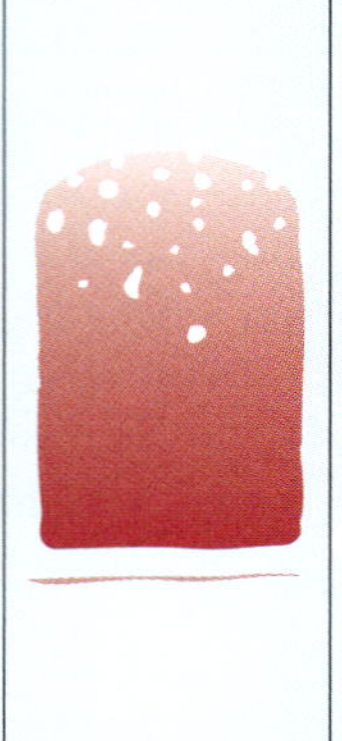

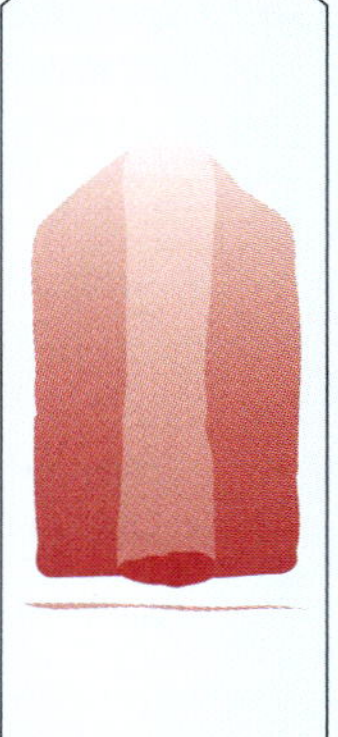

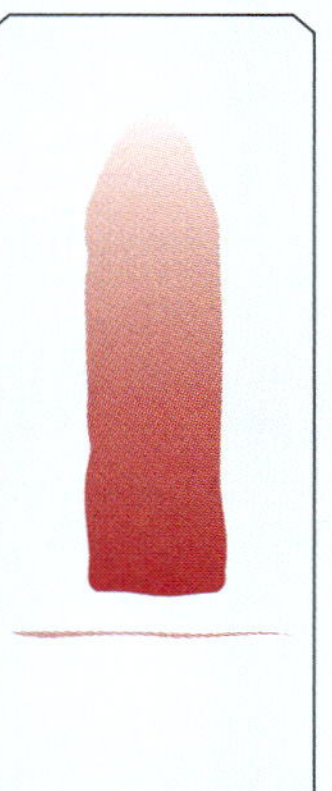

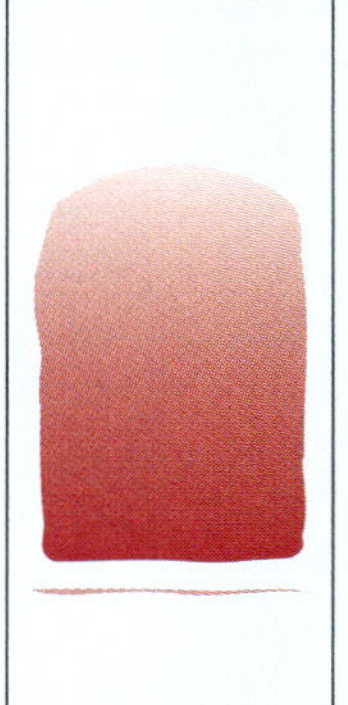

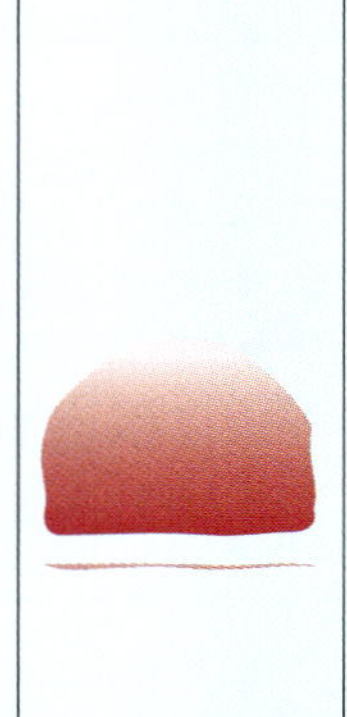

Improperly prepared blood smears. (Modified from Rodak BF: *Hematology: clinical principles and applications*, ed 4, St. Louis, 2012, Elsevier.)

PROCEDURE 32.2 Preparation of a Blood Smear for a WBC Differential Count—cont'd

Principle. An angle of more than 30 degrees causes the smear to be too thick; the cells overlap, do not stain well, and are smaller than normal, making them difficult to count. If the angle is smaller than 30 degrees, the smear will be too thin, and the cells will be spread out, increasing the time needed to count them.

5. **Procedural Step.** Dispose of the spreader slide in a biohazard sharps container.
6. **Procedural Step.** Lay the blood smears on a flat surface, and allow them to air-dry. Never blow on the slides to dry them.

   Principle. The blood smears must be dried immediately to prevent shrinkage of the blood cells, which makes them difficult to identify. Blowing on the slide might cause exhaled water droplets to make holes in the smears.
7. **Procedural Step.** Once the slides are completely dry, apply gloves and place them in a protective slide container. Prepare the slides for transport to the outside laboratory.
   a. Place slide container in a biohazard specimen bag.
   b. If a blood specimen was collected for a CBC, place the lavender closure tube in the specimen bag.
   c. Seal the bag and place the laboratory request in the outside pocket of the specimen bag (or transmit it electronically).
   d. Properly store the specimen while awaiting pickup by a laboratory courier.
8. **Procedural Step.** Remove your gloves, and sanitize your hands.
9. **Procedural Step.** Document the procedure in the patient's medical record.
   a. *Electronic medical record:* Document the type of collection and the date the specimen was transported to the laboratory using the appropriate radio buttons, drop-down menus, and free text fields.
   b. *Paper-based patient record:* Document the date and time, the type of collection and the date the specimen was transported to the laboratory (refer to the PPR documentation example).

9b

DOCUMENTATION EXAMPLE

Date	
5/05/XX	11:15 a.m. Venous blood specimen collected
	from Ⓡ arm. Specimen to Medical Center
	Laboratory for CBC c̄ diff on 5/05/XX. ———
	————————— L. Sharpe, CMA (AAMA)

10. **Procedural Step.** Place the specimen bag in the appropriate location for pickup by a laboratory courier.

PROCEDURE 32.2

33 Blood Chemistry and Immunologic Testing

Check out the Evolve site at http://evolve.elsevier.com/Bonewit/today to access additional interactive activities and exercises to help you study and prepare for success.

LEARNING OBJECTIVES

Blood Chemistry Testing

1. Explain the purpose of a blood chemistry test.
2. State the use of a comprehensive metabolic panel (CMP).

Quality Control

3. Describe the purpose of the test reagent area on a test strip.
4. Explain the purpose of the calibration and control procedures.
5. List factors that can result in the failure of a control to produce expected results.
6. Identify when a control procedure should be performed.

Blood Chemistry Tests

7. State the purpose of blood chemistry testing.
8. Explain the functions of glucose and insulin in the body.
9. Describe the difference between type 1 diabetes and type 2 diabetes.
10. Identify the risk factors for type 2 diabetes.
11. List and describe the various insulin delivery methods.
12. State the purpose of each of the following tests: random blood glucose test, fasting blood glucose test, 2-hour postprandial glucose test, and oral glucose tolerance test.
13. State the patient preparation for a fasting blood glucose test.
14. Identify the ADA guidelines for interpretation of FBG test results.
15. Describe the procedure for a 2-hour postprandial blood glucose test.
16. Identify test requirements for an oral glucose tolerance test (OGTT).
17. State the restrictions that must be followed by the patient during an OGTT.
18. Explain the purpose of the hemoglobin A_{1c} test.
19. State the hemoglobin A_{1c} level for an individual without diabetes.
20. Identify the ADA guidelines for interpretation of hemoglobin A_{1c} test results
21. List advantages of self-monitoring of blood glucose by diabetic patients.
22. Describe the functions of LDL, HDL, and VLDL.
23. State the desirable ranges for each of the following tests: total cholesterol, LDL cholesterol, and HDL cholesterol.
24. State the patient preparation for a triglycerides test.

Immunologic Testing

25. Explain the purpose of each of the following immunologic tests: hepatitis, HIV, syphilis, rheumatoid factor, antistreptolysin O, C-reactive protein, cold agglutinins, *H. pylori*, and mononucleosis.
26. List the symptoms of infectious mononucleosis.
27. Explain the purpose of the Rh antibody titer test and ABO and Rh blood typing.

PROCEDURES

Collect a specimen for a blood chemistry test for transport to an outside laboratory.

Perform a fasting blood glucose test using a CLIA-waived glucose meter.

Perform a hemoglobin A_{1c} test using a CLIA-waived analyzer.

Perform a CLIA-waived rapid mononucleosis test.

CHAPTER OUTLINE

KEY TERMS

agglutination (ah-gloo-ti-NAY-shun)
antibody (AN-ti-bod-ee)
antigen (AN-ti-jen)
blood chemistry testing
cholesterol
glucose
glycogen (GLIE-koe-jen)
glycosylation
HDL
hemoglobin A_{1c}
hyperglycemia (hie-per-glie-SEE-me-ah)
hypoglycemia (hie-poe-glie-SEE-me-ah)
immunologic testing
insulin
LDL
lipoprotein (lie-poe-PROE-teen)
prediabetes
VLDL

INTRODUCTION TO BLOOD CHEMISTRY AND IMMUNOLOGIC TESTING

Blood chemistry and immunologic tests are frequently ordered by the provider to assist in the diagnosis, treatment, and management of disease. There are certain blood chemistry and immunologic laboratory tests that can be performed in the medical office. Advances in CLIA-waived automated analyzers and test kits designed specifically for use in the medical office have made this possible. CLIA-waived test systems can perform these tests in a short time with accurate test results. This allows the provider to make decisions immediately regarding a patient's health care without having to wait for the results from an outside laboratory.

This chapter is divided into two units. The first unit presents blood chemistry testing and the second unit presents immunologic testing; each unit focuses on CLIA-waived tests and conditions causing abnormal test results.

BLOOD CHEMISTRY TESTING

Blood chemistry testing involves the quantitative measurement of chemical substances or analytes dissolved in the plasma of the blood. An *analyte* is a body substance that is being identified or measured in a laboratory test. There are many different types of blood chemistry tests; the type of test (or tests) the provider orders depends on the patient's clinical diagnosis. Table 33.1 lists common blood chemistry tests, including the purpose of the test, reference range, and conditions that cause abnormal test results.

A blood chemistry panel frequently ordered on patients is the *comprehensive metabolic panel* (CMP). A CMP contains numerous blood chemistry tests that provide information on the kidneys, liver, acid–base balance, blood glucose level, and blood proteins. It is used primarily for the routine health screening of a patient to detect any changes in the body's biologic processes that may be present, although the patient may not have had any symptoms to indicate that these changes have occurred. A CMP is also ordered when the patient's symptoms are so vague that the provider does not have

Table 33.1 Common Blood Chemistry Tests

Name of Test	Purpose of Test	Reference Range	Increased With	Decreased With
Albumin	To monitor and treat liver and kidney disease	3.6–5.1 g/dL	Dehydration	Liver disease Nephrotic syndrome Crohn disease Thyroid disease Heart failure
Alanine aminotransferase (ALT)	To detect liver disease	45 U/L or less	Hepatocellular disease Active cirrhosis Metastatic liver tumor Obstructive jaundice Pancreatitis	
Alkaline phosphatase (ALP)	Assists in diagnosis of liver and bone diseases	25–140 U/L	Liver disease Bone disease Hyperparathyroidism Infectious mononucleosis	Hypophosphatasia Malnutrition Hypothyroidism Chronic nephritis
Aspartate aminotransferase (AST)	To detect tissue damage	40 U/L or less	Myocardial infarction Liver disease Acute pancreatitis Acute hemolytic anemia	Beriberi Uncontrolled diabetes with acidosis
Bilirubin, Total (TB)	To evaluate liver functioning and hemolytic anemia	0.2–1.3 mg/dL	Liver disease Obstruction of bile ducts Hemolytic anemia	
Protein, Total (TP)	To screen for diseases that alter protein balance To assess body hydration	6–8.5 g/dL	Dehydration Chronic infections Acute liver disease Multiple myeloma Lupus erythematosus	Severe hemorrhaging Hodgkin disease Severe liver disease Malabsorption
Blood urea nitrogen (BUN)	To screen for kidney disease To monitor the effectiveness of dialysis	7–25 mg/dL	Kidney disease Urinary obstruction Dehydration	Liver failure Malnutrition Impaired absorption
Calcium (Ca)	To assess parathyroid functioning and calcium metabolism To evaluate malignancies	8.5–10.8 mg/dL	Hypercalcemia Hyperparathyroidism Bone metastases Multiple myeloma Hodgkin disease Addison's disease Hyperthyroidism	Hypocalcemia Hypoparathyroidism Acute pancreatitis Renal failure
Carbon dioxide (CO_2)	To diagnose and treat disorders associated with changes in acid-base balance in the body	20–32 mmol/L	Severe, prolonged vomiting and/or diarrhea Cushing syndrome Metabolic alkalosis	Addison disease Diabetic ketoacidosis Metabolic acidosis Respiratory alkalosis Chronic diarrhea
Chloride (Cl)	Assists in diagnosing disorders of acid-base and water balance	96–109 mmol/L	Dehydration Cushing syndrome Hyperventilation Preeclampsia Anemia	Severe vomiting Severe diarrhea Ulcerative colitis Pyloric obstruction Severe burns Heat exhaustion
Cholesterol (Chol)	To screen for atherosclerosis related to CVD To monitor the effectiveness of lipid-lowering medication.	Less than 200 mg/dL	Atherosclerosis Cardiovascular disease Obstructive jaundice Hypothyroidism Nephrosis	Malabsorption Liver disease Hyperthyroidism Anemia
Creatinine (Creat)	Screening test of kidney functioning	0.6–1.5 mg/dL	Impaired renal function Chronic nephritis Obstruction of urinary tract Muscle disease	Muscular dystrophy

Table 33.1 Common Blood Chemistry Tests—cont'd

Name of Test	Purpose of Test	Reference Range	Increased With	Decreased With
Globulin (Glob)	To identify abnormalities in rate of protein synthesis and removal	2–3.5 g/dL	Brucellosis Chronic infections Rheumatoid arthritis Dehydration Hepatic carcinoma Hodgkin disease	Agammaglobulinemia Severe burns
Glucose	To detect disorders of glucose metabolism	*FBG:* 70–99 mg/dL *OGTT:* Less than 140 mg/dL	*Hyperglycemia* Diabetes	*Hypoglycemia* Excess insulin
Lactate dehydrogenase, 30°C (LD)	Assists in confirming myocardial or pulmonary infarction Differential diagnosis of muscular dystrophy and pernicious anemia	240 U/L or less	Acute myocardial infarction Acute leukemia Muscular dystrophy Pernicious anemia Hemolytic anemia Hepatic disease Extensive cancer	
Phosphorus (P)	To evaluate and interpret calcium levels To detect disorders of endocrine system, bone diseases, and kidney dysfunction	2.5–4.5 mg/dL	Hyperphosphatemia Renal insufficiency Severe nephritis Hypoparathyroidism Hypocalcemia Addison disease	Hypophosphatemia Hyperparathyroidism Rickets and osteomalacia Diabetic coma Hyperinsulinism
Potassium (K)	To diagnose disorders of acid–base and water balance in the body To monitor kidney disease To monitor treatment for high BP	3.5–5.3 mmol/L	Hyperkalemia Renal failure Cell damage Acidosis Addison's disease Internal bleeding	Hypokalemia Diarrhea Pyloric obstruction Starvation Malabsorption Severe vomiting Severe burns Diuretic administration Chronic stress Liver disease with ascites
Sodium (Na)	To detect changes in water and salt balance in the body	135–147 mmol/L	Hypernatremia Dehydration Conn syndrome Primary aldosteronism Coma Cushing disease Diabetes insipidus	Hyponatremia Severe burns Severe diarrhea Addison disease Severe nephritis Pyloric obstruction
Total thyroxine (Total T_4)	To assess thyroid functioning To evaluate thyroid replacement therapy	4.5–12 μg/dL	Hyperthyroidism Graves disease Thyrotoxicosis Thyroiditis	Hypothyroidism Cretinism Goiter Myxedema Hypoproteinemia
Triglycerides (Trig)	To evaluate patients with suspected atherosclerosis	*Desirable:* Less than 150 mg/dL	Liver disease Kidney disease Obesity Hypothyroidism Pancreatitis	Malnutrition Congenital lipoproteinemia Hyperthyroidism
Uric acid (UA)	To evaluate renal failure, gout, and leukemia	*Male:* 3.9–9 mg/dL *Female:* 2.2–7.7 mg/dL	Renal failure Gout Leukemia Severe eclampsia Lymphomas	Patients undergoing treatment with uricosuric drugs

enough concrete evidence to support a clinical diagnosis of a specific organ or disease state. Abnormal CMP test results are usually followed up with more specific tests before a diagnosis is made. Another important use of a CMP is to monitor and manage a variety of diseases and conditions such as kidney disease, liver disease, hypertension, and diabetes

SPECIMEN COLLECTION FOR BLOOD CHEMISTRY TESTS

Most blood chemistry tests are moderate complexity tests and are performed by an outside laboratory. The medical assistant may be required to collect a blood specimen for blood chemistry testing following the information presented in the laboratory test directory of the outside laboratory. The specimen collection and handling requirements for a CMP as presented in a laboratory test directory are outlined in Fig. 33.1.

Blood chemistry tests usually require a serum specimen collected in a SST (serum separator tube). General guidelines for the collection of a serum specimen for transport to an outside laboratory include the following:

1. Collect the blood specimen in a SST (gold or marbled red/gray closure tube). The tube selected should have a capacity of 2½ times the amount of serum required.
2. Completely fill the collection tube to the exhaustion of the vacuum to obtain an adequate amount of serum.
3. Gently invert the tube 5 times immediately after collection to mix the clot activator with the blood specimen.

LABORATORY TEST DIRECTORY Comprehensive Metabolic Panel	
CPT Code:	80053
Synonyms:	CMP
Type of Specimen:	Serum
Amount of Specimen:	2 mL
Collection Container:	SST (send entire tube)
Tests Included:	Albumin, ALT, ALP, AST, total bilirubin, BUN, calcium, carbon dioxide, chloride, creatinine, glucose, potassium, total protein, sodium
Patient Preparation:	Fasting for 8 to 12 hours prior to collection.
Collection and Processing:	1. Collect and label specimen. 2. Gently invert tube 5 times immediately after collection. 3. Place specimen in a vertical position and allow to clot for a minimum of 30 minutes and a maximum of 2 hours. 4. Centrifuge specimen for 10 minutes.
Storage and Transport:	Store at RT or refrigerate until pickup by lab courier.
Specimen Stability:	RT 59° F - 86° F (15° C - 30° C): 72 hours Refrigerated: 36° F - 46° F (2° C - 8° C): 72 hours Frozen: Unacceptable
Causes for Rejection:	Nonfasting specimen Specimen other than serum Improper labeling of specimen Hemolysis
Reference Range:	Values given with laboratory report.
Uses:	To determine a patient's general health status; to monitor a variety of diseases and conditions such as kidney disease, liver disease, hypertension, and diabetes; and to monitor the use of specific medications that may affect kidney or liver functioning.
Limitations:	See individual tests for limitations.
Forms:	Order electronically or print the lab request form and submit with specimen.
Methodology:	See individual tests for methodologies.

Fig. 33.1 Comprehensive metabolic panel (CMP) specimen collection and handling requirements as presented in a laboratory test directory.

4. Place the blood specimen tube in an upright position in a test tube rack for 30 to 45 minutes to permit clot formation of the blood cells and avoid the formation of a fibrin clot in the serum.
5. Centrifuge the specimen for 10 minutes. During centrifugation, the gel in the SST temporarily becomes fluid and moves to the dividing point between the serum and the clotted blood cells, where it re-forms into a solid gel, serving as a physical barrier between the serum and the clot (Fig. 33.2). Inspect the tube carefully to ensure that the gel barrier is firmly attached to the glass wall. The serum can be transported to an outside laboratory in the serum separator tube.
6. Store the specimen at room temperature while awaiting pickup by a laboratory courier. The specimen is stable for 3 days at room temperature.

AUTOMATED BLOOD CHEMISTRY ANALYZERS

Automated blood chemistry analyzers are used to perform blood chemistry tests. The analyzer consists of a reflectance photometer that quantitatively measures the amount of chemical substances, or analytes, in a blood specimen. Specifically, a reflectance photometer measures light intensity to determine the exact amount of an analyte present in a specimen.

Outside laboratories use highly sophisticated automated blood chemistry analyzers for performing blood chemistry tests (Fig. 33.3) which provide fast and reliable test results. CLIA-waived automated analyzers have been developed for performing blood chemistry tests in the POL using a capillary blood specimen from a finger puncture. CLIA-waived analyzers are continually increasing in number as new technology becomes available. Medical offices typically use a combination of a POL and an outside laboratory to fulfill their blood chemistry testing requirements. The remainder

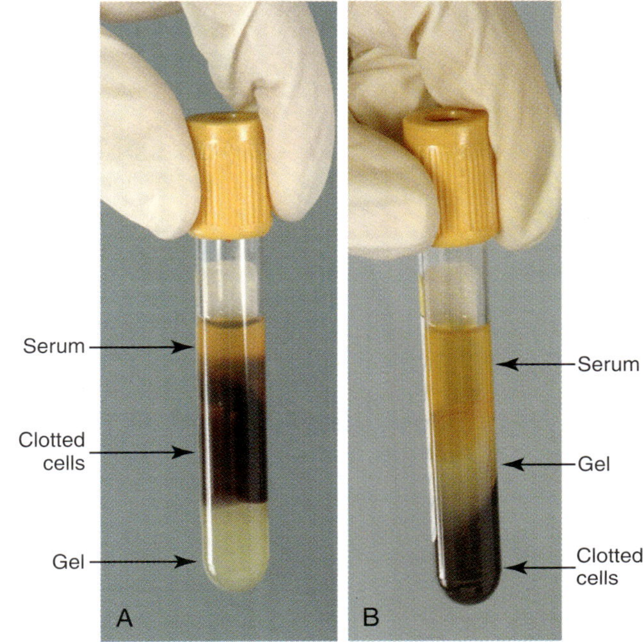

Fig. 33.2 (A) SST before it is centrifuged with the gel barrier at the bottom of the tube. (B) After centrifuging, the gel barrier provides a physical barrier between the serum and the clot. (From Garrels M: *Laboratory and diagnostic testing in ambulatory care*, ed 4, St. Louis, 2019, Elsevier.)

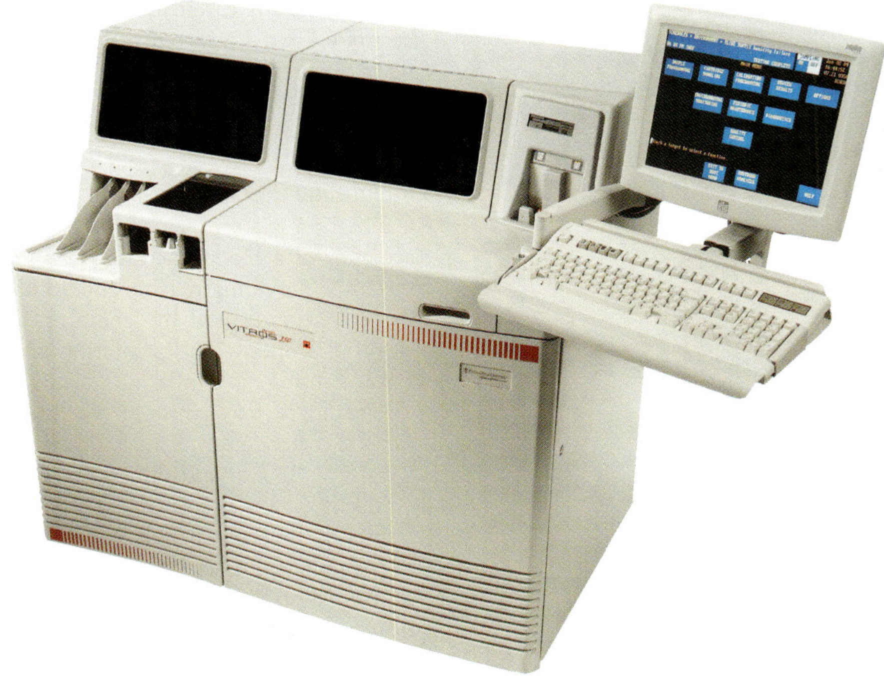

Fig. 33.3 Blood chemistry analyzer used in an outside laboratory. (Courtesy of Holzer Health Systems, Athens, OH.)

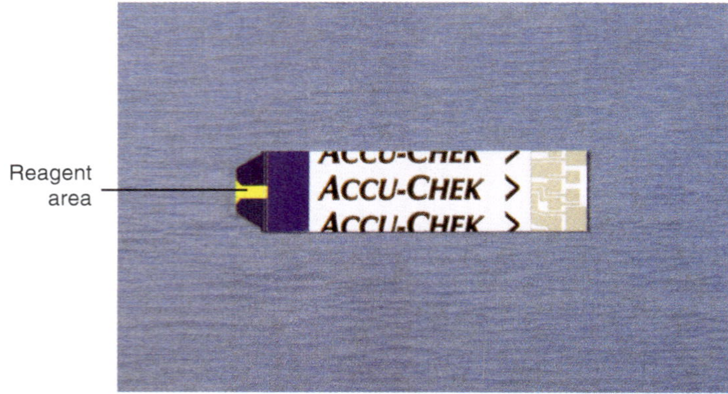

Fig. 33.4 Reagent area of a test strip.

of this section focuses on CLIA-waived analyzers used to perform blood chemistry tests in the medical office.

CLIA-WAIVED AUTOMATED ANALYZERS

CLIA-waived blood chemistry analyzers consist of compact portable devices that permit the testing of a capillary blood specimen in a short time with accurate test results. Test strips, test cassettes, or test cartridges are typically used with these analyzers; the testing device contains a reagent area that contains chemicals which react with the blood specimen (Fig. 33.4). The chemical reaction enables the analyzer to quantitatively measure the amount of an analyte in the blood specimen and display the results as a direct readout (Fig. 33.5).

It is important that the medical assistant become familiar with all aspects of a CLIA-waived blood chemistry analyzer.

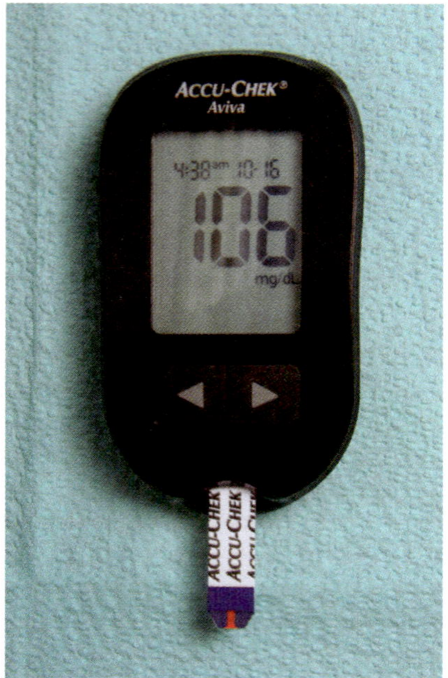

Fig. 33.5 Test results displayed on a CLIA-waived blood chemistry analyzer.

The medical assistant is required to follow the manufacturer's instructions *exactly* for each test procedure. Instructions include information needed to perform quality control procedures, collect and handle the specimen, and test the specimen. Quality control procedures are of particular importance to ensure that the analyzer is functioning properly and that the test results are reliable and accurate. An overview of quality control procedures for CLIA-waived blood chemistry analyzers is presented next while more detailed information on quality control procedures is presented in Chapter 29.

Quality Control

The ultimate goal when performing a blood chemistry test is to ensure that the test accurately measures what it is supposed to measure; this involves practicing and maintaining a quality control program. Quality control consists of methods and means to ensure that test results are reliable and accurate. Two important quality control procedures must be performed routinely when a blood chemistry analyzer is used: these procedures include a calibration procedure and a control procedure.

Calibration Procedure

Calibration is a mechanism used to check the precision and accuracy of a blood chemistry analyzer to determine if the system is providing reliable and accurate results. Calibration detects errors caused by laboratory equipment that is not working properly. The calibration procedure is typically performed using a calibration device known as a *standard.* The standard may come in the form of a calibration strip, cassette, or code key. The standard is inserted into the analyzer (Fig. 33.6A) and the calibration results are printed out or displayed on the screen of the analyzer. The calibration results are then compared with the expected results provided in the package insert accompanying the calibration device or on the calibration device itself (Fig. 33.6B). If the calibration procedure does not perform as expected, patient testing should not be conducted until the problem has been identified and resolved. The frequency of performing the calibration procedure is indicated in the manufacturer's instructions.

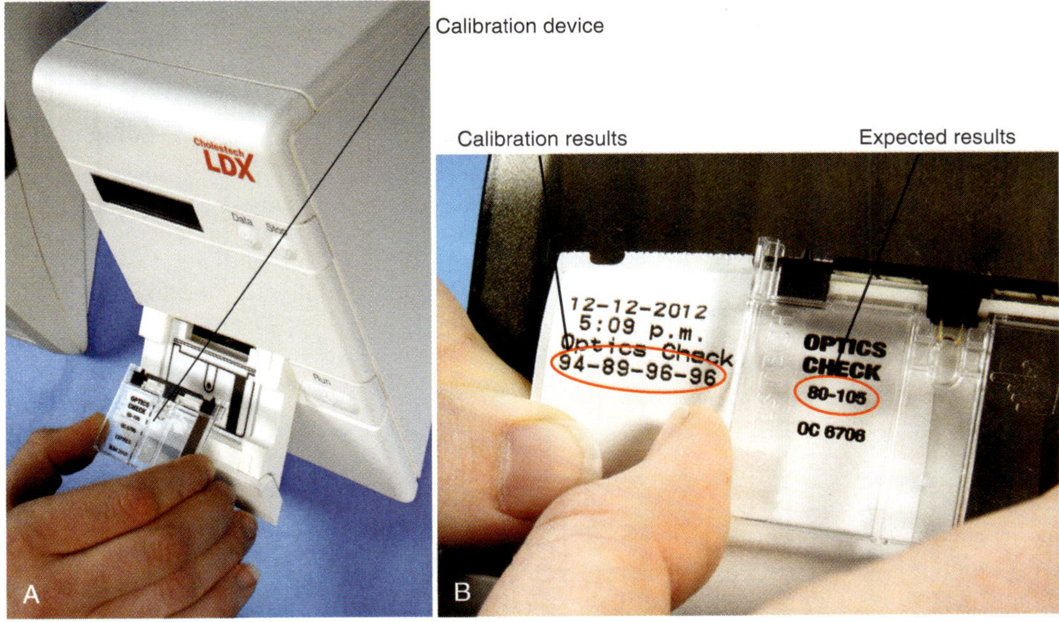

Fig. 33.6 (A) Calibrating a blood chemistry analyzer using a calibration standard. (B) The printed calibration results are compared with the expected results on the calibration standard.

At a minimum, the calibration procedure should be performed when a new lot number of test reagents is put into use.

Some blood chemistry analyzers, such as blood glucose meters, are manufactured with *no-code* technology. This means that the glucose meter does not require manual calibration; the meter automatically calibrates itself when a test strip is inserted into the meter. A no-code glucose meter eliminates having to perform the calibration procedure which saves time and eliminates errors in technique when calibrating the meter.

Control Procedure

A blood chemistry control is a solution with a known value used to monitor a blood chemistry analyzer to ensure reliable and accurate test results. It typically comes with a package insert, which lists expected ranges for control results (Fig. 33.7); however, expected ranges may sometimes be printed on the test reagent container. Controls are used to determine if the test reagents are performing properly and to detect any errors in technique by the individual performing the test.

Generally, two levels of controls must be performed on a blood chemistry analyzer. A *low-level control* (also known as a *Level 1 control*) produces results that fall below the reference range for the test; whereas, a *high-level control* (also known as a *Level 2 control*) produces results that fall above the reference range for the test. The control procedure is performed using the same procedure for performing the test on a patient; however, instead of adding the patient specimen to the test device, the control is added to it (Fig. 33.8). The control results are compared with expected results provided in the package insert or on the test reagent container label (Fig. 33.9).

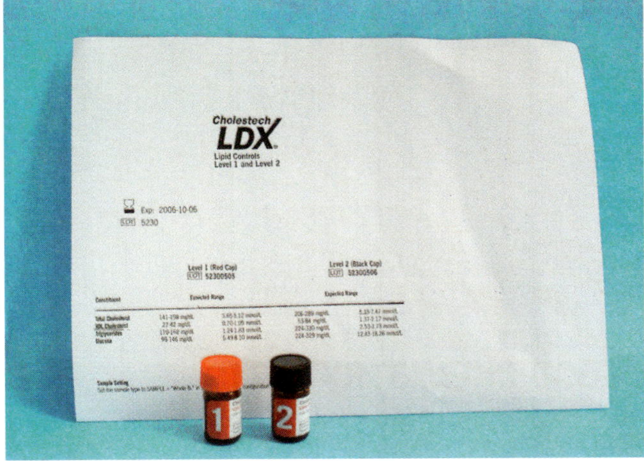

Fig. 33.7 Controls come with a package insert, which lists the expected ranges for control results.

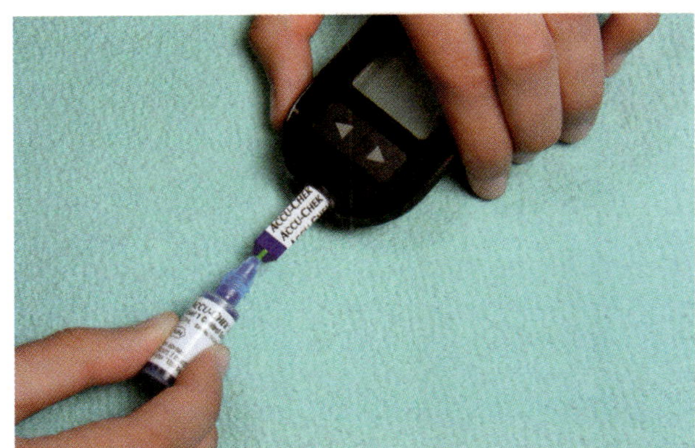

Fig. 33.8 The control solution is added to a test strip.

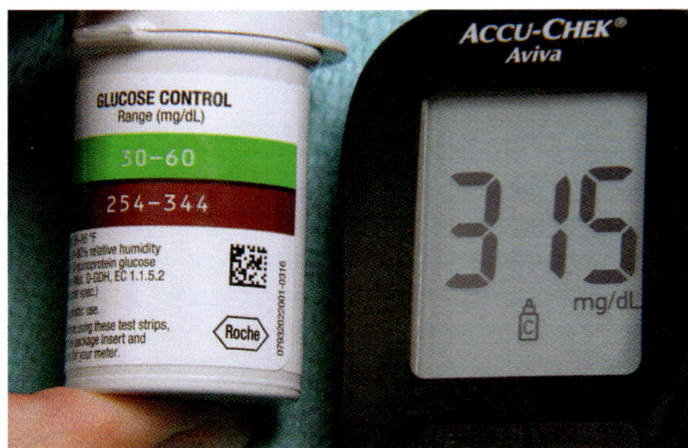

Fig. 33.9 The high-level control result is compared with the expected results.

Failure of a control to produce expected results may be due to the following: expired test components (e.g., test strips, control solutions) improper storage of test components, improper environmental testing conditions, and errors in the technique used to perform the procedure. If the controls do not perform as expected, patient testing should not be conducted until the problem has been identified and resolved.

The frequency of performing the control procedure is specified in the manufacturer's instructions accompanying the test system and usually includes:

- When first receiving the test system
- For periodic routine checking of analyzers and test reagents
- When a new lot number of test reagents is used
- When the test system does not seem to be working properly
- When the test results do not seem to be accurate
- When the test components have been improperly stored
- When an analyzer has been dropped or damaged

BLOOD CHEMISTRY TESTS

Blood chemistry tests quantitatively measure chemical substances dissolved in the plasma of the blood. The most common CLIA-waived blood chemistry tests performed in the medical office include random blood glucose, fasting blood glucose, hemoglobin A_{1c}, and cholesterol which are described in more detail in this section.

BLOOD GLUCOSE

Glucose is the end product of carbohydrate metabolism and is the chief source of energy for the body. Energy is needed for normal body functioning and for maintaining body temperature. The body maintains a constant blood glucose level to ensure a continuous source of energy for the body. Ingested glucose that is not needed for energy can be stored for later use in the form of **glycogen** in muscle and liver tissue. When no more tissue storage is possible, excess glucose is converted to triglycerides (a form of fat) and is stored as adipose tissue.

Function of Insulin

Insulin is a hormone produced and secreted by the beta cells of the pancreas. The pancreas is a gland located behind and below the stomach and is about the size of a hand. Insulin is required for the normal utilization of glucose in the body. Through the process of digestion, carbohydrates are broken down into glucose. Shortly after a meal containing carbohydrates is consumed, glucose levels in the blood begin to increase. This sends a message to the pancreas to secrete insulin. Insulin acts like a key to "unlock" the cells of the body and allow glucose to enter the cells which lowers the glucose level in the blood. Inside the cells, glucose is converted into energy. Glucose is the main source of energy for the body and is needed to carry out normal body functions and to assist in maintaining body temperature. Insulin is also needed for the proper storage of glycogen in liver and muscle cells.

Diabetes

Diabetes is a lifelong condition that occurs when the body is not able to utilize glucose for energy because of a problem with insulin. Diabetes develops when the body produces little or no insulin or when the body cannot use the insulin it does produce (known as *insulin resistance*). According to the American Diabetes Association, more than 38 million Americans have diabetes (1 in 10 individuals); of these, nearly 8.5 million are not yet diagnosed and are unaware that they have diabetes. An additional 96 million people have prediabetes. **Prediabetes** is a condition in which glucose levels are higher than normal, but not high enough to be classified as diabetes. An individual with prediabetes has an increased risk of developing diabetes. According to the American Diabetes Association, 70% of those individuals with prediabetes eventually develop diabetes.

Failure to treat or control diabetes can eventually result in progressive damage to body organs which lead to long-term complications. These include the following: cardiovascular disease, diabetic retinopathy (blindness), hearing impairment, neuropathy (nerve damage), nephropathy (kidney damage), skin conditions, and poor circulation, which can result in amputation of a limb.

Diabetes can be treated but it cannot be cured. The outlook for individuals with diabetes is improving due to better patient education, advances in blood glucose monitoring, and newer methods of insulin delivery that help simplify management of the disease. Today, most individuals with diabetes under good control have life expectancies comparable with those of individuals without diabetes.

Symptoms of Diabetes

Without insulin or proper insulin utilization, glucose cannot enter the cells of the body, causing it to build up in the bloodstream. This results in an abnormally high level of glucose in the blood known as **hyperglycemia**. Although the blood glucose levels are increased, the body is unable to use glucose for energy because it cannot enter the cells to be converted to energy. This results in increased hunger, weight loss, and fatigue. The body attempts to get rid of the excess glucose by expelling it in the urine. To be excreted, the glucose must be diluted in large amounts of water. This results in frequent urination and increased thirst to replace the water being lost. A summary of the symptoms of diabetes include:

- Frequent urination
- Increased thirst
- Unintended weight loss
- Increased hunger
- Nausea and vomiting
- Abdominal pain
- Fatigue
- Blurred vision
- Numbness or tingling in the hands or feet
- Slow healing sores

Types of Diabetes

There are two main types of diabetes: type 1 diabetes and type 2 diabetes. Type 2 diabetes is the most common type; approximately 95% of individuals with diabetes have type 2 diabetes.

Type 1 Diabetes

Type 1 diabetes can occur at any age but is most apt to begin in childhood, adolescence, or early adulthood (before age 30). Type 1 diabetes is an autoimmune disease in which the body produces antibodies that attack and gradually destroy the insulin-producing beta cells of the pancreas. This results in an inability of the body to produce any insulin at all, or it may produce very little insulin. The symptoms are usually severe and occur rapidly—typically over weeks or months. Individuals with type 1 diabetes require insulin injections for the rest of their lives to maintain normal blood glucose levels.

Type 2 Diabetes

Most individuals with diabetes (90% to 95%) have type 2 diabetes. Type 2 diabetes is usually caused by insulin resistance, meaning the pancreas can produce insulin, but the cells are unable to use the insulin resulting in hyperglycemia. In response to the high blood glucose levels, the pancreas responds by making extra insulin to maintain normal blood glucose levels. Over time, the body's insulin resistance becomes worse. Eventually the pancreas becomes exhausted and cannot continue to keep up with the demand for more and more insulin, resulting in high blood glucose levels.

Type 2 diabetes can affect people at any age, but the chance of developing it increases with age, and is more likely to occur in individuals who 45 years of age and older. The biggest risk factor for developing type 2 diabetes is excess body weight. As a result of the recent increase in childhood obesity combined with a sedentary lifestyle, type 2 diabetes is beginning to appear in younger age groups (children, teens, and young adults).

Type 2 diabetes almost always has a slow onset with mild symptoms that appear gradually over a long time (often years). Some individuals have no symptoms at all (except for elevated glucose levels). Because of this, they may be unaware that they have diabetes until a complication from prolonged hyperglycemia occurs, such as a vision problem or foot pain.

Type 2 diabetes is first treated by dietary adjustments, weight reduction, and exercise. These changes can sometimes restore insulin sensitivity, even if the weight loss is modest. Approximately 20% of cases of type 2 diabetes can be managed by lifestyle changes alone. The next step, if necessary, is treatment with non-insulin medications (e.g.; oral hypoglycemics) to lower blood glucose levels. If this treatment becomes ineffective over time, insulin therapy is required to maintain normal or near-normal glucose levels.

Risk Factors for Type 2 Diabetes

The cause of type 2 diabetes is unknown, although certain factors, known as *risk factors*, make a person more prone to developing it. The more risk factors present, the more likely it is that an individual will develop type 2 diabetes. Some of these factors can be controlled, and others cannot.

Risk Factors That Can Be Controlled

1. *Excess body weight.* The risk factor that contributes most to the development of type 2 diabetes is excess body weight. Approximately 90% of individuals with type 2 diabetes are overweight or obese. Being overweight or obese (body mass index of 25 or greater) makes it harder for the body to use insulin. Research shows that people who followed a low-fat, low-calorie diet, lost a moderate amount of weight; and engaged in regular physical activity (five times a week for 30 minutes) sharply reduced their chances of developing type 2 diabetes.
2. *Fat distribution.* Storing fat primarily in the abdomen, rather than the hips and thighs, is a risk factor for diabetes. Men with a waist measurement above 40 inches (101.6 cm) and women with a waist measurement above 35 inches (88.9 cm) are at increased risk for type 2 diabetes.
3. *Smoking.* Smoking makes it harder for the body to regulate insulin levels. High levels of nicotine decrease the effectiveness of insulin, causing the body to require more insulin to regulate the blood glucose level.
4. *Lack of physical activity.* Regular exercise helps the body to use insulin normally, whereas a sedentary lifestyle contributes to insulin resistance.
5. *Prediabetes.* Left untreated, prediabetes often progresses to type 2 diabetes.
6. *High blood pressure, abnormal lipid panel, or both.* The following factors contribute to insulin resistance: a blood pressure greater than 130/80 mmHg, HDL cholesterol less than 40 mg/dL for a man and less than 50 mg/dL for a woman, and a triglycerides level of 150 mg/dL or greater. Decreasing blood pressure can also reduce the risk of cardiovascular complications.

Risk Factors That Cannot Be Controlled

1. *Family history.* The risk of developing type 2 diabetes is increased if a close relative (parent or sibling) has type 2 diabetes.

2. *Gestational diabetes or giving birth to a large infant.* Women who have diabetes during pregnancy or gave birth to an infant weighing more than 9 lb are at greater risk for developing type 2 diabetes.
3. *Age.* Type 2 diabetes is more common in people 45 years and older.
4. *Ethnic group.* The following ethnic groups are more likely to develop type 2 diabetes: African Americans, Hispanic and Latino Americans, Native Americans, Asian Americans, and Pacific Islanders.

Insulin Delivery Methods

Insulin was discovered by Frederick Banting in 1921. Insulin was initially extracted from the pancreases of cows and pigs. In the early 1980s, technology became available to produce human insulin synthetically through genetic engineering.

Insulin dosage is measured in units. The standard and most commonly used strength of insulin in the United States is U-100, which means it has a concentration of 100 units of insulin per milliliter of fluid. There are different types of insulin categorized according to how long it takes the insulin to begin working (onset) and how long it works in the body (duration); they include rapid-acting, intermediate-acting, and long-acting.

As previously discussed, all patients with type 1 diabetes require insulin therapy while approximately 30% of individuals with type 2 diabetes require insulin therapy. Insulin can be administered through several different delivery methods which are described in this section. Regardless of the delivery method, the insulin is delivered into the subcutaneous tissue located just under the skin.

Vial/Syringe

Insulin can be administered through the traditional delivery method using a vial of insulin and an insulin syringe (Fig. 33.10). With the vial/syringe method, the patient must draw up the prescribed amount of insulin into an insulin syringe. The type of syringe used is a U-100 insulin syringe, which is calibrated into 100 units in increments of 2.

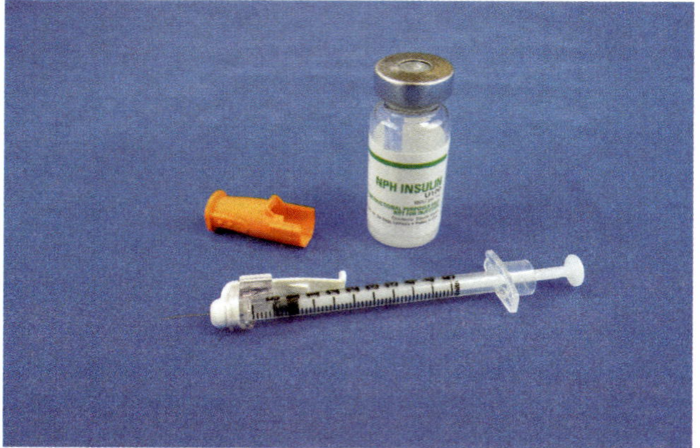

Fig. 33.10 Insulin vial and syringe. (From Melton Stein LN, Hollen CJ: *Concept-based clinical nursing skills: fundamentals to advanced competencies*, ed 2, St. Louis, 2024, Elsevier.)

The insulin is administered through a subcutaneous injection as was previously presented in Chapter 26: *Administration of Medication.*

Insulin Pen

An insulin pen is a newer type of delivery method that is growing in popularity. An insulin pen makes it easier and more convenient for a diabetic patient to administer insulin. Currently, more than 60% of insulin-dependent diabetics now use an insulin pen to administer their insulin.

An insulin pen consists of a cartridge of insulin, a disposable needle, a dial to select the proper dosage of insulin (in units), a dose display window to indicate the number of insulin units selected, an injection button to inject the medication and a pen cap (Fig. 33.11A). Most insulin pens hold 3mL of medication which is equivalent to 300 units of U-100 insulin.

To administer the injection, the patient removes the pen cap and attaches a disposable needle to the needle attachment area. The patient then selects the prescribed dose of insulin using the dial (Fig. 33.11B); the number of units selected is indicated on the dose display window of the pen (Fig. 33.11C). The insulin is then injected into subcutaneous tissue (usually of the lower abdomen or anterior thigh) by depressing and holding the injection button. Following the injection, the needle is discarded into a sharps container.

An insulin pen can be either disposable or reusable. A *disposable insulin pen* contains a prefilled insulin cartridge. After the insulin supply is gone, the entire pen is discarded. A *reusable inulin pen* contains a replaceable insulin cartridge. Once the insulin is gone, the patient removes and discards the empty cartridge and then replaces it with a new cartridge.

Insulin Pump

Insulin can be administered through an insulin pump, also known as a *continuous subcutaneous insulin infusion (CSII) device.* An insulin pump is a small, computerized device that is clipped to a belt or carried in a pocket (Fig. 33.12). The insulin pump is preprogrammed according to the patient's insulin needs; it continually delivers small doses of rapid-acting insulin every few minutes into the subcutaneous tissue of the patient's abdomen. This is accomplished through a length of tubing leading from the pump to a thin cannula placed under the patient's skin. An insulin pump can also be programmed to deliver varying doses of insulin as a patient's need for insulin changes during the day (e.g., before exercise or meals).

Blood Glucose Tests

Measuring the amount of glucose in a blood specimen is one of the most commonly performed blood chemistry tests. It is used to detect abnormalities in carbohydrate metabolism such as those that occur with prediabetes, diabetes, gestational diabetes, hypoglycemia, and liver and adrenocortical dysfunction.

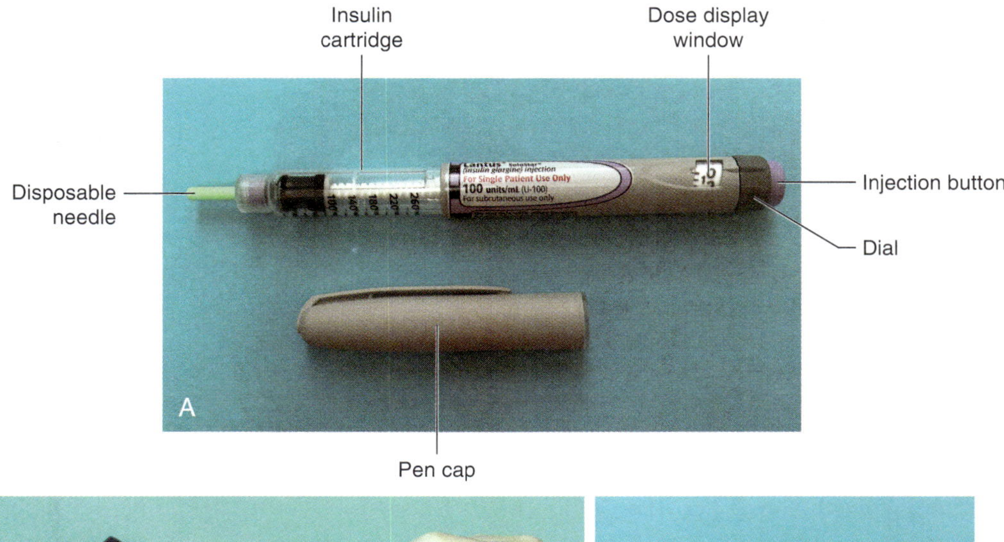

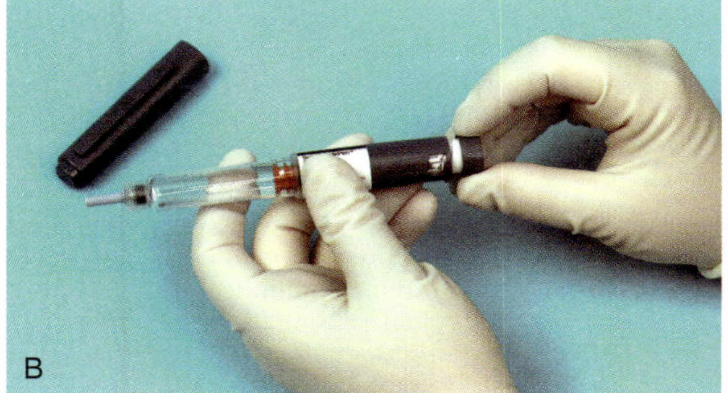

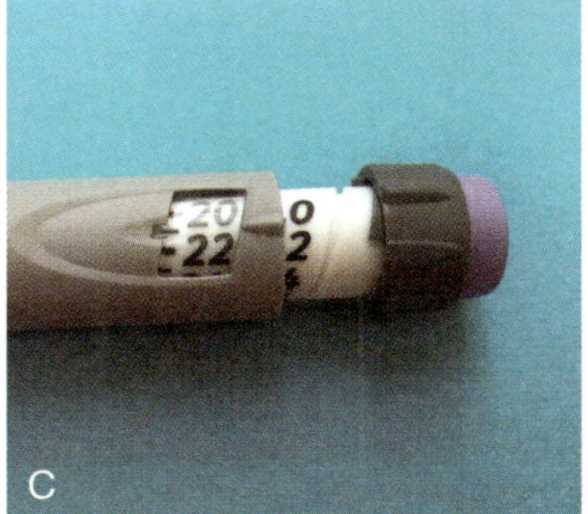

Fig. 33.11 (A) Insulin pen with parts labeled. (B) The patient selects the prescribed dose of insulin using the dial. (C) The number of insulin units selected is indicated in the dose display window. (From Williams PA: *Fundamental concepts and skills for nursing*, ed 6, Philadelphia, 2022, Elsevier Saunders.)

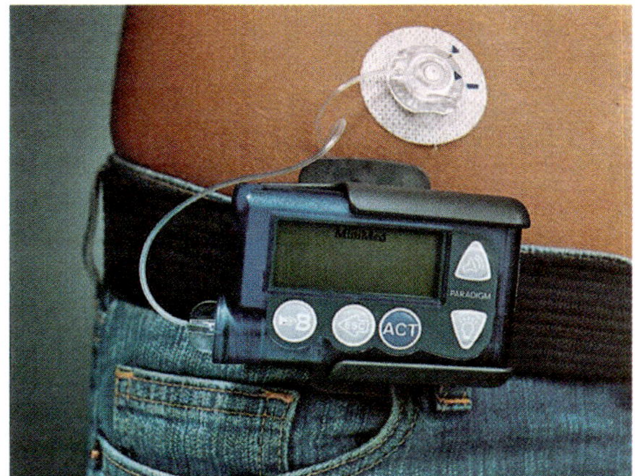

Fig. 33.12 Insulin pump. (From Lewis S: *Medical-surgical nursing*, ed 9, St. Louis, 2014, Mosby.)

Blood glucose is measured by several different types of tests. Each of these tests serves a specific role in diagnosing and evaluating abnormalities in carbohydrate metabolism. Glucose tests include the following: random blood glucose test, fasting blood glucose test, 2-hour postprandial blood glucose test, and the oral glucose tolerance test.

Random Blood Glucose Test

There is no preparation needed for a random blood glucose test. It can be performed at any time of day on a nonfasting patient. In the medical office, this test is performed using a CLIA-waived glucose meter to screen patients for hyperglycemia and hypoglycemia. **Hypoglycemia** refers to an abnormally low level of glucose in the blood. A random blood glucose test result of 200 mg/dL or higher typically means the patient has diabetes; however, more specific tests must be performed to make a diagnosis. Random blood glucose testing is frequently performed by diabetic patients at home as part of their diabetes management plan.

Fasting Blood Glucose Test

Blood glucose is often measured when the patient is in a fasting state. This type of test is known as a *fasting blood glucose* (FBG) test. Fasting requires that a patient not have anything to eat or drink except water for 8 to 12 hours preceding the test. The patient is typically scheduled for the test in the morning to minimize the inconvenience of abstaining from food and fluid. The FBG test provides more specific information as compared with a random blood glucose test.

The FBG test may be performed in the medical office using a CLIA-waived glucose meter to screen patients for

Table 33.2 ADA Guidelines for the Interpretation of FBG Test Results

FBG Test Result	Interpretation
70–99 mg/dL	Normal
100–125 mg/dL	Prediabetes (also termed *impaired fasting glucose*)
126 mg/dL or above	Diabetes (confirm by repeating the FBG test on another day)

prediabetes and diabetes. Guidelines recommended by the American Diabetes Association (ADA) for interpretation of FBG test results are outlined in Table 33.2. A FBG test is routinely performed (along with random glucose testing) by diabetic patients at home to evaluate their progress and regulate treatment. Procedure 33.1 presents the procedure for performing a fasting blood glucose test using a CLIA-waived glucose meter.

Two-Hour Postprandial Blood Glucose Test

The two-hour postprandial blood glucose (2-hour PPBG) test is used to screen for diabetes and may also be performed by diabetic patients at home to regulate their insulin dosage. The patient is required to fast, beginning at midnight preceding the test and continuing until breakfast. For breakfast, the patient must consume a prescribed meal that contains 100 grams of carbohydrate, which consists of orange juice, cereal with sugar, toast, and milk. An alternative to this is the consumption of a 100-gram test-load glucose solution. A blood specimen is collected from the patient exactly 2 hours after consumption of the meal or glucose solution.

In a nondiabetic patient, the glucose level returns to the fasting level within 1½ to 2 hours of glucose consumption, whereas the glucose level in a diabetic patient does not return to the fasting level. A postprandial glucose level of 140 g/dL or higher suggests diabetes and warrants further testing, such as the oral glucose tolerance test or the hemoglobin A_{1c} test.

Putting It All Into Practice

My name is Michelle, and I work for a physician in an internal medicine medical office. My responsibilities include working up patients, running electrocardiograms, applying Holter monitors, and performing pulmonary function tests. I also draw blood and perform CLIA-waived laboratory tests. When performing a venipuncture, you need to make sure all the necessary supplies are on hand and ready for use. Sometimes you may have a tube that has no vacuum in it. In cases like this, it is always better to have a couple of spare tubes on hand. I recently had an experience in which I was collecting a blood specimen for a blood chemistry panel and my SST had no vacuum. Luckily, I had extra tubes within arm's reach, so I did not have to interrupt the procedure to get a new one. I have learned that you can never be too prepared. ■

Oral Glucose Tolerance Test

The oral glucose tolerance test (OGTT) provides more detailed information about the ability of the body to metabolize glucose by assessing the insulin response to a glucose load. The OGTT is used to assist in the diagnosis of prediabetes, diabetes, gestational diabetes, hypoglycemia, and liver and adrenocortical dysfunction. It provides a more thorough analysis of glucose utilization than is provided by the FBG test or the 2-hour PPBG test. The OGTT is usually performed at an outside laboratory; however, the medical assistant is often responsible for providing the patient with instructions regarding this test.

Test Requirements

The patient is required to consume a high-carbohydrate diet, consisting of 150 grams of carbohydrate per day, for 3 days before the OGTT. High carbohydrate foods include bread, pasta, cereal, rice, potatoes, and crackers. The provider will relay to the patient what medication (if any) to discontinue before the test. The patient must be instructed not eat or drink anything except water for 8 to 12 hours before the test.

When the patient arrives at the test site, a blood specimen is drawn from the patient for a FBG test. The patient is then instructed to drink a very sweet solution containing 75 grams of glucose within a 5-minute time frame. At regular intervals (60-, 120-, and 180-minutes), a blood specimen is collected to determine the patient's ability to handle the increased amount of glucose. Each blood specimen is carefully labeled with the exact time of collection. The patient is permitted to eat and drink normally after completion of the test.

It is important that the patient adheres to certain restrictions during the test to ensure accurate test results. Because food and fluid affect blood glucose levels, the patient must not eat or drink anything except small sips of water during the test. Smoking is not permitted during the test because tobacco is a stimulant that increases the blood glucose level. The patient must remain at the test site for 3 to 4 hours to be available for the collection of blood specimens and to minimize activity. Activity affects the test results by using up glucose; the patient should remain relatively inactive during the test. Sitting and reading is an activity that would be recommended.

Side Effects

During the test, the patient may experience some normal side effects, including weakness, a feeling of faintness, and perspiration. These are considered normal reactions of the body to a decrease in the glucose level (hypoglycemia) as insulin is secreted in response to the glucose load. The patient should be reassured that this is a temporary condition. Serious symptoms of severe hypoglycemia that should be reported immediately include headache; pale, cold, and clammy skin; irrational speech or behavior; profuse perspiration; and fainting.

Interpretation of Results

As glucose is absorbed into the bloodstream, the blood glucose level of a nondiabetic individual increases to a peak level of 160 to 180 mg/dL approximately 30 to 60 minutes

Table 33.3 ADA Guidelines for the Interpretation of OGTT Results

OGTT Test Result	Interpretation
Less than 140 mg/dL	Normal
140–199 mg/dL	Prediabetes (also known as *impaired glucose tolerance*)
200 mg/dL or above	Diabetes (confirm by repeating the OGTT test on another day)

after the glucose solution is consumed. The pancreas secretes insulin to compensate for this rise, and the blood glucose returns to the fasting level within 2 hours of ingestion of the glucose solution.

An individual with diabetes does not exhibit the normal use of glucose just described. This is because patients with diabetes are unable to remove glucose from the bloodstream at the same rate as nondiabetic individuals. The blood glucose peaks at a much higher level. In addition, blood glucose levels are above normal throughout the test because of the lack of insulin or the inability of the body to use the insulin it does produce (insulin resistance). Two hours after the glucose solution is consumed, the test results are interpreted according to guidelines set forth by the American Diabetes Association (ADA), as outlined in Table 33.3.

The OGTT is also used to diagnose hypoglycemia. During the OGTT, individuals with hypoglycemia exhibit an abnormally low blood glucose level, beginning at the 2-hour interval and continuing for 4 or 5 hours. Hypoglycemia results from the removal of glucose from the blood at an excessive rate, or from an increased secretion of insulin into the blood. Hypoglycemia can be caused by prediabetes, anorexia, bacterial sepsis, carcinoma of the pancreas, hepatic necrosis, or hypothyroidism.

What Would You Do? What Would You *Not* Do?

Case Study 1

Bianca Diaz previously came to the medical office complaining of symptoms that typically occur with diabetes. A random blood glucose test was performed on Bianca at the medical office and the test results indicated an elevated blood glucose level. The provider ordered an OGTT for Bianca to be performed at an outside laboratory. The instructions for the test were explained to Bianca and she was provided with an information sheet to take home. Bianca returns to the office one week later for her OGTT results. Bianca says that she tried to fast but got extremely hungry while driving to the test site and stopped at McDonald's for a sausage biscuit and orange juice. Bianca says she got quite upset when the test could not be performed requiring her to return to the lab a second time. She demands to know why this test takes so long and why she can't have anything to eat before the test. Bianca also wants to know why she was not allowed to go outside to take a walk and smoke during the test. She says that it's boring to sit so long at the test site and that she's a "nicotine" addict and it's hard to go very long without smoking. Bianca says that she felt weak and perspired a little during the test but did not say anything and wants to know if that was normal. ■

Hemoglobin A_{1c} Test

The hemoglobin A1c test (commonly referred to as the A1c test) is used to determine whether a diabetic patient's blood glucose level is under good control. The A1c test supplies the provider with an assessment of the average amount of glucose in the blood over a 3-month period. The A1c test can also be used to aid in the diagnosis of prediabetes and diabetes, depending on the product's labeling.

When an individual consumes food containing glucose, the glucose is absorbed from the digestive tract and into the circulatory system. Glucose (sugar) has a "sticky" quality to it and thus has a tendency to stick to protein in the body. One of the proteins it attaches to is the protein making up hemoglobin. Hemoglobin is found in red blood cells and functions in transporting oxygen in the body. The process of glucose attaching to hemoglobin is known as **glycosylation**.

When glucose attaches or glycosylates to the protein in hemoglobin, it forms a compound known as **hemoglobin A_{1c}**. Glycosylation occurs in all individuals—hemoglobin A_{1c} is formed in diabetic patients and healthy individuals. The amount of glucose that attaches to hemoglobin is proportional to the amount of glucose in the blood; the more glucose in the blood, the more hemoglobin becomes glycosylated and the higher the A_{1c} level. Individuals with undiagnosed or poorly controlled diabetes have a higher-than-normal blood glucose level, and more hemoglobin A_{1c} forms in these individuals. The percentage of hemoglobin A_{1c} in the blood can be measured by the A_{1c} test. The attachment of glucose to hemoglobin is permanent for the life of the red blood cell (90 to 120 days); because of this, the A_{1c} test result is able to provide an overall picture of the patient's blood glucose level for the past 3 months. CLIA-waived analyzers are available for performing a hemoglobin A_{1c} test in the medical office; an example is the A1CNow (PTS Diagnostics, Whitestown, IN), which is illustrated in Fig. 33.13.

Test Results

The A_{1c} test results are reported as a percentage, the higher the percentage, the higher the blood glucose level. The ADA guidelines for the interpretation of A_{1c} test results are outlined in Table 33.4.

The A_{1c} test is also used to evaluate the effectiveness of a patient's diabetes management plan. The normal A_{1c} level for an individual without diabetes is less than 5.7%. Patients with diabetes usually have a higher A_{1c} level than this. The American Diabetes Association (ADA) strongly recommends that patients with diabetes maintain an A_{1c} level of less than 7%. Table 33.5 shows the correlation between hemoglobin A_{1c} percentages and average blood glucose levels. A change in a patient's diabetes management plan is almost always required if the A_{1c} test result is greater than 8%. Patients with diabetes who keep their A_{1c} levels less than 7% have a much better chance of delaying or preventing diabetic complications than do patients with A_{1c} levels that are 8% or higher.

For stable diabetic patients under good control, the A_{1c} test is typically ordered at least two times a year

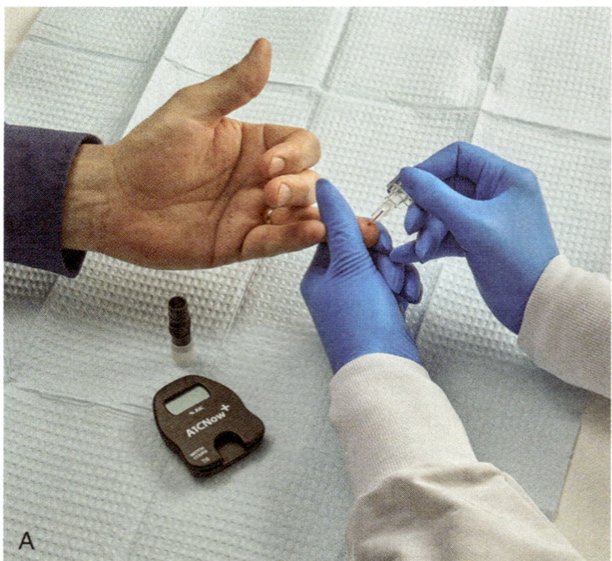

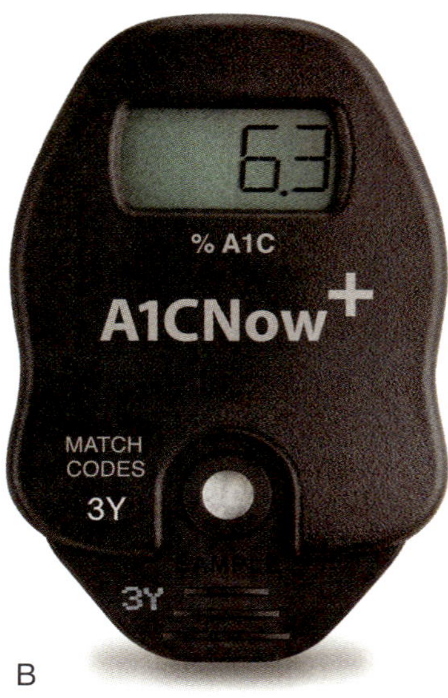

Fig. 33.13 CLIA-waived hemoglobin A1CNow analyzer. (A) Specimen collection for a hemoglobin A_{1c} test. (B) The result on this monitor is 6.3%. (Courtesy of PTS Diagnostics.)

Table 33.4 ADA Guidelines for the Interpretation of Hemoglobin A_{1c} Test Results

A_{1c} Test Result	Interpretation
Less than 5.7%	Normal
5.7% to 6.4%	Prediabetes (also known as *impaired glucose tolerance*)
6.5% or higher	Diabetes

Table 33.5 Comparison of Hemoglobin A_{1c} Percentages with Blood Glucose Levels

Hemoglobin A_{1c} (%)	Average Daily Blood Glucose Level (mg/dL)
5	100
6	126
6.5	140
7	154
7.5	169
8	183
8.5	197
9	212
9.5	226
10	240
10.5	254

(every 6 months). The test is ordered on a more frequent basis for patients who have difficulty maintaining control of their blood glucose levels. The A_{1c} test is also ordered when the provider makes an adjustment to a patient's diabetes management plan to assess the effectiveness of the change in treatment.

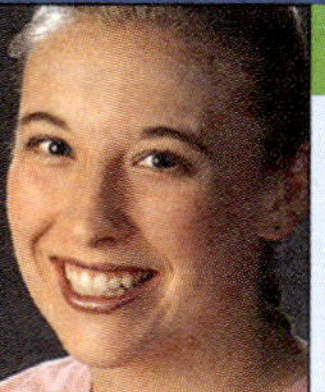

Memories *from* Practicum

Michelle: During my practicum experience, I was assigned to a four-physician pediatric practice. The office was constantly busy with screaming children. As if I were not nervous enough, I was asked to assist in the removal of sutures. When I walked into the room with the physician, beads of sweat began to form on my forehead. A child was laying on the examining table—a little boy no more than 7 years old. He was there to have sutures removed from a recent surgery. The sutures had been tied very well, and it was difficult for the physician to remove them. The little boy lay there with tears streaming down his cheeks. I reassured him and talked to him, and his tears began to subside. "A few more minutes and it will be all over," I told him. And within those next few minutes, the physician cut the last suture. The little boy eagerly hopped down off the examining table and gave me a big hug. I learned that day how a little reassurance can make everyone involved feel better. ■

What Would You Do? What Would You *Not* Do?

Case Study 2

Jackson Williams has recently been diagnosed with type 1 diabetes and is taking insulin. He has come to the office for an FBG test. A finger puncture is performed to collect the specimen and a glucose meter is used to test the specimen. Jackson has been performing this test on himself at home now for 2 weeks and wants to know whether he can stick his own finger and have someone watch him to make sure he is doing it correctly. Jackson says that he's been having a few problems giving himself his insulin injections. He says that he has been getting some very large air bubbles in his syringe when he draws up the insulin. He says he's been having trouble getting them out and wants to know how important that is. Jackson says he is on a limited income and wants to know whether he could use his needle and syringe for more than one injection. ■

Management of Diabetes

It is important that individuals with diabetes manage their condition effectively. This is best accomplished by keeping blood glucose levels as close to normal as possible. Diabetic patients who maintain good blood glucose control generally experience fewer symptoms and delay or prevent long-term complications of the disease leading to a longer and healthier life.

Two methods are used for the management of diabetes: self-monitoring of blood glucose and the hemoglobin A_{1c} test. Self-monitoring of blood glucose (SMBG), which diabetic patients perform at home using a glucose meter, measures day-to-day fluctuations in blood glucose levels. The hemoglobin A_{1c} test must be ordered by the provider and provides an average or overall picture of the patient's blood glucose levels over time. These testing methods assist the patient and the provider in determining whether the diabetes management plan is working or whether it needs to be adjusted. SMBG is described in more detail as follows.

Self-Monitoring of Blood Glucose

Individuals with diabetes cannot usually tell by the way they feel whether or not their blood glucose levels are within normal range. The only way for them to know for certain is by self-monitoring of blood glucose. SMBG not only provides diabetic patients with feedback for maintaining normal blood glucose levels, but it also assists them in anticipating and treating day-to-day, or even hour-to-hour, fluctuations in glucose levels brought on by food, exercise, stress, and illness.

Insulin-dependent diabetic patients must monitor their blood glucose levels each day. Based on the results of SMBG, decisions can be made regarding insulin and dietary adjustments that may be necessary to maintain normal glucose levels and to avoid the extremes of hypoglycemia and hyperglycemia. Satisfactory control of the blood glucose level on a day-to-day basis through SMBG reduces symptoms of the disease and helps delay or prevent long-term complications that can occur with diabetes.

Frequency of Monitoring

The frequency of blood glucose monitoring is determined by a patient's provider and depends on the following factors: the severity of the diabetes, type of treatment, diet, activity level, and special conditions such as pregnancy. Ideally, the blood glucose level for an insulin-dependent diabetic patient should be monitored 4 times a day: in the morning (after an 8-hour fast), before lunch, before dinner, and at bedtime. The blood glucose level should also be monitored if the patient is experiencing symptoms indicative of hyperglycemia or hypoglycemia. The FBG measurement (obtained in the morning) is the best overall indicator of control, and the other glucose determinations provide guidance for adjusting insulin dosage, diet, and exercise.

Glucose Monitoring Devices

Blood glucose levels can be monitored by a patient with diabetes with a glucose meter or a continuous glucose monitor (CGM).

- *Glucose Meter:* A glucose meter is a small, portable, battery-operated device that quantitatively measures the blood glucose level in a capillary blood specimen. The medical assistant may be responsible for instructing the patient in the procedure for using a glucose meter, which is outlined in Procedure 33.1.
- *Continuous glucose monitor:* A CGM measures a patient's blood glucose level continuously throughout the day and night using a small wire catheter known as a *sensor* inserted under the patient's skin. CGM brand names include the Dexcom system (Dexcom, Inc., San Diego, CA) and the FreeStyle Libre system (Abbott, Santa Clara, CA). The CGM provides real-time measurements and reduces the need for a finger puncture. The CGM also sends an alert to the patient if the blood glucose level becomes high or low. Depending on the CGM brand, the sensor can last up to 2 weeks before needing to be replaced. The glucose readings are viewed by the patient on a smartphone app or a handheld receiver (Fig. 33.14).

Target Blood Glucose Levels

Target blood glucose levels for a patient with diabetes are determined by a patient's provider. The ADA recommends the following general guidelines for target blood glucose levels:

- Before meals and snacks: 80 to 130 mg/dL
- 1 to 2 hours after meals: Less than 180 mg/dL

Diabetic patients should maintain a cumulative record of their daily SMBG monitoring results for periodic review by the provider. This record assists the provider in making decisions regarding the patient's diabetes management plan. Most glucose meters have a built-in memory system

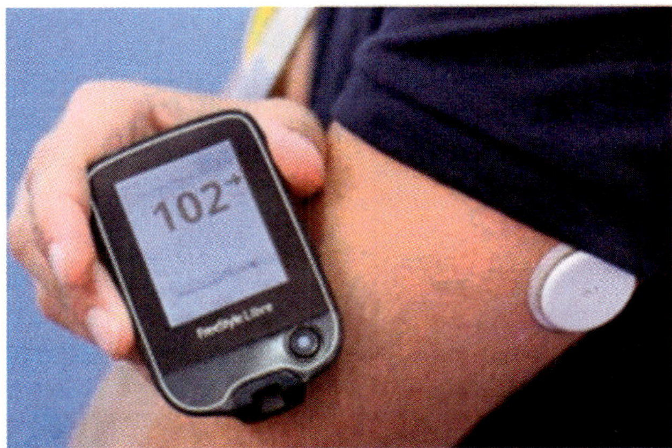

Fig. 33.14 Continuous glucose monitor. (FreeStyle Libre is a trademark of Abbott or its related companies. Reproduced with permission of Abbott, © 2024. All rights reserved.)

that stores test results along with the time and date and can transfer this data electronically to a computer. This provides for the tracking of blood glucose fluctuations over time.

Advantages

Research shows that SMBG is the most effective way for a diabetic patient to maintain normal blood glucose levels. Advantages of SMBG include the following:

1. *Delay or prevention of long-term complications.* High blood glucose levels (greater than 180 mg/dL) for a long period of time can cause progressive damage to the body organs. SMBG can delay or prevent long-term complications associated with diabetes.
2. *Prevention of hypoglycemia.* Hypoglycemia is a short-term complication of diabetes caused by too much insulin in the body which can be due to the administration of too much insulin, skipping meals, and unexpected or unusual exercise. The symptoms of hypoglycemia occur rapidly, usually over 5 to 20 minutes after the blood glucose level begins to decrease. Symptoms begin with sweating or cold, clammy skin, shakiness, dizziness, headache, and tachycardia If not treated, the blood glucose level continues to drop and the patient may experience confusion, irritability, sleepiness, anxiety, problems with speaking (e.g., slurring words), and problems with vision (e.g., double-vision and blurred vision). Without treatment, serious life-threatening symptoms may occur which include seizures, loss of consciousness, and coma. Because the brain requires a constant supply of glucose for proper functioning, permanent brain damage or death can result from severe hypoglycemia (also known as insulin shock). Refer to Chapter 37 for a more thorough discussion of diabetic emergencies and the treatment required.
3. *Convenience of monitoring.* Patients are able to monitor their blood at any time of the day without a laboratory order from the provider. This allows patients to check their blood glucose level when a side effect common to diabetes occurs, such as hypoglycemia. In these situations, treatment can be instituted immediately to prevent the problem from getting worse.
4. *Greater involvement in self-management decisions.* The patient is able to become more involved in self-management decisions regarding insulin dosage, meal planning, and physical activity. More reliable decisions regarding insulin needs can be made during situations that affect the blood glucose level, such as illness, emotional stress, increased physical activity, and hypoglycemia. Initially some patients may lack confidence in making insulin and dietary adjustments based on the blood glucose results. The medical assistant should provide encouragement and emphasize the benefits to be derived in terms of improved regulation of the blood glucose level.

CHOLESTEROL TEST

Cholesterol is a white, waxy, fat-like substance (lipid) that is essential for the normal functioning of the body. It is an important component of all cell membranes in the body and is used in the production of essential hormones and bile. Most of the cholesterol circulating in the blood is manufactured by the liver; however, a small portion of it comes from an individual's diet and is known as *dietary cholesterol.* Dietary cholesterol is found only in animal products, such as organ meats, egg yolk, and dairy products.

A high blood cholesterol level means an excessive amount of cholesterol is present in the blood. An individual's cholesterol level is determined by their genetic makeup and by the amounts of saturated fat and dietary cholesterol consumed. High blood cholesterol may cause fatty deposits, or plaque, to build up on the walls of the arteries, a condition known as *atherosclerosis.* As the atherosclerosis progresses, the arteries become more occluded, which eventually could lead to a heart attack or stroke. Because of this, high blood cholesterol is considered a risk factor for cardiovascular disease (CVD). Refer to *Highlight on Cardiovascular Disease* for more information on CVD.

Lipoproteins

A **lipoprotein** is a complex molecule consisting of protein that combines with and transports lipids (cholesterol and triglycerides) in the plasma of the blood. Lipids are not soluble in the plasma of the blood and therefore must picked up and be transported by lipoproteins. There are different types of lipoproteins that transport lipids in the circulatory system; these include low-density lipoproteins (LDL), high-density lipoproteins (HDL), and very-low-density lipoproteins (VLDL).

LDL picks up cholesterol from ingested fats and the liver and carries it in the plasma of the blood for use by the body's cells. When there is too much LDL cholesterol in the blood, it combines with other substances to form plaque deposits on the walls of arteries resulting in atherosclerosis. Atherosclerosis is a risk factor for CVD, and because of this, LDL cholesterol is often referred to as "bad" cholesterol.

HDL picks up excess cholesterol from cells and carries it to the liver for removal by the body. Because HDL is able to remove excess cholesterol from the walls of the arteries, it is protective and beneficial to the body and is often called "good" cholesterol. A high HDL cholesterol level has been shown to reduce the risk of CVD whereas a low level of HDL cholesterol is a risk factor for CVD.

VLDL picks up triglycerides and delivers them to the cells so that they cane be used for energy by the body or stored for later use. VLDL cholesterol is considered a "bad" form of cholesterol. This is because a high level of VLDL contributes to the formation of plaque deposits on the walls of the arteries (atherosclerosis) which is a risk factor for CVD.

HIGHLIGHT on Cardiovascular Disease

The cardiovascular or circulatory system supplies the body with blood and consists of the heart, arteries, veins, and capillaries. *Cardiovascular disease (CVD)* is a general term used to refer to a variety of conditions that affect the heart and blood vessels and interfere with the flow of blood to the heart. CVD is the leading cause of death in the United States for both men and women.

Types of CVD

Types of cardiovascular disease include the following:

- ***Coronary artery disease (CAD):*** A condition in which there is a build-up of plaque in the arteries supplying blood to the heart which narrows the lumen of the arteries and reduces the flow of blood to the heart.
- ***High blood pressure:*** A condition in which there is an increased force of circulating blood against the walls of blood vessels which damages them and increases the risk of a heart attack or heart failure, stroke, or aneurysm.
- ***Heart attack:*** A condition in which there is a sudden blockage of the blood flow to a part of the heart. If the blood flow is cut off completely, the muscle tissue in that part of the heart dies.
- ***Stroke:*** A condition in which the blood supply to a part of the brain is cut off which could result in brain damage and possibly death.
- ***Heart failure:*** A condition in which the heart cannot pump as well as it should due to weakened heart muscle. It may be due to an injury to the heart muscle (e.g., uncontrolled high blood pressure), a heart attack, or a heart valve that does not work properly.
- ***Congenital heart disease:*** A condition in which the heart does not function properly because the heart did not develop normally before birth.
- ***Rheumatic heart disease:*** A condition in which the heart valves have been permanently damaged by rheumatic fever.
- ***Cardiomyopathy:*** A condition in which the heart enlarges and is unable to pump blood efficiently.
- ***Aortic aneurysm:*** A condition in which the aorta becomes weakened and bulges outwards. It may burst and cause life-threatening bleeding.
- ***Cardiac arrhythmias:*** Abnormal heart rhythms which may prevent the heart from pumping enough blood to meet the body's needs.
- ***Heart valve disease:*** A condition in which one or more of the heart valves does not work properly interfering with the flow of blood through the heart.
- ***Peripheral artery disease:*** The build-up of plaque in the arteries supplying blood to the limbs (usually the legs) which interferes with the flow of blood to the limbs.
- ***Venous thrombosis:*** A condition in which a clot forms in a vein which interferes with the flow of blood. If a clot forms in the leg (DVT), part of the clot may break off and cause a pulmonary embolism.

CVD Risk Factors

Not everyone is equal when it comes to CVD. Some individuals have a much higher risk of developing CVD than others. The following are risk factors for CVD:

- High total blood cholesterol (200 mg/dL or higher)
- High blood pressure
- Cigarette smoking
- Atherosclerosis
- Family history of CVD
- Unhealthy diet
- Lack of physical activity
- Diabetes
- Being overweight or obese: High LDL cholesterol (130 mg/dL or higher)
- High LDL cholesterol (130 mg/dL or higher)
- Low HDL cholesterol (less than 40 mg/dL for men and 50 mg/dL for women): High VLDL level (30 mg/dL or higher)
- High VLDL level (30 mg/dL or higher)
- Elevated triglycerides level (150 mg/dL or higher)
- Being a man older than 45 years
- Being a woman older than 55 years or postmenopausal

Some of these risk factors can be modified; others, such as age, gender, and a family history of CVD, cannot be modified or controlled. Each person's overall risk of CVD must be assessed individually by the provider, based on the type and number of risk factors present. A 47-year-old man with a total blood cholesterol level of 220 mg/dL who smokes a pack of cigarettes a day and is overweight is at greater risk than a 28-year-old man who has a normal weight, does not smoke, and exercises regularly but has a total blood cholesterol level of 250 mg/dL.

Coronary Artery Disease

The most common type of CVD in the U.S. is coronary artery disease (CAD) which is also known as coronary heart disease. Coronary artery disease is due to atherosclerosis of the coronary arteries, which are the blood vessels that supply the heart with oxygen. *Atherosclerosis* of the coronary arteries is a condition in which fibrous plaques of fatty deposits and cholesterol build up on the inner walls of the coronary arteries. This causes narrowing and partial blockage of the lumen of these arteries, along with hardening of the arterial wall. CAD results in a reduction of oxygenated blood flow to the heart muscle. Despite the narrowing, enough oxygen may still reach the heart muscle for normal needs. More oxygen is needed, however, when situations occur that increase the workload of the heart, such as physical activity, emotional stress, a heavy meal, and exposure to cold weather. If the coronary arteries cannot deliver enough oxygen to the heart muscle during these times of increased need, angina pectoris may result. Angina pectoris occurs when the muscle tissue of the heart does not receive enough oxygenated blood, resulting in discomfort or pain under the sternum. Severe and prolonged angina pain generally suggests a myocardial infarction (heart attack) caused by complete blockage of the coronary arteries and requires immediate medical attention.

Continued

HIGHLIGHT on Cardiovascular Disease—cont'd

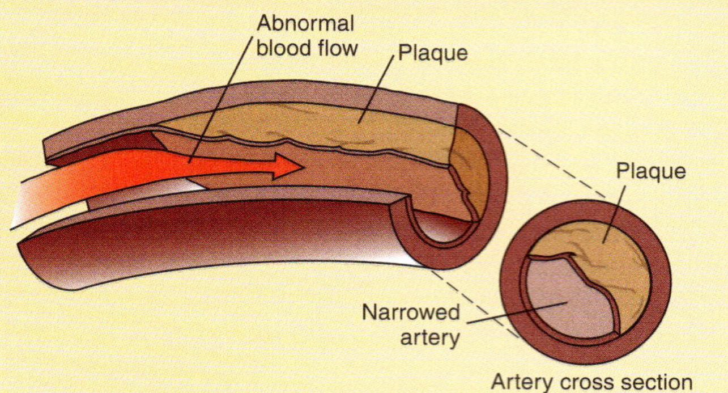

Atherosclerosis. (From Workman ML, LaCharity L: *Understanding pharmacology essentials for medication safety*, ed 2, St. Louis, 2018, Elsevier.)

Prevention of CVD

It is estimated that up to 90% of cases of CVD can be prevented by following a healthy lifestyle. This includes a healthy diet, maintaining a healthy weight, quitting smoking, limiting alcohol consumption, and exercising regularly. Individuals who have a particularly high risk of developing CVD may be prescribed medication to reduce their risk. Depending on the patient's health status, they may be prescribed cholesterol-lowering medication or antihypertensive medication. ■

Cholesterol Testing

The American Heart Association recommends that adults older than 20 years of age have a cholesterol test every 4 to 6 years to assist in determining an individual's risk for CVD. Because an elevated cholesterol level does not have symptoms, the only way to know for sure if an individual has high blood cholesterol is to get tested.

The recommended cholesterol screening test is a lipid panel which includes a determination of the following: total cholesterol, triglycerides, HDL cholesterol, LDL cholesterol, VLDL, and the cholesterol/HDL ratio. *Total cholesterol* is a combined measurement of the LDL cholesterol and HDL cholesterol in the blood. The *cholesterol/HDL ratio* is the ratio of total cholesterol to HDL cholesterol and is obtained by dividing the total cholesterol level by the HDL cholesterol level. This ratio provides information regarding heart health and helps determine an individual's risk of developing heart disease. The LDL cholesterol level is usually determined as a calculation from the triglycerides and HDL cholesterol levels.

A lipid panel is often performed by an outside laboratory and the medical assistant may be responsible for collecting the blood specimen for transport to the laboratory. Most providers prefer that the patient fast for a lipid panel since the triglycerides test is affected by the consumption of food and beverages. CLIA-waived analyzers are available for performing cholesterol testing in the medical office; an example is the Cholestech LDX System (Cholestech Corporation, Hayward, CA) which can perform a lipid panel as well as a glucose test (Fig. 33.15). It is important to follow the manufacturer's instructions *exactly* for performing the test. Quality control procedures are of particular importance to ensure that the analyzer is functioning properly, and that the test results are reliable and accurate.

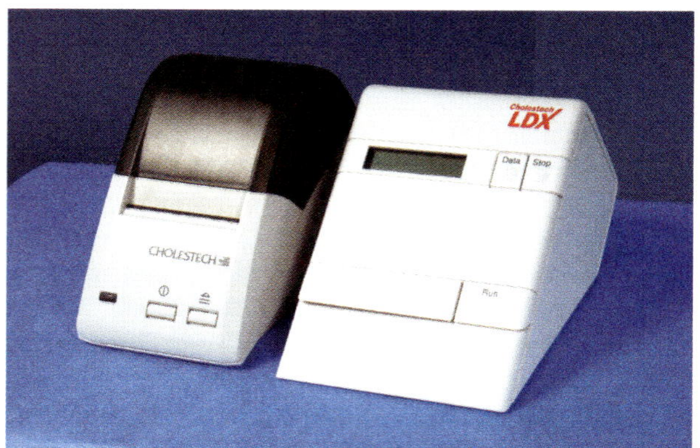

Fig. 33.15 Cholestech LDX Cholesterol System.

Table 33.6 Interpretation of Cholesterol Test Results

Total Cholesterol Test Result (mg/dL)	Interpretation
Less than 200	Desirable
200–239	Borderline high
240 or above	High
LDL Cholesterol Test Result (mg/dL)	**Interpretation**
Less than 100	Optimal
100–129	Near optimal
130–159	Borderline high
160–189	High
190 or above	Very high
HDL Cholesterol Test Result (mg/dL)	**Interpretation**
60 or above	Optimal
Men: 40–50 Women: 50–60	Desirable
Men: Less than 40 Women: Less than 50	Increased risk for CVD

Interpretation of Results

The results of a lipid panel assist in determining the patient's risk for CVD. The interpretation of these results is outlined in Table 33.6. A total cholesterol test result of less than 200 mg/dL and an LDL cholesterol test result of less than 100 mg/dL are desirable. Individuals in the high category for total cholesterol and LDL cholesterol are at increased risk for CVD, and individuals in the borderline high category are at increased risk if they have other CVD risk factors, such as being overweight or smoking. According to the American Heart

Association, an HDL cholesterol level less than 40 mg/dL for men and less than 50 mg/dL for women is considered a risk factor for CVD. An HDL cholesterol level of 60 mg/dL or higher is considered optimal and provides some protection against CVD. An optimal level for VLDL is less than 30 mg/dL. A desirable cholesterol/HDL ratio is below 5.0 and an optimal ratio is below 3.5. A ratio of 5 or more is considered a risk factor for CVD. Refer to Fig. 33.16 for a lipid panel laboratory report.

What Would You Do? What Would You *Not* Do?

Case Study 3

Karen Scrimshaw is at the office. She is 20 years old and is mildly obese. Karen had her cholesterol tested at a health fair, and it was 325. The physician orders a CBC, lipid panel, and thyroid panel on Karen and tells her to return in 1 week for a follow-up visit to discuss the test results. Karen is very concerned about her cholesterol. She says that she had a candy bar and some potato chips before going to the health fair and wants to know whether that could have caused her cholesterol to be so high. She also wants to know the accuracy of machines that are used at health fairs. Karen says that if she has to go on cholesterol medication, it would be hard to decide between Lipitor and Crestor. She says she has seen them advertised on television, and they both seem pretty good to her. ■

TRIGLYCERIDES TEST

Triglycerides are the chemical form in which most fat exists in food, as well as in the body. Triglycerides are derived from two sources. The first is synthesis by the body. Ingested glucose that is not needed for energy can be stored in the form of *glycogen* in muscle and liver tissue for later use. When no more tissue storage is possible, most of the excess glucose is synthesized by the liver into triglycerides and stored as adipose tissue. Excess ingested protein is also synthesized by the liver into triglycerides and stored as adipose tissue. The second source of triglycerides is food. Excess triglycerides consumed by eating foods containing fat (butter, cream, bacon) are also stored as adipose tissue.

Some of the triglycerides in the body are not stored as adipose tissue, but remain in the bloodstream, specifically in the plasma. Triglycerides in the plasma are carried by VLDL to the cells of the body. In normal amounts, triglycerides are essential to good health, serving as a major source of energy for the body.

An excess of blood triglycerides places an individual at increased risk for CVD, particularly when the LDL cholesterol is high, and the HDL cholesterol is low. Triglycerides levels in the blood are measured as part of a lipid panel. The interpretation of triglycerides test results is outlined in Table 33.7. Conditions that result in elevated blood triglycerides levels include obesity, type 2 diabetes, being physically inactive,

LABORATORY REPORT Lipid Panel					
Patient Elsie Mendelssohn 2963 Flint Dr. Clearwater, FL 33759 PH:740-541-3575	ID #: 336879 DOB: 4/28/1970 Age: 66 Gender: F	**Ordered by** Thomas Murphy, MD Pinellas Medical Office 3477 Arrowhead Ave Clearwater, FL 33759		**Results provided by** Medical Center Laboratory 33 West Main St Clearwater, FL 33759	
Specimen Coll. Date	11/25/20XX	Fasting/Nonfasting		Fasting	
Specimen Coll. Time	08:00 am	Accession Number		3380837	
Specimen Received Date/Time	11/25/20XX 05:30 pm	Lab ID Number		773978	
Results Reported Date/Time	11/26/20XX 10:00 am	Test(s) Ordered		CPT: 7600 Lipid Panel	
Test		**Result**	**Reference Range**	**Units**	**Flag**
Cholesterol, Total		**230**	**<200**	**mg/dL**	**H**
HDL cholesterol		64	≥50	mg/dL	
Triglycerides		98	<150	mg/dL	
LDL Cholesterol (Calculated)		**130**	**<100**	**mg/dL**	**H**
VLDL		24	<30	mg/dL	
Cholesterol/HDL ratio		3.6	<5.0		

Fig. 33.16 Lipid panel laboratory report.

Table 33.7 Interpretation of Triglycerides Test Results

Triglycerides Test Result (mg/dL)	Interpretation
Less than 150 mg/dL	Normal
150 to 199 mg/dL	Borderline high
200 to 499 mg/dL	High
500 mg/dL or higher	Very high

excessive alcohol consumption, smoking, hypothyroidism, kidney disease, and liver disease.

BLOOD UREA NITROGEN TEST

The blood urea nitrogen (BUN) test is a kidney function test. Urea is the end product of protein metabolism and is normally present in the blood. Certain kidney diseases may interfere with the ability of the body to excrete the urea properly, causing an increased level of urea in the blood. See Table 33.1, presented earlier, for a list of specific conditions that cause abnormal BUN test results.

IMMUNOLOGIC TESTING

Immunologic testing uses antigen-antibody reactions to determine the presence of a specific substance in the body (e.g., RA factor) or to assist in the diagnosis of an infectious disease (e.g., mononucleosis). An **antigen** is a substance that is capable of stimulating the formation of antibodies in an individual. Antigens may consist of protein, glycoprotein, complex polysaccharides, or nucleic acid. Specific examples of antigens include bacteria and viruses, bacterial toxins, and allergens. An **antibody** is a substance that is capable of combining with an antigen, resulting in an antigen-antibody reaction.

IMMUNOLOGIC TESTS

Specific examples of immunologic tests are described next.

Hepatitis Tests

Hepatitis tests are performed to detect viral hepatitis. There are five types of viral hepatitis—A, B, C, D, and E. Hepatitis testing not only detects the presence of viral hepatitis; it also determines the type of hepatitis present.

HIV Test

The enzyme immune assay (EIA) test and the enzyme-linked immunosorbent assay (ELISA) test are used as screening tests for the presence of human immunodeficiency virus (HIV). CLIA-waived rapid screening test kits are also available to detect the presence of antibodies to HIV; brand names include Uni-Gold Recombigen HIV (Trinity Biotech, Bray, Ireland), and OraQuick Rapid HIV test (OraSure Technologies, Bethlehem, PA). Because of the possibility of a false-positive result, a second screening test is always performed if a blood specimen tests positive. If the second test also is positive, a more specific antigen/antibody test or a nuclei acid test (NAT) is performed by an outside laboratory to confirm the results.

A negative HIV test is not conclusive for the absence of HIV infection. If an individual has recently been infected with HIV, the antibodies may not have had time to develop. It generally takes 2 to 12 weeks (but possibly as long as 6 months) for the HIV antibodies to appear in the blood.

Syphilis Test

Syphilis is a sexually transmitted disease (STD) caused by the microorganism *Treponema pallidum.* The most common tests used to detect the presence of syphilis are the Venereal Disease Research Laboratories (VDRL) test and the rapid plasma reagin (RPR) test. Test results are reported as nonreactive, weakly reactive, or reactive. Weakly reactive and reactive results are considered positive for the presence of syphilis antibodies in the blood. These tests are screening tests, and a positive result warrants more specific tests to arrive at a diagnosis of syphilis.

Rheumatoid Factor Test

Rheumatoid arthritis is a chronic inflammatory disease that affects the joints of the body. The blood of patients with rheumatoid arthritis contains a type of antibody called *rheumatoid factor* (RF). This test detects the presence of rheumatoid factor antibodies and assists in the diagnosis of rheumatoid arthritis.

Antistreptolysin O Test

The antistreptolysin O (ASO) test is used to detect ASO antibodies in the serum; ASO antibodies are common antibodies produced by the immune system in response to a strep infection. The ASO test is the most widely used immunologic test for the detection of conditions resulting from streptococcal infections and diseases that occur secondary to a streptococcal infection. This test is useful in assisting in the diagnosis of rheumatic fever, glomerulonephritis, bacterial endocarditis, and scarlet fever.

C-Reactive Protein Test

During inflammation and tissue destruction, an abnormal protein called *C-reactive protein* (CRP) appears in the blood. Patients with inflammatory conditions or disorders accompanied by tissue destruction have positive results to this test. Because of this, the CRP test is used to assist in diagnosing or documenting the progress of rheumatoid arthritis, acute rheumatic fever, widespread malignancy, and bacterial infections.

Cold Agglutinins Test

The cold agglutinins test is used to detect the presence of antibodies called *cold agglutinins.* This test is performed by incubating the patient's serum with erythrocytes at cold temperatures. If cold agglutinins are present, this causes agglutination of the erythrocytes. **Agglutination** refers to the clumping of red blood cells. Cold agglutinins are found in patients with infectious mononucleosis, mycoplasmal pneumonia, chronic parasitic infections, and lymphoma.

H. pylori Test

Helicobacter pylori (*H. pylori*) is a bacteria that infects the digestive system. Approximately two-thirds of the world's population has *H. pylori* in their body; however, for most individuals, it does not cause a problem. In some people, the bacteria cause a variety of digestive disorders which include gastritis, ulcers of the stomach, small intestine, or esophagus, and certain types of stomach cancer. A blood test can be performed to check for the presence of antibodies to *H. pylori*. CLIA-waived rapid testing kits are available to perform this test in the medical office; brand names include Clearview *H. pylori* One Step (Abbott, Santa Clara, CA) and QuickVue H. pylori Test (Quidel Corporation, San Diego, CA).

Mononucleosis Test

A mononucleosis test ("mono test") is used to detect the presence of infectious mononucleosis which is an acute infectious disease caused by the Epstein–Barr virus (EBV). Infectious mononucleosis most frequently affects children and young adults. It is transmitted through saliva through direct oral contact, and because of this, it is often called the "kissing disease." Symptoms of infectious mononucleosis include extreme fatigue, fever, sore throat, loss of appetite, muscle aches and weakness, headache, rash, and swollen lymph nodes.

The mononucleosis test may be performed in the medical office using a CLIA-waived rapid testing kit. A rapid mononucleosis test is easy to perform and provides reliable results in a short time. Patients with infectious mononucleosis produce an antibody called *heterophile antibody*, usually by 6 to 10 days into the illness. Rapid mono tests detect this antibody. The presence of the heterophile antibody, along with patient symptoms, provide the basis for the diagnosis of infectious mononucleosis.

Fig. 33.17 illustrates the QuickVue+ Mononucleosis Test setup (Quidel Corporation, San Diego, CA) and Fig. 33.18 outlines the procedure for performing a rapid mono test using the QuickVue+ Mononucleosis Test. Fig. 33.19 illustrates positive and negative test results for the QuickVue+ Mononucleosis Test.

IMMUNOHEMATOLOGIC TESTS

Immunohematology is a branch of immunology and is the study of red blood cell antigens and antibodies; it is also known as blood banking. Immunohematologic tests include the following.

Rh Antibody Titer Test

The Rh antibody titer test detects the amount of circulating Rh antibodies in the blood. These antibodies can occur in a pregnant woman who is Rh-negative and is carrying an Rh-positive fetus. This test is most frequently used to detect the presence of an Rh incompatibility problem with a mother and her unborn child.

ABO and Rh Blood Typing

Blood typing is performed to determine an individual's ABO and Rh blood type. Knowledge of blood type helps to prevent transfusion and transplant reactions and helps to identify problems such as hemolytic disease of the newborn.

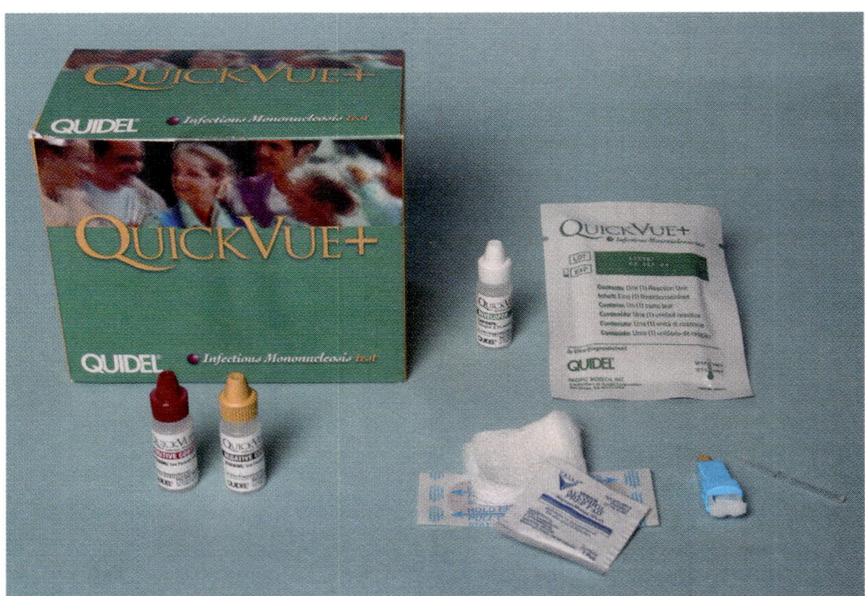

Fig. 33.17 QuickVue+ Mononucleosis Test setup. (From Garrels M, Oatis CS: *Laboratory testing for ambulatory settings*, ed 3. St. Louis, 2015, Elsevier.)

QuickVue+ Infectious Mononucleosis Test

FOR INFORMATIONAL USE ONLY ■ FOR INFORMATIONAL USE ONLY ■ FOR INFORMATIONAL USE ONLY

Not to be used for performing assay. Refer to most current package insert accompanying your test kit.

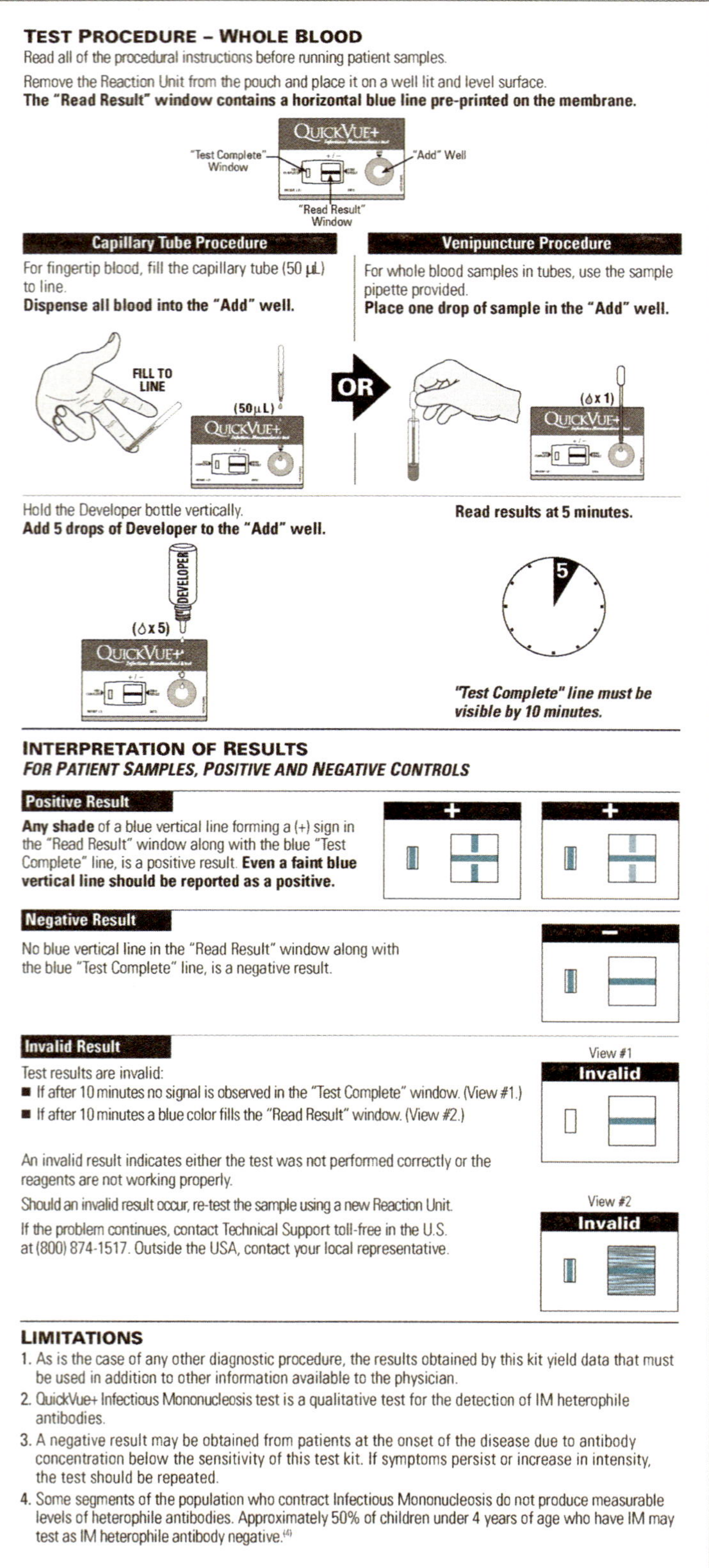

TEST PROCEDURE – WHOLE BLOOD

Read all of the procedural instructions before running patient samples.

Remove the Reaction Unit from the pouch and place it on a well lit and level surface.
The "Read Result" window contains a horizontal blue line pre-printed on the membrane.

Capillary Tube Procedure

For fingertip blood, fill the capillary tube (50 µL) to line.
Dispense all blood into the "Add" well.

Venipuncture Procedure

For whole blood samples in tubes, use the sample pipette provided.
Place one drop of sample in the "Add" well.

Hold the Developer bottle vertically.
Add 5 drops of Developer to the "Add" well.

Read results at 5 minutes.

"Test Complete" line must be visible by 10 minutes.

INTERPRETATION OF RESULTS

FOR PATIENT SAMPLES, POSITIVE AND NEGATIVE CONTROLS

Positive Result

Any shade of a blue vertical line forming a (+) sign in the "Read Result" window along with the blue "Test Complete" line, is a positive result. **Even a faint blue vertical line should be reported as a positive.**

Negative Result

No blue vertical line in the "Read Result" window along with the blue "Test Complete" line, is a negative result.

Invalid Result

Test results are invalid:

- If after 10 minutes no signal is observed in the "Test Complete" window. (View #1.)
- If after 10 minutes a blue color fills the "Read Result" window. (View #2.)

An invalid result indicates either the test was not performed correctly or the reagents are not working properly.

Should an invalid result occur, re-test the sample using a new Reaction Unit.

If the problem continues, contact Technical Support toll-free in the U.S. at (800) 874-1517. Outside the USA, contact your local representative.

LIMITATIONS

1. As is the case of any other diagnostic procedure, the results obtained by this kit yield data that must be used in addition to other information available to the physician.
2. QuickVue+ Infectious Mononucleosis test is a qualitative test for the detection of IM heterophile antibodies.
3. A negative result may be obtained from patients at the onset of the disease due to antibody concentration below the sensitivity of this test kit. If symptoms persist or increase in intensity, the test should be repeated.
4. Some segments of the population who contract Infectious Mononucleosis do not produce measurable levels of heterophile antibodies. Approximately 50% of children under 4 years of age who have IM may test as IM heterophile antibody negative.[4]

Fig. 33.18 Procedure for performing the QuickVue+ Mononucleosis Test. (Courtesy of and modified from Quidel Corporation, San Diego, CA.)

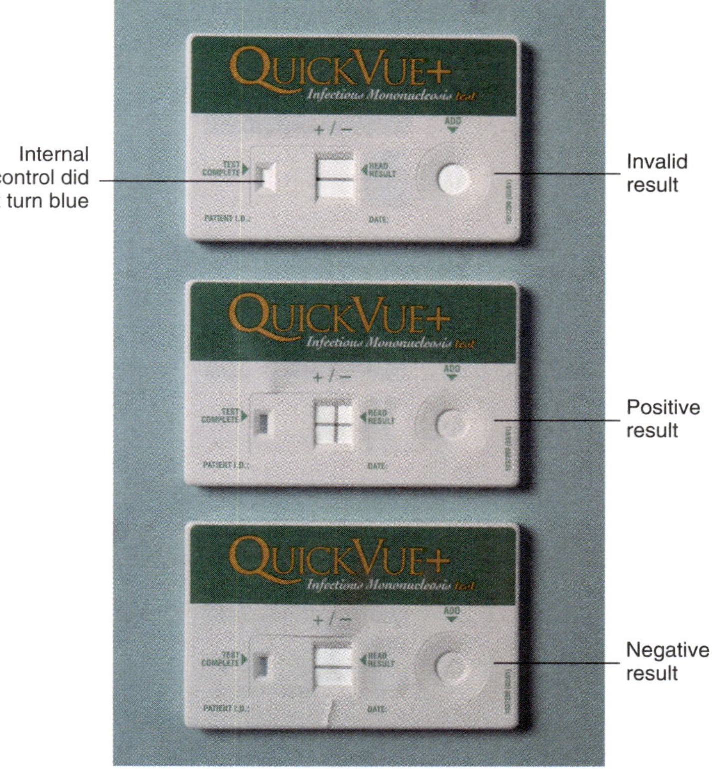

Fig. 33.19 QuickVue+ Mononucleosis Test results. (Modified from Garrels M, Oatis CS: *Laboratory testing for ambulatory settings*, ed 3, St. Louis, 2015, Elsevier.)

What Would You Do? What Would You *Not* Do? RESPONSES

Case Study 1

Page 893

What Did Michelle Do?

- ❑ Empathized with Bianca that it is hard to fast but eating and drinking causes an increase in the blood sugar level which causes the test results to be inaccurate.
- ❑ Empathized with Bianca for having to be at the test site so long. Explained to her that it takes 3 to 4 hours to run an OGTT because several specimens must be collected over time to see how her body handles sugar.
- ❑ Told Bianca that walking burns up sugar in the body which affects the test results.
- ❑ Explained to Bianca that smoking elevates the blood sugar level causing the test results to be inaccurate.
- ❑ Explained to Bianca that weakness and slight perspiration are considered normal side effects of an OGTT.
- ❑ Notified the physician of the side effects experienced by Bianca during the test and documented this information in Bianca's medical record.

What Did Michelle Not *Do?*

- ❑ Did not become defensive or intimidated by Bianca's behavior but tried to understand that patients often become fearful and anxious when faced with a health concern.
- ❑ Did not scold Bianca for not paying attention to the verbal and written instructions that were given to her at the medical office.

Case Study 2

Page 894

What Did Michelle Do?

- ❑ Told Jackson that it would be fine for him to perform his own finger stick.
- ❑ Made sure that Jackson cleansed his finger with an antiseptic wipe before making the finger puncture.
- ❑ Observed the finger puncture performed by Jackson and offered suggestions if needed.
- ❑ Explained to Jackson that the air bubbles take up space that the insulin should occupy, and that if he does not get rid of them he will not get his full dose of insulin.
- ❑ Demonstrated how to remove air bubbles, and had Jackson practice it at the office.
- ❑ Told Jackson he must not reuse his needle and syringe. Explained that a used needle could cause him to get an infection.
- ❑ Asked Jackson if he had checked to see if his insurance would cover the cost of the needles and syringes.

Continued

What Would You Do? What Would You *Not* Do? RESPONSES—cont'd

What Did Michelle* Not *Do?

- ❑ Did not tell Jackson he didn't need to worry about the air bubbles in the syringe.

Case Study 3

Page 899

What Did Michelle Do?

- ❑ Tried to calm and reassure Karen.
- ❑ Explained to Karen that the cholesterol results are not affected by food, so eating before the health fair should not have affected her results.
- ❑ Told Karen that before a cholesterol analyzer is used, it is usually checked to ensure that it is working properly.
- ❑ Reassured Karen that the physician was checking her cholesterol again and was running some additional tests to determine whether she is having any problems.
- ❑ Told Karen that if she must take medication, the physician will determine what drug is best for her.

What Did Michelle* Not *Do?

- ❑ Did not tell Karen that her cholesterol is extremely high.
- ❑ Did not tell Karen that she should be more careful about what she eats because she is overweight.
- ❑ Did not tell Karen that there was no way to know whether the cholesterol analyzer used at the health fair was calibrated and had controls run on it.

TERMINOLOGY REVIEW

Medical Term	Word Parts	Definition
Agglutination (as it pertains to blood)	*agglutin-:* clumping *-ation*: action or process	Clumping of blood cells.
Antibody	*anti-:* against	A substance that is capable of combining with an antigen, resulting in an antigen–antibody reaction.
Antigen	*anti-:* against *-gen:* substance or agent that produces or causes	A substance capable of stimulating the formation of antibodies.
Blood chemistry testing		Testing that involves the quantitative measurement of chemical substances dissolved in the plasma of the blood.
Cholesterol		A white, waxy, fatlike substance (lipid) that is essential for normal functioning of the body.
Glucose	*gluco-:* glucose *-ose*: full of	The end product of carbohydrate metabolism which serves as the chief source of energy for the body.
Glycogen	*glyco-:* sugar *-gen:* substance or agent that produces or causes	The form in which glucose is stored in the body for later use.
Glycosylation	*glyco-:* sugar	The process of glucose attaching to hemoglobin.
HDL (High-density lipoprotein)		A lipoprotein that removes excess cholesterol from the walls of the arteries and carries it to the liver for removal by the body; known as "good" cholesterol because it is protective and beneficial to the body.
Hemoglobin A_{1c}	*hemo-:* blood	A compound formed when glucose attaches or glycosylates to the protein in hemoglobin.
Hyperglycemia	*hyper-:* above, excessive *glyc/o:* sugar *-emia:* blood condition	An abnormally high level of glucose in the blood.
Hypoglycemia	*hypo-:* below, deficient *glyc/o:* sugar *-emia:* blood condition	An abnormally low level of glucose in the blood.
Immunologic testing	*Immun/o:* immune; protection	Testing that uses antigen–antibody reactions to assess the presence of a specific substance in the body or to assist in the diagnosis of an infectious disease.
Insulin		A hormone secreted by the beta cells of the pancreas required for the normal use of glucose in the body.
LDL (Low-density lipoprotein)		A lipoprotein that picks up cholesterol from ingested fats and the liver and carries it in the plasma of the blood for use by the body's cells; known as "bad" cholesterol because a high level contributes to atherosclerosis.

TERMINOLOGY REVIEW—cont'd

Medical Term	Word Parts	Definition
Lipoprotein	*lipo-:* fat	A complex molecule consisting of protein that combines with and transports lipids (cholesterol and triglycerides) in the plasma of the blood.
Prediabetes	*pre:* before	A condition in which glucose levels are higher than normal, but not high enough to be classified as diabetes.
VLDL (Very-low-density lipoprotein)		A lipoprotein that picks up triglycerides and delivers them to the cells so that they can be used for energy by the body or stored for later use; known as "bad" cholesterol because a high level contributes to atherosclerosis.

PROCEDURE 33.1 CLIA-Waived Blood Glucose Test

Outcome Perform a FBG test using an Accu-Chek Aviva glucose meter.

Equipment/Supplies

- Disposable gloves
- Accu-Chek Aviva glucose meter (Roche Diabetes Care, Inc.)
- Accu-Chek Aviva test strips
- Control solutions
- Lancet
- Antiseptic wipe
- Gauze pad
- Biohazard sharps container

1. Procedural Step. Sanitize your hands. Assemble the equipment. Check the expiration date (Use By date) on the container of test strips. Check the expiration date on the control solution bottle. The control solution is effective for 3 months from the date it is opened. When opening a new bottle of control solution, write the date on the container label. The control solution can then be used for 3 months from this date or until the manufacturer's expiration date (stamped on the container) is reached, whichever comes first. Make sure the environmental room temperature falls between 57°F (14°C) and 100°F (38°C).

Principle. Test strips or controls past their expiration can cause inaccurate test results. If the environmental temperature is outside of the required range, the glucose meter is unable to perform the test, causing an error message to appear on the screen of the analyzer.

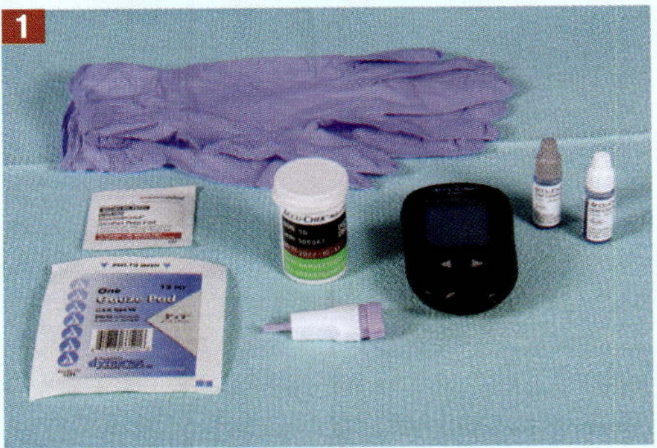

Assemble the equipment.

2. Procedural Step. Insert a test strip into the glucose meter as follows:

a. Remove a test strip from the container and immediately recap the container to prevent the strips from being exposed to moisture.

b. Insert the test strip into the meter in the direction of the arrows with the yellow window facing up. This automatically turns on the meter and a beep sounds.

c. Place the meter on a flat surface.

d. When the strip is ready to accept the control solution or a blood specimen, a symbol of a test strip and a flashing blood drop appear on the display screen.

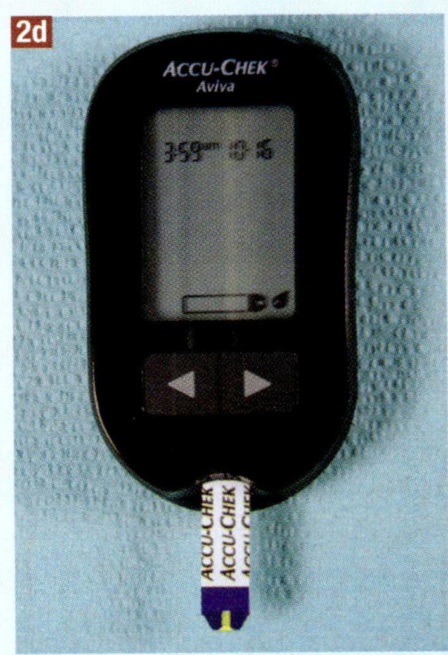

Symbol of the test strip and blood drop.

Continued

PROCEDURE 33.1 CLIA-Waived Blood Glucose Test—cont'd

Principle. Moisture results in deterioration of the chemical reagents on the test strips leading to inaccurate test results. If the meter is tilted the control solution may drip into the meter and damage it.

3. Procedural Step. Perform a Level 1 and 2 control procedure as follows:

a. Remove the cap from the Level 1 (low) control solution bottle and wipe the tip of the bottle with a tissue.

b. Squeeze the bottle until a tiny drop forms at the tip of the bottle.

c. Touch and hold the drop of control solution to the front edge of the yellow window of the test strip. Do not put the control solution on top of the test strip. The meter will beep and an "hourglass" symbol flashes when there is enough control solution on the test strip. The meter automatically recognizes the difference between the control solution and a blood specimen.

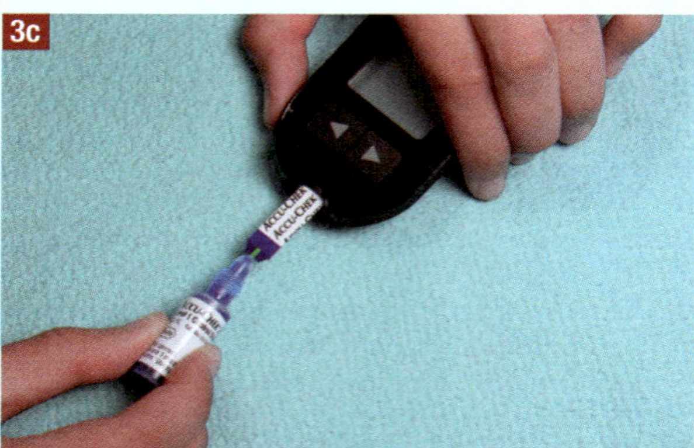

3c

Apply the control solution.

d. Wipe the tip of the bottle with a tissue and recap the bottle tightly.

e. After a short time, the control result appears on the display screen along with a control bottle symbol and a flashing "L". Press and release the right arrow key once to mark the control result as a Level 1 control. Press the Power/Set Button (located on the top of the meter) to set the control level in the meter.

f. If the Level 1 control result is within the acceptable range, the control result will alternate with the word "OK" on the display screen. The control result can also be compared with the expected Level 1 range stamped on the test strip container label. The word "Err" and the control result will alternate on the display if the control result is not within the expected range.

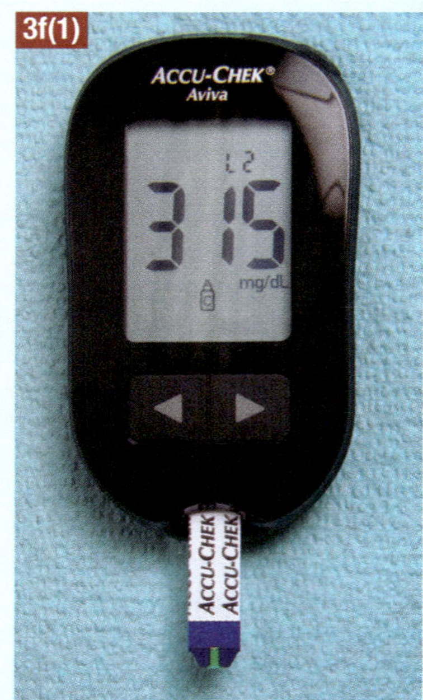

3f(1)

The control results alternate with the word "OK."

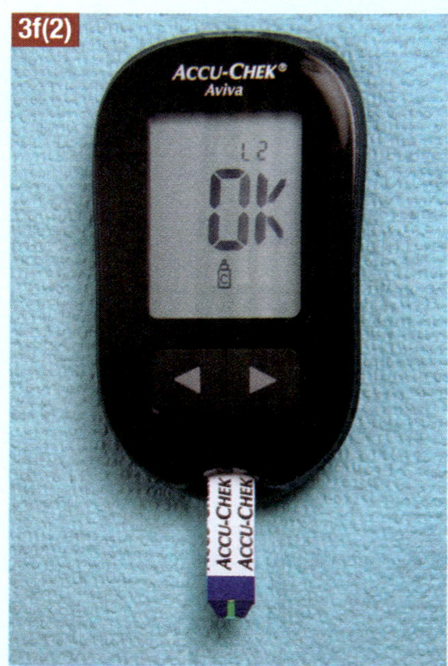

3f(2)

The control results alternate with the word "OK."

g. If the control result is not within the expected range, review the technique used to run the control to make sure it was performed correctly. Any errors should be corrected, and the control should be run again. If the results are still not within the expected range, the manufacturer of the glucose meter should be contacted.

PROCEDURE 33.1

PROCEDURE 33.1 CLIA-Waived Blood Glucose Test—cont'd

h. Remove and discard the used test strip.
i. Repeat the control procedure outlined above using a Level 2 (high) control. When the control result and the flashing "L" appear on the display, press and release the right arrow key twice to mark the control result as a Level 2 control.
j. Document the control results in the quality control log.

Principle. Running a Level 1 and a Level 2 control procedure ensures that the test results are reliable and accurate. Gloves do not need to be worn because the control consists of a glucose solution.

4. Procedural Step. Sanitize your hands. Greet the patient and introduce yourself. Identify the patient by full name and date of birth. Explain the procedure.

5. Procedural Step. Ask the patient whether they have had anything to eat or drink (besides water) for the past 8 to 12 hours.

Principle. Consumption of food or fluid increases the blood glucose level, leading to an inaccurate interpretation of the test results.

6. Procedural Step. Perform the blood glucose test as follows:
a. Insert the test strip into the glucose meter (as previously presented).
b. Cleanse the puncture site with an antiseptic wipe and allow it to air-dry.
c. Apply gloves and perform a finger puncture. Dispose of the lancet in a biohazard sharps container.
d. Wipe away the first drop of blood with a gauze pad.
e. Place the patient's hand in a dependent position (palm facing down), and gently massage the finger around the puncture site until a drop of blood forms.
f. Touch and hold the drop of blood to the front edge (not the top) of the yellow window of the test strip. The meter will beep and an "hourglass" symbol flashes when there is enough blood on the test strip.

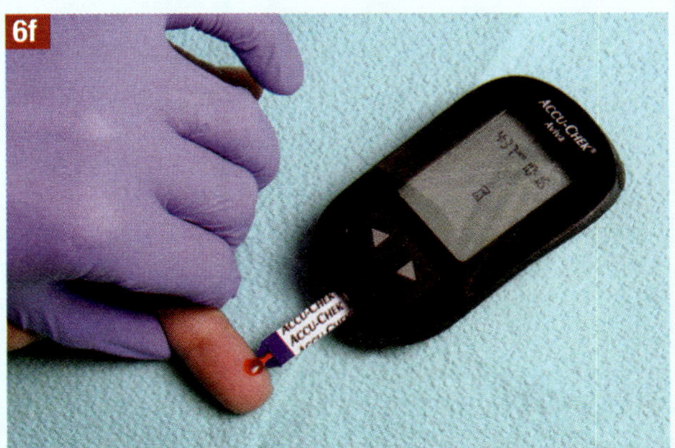

Apply a drop of blood.

g. Have the patient hold a gauze pad over the puncture site and apply pressure until the bleeding stops.
h. An hourglass is displayed on the screen while the meter analyzes the blood specimen. After a short time, the glucose value is displayed in milligrams per deciliter (mg/dL). (The glucose result indicated on this glucose meter is 106 mg/dL.) If the glucose value is higher or lower than the measurement range of the meter, or if the screen displays something other than the glucose value (e.g., an error code), refer to the Troubleshooting Guide section of the operator's manual to obtain instructions for correcting the problem.

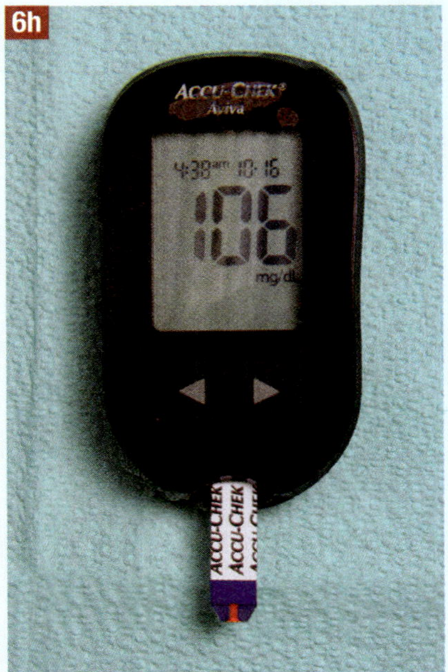

Read the glucose results.

i. Remove the test strip from the meter and discard it in a biohazard waste container. The meter automatically turns off 5 seconds after the test strip is removed.
j. Check the puncture site and apply an adhesive bandage to the patient's finger if needed.

Principle. The antiseptic must be allowed to dry to prevent it from reacting with the chemicals on the reagent pad, which would lead to inaccurate test results. Gloves provide a barrier against bloodborne pathogens. The first drop of blood contains a large amount of tissue fluid, which dilutes the specimen and leads to inaccurate test results.

7. Procedural Step. Remove gloves and sanitize your hands.

Continued

PROCEDURE 33.1 CLIA-Waived Blood Glucose Test—cont'd

8. Procedural Step. Document the results in the patient's medical record.

a. *Electronic health record:* Document the type of glucose test (i.e., FBG), the glucose test results, and when the patient last ate. If the patient has diabetes, also document the time of his or her last insulin injection or last consumption of oral hypoglycemic medication using the appropriate radio buttons, drop-down menus, and free text fields.

b. *Paper-based patient record:* Document the date and time, the type of glucose test (i.e., FBG), the glucose test results, and when the patient last ate. If the patient has diabetes, also document the time of their last insulin injection or last consumption of oral hypoglycemic medication.

8b

DOCUMENTATION EXAMPLE

Date	
5/18/XX	8:30 a.m. FBG: 106 mg/dL. Pt last ate on
	5/17 @ 7:00 p.m.———————
	———————M. Villers, CMA (AAMA)

9. Procedural Step. Clean and disinfect the glucose meter according to the information in the operating manual.

Medical Microbiology

Check out the Evolve site at http://evolve.elsevier.com/Bonewit/today to access additional interactive activities and exercises to help you study and prepare for success.

LEARNING OUTCOMES	PROCEDURES
Microorganisms and Disease	
1. List and describe the three classifications of bacteria based on shape.	
2. Give examples of infectious diseases caused by the following types of cocci: • Staphylococci • Streptococci • Diplococci	
3. State examples of infectious diseases caused by bacilli, spirilla, and viruses.	
4. Explain how droplet transmission spreads infectious respiratory diseases.	
5. List and describe the stages of an infectious disease.	
Microscope	
6. Explain the function of each of the following parts of a compound microscope: base, arm, stage, illuminator, condenser, diaphragm, eyepieces, objectives, and adjustment knobs.	Operate a microscope.
7. Identify the function of each of the following microscope lenses: low power, high power, and oil immersion.	Properly handle and care for a microscope.
8. List the guidelines for proper care of the microscope.	
Microbiologic Specimen Collection	
9. Explain the purpose of obtaining a specimen and identify body areas from which a specimen can be taken for microbiologic examination.	Collect a throat specimen.
10. List ways to prevent contamination of a specimen by extraneous microorganisms.	Collect a nasopharyngeal specimen.
11. Explain the precautions a medical assistant should take to prevent infection from a pathogenic specimen.	
CLIA-Waived Microbiologic Testing	
12. Describe the symptoms of strep throat.	Perform CLIA-waived streptococcus test.
13. Explain the importance of the early diagnosis of streptococcal pharyngitis.	
14. Explain the advantage of using a rapid strep test to diagnose group A streptococcus.	Perform a CLIA-waived influenza test.
15. List and describe the three different types of influenza viruses.	
16. Describe the symptoms, treatment, and potential complications of influenza.	
17. Explain why a new influenza vaccine must be produced each year.	
18. State the purpose of influenza viral medications.	
19. State the symptoms of COVID-19.	
20. List the measures that can be taken to prevent the spread of COVID-19.	
21. State the purpose of COVID-19 antiviral medications.	
22. List and describe the two types of tests that are used to diagnose COVID-19.	
Culture and Sensitivity Testing	
23. State the purpose of culturing a microbiologic specimen.	
24. Explain the difference between a mixed culture and a pure culture.	
25. Explain the purpose of and describe the procedure for a sensitivity test.	
26. List examples of methods to prevent and control infectious diseases in the community.	

CHAPTER OUTLINE

KEY TERMS

bacilli (bah-SILL-ie)
cocci (KOK-sie)
contagious disease
culture
culture medium
false-negative result
incubate (IN-kyoo-bate)
incubation period
infection
infectious disease
inoculate
microbiology (mie-kroe-bie-OL-oe-jee)
microorganism
normal flora
specimen (SPESS-ih-men)
spirilla (spa-RILL-ah)

INTRODUCTION TO MICROBIOLOGY

Microbiology is the scientific study of microorganisms and their activities. **Microorganisms** are tiny living plants and animals that cannot be seen by the naked eye but must be viewed under a microscope. Anton van Leeuwenhoek (1632–1723) designed a magnifying glass strong enough for viewing microorganisms. He was the first individual to observe and describe protozoa and bacteria (Fig. 34.1). Leeuwenhoek's magnifying glass was the precursor of modern microscopes used today to study microorganisms. A microscope allows the observer to see individual microbial cells and to differentiate and identify microorganisms.

For the most part, microbiology deals with unicellular, or one-celled, microscopic organisms. All of the life processes necessary to sustain the microbe are performed by one cell. Among them are the ingestion of food substances and their use for energy, growth, reproduction, and excretion.

Microorganisms are *ubiquitous*; they are found almost everywhere—in the air, in food and water, in the soil, and in association with plants, animals, and human life. Although vast numbers of microorganisms exist, only a relatively small number are pathogenic and capable of causing disease.

When a pathogen infects a host, it often produces a set of symptoms peculiar to that disease. Scarlet fever is characterized by a sore throat, swelling of the lymph nodes in the neck, a red and swollen tongue, and a bright red rash covering the body. These symptoms assist the provider in diagnosing the disease. The medical assistant must be alert to all symptoms that the patient describes and must relay this information to the provider through careful and concise documentation of these symptoms in the patient's medical record.

If the provider is not able to diagnose the disease from the patient's clinical signs and symptoms, laboratory tests may be

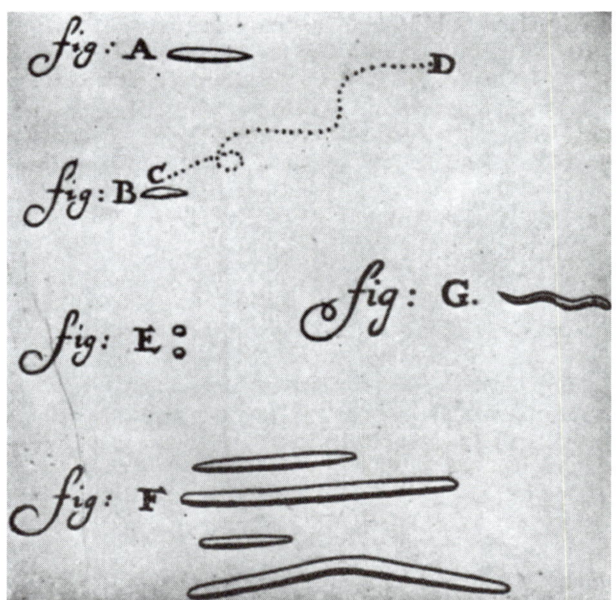

Fig. 34.1 Bacteria drawn by van Leeuwenhoek in 1684. (From Fuerst R: *Frobisher and Fuerst's microbiology in health and disease*, ed 15, Philadelphia, 1983, Saunders.)

used to identify the pathogen causing the disease. Identification of the pathogen leads to proper diagnosis and treatment of the disease. Laboratory tests used to identify a pathogen include rapid antigen tests, PCR tests, and microbial culture tests.

This chapter provides an introduction to microbiology and infectious diseases, including a description of proper microbiologic collection, handling, and transportation procedures that must be followed to ensure a quality specimen. A **specimen** refers to a small sample or part taken from the body to represent the whole. This chapter also presents CLIA-waived tests that can be performed in the medical office to assist in the diagnosis of infectious respiratory diseases. Before undertaking this study, the medical assistant should review Chapter 17, which discusses introductory concepts that are basic to this chapter.

MICROORGANISMS AND DISEASE

The groups of microorganisms known to contain species capable of causing human disease include bacteria, viruses, protozoa, fungi (including yeasts), and animal parasites. Bacteria and viruses are most frequently responsible for causing human diseases and are discussed next.

BACTERIA

Bacteria are microscopic single-celled organisms. Most species of bacteria that reside in humans are harmless, but others can cause human diseases and are known as *pathogens*. The number of pathogenic bacterial species affecting humans is estimated to be less than a hundred. The discovery of antibiotics has helped immensely in combating and controlling bacterial infections. Antibiotics are not effective against viral infections, however.

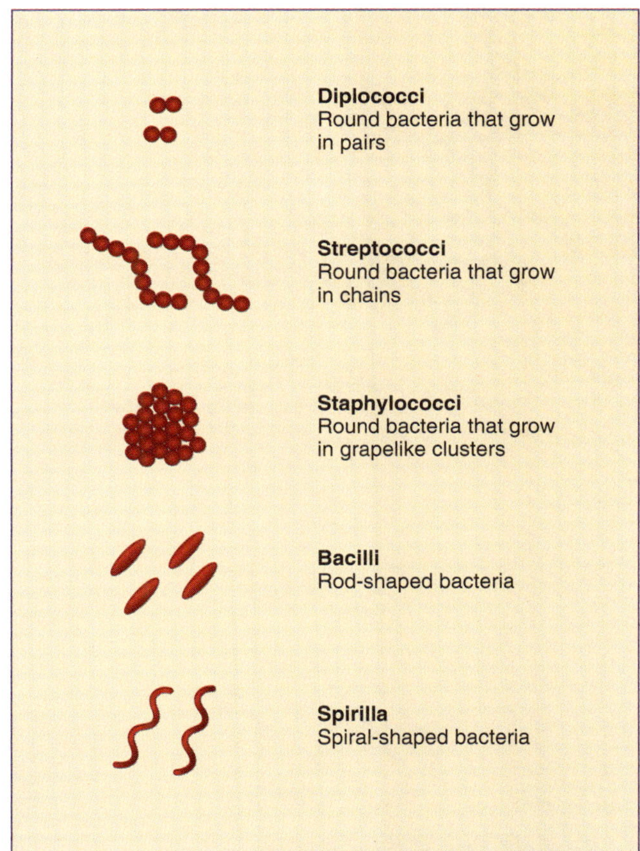

Fig. 34.2 Classification of bacteria based on shape.

Bacteria can be classified according to their shape into three basic groups (Fig. 34.2). Round bacteria are known as **cocci**. Cocci can be categorized further as diplococci, streptococci, or staphylococci, depending on their pattern of growth. Rod-shaped bacteria are **bacilli**. Spiral and curve-shaped bacteria are **spirilla**, and they include spirochetes and vibrios.

Cocci

Staphylococci are round bacteria that grow in grapelike clusters (Fig. 34.3A). The species *Staphylococcus epidermidis* is widely distributed and is normally present on the surface of the skin and the mucous membranes of the mouth, nose, throat, and intestines. *S. epidermidis* is usually nonpathogenic; however, a cut, abrasion, or other break in the skin can allow invasion of the tissues by the organism, resulting in a mild infection.

Staphylococcus aureus is commonly associated with pathologic conditions such as boils, carbuncles, pimples, impetigo, abscesses, *Staphylococcus* food poisoning, and wound infections. Infections caused by staphylococci usually cause much pus formation (suppuration) and are termed *pyogenic* infections.

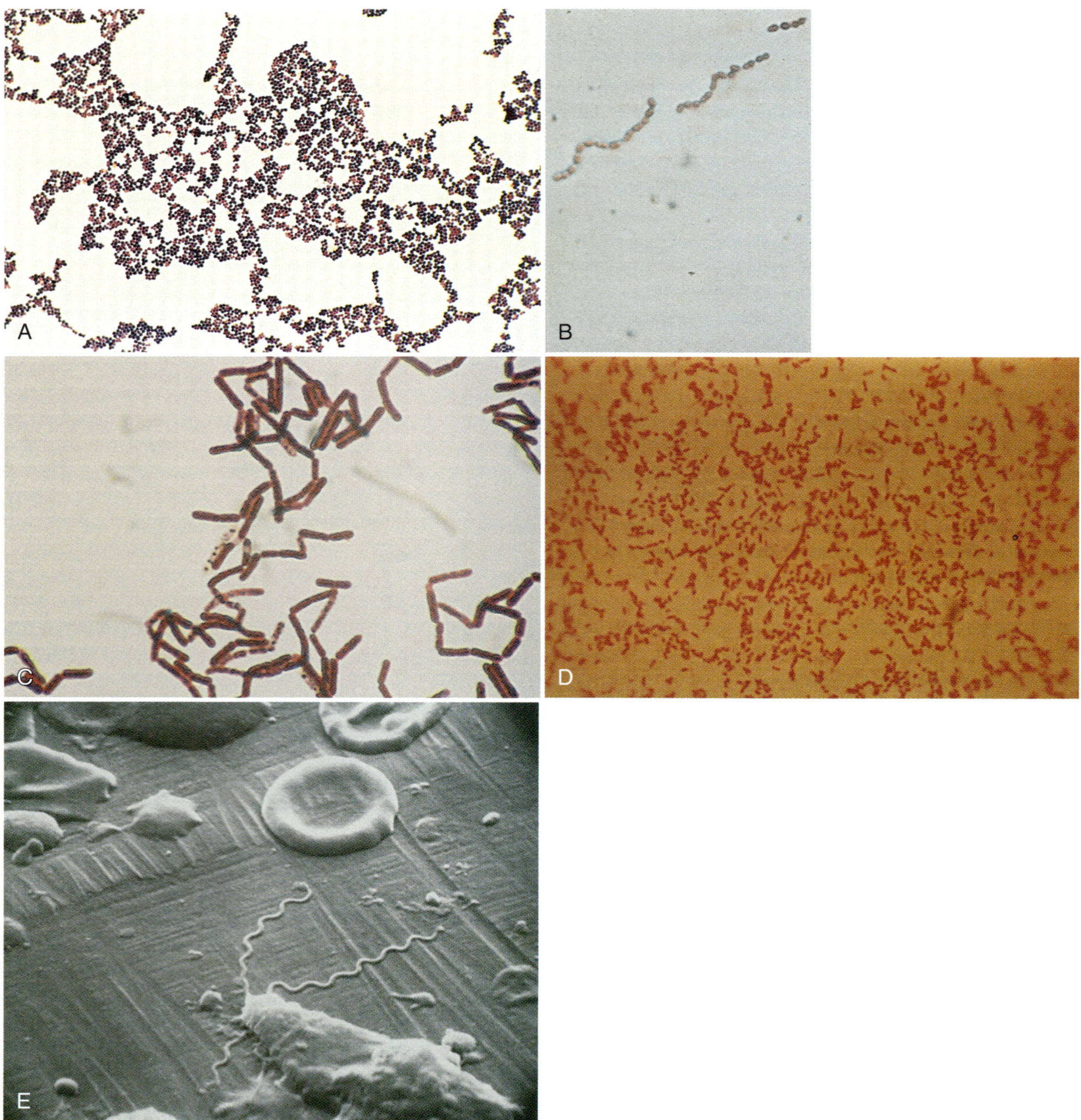

Fig. 34.3 Types of bacteria. **A,** Staphylococci. **B,** Streptococci. **C,** Bacilli. **D,** *Escherichia coli.* **E,** Spirilla. (A, B, and D from Mahon CR, Lehman DC, Manuselis G Jr: *Textbook of diagnostic microbiology*, ed 4, Philadelphia, 2010, Saunders; C, courtesy of Cathy Bissonette; E, courtesy of Dr. Andrew G. Smith.)

Streptococci are round bacteria that grow in chains (Fig. 34.3B). Before the advent of antibiotics, streptococcal infections were a major cause of human death. Diseases caused by streptococci include streptococcal sore throat ("strep throat"), scarlet fever, rheumatic fever, pneumonia, puerperal sepsis, erysipelas, and skin conditions such as carbuncles and impetigo.

Diplococci are round bacteria that grow in pairs. Pneumonia, gonorrhea, and meningitis are infectious diseases caused by diplococci.

Bacilli

Bacilli are rod-shaped bacteria that are frequently found in the soil and air (Fig. 34.3C). Some bacilli are able to form spores, a characteristic that enables them to resist adverse conditions such as heat and disinfectants. Diseases caused by bacilli include botulism, tetanus, gas gangrene, gastroenteritis produced by *Salmonella* food poisoning, typhoid fever, pertussis (whooping cough), bacillary dysentery, diphtheria, tuberculosis, leprosy, and plague.

Escherichia coli is a species of bacillus that is found among the normal flora of the large intestine in enormous numbers (Fig. 34.3D). It is normally a harmless bacterium; however, if it enters the urinary tract as a result of lowered resistance, poor hygiene practices, or both, it may cause a urinary tract infection.

Spirilla

Spirilla are spiral or curve-shaped bacteria. *Treponema pallidum*, a spirochete, is the causative agent of syphilis (Fig. 34.3E). This microorganism cannot be grown in commonly available culture media; the diagnosis of syphilis is generally made using serologic tests. A serologic test is performed on the serum of the blood. Cholera is caused by another type of spirillum, *Vibrio cholerae.* Immunization and proper methods of sanitation and water purification have all but eliminated cholera in the United States.

VIRUSES

Viruses are the smallest microorganisms. They are so small that an electron microscope must be used to view them. A virus can only replicate (make copies of itself) inside the cells of a host using components of the host cells. When a virus enters a host cell, it forces the cell to produce thousands of copies of the original virus. Often, the virus ends up killing the host cell in the process. After replicating, the viruses infect nearby cells and repeat the process. Although viruses are usually classified as microorganisms, they are alive only when replicating inside the host cells. Infectious diseases caused by viruses include the common cold, influenza, COVID-19, hepatitis, AIDS, varicella (chickenpox), rubeola (measles), rubella (German measles), mumps, poliomyelitis, smallpox, rabies, and herpes viruses.

NORMAL FLORA

Every individual has a **normal flora**, which consists of the harmless microorganisms that normally reside in many parts of the body but do not cause disease. The surface of the skin, the mucous membrane of the gastrointestinal tract, and parts of the respiratory and genitourinary tracts all have an abundant normal flora. Some microorganisms that make up the normal flora are beneficial to the body, such as those that inhabit the intestinal tract that feed on other potentially harmful microscopic organisms. Another example is microorganisms found in the intestinal tract that synthesize vitamin K, an essential vitamin needed by the body for proper blood clotting. In rare instances, if the opportunity arises (e.g., lowered body resistance), certain microorganisms of the normal flora can become pathogenic and cause disease.

INFECTION

Invasion of the body by pathogenic microorganisms is known as **infection.** Under conditions favorable to the pathogens, they grow and multiply, resulting in an **infectious disease** that produces harmful effects in the host. Not all pathogens that enter a host are able to cause disease, however. When a pathogen enters the body, it attempts to invade the tissues so that it can grow and multiply. The body tries to stop the invasion with its second line of natural defense mechanisms,[a] which includes inflammation, phagocytosis by white blood cells, and the production of antibodies. These defense mechanisms work to destroy pathogens and remove them from the body. If the body is successful, the pathogens are destroyed, and the individual experiences no adverse effects. If the pathogens are able to overcome the body's natural defense mechanisms, an infectious disease results.

Droplet transmission is the primary mode of transmission for the infectious respiratory disease presented in this chapter (strep throat, influenza, and COVID-19). Respiratory droplets consist of secretions of mucus and saliva that are exhaled by both healthy individuals and those with infectious respiratory diseases. Droplet transmission occurs when infectious pathogens carried by respiratory droplets are transmitted from an infected person to a noninfected person. Millions of respiratory droplets loaded with infectious agents are expelled into the air each time an infected individual breathes, speaks, coughs, sneezes, sings, or shouts. These infectious droplets travel a short distance from the infected host where they can be inhaled into the respiratory tract of a susceptible host. The droplets can also be deposited on the mucosal surfaces of the eyes, nose, or mouth of a susceptible host. Respiratory droplets cannot usually travel more than 6 feet (2 meters) after leaving an infected host, with most droplets traveling less than 3 feet (1 meter). Because of this, droplet transmission requires close proximity between an infected individual and a noninfected individual.

STAGES OF AN INFECTIOUS DISEASE

When a pathogen becomes established in the host resulting in an infectious disease, a series of events occur in stages. The stages of an infectious disease are as follows:

1. The *infection* is the invasion of the body by pathogenic microorganisms.
2. The *incubation period* is the interval of time between the invasion by pathogenic microorganisms and the appearance of the first symptoms of the disease. Depending on

[a]The first line of natural defense mechanisms, which work to prevent the entrance of pathogens into the body (e.g., coughing, sneezing), is described in Chapter 17.

the type of disease, the **incubation period** may range from a few days to several months. During this time, the pathogens are multiplying.

3. The *prodromal period* is a short period in which the first symptoms that indicate an approaching disease occur. Headache and a feeling of illness are common prodromal symptoms.
4. The *acute period* is when the disease is at its peak and symptoms are fully developed. Fever is a symptom of many infectious diseases during the acute period.
5. The *decline period* is when symptoms of the disease begin to subside.
6. The *convalescent period* is the stage in which the patient regains strength and returns to a state of good health.

What Would You Do? What Would You *Not* Do?

Case Study 1

John Seimer calls the medical office. He says that he is not a patient of the office but would like some assistance. He says that for the past 3 days he has had a headache, fever, chills, and aching muscles. He says that a week ago he pulled a tick off his lower leg, and several days later he found a red rash around the tick bite. He says that he went on the internet and looked up his symptoms, and he is sure that he has Lyme disease. The internet site recommended taking doxycycline for 3 weeks to treat Lyme disease. John says that he does not like to go to the doctor and has not been to see a doctor for more than 10 years. He wants to know whether the doctor could call in a prescription for doxycycline for him. He says that he has health insurance, and the doctor could bill him for an appointment, just as long as he does not have to come in. ■

MICROSCOPE

Different types of microscopes are available, but the type used most often for office laboratory work is the *compound microscope*. The compound microscope consists of a two-lens system, and the magnification of one system is increased by the other. A source of bright light is required for proper illumination of the object to be viewed. This combination of lenses and light permits visualization of structures that cannot be seen with the unaided eye, such as microorganisms and cellular forms. The compound microscope consists of two main components: the support system and the optical system. The medical assistant should be able to identify the parts of a microscope (Fig. 34.4) and should be able to operate and care for it properly. Procedure 34.1 outlines the correct operation and care of a microscope.

SUPPORT SYSTEM

Frame

The working parts of the microscope are supported by a sturdy frame consisting of a *base* for support and an *arm* for carrying it without damaging the delicate parts. The arm also is needed to support the magnifying and adjusting systems.

Stage

The *stage* of a microscope is the flat, horizontal platform on which the microscope slide is placed. It is located directly over the condenser and beneath the objective lenses. The stage has a small round opening in the center that permits light from a light source below to pass through the object being viewed and up into the magnifying lenses above. The slide should be placed on the stage; the object to be viewed is positioned over this opening so that it is satisfactorily illuminated by the light source below.

Most microscopes have a *mechanical stage* that allows movement of the slide in a vertical or horizontal position using adjustment knobs. The mechanical stage has a slide holder that secures the slide and provides precise positioning of the slide. This is essential for performing certain procedures, such as WBC differential counts (manual method) and inspection of Gram-stained smears. *(Note: Bacteria are colorless and usually difficult to identify under a microscope unless some type of staining is used. Gram staining allows for the direct viewing of the size, shape, and growth patterns of bacteria under a microscope.)*

Standard microscope stages have metal clips attached to the stage to hold the glass slide securely in place. With this type of stage, the slide must be moved by hand for examination of various areas on it.

Illuminator

The *illuminator* is at the base of the microscope and consists of a built-in light source, along with a switch for turning it on and off. Light from the illuminator is directed to the diaphragm above it and then through the specimen and the objective and ocular lenses to be viewed. An intensity dial is used to increase or decrease the brightness of the illuminator.

Diaphragm

The amount of light focused on the specimen also can be controlled by the *diaphragm*, located above the illuminator and beneath the stage. The diaphragm consists of a series of horizontally arranged interlocking plates with a central opening. The diaphragm has a lever that is used to increase or decrease the amount of light focused on the specimen by increasing or decreasing the size of the opening.

Appropriate light intensity is essential for proper viewing of the specimens, especially at a higher magnification. A general rule is that as the desired magnification increases, the more intense the light must be. Increased light intensity is required for good visualization of a specimen with the oil-immersion objective. With the low-power objective, the light intensity must be diminished to produce the appropriate contrast for specimen detail and to reduce glare.

OPTICAL SYSTEM

Compound microscopes have a two-lens magnification system. *Magnification* is defined as the ratio of the apparent size of an object viewed through the microscope to the actual size of the object.

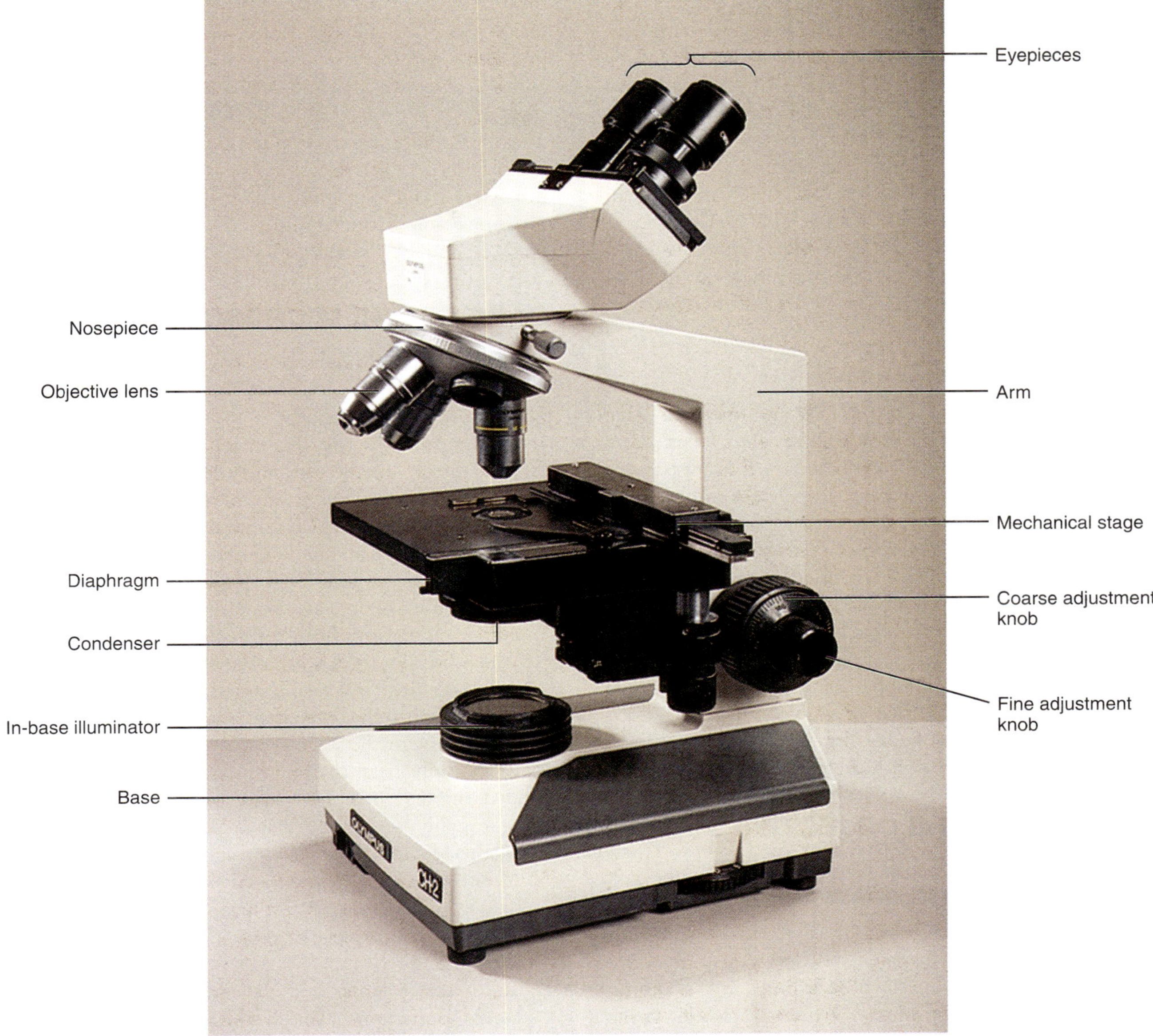

Fig. 34.4 Parts of the microscope.

Eyepiece

The first lens system is the *eyepiece*, or ocular lens, located at the top of the microscope and marked 10×, meaning that it magnifies 10 times. Microscopes that have one eyepiece only are called *monocular* microscopes, and microscopes with two eyepieces are called *binocular*. A binocular microscope is recommended for medical office laboratory work because it causes less eye fatigue than the monocular type. The binocular eyepieces can be adjusted to the individual by moving the eyepieces apart or together as needed.

Objective Lenses

The second lens system consists of three *objective lenses* mounted on a rotating *nosepiece*, each with a different degree of magnification. The nosepiece is used to rotate the different objective lenses into position for viewing the specimen at different magnifications. The metal shafts of the objective lenses differ in length and are identified by power of magnification. The objective with the shortest shaft is known as the *low-power objective* and has a magnification of 10×. The objective with a mid-length shaft is the *high-power objective*; it has a magnification of 40×. The objective with the longest shaft is the *oil-immersion objective*; it has the highest power of magnification, which is 100×.

The degree of magnification is engraved onto the metal shaft of each objective. In addition, some microscope manufacturers identify each objective lens by colored rings that encircle the metal shaft of the objective. Yellow is used for low power, blue for high power, and white for oil immersion. If the objective is not color coded, it can be identified by the length of the metal shaft.

The objective lens magnifies the specimen, and the ocular lens magnifies the image produced by the objective lens. The *total magnification* of each objective is determined by multiplying the ocular lens magnification by the objective lens magnification. The total magnification of the low-power objective is 100 times (100×) the actual size of the object being viewed (10 × 10). The total magnification of the high-power objective is 400× (10 × 40), and that of the oil-immersion objective is 1000× (10 × 100). Some microscopes also have a *scanning objective lens* that has a magnification of 4× and a total magnification of 40× which provides an initial overview or scan of the specimen on the slide.

Focusing System

Two adjustment knobs are used to raise and lower the stage of the microscope to bring the specimen into focus: these include the coarse adjustment knob and the fine adjustment knob. The *coarse adjustment knob* is used first to obtain an approximate focus. The *fine adjustment knob* is then used to obtain the precise focusing necessary to produce a sharp, clear image. On some microscope models, the adjustment knobs are mounted as two separate knobs; on others, they are placed together with the smaller fine adjustment knob extending from a larger coarse adjustment wheel.

Most compound microscopes are *parfocal.* This means that once the specimen is focused with the low-power objective, the nosepiece can be rotated to a higher-power objective and focused simply with the fine adjustment knob.

FUNCTION OF THE OBJECTIVE LENSES

Low- and High-Power Objectives

The low-power objective is used for the initial focusing and light adjustment of the specimen. The low-power objective also is used for the initial observation and scanning requirements needed for most microscopic work. Urine sediment is first examined using the low-power objective to scan the specimen for the presence of casts.

The high-power objective is used for a more thorough study of the specimen, such as observing cells in greater detail. The *working distance*, defined as the distance between the tip of the lens and the slide, is short when using the high-power objective. Because of this, care must be taken in focusing this objective to prevent it from striking and breaking the slide or damaging the lens.

Oil Immersion Objective

The oil-immersion objective provides the highest magnification and is used to view very small structures or the detail of larger structures, such as microorganisms and blood cells. The oil-immersion objective has a very short working distance, and when it is in use, the objective lens nearly rests on the microscope slide itself. A special grade of oil, known as *immersion oil*, must be used with this lens. Oil has the advantage of not drying out when exposed to air for a long time. A drop of oil is placed on the slide and resides between the oil-immersion objective and the slide. The oil provides a path for the light to travel on between the slide and the objective lens and prevents the scattering of light rays, which permits clear viewing of very small structures. The oil also improves the resolution of the objective lens, that is, its ability to provide sharp detail, which is particularly necessary at high magnifications. Procedures that require oil immersion include WBC differential counts (manual method) and examination of Gram-stained smears.

CARE OF THE MICROSCOPE

The microscope is a delicate instrument and must be handled carefully. These guidelines should be followed to care for the microscope properly:

1. Always carry the microscope with two hands. Place one hand firmly on the arm and the other hand under the base for support. Place the microscope down gently to prevent jarring it, which could damage delicate parts.
2. Always handle the microscope so that your fingers do not touch the lenses and leave fingerprints on them. When using a microscope, avoid wearing mascara because it is difficult to remove from the ocular lens.
3. When it is not in use, keep the microscope covered with its plastic dust cover and stored in a case or cupboard. Store it with the nosepiece rotated to the low-power objective with the stage at its lowest position.
4. Periodically clean the microscope by washing the enameled surface with mild soap and water and drying it thoroughly with a soft cloth. Never use alcohol on the enameled surface because it might remove the finish.
5. After each use, wipe the metal stage clean with gauze or tissue. If immersion oil comes in contact with the stage, remove it with a piece of gauze that is slightly moistened with xylene.
6. The eyepiece lenses and the objective lenses consist of hand-ground optical lenses, which must be kept spotlessly clean by using clean, dry lens paper. Optical glass is softer than ordinary glass; to prevent scratching the lens, do not use tissues or gauze. If the lenses are especially dirty, use a commercial lens cleaner in the cleaning process.
7. Keep the illuminator free of dust, lint, and dirt by periodic polishing with lens paper.
8. A malfunctioning microscope should be repaired only by a qualified service person. Attempting to fix the microscope yourself may result in further damage.

MICROBIOLOGIC SPECIMEN COLLECTION

The medical assistant is often responsible for collecting specimens from certain areas of the body, such as the throat, nose, and wounds. The medical assistant may be responsible for assisting the provider in the collection of specimens from other areas, such as the cervix, vagina, urethra, and rectum. In most instances, a sterile swab is used to collect the specimen. A *swab* is a small piece of cotton wrapped around the end of a slender wooden or plastic stick. It is passed across a body surface or opening to obtain a specimen for microbiologic analysis.

If the provider suspects that a particular disease is caused by a pathogen, a specimen may be collected for transport to an outside laboratory for analysis. This analysis identifies the pathogen causing the disease and aids in diagnosis. For example, if a urinary tract infection is suspected, a urine specimen may be obtained and sent to an outside laboratory for a urine culture to identify the pathogen causing the infection. In this instance, a clean-catch midstream collection is required to obtain a specimen that excludes the normal flora of the urethra and urinary meatus.

To prevent inaccurate test results, good techniques of medical and surgical asepsis must be practiced when a specimen is collected. The medical assistant must be careful not to contaminate the specimen with *extraneous microorganisms.* These are undesirable microorganisms (e.g., normal flora) that can enter the specimen in various ways; they grow and multiply and possibly obscure and prevent visualization and identification of pathogens that might be present. To prevent extraneous microorganisms from contaminating the specimen, all supplies used to obtain the specimen (e.g., swabs, inside of specimen containers) must be sterile. In addition, the specimen should not contain microorganisms from areas surrounding the collection site. For example, when obtaining a throat specimen, the swab should not be allowed to touch the inside of the mouth.

After collection, the specimen must be placed in its proper container with the lid securely fastened. The container must be clearly labeled with the patient's name and date of birth, the date, the source of the specimen, the medical assistant's initials, and any other required information. Procedure 34.2 outlines the procedure for collecting a throat specimen for transport to an outside laboratory.

SPECIMEN COLLECTION PRECAUTIONS

The OSHA Bloodborne Pathogens Standard presented in Chapter 17 should be carefully followed when collecting a microbiologic specimen to prevent the medical assistant from becoming infected with a pathogen. Specifically, the medical assistant must wear gloves when it is reasonably anticipated that hand contact might occur with potentially infectious materials. Eating, drinking, handling contact lenses, and applying cosmetics are strictly forbidden when working with microbiologic specimens because pathogens can be transmitted to the medical assistant. If the medical assistant accidentally touches the specimen, the area of contact should be washed immediately and thoroughly with soap and water. If the specimen comes in contact with the worktable, the table should be cleaned immediately with soap and water, followed by a suitable disinfectant. The worktable also should be cleaned with a disinfectant at the end of each day.

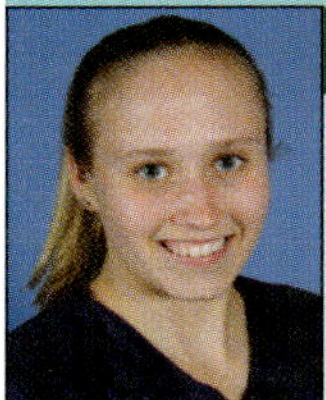

Putting It All Into Practice

My name is Alexandra, and I work for a physician who specializes in family practice. Working as a medical assistant, one can encounter many challenges. One experience that I had involved a 4-year-old boy. The little boy came into the office with a very sore throat and a high fever. He did not think that his office visit had gone too badly until he found out that the physician had ordered a rapid streptococcus test to check for strep throat. That's when he decided he did not care for me, my tongue depressor, or my swab. He decided to protest by keeping his mouth tightly shut. Rather than forcing the procedure on the child, I took my time and kept my patience. I managed to convince him that even though the procedure was uncomfortable and tasted bad, it was the only way we would know if he was really sick or not. I also explained that the test was the only way the doctor would know what kind of medicine to prescribe so he could get well and feel like playing again. It took a while, but we got our specimen. The strep test was positive and the little boy got the right antibiotic that he needed to get better. After the procedure, he gave me a smile and said "I am so glad that is over!" ■

HANDLING AND TRANSPORTING MICROBIOLOGIC SPECIMENS

After a microbiologic specimen has been collected, care should be taken in handling the specimen and preparing it for transport to an outside laboratory. Delay in processing a specimen may cause the death of any pathogens present in the specimen.

Specimens transported to an outside medical laboratory are often placed in a transport medium. The transport medium prevents drying of the specimen and preserves it in its original state until it reaches its destination. Transport media are discussed in greater detail in the section on *Collection and Transport Systems.*

Outside laboratories provide the medical office with a printed or online laboratory test directory with specific instructions on the collection, handling, and storage of specimens being transported to them. These specimens must be accompanied by a laboratory requisition that designates the provider's name and address; the patient's name, age, and gender; the date and time of collection; the type of microbiologic examination requested; the source of the specimen (e.g., throat, wound, urine); and the provider's clinical diagnosis. The form usually includes a space to indicate whether the patient is receiving antibiotic therapy. Antibiotics may suppress the growth of bacteria, a factor that could produce a false-negative test result. A **false-negative result** denotes a condition is absent when it is actually present.

It is important to properly store specimens awaiting pickup following the storage requirements outlined in the laboratory test directory. Some specimens can be stored at room temperature while others may need to be refrigerated or frozen.

Wound Specimens

Wound specimens are collected using many of the techniques described previously. In many cases, two swabs are used to collect the specimen. The specimen is obtained by inserting the swab into the area of the wound that contains the most drainage and gently rotating the swab from side to side to allow it to absorb completely any microorganisms present. The swab is placed in the specimen container, and the process is repeated using a second swab. To obtain accurate and reliable test results, it is important to collect a specimen from within the wound, rather than from the surface.

COLLECTION AND TRANSPORT SYSTEMS

Microbiologic collection and transport systems are available to facilitate the collection of a bacterial specimen to be transported to an outside laboratory for analysis; examples include Culturette (Becton Dickinson, Franklin Lakes, NJ) and Starswab II (Starplex Scientific, Cleveland, TN) (Fig. 34.5). These systems consist of a sterile swab and a plastic tube that contains a transport medium. The transport medium prevents drying of the specimen and preserves it in its original state until it reaches its destination. The collection and transport system comes packaged in a transparent peel-apart envelope and should be stored at room temperature. The procedure for the use of a microbiologic collection and transport system is outlined in Box 34.1.

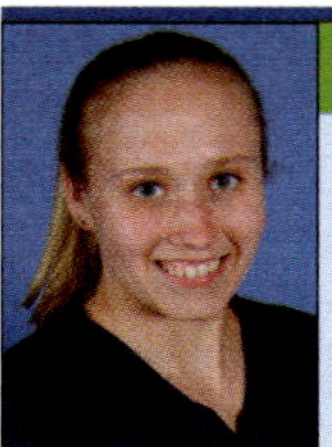

Memories *from* Practicum

Alexandra: Terrified and excited at the same time to be experiencing my first practicum, I found myself in a busy pediatric office. After a few days of watching and learning, I prepared to work up an infant for a well-child examination. Before entering the room, I was told by a staff member that the HIV status of the infant's mother was questionable. Alarmed at first as to how I would feel in this situation, I immediately remembered all the precautions we had been taught in class. As I took the infant from the mother to weigh and measure him, I have to admit many thoughts ran through my mind, but again I was calm because of all the information we had learned in school regarding HIV and OSHA precautions. Faced with that situation today, after practicing wisely and safely for 5 years, I would not think twice about it because I know from my education and experience that these types of situations can be handled without alarm. ■

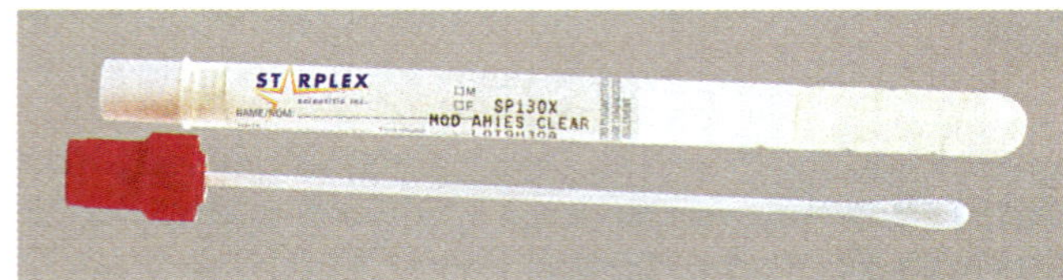

Fig. 34.5 Starswab II Collection and Transport System.

BOX 34.1 Use of a Microbiologic Collection and Transport System

1. Assemble the equipment. Check the expiration date on the collection and transport system envelope containing the transport tube and a sterile swab.
2. Open the peel-apart envelope of the collection and transport system. Remove the transport tube and label it with the patient's full name and date of birth, the collection date, the source of the specimen (e.g., throat, wound), and your initials.
3. Complete a laboratory requisition.
4. Sanitize your hands and apply gloves.
5. Position the patient as required to collect the specimen.
6. Remove the cap/swab unit from the peel-apart envelope. The cap is permanently attached to the sterile swab.
7. Using aseptic technique, collect the specimen. Do not allow the swab to touch any area other than the collection site.
8. Remove the cap from the transport tube and insert the swab into the tube.
9. Push the cap/swab in as far as it will go to completely immerse the swab in the transport medium. Make sure the cap is tightly in place.
10. Remove gloves and sanitize your hands.
11. Place the transport tube in a biohazard specimen bag and transport it to an outside laboratory within 24 hours. If the specimen cannot be transported within 24 hours, it can be refrigerated for up to 72 hours.
12. Document the procedure in the patient's medical record.

CLIA-WAIVED RAPID ANTIGEN TESTS

A microbiologic specimen may be collected and tested in the medical office to detect the presence of an infectious disease using a CLIA-waived *rapid antigen test* (RAT). A RAT is a diagnostic test that is able to detect the presence of the antigen of a pathogen such the influenza virus. The RAT is commonly used to detect respiratory pathogens.

When performing a RAT, a specimen is collected from the patient and then tested using a unitized test device. A unitized test device is a self-contained device, such as a test cassette or test card, to which a specimen is added directly and in which all of the steps of the testing procedure occur. If the pathogen (antigen) is present, a color change occurs next to the letter **T** in the test result window of the test device. This indicates the presence of the pathogen (antigen)

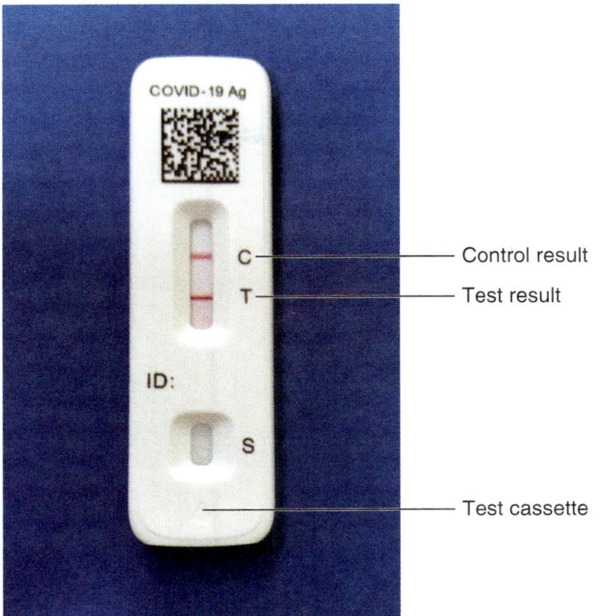

Fig. 34.6 COVID-19 rapid antigen test cassette exhibiting a color change (pink line) next to the letter **T** (test). This indicates the presence of the virus antigen causing COVID-19 and is interpreted as a positive test result. The pink line next to the letter **C** (control) indicates that the test is working properly.

and is interpreted as a positive result. The control (**C**) line is an internal quality control indicator designating that a sufficient sample was added to the test device and that the test is working properly (Fig. 34.6).

There is a higher incidence of false-negative test results with rapid antigen tests as compared to more specific tests performed by outside laboratories. Because of this, an individual may test negative on a RAT but still be infected with the pathogen. The most common CLIA-waived RAT tests performed in the medical office include rapid strep tests, rapid influenza tests, and rapid COVID-19 tests, which are described in detail in this section.

STREPTOCOCCAL PHARYNGITIS (STREP THROAT)

The most common streptococcal condition is streptococcal pharyngitis, or strep throat, which is a bacterial infection of the back of the throat and tonsils. The causative agent of strep throat is group A streptococcus, known as *Streptococcus pyogenes.* Strep throat is seasonal in nature with the highest prevalence occurring during the winter and early spring. Strep throat occurs most frequently in children ages 5 to 15 years old.

Symptoms

The symptoms of strep throat include the following:

- Severe and sudden sore throat
- Fever of 101°F (38.3°C) or higher
- Red and swollen tonsils
- White patches or streaks on the throat and tonsils
- Severe pain and difficulty upon swallowing
- Tender and swollen lymph nodes on the sides of the neck
- Tiny red spots at the back of the roof of the mouth
- Headache

Strep throat can easily be spread from one person to another through droplet transmission and by sharing personal items with an infected person, such as eating utensils. The incubation period for strep throat ranges from 1 to 3 days, with most patients recovering within 7 to 10 days.

Strep throat is a potentially serious condition because (although rare) some patients develop a poststreptococcal complication. A poststreptococcal complication is a morbid secondary condition that occurs as a result of a less serious primary infection. Occasionally a patient with strep throat (primary infection) develops rheumatic fever or acute glomerulonephritis. Owing to the risk of a poststreptococcal complication, early diagnosis and treatment of strep throat with antibiotics is important.

CLIA-Waived Streptococcus Test

In the medical office, a CLIA-waived RAT (rapid antigen test) is often used for identification of group A strep bacteria (antigens) in a throat specimen. Most rapid strep tests require only 10 to 20 minutes to process. This means that a diagnosis can often be made, and antibiotics prescribed, if necessary, before the patient leaves the office. This is in contrast to the more time-consuming throat culture test performed at an outside laboratory which requires 2 to 5 days to generate the test results.

Specific instructions are included with every commercially available CLIA-waived rapid strep test; examples of these tests include QuickVue In-Line Strep A (QuidelOrtho Corporation, San Diego, CA), OSOM Strep A Test (Sekisui Diagnostics, San Diego, CA), and BinaxNOW Strep A Test (Abbott Diagnostics, Santa Clara, CA). The procedure for performing a CLIA-waived rapid strep test is presented in Procedure 34.3.

What Would You Do? What Would You *Not* Do?

Case Study 2

Paula Holmes brings her 8-year-old daughter Caitlin to the medical office. Caitlin has had a fever, sore throat, and difficulty eating for the past 2 days. The physician orders a rapid strep test. Caitlin refuses to open her mouth so that the specimen can be collected. She says that she doesn't want that "stick thing" in her mouth because she's afraid it will make her throw up. Paula wants to know why the strep test must be run. She says that Caitlin's throat is very red with white patches and wants to know why the physician doesn't just prescribe an antibiotic for her without running the test. ■

INFLUENZA

Influenza (commonly called the flu) is a highly contagious acute infectious disease caused by viruses that infect the respiratory tract (nose, throat, and lungs). According to the Centers for Disease Control (CDC), approximately 5% to 20% of the U.S. population will contract influenza each year. Influenza outbreaks are most apt to occur between late fall and early spring (November through April). There are three different types of influenza viruses (A, B, and C), which are described as follows:

- *Influenza type A virus:* This virus type is most prevalent and is responsible for most annual influenza outbreaks. It causes moderate to severe illness, and at times it can lead to serious complications. Influenza A can be further divided into numerous subtypes; for example, H3N2 (Hong Kong flu) and H1N1 (swine flu) are subtypes of influenza type A.
- *Influenza type B virus:* This virus type can cause influenza outbreaks but is usually associated with a less severe infection than type A.
- *Influenza type C virus:* This virus type only causes a mild upper respiratory illness and occurs much less frequently than types A and B.

Transmission and Incubation Period

Influenza spreads easily from one person to another. It is spread primarily through droplet transmission from the respiratory tract of an infected individual when they cough, sneeze, or talk. Influenza is less frequently transmitted through indirect contact such as when a person touches an object or surface contaminated with the influenza virus and then touches their mouth, eyes, or nose. An individual usually becomes infected with either type A or type B influenza, but in rare instances an individual may become infected with both type A and type B influenza at the same time.

The incubation period for influenza is usually 2 days but it can range from 1 to 4 days. An infected individual is most contagious in the first 3 to 4 days after symptoms appear. A **contagious disease** refers to a disease is capable of being transmitted directly or indirectly from one person to another.

Symptoms

In the early stages of influenza, symptoms may be difficult to distinguish from those of the common cold; however, colds usually develop slowly, whereas the flu has a more sudden onset and the symptoms are much worse. Symptoms of influenza vary by age but commonly include the following:

- Fever and chills
- Muscle aches and joint pain
- Sore throat
- Runny nose
- Nasal congestion
- Dry cough
- Headache
- Joint pain
- Anorexia
- Fatigue
- Gastrointestinal symptoms such as nausea, vomiting, and diarrhea (more common in children)

Complications

Influenza can occur among people of all ages. Most individuals with healthy immune systems recover within 7 to 14 days, with the worst symptoms lasting 3 to 4 days. There are certain factors that can increase an individual's risk of developing serious and even life-threatening complications from influenza. These risk factors can be categorized into *health-related factors* and *age-related factors* and are presented in Box 34.2.

Influenza complications range in severity and can include the following: viral pneumonia, a worsening of a chronic medical condition, and secondary bacterial infections such as bacterial pneumonia, bronchitis, sinusitis, and otitis media. Some of these complications can lead to hospitalization and even death. Because of this, individuals with risk factors should seek prompt medical attention at the first sign of flu-like symptoms. Most, but not all, of flu-related deaths occur in individuals 65 years of age and older.

BOX 34.2 Factors That Increase the Risk of Influenza Complications

Individuals with the following health-related and age-related factors are at an increased risk of developing influenza complications and should seek prompt medical attention at the first sign of flu-like symptoms.

Health-Related Factors

Chronic Medical Conditions

- Asthma
- Chronic bronchitis
- Emphysema
- Cystic fibrosis
- Diabetes
- Heart disease
- Kidney or liver disorders
- Blood disorders (e.g., sickle cell disease)
- Very severely obese (body mass index [BMI] of 40 or more)

Diseases or Treatments that Weaken the Immune System

- HIV/AIDS
- Treatment with corticosteroids, immunosuppressants, or chemotherapy

Age-Related Factors

- Adults age 65 years and older
- Young children under 5 years of age, but especially children younger than 2 years of age

Additional Factors

- Individuals with severe influenza symptoms
- Pregnant women
- Residents of nursing homes and other long-term care facilities
- Native Americans and Alaska Natives

Influenza Vaccine

The best means of preventing influenza and its complications is through an annual influenza vaccination. The vaccine is recommended for all individuals ages 6 months and older who do not have contraindications to receiving the vaccine (e.g., severe egg allergy). The vaccine provides protection against both the type A and type B influenza viruses. As previously discussed, there are numerous subtypes of influenza type A. Small changes continuously take place in the genetic material of these subtype viruses resulting in new strains developing that replace the older strains. Because of this, a new vaccine must be produced each year to provide protection against the most recent strains predicted to be circulating during that year's flu season.

It takes approximately 2 weeks following vaccination for the antibodies to develop that provide protection against the virus strains included in the vaccine. The flu vaccine provides reasonable protection among healthy adults. Vaccination is most effective when the circulating virus strains are well matched with the virus strains included in the vaccine. Even if the vaccine does not prevent the flu, however, it can reduce the severity of symptoms and decrease the risk of complications.

The influenza vaccine has only mild side effects or none at all, and it is available as an intramuscular injection (e.g., Fluarix), an intradermal injection (e.g., Fluzone Intradermal), or a nasal spray (e.g., FluMist). Flu vaccination is offered in many locations within a community such as medical offices, health departments, pharmacies, college health centers, workplaces, and even schools. Many communities have programs that offer the vaccine free of charge or at a reduced cost.

Treatment

Treatment for influenza primarily involves home care measures to ease the symptoms but may occasionally involve the use of an antiviral medication. These treatment measures are discussed in more detail as follows:

Home Care

Most people who contract influenza recover on their own without medical intervention. Home care is usually all that is necessary to treat the symptoms of influenza. These measures are outlined as follows:

- Get plenty of rest.
- Increase fluid intake to stay hydrated.
- Avoid the use of alcohol and tobacco.
- Take over-the-counter medications to relieve the symptoms of the disease.

Influenza Antiviral Medications

Influenza antiviral medications are available through a prescription and work by limiting the multiplication of the influenza virus. Antiviral medications lessen the severity of influenza and shorten the duration of the disease by 1 to 2 days. They are not intended, however, to serve as a substitute for an annual influenza immunization. Antiviral medications are recommended primarily for unvaccinated individuals infected with influenza who are at risk of developing complications from influenza (see Box 34.2).

There are four influenza antiviral medications recommended by the CDC for the treatment of influenza. They include Tamiflu (oseltamivir phosphate), Relenza (zanamivir), Rapivab (peramivir), and Xofluza (baloxavir marboxil). These antiviral medications are effective against both influenza virus types A and B and must be started within the first 48 hours of developing symptoms to be most effective. Because of this, individuals at risk for influenza complications are encouraged to contact their providers at the first sign of flu-like symptoms.

CLIA-Waived Influenza Test

In the majority of cases, influenza is diagnosed solely by the clinical signs and symptoms exhibited by the patient. This is because flu symptoms are self-limiting, and most individuals recover without requiring medical treatment. An influenza test may be ordered for a patient who is at high risk for developing influenza complications as a basis for prescribing antiviral medication.

In the medical office, a CLIA-waived rapid influenza test may be used to diagnose influenza. A rapid influenza test is a rapid antigen test (RAT) for the detection of the influenza virus antigen. It is easy to perform and provides results in a short period of time (10 to 30 minutes). It is important to perform a rapid influenza test as close as possible to the onset of symptoms. This is because a patient infected with the influenza virus is most apt to show a positive test result within the first 3 to 4 days after the appearance of symptoms.

Rapid influenza tests vary in their ability to detect type A and type B influenza viruses. The test detects the influenza virus in one of the following ways:

1. Detects the presence of the influenza virus without identifying the type
2. Detects only influenza type A virus
3. Detects the presence of type A and B influenza virus, but does not distinguish between the two types
4. Detects and distinguishes between the presence of type A and type B influenza virus

The main disadvantage of a rapid influenza test is that there is a high rate of false-negative test results. Because of this, the CDC recommend that anticipated treatment not be withheld from patients with suspected influenza, even if the patient tests negative. More specific tests are available (e.g., viral culture) that can be performed by an outside laboratory; however, it can take from 2 to 10 days to perform the test and obtain the results.

The specimen required to perform a rapid influenza test depends on the brand of test being utilized and includes one or more of the following: nasopharyngeal swab specimen, nasal swab specimen, nasal wash, nasal aspirate, and throat specimen. The influenza virus is most likely to be found in the nasopharynx; therefore, a nasopharyngeal swab specimen is considered the preferred specimen for a rapid influenza test and is discussed in more detail next.

Nasopharyngeal Swab Specimen

The nasopharynx is the part of the pharynx above the soft palate that is directly continuous with the nasal passages. This is the area from which a nasopharyngeal swab specimen is collected for the detection of the influenza virus. The influenza virus invades epithelial cells in the nasopharynx; therefore, a specimen obtained from this area is preferred for rapid influenza testing.

The preferred specimen collection device for a nasopharyngeal specimen is a flocked swab. A nasopharyngeal flocked swab consists of a flexible shaft with a small brushlike tip (Fig. 34.7). The shaft of the swab has a thicker diameter at one end (where it is held) and progressively narrows to a thinner end, culminating in the soft brush tip. The tip is coated with short nylon fibers that are arranged in a perpendicular manner. This arrangement results from a process called *flocking*, in which nylon fibers are sprayed onto the tip of the swab. Flocking results in a more abrasive swab tip than a cotton-tipped swab and leads to the removal of a greater number of epithelial cells from the nasopharynx.

The depth to which the swab should be inserted is specific to each patient. For example, in order to reach the nasopharyngeal mucosa, the swab must be inserted to a greater depth in an adult than that of a child. It is possible to determine the distance to which the swab should be inserted by visually estimating the distance between the corner of the nose and the earlobe. The swab should be inserted approximately one-half this distance (Fig. 34.8). This depth usually falls between 4 to 6 centimeters (approximately 1½ to 2½ inches). The procedure for collecting a nasopharyngeal swab specimen and performing a CLIA-waived rapid influenza test is presented in Procedure 34.4.

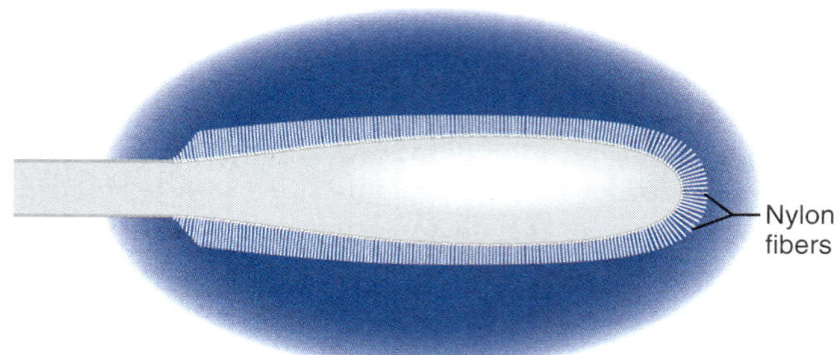

Fig. 34.7 A nasopharyngeal flocked swab consists of a flexible shaft with a small brushlike tip made of nylon fibers.

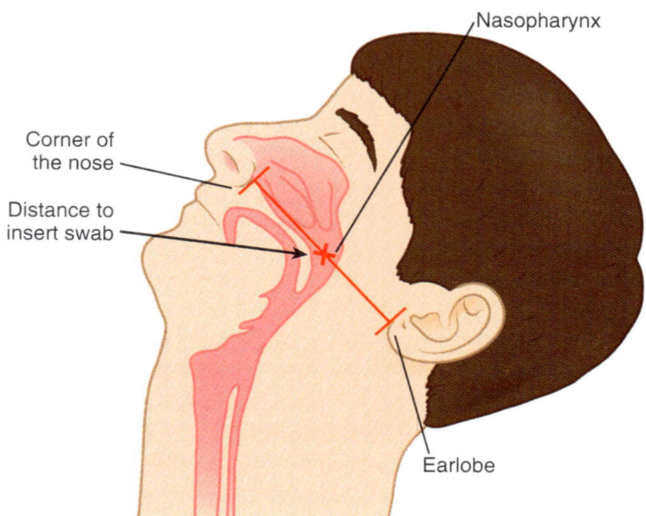

Fig. 34.8 A swab used to collect a nasopharyngeal specimen should be inserted approximately one-half the distance between the corner of the nose and the earlobe.

What Would You Do? What Would You *Not* Do?

Case Study 3

Hollie Dolley, age 18, is at the medical office complaining of fatigue, fever, headache, muscle aching, runny nose, and a sore throat that began a day ago. Hollie also has severe problems with asthma, which began when she was a child. Hollie just enrolled in a medical assisting program at a local college and has been really worried about doing well in her classes. The physician orders a rapid influenza test on Hollie, and it is positive. The physician writes a prescription for an antiviral medication and advises Hollie to get plenty of rest, increase her fluid intake, and to stay at home for at least 24 hours after the fever has subsided. Hollie wants to know how the antiviral medication is going to help her. She says she doesn't know why she has the flu because she got a flu vaccine a week ago. Hollie also wants to know why the physician did not prescribe an antibiotic for her so that she could get well sooner and not have to miss many classes. ■

COVID-19

COVID-19 (*coronavirus disease*) is an acute respiratory disease caused by a novel (or new) strain of coronavirus known as *SARS-CoV-2* (*severe acute respiratory syndrome coronavirus 2*) (Fig. 34.9). The virus is considered novel because it is a new coronavirus that has not been previously identified in humans and the 19 in COVID-19 represents the year in which the virus first appeared. COVID-19 was first detected in China and then quickly spread worldwide resulting in a pandemic.

The primary sites of infection of SARS-CoV-2 are the upper and lower respiratory tracts, especially the lungs. The virus can also infect other parts of the body, such as the heart and blood vessels, kidneys, and brain. The potential of the virus to infect multiple areas of the body helps to explain the wide range of symptoms experienced by COVID-19 patients.

Transmission

COVID-19 is primarily spread by respiratory droplets carrying SARS-CoV-2 exhaled by an infected person during breathing, speaking, coughing, sneezing, singing, and shouting. These infectious droplets travel a short distance from the infected individual where they can be inhaled into the respiratory tract of a susceptible host. An infected person can

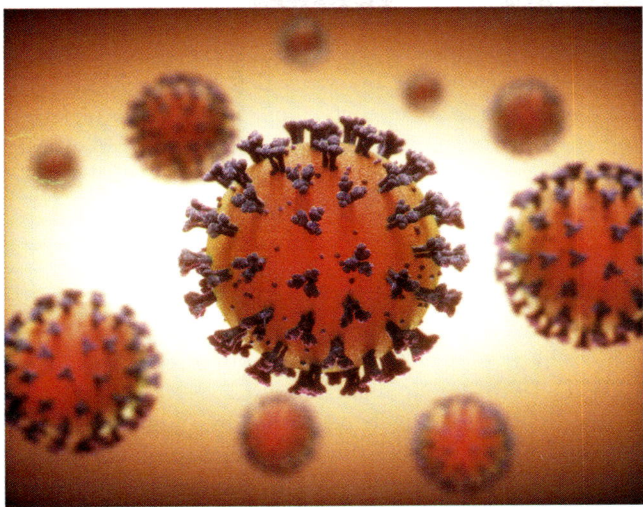

Fig. 34.9 SARS-COV-2 is the virus that causes COVID-19. (ktsimage/ iStock.com)

transmit the virus for up to 2 days before exhibiting symptoms without knowing it. An individual is contagious for up to 10 days following the onset of symptoms and in severe cases, may be contagious for up to 20 days. An infected individual is most contagious during the first week of their illness, meaning they are most contagious shortly before and shortly after symptoms appear.

Symptoms

Symptoms of COVID-19 begin anywhere from 2 to 14 days (incubation period) following infection with the virus and can range from mild to severe. Approximately one-third of individuals infected with COVID-19 do not develop any symptoms at all but are still able to transmit the infection to others. Most symptomatic individuals infected with COVID-19 develop mild to moderate flu-like symptoms and get better on their own within 2 weeks following infection. Symptoms of mild to moderate of COVID-19 vary among individuals and include the following:

- Fever
- Sore throat
- Cough
- Congestion
- Headache
- Fatigue
- Muscle or body aches
- Breathing difficulties
- Loss of smell and taste
- Nausea or vomiting
- Diarrhea

Serious COVID-19 Illness

Some individuals infected with COVID-19 may experience mild to moderate symptoms at first but then go on to develop a serious COVID-19 illness that could be life-threatening. Older adults, and individuals of any age with underlying medical conditions or weakened immune systems, are at a higher risk for progression of the disease to a serious COVID-19 illness. Underlying medical conditions that may increase the risk for serious illness include obesity, diabetes, chronic lung disease, heart disease, and cancer.

Critical symptoms of serious COVID-19 illness include extreme shortness of breath, rapid breathing, tachycardia, pale, gray, or blue-colored skin, lips or nail beds, confusion, and persistent pain or pressure in the chest. These symptoms are caused by a build-up of fluid in the alveoli of the lungs preventing enough oxygen from reaching the circulatory system which could eventually result in organ failure and death. Individuals with severe symptoms should immediately seek emergency medical care.

Prevention of COVID-19

The following measures are recommended by public health authorities to help prevent the spread of COVID-19:

- Stay up to date with COVID-19 vaccines.
- Avoid touching your eyes, nose, and mouth with unwashed hands to prevent the virus that causes COVID-19 from gaining entrance into your body.
- Cover your nose and mouth when you cough or sneeze. To avoid contaminating the hands, cough or sneeze into a tissue or the crook of your elbow.
- Sanitize your hands frequently, either with soap and water for 20 seconds or with an alcohol-based hand sanitizer.
- Avoid crowds and poorly ventilated areas.
- Avoid contact with people who have suspected or confirmed COVID-19.
- Get tested for COVID-19, if necessary. Get tested immediately if you have COVID-19 symptoms. If you have been exposed to COVID-19 and do not have symptoms, wait 5 days to get tested to ensure an accurate test result. Testing too soon after exposure could lead to a false-negative test result.
- If you have been exposed to COVID-19, wear a high-quality mask (N95) when indoors and around others for 10 days. During this time, you should get tested and monitor yourself for symptoms.
- Regardless of vaccination status, if you have confirmed COVID-19, isolate yourself at home and take precautions to avoid infecting others until you recover. Obtain follow-up care with your provider. Seek medical attention immediately if your symptoms become severe.
- Seek antiviral medication treatment if you have mild to moderate COVID-19 and are at a higher risk for developing serious illness.

COVID-19 Vaccine

The COVID-19 vaccine provides the best defense against the virus that causes COVID-19. Although individuals who have been vaccinated may still get infected with the virus, the vaccine is highly effective in preventing serious illness, hospitalization, and death. The COVID-19 vaccine is recommended for all individuals ages 6 months and older. COVID-19 vaccines authorized by the FDA for use in the

United States include Pfizer-BioNTech, Moderna and Novavax.

Side effects of the COVID-19 vaccine vary from one person to another and tend to be mild and temporary. The most common side effects include pain, swelling, and redness at the injection site, headache, fatigue, muscle pain, and fever.

The CDC recommends that all individuals (6 months and older) stay up to date on the COVID-19 immunization schedule. The COVID-19 immunization schedule depends on a person's age, health status, and previous COVID-19 vaccinations and is available for review on the CDC website (www.cdc.gov).

Treatment

Treatment for mild to moderate COVID-19 primarily involves home care measures to ease the symptoms but may occasionally involve the use of antiviral medications. These treatment measures are discussed in more detail as follows:

Home Care

Most people who contract mild to moderate COVID-19 recover on their own without medical intervention. Home care is usually all that is necessary to treat the symptoms of mild to moderate COVID-19. These measures include getting plenty of rest, increasing fluid intake, avoiding smoking, and taking OTC medications to relieve the symptoms of the disease.

COVID-19 Antiviral Medication

Antiviral medications are available through a prescription to treat COVID-19. Antiviral medications are recommended for individuals with mild to moderate COVID-19 who are at high risk for progression of the disease to a serious COVID-19 illness (e.g., individuals with diabetes, chronic lung deisease, heart disease). Studies show that antiviral medications help to lower the risk of serious illness, hospitalization, and death. An antiviral medication approved by the FDA commonly used to treat COVID-19 is Paxlovid (nirmatrelvir with ritonavir) (Fig. 34.10). To be most effective, this medication must be started within the first 5 days after the onset of symptoms.

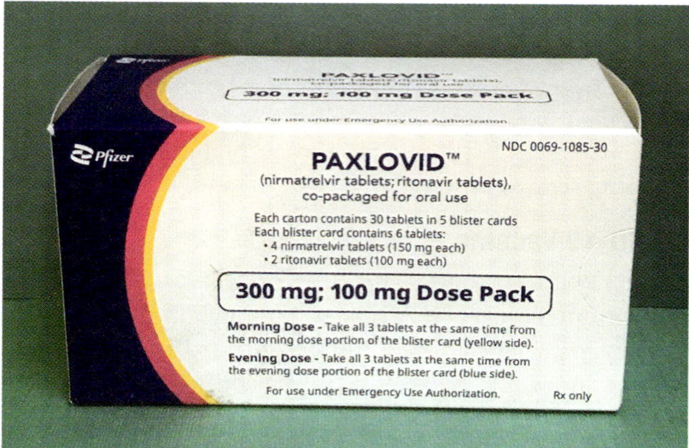

Fig. 34.10 Paxlovid is an antiviral medication used to treat COVID-19.

COVID-19 Tests

There are two different types of COVID-19 tests used to detect the presence of the virus that causes COVID-19. They include a PCR test (also known as a molecular test) and a rapid antigen test. The PCR test is not a CLIA-waived test, however it is frequently used to assist in the diagnosis of COVID-19 and therefore is included in this section.

COVID-19 PCR Test

The PCR (polymerase chain reaction) test for COVID-19 is considered the "gold standard" for COVID-19 testing. It is more likely to detect the presence of the virus that causes COVID-19 than a rapid antigen test.

The PCR test is usually performed by an outside laboratory and works by detecting the presence of the genetic material (called RNA) of the virus. The medical assistant is often responsible for collecting the specimen at the medical office for transport to the outside laboratory for testing. The PCR test is usually performed on an anterior nasal (nares) swab specimen. Other types of specimens that can be used include a nasopharyngeal swab specimen and a saliva specimen. The procedure for collecting an anterior nasal swab specimen for transport to an outside laboratory is outlined in Box 34.3. Although the PCR test is highly accurate, it is time-consuming to perform; it sometimes takes between 1 to 3 days to receive the test results from the laboratory.

CLIA-Waived COVID-19 Test

In the medical office, a CLIA-waived COVID-19 rapid antigen test (RAT) is often performed to assist in the diagnosis of COVID-19 (Fig. 34.11). Rapid COVID-19 tests are easy to perform and provide results in a short period of time (15 to 30 minutes). The specimen required to perform a rapid COVID-19 test depends on the brand of test being utilized. Most tests require the collection of an anterior nasal swab specimen to perform the test (outlined in Box 34.3). Proper collection and handling of the specimen are essential for accurate test results.

Positive test results on a rapid COVID-19 test are very accurate and reliable; therefore, an individual who tests positive is very likely to be infected with the virus that causes COVID-19. Unfortunately, there is a higher rate of false-negative test results with RATs as compared with the PCR test. This means that an individual could test negative on a RAT but still be infected with COVID-19. Because of this, the provider may order a PCR test on a negative RAT to reduce the risk of a false-negative test result.

There are numerous CLIA-waived rapid COVID-19 tests available. Examples include BinaxNOW (Abbott Diagnostics, Santa Clara, CA), Sofia (QuidelOrtho Corporation, San Diego, CA), InteliSwab (OraSure Technologies, Bethlehem, PA) and FlowFlex (ACON Laboratories, San Diego, CA). Rapid antigen tests are also available without a prescription for self-testing by individuals at home. If the virus that causes COVID-19 is detected by a rapid COVID-19 test, a color change occurs in the result window of the test device. This color change is interpreted as a

BOX 34.3 Collection of an Anterior Nasal Swab Specimen

1. Sanitize your hands and assemble equipment. Check the expiration date on the collection kit envelope containing the transport tube and sterile swab.
2. Open the peel-apart envelope and remove the transport tube. Label the tube with the patient's full name and date of birth, the collection date, the source of the specimen (i.e., anterior nasal specimen), and your initials.
3. Complete a laboratory requisition.
4. Apply personal protective equipment including a face mask, protective eyewear, and clean disposable gloves. Perform this step before entering the patient's room.
5. Greet and identify the patient.
6. Ask that patient to tilt their head back slightly (about 70 degrees).
7. Remove the sterile swab from the peel-apart envelope, being careful not to contaminate it.
8. Gently insert the entire soft tip of the swab approximately ½ to ¾ inch (1 to 1.5 cm) into one nostril.
9. Firmly rub the swab against the inside wall of the nostril 5 times or more in a circular motion for at least 15 seconds. This dislodges and collects epithelial cells onto the swab. Failure to collect enough cells may cause a false-negative test result. Do not touch the swab tip to anything other than the inside of the nostril.

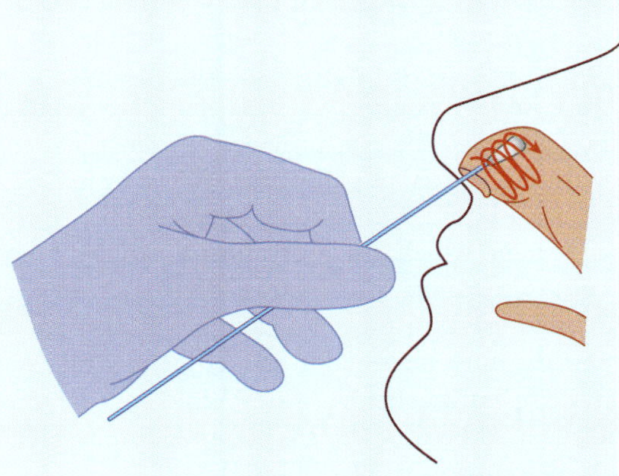

10. Gently remove the swab from the patient's nostril and insert it into the other nostril. Collect a specimen from the other nostril following the same technique outlined in Step 9. This means that a specimen is collected from both nostrils with the same swab.

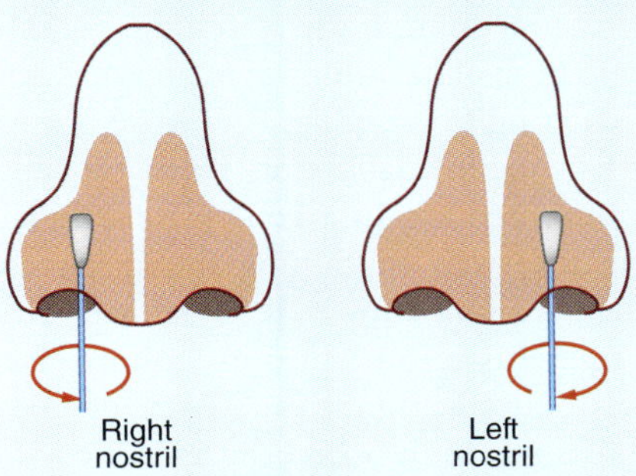

11. While holding the swab, remove the cap from the transport tube and insert the swab into the tube.
12. Carefully break the swab shaft at the score-line by leaning the shaft against the tube rim and applying gentle pressure. Dispose of the top of the swab shaft in a waste container.

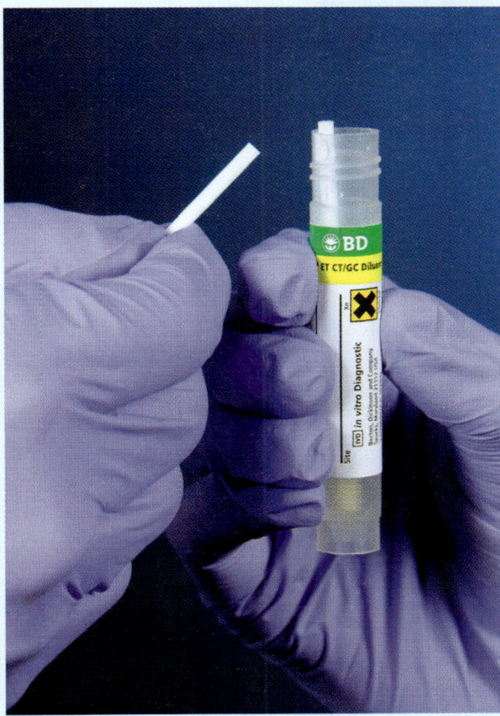

13. Replace the cap on the transport tube and securely tighten it.
14. Offer the patient tissues to blow the nose, if needed.
15. Place the transport tube in a biohazard specimen bag and transport it to an outside laboratory within 24 hours. If the specimen cannot be transported within 24 hours, it can be refrigerated for up to 72 hours.
16. Remove personal protective equipment and sanitize your hands.
17. Document the procedure in the patient's medical record.

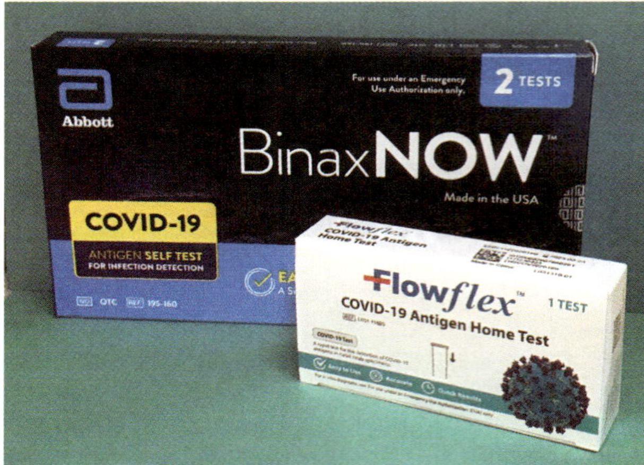

Fig. 34.11 COVID-19 rapid antigen tests.

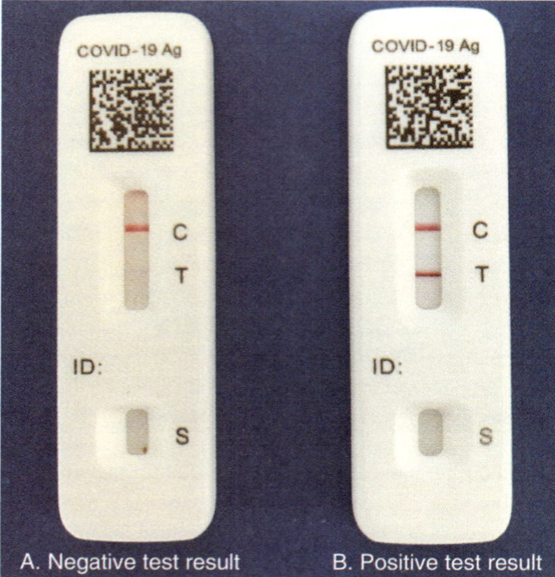

Fig. 34.12 Interpretation of COVID-19 test results on a rapid antigen test. (A) **Negative:** At the proper reading time, there is no pink line next to the letter **T** in the test result window. This means that no virus antigens for COVID-19 were detected. To be considered a valid test result, the test result window must exhibit a pink procedural control line next to the letter **C.** (B) **Positive:** At the proper reading time, the test result window exhibits any shade of a pink test line next to the letter **T**. This means that virus antigens for COVID-19 were detected. To be considered a valid test result, the test result window must exhibit a pink procedural control line next to the letter **C.**

positive test result. If the color change does not occur, the results are interpreted as a negative test result. The method for interpreting test results on a rapid COVID-19 test is presented in Fig. 34.12.

When using a rapid COVID-19 test, the medical assistant should carefully read the package insert accompanying the test and follow the instructions *exactly* to ensure accurate and reliable test results. These instructions include:

- Proper storage of the test kit
- Adherence to expiration dates
- Proper collection and handling of the specimen
- Performance of quality control procedures
- Proper testing of the specimen
- Correct interpretation of test results
- Accurate documentation of test results

CULTURE AND SENSITIVITY TESTING

MICROBIAL CULTURES

After a microbiologic specimen is collected and transported to an outside laboratory, it is analyzed to determine the type of pathogen present. Because most specimens generally contain a limited number of pathogens, it is often desirable to induce any pathogens that are present to grow and multiply.

Most microorganisms, especially bacteria, can be grown on a culture medium. A **culture medium** is a mixture of nutrients on which microorganisms are grown in the laboratory. The culture medium and the environment in which it is placed must meet the requirements to support and encourage the growth of the suspected pathogen. These growth requirements include the presence or the absence of oxygen (depending on the microorganism); proper nutrition, temperature, and pH; and moisture.

The culture medium may be solid or liquid. Blood agar is one of the most frequently used solid culture media because it allows for the growth of a wide range of pathogenic microorganisms. Blood agar is prepared by adding sheep's blood to a substance known as *agar*, which is transparent and colorless. Blood added to the agar provides nutrients that support the growth of a variety of pathogens. When heated, it melts and becomes a liquid. On cooling, agar solidifies, forming a firm surface on which microorganisms can be grown. A liquid culture medium is often referred to as a *broth* and is usually contained in a tube; an example is nutrient broth. Culture media must be stored in the refrigerator and warmed to room temperature before use. A cold culture medium must not be used because the cold temperature results in the death of microorganisms placed on it.

A *Petri plate* is frequently used to hold solid culture medium. The plate consists of a shallow circular dish made of glass or clear plastic with a cover, the diameter of which is greater than that of the base. Microorganisms can be cultured on the surface of the medium in the plate (Fig. 34.13). Petri plates allow examination of a culture while preventing microorganisms from entering or escaping. A **culture** is a mass of microorganisms growing in a laboratory culture medium.

The solid culture medium in a Petri plate is inoculated by lightly rolling the swab containing the specimen over the surface of the medium. **Inoculate** is defined as the introduction of microorganisms into a culture medium for growth and multiplication. The cover of the Petri plate should be removed only when the specimen is being spread on the culture medium. Unnecessary removal of the cover results in contamination of the medium with extraneous microorganisms. The culture is then incubated for 24 to 48 hours **Incubate** refers to placing a culture in a chamber that provides optimal growth requirements for multiplication of the suspected pathogen.

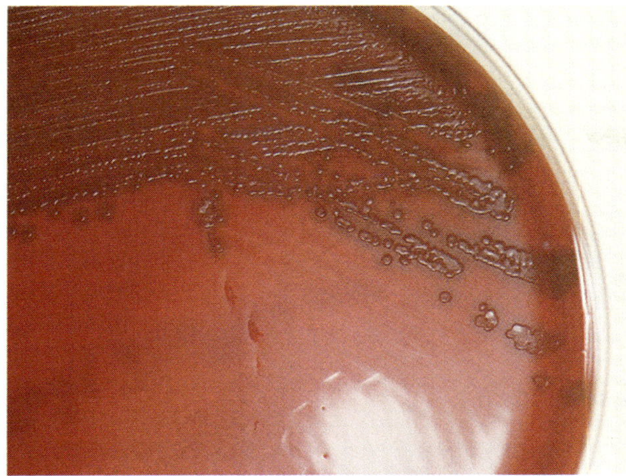

Fig. 34.13 Streptococcal colonies growing on a blood agar culture medium contained in a Petri plate. (From Mahon CR, Lehman DC, Manuselis G Jr: *Textbook of diagnostic microbiology*, ed 4, Philadelphia, 2010, Saunders.)

Most specimens taken for analysis contain a mixture of organisms because of the presence of normal flora in most parts of the body. When this is the case, the resulting culture is known as a *mixed culture*, or one that contains two or more types of microorganisms. To analyze most microbiologic specimens, the suspected pathogen must be separated from the mixed culture and permitted to grow alone. This establishes a *pure culture*, or a culture that contains only one type of microorganism. After the culture has grown sufficiently, the appropriate tests are performed to identify the pathogen. It is impossible to grow viruses by this method; rather, they must be cultured on living tissue or identified using serologic tests.

SENSITIVITY TESTING

The provider may request not only that the laboratory identify the infecting pathogen, but also that a sensitivity test be performed on it to determine the best antibiotic to treat the condition. The test is always performed on a pure rather than a mixed culture. A sensitivity test determines the susceptibility of pathogenic bacteria to various antibiotics; only the growth of the infectious pathogen is desired on the culture.

A common method for sensitivity testing is the *disc-diffusion method* (Fig. 34.14). Commercially prepared disks impregnated with known concentrations of various antibiotics are dropped on the surface of a solid culture medium in a Petri plate inoculated with the pathogen. The culture is incubated, allowing the antibiotics to diffuse into the culture medium. If the pathogen is susceptible or sensitive to an antibiotic, a clear zone without bacterial growth surrounds the disk. This indicates that the antibiotic was effective in destroying the pathogen. If the pathogen is unaffected by or resistant to the antibiotic, no clear zone is seen around the disk, indicating that the antibiotic was unable to kill the pathogen. Sensitivity testing enables the provider to decide which antibiotics would most likely be effective against the infectious disease in question.

PREVENTION AND CONTROL OF INFECTIOUS DISEASES

Individuals in the community can help prevent and control infectious diseases by practicing good techniques of medical asepsis, by obtaining proper nutrition and rest, and by using good hygienic measures. In addition, infected individuals should contact their providers in an effort to ensure early diagnosis and treatment of the infectious disease. Immunizations are available to prevent a wide range of infectious diseases. The medical assistant has a responsibility to help educate community members about practices that reduce the transmission of pathogens and help control and prevent infectious diseases.

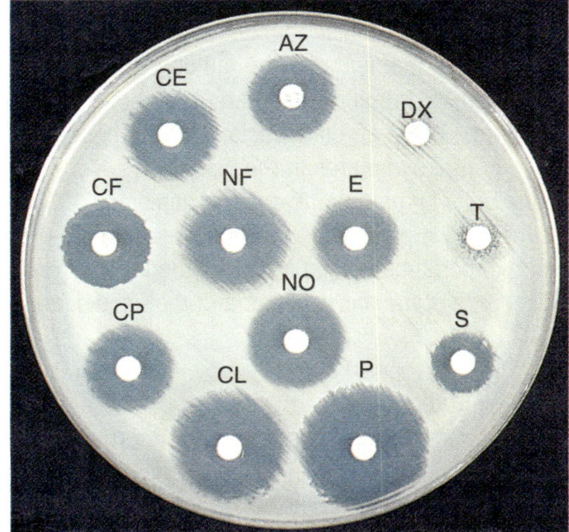

AZ: Azithromycin
CE: Cephalothin
CF: Ciprofloxacin
CL: Clarithromycin
CP: Ciprozil
DX: Doxycycline
E: Erythromycin
NF: Nitrofurantoin
NO: Norfloxacin
P: Penicillin
S: Sulfisoxazole
T: Tetracycline

Fig. 34.14 Sensitivity testing. (From Mahon CR, Lehman DC, Manuselis G Jr: *Textbook of diagnostic microbiology*, ed 4, Philadelphia, 2010, Saunders.)

What Would You Do? What Would You *Not* Do? RESPONSES

Case Study 1
Page 914

What Did Alexandra Do?
- ❑ Empathized with John and told him that a lot of people do not like coming to see the doctor. Told him that the doctor could not legally or ethically prescribe medication for him without seeing him.
- ❑ Told John that the office could not bill him for an appointment that he did not have.
- ❑ Asked John whether he wanted to make an appointment to see the doctor.

What Did Alexandra Not Do?
- ❑ Did not tell John he should not be diagnosing himself with information he found on the internet.

Case Study 2
Page 919

What Did Alexandra Do?
- ❑ Told Paula that it is important that the physician find out whether Caitlin has strep throat because strep can sometimes develop into a more serious infection.
- ❑ Talked with Caitlin about the reason for the test. Explained that it will help the doctor find the best way to treat her so that she starts feeling better as soon as possible.
- ❑ Reassured Caitlin that the procedure would be quick and it would be over before she knew it. Told Caitlin that after the specimen was obtained, she could choose a prize from the treasure box.
- ❑ Explained to Paula that the physician must first determine if Caitlin has strep throat before antibiotics can be prescribed.

What Did Alexandra Not Do?
- ❑ Did not force the collection swab into Caitlin's mouth.

Case Study 3
Page 922

What Did Alexandra Do?
- ❑ Explained to Hollie that the antiviral medication should lessen the severity of her flu and shorten the duration of it by 1 to 2 days.
- ❑ Explained to Hollie that it takes approximately 2 weeks following vaccination for the flu vaccine to be effective.
- ❑ Explained to Hollie that influenza is caused by a virus and that antibiotics do not work against viruses.
- ❑ Empathized with Hollie and made sure she understood the home measures she could take to treat the symptoms of influenza.

What Did Alexandra Not Do?
- ❑ Did not ignore or minimize Hollie's concerns. ■

TERMINOLOGY REVIEW

Medical Term	Word Parts	Definition
Bacilli (*sing.* bacillus)		Bacteria that have a rod shape.
Cocci (*sing.* coccus)	*-cocci:* berry shaped	Bacteria that have a round shape.
Contagious disease		A disease that is capable of being transmitted directly or indirectly from one person to another.
Culture		The propagation of a mass of microorganisms in a laboratory culture medium.
Culture medium		A mixture of nutrients on which microorganisms are grown in the laboratory.
False-negative result		A test result denoting that a condition is absent when it is actually present.
Incubate		In microbiology, the act of placing a culture in a chamber (incubator) that provides optimal growth requirements for the multiplication of the organisms, such as the proper temperature, humidity, and darkness.
Incubation period		The interval of time between the invasion by a pathogenic microorganism and the appearance of first symptoms of the disease.
Infection		Invasion of the body by pathogenic microorganisms.
Infectious disease		A disease caused by a pathogen that produces harmful effects to its host.
Inoculate		To introduce microorganisms into a culture medium for growth and multiplication.
Microbiology	*micro-:* small *bi/o:* life *-ology:* study of	The scientific study of microorganisms and their activities.
Microorganism		A microscopic plant or animal.
Normal flora		Harmless, nonpathogenic microorganisms that normally reside in many parts of the body but do not cause disease.
Specimen		A small sample or part taken from the body to represent the whole.
Spirilla (*sing.* spirillum)		Bacteria that have a spiral or curved shape.

PROCEDURE 34.1 Operate a Compound Microscope

Outcome Operate a compound microscope.

Equipment/Supplies

- Compound microscope with mechanical stage
- Lens paper
- Specimen slide
- Tissue or gauze
- Immersion oil
- Xylene
- Soft cloth

1. **Procedural Step.** Clean the eyepiece and objective lenses with lens paper using a circular motion.

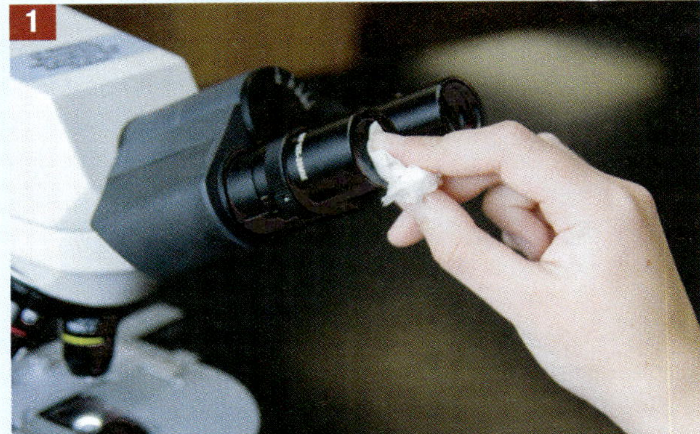

Clean the eyepiece lenses.

2. **Procedural Step.** Turn on the illuminator.
3. **Procedural Step.** Lower the stage all the way down using the coarse adjustment knob. Rotate the nosepiece to the low-power objective (10×) and click it into place. Lowering the stage all the way down provides sufficient working space for placing the slide on the stage and also avoids damaging the objective lens.
4. **Procedural Step.** Place the slide on the mechanical stage specimen side up, and use the slide holder to secure it.

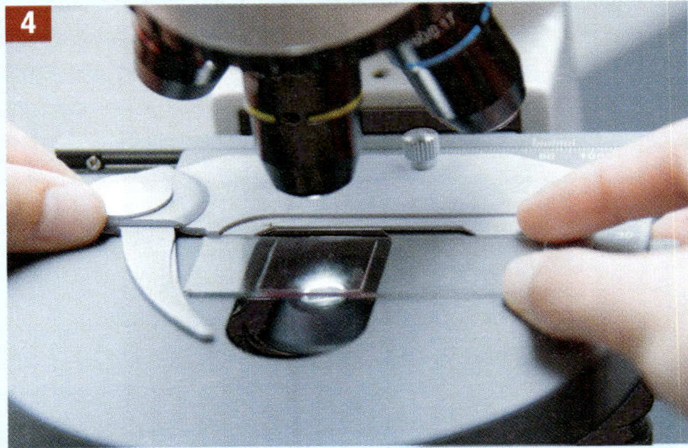

Place the slide on the stage.

5. **Procedural Step.** Using the coarse adjustment knob, raise the stage as far as it will go without letting the slide touch the low-power objective. Be sure to observe this step to prevent the objective from striking the slide.
6. **Procedural Step.** Look through the eyepiece(s). If a monocular microscope is being used, keep both eyes open to prevent eyestrain. With a binocular microscope, adjust the two eyepieces to the width between your eyes until a single circular field of vision is obtained.
7. **Procedural Step.** Slowly lower the stage using the coarse adjustment knob. Observe the specimen through the eyepieces until it comes into focus.

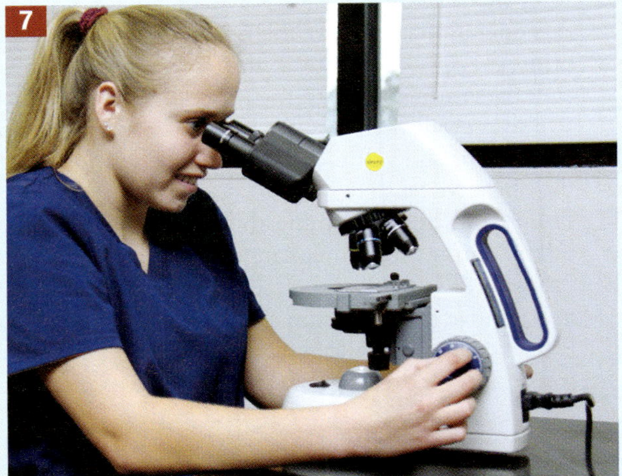

Focus the specimen.

8. **Procedural Step.** Use the fine adjustment knob to bring the specimen into a sharp, clear focus. Use the mechanical stage adjustment knobs to center the specimen as needed for optimal viewing.
9. **Procedural Step.** Adjust the light as needed, using the intensity dial of the illuminator and the diaphragm lever to provide maximal focus and contrast.

Continued

PROCEDURE 34.1 Operate a Compound Microscope—cont'd

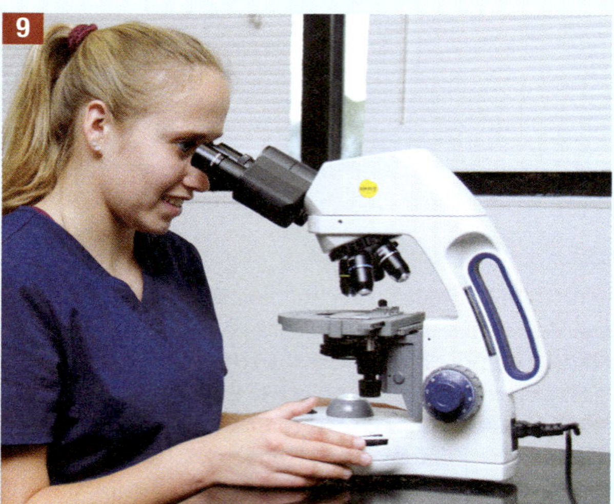

Adjust the light.

10. **Procedural Step.** Rotate the nosepiece to the high-power objective, making sure it clicks into place. Proper focusing with the low-power objective ensures that the objective does not hit the slide during this operation. Use only the fine adjustment knob to bring the specimen into a precise focus. Do not use the coarse adjustment to focus the high-power objective to prevent the objective from moving too far and striking the slide. This can break the slide and damage the objective lens.
11. **Procedural Step.** Examine the specimen as required by the test or procedure being performed.
12. **Procedural Step.** Turn off the illuminator after use and remove the slide from the stage.
13. **Procedural Step.** Clean the stage with a tissue or gauze. Lower the stage all the way down and rotate the nosepiece to the low-power objective.
14. **Procedural Step.** Properly care for and store the microscope.

Using the Oil-Immersion Objective

1. **Procedural Step.** Perform the steps listed above to bring the specimen into focus with first the low-power objective and then with the high-power objective. Rotate the nosepiece to the oil-immersion objective. Do not click it into place, but move it to one side.
2. **Procedural Step.** Place a drop of immersion oil on the slide directly over the center opening in the stage.

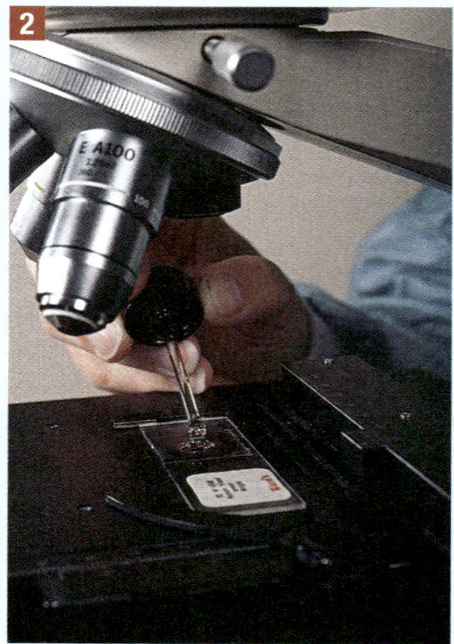

Place a drop of oil on the slide.

3. **Procedural Step.** Move the oil-immersion objective until it clicks into place.
4. **Procedural Step.** Using the fine adjustment knob, slowly position the oil-immersion objective until the tip of the lens just touches the oil but does not come in contact with the slide. A "pop" of light is observed. Be sure to observe carefully this step of the procedure.

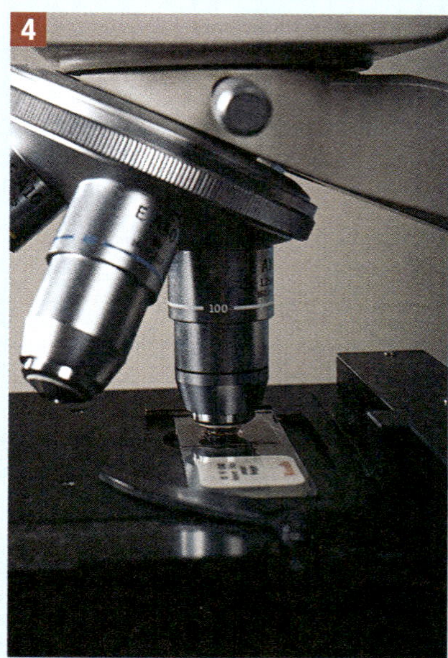

Move the lens until it just touches the oil.

PROCEDURE 34.1 Operate a Compound Microscope—cont'd

5. **Procedural Step.** Look through the eyepieces, and focus slowly using the fine adjustment knob. Bring the specimen into a sharp clear focus to view fine details.
6. **Procedural Step.** Adjust the light as needed, using the diaphragm lever to provide maximal focus and contrast. Increased light intensity is required for good visualization of the specimen with the oil-immersion objective.
7. **Procedural Step.** Examine the specimen as required by the test or procedure being performed.
8. **Procedural Step.** Turn off the illuminator after use. Remove the slide from the stage, being careful not to get oil on the high-power objective lens. Immersion oil can damage the lens of the high-power objective.
9. **Procedural Step.** Using a piece of clean, dry lens paper, gently clean the oil-immersion objective. The lens must be cleaned immediately after use to prevent oil from drying on the lens surface. In addition, the oil may seep into the lens and perhaps loosen it.

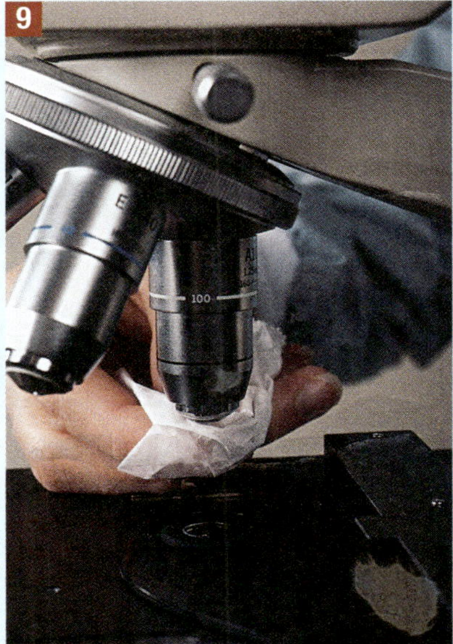

Clean the oil from the lens.

10. **Procedural Step.** Clean the oil from the slide by immersing it in xylene and wiping it off with a soft cloth.

PROCEDURE 34.2 Collecting a Throat Specimen

Outcome Collect a throat specimen for transport to an outside laboratory.

A throat specimen (also known as an oropharyngeal specimen) is obtained by using a sterile swab. It is commonly collected to aid in the diagnosis of infectious diseases such as streptococcal sore throat, pharyngitis, and tonsillitis. Less frequently, it is used to diagnose whooping cough and diphtheria. These latter diseases are not prevalent today because of the availability of vaccines against them. This procedure outlines the steps necessary to collect a throat specimen for transport to an outside laboratory.

Equipment/Supplies

- Disposable gloves
- Tongue depressor
- Sterile swab
- Transport tube
- Laboratory request form
- Biohazard specimen bag
- Waste container

1. **Procedural Step.** Sanitize your hands and assemble the equipment. Check the expiration date of the collection kit envelope containing the transport tube and sterile swab.
2. **Procedural Step.** Open the peel-apart envelope and remove the transport tube. Label the transport tube with the patient's full name and date of birth, the collection date, the source of the specimen, your initials, and any other required information. Complete a laboratory requisition.
3. **Procedural Step.** Greet the patient and introduce yourself. Identify the patient by full name and date of birth and explain the procedure.
4. **Procedural Step.** Position the patient and adjust the light to provide clear visualization of the throat.
   Principle. The throat must be clearly visible so that the medical assistant is able to determine the proper area for obtaining the specimen.
5. **Procedural Step.** Apply gloves. Remove the sterile swab from the peel-apart envelope, being careful not to contaminate it.
   Principle. Contamination of the swab may lead to inaccurate test results.

Continued

PROCEDURE 34.2

PROCEDURE 34.2 Collecting a Throat Specimen—cont'd

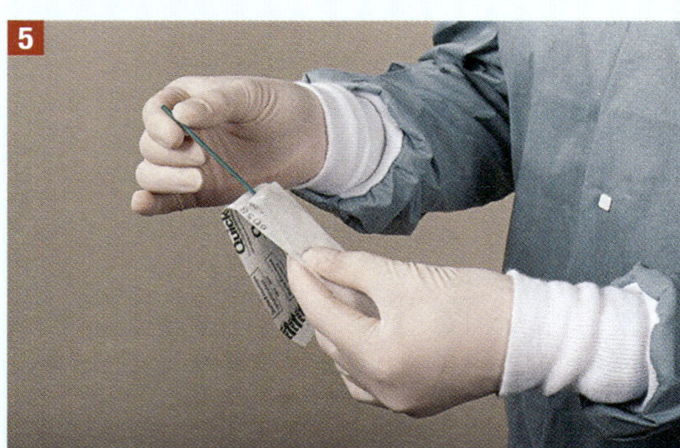

5 Remove the swab.

6. **Procedural Step.** Depress the anterior third of the tongue with the tongue depressor and ask the patient to say "ah". If the patient gags, remove the tongue depressor and allow the patient to relax before reinserting it.
   Principle. The tongue depressor holds the tongue down and facilitates access to the throat. Placing the tongue depressor at the back of the tongue is likely to illicit a gag reflex.
7. **Procedural Step.** Observe the patient's throat for any inflamed areas of the pharynx and tonsils. Place the swab at the back of the throat (posterior pharynx). Do not allow the swab to touch any areas other than the throat, such as the lips, teeth, or inside of the mouth.
8. **Procedural Step.** Firmly rub the swab from side-to-side over any lesions or white or inflamed areas of the mucous membrane of the tonsillar area and posterior pharyngeal wall. Rotate the swab constantly as you collect the specimen, making sure there is good contact with the tonsillar area.
   Principle. The swab should be rubbed over suspicious-looking areas where pathogens are likely to be found. A rotating motion is used to deposit the maximal amount of material possible on the swab. Touching the swab to any areas other than the throat contaminates the specimen with extraneous microorganisms.

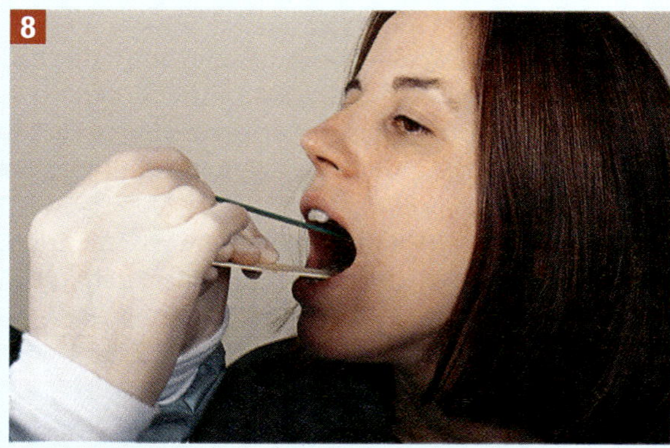

8 Collect the specimen.

9. **Procedural Step.** Keeping the patient's tongue depressed, withdraw the swab, and remove the tongue depressor from the patient's mouth without touching the inside of the mouth.
10. **Procedural Step.** Properly dispose of the tongue depressor in a regular waste container to prevent transmission of microorganisms.
11. **Procedural Step.** While holding the swab, remove the cap of the transport tube and insert the swab into it. Be careful not to touch the swab to any surface prior to placing it in the transport tube. Replace the cap on the transport tube and securely tighten it.
12. **Procedural Step.** Place the transport tube in a biohazard specimen bag and transport it to an outside laboratory within 24 hours. If the specimen cannot be transported within 24 hours, it can be refrigerated for up to 72 hours.
13. **Procedural Step.** Remove gloves and sanitize your hands.
14. **Procedural Step.** Document the information.
    a. *Electronic health record:* Document the type and source of the specimen, the laboratory test(s) ordered by the provider, and information indicating its transport to the outside laboratory using the appropriate radio buttons, drop-down menus, and free-text entry.
    b. *Paper-based patient record*: Document the date and time of collection, the type and source of the specimen, the laboratory test(s) ordered by the provider, and information indicating its transport to the outside laboratory, including the date the specimen was sent (refer to the PPR charting example).

14b

DOCUMENTATION EXAMPLE

Date	
7/12/XX	10:30 a.m. Throat specimen collected for
	culture and sensitivity. Picked up by Medical
	Center Laboratory on 7/12/XX. ___________
	___________ A. Schostek, CMA (AAMA)

PROCEDURE 34.3 Perform a CLIA-Waived Rapid Strep Test

Outcome Collect a throat specimen and perform a CLIA-waived rapid strep test.

Equipment/Supplies

- CLIA-waived QuickVue rapid strep test kit
- Sterile throat swab
- Disposable gloves
- Tongue depressor
- External controls
- Manufacturer's instructions
- Quality control log
- Biohazard waste container

1. **Procedural Step.** Sanitize your hands and assemble the equipment. Check the expiration date on the test kit. It should not be used if the expiration date has passed.
   Principle. An expired strep test may produce inaccurate test results.

Perform the Control Procedure

2. **Procedural Step.** If necessary, apply gloves and perform an external positive and negative control procedure. When a new testing kit is opened (and thereafter on a monthly basis), external positive and negative controls should be performed according to the instructions in the product insert accompanying the controls. If the controls do not perform as expected, patient testing should not be conducted until the problem is identified and resolved.
   Principle. Running positive and negative external controls ensures that the test results are valid and reliable. Factors that can cause abnormal external control results include outdated controls or testing reagents, improper storage of testing components, and an error in the technique used to perform the procedure.
3. **Procedural Step.** Dispose of the test cassettes and control swabs in a biohazard waste container. Remove gloves and sanitize hands.
4. **Procedural Step.** Document the control results in a quality control log.

Collect a Throat Specimen

5. **Procedural Step.** Sanitize hands. Greet the patient and introduce yourself. Identify the patient by full name and date of birth and explain the procedure.
6. **Procedural Step.** Position the patient in a sitting position and adjust the light to provide clear visualization of the throat.
   Principle. The throat must be clearly visible so that the medical assistant is able to determine the proper area for obtaining the specimen.
7. **Procedural Step.** Apply gloves. Remove the test cassette from its foil pouch and place it on a clean, dry, level surface.
   Principle. The foil pouch should not be opened until it is time to perform the test.

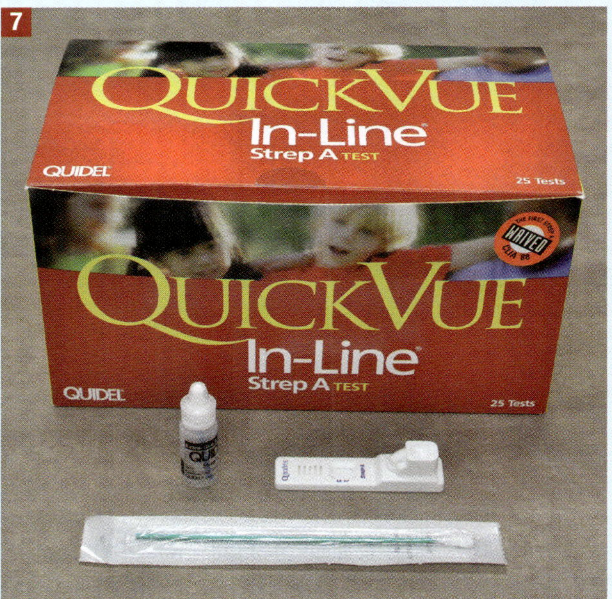

Remove the test cassette from its foil pouch. (From Proctor et al: *Kinn's the medical assistant: an applied learning approach*, ed 13, St. Louis, 2017, Elsevier.)

8. **Procedural Step.** Remove the sterile swab from its peel-apart package being careful not to contaminate it.
   Principle. Contamination of the swab may lead to inaccurate test results.
9. **Procedural Step.** Depress the tongue with the tongue depressor and collect a throat specimen (following the steps outlined in Procedure 34.2: Collecting a Throat Specimen).

Perform the QuickVue Strep Test

10. **Procedural Step.** Using the notch at the back of the chamber as a guide, insert the swab completely into the swab chamber.

Continued

PROCEDURE 34.3 Perform a CLIA-Waived Rapid Strep Test—cont'd

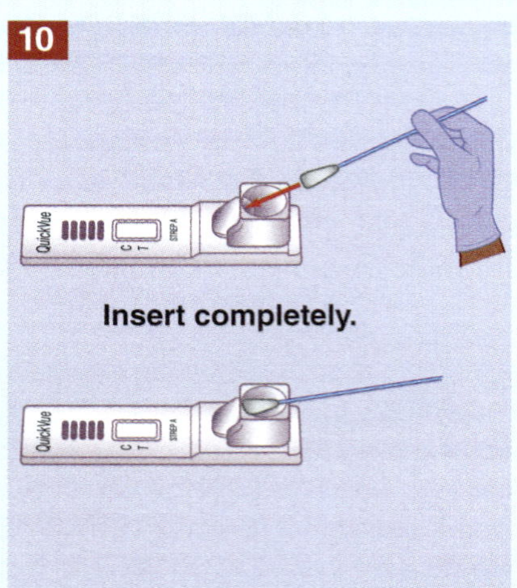

Insert the swab completely into the swab chamber. (Courtesy of Quidel Corporation, San Diego, CA.)

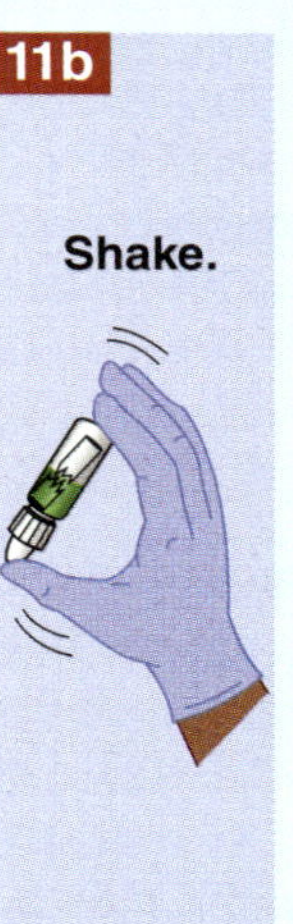

Vigorously shake the bottle five times. (Courtesy of Quidel Corporation, San Diego, CA.)

11. Procedural Step. Squeeze the extraction bottle once to break the glass ampule inside the bottle. Vigorously shake the bottle five times to mix the solutions in the bottle. The solution should turn green after the ampule is broken. (*Note:* Do not use the extraction solution if it is green prior to breaking the ampule.)

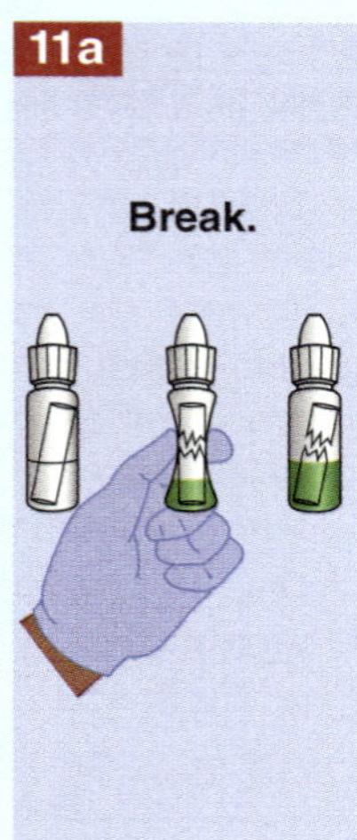

Break the glass ampule inside the bottle. (Courtesy of Quidel Corporation, San Diego, CA.)

12. Procedural Step. Remove the cap of the extraction bottle. Hold the bottle in a vertical position and quickly fill the swab chamber to the rim with the extraction solution (approximately 8 drops).

Principle. The purpose of the extraction solution is to extract the specimen from the swab. Invalid results may occur if too little sample is added to the chamber.

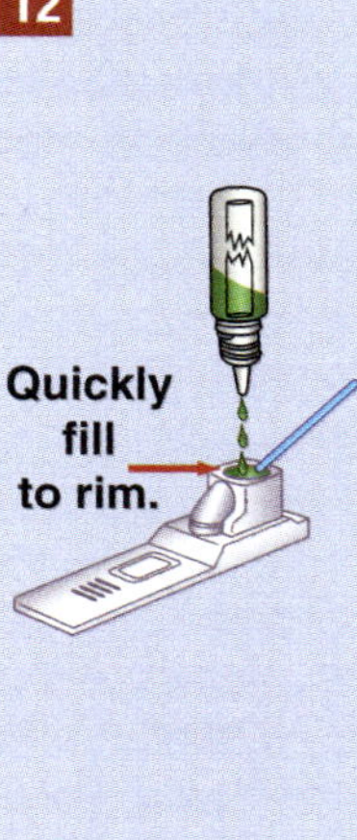

Quickly fill the swab chamber to the rim. (Courtesy Quidel Corporation, San Diego, CA.)

PROCEDURE 34.3 Perform a CLIA-Waived Rapid Strep Test—cont'd

13. **Procedural Step.** Start the timer for 5 minutes. Do not move the test cassette until the procedure is completed. If the liquid has not moved across the result window in 1 minute, completely remove the swab and reinsert it into the chamber. If the liquid still does not move across, repeat the test with a new specimen, test cassette, and bottle of extraction solution.
14. **Procedural Step.** Wait 5 minutes, and read the results by observing the test result window.
    Principle. Reading the results before or after 5 minutes has elapsed may result in inaccurate test results.
15. **Procedural Step.** Interpret the test results as follows:

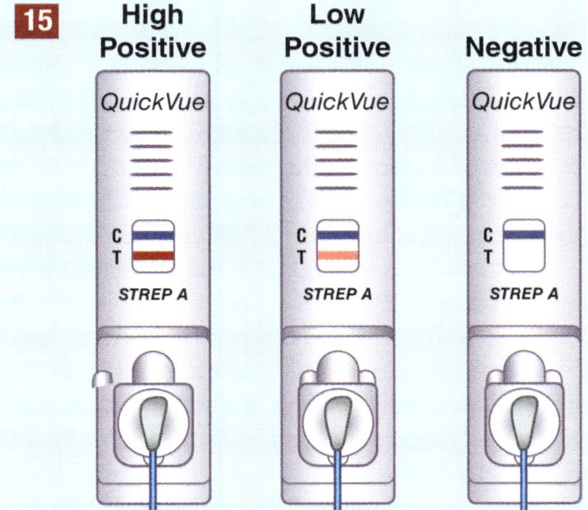

Interpret the test results. (Courtesy of Quidel Corporation, San Diego, CA.)

Negative: The test result window exhibits a blue procedural control line next to the letter **C.** It is presumed that the test is negative for strep but the provider may order further testing to verify this. In addition, there should be a clearing of the background color in the test result window. This area should be white to light pink within 5 minutes and not interfere with the ability to read test results.

Positive: The test result window exhibits any shade of a pink to red test line next to the letter **T** along with a blue procedural control line next to the letter **C.** This means the test is positive for group A streptococcus. In addition, there should be a clearing of the background color in the test result window. This area should be white to light pink within 5 minutes and not interfere with the ability to read test results.

Invalid results: The blue procedural control line does not appear next to the letter **C** at 5 minutes, or the background of the test result window interferes with reading the results. This means the test result is invalid. The test should be repeated with a new specimen and test cassette.

Principle. The blue control line is a positive internal quality control indicator designating that sufficient sample was added to the test device and that the test is working properly. A background in the test result window that is clear and does not interfere with reading the test results is a negative internal quality control indicator and signifies that the test has been performed properly.

16. **Procedural Step.** Dispose of the test cassette in a biohazard waste container. Remove gloves and sanitize your hands.
17. **Procedural Step.** Document the results in the patient's medical record.
    a. *Electronic health record:* Document the name of the test and the test results using the appropriate radio buttons, drop-down menus, and free text fields.
    b. *Paper-based patient record:* Document the date and time, the name of the test, and the test results as positive or negative.

17b

DOCUMENTATION EXAMPLE

Date	
7/12/XX	10:30 a.m. QuickVue Strep Test: Positive. ___
	___ A. Schostek, CMA (AAMA)

PROCEDURE 34.4 Perform a CLIA-Waived Rapid Influenza Test

Outcome Collect a nasopharyngeal specimen and perform a CLIA-waived rapid influenza test.

Equipment/Supplies

- CLIA-waived BinaxNOW Influenza A and B test kit
- Sterile nasopharyngeal flocked swab
- Disposable gloves
- Face mask
- Protective eyewear
- External controls
- Manufacturer's instructions
- Quality control log
- Tissues
- Biohazard waste container

1. **Procedural Step.** Sanitize your hands and assemble the equipment. Check the expiration date on the testing kit. It should not be used if the expiration date has passed.
   Principle. An expired influenza test may produce inaccurate test results.

Perform the Control Procedure

2. **Procedural Step.** If necessary, apply gloves and perform an external positive and negative control procedure. When a new testing kit is opened (and thereafter on a monthly basis), external positive and negative controls should be performed according to the instructions in the product insert accompanying the controls. If the controls do not perform as expected, patient testing should not be conducted until the problem is identified and resolved.
   Principle. Running positive and negative external controls ensures that the test results are valid and reliable. Factors that can cause abnormal external control results include outdated controls or testing reagents, improper storage of testing components, and an error in the technique used to perform the procedure.
3. **Procedural Step.** Dispose of test devices and swabs used to perform the control procedure in a biohazard waste container. Remove gloves and sanitize hands.
4. **Procedural Step.** Document the control results in a quality control log.

Collect a Nasopharyngeal Swab Specimen

5. **Procedural Step.** Sanitize the hands and apply personal protective equipment including a face mask, protective eyewear, and clean disposable gloves. Perform this step before entering the patient's room.
   Principle. Personal protective equipment shields the medical assistant from pathogens that may be released into the environment if the patient coughs or sneezes during the collection procedure.
6. **Procedural Step.** Greet the patient and introduce yourself. Identify the patient by full name and date of birth and explain the collection procedure. Explain to the patient that the collection procedure may cause coughing, sneezing, or tearing of the eyes.
7. **Procedural Step.** Position the patient in a sitting position. Ask the patient to blow their nose to remove excess mucous secretions from the nasal passages.
   Principle. The nasal passages should be clear of mucus, prior to the insertion of the swab. The influenza virus is located in epithelial cells that line the nasal cavity and not in mucous secretions.
8. **Procedural Step.** Ask the patient to tilt their head back slightly (about 70 degrees).
   Principle. Tilting the head back makes the nasal passages more accessible and straightens the passage from the front of the nose to the nasopharynx, making insertion of the swab easier.
9. **Procedural Step.** Remove the cap from the extraction vial using a twisting motion and place it in its cardboard holder. Remove the sterile swab from its peel-apart envelope, being careful not to contaminate it.
   Principle. Contamination of the swab may lead to inaccurate test results.
10. **Procedural Step.** Estimate the depth for insertion of the swab by visually determining the distance from the corner of the nose to the earlobe. The swab should be inserted approximately one-half this distance.
    Principle. Estimating the depth for insertion helps to ensure that the swab is inserted to the proper depth for adequate specimen collection.
11. **Procedural Step.** Gently insert the swab into one nostril along the floor of the nasal passage. The swab should be inserted straight back and not in an upward direction. Slowly push the swab forward into the nasal passage until resistance is encountered, indicating the swab has reached the nasopharyngeal mucosa. The depth of insertion should be equal to approximately one-half the distance from the corner of the nose to the ear lobe (as previously estimated). Do not force the swab. If an obstruction or resistance is encountered before reaching the nasopharynx, remove the swab. Obtain a new sterile swab and try the other nostril.
    Principle. The swab must reach the nasopharyngeal mucosa in order to obtain an adequate specimen.

PROCEDURE 34.4 Perform a CLIA-Waived Rapid Influenza Test—cont'd

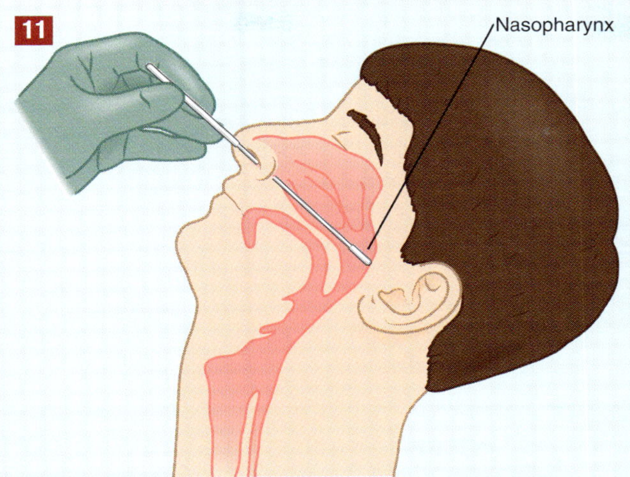

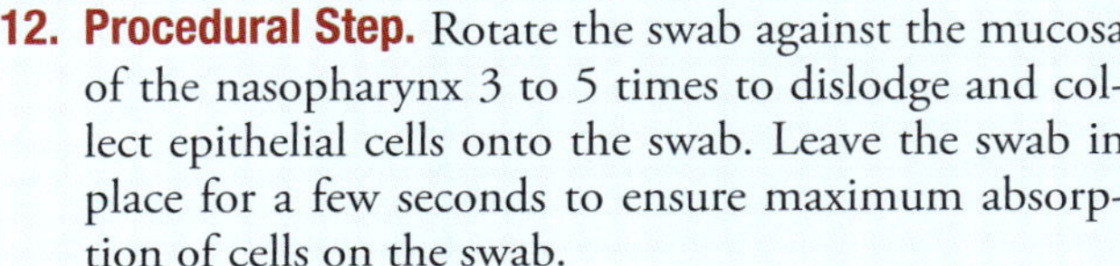

Insert the swab.

12. **Procedural Step.** Rotate the swab against the mucosa of the nasopharynx 3 to 5 times to dislodge and collect epithelial cells onto the swab. Leave the swab in place for a few seconds to ensure maximum absorption of cells on the swab.
    Principle. A rotating motion is used to deposit the maximal amount of material possible on the swab. Failure to collect a sufficient number of cells may cause a false-negative test result.
13. **Procedural Step.** Gently remove the swab from the patient's nose with a rotating motion. Offer the patient tissues to blow their nose.

Perform the BinaxNOW Influenza A and B Test

14. **Procedural Step.** Insert the swab into the solution in the extraction vial. Rinse the swab in the extraction solution by vigorously rotating it three times without creating a lot of bubbles.
    Principle. The purpose of the extraction solution is to extract or remove the specimen from the swab. Vigorous rotation of the swab facilitates the removal of the specimen from the swab.

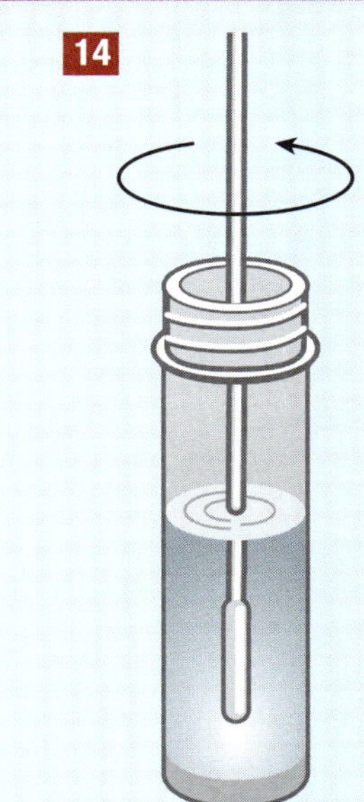

Rinse the swab in the extraction solution.

15. **Procedural Step.** Remove the swab from the vial by rolling it with pressure against the inside of the vial to further extract as much of the specimen as possible from the swab to ensure adequate specimen collection. Properly dispose of the swab in a biohazard waste container.
    Principle. Inadequate specimen collection may lead to a false-negative test result.
16. **Procedural Step.** Remove the cardboard test device from its foil pouch and lay it on a clean, dry, level surface.
    Principle. The foil pouch should not be opened until it is time to perform the test.
17. **Procedural Step.** Fill the pipette by firmly squeezing the top bulb and then placing the pipette tip into the extraction solution. Fill the pipette by slowly releasing pressure from the bulb while the tip is still in the solution.

Continued

PROCEDURE 34.4 Perform a CLIA-Waived Rapid Influenza Test—cont'd

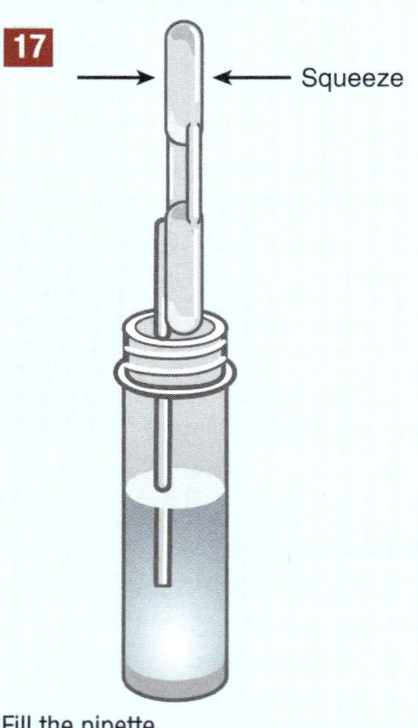

Fill the pipette.

18. Procedural Step. Check to make sure the pipette is full and that there are no air spaces in the lower part of the pipette. If air spaces occur, squeeze the sample back into the specimen container and redraw the sample from the vial. Air spaces take up space that the sample should occupy.

Principle. Invalid results may occur if too little sample is added to the test.

19. Procedural Step. Locate the arrow on the test device to find the white pad at the top of the test strip. Slowly (drop by drop) add the contents of the pipette to the middle of this pad by squeezing the bulb until the entire sample is absorbed into the pad. Do not allow the pipette to touch the pad.

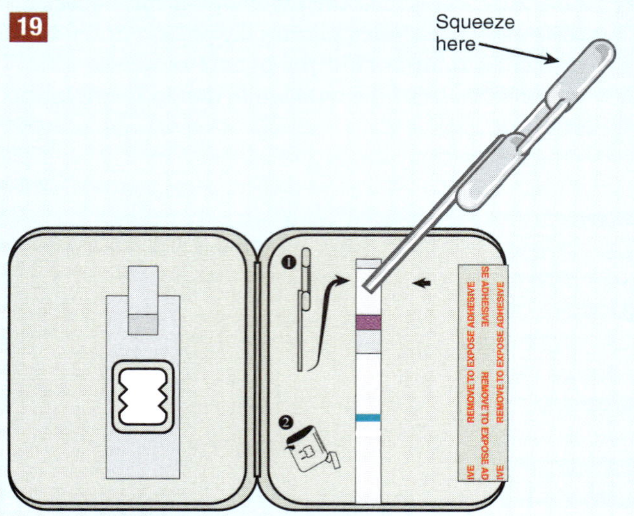

Add the extraction solution to the pad.

20. Procedural Step. Immediately peel off the adhesive liner from the test device. Close and securely seal the test device.

21. Procedural Step. Wait 15 minutes, and read the results by observing the test result window.

Principle. Reading the results before or after 15 minutes has elapsed may result in inaccurate test results.

22. Procedural Step. Interpret the test results according to the *Interpretation of Results* chart. The pink to purple control line is an internal quality control indicator designating that sufficient sample was added to the test device and that the test is working properly.

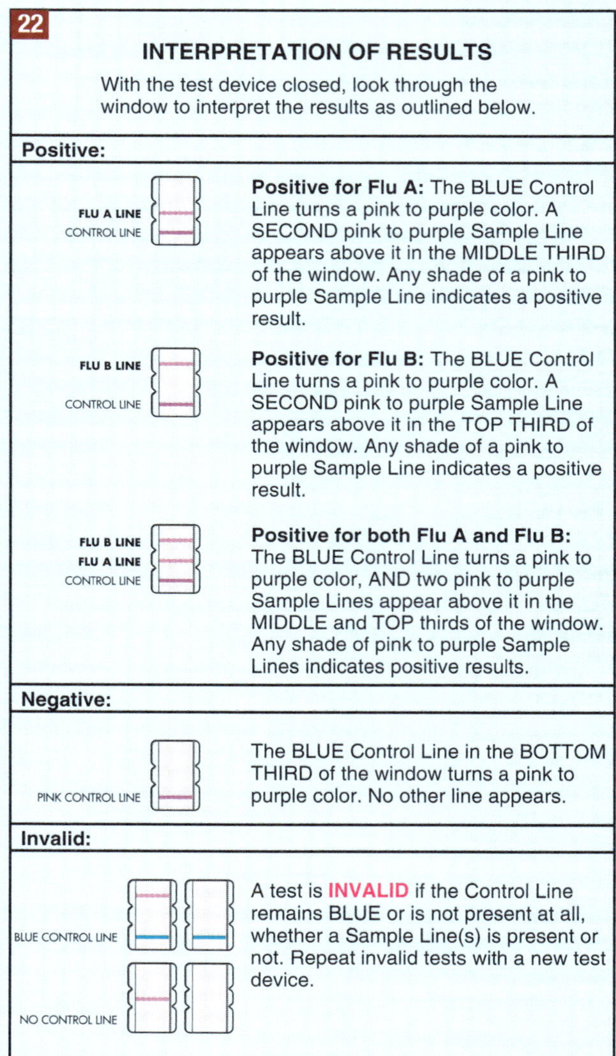

23. Procedural Step. Dispose of the test device in a biohazard waste container. Remove personal protective equipment and sanitize your hands.

PROCEDURE 34.4 Perform a CLIA-Waived Rapid Influenza Test—cont'd

24. Procedural Step. Document the results in the patient's medical record.

a. *Electronic health record:* Document the name of the test and the test results using the appropriate radio buttons, drop-down menus, and free-text fields.

b. *Paper-based patient record:* Document the date and time, the name of the test, and the results as follows:

For negative results: Influenza A and B virus not detected.

For positive results:

Depending on the results document one of the following:

- Positive for influenza A.
- Positive for influenza B.
- Positive for influenza A and B.

24b

DOCUMENTATION EXAMPLE

Date	
3/25/XX	11:30 a.m. BinaxNOW influenza A and B
	test: Positive for influenza A__________
	__________ A. Schostek, CMA (AAMA)

Nutrition

Check out the Evolve site at http://evolve.elsevier.com/Bonewit/today to access additional interactive activities and exercises to help you study and prepare for success.

LEARNING OBJECTIVES/ PROCEDURES

Nutrients

1. List the six classes of nutrients.
2. Explain the difference between a macronutrient and a micronutrient.
3. State the number of kilocalories provided by 1 gram of each of the following: carbohydrate, fat, and protein.
4. Explain the difference between simple carbohydrates and complex carbohydrates. List food sources of each.
5. State the function of fat in the body.
6. Describe the different types of fat found in food.
7. State the function of protein in the body.
8. Explain the difference between essential amino acids and nonessential amino acids.
9. Describe the difference between complete protein and incomplete protein. List food sources of each.
10. Identify the water-soluble vitamins and state the function, food sources, and deficiency diseases of each.
11. Identify the fat-soluble vitamins and state the function, food sources, and deficiency diseases of each.
12. Identify the major minerals and state the function, food sources, and deficiency diseases of each.
13. Identify the trace minerals and state the function, food sources, and deficiency diseases of each.
14. State the function of water in the body.
15. Identify methods by which water is lost from the body.

Tools for Healthy Nutrition

16. Identify the MyPlate food groups and their recommended proportions on the plate.
17. State the purpose of the Dietary Guidelines for Americans.
18. List the four guidelines included in the 2020–2025 Dietary Guidelines for Americans.
19. State the purpose of food labeling.
20. List and describe the five basic sections of the Nutrition Facts label.

Nutrition Therapy

21. Explain the purpose of weight management.
22. List and describe the three components included in a treatment plan for obesity.
23. Identify the elements of the TLC diet plan for a heart healthy diet.
24. Identify the elements of the DASH diet plan to lower hypertension.
25. List examples of foods that are high and low in sodium.
26. Explain the difference between type 1 and type 2 diabetes.
27. Explain the recommended nutrition therapy for type 1 and type 2 diabetes.
28. List the symptoms of lactose intolerance and identify the recommended nutrition therapy.
29. Explain the difference between celiac disease and non-celiac gluten sensitivity.
30. Identify the symptoms and describe the recommended treatment for gluten intolerance.
31. List the common food allergens.
32. Describe the common methods of treatment for food allergies.

Procedures: Instruct a patient according to patient's special dietary needs.

CHAPTER OUTLINE

KEY TERMS

added sugars
antioxidant (an-tee-OCKS-i-dent)
atherosclerosis (ath-er-oh-skleh-ROH-sis)
bariatrics
cholesterol (ko-LES-ter-ol)
complete protein
dietary pattern
disaccharide (die-SAK-a-ride)
empty calorie food
essential amino acid
gluten (GLOO-ten)
glycogen (GLIE-koe-jen)
incomplete protein
kilocalorie (KIL-o-cal-or-ee)
lactose (LAK-tos)
macronutrient (MAK-ro-noo-tree-ent)
micronutrient (MY-crow-noo-tree-ent)
mineral
monosaccharide (mah-no-SAK-a-ride)
natural sugars
nonessential amino acid
nutrient (NOO-tree-ent)
nutrition (noo-TRI-shun)
nutrition therapy
obesity (oh-BEE-si-tee)
percent daily value
polysaccharide
saturated fat
triglycerides (tri-GLIS-eh-rides)
unsaturated fat
vitamin

INTRODUCTION TO NUTRITION

Nutrition is the study of nutrients in food including how the body uses them and their relationship to health. A **nutrient** is a chemical substance found in food that is needed by the body for survival and well-being. Good nutrition is an important component of the health and well-being of an individual. Inadequate nutrition can result in poor health and even disease. Some of the specific benefits derived from good nutrition include the following:

- Supports good physical and mental well-being
- Helps to maintain a healthy weight
- Boosts the functioning of the immune system
- Delays the effects of aging
- Lowers the risk of certain conditions and diseases (e.g., obesity, heart disease, cancer, diabetes)

The medical assistant should have a knowledge of basic nutrition principles and the recommended nutrition therapy for common conditions and diseases. The medical assistant uses this information when scheduling a patient for an appointment with a dietitian, relaying information to patients on dietary restrictions required for tests and procedures, providing patients with nutrition education handouts, and answering basic questions a patient may have regarding nutrition.

Medical assistants are not qualified to conduct nutritional assessments or recommend nutrition therapy. This is the responsibility of a registered dietitian. Medical assistants should make sure to adhere to these guidelines to stay within the scope of practice for a medical assistant.

DEFINITION OF TERMS

Terms that aid in understanding this chapter are listed and defined here.

Diet: A diet consists of the food and drink an individual consumes each day. To promote sound nutrition, an individual's diet should include the proper balance of nutrients.

Dietitian: A dietitian is a professional specially trained to assess the nutritional status of an individual and recommend appropriate nutrition therapy.

Digestion: The process by which food is broken down in the gastrointestinal tract into smaller components that can be absorbed by the bloodstream for use by the body.

Enriched food: A food to which vitamins and minerals have been added to replace those lost during the processing of that food.

Fortified food: A food to which vitamins and minerals that were not there originally have been added to increase the nutritional quality of the food.

Malnutrition (or poor nutrition): An imbalance between the nutrients your body needs to function and the nutrients it gets. Malnutrition is caused by a deficiency of one or more nutrients (undernutrition) or an overconsumption of nutrients (overnutrition) resulting in an overweight or obese individual.

Nutrient density: Refers to the amount of nutrients in a food compared with the amount of calories. A food with a high nutrient density (known as a nutrient-dense food) is high in nutrients compared to the number of calories in the food. A food with a low nutrient density is low in nutrients compared to the number of calories in the food.

NUTRIENTS

Nutrients can be categorized into six classes according to their chemical structure and the role they play in nourishing the body. The six classes of nutrients include carbohydrates, fat, protein, vitamins, minerals, and water and are described in more detail in this section.

Each of the six classes of nutrients plays an important role in supporting good nutritional health. Nutrients provide three primary functions in the body as follows:

- Provide energy for the body
- Build, repair, and maintain body tissue
- Assist in the regulation of body processes

The National Academy of Medicine developed Dietary Reference Intake (DRI) tables to assist individuals in determining their recommended daily intake of essential nutrients. Nutrient recommendations in the DRI tables are based on gender, age, and life stage and also allow for individual variation. The DRI tables can be accessed on the National Academies website.

CLASSIFICATION OF NUTRIENTS

Nutrients can be further classified as macronutrients or micronutrients.

Macronutrients

Macronutrients are nutrients needed in relatively large amounts by the body and include carbohydrates, fats, and proteins. Macronutrients provide kilocalories to the body to yield energy in addition to performing other important body functions, which are discussed in this section. A **kilocalorie** (kcal), often referred to simply as a *calorie*, is a measurement unit of energy. A kilocalorie is defined as the amount of heat needed to raise the temperature of 1 kilogram of water 1° Celsius. The energy value provided by each of the macronutrients is outlined in Table 35.1.

The body uses carbohydrate as a short-term energy fuel and uses fat as a long-term fuel. Although protein provides 4 kcal of energy per gram and can be used as an energy source, the body would rather *not* use protein as an energy source. Instead, the body prefers to use carbohydrate as an energy source to "spare" protein for its more important functions of building, maintaining, and repairing body tissues. Refer to Table 35.1, which outlines the function and food sources of the macronutrients.

The Institute of Medicine recommends guidelines for the optimal intake ranges for the macronutrients (carbohydrates, fats, and proteins) known as the AMDR (Acceptable Macronutrient Distribution Ranges). The AMDR are associated with reduced risk of chronic disease while providing an adequate intake of the macronutrients.

Table 35.1 Macronutrients

Macronutrient	EnergyValue	Function	Food Sources
Carbohydrate	4 kcal/gram	Chief source of energy for the body Primary source of energy for the central nervous system	Pasta, rice, bread, cereal, fruits, vegetables
Fat	9 kcal/gram	Provides energy for the body Transports fat-soluble vitamins in the body Provides essential fatty acids for the body	Fatty meats, butter, cheese, cream, whole milk, egg yolk, vegetable oils, nuts, avocados
Protein	4 kcal/gram	Builds, maintains, and repairs body tissue Makes up enzymes, antibodies, and most hormones	Meat, fish, poultry, potatoes, eggs, milk, cheese, legumes, nuts

Micronutrients

Micronutrients are nutrients required in very small amounts by the body and include vitamins and minerals. Vitamins and minerals are not broken down by the body and are used in the form in which they are absorbed. Micronutrients do not provide calories to yield energy for the body; however, they do perform a variety of other very important functions, which are discussed later in this section.

CLASSES OF NUTRIENTS

CARBOHYDRATES

Carbohydrates are macronutrients made up of organic compounds consisting of carbon, hydrogen, and oxygen. According to the AMDR, approximately 45% to 65% of the total daily caloric intake of an individual should come from carbohydrates.

Through the process of digestion, most carbohydrates are broken down into sugar units and converted into glucose by the body. Glucose is the chief source of energy for the body and the preferred source of energy for the central nervous system. Energy is needed to perform all body functions such as breathing, contraction of the heart, blood circulation, digestion, maintenance of body temperature, and voluntary muscle movement such as walking, running, and lifting.

The body must maintain a constant blood glucose level to ensure a continuous source of energy for the body. Ingested glucose that is not needed for energy is stored for later use in the form of **glycogen** in muscle and liver tissue. *Insulin* is a hormone secreted by the beta cells of the pancreas that is required for normal utilization of glucose in the body. Insulin enables glucose to enter the body cells and be converted to energy. Insulin also is needed for the proper storage of glycogen in muscle and liver tissue.

Classification of Carbohydrates

Carbohydrates are classified into simple and complex carbohydrates.

Simple Carbohydrates

Simple carbohydrates are made up of just one or two sugar units. Simple carbohydrates consisting of one sugar unit are termed **monosaccharides**; they include glucose, fructose (fruit sugar), and galactose. Simple carbohydrates consisting of two sugar units are known as **disaccharides**; they include sucrose (table sugar), lactose (milk sugar), and maltose. Simple carbohydrates provide an immediate source of energy for the body because they can be broken down quickly through digestion for use as energy. Simple carbohydrates are found in processed foods and refined sugars such as candy, cake, cookies, pastries, sweetened beverages, table sugar, syrup, and honey. These foods have a low-nutrient density and are known as **empty calorie foods** because they provide calories but very few or no nutrients (Fig. 35.1A). Simple carbohydrates are also found naturally in foods and beverages such as milk, fruits, and vegetables. Natural sugars are considered a healthier food choice because they typically occur in foods that are also rich in vitamins, minerals, and fiber.

Complex Carbohydrates

Complex carbohydrates, also known as **polysaccharides**, are made up of many sugar units strung together into a long chain. Because complex carbohydrates consist of many sugar units, they take more time for the body to break down for use as energy. This leads to a less dramatic rise in the blood sugar level and provides a more steady supply of energy for the body. Complex carbohydrates come from plant-based foods; examples include pasta, rice, bread, cereal, potatoes, and legumes (Fig. 35.1B).

Dietary Fiber

Dietary fiber is a complex carbohydrate consisting of many sugar units; however, unlike most complex carbohydrates, fiber does not provide energy (calories) for the body. This is because the human body lacks the digestive enzymes necessary to break fiber down so that it can be used as an energy source. Fiber serves some very important functions in the body, which are discussed in this section. The daily recommended amount of fiber and the fiber content of common foods are presented in Table 35.2.

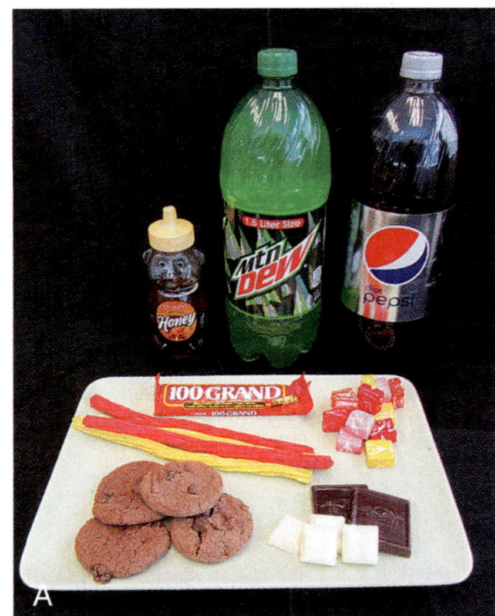

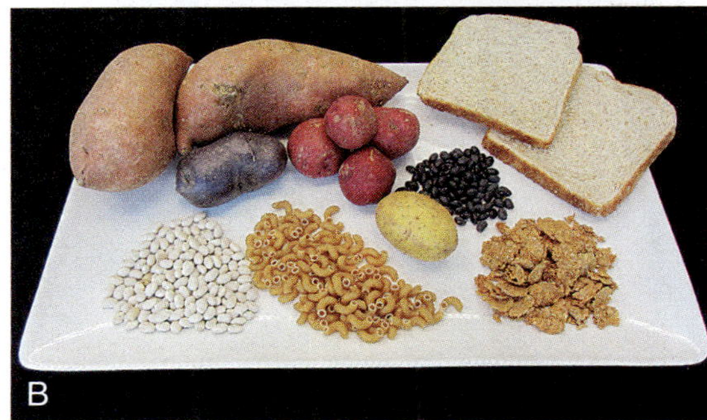

Fig. 35.1 (A) Simple carbohydrate food sources. (B) Complex carbohydrate food sources.

Table 35.2 Fiber Recommendations and Food Sources

FIBER RECOMMENDATIONS		
Age	**Women**	**Men**
Under age 50	25 grams/day	38 grams/day
Over age 50	21 grams/day	30 grams/day
FIBER CONTENT OF COMMON FOODS		
Food	**Serving Size**	**Grams of Fiber**
Navy beans (cooked)	1 cup	19.2
Split peas (cooked)	1 cup	16.3
Black beans (cooked)	1 cup	15
Bran flakes	3/4 cup	5.3
Broccoli (boiled)	1 cup	5.1
Apple with skin	1 medium	4.4
Oatmeal (instant, cooked)	1 cup	4.0
Popcorn (air-popped)	3 cups	3.5
Brown rice (cooked)	1 cup	3.5
Almonds	1 ounce	3.5
Banana	1 medium	3.1
Potato (with skin, baked)	1 medium	2.9
Carrot (raw)	1 medium	1.7

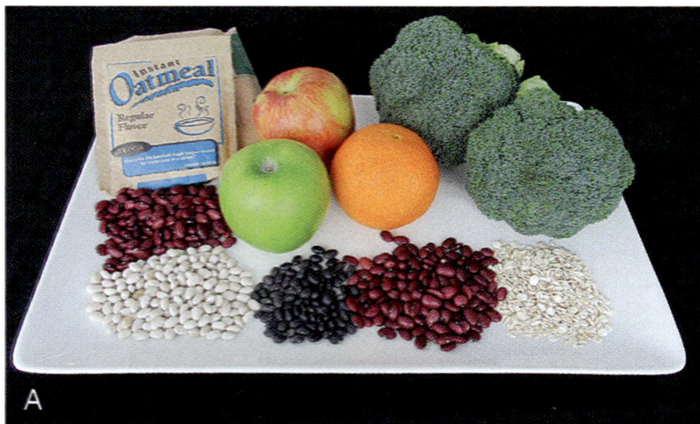

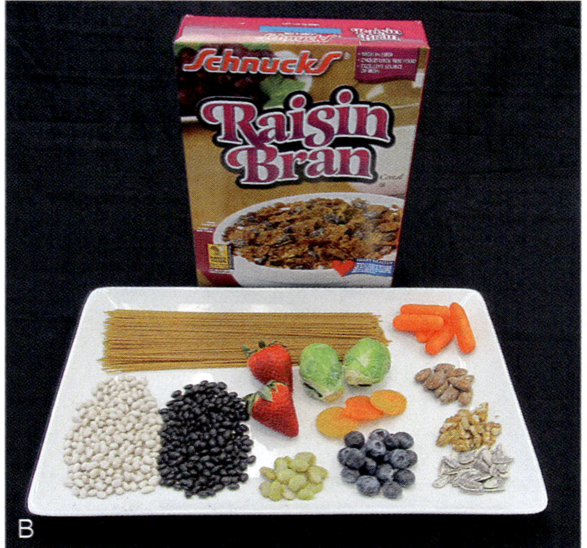

Fig. 35.2 (A) Soluble fiber food sources. (B) Insoluble fiber food sources.

Based on chemical, physical, and functional properties, fiber can be classified as soluble or insoluble. Both types of fiber are important to an individual's health, as is described in more detail as follows.

Soluble Fiber

Soluble fiber dissolves in water after it has been consumed, forming a gel-like material that slows down digestion. This delays the emptying of the stomach and makes an individual feel full longer, which assists in weight control. Soluble fiber also functions to lower blood cholesterol, which helps to protect against heart disease. Good sources of soluble fiber include oatmeal, oat bran, barley, some fruits (e.g., apples, pears, oranges), broccoli, and legumes (Fig. 35.2A).

Insoluble Fiber

Insoluble fiber is found in the rough, fibrous structures of plants such as the outer coverings, leaves, stems, and seeds. It does not dissolve in water and passes through the gastrointestinal (GI) tract relatively intact. Because of this, insoluble fiber provides roughage or bulk to the diet, which helps promote normal elimination and prevents constipation. It may also reduce the risk of diverticular disease and some forms of cancer. Good food sources of insoluble fiber include whole grains, wheat and corn bran, legumes, most fruits and vegetables, and nuts and seeds (Fig. 35.2B).

FATS

Fats, also known as lipids, are macronutrients that do not dissolve in water. Fats are organic compounds composed of carbon, hydrogen, and oxygen. These are the same elements that make up carbohydrates; however, fats are lower in oxygen content than carbohydrates. The body uses fat as a long-term energy fuel and can store it in unlimited quantities in the body.

Despite the misconception that fat is bad for the body and only leads to weight gain, fat serves a number of very important functions. In addition to providing energy for the body, fat functions in transporting fat-soluble vitamins, providing essential fatty acids for the body, assisting in the transmission of nerve impulses, and insulating and cushioning the body. Because fat contains the most calories per gram (9 kcal/gram) among the macronutrients, moderation in fat consumption should be practiced to maintain a healthy weight and a healthy heart. According to the AMDR, no more than 20% to 35% of the total daily caloric intake of an adult should come from fat.

Types of Dietary Fat

Different types of fat are found in foods (dietary fat) and can be classified as follows.

Saturated Fat

Saturated fat is a type of fat that is solid at room temperature and comes primarily from animal sources. It can be found in high amounts in fatty animal products such as bacon, sausage, heavily marbled beef and pork, and the skin

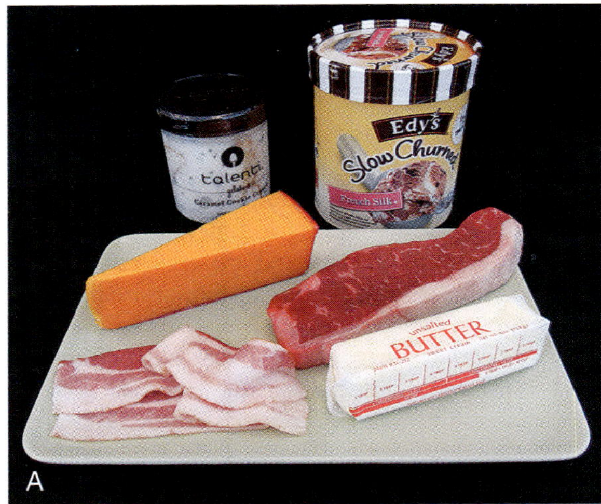

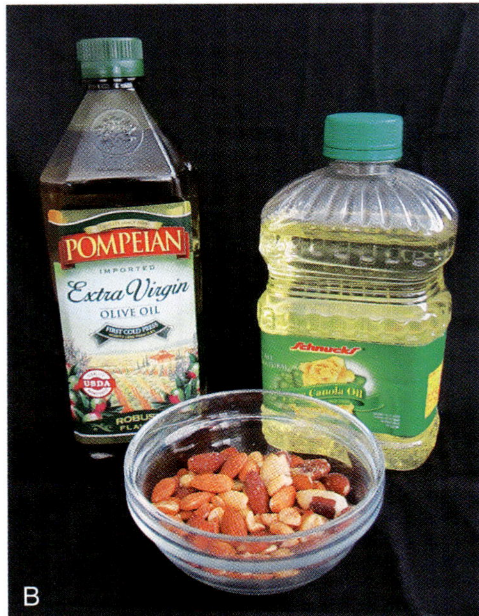

Fig. 35.3 (A) Saturated fat food sources. (B) Unsaturated fat food sources.

of poultry. Whole-fat milk products such as cheese, butter, heavy cream, cream cheese, and ice cream are also high in saturated fat (Fig. 35.3A). Plant sources that are high in saturated fat include palm oil and coconut oil. Saturated fat raises the total blood cholesterol level, which can increase the risk of heart disease. Because of this, the AMDR recommends limiting saturated fat to less than 10% of the total calories consumed each day.

Unsaturated Fat

Unsaturated fat is a type of fat that is liquid at room temperature and comes primarily from plant sources (Fig. 35.3B). Unsaturated fat tends to have a protective effect against heart disease and should make up approximately two-thirds or more of the total fat percentage consumed each day. Unsaturated fat includes monounsaturated fat and polyunsaturated fat. *Monounsaturated* fat is considered to be the most protective against heart disease. Good food sources of monounsaturated fat include olives and olive oil, canola oil, peanut oil, nuts, and avocados. *Polyunsaturated* fat is found primarily in plant-based foods and oils. Good food sources include walnuts, flax seeds, corn oil, soybean oil, sunflower oil, and vegetable oil. Vegetable oil typically consists of a blend of corn oil and soybean oil. Fatty fish and fish oils are polyunsaturated fats that are high in omega-3 fatty acids.

Trans Fat

Trans fat is a form of unsaturated fat. There are two types of trans fat, which include natural trans fat and artificial trans fat. *Natural trans fat* is found in small amounts in certain foods such as beef, lamb, and butter. *Artificial trans fat* is formed as a result of a food-processing method known as hydrogenation. Hydrogenation works by adding hydrogen ions to unsaturated fat to form a semi-solid product known as *partially hydrogenated oil.* Artificial trans fat is more stable and less likely to turn rancid than other types of fat and was developed to preserve food items and increase their shelf-life. It also gives food a more desirable taste and texture. However, studies showed that artificial trans fat increases the level of LDL (bad) cholesterol and decreases the level of HDL (good) cholesterol in the body which, in turn, increases the risk of cardiovascular disease (CVD). Based on these findings, the FDA ruled that artificial trans fat was not generally recognized as safe and banned the use of it in all foods sold in grocery stores and restaurants after June 18, 2018.

Cholesterol

Cholesterol is not a true fat, but rather a white, waxy, fat-like substance that is essential for normal functioning of the body. It is an important component of cell membranes and is used in the production of hormones and bile. Most of the cholesterol circulating in the blood is manufactured by the liver; however, a portion of it comes from an individual's diet and is known as *dietary cholesterol.* Dietary cholesterol is found only in animal products, such as organ meats, egg yolks, and dairy products. Although cholesterol serves some very important functions in the body, a high blood cholesterol level may cause plaque to build up on the inner walls of the arteries, a condition known as **atherosclerosis.** As the atherosclerosis progresses, the arteries become more occluded, which eventually could lead to a heart attack or stroke. Because of this, high blood cholesterol is considered a risk factor for CVD. Total blood cholesterol levels are interpreted as outlined in Table 35.3.

Table 35.3 Interpretation of Total Blood Cholesterol Levels

Total Blood Cholesterol Level	Interpretation
Less than 200 mg/dL	Desirable
200–239 mg/dL	Borderline high
240 mg/dL or above	High

Triglycerides

Triglycerides are the chemical form in which most fat exists in food, as well as in the body. In normal amounts, triglycerides are essential to good health. Triglycerides are derived from two sources. The first is synthesis by the body. Excess carbohydrates, fat, and protein not needed by the body are synthesized into triglycerides and stored as adipose tissue. The second source of triglycerides is food. Excess triglycerides consumed by eating foods containing saturated fat (e.g., butter, cream, bacon) are also stored as adipose tissue.

Some of the triglycerides in the body are not stored as adipose tissue but remain in the bloodstream, specifically in the plasma of the blood. Most triglycerides in the blood are carried by VLDL (*very-low density lipoprotein*) to the cells of the body. Triglycerides carried by VLDL serve as an important source of energy for the cells of the body. An excess of blood triglycerides, however, places an individual at increased risk for CVD, particularly if their LDL (bad) cholesterol is high and their HDL (good) cholesterol is low. Triglycerides levels in the blood are interpreted as outlined in Table 35.4. Conditions that result in elevated blood triglycerides levels include obesity, type 2 diabetes, a physically inactive lifestyle, excessive alcohol consumption, smoking, hypothyroidism, kidney disease, and liver disease.

Table 35.4 Interpretation of Blood Triglycerides Levels

Blood Triglycerides Level	Interpretation
Less than 150 mg/dL	Normal
150–199 mg/dL	Borderline high
200–499 mg/dL	High
500 mg/dL or above	Very high

PROTEINS

Protein is often considered the "special force" macronutrient. Protein contains not only carbon, hydrogen, and oxygen (like carbohydrates and fats), but also nitrogen. The nitrogen provides protein with a special force that enables it to build, maintain, and repair body tissue.

Protein has many important functions in the body. Protein is the primary structural material making up all body tissues such as muscle, bone, skin, and hair. In addition, protein is a major component of enzymes, antibodies, and many hormones that are essential to proper functioning of the body. Protein also plays a role in fluid balance and muscle contractions. According to the AMDR, 10% to 35% of the total daily caloric intake of an individual should come from protein. Rich food sources of protein include meat, fish, poultry, milk, cheese, eggs, legumes, soybeans, and nuts. Grains and soy products also contain moderate amounts of protein and are very useful in a vegetarian diet.

Protein plays an important role in physical activity because exercise breaks down muscle protein, which then requires repair and restoration. The amount of activity performed in a day assists in determining how much protein is needed by an individual. The average adult requires approximately 0.8 grams of protein per kilogram of body weight per day (or 0.36 grams per pound). For a 160-pound man, this translates to about 58 grams of protein. That amount of protein could be easily obtained by consuming 2 cups of milk; 5 ounces of meat, fish, or poultry; and three servings of grain. Protein needs for athletes increase to about 1.2 to 1.8 grams per kilogram of body weight per day. The additional protein needed by an athlete can easily be obtained by an adequate, balanced diet, and the addition of protein supplements is not necessary. In fact, the American diet typically contains too much dietary protein leading to adverse effects. The consequences of excessive protein intake include calcium loss in the urine, increased risk of kidney stones, and dehydration.

HIGHLIGHT on Vegetarianism

What is a Vegetarian?

A vegetarian is an individual who adopts a style of eating in which one or more types of animal protein are omitted from the diet. An individual may choose to become vegetarian for a variety reasons, including religious beliefs, concerns about animal welfare or the use of antibiotics and hormones in livestock, or a desire to conserve environmental resources. Additional factors that influence an individual's decision to become a vegetarian include the healthfulness of a vegetarian diet or simply a dislike of animal protein. The foundation of a vegetarian diet includes plant-based foods such as grains, legumes, nuts, seeds, and fruits and vegetables. Research shows that there are many health benefits to be derived from a vegetarian diet. Vegetarians have a lower risk of developing chronic diseases such as CVD, diabetes, and certain types of cancer. Vegetarians also tend to maintain a healthy weight range throughout their lives. Health professionals recognize that a vegetarian diet may not be suitable for everyone but will encourage the general population to lean in that direction when possible because of the proven health benefits.

What are the Different Types of Vegetarians?

There are different types of vegetarianism, as follows:

- *Vegan*: A vegetarian who does not consume any type of animal products including meat, eggs, and dairy. Many vegans also avoid using anything made from animal products, such as leather, fur, and wool.

HIGHLIGHT on Vegetarianism—cont'd

- *Lacto vegetarian*: A vegetarian who consumes dairy products.
- *Ovo vegetarian:* A vegetarian who consumes eggs.
- *Lacto-ovo vegetarian:* A vegetarian who consumes dairy products and eggs.
- *Pescetarian*: A vegetarian who consumes fish and shellfish.
- *Pollo vegetarian:* A vegetarian who consumes poultry.
- *Fruitarian:* An individual who consumes only fruits, nuts, and seeds.
- *Flexitarian:* An individual who primarily follows a vegetarian diet but occasionally makes exceptions.

For What Nutrient Deficiencies is a Vegetarian at Risk?

Vegetarians (particularly vegans) should have a knowledge of menu planning principles so that their nutritional status remains optimal. Careful menu planning is of particular importance for the following nutrients:

- *Calcium:* Individuals who omit dairy products from their diet may consume marginal levels of calcium. Good alternatives to include in the diet include some green vegetables such as broccoli and kale, legumes, and calcium-fortified products such as orange juice.
- *Vitamin D:* Vegetarians who omit cow's milk from their diet may have a low intake of vitamin D. This can be avoided by supplementing the diet with soy milk that is fortified with vitamin D. The body also manufactures vitamin D when it is exposed to the ultraviolet rays of the sun.
- *Vitamin B_{12}*: Vitamin B_{12} is found only in animal-based foods. The old saying "If it doesn't oink, it doesn't cluck, or it doesn't moo, it doesn't have any B_{12}" holds true. A vitamin B_{12} deficiency can be avoided by supplementing the diet with vitamin B_{12}–fortified soy milk, almond milk, and rice milk. Fortified breakfast cereals are also an excellent source of vitamin B_{12}.
- *Iron:* Iron is found in a variety of foods including red meat, poultry, fish, legumes, dark greens, and dried fruit. Even though a plant-based diet does provide some iron to the diet, the body is unable to absorb it as well as the iron found in animal products. Vitamin C helps to increase the absorption of iron. It is recommended that a vegetarian consume foods rich in vitamin C (e.g., citrus fruits) along with plant-based foods containing iron (e.g., dark green leafy vegetables). ■

Amino Acids

Protein is made up of smaller units known as *amino acids*. The dietary protein consumed by an individual is broken down into amino acids through the process of digestion. These amino acids are then arranged into different combinations to create the various proteins needed by the body (e.g., by cells, tissues, hormones, and enzymes). This can be compared to forming different words using the letters of the alphabet; because of this, amino acids are known as the "building blocks" of life. There are 20 different amino acids that join together to make all types of protein in the body.

Classification of Amino Acids

Amino acids can be classified into two categories: essential and nonessential amino acids.

Essential Amino Acids

Essential amino acids are required by the body; however, they cannot be manufactured by the body and must be obtained from food. Of the 20 amino acids that make up the proteins in the body, nine of these are essential amino acids.

Nonessential Amino Acids

Nonessential amino acids are required by the body; however, they can be synthesized by the body in sufficient quantities to meet its needs. Although nonessential amino acids are required for good health, it is not necessary that they be obtained from food because the body can manufacture them.

Classification of Protein

Proteins can be classified as complete or incomplete.

Complete Protein

A **complete protein** is a protein that contains all the essential amino acids needed by the body. Food sources that contain complete protein include animal-based foods such as meat, poultry, fish, milk, eggs, and cheese (Fig. 35.4A).

Incomplete Protein

An **incomplete protein** is a protein that lacks one or more of the essential amino acids needed by the body. Food sources that contain incomplete protein include plant-based foods such as fruits, vegetables, grains, legumes, and nuts (Fig. 35.4B). *Complementary proteins* are two or more incomplete protein sources that together provide adequate amounts of all the essential amino acids. Examples of complementary proteins include beans and rice, tofu and rice, and humus and pita bread. Vegetarians can obtain all of their essential amino acids through careful planning and use of complementary proteins.

VITAMINS

A **vitamin** is an organic compound that is required in small amounts by the body for normal growth and development. Vitamins are micronutrients that occur naturally in foods and may be added to processed foods to increase their nutritional value. Most vitamins cannot be produced by the body and therefore must be obtained from food.

Classification of Vitamins

Vitamins can be classified into two groups: water-soluble vitamins and fat-soluble vitamins.

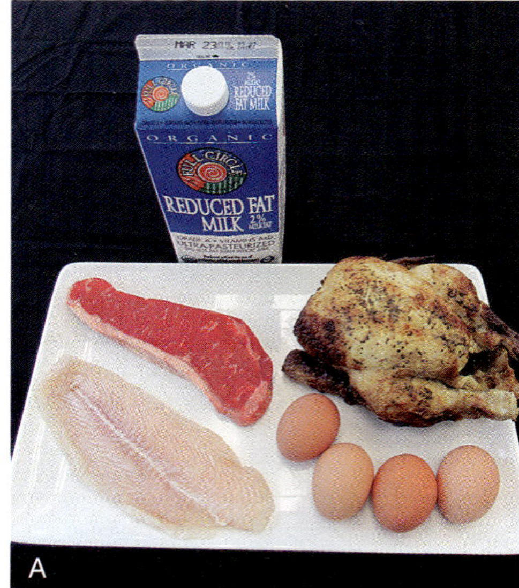

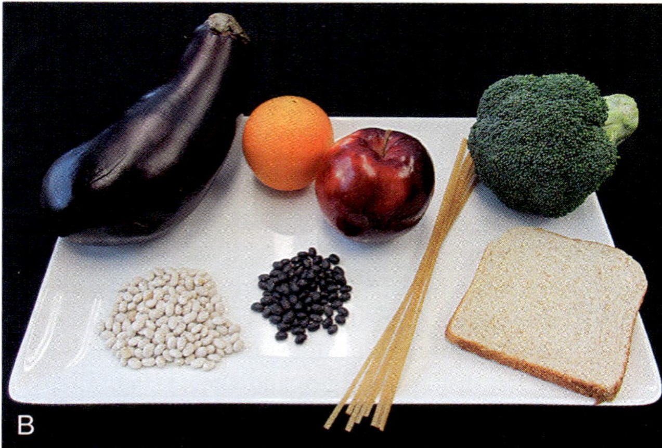

Fig. 35.4 (A) Complete protein food sources. (B) Incomplete protein food sources.

Water-Soluble Vitamins

Water-soluble vitamins derive their name because they dissolve in water. They cannot be stored by the body; water-soluble vitamins consumed in excess of the body's needs are removed through the urine. To maintain good nutritional health, these vitamins should be consumed daily. Water-soluble vitamins include vitamins B_1, B_2, B_3, B_5, B_6, B_7, B_9, B_{12}, and C.

The overall function of the B vitamins is to regulate metabolism, facilitate nervous system functions, and maintain healthy skin. Many of the B vitamins function as coenzymes in energy metabolism. This means that they assist important enzymes in converting food into fuel or energy for the body. Rich food sources of many of the B vitamins include whole grains, legumes, dark green leafy vegetables, pork, beef, and liver (Fig. 35.5). Refer to Table 35.5 for the specific function, food sources, and deficiency diseases of the water-soluble vitamins.

Fat-Soluble Vitamins

Fat-soluble vitamins dissolve in fat. They can be stored by the body; because of this, they do not need to be consumed as often as water-soluble vitamins. In fact, consuming an excessive amount of the fat-soluble vitamins can result in toxicity symptoms leading to health problems. The fat-soluble vitamins include A, D, E, and K. Refer to Table 35.6 for the specific function, food sources, deficiency diseases, and toxicity symptoms (caused by an excessive intake) of the fat-soluble vitamins.

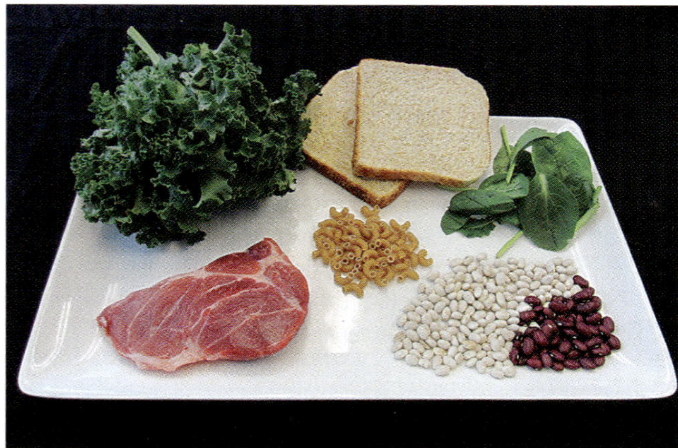

Fig. 35.5 Food sources of the B vitamins.

Antioxidant Vitamins

Vitamins A, C, and E are known as the antioxidant vitamins. An **antioxidant** is a molecule that inhibits the oxidation of other molecules. Oxidation reactions can produce free radicals that can damage body cells. These damaged cells are thought to contribute to aging and certain diseases such as cancer and heart disease. Rich food sources of vitamins A and C include brightly colored fruits and vegetables such as sweet potatoes, citrus fruits, tomatoes, and spinach (Fig. 35.6), while vegetable oils, margarine, and nuts are rich in vitamin E.

MINERALS

A **mineral** is a naturally occurring inorganic substance that is essential to the proper functioning of the body. Minerals are micronutrients that tend to be highly concentrated in foods of animal origin and are absorbed better by the body in this form. Vegetarians can obtain an adequate intake of minerals by emphasizing the following foods in their diet: grains, nuts, and dark green leafy vegetables. A mineral deficiency can lead to poor health and serious illness that affects numerous body systems.

Classification of Minerals

Minerals are divided into two classifications based on the amount required by the body; these classifications include major minerals and trace minerals. Major minerals are required in the body in larger quantities, whereas trace minerals are required in very small amounts. Each of these mineral classifications is described in more detail in the following sections.

Table 35.5 Water-Soluble Vitamins

Vitamin	Function	Food Sources	Deficiency Diseases and Conditions
Vitamin B_1 (thiamine)	Coenzyme in energy metabolism Normal functioning of the nervous system	Pork, beef, liver, eggs, fish, whole-grain and enriched breads, legumes	Beriberi Problems with the GI tract, nervous system, and cardiovascular system
Vitamin B_2 (riboflavin)	Coenzyme in energy metabolism Normal vision and skin health	Milk, meats, green leafy green vegetables, whole-grain and enriched bread and cereals	Cheilosis Eye sensitivity Dermatitis Glossitis
Vitamin B_3 (niacin)	Coenzyme in energy metabolism Healthy skin Healthy nervous and digestive systems Skin health	Milk, eggs, meat, fish, poultry, whole-grain and enriched breads and cereals	Pellagra (dermatitis, neuritis, diarrhea)
Vitamin B_5 (pantothenic acid)	Coenzyme in energy metabolism Synthesis of fatty acids, cholesterol, steroid hormones	Eggs, liver, salmon, poultry, mushrooms, cauliflower, peanuts	Burning feet and other neurologic symptoms
Vitamin B_6 (pyridoxine)	Coenzyme in protein metabolism Assists in making red blood cells	Meat, fish, poultry, liver, milk, eggs, whole grains, legumes, soy products	Cheilosis Glossitis Dermatitis Confusion Depression Irritability
Vitamin B_7 (biotin)	Coenzyme in carbohydrate and protein metabolism	Milk, liver, egg yolk, legumes, yeast, soy flour, cereals, fruit	Dermatitis Nausea Anorexia Depression Hair loss
Vitamin B_9 (folic acid)	Synthesis of red blood cells Synthesis of DNA Development of fetal nervous system	Liver, leafy green vegetables, legumes, seeds, fruit, cereal and bread fortified with folate	Megaloblastic anemia Neural tube birth defects (anencephaly and spina bifida)
Vitamin B_{12} (cobalamin)	Synthesis of red blood cells Maintenance of myelin sheaths	Meat, poultry, fish seafood, liver, eggs, milk, cheese	Pernicious anemia Degeneration of myelin sheaths Sore mouth and tongue Neurologic disorders
Vitamin C (ascorbic acid)	Building and maintenance of strong tissues through collagen synthesis Wound healing Assists in absorption of iron Resistance to infection Antioxidant	Citrus fruits, broccoli, melons, strawberries, tomatoes, Brussels sprouts, potatoes, cabbage, green peppers	Scurvy Muscle cramps Bleeding and loose gums Tendency to bruise easily Poor wound healing Weakened bones

GI, Gastrointestinal.

Major Minerals

Major minerals are required in the adult diet in amounts greater than 100 mg/day and are found in the body in levels of 5 grams or higher. They play important roles in bone and tooth health, blood pressure regulation, and water and acid–base balance. The major minerals include calcium (Fig. 35.7), magnesium phosphorus, potassium, chloride, and sodium. Refer to Table 35.7 for the specific function, food sources, and deficiency diseases of major minerals.

Trace Minerals

Trace minerals are required in the adult diet in amounts less than 50 mg/day and are found in the body in levels of less than 5 grams. They are a diverse group of minerals that assist in proper metabolism and structure as well as immune and blood system functions. Trace minerals include iron, copper, zinc, manganese, fluoride, selenium, iodine, chromium, and molybdenum. Refer to Table 35.8 for the specific function, food sources, and deficiency diseases of trace minerals.

WATER

Water is usually classified as a macronutrient since it is needed in large amounts by the body, however unlike carbohydrates, fats, and proteins, it does not provide

Table 35.6 Fat-Soluble Vitamins

Vitamin	Function	Food Sources	Deficiency Diseases and Conditions, and Toxicity Symptoms
Vitamin A (retinol)	Maintenance of vision in dim light Maintenance of mucous membranes and healthy skin Antioxidant	Liver, whole milk, butter, cream, fish liver oils, dark green leafy vegetables, deep orange fruits and vegetables	*Deficiency:* Night blindness Xerosis Xerophthalmia *Toxicity Symptoms:* Bone pain Dry skin Loss of hair Fatigue Anorexia
Vitamin D (calciferol)	Regulation of the absorption of calcium and phosphorus Calcification of bones and teeth	Fortified milk and margarine, liver, oily fish, fish liver oils Synthesized by the body using the ultraviolet rays of the sun	*Deficiency:* Rickets (in children) Osteomalacia Poorly developed bones and teeth Muscle spasms *Toxicity Symptoms:* Kidney stones Fragile bones Calcification of soft tissue
Vitamin E (tocopherol)	Protection of red blood cells Antioxidant	Vegetable oils, margarine, salad dressing, wheat germ, nuts, avocados	*Deficiency:* Hemolysis of red blood cells
Vitamin K (phylloquinone)	Formation of prothrombin for normal blood clotting Bone development	Green leafy vegetables, milk, meats, cabbage, broccoli, Brussels sprouts Synthesized by intestinal bacterial	*Deficiency:* Bleeding tendencies Poor bone growth *Toxicity Symptoms:* Prolonged blood clotting

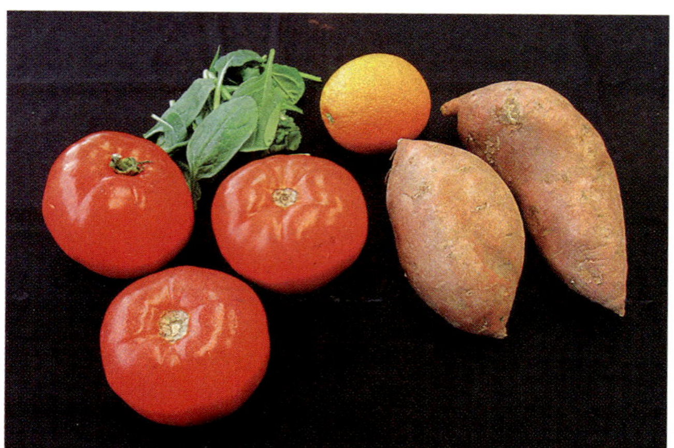

Fig. 35.6 Antioxidant vitamins A and C food sources.

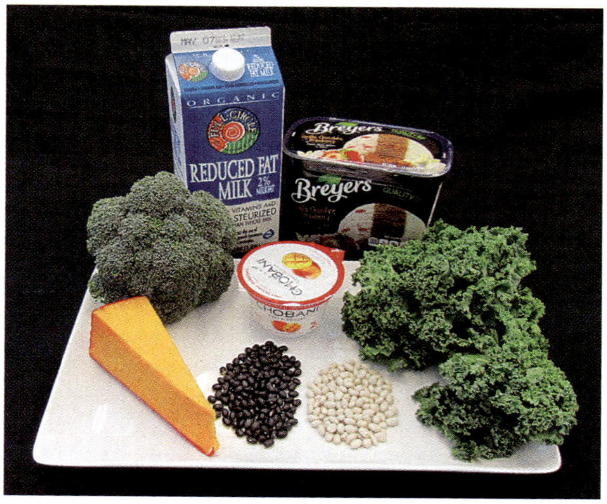

Fig. 35.7 Calcium food sources.

energy (calories) for the body. Water is essential to the survival of an individual. This old adage still holds true: man can survive in the desert without food for more than 30 days but can live only about 3 days without water. Water makes up approximately 60% to 65% of an adult's total body weight, and that percentage is even higher in young children.

Water serves many important functions in the body. Water is the universal solvent of the body; it allows nutrients such as glucose, vitamins, and minerals to dissolve in water and be transported by the circulatory system to the cells of the body. Water allows for transport of substances in and out of cells and is the basis of many chemical reactions in the body. In addition, water provides a solvent for

Table 35.7 Major Minerals

Mineral	Function	Food Sources	Deficiency Diseases and Conditions
Calcium	Healthy bones and teeth Muscle and nerve functioning Proper blood clotting Blood pressure regulation	Milk and milk products, canned fish containing bones (salmon, sardines), some green vegetables such as broccoli and kale, legumes	Osteomalacia Osteoporosis Muscle cramps
Magnesium	Healthy bones and teeth Building protein Muscle and nerve functioning Blood pressure regulation Healthy immune system	Nuts and seeds, whole grains, legumes, dark green vegetables, seafood, chocolate	Muscle weakness and twitching Irritability Fatigue
Phosphorus	Healthy bones and teeth Normal cell membranes Energy production	Meats, milk, nuts, seeds, and legumes	Bone weakness Loss of appetite
Potassium	Normal fluid and electrolyte balance Muscle and nerve functioning Normal cardiac rhythms	Fruits (especially bananas, dried fruit, fruit juices, orange juice), vegetables, grains, legumes	Muscle weakness, twitching or spasms Cardiac arrhythmias Respiratory failure
Chloride	Normal fluid and electrolyte balance Component of gastric juice (hydrochloric acid in the stomach)	Salt, soy sauce, processed foods	Loss of appetite Muscle weakness and cramps
Sodium	Normal fluid and electrolyte balance Muscle and nerve functioning	Salt, soy sauce, processed foods	Muscle weakness and cramps Nausea and vomiting Dizziness Apathy

Table 35.8 Trace Minerals

Mineral	Function	Food Sources	Deficiency Diseases and Conditions
Iron	Makes up hemoglobin (carries oxygen to the body) Makes up myoglobin (carries oxygen to muscles) Assists in energy metabolism	Red meat, liver, dark green leafy vegetables, egg yolk, whole grains, dried fruits	Anemia Irritability Inability to concentrate Pallor Cold sensitivity Lethargy
Copper	Helps form hemoglobin Part of many enzymes	Organ meats, seafood, whole grains, legumes, nuts, seeds, drinking water	Anemia Bone abnormalities
Zinc	Part of many enzymes Functions in taste perception, wound healing, sperm production, normal fetal development, healthy immune system	Meat, fish, poultry, seafood, egg yolk, whole-grain and enriched breads and cereals	Decreased wound healing Decreased taste perception Impaired immune function Growth failure in children
Manganese	Part of many enzymes involved in protein and energy metabolism Bone growth Healthy immune system	Whole-grain breads and cereals, legumes, fruits, vegetables, tea	Impaired bone growth Skeletal abnormalities Depressed growth of hair and nails
Fluoride	Helps to make bones and teeth stronger Increased resistance to cavities	Seafood Fluoridated drinking water, tea	Badly formed or weak teeth Increase in dental cavities
Selenium	Antioxidant Proper functioning of the thyroid gland	Brazil nuts, seafood, organ meats, whole grains	Impaired thyroid function Muscle weakness and tenderness Poor heart function Weakened immune system
Iodine	Proper functioning of the thyroid gland Synthesis of thyroid hormones Energy metabolism	Seafood Iodized salt	Goiter Hypothyroidism Cretinism
Chromium	Normal glucose metabolism	Insulin resistance Glucose intolerance Meat, poultry, fish, whole grains, egg yolks, mushrooms, onions	Insulin resistance Glucose intolerance

ridding the body of waste products in the form of urine. Water also cushions the shock to bones and joints and functions to cool the body's internal temperature through perspiration.

Balancing the amount of water coming into and going out of the body is extremely important to life. Water is obtained primarily from the consumption of fluids and foods. It is also obtained from chemical reactions that take place in the body that produce water as a by-product. Daily fluid needs can be met by drinking water or beverages such as tea, coffee, juices, and milk. A portion of the body's fluid needs can be met by consuming foods that have a high water content such as fresh fruits and vegetables and dairy products.

Water is lost from the body primarily through urine but can also be lost through other means including perspiration, breathing, and defecation. Illness can cause an individual to lose an excessive amount of water through perspiration (associated with a fever), diarrhea, and vomiting which may result in dehydration. Signs and symptoms of dehydration may begin to occur when the amount of fluid lost reaches 2% of the body weight. Dehydration can be fatal when 9% to 12% of the body weight is lost through water. Symptoms of dehydration in adults include increased thirst, dry mouth, decreased urine output, dry skin, headache, weakness, and dizziness.

DIETARY SUPPLEMENTS

The best way to obtain all the nutrients needed by the body is to consume a balanced, healthy diet consisting of nutrient-dense foods that meet nutrient needs. A nutrient-dense food is a food that is high in nutrients compared to the number of calories in the food. Examples of nutrient-dense foods include fruits, vegetables, whole grains, low-fat or fat-free dairy products, lean cuts of meat, and beans, nuts, and seeds (Fig. 35.8).

More than half of the American population takes a dietary supplement, the most common one being a multivitamin and mineral (MVM) supplement. Although MVM supplements can help to fill minor nutritional gaps in the American diet, they do not serve as a substitute for an unhealthy diet. This is because MVM supplements do not compare with the wide variety of vitamins, minerals, phytochemicals, and fiber found in foods. On the other hand, there are certain conditions or diseases that may warrant the use of a vitamin and mineral supplement, as follows:

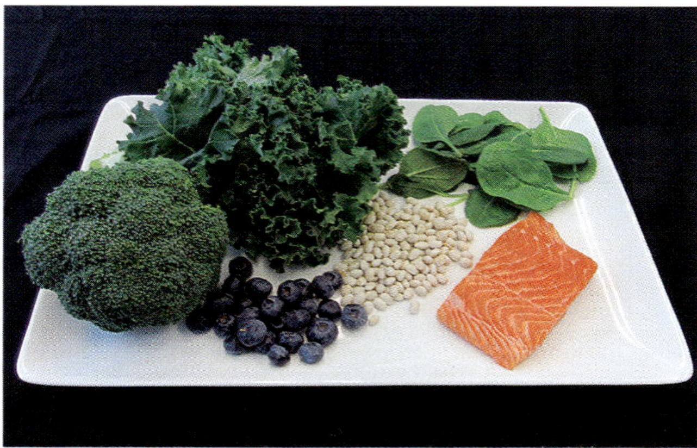

Fig. 35.8 Nutrient dense foods.

- *Individuals consuming less than 1200 kcal/day.* A calorie intake of 1200 kcal/day is the lowest calorie level that an individual can consume and still obtain all their necessary nutrients. Individuals who consume less than this amount may need an MVM supplement to ensure adequate nutrition.
- *Individuals with conditions or diseases that interfere with the absorption of vitamins and minerals.* Certain diseases, such as Crohn disease, celiac disease, chronic liver disease, cystic fibrosis, and chronic pancreatitis, may interfere with the proper absorption of vitamins and minerals from food. A vitamin and mineral supplement may be prescribed by the provider for patients with these diseases. Smoking can interfere with the absorption of some vitamins such as vitamin C and D.
- *Individuals who are pregnant or lactating.* Pregnant and lactating women benefit from taking an MVM supplement because of their increased need for vitamins and minerals. It is important for a pregnant woman to obtain an adequate amount of folic acid to help prevent neural tube defects in the infant. The MVM supplement is prescribed by a provider and is specially formulated to meet the requirements of the pregnant or lactating woman.
- *Individuals who practice a vegetarian lifestyle.* Vegetarians may be at risk for an inadequate intake of certain nutrients and therefore may benefit from an MVM supplement.
- *Elderly individuals.* Elderly individuals often experience a decrease in the absorption of nutrients because of an aging GI tract and therefore may require an MVM supplement. The elderly may also be at risk for an inadequate intake of nutrients because of illness or socioeconomic factors.

There are certain disadvantages to taking an excessive amount of a vitamin supplement. As previously discussed, water-soluble vitamins consumed in excess of the body's needs are removed from the body through the urine. On the other hand, the fat-soluble vitamins (A, D, E, and K) can be stored by the body. Consuming an excessive amount of fat-soluble vitamins can cause of buildup of these vitamins in the body, resulting in toxicity symptoms. These symptoms may be relatively mild such as itching, headache, flushed skin, and nausea. They may also be more severe and include symptoms such as loss of hair, bone pain, kidney stones, hemolysis of blood cells, and prolonged blood clotting. (Refer to Table 35.6 for a list of the fat-soluble vitamins and the toxicity symptoms that can occur from an excessive intake of these vitamins.)

TOOLS FOR HEALTHY NUTRITION

NUTRITION GUIDES

MyPlate and the *Dietary Guidelines for Americans* (DGA) are nutrition guides developed by the U.S. Department of Agriculture (USDA) and the U.S. Department of Health and Human Services (HHS). The major objective of these guides is to achieve and maintain a healthy weight through a balanced nutritious diet, which assists in preventing and reducing chronic diseases such as cardiovascular disease, type 2 diabetes, obesity, and some types of cancer. Studies show that approximately 60% of all American adults have one or more preventable chronic diseases relating to poor-quality eating patterns and physical inactivity. The MyPlate and the DGA nutrition guides are described in more detail in this section.

MyPlate

MyPlate is an easy-to-follow nutrition guide (published by the USDA) that is available online at www.myplate.gov. MyPlate consists of a food circle or pie chart that illustrates a place setting with a plate and glass divided into five food groups (Fig. 35.9). The MyPlate nutrition guide encourages Americans to practice portion control by including specific proportions of the following food groups on their plate:

- *Fruits and vegetables:* Half the plate should include fruits and vegetables, with the vegetable portion being a bit bigger. Fruits and vegetables contribute carbohydrate, vitamins A and C, potassium, folate, and fiber to the diet.
- *Protein:* One quarter of the plate should be made up of the protein group. Dried beans, peas, nuts, and seafood should be incorporated into this group, which reduces a heavy reliance on animal-based proteins. This food group provides protein, iron, vitamins B_6 and B_{12}, zinc, and magnesium to the diet.
- *Grains:* One quarter of the plate should consist of grains. Whole-grain breads and cereals should make up at least half of the total grain intake. This food group provides rich sources of carbohydrate, fiber, B vitamins, and iron to the diet.
- *Dairy:* One serving of low-fat dairy foods such as skim milk or yogurt should accompany the meal. This food group contributes protein, calcium, vitamin D, riboflavin, and vitamin B_{12} to the diet.

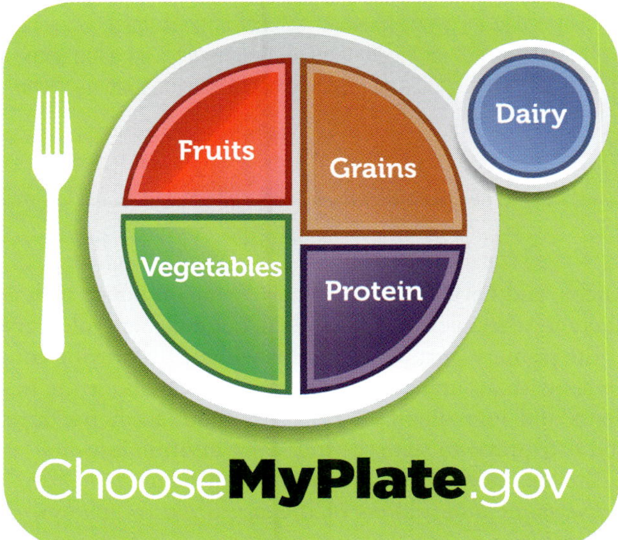

Fig. 35.9 MyPlate nutrition guide. (From U.S. Department of Agriculture: MyPlate, 2011, www.myplate.gov.)

Numerous resources are available on the MyPlate website. It provides the user with individualized nutritional guidance that allows tracking of daily food intake and physical activity (SuperTracker), access to calorie and food group information for specific foods (Food-A-Pedia), and a personalized nutrition plan based on gender, age, and physical activity (My Plan). One of the most important messages promoted by the MyPlate guide is to avoid oversized portions. It can often be difficult to understand what standard serving sizes for specific foods are. The MyPlate website features a section that contains an extensive reference about the specific food groups and related serving sizes.

Dietary Guidelines for Americans

The Dietary Guidelines for Americans provide important guidelines that support sound nutrition. The goal of the DGA is to promote health, reduce the risk of diet-related chronic disease, and meet nutrient needs. The information in the DGA is also used to develop, implement, and evaluate Federal food, nutrition, and health policies and programs in the United States. The DGA is updated at least every 5 years by the USDA and HHS to reflect the most recent scientific research about nutrition and health. The 2020–2025 DGA consists of four primary dietary guidelines for healthier living. A summary of the 2020–2025 DGA is presented in Box 35.1 while the comprehensive document is available at www.dietaryguidelines.gov.

The 2020–2025 DGA focuses on achieving and maintaining a healthy dietary pattern at every stage of life from infancy through older adulthood. A **dietary pattern** is defined as the combination of food and beverages that constitute an individual's complete dietary intake over time. It has been determined that a dietary pattern is more predictive of overall health status than a focus on individual nutrients. For most individuals, achieving a healthy dietary pattern may require adjustments in their food and beverage choices. Examples of healthy dietary patterns recommended by the DGA include the Mediterranean Diet plan and the Dietary Approaches to Stop Hypertension (DASH) diet plan. The DASH diet plan is discussed in more detail later in this chapter.

The 2020–2025 DGA also provides guidance on choosing nutrient-dense foods and beverages in place of less healthy choices. Nutrient-dense foods and beverages provide vitamins and minerals and other health-promoting components and have little or no added sugars, saturated fat, and sodium.

BOX 35.1 Summary: 2020-2025 Dietary Guidelines for Americans

Make every bite count with the Dietary Guidelines for Americans. Here's how:

1. Follow a healthy dietary pattern at every life stage.
   At every life stage—infancy, toddlerhood, childhood, adolescence, adulthood, pregnancy, lactation, and older adulthood—it is never too early or too late to eat healthfully.
   - For about the first 6 months of life, exclusively feed infants human milk. Continue to feed infants human milk through at least the first year of life, and longer if desired. Feed infants iron-fortified infant formula during the first year of life when human milk is unavailable. Provide infants with supplemental vitamin D beginning soon after birth.
   - At about 6 months, introduce infants to nutrient-dense complementary foods. Introduce infants to potentially allergenic foods along with other complementary foods. Encourage infants and toddlers to consume a variety of foods from all food groups. Include foods rich in iron and zinc, particularly for infants fed human milk.
   - From 12 months through older adulthood, follow a healthy dietary pattern across the lifespan to meet nutrient needs, help achieve a healthy body weight, and reduce the risk of chronic disease.
2. Customize and enjoy nutrient-dense food and beverage choices to reflect personal preferences, cultural traditions, and budgetary considerations.
   A healthy dietary pattern can benefit all individuals regardless of age, race, ethnicity, or current health status. The Dietary Guidelines provides a framework intended to be customized to individual needs and preferences, as well as the foodways of the diverse cultures in the United States.
3. Focus on meeting food group needs with nutrient-dense foods and beverages, and stay within calorie limits.
   An underlying premise of the Dietary Guidelines is that nutritional needs should be met primarily from foods and beverages—specifically, nutrient-dense foods and beverages. Nutrient-dense foods provide vitamins, minerals, and other health-promoting components and have no or little added sugars, saturated fat, and sodium. A healthy dietary pattern consists of nutrient-dense forms of foods and beverages across all food groups, in recommended amounts, and within calorie limits.
   The core elements that make up a healthy dietary pattern include:
   - Vegetables of all types—dark green; red and orange; beans, peas, and lentils; starchy; and other vegetables
   - Fruits, especially whole fruit
   - Grains, at least half of which are whole grain
   - Dairy, including fat-free or low-fat milk, yogurt, and cheese, and/or lactose-free versions and fortified soy beverages and yogurt as alternatives
   - Protein foods, including lean meats, poultry, and eggs; seafood; beans, peas, and lentils; and nuts, seeds, and soy products
   - Oils, including vegetable oils and oils in food, such as seafood and nuts
4. Limit foods and beverages higher in added sugars, saturated fat, and sodium, and limit alcoholic beverages.
   At every life stage, meeting food group recommendations—even with nutrient-dense choices—requires most of a person's daily calorie needs and sodium limits. A healthy dietary pattern doesn't have much room for extra added sugars, saturated fat, or sodium—or for alcoholic beverages. A small amount of added sugars, saturated fat, or sodium can be added to nutrient-dense foods and beverages to help meet food group recommendations, but foods and beverages high in these components should be limited. Limits are:
   - Added sugars—Less than 10% of calories per day starting at age 2. Avoid foods and beverages with added sugars for those younger than age 2.
   - Saturated fat—Less than 10% of calories per day starting at age 2.
   - Sodium—Less than 2300 milligrams per day—and even less for children younger than age 14.
   - Alcoholic beverages—Adults of legal drinking age can choose not to drink, or to drink in moderation by limiting intake to 2 drinks or less in a day for men and 1 drink or less in a day for women, when alcohol is consumed. Drinking less is better for health than drinking more. There are some adults who should not drink alcohol, such as women who are pregnant.

The 2020–2025 DGA emphasizes that the dietary guidelines are not intended to be a rigid prescription, but rather an adaptable framework within which individuals make nutrient-dense food and beverage choices to reflect their personal preferences, cultural traditions, and budgetary considerations.

FOOD LABELS

Food labels are required by the FDA for most packaged foods such as breads, cereals, canned and frozen foods, snacks, desserts, and beverages. Food labels for raw produce such as fruits and vegetables are not required, but rather are voluntary.

The primary purpose of food labeling is to provide consumers with accurate and valid information about the nutrients and ingredients in packaged food. Each packaged food is required to state the following information:

- The common or usual name of the product
- The name and address of the manufacturer, packer, or distributor
- The net quantity of contents in terms of weight, measure, or numeric count

- The nutrient contents of the food item (Nutrition Facts label)
- The ingredients in descending order of predominance by weight (ingredient list)

Two important components of the food label are the Nutrition Facts label and the ingredients list. These components provide guidance to the consumer for making healthy food choices and are discussed in more detail in the following sections.

Nutrition Facts Label

The Nutrition Facts label provides detailed information about the nutrient content of a food, which serves as a nutrition guide to consumers for making informed choices when purchasing packaged foods. The Nutrition Facts label is especially beneficial to individuals with health conditions, such as hypertension and diabetes, that require them to follow a specialized diet.

The Nutrition Facts label is illustrated in Fig. 35.10. It is divided into five basic sections which are color-coded in Fig. 35.10 for ease in identifying each section.

1. Serving Information

This section of the label (highlighted in blue) indicates the total number of servings included in the package and the size of a single serving. The serving size is in large bold letters and numbers and reflects the amount that people typically eat or drink at one time. It is not a recommendation of how much a person should eat or drink. A packaged food frequently contains more than one serving. The serving size is presented in familiar units, such as cup, tablespoon, piece, or slice, followed by the metric amount in grams. The amount of calories and nutrients listed on the label are based on one serving. This section assists consumers in comparing similar foods with the same serving size to determine which is a healthier choice.

2. Calories

This section of the label (highlighted in pink) indicates the total number of calories in one serving in large, bold letters and numbers. It is important to note that an individual must pay attention to the number of servings consumed. If an individual consumes two servings, this in turn doubles the amount of calories and nutrients consumed. For example, if the calories per serving equals 250 but there are two servings per package, the consumer would actually be taking in 500 calories if the entire package was consumed.

3. Percent Daily Value

There is a column on the right side of the label (highlighted in purple) that lists the **percent daily value** (% DV). This is defined as the percentage of a nutrient provided by a single

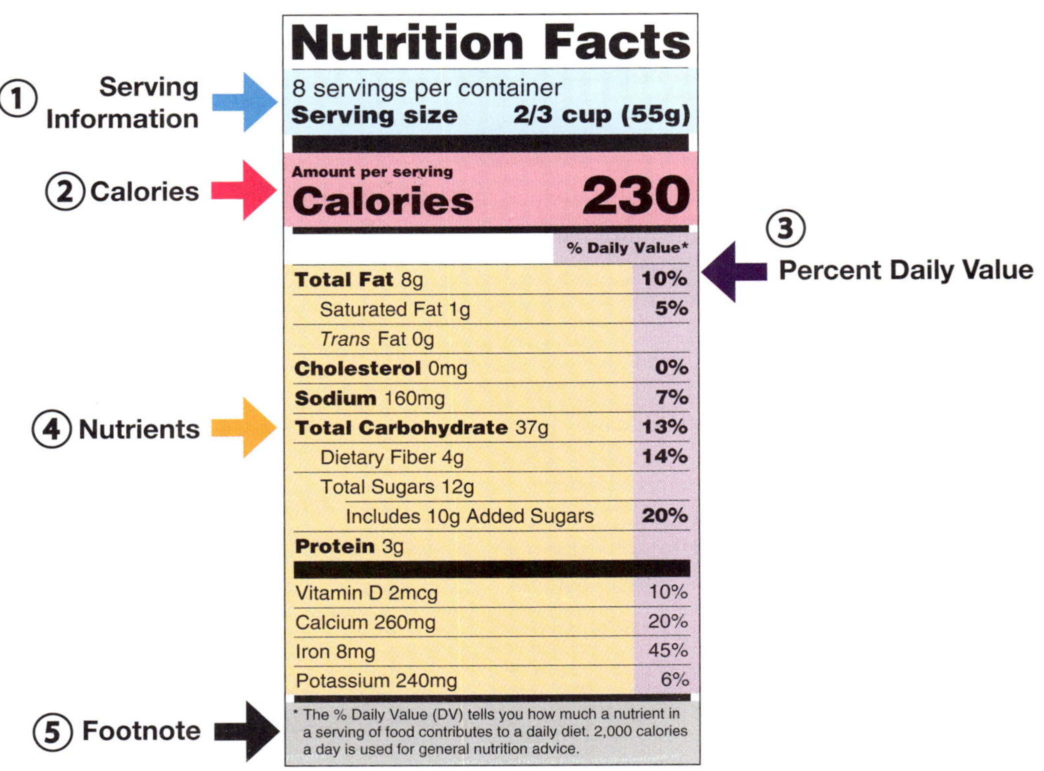

Fig. 35.10 Nutrition Facts Label. (From U.S. Food and Drug Administration, www.fda.gov.)

serving of a food item compared with how much is required for the entire day. This section of the label provides information on whether a nutrient in one serving of food contributes "a little" or "a lot" of that nutrient to the total daily diet.

The % DV is based on a 2000-kcal/day diet, and each nutrient is based on 100% of the recommended daily amount for that nutrient. For example, a food item with a 20% DV of iron provides 20% of the daily iron needed by an individual on a 2000-kilocalorie diet. For the individual to meet the recommended daily goal of 100%, the remaining 80% DV of iron would need to come from other foods containing iron. These percentages should be modified appropriately if an individual consumes more or less than 2000 kcal/day.

The % DV also allows consumers to make informed food choices to meet their specific dietary requirements by following these interpretation guidelines:

- Low nutrient level: 5% DV or less
- High or rich nutrient level: 20% DV or more

For example, if individuals want to include foods in their diet to assist them in decreasing their risk of osteoporosis, they should look for labels that indicate a 20% DV or more for calcium. Other individuals might be trying to lower their risk of heart disease and should look for labels that indicate a 5% DV or less in saturated fat.

4. Nutrients

The nutrients section of the label (highlighted in orange) includes key nutrients that impact on an individual's health. Individuals can use this section to support their personal dietary needs. Using this section, individuals can limit foods in their diet that contain nutrients that contribute to health problems. Individuals can also use this section to choose foods that contain nutrients they need to get more of in their diet.

a. Nutrients That Should Be Limited

There are certain nutrients presented on the Nutrition Facts label that should be limited in the diet because they contribute to health problems such as heart disease, some cancers, obesity, and hypertension. These nutrients include saturated fat, trans fat, cholesterol, sodium, and added sugars. *Added sugars* include sugars that are either added during the processing of foods (e.g., sucrose and dextrose), or are packaged as sweeteners (e.g., table sugar), and also includes sugars from syrups and honey, and sugars from concentrated fruit or vegetable juices. The recommended goal is to stay below 100% DV for each of these nutrients every day. To consume less of these nutrients, individuals should select foods that have a low % DV of these nutrients listed on the label; 5% DV or less is considered low. There is no recommended % DV for trans fat on a food label since artificial trans fat is now banned in all foods sold in grocery stores and restaurants. Because natural trans fat is found in small amounts in certain foods, the grams of trans fat in a food item must be listed on the label to alert the consumer of its presence.

b. Nutrients That Should Be Obtained in Adequate Amounts

There are certain nutrients that are especially important to health and should be obtained in adequate amounts. These nutrients include dietary fiber, vitamin D, calcium, iron, and potassium. The actual amount (in mg or mcg) and the % DV must be listed for each of these nutrients. An individual should strive to achieve a 100% DV of each of these nutrients every day. Consuming adequate amounts of these nutrients improves health and helps reduce the risk of certain diseases and conditions. To consume adequate amounts of these nutrients, individuals should select foods that have a high % DV of these nutrients listed on the label; 20% DV or more is considered high.

c. Additional Nutrients

Additional nutrients presented on the label include total carbohydrate and protein.

- Total Carbohydrate: The total carbohydrate value featured on the label consists of both simple and complex carbohydrates. *Total sugars* include both natural and *added sugars*, while the added sugars value on the label includes just the added sugars. This helps the consumer to see how much of the total sugar in the food comes from added sugars.
- Protein: Most Americans consume the recommended amount of protein to meet their daily needs; therefore a % DV for protein is not required on the Nutrition Facts label. Individuals are encouraged to consume moderate portions of foods containing protein such as meat, poultry, milk, eggs, cheese, legumes, and nuts.

5. Footnote

The footnote (highlighted in gray) explains the meaning of % Daily Value and identifies the number of calories used (2000) for general nutrition advice.

Ingredients List

The ingredients list is an important component of food labeling. Ingredients are listed in descending order of weight from highest to lowest (Fig. 35.11). This means that the first ingredient makes up the largest proportion of the food by weight compared with any other ingredients.

A

Ingredients: Whole grain wheat, wheat bran, raisins, oat fiber, sugar, sea salt.

B

Ingredients: Corn flour, high-fructose corn syrup, oat flour, brown sugar, partially hydrogenated vegetable oil, salt, sodium citrate, natural and artificial flavor, trisodium phosphate, fruit juice concentrate, malic acid, red 40, niacinamide, yellow 5, blue 1, thiamin mononitrate, pyridoxine hydrochloride, BHT.

Fig. 35.11 Ingredients list. A, Short ingredients list. B, Lengthy ingredients list.

Consumers can use the information in the ingredients list to make healthy food choices. For example, the 2020–2025 DGA recommends limiting the amount of added sugars in the diet to reduce the incidence of obesity and heart disease. A good guideline to follow is to avoid foods that list added sugars as the first or second ingredient. Added sugars appears in the ingredients list under a number of different terms. Refer to Fig. 35.12 for a list of names used to describe sugars and to the *Patient Coaching: Added Sugars* box for more detailed information on added sugars.

The ingredients list also allows consumers to quickly scan for ingredients that may cause food allergies (e.g., peanuts) or food intolerances (e.g., lactose) or that should be avoided for religious or cultural reasons.

Another benefit of the ingredients list is to assist individuals in selecting fresh or unprocessed foods that promote good health and prevent disease. These foods typically have an ingredients list that is short and simple (see Fig. 35.11A), and "fresh" terms are found in the list of ingredients such as *whole oats*, *whole-grain flour*, *diced tomatoes*, *chicken broth*, and *vegetable oil*. On the other hand, processed foods typically have a lengthy list of ingredients (see Fig. 35.11B) and include chemical terms such as *sodium citrate*, *trisodium phosphate*, *benzoic acid*, *sodium nitrate*, and *monosodium glutamate*.

TERMS FOR ADDED SUGARS	
• Anhydrous dextrose • Brown sugar • Cane crystals • Confectioner's powdered sugar • Corn sweetener • Corn syrup • Dextrose • Evaporated can juice • Fructose • Fruit juice concentrate	• Granulated sugar • High-fructose corn syrup • Honey • Lactose • Malt syrup • Maple syrup • Molasses • Raw sugar • Sucrose • Sugars

Fig. 35.12 Names that describe sugar.

PATIENT COACHING Added Sugars

Answer questions that patients have on added sugars.

What is the Difference Between Natural Sugars and Added Sugars?

Natural sugars are sugars that occur naturally in foods and beverages; examples include fructose in fruit and lactose in milk and dairy products. **Added sugars** include sugars and syrups that are added to foods and beverages at home or during the commercial preparation of food known as *processing*. Examples include the sugar individuals add to their coffee or cereal at home and the sugar added to ketchup during commercial food processing.

What Role Does Sugar Play in the Diet?

All sugar—whet er natural or added–is classified as a simple carbohydrate. Simple carbohydrate is used as a source of energy by the body. Natural sugars are considered a healthier food choice because they typically occur in foods that are also rich in vitamins, minerals, and fiber such as fruits and vegetables. Added sugars contribute "empty calories" to foods because they provide additional calories to a food without adding any nutritional value. Added sugars are often found in processed foods such as baked goods, sauces, and salad dressings.

Why is Sugar Added to Foods and Beverages?

Sugar is added to foods for a variety of reasons which include the following:

- **Taste:** Sugar provides sweetness to improve the taste of foods such as breakfast cereal.
- **Color and Flavor:** Sugar improves the color and flavor of many foods such as baked goods and chocolate.
- **Bulk and Texture:** Sugar contributes bulk to certain foods which improves the texture of the food such as baked goods and ice cream.
- **Fermentation:** Sugar assists in the fermentation of many common foods such as yogurt, vinegar, sour cream, cheese, soy sauce, sauerkraut, wine and beer. Sugar is also involved in a chemical reaction (along with yeast) that allows bread to rise.
- **Preservation:** Sugar assists in preserving and extending the shelf-life of certain foods such as jams, jellies, and baked goods.

What are the Primary Sources of Added Sugars Consumed By Americans?

According to the American Cancer Society, the sources of sugar in the typical American diet are broken down as follows:

1. Approximately 50% of sugar comes from sweetened beverages such as:
   - Regular (non-diet) soft drinks
   - Sweetened fruit drinks
   - Sugary specialty coffees and teas
   - Sports and energy drinks
2. Another 25% of sugar comes from sweet treats such as:
   - Candy
   - Pies and cakes
   - Cookies
   - Doughnuts, pastries, and sweet rolls

Continued

PATIENT COACHING Added Sugars —cont'd

- Ice cream and sweetened yogurt
- Sugary breakfast cereal

3. The remaining 25% of sugar comes from:
   - Sugar used in cooking
   - Sugar added at the table
   - Sugar present in processed foods such as crackers, salad dressing, and spaghetti sauce

Why should Added Sugars be Limited?

Consuming a diet high in added sugars can make it difficult for individuals to meet their nutrient requirements while staying within their caloric limits. The 2020–2025 DGA recommends that individuals should limit total daily consumption of added sugars to less than 10% of calories per day from added sugars. This equates to no more than 200 calories of added sugars each day for an individual following a 2000 calories per day dietary pattern. Studies suggest that consuming too much added sugar can lead to the following health problems:

- Obesity
- Increased risk of heart disease
- Suppression of the immune system
- Increased risk of hypertension
- Difficulty in controlling type 2 diabetes
- Tooth decay

How can I Reduce Added Sugars in My Diet?

Tips for reducing added sugars in the diet include the following:

- Drink water instead of sugary beverages such as regular (non-diet) soft drinks, sports drinks, and specialty coffees and teas
- Limit foods that are high in added sugars such as sugary breakfast cereals, candy, baked goods, and sweet desserts
- Cut back on the amount of sugar added to foods and beverages such as cereal, pancakes, coffee and tea.
- Buy fresh fruit or fruit packed in water or natural juice. Avoid those packed in syrup.
- Limit condiments that are high in added sugars such as ketchup, barbecue sauce, relish, and salad dressing. Instead use herbs and spices to provide flavor.
- Choose heart healthy snacks such as fruits, vegetables, and low-fat cheese instead of candy, pastries, and cookies.
- Reduce the amount of sugar used in recipes for foods prepared at home such as cookies, cakes and brownies.
- Choose fruit for dessert instead of cakes, cookies, pies, ice cream and other sweets

NUTRITION THERAPY

Nutrition therapy is the application of the science of nutrition to promote optimal health and treat illness. Nutrition therapy is an important component of the medical treatment plan for managing certain diseases and conditions. As previously discussed, the medical assistant should have a basic knowledge of the type of nutrition therapy prescribed for common conditions and diseases; however, the medical assistant is not qualified to recommend or provide nutrition therapy to patients. This is the responsibility of a registered dietitian, who is specially trained to assess the nutritional status of a patient and recommend appropriate nutrition therapy.

Common conditions and diseases that require nutrition therapy are discussed in this section.

WEIGHT MANAGEMENT

Weight management involves following a set of practices and behaviors that keep an individual's weight at a healthy level. The basis of weight management depends on the number of calories consumed ("calories in") compared with the number of calories used ("calories out") over a period of time. Individuals who consume roughly the same number of calories that they use will remain at the same weight. On the other hand, individuals who consume more calories than they use over a period of time will gain weight, and individuals who consume fewer calories than they use over a period of time will lose weight. Weight management is particularly important in the prevention and treatment of obesity.

Obesity

Obesity is a medical condition in which there is an excessive accumulation of body fat to the extent where it may have an adverse effect on the health and well-being of an individual.

The incidence of obesity in the United States has increased markedly, and obesity is now one of the most common chronic health problems encountered by primary care providers. Approximately 70% of adults in the United States are either overweight or obese. That means that two out of every three Americans are overweight or obese. Obesity is not just an appearance or body image concern. It is associated with premature death and, after smoking, is the second leading cause of preventable death in the United States today. The primary causes of obesity include an excessive food intake and a lack of physical exercise.

The body mass index (BMI) strongly correlates with total body fat and therefore is used as a screening tool to identify patients who may be at risk for diseases that occur with overweight and obesity. As previously discussed in Chapter 20, an adult patient's weight and height are used to determine their BMI. The BMI of an adult is then interpreted using the weight status categories outlined in Table 35.9. It has been determined that as the BMI increases to greater than 25, there is an increased risk of developing certain diseases associated with overweight and obesity such as hypertension, heart disease, stroke, type 2 diabetes, sleep apnea and respiratory problems, and osteoarthritis.

Table 35.9 Interpretation of Body Mass Index (BMI)

BMI	Weight Status Category
Less than 15	Very severely underweight
15–15.9	Severely underweight
16–8.49	Underweight
18.5–24.9	Healthy weight
25–29.9	Overweight
30–34.9	Obese Class I (Moderately obese)
35.0–39.9	Obese Class II (Severely obese)
40 or more	Obese Class III (Very severely obese)

Treatment of Obesity

Obesity is considered a chronic condition that requires a multiple treatment approach consisting of the following three components: nutrition therapy, a physical exercise program, and a behavior modification plan. These three components are also key elements for the long-term maintenance of weight loss. Additional methods of treatment for obesity include prescription weight loss medications and bariatric surgery. Studies show that even a modest loss of weight results in improved health and the prevention of problems associated with obesity.

It should be emphasized that it is important for an individual to consult with their provider before beginning treatment for obesity. Primary care providers often manage individuals with Class I obesity and Class II obesity, but patients with Class III obesity are usually referred to a bariatric specialist. **Bariatrics** is the branch of medicine that deals with the treatment and control of obesity and diseases associated with obesity.

Nutrition Therapy

Nutrition therapy for obesity involves the selection of an appropriate dietary plan for weight loss. It is essential that the dietary plan selected ensures an adequate intake of nutrients. The MyPlate nutrition guide and the Dietary Guidelines for Americans (previously discussed in this chapter) provide valuable recommendations for a healthy and balanced dietary plan.

Before beginning a weight reduction program, it is important to first set reasonable and safe weight loss goals. Most weight loss authorities recommend a slow steady weight loss of no more than 1 to 2 pounds per week. This is accomplished by a moderate reduction in the total number of calories consumed to create what is known as a *caloric deficit.* A caloric deficit occurs when more calories are used for energy by the body (calories out) than are consumed (calories in), resulting in the burning of body fat, which leads to a loss of weight.

To completely understand the concept of a caloric deficit, it is important to have a knowledge of the relationship between calories and body fat. One pound of body fat is equal to 3500 kilocalories. Therefore, a decrease of 500 kilocalories each day typically results in a loss of 1 pound each week ($500 \times 7 = 3500$ kilocalories, or 1 pound). A decrease of 1000 kilocalories each day is needed to lose about 2 pounds each week ($1000 \times 7 = 7000$ kilocalories, or 2 pounds). The total number of kilocalories consumed each day, however, should not fall below 1200 kilocalories to ensure an individual is obtaining all the required nutrients. Most women lose weight safely on a diet plan consisting of 1200 to 1500 kcal/day, and most men lose weight safely by consuming 1500 to 1800 kcal/day.

Numerous weight loss programs are available to assist individuals in achieving their weight loss goals; examples include the DASH (Dietary Approaches to Stop Hypertension) diet plan, the Weight Watchers diet plan, and the Mediterranean Diet plan. When choosing a weight loss diet plan, it is important for individuals to choose a program that is medically proven and is best suited to their particular needs and lifestyle. Fad diets should be avoided because they can be harmful to health and do not typically result in good long-term results; examples include the grapefruit diet, the cabbage soup diet, and the Scarsdale diet. Characteristics of fad diets typically include no exercise, a promise of quick and easy weight loss, a guarantee of a large amount of weight loss, and the elimination of one or more food groups.

Physical Exercise Program

Physical exercise plays a key role in the treatment of obesity. Exercise increases the number of calories the body burns for energy (calories out), contributing to a caloric deficit and loss of weight. Physical exercise offers additional benefits such as increased lean body mass, improved cardiorespiratory functioning, and an improved quality of life and general well-being. Studies show that individuals who exercise are also less likely to regain their weight after having lost it.

The AHA recommends that healthy adults spend at least 150 minutes per week in moderate-intensity aerobic exercise. The AHA further recommends that adults perform muscle-strengthening activities at least 2 days per week. Refer to the Patient Coaching box *Aerobic Exercise* in Chapter 19 for a more thorough discussion of physical exercise recommendations for adults.

Behavior Modification Plan

A behavior modification plan is an important component in the treatment of obesity. The purpose of such a plan is to assist individuals in changing behaviors that have contributed to their weight gain. An individual must first identify the behaviors that have contributed to their weight gain; examples include eating too fast, eating when not hungry, using food as a reward, eating while standing or watching television, and eating to relieve stress or boredom. Once an individual identifies these behaviors, they can then take steps to replace these unhealthy behaviors with behaviors that encourage weight loss such as chewing food more slowly, keeping tempting foods out of the house, using nonfood incentives as a reward, eating only while sitting at a table, and using techniques other than food to relieve stress and boredom.

PATIENT COACHING Eating Disorders

Answer questions that patients have on eating disorders.

What is an Eating Disorder?

Eating disorders are characterized by severe disturbances in eating behaviors, thoughts, and emotions. They can cause serious health problems and may even become life-threatening. Eating disorders affect approximately 29 million people in the United States. Eating disorders include anorexia nervosa (AN), bulimia nervosa (BN), and binge eating disorder (BED). Despite having significant nutritional implications, all of these conditions have been classified as psychological disorders. Some of the underlying problems that may be associated with an eating disorder include low self-esteem, depression, feelings of worthlessness and loss of control, troubled family and personal relationships, and a history of physical and sexual abuse.

Anorexia Nervosa

What is Anorexia Nervosa?

AN is characterized by a distorted body image, self-starvation, and extreme weight loss that usually stem from underlying emotional problems. Approximately 90% of those affected with AN are girls and young women between 12 and 25 years of age.

Individuals diagnosed with AN often become preoccupied with weight and an intense fear of becoming fat. Rituals surrounding food are common with AN—for example, where food is positioned on the plate and how the napkin is folded. Affected individuals often spend a lot of time cutting and rearranging the food on the plate. They typically are very knowledgeable about the caloric and nutritional content of food and may exclude themselves from social gatherings or activities where food is served. Individuals with AN are often high achievers who experience anxiety and depression. They are also typically raised in families where pressure to succeed exists and where criticism (particularly of physical appearance) is commonplace.

What are the Signs and Symptoms of Anorexia Nervosa?

The physical signs and symptoms of AN include very thin arms and legs, dry skin, loss of muscle, brittle pluckable hair, frequently being cold, sunken dark eyes, and amenorrhea. The presence of lanugo or fine "peach fuzz" hair may develop as the body attempts to trap heat and maintain an adequate body temperature. Other symptoms may include irregular heart rhythms, low blood pressure, a decreased heart and respiratory rate, abdominal pain, and an impaired immune response.

What is the Treatment for Anorexia Nervosa?

Treatment for AN is best provided by a team of professionals (provider, nurse, dietitian, counselor, and social worker) in a specialized treatment facility. Cognitive behavior therapy (CBT) is considered the counseling method of choice for AN. This counseling technique encourages the individual to carefully explore her or his beliefs surrounding body image, food, and self-esteem. Once these irrational beliefs are identified, healthful eating behaviors may then be pursued and reinforced. Counseling related to the patient's family dynamics is also considered a vital part of the recovery process. Nutrition therapy focuses on a gradual increase in the caloric intake that includes mandatory nutrition supplements. Meals and snacks are frequent and small to minimize feelings of fullness.

Bulimia Nervosa

What is Bulimia Nervosa?

BN is an eating disorder characterized by the rapid consumption of a large amount of food in a short period of time (binging) then immediately ridding the body (purging) of that food through self-induced vomiting, laxative abuse, or over-exercising. The binge–purge cycle may occur anywhere from many times each day to several times per week.

Individuals with BN often come from families where emotional connections are minimal and criticism is common. As a result, bulimics frequently exhibit a negative self-image, which triggers the binge–purge cycle. In addition, individuals diagnosed with BN may have a history of physical or sexual abuse. Bulimia is similar to AN in that individuals may be overachievers and may have obsessive–compulsive tendencies. Bulimics often have feelings of shame, disgust, and guilt after a binge episode, which stimulates the desire to purge. The body weight of an individual with BN is usually within the normal range; however, intense dissatisfaction about body weight and shape is usually present.

What are the Dangers of Purging?

Continued purging results in damage and irritation to the lining of the esophagus as well as erosion of the tooth enamel. Self-induced vomiting also causes broken capillaries of the face and eyes and swollen salivary glands or "chipmunk cheeks." Individuals with BN may also develop sores, scars, or calluses on their knuckles from self-induced vomiting. Excessive loss of fluid from vomiting and diarrhea (from laxative abuse) can lead to an electrolyte imbalance and dehydration.

What is the Treatment for Bulimia Nervosa?

Treatment of BN consists of a multidisciplinary team approach of medical, nutritional, individual, and family counseling. The goal of recovery is to explore the underlying causes of the binge–purge cycle and to identify any irrational beliefs that may be present. Nutrition therapy focuses on returning the individual to normal eating behaviors. Patients are taught to focus on their "hunger and fullness signals" and to pay attention to proper portion control. Meals and snacks should be consumed by the patient at a relaxed pace.

Binge Eating Disorder

What is Binge Eating Disorder?

BED is the most common eating disorder in the United Stages, affecting more individuals than AN and BN combined. BED occurs when an individual engages in recurrent episodes of binging and experiences marked distress about the binge episode. Unlike bulimia, an individual with BED does not purge following a binging episode. Individuals with BED report feeling "out of control"

PATIENT COACHING **Eating Disorders —cont'd**

during eating binges. They spend large amounts of time thinking about food, planning their binge, and shopping for it. Uncontrolled eating behaviors of BED typically occur in a rapid and frenzied manner and in private. An individual with BED may often continue to eat even after they become uncomfortably full. Like the bulimic, a binge eater feels shame, disgust, embarrassment, and guilt after a binge episode. If left untreated, BED can lead to obesity and increase the risk of chronic diseases such as type 2 diabetes, high blood pressure, and heart disease. Depression and sleep apnea are also seen in these individuals.

What are the Risk Factors for BED?

BED is more common in women than in men. Individuals of any age can have BED, however it is most likely to begin in the late teens or early twenties. People with a history of dieting are more likely to develop BED. Individuals with BED frequently experience a negative self-image which can trigger a binge episode. Studies suggest that people with BED may use overeating to deal with emotions such as anger, sadness, boredom, anxiety, or stress.

Orthorexia

Orthorexia is defined as an extreme preoccupation with the healthfulness of food. It is a "proposed" eating disorder, meaning it has not yet been classified as a true eating disorder. Individuals with orthorexia often impose strict eating rules on themselves such as consuming only organic, raw, or plant-based foods. Ironically, such restrictive behavior often leads to an unbalanced and inadequate intake of nutrients. Patients with this disorder typically exhibit low self-esteem and a negative body image and often become increasingly socially isolated.

Recovery and Prevention

What is the Prognosis for Eating Disorders?

Recovery from an eating disorder is a gradual process, with relapses often occurring. Approximately 50% of individuals with an eating disorder recover completely, and another 30% attain partial recovery. The remaining 20% continue to struggle with disordered eating throughout their lives. Suicide rates are higher in individuals with eating disorders than in the general population. If the medical assistant observes that a patient is exhibiting any of the physical or psychological symptoms of an eating disorder, they should inform the provider.

Are There Methods for Preventing Eating Disorders?

There are many strategies that help to decrease the risk of developing an eating disorder. These include the following:

- Strive for body acceptance. Focus on what your body can do, not how it looks.
- Avoid physical comparisons with others.
- Be mindful of your genetic influences on body type and embrace them.
- Avoid caloric restrictions that are below 1200 kcal daily.
- Be realistic with weight loss goals. The rate of healthy weight loss is 1 to 2 pounds weekly.
- Adopt a grazing type of eating style. Avoid going more than 4 hours without a meal or snack.
- Listen to your body. Eat when you are hungry and stop when you are full.

CARDIOVASCULAR DISEASE

The leading cause of death in the United States is cardiovascular disease (CVD). The most common cause of CVD is atherosclerosis of the coronary arteries. As previously described, atherosclerosis of the coronary arteries is a condition in which fibrous plaques of fatty deposits and cholesterol build up on the inner walls of the coronary arteries. This causes narrowing and partial blockage of the lumen of these arteries, along with hardening of the arterial wall, leading to coronary artery disease (CAD). As the atherosclerosis progresses, the coronary arteries become more occluded, which eventually could lead to a heart attack.

Research has shown that high total blood cholesterol is a major risk factor for CAD, and the higher the cholesterol, the greater the risk. The National Cholesterol Educational Program (NCEP) was established by the federal government to reduce the prevalence of elevated blood cholesterol levels in the United States by educating the public about the health risks associated with high blood cholesterol and to make recommendations for helping individuals reduce their cholesterol levels. The NCEP recommendations are published as a set of guidelines known as the TLC (Therapeutic Lifestyle Changes) diet plan. The TLC diet plan provides numeric recommendations for a heart-healthy diet, which is presented in Table 35.10 and is described in more detail in the following section.

Nutrition Therapy

TLC Diet Plan

Nutrition therapy is the first line of treatment for high blood cholesterol. The TLC diet plan recommends that all individuals older than 2 years reduce dietary cholesterol and saturated fats and increase their dietary fiber. Many foods high in fat tend to be high in cholesterol. Nutrition labels on packaged products provide information on the cholesterol, fat, and fiber content of a food. Following the nutrition therapy measures discussed later can help individuals reduce their level of "bad" LDL cholesterol and increase their level of "good" HDL cholesterol.

Dietary Cholesterol

The body manufactures all the cholesterol it needs for normal functioning, and dietary intake of cholesterol (in foods) serves only to increase the blood cholesterol. According to the TLC diet plan, dietary cholesterol should be limited to less than 200 mg each day. Cholesterol is found only in animal foods and shellfish. Egg yolks, dairy products, and organ meats such as liver and kidneys are especially high in cholesterol.

Saturated Fat

The intake of saturated fat is the most important dietary factor leading to high blood cholesterol, even more so than consuming dietary cholesterol. This is because a diet that is high in saturated fat raises the LDL cholesterol and lowers the HDL cholesterol. In general, the more saturated a fat is, the harder and more solid it is at room temperature. The main source of saturated fat is animal products, including meat fat, poultry skin, and the fat in dairy products (butter, cream, ice cream, cheese, whole milk). Plant sources that are high in saturated fat include palm oil and coconut oil.

The TLC diet plan recommends that no more than 25% to 35% of the calories consumed each day come from total fat, with less than 7% of calories coming from saturated fat and with the remaining fat coming from unsaturated (monounsaturated and polyunsaturated) fat. Refer to Table 35.10 for a summary of the TLC recommendations for daily fat consumption.

Soluble Fiber

Soluble fiber, in particular, has been shown to lower the cholesterol level by keeping the cholesterol consumed in food from being absorbed through the intestinal wall and into the body. Examples of foods high in soluble fiber include oatmeal, oat bran, barley, some fruits (e.g., apples and oranges), broccoli, and legumes. The TLC diet plan recommends that an individual consume 20 to 30 grams of dietary fiber each day, with 10 to 25 grams of that amount consisting of soluble fiber.

In general, the cholesterol level begins to decrease 2 to 3 weeks after a cholesterol-lowering diet and other cholesterol-lowering measures (such as exercise and weight loss) are begun. Over time, it is possible to reduce the total cholesterol level by 30 to 55 mg/dL or even more through these lifestyle changes. If the blood cholesterol level cannot be lowered to an acceptable level, the provider may prescribe cholesterol-lowering medications along with continuation of the aforementioned measures.

Table 35.10 Therapeutic Lifestyle Changes (TLC) Diet Plan

Nutrient	Daily Recommended Intake
Total fat	25% to 35% of total calories
Saturated Fat	Less than 7% of total calories
Polyunsaturated fat	Up to 10% of total calories
Monounsaturated fat	Up to 20% of total calories
Carbohydrate	50% to 60% of total calories
Dietary fiber	20–30 g/day (10–25 g/day should consist of soluble fiber)
Protein	15% to 25% of total calories
Cholesterol	Less than 200 mg/day
Sodium	Less than 2300 mg/day

HYPERTENSION

Hypertension is the most common life-threatening disease among Americans. It is estimated that 116 million Americans adults have high blood pressure but only 1 in 4 of these adults have their high blood pressure under control. The incidence of hypertension in the United States has increased dramatically as a result of a sedentary lifestyle and an increased incidence of obesity.

If hypertension is not brought under control, over time it can cause severe damage to the blood vessels of vital organs, such as the heart, brain, kidneys, and eyes. This damage increases the risk of a heart attack or heart failure, stroke, aneurysm, kidney damage, and damaged vision. Early detection and treatment of hypertension can prevent these complications.

Nutrition Therapy

DASH Diet Plan

Hypertension can be prevented and controlled by following the DASH (Dietary Approaches to Stop Hypertension) diet plan. The DASH diet plan is a lifelong approach to healthy eating that is recommended not only for individuals who have hypertension, but for all individuals. The DASH plan consists of a flexible and balanced diet plan that focuses on fruits, vegetables, whole grains, and low-fat dairy products. The DASH diet plan is low in saturated fat and sodium and limits sweets and sugar-sweetened beverages. In addition to lowering blood pressure, the DASH diet plan can help prevent the development of certain conditions such as obesity, osteoporosis, diabetes, cancer, heart disease, and stroke. The comprehensive DASH diet plan is available on the National Heart, Lung, and Blood Institute website and is summarized in Table 35.11.

Table 35.11 Dietary Approaches to Stop Hypertension (DASH) Diet Plan

Food Group	Frequency*
Whole grains	6 to 8 servings per day
Vegetables	4 to 5 servings per day
Fruits	4 to 5 servings per day
Low-fat or fat-free dairy products	2 to 3 servings per day
Lean meats, poultry, and fish	6 or fewer servings per day
Nuts, seeds, and legumes	4 to 5 servings per week
Fats and oils	2 to 3 servings per day
Sweets and added sugars	5 or fewer servings per week
Sodium	Limit sodium intake to less than 2300 mg daily

*Based on a 2000 kcal per day diet.

BOX 35.2 Sodium Content of Food

High-Sodium Foods
- Many restaurant and fast food meals
- Cured meats such as ham, bologna, and hot dogs
- Canned foods such as soups, vegetables, vegetable juices, and meats
- Frozen meals
- Snack foods including pretzels, potato chips, salted crackers, and nuts
- Many condiments such as soy sauce, steak sauce, onion salt, garlic salt, salad dressings, marinades, and catsup
- Pickled foods such as pickles, relish, and sauerkraut

Low-Sodium Foods
- Fresh or frozen fruits and vegetables
- Dried beans, peas, and legumes
- Whole-grain products
- Fresh meat, fish, and poultry
- Dairy products including milk, yogurt, hard cheeses, and ice cream and frozen yogurt
- Most beverages including fruit juices and carbonated beverages
- Unsalted nuts and seeds
- Condiments such as herbs, spices, citrus, Tabasco, salsa, mustard, and chili sauce

Sodium Intake

A small amount of sodium is needed in the diet; however, most Americans consume too much sodium. It is particularly important for individuals with hypertension to limit the amount of sodium in their diet, which assists in lowering blood pressure.

The relationship between sodium and water can be summarized as follows: "Where sodium goes, water follows." Because the plasma of the blood consists primarily of water, a decrease in sodium in the diet causes a decrease in the blood volume. When the blood volume is reduced, there is less resistance or force of the blood against artery walls. Less resistance translates into a lowered blood pressure. Refer to Box 35.2 for a list of foods that are high and low in sodium content.

DIABETES

Diabetes is a lifelong condition that occurs when the body is not able to use glucose for energy because of a problem with insulin. Diabetes develops when the body produces little or no insulin, or when the body cannot use the insulin it does produce effectively (known as *insulin resistance*). According to the American Diabetes Association, more than 37 million Americans have diabetes; of these, nearly 8.5 million are not yet diagnosed and are unaware that they have diabetes. An additional 96 million people have prediabetes. *Prediabetes* is a condition in which the glucose levels of an individual are higher than normal but not high enough to be classified as diabetes. An individual with prediabetes has an increased risk of developing type 2 diabetes. Refer to Chapter 33 of your textbook for a more in-depth discussion of diabetes.

Type 1 Diabetes

Type 1 diabetes is caused by an autoimmune defect that destroys the insulin-producing cells or beta cells of the pancreas. As a result, the body can no longer produce insulin and therefore it must be administered by injection.

Nutrition Therapy

The nutrition therapy for type 1 diabetes focuses on maintaining good control of the blood glucose level. This is accomplished by keeping track of the amount and type of carbohydrate consumed and when (time of day) the carbohydrate is consumed. Nutrition therapy for controlling a patient's blood glucose level includes the following methods: exchange lists, carbohydrate counting, and MyPlate. These methods are described here.

Exchange List System

The exchange list system categorizes foods into six groups according to their carbohydrate, protein, and fat content. The six food groups include starch, fruits, vegetables, meat, milk, and fat. Each food group lists examples of specifically portioned foods belonging to that group. An example of an exchange list for fruits is illustrated in Fig. 35.13.

The term *exchange* is actually the same as a food serving. Each exchange or serving has a known or predictable blood glucose response. Any food within a given food group can be exchanged for another one in that group. For example, in the fruit group, a small orange is equivalent to or can be exchanged with one small banana (refer to Fig. 35.13). Because of this, patients following the exchange system must become familiar with food serving sizes. The patient is provided with an individualized plan that specifies the number and type of exchanges that should be included for both meals and snacks. The exchange method provides a balanced and portion-controlled nutrition plan that assists in nourishing the individual while controlling their blood glucose level.

Carbohydrate Counting Method

The carbohydrate counting method offers more flexibility in meal planning than the exchange method. With this method, the carbohydrate content of a food measured in grams is balanced against the amount of insulin administered. Typically, 1 unit of insulin helps to process or metabolize 15 grams of carbohydrate. To balance the amount of insulin administered, women usually need to consume 45 to 60 grams of carbohydrate at each meal and men need 60 to 75 grams at each meal.

Individuals following the carbohydrate counting method must determine the carbohydrate content (in grams) of all

Fruit Each fruit exchange (one serving) contains about 15 grams of carbohydrate.	Serving Size
Apple with skin (fresh)	1 small
Applesauce (unsweetened)	½ cup
Apricots (fresh)	4 apricots
Banana (fresh)	1 small
Blackberries (fresh)	¾ cup
Blueberries (fresh)	¾ cup
Cantaloupe (fresh)	1 cup
Cherries (fresh)	12 cherries
Grapefruit (fresh)	½ medium
Grapes	17 grapes
Orange (fresh)	1 small
Peaches (fresh)	1 medium
Peaches (canned)	½ cup
Pear (fresh)	½ large
Pears (canned)	½ cup
Pineapple (fresh)	¾ cup
Plums (fresh)	2 small
Raspberries (fresh)	1 cup
Strawberries (fresh)	1 ¼ cups
Tangerine	2 small
Watermelon (cubes)	1 ¼ cups

Fig. 35.13 Diabetic exchange list for fruit.

of the foods they consume. This information can be obtained by referring to the data provided in the diabetic exchange lists or by referring to food labels and noting the total carbohydrate content of each food item consumed.

MyPlate Method

The MyPlate method (discussed earlier in this chapter) is the most basic dietary approach for controlling blood glucose (refer to Fig. 35.9). It is ideal for the patient who has low literacy skills or may be mentally challenged. Patients are taught to visually divide their dinner plate in half. Fruits and vegetables should occupy 50% of the plate. The remaining 50% of the plate is then divided into two parts, one for the protein group, and the other for the starchy foods (grains). Starchy foods produce the highest blood glucose response and include grain-based foods such as pasta, rice, and bread. Starchy vegetables such as corn, peas, potatoes, winter squash, and lima beans are also included under this classification. By limiting the intake of starchy foods to one quarter of the plate, the individual can control the blood glucose level.

Type 2 Diabetes

Type 2 diabetes can affect people at any age, but the chance of developing it increases with age, and it is more likely to occur in individuals who are 45 years of age or older. The biggest risk factor for developing type 2 diabetes is excess body weight. As a result of the recent increase in childhood obesity combined with a sedentary lifestyle, type 2 diabetes is starting to appear in younger age groups.

Type 2 diabetes is usually caused by insulin resistance. Insulin resistance is a condition in which the body produces insulin but does not use it effectively. Normally, when the blood glucose level rises in the body, insulin is released by the pancreas. Insulin binds to the surface of the cells at a special receptor site, similar to a lock-and-key system. The cell recognizes the insulin and opens up so that the glucose in the blood can flow into the cell and be converted to energy. Obesity can interfere with this lock-and-key system, causing the cell to become insensitive or resistant to the presence of insulin. When this occurs, the pancreas produces more insulin in an attempt to lower the blood glucose level. Over time, the pancreas is unable to keep up with the increased demand for insulin. Without enough insulin, the blood glucose level rises above normal, resulting in hyperglycemia.

Nutrition Therapy

Weight management and carbohydrate control are the keys for the dietary management of type 2 diabetes. Individuals with type 2 diabetes should consume well-balanced meals and snacks that provide an even distribution of carbohydrates throughout the day. These individuals can also maintain good blood glucose levels by controlling portion size, limiting concentrated sweets, emphasizing low glycemic index foods, and increasing the amount of soluble fiber in the diet. Soluble fiber slows down the absorption of glucose, which helps in controlling blood glucose levels.

Another very important aspect of blood glucose management in individuals with type 2 diabetes is attaining a healthy body weight through caloric restriction and daily exercise. Lowering the calorie intake by 500 kcal each day usually results in a weight loss of about 1 pound each week. Caloric restriction should not fall lower than 1200 kcal/day, however, to ensure an adequate intake of nutrients.

LACTOSE INTOLERANCE

Lactose intolerance is not a food allergy but rather a condition in which the body is unable to fully digest lactose. **Lactose** (milk sugar) is a disaccharide that consists of two sugar units and is found in milk and milk products.

Lactose intolerance is caused by a deficiency of lactase, which is an enzyme produced by the lining of the small intestine. Lactase is needed to break down lactose into glucose and galactose, which are then absorbed into the bloodstream for use by the body. When the small intestine does not produce enough of the lactase enzyme, lactose is unable to be broken down and moves through the intestines in an undigested form. When this undigested lactose reaches the large intestine, it is broken down and used as a food source by bacteria normally found in the large intestine. The by-products that result from this breakdown include copious amounts of gas that cause the symptoms of lactose intolerance.

Lactose intolerance usually begins during late adolescence or adulthood. This is because the amount of lactase produced by the body gradually declines after childhood. Lactose intolerance can also be caused by intestinal disease or injury. Lactose intolerance is most common in individuals of Asian, African American, and Hispanic descent and much less common in individuals of European descent.

The symptoms of lactose intolerance vary based on the amount of lactose an individual can tolerate. Some individuals may be able to tolerate only very small amounts of lactose before they begin experiencing symptoms, whereas others may be able to consume larger amounts of lactose before experiencing symptoms. The symptoms of lactose intolerance can range from mild to severe and usually begin 30 minutes to 2 hours after consumption of foods containing lactose.

Common signs and symptoms of lactose intolerance include the following:

- Abdominal bloating and cramping
- Flatulence
- Diarrhea
- Borborygmi (gurgling or rumbling sounds in the abdomen)
- Nausea

Nutrition Therapy

Lactose intolerance is treated by limiting or avoiding foods containing lactose such as milk and milk products (Fig. 35.14). Consuming a food containing lactose with a meal, instead of by itself, may help prevent or reduce symptoms. Other forms of treatment include consuming lactose-free dairy products (Fig. 35.15) and substituting nut milk, oat milk, rice milk, soy milk, and soy cheese for milk and milk products. Cultured milk products such as yogurt contain bacteria that produce the enzyme for breaking down lactose. These products can usually be consumed by a lactose-intolerant individual without triggering symptoms. There are also over-the-counter lactase enzyme supplements available (e.g., Dairy Ease capsules, Lactaid Chewables) that assist in digesting lactose. These supplements must be taken before consuming foods that contain lactose. Although there is no cure for lactose intolerance, it is not a serious condition and can be treated effectively through careful dietary planning.

Consuming milk and milk products provides a convenient way to obtain enough calcium and vitamin D in the diet. Individuals who are lactose intolerant may need to ensure they are obtaining enough of these nutrients through careful menu planning. Nondairy foods that contain calcium include

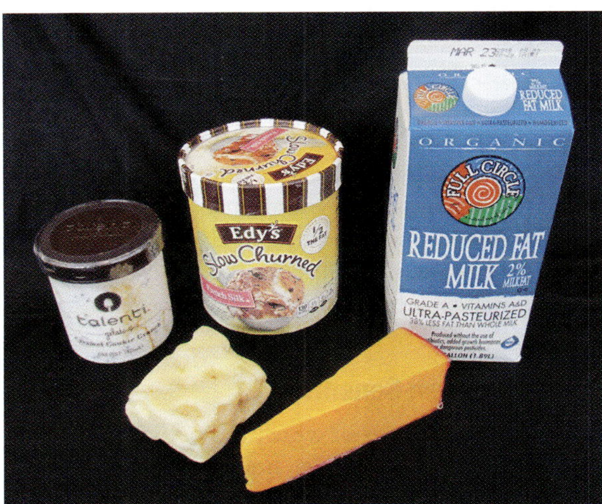

Fig. 35.14 Foods containing lactose.

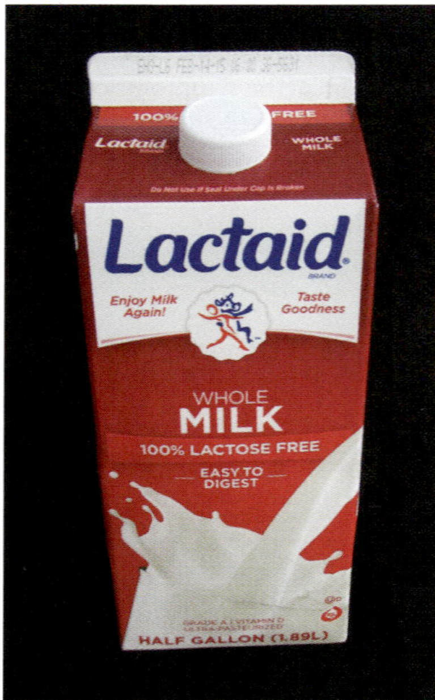

Fig. 35.15 Lactose-free milk.

canned fish containing bones (e.g., salmon, sardines), broccoli, spinach, legumes, and calcium-fortified breads and cereals. Nondairy foods that contain vitamin D include fish liver oil, liver, and fortified cereals. The body also manufactures vitamin D when it is exposed to the ultraviolet rays of the sun.

GLUTEN INTOLERANCE

Gluten intolerance is a condition in which an individual cannot tolerate the ingestion of a substance known as gluten. **Gluten** consists of a protein found in certain grains such as wheat, rye, barley, and triticale (a cross between wheat and rye). Gluten intolerance most commonly occurs with celiac disease and non-celiac gluten sensitivity (NCGS), which are discussed in more detail in the following sections.

Celiac Disease

Celiac disease is an autoimmune disorder of the digestive tract in which the immune system launches an attack against gluten. The ingestion of gluten irritates the small intestine, which causes damage to the villi. Villi are fingerlike extensions that line the small intestine and increase its surface area, providing for increased absorption of nutrients into the bloodstream. Damage to the villi results in a decreased surface area for absorption, which leads to malabsorption of nutrients.

Non-Celiac Gluten Sensitivity

NCGS is also a disorder in which the body cannot tolerate gluten. Unlike celiac disease, however, NCGS does not cause damage to the villi of the small intestine. Before a diagnosis of NCGS is made, the patient is first tested for celiac disease to rule out that condition. Research estimates that approximately 18 million individuals in the United States have NCGS, which is six times the number of individuals with celiac disease.

Symptoms of Gluten Intolerance

Celiac disease and NCGS share many of the same symptoms; however, the symptoms of NCGS are usually less severe. Symptoms of gluten intolerance tend to vary widely among patients and can include the following:

- Abdominal bloating
- Abdominal pain
- Weight loss
- Flatulence
- Diarrhea
- Constipation
- Foul-smelling stools
- Headache
- Fatigue
- Joint pain
- Brain fog
- Depression

Nutrition Therapy

The treatment for gluten intolerance is to follow a gluten-free diet, which excludes the consumption of all foods containing wheat, barley, rye, and triticale. Foods that frequently contain gluten include bread, cereal, crackers, pasta, salad dressing, baked goods, soups, sauces, and beer (Fig. 35.16A). Foods that are gluten free include beans, seeds, nuts, eggs, meat, poultry, fish, seafood, fruits, vegetables, and dairy products (Fig. 35.16B). Grains that are gluten free include buckwheat, cornmeal, flax, quinoa, rice, soy, and gluten-free oats. There are also many gluten-free food products available that can be used as alternatives to foods that contain gluten.

FOOD ALLERGIES

In the United States, food allergies affect approximately 33 million individuals; this includes 5.6 million children under the age of 18. Common food allergens include milk, eggs, wheat, fish and shellfish, peanuts, soybeans, and tree nuts (Fig. 35.17). Examples of tree nuts include cashews, pecans, walnuts, Brazil nuts, hazelnuts, almonds, and coconut. Food allergies may also be triggered by certain fruits and vegetables such as strawberries, tomatoes, and peppers.

It is important to recognize the signs and symptoms of food allergies so that proper treatment can be obtained. The symptoms of a food allergy commonly occur within 2 hours after ingestion of the food. The skin and the respiratory and GI systems are often affected. Common symptoms include skin rash, hives, and swelling. In addition, swelling and itching of the face, tongue, ears, eyelids, and lips may occur. Respiratory symptoms include wheezing, shortness of breath, or difficulty breathing. GI symptoms

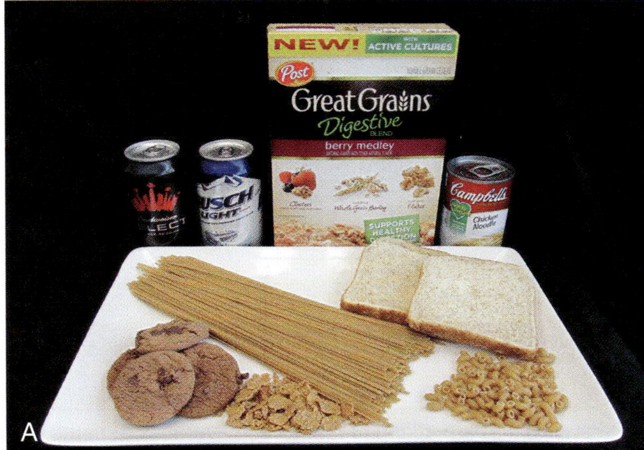

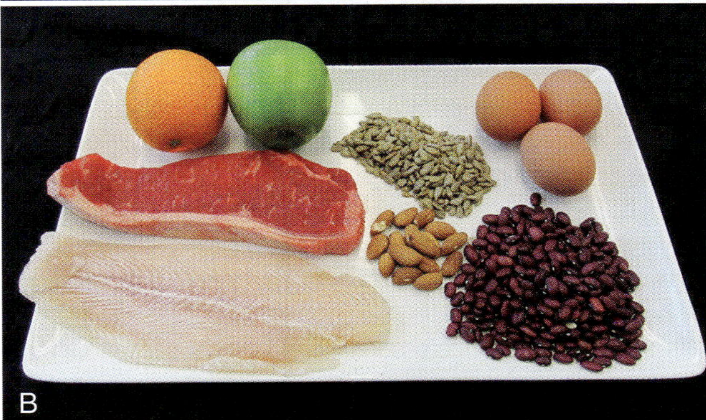

Fig. 35.16 (A) Foods containing gluten. (B) Gluten-free foods.

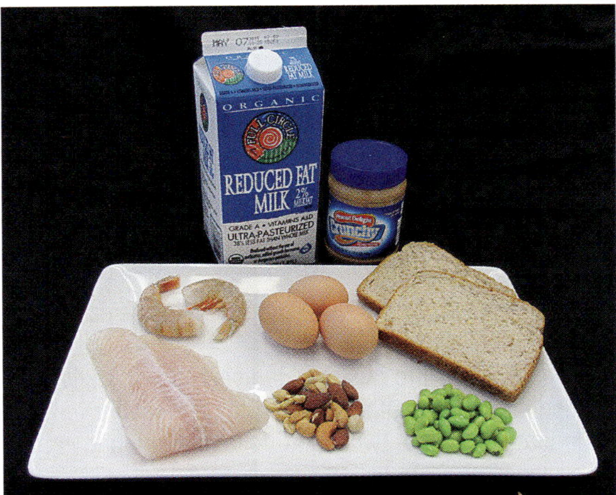

Fig. 35.17 Common food allergens.

may occur, such as abdominal cramping and pain, nausea, vomiting, or diarrhea.

Nutrition Therapy

Food allergies are most commonly treated with special diets. The response of the body to a food allergen can range from mild to moderate to severe. The specific treatment recommended depends, in large part, on the severity of the allergy.

Common Methods of Treatment for Food Allergies are as Follows

Elimination Diet

An elimination diet involves removing the offending food from the diet and is typically recommended when an individual is allergic to only one or two foods. Removing the offending food(s) from the diet is an easy way to prevent an allergic reaction. An elimination diet is also necessary when an individual has a very severe allergy to a food (e.g., peanuts) that might result in an anaphylactic reaction if the food were consumed. Food allergies are typically more severe earlier in life and tend to diminish in intensity as aging occurs. Reintroduction of that food allergen should be conducted only under a provider's guidance.

Rotation Diet

The allergic response to a food is often increased when a food is repeatedly consumed. A rotation diet (use of a rotation schedule) limits the number of times a food is ingested. This typically leads to a gradual desensitization to the food allergen, which lowers the allergic response to that food. A rotation diet is usually recommended for mild or moderate food allergies.

The most commonly used food rotation interval is 4 to 5 days. This means that the problem food (as well as foods belonging to the same food family) are consumed only every 4 to 5 days. A rotational schedule not only allows for the consumption of a known food allergen on a rotational basis, but may also minimize the development of a new food allergy.

Denaturation

Exposing a food to heat will denature or alter the chemical structure of the food allergen protein, so that the body no longer recognizes it as an invader. A child who is allergic to milk may be able to tolerate milk if it is heated in hot chocolate because of this denaturing process. An individual's tolerance to cooked or canned fruits and vegetables is typically much better than to fresh fruits and vegetables. Exposing the food allergen to acid has the same result. For example, adding tomato or lemon juice to food allergens may significantly reduce the allergic response.

Medication and Supplements

Medications that suppress the allergic response may be prescribed to treat the food allergy. Because such medications treat only the symptoms and not the cause of the allergy, the food allergy may actually become worse over time.

The oral intake of supplemental digestive enzymes can assist in treating food allergies. Digestive enzymes help break down the food into smaller, less allergenic molecules. This, in turn, decreases the allergenic response of the body. With continued intake, however, the individual may actually become allergic to the enzymes themselves.

Antacids that contain bicarbonate are used to treat food reactions. The pH of the blood becomes more acidic during an allergic reaction. Bicarbonate antacids cause the blood to become more alkaline, which works to neutralize the acid pH and helps to relieve the allergic symptoms.

There are several vitamins that assist in controlling food allergies; they include vitamin C and vitamin B_5 (pantothenic acid). Vitamin C exerts a stabilizing effect on mast cells, resulting in a reduction in the amount of histamine released by the body. Vitamin B_5 (pantothenic acid) functions in steroidal hormone production, which can lower the allergic response. Both of these vitamins are water soluble and therefore can be administered as a supplement without danger of toxicity or overdose.

TERMINOLOGY REVIEW

Key Term	Word Parts	Definition
Added sugars		Sugar and syrups that are added to foods and beverages at home or during the commercial preparation of food.
Antioxidant	*anti-:* against *ox/i:* oxygen	A molecule that inhibits the oxidation of other molecules.
Atherosclerosis	*ather/o:* yellowish, fatty plaque *-sclerosis:* hardening	Buildup of fibrous plaques of fatty deposits and cholesterol on the inner walls of an artery that causes narrowing, obstruction, and hardening of the artery.
Bariatrics	*bar/o:* weight *-iatrics:* a branch of medicine	The branch of medicine that deals with the treatment and control of obesity and diseases associated with obesity.
Cholesterol		A white, waxy, fatlike substance that is essential for normal functioning of the body.
Complete protein		A protein that contains all the essential amino acids needed by the body.
Dietary pattern		The combination of food and beverages that constitute an individual's complete dietary intake over time.
Disaccharide	*di-:* two *-saccharide:* containing sugar	A simple carbohydrate consisting of two sugar units.
Empty calorie food		A food that provides calories but few or no nutrients. Also known as a low–nutrient density food.
Essential amino acid		An amino acid that is required by the body but cannot be manufactured by the body and must be obtained from food.
Gluten		A type of protein found in certain grains such as wheat, rye, and barley.
Glycogen	*glyc/o-:* sugar *-gen:* substance or agent that produces or causes	The form in which glucose is stored in the body for later use.
Incomplete protein		A protein that lacks one or more of the essential amino acids needed by the body.
Kilocalorie	*kilo-:* thousand	The amount of heat needed to raise the temperature of 1 kilogram of water 1 degree Celsius. (Often referred to as a *calorie.*)
Lactose	*lact/o:* milk *-ose:* full of (sugar)	A disaccharide that consists of two sugar units that is found in milk and milk products.
Macronutrient	*macro-:* large *nutriti/o:* nourishing	A nutrient required in relatively large amounts by the body. Includes carbohydrates, fat, and protein.
Micronutrient	*micro-:* small *nutriti/o:* nourishing	A nutrient required in very small amounts by the body. Includes vitamins and minerals.
Mineral		A naturally occurring inorganic substance that is essential to the proper functioning of the body.
Monosaccharide	*mono-:* one	A simple carbohydrate consisting of one sugar unit.
Natural sugars		Sugars that occur naturally in foods and beverages.
Nonessential amino acid	*non-:* not	An amino acid required by the body that can be synthesized by the body in sufficient quantities to meet its needs.

TERMINOLOGY REVIEW —cont'd

Key Term	Word Parts	Definition
Nutrient	*nutriti/o:* nourishing	A chemical substance found in food that is needed by the body for survival and well-being.
Nutrition	*nutriti/o:* nourishing *-ion:* condition of	The study of nutrients in food including how the body uses them and their relationship to health.
Nutrition therapy	*nutriti/o:* nourishing *-ion:* condition of	The application of the science of nutrition to promote optimal heath and treat illness.
Obesity		A medical condition in which there is an excessive accumulation of body fat to the extent to which it may have an adverse effect on the health and well-being of an individual.
Percent daily value		The percentage of a nutrient provided by a single serving of a food item compared with how much is required for the entire day.
Polysaccharide	*poly-*: many	A complex carbohydrate made up of many sugar units strung together in a long chain.
Saturated fat	*satur-:* full, well-fed	A type of fat that is solid at room temperature and comes primarily from animal sources.
Triglycerides	*tri-:* three	The chemical form in which most fat exists in food, as well as in the body.
Unsaturated fat	*un-:* not *satur-:* full, well-fed	A type of fat that is liquid at room temperature and comes primarily from plant sources.
Vitamin	*vit/a:* life	An organic compound that is required in small amounts by the body for normal growth and development.

Emergency Preparedness and Protective Practices

Check out the Evolve site at http://evolve.elsevier.com/Bonewit/today to access additional interactive activities and exercises to help you study and prepare for success.

LEARNING OBJECTIVES

Disasters

1. State the effects a disaster or serious emergency can have on a health care facility.
2. Explain the difference between a natural disaster and a man-made disaster and list examples of each.

Psychological Effects of Emergencies

3. List the characteristics of a disaster that tend to cause the most serious psychological effects.
4. List and describe the three phases of the generalized adaptation syndrome.
5. List and describe the stages of anxiety and the intervention that should be employed for each.

Emergency Preparedness

6. State the purpose of an emergency action plan.
7. List and describe the six elements that must be included in an emergency action plan.
8. List and describe the three components of an emergency evacuation plan.
9. Identify the information that should be included on an evacuation floor plan.
10. State the duties that may be performed by evacuation wardens in the medical office.

Fire Safety and Prevention

11. List and describe the elements of a fire.
12. State the five elements that must be included in a fire prevention plan.
13. Identify methods of fire prevention for the medical office.
14. List and describe safety measures used for fire protection in the medical office.
15. List and describe the five classes of fire.
16. Identify the steps included in the RACE response.

Employee Training

17. Identify the education and training that must be provided to medical assistants related to medical office emergency situations.
18. State the purpose of emergency practice drills.
19. Describe the role of the medical assistant in disasters and serious emergencies.

PROCEDURES

Develop an emergency action plan for a natural or man-made disaster.

Demonstrate methods of fire prevention in the health care setting.

Demonstrate proper use of a fire extinguisher.

Participate in a mock exposure event, and document the steps taken.

CHAPTER OUTLINE

KEY TERMS

anxiety
disaster
emergency action plan
emergency preparedness
evacuation
evacuation procedures
exit route
fire extinguisher
fire prevention plan
fire protection
HAZMAT
man-made disaster
natural disaster
stress

INTRODUCTION TO DISASTER AND EMERGENCY PLANNING

Every health care facility faces the possibility that a disaster or serious emergency may occur, resulting in injuries, loss of life, property damage, and the inability to provide usual services. Medical offices must plan ahead to minimize the damage from any disaster or serious emergency and facilitate recovery so that services can be restored as efficiently as possible.

This chapter presents an overview of the various types of disasters and serious emergencies that may affect the medical office along with the psychological effects that emergency situations can have on an individual. Also presented in this chapter is a discussion of emergency preparedness and protective practice guidelines including the OSHA requirements for developing an emergency action plan and a fire prevention plan.

CATEGORIES OF DISASTERS

A **disaster** is defined as a sudden adverse event that can cause damage or loss of life. Disasters can be categorized as natural or man-made.

NATURAL DISASTERS

A **natural disaster** is a catastrophic event that is caused by nature or the natural processes of the earth (Fig. 36.1). Examples of natural disasters include floods, tornados, hurricanes, earthquakes, tsunamis, blizzards, volcanic eruptions, and epidemics. Natural disasters may cause injuries and loss of life as well as significant damage to the environment. Natural disasters may occur with or without warning. For example, a hurricane develops over a period of days, which allows for some preparation. On the other hand, an earthquake usually occurs without warning. The impact of a natural disaster may be random. For example, the exact strength and path of a hurricane are difficult to predict. This often requires numerous communities to prepare for this type of disaster in the event the hurricane hits their community.

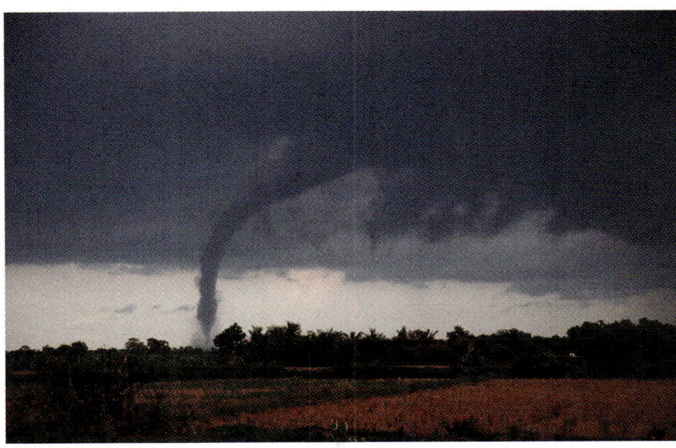

Fig. 36.1 A tornado is an example of a natural disaster.

MAN-MADE DISASTERS

A **man-made disaster** is an event that causes serious damage through intentional or negligent human actions or the failure of a man-made system (Fig. 36.2). Examples of man-made disasters include fire, power outages, bomb explosions, terrorism, structural collapse, radiation accidents, chemical spills, and bioterrorism.

The amount of threat or damage from man-made disasters can vary considerably. For example, a fire in a wastebasket is

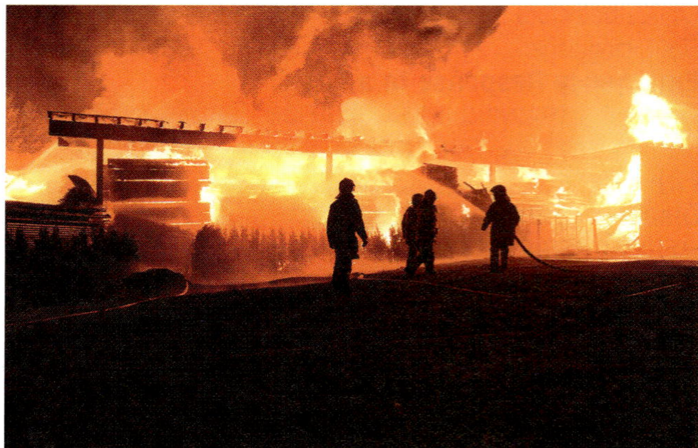

Fig. 36.2 A fire is an example of a man-made disaster.

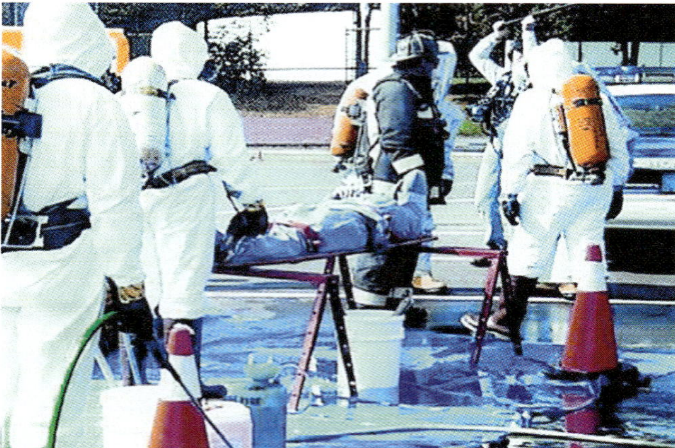

Fig. 36.3 Teams responding to disasters involving a hazardous material (HAZMAT) must wear protective clothing and initiate decontamination of casualties.

usually quickly contained. On the other hand, a hazardous chemical spill may involve an entire city or area. The type of emergency personnel who respond to a man-made disaster depends on the nature of the disaster. Municipal fire departments and police departments provide rapid assistance for fires, injury, structural collapse, and criminal activity. The National Response Center of the Environmental Protection Agency (EPA) responds to the release, or potential release, of oil, radioactive materials, or hazardous chemicals into the air, land, or water (Fig. 36.3).

PSYCHOLOGICAL EFFECTS OF EMERGENCIES

Whenever an emergency situation occurs that causes serious damage or interruption of the normal daily routine, individuals react positively and negatively to the loss of property or disruption of service. Positive reactions involve the triggering of resources, both internal and external, to meet the challenges. For example, when a serious flood threatens an area, individuals usually mobilize quickly to fill and place sandbags to minimize the anticipated damage. When physical and emotional resources are depleted, however, individuals react negatively. Disasters that tend to cause the most serious psychological effects include those with the following characteristics:

- Occur without warning
- Pose a serious threat to personal safety or have unknown health effects
- Have an uncertain duration (such as serious floods of major rivers)
- Result from malicious intent or human error
- Have symbolic significance (such as the 9/11 attacks)

THE STRESS RESPONSE

Stress is the body's response to threat or change. When a disaster or serious emergency occurs, individuals who are affected by it frequently experience stress. Hans Selye was an Austrian physician who practiced medicine in the middle of the 20th century. Selye described the body's reaction to stress as a three-part general adaptation syndrome (GAS), which is illustrated in Fig. 36.4. The three stages of the GAS include the alarm phase, the resistance phase, and the recovery or exhaustion phase.

Alarm Phase

This phase is often called the *fight-or-flight response.* In this phase, the body senses a stressor and begins to react to combat it. Epinephrine is released from the adrenal medulla, which stimulates the sympathetic nervous system, triggering the following changes in the body: dilation of the pupils, increase in heart rate, increase in respirations and perspiration, and increase in the blood pressure. These changes prepare the body to fight or to run away. In addition, the muscles tense in preparation for action, and the attention becomes narrowly focused on the perceived threat or significant task. This phase does not last very long; in some instances it may only last a matter of seconds. Some people experience the alarm phase as energizing, whereas others quickly become extremely anxious.

Example: If a serious fire erupts in a medical office, employees typically experience the alarm phase. The fight-or-flight response helps employees to remain focused and allows them to quickly and effectively evacuate themselves and others from the burning building and perform other types of rescue duties.

Resistance Phase

The resistance phase begins almost immediately after the alarm phase. In this phase, the stress remains but the body adapts in an effort to cope with the stressor. The resistance phase may last hours, days, or even months depending on the circumstances. During this phase, the adrenal cortex secretes cortisol. Cortisol increases the blood glucose level to sustain energy because more energy is required to maintain the stage of resistance than the normal state. The body

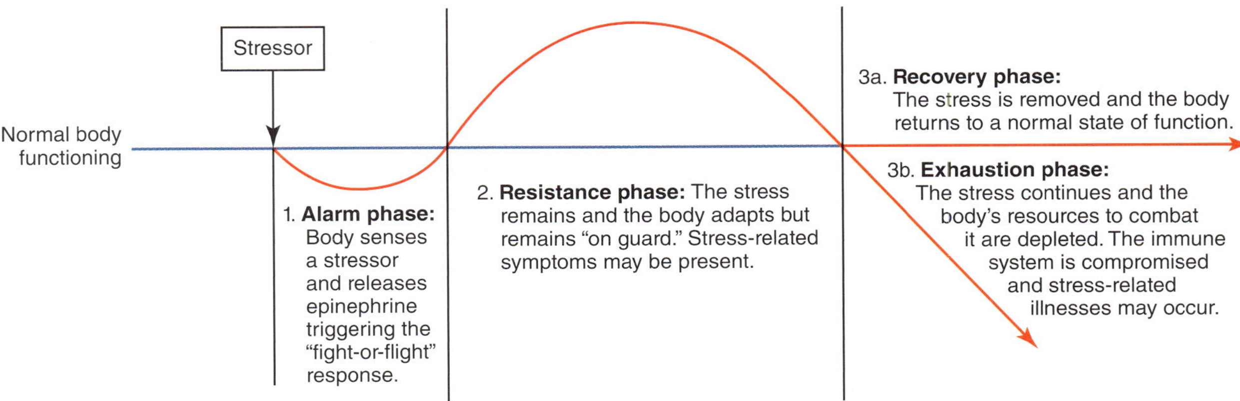

Fig. 36.4 The general adaptation syndrome (GAS) developed by Hans Selye.

constantly remains "on guard" and is not in a state of balance (homeostasis) but is able to carry on its normal functions. Individuals may experience a number of stress-related symptoms during this phase such as fatigue, irritability, lethargy, and lapses in concentration.

Example: If a medical office employee temporarily becomes trapped by the fire (described in the earlier example), he or she may be unable to cope with the stress of that experience. In this case, the employee enters the resistance phase and constantly feels on guard but is still able to function normally. If the resistance phase lasts for a period of time, the employee may begin experiencing stress-related symptoms.

Recovery or Exhaustion Phase

If the stress is removed, the body enters the recovery phase. However, if the stress continues, the body's ability to resist stress is lost and the individual enters the exhaustion phase.

a. *Recovery phase*: In the recovery phase, the stress has been removed and the parasympathetic nervous system begins to regain control. Eventually the body returns to its normal level of function (homeostasis).
b. *Exhaustion phase*: If stress is chronic and excessive, the body's resources to combat it become depleted. Eventually the immune system is compromised, and the individual becomes more susceptible to a variety of illnesses ranging all the way from colds and flu to cancer.

Example: If the employee learns to cope with the stress of being trapped in the fire, the body enters the recovery phase and returns to a normal level of functioning. If the employee is unable to cope, the stress becomes chronic and the employee will enter the exhaustion phase and begin to experience stress-related illnesses (Fig. 36.5).

MANAGING ANXIETY

Anxiety is defined as a feeling of worry or uneasiness, often triggered by an event that is perceived as having an uncertain outcome. There are four levels of anxiety that range in

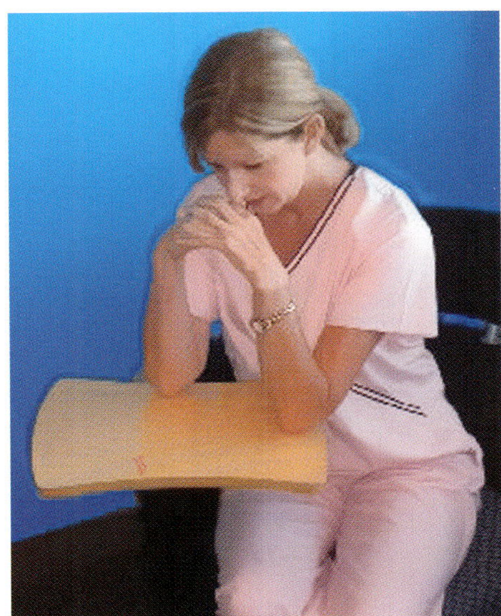

Fig. 36.5 In the exhaustion phase, the body's resources to combat stress become depleted.

degree from fleeting worried thoughts to a full-blown panic attack. The four levels of anxiety are outlined Fig. 36.6.

An individual's level of anxiety has a direct influence on their ability to function effectively in an emergency situation. For example, a medical assistant with moderate anxiety is not able to notice details and think as clearly in an emergency situation. However, emergency procedures that have been thoroughly learned through practice drills help the medical assistant decide what to do without having to think through all the possibilities. In addition, practice drills tend to keep the anxiety level from rising because the medical assistant feels more confident when there is a structured plan to respond to in an emergency situation.

Severe anxiety can be problematic in an emergency situation because it tends to immobilize an individual and stimulate anxiety in others. Symptoms of severe anxiety include the following: hyperventilation, rapid pulse rate, excessive

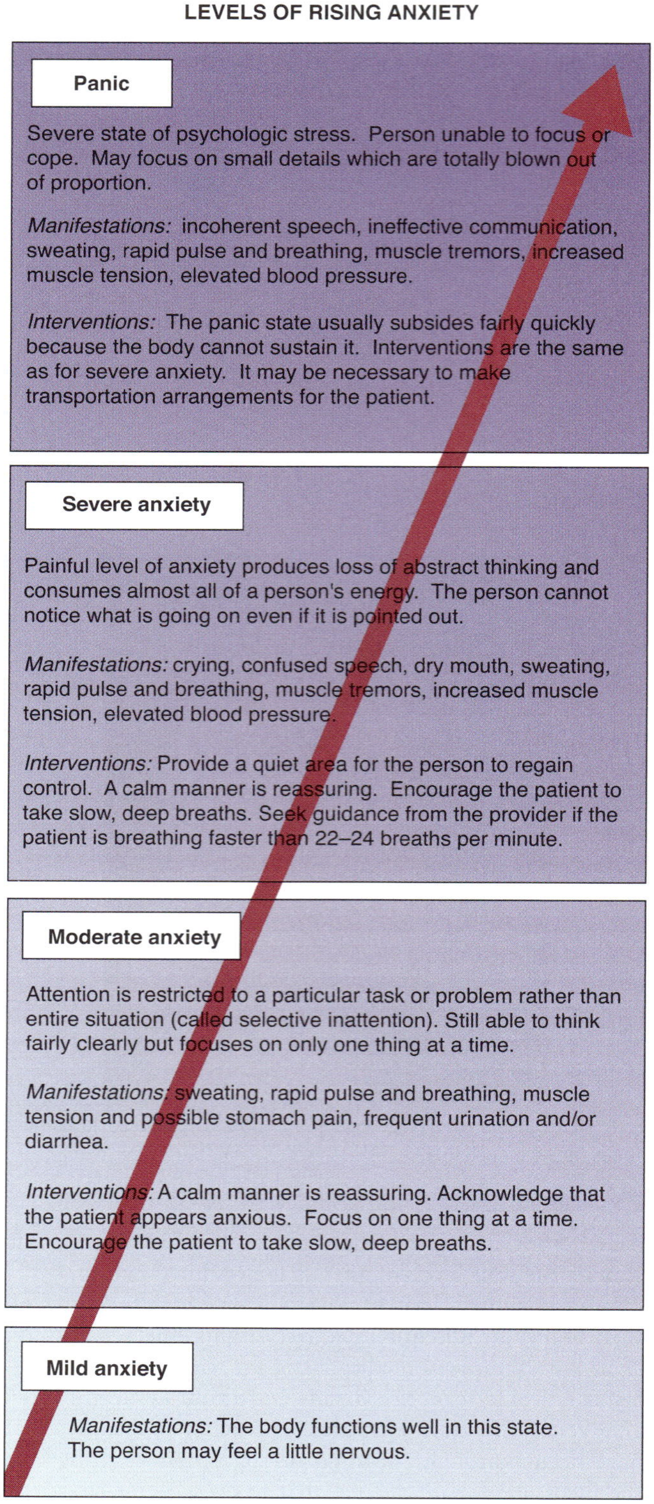

LEVELS OF RISING ANXIETY

Panic

Severe state of psychologic stress. Person unable to focus or cope. May focus on small details which are totally blown out of proportion.

Manifestations: incoherent speech, ineffective communication, sweating, rapid pulse and breathing, muscle tremors, increased muscle tension, elevated blood pressure.

Interventions: The panic state usually subsides fairly quickly because the body cannot sustain it. Interventions are the same as for severe anxiety. It may be necessary to make transportation arrangements for the patient.

Severe anxiety

Painful level of anxiety produces loss of abstract thinking and consumes almost all of a person's energy. The person cannot notice what is going on even if it is pointed out.

Manifestations: crying, confused speech, dry mouth, sweating, rapid pulse and breathing, muscle tremors, increased muscle tension, elevated blood pressure.

Interventions: Provide a quiet area for the person to regain control. A calm manner is reassuring. Encourage the patient to take slow, deep breaths. Seek guidance from the provider if the patient is breathing faster than 22–24 breaths per minute.

Moderate anxiety

Attention is restricted to a particular task or problem rather than entire situation (called selective inattention). Still able to think fairly clearly but focuses on only one thing at a time.

Manifestations: sweating, rapid pulse and breathing, muscle tension and possible stomach pain, frequent urination and/or diarrhea.

Interventions: A calm manner is reassuring. Acknowledge that the patient appears anxious. Focus on one thing at a time. Encourage the patient to take slow, deep breaths.

Mild anxiety

Manifestations: The body functions well in this state. The person may feel a little nervous.

Fig. 36.6 Levels of anxiety.

perspiration, and confused speech. In an emergency situation, a patient with severe anxiety may lose control their emotions and cry or scream. This behavior can be minimized by the medical assistant giving the patient directions in a calm and reassuring voice. It may first be necessary to touch the patient to gain their attention, and then directions should be given in short sentences, speaking a little more slowly than usual. Helping the patient to breathe deeply helps to reduce anxiety, but it is also important to direct the person exactly where to go if a dangerous area must be evacuated.

If an emergency occurs in the workplace, the medical assistant should immediately focus on responding to the situation, implementing established procedures, and helping others. Deep breaths will help to control anxiety, which should be seen as a normal response. Even in disasters that have caused enormous amounts of damage, lives have been saved and injury has been minimized when people have been able to stay reasonably calm and follow established emergency procedures.

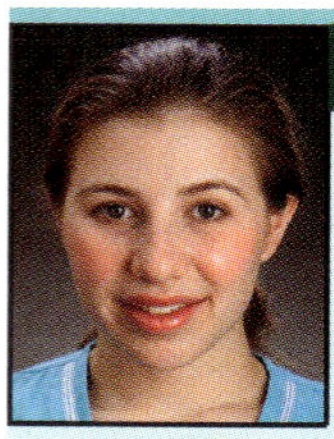

Putting It All Into Practice

My name is Beth Ann, and I am a Certified Medical Assistant. I have been assisting the office manager in updating the equipment and supplies in our office that might be used in case of a disaster such as a fire or tornado. We recently purchased an additional fire extinguisher for the staff break room, where we have a microwave and coffee maker. In addition, we have purchased an office disaster kit which has emergency supplies for 10 people for a few days, including food, water, flashlights, a radio, batteries, a first aid kit, and other supplies that would be useful in a disaster. Of course, we hope that we will never have to use these things. I was also one of the staff members from our office who participated recently as a "victim" in a mock disaster drill that was held for emergency personnel in our town. I played the role of a victim with a fracture of both my arm and my leg. I had never been in a situation where there were many people injured or been transported in an ambulance. The experience increased my understanding of the problems that emergency personnel face, and now I have a more personal understanding of how important it is to be prepared with training and equipment. ■

What Would You Do? What Would You *Not* Do?

Case Study 1

Julie Manning, who is sitting in the waiting room, receives a phone call, speaks on the telephone for a few minutes, and rushes to the front desk window. She tells Beth Ann that she has to leave immediately because she has just learned that there is a fire at her son's school. Mrs. Manning speaks very quickly, but her story seems disconnected. It is also clear that she is breathing very rapidly and is perspiring excessively. ■

EMERGENCY PREPAREDNESS IN THE MEDICAL OFFICE

Large clinics and small medical offices alike may experience emergencies such as fires, floods, earthquakes, power outages, workplace violence, and a variety of other emergency situations. **Emergency preparedness** is the process of making plans to prevent, respond, and recover from an emergency situation. To protect employees from fire and other emergencies and to prevent property loss, medical offices must develop emergency preparedness plans. Emergency preparedness plans, as stipulated by OSHA, must include an emergency action plan (EAP) and a fire prevention plan. These plans are discussed in more detail on the following pages.

EMERGENCY ACTION PLAN

An **emergency action plan** (EAP) is a written document that describes the actions that employees should take to ensure their safety if a fire or other emergency situation occurs. The purpose of an EAP is to prepare employees for potential emergency situations to prevent fatalities, injuries, and property damage. Almost all medical offices are required by OSHA to develop an EAP. The EAP must be in writing, be kept in the workplace, and be available for employee review.

Before development of the EAP, an assessment must be performed by the medical office to determine the potential emergencies that could affect the office. Some emergencies may occur within the medical office; examples include a fire, workplace violence, or a medical emergency (e.g., patient having a heart attack). Other emergencies may arise from situations occurring outside of the facility; examples include a flood, tornado, and earthquake. The EAP should outline the actions that should be taken for each of the potential emergency situations identified by the office.

Components of an Emergency Action Plan

There are six elements (as required by OSHA) that must be included in an EAP; these are listed and described in the following paragraphs.

The six elements required in an EAP are as follows.

1. *The preferred means of reporting fires and other emergencies*
   In the event of an emergency situation, it is important to report the situation and alert employees immediately. Emergency situations, such as fires, can reach dangerous levels very quickly, and a delay in summoning emergency responders and alerting employees may result in the loss of life and property. One or more of the following methods are typically used to report an emergency and/or alert employees to the presence of an emergency situation:
   a. *Dialing 911:* This is a common and preferred method for reporting emergencies.
   b. *Dialing an internal emergency phone numbers:* If internal ("in-house") numbers are used for reporting emergencies, they should be posted on or near each phone. Internal emergency numbers are sometimes connected to an intercom system so that coded announcements may be made throughout the facility. For example, a facility may indicate a patient is having a heart attack by an announcement of "Code Blue" or that there is a fire in the facility by an announcement of "Code Red."
   c. *Activation of a manual alarm system:* OSHA requires that employers provide an early warning system so that employees can safely escape the workplace. The most common means to alert employees (and other building occupants) are audible and visual alarms. In offices with 10 or fewer employees, it is acceptable to use direct voice communication for alerting employees, provided that all employees can hear the voice alarm. OSHA requires that the alarm be distinctive and recognized by all employees as a signal to evacuate the workplace or to begin implementing emergency actions.
2. *Emergency evacuation plan*
   An **evacuation** is a planned systematic retreat of people to safety in an emergency situation. According to OSHA, the emergency evacuation plan for the medical office must include the following three components:
   a. *Emergency evacuation procedures:* **Evacuation procedures** consist of clear step-by-step procedures for the rapid, efficient, and safe removal of individuals from a building during an emergency. It is recommended that an *emergency evacuation coordinator* be assigned to take charge of and manage the evacuation procedures during an emergency. In high-rise buildings, the office evacuation procedures should coordinate with the building evacuation procedures. Evacuation procedures should include the following:
      - The conditions that would require evacuation of the area
      - The chain of command showing who can authorize an evacuation
      - The actions employees should take during the evacuation (e.g., shutting windows, turning off equipment, closing doors)
      - Procedures for evacuating individuals with disabilities or who do not speak English
   b. *Type of evacuation:* The type of evacuation ordered during an emergency depends on the type of emergency situation. For example, the immediate and complete evacuation of a building to a safe area is typically required in the event of a large fire On the other hand, a small fire in a wastebasket may require only a partial evacuation of employees from the immediate area. In some instances, the evacuation of occupants from the building may not be the best response. In the event of a tornado, for example, employees are typically required to evacuate to a safe part of the building such as a designated shelter area (known as a *shelter-in-place* evacuation). The EAP should specify the type of evacuation recommended for each type of emergency identified in the plan.
   c. *Exit routes:* An **exit route** is a continuous and unobstructed path of travel from any point within a

workplace to a place of safety. OSHA requires that specific guidelines be followed with respect to exit routes. Some of these guidelines (that most affect the medical office) are as follows:

- Exits should be clearly marked and well lit.
- Exit routes must be at least 28 inches wide at all points.
- Exit routes should be unobstructed and free of clutter at all times.
- Exit signs should be posted indicating the nearest emergency exit.
- Exit doors must be free of decorations or signs that obscure visibility of the exit route door.
- Doors that cannot be used to leave the facility should be clearly labeled "Not an Exit" or identified by a sign indicating the door's actual use (e.g., "Storeroom").
- An exit door must be unlocked from the inside.
- An exit door must open outward.

d. *Evacuation floor plan:* Exit routes should be clearly identified and marked on an evacuation floor plan (Fig. 36.7). It is recommended (if possible) that both a primary and a secondary exit route be identified on the floor plan. A *primary exit route* is the quickest and easiest way to exit a building during an evacuation and is usually represented on the floor plan by a continuous solid

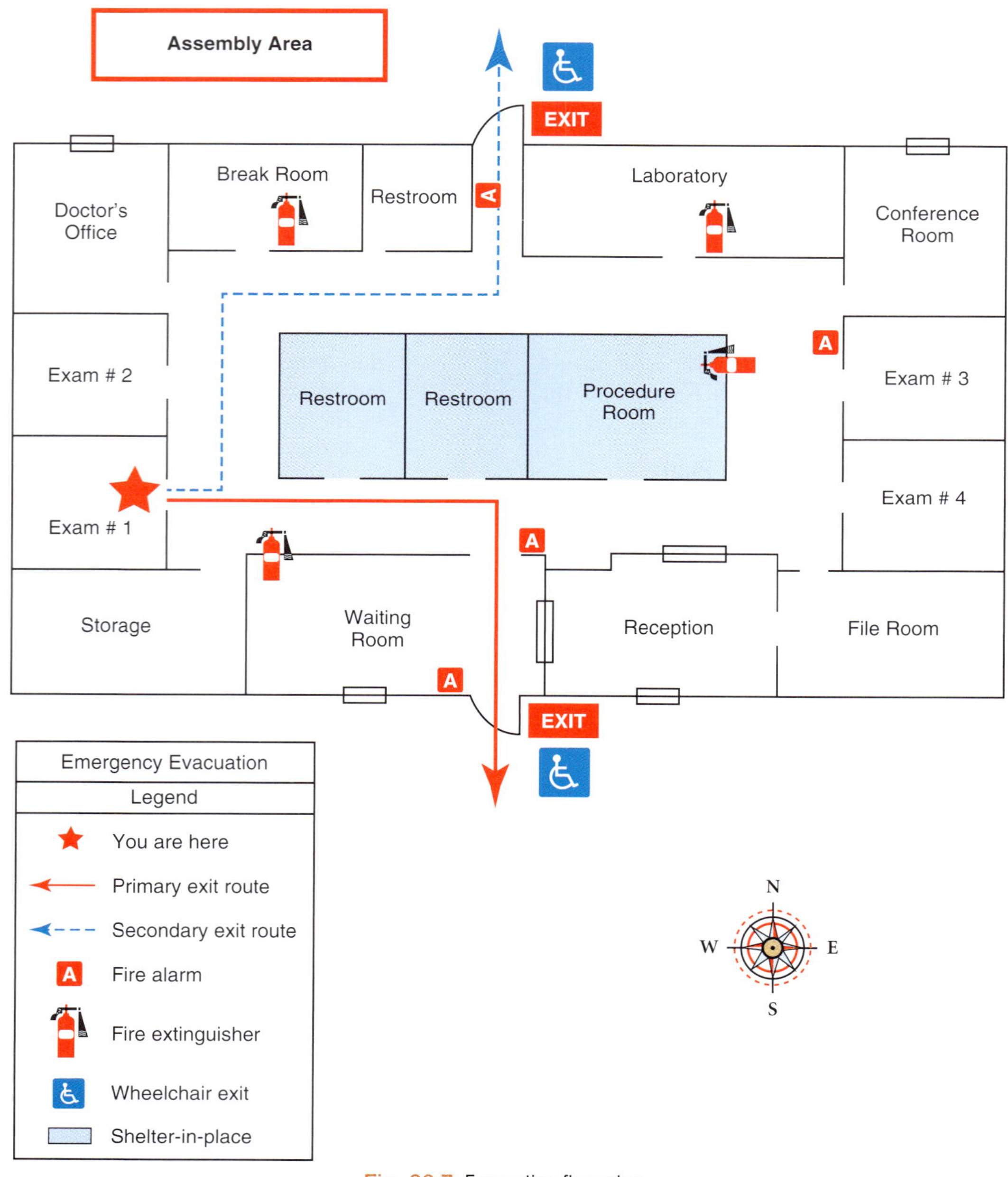

Fig. 36.7 Evacuation floor plan.

red line with a directional arrow. A *secondary exit route* provides a secondary means of escape in the event the primary route becomes blocked by smoke or fire. It is often represented by a continuous dashed blue line with a directional arrow on the evacuation floor plan.

The floor plan of a multiple-story building should show the locations of stairways and elevators and must indicate that the stairs (not the elevators) should be used as a means of exit in an emergency. Evacuation floor plans should be posted in multiple locations throughout the medical office including each examining room, the waiting room, rest rooms, the break room, and offices.

An evacuation floor plan should include the location of the following:

- Occupant's current location
- Primary and secondary exit routes
- Manual fire alarm boxes
- Portable fire extinguishers
- Emergency exit doors
- Wheelchair accessible exits
- Shelter-in-place areas
- Assembly areas

3. *Procedures for employees who remain behind to perform critical operations before evacuation*

   If necessary, some employees may be designated to stay behind briefly to operate fire extinguishers or shut down electrical equipment or special equipment that could be damaged if left operating or create additional hazards to emergency responders. The EAP should identify each of these employees and describe in detail the procedure that each is to perform. Any employee remaining behind must be capable of recognizing when to abandon the operation or task and evacuate to a safe area.

4. *Procedures to account for all employees after an evacuation*

   The EAP should identify an assembly area for employees to meet after an evacuation. The assembly area should be a safe distance from the building and have enough space to accommodate all of the employees. Assembly areas typically include parking lots and other open areas away from busy streets.

   The EAP should include a mechanism for accounting for all employees after an evacuation. The purpose of accounting for building occupants following an evacuation is to help determine if someone is still in the building in need of rescue. This can be accomplished by taking a head count or through the use of an employee roster checklist. A mechanism also needs to be established for accounting for non-employees such as patients and visitors (e.g., pharmaceutical company representatives). Most offices designate the patient log-in sheet as a means of accounting for patients in the event of an evacuation. The name and last known location of any individual not accounted for need to be relayed to an emergency official. It is important that the building occupants be instructed not to leave the assembly area until everyone has been accounted for and dismissed.

5. *Procedures for employees performing rescue or medical duties*

   During an emergency situation, various rescue or medical duties may need to be performed by employees. These employees are often referred to as *evacuation wardens.* The type of duties vary depend on the emergency situation. The EAP should specify these duties, including the type of duty to be performed and the name of the employee who is to perform it. Employee evacuation wardens must be thoroughly trained in the duties they are to perform. Duties that need to be performed by evacuation wardens during a fire are discussed later in this chapter.

6. *The names or job titles of individuals who can be contacted for further information or explanation of duties under the plan*

   At times, an employee may need additional information or further clarification of the duties to be performed that are included in the plan. The EAP should list the names or job titles of the individuals, both within and outside of the facility, who can be contacted to provide this information.

FIRE SAFETY IN THE MEDICAL OFFICE

Fire is the most common type of emergency situation that occurs in the workplace. Each year there are approximately 70,000 to 80,000 serious workplace fires in the United States that result in the deaths of more than 200 workers and injure 5000 more workers. It has been shown that approximately 85% of workplace fires are the result of human behavior, whereas only 15% are caused by catastrophic failure of equipment. Overall, fire is third leading cause of accidental death in the United States. In addition to the human cost, a fire can also cause structural damage to the medical facility as well as the loss of valuable documents and information.

There are numerous ways for fires to start in the medical office. Examples include overloaded electrical outlets; heat-producing equipment that is too close to combustible materials; improper use of appliances (e.g., coffee makers, microwave ovens, stoves); improper handling and storage of chemicals, cleaning supplies, and other combustible materials; and arson. If the medical office processes its own laundry, poorly maintained washers and dryers can also cause fires, especially if the dryer is vented improperly or if the lint trap is not kept clean.

ELEMENTS OF A FIRE

A fire is a chemical reaction that involves the rapid burning of a fuel. A fire needs three elements to occur: a fuel source, an ignition source (heat), and oxygen. Once a fire has started, it will grow hotter and it will not stop until at least one of these three elements has been removed.

FUEL SOURCE

A fuel source consists of any flammable or combustible material. A *flammable* material catches on fire easily (e.g., propane, gasoline), whereas a *combustible* material is any material that will burn (e.g., paper, wood). All flammable materials are combustible, but not all combustible materials are flammable. A tiny spark may cause a flammable material to ignite but would not cause a combustible material to ignite. Many items can provide fuel for a fire, such as paper, cardboard, wood, plastic, fabric, and flammable liquids. Common examples of fuel sources found in the medical office include the following:

- Patient medical records
- Furniture
- Drapes and rugs
- Office equipment
- Chemicals used for sterilization and disinfection
- Laboratory testing chemicals
- Trash

IGNITION SOURCE (HEAT)

An ignition source provides the energy necessary to increase the temperature of the fuel source to a point at which it ignites. Once the fuel source has ignited, it produces heat. As long as enough fuel and oxygen are present, the heat generated by the fuel source will continue the combustion process. Examples of common ignition sources include the following:

- Open flames (e.g., burning candle)
- Faulty electrical equipment
- Hot surfaces (e.g., examination light)
- Sparks (e.g., burning cigarette)

OXYGEN

The air around us has about a 21% oxygen content, and most fires only require an atmosphere of 16% oxygen to burn. Many medical offices store oxygen in their facilities to administer to patients if necessary. This stored oxygen is a safe gas as long as it is stored and used properly. Oxygen stored in the medical office is not flammable, nor will it explode; however, it greatly increases the combustion rate of a fire. If something catches fire, oxygen will make the flame hotter and cause it to burn faster and more vigorously. The result is that a fire involving oxygen can appear explosive-like.

FIRE PREVENTION PLAN

A **fire prevention plan** is a written document that identifies flammable and combustible materials stored in the workplace and ways to control workplace fire hazards. A fire prevention plan reduces the probability that a workplace fire will ignite or spread, which helps prevent injury or death, keeps the workplace safe, and helps to prevent financial losses to the medical office. Almost all medical offices are required by OSHA to develop a fire prevention plan. The fire prevention plan must be in writing, be kept in the workplace, and be available for employee review.

COMPONENTS OF A FIRE PREVENTION PLAN

Five elements (as required by OSHA) must be included in a fire prevention plan; these are as follows:

1. A list of all major fire hazards including:
   a. Proper handling and storage of fire hazards
   b. Potential ignition sources and controls
   c. Type of fire protection equipment necessary to control each fire hazard
2. Procedures to control accumulation of flammable and combustible waste materials
3. Procedures for regular maintenance of safeguards installed on heat-producing equipment to prevent accidental ignition of combustible materials
4. Name or job title of employees responsible for maintaining equipment to prevent or control ignition sources or fires
5. Name or job title of employees responsible for the control of fuel source hazards

Methods of fire prevention for the medical office (which incorporate many of the elements listed above) are presented in Box 36.1.

FIRE PROTECTION IN THE MEDICAL OFFICE

Fire protection involves the implementation of safety measures to reduce the unwanted effects of fire. The purpose of fire protection is to prevent the spread of fire from one area of a building to another, allow for the safe exit of building occupants, and prevent or reduce the amount of property damage. Fire protection for an office building is specified by fire code requirements and is the responsibility of the owner of the building; however, fire protection for the contents of the office is the responsibility of office staff. Some of the important safety measures employed in fire protection are listed and described in the following paragraphs.

Sprinkler Systems

Sprinkler systems are one of the best measures available to extinguish a fire in its early stages. Sprinkler systems are usually located at ceiling level and use water to put out or slow the progress of a fire. Sprinklers are activated by the build-up of heat in the fire area, which causes a glass component in the sprinkler head to melt or break, releasing water from the sprinkler. Only those sprinklers closest to the fire area are activated, which reduces water damage to the contents of the building. For example, just one or two activated sprinklers may be able to quickly extinguish a fire that has just started in an office laboratory. Most sprinkler

BOX 36.1 Methods of Fire Prevention in the Medical Office

Flammable and Combustible Materials

1. Keep the medical office free of clutter.
2. Keep flammable and combustible materials away from ignition sources.
3. Read the label and safety data sheet (SDS) accompanying medical office supplies (e.g., laboratory testing kits, hazardous chemicals, printer toner cartridges) to determine how to properly handle, store, and use these items.
4. Do not allow trash to accumulate.
5. Store trash awaiting removal in a safe location away from heat-producing equipment.
6. Safely dispose of flammable and combustible waste.
7. Clean up any spill of flammable liquids immediately.
8. Do not allow the use of open flames (e.g., burning candles) in the medical office.
9. Ensure that smoking bans are enforced in the workplace.
10. Designate an area outside the building for smoking, with fire-resistant containers.

Electrical Equipment and Appliances

1. Make sure equipment and appliances are properly plugged into wall outlets.
2. Use only grounded appliances plugged into grounded outlets (three-prong plug).
3. Do not overload electrical outlets.
4. Promptly disconnect and replace cracked, frayed, or broken electrical cords.
5. Keep heat-producing equipment (e.g., coffee makers, copy machines) away from flammable or combustible materials.
6. Turn off all heat-producing equipment (e.g., examination lights, autoclave) and appliances (e.g., coffee makers) at the end of each work day.
7. Shut down electrical equipment that malfunctions or gives off a strange odor.
8. Avoid the use of extension cords.
9. Avoid the use of space heaters.

Inspection and Maintenance

1. Store oxygen in a clean, dry, well ventilated room.
2. Keep compressed oxygen cylinders and liquid oxygen tanks upright at all times.
3. Ensure that fire alarms and fire extinguishers are clearly visible and not blocked by equipment, decorations, coats, or other objects.
4. Ensure that fire extinguishers are properly stored in their designated locations.
5. Ensure that authorized personnel perform yearly inspections and maintenance of medical equipment (e.g., autoclave, electrocardiograph).
6. Test smoke detectors every month and replace batteries every 6 months.
7. Have authorized personnel perform regular inspections, maintenance, and testing of fire alarms, sprinkler systems, and fire extinguishers.
8. Report fire hazards you cannot correct yourself.

systems include an alarm system that alerts both building occupants and emergency responders when sprinkler activation occurs.

Many states require sprinkler systems in commercial and office buildings. Some states that require sprinklers for larger office buildings do not require them for smaller offices (e.g., provider's office that has been converted from a house).

Fire Doors

A fire door is a fire-resistant door that is designed to prevent the spread of fire from one area of a building to another (Fig. 36.8). Fire doors assist in the safe escape of occupants from a building during a fire and help to reduce property damage. In a large office or freestanding clinic, fire doors are typically located at certain points in the corridors. Fire doors should never be propped open; instead they should be allowed to shut to their naturally closed position.

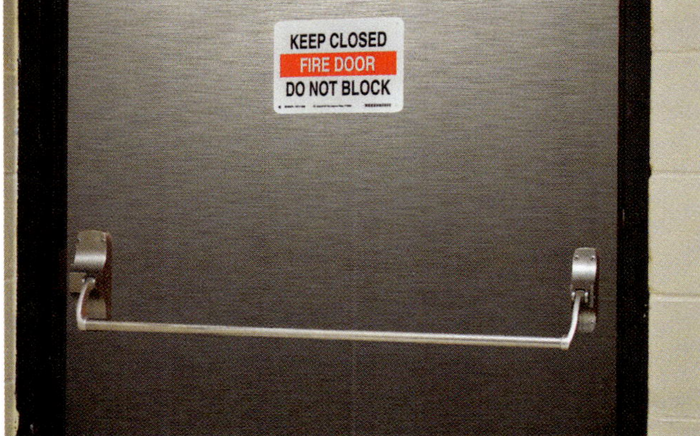

Fig. 36.8 A fire door prevents the spread of fire from one area of a building to another.

Fire-Resistant Cabinets

Whenever possible, records should be stored in fire-resistant file cabinets. If the office uses a physical system to back up computer files (instead of a network or an internet system), the backup drives should be stored in a fire-resistant file cabinet or fire-resistant box-type safe. It is always preferable to store a backup copy on the internet or at another location.

Fire Alarms

A fire alarm is a device that warns building occupants of the presence of a fire (Fig. 36.9). Once a fire alarm has been

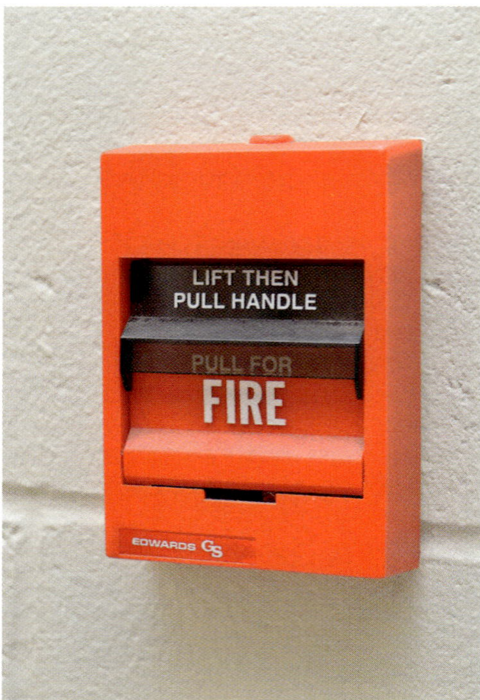

Fig. 36.9 Fire alarm pull stations are commonly found in the corridors of an office building.

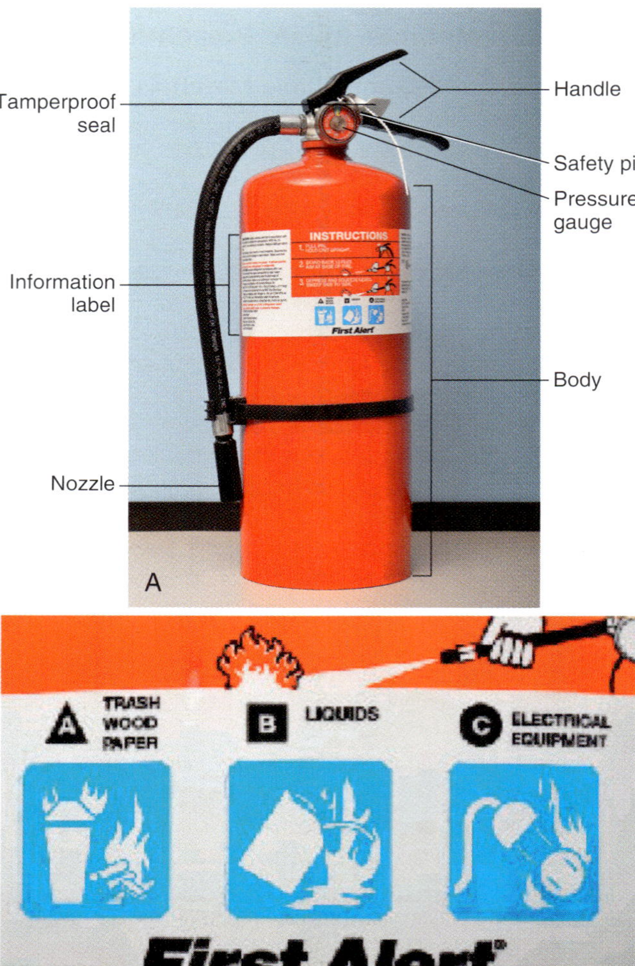

Fig. 36.10 (A) Fire extinguisher with parts labeled. (B) A multipurpose fire extinguisher is labeled with three pictograms indicating the A, B, and C fire classifications it is designed to extinguish.

activated, a loud noise and flashing lights are broadcasted to alert building occupants of the fire and to provide them with enough time to safely evacuate the building. The alarm also notifies the fire department so that firefighters can quickly respond to the fire. Fire alarm pull stations are frequently located in the corridors of buildings. It is important for employees to be trained in the proper activation of a fire alarm and what conditions necessitate activating the alarm.

Smoke Detectors

A smoke detector is a device that detects and automatically provides a warning of the presence of smoke. Smoke detector laws vary by state in terms of how many must be in an office and where they must be located. In many buildings, smoke detectors are wired into the building's security and fire alarm system. If the office has battery-operated smoke detectors, these should be tested monthly by pressing the test button. Batteries should be changed every 6 months, and the date should be noted on the detector.

Fire Extinguisher

A **fire extinguisher** is a portable device that discharges an agent designed to extinguish a fire (Fig. 36.10A. Common examples of extinguishing agents include dry chemicals, foam, carbon dioxide, and water. Portable fire extinguishers are considered a first line of defense in the early stages of a fire and have two primary functions: to control or extinguish a small fire that has just started and to protect an evacuation route that a fire may block with smoke or burning materials. A fire extinguisher should never be used to fight a large fire that is out of control; instead, the building occupants should evacuate the premises immediately and call the fire department.

Fires are classified into five categories according to the type of fuel that is burning. For example, a class A fire involves the burning of ordinary combustible materials. Fire extinguishers are marked with a label indicating the type of fire classification they are designed to handle. Newer types of fire extinguishers are labeled with a pictogram illustrating the type of fuel that can be extinguished by that particular extinguisher. Older types of extinguishers are labeled with colored geometric shapes with letter designations. Table 36.1 lists and describes the five fire classifications along with the type of extinguisher (by label) that can be used to extinguish each class of fire. Most fire extinguishers are designed to handle more than one fire classification. For example, a multipurpose fire extinguisher is labeled with three pictograms (Fig. 36.10B) and is designed to extinguish class A, B, and C fires. Most medical offices have multipurpose fire extinguishers in

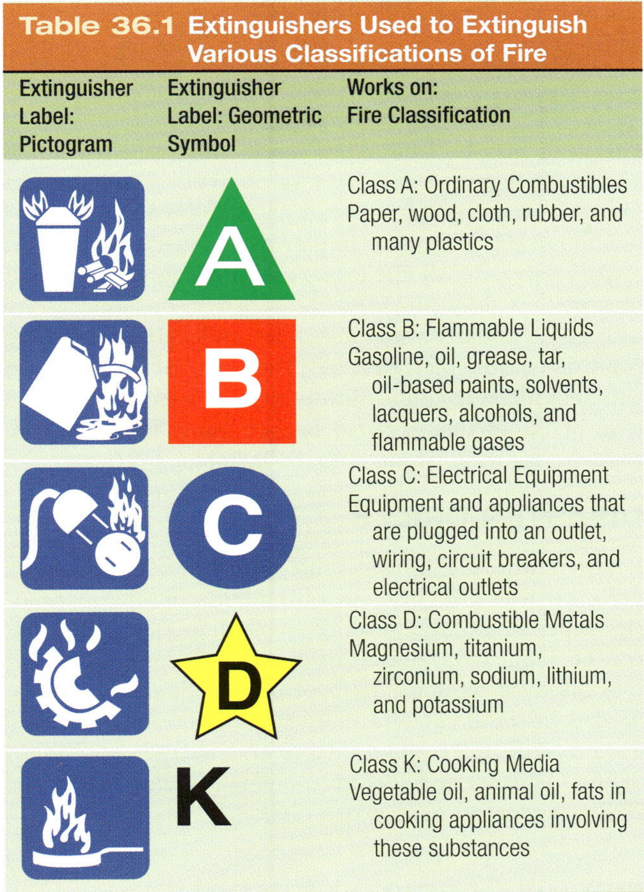

Table 36.1 Extinguishers Used to Extinguish Various Classifications of Fire

Extinguisher Label: Pictogram	Extinguisher Label: Geometric Symbol	Works on: Fire Classification
	A	Class A: Ordinary Combustibles Paper, wood, cloth, rubber, and many plastics
	B	Class B: Flammable Liquids Gasoline, oil, grease, tar, oil-based paints, solvents, lacquers, alcohols, and flammable gases
	C	Class C: Electrical Equipment Equipment and appliances that are plugged into an outlet, wiring, circuit breakers, and electrical outlets
	D	Class D: Combustible Metals Magnesium, titanium, zirconium, sodium, lithium, and potassium
	K	Class K: Cooking Media Vegetable oil, animal oil, fats in cooking appliances involving these substances

their facilities because this type of extinguisher can put out most types of fire.

Fire extinguishers must be properly identified (Fig. 36.11) and readily accessible in an emergency situation. Fire code requirements specify the size, number, location, and type of fire extinguishers within a facility. These requirements are based on the protection level that is appropriate for the hazard class of the building and the types (classes) of fire most likely to occur in that facility. Fire extinguishers are mounted on brackets or installed in wall cabinets (see Fig. 36.11) and are usually located along normal paths of travel and near building exits. If a fire extinguisher is mounted in a room, it is placed near the door so that the fire does not get between an individual and an exit. There should always be a fire extinguisher within a 50-foot travel distance of flammable liquids that are stored in containers. Fire extinguishers must be stored in their designated place at all times except during operation.

Fire extinguishers must be properly maintained to ensure that they are safe to use and will operate properly when needed. Most medical offices use maintenance personnel and a certified fire extinguisher agency to inspect, maintain, and test their fire extinguishers on a regular basis (monthly and yearly). A durable tag is attached to each fire extinguisher to document each service check, including the date of the service and the signature of the individual performing the service.

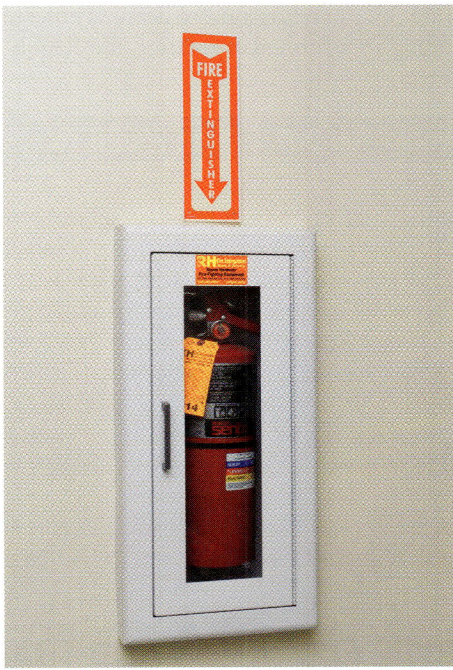

Fig. 36.11 A fire extinguisher installed in a wall cabinet.

Small fires can often be put out quickly by an employee using a portable fire extinguisher, ending the threat of a major fire. To do this safely, however, the employee must know how to properly operate a fire extinguisher. OSHA requires that any employee responsible for operating a portable fire extinguisher be thoroughly trained in the use of the fire extinguisher as well as the hazards associated with fighting a fire. The acronym *PASS* is used to help remember the steps involved in operating a fire extinguisher:

P: Pull out the pin.
A: Aim the nozzle at the base of the fire.
S: Squeeze the handle.
S: Sweep the nozzle from side to side at the base of the fire.

Procedure 36.1 outlines in more detail the procedure for operating a fire extinguisher.

EMERGENCY RESPONSE TO A FIRE

It is important to respond immediately to a fire. Most fires start out small but can quickly increase in size and intensity and become life-threatening in just a matter of minutes. The heat, smoke, and toxic gases from a fire that is spreading are often more dangerous than the flames.

The acronym *RACE* can be used to identify the basic steps to follow in responding to a fire (RACE against fire). These steps are as follows:

R: Rescue anyone in immediate danger of the fire.
A: Activate the alarm.
C: Confine the fire by closing doors and windows.
E: Extinguish the fire or evacuate the area. If the fire is small, use a fire extinguisher to put the fire out. If the fire cannot be extinguished, evacuate the area.

Procedure 36.2 presents a more detailed emergency plan for responding to a fire, incorporating the RACE response outlined here.

What Would You Do? What Would You *Not* Do?

Case Study 2

Brie Matthews is at the medical office for an evaluation of her diabetes. Mary Beth enters the examining room to measure Brie's vital signs. As Mary Beth enters the room, she notices that Brie is studying the fire extinguisher mounted on brackets near the door and turning the service tag over to read the information on it. Brie indicates that she needs to get a fire extinguisher for her home and wants to know the meaning of the three pictures on the extinguisher and why the extinguisher has a tag attached to it. Brie wants to know who is allowed to operate the fire extinguisher and how long the extinguisher lasts before it gets "used up." Brie also wants to know why there are fire extinguishers in the office, because she noticed that the office has sprinklers in the ceiling. ■

EMPLOYEE EDUCATION AND TRAINING

Medical assisting employees must know what types of emergencies may occur in their medical office and what course of action they should take. OSHA requires that employees be provided with education and training on the EAP. The training should include the following:

- Individual roles and responsibilities
- Threats, hazards, and protective actions
- Location and operation of manually activated pull stations and communication equipment
- Emergency response procedures
- Evacuation, shelter, and accountability procedures
- Location and use of common emergency equipment
- Emergency shutdown procedures

The EAP must be reviewed with each employee at the following times:

- When the initial plan is developed
- When new employees are hired
- When the employee's responsibilities or designated actions under the plan change
- Whenever the plan is changed

EMERGENCY PRACTICE DRILLS

Once employees have reviewed and been trained in the EAP, it is important to hold emergency practice drills. The purpose of a practice drill is to provide employees with the opportunity to practice their assigned duties in a simulated emergency situation. This increases the probability that employees will perform their duties safely and effectively in the event of an actual disaster or serious emergency. Emergency practice drills also provide the opportunity to evaluate the effectiveness of the EAP and determine any necessary changes or adjustments needed for improving performance. There are two types of emergency practice drills—fire drills and disaster drills—which are discussed in more detail in the following sections.

FIRE DRILLS

Fire drills may be required at specific intervals depending on the municipal or state laws for the type of building and insurance requirements. Fire drills may be announced or unannounced. They assist employees of a medical facility to review emergency escape routes and procedures to respond to a fire. Fire drills provide employees with the opportunity to become familiar with exit routes under nonthreatening conditions. This increases the probability of an organized and smooth evacuation during an actual emergency. The type of duties that need to be performed by evacuation wardens during a fire are outlined in Table 36.2.

DISASTER DRILLS

Disaster drills are usually more comprehensive than fire drills. Disaster drills often involve several community agencies depending on the severity of the disaster scenario that will be simulated. Disaster drills are time-consuming, but they allow all participants to practice skills that would be needed in the event of a disaster. In addition, they allow organizations and communities to evaluate the effectiveness of their systems and identify potential weaknesses in the ability to respond to an actual disaster.

MEDICAL ASSISTANT'S ROLE

The medical assistant is an important team member in developing and implementing the EAP for a health care setting and can also contribute to emergency preparedness in the community. The medical assistant may make recommendations to supplement emergency equipment or facilities in the office, serve on a committee to review or revise the emergency plan, participate actively in all fire drills and disaster drills, and participate in the review of the effectiveness of any drill. In addition, the medical assistant must be prepared to provide emergency first aid or cardiopulmonary resuscitation (CPR), both in the workplace and in the community (see Chapter 37). In an actual disaster, medical assistants might assist by providing emergency first aid, conducting patient interviews, helping to calm victims, documenting services provided, and performing phlebotomy or other procedures as directed.

The medical assistant should be aware of community resources for emergency preparedness. The medical office may keep a list of local organizations with telephone numbers or other contact information in the following areas:

- Emergency Medical Services (911)
- Poison Control Center
- Telephone numbers of local hospitals
- Telephone numbers of local and state health departments
- Telephone number for the state HAZMAT response team (**HAZMAT** is an acronym constructed from "*haz*ardous

Table 36.2 Duties Performed by Evacuation Wardens During a Fire

Duties	Guidelines and Key Points
Activate the nearest fire alarm pull station	The employee who first discovers the fire should activate the nearest fire alarm pull station.
Operate a fire extinguisher	A fire extinguisher can be used to extinguish a small fire in the beginning stages. *Do not* attempt to extinguish a fire if it is too large or if there is excessive smoke or heat.
Alert patients to the presence of a fire	Alert patients using a calm and firm manner so as not to cause panic. Use a clear and distinct voice to instruct patients during the evacuation.
Evacuate patients and visitors from each room and close windows and doors in each room	Closing windows and doors reduces the amount of oxygen that is able to get to the fire and helps to limit the spread of smoke and fire throughout the building.
Escort patients and visitors to the nearest exit and assembly area according to the evacuation floor plan	Use the primary exit route if available. If the primary exit route is blocked, use the secondary exit route. If smoke is present, stay low and close to the floor while evacuating because the air is fresher nearer to the ground. Proceed (walk, do not run) through the escape route in a quiet, orderly manner.
Assist patients with disabilities	If it is not possible to evacuate a disabled patient, take the patient to a shelter-in-place area and notify emergency personnel of the patient's location.
Direct patients to stairways that are free of smoke	Instruct individuals to not push, rush, or jostle other individuals when exiting by way of a stairway.
Keep people out of elevators	Elevators should not be used during a fire because: a. Elevator may fail during a fire, trapping the occupants. b. Elevator shafts may fill with smoke. c. Elevators need to be available to emergency responders.
Perform a final check of each room (examining rooms, rest rooms, offices, break room, storage rooms) to make sure everyone has been evacuated	A final check ensures that all occupants have been evacuated from the building.
Make sure fire doors are closed when exiting	Fire doors prevent spread of fire from one area to another.
Instruct building occupants not to leave the assembly area or to go back into the building	Building occupants need to remain in the assembly area so that they can be accounted for by the emergency evacuation coordinator. Occupants should not go back into the building until given permission to do so by emergency officials.
Direct emergency responders to the location of the fire	Use a clear and distinct voice to direct emergency responders to the location of the fire.
Notify emergency responders of hazardous materials (e.g., oxygen tanks, hazardous chemicals) in the building	Providing information on hazardous materials is essential to the safety of emergency responders.

*mat*erials." It refers to materials that pose a danger to health or the environment and for which protective clothing is required for cleanup.)

The medical assistant should also be aware of community disaster plans and community organizations that might assist in a disaster. The website of the state emergency medical agency often includes helpful articles related to the disasters that occur most frequently in that state. It is helpful to develop a list of useful resources for the medical office and update it regularly.

What Would You Do? What Would You *Not* Do?

Case Study 3

Jordan Mendels, 32 years of age, is at the medical office complaining of headaches, fatigue, and insomnia. Jordan tearfully relays that her brother's house burned down 2 weeks ago. Jordan is now concerned about a fire in her own home. She wants to know the best way to prevent that from happening and also wants to know if her family should hold fire drills. Jordan says that she knows she should get a fire extinguisher but she doesn't know how to use one. ■

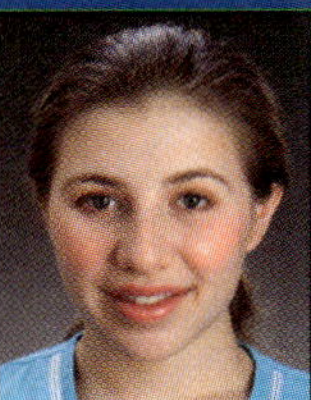

Memories *from* Practicum

Beth Ann: The office where I did my practicum was a clinic in a large city hospital. While I was there, I was allowed to attend a hands-on fire training session for hospital employees. We met at a training facility at the fire department where we saw two training videos. One of them showed how to test a door for warmth and emphasized that a warm door or a door with smoke leaking around the edge should never be opened. In the film, a fireman did open the door, and we saw how the flames and smoke gushed out when the fire received the new supply of oxygen. Someone asked what you should do if you knew there was a patient in the room behind a warm door. The fireman answered that if possible, you should wait for a firefighter, who would be prepared to handle the flame and smoke. After the videos, we were dressed in protective equipment and allowed to discharge fire extinguishers to put out small fires. Even though the fires were small, it was still a scary experience. I hope I never have to deal with a fire, even a small one, but I know that this experience helped to prepare me if it ever happens. ■

What Would You Do? What Would You *Not* Do? RESPONSES

Case Study 1

Page 974

What Did Beth Ann Do?

- ❑ Told Mrs. Manning to stop and breathe, and encouraged her to take several deep breaths.
- ❑ Recognized that Mrs. Manning was showing signs of severe anxiety, which would make it difficult for her to focus on driving safely.
- ❑ Told Mrs. Manning that she seemed very upset by the news, reassured her that the fire department would respond promptly, and encouraged her to sit down and relax for a minute until she collects herself.
- ❑ Asked Mrs. Manning if there was a family member or friend she could call to pick her up and drive her to her son's school.
- ❑ Listened attentively to Mrs. Manning's concerns.

What Did Beth Ann Not Do?

- ❑ Did not allow Mrs. Manning to leave and drive an automobile while in a state of severe anxiety.
- ❑ Did not tell Mrs. Manning to calm down because she was overreacting.
- ❑ Did not give Mrs. Manning a detailed explanation of the effects of anxiety.

Case Study 2

Page 982

What Did Beth Ann Do?

- ❑ Told Brie that the pictures indicate the type of fires the extinguisher can handle and that this extinguisher is a multipurpose extinguisher and can put out fires caused by ordinary combustibles such as paper or wood, flammable liquids, and electrical equipment.
- ❑ Explained to Brie that each fire extinguisher must be inspected and maintained on a regular basis and the tag documents the date of each service check.
- ❑ Informed Brie that only employees with the proper training and knowledge are permitted to operate the fire extinguishers in the office in the event of a fire.
- ❑ Told Brie that fire extinguishers use up their extinguishing agent within 10 to 30 seconds depending on the size of the extinguisher.
- ❑ Relayed to Brie that fire code requirements, which often include a variety of safety measures, specify the type of fire protection safety measures that must be present in a building.

What Did Beth Ann Not Do?

- ❑ Did not let Brie remove the fire extinguisher from its mounting brackets.
- ❑ Did not scold Brie for not already having a fire extinguisher in her home.

Case Study 3

Page 983

What Did Beth Ann Do?

- ❑ Listened empathetically to Jordan and allowed her to express her fears and concerns.
- ❑ Reassured Jordan that practicing fire prevention methods in the home is the best way to reduce the possibility of a fire.
- ❑ Provided Jordan with the names of websites (FEMA, American Red Cross, National Fire Protection Association, ready.gov) that she could use to access information on fire prevention and protective measures in the home.
- ❑ Told Jordan that it is a very good idea to hold fire drills in the home to make sure everyone knows what to do in the event of a fire and how to evacuate quickly and safely.
- ❑ Explained to Jordan that fire extinguishers are not difficult to operate and that each fire extinguisher comes with step-by-step instructions.
- ❑ Informed the physician of the situation so that he could provide the best treatment for Jordan.
- ❑ Reminded Jordan that fires in the home do happen, but they are not regular occurrences.

What Did Beth Ann Not Do?

- ❑ Did not say or imply that Jordan was overreacting or worrying for no reason.
- ❑ Did not push Jordan to accept her suggestions, but rather just offered information.
- ❑ Did not alarm Jordan about the possibility of a home fire.

TERMINOLOGY REVIEW

Key Term	Definition
Anxiety	A feeling of worry or uneasiness, often triggered by an event that is perceived as having an uncertain outcome.
Disaster	A sudden event that causes damage or loss of life.
Emergency action plan	A written document that describes the actions that employees should take to ensure their safety if a fire or other emergency situation occurs.
Emergency preparedness	The process of making plans to prevent, respond to, and recover from an emergency situation.
Evacuation	A planned systematic retreat of people to safety in an emergency situation.
Evacuation procedures	Clear step-by-step procedures for the rapid, efficient, and safe removal of individuals from a building during an emergency.
Exit route	A continuous and unobstructed path of travel from any point within a workplace to a place of safety.
Fire extinguisher	A portable device that discharges an agent designed to extinguish a fire.
Fire prevention plan	A written document that identifies flammable and combustible materials stored in the workplace and ways to control workplace fire hazards.
Fire protection	The implementation of safety measures to reduce the unwanted effects of fire.
HAZMAT	An acronym constructed from the beginnings of the two words "*haz*ardous *mat*erials." It refers to materials that pose a danger to health or the environment and must be handled with protective equipment.
Man-made disaster	An event that causes serious damage through intentional or negligent human actions or the failure of a man-made system.
Natural disaster	A catastrophic event that is caused by nature or the natural process of the earth.
Stress	The body's response to threat or change.

PROCEDURE 36.1 Demonstrating Proper Use of a Fire Extinguisher

Outcome Demonstrate proper use of a fire extinguisher in a role-playing situation.

Equipment/Supplies

- Portable office-size multipurpose (ABC) fire extinguisher that has been discharged

1. **Procedural Step.** Identify a safe evacuation route before approaching the fire.
   Principle. A clear evacuation route allows for immediate escape if the fire gets worse.
2. **Procedural Step.** Remove the multipurpose fire extinguisher from its mounting device and hold it upright with the nozzle pointing away from you. Stand 6 to 8 feet from the fire, keeping your back to the exit at all times.
   Principle. Standing at 6 to 8 feet prevents being burned or being hit by splattering material or sparks. Keeping the back to the exit allows for constant monitoring of the situation and immediate awareness if the fire begins to flare up or spread.
3. **Procedural Step.** Perform a quick assessment of the fire to determine if it is small enough to extinguish with a fire extinguisher (while continuing to stand at a distance of 6 to 8 feet). *Do not* attempt to extinguish the fire if it is too large or if there is excessive smoke or heat. In these instances, close the door to contain the fire then evacuate immediately.
   Principle. A fire extinguisher is designed to handle only small fires in the beginning stages.
4. **Procedural Step.** Operate the fire extinguisher using the PASS technique:
   a. *Pull* the safety pin straight out from the handle located at the top of the extinguisher. This will also break the tamper-proof seal. Make sure the fire extinguisher is held in an upright position at all times.
   Principle. The tamper-proof seal holds the safety pin in place. The safety pin provides a locking mechanism that prevents the fire extinguisher from accidentally discharging.

Continued

PROCEDURE 36.1 Demonstrating Proper Use of a Fire Extinguisher—cont'd

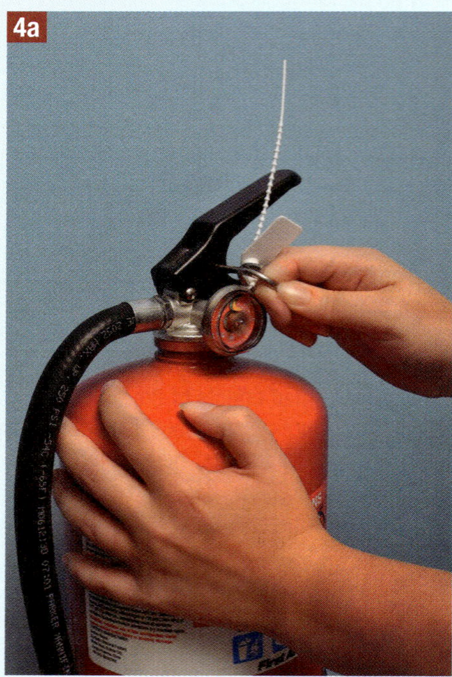

Pull the safety pin straight out from the handle.

b. *Aim* the nozzle at the base of the fire (not the flames) with your dominant hand.
Principle. Aiming the nozzle at the base of the fire allows the extinguishing agent to deprive the fire of fuel. Aiming the nozzle at the flames causes the extinguishing agent to pass through the flames without stopping the fire.

c. *Squeeze* the handle slowly and continuously to release the extinguishing agent. Letting go of the pressure on the handle causes the discharge of the extinguishing agent to cease.
Principle. Squeezing the handle opens a valve that releases the pressurized extinguishing agent from the fire extinguisher.

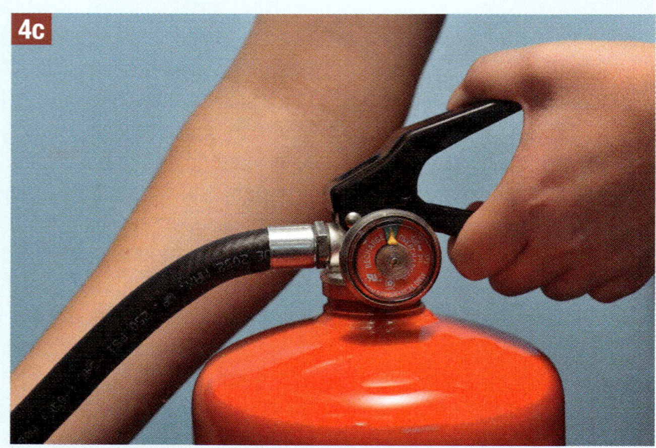

Squeeze the handle slowly and continuously.

d. *Sweep* the nozzle of the extinguisher evenly from side to side at the base of the fire. Gradually move closer to the fire as it begins to smolder. Continue to discharge the extinguishing agent until the fire is completely out. Evacuate immediately if the fire grows larger or if the extinguisher is empty and the fire is not out. Fire extinguishers use up their extinguishing agent within 10 to 30 seconds, depending on the size of the extinguisher.
Principle. A sweeping motion helps to extinguish the fire. Even distribution of the agent helps to put out the fire at a faster rate.

5. **Procedural Step.** Back away from the extinguished fire in case it flares up again. Continue to watch the area to be sure that flames do not recur after having been extinguished.
Principle. Material that has been burning can remain hot enough that flames will reignite.

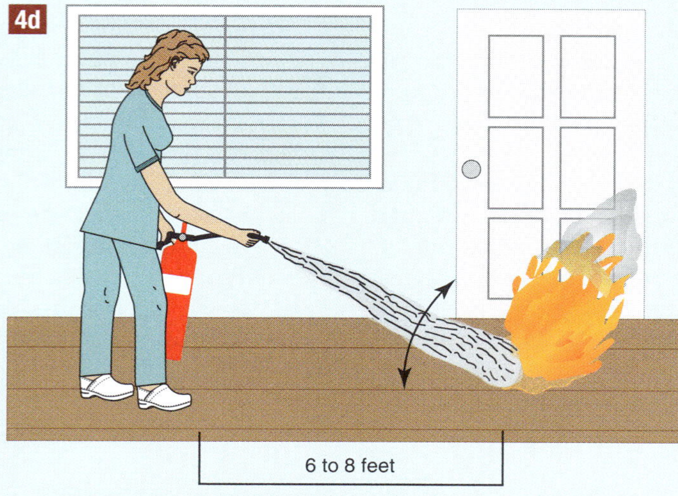

Sweep the nozzle of the extinguisher at the base of the fire.

PROCEDURE 36.2 Participating in a Mock Exposure Event

Outcome Participate in a mock environmental exposure event and document the steps taken.

Scenario

A fire has erupted in an examining room at your medical office. The fire, caused by faulty electrical wiring, has ignited several boxes of disposable drapes. (Place a poster, flashing light, or other indicator at the location of the "fire".) A disabled patient in a wheelchair is located in the room where the fire erupts. The emergency evacuation coordinator determines that an evacuation of the facility is necessary.

Equipment/Supplies

- Scenario
- Emergency evacuation floor plan
- Employee roster
- Patient log-in sheet
- Pen and paper

Predrill Activities

1. **Procedural Step.** Make a list of the names and phone numbers of the following resources that may be needed in the event of a fire:
   a. Emergency responders (911)
   b. Fire department
   c. Police department
   d. Local hospital
   e. Insurance carrier
2. **Procedural Step.** Review the location and purpose of fire protection safety measures.
   a. Locate and review the purpose of the following in your facility using the evacuation floor plan as a reference:
      - Manual fire alarm pull stations
      - Portable fire extinguishers
      - The path of the primary exit route
      - The path of the secondary exit route
      - Emergency exit doors
      - Wheelchair accessible exits
      - Assembly area
      - Shelter-in-place areas

2a

EVACUATION PLAN

THIRD FLOOR

Locate the path of the primary and secondary exit routes.

   b. Locate and review the purpose of the following through visual inspection of the facility:
      - Sprinklers
      - Smoke detectors
      - Fire doors
      - Exit signs

   Principle. The medical assistant should know the location and purpose of the fire protection safety measures in his or her facility.
3. **Procedural Step.** Evaluate primary and secondary exit routes for the following:
   a. Exits are clearly marked and well lit.
   b. Exit routes are unobstructed and free of clutter.
   c. Exit doors are free of decorations or signs that obscure the visibility of the exit.
   d. Exit doors are unlocked from the inside.
   e. Exit doors open outward.
   f. Fire extinguishers are in place and clearly identified.
   g. Evacuation floor plans are posted in multiple locations throughout the facility.
4. **Procedural Step.** Assign an emergency evacuation coordinator to assume overall charge and responsibility for the evacuation process including the following:
   a. Calling emergency responders (911)
   b. Identifying safe evacuation routes
   c. Ensuring that evacuation wardens are performing their duties
   d. Coordinating with the emergency responders

   Principle. The emergency evacuation coordinator is responsible for taking charge of the evacuation process.
5. **Procedural Step.** Compile an employee roster and assign evacuation wardens to perform one or more of the duties outlined in Table 36.2. Make sure each evacuation warden understands his or her roles and responsibilities and is well trained in his or her assigned duties.

   Principle. Evacuation wardens are responsible for performing rescue duties during an evacuation.

Continued

PROCEDURE 36.2 Participating in a Mock Exposure Event—cont'd

6. **Procedural Step.** Assign individuals to play the role of patients and compile a patient log-in sheet. Patients with special needs should be included, such as:
   a. Mother with a young child with an illness
   b. Patient with emphysema on oxygen
   c. Pregnant patient in the last trimester of her pregnancy
   d. Patient with crutches wearing a leg cast
   e. Elderly patient with a heart condition
   f. Patient with dementia
   g. Disabled patient in a wheelchair
   h. Patient with severe anxiety
   i. Hearing-impaired patient
   j. Patient with a visual impairment

Conduct the Fire Drill

(The emergency evacuation coordinator and evacuation wardens should perform their assigned duties concurrently during the fire drill.)

1. **Procedural Step**. Rescue anyone in immediate danger of the fire. If an individual's clothes catch on fire, the following can be performed to extinguish the flames:
   a. Instruct the person to stop, drop, and roll.
   b. Cover the person with a blanket or clothing to help extinguish the flames.

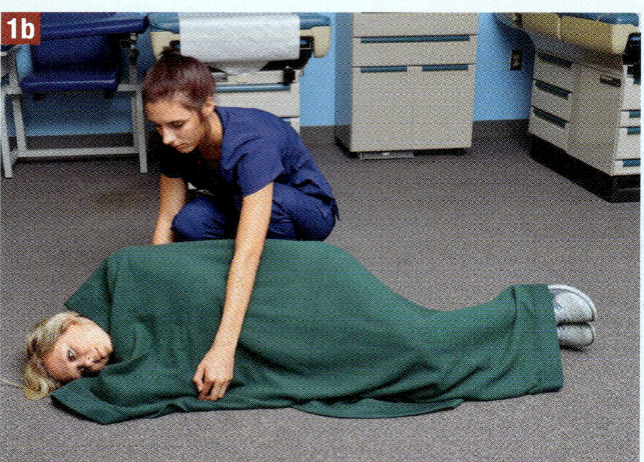
1b

Cover the person with a blanket or clothes to extinguish flames.

2. **Procedural Step.** Activate the fire alarm to warn building occupants of the presence of the fire and to provide them with enough time to safely evacuate the building. The employee who first discovers the fire should activate the nearest fire alarm pull station by pulling down on the lever.

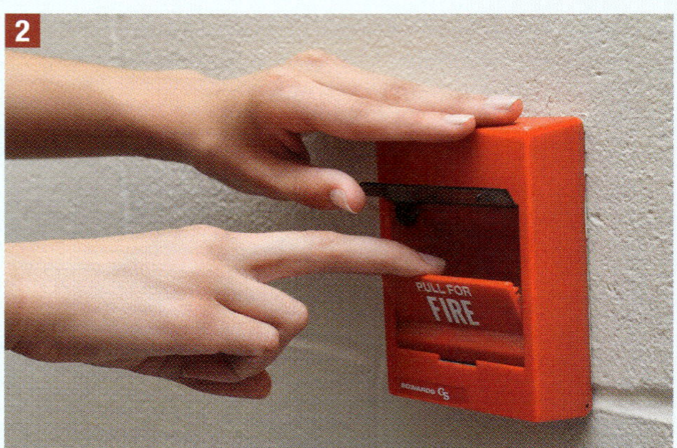

2

Activate the alarm.

3. **Procedural Step.** Immediately notify emergency responders by dialing 911. Speak clearly and calmly to the emergency medical dispatcher. Identify the problem as accurately and concisely as possible so that proper equipment and personnel can be sent. Do not hang up until the dispatcher gives you permission to do so. Information that should be relayed (if known) to the emergency dispatcher includes the following:
   a. Type of fire (e.g., electrical, combustibles, flammable liquids)
   b. Exact location of the fire
   c. Extent of the fire
   d. Whether an evacuation is in process
   e. Other information requested by the dispatcher

   Principle. Calling 911 allows the fire department to be on its way while other activities are being performed. Any delay may allow the fire to grow and further endanger the building occupants and property.
4. **Procedural Step.** Extinguish the fire with a portable fire extinguisher if it is small and confined, following the steps outlined in Procedure 36.1. *Do not* attempt to extinguish the fire if it is too large or if there is excessive smoke or heat. In these instances, close the door to contain the fire then evacuate immediately.
5. **Procedural Step.** Evacuate the area immediately. The evacuation wardens should perform their evacuation duties as assigned in Table 36.2. Important evacuation guidelines include the following:
   a. Evacuate patients and visitors from each room of the medical office (e.g., examining rooms, rest rooms).
   b. Use the primary exit route if possible. If the primary exit route is blocked by fire or smoke, use the secondary exit route.
   c. Exit by stairways only. Do not use elevators.

PROCEDURE 36.2 Participating in a Mock Exposure Event—cont'd

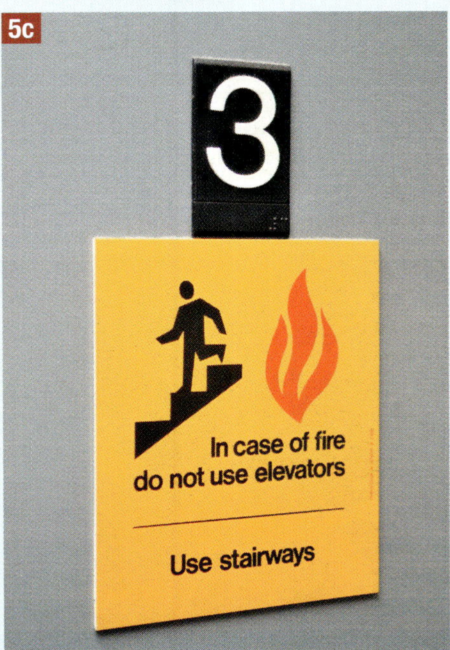

5c
3
In case of fire
do not use elevators
Use stairways
Do not use elevators.

d. Close the door after a room is evacuated and place an X on the door with chalk or a marker to indicate the room has been evacuated.

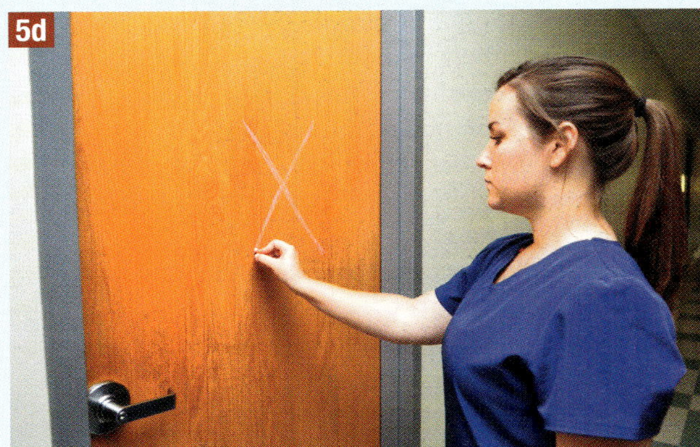

Place an X on the door.

e. Perform a final check to make sure everyone has been evacuated.

f. Make sure all fire doors are closed.

Principle: The size of a fire can double every 30 seconds; therefore it is important to evacuate immediately. The primary exit route is the quickest and easiest way to exit a building during an evacuation. Elevators may fail during a fire trapping occupants.

6. Procedural Step. Before exiting a room with a closed door, feel the door with the back of your hand. If the door is warm:

- Do not open the door.
- Call 911 to report your location or place a signal in the window.
- Place clothing or towels along the bottom of the door to keep out smoke.
- Stay calm and wait to be rescued.
- Do not break the window. Smoke entering from the outside may hamper rescue.

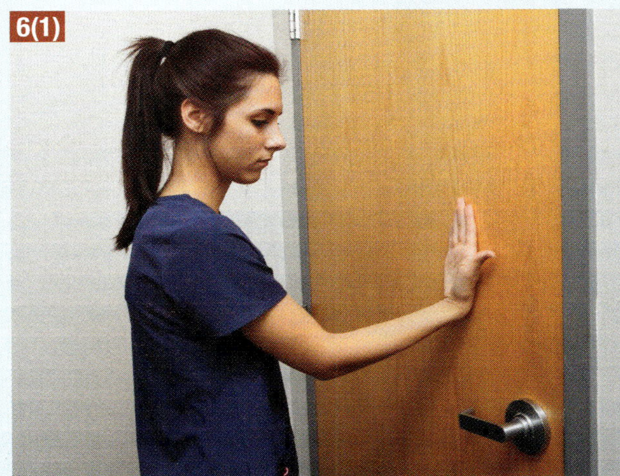

Feel the door with the back of your hand before exiting the room.

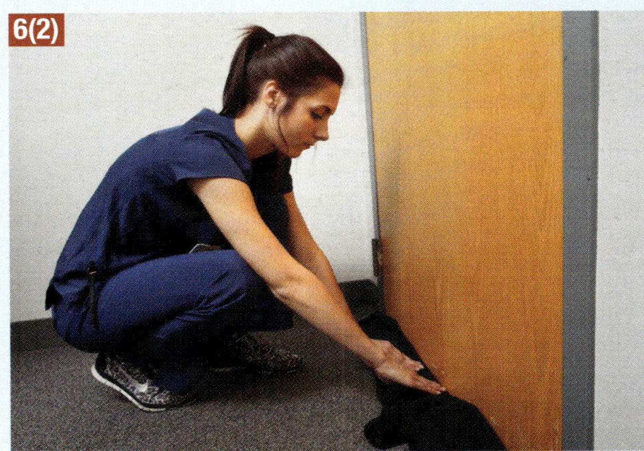

Place clothing along the bottom of the door.

7. Procedural Step. Escort patients and visitors to the designated assembly area. Check to make sure everyone is accounted for by completing the following:

a. Account for all employees using the employee roster checklist.

Continued

PROCEDURE 36.2 Participating in a Mock Exposure Event—cont'd

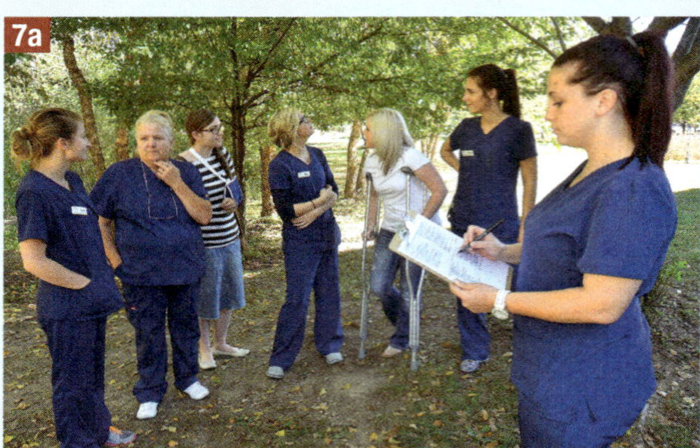

7a Account for all employees.

b. Account for all patients using the patient log-in sheet.

Principle. Accounting for building occupants helps to determine if someone is still in the building and in need of rescue.

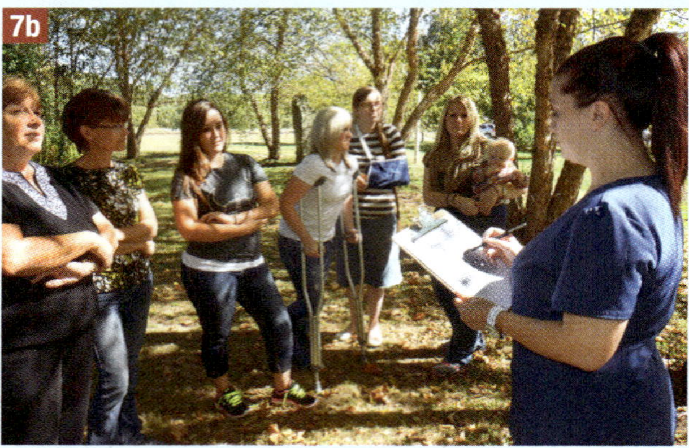

7b Account for all patients.

8. **Procedural Step.** Keep the building occupants together in the assembly area at a safe distance from the building. Make sure that occupants do not block access to the building by emergency responders. Do not allow anyone to reenter the building unless directed to do so by emergency officials. Instruct occupants not to leave until everyone has been accounted for and dismissed.

9. **Procedural Step.** Direct emergency responders to the location of the fire. Provide emergency responders with the following information:
   a. The name and last known location of any individual not accounted for during the head count.
   b. Special hazards in the building that may endanger emergency responders such as oxygen tanks and hazardous chemicals.

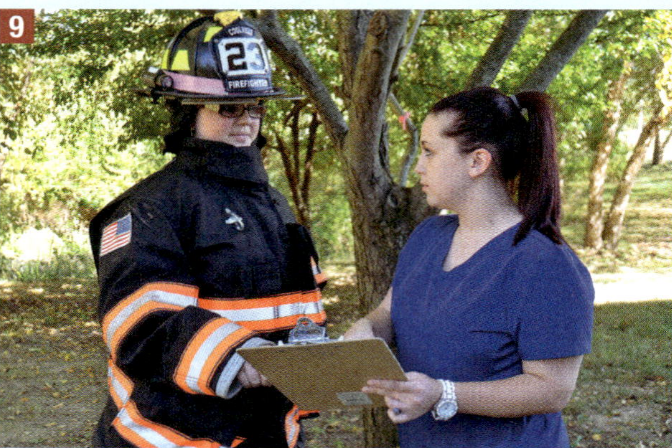

9 Provide emergency responders with information.

Postdrill Activities

1. **Procedural Step.** Critique the effectiveness of the fire drill (in terms of strengths, concerns, and means of improvement) by evaluating the following:
   a. The evacuation was completed in an orderly, efficient, and timely manner.
   b. Building occupants and emergency responders were immediately alerted of the situation.
   c. Evacuation wardens effectively completed their duties.
   d. Patients and visitors were escorted to the nearest exit and assembly area.
   e. Each building occupant was accounted for after the evacuation.
   f. Emergency responders were provided with appropriate information.
2. **Procedural Step.** Document the results of the fire drill including your role and the effectiveness of the group as a whole in carrying out the evacuation.

   Principle. Evaluation of the fire drill identifies strengths, concerns, and means of improvement.

Emergency Medical Procedures and First Aid

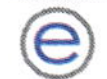 Check out the Evolve site at http://evolve.elsevier.com/Bonewit/today to access additional interactive activities and exercises to help you study and prepare for success.

LEARNING OBJECTIVES

First Aid

1. State the purpose of first aid.
2. Explain the purpose of the emergency medical services (EMS) system.
3. List the OSHA standards for administering first aid.
4. List the guidelines that should be followed when providing emergency care.

Common Emergency Situations

5. List and describe conditions that cause respiratory distress.
6. List the symptoms of a heart attack and a stroke.
7. Explain the causes of each of the following types of shock: cardiogenic, neurogenic, anaphylactic, and psychogenic.
8. Identify and describe the three classifications of external bleeding.
9. Explain the difference between an open wound and a closed wound.
10. Describe the characteristics of each of the following fractures: impacted, greenstick, transverse, oblique, comminuted, and spiral.
11. Identify the characteristics of each of the following burns: superficial, partial thickness, and full thickness.
12. Explain the difference between a partial seizure and a generalized seizure.
13. List examples of each of the following types of poisoning: ingested, inhaled, absorbed, and injected.
14. Identify factors that place an individual at higher risk for developing heat-related and cold-related injuries.
15. Describe the differences between type 1 and type 2 diabetes mellitus.
16. Explain the causes of insulin shock and diabetic coma.
17. Identify the symptoms and describe emergency care for each of the following conditions: respiratory distress, heart attack, stroke, shock, bleeding, wounds, musculoskeletal injuries, burns, seizures, poisoning, heat and cold exposure, and diabetic emergencies.

PROCEDURES

Respond to common emergency situations.

CHAPTER OUTLINE

KEY TERMS

burn
crash cart
crepitus (KREP-it-us)
dislocation
emergency medical services (EMS) system
first aid
fracture (FRAK-shur)
hypothermia (hie-poe-THER-mee-ah)
poison
pressure point
seizure (SEE-zhur)
shock
splint
sprain
strain
wound

INTRODUCTION TO EMERGENCY MEDICAL PROCEDURES

Medical emergencies often arise inside and outside of the workplace and can result in sudden loss of life or permanent disability. If an emergency situation occurs in the medical office, the provider provides immediate medical care for the patient. Some medical offices maintain a **crash cart** for this purpose. In these situations, the medical assistant may be required to assist the provider in providing emergency medical care.

The medical assistant may need to administer first aid for medical emergencies that occur outside of the medical office environment. **First aid** is defined as the immediate care administered before complete medical care can be obtained to an individual who is injured or suddenly becomes ill. The medical assistant is most likely to administer first aid to a family member or friend. The purposes of first aid are to save a life, reduce pain and suffering, prevent further injury, reduce the incidence of permanent disability, and increase the opportunity for an early recovery.

This chapter focuses on common emergency situations that the medical assistant may encounter and the first aid required for each. It is not intended, however, as a substitute for thorough first aid instruction through the American Red Cross, National Safety Council, or American Heart Association.

OFFICE CRASH CART

A crash cart is a specially equipped cart for holding and transporting medications, equipment, and supplies needed to perform lifesaving procedures in an emergency. A growing number of providers are incorporating crash carts into their medical offices. Patients who are injured or suddenly become ill might be brought to the medical office for emergency medical care. In addition, a patient might develop a sudden illness at the medical office that requires emergency medical care. Examples of these situations include life-threatening cardiac dysrhythmias, shock, cardiac arrest, poisoning, and traumatic injury.

The items on an office crash cart vary widely among medical offices depending on the extent of the emergency medical care that is likely to be administered. This is directly related to the time it takes for emergency medical personnel to arrive and the location of the nearest hospital. The medical assistant may be responsible for regularly checking the crash cart to replenish supplies and to check the expiration dates on medications.

EMERGENCY MEDICAL SERVICES SYSTEM

The **emergency medical services (EMS) system** is a network of community resources, equipment, and emergency medical technicians (EMTs) that provides emergency care to victims of injury or sudden illness. An *EMT* is a professional provider of prehospital emergency care, which includes care at the scene and during transportation to the hospital. An EMT-Basic (EMT-B) has received formal training and is certified to provide basic life support measures. An *EMT-Paramedic* (EMT-P) is qualified to provide advanced life support care, including advanced airway maintenance, initiation of intravenous drips, administration of medication, cardiac monitoring and interpretation, and cardiac defibrillation.

Activating the EMS system is often the most important step in an emergency. Rapid arrival of EMTs increases the patient's chances of surviving a life-threatening emergency. In most urban and in some rural areas in the United States, the medical assistant can activate the local EMS system by dialing 911 on the telephone. Other areas have a local seven-digit number, in which case it is important to keep the number at hand.

When calling local EMS, the medical assistant speaks with an *emergency medical dispatcher* (EMD). An EMD has had formal training in handling emergency situations over the phone. The responsibility of the EMD is to answer the emergency call, listen to the caller, obtain critical information, determine what help is needed, and send the appropriate personnel and equipment. The EMD also is responsible for relaying instructions to the caller about providing emergency care until the EMTs arrive.

These guidelines should be followed when calling EMS:

- Speak clearly and calmly to the EMD. Identify the problem as accurately and concisely as possible so that proper equipment and personnel can be sent. The EMD needs to know the number of victims, the condition of the victim or victims, and the emergency care that has already been administered.
- The EMD will ask you for your phone number and address. In responding, relay to the dispatcher the exact location of the victim, including the correct street name and house number and (if applicable) the building name, floor, and room number. With the 911 enhanced emergency system, the address automatically appears on a monitor; however, there is a chance that the address will not show up on the monitor. In addition, the emergency may not be happening in the same location as the caller. If possible, have someone meet the ambulance personnel and direct them to the scene.
- Do not hang up until the EMD gives you permission to do so. The dispatcher may need additional information or may give you instructions on treating the patient until EMTs arrive.

FIRST AID KIT

The medical office should acquire and maintain a first aid kit. A first aid kit contains basic supplies to provide emergency care to individuals who have been injured or become suddenly ill (Fig. 37.1). It is recommended that a first aid kit be kept at home and in the car.

First aid kits are available at most drug stores. It also is possible to make your own. Along with the items shown in Fig. 37.1, the first aid kit should include the phone numbers of the local EMS, the Poison Help center, and the police and fire departments. It is important to check the first aid kit regularly and replace supplies as needed.

OSHA SAFETY PRECAUTIONS

To prevent exposure to bloodborne pathogens and other potentially infectious materials, the OSHA Bloodborne Pathogens Standard presented in Chapter 17 should be followed when performing first aid. The following guidelines help reduce or eliminate the risk of infection:

1. Make sure that your first aid kit contains personal protective equipment, such as gloves, a face shield and mask, and a pocket mask.
2. Wear gloves when it is reasonably anticipated that your hands will come into contact with the following: blood and other potentially infectious materials, mucous membranes, nonintact skin, and contaminated articles or surfaces.
3. Perform all first aid procedures involving blood or other potentially infectious materials in a manner that minimizes splashing, spraying, spattering, and generation of droplets of these substances.
4. Wear protective clothing and gloves to cover cuts or other lesions of the skin.
5. Sanitize your hands as soon as possible after removing gloves.
6. Avoid touching objects that may be contaminated with blood or other potentially infectious materials.
7. If your hands or other skin surfaces come in contact with blood or other potentially infectious materials, wash the area as soon as possible with soap and water.
8. If your mucous membranes (in eyes, nose, and mouth) come in contact with blood or other potentially infectious materials, flush them with water as soon as possible.
9. Avoid eating, drinking, and touching your mouth, eyes, and nose while providing emergency care or before you sanitize your hands.
10. If you are exposed to blood or other potentially infectious materials, report the incident as soon as possible to your provider so that postexposure procedures can be instituted.

GUIDELINES FOR PROVIDING EMERGENCY CARE

The remainder of this chapter presents specific emergency situations that may be encountered by the medical assistant

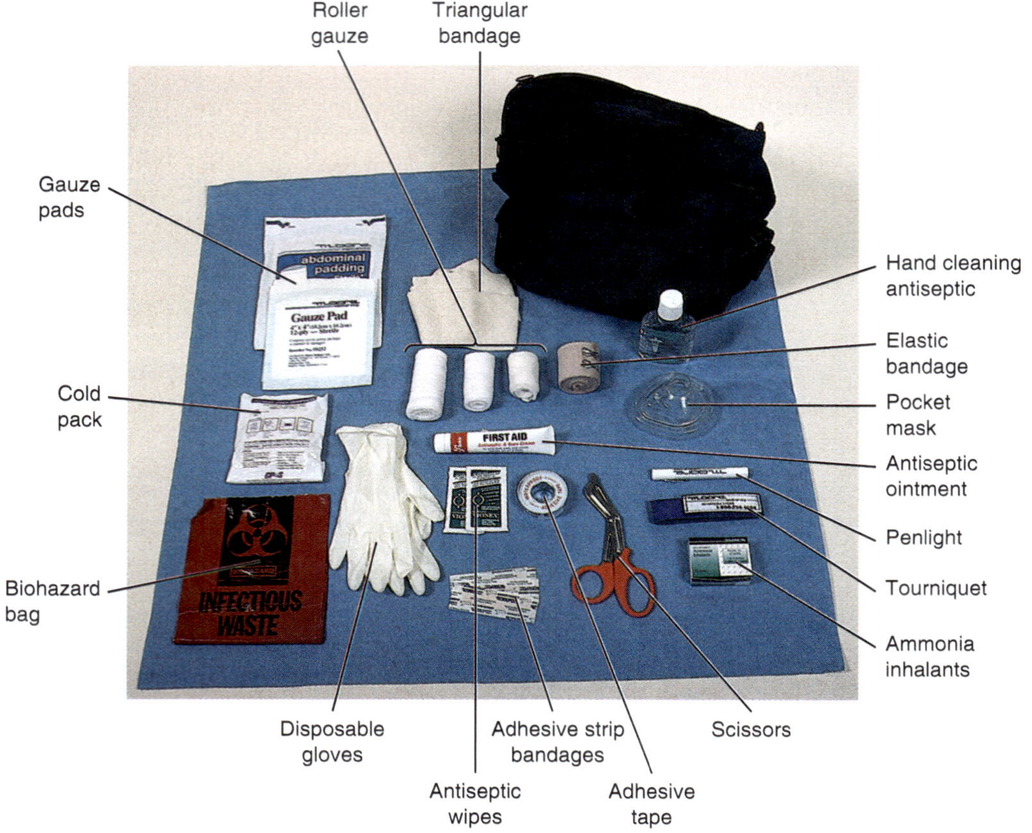

Fig. 37.1 First aid kit.

and the emergency care required for each. These guidelines should be followed when providing emergency care:

1. Remain calm and speak in a normal tone of voice. These measures help calm and reassure the patient.
2. Make sure that the scene is safe before approaching the patient. It is important that you protect yourself from harm in an emergency situation.
3. Before administering emergency care to a conscious patient, you must first have permission or consent. To obtain consent, you must inform the patient who you are, your level of training, and what you are going to do to help. *Never* administer care to a conscious patient who refuses it. When a life-threatening condition exists and the patient is unconscious or otherwise unable to give consent, consent is assumed or implied. Under law, it is implied that if the patient could give consent to care, the patient would.
4. Follow the OSHA standards when providing emergency care to reduce or eliminate exposure to bloodborne pathogens or other potentially infectious materials.
5. Know how to activate your local EMS system. Activating the EMS is often the most important step you can take to help a patient who has experienced an injury or sudden illness.
6. Do not move the patient unnecessarily. Unnecessary movement can result in further injury or can be life-threatening to a patient with a serious condition.
7. Obtain information as to what happened from the patient, family members, co-workers, or bystanders.
8. Look for a medical alert tag on the patient's wrist, neck, or ankle. A medical alert tag provides information on a medical condition the patient may have.

HIGHLIGHT on Good Samaritan Laws

In all 50 states and the District of Columbia, Good Samaritan laws have been enacted to provide immunity to individuals, such as the medical assistant who administers first aid at the scene of an emergency. These laws were enacted to encourage individuals to help others in an emergency. They assume that an individual would do her or his best to save a life or prevent further injury.

The legal immunity provided by Good Samaritan laws protects an individual from being sued and found financially responsible for a patient's injury. The individual is immune from liability (except for "gross negligence") if the individual acts in good faith and uses a reasonable level of skill that does not exceed the scope of their training.

Good Samaritan laws do not mean that an individual cannot be sued for administering first aid. An individual is not protected from liability if they are grossly careless or reckless in handling the situation. Because the components of Good Samaritan laws vary from state to state, the medical assistant must become familiar with the laws that govern the state in which they work. ■

9. Continue caring for the patient until more highly trained personnel arrive. On the arrival of emergency medical personnel or a provider, relay the condition in which you found the patient and the emergency care that has been administered.

RESPIRATORY DISTRESS

Respiratory distress indicates that the patient is breathing but is having great difficulty doing so. Respiratory distress sometimes may lead to respiratory arrest. It is important that the medical assistant be alert for the signs and symptoms of respiratory distress, which may include noisy breathing, such as gasping for air or rasping, gurgling, or whistling sounds; breathing that is unusually fast or slow; and breathing that is painful. The general care for respiratory distress is to place the patient in a comfortable position that facilitates breathing. Most patients prefer a sitting or semireclining position. Remain calm and reassure the patient to help reduce anxiety. Calming the patient may help the patient breathe easier. If the patient's condition worsens or does not resolve within a few minutes, activate the local EMS system. Examples of conditions that frequently cause respiratory distress are described next.

Asthma

Asthma is a chronic inflammatory lung disease that affects the airways of the lungs. Asthma is characterized by recurrent episodes of coughing, chest tightness, shortness of breath, and wheezing known as an *asthma attack*. During an asthmatic attack, the bronchioles constrict and become clogged with mucus, which accounts for many of the symptoms of asthma.

Asthma may occur at any age, but it is more common in children and young adults. If the condition is not treated, it can lead to serious complications, such as permanent lung damage. It is frequently, but not always, associated with a family history of allergies. Any of the common allergens, such as dust mites, pollens, molds, animal dander, and cockroaches may trigger an asthmatic attack. Asthma attacks can also be triggered by environmental irritants, activities, or events, including air pollutants, tobacco smoke, chemical fumes (e.g., perfume, paint, and gasoline), vigorous physical exercise, upper respiratory viral infections, exposure to cold, and emotional stress. In normal circumstances an individual with asthma controls attacks with medications. These medications stop the muscle spasms and open the airway, making breathing easier.

Some patients may develop a severe prolonged asthmatic attack that is life-threatening, which is known as *status asthmaticus*. These patients can move only a small amount of air. Because so little air is being moved, the typical breathing sounds associated with asthma may not be audible. The patient may have a bluish discoloration of the skin and extremely labored breathing. Status asthmaticus is a true emergency and requires immediate transportation of the patient to an emergency care facility by the fastest way possible.

Emphysema

Emphysema is a progressive lung disorder in which the terminal bronchioles that lead into the alveoli become plugged with mucus. Because of this problem, the alveoli become damaged, resulting in less surface area to diffuse oxygen into the blood. Eventually this condition results in loss of elasticity of the alveoli, causing inhaled air to become trapped in the lungs. This makes breathing difficult, particularly during exhalation. Symptoms of emphysema include shortness of breath, coughing, wheezing and chest tightness.

Emphysema usually develops over many years and is found most frequently in heavy smokers. It also occurs in patients with chronic bronchitis and in elderly patients whose lungs have lost their natural elasticity. Chronic emphysema is one of the major causes of death in the United States. As the lungs progressively become less efficient, breathing becomes more and more difficult. Patients with advanced cases may go into respiratory or cardiac arrest.

Hyperventilation

Hyperventilation literally means "overbreathing." Hyperventilation is a manner of breathing in which the respirations become rapid and deep, causing an individual to exhale too much carbon dioxide. Low carbon dioxide levels in the body account for many of the symptoms of hyperventilation. Hyperventilation is often the result of fear or anxiety and is more likely to occur in individuals who are tense and nervous. It also is caused by serious organic conditions, such as diabetic coma, pneumonia, pulmonary edema, pulmonary embolism, head injury, high fever, and aspirin poisoning.

In addition to rapid and deep respirations, the signs and symptoms of hyperventilation include dizziness, faintness, and light-headedness; visual disturbances; chest pain; tachycardia; palpitations; fullness in the throat; and numbness and tingling of the fingers, toes, and the area around the mouth. Despite their rapid breathing efforts, patients complain that they cannot get enough air. They often think they are having a heart attack.

Treatment for hyperventilation caused by emotional factors is as follows: Calm and reassure the patient, and encourage them to slow the respirations, allowing the carbon dioxide level to return to normal. In the past, breathing into a paper bag was advocated as a remedy for hyperventilation. More recent studies no longer recommend this practice because it could be harmful if an underlying medical condition exists or if the patient is not actually hyperventilating. If the medical assistant suspects that hyperventilation has been caused by an organic problem, EMS should be activated immediately.

HEART ATTACK

A heart attack, also known as a *myocardial infarction* (MI), is caused by partial or complete obstruction of one or both of the coronary arteries or their branches. In most cases, the severity of the attack depends on the size of the obstructed artery and the amount of myocardial tissue nourished by that artery. If a small branch of a coronary artery is obstructed, myocardial damage and symptoms may be mild, whereas the damage is usually extensive and the symptoms intense if a coronary artery is completely blocked.

The principal symptom of a heart attack is chest pain or discomfort. Patients describe the chest pain as squeezing or crushing pressure, severe indigestion or burning, heaviness, or aching. Chest discomfort can range in severity from only mildly uncomfortable to intense and accompanied by a feeling of suffocation and doom. The pain is usually felt behind the sternum and may radiate to the neck, throat, or jaw or to both shoulders and both arms. The pain associated with a heart attack is prolonged and usually is not relieved by resting or taking nitroglycerin. Other signs and symptoms of a heart attack include shortness of breath, profuse perspiration, nausea, and fainting.

If the medical assistant suspects that the patient is having a heart attack, EMS should be activated immediately. Meanwhile, loosen tight clothing and have the patient rest in a comfortable position that facilitates breathing. If cardiac arrest occurs, the medical assistant should begin cardiopulmonary resuscitation (CPR) immediately.

STROKE

A stroke, also called a *cerebrovascular accident* (CVA), results when an artery to the brain is blocked or ruptures, causing an interruption of blood flow to the brain. The signs and symptoms of a stroke include sudden weakness or numbness of the face, arm, or leg on one side of the body; difficulty in speaking; dimmed vision or loss of vision in one eye; double vision; dizziness; confusion; severe headache; and loss of consciousness.

If the medical assistant suspects that the patient is having a stroke, EMS should be activated immediately. Meanwhile, loosen tight clothing and have the patient rest in a comfortable position. If respiratory arrest, cardiac arrest, or both occur, begin rescue breathing and CPR as required.

SHOCK

For the body to function properly, adequate blood flow must be maintained to all of the vital organs. This is accomplished by the three important cardiovascular functions, as follows:

- Adequate pumping action of the heart
- Sufficient blood circulating in the blood vessels
- Blood vessels being able to respond to blood flow

When an individual experiences a severe injury or illness, one or more of these cardiovascular functions may be affected, which can lead to shock.

Shock is defined as the failure of the cardiovascular system to deliver enough blood to all of the body's vital organs. Shock accompanies different types of emergency situations, such as hemorrhaging, MI, and severe allergic reaction. The five major types of shock are categorized according to cause: hypovolemic, cardiogenic, neurogenic, anaphylactic, and psychogenic. Each type of shock is described in this section. If not treated, most types of shock become life-threatening. This is because shock is progressive—when it reaches a certain point, it becomes irreversible, and the patient's life cannot be saved.

The signs and symptoms of shock are caused by the failure of the vital organs to receive enough oxygen and nutrients. The organs most affected are the heart, brain, and lungs, which can be irreparably damaged in 4 to 6 minutes. The general signs and symptoms of shock are weakness, restlessness, anxiety, disorientation, pallor, cold and clammy skin, rapid breathing, and rapid pulse.

If not treated, these symptoms can progress rapidly to a significant drop in blood pressure, cyanosis, loss of consciousness, and death. The signs and symptoms of shock may be subtle or pronounced. In addition, no single sign or symptom determines accurately the presence or severity of the shock. Because of this, it is crucial to consider the nature of the illness or injury in determining whether the patient is a possible victim of shock. If a patient has a traumatic injury to the abdomen, shock should be considered a possibility, even if the patient's signs and symptoms do not suggest shock.

Shock (with the exception of psychogenic shock) requires immediate medical care. The medical assistant should activate EMS without delay so that proper medical care can be obtained as soon as possible.

Hypovolemic Shock

Hypovolemic shock is caused by loss of blood or other body fluids. Conditions that result in this type of shock include external and internal hemorrhaging; plasma loss from severe burns; and severe dehydration from vomiting, diarrhea, or profuse perspiration. The first priority in hypovolemic shock is to control bleeding. A patient in hypovolemic shock must have the volume of fluid that was lost replaced and must be transported to an emergency care facility immediately.

Cardiogenic Shock

Cardiogenic shock is caused by the failure of the heart to pump blood adequately to all of the body's vital organs. This type of shock occurs when the heart has been injured or damaged. Cardiogenic shock is most frequently seen with MI. Other causes include dysrhythmias, severe congestive heart failure, acute valvular damage, and pulmonary embolism. When a patient develops cardiogenic shock, it is difficult to reverse and has a high fatality rate (80% to 90%).

Neurogenic Shock

Neurogenic shock occurs when the nervous system is unable to control the diameter of the blood vessels. In normal situations, the nervous system instructs the blood vessels to constrict or dilate, which controls blood pressure. In neurogenic shock, that control is lost, and the blood vessels dilate, causing the blood to pool in peripheral areas of the body away from vital organs.

This type of shock is most often seen with brain and spinal injuries. The blood vessels become dilated, and not enough blood is present in the circulatory system to fill the dilated vessels, which causes the blood pressure to drop significantly.

Anaphylactic Shock

Anaphylactic shock is a life-threatening reaction of the body to a substance to which an individual is highly allergic. Allergens that are most apt to result in anaphylaxis are drugs (e.g., penicillin), insect venoms, foods, and allergen extracts used in hyposensitization injections.

An anaphylactic reaction causes the release of large amounts of histamine, resulting in dilation of the blood vessels throughout the entire body and a decrease in blood pressure. The symptoms of anaphylactic shock begin with sneezing, hives, itching, angioedema, erythema, and disorientation and progress to difficulty in breathing, dizziness, fainting, and loss of consciousness. Medical care should be obtained immediately because most fatalities occur within the first 2 hours.

The emergency care for anaphylactic shock is the administration of epinephrine. Because time is a factor, individuals known to have a severe allergy carry an anaphylactic emergency treatment kit that contains injectable epinephrine (Fig. 37.2) and oral antihistamines. With the kit, treatment for a severe allergic reaction can be started immediately.

Psychogenic Shock

Psychogenic shock is the least serious type of shock. It is caused by unpleasant physical or emotional stimuli, such as pain, fright, and the sight of blood. With psychogenic shock, sudden dilation of the blood vessels causes blood to pool in the abdomen and extremities. This temporarily deprives the brain of blood, causing a temporary loss of consciousness (fainting), usually lasting 1 to 2 minutes. In general, fainting occurs when an individual is in an upright position. Before fainting, the patient usually experiences some warning signals such as sudden lightheadedness, pallor, nausea, weakness, yawning, blurred vision, a feeling of warmth, and sweating.

An individual who is about to faint should be placed in a position that facilitates blood flow to the brain and told to breathe deeply. The preferred position is to move the patient into a supine position with the legs elevated approximately 12 inches and the collar and clothing loosened (Fig. 37.3). This position is not always possible, such as when a patient is seated; in this case, the patient's head should be lowered between the legs (Fig. 37.4). A patient who has fainted should be placed in the supine position with the legs elevated. It is recommended that a patient who has fainted should contact her or his provider for further evaluation.

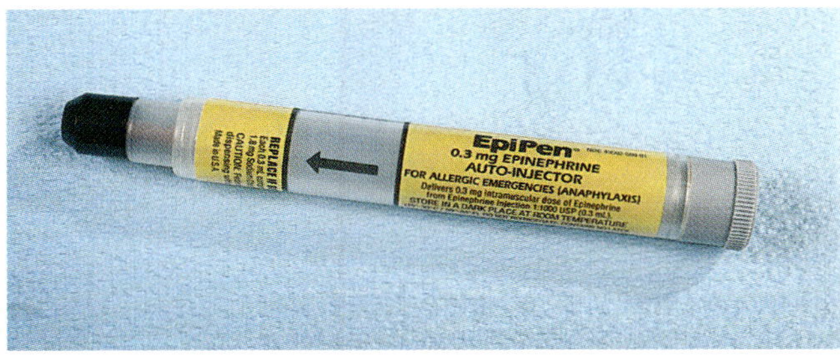

Fig. 37.2 Anaphylactic emergency epinephrine injector.

BLEEDING

Bleeding, or hemorrhaging, is the escape of blood from a severed blood vessel. Bleeding can range from very minor to very serious, leading to shock and death. The amount of blood that can be lost before bleeding becomes life-threatening varies according to each individual. In general, loss of 25% to 40% of an individual's total blood volume can be fatal. This equates to approximately 2 to 4 pints of blood for the average adult.

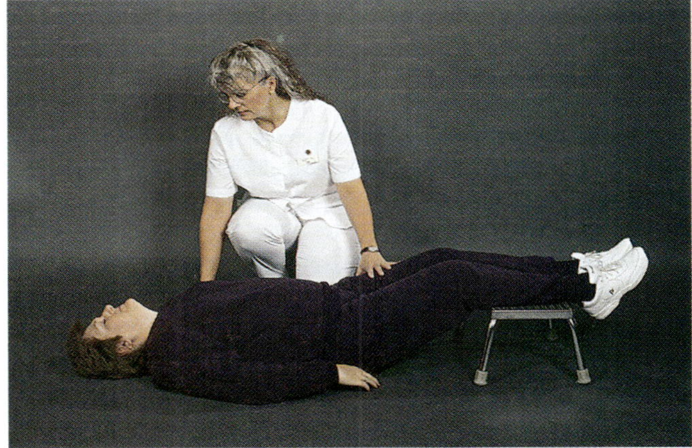

Fig. 37.3 Prevention and treatment of fainting.

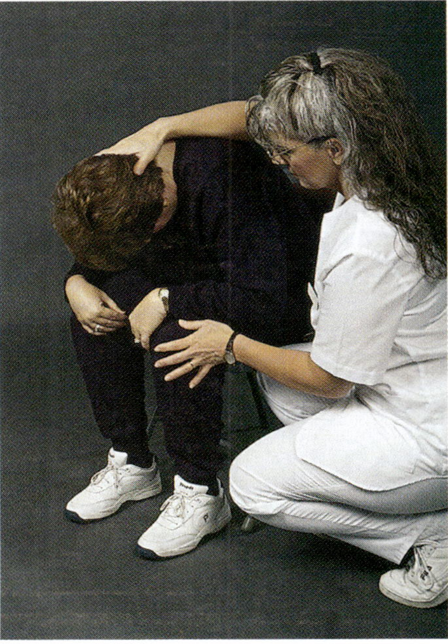

Fig. 37.4 Prevention of fainting.

External Bleeding

External bleeding is bleeding that can be seen coming from a wound. Common examples of external bleeding include bleeding from open fractures, lacerations, and the nose. Individuals with serious external bleeding exhibit the following symptoms: obvious bleeding, restlessness, cold and clammy skin, thirst, increased and thready pulse, rapid and shallow respirations, a drop in blood pressure (a late symptom), and decreasing levels of consciousness. Three types of external bleeding can be classified according to the type of blood vessel that has been injured: capillary, venous, and arterial.

Capillary Bleeding

Capillary bleeding, the most common type of external bleeding, consists of a slow oozing of bright red blood. This type of bleeding occurs with minor cuts, scratches, and abrasions.

Venous Bleeding

Venous bleeding occurs when a vein has been punctured or severed. This type of bleeding is characterized by a slow and steady flow of dark red blood.

Arterial Bleeding

Arterial bleeding, the most serious type of external bleeding, occurs when an artery is punctured or severed. It is the least common type of bleeding because arteries are situated deeper in the body and are protected by bone. Arterial bleeding is characterized by bright red blood that spurts. The arteries most frequently involved in accidents are the carotid, brachial, radial, and femoral arteries.

Emergency Care for External Bleeding

The most effective way to control bleeding is to apply direct pressure to the bleeding site. The pressure functions by slowing down or stopping the flow of blood. The amount of pressure required depends on the type of bleeding. A small amount of pressure is usually sufficient to control capillary bleeding, whereas significant pressure is often required to control arterial bleeding.

If bleeding cannot be controlled with direct pressure, a pressure point can be used. A **pressure point** is a site on the body where an artery lies close to the surface of the skin and can be compressed against an underlying bone. Fig. 37.5 illustrates pressure points. Using a pressure point helps slow

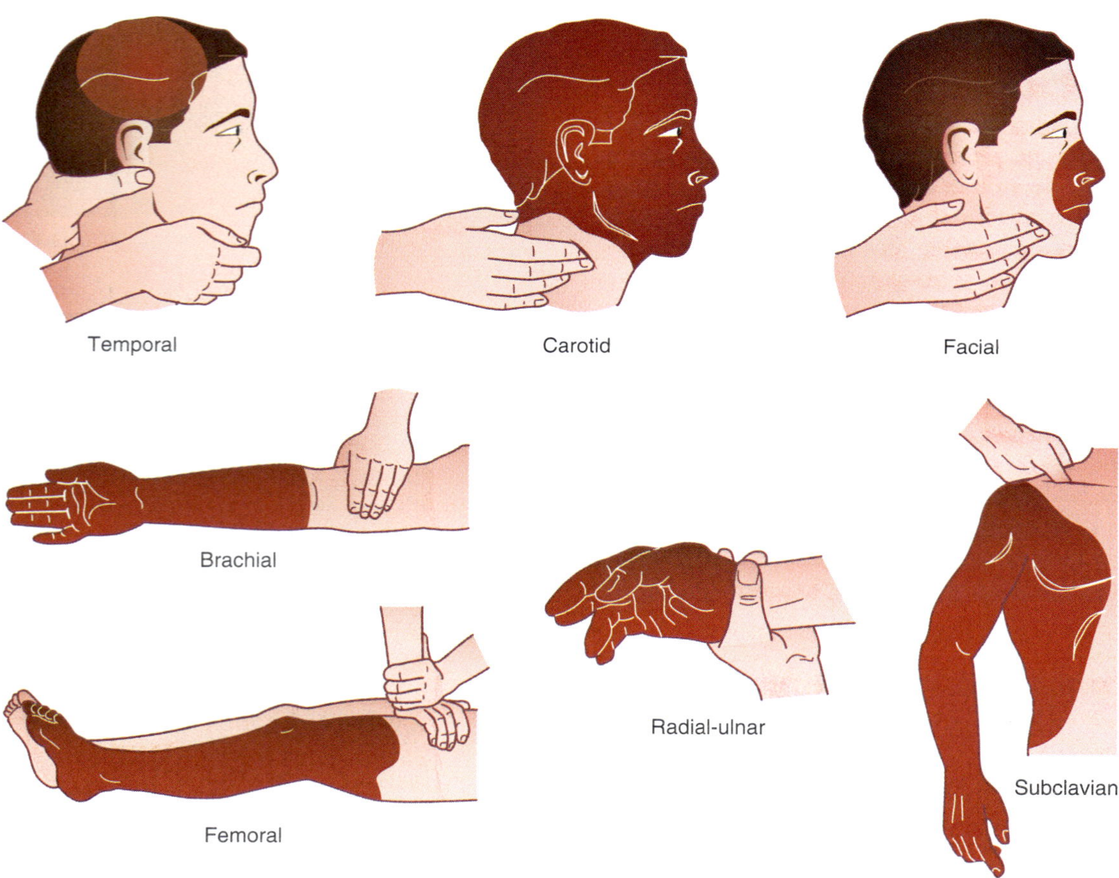

Fig. 37.5 Locations of pressure points. Shaded areas show the regions in which bleeding may be controlled by pressure at the points indicated. (From Miller BF, Keane CB: *Encyclopedia and dictionary of medicine, nursing, and allied health*, ed 7, Philadelphia, 2003, Saunders.)

or stop the flow of blood from the wound. The pressure points used most often are found on the brachial and femoral arteries. The brachial artery is located on the inside of the upper arm midway between the elbow and the shoulder. Squeezing the brachial artery helps control severe bleeding in the arm. The femoral artery is located in the groin, and squeezing helps control severe bleeding in the leg.

The specific steps for controlling bleeding are as follows:

1. Apply direct pressure to the wound with a clean covering such as a large, thick gauze dressing (Fig. 37.6A). If gauze is unavailable, a clean material such as a sanitary napkin, washcloth, handkerchief, or sock can be used. If the wound is located on an extremity, elevate the limb while continuing to apply direct pressure.
2. Apply additional dressings if needed. If the dressing soaks through, apply another dressing over the first one, and continue to apply pressure (Fig. 37.6B). (Never remove a dressing after it has been applied because this could result in more bleeding.) If bleeding cannot be controlled with direct pressure, apply pressure to the appropriate pressure point while continuing to apply direct local pressure.
3. Apply a pressure bandage. When bleeding has been controlled, apply a bandage snugly over the dressing to maintain pressure on the wound (Fig. 37.6C).
4. Transport the patient to an emergency care facility, or, if the case is serious enough, activate the local EMS system.

Nosebleeds

A nosebleed, or epistaxis, is a common form of external bleeding that usually is not serious but is more of a nuisance. Nosebleeds are usually caused by an upper respiratory infection but can result from a direct blow from a blunt object, hypertension, strenuous activity, and exposure to high altitudes.

Emergency Care for a Nosebleed

1. Position the patient in a sitting position with the head tilted forward. This prevents the blood from running down the back of the throat, which may result in nausea.
2. Apply direct pressure by pinching the nostrils together (Fig. 37.7A). Do not release the pressure too soon because the bleeding may resume. Adequate clot formation usually takes about 15 minutes. An ice pack can be applied to the bridge of the nose to help control the bleeding (Fig. 37.7B). After the bleeding has stopped, tell the patient not to blow the nose for several hours because this could loosen the clot, causing the bleeding to start again.
3. If bleeding cannot be controlled, transport the patient to an emergency care facility for further treatment.

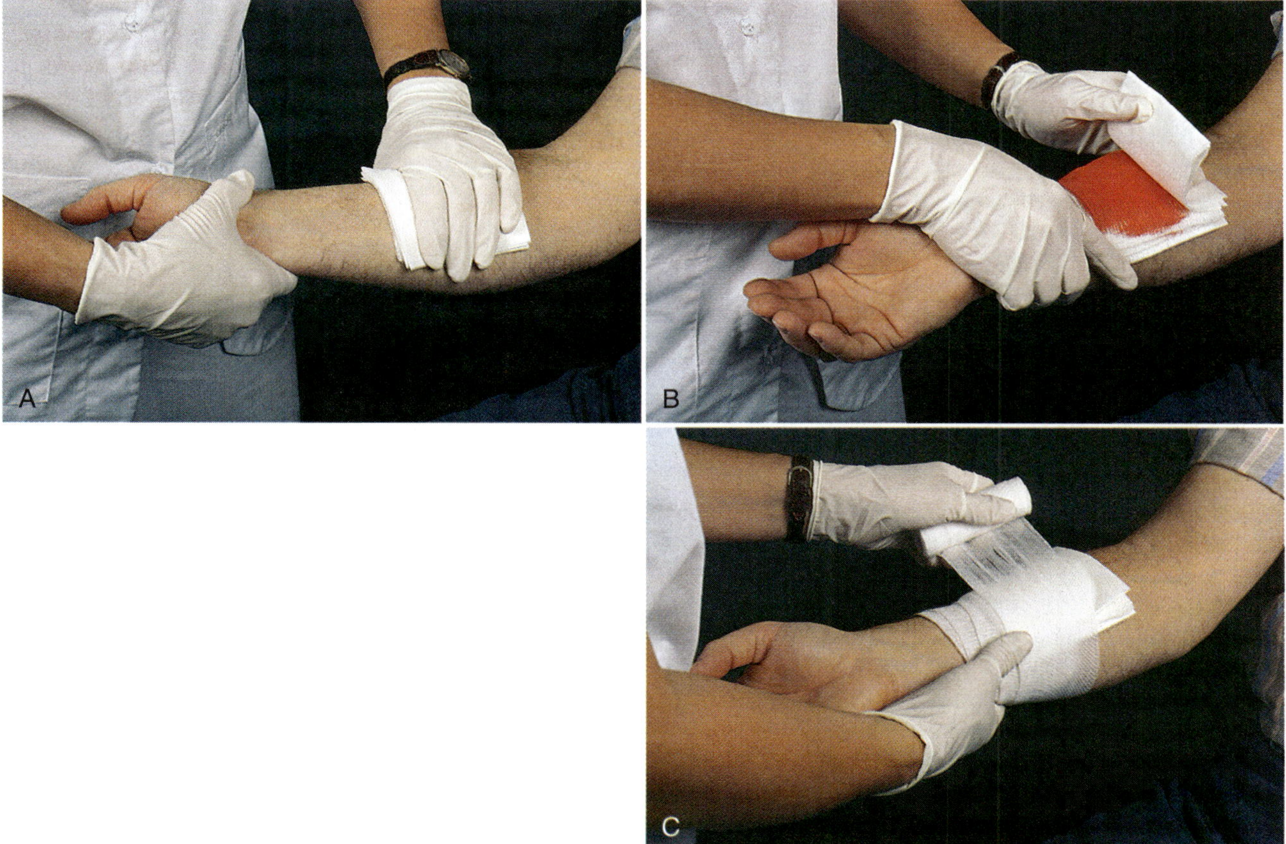

Fig. 37.6 Control of bleeding. (A) Apply direct pressure to the wound with a large, thick gauze dressing. (B) If blood soaks through the dressing, apply another dressing over the first one, and continue to apply pressure. (C) When bleeding has been controlled, apply a pressure bandage.

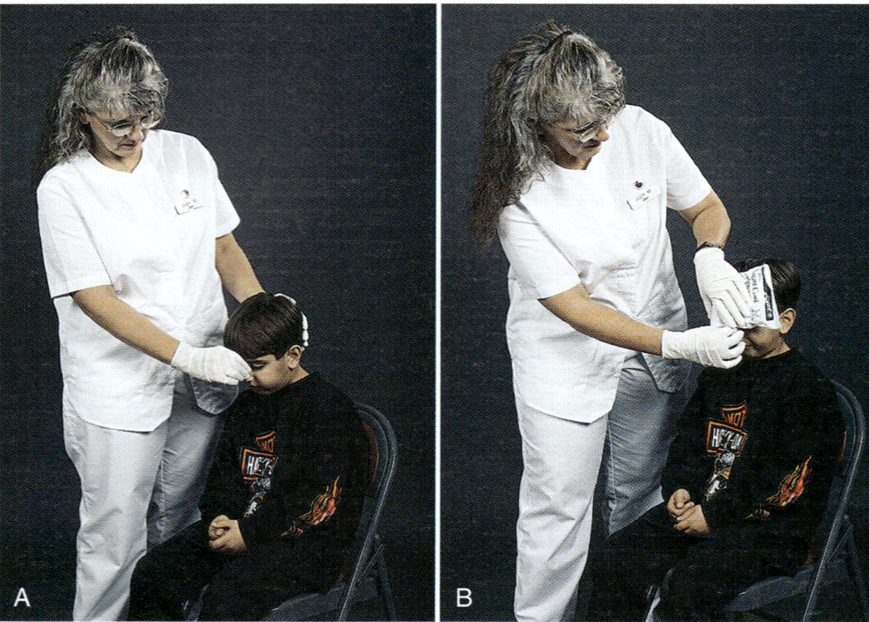

Fig. 37.7 Care of a nosebleed. (A) Apply direct pressure by pinching the nostrils together. (B) An ice pack can be applied to the bridge of the nose to help control the bleeding.

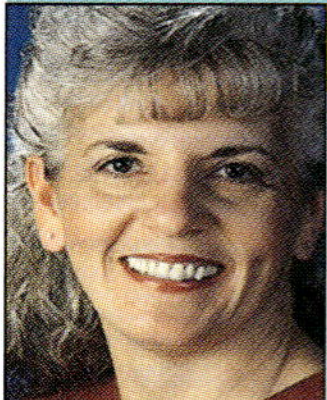

Putting It All Into Practice

My name is Judy Markins, and I work at a large clinic in the family medicine department with 12 physicians. We also have 6 to 10 physicians who do their internships and residency programs with us.

One day as I was performing my usual morning duties of getting the office ready for that day's patients, the office door opened. There stood a mother with her very ill child. I immediately took them back to a room. When I took the boy's temperature, it was 104° F. I asked the mother if she had been giving him any type of fever reducer. She said she had, but that it was not helping. Under the direction of our physician, I immediately started trying to reduce the fever. The fever started to come down, and the look of relief on the mother's face was beyond words. That was one of the many days that reinforced how satisfied I am with my career choice. ■

Internal Bleeding

Internal bleeding is bleeding that flows into a body cavity or an organ, or between tissues. It may be minor, as in the case of a contusion, or it may be very serious, such as with a severe, blunt blow to the abdomen.

Severe internal bleeding is a life-threatening emergency. Because no obvious blood flow occurs, the nature of the injury and the signs and symptoms of bleeding must be used to recognize internal bleeding. Signs and symptoms include bruises, pain, tenderness, or swelling at the site of the injury; rapid weak pulse; cold, clammy skin; nausea and vomiting; excessive thirst; a drop in blood pressure; and a decreased level of consciousness.

If a patient is suspected to have internal bleeding, the local EMS system should be activated immediately. Until emergency medical personnel arrive, the patient should be kept quiet and treated for shock.

WOUNDS

A **wound** is a break in the continuity of an external or internal surface, caused by physical means. Wounds may be open or closed.

Open Wounds

An open wound is a break in the skin surface or mucous membrane that exposes the underlying tissues. Because the skin is broken, hemorrhaging and wound contamination are primary concerns with open wounds. Open wounds include incisions, lacerations, punctures, and abrasions (Fig. 37.8). An individual with an open wound should receive prompt medical attention from a provider if any of the following occur: spurting blood; bleeding that cannot be controlled; a break in the skin that is deeper than just the outer skin layers; embedded debris or an embedded object in the wound; involvement of nerves, muscles, or tendons; and occurrence on the mouth, tongue, face, genitals, or other area where scarring would be apparent.

Incisions and Lacerations

An **incision** is a clean, smooth cut caused by a sharp cutting instrument, such as a knife, a razor, or a piece of glass. Deep incisions are accompanied by profuse bleeding; in addition,

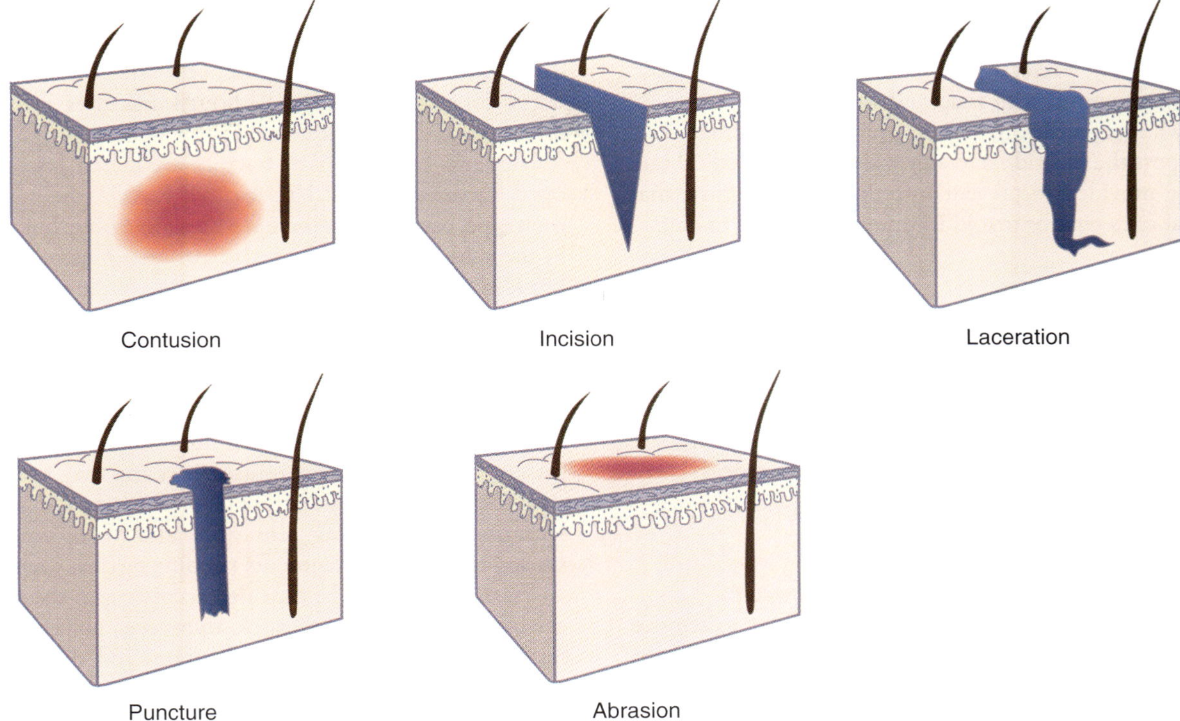

Fig. 37.8 Types of wounds.

damage to muscles, tendons, and nerves may occur. Because the edges of the wound are smooth and straight, incisions usually heal better than lacerations.

A **laceration** is a wound in which the tissues are torn apart, rather than cut, leaving ragged and irregular edges. Lacerations are caused by dull knives, large objects that have been driven into the skin, and heavy machinery. Deep lacerations result in profuse bleeding, and a scar often results from jagged tearing of the tissues.

Emergency Care for Incisions and Lacerations

Minor Incisions and Lacerations

1. Assess the length, depth, and location of the wound.
2. Control bleeding by covering the wound with a dressing and applying firm pressure.
3. Clean the wound with soap and water to remove dirt and other debris (Fig. 37.9).
4. Cover the wound with a dry, sterile dressing. Instruct the patient to check the wound for redness, swelling, discharge, or an increase in pain and to contact a provider if any of these problems occur.

Serious Incisions and Lacerations

1. Control bleeding by covering the wound with a large, thick gauze dressing and applying firm pressure. Do not clean or probe the wound because this may result in more bleeding.
2. Transport the individual to a provider, or, if the wound is serious enough, activate the local EMS system.

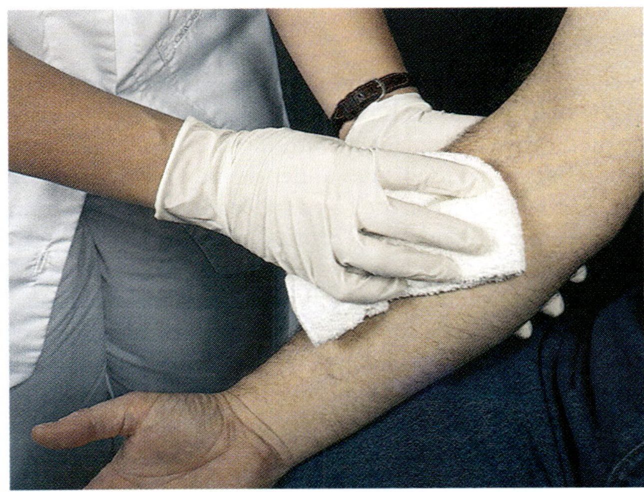

Fig. 37.9 Minor incisions and lacerations should be cleaned with soap and water to remove dirt and other debris.

Punctures

A **puncture** is a wound made by a sharp, pointed object piercing the skin layers and sometimes the underlying structures. Objects that cause a puncture wound include a nail, splinter, needle, wire, knife, bullet, and animal bite. A puncture wound has a very small external skin opening, and for this reason bleeding is usually minor. A tetanus booster may be administered because the tetanus bacteria grow best in a warm, anaerobic environment, as would be found in a puncture wound.

Emergency Care for Puncture Wounds

1. Allow the wound to bleed freely for a few minutes to help wash out bacteria.
2. Clean the wound with soap and water.
3. Apply a dry, sterile dressing to prevent contamination.
4. Transport the individual to a provider so that medical care can be provided to prevent infection and to ensure that the patient's tetanus toxoid immunization is up to date.

Abrasions

An **abrasion**, or scrape, is a wound in which the outer layers of the skin are scraped or rubbed off. Blood may ooze from ruptured capillaries; however, the bleeding usually is not severe. Abrasions are caused by falls, resulting in floor burns and skinned knees and elbows. Dirt and other debris are frequently rubbed into the wound; it is important to clean scrapes thoroughly to prevent infection.

Emergency Care for Abrasions

1. Rinse the wound with cool to lukewarm water.
2. Wash the wound gently with soap and water to remove dirt and other debris. A provider should remove embedded debris.
3. Cover large abrasions with a dry, sterile dressing. Small minor abrasions do not require a dressing.
4. Instruct the patient to check the wound for signs of inflammation, including redness, swelling, discharge, or increased pain, and to contact a provider if they occur.

Closed Wounds

A closed wound involves an injury to the underlying tissues of the body without a break in the skin surface or mucous membrane; an example is a contusion or a bruise. A contusion results when the tissues under the skin are injured (see Fig. 37.8); it is often caused by a sudden blow or force from a blunt object. Blood vessels rupture, allowing blood to seep into the tissues, which results in a bluish discoloration of the skin and swelling. Most contusions heal without special treatment, but cold compresses may reduce bleeding, reduce swelling and discoloration, and relieve pain. After several days, the color of the contusion turns greenish or yellow owing to oxidation of blood pigments. Contusions commonly occur with injuries such as fractures, sprains, strains, and black eyes. These injuries, along with the corresponding emergency care, are discussed next.

MUSCULOSKELETAL INJURIES

The musculoskeletal system consists of all the bones, muscles, tendons, and ligaments of the body. Injuries that affect the musculoskeletal system include fractures, dislocations, sprains, and strains.

Fracture

A **fracture** is any break in a bone. The break may range in severity from a simple chip or a crack to a complete break or shattering of the bone. Fractures can occur anywhere on the surface of the bone, including across the surface of a joint such as the wrist or ankle. Fractures result from a direct blow, a fall, bone disease, or a twisting force as may occur in a sports injury. Although fractures often cause severe pain, they are seldom life-threatening.

The two basic types of fracture are closed fractures and open fractures (Fig. 37.10). A *closed fracture,* the most common type, occurs when there is a break in a bone but no break in the skin over the fracture site. An *open fracture* involves a break in the bone along with penetration of the overlying skin surface. Open fractures are more serious owing to the risk of blood loss and contamination leading to infection.

The signs and symptoms of a fracture include pain and tenderness, deformity, swelling and discoloration, loss of function of the body part, and numbness or tingling. The patient usually guards the injured part and may relay to you that they heard the bone break or snap or felt a grating sensation. This grating sensation, known as **crepitus**, is caused by the bone fragments rubbing against each other.

Fractures also can be classified according to the nature of the break: impacted, greenstick, transverse, oblique, comminuted, and spiral. Fig. 37.11 illustrates and describes these types of fracture.

Dislocation

A **dislocation** is an injury in which one end of a bone making up a joint is separated or displaced from its normal position. A dislocation is caused by a violent pulling or pushing force

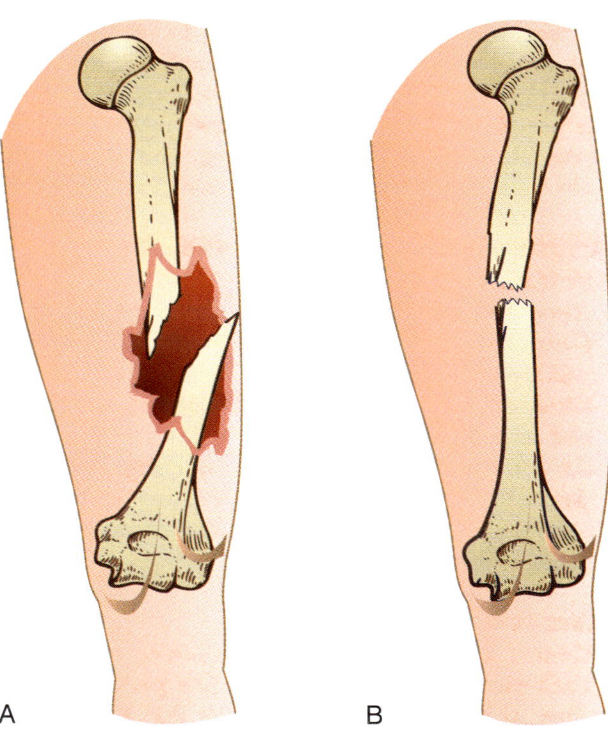

Fig. 37.10 Fractures. (A) Open fracture. (B) Closed fracture. (From Connolly JF: *DePalma's The management of fractures and dislocations: an atlas*, Philadelphia, 1981, Saunders.)

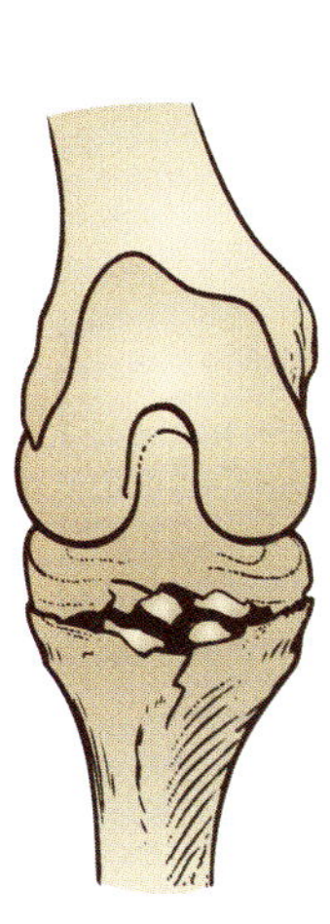

Impacted fracture
The broken ends of the bones are forcefully jammed together.

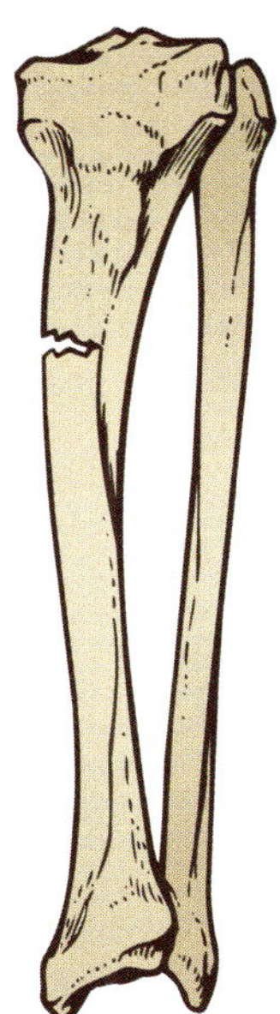

Greenstick fracture
The bone remains intact on one side, but broken on the other, in much the same way that a "green stick" bends; common in children, whose bones are more flexible than those of adults.

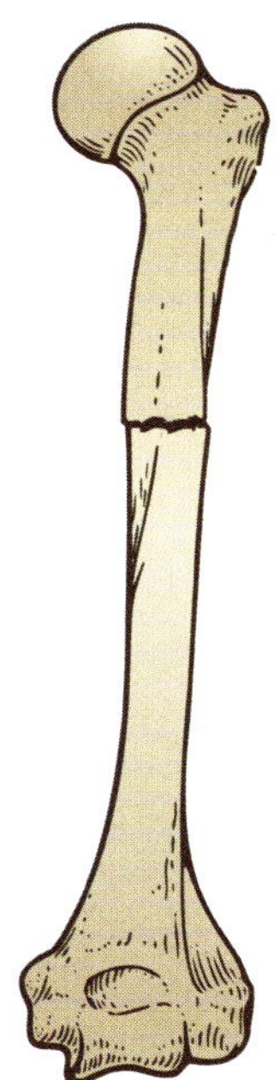

Transverse fracture
The break occurs perpendicular to the long axis of the bone.

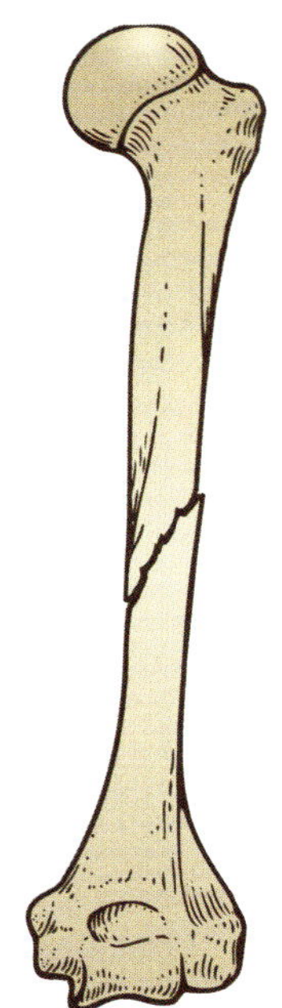

Oblique fracture
The break occurs diagonally across the bone; generally the result of a twisting force.

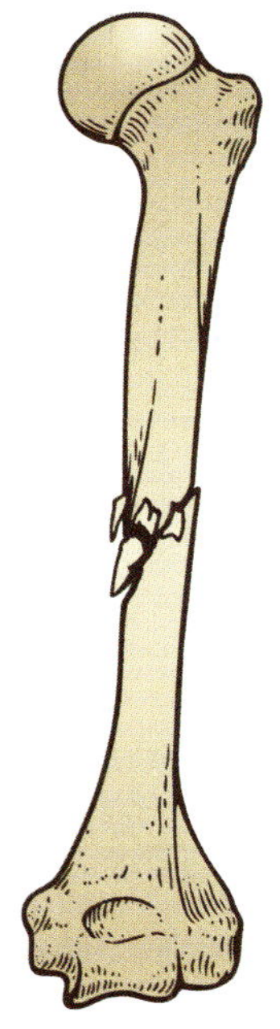

Comminuted fracture
The bone is splintered or shattered into three or more fragments; usually caused by an extremely traumatic direct force.

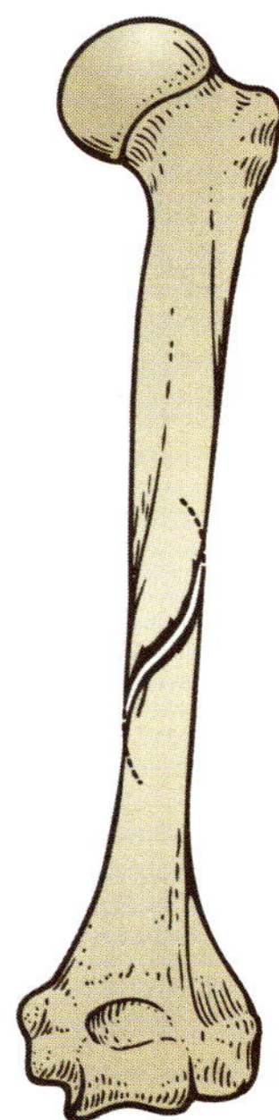

Spiral fracture
The bone is broken into a spiral or S-shape; caused by a twisting force.

Fig. 37.11 Types of fractures.

that tears the ligaments. Dislocations usually result from falls, sports injuries, and motor vehicle accidents. Signs and symptoms of a dislocation include significant deformity of the joint, pain and swelling, and loss of function.

Sprain

A **sprain** is the tearing of ligaments at a joint. Sprains may result from a fall, a sports injury, or a motor vehicle accident. The joints most often sprained are the ankle, knee, wrist, and fingers. Signs and symptoms of a sprain include pain, swelling, and discoloration. Sprains can vary in seriousness from mild to severe, depending on the amount of damage to the ligaments.

Strain

A **strain** is the stretching and tearing of muscles or tendons. Strains are most likely to occur when an individual lifts a heavy object or overworks a muscle, as during exercise. The muscles most commonly strained are those of the neck, back, thigh, and calf. Signs and symptoms of a strain are pain and swelling. Strains do not usually cause the intense symptoms associated with fractures, dislocations, and sprains.

Emergency Care for a Fracture

It is often difficult to determine whether a patient has a fracture, a dislocation, or a sprain because the symptoms of these injuries are similar. Because of this, any serious musculoskeletal injury to an extremity should be treated as though it were a fracture.

The primary goal of emergency care for a fracture is to immobilize the body part. Immobilization reduces pain and prevents further damage. A **splint** is any item that immobilizes a body part. In an emergency situation, items such as a length of wood, cardboard, or rolled newspapers or magazines can be used for splinting. The splint should be padded with a soft material such as a rolled-up towel.

The body part should be splinted in the position in which you found it. Severely angulated fractures may have to be straightened before splinting, however. If you attempt to straighten an angulated fracture, be careful not to force the affected part. A dislocated bone end can become "locked" and would have to be realigned at the hospital. If you straighten an angulated bone and encounter pain, stop and splint it in the position in which you found it. The splint also should immobilize the area above and below the injury. In splinting an injured wrist, the hand and forearm also should be immobilized (Fig. 37.12A). In splinting an injury to the shaft of the bone, the joints above and below the injury should be immobilized. In splinting the forearm, the elbow joint and the wrist joint should be immobilized.

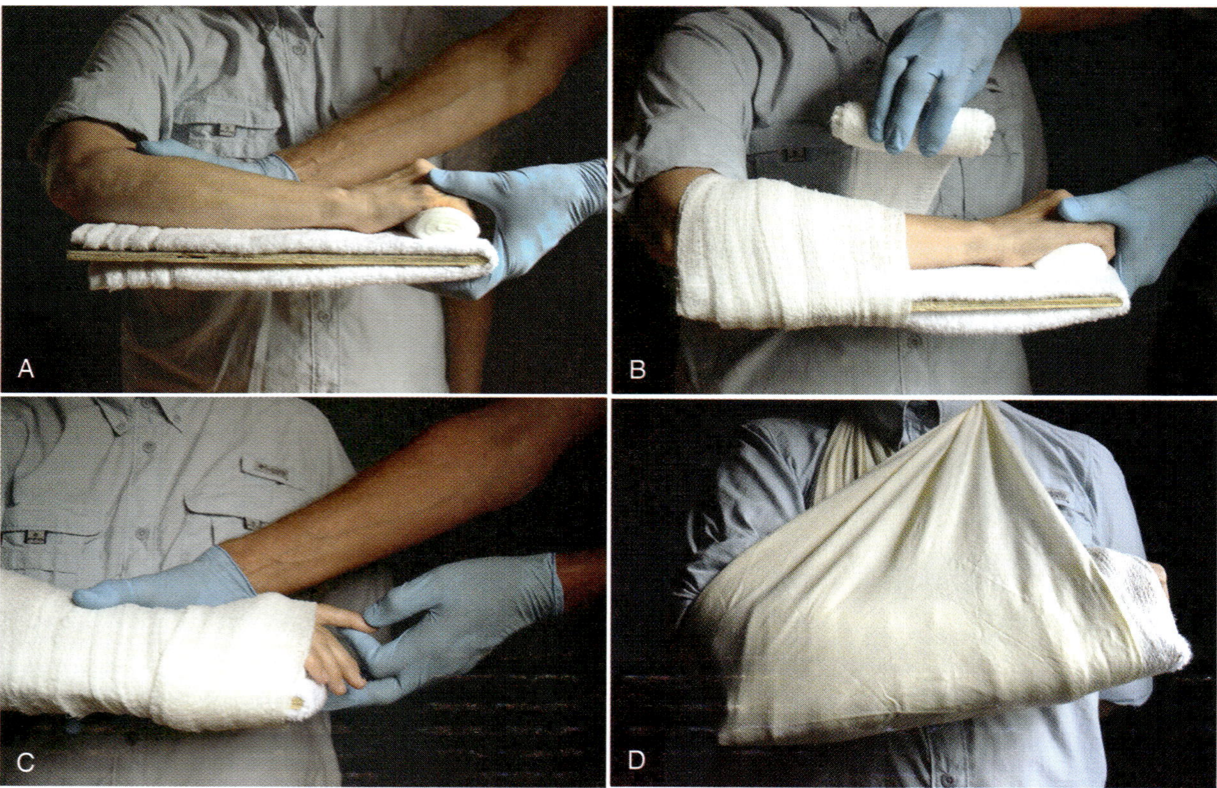

Fig. 37.12 Emergency care of a fracture. (A) The splint should immobilize the area above and below the injury. (B) The splint is held in place with a roller gauze bandage. (C) After the splint is applied, the pulse below the splint should be checked to ensure that the splint has not been applied too tightly. (D) A sling can be used to elevate the extremity to reduce swelling.

The splint should be held in place with a roller gauze bandage or other suitable material, such as neckties, scarves, or strips of cloth (Fig. 37.12B). The splint should be applied snugly, but not so tightly that it interferes with proper circulation. After applying the splint, check the pulse below the splint to ensure the splint has not been applied too tightly. If you cannot detect a pulse, immediately loosen the splint until you can feel the pulse (Fig. 37.12C).

Whenever possible, elevate an injured extremity after it has been immobilized to reduce swelling (Fig. 37.12D). An ice pack also can be applied to the injured part. Cold limits the accumulation of fluid in the body tissues by constricting blood vessels and reducing leakage of fluid into the tissues. In addition, cold temporarily relieves pain through its anesthetic or numbing effect, which reduces stimulation of nerve receptors.

After you have properly immobilized the injury, transport the patient to an emergency care facility, or if the injury is serious enough, activate the local EMS system. In any situation in which an injury to the spine is suspected, activate EMS.

BURNS

A **burn** is an injury to the tissues caused by exposure to thermal, chemical, electrical, or radioactive agents. The severity of a burn depends on the depth of the burn, the percentage of the body involved, the type of agent causing the burn, the duration and intensity of the agent, and the part of the body affected. Burns are classified according to the depth of tissue injury, as illustrated in Fig. 37.13.

Superficial (First-Degree) Burn

A superficial burn is the most common type of burn. It involves only the top layer of skin, the epidermis. With this type of burn, the skin appears red, is warm and dry to the touch, and is usually painful. Sunburn is a common example of a superficial burn. A superficial burn heals in 2 to 5 days of its own accord and does not cause scarring.

Partial-Thickness (Second-Degree) Burn

A partial-thickness burn involves the epidermis and extends into the dermis but does not pass through the dermis to the underlying tissues. The burned area usually appears red, mottled, and blistered. In most cases, the blisters should not be broken because they provide a protective barrier against infection. Partial-thickness burns are usually very painful, and the area often swells. This type of burn usually heals within 3 to 4 weeks and may result in some scarring.

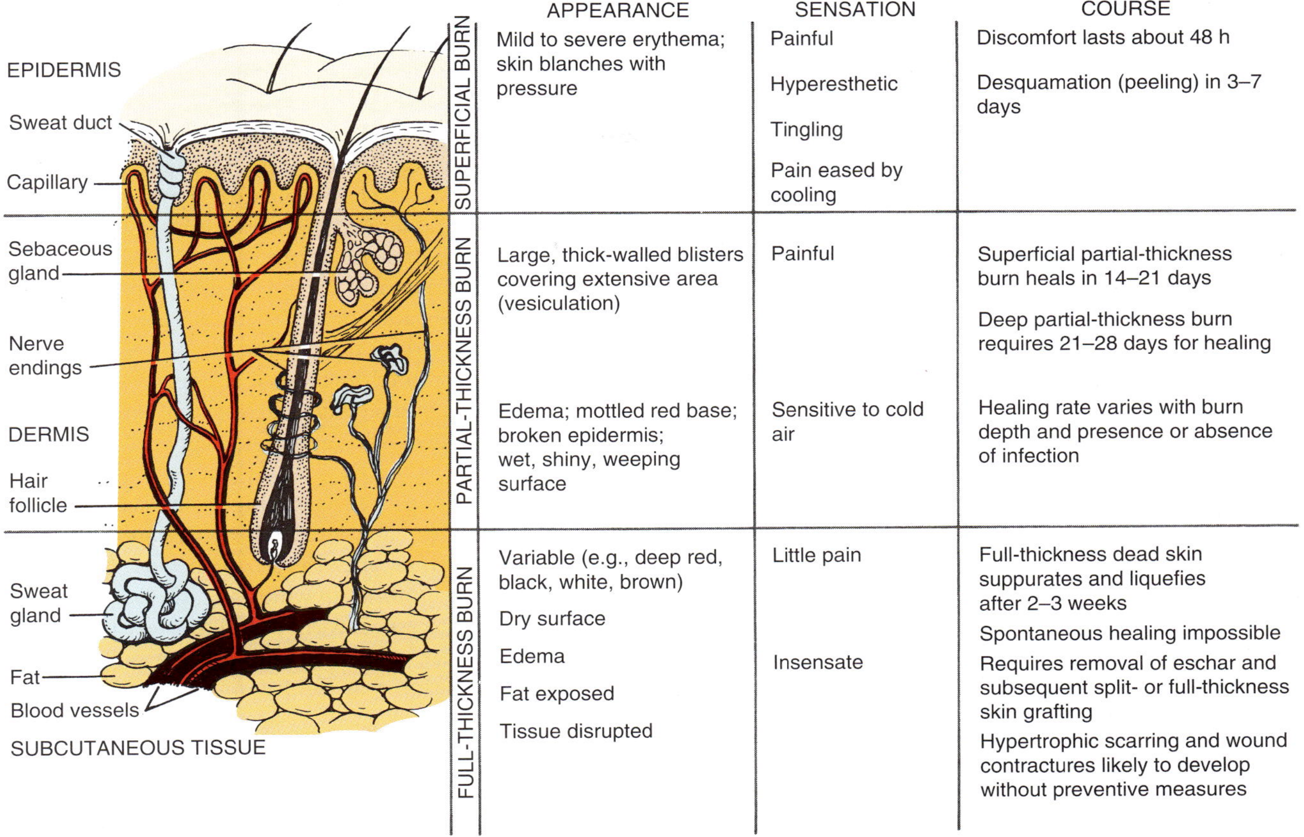

	APPEARANCE	SENSATION	COURSE
SUPERFICIAL BURN	Mild to severe erythema; skin blanches with pressure	Painful Hyperesthetic Tingling Pain eased by cooling	Discomfort lasts about 48 h Desquamation (peeling) in 3–7 days
PARTIAL-THICKNESS BURN	Large, thick-walled blisters covering extensive area (vesiculation)	Painful	Superficial partial-thickness burn heals in 14–21 days Deep partial-thickness burn requires 21–28 days for healing
	Edema; mottled red base; broken epidermis; wet, shiny, weeping surface	Sensitive to cold air	Healing rate varies with burn depth and presence or absence of infection
FULL-THICKNESS BURN	Variable (e.g., deep red, black, white, brown) Dry surface Edema Fat exposed Tissue disrupted	Little pain Insensate	Full-thickness dead skin suppurates and liquefies after 2–3 weeks Spontaneous healing impossible Requires removal of eschar and subsequent split- or full-thickness skin grafting Hypertrophic scarring and wound contractures likely to develop without preventive measures

Fig. 37.13 Types of burns. (From Polaski AL, Tatro SE: *Luckmann's Core principles and practice of medical-surgical nursing*, Philadelphia, 1996, Saunders.)

Full-Thickness (Third-Degree) Burn

A full-thickness burn completely destroys the epidermis and the dermis and extends into the underlying tissues, such as fat, muscle, bone, and nerves. The affected area appears charred black, brown, and cherry red, with the damaged tissues underneath often pearly white. The patient may experience intense pain; however, if damage to the nerve endings is substantial, the patient may feel no pain at all. During the healing process, dense scars typically result. Infection is a major concern, and the patient must be carefully monitored.

Thermal Burns

Thermal burns usually occur in the home, often as a result of fire, scalding water, or coming into contact with a hot object such as a stove or curling iron.

Emergency Care for Major Thermal Burns

1. Stop the burning process to prevent further injury. If the individual is on fire, wrap them in a blanket, rug, or heavy coat and push them to the ground to help smother the flames. If a covering is unavailable, shout at the individual to drop to the ground and roll around to smother the flames.
2. Cool the burn, using large amounts of cool water from a faucet or garden hose. Do not use ice or ice water because this may result in further tissue damage; it also causes heat loss from the body. If the burn covers a large surface area (greater than 20%), do not use water. The loss of a large amount of skin surface places the patient at risk for hypothermia (generalized body cooling). With large surface area burns, you may cool the most painful areas, but not an area greater than 20% of the body (e.g., two arms, one leg).
3. Activate the local EMS system.
4. Cover the patient with a clean, nonfuzzy material such as a tablecloth or sheet. The cover maintains warmth, reduces pain, and reduces the risk of contamination. Do not apply any type of ointment, antiseptic, or other substance to the burned area.

Emergency Care for Minor Thermal Burns

1. Immerse the affected area in cool water for 2 to 5 minutes. Be careful not to break any blisters because they provide a protective barrier against infection.
2. Cover the burn with a dry sterile dressing.

Chemical Burns

Chemical burns occur in the workplace and at home. The severity of the burn depends on the type and strength of the chemical and the duration of exposure to the chemical. The main difference between a chemical burn and a thermal burn is that the chemical continues to burn the patient's tissues as long as it is on the skin. Because of this factor, it is important to remove the chemical from the skin as quickly as possible and then to activate the local EMS system.

Liquid chemical burns should be treated by flooding the area with large amounts of cool running water until emergency personnel arrive. If a solid substance such as lime has been spilled on the patient, it should be brushed off before flooding the area with water. This is because a dry chemical may be activated by contact with water.

SEIZURES

A **seizure** is a sudden episode of involuntary muscular contractions and relaxation, often accompanied by changes in sensation, behavior, and level of consciousness. A seizure results when the normal electrical activity of the brain is disturbed, causing the brain cells to become irritated and overactive. Specific conditions that trigger a seizure include epilepsy, encephalitis, a recent or old head injury, high fever in infants and young children, drug and alcohol abuse or withdrawal, eclampsia associated with toxemia of pregnancy, diabetic conditions, and heatstroke.

Seizures are classified as partial or generalized according to the location of the abnormal electrical activity in the brain. *Partial seizures* are the most common type, occurring in approximately 80% of individuals who have seizures. With a partial seizure the abnormal electrical activity is localized into specific areas of the brain; only the brain functions in those areas are affected.

Partial seizures are further classified as simple or complex, depending on whether the patient's level of consciousness is affected. The symptoms of a *simple partial seizure* include twitching or jerking in just one part of the body. This type of seizure lasts less than 1 minute, and the patient remains awake and alert during the seizure. With a *complex partial seizure* the patient's level of consciousness is affected, and the patient has little or no memory of the seizure afterward. Symptoms of this type of seizure include abnormal behavior such as confusion, a glassy stare, aimless wandering, lip smacking or chewing, and fidgeting with clothing, which lasts from a few seconds to a minute or two. A simple and a complex partial seizure can progress to a generalized seizure.

With a *generalized seizure* the abnormal electrical activity spreads through the entire brain. The best-known type of generalized seizure is a *tonic-clonic seizure* (formerly known as a *grand mal seizure*). With this type of seizure, the patient exhibits tonic-clonic activity followed by a postictal state. During the tonic phase, the patient suddenly loses consciousness and exhibits rigid muscular contractions, which result in odd posturing of the body. Respirations are inhibited, which may cause cyanosis around the mouth and lips. The patient may lose control of the bladder or bowels, resulting in involuntary urination and defecation. The tonic phase lasts 30 seconds, followed by the clonic phase. During the clonic phase, the patient's body jerks about violently. The patient's jaw muscles contract, which may cause the patient to bite the tongue or lips. The final phase of the seizure is the postictal state, lasting 10 to 30 minutes, in which the patient exhibits a depressed level of consciousness, is disoriented, and often has a headache. The patient typically has little or no memory of the seizure and feels confused and exhausted for several hours after the seizure.

In some instances of seizures, particularly in patients with epilepsy, an aura precedes the seizure. An *aura* is a sensation perceived by the patient that something is about to happen; examples include a strange taste, smell, or sound; a twitch; or a feeling of dizziness or anxiety. An aura provides the patient with a warning signal that a seizure is about to begin.

Although seizures are frightening to observe, they usually are not as bad as they look. Most patients fully recover within a few minutes after the seizure begins. An exception to this is *status epilepticus*, in which seizures are prolonged or come in rapid succession without full recovery of consciousness between them. Status epilepticus is a potentially life-threatening situation that requires immediate medical care.

Emergency Care for Seizures

The most important criterion in caring for a patient in a seizure is to protect the patient from harm. Remove hazards from the immediate area to protect the patient from injury sustained by striking a surrounding object. Do not restrain the patient. Loosen restrictive clothing that may interfere with breathing, such as collars, neckties, scarves, and jewelry. The seizure will occur no matter what you do; restraining the patient could seriously injure the patient's muscles, bones, or joints. Do not insert anything into the patient's mouth during the seizure because this could damage the teeth or mouth or interfere with breathing. In addition, it could trigger the gag reflex, causing the patient to vomit and possibly aspirate the vomitus into the lungs. If the patient vomits, roll them onto one side so that the vomitus can drain from the mouth.

If you are uncertain as to the cause of the seizure, or if you suspect that the patient is having status epilepticus, activate your local EMS system immediately. Otherwise, transport the patient to an emergency medical care facility for further evaluation and treatment after the seizure is over.

POISONING

A **poison** is any substance that causes illness, injury, or death if it enters the body. Most poisoning episodes occur in the home, are accidental, and occur in children younger than 5 years. Poisoning usually involves common substances, such as cleaning agents, medications, and pesticides. For most poisonous substances, the reaction is more serious in children and the elderly than in adults. A poison can enter the body in four ways: ingestion, inhalation, absorption, or injection.

Poison control centers are valuable resources that are easily accessible to medical personnel and the community. More than 500 regional poison control centers have been established across the United States; most are located in the emergency departments of large hospitals. These centers are staffed by personnel who have access to information about almost all poisonous substances. Most centers are staffed 24 hours a day, and calls are toll-free. In addition, a national Poison Help number (1-800-222-1222) can be called 24 hours a day.

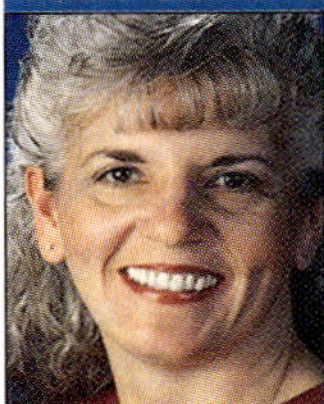

Memories *from* Practicum

Judy Markins: As it turned out, one of my most terrible moments during my practicum was a great learning experience. I was drawing blood (which was not my favorite procedure) and missed the vein—not once, but twice. You could see the sweat under my gloves. My stomach was in my throat, and I did not want to try again. Thank goodness my patient was understanding, and I had an excellent practicum supervisor. She insisted that I try again, encouraging me that I could do it and suggesting some techniques that she had learned from her many years of experience. I got the blood specimen, along with some new-found confidence.

In most situations, someone can help you if you have questions. Use your resources when you need to. Be honest, know your procedure, and have confidence in yourself. ■

What Would You Do? What Would You *Not* Do?

Case Study 1

Beth Eaton calls the office. She says that she thinks her 3-year-old daughter, Olivia, has eaten some chewable vitamins. Beth was taking a shower, and when she came out, Olivia was holding an empty vitamin bottle and saying "Good candy." Beth says she does not know how Olivia got the childproof top off. She thinks the bottle was about a third of the way full. Beth says that Olivia is complaining that her tummy hurts. Beth says she has syrup of ipecac and wants to know whether she should give some to Olivia. ■

Ingested Poisons

Poisons that are ingested enter the body by being swallowed. Ingestion is the most common route of entry for poisons. Examples of poisons that are often ingested include cleaning products, pesticides, contaminated food, petroleum products (e.g., gasoline, kerosene), and poisonous plants. Abuse of drugs, alcohol, or both also can result in poisoning from an accidental or intentional overdose. Signs and symptoms of poisoning by ingestion are based on the specific substance that has been consumed but often include strange odors, burns or stains around the mouth, nausea, vomiting, abdominal pain, diarrhea, difficulty in breathing, profuse perspiration, excessive salivation, dilated or constricted pupils, unconsciousness, and convulsions.

Emergency Care for Poisoning by Ingestion

1. Acquire as much information as possible about the type of poison, the amount ingested, and when it was ingested.
2. Call your poison control center or local EMS. *Never* induce vomiting unless directed to do so by a medical authority. Vomiting is often contraindicated—for instance, when an individual is unconscious, has swallowed a petroleum product, or has swallowed a corrosive poison such as a strong acid or base. Corrosive poisons may cause more injury to the esophagus, throat, and mouth if they are vomited back up. If it is available, you may be directed by the poison control center to administer activated charcoal. Activated charcoal is used to absorb the poison that remains in the stomach and prevents absorption by the intestine.
3. If the individual vomits, collect some of the vomitus for transport with the patient to the hospital for analysis by a toxicologist, if necessary. In addition, bring along containers of any substances ingested, such as empty medication bottles and household cleaner containers, because the label of the container often lists the ingredients in the product.

Inhaled Poisons

A poison that is inhaled is breathed into the body in the form of gas, vapor, or spray. The most commonly inhaled poison is carbon monoxide, such as from car exhausts, malfunctioning furnaces, and fires. Other inhaled poisons include carbon dioxide from wells and sewers and fumes from household products such as glues, paints, insect sprays, and cleaners (e.g., ammonia, chlorine). Signs and symptoms of inhaled poisoning often include severe headache; nausea and vomiting; coughing or wheezing; shortness of breath; chest pain or tightness; facial burns; burning of the mouth, nose, eyes, throat, or chest; cyanosis; confusion; dizziness; and unconsciousness.

Emergency Care for Inhaled Poisons

1. Determine whether it is safe to approach the patient. Toxic gases and fumes also can be dangerous to individuals helping the patient.
2. Remove the individual from the source of the poison and into fresh air as quickly as possible.
3. Call your poison control center or local EMS.
4. If oxygen is available, you may be directed to administer it under the supervision of a provider. Oxygen is the primary antidote for carbon monoxide poisoning.

Absorbed Poisons

A poison that is absorbed enters the body through the skin. Examples of absorbed poisons include fertilizers and pesticides used for lawn and garden care. Signs and symptoms of absorbed poisoning include irritation, burning and itching, burning of the skin or eyes, headache, and abnormal pulse or respiration or both.

Emergency Care for Absorbed Poisons

1. Remove the patient from the source of the poison. Avoid contact with the toxic substance.
2. Call your poison control center or local EMS. In most cases, you will be instructed to flood the area that has been exposed to the poison with water. Dry chemicals should be brushed from the skin before flooding with water.

What Would You Do? What Would You *Not* Do?

Case Study 2

Anita Alland calls the office and says that her son, Garon, was stung by a yellow jacket about an hour ago while mowing the grass. She says that his entire arm and back are red and swollen, and that he has a lot of redness and swelling around his eyes. Garon is itching all over and seems fuzzy headed. Anita says she has never seen anyone do this after being stung. She says she had Garon take a cold shower to see if it would help. After the shower, he started feeling faint and dizzy, and now he is having trouble breathing. Anita wants to know whether she can bring him to the office so that he can be seen by the physician. ■

Injected Poisons

An injected poison enters the body through bites, through stings, or from a needle. Examples of injected poisons include the venom of insects, spiders, snakes, and marine creatures such as jellyfish and substances from the bite of a rabid animal. The poison also may be a drug that is self-administered with a hypodermic needle, such as heroin. General signs and symptoms of injected poisoning include an altered state of awareness; evidence of stings, bites, or puncture marks on the skin; mottled skin; localized pain or itching; burning, swelling, or blistering at the site; difficulty in breathing; abnormal pulse rate; nausea and vomiting; and anaphylactic shock.

Insect Stings

It is estimated that 1 of every 125 Americans is allergic to insect stings. Approximately 40 people in the United States die every year from a severe allergic reaction to insect stings. The incidence of deaths is low because most people know they need to obtain medical attention immediately if an allergic reaction begins.

Almost all of the insects whose venom can cause allergic reactions belong to a group called *Hymenoptera*, which includes honeybees and bumblebees, wasps, yellow jackets, and hornets. When a honeybee stings, its stinger remains embedded in the victim's skin, causing the bee to die as it tries to tear itself away. Wasps, yellow jackets, and hornets are more aggressive than bees and can sting repeatedly. Hornets are the most aggressive of the group and may sting even when not provoked. Yellow jackets are close behind in aggressiveness, and wasps usually sting only if someone interferes with them near their nest.

If an insect sting does not cause an allergic reaction within 30 minutes, chances are excellent that no problem will occur. A normal reaction to an insect sting includes localized pain, redness, swelling, and itching lasting 1 to 2 days. Any generalized reaction not arising directly from the area of the sting is almost certain to be an allergic reaction, which begins with symptoms such as sneezing, hives, itching, angioedema, erythema, and disorientation and progresses to difficulty in breathing, dizziness, faintness, and loss of consciousness.

Medical care should be sought immediately because these are the symptoms of an anaphylactic reaction, and most fatalities occur within 2 hours of the sting. Because time is a factor, individuals known to have a severe allergy to insect stings carry an anaphylactic emergency treatment kit containing injectable epinephrine and oral antihistamines (see Fig. 37.2). With this kit, treatment for a severe allergic reaction can be started immediately.

Emergency Care for Insect Stings

1. Remove the stinger and attached venom sac. Scrape the stinger off the patient's skin with your fingernail or a plastic card such as a credit card (Fig. 37.14). Do not use tweezers or forceps because squeezing the venom sac may cause more venom to be injected into the patient's tissues.
2. Wash the site with soap and water.
3. Apply a cold pack to the affected area to reduce pain and swelling.
4. Observe the patient for signs of an anaphylactic reaction.

Spider Bites

Although spiders are numerous throughout the United States, most do not cause injuries or serious complications. Only two

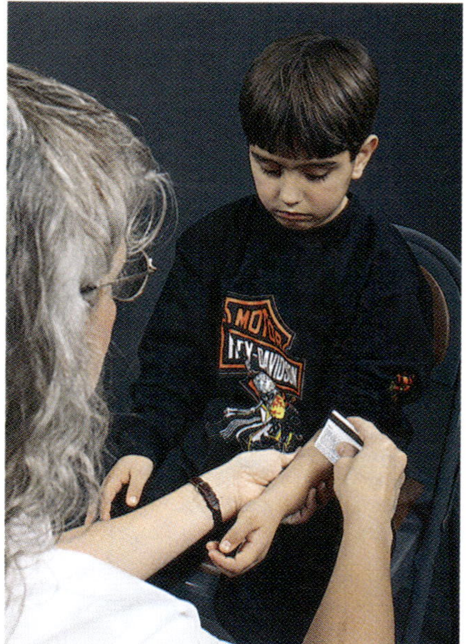

Fig. 37.14 Removing a honeybee stinger and venom sac using the edge of a credit card.

spiders have bites that cause serious or life-threatening reactions: the black widow spider and the brown recluse spider. Both of these spiders prefer dark, out-of-the-way places such as in woodpiles, in brush piles, under rocks, and in dark garages and attics. Because of this, bites usually occur on the hands and arms of individuals reaching into places where the spiders are hiding. Often the individual does not know that they have been bitten until they begin to feel ill or notice swelling and a bite mark on the skin.

The black widow spider is approximately 1 inch long and is black with a distinctive bright-red hourglass shape on its abdomen. The venom injected when this spider bites an individual is toxic to the central nervous system. Signs and symptoms of a black widow bite include swelling and a dull pain at the injection site; nausea and vomiting; a rigid, boardlike abdomen; fever; rash; and difficulty in breathing or swallowing. Although the symptoms are severe, they are not usually fatal. An antivenin is available; however, because of its undesirable and frequent side effects, it usually is administered only to individuals with severe bites and to those who may have a heightened reaction, such as elderly individuals and children younger than 5 years.

The brown recluse spider is light brown with a dark-brown violin-shaped mark on its back. The bite of a brown recluse causes severe local effects, including tenderness, redness, and swelling at the injection site. Systemic effects, such as difficulty in breathing or swallowing, seldom occur.

Emergency Care for Spider Bites

1. Wash the wound.
2. Apply a cold pack to the affected area to reduce pain and swelling.
3. Obtain medical help immediately if you suspect the individual has been bitten by a black widow spider or a brown recluse spider, or if a severe reaction begins to occur.

Snakebites

Snakebites kill very few people in the United States. Every year, approximately 45,000 persons are bitten by a snake; however, only 7000 of these bites involve a poisonous snake, and fewer than 15 of the individuals die. Species of poisonous snakes in the United States include rattlesnakes, copperheads, cottonmouths (water moccasins), and coral snakes. Individuals, zoos, or laboratories may own other poisonous species, however. Rattlesnakes account for most snakebites and nearly all fatalities from snakebites. Most snakebites occur near the home, as opposed to in the wild. Because it is often difficult to identify a snake, any unidentified snake should be considered poisonous. General signs and symptoms of a bite from a poisonous snake include puncture marks on the skin, pain and swelling at the puncture site, rapid pulse, nausea, vomiting, unconsciousness, and convulsions.

Emergency Care for Snakebites

1. Wash the bite area gently with soap and water.
2. Immobilize the injured part, and position it below the level of the heart.
3. Call emergency personnel. Do not apply ice to a snakebite. Do not apply a tourniquet, and do not cut or suction the wound.
4. If the snake is dead, inform emergency personnel of its location so that it can be transported to the hospital for identification.

Animal Bites

Bites and other injuries from animals range in severity from minor to serious and fatal. Most people who are bitten by animals do not report the bite to a provider. Because of this factor, the incidence of animal bites in the United States each year is unknown but has been estimated at approximately 5 to 6 million for dog bites and 400,000 for cat bites.

The most serious type of bite is one from an animal with rabies. Rabies is a viral infection transmitted through the saliva of an infected animal. If the condition is not treated, rabies is usually fatal. Certain animals tend to have a higher incidence of rabies than others. These include skunks, bats, raccoons, cats, dogs, cattle, and foxes. Hamsters, gerbils, guinea pigs, chipmunks, rats, mice, gophers, and rabbits are rarely infected with the rabies virus.

An individual who has been bitten by an animal that has rabies or is suspected of having rabies must obtain medical care. To prevent rabies, a rabies vaccine, which produces antibodies to fight the rabies virus, is administered to the individual.

Emergency Care for Animal Bites

Minor Animal Bites

Wash the wound with soap and water. Apply an antibiotic ointment and a dry sterile dressing. Transport the individual to a provider so that medical care can be provided to prevent infection and to ensure that the patient's tetanus toxoid immunization is up-to-date.

Serious Bites

If the wound is bleeding heavily, first control the bleeding with direct pressure. Do not clean the wound because this may result in more bleeding. Transport the patient to a provider, or if the bite is serious enough, call the local EMS system.

All Animal Bites

If you suspect that the animal has rabies, relay this information to the appropriate authorities, such as medical personnel, the police, or animal control personnel. If possible, try to remember what the animal looked like and the area in which you last saw it.

HEAT AND COLD EXPOSURE

Exposure to excessive environmental heat or cold can result in injury to the body ranging in severity from minor to life-threatening. Heat-related injuries are most apt to occur on very hot days that are accompanied by high humidity with little or no air movement. The three conditions caused by overexposure to heat are heat cramps, heat exhaustion, and heatstroke.

The two major types of cold-related injury are frostbite and hypothermia. Although cold-related injuries are most apt to occur in the winter months, they can occur at other times of the year, such as when an individual is exposed to cold water in a near-drowning incident.

Certain individuals are at higher risk for developing heat-related and cold-related injuries, as follows:

- Elderly individuals
- Young children, particularly infants
- Individuals who work or exercise outdoors
- Individuals with medical conditions that cause poor blood circulation, such as diabetes mellitus and cardiovascular disease
- Individuals who have had heat-related or cold-related injuries in the past
- Individuals under the influence of drugs or alcohol

Heat Cramps

Heat cramps are the least serious of the three types of heat-related injury. Heat cramps are most apt to occur when an individual is exercising or working in a hot environment and fails to replace lost fluids and electrolytes. Lost electrolytes can be replaced with a commercial sports drink (e.g., Gatorade).

Signs and symptoms of heat cramps include painful muscle spasms, particularly of the legs, calves, and abdomen; hot, sweaty skin; weakness; and a rapid pulse. These symptoms are a warning that an individual is having a problem with the heat. If the problem is ignored, heat cramps may progress to a more serious condition, such as heat exhaustion or heatstroke.

Treatment of heat cramps consists of removal of the patient to a cool environment, rest, and replacement of fluids and electrolytes. If the patient's condition does not improve, they should be transported to an emergency care facility for further treatment.

Heat Exhaustion

Heat exhaustion is the most common heat-related injury. It occurs most often in individuals involved in vigorous physical activity on a hot and humid day, such as athletes and construction workers. It also can occur in people who are wearing too much clothing on a hot and humid day. Signs and symptoms of heat exhaustion are similar to those of influenza: cold and clammy skin that is pale or gray, profuse sweating, headache, nausea, dizziness, weakness, and diarrhea.

Treatment of heat exhaustion consists of removal of the patient to a cool environment, replacement of fluids and electrolytes, application of a cold compress to the forehead, and rest (Fig. 37.15). Tight clothing should be loosened, and excessive layers of clothing should be removed. In most cases, these measures improve the patient's condition in approximately 30 minutes. If the patient's condition does not improve, however, they should be transported to an emergency care facility.

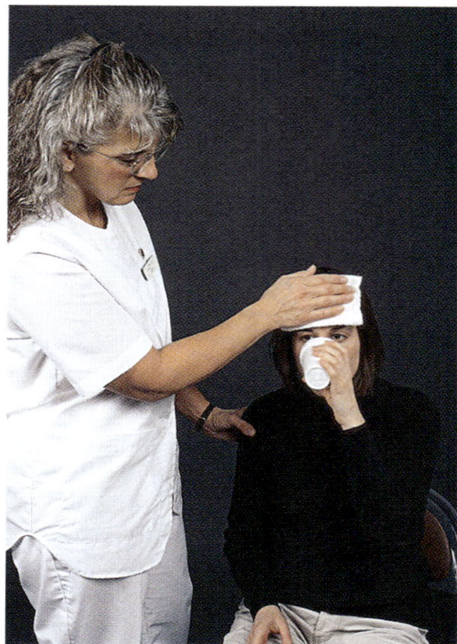

Fig. 37.15 Treatment of heat exhaustion consists of moving the patient to a cool environment, replacing fluids and electrolytes, and applying a cold compress to the forehead; the patient should then rest.

Heatstroke

Heatstroke is the least common, but most serious, of the three heat-related injuries. Heatstroke is most apt to occur in elderly people during a heat wave and in athletes who overexert in a hot and humid environment. Heatstroke can occur in a very short time, as when a child has been left to wait in a closed car on a hot day.

During heatstroke, the body becomes so overheated that the heat-regulating mechanism breaks down and is unable to cool the body. The body temperature increases to a dangerous level, causing destruction of tissues. Signs and symptoms of heatstroke include a body temperature of 105°F (40°C) or greater; red, hot, dry skin; a rapid, weak pulse; dizziness and weakness; rapid, shallow breathing; decreased levels of consciousness; and seizures.

Heatstroke is a life-threatening emergency that requires immediate transport of the patient to an emergency care facility by the fastest way possible. If not treated, heatstroke is always fatal. During transport, every attempt should be made to lower the body temperature, such as setting the air conditioner to its maximal capacity; covering the victim with cool, wet sheets; and fanning the victim.

What Would You Do? What Would You *Not* Do?

Case Study 3

David Brently has come to the medical office. He is a member of Kiwanis, and this year it was his turn to deliver Easter candy and flowers to patients at the local hospital and nursing home while wearing a bunny costume. It is a very warm day, and David says that he got really hot and sweaty in his costume and then started feeling dizzy and nauseous. He got a little worried and decided to drive himself to the medical office. David says he cannot get his costume off because the zipper is stuck. He does not want to cut it off because that would ruin it and Kiwanis would not be able to use it next year. He is hoping the physician can fix him up well enough so that he can drive home. David says he is sure his wife can get the costume off without damaging it. ■

Frostbite

Frostbite is the localized freezing of body tissue as a result of exposure to cold. The severity of frostbite depends on the environmental temperature, the duration of exposure, and the wind-chill factor. Frostbite most commonly affects the hands, fingers, feet, toes, ears, nose, and cheeks. Although frostbite is not life-threatening, it can cause severe tissue damage that may require amputation of the affected body part. Signs and symptoms of frostbite include loss of feeling in the affected area; cold and waxy skin; and white, yellow, or blue discoloration of the skin.

Treatment of frostbite requires rewarming of the affected body part to prevent permanent damage. This is best accomplished in an emergency care facility because improper rewarming can result in further tissue damage. To transport the patient, loosely wrap warm clothing or blankets around the affected body part. The frozen area also can be placed in contact with another body part that is warm. It is important to handle the affected area gently. Do not rub or massage the affected area because this can damage frozen tissue further.

Hypothermia

Hypothermia is a life-threatening emergency in which the temperature of the entire body falls to a dangerously low level. Hypothermia can occur rapidly, such as when an individual falls through the ice on a frozen lake. It also can occur slowly when an individual is exposed to a cold environment for a long time, such as when a hiker is lost in the woods.

When the core body temperature decreases too much, the body loses its ability to regulate its temperature and to generate body heat. Signs and symptoms of hypothermia include shivering, numbness, drowsiness, apathy, a glassy stare, and decreased levels of consciousness.

Treatment of hypothermia should focus on preventing further heat loss. Remove the patient from the cold, or, if this is impossible, wrap them in blankets. Do not attempt to rewarm the patient such as through immersion in warm water. Rapid rewarming can result in serious respiratory and cardiac problems. The patient should be transported immediately to an emergency care facility.

DIABETIC EMERGENCIES

Glucose is the end product of carbohydrate metabolism. It serves as the chief source of energy to perform normal body functions and to assist in maintaining body temperature. The body maintains a constant blood glucose level to ensure a continuous source of energy for the body. Glucose that is not needed for energy can be stored in the form of glycogen in muscle and liver tissue for later use. When no more tissue storage is possible, excess glucose is converted to fat and stored as adipose tissue.

Insulin, a hormone secreted by the beta cells of the pancreas, is required for normal use of glucose in the body. Insulin enables glucose to enter the body's cells and be converted to energy. Insulin also is needed for proper storage of glycogen in liver and muscle cells.

Diabetes mellitus is a disease in which the body is unable to use glucose for energy because of a lack of insulin in the body. There are two types of diabetes—a severe form, usually appearing in childhood, known as *type 1 diabetes*, and a mild form, usually appearing in adulthood, known as *type 2 diabetes*. Most individuals with diabetes (90%) have type 2 diabetes. No cure for diabetes mellitus is known, but significant advances have been made in controlling the disease through a combination of drug therapy, diet therapy, and activity. The goal for the diabetic patient is to balance food intake and level of activity with the body's insulin.

A diabetic patient can experience two types of emergency: *hypoglycemia*, commonly referred to as "insulin shock," and *diabetic ketoacidosis*, commonly known as "diabetic coma." Insulin shock (hypoglycemia) occurs when there is too much insulin in the body and not enough glucose. Insulin shock can be caused by administration of too much insulin, skipping meals, and unexpected or unusual exercise. Symptoms of insulin shock include normal or rapid respirations; pale, cold, and clammy skin; sweating; dizziness and headache; full, rapid pulse; normal or high blood pressure; extreme hunger; aggressive or unusual behavior; fainting; and seizure or coma. The onset of insulin shock occurs rapidly, usually over 5 to 20 minutes, after the blood glucose level begins to decrease. Because the brain requires a constant supply of glucose for proper functioning, permanent brain damage or death can result from severe hypoglycemia.

Diabetic coma (diabetic ketoacidosis) occurs when there is not enough insulin in the body. This causes the blood glucose level to increase, resulting in hyperglycemia. When glucose cannot be used for energy, fat is broken down. This results in a buildup of acid waste products in the blood, known as *ketoacidosis*. The combined effect of the hyperglycemia and the ketoacidosis causes the following symptoms: polyuria; excessive thirst and hunger; vomiting; abdominal pain; dry, warm skin; rapid, deep sighing respirations; a sweet or fruity (acetone) odor to the breath; and a rapid, weak pulse.

If the condition is not treated, diabetic coma can progress to dehydration, hypotension, coma, and death. In contrast to insulin shock, however, the onset of diabetic coma is gradual, usually developing over 12 to 48 hours. Diabetic coma can be caused by illness and infection, overeating, forgetting to administer an insulin injection, or administering an insufficient amount of insulin.

Most individuals with diabetes have a thorough knowledge of their disease and manage it effectively. Because of this, diabetic emergencies are most apt to occur when there is an unusual upset in the insulin-glucose balance in the body, such as might be caused by illness or infection. An emergency situation also may arise in an individual who has diabetes but in whom the condition has not yet been diagnosed.

It may be difficult to tell the difference between insulin shock and diabetic coma because the symptoms are similar. Often a patient with either of these conditions seems to be intoxicated. If conscious, the diabetic patient usually

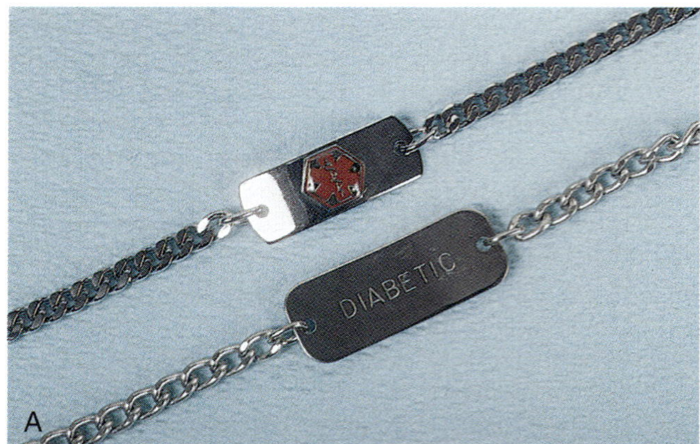

ALERT

I HAVE TYPE I DIABETES

If I appear to be intoxicated or am unconscious, I may be having a reaction to diabetes or its treatment.

EMERGENCY TREATMENT

If I am able to swallow, please give me a beverage that contains sugar, such as orange juice, cola or even sugar in water. Then please send me to the nearest hospital **IMMEDIATELY.**

B

Fig. 37.16 Diabetic medical identification. (A) Diabetic medical alert bracelet. **(B)** Diabetic wallet card.

knows what the trouble is; you should listen carefully to the patient to determine what may have caused the problem (e.g., not eating, forgetting to administer an insulin injection). If the patient is unconscious and unable to communicate, you should observe the patient's respirations. A patient in insulin shock has normal or rapid respirations, whereas a patient in diabetic coma has deep, labored respirations. Most diabetic patients carry an emergency medical identification, such as a medical alert bracelet or necklace and a wallet card (Fig. 37.16), to alert others to their condition when they cannot.

Emergency Care in Diabetes

Insulin Shock (Hypoglycemia)

A patient in insulin shock needs sugar immediately. For a conscious patient, glucose should be administered by

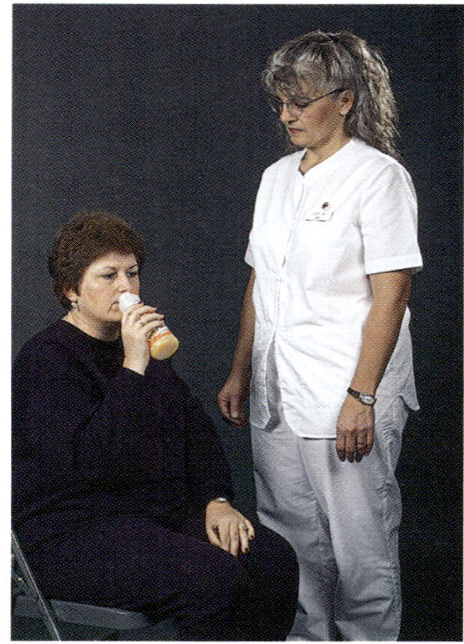

Fig. 37.17 Orange juice is administered to a diabetic patient showing signs and symptoms of insulin shock.

mouth in the form of fruit juice (e.g., orange juice), nondiet soft drinks, candy, honey, or table sugar dissolved in water (Fig. 37.17). Improvement is usually rapid after the glucose has been consumed. If the patient is unconscious, do not give anything by mouth because it may be aspirated into the lungs. Instead, provide the fastest possible transportation of the patient to an emergency care facility.

Diabetic Coma (Diabetic Ketoacidosis)

A patient in diabetic coma needs insulin and must be transported as soon as possible to an emergency care facility.

Doubtful Situations

If you are ever in doubt as to whether a patient is developing insulin shock or diabetic coma, give sugar, even though the final diagnosis may be diabetic coma. This is because insulin shock develops much more rapidly than diabetic coma and can quickly cause permanent brain damage or death. If you give sugar to a patient in diabetic coma, there is little risk of making the condition worse because a patient can withstand a high blood glucose level longer than they can tolerate a low blood glucose level.

What Would You Do? What Would You *Not* Do? RESPONSES

Case Study 1
Page 1007

What Did Judy Do?

- ❑ Gave Beth the national Poison Help number (1-800-222-1222) and told her to call it immediately. Explained that was the fastest way to obtain information on what to do.
- ❑ Told Beth not to give the syrup of ipecac to Olivia unless she was told to do so by the Poison Help operator.
- ❑ Told Beth to have the vitamin bottle in her hand when she calls. Told her that the Poison Help operator would want to know information from the label and would especially want to know whether the vitamins contained iron.

What Would You Do? What Would You *Not* Do? RESPONSES—cont'd

- ❑ Told Beth to call the office back if she needs any more help after talking with Poison Help.

What Did Judy Not Do?

- ❑ Did not tell Beth she should give Olivia syrup of ipecac, because some poisons can cause additional problems if they are brought back up.

Case Study 2

Page 1008

What Did Judy Do?

- ❑ Told Anita that Garon needs to get to the hospital as soon as possible. Explained that he is having a very serious allergic reaction that could be life-threatening.
- ❑ Told her to stay calm and call 911 immediately.
- ❑ Notified the physician of the situation.

What Did Judy Not Do?

- ❑ Did not tell her to bring Garon to the office, because he may need special life-support equipment available only at the hospital.

Case Study 3

Page 1010

What Did Judy Do?

- ❑ Took David to an examining room that was cool and gave him a glass of water.
- ❑ Told David she needed to get his costume off as soon as possible. Explained that if his condition gets worse, it could become life-threatening.
- ❑ Helped David out of the costume and gave him another glass of water.

What Did Judy Not Do?

- ❑ Did not tell David to keep the costume on.

TERMINOLOGY REVIEW

Key Term	Word Parts	Definition
Burn		An injury to the tissues caused by exposure to thermal, chemical, electrical, or radioactive agents.
Crash cart		A specially equipped cart for holding and transporting medications, equipment, and supplies needed for lifesaving procedures in an emergency.
Crepitus		A grating sensation caused by fractured bone fragments rubbing against each other.
Dislocation	*dis-:* to undo, free from	An injury in which one end of a bone making up a joint is separated or displaced from its normal anatomic position.
Emergency medical services (EMS) system		A network of community resources, equipment, and personnel that provides care to victims of injury or sudden illness.
First aid		The immediate care administered before complete medical care can be provided to an individual who is injured or suddenly becomes ill.
Fracture		Any break in a bone.
Hypothermia	*hypo-:* below, deficient *therm/o:* heat *-ia:* condition of diseased or abnormal state	A life-threatening condition in which the temperature of the entire body falls to a dangerously low level.
Poison		Any substance that causes illness, injury, or death if it enters the body.
Pressure point		A site on the body where an artery lies close to the surface of the skin and can be compressed against an underlying bone to control bleeding.
Seizure		A sudden episode of involuntary muscular contractions and relaxation, often accompanied by changes in sensation, behavior, and level of consciousness.
Shock		The failure of the cardiovascular system to deliver enough blood to all of the vital organs of the body.
Splint		Any device that immobilizes a body part.
Sprain		Trauma to a joint that causes tearing of ligaments.
Strain		A stretching or tearing of muscles or tendons caused by trauma.
Wound		A break in the continuity of an external or internal surface, caused by physical means.

ON THE WEB

For information on emergency medicine:

American Red Cross: www.redcross.org

Federal Emergency Management Agency: www.fema.gov

The Medical Record

Check out the Evolve site at http://evolve.elsevier.com/Bonewit/today to access additional interactive activities and exercises to help you study and prepare for success.

LEARNING OBJECTIVES	PROCEDURES
Types of Medical Records	
1. Explain the difference between a paper-based medical record and an electronic health record (EHR).	
2. List the general functions of EHR software.	
Medical Record Formats	
3. Describe the organization of a source-oriented medical record and a problem-oriented medical record.	
4. List and define the four subcategories included in the progress notes of a problem-oriented record (POR).	
5. Describe the usual format of an EHR.	
Administrative Section of the Medical Record	
6. List the categories of information obtained on the new patient information form.	Completion of a procedure consent form.
7. Describe the function of the Notice of Privacy Practices.	Release of medical information.
8. Identify the information obtained in each of the following consent documents: procedure consent and release of medical information.	
9. Give examples of correspondence and telephone messages often found in the medical record.	
Clinical Section of the Medical Record	
10. List and describe the components of the medical record database.	
11. Describe how the problem list is coordinated with billing in the EHR.	
12. Explain the necessity to finalize progress notes in the EHR.	
13. Compare storage of laboratory reports, diagnostic tests, and reports of diagnostic tests in the paper-based medical record and the EHR.	
14. List and describe other clinical reports that may be found in a medical record.	
Health History	
15. List and describe the seven sections of the health history.	Obtaining patient history and formulate chief complaint.
16. List the guidelines that should be followed in recording the chief complaint.	
Documentation	
17. List and describe the guidelines to follow to ensure accurate and concise documentation.	
18. List and describe the types of progress notes that may be documented by the medical assistant.	
19. List examples of subjective symptoms and objective symptoms.	
20. List and describe common symptoms.	

CHAPTER OUTLINE

KEY TERMS

attending provider/hospitalist
chief complaint
consultation report
diagnosis (dye-ag-NOE-sis)
diagnostic procedure
digital image
discharge summary report
documenting
electronic health record (EHR)
electronic medical record (EMR)
familial (fah-MIL-yul)
flow sheet
health history
home health care
inpatient
medical record
medical record format
objective symptom
paper-based patient record
physical examination
problem
problem-oriented record (POR)
reverse chronological order
SOAP
source-oriented record (SOR)
subjective symptom
symptom (SIMP-tum)

INTRODUCTION TO THE MEDICAL RECORD

Medical records are a crucial part of a medical practice. A **medical record** is a written or electronic record of the important information regarding a patient, including the care of that individual and the progress of their condition.

The patient's medical record serves many important functions. The provider uses the information in the medical record as a basis for decisions regarding the patient's care and treatment. The medical record documents the results of treatment and the patient's progress. The medical record provides an efficient and effective method by which information can be communicated to authorized personnel in the medical office.

The medical record also serves as a legal document. The law requires that a record be maintained to document the care and treatment being received by a patient. If something goes wrong, good documentation works to protect the provider and the medical staff legally. Incomplete records could be used as evidence in court to show that a patient did not receive the quality of care that meets generally accepted standards.

The medical assistant must always keep in mind that the information contained in a patient's medical record is strictly confidential and must not be read by or discussed with anyone except the provider or medical staff involved with the care of the patient (see *Highlight on the Health Insurance Portability and Accountability Act [HIPAA] Privacy Rule*).

HIGHLIGHT on the Health Insurance Portability and Accountability Act Privacy Rule

What Is the HIPAA Privacy Rule?

The acronym *HIPAA* stands for the *Health Insurance Portability and Accountability Act.* HIPAA is a federal law consisting of several components, one of which contains provisions to protect a patient's privacy, known as the *HIPAA Privacy Rule.*

The HIPAA Privacy Rule went into effect on April 14, 2003. The primary purpose of this rule is to provide patients with better control over the use and disclosure of their health information. All health care providers, health plans, and health care clearinghouses (e.g., billing services) that use, store, maintain, or transmit health information must comply with this rule. Privacy protections were strengthened in 2013 with modifications to the HIPAA rules to implement statutory amendments under the Health Information Technology for Economic and Clinical Health Act (HITECH).

What Is Included in the HIPAA Privacy Rule?

The HIPAA Privacy Rule is outlined here as it relates to the medical office:

1. The medical office must develop a written document known as a *Notice of Privacy Practices* (NPP). The NPP must explain to patients how their *protected health information* (PHI) will be used and protected by the medical office. PHI includes health information in any form (written, electronic, or oral) that contains patient-identifiable information (e.g., name, social security number, telephone number). The medical office must make a reasonable effort to provide an NPP to each patient and to obtain and keep on file a signed acknowledgment from the patient that they have received an NPP.
2. A patient's written consent is not required for the use or disclosure of PHI for the following:
   - Medical treatment. *Examples:*
     - Patient referral to a specialist
     - Emergency care provided at a hospital
     - Tests on a patient performed by the laboratory
   - Payment. *Examples:*
     - Determination of eligibility for insurance benefits
     - Review of services provided for medical necessity
     - Utilization review activities
   - Health care operations. *Examples:*
     - Quality assessment activities
     - Contacting patients with information about care or treatment
     - Employee review activities
     - Training of health care students
   - Legally mandated reports. *Examples:*
     - Reports of child or elder abuse
     - Reportable diseases
     - Reports of injuries that may be a result of a crime
3. Patients have the right to access their medical records and to request changes to the records if they believe them to be inaccurate.
4. To prevent unnecessary or inappropriate access to PHI, the medical office must make an effort to limit the use of, disclosure of, and requests for PHI to the minimum necessary to accomplish the intended purpose (e.g., a request from an insurance company for procedures performed on a patient). This requirement does not apply, however, to the use of PHI for the routine practice of medicine within the medical office.
5. Patients have a right to request an accounting of the transfer of their information for purposes other than treatment, payment, or health care operations.
6. Business associates to whom the medical office may disclose PHI must respect the HIPAA Privacy Rule. The medical office must execute a written agreement with each business associate and/or subcontractor to handle PHI in accordance with HIPAA. Business associates may include the following organizations and firms:
   - Medical laboratories
   - Transcription services
   - Law firms
   - Accounting firms
   - Software and hardware consultants
   - Billing services
7. The medical office must implement for all employees a basic training program on privacy and security of PHI.
8. The medical office is required to put in place appropriate administrative, physical, and technical security safeguards to protect the privacy of PHI from accidental use or disclosure or violation of the aforementioned requirements.
9. The medical office is required to notify affected individuals following a breach of unsecured PHI.

What If a Medical Office Does not Comply With the HIPAA Privacy Rule?

There are severe penalties if a medical office fails to comply with the HIPAA Privacy Rule, which can include civil and criminal penalties. An employee who knowingly violates HIPAA can be fined or imprisoned, depending on the severity of the violation.

Where Can More information on the HIPAA Privacy Rule Be Found?

The following websites contain current information on HIPAA:
www.cms.gov and enter search term: HIPAA
https://www.hhs.gov/hipaa/for-professionals/privacy/laws-regulations/index.html ■

TYPES OF MEDICAL RECORDS

PAPER-BASED PATIENT RECORD

Medical offices may rely on the use of paper medical records, known as **paper-based patient records** (also called *paper-based medical records*). Historically, this type of medical record system was a collection of data related to the medical care of the patient with patient registration information, patient scheduling information, and billing information kept separately. Originally, administrative record keeping was also paper based, but computer programs for scheduling and billing have been widely used for several decades. Because all information in the paper-based patient record is in printed format, the physical management of the record is time-consuming, and significant storage space is required. Procedures for creating paper-based records, adding documents, and filing are discussed in Chapter 43.

ELECTRONIC HEALTH RECORD

Most medical offices have converted to an **electronic health record (EHR)** for maintaining patient health information. The EHR is a computerized record of the important health information regarding a patient, including the care of that individual and the progress of the patient's condition. In addition, EHR software allows for the creation, storage, organization, editing, and retrieval of medical records on a computer. The EHR software is usually linked to or incorporates software for scheduling, billing, and filing insurance claims. This allows the EHR to include more information than a traditional medical record. Information entered when scheduling a patient's first appointment becomes available as part of the patient medical record and can be accessed for both clinical and administrative functions.

Making the transition to an EHR is a major undertaking for a medical office. The HITECH Act, which was part of the 2009 stimulus package, accelerated the adoption of EHRs because of financial incentive payments to those who adopted and used them. In addition, the language of the HITECH Act has blurred the previous distinction between the **electronic medical record (EMR)**, which designates an electronic form of a paper medical record generated by an individual health care provider or organization, and the **electronic health record (EHR)**. The EMR designates a patient health record generated by an individual health care provider or organization that is stored on a computer. The EHR refers to an electronic record that contains more information than a traditional paper medical record and that also has the capacity to be shared among health care organizations. The Office of the National Coordinator for Health Information Technology (ONC) uses only the term *EHR* to designate any digital "real-time, patient-centered" record.

MEDICAL RECORD FORMATS

The way a medical record is organized is known as its *format.* The two traditional types of **medical record formats** are the *source-oriented record* and the *problem-oriented record* (POR). The EHR uses a functional format that combines elements of these traditional formats for clinical information but also includes separate sections for scheduling and billing.

SOURCE-ORIENTED RECORD

The **source-oriented record (SOR)** format, or a source-oriented medical format (SOMR), is used most often in the medical office for organizing a paper-based patient record. The documents in a SOR are organized into sections based on the department, facility, or other source that generated the information (e.g., laboratory, hospital, consultant). Because documents from each source are filed together, it is easy to compare information from laboratory and diagnostic test results, assessments, and treatments.

Each section in a paper SOR is usually separated from the other sections by a chart divider. Attached to each divider is a color-coded tab labeled with the title of its section (Fig. 38.1). Within each of these sections, the documents are arranged according to date. Most offices use reverse chronological order to arrange the documents. **Reverse chronological order** means that the most recent document is placed on top or in front of the others, and thus the oldest document is on the bottom or at the end of that section.

Some parts of an EHR may also be arranged in a source-oriented format using tabs to identify laboratory reports or correspondence, but the bulk of the EHR is arranged in a more problem-oriented format, which is discussed next.

PROBLEM-ORIENTED RECORD

The documents in a **problem-oriented record (POR)**, or problem-oriented medical record (POMR), are organized

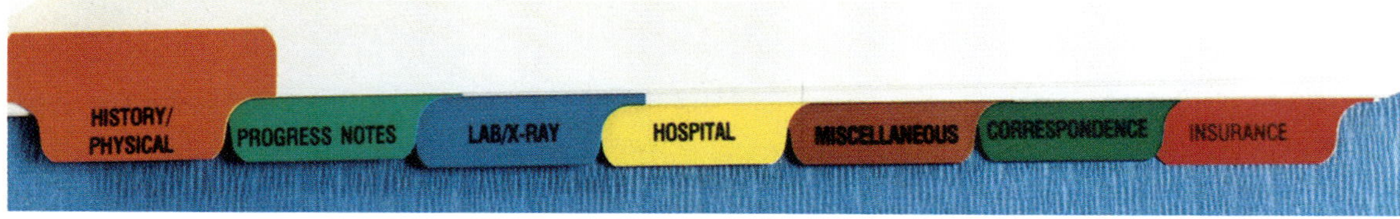

Fig. 38.1 Chart dividers in a source-oriented record.

according to the patient's health problems. This medical record format was initially developed by Lawrence Weed as a functional way to organize information. The advantage of using the POR is that each of the patient's problems can be defined and followed individually. The POR is developed in four stages:

1. Establishing a *database*
2. Compiling a *problem list*
3. Devising a *plan* of action for each problem
4. Following each problem with *progress notes*

Database

The first step in developing a POR is to establish a database. The database consists of a collection of subjective and objective data including the health history report, the physical examination report, and the results of baseline laboratory and diagnostic tests. The information in the database is used to identify and compile a problem list.

Problem List

The problem list is developed shortly after the database is completed and lists all the patient's problems (Fig. 38.2). A **problem** is defined as any patient condition that requires observation, diagnosis, management, or patient education. This includes not only medical problems but also psychological and social problems. The problem list is a crucial part of the POR and is located in the front of the paper-based patient record and on a separate tab in the EHR.

The problem list should be thought of as a table of contents for the record. Each problem in the list is numbered and titled. The problem title is stated as a diagnosis, a physiologic finding, a symptom, or an abnormal test result. All subsequent data (plans and progress notes) added to the medical record are cross-referenced to these numbered problems.

The problem list is modified as needed. If a new problem is identified, it is added to the list and dated accordingly. When a problem is resolved, it is marked as such, and the date is recorded.

Plan

After examining the problem list, the provider develops the third section of the POR. This involves devising a plan of action for further evaluation and treatment of each problem. Each plan begins with a heading that identifies the number of the problem, followed by the plan of action for the problem. This may include plans for laboratory and diagnostic tests, medical or surgical treatment, therapy, and patient education.

Progress Notes

The last stage in the development of the POR is the follow-up for each problem, or the progress notes (Fig. 38.3). The progress notes include the following four categories:

- *Subjective data:* Subjective data obtained from the patient
- *Objective data:* Objective data obtained by observation, physical examination, and laboratory and diagnostic tests
- *Assessment:* The provider's interpretation of the current condition based on analysis of the subjective and objective data
- *Plan:* Proposed treatment for the patient

The acronym for this method of documentation is **SOAP**, and this method of creating progress notes is now widely used in all medical record formats.

FORMAT OF THE ELECTRONIC HEALTH RECORD

Most modern medical records combine elements of both traditional medical record formats. Paper-based patient records are primarily clinical, and they include elements from the POR such as a problem list and progress notes in SOAP format. The entire record is rarely organized by patient problem, however. Elements from the SOR format include separate sections for laboratory data and/or diagnostic tests, correspondence, and telephone messages.

The general format for an EHR usually includes major divisions into clinical, scheduling, and billing functions. Within the clinical section, there are tabs that allow the

Problem List

Showing 1 to 2 of 2 entries — First Previous 1 Next Last

No.	Encounter Type	Problem	ICD-9 Code	ICD-10 Code	Status	Entry By	Action
1	Office Visit - New Patient Visit 04/03/20XX	Hypertension	- -	I10	Active	Sue Hunt	
2	Office Visit - New Patient Visit 04/03/20XX	Diabetes mellitus, Type II without complications	- -	E11.9	Active	Sue Hunt	

Add Problem

Fig. 38.2 Problem list in SimChart for the Medical Office.

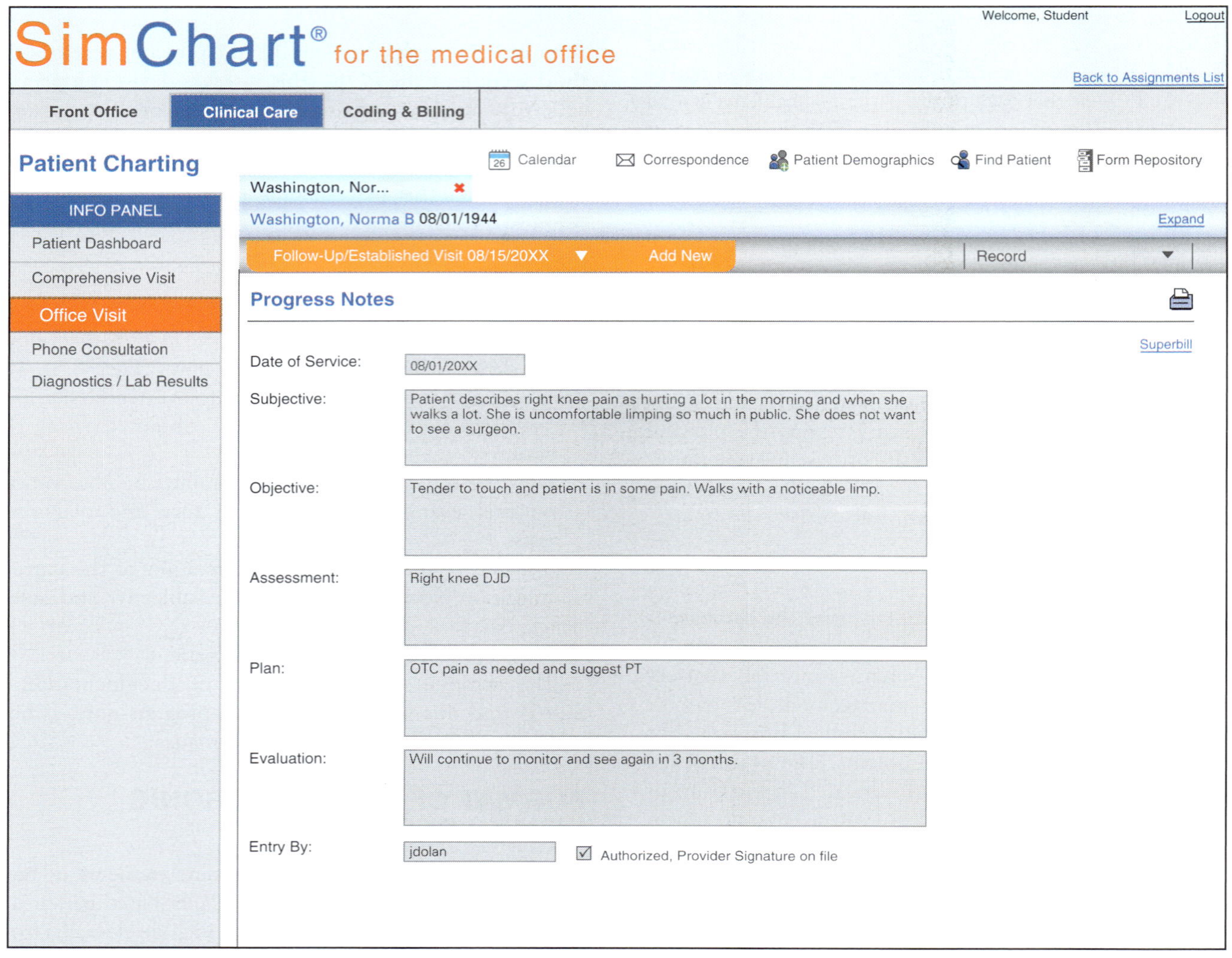

Fig. 38.3 SOAP progress note in SimChart for the Medical Office.

clinician to link easily to the health history, lists of problems, medications, allergies, and immunizations, as well as to vital signs and progress notes.

What Would You Do? What Would You *Not* Do?

Case Study 1

Moira Celeste, an account executive for a large insurance company, comes to the office complaining of insomnia and depression. Three months ago, her husband of 27 years left, and now they are legally separated. Since then, Moira has had a lot of trouble sleeping at night. She also feels lethargic during the day and has not been eating much. Moira says that she has been having some problems with alcohol. She wants to know of any community agencies that could help her with her problem but that would be bound to keep the information confidential. She has a very responsible job with her firm and does not want anyone to know about her alcohol problem. She also does not want any information about her problem put in her chart, and she especially does not want the provider to know about it because he is friends with many of her colleagues at work. ■

ADMINISTRATIVE SECTION OF THE MEDICAL RECORD

PATIENT REGISTRATION RECORD

The patient registration record consists of demographic and billing information. Although a new patient may have given much of the information by telephone before the first appointment, the patient usually fills out a patient registration form at the first visit. At this time, the medical assistant enters the information into the computer or verifies the information in the computer system. Most medical offices now ask the patient to provide information about ethnicity, race, and preferred language. These were introduced in order to qualify for Medicare incentive payments under the HITECH Act (see *Highlight on MACRA*). Demographic and billing information is used for numerous computerized functions, such as scheduling appointments, posting patient transactions, and processing patient statements and insurance claims. With a paper-based patient record, the original patient registration record is then usually placed in the front of the patient's medical record. After patient registration information has been entered into the EHR, it can usually be viewed on a single screen (sometimes called a *patient dashboard*) with other important information about patients such as their medications and allergies. With an EHR, the original registration record is usually shredded.

HIGHLIGHT on MACRA and Promoting Interoperability Programs for Hospitals

What Is MACRA?

MACRA refers to the Medical Access and CHIP Reauthorization Act of 2015 which established new guidelines for verifying quality and use of EHR technology for Medicare-enrolled practitioners. Practitioners must verify that they meet evidence-based, specialty-specific standards and practice improvement activities in addition to the use of a certified EHR as part of the Quality Payment Program.

What Is Promoting Interoperability Programs for Hospitals?

Promoting Interoperability Program was previously known as Medicare and Medicaid EHR Incentive Program. The main purpose is to show meaningful use of EHRs with additional focus of interoperability and improving patient access to health information. The focus of this program is that providers need to show how they are using EHR technology to provide the best care to patients. To do this, providers must show that they are using certified EHR technology to:

- Improve quality, safety, and efficiency
- Engage patients and families
- Improve care coordination
- Improve public and population health
- Ensure privacy and security for protected health information

OTHER ADMINISTRATIVE FORMS

Notice of Privacy Practices (NPP)

An NPP is a written document that explains to patients how their PHI will be used and protected by the medical office. The patient must sign a form acknowledging that they have received the NPP. Many medical offices give the patient a paper consent form to sign, and then the form is scanned into the computer and filed in the patient's EHR.

Advance Directives

Patients are encouraged to fill out a form or provide a copy of their existing advance directives. Advance directives may name an individual to make medical decisions for the patient if they become incapacitated and/or state the patient's wishes if they become unable to direct care.

Consent Forms

Patient consent may be obtained on a paper form that is scanned into the EHR, or the patient may be asked to sign on an electronic form viewed on an electronic device such as a tablet or laptop computer. For example, the consent to treatment and billing section on the new patient information form is usually scanned into the computer and attached to the individual patient record. Consent forms are legal documents required to perform certain procedures or to release information contained in the patient's medical record.

Completion of a procedure consent form (Procedure 38.1) is required for all surgical operations and nonroutine therapeutic and diagnostic procedures (e.g., sigmoidoscopy) performed in the medical office. The form must be signed by the patient or their legally authorized representative and must provide written evidence that the patient agrees to the procedure or procedures listed on the form (Fig. 38.4).

The procedure consent form should not be signed until the patient has been provided with all necessary information related to the procedure. (See Chapter 3 for a full discussion of informed consent.) The patient's signature must be witnessed; this is usually the responsibility of the medical assistant. *Witnessing a signature* means only that the medical assistant verified the patient's identity and watched the patient sign the form; it *does not* mean that the medical assistant is attesting to the accuracy of the information provided.

The procedure consent form outlines the details of the discussion with the patient and includes the following information:

- The patient's full name
- Name of the procedure to be performed
- A statement indicating that the patient agrees to receive the procedure
- Acknowledgment that a disclosure of information has been made
- Acknowledgment that all questions were answered in a satisfactory manner
- A statement that no guarantee as to the outcome has been made
- Signature of the patient or their legal representative
- Signature of the witness and date obtained

Medical Records Release Form

As previously explained in the box entitled *Highlight on the Health Insurance Portability and Accountability Act [HIPAA] Privacy Rule*, a patient's written consent is not required for the use or disclosure of PHI for the purpose of medical treatment, payment, and health care operations. If a request for PHI is required for other purposes, however, a detailed form must be completed, known as a *medical records release form* (Fig. 38.5). If a patient is moving to another state and wants to transfer their medical record to a new provider, a release of medical information form must be completed.

The medical records release form must be signed by the patient authorizing the disclosure of their PHI (Procedure 38.2). If the patient is a minor, the form must be signed by the parent or legal guardian of the minor. The release of medical information form must stipulate the following:

WALDEN-MARTIN

FAMILY MEDICAL CLINIC
1234 ANYSTREET ANYTOWN, ANYSTATE 1234
PHONE 123-123-1234 FAX 123-123-5678

General Procedure Consent

Patient Name: ______________________ **Date:** ______________________

The Doctor has discussed with you your condition and the recommended surgical or medical procedures to be performed. This discussion was intended to ensure that you had the opportunity to receive the information necessary to make a reasoned and informed decision whether or not to consent to the procedure. This document is written confirmation of the discussion and contains some of the more significant medical information discussed.

1. Based on this discussion, I understand the following condition may exist in my case:

2. I understand the procedure proposed for treating or diagnosing my condition is:

3. I have been informed of the purpose and reasonable expected benefits of the proposed procedure, the possibility of success or failure, major problems of recuperation, the reasonably anticipated consequences if the procedure is not performed, and the available alternatives.

4. I understand that all surgical and therapeutic procedures involve some risks including pain, scarring, bleeding and infection.

5. I am aware that in the practice of medicine, other unexpected risks or complications not discussed may or may not further acknowledge that no guarantees or promises have been made to me concerning the results of any procedures. Although the benefits are judged to outweigh the risks, should any complications occur, any one of them could be permanent. I hereby voluntarily give my authority and consent to the doctor to perform the proposed procedure described above.

6. I have been given the opportunity to ask questions about my condition, alternative forms of treatment, risk treatment, the procedure to be used, and the risks and hazards involved. I believe I have sufficient information to give this informed consent.

I understand I have read and fully understand the contents of this form, that the disclosures referred to above were made to me and that all blanks and statements requiring insertion or completion were filled in before I signed my name below.

Patient Signature: ______________________ **Date:** ______________________

If a patient is a minor or unable to give consent,
Signature of person authorized to consent for patient:

Relationship to Patient: ______________________

Witness: ______________________ **Date:** ______________________

Fig. 38.4 General procedure consent form from SimChart for the Medical Office.

WALDEN-MARTIN

FAMILY MEDICAL CLINIC
1234 ANYSTREET ANYTOWN, ANYSTATE 1234
PHONE 123-123-1234 FAX 123-123-5678

Medical Records Release

Patient Name: ______________________ **Date of Birth:** ______________________

SSN: ______________________ **Phone:** ______________________

Address:

I, ______________________ authorize ______________________

Walden-Martin Family Medical Clinic to disclose/release the following information (check all applicable):

- ☐ All records
- ☐ Laboratory/pathology records
- ☐ X-ray/radiology records
- ☐ Billing records
- ☐ Abstract/summary
- ☐ Pharmacy/prescription records
- ☐ Other

***Note**: If these records contain any information from previous providers or information about HIV/AIDS status, cancer diagnosis, drug or alcohol abuse, or sexually transmitted disease, you are hereby authorizing disclosure of this information. A copy of this signed authorization must be given to the individual.*

These records are for services provided on the following date(s):

Please send the records listed above to (use additional sheets if necessary):

Name: ______________________ **Phone:** ______________________

Address: **Fax:** ______________________

The information may be used/disclosed for each of the following purposes:

- ☐ At patient's request
- ☐ For patient's health care
- ☐ For payment/insurance
- ☐ For employment purposes
- ☐ Other

This authorization shall expire no later than: __________or upon the following event __________, and may not be valid for greater than one year from the date of signature for medical records.

I understand that after the custodian of records discloses my health information, it may no longer be protected by federal privacy laws. I understand that this authorization is voluntary and I may refuse to sign this authorization which will not affect my ability to obtain treatment; receive payment; or eligibility for benefits unless allowed by law. By signing below I represent and warrant that I have authority to sign this document and authorize the use or disclosure of protected health information and that there are no claims or orders that would prohibit, limit, or otherwise restrict my ability to authorize the use or disclosure of this protected health information.

Patient signature
(or patient's personal representative)

Date:

Printed name of patient representative

Representative's authority to sign for patient
(i.e. parent, guardian, power of attorney, executor)

Fig. 38.5 Medical records release form from SimChart for the Medical Office.

- The patient's full name and address
- Name of the medical practice releasing the information
- Name of the individual or facility to receive the information
- Specific information to be released
- The purpose of or need for the information
- Method of release of the information
- Signature of the patient or their legal representative
- Date that the consent form was signed
- Expiration date of the consent form

Most medical offices require that the patient come to the office to sign the medical records release form; however, this may not always be possible. An example is a patient who has moved away and is requesting the transfer of their medical records to a new provider. In this instance, the patient may fill out a medical records release form and mail it or fax it to the medical office. The procedure for processing this type of request is outlined at the end of Procedure 38.2.

Correspondence and Messages

Correspondence regarding a patient may be received from a number of individuals or facilities. Examples include the patient's insurance company, the patient's attorney, or the patient themselves. If the correspondence is transmitted electronically to the medical office, it will already be in a digital format and can be transferred to the patient's EHR. An example of this is a letter from an insurance company sent as an attachment to an e-mail. If the correspondence is received in a paper format, the medical assistant must first convert the correspondence into a digital format by scanning it into the computer. The medical assistant then transfers the correspondence to the patient's EHR and (if office policy dictates) shreds the paper document. Correspondence also includes copies of letters that are sent from the office; examples are a new patient welcome letter or a collection letter sent to the patient. These letters may be generated by the office in an electronic format through word processing with a copy transferred to the patient's EHR, or it is often possible to create letters directly through the EHR.

Telephone messages are also usually filed or documented in a patient's medical record because they often contain important information related to patient care. If an EHR is used, there is usually a function to record messages using a form or tab in the medical record. Patient information (such as medication information) can often be transferred into the message, and it may also be possible to create a chart note of the message. The EHR may also have an internal message system (sometimes called *clinical messaging*) to securely relay information that relates to patients. For example, a medical assistant may send a patient's medical question as a message to the provider through the EHR.

Schedule and Billing Information

The EHR may maintain the schedule and perform billing, or there may be an interface among the scheduling program, the billing program, and the EHR. The schedule is discussed in Chapter 42, and billing is discussed in Chapter 45.

What Would You Do? What Would You *Not* Do?

Case Study 2

Tessa Walsh, her husband, and their two children are moving to another state. They will be leaving in 2 days. Tessa calls the office to have their medical records transferred to their new provider. Tessa's daughter has type 1 diabetes, so it is important that this be done as soon as possible. Tessa is quite annoyed to learn that she has to come in and sign a special form. She says that their medical records belong to them. Tessa says that the whole family has been coming there for the past 8 years and is well known by the provider and staff. She says that they have been good patients, have followed the provider's advice, and have always paid their bills on time. Tessa thinks that verbal permission should be enough. She is extremely busy packing and taking care of other moving details and does not have a minute to spare. ■

Putting It All Into Practice

My name is Dawn Bennett, and I work for an orthopedic surgeon. When our practice joined with a large medical group a few years ago, we had to adopt the electronic health record (EHR) used by all the other practices in that group. It was a difficult transition. Because we are a specialty practice, we used special forms in our paper-based medical record that were not part of the EHR which we had to adopt. We had to improvise at first and later have forms built for our use. Our providers were not used to the challenges of an EHR, and in the beginning they were always asking me for help. Things go more smoothly now, although the providers still complain about having to select the "correct" diagnosis code using the EHR every time they identify a new problem. The front office finds it helpful that the correct codes are already entered in the EHR by the time the patient visit is complete. The providers have also become accustomed to dictating progress notes directly into the EHR using speech recognition software. Another advantage is the increased space in the office because we do not have to store the paper charts anymore. Fortunately, the main medical group is responsible for submitting the paperwork needed to verify that we (and the other offices) are using the EHR according to specified guidelines. ■

CLINICAL SECTION OF THE MEDICAL RECORD

The clinical section of the medical record includes a variety of records and reports that assist the provider in the care and treatment of the patient. Common clinical records are listed and described next. Paper forms filled out by the patient or received in the mail are always filed in a patient's paper-based medical record. If there is an EHR, paper records, or at least some part of them, are usually scanned into it when it is adopted, and the original is either shredded or retained in a patient file with other paper records.

DATABASE

Health History

A **health history** is a collection of subjective data about the patient. Most of this information is obtained by having the patient complete a preprinted form that is then reviewed for completeness by the medical assistant. Some of the information included in the health history is obtained by the provider or medical assistant by interviewing the patient. Computer-guided questionnaires are available so that patients can enter their own health histories. The medical office must provide a private area for the patient to complete the questionnaire, and the medical assistant must be available to answer questions.

Along with the physical examination and laboratory and diagnostic tests, the health history is used for the following reasons: to determine the patient's general state of health, to arrive at a diagnosis and to prescribe treatment, and to document any change in a patient's illness after treatment has been instituted. The term **diagnosis** refers to the scientific method of determining and identifying a patient's condition. Before there is enough information to make a definitive diagnosis, the provider uses terms such as *medical impression*, *provisional diagnosis*, *preliminary diagnosis*, or *tentative diagnosis*.

A thorough history of personal health is obtained for each new patient, and subsequent office visits provide additional information regarding changes in the patient's condition or treatment. A complete discussion of the health history is presented later in this chapter.

Physical Examination

A **physical examination** is an assessment of each part of the patient's body. The purpose of the physical examination is to obtain objective data about the patient, which assists the provider in determining the patient's state of health. (The physical examination is described in detail in Chapter 20.)

The provider's findings from the head-to-toe assessment of each part of the patient's body are included in the paper medical record as a history and physical examination report. In the EHR, there may be a separate section to document the results of the physical examination, or it may be documented as a progress note. Each type of EHR is set up individually, and there are many methods to enter information.

Allergies

The patient usually includes all known allergies on the patient history form. For paper-based patient records, serious allergies are often noted on the chart folder using red or orange stickers. The EHR usually has an easily accessible record of patient allergies including medication, food, and environmental allergies. This is found in the database section of the record. For each allergen, it is noted if the allergy is active, the reaction type, and the severity of reactions. This should be updated at every visit as needed. There may be a checkbox in the EHR to indicate that the medical assistant has reviewed allergies with the patient.

One of the advantages of the EHR related to allergies is its ability to cross-check allergies with new medications that might be ordered, including immunizations. For example, if a patient has a recorded allergy to eggs, an alert will be issued if the provider orders an immunization that contains (or may contain) egg proteins. An alert is also triggered for new prescriptions if they contain medications or food products to which the patient is allergic.

Medication Record

A medication record consists of detailed information related to a patient's medications. The record usually includes one or more of the following categories: prescription medications, over-the-counter (OTC) medications, herbal and natural remedy products, immunizations, and other medications administered at the medical office. In the paper-based medical record, most medical offices use separate forms to record current prescription and OTC medications and immunizations and an additional form to keep a record of medications administered to the patient at the medical office. In the EHR, there will be separate screens for each of these areas depending on the type of EHR used. If a new medication is added, the program often has drop-down menus that facilitate this (Fig. 38.6). The record of immunizations includes the name of the vaccine, type, dose, date, provider, route and site, manufacturer and lot number, expiration date, and any reaction.

EHR software includes a prescription program, which greatly reduces the amount of time needed to prescribe and refill medication. The prescription program can print a prescription for the provider to sign, or it can transmit the prescription electronically (by e-fax or e-mail) to the patient's pharmacy. Both these features eliminate the need of the pharmacist to decipher the provider's handwriting. If the medical office uses a paper medical record, providers may still have the ability to send prescriptions directly to the patient's pharmacy by using a handheld device, such as a smartphone.

The EHR automatically checks any new medication against any drug allergies the patient may have. It also checks for potential interactions with other medications the patient is taking. Once the provider has entered the prescription into the computer, the medication is recorded in the patient's medication list. The EHR usually provides access to extensive and current product information on all medications approved by the U.S. Food and Drug Administration (FDA). It may also have the capability of comparing the prescription with the formulary or list of drugs covered by the patient's insurance plan. If the prescription is not in the patient's formulary, the provider is advised of alternative drugs that are covered by the patient's insurance plan.

PROBLEM LIST

The problem list is updated at every visit so that active problems can be identified. In the EHR, it is often required to add the diagnosis code directly on the problem list to

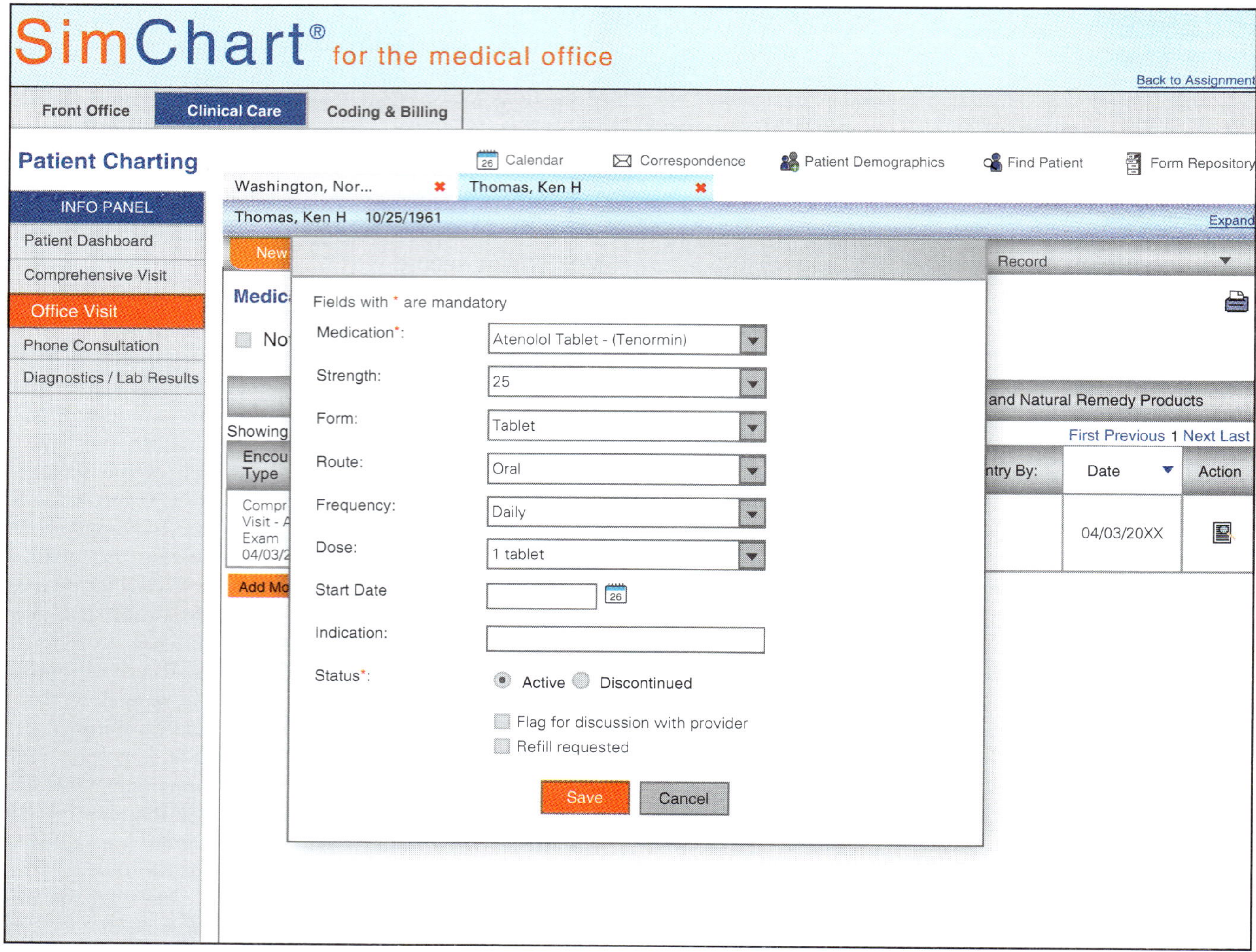

Fig. 38.6 Adding a medication in SimChart for the Medical Office.

assist with billing. There is usually a separate screen for active and inactive problems. The problem list helps the provider organize and plan appropriate care for the patient.

PROGRESS NOTES

Progress notes update the medical record with new information each time the patient visits or telephones the medical office. With an EHR, the provider or medical assistant enters this information directly into the computer using free text entry, drop-down lists, checkboxes, or dictates a progress note using voice-recognition software. Most EHR programs require a person entering data to finalize each entry. This may be done automatically when information is saved, or an additional step may be required such as checking a box or entering a digital signature (such as a password). Once the entry is finalized, it is automatically linked to a specific date and time, and it cannot be changed. (See Chapter 40 for a more complete discussion of computer features and passwords.) It is important that the date and time be included with each progress note in the paper-based medical record, along with the signature and credentials of the individual making the entry. A thorough discussion of documenting progress notes is presented later in this chapter.

LABORATORY DATA

In the POR, laboratory data obtained at the initial visit and the physical examination findings are considered part of the database, whereas laboratory reports related to specific problems are to be filed with other reports related to the problem. Laboratory reports are usually filed together in a paper-based medical record and accessed from one tab in an EHR. Many medical offices already communicate with outside laboratories electronically using a computer system that interfaces with the computer of the outside laboratory. This provides distinct advantages for the medical office using an EHR. Laboratory requisition forms can be completed on a request form displayed on the computer screen using fill-in boxes, drop-down lists, and checkboxes. The form can then be transmitted electronically to the medical laboratory. Once the patient's tests have been completed, the laboratory test results can be sent electronically to the patient's medical record in the medical office. At the same time, a notification that there are new laboratory data is placed in the provider's "electronic review bin" for their review and electronic signature. Abnormal values are highlighted on the report; for example, a high value may be highlighted in red and a low value in green. If a critical result appears on the laboratory report, an urgent message is e-mailed to the provider.

An advantage of the EHR is the ability to quickly view laboratory results in a chronological order. In addition, the results of laboratory tests performed on a routine basis (e.g., blood glucose) can usually be accessed by the computer and graphed. This permits an abnormal trend to be identified early so that appropriate action can be taken.

If the medical office is not networked through computers with an outside laboratory, the laboratory reports received by the office must either be scanned into the computer or filed in the patient's paper-based medical record.

DIAGNOSTIC PROCEDURES

A **diagnostic procedure** is a type of procedure performed to assist in the diagnosis, management, or treatment of a patient's condition. The procedure may be performed by a provider, the medical assistant, or a technician specially trained in the procedure. A provider is responsible for interpreting the results of the diagnostic procedure and completing the written report. In the paper-based medical record, a report is filed in the record with a paper copy of test results that can be printed on paper (such as electrocardiogram [ECG], spirometry results). The image of a diagnostic procedure (e.g., x-ray study, computed tomography [CT] scan, magnetic resonance imaging [MRI] scan, ECG) can be stored in the EHR as a digital image. A **digital image** is a picture that is stored electronically to allow viewing on a computer. EHR software can then display the digital image. The machine used for a procedure performed in the medical office (e.g., ECG, spirometry) must be interfaced with the office's computer system for the image to be directly transmitted to the EHR.

A diagnostic procedure report consists of a narrative description and interpretation of a diagnostic procedure. Diagnostic procedure reports completed by an outside facility may be sent electronically to the medical office.

Electrocardiogram Report

An ECG report is a narrative description of a cardiologist's interpretation of an ECG, including the implications for the patient. The graphic tracing is usually included with the report either in paper form or as a digital image.

Holter Monitor Report

A Holter monitor report is a narrative description of the interpretation of a 24- to 48-hour ambulatory ECG, including the evaluator's impressions. Portions of the graphic tracing are usually included with the report.

Spirometry Report

A spirometry report is a narrative and graphic description of the interpretation of a patient's breathing capacity as measured with a spirometer.

Radiology Report

A radiology report is a narrative description of a diagnostic or therapeutic radiologic procedure. If the procedure is done outside the medical office, a radiologist examines the radiograph and provides a written report, which includes a detailed interpretation of the radiograph and their impressions. If the office EHR has an interface to the facility where the study was done, the digital image will also be available in the patient's record.

Diagnostic Imaging Report

A diagnostic imaging report is a narrative description of a diagnostic imaging procedure. The report includes a detailed interpretation of the diagnostic image, along with the practitioner's impressions. Examples of common diagnostic imaging procedures include ultrasonography, CT scan, and MRI.

CONTINUITY OF CARE

Continuity of care measures are part of the meaningful use measures for the EHR. Core objectives for Stage 2 include a requirement for a summary care record when patients are referred to another setting of care or provider of care. A percentage of these records must be electronically transmitted to the recipient following specified guidelines. Other data must also be transferred electronically, including immunization data to immunization registries and clinical data related to public health (e.g., reporting cancer cases to a public health central cancer registry).

Reports of services received from other providers, hospitals, home health agencies, or other health care providers may be included in a paper-based medical record or an EHR in the office of the primary care provider. This also facilitates continuity of care for the patient.

Consultation Report

A **consultation report** is a narrative report of a clinical opinion about a patient's condition by a practitioner other than the primary provider, known as a *consultant.* The consultant is usually a specialist in a certain field of medicine (e.g., cardiology, endocrinology, urology). The consultant's opinion of the patient's condition is based on a review of the patient's record and an examination of the patient. The consultation report must include the following:

- Documentation that the consultant reviewed the patient's health history
- Documentation that the consultant examined the patient
- A report of the consultant's impressions
- Any care or treatment provided by the consultant
- A report of the consultant's recommendations

Home Health Care Report

Home health care is the provision of medical and nonmedical care in a patient's home or place of residence. The purpose of home health care is to minimize the effect of disease or disability by promoting, maintaining, and restoring the patient's health. There is a growing preference for home health care over equivalent health care options. Research shows that familiar surroundings contribute positively to a patient's emotional and physical well-being.

Home health care must be ordered by the patient's provider and is provided by skilled professionals. Home health care professionals include nurses, home health aides, dietitians, physical therapists, occupational therapists, speech therapists, and social workers. Examples of specialized services available through home health care include cardiac home care, intravenous (IV) therapy, respiratory therapy, pain management, diabetes management, rehabilitation, and maternal–child care. Home health care providers must periodically provide a summary report to the patient's provider that includes the following:

- Observations and evaluations
- Type of care or service provided
- Instructions given to the patient on medications
- Safety measures recommended for the home
- Diet
- Activities permitted

Therapeutic Service Documents

A therapeutic service report documents the assessments and treatments designed to restore a patient's ability to function. Examples of therapeutic services are physical therapy, occupational therapy, and speech therapy.

Physical therapy involves the use of therapeutic exercise, thermal modalities, cold, hydrotherapy, electrical stimulation, massage, and other physical agents to restore function and promote healing after an illness or injury. A physical therapist might help a football player with a knee injury to regain normal functioning of the knee or assist a patient recovering from a stroke to use their legs to walk again.

Occupational therapy helps a patient learn new skills to adapt to a physically, developmentally, emotionally, or mentally disabling condition. This enables the patient to perform activities of daily living and to achieve as much independence as possible. An occupational therapist might help an individual with a physical disability learn how to get dressed and how to prepare meals.

Speech therapy refers to treatment for the correction of a speech impairment resulting from birth, disease, injury, or previous medical treatment.

Hospital Documents

Hospital documents are prepared by the provider responsible for the care of a patient while at the hospital; this provider is known as the **attending provider** or **hospitalist**. The attending provider may be the patient's regular provider or a different provider. An example of the latter is a provider attending a patient at an urgent care center or in the emergency department of a hospital.

Hospital documents are prepared by the attending provider at the hospital. The original document is filed in the patient's hospital medical record, and a copy is sent to the patient's primary care provider. Hospital documents assist the patient's provider in reviewing the patient's hospital visit and in providing follow-up care. They include a history and the physical examination findings from the inpatient stay, a discharge summary, and any operative reports. If a patient is seen at an emergency department, a copy of the emergency department report will also be sent to the patient's primary care provider.

The term **inpatient** refers to a patient who has been admitted to the hospital for at least one overnight stay. A health history must be obtained and a physical examination performed on all inpatients. There is one exception to this: If a patient history was obtained and a physical examination performed at the medical office within 1 week before admission, a copy of these documents may be used. In the event that a reliable health history cannot be obtained from the patient, it must be obtained from the person best able to relay the facts.

An operative report must be completed for all patients who have undergone a surgical procedure. This report describes the surgical procedure and must be completed and signed by the surgeon who performed the operation. If tissue was removed for microscopic examination, a pathology report will also be generated.

The **discharge summary report** is a brief (usually one-page) summary of the significant events of a patient's hospitalization. The report must be completed and signed by the attending provider. The discharge summary report includes a concise account of the patient's illness, course of treatment, and response to treatment, as well as the condition of the patient at the time of discharge from the hospital. The purpose of this report is to document information needed by the patient's provider to provide for the continuity of future care. It also is used to respond to authorized requests for information regarding the patient's hospitalization.

The emergency department report is a record of the significant information obtained during an emergency department visit. The report is prepared and signed by the emergency department provider, and a copy is sent to the primary care provider for the purpose of providing follow-up care.

TAKING A HEALTH HISTORY

The health history is a collection of subjective health data obtained by interviewing. A thorough history is taken for each new patient as a baseline. Progress notes recorded at subsequent office visits provide information regarding changes in the patient's illness or treatment, but the health history is usually reviewed and updated annually. A quiet, comfortable room that allows for privacy encourages the

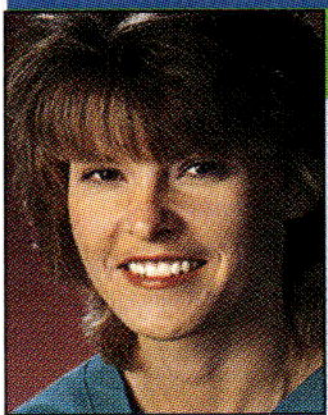

Memories *From* Practicum

Dawn Bennett: During my practicum as a medical assisting student, I was placed in a family practice clinic. I was very nervous my first day, wondering how in the world I would be able to remember everything I had learned in school. My first patients were an elderly couple. The wife was there for some test results for cancer. I looked at the results, and they were positive. After the provider relayed the results, the husband broke down. He had just lost his granddaughter after a car accident and his son-in-law to a stroke. You could tell that he just could not bear losing his wife too.

One week later, the elderly man's wife was placed in a nursing home. He came into our office for an appointment. As I was working him up, he was telling me stories about himself and his wife when they were first married. He looked so sad. I sat with him for a few minutes after completing his workup and gave his stories my full attention. As I was leaving the room, a smile came across his face, and he thanked me for listening to him. I realized that working in a provider's office is more than just knowing what I learned in school. Compassion and showing patients you really do care about them are just as important. I felt good about myself that day. ■

patient to communicate honestly and openly. Showing genuine interest in and concern for the patient reduces apprehension and facilitates the collection of data.

COMPONENTS OF THE HEALTH HISTORY

The health history is taken before the physical examination is performed, providing the provider the opportunity to compare findings. The health history consists of several parts or sections.

Identification Data

The identification data section is included at the beginning of a paper health history form to obtain basic demographic data regarding the patient (see Fig. 38.7A). The patient completes the identification data section. If the office uses an EHR, selecting the correct patient automatically links history information to the patient demographic data.

Chief Complaint

The **chief complaint** (CC) identifies the patient's reason for seeking care—that is, the symptom that is causing the patient the most trouble. The CC is used as a foundation for the more detailed information obtained for the present illness (PI) and review of systems (ROS) sections of the health history. The medical assistant is usually responsible for obtaining the CC from the patient and recording it in the patient's chart. This information may be recorded on a paper form or entered directly into an EHR (Fig. 38.8). Certain guidelines must be followed in obtaining and recording the CC, as follows:

- An open-ended question should be used to elicit the CC from the patient: What seems to be the problem? How can we help you today? What brings you to the doctor today?
- The CC should be limited to one or two symptoms and should refer to a specific rather than a vague symptom.
- The CC should be recorded concisely and briefly, using the patient's own words as much as possible.
- The duration of the symptom (onset) should be included in the CC.
- The medical assistant should avoid using names of diseases or diagnostic terms to record the CC.

Recording Chief Complaints

Following are correct and incorrect examples of recording chief complaints.

Correct Examples

- Burning during urination that has lasted for 2 days
- Pain in the right shoulder that started 2 weeks ago
- Shortness of breath for the past month

Incorrect Examples

- Has not felt well for the past 2 weeks. (This statement refers to a vague rather than a specific complaint.)
- Ear pain and fever. (The duration of the symptoms is not listed.)
- Pain on urination indicative of a urinary tract infection. (Names of diseases should not be used to record the chief complaint; the duration of the symptom is not listed.)

Present Illness

The PI is an expansion of the chief complaint and includes a full description of the patient's current illness from the time of its onset. The medical assistant is often responsible for completing this section of the health history, which is recorded on the same form as the chief complaint in the EHR (see Fig. 38.8). To complete this section of the health history, the medical assistant asks the patient questions to obtain a detailed description of the symptom causing the greatest problem. The medical assistant is encouraged to use the patient's own words if possible. Much skill and practice in asking the proper questions are required to elicit detailed information.

Allergies, Current Medications, and Immunizations

The lists of allergies, current medications, and immunizations, as discussed earlier, are usually on separate screens in the EHR. The information is often collected from patients on a paper patient history form.

Past History

The past medical history is a review of the patient's past medical status (Fig. 38.7B). Obtaining information on past medical care assists the provider in providing optimal care for the current problem. Most medical offices ask the patient

PATIENT HEALTH HISTORY

A

IDENTIFICATION DATA Please print the following information.

Today's date ______

Name ______ ___ Male ___ Female

Address ______ ___ Married ___ Separated ___ Divorced ___ Widowed ___ Single

______ Date of Birth ______

Telephone ______ ______
Home number Work number

B

PAST HISTORY

Have you ever had the following: (Circle "no" or "yes", leave blank if uncertain)

Measles ___ no yes	Heart Disease ___ no yes	Diabetes ___ no yes	Hemorrhoids ___ no yes
Mumps ___ no yes	Arthritis ___ no yes	Cancer ___ no yes	Asthma ___ no yes
Chickenpox ___ no yes	Sexually Transmitted Disease ___ no yes	Polio ___ no yes	Allergies ___ no yes
Whooping Cough ___ no yes	Anemia ___ no yes	Glaucoma ___ no yes	Eczema ___ no yes
Scarlet Fever ___ no yes	Bladder Infections ___ no yes	Hernia ___ no yes	AIDS or HIV+ ___ no yes
Diphtheria ___ no yes	Epilepsy ___ no yes	Blood or Plasma Transfusions ___ no yes	Infectious Mono ___ no yes
Pneumonia ___ no yes	Migraine Headaches ___ no yes	Back Trouble ___ no yes	Bronchitis ___ no yes
Rheumatic Fever ___ no yes	Tuberculosis ___ no yes	High Blood Pressure ___ no yes	Mitral Valve Prolapse no yes
Stroke ___ no yes	Ulcer ___ no yes	Thyroid Disease ___ no yes	Any other disease ___ no yes Please list: ______
Hepatitis ___ no yes	Kidney Disease ___ no yes	Bleeding Tendency ___ no yes	

MAJOR HOSPITALIZATIONS: If you have ever been hospitalized for any major medical illness or operation, write in your most recent hospitalizations below.

Hospitalizations	Year	Operation or illness	Name of hospital	City and state
1st Hospitalization				
2nd Hospitalization				
3rd Hospitalization				
4th Hospitalization				

TESTS AND IMMUNIZATIONS: Mark an X next to those that you have had.

Tests:
- ☐ TB Test
- ☐ Rectal/Hemoccult
- ☐ Sigmoidoscopy
- ☐ Colonoscopy
- ☐ Electrocardiogram
- ☐ Chest x-ray
- ☐ Mammogram
- ☐ Pap Test

Immunizations:
- ☐ Influenza
- ☐ Hepatitis B
- ☐ Tetanus
- ☐ MMR
- ☐ Polio

CURRENT MEDICATIONS: List the following that you are currently taking: Prescription medications, over-the-counter (OTC) medications, vitamin supplements, and herbal supplements. ☐ None

Medication Frequency

______

ALLERGIES: List all allergies (foods, drugs, environment). ☐ None

______

ACCIDENTS/ INJURIES: Describe all serious accidents, severe injuries, head injury, or fractures. Include the date each occurred. ☐ None

Accident/Injury: Date:

______

Fig. 38.7 (A–D) Health history form.

C

FAMILY HISTORY

For each member of your family, follow the purple or blue line across the page and check boxes for:
1. His or her present state of health
2. Any illnesses he or she has had

	Good Health	Poor Health	Deceased	If deceased, write in age and cause of death.	Allergies or Asthma	Diabetes	Heart Disease	Stroke	Cancer	High Blood Pressure	Glaucoma	Arthritis	Ulcer	Kidney Disease	Mental Health Problems	Alcohol/Drug Abuse	Obesity	High Cholesterol	Thyroid Disease
Father:																			
Mother:																			
Brothers/Sisters:																			

D

SOCIAL HISTORY

EDUCATION ______ High school ______ College ______ Postgraduate

Occupation ______ Years ______

Previous occupations ______ Years ______

______ Years ______

Have you ever been exposed to any of the following in your environment?

- ☐ Excess dust (coal, lime, rock)
- ☐ Sand
- ☐ Chemicals
- ☐ Cleaning fluids/solvents
- ☐ Hair spray
- ☐ Smoke or auto exhaust fumes
- ☐ Radiation
- ☐ Insecticides
- ☐ Paints
- ☐ Other toxic materials

Please answer the following questions by placing an X in the box in front of the word Yes or No, except where you are asked for specific information. This information is obviously highly confidential and will be released to other healthcare professionals or insurance carriers ONLY with your consent.

DIET:

- Do you eat a good breakfast? ☐ Yes ☐ No
- Do you snack between meals (soft drinks, chips, candy bars)? ☐ Yes ☐ No
- Do you eat fresh fruits and vegetables each day? ☐ Yes ☐ No
- Do you eat whole grain breads and cereals? ☐ Yes ☐ No
- Is your diet high in fat content? ☐ Yes ☐ No
- Is your diet high in cholesterol content? ☐ Yes ☐ No
- Is your diet high in salt content? ☐ Yes ☐ No
- Are you allergic to any foods? ☐ Yes ☐ No
- How many glasses of water do you drink each day? ______
- How would you describe your overall eating habits? ☐ Excellent ☐ Good ☐ Fair ☐ Poor

PERSONAL HISTORY:

- Do you find it hard to make decisions? ☐ Yes ☐ No
- Do you find it hard to concentrate or remember? ☐ Yes ☐ No
- Do you feel depressed? ☐ Yes ☐ No
- Do you have difficulty relaxing? ☐ Yes ☐ No
- Do you have a tendency to worry a lot? ☐ Yes ☐ No
- Have you gained or lost much weight recently? ☐ Yes ☐ No
- Do you lose your temper often? ☐ Yes ☐ No
- Are you disturbed by any work or family problems? ☐ Yes ☐ No
- Are you having sexual difficulties? ☐ Yes ☐ No
- Have you ever considered committing suicide? ☐ Yes ☐ No
- Have you ever desired or sought psychiatric help? ☐ Yes ☐ No

EXERCISE:

- Do you exercise on a regular basis? ☐ Yes ☐ No
- Does your job require strenuous, sustained physical work? ☐ Yes ☐ No

SLEEP PATTERNS:

- Do you seem to feel exhausted or fatigued most of the time? ☐ Yes ☐ No
- Do you have difficulty either falling asleep or staying asleep? ☐ Yes ☐ No

USE OF TOBACCO/ALCOHOL/CAFFEINE/DRUGS: Amt:

- How much do you smoke per day? ☐ Cigarettes ___ ☐ Cigars/pipes ___ ☐ Don't smoke
- Do you take two or more alcoholic drinks per day? ☐ Yes ☐ No
- Do you drink six or more cups of coffee or tea per day? ☐ Yes ☐ No
- Are you a regular user of sleeping pills, marijuana, tranquilizers, pain killers, etc? ☐ Yes ☐ No
- Have you ever used heroin, cocaine, LSD, PCP, etc? ☐ Yes ☐ No

List any country outside the USA you have visited in the past six months. ______

When did you have your last physical examination? ______

Fig. 38.7, cont'd

Chief Complaint *:

Dizziness when standing up X 2 weeks

History of Present Illness

Location:	Generalized	Timing:	"It happens when I stand up"
Quality:	"I feel dizzy and weak"	Context:	"If I have been sitting or lying down"
Severity:	Moderate dizziness for a few seconds	Modifying Factors:	"It is worse if I stand up fast"
Duration:	2 weeks	Associated Signs and Symptoms:	None

Fig. 38.8 Recording the chief complaint and history of present illness in SimChart for the Medical Office.

to complete this section of the health history through a checklist type of form. The medical assistant should assist the patient with this section as necessary by offering to answer any questions regarding the information required. The information may be transferred to an EHR either at the beginning of the visit or during the patient visit. The past history includes the following areas:

- Major illnesses and/or previous health problems
- Childhood diseases
- Unusual infections
- Accidents and injuries
- Hospitalizations and operations
- Previous medical tests, immunizations, allergies
- Previous surgeries

Family History

The family history is a review of the health status of the patient's blood relatives (Fig. 38.7C). This section of the health history focuses on diseases that tend to be familial. A **familial** disease is one that occurs in or affects blood relatives more frequently than would be expected by chance. Examples of familial diseases include hypertension, heart disease, allergies, and diabetes mellitus. The patient usually completes this section of the health history and is asked to provide the following information about each blood relative:

- State of health
- Presence of any significant disease
- If deceased, cause of death

Paternal relatives include a patient's father and his parents and/or siblings. Maternal relatives include a patient's mother and her parents and/or siblings. The patient's own siblings should also be entered. Aunts and uncles are usually entered only if they have familial or hereditary diseases.

Social History

The social history section of the health history includes information on the patient's lifestyle, such as health habits and living environment (Fig. 38.7D). The social history is important because the patient's lifestyle may have an impact on their condition and may influence the course of treatment chosen by the provider. The social history also provides the provider with information regarding the effect that the illness may have on the patient's daily living pattern. If it is necessary for the individual to make a major lifestyle adjustment (e.g., stop smoking, reduce working hours), the provider may recommend support services to assist in this transition. This section of the history is usually completed by the patient and includes the following areas:

- Education
- Occupation (past and present)
- Living environment (including whether the patient feels safe at home)
- Diet
- Personal history
- Use of tobacco, caffeine, drugs
- Exercise

Review of Systems

A review of systems (ROS) is a systematic review of each body system to detect any symptoms that have not yet been revealed. The importance of the ROS is that it assists in identifying symptoms that might otherwise remain undetected. The provider usually completes the ROS by asking a series of detailed and direct questions related to each body system; the results of this section of the health history assist the provider in a preliminary assessment of the type and extent of physical examination required. If an EHR is being used, the information is usually entered into the computer as the questions are asked (Fig. 38.9).

What Would You Do? What Would You *Not* Do?

Case Study 3

Brett Oberlin is 21 years old and lives at home. He commutes to a local college and is a junior majoring in art education. His mother and father have come to the medical office asking to see his medical record. The provider is attending a medical conference and will not return for another 4 days. Mr. and Mrs. Oberlin found some medications in Brett's room and looked them up on the internet. They found out that they are used to treat human immunodeficiency virus (HIV) infection. Brett would not talk to them about the medications and told them he is an adult and it is none of their business. Mr. and Mrs. Oberlin are very concerned about Brett's health and well-being. They say that because they are supporting him, they should be allowed to see his record. ■

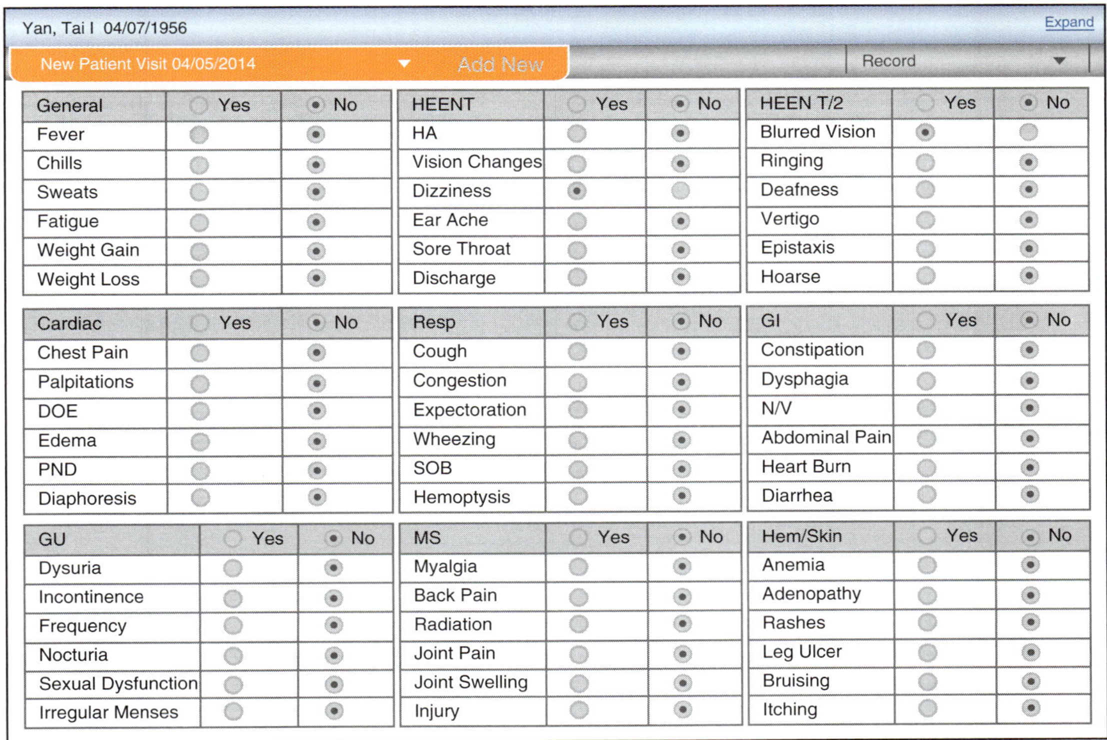
Yan, Tai I 04/07/1956 Expand

New Patient Visit 04/05/2014 Add New Record

General	Yes	No	HEENT	Yes	No	HEENT T/2	Yes	No
Fever	○	●	HA	○	●	Blurred Vision	●	○
Chills	○	●	Vision Changes	○	●	Ringing	○	●
Sweats	○	●	Dizziness	●	○	Deafness	○	●
Fatigue	○	●	Ear Ache	○	●	Vertigo	○	●
Weight Gain	○	●	Sore Throat	○	●	Epistaxis	○	●
Weight Loss	○	●	Discharge	○	●	Hoarse	○	●

Cardiac	Yes	No	Resp	Yes	No	GI	Yes	No
Chest Pain	○	●	Cough	○	●	Constipation	○	●
Palpitations	○	●	Congestion	○	●	Dysphagia	○	●
DOE	○	●	Expectoration	○	●	N/V	○	●
Edema	○	●	Wheezing	○	●	Abdominal Pain	○	●
PND	○	●	SOB	○	●	Heart Burn	○	●
Diaphoresis	○	●	Hemoptysis	○	●	Diarrhea	○	●

GU	Yes	No	MS	Yes	No	Hem/Skin	Yes	No
Dysuria	○	●	Myalgia	○	●	Anemia	○	●
Incontinence	○	●	Back Pain	○	●	Adenopathy	○	●
Frequency	○	●	Radiation	○	●	Rashes	○	●
Nocturia	○	●	Joint Pain	○	●	Leg Ulcer	○	●
Sexual Dysfunction	○	●	Joint Swelling	○	●	Bruising	○	●
Irregular Menses	○	●	Injury	○	●	Itching	○	●

Fig. 38.9 Review of systems in SimChart for the Medical Office.

DOCUMENTATION IN THE MEDICAL RECORD

Documenting is the process of making written or electronic entries about a patient in the medical record and is performed by medical office personnel who are directly involved with the health care of the patient. The medical record is considered a legal document; the information must be documented as completely and accurately as possible. Developing good documentation skills requires a thorough knowledge of the guidelines combined with much repeated practice. To provide guidance in attaining this important skill, general guidelines for documenting in both the EHR and the paper-based medical record are presented in this section, followed by specific guidelines with examples of entries documented properly.

GENERAL GUIDELINES FOR DOCUMENTATION

To ensure accurate and concise documentation, specific guidelines must be followed. These are listed and described as follows:

1. *Check the name and date of birth on the EHR or paper chart before making an entry to ensure you have the correct record.* If the medical assistant records in the wrong patient's record by mistake, information such as a procedure that was performed on a patient may be excluded from the correct patient's record. As previously stated, from a legal standpoint, a procedure not documented will be considered not to have been performed.
2. *Document information accurately in a logical order, using clear and concise phrases.*
   - The medical assistant should be brief but thorough and should avoid vagueness and duplication of information.
   - It is not necessary to include the patient's name in the entry because the entire medical record centers on one patient; it is assumed the information refers to that patient.
   - Each phrase should begin with a capital letter and end with a period.
   - Standard abbreviations, medical terms, and symbols can be used to help save time and space. It is *crucial* that the medical assistant first check the office policy to determine the abbreviations, medical terms, and symbols that are commonly used in that office. Using abbreviations that can be substantiated in a medical dictionary avoids confusing others who read the record. A list of abbreviations and symbols commonly used in medical offices is presented in Table 38.1.
3. *Spell correctly.* Correct spelling is essential for accuracy in documentation. A dictionary should be consulted as needed.
4. *Document immediately after performing a procedure.* When a procedure has been performed, it should be documented without delay. The name of the provider who ordered the procedure or who is going to be cosigning the note must be included. If a time lapse occurs between performing the procedure and documenting it, the medical assistant may not remember certain aspects

Table 38.1 Abbreviations and Symbols Commonly Used in the Medical Office

Abbreviations Used to Document Symptoms and Procedures

Abbreviation	Meaning
$\overline{aa}$	of each
Ab	abortion
ac	before meals
ad lib	as desired
AM or a.m.	before noon
amt	amount
AP	apical pulse
approx	approximately
appt	appointment
ASAP	as soon as possible
BA	backache
BC	birth control
bid	twice a day
BM	bowel movement
BP	blood pressure
BPM	beats per minute
BSE	breast self-examination
$\overline{c}$	With
caps	capsules
cath	catheter, catheterize
CC	chief complaint
chemo	chemotherapy
CMA (AAMA)	certified medical assistant (American Association of Medical Assistants)
c/o	complains of
CS	cesarean section
Cx	cervix
d	day
/d	per day
disch	discharge
DNKA	did not keep appointment
DOB	date of birth
DRE	digital rectal examination
DTaP	diphtheria and tetanus toxoids and acellular pertussis vaccine
DVA	distance visual acuity
ED	emergency department
EDD	expected date of delivery
Fe	iron
F/U	follow-up
Fx	fracture
GYN	gynecology
h or hr	hour
H/A	headache
HBP	high blood pressure
Hep B	hepatitis B vaccine
Hg	mercury
H_2O	water
HR	heart rate
HRT	hormone replacement therapy
ht	height
ID	intradermal
IM	intramuscular
IPV	inactivated polio vaccine
IV	intravenous
lab	laboratory
lac	laceration
lat	lateral
lax	laxative
liq	liquid
LMP	last menstrual period
med, meds	medication, medications
min	minute
MMR	measles, mumps, and rubella
mod	moderate
N/A	not applicable
neg	negative
NICU	newborn intensive care unit
NKA	no known allergies
NKDA	no known drug allergies
noct	nocturnal
NS	normal saline
N&V	nausea and vomiting
NVA	near visual acuity
OB	obstetrics
occ	occasionally
oint	ointment
OR	operating room
OT	occupational therapy
OTC	over-the-counter (nonprescription medication)
OV	office visit
P	pulse
Pap	Papanicolaou (Pap) test
path	pathology
pc	after meals
peds	pediatrics
per	by or through
pharm	pharmacy
PM or p.m.	afternoon
PMS	premenstrual syndrome
po or PO	by mouth
pos	positive
postop	postoperative (after surgery)
preop	preoperative (before surgery)
prep	preparation
prn	as needed
PT	physical therapy, prothrombin time
Pt or pt	patient
qh	every hour
q(2,3,4)h	every (2, 3, 4) hours
qid	four times a day

Table 38.1 Abbreviations and Symbols Commonly Used in the Medical Office—cont'd

R	respiration
reg	regular
rehab	rehabilitation
RMA	registered medical assistant
Rx	prescription
s̄	without
S/E	side effects
SOB	shortness of breath
sol	solution
spec	specimen
STAT	immediately
surg	surgery
T	temperature
tab, tabs	tablet, tablets
temp	temperature
tid	three times a day
TLC	total lung capacity, tender loving care
TPR	temperature, pulse, and respiration
tr	trace
TSE	testicular self-examination
VO	verbal order
VS	vital signs
WNL	within normal limits
WO	written order
w/o	without
wt	weight
Abbreviations Used to Document Body Parts and Locations	
abd	abdomen
EENT	eye, ear, nose, and throat
GI	gastrointestinal
GU	genitourinary
Ⓛ or lt	left
(LA)	left arm
(LL)	left leg
LLQ	lower left quadrant
LRQ	lower right quadrant
LUQ	left upper quadrant
Ⓡ or rt	right
(RA)	right arm
(RL)	right leg
RLQ	right lower quadrant
RUQ	right upper quadrant
Abbreviations Used to Document Measurement	
C	Celsius
cm	centimeter
dL	deciliter
F	Fahrenheit
g	gram
kg	kilogram
L	liter
lb	pound
m	meter
mcg	microgram
mg	milligram
mL or ml	milliliter
mm	millimeter
oz	ounce
pt	pint
qt	quart
ss	one half
T	Tablespoon
tsp	teaspoon
Miscellaneous Abbreviations	
Patient Examination	
Dx	diagnosis
H/O	history of
H&P	history and physical
Hx	history
PE or Px	physical examination
Sx	Symptoms
Tx	treatment
Conditions	
BPH	benign prostatic hyperplasia
CA	cancer
CAD	coronary artery disease
CHF	congestive heart failure
COPD	chronic obstructive pulmonary disease
CRC	colorectal cancer
CVA	cerebrovascular accident
DM	diabetes mellitus
DVT	deep vein thrombosis
GC	Gonorrhea (gonococcus)
GDM	gestational diabetes mellitus
HTN	hypertension
IBS	irritable bowel syndrome
MI	myocardial infarction
MS	multiple sclerosis
OA	osteoarthritis
OM	otitis media
PID	pelvic inflammatory disease
RA	rheumatoid arthritis
RF	rheumatic fever
STD (STI)	sexually transmitted disease (sexually transmitted infection)
TB	tuberculosis
URI	upper respiratory infection
UTI	urinary tract infection
Diagnostic Procedures	
CT, CAT	computed axial tomography

Continued

Table 38.1 Abbreviations and Symbols Commonly Used in the Medical Office—cont'd

CXR	chest x-ray	PT, PT/INR	prothrombin time, prothrombin time/international normalized ratio
ECG	electrocardiogram	RBC	red blood cell
Echo	echocardiogram	RBS	random blood sugar
EEG	electroencephalogram	SG	specific gravity
FOBT	fecal occult blood test	UA	Urinalysis
IVP	intravenous pyelogram	WBC	white blood cell
LP	lumbar puncture		
MRI	magnetic resonance imaging	***Symbols***	
NST	nonstress test	Ø	none, no
PET	positron emission tomography	✓	check
PFT	pulmonary function test	↑	increase
US	ultrasound	↓	decrease
Laboratory Tests		♀	female
ABG	arterial blood gas	♂	male
BG	blood glucose	°	degree
Bx	biopsy	×	times
CBC	complete blood count	$\bar{p}$	after
C&S	culture and sensitivity	#	number
diff	differential	1°	primary
ESR	erythrocyte sedimentation rate	2°	secondary
FBG	fasting blood glucose	+	positive
FBS	fasting blood sugar	−	negative
GCT	glucose challenge test	Ⓡ	rectal temperature
GTT	glucose tolerance test	Ⓐ	axillary temperature
Hct	hematocrit	″	inches
Hgb	hemoglobin	′	feet
PSA	prostate-specific antigen		

Note: This table follows The Joint Commission's list of "Do Not Use" abbreviations and symbols. The Joint Commission requirements do not currently apply to preprogrammed health information technology systems such as electronic health records.

of the procedure, such as the results of the treatment or the patient's reaction.

5. *Procedures should never be documented in advance.* The individual performing the procedure should be the one to document it after the procedure has been completed.

DOCUMENTING IN THE PAPER-BASED MEDICAL RECORD

1. *Use black ink to make entries in the paper medical record.* Black ink must be used to provide a permanent record. In addition, entries made in black ink are easier to reproduce when a record must be duplicated for insurance company purposes and patient referral.
2. *Write in legible handwriting or print.* For the medical record to be meaningful to others, the medical assistant must document information legibly. If the medical assistant's cursive script is not legible, the information should be printed.
3. *Begin each new entry on a separate line but do not leave blank lines.* Each new entry should begin on a separate line and be dated with the month, day, year, and time (either AM/PM [a.m./p.m.] or military time [24-hour clock]). If the entire line is not needed, draw a single line through unneeded space so that nothing can be added at a later date.
4. *Each entry should be signed by the person making it.* The signature should include the medical assistant's first initial, full last name, and title (e.g., D. Bennett, CMA [AAMA]). The following title abbreviations are often used for medical assistants, although medical assistants with other credentials may use other appropriate abbreviations:
   CMA (AAMA): certified medical assistant
   RMA: registered medical assistant
   MA: medical assistant
   SMA: student medical assistant
5. *Never erase or obliterate an entry.* If an error is made in a paper record, the medical assistant must never erase or obliterate it. Should the provider or medical staff be involved in litigation, erased or obliterated entries tend to reduce credibility. If incorrect information is documented, the medical assistant should draw a single line through the incorrect information, permitting it to remain legible. The word *error* or *correction* is then written above the incorrect data, including the date

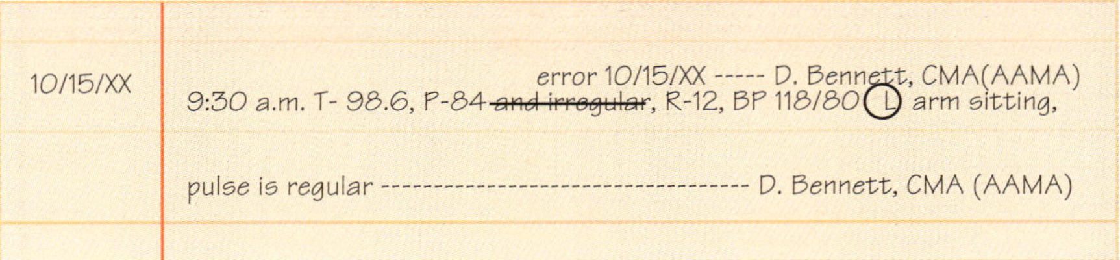
10/15/XX | 9:30 a.m. T- 98.6, P-84 ~~and irregular~~, R-12, BP 118/80 Ⓛ arm sitting,
error 10/15/XX ----- D. Bennett, CMA(AAMA)
pulse is regular ---------------------------------- D. Bennett, CMA (AAMA)

Fig. 38.10 Correction of handwritten documentation error.

and the medical assistant's first initial, last name, and credentials. If the correct information can be entered on the same line, it can be added next to the deleted entry. Otherwise, it should be entered on the next blank line (not above or below the line). It is impossible to know when a correction that is not on the main line of writing was actually made (Fig. 38.10).

UPDATING ALLERGIES AND MEDICATIONS

At the beginning of every office visit, the medical assistant should review a patient's allergies and current medications with a patient and record any changes. A list of current medications is often printed from the EHR, and the patient is asked to review and update the list. The medical assistant may update the list of current medications either on the paper printout or in the EHR, but in many offices the provider must review and approve any updates. It is important for the provider to be aware of any changes in the medications that the patient is actually taking.

DOCUMENTING ON FLOW SHEETS

Much of the documenting done by medical assistants in the EHR is done on **flow sheets**, records or computer screens that allow similar data to be recorded and viewed chronologically. These data include vital signs, growth charts, and immunization records. Complete information should be entered on these screens (Fig. 38.11). For example, a drop-down box must be selected when entering a temperature to identify the method used to measure the temperature.

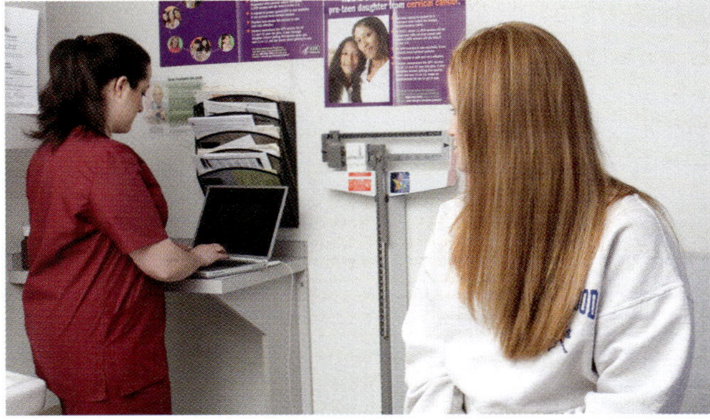

Fig. 38.11 Medical assistant documenting patient vital signs in the electronic health record.

DOCUMENTING IN PROGRESS NOTES

After completion of the initial health history, a system is needed to update the medical record with new information each time the patient visits the medical office. Most offices use progress notes to fulfill this function. Progress notes document the patient's health status and the care and treatment being received by the patient in chronological order. Progress notes provide effective communication among medical office personnel and serve as a legal document.

The medical assistant is frequently responsible for creating progress notes in the medical record. They are entered in SOAP format on progress note screens in the EHR. They are usually entered on special preprinted lined sheets known as *progress note sheets* in paper-based patient records. These sheets have a column for the date and a column for patient information. Types of notes that may be documented by the medical assistant are presented next, along with an example of each.

DOCUMENTING PATIENT SYMPTOMS

The medical assistant records patient symptoms during office visits and telephone conversations. Information conveyed during a telephone conversation helps the medical assistant determine whether the patient needs to be seen and the immediacy of the situation.

A **symptom** is any change in the body or its functioning that indicates the presence of disease. Symptoms can be classified as subjective or objective. A **subjective symptom** is one that is felt by the patient and cannot be observed by another person. Pain, pruritus, vertigo, and nausea are examples of subjective symptoms. An **objective symptom** is one that can be observed by another person and by the patient. Rash, coughing, and cyanosis are objective symptoms. The medical assistant should have a thorough knowledge of common symptoms and should be able to recognize them. Table 38.2 lists and describes common symptoms.

Taking patient symptoms during an office visit consists of the following:

1. Obtaining a chief complaint (see earlier discussion)
2. Obtaining additional information about the chief complaint

If the patient complains of pain in the abdomen that has lasted for 2 days (chief complaint), additional information is needed to describe the pain, including its location, quality, severity, duration, timing, and context; modifying factors; and associated signs and symptoms. The procedure for

Table 38.2 Common Symptoms

Symptom	Definition
Integumentary System	
Diaphoresis	Excessive perspiration.
Flushing	A red appearance to the skin, which typically affects the face and neck. A flushed appearance is commonly present with a fever.
Jaundice	A yellow appearance to the skin, first evident in the whites of the eyes.
Rash	An eruption on the skin.
Circulatory System	
Bradycardia	An abnormally slow pulse rate.
Dehydration	A decrease in the amount of water in the body. The patient has a flushed appearance, dry skin, and decreased output of urine.
Edema	The retention of fluid in the tissues, resulting in swelling. Skin over the area is tight. Edema is most easily observed in the extremities.
Tachycardia	An abnormally fast pulse rate.
Gastrointestinal System	
Anorexia	A loss of appetite and a lack of interest in food.
Constipation	A condition in which the stool becomes hard and dry, resulting in difficult passage from the rectum. The consistency of the stool, rather than the frequency of defecation, is used as a guide in determining the presence of constipation. (Frequency of bowel movements varies with the individual; some people have a bowel movement only every 2 to 3 days but are not constipated.) Other symptoms of constipation include headache, nausea, and general malaise.
Diarrhea	The passage of an increased number of loose, watery stools. The fecal material moves rapidly through the intestinal tract, resulting in decreased absorption by the body of water, electrolytes, and nutrients. Other symptoms usually associated with diarrhea are intestinal cramping and general weakness.
Flatulence	The presence of excessive gas in the stomach or intestines.
Nausea and vomiting	Nausea is a sensation of discomfort in the stomach with a feeling that vomiting may occur. Vomiting is the ejection of the stomach contents through the mouth, also known as *emesis.* The ejected content is known as *vomitus.*
Respiratory System	
Cough	An involuntary and forceful exhalation of air followed by a deep inhalation. A cough may be productive (meaning a discharge is produced) or nonproductive (no discharge is present).
Cyanosis	A bluish discoloration of the skin caused by lack of oxygen.
Dyspnea	Labored or difficult breathing.
Epistaxis	Hemorrhaging from the nose (nosebleed).
Nervous System	
Chills	A feeling of coldness accompanied by shivering. In general, chills are present with a fever.
Convulsions	Involuntary contractions of the muscles.
Fever or pyrexia	A body temperature that is higher than normal.
Headache	A feeling of pain or aching in the head. It is a common symptom that accompanies many illnesses. Tension, fatigue, and eyestrain can result in a headache.
Malaise	A vague sense of body discomfort, weakness, and fatigue, often marking the onset of a disease and continuing through the course of the illness.
Pain	Irritation of pain receptors, resulting in a feeling of distress or suffering. Pain is an important indication that a part of the body is not working properly.
Pruritus	Severe itching.
Vertigo	A feeling of dizziness or lightheadedness.

taking and recording the patient's chief complaint during an office visit is outlined in Procedure 38.3. Additional skills and practice in taking patient symptoms are included in Chapter 38 of the *Study Guide*.

OTHER ACTIVITIES THAT NEED TO BE DOCUMENTED

Procedures

The medical assistant frequently documents procedures performed on the patient, including vital signs, weight and height, visual acuity, and ear irrigations. Procedures should be documented immediately after they are performed; as has been stated, from a legal standpoint any procedure not documented was not performed. In the EHR, procedures are usually documented as orders instead of notes. In general, the following information should be included: the type of procedure, the ordering provider, the outcome, and the patient reaction. In a paper record, the date and time should also be recorded. The specific information to be documented is included with each procedure presented in this text.

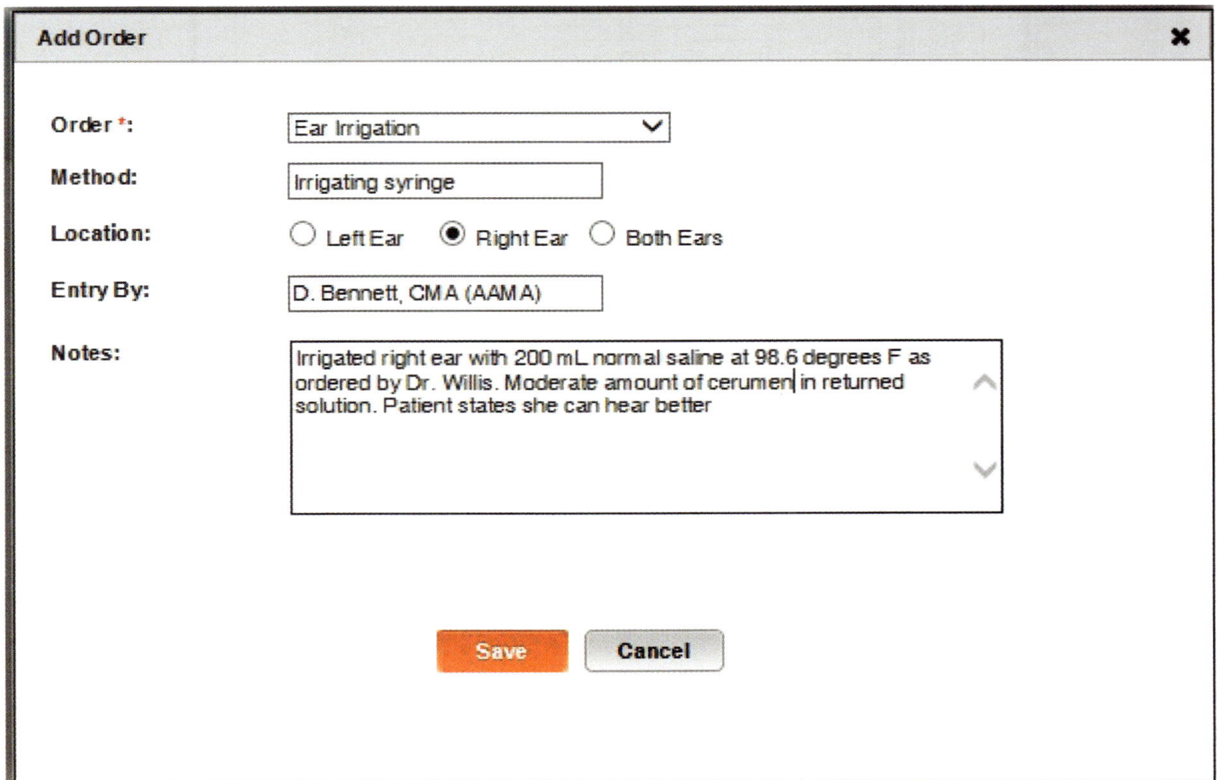

Procedure.

Administration of Medication

Documenting medications and immunizations administered to the patient is an important responsibility in the medical office. The recording should include the name of the medication, the ordering provider, the lot number (if required), the dosage given, the route of administration, the injection site used (for parenteral medication), and any significant observations or patient reactions. In a paper record, the date and time should be recorded. In an EHR, the information may be entered on a flow sheet or in a progress note depending on the type of EHR used by the medical office.

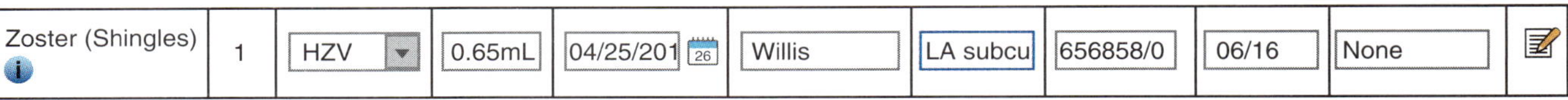

Administration of immunization.

Specimen Collection

Each time a specimen is collected from a patient, the medical assistant should document the date and time of the collection, the type of specimen, and the area of the body from which the specimen was obtained. If the specimen is to be sent to an outside laboratory for testing, this information also should be recorded, including the tests requested, the ordering provider, the date the specimen was sent, and where it was sent. Thus, the provider would know that the specimen was collected and sent to the laboratory when test results are not back yet.

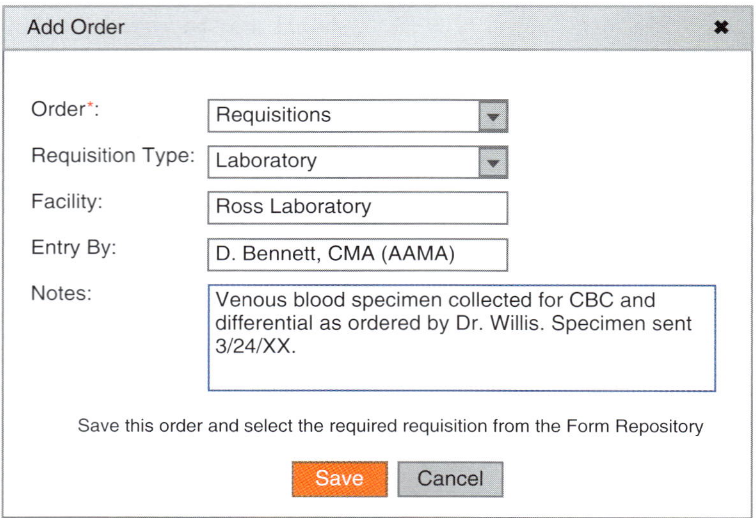

Specimen collection.

Diagnostic Procedures and Laboratory Tests

Diagnostic procedures and laboratory tests ordered for a patient should always be documented in the medical record. If the patient does not undergo the test, documented proof exists that the test was ordered. Recording that diagnostic procedures and laboratory tests were ordered protects the provider legally and refreshes the provider 's memory of the procedures and tests being run on the patient when results are not yet back from the testing facility. Information to include in the entry consists of the date and time, the type of procedure or test ordered, the ordering provider, the scheduling date, and where the procedure is being performed.

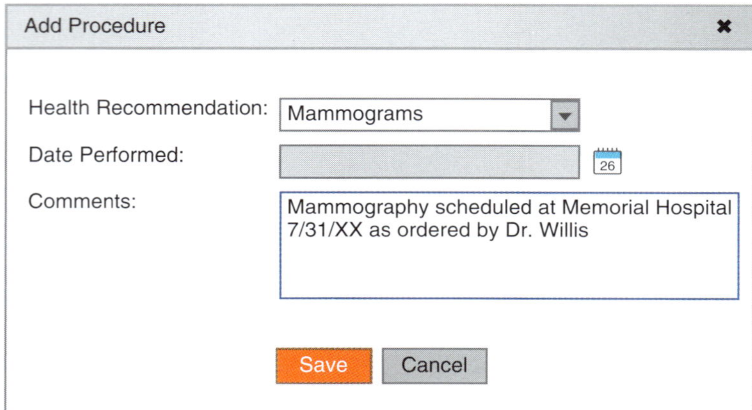

Diagnostic or laboratory tests.

Results of Laboratory Tests

It is usually unnecessary to document results from laboratory reports returned from outside laboratories because the report itself is filed in the patient's record. In case of a STAT request or critical findings, the test results may be telephoned to the medical office, requiring the medical assistant to record the results on a report form. Careful recording is essential to avoid errors, which could affect the patient's diagnosis. Results of laboratory tests performed by the medical assistant in the office should be documented in the medical record. Sometimes laboratory tests performed by the medical assistant must be entered as orders and be signed by the provider before results can be entered. There are usually specific screens to enter test results in the EHR. The EHR identifies all entries by date, time, and person entering the information.

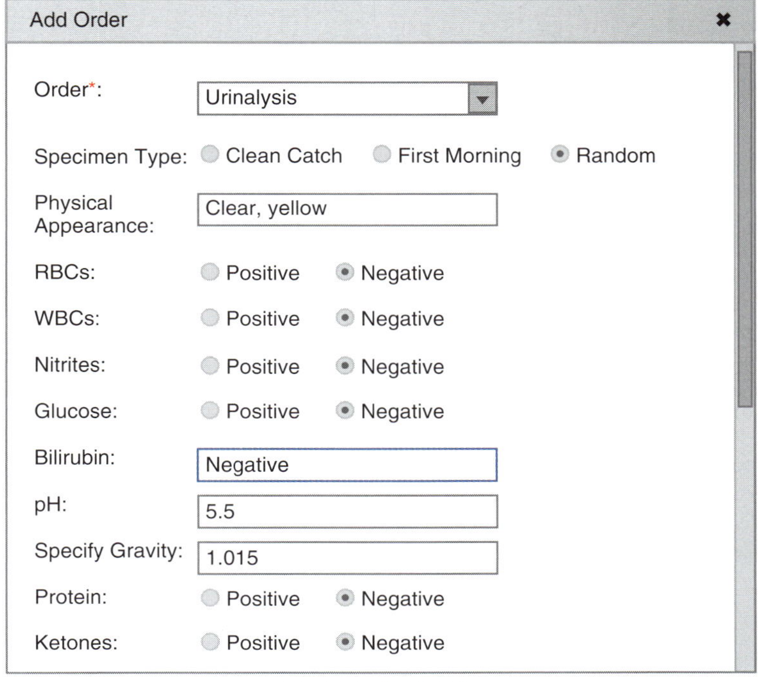

Laboratory test results.

Patient Instructions

It often is necessary to relay instructions to a patient regarding medical care (e.g., wound care, cast care, care of sutures). The medical assistant should document this information, taking care to include the date and time and the type of instructions relayed to the patient. Many medical offices have printed instruction sheets that are given to the patient. The patient may be asked to sign a form, which is filed in or scanned into the patient's record, indicating that they have read and understands the instructions (Fig. 38.12). The form also should be signed by the medical assistant, who functions as a signature witness. This protects the provider legally in the event that the patient fails to follow the instructions and causes further harm or damage to a body part.

Other items that the medical assistant is responsible for documenting in the medical record include missed or canceled appointments, telephone calls from patients, medication refills, and changes in medication or dosage ordered by the provider. Information related to routine teaching can usually be entered on a patient instruction screen in the EHR. Information related to telephone calls from patients or medication refills can usually be entered into a message screen.

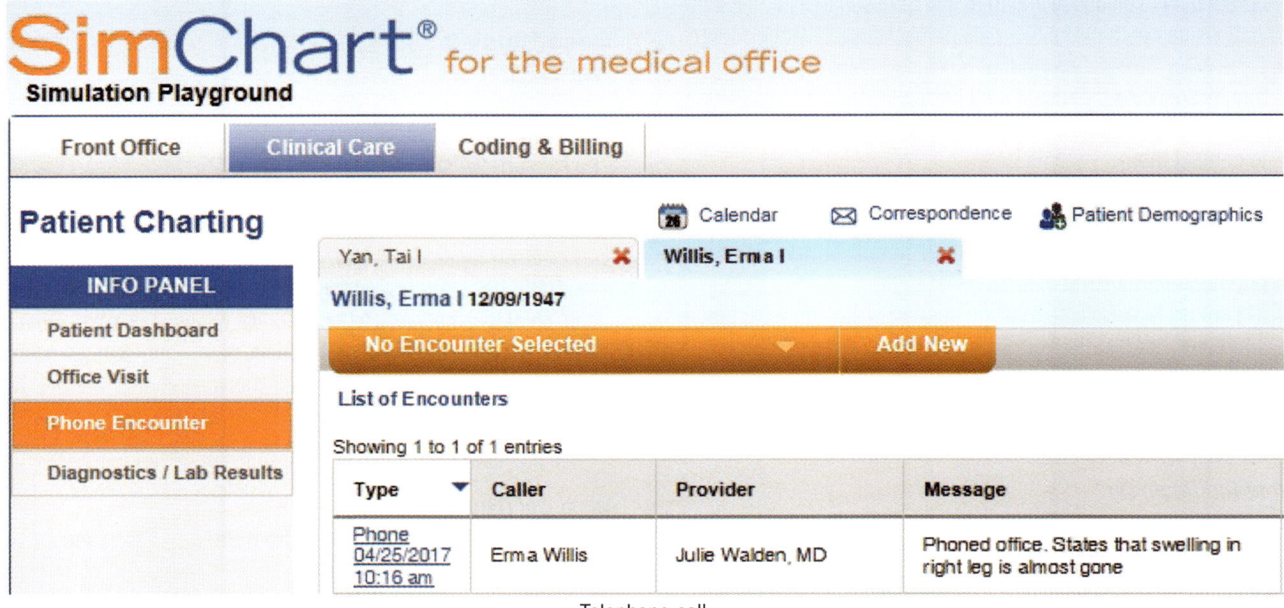

Telephone call.

PATIENT INSTRUCTIONS FOR WOUND CARE

Name of patient: ______________________________

Follow the instructions indicated below for care of your wound:

1. Use ice bag and elevate to reduce swelling and pain. Elevate higher than your heart.
2. You may take aspirin/Tylenol for pain.
3. Keep the dressing clean and dry.
4. Replace the dressing within __________ days.
5. Discard the dressing within __________ days.
6. Cleanse the wound daily as instructed.
7. Stitches should be removed in __________ days.
8. Despite the greatest of care, any wound can become infected. If your wound becomes red or swollen, shows pus or red streaks, or feels more sore instead of less sore, contact the physician **immediately.**

I have received and understand the above instructions:

Patient (or representative): ______________________________

Relationship to patient: ______________________________

Witness: ______________________________ Time and date: ______________

Fig. 38.12 Instruction sheet for patients.

What Would You Do? What Would You *Not* Do? RESPONSES

Case Study 1

Page 1020

What Did Dawn Do?

- ❑ Listened carefully to Mrs. Celeste and relayed concern through both verbal and nonverbal behavior.
- ❑ Reassured Mrs. Celeste that her information would be kept completely confidential. Explained to Mrs. Celeste that health care professionals are required by law to keep all patient information confidential.
- ❑ Told Mrs. Celeste how important it is to record information that relates to her health. Explained that the provider must have accurate data to diagnose and treat her. Stressed that certain medications can be harmful to a patient if consumed with alcohol.
- ❑ Gave Mrs. Celeste information (including brochures) on community agencies that could help her. Explained that these agencies are required to maintain confidentiality and encouraged her to contact them.

What Did Dawn Not Do?

- ❑ Did not tell Mrs. Celeste to go to a different provider to ensure that her information remained private.
- ❑ Did not tell Mrs. Celeste that she needed to stop drinking before it affected her health.

Case Study 2

Page 1024

What Did Dawn Do?

- ❑ Reassured Tessa that she and her family have been good patients and apologized for the inconvenience.
- ❑ Told Tessa that it is against the law to transfer medical records without the patient's written authorization. Explained that the reason for the law is to safeguard a patient's privacy.
- ❑ Asked Tessa if she had a fax machine because the forms could be faxed to her for signing and then faxed back to the office. If not, explained that Tessa and her husband would need to come to the office to sign release forms.

What Did Dawn Not Do?

- ❑ Did not get defensive about Tessa being so annoyed.
- ❑ Did not send the family's medical records to the new provider without the signed release forms.

Case Study 3

Page 1032

What Did Dawn Do?

- ❑ Listened to and empathized with Mr. and Mrs. Oberlin's concerns.
- ❑ Told Mr. and Mrs. Oberlin that because Brett is of adult age, it would be against the law to let them see his medical record without his written authorization. Explained that the law is there to protect a patient's right to privacy, and just as it protects Brett's right, the law also protects their right, so that no one can obtain information from their medical records without their authorization.
- ❑ Suggested that they talk with Brett again regarding the situation.

What Did Dawn Not Do?

Did not give them any information from Brett's medical record. ■

TERMINOLOGY REVIEW

Key Term	Word Parts	Definition
Attending provider/hospitalist		The provider responsible for the care of a hospitalized patient.
Chief complaint		A statement of the most important symptom or symptoms for which a patient is seeking care.
Consultation report		A narrative report of an opinion about a patient's condition by a practitioner other than the attending provider.
Diagnosis	*dia-:* thorough, complete *-gnosis:* knowledge	The scientific method of determining and identifying a patient's condition.
Diagnostic procedure	*dia-:* thorough, complete *gnos/o:* knowledge *-ic:* pertaining to	A procedure performed to assist in the diagnosis, management, or treatment of a patient's condition.
Digital image		A picture that is stored electronically to allow viewing on a computer.
Discharge summary report		A brief summary of the significant events of a patient's hospitalization.
Documenting		The process of making written or electronic entries about a patient in the medical record.
Electronic health record (EHR)		A computerized record of the important health information regarding a patient. This term is preferred over *electronic medical record.*
Electronic medical record (EMR)		A patient health record generated by a single provider or organization that is stored on a computer.
Familial	*famil:* family *-al:* pertaining to	Occurring in or affecting members of a family more frequently than would be expected by chance.
Flow sheet		A paper document or electronic screen that allows similar data to be recorded and viewed chronologically.
Health history		A collection of subjective data about a patient.
Home health care		The provision of medical and nonmedical care in a patient's home or place of residence.
Inpatient		A patient who has been admitted to a hospital for at least one overnight stay.
Medical record		A written or electronic record of important information regarding a patient, including the care of that individual and the progress of the patient's condition.
Medical record format		The way a medical record is organized. The two main types of medical record formats are the source-oriented record and the problem-oriented record.
Objective symptom		A symptom that can be observed by an examiner and the patient.
Paper-based patient record		A medical record in paper form.
Physical examination		An assessment of each part of the patient's body to obtain objective data about the patient that assists the provider in determining the patient's state of health.
Problem		Any condition that requires further observation, diagnosis, management, or patient education.
Problem-oriented record		A medical record organized according to the patient's health problems.
Reverse chronological order		Arranging documents with the most recent document on top or in the front, which means that the oldest document is on the bottom or at the back of a section or file.
SOAP		A method of organization for recording progress notes. The SOAP note includes the following categories: subjective data, objective data, assessment, and plan.
Source-oriented record		A medical record that is organized into sections based on the department, facility, or other source that generated the information.
Subjective symptom		A symptom that is felt by the patient but is not observable by an examiner.
Symptom		Any change in the body or its functioning that indicates the presence of disease.

PROCEDURE 38.1 Completion of a Procedure Consent Form

Outcome Complete procedure consent form

Equipment/Supplies

- Procedure consent form
- Clipboard
- Black pen

1. **Procedural Step.** Type or print all required information on the procedure consent form in the spaces provided (e.g., patient's full name, name of the procedure to be performed).
2. **Procedural Step.** Ensure that the provider has had a discussion to give the patient complete information about the procedure to be performed.
   Principle. For the patient's consent to be valid, it must be informed consent. Full understanding of procedures and their possible outcomes is an important patient right.
3. **Procedural Step.** Greet the patient and introduce yourself. Identify the patient by their full name and date of birth. Explain to the patient the purpose of the consent form.
4. **Procedural Step.** Give the consent form to the patient and ask them to read it. Ask the patient whether they have any questions. Listen carefully to the patient's questions to be sure that the patient understands the procedure. If there are questions or if the patient appears confused or to have reservations about having the procedure, refer the patient back to the provider before obtaining a signature.
   Principle. It is beyond the medical assistant's scope of practice to explain a procedure or answer specific questions about a procedure that will be performed by a provider. A patient has a right to refuse to undergo a procedure.
5. **Procedural Step.** Ask the patient or the patient's representative to sign the consent form.
6. **Procedural Step.** Witness the patient's signature by signing your name in the appropriate space on the form. Include today's date.
   Principle. Witnessing a signature means that the medical assistant verified the identity of the patient and watched the patient sign the form; it does not mean that the medical assistant is attesting to the accuracy of the information provided.
7. **Procedural Step.** Provide the patient with a copy of the completed consent form for their files.
8. **Procedural Step.** File the form in a paper medical record or scan the completed form into the patient's electronic health record.
   Principle. Maintaining the form provides legal documentation that the patient gave permission for treatment.

PROCEDURE 38.2 Release of Medical Information

Outcomes

1. Assist a patient in the completion of a medical records release form
2. Release medical information according to a completed medical records release form

Equipment/Supplies

- Medical records release form
- Pen (as needed)
- Clipboard (as needed)
- Patient's medical record

1. **Procedural Step.** Greet the patient and introduce yourself. Identify the patient by their full name and date of birth. Explain the purpose of the medical records release form. (*Note:* If you do not recognize the patient, ask them to provide photo identification such as a driver's license.)
2. **Procedural Step.** Provide the patient with the medical records form and ask the patient or the patient's representative to complete the form. Provide assistance if needed.
   Principle. Information from a patient's medical record can be released only on written authorization of the

PROCEDURE 38.2 Release of Medical Information—cont'd

patient or the patient's representative (except when permitted by law).

3. **Procedural Step.** Check to ensure that all information requested on the form has been completed.
4. **Procedural Step.** Ask the patient or the patient's representative to sign the form. Include today's date. If required by your medical office policy, witness the patient's signature by signing your name in the appropriate space on the form.
   Principle. For information to be released, the form must be signed by the patient or patient's representative authorizing the disclosure of medical information. The signature validates the required patient consent under the Health Insurance Portability and Accountability Act (HIPAA).
5. **Procedural Step.** Provide the patient with a copy of the medical records release form for their files.
6. **Procedural Step.** Copy the information requested on the form or print the information from the electronic health record (EHR). Release only the information requested. Include a copy of the completed release form with the medical information.
7. **Procedural Step.** Document what information is being released and the date of its release on the medical records release form or in a progress note in the medical record. Sign the release of information form with your name and credentials verifying you were the individual releasing the information.
8. **Procedural Step.** File the original document and the release of medical information form in the paper medical record or scan into the EHR.
   Principle. Maintaining the release form provides legal documentation that the patient gave permission for the release of their medical information.
9. **Procedural Step.** Send the medical information to the appropriate site according to your medical office policy.

Mailed or Faxed Requests for Release of Medical Information

These steps should be followed when a completed medical records release form has been mailed or faxed to the medical office:

1. **Procedural Step.** Check the expiration date on the medical records release form. If the authorization is outdated, a new release form needs to be completed.
2. **Procedural Step.** Verify the authenticity of the signature on the form. This can be accomplished by comparing the patient's signature on the form with the patient's signature in their medical record. If you have any doubt as to the authenticity of the signature, do not release the records.
3. **Procedural Step.** Copy or print the information requested on the form. Release only the information requested. Include a copy of the completed release form with the medical information.
4. **Procedural Step.** Document what information is being released and the date of its release on the release of information form.
5. **Procedural Step.** File the release of medical information form or scan it and save it in the patient's medical record.
6. **Procedural Step.** Send the medical information according to your medical office policy.

PROCEDURE 38.3

PROCEDURE 38.3 Obtaining Patient History and Formulating Chief Complaint

Outcomes

1. Obtain a patient history using reflection, restatement, and clarification techniques
2. Formulate and document the patient's chief complaint and/or patient symptoms

Equipment/Supplies

- Medical record of the patient to be interviewed
- Patient history form
- Black ink pen
- Computer or laptop with access to electronic medical record (EHR)

1. **Procedural Step.** Assemble the equipment. Ensure that you have the correct patient's record in the form of either an electronic record or a paper record. If using a paper record, be sure you have a black ink pen for entering patient information.
   Principle. Black ink must be used to provide a permanent record.
2. **Procedural Step.** Escort the patient to a quiet examination room or other room.

Continued

PROCEDURE 38.3 Obtaining Patient History and Formulating Chief Complaint—cont'd

Principle. Information related to patient health should be taken in a room that encourages communication and maintains privacy.

3. **Procedural Step.** In a calm and friendly manner, greet the patient and introduce yourself. Identify the patient by their full name and date of birth.
   Principle. A warm introduction sets a positive tone for the remainder of the interview.
4. **Procedural Step.** Ask the patient to be seated. You should seat yourself so that you face the patient at a distance of 3–4 feet.
   Principle. This type of seating arrangement facilitates open communication and respects a patient's personal boundaries.
5. **Procedural Step.** Use effective communication skills to interact with the patient. These include the following:
   a. Use the patient's name of choice.
   b. Show genuine interest and concern for the patient.
   c. Maintain appropriate eye contact.
   d. Adjust terminology based on the patient's age, education, and English competency.
   e. Listen carefully and attentively to the patient.
   f. Pay attention to the patient's nonverbal messages.
   g. Avoid judgmental comments.
   h. Avoid rushing the patient.
   i. Use reflection, restatement, and clarification techniques as necessary.
6. **Procedural Step.** If it is a new patient or a physical examination, record or review the following information on the patient history form (paper-based medical record) or in the EHR: past history, family history, social history, and pregnancy history (for a female patient). Be sure to include information about the use of tobacco products and smoking status. If using SimChart for the Medical Office, fill in or review each field and save your work on each screen before progressing to the next part of the history.
   Principle: A complete medical history is obtained from a new patient and updated during the physical examination of an established patient. Smoking status is required to demonstrate meaningful use of the EHR.
7. **Procedural Step.** Ask the patient if they have any allergies to medications or other substances; record the patient's allergies for a new patient, or review them for an established patient and add any new allergies. If using a paper-based medical record, allergies may be recorded in red, and a sticker is usually applied to the front of the medical record that contains the name of the allergen. If using SimChart for the Medical Office, click the *Add Allergy* button on the *Allergy* screen to add each allergy and follow directions, saving every screen as indicated.
8. **Procedural Step.** Review the patient's current medications and repeat that all prescription medications, over-the-counter medications, and vitamins or supplements should be included. If using SimChart for the Medical Office, click the *Add Medication* button on the *Medication* screen to add each medication, saving entries as indicated.
9. **Procedural Step.** Locate the screen for chief complaint in the EHR or the progress note sheet in the paper medical record. If documenting in a paper record, write the date and time and the abbreviation for chief complaint (CC).
10. **Procedural Step.** Use an open-ended question to elicit the chief complaint, such as "What seems to be the problem today?"
    Principle. An open-ended question allows the patient to verbalize freely.
11. **Procedural Step.** Document the chief complaint while following the documentation guidelines that are outlined beginning on the next page. In addition, these guidelines should be followed:
    a. Limit the chief complaint to one or two symptoms and refer to a specific rather than a vague symptom.
    b. Document the chief complaint concisely and briefly, using the patient's own words as much as possible.
    c. Fill in boxes.
    d. Avoid using names of diseases or diagnostic terms to record the chief complaint.
    Principle. Medical assistants should use correct terminology but may not use diagnostic terms in documentation.
12. **Procedural Step.** Obtain additional information regarding the chief complaint using *what*, *when*, and *where* questions. Fill in boxes in the EHR for location, quality, severity, duration, timing, context, modifying factors, associated signs and symptoms in the EHR or summarize this information in a paper medical record.

What Questions

- What does it feel like when the symptom occurs?
- Does the symptom occur suddenly or gradually?
- Does anything make it worse? Or better?
- What else do you experience when the symptom occurs?

Where Question

- Where is the symptom located?

When Questions

- When did the symptom first occur?
- How long does it last?
- How frequently does it occur?

PROCEDURE 38.3 Obtaining Patient History and Formulating Chief Complaint—cont'd

Principle. This information provides a complete description of the chief complaint.

13. **Procedural Step.** Clarify as needed using reflection, restatement, or summarizing what the patient has said. Repeat in simpler language if the patient does not seem to understand you.
Principle. Effective communication requires continuous feedback to be sure that there is mutual understanding of what is being communicated.

14. **Procedural Step.** Thank the patient and proceed to the next step in the patient workup. (This may include measuring vital signs and height and weight and preparing the patient as needed for the physical examination [see Chapters 19 and 20].)

15. **Procedural Step.** Inform the patient approximately how long they will have to wait for the provider.
Principle. Patients have a right to a realistic estimate of projected waiting time.

39 Patient Reception

Check out the Evolve site at http://evolve.elsevier.com/Bonewit/today to access additional interactive activities and exercises to help you study and prepare for success.

LEARNING OBJECTIVES

1. Describe how to open the medical office and prepare for the day's activities.
2. Compare and contrast the tasks necessary to open and close the medical office.
3. Discuss measures to protect the confidentiality of patients in the reception areas.
4. List information that must be obtained from new patients.
5. Describe the proper procedure to check in a new or established patient.
6. Discuss procedures that are necessary to validate that a patient's insurance will pay the bill.
7. List information that must be given to a new patient about the practice.
8. Describe different types of informational materials for new and prospective patients.

PROCEDURES

Opening the medical office.
Closing the medical office.

Obtaining new patient information.

Explaining office policies and procedures.

CHAPTER OUTLINE

KEY TERMS

assignment (ah-SIGN-ment) of benefits
call-in times
copayment
Medicaid (MEH-dih-kayed)
tickler file

INTRODUCTION TO PATIENT RECEPTION

The medical assistant may be responsible for opening the office, preparing for patients, and processing patients as they arrive for appointments. It is important to be sure that all parts of the office are prepared for patients because there is little time to pick up or arrange facilities once patient appointments begin. There are several forms that new patients must fill out, and the patient signature must be kept on file as permission to provide treatment, bill insurance, and verify that the patient has been given the office's Notice of Privacy Practices. At the end of the day, the medical assistant must prepare for the next day and close the medical office. The activities covered in this chapter mainly pertain to administrative medical assisting. Although they may not be performed by clinical medical assistants, it is still important to have knowledge of these activities, especially for those who intend to obtain certification.

PREPARING FOR PATIENTS

OPENING THE MEDICAL OFFICE

Office staff need to arrive at the medical office early enough to make sure the office is prepared for the patients. The medical assistant is often responsible for opening the office (Procedure 39.1). Several activities must be performed immediately:

- Disarming the alarm system
- Turning on the lights
- Unlocking the door through which patients enter
- Unlocking file cabinets, medication cabinets, and medical record files (if paper records are used)
- Turning on all of the office equipment that will be used during the day, such as computers and copy machines

Depending on the way the medical office is organized, there may be several other tasks that should be completed before the first patient arrives.

Checking for Messages and/or Faxes

Someone must review messages and prepare the telephone system for the day's activities. The telephone message must be switched from the night and weekend message to the telephone system used during the day. Usually the night and weekend message states that the office is closed, suggests calling 911 if it is an emergency, gives a telephone number to contact the provider on call for an urgent situation, and directs the caller to leave a message if the matter is not urgent. During the day, the medical assistant may answer the telephone directly or the caller may have to select an option from a menu before being connected to a member of the office staff.

If the medical office uses an answering service, the medical assistant should call the service to indicate that the office is open. The medical assistant must also obtain any messages that have come in within the past hour or nonurgent messages left during the night. For calls relating to illness, the answering service would have contacted the provider on call overnight.

After checking the message mailbox or answering machine, the medical assistant usually checks for faxes that have arrived overnight and routes the messages and faxes to the appropriate person.

A separate mailbox or answering machine may be used for prescription refill requests. If this is the case, the medical assistant should retrieve the messages from this mailbox before the physician arrives.

Preparing for the Day's Activities

It is helpful to take a minute at the beginning of the day to organize the day's tasks. This includes reviewing the appointment schedule and noting deviations from the routine schedule, such as providers who are out of the office for all or part of the day. Reminders about the day's activities may be stored using an electronic task system and/or a physical **tickler file**. A manual tickler file is a set of 43 file folders, one for each month (for a total of 12 folders) and an additional set of 31 folders for the days of the current month. Written notes, bills to be paid, receipts, or other items are filed in these folders to "tickle" the memory at the time when they must be handled (tickler files are also discussed in Chapter 43). Electronic reminders are usually handled using an electronic calendar.

The medical assistant usually counts the cash in the cash drawer, this is a fixed amount of money used to make change when patients pay in cash. The cash drawer (change fund) is usually kept locked except when the medical assistant is actually sitting at the reception desk. Some offices may not accept cash payments from patients at the reception desk, especially if there is a centralized cashier.

Making Sure Patient Records Are Prepared

Paper-based patient records are usually pulled the evening before the next appointment day or are prepared in the morning before the patients arrive. Even if the office uses an electronic health record (EHR), some providers may want to be able to consult a patient's old paper medical record (depending on how old the EHR system is). If used, paper charts must be arranged for each physician in order of the arrival of the patient. A separate appointment schedule is usually prepared for each physician. A charge slip may be created for each person before the visit, or more commonly the entire billing and charging system may be electronic. Some offices also print other sheets, for example, a list of medications for the patient to review and update.

Copies of the appointment schedule(s) are usually printed and placed at designated locations, although staff members and providers are more likely to refer to the schedule on the computer. The medical assistant usually places a schedule in each provider's office, at the reception desk, and at the medical assistant's desk. The schedule may be printed the evening before in case of a power outage or server problem, but it is usually updated with new appointments in the early morning and if appointments change or are added.

Checking the Office and Waiting Room

The waiting room, reception area, and examination and treatment rooms all need to be checked for the following: cleanliness, neatness, correct temperature, and appropriate reading material. The medical assistant should make sure that the cleaning service has cleaned all parts of the office and emptied the trash. The medical assistant may need to turn on a television or radio, in the patient waiting room. Magazines should be stored neatly and replaced with current issues as needed. If there are toys in the waiting room, they should be cleaned regularly and stored neatly. Holders in the waiting room that contain information brochures for patients should be restocked and arranged neatly (Fig. 39.1).

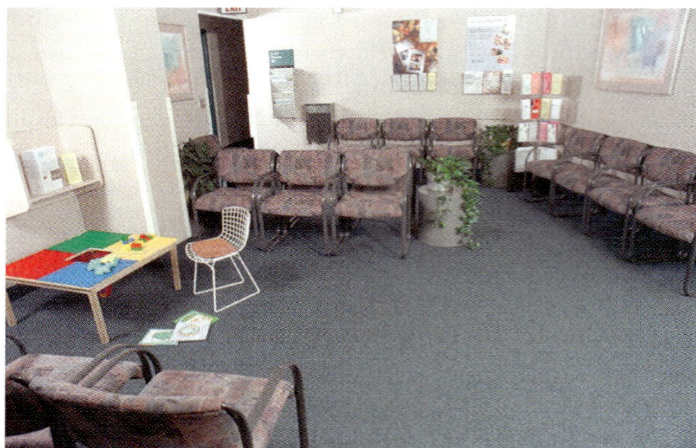

Fig. 39.1 The waiting area should be kept tidy for patients.

Checking Equipment and Supplies

The medical assistant should perform a visual safety check of the medical office daily. This includes removing any hazards that might block hallways or exits and making sure that all equipment is performing correctly. It is helpful to fill the paper trays of the copier, printer, and fax machine every morning.

The reception area and examination rooms should be tidied and restocked daily, either in the morning or at closing and sometimes again at a specified time during the day. Biohazard waste containers should be checked, and waste discarded properly if necessary. The medical assistant may need to turn on or set up equipment used for clinical procedures, run controls in the laboratory, and/or remove items from a battery charger. It may also be necessary to unload the autoclave and put away items that were sterilized the evening before.

CLOSING THE MEDICAL OFFICE

At the end of the day, the activities of the morning are reversed. Many medical offices run the autoclave in the afternoon so that items can dry thoroughly overnight. If paper-based medical records are used, they are usually prepared for new patients and removed from the files for established patients in the late afternoon because it leaves more time in the morning. Before leaving the office, the medical assistant may perform the following tasks (Procedure 39.2):

- Prepare the bank deposit and balance the cash drawer. At the end of the day, the money in the cash drawer must be balanced against cash receipts. Any amount above the usual change fund is added to the bank deposit (see Chapter 45).
- Make a backup copy of the main computer hard drive if the office does not subscribe to an online computer backup service or if backups are not handled by a separate department.
- Check the fax machine for faxes that have come in during the day.
- Turn off computers, printers, copiers, and other equipment (with the exception of the fax machine).
- Change the telephone to the night message or call the answering service to tell them the office is closing.
- Lock the door through which patients enter.
- Lock file cabinets, medical record files, and medication cabinets.
- Make sure the coffee machine or other kitchen equipment is turned off.
- Unplug equipment, such as a toaster, that might be a fire hazard.
- Turn off the lights.
- The last person to leave the medical office makes sure the door is locked and sets the alarm system.

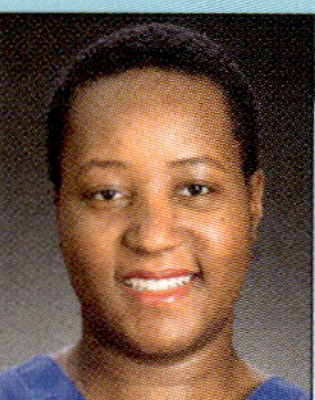

Putting It All Into Practice

My name is Keisha White, and I work in a small office with two internists. We are the primary care providers for most of our patients. I am responsible for opening the office every day, and I usually arrive at about 8:00 a.m. I leave before the office closes every day except Friday. Gerri, another medical assistant, is responsible for closing the office. We had an alarm system put in several years ago, so as soon as I enter the office, I go to the keypad and enter the code so that the alarm won't go off. Then I have a look around as I turn on the lights. Sometimes the air seems a little stale, so I either open a window or turn up the air conditioning, depending on how hot it is outside. After I turn on the copier and the computers, I switch the telephone to the day message. I take down any messages from voicemail and put the messages where they will be handled once the office has been opened up. Next, I turn on the lights in the patient waiting area, make sure everything is tidy, and unlock the door for patients. We have a television in the waiting room, and I turn it on. We have shifted over to an electronic health record. In the morning we print a medication list from the medical record of each scheduled patient. Once the computers are warmed up, I check the electronic calendar to see if there is anything special to do that day, and I print appointment schedules. We keep one schedule at the front desk, and I put one on each physician's desk. When patients arrive, we give them their medication list to review. Then we call the patient to escort them to the examination room and prep them for the provider. The first appointment is scheduled for 8:30, so I really have to keep moving to be ready for the day. ■

PATIENT CHECK-IN

It is important to acknowledge each person who enters the office as soon as possible to prevent that person from feeling awkward. The medical assistant or a receptionist usually sits at the reception desk. This person should greet everyone who enters the office. If a sign-in sheet is used, it is recommended that this sign-in sheet have adhesive peel-off strips for each line so that the medical assistant can remove the patient's name immediately after check-in.

MAINTAINING CONFIDENTIALITY

Many offices have a sliding glass window. This prevents people in the waiting room from hearing telephone conversations or other discussions in the reception area. In some facilities, the medical assistant sits behind a reception desk that is recessed but open (Fig. 39.2). Because patients standing near the desk can hear any conversation behind the desk, these offices may have a separate room or area for scheduling appointments in person and by telephone. When a patient is at the desk, the medical assistant should not carry on a telephone conversation with another patient. Only one patient should be at the desk or window at a time. The medical assistant can instruct other patients and/or family members to have a seat in the waiting room or line up at a distance from the desk.

If it is necessary to discuss sensitive or personal information, the patient should be taken to a private area.

NEW PATIENTS

The office must obtain several types of information about new patients. Personal and insurance information is obtained either when the appointment is made or at the first visit. It may be obtained on a paper form, the patient may be asked to call a specific telephone number to register, or the information may be taken by a staff member at a computer. It is important to maintain patient confidentiality when discussing personal information. The information is entered into the office practice management system. It is important to remember that many office computer systems combine a practice management system (for patient demographic data, appointments, and billing) with an EHR for medical information either in one program or using two programs that interact.

The patient is usually asked to sign a statement that allows the office to release information to the insurance company for billing purposes. This consent may be part of the patient information form or may be a separate sheet. For the office to receive payments directly from the insurance company (called **assignment of benefits**), the patient must also sign a form authorizing this. The assignment of benefits statement is usually included with the consent to release information to insurance companies. The patient signature authorizes the provider or medical practice to release information to the insurance company and authorizes the insurance company to pay the medical practice directly. In addition, the patient usually agrees to be responsible for charges not covered by insurance.

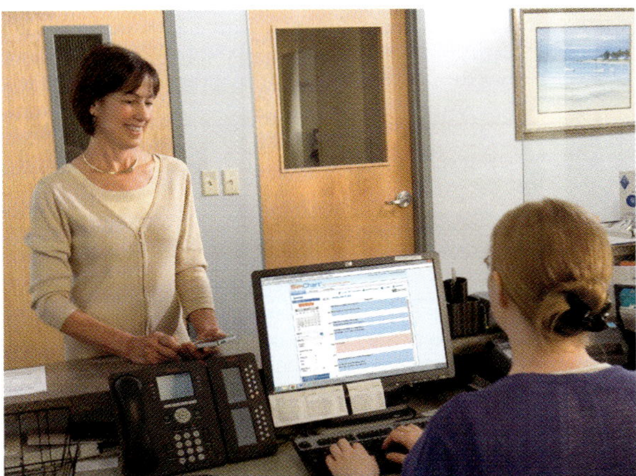

Fig. 39.2 If an open desk is used for reception, the waiting room should be large enough to prevent other patients from overhearing the conversation at the desk.

If a paper form is used to obtain information it includes the following:

- Patient information (personal and demographic)
- Guarantor information (personal and employment information for the individual who will be financially responsible)
- Provider information (primary care provider and/or referring provider)
- Insurance information (insurance company, policy holder, ID number and group number for primary and any other insurance)
- Assignment of benefits consent
- Authorization to release information to insurance
- Agreement to pay costs that insurance does not cover

In addition to the new patient information form (Fig. 39.3), the medical office may also use an additional form to obtain other information as needed. For example, to meet criteria for meaningful use of the EHR, an office must collect demographic data about patients related to ethnicity, race, and preferred language that may not be requested on traditional patient information forms. Until new forms are ordered, the office may collect these and other data on an additional form (Fig. 39.4). Paper forms may be scanned into the office computer system to preserve the patient's signature (Fig. 39.5).

The Forms Repository in SimChart for the Medical Office contains a Patient Information Form and Notice of Privacy Practices that can be printed for patients.

Acknowledgement of Receipt of Notice of Privacy Practices

The Health Insurance Portability and Accountability Act (HIPAA) requires that patients sign a form acknowledging that they were given the opportunity to read or were given a copy of the office Notice of Privacy Practices (Fig. 39.6). The Notice of Privacy Practices itself is usually very detailed. It is usually given to patients at their first visit and is also posted in an accessible location.

Patient History Form

Most offices also have a history form for the patient to fill out before being seen by the physician (see Chapter 38). It may be mailed to the new patient before the first appointment, or the patient may fill it out in the waiting room. The medical assistant goes over this form with the patient in the examination room to be sure that all of the relevant information has been included. Medical information should not be discussed at the front desk.

REGISTRATION
(PLEASE PRINT)

Home Phone: ________________ Today's Date: ________________

PATIENT INFORMATION

Name ______________________________ Soc. Sec.# ________________
Last Name First Name Initial

Address ______________________________

City ____________________ State ____________ Zip ____________

Single ___ Married ___ Widowed ___ Separated ___ Divorced ___ Sex M___ F___ Age___ Birthdate ____________

Patient Employed by ______________________________ Occupation ____________

Business Address ______________________________ Business Phone ____________

By whom were you referred? ______________________________

In case of emergency who should be notified? ______________________________ Phone ____________
Last Name Relationship to Patient

PRIMARY INSURANCE

Person Responsible for Account ______________________________
Last Name First Name Initial

Relation to Patient ____________ Birthdate ____________ Soc. Sec.# ____________

Address (if different from patient's) ______________________________ Phone ____________

City ____________________ State ____________ Zip ____________

Person Responsible Employed by ______________________________ Occupation ____________

Business Address ______________________________ Business Phone ____________

Insurance Company ______________________________

Contract # ____________ Group # ____________ Subscriber # ____________

Name of other dependents covered under this plan ______________________________

ADDITIONAL INSURANCE

Is patient covered by additional insurance? ___ Yes ___ No

Subscriber Name ____________ Relationship to Patient ____________ Birthdate ____________

Address (if different from patient's) ______________________________ Phone ____________

City ____________________ State ____________ Zip ____________

Subscriber Employed by ______________________________ Business Phone ____________

Insurance Company ______________________________

Contract # ____________ Group # ____________ Subscriber # ____________

Name of other dependents covered under this plan ______________________________

ASSIGNMENT AND RELEASE

I, the undersigned, certify that I (or my dependent) have insurance coverage with ______________________________
Name of Insurance Company(ies)

and assign directly to Dr. ____________ insurance benefits, if any, otherwise payable to me for services rendered. I understand that I am financially responsible for all charges whether or not paid by insurance. I hereby authorize the doctor to release all information necessary to secure the payment of benefits. I authorize the use of this signature on all insurance submissions.

____________________ ____________________ ____________________
Responsible Party Signature Relationship Date

Fig. 39.3 New patient information form. (Courtesy Bibbero Systems, Petaluma, CA.)

WALDEN-MARTIN
FAMILY MEDICAL CLINIC
1234 ANYSTREET ANYTOWN, ANYSTATE 1234
PHONE 123-123-1234 FAX 123-123-5678

PATIENT INFORMATION FORM – ADDITIONAL INFORMATION

Patient Name: ______________________________ Date: ______________

1. Do you have a written Advanced Directive/Living Will or Healthcare Power of Attorney in place? If yes, please plan to bring a copy with you to your next appointment for us to scan into your record.

☐ YES ☐ NO

If no, would you like information regarding your patient rights in making healthcare decisions?

☐ YES ☐ NO

2. May we send you email or text messages?

☐ YES ☐ NO

Email address: ______________________________

Cell phone # for text messages: ______________________________

3. What is your Ethnicity?
   - ☐ Hispanic or Latino
   - ☐ Not Hispanic or Latino
   - ☐ Decline to Specify

4. What is your race?
   - ☐ American Indian or Alaska Native
   - ☐ Asian
   - ☐ Black or African American
   - ☐ Native Hawaiian/Other Pacific Islander
   - ☐ White
   - ☐ Decline to Specify

5. What is your preferred language for communication?

Patient Signature: ______________________________ Date: ______________

Fig. 39.4 Patient information form for additional information.

What Would You Do? What Would You *Not* Do?

Case Study 1

Angela Harris is a 62-year-old new patient. When she comes to the reception desk to check in, she gives Keisha the completed patient history form that had been mailed to her. Keisha hands her a Notice of Privacy Practices and a clipboard and pen. She asks her to fill out a new patient information form and sign the form acknowledging the receipt of the Notice of Privacy Practices. Ms. Harris seems reluctant to take the clipboard. She says, "I'm sorry, I don't have my reading glasses with me. I didn't know I would need them. Besides, I gave you all that information on the telephone, didn't I?" ■

Verifying Insurance and Obtaining Authorizations

After a new patient has filled out the patient information sheet, the medical assistant should ask for their insurance card. After making a photocopy of both sides or scanning the card, the medical assistant stores the copy with the patient's medical record. The card verifies the information given by the patient and sometimes gives additional information needed for billing. An insurance card scanner at the front desk may be used to read both sides of the insurance card and scan it into the computer. Information from the card can be transferred to the practice management software, and an image of the card can be saved to the patient's EHR.

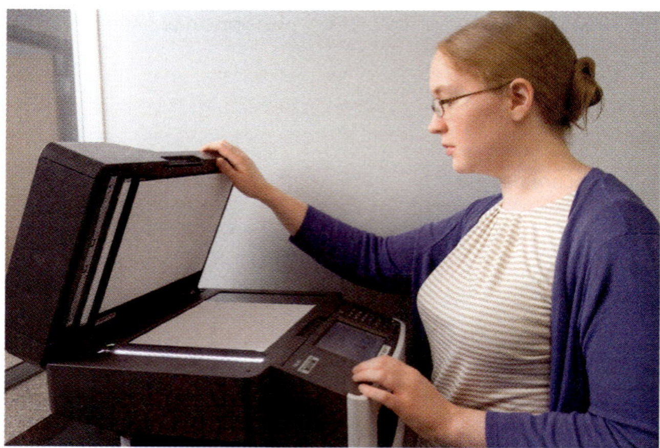

Fig. 39.5 Medical assistant scanning information for the electronic health record.

It may also be office policy to verify a patient's identity at every visit by asking for photo ID or two other forms of identification and retaining photocopies. Medical identity theft has become a more common problem in the past decade. It can result in incorrect information in the medical record as well as fraudulent charges to insurance companies.

Some types of insurance require authorization every time the patient visits the primary care physician. Patients with Medicaid must usually have their coverage verified and/or must receive prior authorization for each visit. **Medicaid** is an insurance program established by the federal government that pays for low-income patients' medical needs. Each state administers Medicaid independently, and the program has a different name in each state. The cost is split between the state and the federal governments. In some states, some patients on Medicaid receive new identification cards each month; in other states, patients' insurance coverage can be verified by telephone, fax, or an electronic card reader. An electronic card reader is a small machine in the physician's office that is connected via telephone to the insurance company's database and can verify insurance benefits while the patient is in the office. Many offices use a card reader that can read not only the patient's insurance card, but also several types of credit cards (Fig. 39.7).

Acknowledgement of Receipt of the Notice of Privacy Practices

Please Review Carefully

The Notice of Privacy Practices tells you how **[Practice Name]** uses and discloses information about you. Not all situations will be described. We are required to give you a notice of our privacy practices for the information we collect and keep about you. We reserve the right to revise this notice, and you can obtain a copy of any revision upon written request.

I, ________________________________, have been given a copy of the **Notice of Privacy Practices.**

______________________ ________ ______________________
Patient or Legal Guardian's Signature | Date | Relationship to Patient

______________________ ______________________
Print Patient's Name | Print Name of Legal Guardian (if any)

______________________________ ________
Signature of Witness (If signed with an "X" or mark) | Date

Effective Date: April 14, 2003

Fig. 39.6 The Health Insurance Portability and Accountability Act requires new patients to sign a form acknowledging receipt of a medical office's Notice of Privacy Practices.

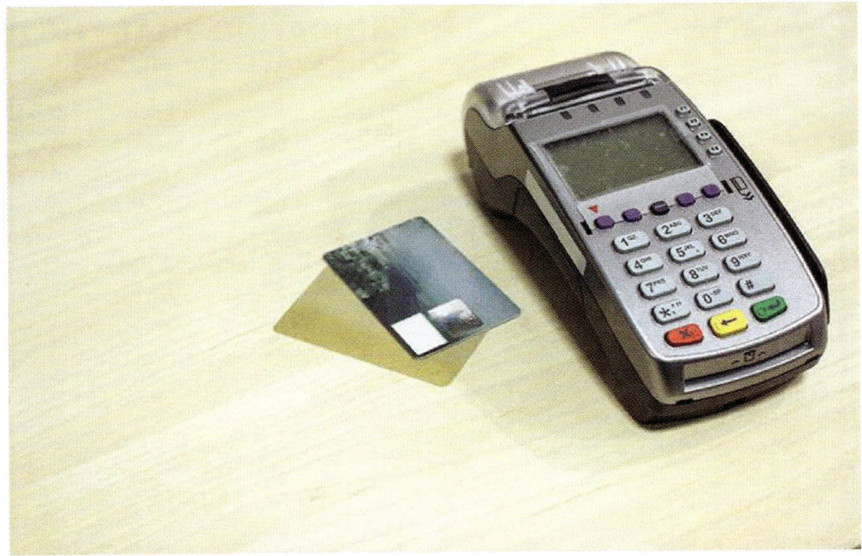

Fig. 39.7 Card reader used to validate insurance coverage for Medicaid and other insurance plans. (From Niedzwiecki B, Pepper J: *Kinn's The medical assistant*, ed 14, St. Louis, Elsevier, 2020.)

For other types of insurance, it may be necessary to call the patient's insurance company to obtain authorization for treatment (especially if the patient needs minor surgery or a special treatment). This may be done when the patient makes the appointment, when the patient checks in, or after the first visit, when the physician has identified what treatment is necessary and how many visits are anticipated.

Each office has its own procedure for verifying insurance. If possible, insurance should be verified for a new patient before the appointment using either an insurance company or managed care website or an online service that is purchased to perform the electronic verification and eligibility for all the office's patients. If there is a question about whether a patient has insurance coverage or whether the service will be covered, the medical assistant should always contact the insurance company before the service is provided (Procedure 39.3).

Verifying a Managed Care Referral

If the patient has been referred by another provider through a managed care plan, it is important to validate that the patient has a completed referral form from the primary care provider. This may be a paper form. Sometimes the referring provider has sent it in advance, but the patient may bring it personally to the visit. For most managed care plans, it will be possible to access the referral form using the internet. If there is no valid referral form, the insurance company may not pay for the visit.

The referral form will state how many visits are allowed (how many will be paid for by the managed care plan) and the problem for which the patient is being referred. Depending on the patient's insurance, the patient may also be required to sign a statement promising to pay any charges that the insurance does not cover. If the patient is part of a managed care plan, however, and a referral form was not obtained, the patient cannot usually be billed, so the visit becomes a write-off for the office.

Although the medical office is allowed to bill for services that the patient's insurance does not cover, managed care plans usually do not allow providers who accept referrals to bill the patient for excess charges (a practice known as *balance billing*). Medicare also does not allow balance billing from participating providers.

If the patient has not yet obtained a referral authorization, or if it is uncertain that the insurance will cover the services, the patient must be informed before any service is provided that they will be responsible for payment of the bill.

ESTABLISHED PATIENTS

If the patient has been seen in the office before, it is necessary to verify that the billing information is still correct. When checking a patient in, the medical assistant should first identify the patient by asking the patient to state their name, spell the last name, and state the date of birth. Then the patient's personal information is verified in the computer system including address, telephone number, and insurance information. Patients who have moved may assume that the office is aware of the change, so it is recommended to ask, "Is your address still...?" and "Is your telephone number still...?" The patient should also be asked for their insurance card. If any information has changed, the new card should be photocopied and the updated information should be entered into the computer billing system and into the medical record, whether paper or electronic. As stated previously, established patients may also be asked to verify their identity using a photo ID if they are not personally known to the person checking them in.

ACCEPTING COPAYMENTS

A **copayment** is a fixed amount of money that patients are required to pay each time they receive medical treatment. The amount of the copayment is usually printed on the patient's insurance card. If there is any question about the amount of the copayment, it may be easily determined by checking the patient's eligibility on the website of their insurance company or by a telephone call. Many offices collect the copayment before the visit because it is a fixed fee, although this can also be done at the end of the visit. The amount paid is entered on the patient's charge slip or entered directly into the computer. A receipt should be given to the patient at the time the copayment is made. It may be generated by the computer when the payment is entered. Most offices use a numbered receipt system for handwritten receipts so that payments are accounted for.

What Would You Do? What Would You *Not* Do?

Case Study 2

Joseph Ritano is a 38-year-old new patient. After filling out the new patient information form, he comes to the desk and says, "I don't seem to have my insurance card with me today. I must have forgotten to put it back in my wallet when I gave you the information over the telephone last week. I know that the company is Bristol Medical Care, but I don't know my ID number. Do you have it in the computer? I know that my copayment is $20.00." ■

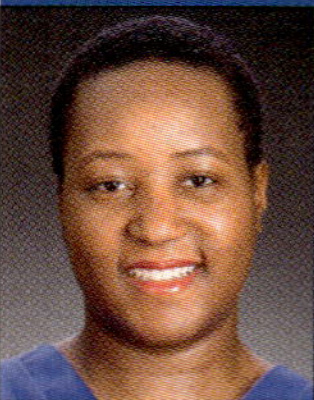

Memories *from* Practicum

Keisha White: When I checked patients in during my practicum, it was a challenge to protect patient confidentiality while also being careful to verify all information about the patient in the computer. I have a fairly loud voice, and it took several reminders for me to learn to speak in a clear tone that was loud enough for the patient to hear, but not so loud that all the patients in the waiting room would hear me. I also had to remember to ask waiting patients to stand back behind the sign that we had placed about 8 feet away from the reception desk. In the office where I work now, we have cubicles at the front desk so that the patient sits within a sort of booth and can't be easily seen or overheard by another patient. Usually, the patient information was entered into the computer or verified when the patient made the appointment, but we still asked new patients to fill out a new patient information form. During my practicum, I asked the patient to state their name and birth date and spell the last name to be sure that I was looking at the information about the correct patient. Then I verified the information in the computer system. I also asked for the insurance card and photocopied it. Where I work now, we scan the insurance card directly into the EHR. During my practicum there were one or two patients who expressed that they were glad we took precautions to protect their privacy. One woman said, "I really don't want everyone to know who I am and why I'm here. You do a great job keeping it between me and you." ■

INDICATING THAT THE PATIENT IS IN THE WAITING ROOM

After the patient has been checked in at the front desk, any paperwork such as a form for patients to update current medications and/or medical history may be located or printed. If paper charge slips are used, these are also printed, and they may be clipped to the patient's paper-based medical record, if that is still used. Any paperwork is placed in the designated space for patients who are ready to be seen. Most offices also automatically print patient labels for use on laboratory requisitions and specimens.

ORIENTING PATIENTS TO THE MEDICAL OFFICE

INFORMATION FOR NEW OR PROSPECTIVE PATIENTS

The medical assistant may be responsible for informing new patients and prospective patients about the medical office and its policies and procedures (Procedure 39.4). The medical assistant should be familiar with all of the following information:

- A brief description of the providers, how long each has been in practice, each provider's credentials, and whether each provider is accepting new patients.
- Specialties of the providers in the practice, types of patients seen, and basic philosophy of the provider(s).
- Information about languages spoken by staff, whether the provider practices alternative therapies (e.g., acupuncture), or whether the provider insists that patients stop smoking.
- Location of the main office and satellite offices, directions to each office, and a description of available parking and access to public transportation, if applicable.
- The types of insurance that the practice accepts, whether the patient's insurance will be accepted, and whether payment is required at each visit.
- How to make appointments and the policy regarding canceling appointments. Patients are normally asked to give 24 hours' notice if possible for a cancellation.
- The telephone procedure and whether the physician has **call-in times** (when the provider takes telephone calls).
- What hospital(s) each provider is affiliated with; some patients might also want to know whether the provider makes nursing home visits.
- How medication refills are handled and whether the patient can request refills through the online patient portal.
- How to sign up to use an online patient portal (which usually includes the EHR and/or an appointment request system).

SELECTING A PROVIDER FOR A NEW PATIENT

New patients are assigned to practice providers who are accepting new patients. If there is more than one, a new patient will appreciate a brief description of each. A physician might not be accepting new patients for a few reasons:

- A provider may have so many patients that they cannot in all fairness accept new patients. If the patient load decreases, the provider may begin to accept new patients again.
- The provider may be returning from a maternity, family, or personal disability leave and be working a reduced schedule.
- The provider may be easing back before retiring.

The medical assistant should also be able to tell prospective patients how much time to allow for a first (new patient) visit. Most providers see new patients only on certain days and at certain times. Medical assistants should be sure to remind new patients to bring a complete list of their medications to the initial appointment, as well as a written list of concerns.

What Would You Do? What Would You *Not* Do?

Case Study 3

Donna Pohl calls the office to ask about the medical practice. An acquaintance has recommended Dr. Sylvia Lawrence. She says that she prefers a female provider. She asks for information about her and her specialty. Dr. Lawrence specializes in general internal medicine. At the current time the doctor is pregnant, and her due date is 2 months away. Although Dr. Lawrence is still seeing established patients, she has instructed Keisha not to make any appointments for her with new patients for the next 4 months. The other provider in the practice, Dr. William Rudner, also specializes in general internal medicine. ■

CONSIDERATIONS TO FACILITATE PATIENT UNDERSTANDING

When coaching new or prospective patients about the medical office, the medical assistant must take into account the patient's cultural or ethnic background, the patient's developmental stage, and any communication barriers that may exist. Depending on the patient's cultural background and preferred language, it may be desirable to have a medical interpreter or translator follow up with the patient to be sure there are no unanswered questions. It may also be necessary to simplify explanations or increase the amount of information provided if the patient appears to be unfamiliar with a typical medical office. If the patient is hard of hearing, the medical assistant should speak clearly, use short sentences, and repeat as needed. At the first office visit, the medical assistant should always speak using language appropriate for the patient's developmental stage and should implement additional safety measures as needed for very young or elderly patients.

PATIENT INFORMATIONAL MATERIALS

An increasing number of practices today have a website that contains the previously mentioned information. There are also often photographs of the office and office staff. Pages on the website usually include information about the practice as well as directions to the main facility and any satellite facilities. There may be a section related to health and wellness with information about specific medical conditions, especially those related to the specialty of the practice. Maintaining the website is usually not the responsibility of the medical assistant, but they can remind the office administrator if certain information needs to be updated. Photographs of patients should be used only if the patient has signed a release form. The Web address of the practice website can be added to the business cards of the practice providers.

In addition to a practice website, there is usually information about each provider available on the website of the hospital(s) where the provider has privileges as well as the website of any large group with which the medical practice is affiliated. Most of these websites have a "find a doctor" feature for all their providers, and these usually link to an information page about each provider. These links may need updating if the provider obtains new credentials or if the provider starts or stops accepting new patients.

Patient information booklets are another very successful marketing and public relations tool, but they must be kept up to date. A patient information booklet should include all the information for new patients that was discussed previously. Patients appreciate having something in writing to which they can refer. A patient information booklet should be given to a new patient at the first visit and should be on display for established patients to request if they want one.

What Would You Do? What Would You *Not* Do? RESPONSES

Case Study 1

Page 1053

What Did Keisha Do?

- ❑ Checked to see if there were other patients in the waiting room. Because there were, she took Ms. Harris to a private area.
- ❑ Asked Ms. Harris for each piece of information on the new patient information form and filled it in for her.
- ❑ Read each statement at the bottom of the form out loud and showed Ms. Harris where to sign the form.
- ❑ Explained that Ms. Harris could read the Notice of Privacy Practices at a later time when she had her glasses, but asked her to sign the form acknowledging receipt of the Notice of Privacy Practices.

Continued

What Would You Do? What Would You *Not* Do? RESPONSES—cont'd

What Did Keisha Not Do?

- ❑ Did not tell the patient that she should have realized she might need her reading glasses.
- ❑ Did not tell the patient to sign any of the consents without reading them to her.
- ❑ Did not ask for protected health information where another patient could hear the conversation.

Case Study 2

Page 1056

What Did Keisha Do?

- ❑ Looked up the policy number for Mr. Ritano in the computer and handed it to him in writing so that he could write it on the form.
- ❑ Attempted to call the insurance company to verify his coverage.
- ❑ Explained that she needed to scan his insurance card and asked him to bring it in as soon as possible.
- ❑ Accepted his check for $20.00 for his copayment.
- ❑ Explained that if it turned out that his insurance did not cover this visit or if he needed an authorization or referral, he would be responsible for paying the charges for the visit.
- ❑ Gave him an estimate of the cost of the visit.
- ❑ Allowed him to reschedule if he wanted to wait until he had his insurance card.

What Did Keisha Not Do?

- ❑ Did not refuse to let Mr. Ritano see the provider until he brought his insurance card.
- ❑ Did not make negative comments about forgetting the insurance card or imply that she does not believe he has insurance.
- ❑ Did not discuss his protected health information in front of other patients.
- ❑ Did not talk to other staff members about the forgotten insurance card unless he stated he would bring the card when she did not expect to be in the office.

Case Study 3

Page 1057

What Did Keisha Do?

- ❑ Explained that Dr. Sylvia Lawrence would be out on leave and could not accept appointments for 4 months.
- ❑ Offered to make an appointment with Dr. Lawrence after the 4-month period.
- ❑ Offered to make an appointment with Dr. Rudner as soon as he had one available.
- ❑ Listened sympathetically if Ms. Pohl was displeased about not being able to be seen more promptly by a female provider.
- ❑ Responded calmly and in a normal speaking voice if the patient became irritated or upset.
- ❑ Made a recommendation about another female provider only if specifically instructed to do so by Dr. Lawrence.

What Did Keisha Not Do?

- ❑ Did not agree to make an appointment with Dr. Lawrence before the end of the 4-month period just this once.
- ❑ Did not become defensive or imply that Ms. Pohl's preference for a female provider is silly.
- ❑ Did not become irritated or upset with Ms. Pohl.
- ❑ Did not talk about the telephone conversation later with other office staff.

TERMINOLOGY REVIEW

Key Term	Definition
Assignment of benefits	Authorization given by the patient to allow the insurance company to make payments directly to the health care provider instead of to the patient.
Call-in times	Blocks of time when a provider accepts telephone calls from patients.
Copayment	A fixed amount of money that the patient is responsible to pay at each visit.
Medicaid	A federal and state insurance program for low-income patients. The Medicaid program has a different name in each state.
Tickler file	A chronological file containing reminders of things to be done.

PROCEDURE 39.1 Opening the Medical Office

Outcome Open the medical office

Equipment/Supplies:

- Medical office

1. **Procedural Step.** Enter the office and disarm any alarm system immediately.
2. **Procedural Step.** Turn on the lights.
3. **Procedural Step.** Adjust heat or air conditioning to a comfortable setting.
4. **Procedural Step.** Unlock the door through which patients and visitors will enter the office.
   Principle. Medical office staff usually enter the office through a different door than patients and visitors.
5. **Procedural Step.** Turn on machines that will be used all day, including computers, printers, and copier.
6. **Procedural Step.** Set the telephone system to the day setting and get messages from the electronic mailbox, telephone answering machine, or answering service.
   Principle. Callers to a business expect calls to be picked up as soon as the business opens. An important telephone message may need attention.
7. **Procedural Step.** Listen to any messages in order, writing down the pertinent information for each message on a message pad. (See Chapter 41, Procedure 41.2: Taking a Telephone Message.) Fill in the information, including the name of the caller, business affiliation (if any), date, time of the call, telephone number including area code, and information the caller wishes to leave about the reason for the call. Place your initials on the message in case there are questions. Messages may also be taken using the computer.
   Principle. Complete information is necessary for the appropriate person to return the call.
8. **Procedural Step.** Arrange the messages in order of importance. Deal with any urgent calls at once, then work through other calls. Pull medical records (if paper records are used) for calls from patients and place the messages in the appropriate locations for various office staff to review.
9. **Procedural Step.** Review the day's activities and note any special tasks that must be completed that day.
10. **Procedural Step.** Count the money in the cash drawer and record the amount.
11. **Procedural Step.** Check the office for safety hazards including frayed wires, items blocking corridors or walkways, and other hazards.
12. **Procedural Step.** Straighten up the waiting room, including reading material; clean children's toys as needed; turn on radio, television, and restock patient information brochures.
13. **Procedural Step.** Print appointment lists and make sure all paper patient medical records have been pulled and arranged in order as needed. Print or stamp today's date on the progress notes and place the medical records in the designated location. If an electronic health record system is used, be sure any necessary paperwork has been printed.
14. **Procedural Step.** If it is office policy, prepare charge slips and clip to each patient's medical record or paperwork.
15. **Procedural Step.** Check biohazard waste containers and discard properly.
16. **Procedural Step.** Check examination rooms to be sure they are clean and contain all needed supplies and equipment.
17. **Procedural Step.** Run the autoclave as needed, or empty the autoclave if it was run the evening before.

PROCEDURE 39.2 Closing the Medical Office

Outcome Close the medical office

Equipment/Supplies:

- Medical office

1. **Procedural Step.** Make sure examination rooms are clean and contain all necessary supplies.
2. **Procedural Step.** Run the autoclave if needed.
   Principle. If the autoclave is run at the end of the day, supplies can dry overnight.
3. **Procedural Step.** Print a patient schedule for the next day, and pull paper medical records if needed. Print charge slips and clip to each patient's medical record if it is office policy.
4. **Procedural Step.** Make sure all cabinets or rooms containing medical records are locked.

Continued

PROCEDURE 39.2 Closing the Medical Office—cont'd

5. **Procedural Step.** Balance the cash drawer and prepare the bank deposit. Lock the cash drawer or place the change fund in the office safe. If possible, make the bank deposit at the end of the day.
   Principle. It is best to leave as little money in the office as possible. The change fund should be kept under lock and key.
6. **Procedural Step.** Make sure the night system for the telephones is activated. Switch the message on the electronic telephone system or answering machine and call the answering service as needed.
7. **Procedural Step.** Turn off all machines throughout the medical office that are used only during the day. Exceptions include the fax machine and telephone system. Unplug machines such as a coffee maker or toaster oven that might pose a fire hazard.
   Principle. Machines that generate heat such as coffee makers can pose a fire hazard. Unplugging these machines is also an extra reminder to make sure they do not remain on overnight.
8. **Procedural Step.** Lock the door through which patients and visitors enter the medical office.
9. **Procedural Step.** Turn the heat or air conditioning to the night setting.
10. **Procedural Step.** Turn off the lights.
11. **Procedural Step.** Arm the security system and make sure the door is securely locked as you leave the medical office.

PROCEDURE 39.3 Obtaining New Patient Information

Outcomes

1. Obtain information from a new patient, obtain consents, and validate insurance coverage
2. Respond to issues of confidentiality
3. Input patient data using a practice management system

Equipment/Supplies:

- Clipboard
- Pen
- New patient information form containing consent to treatment and assignment of benefits consents
- Notice of Privacy Practices
- Receipt of Notice of Privacy Practices form
- Consent for release of protected health information (optional)
- Photocopier
- Insurance card reader (optional)
- Telephone
- Medical record
- Computer
- Scanner

1. **Procedural Step.** Place a new patient information form on a clipboard with a pen and ask a new patient to complete the form and return it to you.
   Principle. Complete information about the patient facilitates the billing and insurance process.
2. **Procedural Step.** Explain why patient confidentiality must be maintained when the patient returns the form, both for the patient being processed and for other patients. Identify and take measures to preserve confidentiality.
   Principle. The Health Insurance Portability and Accountability Act (HIPAA) requires confidentiality in discussions with patients that involve personal information and protected health information.
3. **Procedural Step.** Make sure the form is complete and the patient or authorized representative has signed the form as needed.
   Principle. The patient must consent in writing to treatment, to allowing the office to bill the insurance company, and to allowing the insurance company to pay the physician.
4. **Procedural Step.** Ask to see the insurance card of the patient or other insured person.
5. **Procedural Step.** Scan the insurance card or photocopy both sides of the insurance card and place the copy in the patient's paper medical record if used.
   Principle. The insurance card contains information about the patient's copayment amount, as well as the address and telephone number of the insurance company.
6. **Procedural Step.** Confirm patient eligibility for insurance coverage using a card reader, computer, or telephone if required by the patient's insurance provider, and confirm that there is a complete referral form if necessary. If the visit will not be completely covered

PROCEDURE 39.3 Obtaining New Patient Information—cont'd

by insurance, display sensitivity when discussing the patient's financial responsibility. If personal information is discussed, take the patient to a private area.

Principle. The patient has a right to know what their financial obligation will be before receiving service.

7. **Procedural Step.** Ask to see a photo ID or two other forms of identification if it is office policy.

   Principle. Verifying patient identity may be part of the office's plan to prevent identity theft.

8. **Procedural Step.** Give the patient a copy of the Notice of Privacy Practices and ask the patient to sign the form acknowledging the receipt of the Notice of Privacy Practices. Sign the form as a witness to the patient's signature if it is office policy.

   Principle. HIPAA requires that the patient acknowledge the receipt of the Notice of Privacy Practices in writing.

9. **Procedural Step.** Ask the patient to read and sign any consent for release of protected health information used by the office.

   Principle. A general consent for release of personal health information enables the office to leave messages on the patient's answering machine, to send laboratory results to the patient's home address, and so on.

10. **Procedural Step.** Prepare paperwork to indicate that the patient is ready to be examined. If a paper medical record is used, insert any new forms into the medical record and place it with the paper charge slip. Ask the patient to have a seat and tell them the approximate waiting time for the examination.

    Principle. When the paperwork is complete, it will help the patient feel more in control to know how long they can expect to wait before the examination.

11. **Procedural Step.** Transfer the information from the new patient information form to the patient's computer account, or validate that information obtained by telephone is correct.

    Principle. Demographic information must be entered into the computer system for billing and appointment scheduling, in addition to the recording of health information. An electronic health record (EHR) often includes a practice management system (patient demographic information, billing, scheduling) as well as patients' clinical information.

12. **Procedural Step.** Scan the new patient information form, insurance card, and other consent forms if it is office policy.

    Principle. If the office stores a patient's health information electronically in addition to billing records, all new paper forms must be scanned into the computer.

PROCEDURE 39.4 Explaining Office Policies and Procedures

Outcome Coach a patient regarding office policies and procedures

Equipment/Supplies:

- Patient information booklet (if available)
- Map
- List of points to cover

1. **Procedural Step.** Offer to give or send the patient a patient information booklet if one is available.

   Principle. A patient information booklet provides a handy resource to answer questions about a medical practice.

2. **Procedural Step.** Take a patient's cultural background, developmental life stage, and potential barriers to communication into consideration when coaching the patient about office policies.

3. **Procedural Step.** Identify the name, credentials, and specialties of providers who are accepting patients in the medical office.

   Principle. Some providers may not currently be accepting patients.

4. **Procedural Step.** Offer information as required about languages spoken by staff in the medical office and additional services or specialized complementary practices.

5. **Procedural Step.** Identify the location of the office and/or satellite offices and give directions as needed. Identify where the patient can park if necessary.

6. **Procedural Step.** Tell the patient whether the office accepts their medical insurance plan and discuss expectations for payment of the patient's bill.

   Principle. The patient has a right to know what their financial obligation will be before receiving service.

7. **Procedural Step.** Describe how far in advance to make appointments and the office policy on canceling appointments.

Continued

PROCEDURE 39.4 Explaining Office Policies and Procedures—cont'd

Principle. Most offices reserve the right to charge the patient if the appointment is not cancelled at least 24 hours in advance.

8. **Procedural Step.** Tell the patient when and how to contact the office and notify the patient if the provider has specific call-in times (times when they take telephone calls).
9. **Procedural Step.** Explain how prescriptions and prescription refills are handled as needed.
10. **Procedural Step.** Explain and/or provide written information about how to sign up for and use any patient access to an online health record or appointment request system.
11. **Procedural Step.** Identify the hospital(s) with which each provider is affiliated. Answer any questions about other services (e.g., nursing home visits) that each provider may provide.

Medical Office Computerization

Check out the Evolve site at http://evolve.elsevier.com/Bonewit/today to access additional interactive activities and exercises to help you study and prepare for success.

LEARNING OBJECTIVES

1. Explain the difference between data and a program.
2. Explain the purpose of each of the following parts of the data processing cycle: input, processing, and output.
3. List examples of input and output devices.
4. Explain the difference between software and hardware.
5. Explain the function of an operating system.
6. State the function of application software.
7. List common types of application software and describe how each works.
8. Describe the care and maintenance of the main computer unit.
9. Describe the function, care, maintenance, and ergonomics of the computer monitor.
10. Describe the use of a touchscreen to input data.
11. Describe the care, maintenance, and ergonomics of a computer keyboard.
12. Identify the guidelines to follow in the care and maintenance of a printer.
13. List and describe the storage devices used with microcomputer systems.
14. Explain why it is important to have a foundation in computer concepts before engaging in hands-on computer operations.
15. Identify the medical assistant's role in telehealth.
16. Define and explain the function of an audit trail.
17. List and describe measures that can be taken to promote the efficient running of a computerized medical office.
18. Describe the processes for obtaining information from the internet and sharing information electronically.
19. Describe the methods used to maintain security of the medical office computer system.
20. List and describe methods used to back up computer data in the medical office.
21. Explain the importance of data back-up.
22. State the various types of system maintenance that should be performed on a computer system.

CHAPTER OUTLINE

KEY TERMS

app
application software
backup
broadband
cloud computing
computer system
data
data processing
digital subscriber line (DSL)
e-mail
encryption
firewall
gigabyte (GB)
hard disk drive
hardware
input
input device
internet
kilobyte (KB)
medical practice
megabyte (MB)
network
operating system
output
output device
patient kiosks
patient portal
processing
program
router
server
social media
software
solid state drive
storage capacity
system software
telehealth
terabyte (TB)
touchscreen
URL
USB port
Web browser
WiFi
World Wide Web

INTRODUCTION TO MEDICAL OFFICE COMPUTERIZATION

The computer is the most frequently used piece of equipment in today's medical office. It may be used to schedule appointments, process patient statements and insurance claims, order supplies, maintain computerized medical records, prescribe medications, receive e-mail, create reports, etc. The medical assistant must be very familiar with the computer system used in their office and the programs (e.g., medical practice management program or electronic health record [EHR] program) being run on that computer system.

This chapter presents an overview of the parts of the medical office computer system, as well as important information about maintenance and data storage.

COMPUTER CONCEPTS

A computer is a device consisting of electronic components, which have the ability to process data according to a program to produce a desired result. The primary advantage of using a computer to perform administrative procedures in the medical office is that these tasks are performed with greater speed and accuracy than with other types of devices (e.g., typewriter, pegboard system, or calculator). In addition, computers are versatile: Rather than performing only one function (e.g., typing, posting a payment, or math calculations), a computer can perform many different types of tasks.

Computers are useful tools because they can perform the same tasks repeatedly while maintaining the same level of efficiency. It should always be remembered, however, that the computer does not have a mind of its own. You are always in charge, and the computer will never do anything without your direction.

Most medical offices use personal computers or desktop computers linked together to form a **network,** a collection of computers that can share data and resources (Box 40.1). The number of computers in a network varies based on the size of the medical practice and the type and number of tasks performed on the computer. For example, a two-physician medical office using a practice management program typically has four to eight networked computers.

BOX 40.1 Types of Computers

Desktop Computer
A desktop computer, so named because it can fit on and under a desk, usually consists of a plastic case containing the CPU (central processing unit), storage devices (e.g., hard disk and DVD/CD-ROM discs), other personal computer (PC) components (e.g., video card and sound card), a monitor, a keyboard, and a mouse.

Workstation
A workstation designates a desktop computer that is more powerful than a typical desktop computer and is normally devoted to one task. The term may also be used to indicate an area for a single worker in an office or laboratory setting.

Laptop Computer
A laptop computer (also called a *notebook*) usually weighs less than 5 lb and contains the processor, screen, other PC components, storage devices, and a means to input data, all contained in one portable unit.

Tablet Computer or Tablet
A tablet computer is a complete computer with a touchscreen contained in one portable unit. This may be a modified laptop that folds so that the screen faces out.

Handheld Devices
Smartphones, personal digital assistants (PDAs), and palmtop or handheld PCs are small devices with less powerful computing capabilities but greater portability than other types of computers.

A small network is called a *local area network* (LAN). In a larger system, the computers in a medical office may be linked to a hospital and possibly other offices. LANs may be linked to form larger networks. A *wide area network* (WAN), such as the internet, is a collection of connected LANs. Networks for large systems usually contain one or more **servers,** large computers that store data and manage tasks for the computers on the network.

Increasingly, computer networks use **cloud computing**, a model in which the internet is used to store and access data and programs, and servers are not physically located at the same site as the computer. The term *cloud* is reflected in the cloudlike symbol that is used in network diagrams around entry and exit points when the network architecture is not specifically delineated. The information being accessed is found "in the cloud," and the user can access it from many different locations.

DATA PROCESSING CYCLE

As previously described, computers function by processing data. **Data processing** is the term applied to changing raw facts or data into an organized, recognizable form. To fully comprehend data processing, it is important to have a thorough understanding of the terms *data* and *program.* **Data** is a general term used to describe the raw, unorganized facts presented to the computer for processing. Patients' names, addresses, and telephone numbers are examples of data frequently entered into the computer in the medical office.

A **program** is defined as a set of instructions organized in a logical step-by-step sequence that tells the computer how to perform a specific function. As in cooking, when a recipe is required to explain how to mix ingredients, a computer requires a program to tell it how to process data.

Computers process data in a logical three-part sequence known as the *data processing cycle* (Fig. 40.1). The data processing cycle includes the following phases: input, processing, and output. Each phase of the data processing cycle involves a specific activity, which is described as follows.

The terms *input* and *output* have slightly different meanings depending on how they are used. When referring to the data processing cycle, they are used from the "computer's point of view" as verbs to describe the transfer of information. Input and output are also used as nouns to describe the data that have been entered into the computer (input) and the information that has been generated by the computer (output). As these terms appear throughout this chapter, you will become familiar with their different meanings.

INPUT

The **input** of data is the transfer of data to the computer for processing. Input includes both the entering of data into the computer and the conversion of it into an electronic form that can be understood by the computer. Because computers cannot understand the written word in the form used in communication among humans, the data must first be translated into an electronic code that can then be processed by the computer. Once the computer is finished working on the "electronic" data, the result must be converted back into a form that can be understood by the user.

Data must be entered into the computer through an **input device** (see Fig. 40.1). The most common examples of input devices are the computer keyboard and the mouse, which are usually used together. They convert data into electronic code that can be understood and processed very quickly by the computer. Other examples of input devices include a scanner, a digital camera, and a microphone.

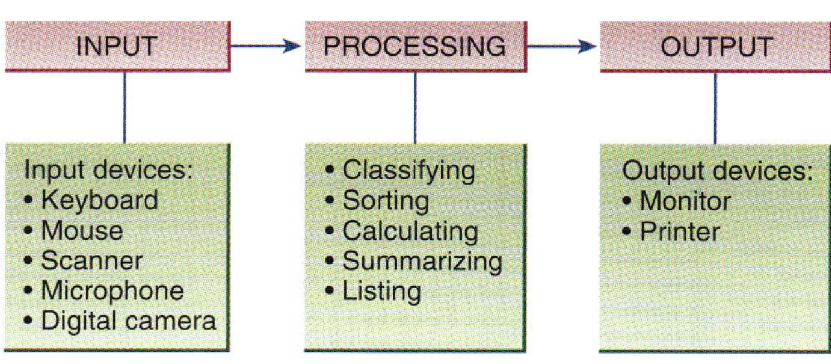

Fig. 40.1 Data processing cycle.

PROCESSING

The **processing** of data is the handling and arranging of the electronic data by the computer according to a program; in other words, the data undergo some type of manipulation or change to produce useful information. Depending on the result, the processing phase may include one or more of the following: classifying, sorting, calculating, summarizing, or listing of the data (see Fig. 40.1).

OUTPUT

The final phase of the data processing sequence is the output of the processed data. **Output** is the transfer of usable information back to the user. Because the computer works with an electronic code, an output device must be used to communicate with the user. The **output device** converts the electronic code into a form that can be understood by the user. The most common output devices are the monitor and the printer (see Fig. 40.1). Sometimes output is attached as a file to a message sent by e-mail.

COMPONENTS OF THE COMPUTER SYSTEM

All of the components making up the computer are collectively known as the **computer system** (Fig. 40.2). Computer systems include two major divisions: software and hardware.

SOFTWARE

Software is a general term for the programs or instructions that tell a computer what to do. Software tells the computer how to perform specific tasks in a series of step-by-step instructions organized in a logical sequence. Two categories of software exist: system software and application software.

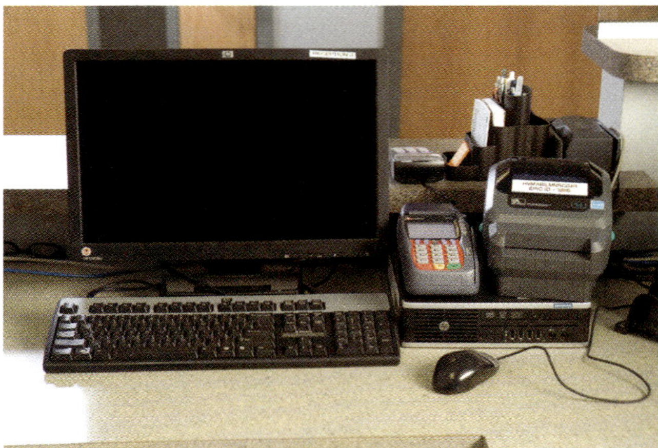

Fig. 40.2 Computer system.

System software assists the computer in carrying out its tasks, whereas application software assists the user in carrying out their computer tasks. Each software category is described in more detail next.

System Software

System software is made up of a group of special programs that control or maintain the operations of a computer. The most important type of system software is the **operating system.** The operating system is installed on the hard disk of the computer and is automatically loaded into the computer's main memory when the computer is turned on. An example of an operating system frequently used in the medical office is Windows (Microsoft Corporation). The operating system performs "housekeeping" chores required by the computer system to operate itself. The most important function performed by an operating system is to serve as an intermediary to tell the hardware how to run an application program. Hence, application programs are useless without an operating system.

HIGHLIGHT on Operating Systems

Almost all of today's medical office computers run on a Windows operating system. The Windows operating system was introduced in the 1980s as a more intuitive system than the command-based interface, the Disk Operating System (DOS), that had been used before. An operating system allows interactions between the computer and the user, between the computer and peripheral equipment, and between computer and computer. The interaction may occur through a direct connection, a wireless network, a telephone line, or the internet. Each time a new operating system is developed, it allows for more complex computer system interactions.

Windows and the Mac OS are based on the concept of the graphical user interface. The theory behind this type of operating system is that it operates the way people think—it is intuitive. When the computer is turned on, a start screen appears. This is the starting place for the user to open and view programs and files, to perform operations, and to create and store files.

An individual item, such as a patient record, a daily appointment list, or a medical record, is called a *file.* A file is a set of computer data that has been saved to disk. Files are collected in folders, indicated by an icon of a file folder. Folders can be displayed individually either within a window or on the desktop. When a folder is opened, it appears as a window, and all the files that reside in the folder are in the window. Files can be moved from one folder to another, just as they might be at a desk with papers, folders, and files.

Arranged on the desktop screen in Windows 11 are icons. Icons are small graphics that provide a link to files, folders, or applications. The start screen in Windows 11 has tiles that link to programs or apps by a touch or mouse click, depending on the type of computer. ■

Application Software

Software designed to allow a user to accomplish a specific task is **application software,** also known as an *application program* or *software program.* Application software constitutes the greatest proportion of the software available for use with a computer. An **app** is a small, specialized program that can run on a computer or a mobile device.

Office suites are collections of programs used to facilitate general tasks in all kinds of offices. They often contain at least four types of application programs: word processing, spreadsheets, telecommunications, and database management. More detail about these application programs is found below.

A **medical practice** management program provides instruction to the computer for performing medical practice management procedures, including appointment scheduling and managing practice finances. It facilitates the day-to-day administrative operations of a medical office. It uses database capabilities to store demographic information about patients, physicians, insurance providers, and procedure and diagnosis codes. It uses spreadsheet and database capabilities to manage financial records, generate patient statements, and perform insurance billing. It also maintains the appointment schedule, which interfaces with patient information. EHRs may be linked to a medical practice management program, or practice management and word processing functions may be embedded in the EHR.

Word Processing

Word processing software allows the user to enter, edit, format, and file (store) text. Microsoft Word is an example of a commercially available word processing application program. A medical practice management program can produce letters, statements, receipts, and insurance forms using data from its database.

Spreadsheet

A spreadsheet is an electronic ledger designed to perform mathematic calculations quickly. Spreadsheet programs are used to produce financial reports and to analyze and process statistics. An example of a commercially available spreadsheet application program is Microsoft Excel. A medical practice management program or EHR can generate financial reports for the office and revise the data quickly in the same way as a spreadsheet application program.

Telecommunications

A telecommunications application provides the means for one computer to "talk" with another computer. Electronic communication between computers greatly reduces the time it takes to send information. A medical practice management program and/or EHR incorporates a telecommunications application for the electronic submission of insurance claims.

In addition, telecommunications software is used to send letters and messages as electronic mail (e-mail). A common telecommunications program is Microsoft Outlook.

Many EHRs have an internal messaging system that allows patient records to be linked with the messages. If the messages stay within the EHR, they are as secure as the EHR itself.

Database Management

Database management is the storing and retrieving of data in and from a database. Database management allows the user to store large amounts of data on a storage device (e.g., hard disk). The data can then be easily retrieved and manipulated. An example of a commercially available database management software program is Microsoft Access. The data in the database of the medical office computers can be accessed by both the medical practice management program and the electronic health record (EHR) system. Database management increases efficiency in recordkeeping and eliminates numerous time-consuming repetitive tasks. The database for a medical practice consists of patient records, patient transactions, diagnosis codes, procedure codes, insurance carriers, and so on. This information is stored on the hard disk of the computer or server for later retrieval and use as needed. A database also provides the ability to add new information, modify existing information, and delete unneeded information. The most significant aspect of a database is that the computer can cross-reference all the information stored in its database. The medical practice database can be thought of as a large pool of information that the computer can access in a multitude of ways according to the task being performed.

Entering Data

There are a variety of methods to enter data into practice management programs and/or EHRs. The user may fill in information in text boxes. Screens may be set up to select one option using a check-box or radio button. When new data, such as a new patient, new appointment, or new medication, are entered, a popup window may appear to allow entry of the information with a save button at the bottom of the window. A drop-down menu allows the user to choose one value from a list, which is usually activated by clicking on a down arrow to the right of the list. Progress notes are usually entered using free text boxes, although it is possible to set up templates with some information already filled in (Fig. 40.3). As stated earlier, it is possible to dictate information for free text boxes using voice recognition software.

Voice Recognition

Voice recognition software or speech recognition software is built into Windows and many mobile devices, or a separate program may be purchased. By speaking into the microphone, the user can give commands that instruct the computer or other device what to do. It is also possible to dictate information that the computer transforms into text. The user must usually work with this feature to learn the commands and to give the computer an opportunity to learn to recognize the user's speech patterns. Many physicians now use this method to dictate progress notes and reports.

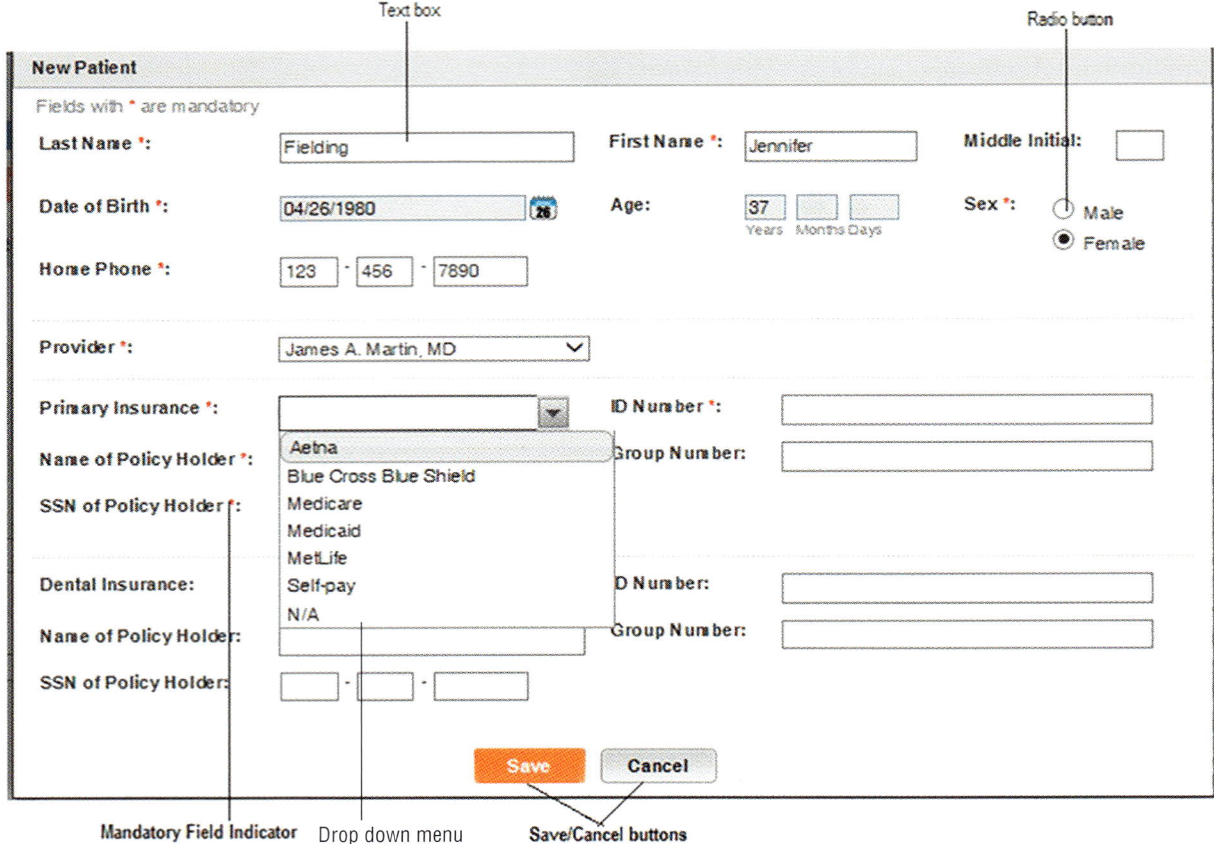

Fig. 40.3 Pop-up window in SimChart for the Medical Office.

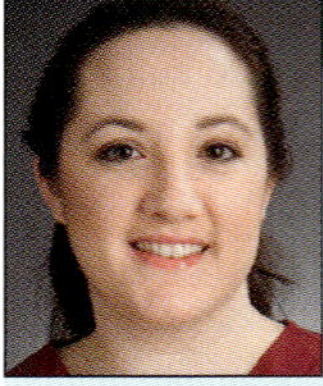

Putting It All Into Practice

My name is Emma Hayes, and I am a Certified Medical Assistant. Since I graduated, I have been working at the main office of an internal medicine practice. Our office manager is very interested in computers, and we have been using integrated practice management and EHR software for a few years now. When a new patient calls for an appointment, we obtain all their personal and insurance information and enter it into the computer during that first conversation. When patients first come to the office, we have them sit at a computer terminal in a private room next to the waiting room and enter their health history. If the patient is not comfortable with the computer, we have the patient complete a paper form, and then I enter the data from the form into the computer. We have a scanner at the front desk to scan the patients' insurance cards and all the forms they sign at the first visit. We keep a folder for each patient with forms that they have signed, but everything is also available in electronic form.

One of the things our patients really like is that our providers send all prescriptions to the pharmacy electronically. At the first visit, we ask patients for the name, address, and telephone number of the pharmacy they want to use. Some patients like to get their prescriptions by mail order, and we can also indicate that. I also ask the patient what medications they are taking and enter them into the computer. After that, the provider can go to the patient's EHR, enter the information about the medication they want to prescribe, and automatically send the prescription directly to the patient's pharmacy. The EHR program checks for drug interactions with all the medications that the patient is taking. Our providers believe that this saves time and is actually more accurate, because the pharmacist doesn't have to read the handwritten prescriptions. ■

HARDWARE

Hardware is the term for the physical equipment making up the computer system—that is, the tangible computer parts. Although a computer system may include a variety of hardware, the following hardware devices are necessary to perform administrative procedures in the medical office: computer (either desktop, laptop, or tablet), monitor, computer keyboard and mouse (if a desktop computer is used), and printer. External devices are connected to the computer with cables that attach to the computer at a specialized port (such as a printer port), a jack (usually for audio components), a USB (Universal Serial Bus) port, or using a wireless connection. A **USB port** is a standard computer cable connection interface that allows several types to devices to be connected to the computer in order to transfer data across short distances. Laptops or tablets may communicate with the network using **WiFi**, a technology for wireless local area networking and connection to the internet.

MAIN COMPUTER UNIT

The main unit of a desktop computer consists of a hard plastic case that is usually rectangular in shape. The main unit houses all the components that make the computer work. These include a primary circuit board; the microprocessor chip that runs the computer; additional circuit boards for memory, graphics, sound, and so on; and storage devices.

STORAGE CAPACITY

Storage capacity (the amount of information that can be stored) is measured in units of storage known as *bytes*. One byte, usually 8 bits, is approximately equal to one character, such as a letter or number. Stating the capacity of random access memory (RAM), in bytes, however, results in astronomically high numbers. Therefore, it is more convenient to use larger units, such as kilobytes, megabytes, gigabytes, and terabytes. A **kilobyte (KB)** is equal to 1024 bytes, which is usually rounded off to 1000 bytes. A **megabyte (MB)** is equal to a little more than 1 million bytes; in terms of kilobytes, 1 MB is equal to 1000 KB. An even larger measure than a megabyte is a **gigabyte (GB);** 1 GB is equal to 1 billion bytes or 1000 MB. The largest measure in current use is a **terabyte (TB)**; 1 TB is equal to 1 trillion bytes or 1000 GB. There are names for even larger units (petabyte—1000^5 bytes; exabyte—1000^6 bytes; zettabyte—1000^7 bytes; yottabyte - 1000^8 bytes), and as storage capacity increases, these units will come into more common usage.

As you would imagine, the larger the capacity of RAM, the more information it can hold at one time. For example, a computer with 2 GB of RAM can hold more than 2 billion bytes. Most microcomputers now come with a main memory of 2 GB or more.

The capacity of a computer's memory correlates directly with the level of complexity of the programs it can run. A program takes up a certain amount of space in memory. A small and simple application program that performs a limited number of tasks occupies much less space than a large, complex, and powerful program that performs numerous complicated tasks, such as an EHR. The amount of memory is an important criterion to consider when working with or purchasing a computer or an application program. A computer with less than the required memory for a particular program would not have enough storage space to hold that program. Hence, the program could not be run on that particular computer. The packaging of the application program is labeled with information on *computer system requirements.* System requirements tell you what your computer system must have (e.g., type of operating system, microprocessor speed, amount of memory, hard disk space) to run the program. Storage devices are discussed later in the chapter. The use of WiFi and servers allows medical facilities to have access to large amounts of information that is not stored within an individual computer.

CARE AND MAINTENANCE OF THE MAIN COMPUTER UNIT

The main computer unit should be placed on a flat, stable surface, such as a computer desk. This prevents excessive vibration during operation, which could loosen the electronic circuit boards. If the main unit is found in a tower, it is designed to be placed in a vertical position. Information on proper positioning is always indicated in the instruction manual accompanying the computer. Laptops should also be placed on a flat, stable surface if possible, and they should be lifted by the base, not the screen.

Computers operate best in a moderately cool environment. Extreme heat and inadequate ventilation increase the chance of malfunction. As a precautionary measure, the main unit should not be placed near a window or other areas that receive direct sunlight. In addition, to prevent overheating, the ventilation slots on the main unit should not be obstructed.

A common cause of improper functioning of the computer is exposure to environmental contaminants, such as dust, dirt, and smoke. For this reason, rooms with computers should be kept clean with no smoking permitted. The casing of the main unit should be periodically wiped with a slightly damp, lint-free cloth to remove dust and dirt. Aerosol sprays, solvents, and abrasives should never be used to clean the casing because they can damage the finish. Liquids should be kept away from the computer. A liquid spilled into the main unit can cause irreparable damage to the electronic circuit boards. In addition, an electrical short may occur and could result in a fire or small explosion.

Any cables attaching a computer to other components should be checked on a regular basis to ensure that they are secure. A loose or disengaged cable can result in temporary malfunctioning of the computer system.

COMPUTER MONITOR

A computer monitor displays images generated by a computer. The monitor permits the user to view the data entered into the computer, and the information produced by the computer as a result of processing.

Viewing the input displayed on the monitor allows the user to check the data for accuracy as they are entered. As an output device, the monitor is often used to review information that needs to be viewed briefly and for which a printed copy (hard copy) is not necessary. For example, if a patient calls your office to inquire when their next appointment is scheduled, you can quickly call up this information, view it on the display screen, and relay it to the patient.

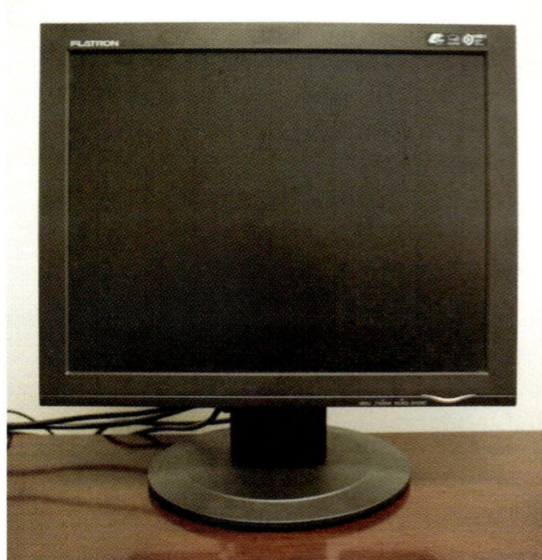

Fig. 40.4 Liquid crystal display flat panel monitor.

Modern liquid crystal display (LCD) flat panel monitors (Fig. 40.4) are small, lightweight, and compact. LCD monitors consume very little power and are, therefore, very energy efficient. LCD monitors or LCDs on tablets or mobile electronic devices create a visual image on the screen by manipulating light within a layer of liquid crystal cells. With an LCD monitor, it is sometimes difficult to view the image on the screen from an angle, which can help to keep patient information private.

MONITOR ERGONOMICS

The monitor should be placed directly in front of the user and at an arm's length distance when sitting back in a chair. This position provides the most comfortable viewing distance. The monitor should be positioned so that the top of the monitor is approximately 2 to 3 inches above eye level. This position helps prevent back and neck tension. It is known that eye muscles must work harder to focus on near objects. Therefore, when working on the computer for a prolonged period of time, occasionally focus your eyes on a distant object (more than 20 feet away) to prevent eyestrain. It is also important to blink frequently while you work to lubricate and moisten the eyes to prevent them from drying out.

To avoid glare, the monitor should be positioned so that the screen does not reflect bright light, which could decrease visibility as well as result in eyestrain. For example, positioning the monitor directly in front of a bright window causes a distracting reflection on the screen. Subdued overhead lighting is considered best for computer use because it causes the least amount of glare. Glare filters are available to help reduce unavoidable reflections, such as from bright overhead fluorescent lights. Privacy filters reduce glare as well as increase privacy of screen information by blurring or blacking out the screen image to anyone who is not directly in front of it.

MONITOR CARE AND MAINTENANCE

The monitor should rest on a flat, stable surface, such as a computer desk.

Monitors collect dust and dirt and, therefore, must be properly maintained. The screen should be cleaned regularly. To clean an LCD monitor, first turn the monitor off. Wipe it gently with a soft, lint-free cloth. Do not use paper towels or tissues because they can scratch the screen. If the dry cloth does not remove all soil, do not press harder because the screen can be damaged. If necessary, use distilled water on a soft cloth or commercial wipes or cleaners for LCD screens. Do not use cleaners that contain chemicals such as ethyl alcohol or acetone, because these can discolor the screen. The cleaner should not be applied directly to the screen or sprayed on the screen because it may run down into the inside of the case and damage the electrical circuits. Keeping the screen clean helps prevent distracting reflections.

The outside casing of the monitor should periodically be wiped with a damp, lint-free cloth to remove dust and dirt. Aerosol sprays, solvents, and abrasives should not be used to clean the casing because they can damage the finish.

INPUT DEVICES

COMPUTER KEYBOARD

The computer keyboard is the most common input device. It contains keys that are pressed to enter data and instructions into the computer. Different brands of computer keyboards vary in size, shape, and layout, but all contain the same basic elements.

The composition of the computer keyboard is alphanumeric—that is, it consists of both alphabetic and numeric keys. Computer keyboards produce both uppercase and lowercase letters and have the standard typewriter *QWERTY* layout, named for the first half row of letters on the keyboard. Some computer keyboards also have a numeric keypad on the right side of the keyboard, which is used for entering numbers quickly.

The keyboard of a desktop computer is either attached by a cable to the main computer unit or is wireless and transmits signals to a receiver that is connected to the computer through a USB port. The user positions the keyboard of a desktop computer according to their preference and comfort. The keyboard is usually built into a laptop computer, whereas tablet devices and handheld devices often use a touchscreen keyboard (see below).

Keyboard Ergonomics

To prevent muscle fatigue of the upper extremities, the computer keyboard should be placed at a level that is lower than that of a conventional desk or table. The feet should be flat on the floor and the hands should rest comfortably at the keyboard with the shoulders relaxed and the elbows flexed at a 90-degree angle or tilted slightly upward. An adjustable chair with good back support is recommended to attain the proper typing height for each individual working with the computer (Fig. 40.5).

For entering data, a light touch should be used and the hands and fingers should be kept as relaxed as possible. If using a mouse, position it at the same height as the keyboard. Be sure to allow adequate workspace to use both the keyboard and mouse comfortably. These measures help prevent strain on the wrists and hands.

An adequate working space should be available to position the material being entered into the computer. The material should be placed so that it can be viewed easily, either by positioning it lying flat on the work surface or vertically in a copy holder.

Keyboard Care and Maintenance

With extended use, residue may build up on the surface of the keyboard. This residue, often referred to as *grime,* should be cleaned with an antiseptic wipe or a slightly damp, lint-free cloth. Aerosol sprays should never be used to clean the keyboard because liquid may drip down into the keyboard, damaging its electrical components. The keyboard interior can be "dusted" by using a compressed inert gas that comes in a pressurized can and is available from computer supply stores. Alternatively, a vacuum cleaner with a small brush attachment may be used to clean the keyboard interior.

The following steps should be followed when cleaning the computer keyboard:

1. Shut down the computer.
2. Disconnect the keyboard cable.
3. Hold the keyboard upside down and shake it to remove any dust, dirt, or crumbs that may be stuck in the keyboard.
4. Clean the keyboard using a can of compressed air following the manufacturer's instructions. Use the can in an upright position. Do not tilt or shake the can.
5. Clean the top and side of the keys with an antiseptic wipe or a damp, lint-free cloth to remove grime. A cotton swab moistened with alcohol can be used to clean between the keys.
6. Allow the keyboard to dry completely (about 30 minutes) before reconnecting it to the computer.

Because of their electronic components, computer keyboards can be damaged if liquids spill into them, particularly liquids that are sweet or sticky, such as soft drinks. Therefore, it is best not to place beverages close to the keyboard. If a liquid is accidentally spilled into the keyboard, the computer should immediately be turned off. If the liquid spilled is thin and clear, such as water, unplug the keyboard, turn it upside down and shake it gently to get as much liquid out as possible. Keep the keyboard inverted to allow additional liquid to drain out, and use a paper towel or cloth to wipe off the top of the keyboard. Let the keyboard dry in an inverted position for 24 hours at room temperature. If after these steps have been taken the keyboard does not work, it should be replaced. A greasy, sweet, or sticky liquid such as a soft drink spilled into the keyboard usually causes permanent damage and the keyboard must be replaced.

MOUSE

After the keyboard, the mouse is the second most commonly used input device. A mouse is a pointing device that fits comfortably under the palm of the hand. The mouse is used to move the pointer on the screen to an object on the screen, such as a menu item, an icon, or a line of text. The mouse must then be "clicked" to perform a certain action associated with that object. The mouse may be wireless or connected directly to the computer. The mousepad is found on a laptop computer. It is usually a touchpad that can be used to move the mouse with the fingertip. To click the mousepad, you would touch it lightly once or twice depending on what you wanted it to do.

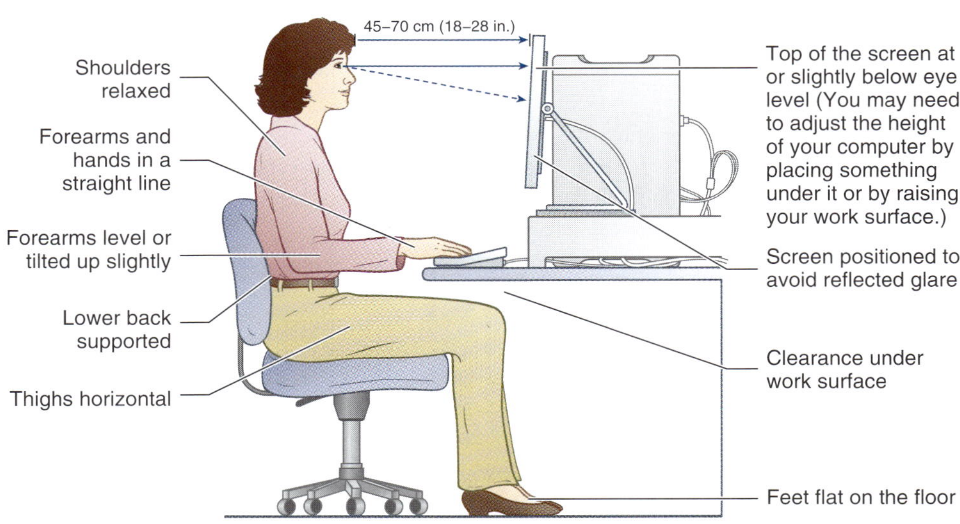

Fig. 40.5 Keyboard ergonomics.

TOUCHSCREEN

Tablets, smartphones, and other mobile devices usually have a **touchscreen,** a visual display unit that the user controls directly using either one or more fingers or a stylus. Different touchscreens have different methods of sensing touch. It is important to use the correct amount of pressure to avoid damaging the screen.

PRINTER

A printer is an output device capable of printing text and graphics on paper. Printers convert processed data from a combination of electronic impulses into a printed form called hard copy. In the medical office, a hard copy of the computer input is frequently required; examples include patient reminders, patient receipts, visit summaries, prescriptions, patient statements, and office reports.

Some printers can also double as fax machines and photocopiers, but this is practical only when there is a small volume of work. A printer can be dedicated to one computer or can be networked to a number of computers.

The printers most commonly used in the medical office are inkjet and laser printers.

INKJET PRINTER

An inkjet printer uses droplets of ink to form text characters and graphics. This type of printer contains nozzles that spray tiny drops of ink onto the paper to create an image. Inkjet printers are lightweight and inexpensive and can produce text and graphics in both black and white and color on a variety of paper types.

Although the initial cost of an inkjet printer is low, operating costs are higher than those of a laser printer. The ink used by an inkjet printer is contained in cartridges, which are expensive and must be replaced frequently. Most inkjet printers have at least two ink cartridges—one containing black ink, and one or more containing colored ink.

LASER PRINTER

The most significant feature of a laser printer (Fig. 40.6) is that it has a "computer of its own" to direct its functioning. Laser printers use a micro-thin beam of light (laser beam), electric charges, and a toner powder to produce each page of text. Under direction of the printer's computer, the laser beam is bounced off a series of mirrors onto a positively charged rotating drum. The pulses of the beam correspond to the characters making up the document being printed. The areas where the laser beam hits the drum become neutral, which enables the toner powder to stick to them and form characters. Finally, the characters are transferred from the rotating drum to paper with the use of pressure and heat to solidify the toner powder on the paper. This process is similar to that of a photocopy machine.

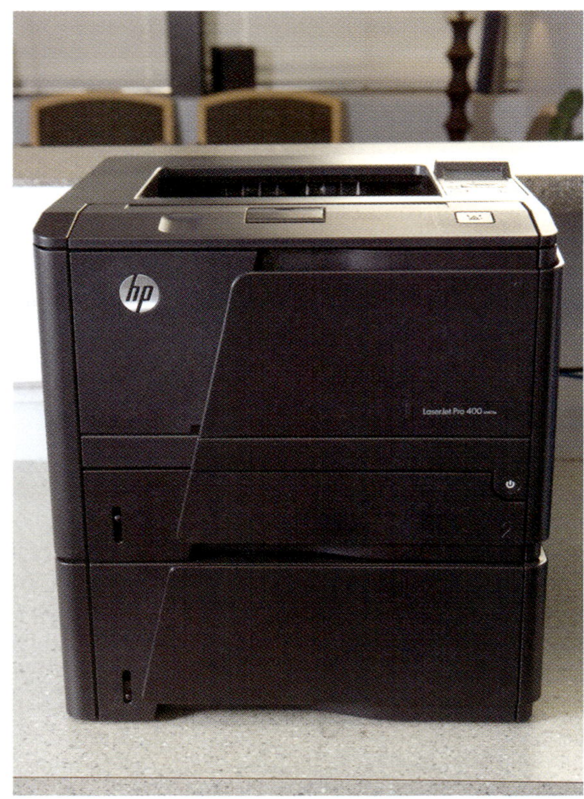

Fig. 40.6 Laser printer.

The toner powder used with a laser printer is housed in a plastic cartridge and must be replaced when it runs out. Although the initial cost of a laser printer is more than that of an inkjet printer, the operating cost is less than that of an inkjet. This is because the cost per page of using toner powder (laser printer) is less than the cost per page of using ink cartridges (inkjet printer).

The print quality of laser printers is superb, nearly attaining the quality of typesetting seen in textbooks. Laser printers are available in both black-and-white and color models. Other advantages of laser printers include their fast printing speed and quiet mode of operation. The printing speed of laser printers is faster than that of inkjet printers. Laser printers do not have as many mechanical moving parts as other types of printers, which usually reduces their frequency of repair.

WIRELESS PRINTING

Many modern printers contain WiFi transceivers and are able to print without a cable connection from any computer connected to the network. The printer must be installed on the wireless network. Smartphones and tablets can also be connected to the network using the requested login credentials so that documents can be printed. It may be necessary to download printing apps such as AirPrint for Apple devices.

PRINTER CARE AND MAINTENANCE

Proper maintenance keeps the printer operating at its best and prolongs its life. Some general guidelines that should be followed to properly care for and maintain an inkjet and a laser printer are as follows:

1. Place the printer on a flat, stable surface.
2. Avoid placing the printer in a location that would expose it to direct sunlight, excessive heat, moisture, or dust.
3. Sufficient room should be left around the printer to allow for easy access for such tasks as adding paper and replacing ink or toner cartridges.
4. Add paper when needed, following the manufacturer's instructions. Inkjet and laser printers use individual sheets of paper stored in a tray in the printer's casing.
5. Replace ink cartridges in inkjet printers and toner cartridges in laser printers as required, following the manufacturer's instructions.
6. After turning off the printer, wait at least 5 seconds before turning it back on. Rapid switching of the power off and on can damage the printer.
7. The printer should be cleaned regularly to remove accumulated dust and dirt. The outside case should be cleaned with a soft clean cloth dampened with a mild detergent solution. Never use strong detergents or solvents on the casing because they could damage the finish. Clean the platen glass, inside of the document cover, and document feeder with a lint-free cloth moistened with water to prevent streaks. The inside of the printer should be cleaned according to the instructions in the printer's user manual.

STORAGE OPTIONS

A storage option permanently stores information for later retrieval by the computer. A storage option retains its information after the power has been removed and is used to store both programs and data. Examples of storage options available for microcomputer systems include hard disks, USB flash drives, and cloud storage, which are discussed below.

Storage capacity varies widely based on the type of storage device and usually is related to the cost of the device. For example, a flash drive can hold up to 2 TB, whereas the hard disk drive of a new computer often has a storage capacity of 500 GB to 4 TB.

HARD DISK DRIVES

A **hard disk drive** is a storage device consisting of one or more rigid, nonflexible platters coated with a magnetically sensitive material and encased in a permanently sealed, airtight container (Fig. 40.7). The composition of a hard disk is designed to maximize its important functions: the storage and retrieval of information. To accommodate the storage of information, hard disks are coated with a magnetically sensitive material. Data are stored on the disk as magnetic particles.

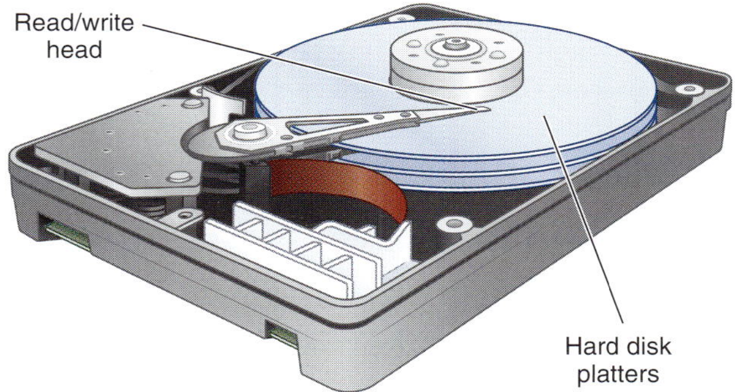

Fig. 40.7 Hard disk drive.

Desktop computers have an internal hard disk drive, meaning it is located inside the main computer unit. Portable hard disk drives can be attached to the computer using a USB port for additional data storage or backups. Because a hard disk is very sensitive to dirt, dust, and smoke, the entire disk unit is encased in a permanently sealed, airtight container to protect it from these contaminants.

SOLID STATE DRIVES

Solid state drives use integrated circuit assemblies to store data permanently, and they have no actual "disks" or motors. They usually use nonvolatile semiconductor-based integrated circuits (flash memory) on a memory chip to store information. Although solid state drives are more expensive than hard disks, they are faster and more durable. They are commonly found in laptop computers and tablets as well as other portable devices.

USB FLASH DRIVE

A USB flash drive is a portable storage device that consists of a small circuit board in a plastic case. Other terms for a flash drive include a *jump drive* and a *thumb drive* (Fig. 40.8). It is called a flash drive because it uses flash memory. For a flash drive to be used, it must be inserted into a USB port on the

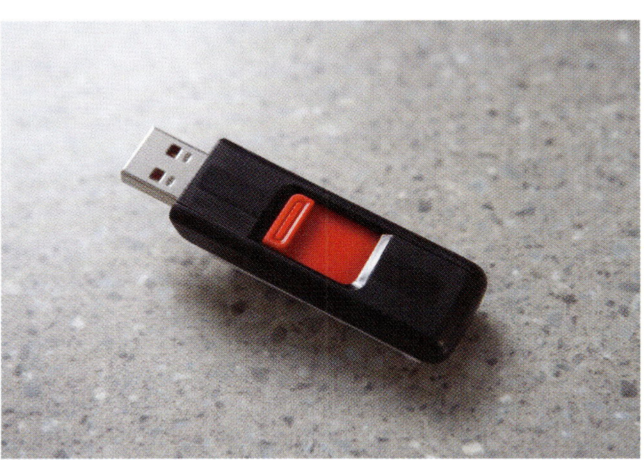

Fig. 40.8 Flash drive.

main unit. A USB flash drive has a storage capacity that usually ranges from 8 GB to 100 GB, although some flash drives have considerably more memory.

CLOUD STORAGE

Cloud storage is when information is stored on servers that are in off-site locations. This type of storage is very beneficial in that if something happens to the onsite storage of information it will be saved and be accessible. Many medical offices have storage in the cloud to make sure that all of the information stored in their onsite computer is also stored in the cloud so that if something were to happen, such as a tornado or hurricane, that information could be accessed at another site on another computer system. There are many cloud storage options available, including Microsoft Onedrive, Dropbox, Google Cloud, Box, and Carbonite.

MEDICAL OFFICE COMPUTERIZATION

Medical office computerization is the use of the computer to perform medical office administrative procedures. With the advent of the microcomputer, medical offices now use computers to perform administrative procedures that were previously performed manually. This, in turn, has increased the demand for qualified individuals trained in medical office computerization, not only to perform the administrative tasks on the computer but also to instruct other staff members in computer operations.

IMPACT OF MEDICAL OFFICE COMPUTERIZATION

Almost all medical offices use computers to perform at least some functions. Although there are distinct advantages to using a computer, it should be realized that there are also some disadvantages that can lead to difficulties, such as temporary loss of computer service. It is important to be aware of these problem areas so that steps can be taken to either prevent them altogether or be better prepared for them if they occur. Adequate preparation will result in the least amount of disruption to the efficient running of a computerized front office.

Telehealth

Telehealth, provision of health care via telecommunication technology, is another method for a health care team to maintain contact with patients without having the patient come into the office. It is usually done online and allows the health care team to provide services and information (Procedure 40.1). Telehealth can also utilize just the phone line for those that are not comfortable using a computer. This could mean that the patient will be talking and viewing the provider, allowing the patient and the provider to send/receive messages, and to use remote monitoring devices to gather information about the patient's health. Telehealth became very popular during the COVID-19 pandemic. It allowed providers to see patients without them coming into the medical office and risk exposure to COVID-19. It allowed all health care providers to become better at providing care without actually physically seeing the patient.

Audit Trail

The computer can keep track of data entry. When new information is entered or existing information is changed, a log is created to record the time and date of the entry, as well as the name of the computer operator. This log is stored and can be retrieved to detect irregularities. If an error was made, the program lists the name of the operator and the date the information was entered. The computer may also keep track of each person that accessed data in a medical record. This capability helps protect patient privacy. If an employee looks up information in a patient's EHR without being authorized to do so, it may be grounds for termination.

What Would You Do? What Would You *Not* Do?

Case Study 1

Olivia Young has moved to the community and has come to the medical office for a new patient appointment for her chronic asthma. Olivia is leaving the office and is quite upset. She says that she doesn't like having computers in the examining rooms—that it's not natural. She feels like the physician and medical assistant are ignoring her and interacting more with the computer than with her. Olivia says it's like there's a barrier between her and the doctor. She says that the medical office she used to go to didn't have computers in the examination rooms and the doctor really paid attention to her and listened to what she had to say. She says she's thinking of looking for another doctor so that she doesn't have to play second fiddle to a computer. ■

What Would You Do? What Would You *Not* Do?

Case Study 2

Kacy Ervin comes to the medical office and is diagnosed with strep throat. The physician uses Kacy's EHR to prescribe an antibiotic and gives her instructions for taking the medication with patient information on strep throat printed on two regular sheets of paper that have been generated by the computer. The next day Kacy calls the office to say that she drove to her pharmacy on the way home from the doctor's appointment. When she pulled the papers from the doctor's office out of her purse, she found a sheet of paper with information about her prescription that was signed by the physician but could not find the prescription form to give to the pharmacist. She says she must have lost the prescription and wants to know if the office can call in the prescription to her pharmacy. ■

COMPUTER SYSTEM MALFUNCTIONS

Even the best hardware and software systems can and will occasionally fail, and one or more of the medical office procedures will come to an abrupt halt. Some problems have no explanations, whereas others are directly related to a specific event, such as operator error, a software bug, or a hardware malfunction. To minimize computer downtime, most medical offices are connected to some kind of network or server that stores information and provides backup systems.

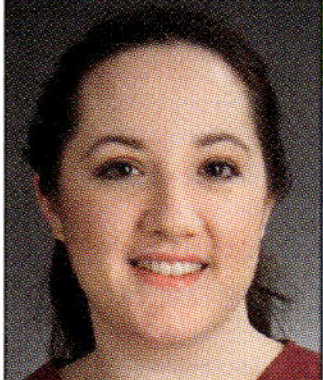

Memories *from* Practicum

Emma Hayes: When I did my practicum, it was the first time I really realized how much a modern medical office relies on its computer system. At that time, the office where I was placed was using a computer program to schedule appointments and manage the patient billing, but they were using a traditional paper medical record. There were four computers in the office, and they were networked together with two laser printers. The night before, we printed a list of patients scheduled for the next day, and we used that list to pull the medical records. In the evening, we also backed up all the computer files from that day. We were using a magnetic tape drive at that time to make a copy of all the files from the financial management software and appointment program. Individuals who did word processing or used a spreadsheet program had to back up their own files. I think that there wouldn't be enough storage space for most offices to do backups this way today. One day, the office computer system was not working, and we couldn't look anything up. It was very frustrating because we didn't know how much the patient's copayment was and we couldn't enter information about the visit. We did have the paper charge slips that the physicians had filled out, and by the next day everything was working again. I think it would be even more difficult now because we are using an electronic medical record as well. ■

ELECTRONIC INFORMATION TRANSFER

One of the major developments of the past 25 years has been the significant increase in the use of the internet to transfer data over great distances. The first network of computers sharing information by telephone lines was set up in 1969, but the internet as we know it first became available to commercial users and the general public in the 1990s. In the medical office, electronic data sharing is primarily used for e-mail, transfer of billing and insurance information, banking, and e-prescribing, in addition to local network capabilities that allow for communication of data within the office itself or between different facilities of the same organization.

INTERNET

The **internet** is a global system of interconnected computer networks that use the transmission control protocol/internet protocol (TCP/IP) to transmit and exchange data. Individual computers or LANs are connected to the internet by **routers,** various types of wired or wireless devices to connect networks. An *internet service provider* (ISP) is a company that provides access to the internet (such as EarthLink, Verizon, or Comcast). Each computer is assigned a specific *internet protocol address* (IP address) for identification and location addressing. Various technologies exist to link a computer or LAN to the internet, but some are considerably faster than others. Modern systems usually use a **broadband** router, which handles a wide range of frequencies. **Digital subscriber line (DSL)** technologies allow for continuous digital connection over the telephone line, which can still be used for voice calls. This type of connection provides very fast transmission. Telephone companies are also providing fiberoptic cables with a glass core that transmit electronic information as light impulses. A method of transmitting electronic information that does not use a telephone line is a cable modem. This type of modem hooks up to a cable television connection. For a business such as the medical office, speed and reliability are major concerns when selecting a means of electronic transmission. Connection to the internet allows a medical office to access the World Wide Web, send and receive e-mail, and transfer data electronically.

The **World Wide Web** is a series of documents, or webpages, that can be accessed by a software application called a **Web browser,** such as Edge, Google Chrome, Safari, or Firefox. To access resources, the user inputs a type of Web address—a uniform resource locator (**URL**)—that identifies the specific page to be located. Many medical offices and other medical facilities maintain websites with information for prospective and current patients.

E-MAIL

E-mail (electronic mail) is a method of composing, sending, receiving, and storing messages that are sent over the internet. Files, such as documents, spreadsheets, and images, can be attached. Security and confidentiality are issues when using e-mail. The medical assistant should assume that an e-mail message may be read by someone else (e.g., a member of the recipient's family). It is also likely that the organization for which the medical assistant works may have access to e-mail messages, even if they have been deleted. In the medical office, e-mail should not be used for private messages or information.

SOCIAL MEDIA

Social media includes websites and applications used by individuals and communities to participate in social networking. Social media sites may facilitate social networking, professional networking, media sharing, knowledge sharing, and other functions. Health professionals may join online communities to network and keep abreast of health care developments. They need to be sure that patient information is never shared without specific authorization. Many health professionals join social community sites in order to network with colleagues. In addition, many health care organizations use social media to enhance their image and communicate with the public through sites like Facebook, X (formerly Twitter), and YouTube. They may also use blogs, podcasts, and webinars to educate both the public and other health professionals.

SECURE MESSAGING WITHIN THE ELECTRONIC MEDICAL RECORD

Most EHRs incorporate some type of messaging system, which can be thought of as e-mail within the EHR. It allows secure communications among health care providers and gives the ability to link directly to clinical and laboratory data regarding patients. When there is an interface with patient insurance information, the provider can often identify which specific medications a patient's insurance will cover. This system is often used for communication between the provider and the medical assistant. It may be used to notify the provider when a patient is ready to be seen or when a patient needs additional services (such as an electrocardiogram or blood draw). In addition, it can be used for messages such as patient requests for medication refills (see Chapter 41).

PATIENT PORTALS

Patients often have access to a variety of services through the **patient portal** of a medical office or larger health care entity. This is an online application that allows patients to interact with and communicate with their health care providers. In addition to access to laboratory reports and health education resources, there is often a secure e-mail system allowing patients to communicate directly with health care providers and other staff members by secure e-mail. These systems are password-protected and must comply with Health Insurance Portability and Accountability Act (HIPAA) regulations. The patient messages and physician replies are automatically incorporated into the patient's EHR. It is important for the office to develop a system to encourage patients to sign up for this service and also to respond promptly to patient messages.

ELECTRONIC TRANSMISSION OF BILLING AND INSURANCE INFORMATION

Insurance and billing information is often transmitted electronically via telephone lines to billing departments, billing affiliates, and/or insurance companies. The HIPAA Security Rule sets standards to safeguard the transmission of patient health information electronically, and each medical office must comply with these standards. This includes maintaining secure networks and using an encryption system, to maintain data security. **Encryption** refers to a process by which electronic information is changed into an unreadable form that requires the original encryption software to reverse the process.

E-PRESCRIBING

Traditionally, patients were given written prescriptions, and prescription refills were often handled either by telephone or by fax. The last 10 years have seen a significant increase in the transmission of prescriptions directly to pharmacies electronically. This is usually accomplished as a function of an EHR. The computer program used by the provider and/or the pharmacy usually can access drug information; information about the patient's history, allergies, and so on; information about the patient's insurance coverage for specific medications; and information about drug interactions. Because the patient's entire medication history is usually available through a national database, it can be an effective way to identify patients who see multiple physicians for the same complaint in an effort to obtain certain medications. E-prescribing is one of the quality measures used as part of the Medicare Quality Payment program.

PATIENT KIOSKS

Many medical offices have added **patient kiosks**, a device that allows patients to digitally check-in for their appointments. The device may include a keyboard and/or a touchscreen that allows the patient to enter the information needed to get checked in. The kiosk is usually located in the waiting area and allows patients to check-in for their appointment, complete forms, provide information to the provider or the patient, allow the patient to make copayments or to make a payment on their account. This can be done without the help of someone else, but if the patient does need help there will be someone who works for the medical office close by.

COMPUTER NETWORK SECURITY

Because all HIPAA regulations apply to the EHR, the medical office must provide secure access to patient demographic and health information stored in the computer's database. If a cloud-based EHR is used, the company providing the health record is responsible for maintaining security of any records stored on its servers. When a centralized system is used in several office locations, there must be extensive security controls. Security of computer networks is accomplished through the following methods.

AUTHENTICATION

Each health care worker with permission to use the computer network must have a password and must log in to access the network. Passwords should be changed at regular intervals, and in fact there may be a system function that requires this. The medical assistant should not share their password with anyone else. Effective passwords include random series of digits, letters, and symbols rather than English words, telephone numbers, or other combinations that have meaning. A separate set of keystrokes is often used as an electronic signature.

LEVELS OF AUTHORIZATION

A computer network has specific levels of authorization so that certain screens and certain functions are available only to users with the correct level of authorization. For example, at the end of a patient visit that has been recorded in the EHR, the provider must electronically sign the record. This closes the visit so that information about that visit cannot be changed at a later date. A medical assistant would not usually be authorized to perform this function.

AUTOMATIC LOGOFF

All users should log out of the computer network when their workstations are unattended. If the user forgets to do this, the software has a feature that automatically logs a user off after a predetermined period of inactivity.

AUDIT CONTROLS

Practice management programs and EHR programs have the ability to track every activity of individuals using the computer system. This can be used to determine if security violations have occurred and to identify the individual with whom those violations may be associated.

ANTIVIRUS SOFTWARE

Antivirus software is a type of system software known as a *utility program.* Antivirus software should be installed on the computer system to scan for computer viruses. The term *computer virus* refers to software designed to penetrate a computer or network without consent. A computer virus can access information and/or cause damage. Once installed, antivirus software operates in the background and monitors all files for viruses. It also updates itself regularly because new computer viruses are developed constantly and can be spread quickly through the internet.

FIREWALL

A **firewall** is a system that protects a computer network from unauthorized access by users on its own network or another network, such as the internet. A firewall takes its name from a wall in a building that is made of a material that will prevent a fire from spreading from one part of the building to another. A firewall may be in the form of a utility software program, or it may be more complex and consist of a firewall hardware device that connects to the computer.

All inquiries and messages entering or leaving the computer system must pass through the firewall, which examines each inquiry or message and blocks those that do not meet the firewall's specified security criteria. If the firewall is unsure about whether or not to grant access, it will display a screen message for the user regarding the access. The computer user is given the following choices: to refuse access, to permit access once, or to permit unlimited access. The firewall does not substitute for antivirus software because it cannot protect against viruses received as e-mail attachments.

BACKUPS

In the medical office, records are permanently stored on the computer's internal hard disk or the network server. A copy of this information, known as a *backup*, should be made at least every day although facilities using an EHR system usually utilize frequent or continuous backups. A **backup** is a duplicate copy of a program or data kept for reference in case the original is damaged, lost, or destroyed. Backups prevent loss of data, which are especially important in the EHR as well as in the scheduling and billing section of the practice management software.

Many medical offices contract with an online backup service that provides secure backups of all files used in the office for a monthly fee. These backups may be performed every few hours or at scheduled times. The information is encrypted using methods similar to those used by banks and financial institutions. Although this service may seem expensive, it ensures that data will not be lost or destroyed.

Large health care facilities may be able to back up information from individual computers using their own network system. These backups usually occur automatically, although it may be necessary for a staff member to initiate the backup.

External hard drives, USB flash drives and cloud storage can be used to create physical backup copies. When a physical copy is used for backup, it should be stored in a secure place that is physically remote from the computer system or in a fireproof safe in the medical office.

SYSTEM MAINTENANCE

The medical office must assign an individual to be responsible for system maintenance. System maintenance involves setting up and overseeing the computer system. In Windows 11, disk cleanup and disk defragmentation processes to remove unnecessary information and consolidate existing information occur automatically. Updates are also usually set up to occur automatically, although all of these processes can be performed manually if needed. In addition, one individual is usually a system administrator who has the authority to assign levels of authorization and perform other system functions to maintain the computer system.

What Would You Do? What Would You *Not* Do?

Case Study 3

John Gurnsey comes to the medical office for a checkup for his psoriasis and clinical depression. John says he likes the computer system used in the office but worries about the security of his medical record. He says that he doesn't want any of his friends or co-workers to know that he has psoriasis or that he is on an antidepressant. John wants to know how the office protects his medical record from people like computer hackers. He says that because there is a computer in every room, how is a patient who has been left alone in a room prevented from looking up patient records on the computer? John says that viruses keep getting into his computer at home and that data on his hard drive have been destroyed three different times. He wants to know if this ever happens at the medical office. ■

What Would You Do? What Would You *Not* Do? RESPONSES

Case Study 1

Page 1074

What Did Emma Do?

- ❑ Listened carefully to what Olivia was saying and agreed that sometimes patients feel as though the computer places a barrier between the patient and the doctor.
- ❑ Reassured Olivia that the doctor and staff always pay attention and listen very closely to what she has to relay about her health.
- ❑ Explained that staff members are very familiar with the computer system, and they may forget that computers in the examination room may seem strange to some patients.
- ❑ Stressed to Olivia that computerized medical records provide better patient care through improved communication, faster access to data, and clearer and better documentation.
- ❑ Relayed Olivia's concern at the next medical office staff meeting.

What Did Emma Not Do?

- ❑ Did not minimize or ignore Olivia's concerns.
- ❑ Did not tell Olivia that she is outdated and needs to adjust to the 21st century.

Case Study 2

Page 1074

What Did Emma Do?

- ❑ Explained that the physician sent the prescription to the pharmacy by computer and instructed Kacy simply to stop by the pharmacy to pick it up.
- ❑ Reassured Kacy that many patients are confused about this until they get used to the new system.

What Did Emma Not Do?

- ❑ Did not imply that Kacy should have realized that the physician was using an e-prescription.
- ❑ Did not promise to call the pharmacy to make sure they have received the prescription.

Case Study 3

Page 1078

What Did Emma Do?

- ❑ Reassured John that it is a legitimate concern to want to make sure his medical information is kept confidential.
- ❑ Explained to John that something called a "firewall" protects the office computers from unauthorized access by computer hackers.
- ❑ Told John that each staff member has to enter a password to log onto the computer and that a patient would not have a password and would not be able to log onto the computer.
- ❑ Explained to John that the office places a lot of emphasis on maintaining security of the computer system and preventing loss of data. Told John that the office has antivirus software running all the time to protect the computer from viruses and that the office also has a backup system so that even if data were lost, there would be a backup of the data.

What Did Emma Not Do?

- ❑ Did not minimize John's concerns.
- ❑ Did not criticize John for not having an antivirus program on his home computer.

TERMINOLOGY REVIEW

Key Term	Word Parts	Definition
App		A specialized program, often small enough to run on a mobile device.
Application software		Software designed to accomplish a specific task (e.g., word processing); also called *application program* and *software program.*
Backup		A duplicate copy of a program or data kept for reference in case the original is damaged, lost, or destroyed.
Broadband		A method of transmitting electronic data that handles a wide range of frequencies.

TERMINOLOGY REVIEW—cont'd

Key Term	Word Parts	Definition
Cloud computing		A model in which the internet is used to store and access data and programs, and servers are not physically located at the same site as the computer.
Computer system		All of the hardware and software components making up the computer.
Data		Raw, unorganized facts about subject matter presented to the computer for processing.
Data processing		The changing of raw facts or data into usable information by following a three-part sequence: input, processing, and output.
Digital subscriber line (DSL)		Technology that allows digital signals to be transmitted over telephone lines at high speed even if the telephone line is also being used for voice transmission.
E-mail		A method of composing, sending, receiving, and storing messages that are sent over the internet.
Encryption	*crypt-:* secret	A process by which electronic information is changed into an unreadable form that requires the original encryption software to reverse the process.
Firewall		A system that protects a computer network from unauthorized access by users on its own network or another network, such as the internet.
Gigabyte (GB)	*giga-*: one billion	A unit of computer storage capacity. One gigabyte is equal to a little more than 1 billion bytes or 1000 megabytes.
Hard disk drive		A storage device consisting of one or more rigid, nonflexible platters coated with a magnetically sensitive material and encased in a permanently sealed, airtight container.
Hardware		The physical devices making up a computer system (e.g., main computer unit, keyboard, monitor, and printer).
Input		1. (noun) Data that have been entered into the computer. 2. (verb) The transfer of data to the computer for processing.
Input device		A device for entering data into the computer (e.g., keyboard, mouse, and scanner).
Internet		A global system of interconnected computer networks that use the internet protocol (TCP/IP) to transmit and exchange data.
Kilobyte (KB)	*kilo-*: one thousand	A unit of computer storage capacity. One kilobyte is equal to 1024 bytes (characters).
Megabyte (MB)	*mega-*: one million	A unit of computer storage capacity. One megabyte is equal to a little more than 1 million bytes or 1000 kilobytes.
Network		A group of computers that share data and resources.
Operating system		A type of system software that performs tasks required by the computer to operate itself.
Output		1. (noun) Information that has been generated by the computer. 2. (verb) The transfer of processed data back to the user.
Output device		A device that transfers processed data to the user (e.g., computer monitor and printer).
Patient kiosks		A device that allows patients to check in electronically.
Patient portal		An online application that allows patients to interact with and communicate with their health care providers.
Processing		The manipulation and reorganization of data according to the instructions in a program.
Program		A set of instructions organized in a logical step-by-step sequence, which tells the computer how to perform a specific function.
Router		A wired or wireless device used to form or connect networks.
Server		A large computer that stores data and manages tasks for other computers on a network.
Social media		Applications and websites used by individuals and communities to participate in social networking.
Software		A general term for the programs or instructions that tell a computer what to do.

Continued

TERMINOLOGY REVIEW—cont'd

Key Term	Word Parts	Definition
Solid state drive		Drive that uses integrated circuits (flash memory) to store data permanently.
Storage capacity		The maximum amount of information that a device can hold, measured in bytes.
System software		A group of programs that control or maintain the operations of a computer.
Telehealth		Providing health care via telecommunication technology.
Terabyte (TB)	*tera-*: one trillion	A unit of computer storage. One terabyte is equivalent to a little more than a trillion bytes or 1000 gigabytes.
Touchscreen		A visual display unit that the user can touch to input data using the fingers or a stylus.
URL		The characters and/or words used to access a specific website or file on the World Wide Web.
USB port		A standard computer cable connection interface that allows several types to devices to be connected to the computer in order to transfer data across short distances.
Web browser		A software program used to access the World Wide Web.
WiFi		A technology for wireless local area networking and connection to the internet.
World Wide Web		A series of interlinked websites or files accessed via the internet.

PROCEDURE 40.1 Telehealth Interaction with a Patient

Outcome Interact with a patient regarding a recent health issue

Equipment/Supplies:

- Computer
- Paper
- Pen or pencil

1. **Procedure Step.** Identify the medical office and give your name. Each practice will have a preferred way for all employees to identify the practice and themselves. Example: "Hello, this is Emma at Primary Care Associates." Do not rush through the greeting. The patient needs to hear the greeting clearly and understand who they are speaking with.
   Principle. The patients involved in a telehealth interaction need to feel comfortable with the process and who they are dealing with.
2. **Procedure Step.** Identify the patient by asking their name and date of birth.
   Principle. It is important to identify the patient so that the information is recorded in the correct patients record.
3. **Procedure Step.** Ask the patient how they have been doing since their last visit in to see the provider. Document the information provided to you.
   Principle. If the patient has developed any new issues, it is important to get it documented in the patient record.
4. **Procedure Step.** Ask the patient to confirm their demographic information.
   Principle. It is important to identify any new demographic information at each visit.
5. **Procedure Step.** Thank the patient for the time spent with you, ask them to wait for the provider. Inform them that the provider will be with them shortly.
   Principle. The patient will be more cooperative if they are kept informed of what the process is for this type of visit.
6. **Procedure Step.** Let the provider know that the patient is ready for them.
   Principle. The provider needs to know that the patient has been prepped for the virtual visit.

Telephone Techniques

Check out the Evolve site at http://evolve.elsevier.com/Bonewit/today to access additional interactive activities and exercises to help you study and prepare for success.

LEARNING OBJECTIVES

1. Describe the importance of effective telephone courtesy and a pleasing telephone personality for the medical assistant.
2. Explain the use of multiline telephones, cell phones, smartphones, and pagers in the medical office.
3. Differentiate between incoming telephone calls the medical assistant can handle and other incoming calls.
4. Describe the correct procedure for screening incoming calls.
5. Describe the correct procedure for taking messages and transcribing messages recorded on an answering machine or voicemail.
6. Identify the correct steps to respond to a telephone call regarding an emergency or urgent medical problem.
7. Describe how to deal with problem calls.
8. Explain how the medical assistant should make outgoing telephone calls.

PROCEDURES

Performing telephone screening.
Taking a telephone message.
Taking requests for medication or prescription refills.

Telephoning a patient for follow-up.

CHAPTER OUTLINE

INTRODUCTION TO TELEPHONE TECHNIQUES
USING THE TELEPHONE EFFECTIVELY
Verbal and Nonverbal Communication
Telephone Courtesy
Telephone Personality
Maintaining Patient Privacy
Effective Telephone Communication
TELEPHONE TECHNOLOGY
Multiline Phones
Special Features
Answering Machines and Voicemail
Cell Phones and Smartphones
Pagers
INCOMING CALLS
Centralized or Electronic Routing
Managing Incoming Calls
Performing Telephone Screening
Calls the Medical Assistant Usually Handles
Taking Messages on a Paper Message Form
Taking Messages on the Computer
Calls From Other Providers
Calls From Salespeople
Urgent or Emergency Calls
Dealing With Problem Calls
The Caller Who Refuses to Give Information
Complaints
Patients With Special Problems
OUTGOING CALLS
Local Calls
Appointment Reminders
Long-Distance and International Calls
Conference Calls

KEY TERMS

enunciation (ee-nun-see-AY-shun)
pager
smartphone
voicemail

INTRODUCTION TO TELEPHONE TECHNIQUES

Contact with a patient takes many forms. In addition to face-to-face contact, medical assistants often speak to patients and other callers over the telephone. The telephone is often the first contact between the medical office and a patient. In addition, the telephone is used throughout the day to make and receive referrals, request laboratory results, and respond to patient questions.

Managing the phone is one of the most important jobs in the office. It is the first chance the medical assistant has to project a positive attitude and image to a patient. One never has a second chance to make a first impression.

USING THE TELEPHONE EFFECTIVELY

VERBAL AND NONVERBAL COMMUNICATION

Communicating well on the telephone is an important skill for every medical assistant to have. It involves both verbal and nonverbal communication skills. What's the difference between the two? Verbal communication is our use of words and nonverbal communication is things like our tone of voice, body gestures, facial expressions, eye contact, and physical proximity. The majority of our communication is nonverbal. It is very important to make sure that we are using the right words, especially on the telephone, but it is important that we pay attention to our nonverbal communication as well.

TELEPHONE COURTESY

The telephone in a medical office should always be answered promptly. Some offices have a policy that every phone call should be answered within three rings. The medical assistant identifies the office, gives their own name, then finds out who is calling. If the call will be transferred, the staff member needs to know who will be on the other end of the call.

The medical assistant should always speak before putting someone on hold. It is not courteous to immediately place a call on hold before speaking to the caller. The caller cannot even be sure that they have reached the correct telephone number. It is far more polite to obtain the caller's name and purpose for calling before putting the caller on hold. It is helpful to keep a written record of each caller's name, with the number of the line on which the caller is holding. A provider should not be placed on hold if it can be avoided. The medical assistant should check back about every 30 seconds or so with a person who is on hold. This reassures the caller that the medical assistant is aware of the call. The medical assistant should also try to give an idea of how long it will take before the call will be answered.

When handling a call, the medical assistant should not chew gum or eat. Paying close attention during the telephone call is also important. A caller can tell if the medical assistant is distracted.

TELEPHONE PERSONALITY

In addition to words or verbal communication, many nonverbal cues or communication are given in the quality of a medical assistant's voice on the telephone. The "telephone personality" is important. It is important to stay focused on the call and smile. The medical assistant should use the same volume as when speaking in person and should speak naturally. An artificial telephone voice may be perceived as cold and "fake."

All words should be spoken clearly so that they are easy to understand. **Enunciation** is the act of speaking so that the message can be easily understood. It may be necessary to speak a little more slowly on the telephone, and it is very important to avoid mumbling. It may be helpful for a medical assistant to record a telephone greeting and analyze the quality of their voice and the personality that is projected.

Qualities such as interest, friendliness, concern, and understanding are clearly communicated over the telephone. So too are boredom, anxiety, and indifference.

MAINTAINING PATIENT PRIVACY

When speaking on the telephone, the medical assistant must take measures to maintain patient privacy and confidentiality as required by the Health Insurance Portability and Accountability Act (HIPAA). When the telephone located at the front desk is used, the privacy window should be closed, if there is one. Otherwise, waiting patients should stand away from the intake area, and the medical assistant's voice should be low enough to avoid being overheard. The telephone used for responding to patient calls and scheduling urgent appointments is often located in a separate area so that patients cannot overhear conversations. The medical assistant should remember to maintain a professional tone in all telephone conversations.

EFFECTIVE TELEPHONE COMMUNICATION

When speaking on the telephone, the medical assistant should try to complete the call without interruption. If it is necessary to put someone on hold, the medical assistant should give a reason and apologize to the caller when the call is resumed. Information and materials should be readily available to handle calls and take messages. These include message slips or a computer messaging system, a pen, the office computer appointment program, and a resource for frequently used telephone numbers. A desk clock, computer clock, or wristwatch should be visible to note the time when taking messages.

The medical assistant begins the conversation by identifying the practice—for example, "Primary Care Associates, Channa speaking." If the caller asks a question or asks for a staff member without identifying himself or herself, the medical assistant asks politely for the caller's name: "With whom am I speaking?" or "May I ask who is calling?" Using complete sentences is important because the medical assistant does not want to sound abrupt or rude.

The medical assistant should use good body mechanics such as, sitting with the back supported and the head in a neutral position (not forward or to one side). The feet should be flat on the floor or supported on a footstool. Fig. 41.1 shows proper body position for answering the telephone. If the receiver is tucked between the head and shoulder, it places strain on the shoulder muscles and may change the voice quality, so this should be avoided. A headset, which consists of an earpiece that fits over the ear and a mouthpiece in front of the mouth, allows for good body posture and leaves the hands free. This is recommended if the medical assistant spends a lot of time on the telephone. Fig. 41.2 shows such a headset.

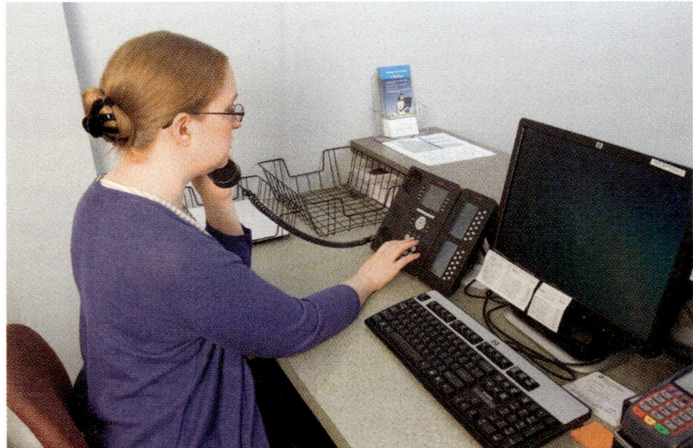

Fig. 41.1 Good posture when answering the telephone improves voice quality and prevents muscle strain.

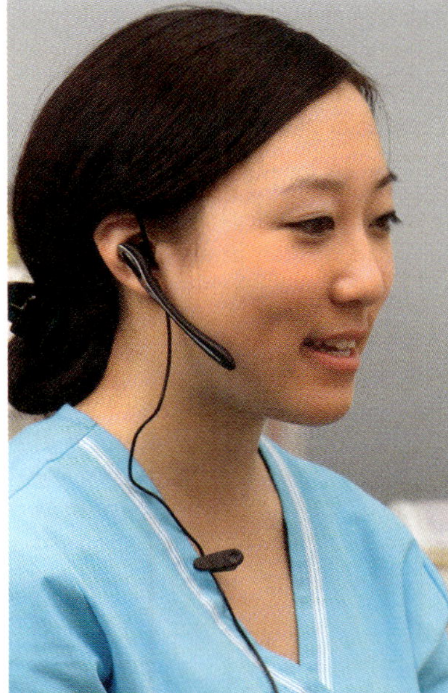

Fig. 41.2 A telephone headset leaves the hands free and facilitates good body posture.

The medical assistant should be clear with callers who leave messages about when they can expect their calls to be returned. Many providers have specific times when they return nonurgent telephone calls, such as late morning, lunch time, or the end of the day.

One should avoid cutting into a person's replies, even if they ramble on and repeat information. When the medical assistant gets the chance to speak, they should try to give a focused answer that lets the caller know what can be done and what the medical assistant is going to do.

TELEPHONE TECHNOLOGY

Advances in telephone technology have given medical offices many options to maintain contact with patients, providers, pharmacies, laboratories, and hospitals.

MULTILINE PHONES

Most offices have a multiline telephone, with several extensions. It is important for the medical assistant to learn how to determine which line is ringing, how to place calls on hold, and how to transfer calls to all parts of the medical office. Fig. 41.3 illustrates a multiline telephone.

A flashing light usually identifies a line that is ringing; it flashes at a different rate on a line where a person is on hold. The medical assistant answers a call by pressing the button on the telephone that corresponds to the line that is ringing. If a second call comes in while the medical assistant is speaking to a caller, the medical assistant should tell the first caller that they need to place the caller on hold, then they press the hold button. The medical assistant answers the second call, identifies the caller, and usually places that caller on hold before returning to the first caller and apologizing for the interruption. The calls are then handled in order.

If the caller asks to be connected to another extension or person, the medical assistant should first obtain the caller's name. To transfer a call, the medical assistant may need to

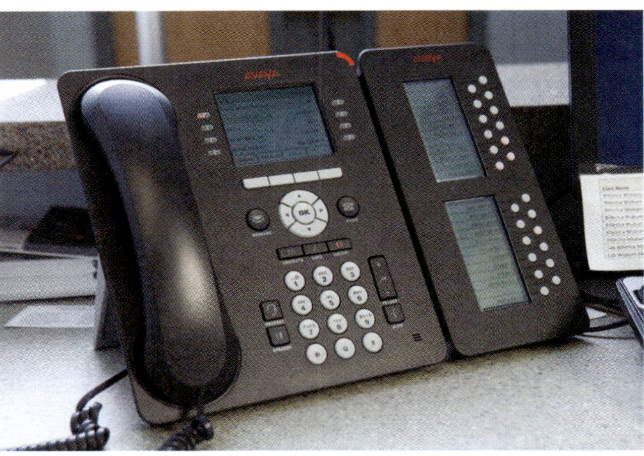

Fig. 41.3 A multiline telephone is commonly used in a medical office.

press another button and/or dial an extension number, depending on the type of telephone system. Knowing the caller's name allows the medical assistant to announce the caller when the call is connected, and it is also helpful if the call is disconnected for some reason.

While a caller is on hold, the light on that line will flash. If the light continues to flash, the medical assistant should pick up that line about every 30 seconds and ask if the person would like to continue holding or leave a message. Sometimes transfers do not go through or the call is not picked up.

Special Features

Multiline telephone systems come with many other features, including speed dialing, call forwarding, call park, and caller ID.

Speed dialing allows storage of frequently called telephone numbers in the telephone system's memory. These numbers can be called by pressing a button or a one- or two-digit code.

Call forwarding allows forwarding of incoming calls to another telephone number. This service is turned on and off by dialing a sequence of numbers and activity keys.

Call park allows a call to be placed on hold and retrieved from another telephone.

Caller ID identifies the caller's telephone number before the telephone is answered. This feature may be available on some, but not all, telephones within a telephone system.

The medical assistant must learn how to use these and other features of the telephone system efficiently.

ANSWERING MACHINES AND VOICEMAIL

Providers have always needed to be available at all times. Some providers' offices still use an answering service for getting messages to providers during hours when the office is normally closed. This is an independent company that answers telephones for a number of clients. Some offices also have an answering machine or voicemail system, which has a message with a number to call outside of office hours and gives people the option to leave a nonurgent message. **Voicemail** is a method for message delivery, storage, and retrieval that is built into the telephone system. It is usually attached to each individual extension. Answering services and answering machines are activated whenever the office is closed, including during lunch break if no one is assigned to take phone calls during that time. The answering service should be notified if the office is closed, although the service will usually pick up phones after a predetermined number of rings.

Increasingly, providers' offices use voicemail systems instead of or in addition to answering machines. Voicemail is a system provided by the office's telephone carrier that allows for messages to be left in a number of "mailboxes" for different people. Each provider might have their own voicemail box as well as each medical assistant, the business manager, and so on. If a call is not answered, many telephone systems will give a caller the option of leaving a message in a voicemail box. Each box has a two- to four-number extension. Many voicemail systems have a directory by which people can find voicemail box numbers by using their touch-tone phone to type in some or all of the letters of the last name of the person with whom they would like to speak.

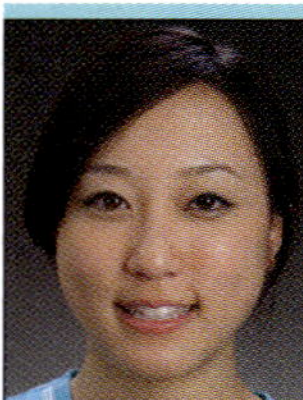

Putting It All Into Practice

My name is Channa Eng, and I am a Certified Medical Assistant. I work for an internal medical practice with two physicians and two nurse practitioners in an urban area. We have many Asian and Hispanic patients. I don't speak much Spanish, but I do speak Cambodian and some Vietnamese. Another medical assistant speaks Spanish, and we both help with translating telephone calls from patients who have difficulty in English. When patients call our office, they get three choices right away. They can hear the message in English, Spanish, or Cambodian. Most patients like this because they can hear the instructions in a language they are comfortable with. On Tuesdays and Thursdays, I spend most of the day on the telephone making appointments and responding to patients who call with medical problems. I don't usually sit at the front desk. Instead, we have a telephone room with three telephones. When it is very busy, there are usually two of us. When a patient calls for an appointment, I ask for their name and date of birth. Then I locate the patient in the electronic health record (EHR). Our system coordinates the clinical record with the appointment system. In addition, I can take messages through the EHR, which are attached to the patient's record and routed to the patient's provider or another staff member. My goal is to handle each call as quickly and efficiently as possible while still making the patients feel that their needs were met. In our office we think that telephone conversations are very important. We try very hard to answer all telephone calls promptly and to avoid putting patients on hold. ■

CELL PHONES AND SMARTPHONES

Cell phones allow two individuals to speak to each other as they would using regular telephones, but the cell phone uses radio signals instead of telephone wires. A **smartphone** is a device that adds computer capabilities to the cell phone, with a drug reference, address book, and other tools; an internet connection; the ability to send and receive e-mails; and sometimes even access to the EHR system used by the health care facility. Many providers use cell phones or smartphones to remain in contact with the medical office when they are in other locations. The providers' cell phone numbers should never be given to patients, but they should be available to office staff so that providers can be contacted as needed.

PAGERS

Pagers may be used in areas with unreliable cell phone service and sometimes in large institutions such as hospitals.

If the providers in a medical practice are affiliated with a large hospital, they may still prefer to be contacted using a pager issued by the institution rather than a personal cell phone. A **pager** (also called a *beeper*) is like a radio that is always tuned in to a single station. When it "hears" its unique access code signal, it lights up, beeps, or vibrates to indicate that a message is being received. Some pagers are also linked to voicemail. Pagers used by physicians or other health professionals are either numeric or alphanumeric. A numeric pager's message is a telephone number (e.g., the answering service, the office, the emergency department, home, a colleague). The provider then returns the call to the number on the display. An alphanumeric pager displays an entire message, so the provider can return a phone call or act on the information that is relayed to the pager. Some pagers also include e-mail so that a return message can be sent. If the providers use pagers, the office staff should have the pager numbers for each provider in the practice.

A simple type of pager may also be used for patients in ambulatory care areas of hospitals or clinics. It is similar to pagers used in restaurants and lights up and/or vibrates to notify patients when it is their turn. Patients can leave the waiting area and be notified when to return. This type of pager provides patient confidentiality because it eliminates the need to call the patient by name.

INCOMING CALLS

An incoming telephone call sounds like a routine event. But breaking down the process, it becomes clear that a number of different elements go into answering a routine call.

CENTRALIZED OR ELECTRONIC ROUTING

Many offices use an electronic routing system to direct calls. If electronic routing is used, the message should be kept up to date and be as clear and concise as possible. The message usually instructs a caller with an urgent problem to contact emergency services at 911 immediately. At each extension, the telephone may be answered or the call will go to voicemail, and the caller can leave a message for office staff members who are not available. By offering the caller several options (e.g., scheduling an appointment, speaking with

HIGHLIGHT on Customer Service

Health care organizations recognize that excellent service is an important part of providing high-quality health care. Because the first contact with a patient is often a telephone contact, it is vital for a medical assistant to be aware of the importance of good customer service.

Internal customers include other departments within the health care facility as well as physician employers and fellow employees. External customers include patients, referring or consulting physicians, visitors, third-party payors, and suppliers. Both types of customers must be treated with respect on the telephone as well as in person. Medical assistants should follow guidelines to be sure that telephone calls are answered promptly, that accurate and complete information is given and received, and that any complaints or concerns are met with an understanding and appropriate response.

There are several service expectations when using the telephone.

- Use a four-part greeting: Answer the telephone using a greeting, introduce yourself, identify your department, and ask how you can help.
- Address the patient by *Miss*, *Mrs.*, *Ms.*, or *Mr.*
- Ask for permission before putting the caller on hold.
- Ask the caller for permission to transfer the call.
- Repeat information such as an appointment date and time before ending the call.
- Ask the caller if there is anything else you can do before ending the call.
- Listen attentively.
- Smile and use a friendly tone of voice.

An acronym that is often recommended to provide excellent customer service to patients is *AIDET*. It stands for Acknowledge, Introduce, Duration, Explanation, Thank You. This is important for telephone calls as well as in all interactions with patients.

- *Acknowledge:* Acknowledge patients or other customers promptly and greet them as the first step in building a connection.
- *Introduce:* Identify yourself and then identify the customer, especially if it is a patient.
- *Duration:* Reduce anxiety by setting time expectations. On the telephone, ask permission before placing a caller on hold, and return to the call at regular intervals. Offer timely appointments.
- *Explanation:* Explain procedures or other information in terms that the patient can understand. Good explanations are a cornerstone of good health care.
- *Thank You:* Thank the caller before ending the call.

If a customer has a complaint, it is important to listen carefully and address the problem. If necessary, staff should have tools available to amend the situation for a patient who is present in person, such as food or parking vouchers. For patients on the telephone, a caring attitude and careful listening are the main tools available to the medical assistant. A four-part service recovery model called *LEAD* is sometimes recommended.

- *Listen:* Allow the patient and/or family to feel heard.
- *Empathize:* Notice and acknowledge feelings.
- *Apologize:* Acknowledge the situation without blame and apologize on behalf of the health care organization.
- *Do the Right Thing:* Determine the best solution and be timely with corrective action.

It may be necessary to report a situation to the manager if it cannot be resolved on the spot. Inform a telephone caller of the action that will be taken and be sure to follow through. ■

the medical assistant, or discussing a billing question), the electronic routing system directs the call to the appropriate part of the office, saving the expense of a staff person who would otherwise be answering the call. It also keeps patients from being put on hold, which some people appreciate.

MANAGING INCOMING CALLS

Performing Telephone Screening

The first step in handling telephone calls is to find out how urgent the call is and what is necessary to handle the call.

Most calls are routine and can be taken in the order in which they come. In most cases a new call is placed on hold while the previous call is handled. However, there are some exceptions:

- Calls from other providers are put through at once.
- Emergency calls are treated as urgent and receive top priority. They will be discussed in detail later in this chapter.
- If the caller is a relative of the provider, the medical assistant either puts the caller through or speaks to the provider via intercom to determine how to handle the call.

When answering calls, it is polite to obtain the caller's name and ask permission to place the caller on hold. This gives the caller the opportunity to identify the call as urgent.

After the caller's name has been obtained, the caller usually states the reason for the call or asks for a staff member or department. When the caller asks for a staff member by name, the medical assistant usually transfers the call. If that staff member is with a patient, the medical assistant may offer to take a message or transfer the call to voicemail. Often the caller asks for the provider. Most providers do not take calls while they are seeing patients. Additional questions may show that the medical assistant can handle the call, or it may be necessary to take a message for the provider (Procedure 41.1).

Calls the Medical Assistant Usually Handles

The medical assistant usually handles four kinds of calls.

1. *Requests to schedule appointments.* The medical assistant will usually schedule appointments and tests, either in the office or at an outside laboratory or the hospital. This topic is discussed in Chapter 42.
2. *Billing inquiries.* The medical assistant may handle inquiries about a patient bill or insurance. For this type of call, the medical assistant refers to the patient account in the computer and gives the caller the information requested. If the caller's question is complicated, the call may be referred to a billing specialist or the office manager.
3. *Receiving diagnostic test and laboratory results.* The medical assistant can also take calls regarding diagnostic test and laboratory results. Most laboratory results today are sent to providers' offices by fax or directly through the computer system. But if a laboratory calls in test results, the medical assistant needs to have a blank laboratory slip so that the results can be filled in, along with the patient's name and the date the tests were taken. After taking the results, the medical assistant places them for the provider to review. If a paper medical record system is used, the report is clipped to the patient's medical record. Taking all results accurately is very important.
4. *Requests for information.* Finally, the medical assistant can handle calls requesting information, such as directions to get to the office, office hours, and the office's medical specialty.

What Would You Do? What Would You *Not* Do?

Case Study 1

Channa has answered a telephone call from Jane Weston, who has called to make a routine appointment. Although the patient has been offered several different appointment days and times, none of the choices has been satisfactory. A low buzz indicates a call on another telephone line. Channa is the only person available to take the call. She tells Mrs. Weston that she will need to put her on hold for a minute. Mrs. Weston says, "Please don't put me on hold. I'll take that last appointment. What time was it for?" ■

Taking Messages on a Paper Message Form

The medical assistant may take messages on a paper message form. Some forms are pressure sensitive so that a copy is created with the original message. The originals stay in the message book and form a telephone log. If the message form does not create a copy, it is helpful to keep a separate telephone log for future reference. In some offices a form is used that has a space for the provider to write orders or desired follow-up on the bottom of the form. The medical assistant should not write in this space when taking the message. If telephone messages are filed in the patient's medical record after the provider or other recipient has responded to the message, a form with a peel-off backing is preferable.

Taking Messages on the Computer

The medical assistant may work in a facility where telephone messages are taken using the computer, either using a stand-alone computer messaging program or using the clinical messaging feature within the EHR. Built-in message templates facilitate taking the message during the telephone call and forwarding the message to one or more recipients. When this feature is part of the EHR, the patient's medical record can be attached to the message, and the transmission is secure. This can be very useful for questions about laboratory results and requests to renew prescriptions.

When taking a message about a patient, include the following information in the message:

- Date and time.
- Name of the physician or staff member.
- Patient's full name and date of birth.
- Name of the caller (if not the patient).
- Message or question that indicates clearly what the patient wants (e.g., prescription, laboratory results, or medical advice).

- Additional information to clarify the message, such as symptoms, medication and pharmacy information, and actions that have already been taken.
- If the patient is ill or requests medication, any medication allergies should be noted.
- Telephone number.
- Initials of the person taking the message.

When a medical assistant transcribes messages from an answering machine or from voicemail, the same paper or electronic message form should be used as for ordinary telephone calls. The time the call was recorded should be used. The medical assistant may need to play the message more than once to record all information (Procedure 41.2).

Patients Requesting Test Results

When a patient calls requesting test results, the medical assistant should find out when and where the test was done and take a message for the provider. Some offices choose to send patients letters about laboratory results, which cuts down on the number of telephone calls requesting information, especially for routine tests. Patients may also see the test results in the patient portal, but may have questions about the results. After reviewing the laboratory or diagnostic test results, the provider may instruct the medical assistant to call the patient back to give the results, to schedule follow-up testing, and/or to ask the patient to schedule an appointment to discuss the results.

Patients Reporting Satisfactory or Unsatisfactory Progress

Providers often tell a patient to call and check at a specified interval after a visit, to report on how a condition is resolving after treatment. If the patient reports satisfactory progress, the medical assistant should take a brief message and leave it for the provider. An unsatisfactory report should generate a more complete message. When a patient gives a progress report on the telephone, either the original message should be filed in the patient record or the medical assistant should document the telephone conversation in the record. Messages taken through the EHR are usually automatically recorded with other information related to an individual patient.

Requests for Medication or Prescription Refills

Often patients or pharmacies call with requests to have prescriptions refilled or renewed. When the pharmacy calls, it is important to get the patient's name and date of birth, name of the medication, dosage, and amount of medication prescribed. When the patient calls, it is important to get the name of the medication, dosage, and how often the patient takes it. In addition, it is important to determine how the patient wants to receive the medication (from the pharmacy or by mail). It is helpful to verify the information in the patient's medical record when an EHR is used. Otherwise, the message should include the name, telephone number, and location of the pharmacy or mail-order company. Usually, a provider transmits the prescription using an EHR, but if this is not the case, a written prescription may be faxed to the pharmacy or sent to the patient. If the medication is an antibiotic or a controlled substance used for pain relief, the medical assistant should ask about symptoms that would require a refill. The medical assistant should tell patients to check with the pharmacy the next day unless they hear from the provider or office. A message to request medication is also attached to the patient's medical record. Providers often follow up directly with the pharmacy, especially if they are using an electronic prescription routing service, but in some offices the provider may write the prescribing information on the bottom of a paper message for the medical assistant to fax or call in to the pharmacy. If a medical assistant telephones a prescription, it should always be noted in the progress notes and/or medication record (Procedure 41.3).

Calls for Referrals or Requesting Laboratory or Diagnostic Tests

A patient may call to say they need a referral (because of a particular insurance company's policy) to see a specialist outside the medical group or to have a laboratory test or diagnostic procedure done.

The medical assistant takes the necessary information (what type of referral, for what, to whom) as a message for the physician. If a referral is approved by the provider, the medical assistant may complete a paper or electronic form. If the patient is asking for a laboratory test, such as a throat culture, the medical assistant may fill out a laboratory form for the patient to pick up or more commonly will enter the information into the computer for the physician to sign. The provider may ask the medical assistant to call the patient and schedule an appointment before authorizing a referral or laboratory test.

Patients With Medical Questions

For patients with medical questions, the medical assistant takes a message for a provider or refers the call to another staff member designated by the office to handle such calls. The office should have written guidelines to follow if a medical assistant screens medical questions. The medical assistant should follow the written guidelines closely and take a message for the provider about any concern or question that falls outside the preset guidelines.

What Would You Do? What Would You *Not* Do?

Case Study 2

Mary Woodward, a 62-year-old woman with hypertension, has called because she has run out of her blood pressure medication. Mrs. Woodward tells Channa that the medication is atenolol and she is pretty sure that the dose is 50 mg every morning. When Channa asks for the pharmacy name, Mrs. Woodward says, "It's the Best Buy Pharmacy in Whittier, but that doesn't matter because I will come in and pick up the prescription." Channa checks the electronic medical record in the computer and finds that the office has a different preferred pharmacy recorded for this patient. ■

Calls From Other Providers

Calls from other providers are usually put through right away, even if the provider is examining a patient. If the medical assistant has to find the provider, this may be given as a reason to place the caller on hold briefly, but the medical assistant should locate the provider as quickly as possible and explain which provider is calling. The provider may ask the medical assistant to transfer the call to another extension to avoid talking in front of a patient.

Calls From Salespeople

Often a sales representative from a pharmaceutical company or equipment company calls before visiting the provider's office. Salespeople are usually seen by the office manager, who gives the information to the provider. Drug company representatives sometimes drop by, but if they hope to talk to the provider they usually must call and ask for an appointment. Providers usually schedule sales representatives during lunch. The provider must agree to see the representative before a medical assistant makes an appointment.

URGENT OR EMERGENCY CALLS

If a patient calls with a medical problem, the medical assistant asks questions to determine how urgent the problem is. After obtaining the caller's name and telephone number and identifying who has the problem (the patient's name, age or date of birth, and relationship to the caller), the medical assistant should obtain the patient's symptoms and current condition. In most offices there is a guide to telephone screening in the office procedure manual. This helps the medical assistant identify which questions to ask to determine how urgent the problem is. In the next chapter, there is a more complete discussion of the kind of appointment to offer a patient based on the symptoms the patient reports.

If the medical assistant determines that the call represents an urgent problem or emergency, they should follow office policy. The call should be referred to a provider if one is in the office; in a group practice, one provider may be assigned at all times to take urgent calls. If there is no physician in the office, a nurse practitioner, physician's assistant, or registered nurse may be assigned to take urgent calls. If no licensed professional is present in the office, the medical assistant must advise the caller or contact the on-call provider. The following are the guidelines for dealing with such a call:

1. If the emergency is serious or life-threatening, the caller should be instructed to call an ambulance by dialing 911. This activates the emergency medical services (EMS) system. If the caller is a child or seems upset or confused, the medical assistant can offer to call an ambulance for the caller.
2. If the emergency is a case of poisoning, the caller should be instructed to call the Poison Control Center number. The Poison Control Center number (1-800-222-1222) should be placed next to every telephone in the medical office. Even if it is not a case of poisoning, if the patient is unconscious or not breathing, the caller should be instructed to call an ambulance.
3. If the patient has a problem that requires treatment in an emergency department but is conscious and able to walk (e.g., a bleeding wound), the caller should be instructed to take the patient to the nearest emergency department or call an ambulance. If the patient is alone, an ambulance should be called.
4. If the patient's problem is usually treated in the office, the patient should be given an appointment for that day.
5. If the condition of the patient is not life-threatening and/or the medical assistant is unsure how urgent the problem is, the provider should be contacted for instructions either by cell phone or pager. If there is any doubt about how serious the patient's condition is, it is safer to instruct the patient to call an ambulance and/or go to the hospital emergency department.

Whenever an urgent call is handled, the medical assistant should fill out a message form to be sure that the information has been written down. Either the message form or the instructions given to the patient should later be documented in the medical record. If a patient has been instructed to go to the emergency department, the provider should be notified promptly.

DEALING WITH PROBLEM CALLS

The Caller Who Refuses to Give Information

When callers ask for a provider and refuse to identify themselves, it is probably because they want to speak to the provider but suspect that if they give a name, they will be asked to leave a message. The medical assistant should explain politely that the provider is not available and offer to take a message. If the caller still refuses to give information, the medical assistant can instruct the caller to write a letter to the physician and mark it "personal."

Complaints

The medical assistant should listen carefully to callers with complaints, avoid getting defensive or angry, and ask for specific information. It is important to remain calm so that a professional demeanor is maintained. The medical assistant should state clearly what they can and will do. It may be necessary to refer the matter to the office manager or the provider, but the medical assistant should get as much information as possible at the initial contact.

It is important to avoid hanging up on an angry caller. It is usually possible to calm a caller down as long as the medical assistant does not raise their voice and does not become defensive. The caller should be told a specific time when they can expect to hear back from someone in the office.

Patients With Special Problems

If a patient calls who is confused or has difficulty with English, the medical assistant should listen carefully and try as hard as possible to understand. The medical assistant may speak more slowly than usual but should not speak more loudly. If it is impossible to communicate, even using simple language, the medical assistant should try to at least obtain the caller's name and telephone number. Then it may be possible to find out from the medical record if the patient speaks a different language or if there is an emergency contact number. If the person seems confused, the medical assistant should ask if there is another person with whom they can speak because this may be a medical emergency. The medical assistant may need to ask for guidance from the provider or office manager.

OUTGOING CALLS

More calls come into the office than go out. But there are certainly many outgoing calls. Medical assistants make many of them. Outgoing calls a medical assistant may make include calls to patients, suppliers, insurance companies, other medical offices, laboratories, pharmacies, and hospitals. In some systems it is necessary to dial the number 9 before the telephone number to get an outside line. Telephone numbers of businesses can be looked up using the internet, but it is helpful to keep an office directory of frequently called numbers.

LOCAL CALLS

Calls to patients, whether the matter is medical or financial, should be made from the front desk only if the privacy window is closed. The medical assistant must prepare information and supplies before making the call. If the medical assistant is calling a patient, the patient's medical record should be at hand with any notes from the physician. If the call is picked up by an answering machine, it is permissible to leave your name, practice name, and telephone number for the patient to call back. Because the patient's family members may have access to the answering machine or voicemail, no medical information should be included in the message (Procedure 41.4).

It may be necessary to call a patient about an overdue account. The medical assistant should not call the patient at work for this type of call or discuss billing information with anyone other than the person responsible for the bill.

For calls to laboratories, hospitals, or suppliers, the medical assistant should be sure to have organized the information necessary to complete the call before dialing the telephone number.

If the medical assistant places a call for one of the office's providers, the provider must be ready to talk before the call is placed. As soon as the person being called is located, the medical assistant connects the office provider placing the call.

Medical assistants and other office staff should not make or receive personal calls using the office telephone system except for emergencies, both to avoid tying up the telephone and because telephone calls take time away from work. The medical assistant can check messages and make outgoing calls during breaks or at lunchtime using a personal cell phone. Although permission may be given to make an urgent call using the office telephone, a personal long-distance call is never appropriate. In most offices medical assistants are not allowed to carry cell phones while they are working even if the phones are set to vibrate instead of ringing. Cell phones can interfere with medical equipment, such as electrocardiographs. They can also be a distraction, even if they do not make a noise.

What Would You Do? What Would You *Not* Do?

Case Study 3

The physician asks Channa to schedule an appointment for Andrew Page, a 35-year-old man whose recent lipid profile shows an elevated cholesterol and triglyceride level. This is a change from previous laboratory work. The physician says to tell the patient that he wants to discuss the recent blood work in person. When Channa calls the patient, his wife answers the telephone. Channa identifies herself and the medical office and asks to leave a message for Mr. Page to return her call. Mrs. Page says, "He's away on a business trip until Thursday. What is this about? Is it really important?" ■

APPOINTMENT REMINDERS

Medical assistants may be asked to place reminder telephone calls to patients 24 to 48 hours before their scheduled appointments. The HIPAA Privacy Rule allows health care providers to call patients and leave messages regarding their care as long as the patient has not requested confidential communication. It is recommended to limit the information left in a message to the minimum required to confirm the appointment.

Medical offices have begun to use computer programs that interface with scheduling programs and call patients automatically 24 to 48 hours before a scheduled appointment. They provide a recorded message about the appointment and will leave a message if no one answers the telephone. It may be possible for the person who answers the call to confirm or cancel the appointment after listening to the recorded message. The patient is instructed to call the office with any questions or to change the appointment.

LONG-DISTANCE AND INTERNATIONAL CALLS

Long-distance calls are almost always dialed directly. The telephone number for a long-distance call can be obtained from directory assistance (411). When calling distant locations, it is important to be aware of the different time zones. To make international calls, the medical assistant should dial 1, then the country code, then the telephone number. To prevent unauthorized international calls, most offices have a code that must be used to access the long-distance system, especially for international calls. Long-distance services may also be limited to one or two extensions.

CONFERENCE CALLS

Some phone systems allow conference calls among three or more parties, such as a provider and other individuals who are being called at different telephone numbers. If the telephone system allows this, the medical assistant should learn how to set up such calls for the providers. Conference calls among several parties are sometimes scheduled using a special service.

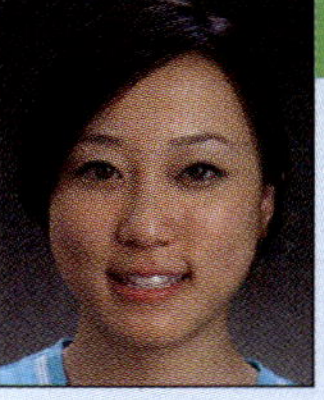

Memories *from* Practicum

Channa Eng: I was terrified of the telephone when I first started my practicum. It was a busy clinic, and I started out in adult medicine. In the morning, I sat at the front desk to check patients in, take copayments, and answer the telephone. I was always afraid that I wouldn't know what to say. We got the callers who wanted to speak to someone in person, so you never knew what to expect. My supervisor told me to answer each call by saying "hello" followed by my name and the name of the clinic, and then ask how I could help the caller. If I didn't know how to handle the call, I was supposed to put the caller on hold and ask Mary Lynn, the other medical assistant, for guidance. One call that I remember particularly was from an older woman who seemed lonely and confused. She asked for her provider, but she was willing to leave a message when I told her that the provider didn't take calls while he was seeing patients. She said that she couldn't remember if she was supposed to take her blood pressure medication once a day or twice a day and she wasn't sure if it was one pill or two pills. She told me that her daughter set up her pills in a pill container every week but she had forgotten if she should take them both in the morning or one in the morning and one at night. I asked her to get the bottle of medication and read the label to me. From the label we determined that she was supposed to take two pills every morning. She thanked me, and I indicated on the message form that we had clarified the problem. After the call, Mary Lynn complimented me for being so helpful and for handling the call by myself. After that I began to feel more confident about taking telephone calls. ■

What Would You Do? What Would You *Not* Do? RESPONSES

Case Study 1
Page 1086

What Did Channa Do?
- ❑ Spoke politely, and told Mrs. Weston that she needed to pick up the other call.
- ❑ Gave Mrs. Weston the choice of being placed on hold or being called back.
- ❑ Assured Mrs. Weston that she would get back to the telephone call with her as soon as possible.
- ❑ Kept her voice calm and friendly.

What Did Channa Not Do?
- ❑ Did not let the second telephone call ring more than three times.
- ❑ Did not promise Mrs. Weston that she would put the other call on hold immediately.
- ❑ Did not try to rush through the call with Mrs. Weston without making sure that she is clear about the appointment date and time.

Case Study 2
Page 1087

What Did Channa Do?
- ❑ Told Mrs. Woodward to get the bottle of pills, which has a record of the dose and exact name of the pharmacy.
- ❑ Told Mrs. Woodward she would place her on hold; instructed Mrs. Woodward to stay on the line after finding the medication bottle.
- ❑ Gave Mrs. Woodward the option of calling back when she had found the bottle of pills.
- ❑ Told Mrs. Woodward that the physician would be glad to send the prescription directly to the pharmacy, and instructed her to check with the pharmacy the next day.
- ❑ Remained calm and friendly.
- ❑ Made sure to follow up and complete the message.
- ❑ Clarified the pharmacy information in the EHR and updated if necessary.

What Did Channa Not Do?
- ❑ Did not become impatient or tell Mrs. Woodward that she should know she needed her bottle of medication ready when she called to ask for a refill.
- ❑ Did not pass on the message without confirming that Mrs. Woodward had asked for the correct dose of medication.
- ❑ Did not pass on the message without confirming the name and location of the pharmacy.

Case Study 3
Page 1089

What Did Channa Do?
- ❑ Reassured Mrs. Page that it was not an urgent matter, but said she hoped Mr. Page would return her call after his trip.
- ❑ Told Mrs. Page politely that she could not discuss the matter with anyone but Mr. Page.

What Did Channa Not Do?
- ❑ Did not tell Mrs. Page exactly why she was calling her husband.
- ❑ Did not tell Mrs. Page that the matter was not important.
- ❑ Did not ask Mrs. Page to contact her husband before he returned from his business trip.
- ❑ Did not tell Mrs. Page that the physician could give her more information about the matter.

TERMINOLOGY REVIEW

Key Term	Definition
Enunciation	The act of speaking clearly and concisely.
Pager	An electronic device that notifies the recipient to receive a message or return a telephone call.
Smartphone	A cell phone with computer capabilities.
Voicemail	A method for delivery, storage, and retrieval of telephone messages that is built into the telephone system.

PROCEDURE 41.1 Performing Telephone Screening

Outcome Screen incoming telephone calls

Equipment/Supplies:

- Telephone
- Message pad
- Pen or pencil
- Computer terminal or manual appointment book
- Clock or watch

1. **Procedural Step.** When answering the telephone identify the medical office and give your name. Each practice will have a preferred way for all employees to answer the telephone. Example: "Hello, this is Channa at Primary Care Associates. How can I help you?" Do not rush through the greeting. The caller needs to hear this greeting clearly.
   Principle. Callers need to know what business they have reached and with whom they are speaking. Good customer service involves an offer to be of assistance.
2. **Procedural Step.** Listen carefully to what the caller says and decide as soon as possible whether this is a call you can handle, whether you need to take a message, or whether the call should be transferred to someone else in the office.
   Principle. The caller does not want to have to repeat all the details if the call must be transferred. If you need to take a message, begin recording it.
3. **Procedural Step.** Ask for the caller's name. "May I ask who is calling?"
   Principle. You will need the caller's name to address the caller by name, to take a message, or to identify the caller when transferring the call.
4. **Procedural Step.** Clarify whether the caller is a patient or calling about a patient. Obtain the patient's name (if not the caller) and date of birth.
5. **Procedural Step.** If you can handle the call, such as a call for an appointment, do so promptly.
6. **Procedural Step.** If you need to take a message, see : Taking a Telephone Message.
7. **Procedural Step.** If you need to transfer the call to someone else in the office, place the caller on hold, noting the caller's name and the extension. Tell the person to whom you are transferring the call who is calling and what extension the call is on.
   Principle. It is a courtesy to tell the person to whom you transfer a call who is calling; the call recipient must be able to locate the call if more than one line has a call on hold.
8. **Procedural Step.** If the caller describes symptoms that require immediate care, ask questions to assess the problem, following guidelines in the office procedure manual. If there is a physician or other licensed professional in the office, transfer the call immediately. Otherwise, assess the urgency of the problem and follow up according to office guidelines. If the patient's health is at risk, instruct the caller to call 911 or assist them by keeping them on the line and calling 911.
   Principle. Patients expect correct medical advice from a health care facility when they have urgent medical problems.
9. **Procedural Step.** If your telephone has more than two lines, it is helpful to keep a list of the names of callers and extensions. When a call is on hold, the light for that telephone line blinks. If you have transferred a call but the caller remains on hold, within 30 to 45 seconds you should determine if the caller is still holding; if so, you should try to transfer the call again or take a message.
   Principle. Sometimes a transfer does not go through or the call is not picked up. The caller has no way to get back in contact with you to leave a message or to ask to speak to someone else.
10. **Procedural Step.** If the telephone rings for another call, ask if you may put the caller to whom you are speaking on hold and wait for the caller to agree. After pressing the hold button, answer the other call and explain that you are speaking to a caller on another line. Give the second caller the option to hold and wait for you or take the caller's number and offer to call back as soon as you are finished.

Continued

PROCEDURE 41.1 Performing Telephone Screening—cont'd

Principle. In general, calls are handled in the order they are received. By asking for permission to put the caller on hold, you give the caller a chance to tell you if it is an emergency. Some callers prefer to hold; others prefer to be called back. Time passes slowly when a caller is on hold, and the caller may become tired of waiting and wish to leave a message.

11. **Procedural Step.** At the end of the call, repeat any information you have discussed (such as the date and time of an appointment). End the call politely by thanking the caller and saying goodbye.
    Principle. Confirmation helps avoid misunderstandings. Thanking the caller and closing the conversation demonstrates good customer service.

PROCEDURE 41.2 Taking a Telephone Message

Outcome Take a telephone message

Equipment/Supplies:

- Telephone
- Computer
- Message pad
- Pen or pencil
- Clock or watch

1. **Procedural Step.** If you determine that the person to whom a telephone caller wants to speak is not available, offer to take a message.
   Principle. A message is a way of communicating with a person who is not available to speak on the telephone.
2. **Procedural Step.** Give the caller a reason why the person cannot take the call. Acceptable reasons are as follows: busy with a patient, not at their desk, not in the office, on another line. In general, providers do not take calls except possibly during specified hours. Patients who ask for the provider are told that the provider is not in the office or that the provider is busy with patients.
   Principle. Most callers are willing to leave a message if they understand why their call is not being answered.
3. **Procedural Step.** Fill in the information in the computer messaging program or on a paper message form, including the name of the caller, business affiliation (if any), patient name (if not the caller) and patient date of birth, date of the call, time of the call, telephone number including area code, and information the caller wishes to leave about the reason for the call. Place your initials on the message in case there are questions. If there is a section at the bottom of a paper message form for a response to the message, leave that area blank.
   Principle. Complete information is necessary for a call to be returned.
4. **Procedural Step.** Verify the information. If possible, give a time when the call might be returned. If the message recipient does not have a scheduled time to return messages, say, "I will give them the message."
   Principle. Callers like to know when to expect a return call.

PROCEDURE 41.2 Taking a Telephone Message—cont'd

4

MESSAGE FROM

For Dr.	Name of Caller	Ref. to pt.	Patient	Pt. Age	Pt. Temp.	Message Date	Message Time	Urgent
Lawler	Anne Richards	mother	Janice	4	101°	10 / 13 / xx	9:00 AM	❑ Yes ❑ No

Message: Child has been on antibiotic for two days – still has fever. Should she come in again?

Allergies: Ø

DOB: 4/2/xx

Respond to Phone #	Best Time to Call	Pharmacy Name / #	Patient's Chart Attached	Patient's chart #	Initials
814-322-6510	any AM PM	West Side 814-754-9817	☒ Yes ❑ No		KJ

DOCTOR - STAFF RESPONSE

Doctor's / Staff Orders / Follow-up Action

Call Back	Chart. Mes.	Follow-up Date	Follow-up Completed-Date/Time	Response By:
❑ Yes ❑ No	❑ Yes ❑ No	/ /	/ / AM PM	

Fill in the information on the message form.

5. **Procedural Step.** End the call politely.
6. **Procedural Step.** If the call is from a patient or concerns a patient, attach the message to the patient medical record in a clinical messaging computer program or attach a paper medical record if a paper record system is used. Be sure to select the correct EHR or paper medical record.
   Principle. This ensures that information about the patient is available, and the action taken on the call can be documented if necessary.
7. **Procedural Step.** Place the message (with the patient record, if needed) where the person for whom it is intended expects to find messages. This may be on a desk or in a mailbox. If a computer messaging program was used, send the message to the intended recipient(s) using secure messaging.
8. **Procedural Step.** Perform follow-up according to office procedure.
   Principle. This ensures that important issues do not fall through the cracks.

PROCEDURE 41.3 Taking Requests for Medication or Prescription Refills

Outcome Take a message requesting medication or a prescription refill

Equipment/Supplies:

- Telephone
- Computer
- Message pad
- Pen or pencil
- Medical record
- Clock or watch

1. **Procedural Step.** Identify the caller and telephone number.
2. **Procedural Step.** Identify whether the caller is a patient or a pharmacy employee.
3. **Procedural Step.** If the caller is a patient, identify the patient and date of birth. Take the information about the medication requested, dose, and number of times a day the patient takes the medication. Write down or enter into the computer the name and telephone number of the patient's preferred pharmacy or mail order supplier.
4. **Procedural Step.** If the caller is a pharmacy employee, usually the medical assistant takes a message, including the name and address of the patient, the medication requested, and the dosage and amount of medication to be prescribed. Inform the pharmacy when the provider is likely to approve the refill so that the pharmacy can tell the patient.

Continued

PROCEDURE 41.3

PROCEDURE 41.3 Taking Requests for Medication or Prescription Refills—cont'd

Principle. Usually, providers have specific times when they review and respond to messages.

5. **Procedural Step.** End the call politely.
6. **Procedural Step.** Follow usual procedures to attach the patient's medical record to the message (either manually or electronically) and place the message where the provider can review it, or send the message electronically.
   Principle. The provider will need to review information about the patient before agreeing to refill or prescribe medication.
7. **Procedural Step.** Usually, the provider fills the prescription directly by computer, indicates on the message slip whether the prescription may be refilled, or writes a new prescription on the message slip for the medical assistant to call or fax the pharmacy with the information. Read the prescription from the message slip exactly as the provider has written it.
   Principle. The medical assistant functions as an agent of the provider in this case. The medical assistant must give the exact information the provider has indicated.

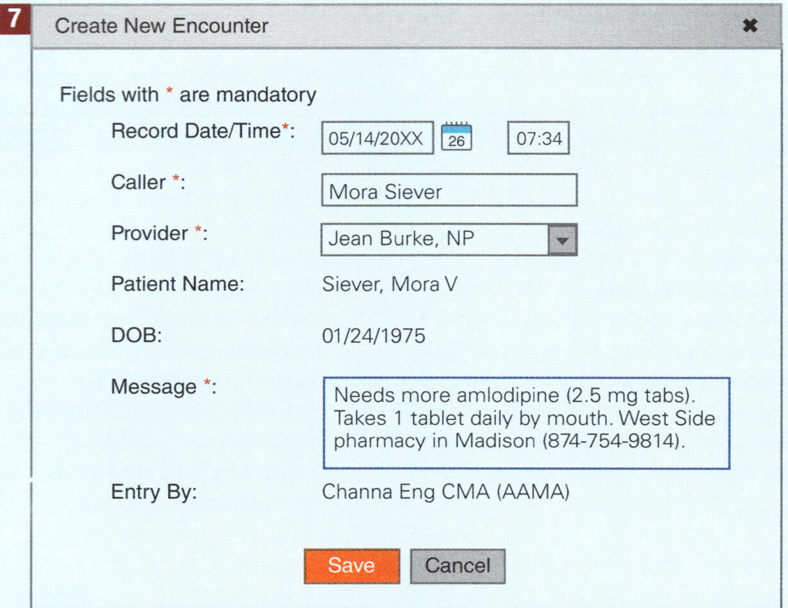

8. **Procedural Step.** Verify that the refill or prescription has been documented in the patient's medical record. In some offices the message itself is filed in the medical record. See Chapter 38 to review common abbreviations used when documenting medications.
   Principle. Any treatment of the patient must be documented in the medical record as part of the continuous record of care given.

PROCEDURE 41.4 Telephoning a Patient for Follow-Up

Outcome Place an outgoing telephone call to a patient for follow-up

Equipment/Supplies:

- Telephone
- Scratch paper
- Pen or pencil or
- Electronic health record
- Material necessary to place the call, including the telephone number, instructions from physician, and/or patient medical record

1. **Procedural Step.** Organize all materials that may be necessary during the telephone call. Schedule calls during business hours.
   Principle. Preparation allows calls to be made more efficiently.
2. **Procedural Step.** Write the telephone number on a piece of paper. Include the area code and a country code, if necessary.
   Principle. It may be difficult to remember the number, especially if you do not reach the number on the first attempt.
3. **Procedural Step.** Place the call. When it is answered, ask for your party. Identify yourself with your practice's name and your name ("This is Channa from Primary Care Associates").
4. **Procedural Step.** If you reach an answering machine, identify yourself with your practice name and your name and ask the intended recipient to call you back. Leave your telephone number with area code.
   Principle. Unless it is an appointment reminder, the subject of the telephone call should not be left on an answering machine to protect patient confidentiality.
5. **Procedural Step.** If you are speaking to the patient, give the information requested by the provider. This may be an instruction to make an appointment or may include laboratory results. Do not give more information than the provider has authorized.
   Principle. As an agent of the provider, you have limited authorization to provide information.
6. **Procedural Step.** If the patient has additional questions, offer to take a message for the provider.
7. **Procedural Step.** Close the call politely. Repeat instructions if any were given.
8. **Procedural Step.** Document the telephone call including the name of the provider who instructed you to make the call (if any). Include any specific instructions given to the patient in the documentation.

Scheduling Appointments

Check out the Evolve site at http://evolve.elsevier.com/Bonewit/today to access additional interactive activities and exercises to help you study and prepare for success.

LEARNING OBJECTIVES

Methods of Scheduling

1. Describe how scheduling appointments efficiently meets the needs of both providers and patients.
2. Compare and contrast manual and computer scheduling systems.
3. Explain why the medical office must retain an official record of patients seen each day (daily appointment schedule).

Types of Scheduling

4. Describe several types of scheduling, including stream scheduling, wave scheduling, modified wave scheduling, double booking, open booking, and patient self-scheduling.
5. Identify types of patient appointments that may be clustered in the appointment schedule.

Setting Up the Appointment Schedule

6. Identify factors to be considered when setting up the appointment schedule.
7. Explain how to set up the appointment schedule.

Procedure: Setting up the appointment schedule.

Making an Appointment

8. Differentiate between the information needed to make an appointment for a new patient and for an established patient.
9. Differentiate among medical conditions that require emergency care, urgent care, and routine care.
10. Describe how to schedule appointments for individuals who are not patients.

Procedure: Making an appointment.

Managing the Appointment Schedule

11. Describe the method for changing or canceling appointments.
12. Describe how to document changes to the appointment schedule and cancelations or no-shows in the medical record.
13. Identify three methods to remind patients to make or keep appointments.
14. Discuss the storage of appointment schedules and/or daily schedules.

Procedure: Managing the appointment schedule.

Scheduling Diagnostic Tests, Procedures, and Admissions

15. Identify how to schedule inpatient and outpatient diagnostic tests and procedures.
16. Identify how to schedule hospital admissions and surgery.

Procedures: Scheduling inpatient and outpatient diagnostic tests or procedures. Scheduling inpatient or outpatient admissions.

CHAPTER OUTLINE

KEY TERMS

appointment matrix (MAY-trix)
blocked
clustering
double booking
established patient
fixed appointment scheduling
hospice (HOSS-piss)
modified wave scheduling
new patient
no-show
open booking
patient self-scheduling
preadmission testing (PAT)
preauthorization (pree-awe-thur-eye-ZAY-shun)/ precertification
referral
single booking
stream scheduling
time-specified scheduling
triage (TREE-ahzh)
wave scheduling

INTRODUCTION TO APPOINTMENT SCHEDULING

Scheduling appointments is one of the most important administrative responsibilities performed in the medical office. Until the 1970s, people went to a medical office expecting to wait as long as an hour or more. Most providers liked to see a full waiting room; it reassured them that their practice was healthy.

In the 21st century, people have little tolerance for waiting in a medical office. Lifestyles have changed, and people have busy lives. Many have to take personal time away from work to go to the medical office, and they feel that their time is as valuable as the provider's time. In the patient-centered medical home (PCMH), one of the key goals is to reduce patient wait time and provide same-day appointments if needed. PCMH is discussed in more detail in Chapter 1.

Scheduling appointments correctly and efficiently is crucial to the smooth operation of the medical office. Many factors must be taken into consideration when scheduling appointments. The patient who has made an appointment weeks or even months in advance wants to be seen within 15 minutes after arriving at the medical office. The provider wants a smooth flow of patients during the time scheduled for seeing patients. Patients who are ill or have accidents want to be able to see their provider on the day of the illness or injury. They prefer to be given a specific time, even if it is later in the day, rather than come into the office and wait for an open moment.

GUIDELINES FOR APPOINTMENT SCHEDULING

When scheduling appointments, it is important for the medical assistant to use good interpersonal skills and minimize the amount of time a patient has to wait to see the provider. To accomplish this, the medical assistant should follow seven guidelines:

1. Maintain the confidentiality of the patient. For example, do not discuss protected health information within hearing distance of other patients.
2. Speak clearly, and do not appear rushed. Make sure the tone of your voice is friendly and courteous.
3. Concentrate only on the person to whom you are speaking.
4. Obtain all the necessary information from the patient. Make sure the information is both correct and complete.
5. Repeat the information relayed to you by the patient. This avoids errors.
6. Schedule the proper amount of time for the type of appointment you are scheduling. For example, a new patient requires more time than an established patient.
7. Document all of the necessary information correctly in the appointment schedule.

TYPES OF APPOINTMENT SYSTEMS

Appointments are almost always scheduled using a computerized appointment scheduling program. Using a computer to schedule appointments offers advantages. The computer allows the medical assistant to designate appointment intervals. The appointment interval can be adjusted to 10, 15, or 20 minutes depending on the needs of the practice. The computer makes it easy to add, delete, or change appointments; set up repeating appointments; and set up a recall system. A recall system identifies patients who need to be contacted when it is time for them to schedule another appointment.

The medical assistant enters the patient's appointment into a data entry screen (Fig. 42.1). This screen requires the entry of the same information as a paper appointment book, although all information linked to an appointment may not be visible on the main screen. The computer also allows the medical assistant to print out a daily appointment schedule of patients to be seen that day.

Disadvantages of a computer appointment schedule are obvious when the computer system is not accessible for some reason. Unless there is a printed schedule, it is impossible to know who is scheduled. Unless there is remote access to the scheduling system, it may also be difficult to contact scheduled patients if the office is closed unexpectedly (such as due to bad weather).

A manual appointment system may offer more flexibility, especially in a small office. Appointments can be made and changed, and the appointment book can accompany one of the office staff, especially if bad weather is predicted. This type of system is cumbersome when the office includes several practitioners and/or several locations, especially if appointment scheduling is centralized for more than one location. Appointment schedules must also be created and revised manually.

Appointment books are usually spiral bound, so they will lie flat when opened. Occasionally a paper appointment book is used in the medical office as a backup to the computer schedule. Appointment books are available in the following formats: pages for a single day, pages that display a week when open (over two pages), or pages with two or three providers' schedules for a single day. The pages are further divided into time intervals. The pages are typically divided into 10- or 15-minute intervals.

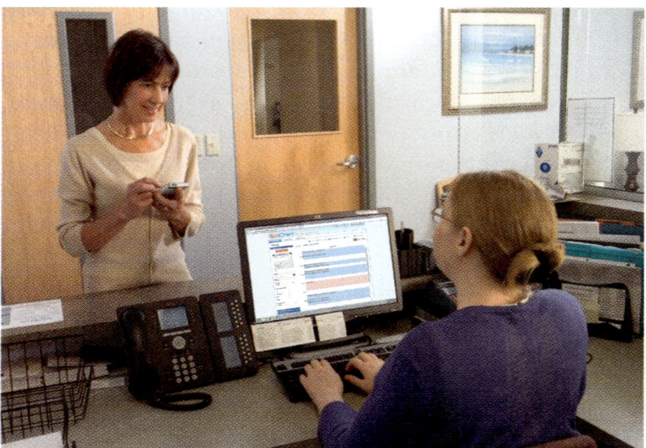

Fig. 42.1 Medical assistant making an appointment.

DAILY APPOINTMENT SCHEDULE

In a computer appointment scheduling program, the daily appointment schedule can be viewed on the computer, and an updated hard copy can be printed as needed. It may be used as a guide for pulling patients' paper medical records or appointment reminder calls. When a manual system is used, usually a daily schedule is created using a word processing program. A printed appointment schedule usually contains the patients' names and telephone numbers and the reasons for their visits (e.g., new patient, physical examination, or recheck) (Fig. 42.2). According to Health Insurance Portability and Accountability Act (HIPAA) requirements, the daily appointment schedule should never be posted in an office area accessible to patients. The office must keep an updated record either on paper or electronically to verify tax returns and insurance claims.

TYPES OF SCHEDULING

Several methods are available to schedule appointments in the medical office. They include time-specified scheduling, wave scheduling, modified wave scheduling, double booking, and open booking. Many offices allow established patients to request appointments or schedule appointments using the internet. In addition, appointments may be clustered or categorized depending on the type of patient or type of examination or treatment. The method an office uses to schedule appointments is based on the needs of the practice and provider preference.

TIME-SPECIFIED (STREAM) SCHEDULING

Time-specified scheduling, also known as **stream scheduling,** involves scheduling appointments at a specific time. Most offices use this method for scheduling appointments. The goal of time-specified appointments is to minimize the waiting time for the patient and at the same time to keep a steady flow of patients moving through the office (like a stream of water). The amount of time allotted for a time-specified appointment depends on the reason for the visit. In general, the following times are allotted:

- New patient: 30 to 45 minutes
- Complete physical examination: 30 to 45 minutes
- Established patient: 10 to 20 minutes

When using the time-specified method, the medical assistant needs to make sure to allow time in the schedule to accommodate urgent visits, such as from ill or injured patients. There are two other terms that may be used for this type of scheduling: **fixed appointment scheduling** and **single booking.**

WALDEN-MARTIN Family Medical Clinic

James Martin, MD
Schedule for May 30, 20XX

Time	Name	Reason	Home Phone	Work Phone
9:00 AM	ROBERT RICIGLIANO	Physical exam	(123) 459-2811	(123) 459-7218
9:15 AM	******************************			
9:30 AM	******************************			
9:45 AM	JUNE ST. JAMES	BP & ECG	(123) 123-5807	(123) 123-9222
10:00 AM	DARLA SISSLE	Influenza vaccine	(123) 268-1156	
10:15 AM	NORMA WASHINGTON	Recheck	(123) 754-4685	
10:30 AM	Catch-up			
10:45 AM	ESTELLE JORDAN	New patient	(123) 459-8249	(123) 459-0419
11:00 AM	******************************			
11:15 AM	******************************			
11:30 AM	ROBIN SOTO	Well-baby check	(123) 459-1349	
11:45 AM	******************************			
12:00 PM	Lunch			
12:15 PM	******************************			
12:30 PM	******************************			
12:45 PM	******************************			
1:00 PM	CELIA TAPIA	Recheck	(123) 858-1545	(123) 858-6603
1:15 PM	THOMAS MAXWELL	Recheck	(123) 459-4123	(123) 459-1062
1:30 PM	LUCILLE MORENA	School physical exam	(123) 268-6677	
1:45 PM	******************************			
2:00 PM	LLOYD RIDLON	Recheck	(123) 220-4242	(123) 220-0419

Fig. 42.2 Daily appointment schedule.

WAVE SCHEDULING

With **wave scheduling,** three or four patients are scheduled every hour and are seen in the order in which they arrive at the office. The goal is for patients to arrive in "waves" so that there is always a patient waiting to be seen. Sometimes, ill patients are seen before those with routine appointments.

This scheduling system assumes that some patients will need to be worked into the schedule. Sometimes patients become uncomfortable when they realize that another patient was given the same appointment time, but a simple explanation can usually reassure the patient. The medical assistant might say, "We schedule all our patients on the hour, and then they are seen in the order they arrive. There is always a patient to be seen, and we find that patients don't really arrive all at once."

MODIFIED WAVE SCHEDULING

The wave system can be changed in several ways. This is called **modified wave scheduling.** The office may schedule patients at specific times during the first half of each hour and keep the second half-hour open for special circumstances. This may include working in patients, seeing patients who arrived late, or finishing up with patients from the first half-hour.

Another modification to the wave system is to schedule one appointment that is expected to take longer (e.g., physical examination) on the hour and to schedule three or four follow-up appointments on the half-hour (Fig. 42.3).

DOUBLE BOOKING

When two patients are given the same appointment time, the practice is called **double booking.** Double booking means that two patients are scheduled into a single time slot. Double booking may be used when a patient can be fitted in around a patient undergoing a diagnostic procedure such as an electrocardiogram (ECG). It is also used for siblings in a pediatric practice or when a patient with an injury or acute illness must be added to an already-full schedule.

OPEN BOOKING

Sometimes patients are not given a specific appointment time but are told to come in during a time range, such as between 9:00 a.m. and 11:00 a.m. The patients are then

Time	Single Booking	Time	Wave Scheduling	Time	Modified Wave Scheduling
9:00	Robert Ricigliano	9:00	Robert Ricigliano	9:00	Robert Ricigliano
	(490) 459-1111		(490) 459-1111		(490) 459-1111
9:10	*Physical exam*		*Physical exam*		*Physical exam*
	↓		June St. James *Re* √		
9:20			(490) 459-1000		
	↓		Robin Soto		
9:30	June St. James *Re* √		(490) 297-1349	9:30	June St. James *Re* √
	(490) 459-1000		*Well-child visit*		(490) 459-1000
9:40	Robin Soto				Robin Soto
	(490) 297-1349				(490) 297-1349
9:50	*Well-child visit*				*Well-child visit*
	↓				

Fig. 42.3 Comparison of single booking, wave scheduling, and modified wave scheduling.

seen in the order in which they arrive. In an **open booking** system, patients with an injury or an acute illness may be seen ahead of patients with less significant complaints.

Sometimes medical offices and clinics have walk-in hours designated for urgent care before regular office hours. In this situation, patients are seen in the order of arrival.

Open booking works best when there is a constant stream of patients or when a practice is not busy. Because patient flow is unpredictable, patients often have to wait a long time.

PATIENT APPOINTMENT REQUESTS AND SELF-SCHEDULING

Many medical practices allow patients to request routine appointments from the practice website. Office staff usually schedule the appointment, making every effort to accommodate the patient's request. After the appointment has been made, staff notify the patient either electronically or by a letter. Some practices even give patients limited access to their appointment scheduling software so that patients can schedule their own appointments if a desired time is available. This is called **patient self-scheduling.**

CLUSTERING OR CATEGORIZATION

Clustering involves scheduling patients with similar problems or conditions into groups. Each group is seen on a certain day or within a certain time block during the day. This scheduling method is also called *categorization.* Examples of conditions that can easily be clustered into a day or portion of a day are as follows:

- Physical examinations
- Prenatal patient visits in an obstetrics and gynecology (OB/GYN) practice
- Diagnostic procedures

MULTIPLE OFFICES

Some providers see patients in more than one office. Appointments may be scheduled in each office or through a central system. In this case, it is important to clarify which office the patient wants to visit. When there are multiple offices, it is an advantage to have an electronic health record (EHR). If a paper record system is used, patients are encouraged to choose one location where their record will be stored.

SETTING UP THE APPOINTMENT SCHEDULE

Appointments are usually scheduled up to 6 months in advance. Before scheduling can begin, the appointment book or computer software must be set up to indicate the times when the provider will see patients. Times when the provider is not available to see patients must be **blocked** out. The appointment schedule showing only available times for appointments is sometimes called the **appointment matrix** because it is the basic pattern of available patient appointment times (Procedure 42.1).

How the times are blocked out depends on the scheduling method used by the office. If the office uses an appointment book, the times are blocked out by drawing lines through the blocked times. If a computer is used to schedule appointments, the times are blocked out by telling the computer to block the specific time and the reason for the blockage. Various types of color-coding are used in a computer scheduling program, but blocked times are different colors than open appointment times (Fig. 42.4).

The appointment schedule must take three variables into consideration: the scheduling system, the provider's preferences and needs, and the facility and equipment requirements. Each of these will be discussed later.

APPOINTMENT INTERVALS

Appointments are usually scheduled at intervals of 10, 15, or 20 minutes. An appointment may be scheduled for more than one block, depending on the type of appointment. For example, if a 10-minute interval is used, an established

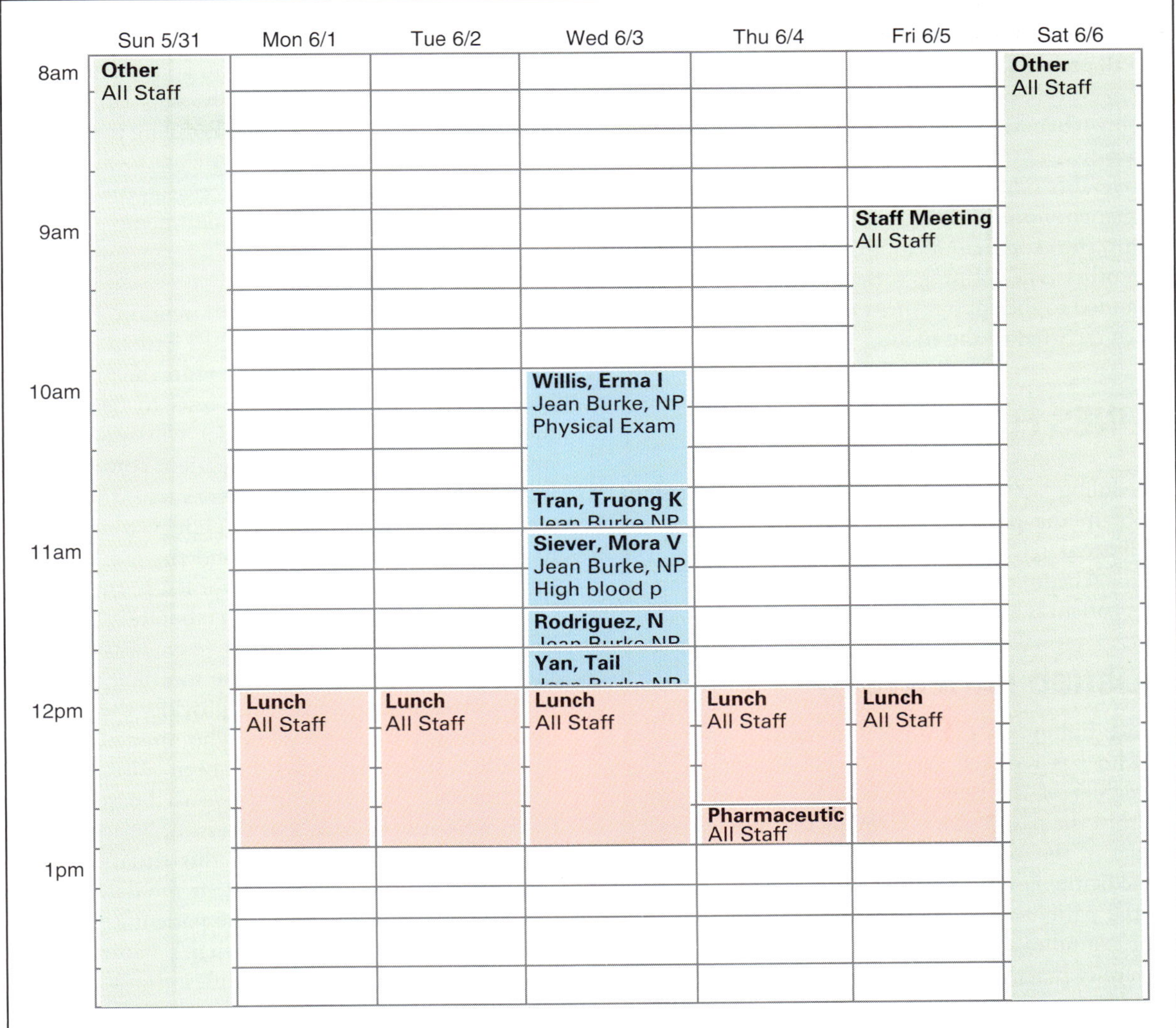

Fig. 42.4 Appointment schedule from SimChart for the Medical Office.

patient coming to have their blood pressure checked might be scheduled for one 10-minute interval and a new patient might be scheduled for three 10-minute intervals. In this case a 10-minute interval uses one line and a new patient uses three lines in the schedule. If a 15-minute interval is used, all appointments are scheduled in multiples of 15 minutes. In general, more time must be allotted for new patients, physical examinations, and special procedures than for routine follow-up visits.

PROVIDER'S PREFERENCES AND NEEDS

The second variable influencing the appointment schedule is the provider's preferences and needs. Providers may prefer to do physical examinations and/or procedures at specific times as well as a certain number of either during a day. The appointment slots for those times would need to indicate the type of visit (such as a physical). If there are multiple providers, their preferences may vary and certain rooms may need to be shared.

At times during the day the provider is not able to see patients, and, therefore, these times must be blocked out on the schedule. Time must be blocked out when the provider has another obligation, such as hospital rounds and nursing-home visits. Time may also need to be blocked out for lunch, pharmaceutical representative visits, and catch-up. Days are also blocked out of the schedule for vacation, days off, attendance at conferences, lectures to be given, and other professional activities. Protocols for each provider should be kept available for those setting up the appointment schedule.

FACILITY AND EQUIPMENT REQUIREMENTS

The third variable affecting the appointment schedule is the availability of facilities and equipment. The appointment schedule must be set up so that examination rooms and rooms with equipment required for certain procedures are available to all providers who are seeing patients. For optimal use of resources, one or more providers should be available to see patients whenever the office is open. Providers like to have at least two examination rooms available for seeing patients, preferably side by side. This improves efficiency and time management for examining patients. In many scheduling programs, the examination room can be scheduled with the visit. In other types of programs, the examination room number is added to the appointment after the patient arrives and has been escorted to the room.

GUIDELINES FOR SCHEDULING

When scheduling an appointment, the medical assistant needs to obtain the proper information from the patient, document it accurately, and confirm it with the patient. The procedure for scheduling appointments varies depending on whether the patient is an established patient or a new patient.

ESTABLISHED PATIENTS

For insurance billing, an **established patient** is defined as a patient who has received services from the provider or another provider of the same specialty in the same group practice within the past 3 years. If the patient has been seen by a provider in the group who specializes in primary care (internal medicine, family practice, or pediatrics), this does not make the patient an established patient for other specialties. For example, a patient has been treated for several years by a family practice provider who refers the patient to an orthopedic surgeon within the group. The patient is a new patient for the orthopedic surgeon. If the patient is seen by a different family practice provider for an urgent care appointment, the patient is an established patient for that provider. Patients who have not been seen within the past 3 years are typically treated as new patients, although their old medical records should be found if possible.

If an established patient is scheduling a return appointment after a visit, the provider usually specifies a time interval for the return visit (e.g., 1 week, 2 weeks, 1 month, or 6 months). The appointment should be scheduled as close as possible to the interval specified by the provider. The appointment must also be scheduled for the length of time preferred by the provider, which is usually 10 to 15 minutes. Before locating available appointment times to offer the patient, the medical assistant should ask what day of the week and what time of day are convenient for the patient. For an established patient, it is necessary to obtain the patient's name, date of birth, and provider. When the correct patient is selected, other demographic information (e.g., telephone number and address) is automatically linked to the appointment.

If the patient is at the office, the medical assistant should complete an appointment reminder card or print an appointment reminder from the computer and give it to the patient. The reminder includes the patient's name, the name of the provider, and the date and time of the new appointment.

If the patient has submitted an appointment request electronically, the medical assistant should attempt to accommodate the patient's wishes when scheduling the appointment or should make the appointment as close to the time requested as possible. The patient should receive an email or letter verifying the date and time of the appointment.

Special Situations

Some situations require special attention when scheduling an appointment for an established patient. The most common situation is when a patient visits the medical office and the provider orders laboratory tests to be performed at a medical laboratory. The provider will want to review the results of these tests before the patient comes in for a return visit. When scheduling the patient's return visit, the medical assistant must be sure to allow enough time for the patient to have these tests performed and the results to be entered into the computer system or returned to the office.

Patients who must undergo a laboratory test at the medical office that requires fasting (e.g., fasting blood sugar) should be scheduled early in the morning and be provided with written instructions. This provides the least amount of inconvenience for the patient, who must not consume food or fluids until the specimen has been collected.

Sometimes the patient needs to be scheduled for an appointment for a date later than can be accommodated by the appointment schedule. In this situation, the medical assistant can either tell the patient the date when they can request the appointment, or the patient's name can be put on a recall list. When the patient's name comes up, the medical assistant either schedules the appointment and notifies the patient or sends a letter reminding the patient to schedule the appointment.

NEW PATIENTS

Specific information needs to be obtained when scheduling an appointment for a **new patient.** This includes the patient's full name and daytime telephone number and the reason for the visit or type of visit (e.g., sick visit, physical examination, or diagnostic procedure). The medical assistant should ask the patient if they have been referred by another provider and determine the patient's insurance and if that insurance requires **preauthorization** (**precertification**). The process for verifying that insurance requirements have been met is discussed later in the chapter.

Most offices schedule new patients for 30 to 45 minutes. The medical assistant should set aside the correct amount of time for the appointment depending on the provider's preference.

The medical assistant may need to relay directions to the office location to the patient. Some offices mail the health history form to new patients and instruct them to bring the completed form to the first appointment. An office brochure containing information about the practice may also be mailed to the patient or given to the patient at the first appointment.

When the patient has been referred by another provider, the patient should be given an appointment as soon as possible, especially if the patient has urgent symptoms or if the patient's primary provider's office is calling to make the appointment (Procedure 42.2).

SAME-DAY APPOINTMENTS

The following problems are usually treated in the medical office and are usually scheduled the same day as the patient calls. The medical assistant should be familiar with office policy because each office varies in the degree of complexity of care it offers.

- Wounds without fracture or dislocation
- Sprains and strains
- Nausea, vomiting, or diarrhea that has persisted for more than 2 or 3 days
- Fever (defined by office guidelines)
- Sudden illness or severe pain without bleeding, fainting, or loss of consciousness
- Sore throat, especially with fever
- Burning, frequency, or urgency associated with urination, especially if accompanied by fever or blood in the urine
- Vaginal bleeding in a pregnant woman (who may also be sent to the emergency department)

If a patient's primary provider's schedule is booked, patients with these types of conditions may need to be scheduled with a practitioner who has more availability. When there are several practitioners in an office, a period of time may be blocked off in one provider's schedule to accommodate same-day appointments.

What Would You Do? What Would You *Not* Do?

Case Study 1

Sandra Meyers has been sitting in the waiting room for several minutes. She arrived at the office at 10:50 a.m. for an appointment scheduled at 11:00 a.m. At 11:15 a.m. she approaches the front desk and asks how long she will have to wait to see the provider. On this day the provider is running about 25 minutes behind schedule, and there are still two patients ahead of Sandra. She appears to be upset, and she says that she needs to be back in her office by 12:30 p.m. to prepare for an important afternoon meeting. ■

URGENT CARE AND EMERGENCIES

The majority of appointments are made well in advance of the date a patient will see the provider, but there are times when urgent or emergency situations occur. A patient calling the office with an emergency presents a challenging situation for the medical assistant. It is important to give a caller a chance to tell you that it is an urgent situation before putting the call on hold. A life-threatening or serious medical problem should be immediately referred to the physician or other licensed practitioner. The practitioner will make the decision about the appropriate course of action to take. If the provider is not present, the caller should be referred to the emergency medical services system, usually activated by calling 911 (Box 42.1). The office procedure manual should be used when responding to emergencies.

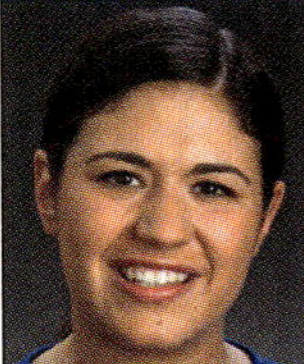

Putting It All Into Practice

My name is Elaine Wyatt, and I am a Certified Medical Assistant. My primary responsibility is to schedule appointments, although sometimes I sit at the front desk and check patients in. I work in an office with five internists and two nurse practitioners. Calls from patients who select "make an appointment" from our telephone menu will end up with me or another medical assistant, or the receptionist may transfer a call to me. I also check patients out after they have been seen and make follow-up appointments using our computer system. Sometimes the telephone is ringing off the hook, and I really have to concentrate to keep track of each call. Our office has a procedure manual with guidelines for handling urgent calls, and we try very hard to give patients appointments the same day if they are sick. We leave several open appointments for this, but even if we have to double book, we will fit them in because our providers want to be sure that everyone receives the care they need. All of our providers are accepting new patients, and we always ask new patients to arrive at the office about 15 minutes early to fill out a patient health history form. Usually, our appointment system works pretty well and patients do not have to wait more than 10 or 15 minutes—at least, that is our goal. There are days, of course, when the providers get behind, but through trial and error, we have developed a system that works pretty well for us. ■

WALK-IN PATIENTS

Sometimes patients come to the office without an appointment and ask to be seen. If the patient is experiencing an emergency or urgent problem, the provider may ask the medical assistant to work the patient into the schedule. However, in routine situations the patient is offered an appointment at a later date. In these situations, the medical assistant should tactfully inform the patient of the medical office policy with respect to scheduling appointments.

INDIVIDUALS WHO ARE NOT PATIENTS

During office hours, the provider may see various individuals who are not patients. Time should be blocked from the schedule to accommodate these appointments. Many offices have a specific time slot, often during the lunch hour, to schedule representatives of pharmaceutical companies or representatives of companies with medical equipment or

BOX 42.1 Medical Conditions Referred to Emergency Medical Services (911)

1. Conditions that may result in damage to body structures. This is especially important for problems that can cause a significant decrease in oxygen to the body because of breathing or circulation disorders:
   - Breathing problems or respiratory arrest
   - Severe chest pain or cardiac arrest
   - Bleeding that cannot be controlled
   - Large open wounds
   - Any condition that raises the suspicion of internal bleeding
   - Potential poisoning or overdose
   - Bleeding in, or injury to, a pregnant woman
2. Conditions that result in very low blood pressure:
   - Shock
   - Serious burns
   - Severe bleeding
3. Conditions that result in a change in the level of consciousness (loss of consciousness, disorientation, confusion, and loss of alertness)
4. Fractures or large wounds that require the equipment found in an emergency department

***HIGHLIGHT* on Triage**

Triage is the process of sorting patients according to their need for care. When a disaster occurs, health care workers choose which patients to treat first, depending both on the severity of their injuries and the likelihood the person will survive.

Victims are sorted into three groups—hence the word *triage*, from a French word meaning "sort." Some victims' injuries are minor and can wait for treatment; some victims have injuries so severe that they will probably not survive no matter what effort is put into their treatment; and some have severe injuries but will probably survive if prompt treatment is given.

This system has been adapted to office and appointment scheduling to decide if a patient can wait for the next available appointment, if the patient should be seen immediately, or if the patient should be sent to the emergency department. Triage in the medical office setting is rarely a case of life or death, and the term *triage* is usually reserved for screening performed by licensed health care personnel with the education needed to assess the medical needs of ill patients.

The medical assistant may screen calls and make decisions based on guidelines established by the providers where they work. The medical assistant must remember that if there is any question about a patient needing immediate care, either the telephone call should be referred to a qualified person in the office or the patient should be directed to an emergency department or other facility where care can be obtained. The medical assistant should be familiar with the policies of their employer and work within them, both to avoid injuring the patient and to protect against liability in a potential lawsuit. ■

computer equipment that the office may be thinking of purchasing. There is usually a maximum of one or two appointments set aside for each provider for this type of appointment each week.

What Would You Do? What Would You *Not* Do?

Case Study 2

On a winter afternoon, there is only one provider in the office. He must leave promptly at 3:45 p.m. because he is scheduled to give a lecture to medical students at a nearby hospital shortly after 4:00 p.m. The provider has been running behind because two extra patients have been worked into the schedule. At 2:30 p.m., in addition to three patients in the waiting room, he still has four established patients scheduled, as well as one new patient scheduled for 3:15 p.m., the last appointment of the day. ■

MANAGING THE APPOINTMENT SCHEDULE

CHANGING APPOINTMENTS

The most frequent modification required in the appointment schedule is to change an appointment from one time slot to another. In the computer appointment schedule, the original appointment can usually be changed by altering the date and time within the appointment pop-up window. In some systems the appointment should be copied and pasted to the new time.

Occasionally an entire block of patients has to be rescheduled. This occurs when the provider is unexpectedly absent or delayed during office hours. The absence or delay may be the result of an emergency, a delay at the hospital, or personal illness. Every effort must be made to accommodate scheduled patients by giving them a new appointment as quickly as possible. If there are patients in the office when a provider is severely delayed or must leave, it is important to tell patients how long they can expect to wait. The patients should be given the option of waiting or rescheduling their appointments.

If the provider is running seriously behind schedule, patients often become impatient. Some may wish to reschedule, and this should be done willingly. Usually, the provider is willing to stay late to finish the day's appointments, but if the provider must leave at a particular time, appointments set for late in the day may need to be rescheduled.

No-shows are patients who simply do not show up for their appointment without letting the office know. No-shows and cancelations on the day of the appointment should be noted on the official appointment schedule. The information should also be documented in the patient's medical record. This provides a permanent record in case the patient's condition becomes worse and the patient claims that the provider would not see them (Procedure 42.3).

Most offices have a policy of reviewing records of patients after three consecutively missed appointments.

If the patient is not motivated to adhere to the treatment plan, the provider may wish to terminate the relationship with the patient.

LATE PATIENTS

The office should have a policy regarding late patients. Traffic problems or other incidents can delay even the most punctual person, and usually the office attempts to work the patient into the schedule. If a patient telephones to say that they will be unexpectedly delayed, either the schedule can be adjusted or the patient can be offered a new appointment. Patients who habitually arrive late can cause delays in the appointment schedule. They may be given the last appointment of the day when the provider is most likely to be running late. In some practices, habitual latecomers are given an appointment time that is 15 to 30 minutes earlier than the appointment is actually scheduled.

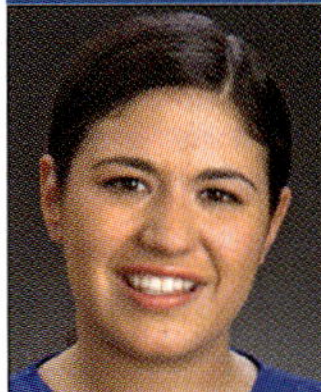

Memories *from* Practicum

Elaine Wyatt: The office where I did my practicum was always very busy. I remember one afternoon when one of the providers had to leave suddenly. She was expected to be gone about 2 hours. I was told to call the list of afternoon patients and tell them that the provider had been called away from the office and would be delayed about 2 hours. If the patient wanted to reschedule, I had to put them on hold and transfer the call to the appointment scheduler. If the patient wanted to be seen that day, I had to give them a time from the revised list. I was surprised that about half of the patients were completely willing to reschedule, so there did end up being enough appointment times for the patients who still wanted to be seen. The major problems occurred when we could not reach the patients by telephone. There were about five of them, and they all came. Two of them were during the 2-hour delay, and both of them decided to reschedule. The other three had appointments after the provider returned. We managed to fit them in close to their original appointment times, and they never even knew that the provider had been out of the office unexpectedly. ■

APPOINTMENT REMINDERS

It is easy to print an appointment reminder for a patient who makes an appointment before leaving the office, or a card may be filled out manually. Appointment reminders help patients to remember the exact date and time of their next appointment.

Most offices also send reminder letters, emails, or text messages and/or call patients 1 or 2 days before the appointment. The patient's preference should be noted and permission obtained if email or text messages are used. The medical assistant may place a personal call to each patient scheduled for an appointment (see Chapter 41), or the office may use a computer-generated appointment reminder system. The computer may also be used to generate letters or emails reminding patients to make appointments for periodic routine examinations such as a physical examination or a mammogram.

Text messages to patients may be used for appointment and laboratory reminders, but text message systems are usually not secure and should not contain protected health information. If a medical office uses text messaging, it should inform patients at the time that cell phone numbers are collected how they will be used and allow patients to opt out of receiving text messages.

STORING APPOINTMENT BOOKS AND DAILY SCHEDULES

When computer appointment schedules are used as official schedules, backups should be made according to the guidelines in Chapter 40. If a paper schedule or appointment book (maintained in ink) is used as the official schedule, it should be stored in a secure area.

SCHEDULING REFERRAL APPOINTMENTS, DIAGNOSTIC TESTS, PROCEDURES, AND ADMISSIONS

REFERRALS

A **referral** is an authorization for a visit to another provider, usually a specialist. A referral is made by the patient's primary care provider. It may be necessary to obtain preauthorization (official permission from the patient's insurance company) before the patient can see the specialist. The provider determines the type and amount of service needed, but the medical assistant usually obtains the necessary insurance authorization (see Chapter 48).

After obtaining all necessary information and insurance authorization, the medical assistant either instructs the patient to make the appointment or calls to make the appointment for the patient. Some managed care plans require the referring provider's office to make the appointment. If the medical assistant calls from the office, the patient may be able to obtain an earlier appointment, but it is important to verify the date and time with the patient. Fig. 42.5 is an example of an approved electronic request for referral to a medical specialist.

For a referral to a community resource, the medical assistant must know the patient's name, address, and telephone number, as well as the needed resource, the diagnosis, and the reason for the service. Community services include home health care and **hospice** care (a range of services provided to an individual with a terminal illness). Most community agencies do an intake evaluation of the patient, but others depend on the primary care or other provider and staff to tell them what resources the patient needs.

SH9999999 Detail Approved			Mary Patient SH123456789		
			Request Information		
Patient	MARY PATIENT	Requesting provider	RICHARD WARNER (1234567890 NPI)	Contact info	(490) 555-6464
Diagnosis	I145.10 RT BUNDLE BRANCH BLOCK	Servicing provider	THOMAS HIGHT (2345678901 NPI)	Contact info	(490) 222-3232
Requested service	Specialist consult			Units	1 visit approved
Procedure code				Procedure date	
Start date	4/5/XX	End date	9/5/XX	Delay reason	
Level of service		Related causes		Release of information	Signed statement/ claims
Remarks	Transaction approved				
Procedures and Services					
Status			Reason	Follow-up	Description
Approved (Transaction approved)					Consult
Additional Information					
Additional information requested			Identification code	Description	
No paper work at this time					
Edit	Cancel				

Fig. 42.5 Approved electronic request for referral to a specialist.

SCHEDULING DIAGNOSTIC PROCEDURES AND HOSPITAL ADMISSIONS

It is often easier for a provider's office to schedule a diagnostic procedure or laboratory test for a patient than to have the patient schedule it. Hospital admissions are always scheduled by the provider's office. Scheduling procedures and admissions can be performed while the patient is at the office or when the patient is at home. If the patient is at home, the details of the appointment and any special patient instructions must be mailed to the patient and confirmed with a follow-up telephone call.

Scheduling a Diagnostic Procedure

Before scheduling a diagnostic procedure for a patient with an outside facility, the medical assistant should compile all of the information that needs to be relayed to the facility. This includes the patient's name and telephone number, the type of procedure being performed, the reason for the procedure, the time frame within which the procedure must be performed, the provider's National Provider Identifier (NPI) number and contact information, and insurance information including any preauthorization number.

After an appointment has been made, the medical assistant must contact the patient to relay when and where the procedure will be performed. The medical assistant may also need to provide directions to the facility. Patients are often required to prepare for a diagnostic procedure. For example, a patient undergoing a colonoscopy needs to perform procedures at home to cleanse the colon of gas and fecal material. These instructions must be relayed to the patient by the medical assistant. If written instructions are available, they should be given or sent to the patient. The medical assistant should document in the patient record the type of verbal and written instructions provided to the patient. After the procedure, the medical assistant should document when and how the patient was notified of the results of the diagnostic procedure. Precise documentation in patient charts is necessary to avoid later claims of malpractice or abandonment (Procedure 42.4).

What Would You Do? What Would You *Not* Do?

Case Study 3

Anna Greene, a 17-year-old girl, came to see the provider for a physical examination. On the basis of her history and physical examination findings, the provider has ordered her to have an echocardiogram (ultrasound of the heart). Anna's mother says that the provider did not really explain why Anna needs this test, and she expresses concern that her insurance will not cover the total cost of the test. She appears to be reluctant to allow the test to be scheduled and says that she will call and schedule it herself in a few days. ■

Scheduling an Inpatient Admission

The medical assistant has several tasks that must be performed when a patient is admitted to the hospital. The medical assistant must contact the patient's insurance company to obtain preauthorization. The next step is to call the hospital's admitting department to schedule the admission.

The medical assistant must provide the admitting department with the patient's name, address, date of birth, admitting diagnosis, insurance information and preauthorization number. A patient must be seen by their provider within the first 24 hours after admission. Because of this, the hospital may ask when the provider is coming to see the patient. In addition, admitting orders must be sent (electronically or by mail) or faxed before the patient is admitted to the hospital.

The procedure for admitting a patient to the hospital is modified somewhat if the patient is first seen in the emergency department and then admitted to the hospital. In this situation the hospital obtains the information from the patient and then contacts the provider to obtain admitting orders (Procedure 42.5).

SCHEDULING SURGERY

Scheduling a surgery is similar to scheduling a diagnostic procedure; however, more information is necessary to schedule a patient for surgery. In addition to the patient's name, date of birth, and telephone number, the medical assistant must also know the type of surgery to be performed, the time frame within which the surgery is to be performed, who the surgeon and any assistant surgeons will be, who the anesthesiologist will be, and the name of the hospital or outpatient center at which the surgery will be performed.

Before scheduling the surgery, the medical assistant must call the patient's insurance company and obtain preauthorization (prior approval by the insurance company). The preauthorization number must be relayed when scheduling surgery. This number facilitates payment by the insurance company for the procedure. The patient's insurance may require the patient to undergo the surgery at specific hospitals or outpatient facilities.

Before a patient undergoes a surgical procedure, **preadmission testing (PAT)** is performed. PAT includes blood tests, an ECG, and a chest x-ray examination. A physical examination must also be performed within 6 months of the surgery and may be done by the provider or as part of PAT. The purposes of PAT are to obtain data about the patient's health before surgery, to be sure that the patient can tolerate the proposed surgical procedure and anesthesia, and to obtain baseline data for comparison during and after the surgical procedure. The medical assistant helps the patient to schedule this testing.

PAT may be performed in the hospital or medical office, depending on the requirements of the facility where the surgery will be done. If performed in the medical office, the PAT is done either at the surgeon's office or at the office of the patient's primary care provider.

A patient may also need to be scheduled to donate one or more units of their own blood. This blood would then be available if a patient needs a transfusion during or after surgery.

Giving a Patient Instructions Before Surgery

The medical assistant is often responsible for providing the patient with specific instructions before the surgery. The office usually gives the patient a set of written instructions so that the patient will remember everything. If the patient is receiving a general anesthetic, they must fast for a period of time before the surgery. Fasting requires that the patient have nothing to eat or drink for approximately 12 hours before the surgery. If the patient takes medication for hypertension or heart problems, the surgeon may allow the patient to take their morning medication with a sip of water. Other examples of preparation that may be required before a surgical operation include washing with an antibiotic soap and removing body piercings. Patients should be instructed not to bring valuables with them on the day of surgery. If they are having outpatient surgery, they need to have someone available to drive them home after the surgery.

Documenting an Appointment for Surgery

It is important for the medical assistant to carefully document all information relayed to the patient regarding the surgery. Other information that should be documented includes the interactions with the surgical team members, patient, and facilities.

What Would You Do? What Would You *Not* Do? RESPONSES

Case Study 1
Page 1103

What Did Elaine Do?
- ❑ Listened to Sandra's concerns without interrupting.
- ❑ Apologized for the delay and agreed that it is difficult to wait when you have other obligations.
- ❑ Informed Sandra that the provider was running behind schedule and that there were two patients ahead of her. Gave her a realistic estimate of when she would be taken to an examination room.
- ❑ Offered to reschedule the appointment if Sandra said that she really could not wait to see the provider that day.

What Did Elaine Not Do?
- ❑ Did not tell Sandra that she would be taken to an examination room in just a minute.
- ❑ Did not give a long explanation about why the provider was delayed.
- ❑ Did not give exaggerated or made-up excuses to imply that this was a one-time crisis.
- ❑ Did not become defensive or interrupt Sandra.

Case Study 2
Page 1104

What Did Elaine Do?
- ❑ Asked the provider if it would be a good idea to reschedule the new patient or some of the other patients for another appointment in the next few days.
- ❑ If instructed to do so, called patients, explained that the provider was going to have to leave the office early, and asked if they would be willing to reschedule.
- ❑ If instructed to do so, explained to the patients in the waiting room that the provider was delayed, and asked if they would like to reschedule.
- ❑ Evaluated all patients carefully to be sure that everything was prepared to make their examinations go smoothly.

What Did Elaine Not Do?
- ❑ Did not reschedule patients without discussing it with the provider.
- ❑ Did not tell the patients specific information about the provider's commitments.

Case Study 3
Page 1107

What Did Elaine Do?
- ❑ Made a general statement that the provider thought the test was important, and it would help the provider to provide the best care for Anna.
- ❑ Asked Mrs. Greene and Anna to wait to see if the provider could give them more information about the reason and need for the test.
- ❑ Offered to call the insurance company to determine whether Mrs. Greene's insurance would cover the cost of the test.
- ❑ Explained that the office preferred to schedule this type of test to be sure that the testing facility had all necessary information from the provider.
- ❑ Documented the interaction with the patient in detail.

What Did Elaine Not Do?
- ❑ Did not give a reason for the test unless authorized by the provider.
- ❑ Did not imply that the mother cared more about the money than her daughter.
- ❑ Did not say that the provider knows what he is doing.
- ❑ Did not insist on scheduling the test even if Mrs. Greene did not agree to it.

TERMINOLOGY REVIEW

Key Term	Definition
Appointment matrix	Basic pattern of available appointment times.
Blocked	Times in the appointment schedule when providers are not available to see patients.
Clustering	Scheduling similar types of patients or examinations on the same day or part of the day.
Double booking	Scheduling two patients for the same appointment time.
Established patient	A patient who has been seen by one of the providers in the practice of the same specialty within the past 3 years.
Fixed appointment scheduling	An appointment scheduling method in which each patient is given a different, specific appointment time. Also called *stream scheduling*, *time-specified scheduling*, or *single booking.*
Hospice	Palliative service provided for patients whose life expectancy is less than 6 months. Services may be provided in the patient's home, a nursing home, or a special hospice facility.

TERMINOLOGY REVIEW—cont'd

Key Term	Definition
Modified wave scheduling	An appointment system that has some fixed appointments and some appointment times during which patients are seen in order of arrival.
New patient	For billing purposes, a patient who has not received services during the previous 3 years from any provider of the same specialty in a medical practice.
No-show	A patient who does not keep a scheduled appointment.
Open booking	Patients are told to come in during a time range.
Patient self-scheduling	The practice of allowing patients to have access to the computer scheduling program so that they can schedule their own appointments.
Preadmission testing (PAT)	A series of diagnostic tests done before surgery to establish the patient's health status and identify any potential problems that may occur during surgery.
Preauthorization/precertification	Permission from a patient's insurance company for a test, procedure, or surgery.
Referral	The directing of a patient to a medical specialist by a primary care provider.
Single booking	An appointment scheduling method in which each patient is given a different, specific appointment time. Also called *stream scheduling* or *fixed appointment scheduling.*
Stream scheduling	An appointment scheduling method in which each patient is given a different, specific appointment time. Also called *fixed appointment scheduling*, *time-specified scheduling*, or *single booking.*
Time-specified scheduling	An appointment scheduling method in which each patient is given a different, specific appointment time. Also called *stream scheduling*, *fixed appointment scheduling*, or *single booking.*
Triage	The process of separating patients by the urgency of their need for care.
Wave scheduling	A method of scheduling appointments in which several patients are given the same appointment time and are seen in the order in which they arrive.

PROCEDURE 42.1 Setting Up the Appointment Schedule

Outcomes

1. Set up an appointment schedule
2. Implement time management principles to maintain effective office functions

Equipment/Supplies:

- Computer appointment schedule or appointment book
- Pen
- Provider schedule
- Office calendar

1. **Procedural Step.** Block times when the office is not open to see patients. This includes times before office hours begin, lunch and/or breaks for all office staff, afternoons or days when the office is closed, and holidays when the office will be closed. Some offices set up the appointment schedule 6 months in advance, whereas others do it for a year in advance. In a computer schedule, either set up the schedule so that only times when the office is open appear on the schedule, or block times when the office is closed. In an appointment book, draw an X through times when the office is closed.
   Principle. In an effective appointment schedule, only available appointment times are blank.
2. **Procedural Step.** Block times when each individual provider is not available to see patients, including lunch (if the office does not close for lunch) and hospital rounds. In addition, block days when each provider will be away from the office for vacations, conferences, or other anticipated absences. If the provider has regular meetings or other regular commitments (such as nursing home visits), mark these also. In a computer schedule, schedule the meeting, vacation, or other anticipated absence, such as an appointment, using color-coding to show that the times are unavailable. In an appointment book, draw an X through the times when the provider is not available.

Continued

PROCEDURE 42.1 Setting Up the Appointment Schedule—cont'd

3. **Procedural Step.** For each provider, mark times when the provider does certain types of examinations, procedures (e.g., physical examinations or obstetric visits), or surgery. In a computer schedule, these times may be set up as if for a separate provider (e.g., "Dr. Gomez" and "Dr. Gomez—OB visits"), or a color-coding system can be used. In an appointment book, these are often highlighted with a marker or given a written title at the beginning of the time block.
4. **Procedural Step.** Depending on office policy, block out as much time as is anticipated for same-day appointments, catch-up time, and unexpected needs. Depending on the practice, catch-up time may be 15 minutes in the morning and afternoon for each provider, and time for same-day appointments may be an hour or longer for all providers or one particular provider on a rotating basis. These times can be marked in various ways as long as it is generally understood that they must be saved until the scheduled day.
Example. On this day, the office will be open from 9 a.m. to 5 p.m., but Dr. Martin will be available to see patients only from 9 a.m. to 12 p.m. because he plans to attend a conference in the afternoon. The appointment interval is 15 minutes. Dr. Warner likes to have 15 minutes set aside for catch-up time at 10:30 a.m.

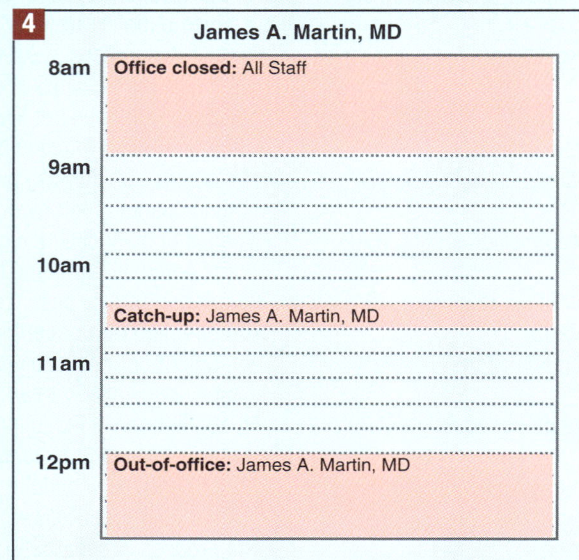

In SimChart for the Medical Office, block times when the provider is not available using a colored background. (*Note*: "Catch-up" may also be called "buffer time.")

PROCEDURE 42.2 Making an Appointment

Outcome Make an appointment for a patient

Equipment/Supplies:

- Computer appointment schedule or appointment book
- Pencil

1. **Procedural Step.** Identify the patient using the full name and date of birth. Obtain information from the patient: the provider, the purpose of the appointment, and any scheduling preference. Referrals are usually offered the first available appointment. If you do not find the patient in the computer database, ask if they have been seen before. New patients may be encouraged to choose a provider who has joined the practice recently if no provider preference is mentioned. Established patients are usually booked with their primary provider, but if it is an urgent problem the patient may accept an appointment with another provider in the practice.
2. **Procedural Step.** Offer the patient a date and time for the appointment. Keep locating appointments until an acceptable date and time have been found. The more urgent the appointment, the more the patient must adapt to the office schedule.
3. **Procedural Step.** For a new patient, obtain the patient's demographic data (e.g., address, telephone number, and date of birth), the name of the patient's insurance company, the name of the insured, the patient's insurance group number and ID number, a prior authorization (precertification) number, or other information related to insurance. Be sure to discuss the cost of the visit or procedure if the patient does not have insurance. Inform the patient if a referral form from the primary provider is necessary. Enter this information directly into the computer as you obtain it from the patient.

PROCEDURE 42.2 Making an Appointment—cont'd

Principle. Before making an appointment for a new patient, it is important to be sure that the patient can pay the bill. Information about insurance and referral provides a basis to inform the patient what their personal financial liability is likely to be.

4. **Procedural Step.** For an established patient, obtain the information to make the appointment. After identifying the patient, this includes the reason for the visit, the provider, and the desired date and time.
5. **Procedural Step.** Repeat the information to the patient to confirm the appointment. Offer to tell a new patient where the office is located.
6. **Procedural Step.** Enter the patient's name, the correct amount of time for the appointment, and the reason for the visit. If using an appointment book, enter the information in pencil and block out the correct amount of time.

Example. The appointment schedule shows a 30-minute appointment for Norma Washington, who complains of back pain; a 30-minute appointment to evaluate shortness of breath for Carl Bowden; and a 45-minute appointment for a new patient, Estelle Jordan.

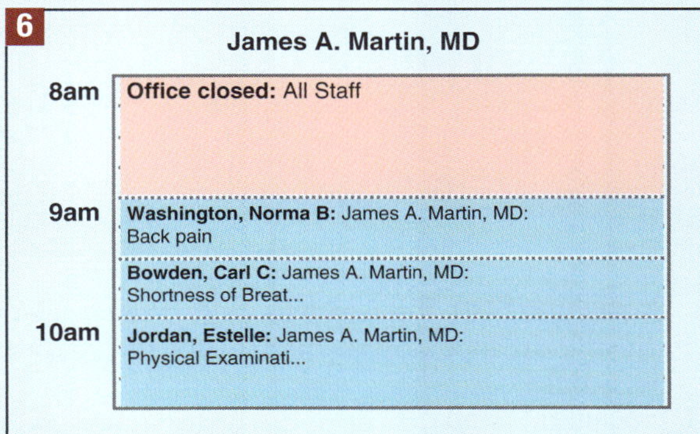

In SimChart for the Medical Office, schedule appointment times for the correct amount of time.

PROCEDURE 42.3 Managing the Appointment Schedule

Outcomes

1. Review the daily appointment schedule
2. Cancel a patient appointment
3. Change a patient appointment
4. Indicate a missed appointment
5. Document cancelations and missed appointments on the day of the appointment

Equipment/Supplies:

- Computer appointment schedule or appointment book
- Pen

1. **Procedural Step.** Review the daily appointment schedule and be sure that all paperwork and/or paper medical records have been prepared.
2. **Procedural Step.** Check patients in as they arrive. Depending on office procedure, you may check them in using the electronic appointment schedule or a paper appointment schedule.
3. **Procedural Step.** If a patient calls to cancel an appointment, locate the appointment on the appointment schedule, in the appointment book, and/or in the computer appointment program. Ask whether the patient wants to reschedule the appointment.

   Principle. The patient may have a schedule conflict with the original appointment.
4. **Procedural Step.** To cancel an appointment without rescheduling, delete the appointment. When using a paper schedule, if the appointment is canceled on the day of the appointment, draw a line through the patient's name on the schedule.

   Principle. If a paper schedule is used as the official schedule, it is a legal document so changes must be made in ink.
5. **Procedural Step.** If the patient cancels an appointment and declines or postpones making a new appointment, document the cancelation in the patient's medical record. This can be done as a telephone message filed in the medical record or as a progress note.

   Principle. Documentation of canceled or missed appointments makes it readily apparent if this behavior is a common pattern for the patient.

Continued

PROCEDURE 42.3 Managing the Appointment Schedule—cont'd

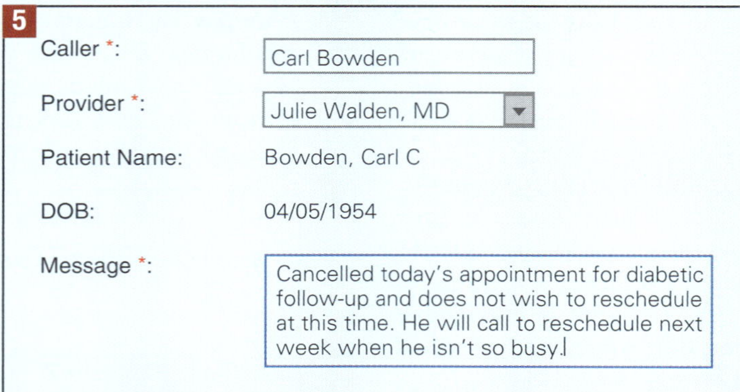

6. **Procedural Step.** If the patient wants to change or reschedule an appointment, find an acceptable time to reschedule.
7. **Procedural Step.** Change the appointment in the computer program by finding the appointment at the originally scheduled date and time and changing to the new date and time. Enter the new appointment in a manual appointment book, then erase the original appointment after checking to make sure all information was copied correctly.
   Principle. Changing the appointment in the computer (instead of deleting) makes it unnecessary to reenter the appointment information.
8. **Procedural Step.** Repeat the information to the patient if speaking on the telephone or fill out an appointment reminder if the patient is present in the office.
9. **Procedural Step.** If the patient misses an appointment without canceling, draw a line in ink through the appointment on the daily appointment sheet and label the appointment "No Show." If the official schedule is maintained in the computer, indicate that the appointment was not kept by marking the appointment as a missed appointment or no-show or adding a comment that the patient did not keep the appointment, depending on the computer program.
   Principle. Computer scheduling programs often provide an opportunity to track no-show or missed appointments. If it becomes a pattern for an individual patient, it is easy to identify the problem.
10. **Procedural Step.** It may be office policy to telephone the patient to determine why the appointment was missed and offer another appointment.
11. **Procedural Step.** Document the no-show appointment in the medical record and indicate whether any follow-up was done.

PROCEDURE 42.4 Scheduling Inpatient or Outpatient Diagnostic Tests or Procedures

Outcome Schedule an inpatient or outpatient diagnostic test or procedure

Equipment/Supplies:

- The patient's computer or paper medical record and insurance information
- Name of the test or procedure to be scheduled
- Telephone
- Telephone number of the facility and name of the appropriate department with which to schedule the test or procedure
- Pen

1. **Procedural Step.** Assemble necessary information about the patient, including the patient's demographic and insurance information.
2. **Procedural Step.** From the patient's medical record and/or a diagnostic test or procedure requisition filled out by the provider, determine the facility and department to call for scheduling. If the office uses a computerized system, be sure the test, procedure, or hospital admission has been ordered in the computer.

PROCEDURE 42.4 Scheduling Inpatient or Outpatient Diagnostic Tests or Procedures—cont'd

Principle. Any admission, diagnostic test, or diagnostic procedure must have a valid provider order. For insurance reimbursement, a facility that participates in the patient's insurance plan must be used.

3. **Procedural Step.** Determine the time frame for scheduling and, if possible, discuss with the patient preferred days and times.
4. **Procedural Step.** Obtain preauthorization from the patient's insurance, if necessary.
   Principle. The patient's medical condition must justify the service requested. Failure to obtain preauthorization required by the insurance company will result in denial of the patient's insurance claim.
5. **Procedural Step.** Call the department of the facility where the procedure will be performed.
6. **Procedural Step.** Provide the patient's name and demographic and insurance information as needed and a preauthorization number if needed. Identify the test or procedure to be scheduled and set up a specific day and time.
7. **Procedural Step.** Inform the patient of the date and time for the test or procedure and provide verbal and written instructions, including preparation for the test, special instructions, and/or dietary restrictions.

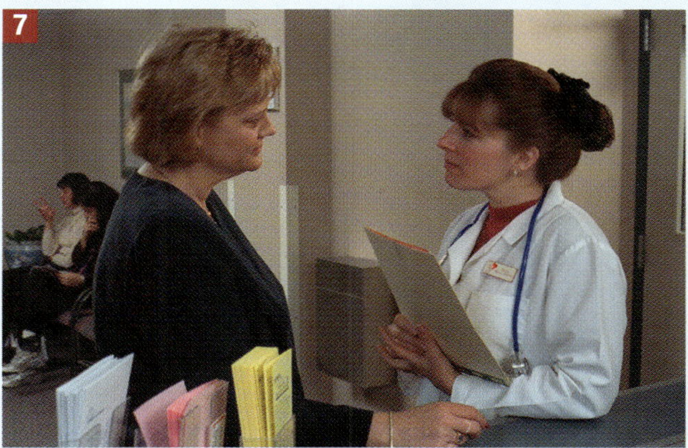
Go over any instructions with the patient before the test.

   Principle. The patient must know how to prepare for the test or procedure. Written instructions reinforce verbal explanations.
8. **Procedural Step.** Send a computer or paper requisition to the facility or give a paper requisition to the patient to take to the test.
9. **Procedural Step.** Document the scheduled diagnostic test or procedure and instructions given to the patient in the patient's medical record.

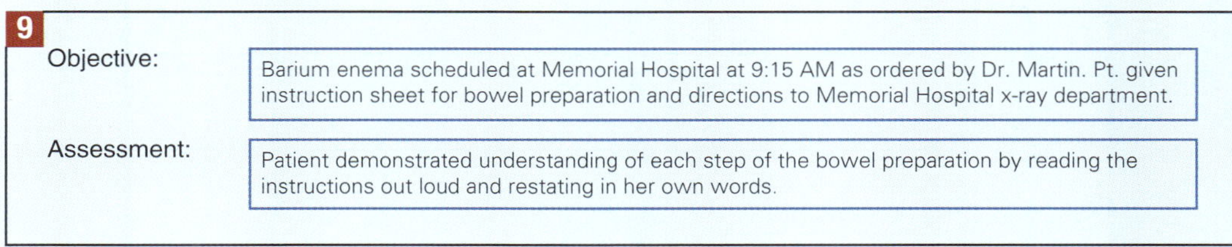
9

Objective: Barium enema scheduled at Memorial Hospital at 9:15 AM as ordered by Dr. Martin. Pt. given instruction sheet for bowel preparation and directions to Memorial Hospital x-ray department.

Assessment: Patient demonstrated understanding of each step of the bowel preparation by reading the instructions out loud and restating in her own words.

PROCEDURE 42.5 Scheduling Inpatient or Outpatient Admissions

Outcome Schedule an inpatient or outpatient admission for a patient

Equipment/Supplies:

- The patient's computer or paper medical record and insurance information
- Name of the procedure to be scheduled or reason for the hospital admission
- Telephone
- Telephone number of the facility and the admitting department
- Pen

1. **Procedural Step.** Assemble necessary information about the patient, including the patient's demographic and insurance information.
2. **Procedural Step.** From the patient's medical record and/or directions from the provider, determine the reason for the inpatient or outpatient admission.
   Principle. Any admission must have a valid provider order. For insurance reimbursement, a facility that participates in the patient's insurance plan must be used.
3. **Procedural Step.** Determine the time frame for the admission. If it is for an elective procedure or surgery, discuss with the patient preferred days and times.

Continued

PROCEDURE 42.5

PROCEDURE 42.5 Scheduling Inpatient or Outpatient Admissions—cont'd

4. **Procedural Step.** Obtain preauthorization from the patient's insurance company.
   Principle. The patient's medical condition must justify the service requested. Failure to obtain preauthorization required by the insurance company will result in denial of the patient's insurance claim.
5. **Procedural Step.** Call the admissions department to schedule the admission.
   Principle. The patient must be entered into the facility's computer system with all demographic and insurance information for an inpatient or outpatient hospital admission.
6. **Procedural Step.** Provide all necessary information including demographic and insurance information about the patient, preauthorization number (if any), diagnosis or reason for the admission, and date of the admission.
7. **Procedural Step.** For an inpatient admission, provide admitting orders as needed or fill out admitting orders according to the patient's medical record and fax to the department or nursing floor.
8. **Procedural Step.** If the patient is to be admitted to the hospital directly from the provider's office, help the patient notify a family member, prepare a patient transfer form, obtain consent forms to release information, and make arrangements for the patient to be transported to the hospital.
9. **Procedural Step.** If the patient is to be admitted for a procedure or surgery in the future, inform the patient of the date and time of the test or procedure and provide verbal and written instructions, including preparation, special instructions, and dietary restrictions.
   Principle. The patient must know how to prepare for the procedure or surgery. Written instructions reinforce verbal explanations.
10. **Procedural Step.** Document in the patient's medical record the admission, other pertinent information, and instructions given to the patient. For a hospital admission, identify any documents sent with the patient.

10

Plan: Apply oxygen at 2 L/min per order Dr. Martin. To be transferred to Memorial Hospital by ambulance. Admitting orders and copies of medical records will be sent with the patient. Patient's son notified and states he will meet his mother at the hospital.

Evaluation:

Entry By: Elaine Wyatt, RMA

Medical Record Management

Check out the Evolve site at http://evolve.elsevier.com/Bonewit/today to access additional interactive activities and exercises to help you study and prepare for success.

LEARNING OBJECTIVES	PROCEDURES
1. Describe how an electronic health record (EHR) system saves time, once it is set up and staff have been trained.	
2. Discuss methods to maintain the integrity of the EHR.	
3. Describe the individuals who are authorized to view a patient's EHR.	
4. Discuss the methods for storage of EHRs.	
5. Identify supplies and equipment needed to create and store paper-based medical records.	
6. Describe how to create a new paper-based medical record.	Preparing a medical record.
7. Describe different types of filing systems.	
8. List principles of alphabetic and numeric filing.	Filing patient records: alphabetic.
9. Describe the process of filing reports and paper-based medical records.	Filing patient records: numeric.
10. Compare and contrast advantages and disadvantages of alphabetic and numeric filing systems for paper-based medical records.	Filing reports.
11. Identify methods for retention and disposition of paper-based medical records.	

CHAPTER OUTLINE

KEY TERMS

acronym
active record
cross-index
electronic signature
filing system
indexing units
medical record management
outguide
sorter
surname
tab
terminal digit filing

INTRODUCTION TO MEDICAL RECORDS

A medical record (also known as a *patient chart* or *health record*) contains the important information related to an individual patient in written or electronic form. It includes the care given to that patient and the progress of the patient's condition. **Medical record management** is the process of controlling and handling medical records from the time a record is created until it is placed in permanent storage or destroyed. In addition to recording the care given to patients, both electronic health records (EHRs) and paper-based records may be used to review the quality of care and for recording statistical information. The medical record is owned by the provider, but the patient has control over who can have access to the information.

It is impossible for a provider or other professional to remember every detail of care, such as the results of a physical examination or doses of particular medications, especially if questions arise after months or years. Many people in the primary care provider's' office have contact with a patient, as well as consulting professionals, laboratories, and hospitals. It is important that each interaction be recorded in the patient's medical record. This provides an ongoing record of both the patient's state of health and the service provided by the medical office.

Medical records are also used as legal documents, available if there are questions about the care given. If a patient sues a provider, the court will require documentary evidence, such as a medical record, to be presented in court. The court will take the position that whatever is documented in the record is the care that was given. If something is not documented, officially it never happened. To protect the legal interests of the provider's office, it is, therefore, important to keep complete medical records. The contents of the medical record (especially the EHR) were discussed in Chapter 38. This chapter focuses on principles of record management. It is important to discuss management of both the EHR and the paper-based medical record because there are still medical offices that have not switched to an EHR format.

STORAGE OF ELECTRONIC HEALTH RECORDS

One of the advantages of electronic records is that they are filed automatically within the computer system. In an office using paper-based medical records, staff spend large amounts of time filing records and reports. Because every report requires a paper document, the medical record can become very bulky, and storage requires large amounts of space. When an EHR is used, data are entered directly into the electronic system, and records are usually stored on *servers*, large computers that store data and manage tasks for other computers on a network. These servers may either be in-house or contracted from an outside company, often the original provider of the EHR.

MAINTAINING THE INTEGRITY OF THE EHR

LEVELS OF ACCESS

EHRs are always password protected, and in addition, users are usually assigned a level of access that specifies what they are able to do within the medical record. For example, medical assistants should be able to indicate medications that a patient would like to have refilled, but they should not be able to order those medications from the patient's pharmacy. These access levels must be managed by a system administrator or specified individual within the department responsible for maintaining the EHR. Usually, a new employee is granted certain access levels appropriate with their job description, but a department head can request additional access. Procedure 43.1 involves setting up an electronic medical record for a new patient.

STAFF TRAINING TO MAINTAIN INTEGRITY

New hires must be trained in an institution's procedures to maintain the integrity of the EHR. This involves closing the EHR or locking the screen before stepping away from a computer, not leaving patients alone in an exam room with their own EHR visible on the computer screen, and never sharing a password with other staff or allowing other staff members to use the EHR when signed in. Staff should be trained in the procedure to release all or part of the medical record. (This is covered in Chapter 38.) New hires should also be aware of the institution's policy regarding unauthorized viewing of a patient's EHR. In general, a staff member involved in the direct care of a patient is authorized to view and make entries in a patient's medical record. If a staff member views the medical record of a patient without a need to do so, it is a violation of the patient's rights under the Health Insurance Portability and Accountability Act

(HIPAA). Audit controls in the EHR make such an action obvious, and the institution should have a policy regarding the consequences of such activity. Information about maintaining the integrity of the computer system as a whole is found in Chapter 40.

UPDATES

The EHR has the flexibility to be adapted to the needs of the medical office using it, and like every program, it will also have updates to keep it current and/or to improve performance. Special features may be added to record information (e.g., a detailed eye examination in an ophthalmology practice). These may be additional modules purchased from the company that originally developed the EHR, or a large institution may have a technology department capable of programming needed additions to the EHR. In addition to initial staff training, there must be training related to updates and/or initiation of new features. This training may be contracted or provided by in-house staff.

STORING COMPUTERIZED RECORDS

EHRs should be backed up regularly and securely. The system administrator is usually responsible for ensuring that the backup system is implemented according to plan. Backups may be done to network storage and/or storage devices, such as hard drives, cloud-based systems, or other devices. It is important to maintain some kind of backup off-site in case of fire or disaster. Inactive electronic records can be transferred to separate storage if the system capacity becomes strained. The system administrator must also be sure that program updates are compatible with previously stored data. Most practices have multiple backup copies to ensure that no data are lost.

PAPER-BASED MEDICAL RECORDS

Some medical offices still rely on paper-based medical records to document care. A manila file folder is created for each patient, containing all documents related to the care of that patient. These records are maintained in files to be available each time the patient is seen at the office. After the transition to an EHR, the old paper record may be destroyed if the entire record has been scanned. In some offices, most of the paper record is scanned into the new electronic record system, and the old record is placed in storage. However, in most offices, only baseline data and very recent information are entered into the new electronic record, because large charts are time consuming to scan and too much information tends to overwhelm the system. For at least 2 to 3 years after the transition to an EHR, the old paper chart is made available to the provider for each patient visit.

EQUIPMENT AND SUPPLIES FOR PAPER-BASED MEDICAL RECORDS

STORAGE EQUIPMENT

Paper-based medical records may be kept in various types of file cabinets or on open shelves. The choice of equipment depends on the following: the number of people who need to access the medical records, the office layout, and the amount of floor space available. Usually, the records are stored with the files side to side. The files may take up part or all of a room. In a rotary system, the medical assistant can move sections of shelving to access other shelves behind. Large offices may even use an automated system, which stores more records and brings the record to the medical assistant. The room(s), cabinets, or shelves where paper-based medical records are stored should be able to be locked separately when not in use or when the office is closed.

Shelf Filing Units

File folders with side tabs (described later in this chapter) must be used with shelf units to permit the patient's name to be visible on the shelf. A record is placed on the shelf with the bottom edges of the folder down and the side tabs facing outward. This means that the record is accessed from the side, rather than the top, as with drawer filing cabinets.

Shelf files are preferred because they allow easier access to records, and a number of people can have access to the shelves at the same time. For example, a medical assistant may need to retrieve the medical records of patients to be seen that day, while at the same time another medical assistant may need to look up information for an insurance company or to document a patient telephone call.

Shelf units are available in two styles: open-shelf units or pull-down front units. As the name suggests, open-shelf units are open to the environment and cannot be closed. They must be in a room that can be locked separately from other parts of the office. The pull-down front units have lids that can be pulled over the front of the shelves and locked. This protects the records from environmental factors and allows each part of the file to be locked. It must always be possible to lock either the entire medical record room or individual shelving units.

FILING SUPPLIES

File Folders

A file folder is a protective cover used to hold paper-based medical record documents in an organized format. Usually, file folders are made of manila card stock. Flexible metal fasteners at the top of the inside of the folder hold documents in place.

Folders are available with tabs. A **tab** is a projection of a folder that extends beyond the top or side edge of the folder. Folders for a file cabinet with drawers have tabs on the top, whereas folders for shelf units have tabs at the side of the file folder. In the medical office with shelf filing cabinets, a folder with a full-cut side tab is used. Indentations at intervals along

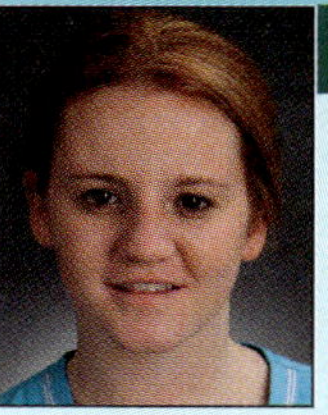

Putting It All Into Practice

My name is Ellen McDonald, and I am a Certified Medical Assistant. I have been working for a cardiologist for about a year. Although our office uses a computer-based billing and appointment system, our patient medical records are still in paper-based format. We file our records alphabetically. The provider plans to retire within 2 years and doesn't want the expense or trouble of changing to an electronic health record. There is always a big stack of reports, correspondence, and other paperwork to be filed. We are not allowed to file any report unless the provider has seen it. In addition, our provider still dictates the progress notes, which are sent electronically to a transcription service. Every day we print the dictation that the transcription service has returned to us electronically, and we stamp them for the provider to initial after he reads them and makes any corrections. I am responsible for making sure the files of medical records are kept in good order. In addition to pulling records and putting them away, I sometimes have to look for misplaced records. If I can't find a patient's medical record, I begin to look for it. First, I check the stacks of records for patients who will be seen that day or the next day. Sometimes a medical record gets caught on another record, so it is important to check through the stacks thoroughly. Next, I check the computer to find out when the patient was last seen. I check on and behind the desks of the provider the patient last saw, as well as the billing desk. I also check through the files looking for a record that has been misfiled. We use color-coded labels, so it is usually easy to see when a record is out of place. These measures are usually enough to find the record, although sometimes it may take as long as a week before the record turns up. One time we looked for a record for 3 weeks before we found it. Whenever I am filing, I am very careful because I remember how much work it is to find a record that has been misfiled. ■

the tab indicate the placement of adhesive labels. This ensures that all the labels on all the medical records are affixed at the same place on the file folders (Fig. 43.1).

Folder Labels

Labels are used to identify the paper-based medical record and are commercially available in rolls or continuous folded strips. Most offices use pressure-sensitive self-adhesive labels. The labels for an alphabetic system assign colors to letters in either the first third or first half of the alphabet, and the remaining letters are assigned the same colors along with some type of distinguishing mark, such as one or two white stripes. If the office uses a numeric filing system, each digit from zero to nine is assigned a specific color. Color-coded year labels are often used to identify the last year a patient was seen at the office. The current year label is placed on a new record and updated the first time a patient has an office visit each year. This allows the records of patients who have not been seen for some time to be removed from the active files and placed in inactive storage.

Chart Dividers

Chart dividers are used to identify each section of the paper-based medical record by subject. Chart dividers are made of a heavy material such as manila card stock. Each divider has a tab for identification. Common categories include Progress Notes, History/Physical, Laboratory Reports, Diagnostic Testing, Hospital Reports, Immunizations/Medications, and Correspondence, but this varies according to medical office requirements.

Mounting Sheets

Laboratory reports, copies of prescriptions, and telephone messages are often filed on mounting sheets with adhesive strips. Usually, several items can be filed on the same sheet. The medical assistant files the first item at the bottom, with each succeeding item shingled up the mounting sheet. With this system the most recent item is always on top. Fig. 43.2 shows this type of mounting sheet.

Other Supplies

An **outguide** is placed in the file to mark the place where a folder has been removed. (Several outguides are shown in Fig. 43.3.) Each guide has a pocket for a card indicating who removed the record and/or items that accumulate while the record is out of its storage area. Another type of outguide is made of heavy cardboard and has lines to write the name of the individual removing the record.

A **sorter** is a device that facilitates placing documents in alphabetic or numeric order. It has pockets or dividers for each letter or number.

What Would You Do? What would You *Not* Do?

Case Study 1

A patient has come to the office to request that a copy of her medical record be sent to another provider. She says that her name is Anna Soubrette and her birth date is April 25, 1962. She says that she has not been seen for 4 years, but her current provider had asked about various medications she had taken for a heart problem in the past. Ellen looks for the medical record in the files for inactive patients under Soubrette, but she does not find any record. ■

PREPARING A PAPER-BASED MEDICAL RECORD FOR A NEW PATIENT

When a patient comes to the medical office for their first visit, a medical record must be prepared for that patient (Procedure 43.2). The method used to prepare the record depends on the following criteria: the format used to organize the record, the filing system, and the type of storage equipment. Most medical offices use the source-oriented format to organize their medical records, the alphabetic filing system to arrange the records, and shelf filing units to

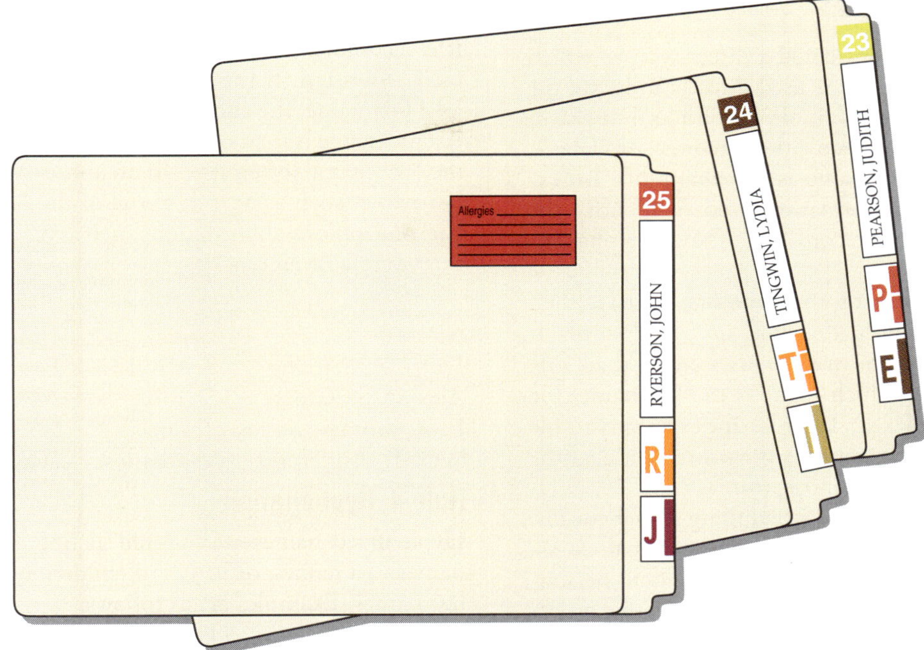

Fig. 43.1 File folders for shelf units have a full-cut side tab. Color labels are affixed in the same position on each folder.

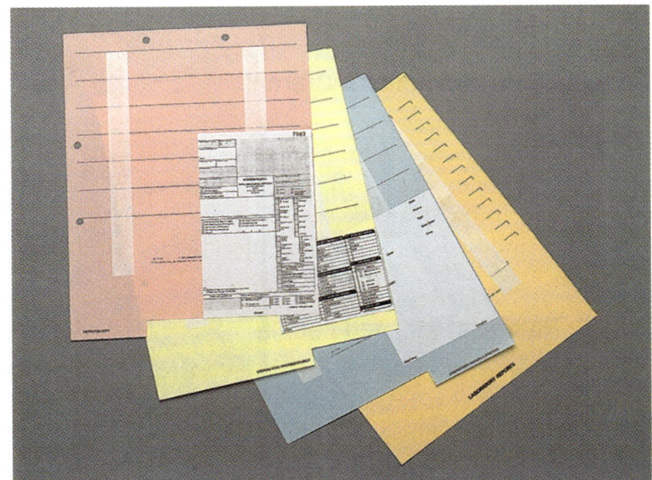

Fig. 43.2 Laboratory reports are often mounted one above another so that the most recent is visible on top. (Courtesy Bibbero Systems, Petaluma, CA, 1-800-242-2376; fax 1-800-242-9330; www.bibbero.com.)

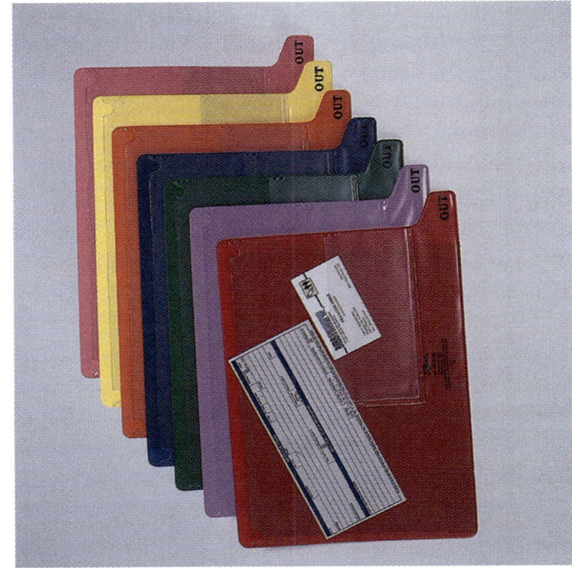

Fig. 43.3 Outguides. (Courtesy Bibbero Systems, Petaluma, CA, 1-800-242-2376; fax 1-800-242-9330; www.bibbero.com.)

store the medical records. Many offices keep partially prepared medical records at the front desk and add the patient's name and labels on the day before or day of a new patient's first appointment.

FILING SYSTEMS

The way in which paper-based records are arranged is referred to as a **filing system.** The primary purpose of a filing system is to facilitate the storage and retrieval of records; a secondary function is to allow for expansion of the records with a minimum of disruption. The two systems most commonly used to arrange paper-based medical records are alphabetic and numeric. Other types of records (such as financial records or office correspondence) can be arranged in chronologic order, by subject, or by geographic location.

ALPHABETIC FILING

The alphabetic system is considered a direct system, which means that the patient's name is used directly to locate the medical record (Procedure 43.3). It is commonly used in medical offices with fewer than 5000 records. Alphabetic filing uses parts of the legal name as indexing units. **Indexing units** are pieces of information used to identify the correct filing location. The records are arranged alphabetically based on the first unit.

All names that have exactly the same first unit are then arranged by the second unit, the third unit, and so on. If the name is unusual, if the patient uses more than one name, or if it is unclear which name is the last name, the record may be cross-indexed. To **cross-index** means to file under one unit and to file a guide or card referring to the primary filing location under another unit.

It is important to follow rules when filing alphabetically. One resource for guidelines is ARMA International, an association for records and information management personnel. The medical assistant must always clarify the procedures followed by any given medical office.

Rule 1: Individual Names

In a patient's name, the **surname** (last name) is the first indexing unit, the given name (first name) is the second unit, and the middle name or middle initial is the third unit. A name with only two units is filed before a name with three units. ("Nothing" always comes before "something.") A unit with only an initial is filed before a unit with a full name beginning with that initial. Business names are indexed in the order of the names in the business (excluding *a*, *an*, and *the*). Examples are as follows:

Name	Unit 1	Unit 2	Unit 3
Alan Stone	Stone	Alan	
Alan C. Stone	Stone	Alan	C.
Alan Charles Stone	Stone	Alan	Charles
Peter H. Stones	Stones	Peter	H.
The Acme Medical Supplies	Acme	Medical	Supplies

Rule 2: Prefixes

If the last name has a prefix, such as *Mc*, *Mac*, *Van*, *de*, *Des*, or *D'*, the prefix is considered part of the last name. Therefore, it begins the first indexing unit. Traditionally these prefixes were lowercase, but nowadays they may be uppercase or lowercase. The prefixes *Mc* and *Mac* are usually filed in regular order. However, in some medical offices, they may all be filed as *Mc*, often as a separate group from other names beginning with *M*. Examples are as follows:

Name	Unit 1	Unit 2	Unit 3
Lyndon A. De Larosa	Delarosa	Lyndon	A.
Stephen P. Dennis	Dennis	Stephen	P.
Mary Ann d'Entremont	Dentremont	Mary	Ann
Joanne McCarthy	Mccarthy	Joanne	

Rule 3: Abbreviations and Nicknames

It is recommended that abbreviated first and last names be filed as written. If the patient commonly uses an abbreviated first name, the abbreviation is used as an indexing unit. If a nickname is used on the record, it is indexed as if it were the legal name (often it is). If an abbreviation is part of the last name (such as *St.*), it is part of the first indexing unit. (In some offices, abbreviations such as *St.* are filed as though they were written out.)

Name	Unit 1	Unit 2	Unit 3
Dottie A. Settland	Settland	Dottie	A.
Alex M. St. Croix	Stcroix	Alex	M.
E. V. Thomas	Thomas	E.	V.
Wm. T. Vanderpost	Vanderpost	Wm.	T.

Rule 4: Hyphenation

Hyphenated names are indexed as one unit, whether first names, last names, or names of children using both parents' last names. Examples are as follows:

Name	Unit 1	Unit 2	Unit 3
Eustace F. Brightfellow	Brightfellow	Eustace	F.
Claire Bryant-Litson	Bryantlitson	Claire	
Ann Marie Smith	Smith	Ann	Marie
Annabelle Smith	Smith	Annabelle	
Ann-Marie Smith	Smith	Annmarie	

Rule 5: Titles and Seniority Terms

Disregard titles unless the complete name is not given or unless they are necessary to distinguish between two individuals with the exact same name. Seniority terms, such as *Jr.*, may be indexed as the last unit. Numeric seniority terms are indexed in numeric order before alphabetic terms.

Rule 6: Names of Married People

Married people may take their spouse's surname, but they retain their own first and middle names. They may also retain their original name or use both their original name and their spouse's name. If two last names are used, they may or may not be hyphenated. It may be necessary to cross-index the name to prevent confusion. Sometimes the hyphenated surname is used only for the couple's children. Examples are as follows:

Name	Unit 1	Unit 2	Unit 3
Mrs. Arlene Sandra Trim	Trim	Arlene	Sandra
Mr. James Walker Trim	Trim	James	Walker
Mrs. John (Sandra A.) Trim	Trim	Sandra	A.
Mrs. Ann Walker	Walker	Ann	
Mrs. Ann R. Walker	Walker	Ann	R.

Rule 7: Companies and Businesses

The names of companies and businesses are indexed in the same order as written. These are not used for medical records, but the medical assistant may use an alphabetic file (either paper or electronic) for telephone numbers. Disregard punctuation, such as commas, apostrophes, or hyphens. Disregard articles such as *a*, *an*, and *the*. When indexing an **acronym** (a word formed in upper case letters using the first letters of all the words in a name, such as NERF, Non Expanding Recreational Foam), the acronym is indexed as one word.

Rule 8: Identical Names

If two names are exactly the same, it is proper to index them first under the name, and then under the location, beginning with the city as the first unit, state as second unit, street as third unit, and street number from lowest to highest. This applies to names of patients and businesses. In the EHR the date of birth is used to distinguish between two patients with exactly the same name.

NUMERIC FILING

In many practices, each new patient is assigned a number. This number is used to identify the patient and file the paper medical record (Procedure 43.4). The patient's number can be accessed with other data in the computer, usually from the name and date of birth, although the patient may also be given a plastic identification card with the medical ID number. A numeric system has two major advantages:

- It is easier to preserve confidentiality.
- In a large practice, it is easier to identify a patient by number when several patients have the same last name.

The main disadvantage of using a numeric system for medical record management is that it is an indirect system. This means a cross-referenced index must be maintained to link the patient's name with the record identification number. Computers can cross-reference information without difficulty, so the EHR is usually linked to a patient identification number as well as the patient's date of birth.

Terminal Digit Filing Systems

A common numeric filing system formerly used in large medical offices and hospitals uses a six-digit number with a hyphen between each group of two digits (e.g., 01-22-19). A system that uses the final group of digits as the first indexing unit is called a **terminal digit filing** system. A terminal digit filing system mixes up **active records** and inactive records in the files, so the numbers of the newest (and usually most active) patients are not all located in the same section of the file shelves, as they tend to be in a consecutive numeric system.

With terminal digit filing, the numbers are indexed by group, working back from the final to the first group (right to left). Within each group the numbers are arranged from lowest to highest. To file the record with the number 01-22-19, the medical assistant would first locate the position of charts that end in 19 (first indexing unit). Assuming that there would be several records that end in -19, the medical assistant would then locate the position of charts that end in -22-19. Finally, the medical assistant would file the record between 00-22-19 and 02-22-19. Examples using two-digit groups are as follows:

Number	Unit 1	Unit 2	Unit 3
89-25-68	68	25	89
48-31-69	69	31	48
48-35-69	69	35	48

Another way to provide nonconsecutive filing is to assign each patient a combination of both letters and numbers. The records are then filed under the letters alphabetically, followed by the numbers.

What Would You Do? What Would You *Not* Do?

Case Study 2

Lorna Bennett, a 45-year-old woman with hypertension, has come to the office for a physical examination. When Ellen takes her to the examination room, the patient says, "I'm glad I had an appointment today because I can take care of two things at once. My husband and I are moving out of state next month, so I guess I will just take my medical record with me today so that I can give it to my new provider out there. That will give me a chance to read it, too. I've always wondered what was in there." ■

Consecutive Filing Systems

In consecutive filing systems, numbers are arranged and filed from the lowest to the highest. When such a system is used for paper-based medical records, zeroes are often assigned or assumed at the beginning of each number. The number of digits is commonly three to six. This depends on the projected number of patients after 5 to 10 years. This type of filing system may be used in a small medical office. In the following example, six digits are used with a consecutive numeric filing system:

Number	Unit 1	Unit 2	Unit 3	Unit 4	Unit 5	Unit 6
000642	0	0	0	6	4	2
000853	0	0	0	8	5	3
001215	0	0	1	2	1	5

SUBJECT FILING

Filing systems for documents (e.g., preprinted forms, invoices, purchase orders, and service agreements) are often arranged according to subject. Within the subject category, documents may be arranged alphabetically or by date. In the medical office, subject filing is often used for insurance, bills, research, or other documents related to running the practice rather than the patient records.

CHRONOLOGIC FILING

In a chronologic filing system, items are filed by date. A tickler file, which is used to "tickle" the memory by serving as a reminder that a specific action must be taken on a specific date, is a type of chronologic system. It may consist of cards or folders. An electronic system is usually linked to a calendar. In a manual system, a card or folder is used for each day of the month, with file guides for each of the 12 months and each day of the month. As each month passes, the day guides are added to items for the current months. A manual system may be useful to identify bills to pay or other activities related to paper documents, but a computer reminder system is often used for daily tasks and/or patient reminders. A chronologic filing system is also useful for filing (or arranging) dated items such as invoices.

ADVANTAGES AND DISADVANTAGES OF FILING SYSTEMS

Alphabetic filing of paper-based medical records is somewhat easier, but numeric systems are best for maintaining privacy. However, numeric systems are more complex because of the need for cross-indexing. When the system is very large, it is easier to prevent confusion if each patient is given a unique number, because many patients may have similar names or even the same name. If several individuals will be filing paper records, a nonconsecutive system such as the terminal digit filing system does make it easier for more than one individual to work comfortably in the filing area, but most large organizations have switched to an EHR. The EHR allows a user to search both alphabetically by a patient's name and numerically by a patient's birth date. The patient also has a medical record number but is not usually expected to be able to identify it.

RETRIEVING OR FILING A PAPER-BASED MEDICAL RECORD

RETRIEVING PATIENT RECORDS

A paper-based patient record has to be removed from its proper location in the file whenever someone in the office wants to look at it (e.g., for an appointment or when a patient leaves a message).

The record is located using the filing guidelines of the particular office. Paper-based medical records needed for patients with appointments on a particular day are usually pulled the afternoon before the appointments, using the printed appointment list. Each time a record is taken from storage, an outguide is placed exactly where the record was removed, as illustrated in Fig. 43.4.

FILING RECORDS

Each day, several records need to be returned to the file when a paper-based record system is used. In most offices, records ready for filing are placed in one location.

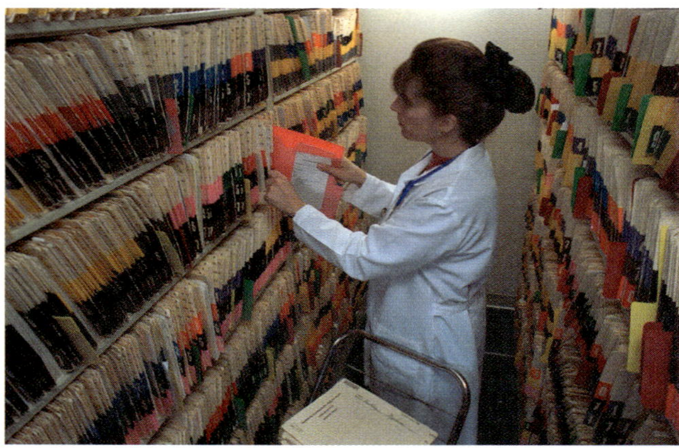

Fig. 43.4 Placing an outguide.

Before filing records or documents, the medical assistant should be sure that the records are ready to file by removing clips or pins and repairing any tears with tape.

A sorter is used to arrange the records so that they can be filed efficiently according to name or medical record number. It is important to locate the correct position to replace the record and remove the outguide. Any items that have been placed in the pocket of the outguide should be filed in the record at this time.

FILING REPORTS AND CORRESPONDENCE

All reports, letters, and other materials that come into the office should be reviewed by the provider, initialed, and then filed in the patient record or scanned into the EHR. A date stamp is often used to identify exactly when a report or letter was received. With the paper medical record, there is no end to the number of papers that the provider must review. Even if an EHR is used, the medical office receives many paper reports and letters that must be reviewed and scanned. The medical assistant must complete any follow-up before filing the report (or record) (Procedure 43.5).

Several steps facilitate filing reports or other items in the paper medical record:

- Each report or note to be filed should be initialed by the provider, and any required action should be completed.
- Reports should be sorted before filing according to name or medical record number.
- Once the correct record has been located, the report is filed at the front of the appropriate section. It may be necessary to remove a section of the record to insert the new item.
- The record should be reassembled before being replaced in the file.
- Reports for items that are not in their correct locations should be set aside. After all other reports have been filed, if time permits, the medical assistant can search for the missing records.

What Would You Do? What Would You *Not* Do?

Case Study 3

When Ellen is pulling paper-based medical records for the next day's appointments, she does not find the medical record for Alan DuBois under "Dubois." The file also has no outguide. Ellen remembers that the patient was seen within the past week or two. She also checks under "Bois," but the record is not filed there either. ■

STORING PAPER MEDICAL RECORDS

The storage area for paper medical records should be well lit and climate controlled. It is important to maintain the relative humidity at 48% to 52% to prevent deterioration of the records. Basement storage is not recommended unless the humidity is well controlled. The records should also be protected from dust, insects, rodents, fires, and floods. As discussed earlier, records should be secure when the office is closed so that unauthorized personnel do not have access to them. The Occupational Health and Safety Administration (OSHA) requires that main aisles leading out of a room or to a fire exit be a minimum of 5 feet wide, and secondary aisles, such as between shelving units, be a minimum of 3 feet wide.

The shelf files should be full enough to allow the folders to stand upright but loose enough to allow folders to be easily stored and retrieved.

HIGHLIGHT on Electronic Signatures

When talking about electronic signatures, it is important to distinguish between actual signatures that are captured electronically and an electronic entry specific to one individual that authenticates identity and can be linked to a specific date and time.

When a medical office uses an electronic health record (EHR), the staff can use two ways to handle actual patient signatures. With the first method, the patient signs a paper consent form and the paper consent form is then scanned into the electronic record. With the second method, the patient reads the consent form, either in a paper version or on a computer screen, and then the patient signs an electronic signature pad that captures an image of the actual signature and inserts it into an electronic version of the form being signed.

Providers and other staff in the medical office usually use an **electronic signature**, an electronic sound, symbol, or process added to an electronic record that indicates intent to sign. These processes are built into the software with safeguards to validate the time of the entry and the identity of the individual making the entry. Electronic signatures are also used for transmitting insurance claims and for validating entries to the EHR. Electronic signatures are valid in all states and are accepted by the Health Insurance Portability and Accountability Act (HIPAA), provided that the software being used validates identity, validates that the document was not altered later, and provides that the user cannot later repudiate the electronic signature.

The term *digital signature* is used for a form of encryption that binds electronic records to an "electronic fingerprint." Digital signatures require validation by private companies called *certification authorities.* The entire document is encrypted and decrypted using public and private keys (mathematic formulas). Digital signatures are used for transferring money and signing legal documents electronically. This level of security is not currently required for EHRs. ■

Memories *from* Practicum

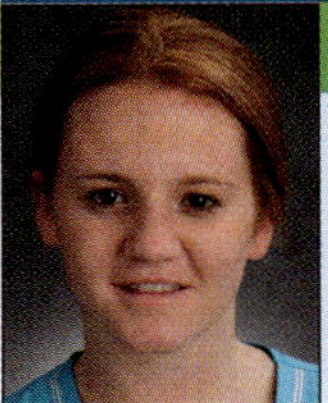

Ellen McDonald: I did my practicum in a clinic affiliated with a large hospital that had made the transition from paper medical records to an electronic health record (EHR). When a patient checked in, we entered the data from the patient information sheet into the computer immediately, and we used a signature pad at the front desk to obtain electronic signatures from the patient for consent to treatment, authorization to disclose information for billing, and acknowledgement of receipt of Health Insurance Portability and Accountability Act (HIPAA) confidentiality information.

Each medical assistant had to log into the system to enter information in the medical record. Even as a student, I was given a password so that I could check patients in, enter vital signs, and enter other information. For example, the machine for electrocardiograms (ECGs) looked like a laptop computer attached to the ECG cables. It was also connected to the EHR. We entered patient information using a computer keyboard. I learned how to print the ECG as a hard copy, but the provider could also view the tracing on the computer.

When the clinic made the transition to the EHR, the records of active patients were scanned into the system, but they kept the paper records for inactive patients. I remember one time when a patient who had not been seen for about 6 years made an appointment. He was experiencing medical problems that he thought might be connected to earlier radiation therapy. I was instructed to create a new electronic record for him, and then I was sent to find the old paper record. Several rooms were full of paper medical records, arranged in order by clinic number. I found it confusing because I was not very familiar with the terminal digit method of filing, but one of the staff members helped me to find the record. After the appointment, I had to return the record to storage. ■

RETENTION OF RECORDS

The length of time for which a medical record must be retained is difficult to determine. Each state has a law limiting the time period for beginning a lawsuit for malpractice. This is known as the *statute of limitations* for medical malpractice. A state may also have a minimum requirement for retaining medical records. In the absence of state regulations, a medical office can review retention guidelines established by the American Medical Association (AMA) in 1994. The AMA recommends that records be retained primarily based on the health needs of the patient, but for at least as long as the state requires or the length of time of the statute of limitations for malpractice claims. For a minor, the time period should be considered to begin at the age of majority. Records of Medicare and Medicaid patients should be retained for at least 5 years after the last contact. Vaccine records should be retained indefinitely.

At the end of the retention period, the inactive paper medical record may be destroyed (by shredding or burning) or put in a final storage place to be kept permanently. The AMA recommends that the patient have an opportunity to claim the record before it is destroyed, if possible. Paper records that are closed (it is known that the patient will not return) may be transferred to microfilm or microfiche. They can also be copied using a laser beam and stored on laser disks. These options are expensive and time-consuming but may be worthwhile for larger practices. Other records that should be kept indefinitely are insurance policies, licenses, and Drug Enforcement Administration (DEA) controlled-substance records. All tax records should also be kept for 7 years; after that, background records used to determine taxes can be destroyed, but copies of tax forms should be kept indefinitely.

What Would You Do? What Would You *Not* Do? RESPONSES

Case Study 1

Page 1118

What Did Ellen Do?

- ❑ Made every possible attempt to find the patient's record.
- ❑ Asked the patient if she could have been seen under another last name.
- ❑ Tried to locate the patient under her maiden name.
- ❑ Attempted to locate the record in the storage area for inactive patients under Soubrette.
- ❑ Even if Ellen was not able to locate the record, she asked Ms. Soubrette to fill out a release of information sheet, took her telephone number, and said she would contact Ms. Soubrette to let her know if she had been able to locate the record.
- ❑ Asked the office manager for other ideas for locating the record.

What Did Ellen Not Do?

- ❑ Did not tell the patient that she must have been thinking about a different practice.
- ❑ Did not assume that the record had been lost or destroyed.
- ❑ Did not tell the patient that after such a long time, the information probably would not be useful anyway.

Case Study 2

Page 1121

What Did Ellen Do?

- ❑ Explained that the office would be glad to send or provide a copy of the medical record to the patient and/or the new provider as soon as Ms. Bennett provided a provider name and address.
- ❑ Encouraged the patient to fill out a release of information sheet for a personal copy of the medical record or to take a form home to mail back when she had selected a new provider.
- ❑ Explained that Ms. Bennett was in charge of the information in the medical record, but the original record belonged to her provider.
- ❑ Notified Ms. Bennett how long it would take to prepare a copy and if any copying fee would be required.

What Did Ellen Not Do?

- ❑ Did not allow the patient to take the original medical record.
- ❑ Did not promise to prepare a copy of the entire medical record that day.

Case Study 3

Page 1123

What Did Ellen Do?

- ❑ Looked up Alan DuBois in the computer to identify the date of his last appointment and who saw him.
- ❑ Checked the provider's' office, as well as the billing desk.
- ❑ Looked behind furniture, especially in the provider's office.
- ❑ Asked other staff members if they had seen this medical record.
- ❑ Created a temporary paper record for the patient if the record was not found before the appointment.

What Did Ellen Not Do?

- ❑ Did not give up looking for the record before she had made an extensive search.
- ❑ Did not accuse any staff member of hiding the medical record.
- ❑ Did not call the patient and change his appointment in case the record could not be located.

TERMINOLOGY REVIEW

Key Term	Definition
Acronym	A word formed from the first letters in a name, written in upper case letters.
Active record	Records that have been used in the last three years.
Cross-index	To file under one unit and use a guide or card filed under another unit that refers to the primary filing location.
Electronic signature	An electronic sound, symbol, or process added to an electronic record that indicates intent to sign.
Filing system	The way in which records are arranged. Common filing systems in the medical office include alphabetic, numeric, by subject, or chronologic.
Indexing units	Pieces of information used to identify a correct filing location.
Medical record management	Activities related to the creation, management, use, and disposition of patient medical records.
Outguide	A cardboard or plastic card to insert in a file when a medical record is removed.
Sorter	A device that facilitates putting papers or records in alphabetic or numeric order.
Surname	Last name or family name of an individual; used as the first indexing unit in alphabetic filing.
Tab	A projection of a folder that extends beyond the top or side of the folder.
Terminal digit filing	A chronologic filing system that uses the last number or number group as the first indexing unit.

PROCEDURE 43.1 Preparing a Electronic Health Record

Outcomes Prepare an electronic health record for a new patient

The following procedure outlines the method for preparing a electronic health record for a new patient.

Equipment/Supplies:

- Computer
- New Patient Information Form

1. **Procedural Step.** Greet the patient when they arrive at the medical office. Introduce yourself and identify the patient. Verify that the patient is a new patient.
2. **Procedural Step.** Ask the patient to complete a patient registration form.
3. **Procedural Step.** When the patient returns the completed form, check the new patient information form for accuracy, and make sure that you can read the patient's handwriting. If you have any questions regarding the information on the form, ask the patient for clarification. Ask the patient for their insurance card and scan it.
   Principle. A copy of the patient's insurance card is used for third-party billing.
4. **Procedural Step.** Enter into the computer program for the electronic health record and enter the data on the completed new patient information form. Search for the patient's name in the computer. If the name does not appear then enter the patient's full name, last name first, into the computer as a new patient. Ensure that the patient's name is spelled correctly.
   Principle. Following these guidelines facilitates the accurate and efficient creation of the patient's electronic health record.
5. **Procedural Step.** Enter all of the patient information needed to create a new patient in the electronic record system. This will include patient information, guarantor information, and insurance information.
   Principle. Ensure that all of the information has been completed on the patient information form.
6. **Procedural Step.** Click on the Save button to save the patient information.
7. **Procedural Step.** Check the electronic health record to ensure that the patient has been registered properly.
8. **Procedural Step.** Print a Notice of Privacy Practices and Acknowledgement form for the patient.

PROCEDURE 43.2 Preparing a Medical Record

Outcomes

1. Prepare a paper-based medical record
2. Organize a patient's paper-based medical record

The following procedure outlines the method for preparing a paper-based medical record for a new patient using the following organization: a source-oriented format stored in shelf files using a color-coded alphabetic filing system.

Equipment/Supplies:

- New Patient Information Form
- Notice of Privacy Practices (NPP)
- NPP acknowledgment form
- File folder with a full-cut side tab
- Metal fasteners
- Name labels
- Color-coded alphabetic bar labels
- Miscellaneous chart labels
- Set of chart dividers
- Blank preprinted forms
- Two-hole punch

1. **Procedural Step.** Greet the patient when they arrive at the medical office. Introduce yourself and identify the patient. Verify that the patient is a new patient.
2. **Procedural Step.** Ask the patient to do the following:
   a. Complete a patient registration form.
   b. Read a Notice of Privacy Practices (NPP).
   c. Sign an NPP acknowledgment form.
3. **Procedural Step.** When the patient returns the completed forms, check the new patient information form for accuracy, and make sure that you can read the patient's handwriting. If you have any questions regarding the information on the form, ask the patient for clarification. Ask the patient for their insurance card and make a copy of it.
   Principle. A copy of the patient's insurance card is used for third-party billing.
4. **Procedural Step.** Enter into the computer the data on the completed new patient information form.
5. **Procedural Step.** Assemble supplies needed to prepare the medical record. Enter the patient's full name into the computer for printing on a name label, following these guidelines:
   a. Enter the patient's name in transposed order as follows: last name, first name, and middle name (or initial).
   b. Enter the patient's name two or three spaces from the left edge of the label and one line down from the top of the label.
   c. Ensure that the patient's name is spelled correctly.
   Principle. Following these guidelines facilitates the accurate and efficient filing of the patient's medical record.
6. **Procedural Step.** Determine the first two letters of the patient's last name and select the appropriate alphabetic color-coded labels. Attach the color-coded labels to the (full-cut) side tab. The labels should be affixed to the folder using the label placement indentations on the tab.
   Principle. Using the label placement indentations ensures that all labels on medical records are affixed at the same place.
7. **Procedural Step.** Affix the name label immediately above the first color-coded alphabetic label.

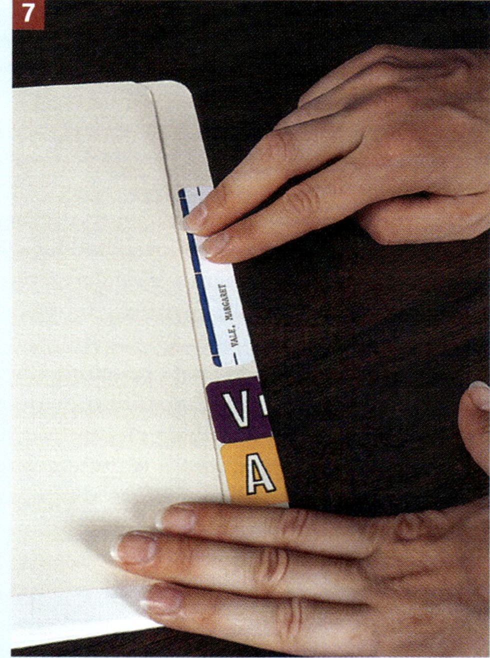

Affix the name label.

8. **Procedural Step.** Attach any additional chart labels, such as a year label and miscellaneous chart labels (e.g., allergy, insurance), to the folder according to the office policy.
9. **Procedural Step.** Insert the chart dividers onto the metal fasteners of the file folder.

PROCEDURE 43.2 Preparing a Medical Record—cont'd

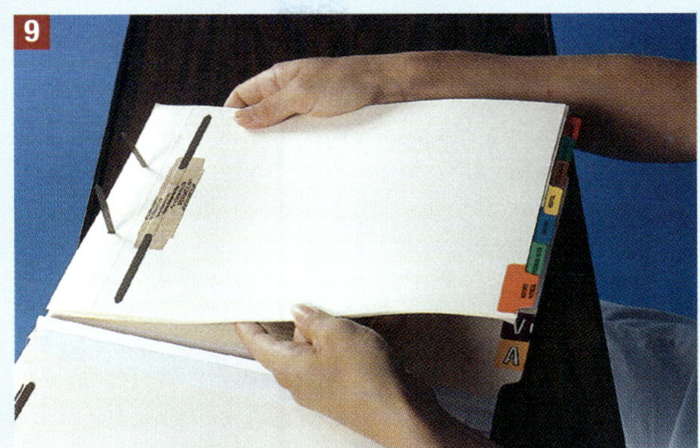
Insert the chart dividers into the metal fasteners.

10. **Procedural Step.** Place the original patient registration form in the front of the medical record. Place the signed NPP acknowledgment form and the copy of the patient's insurance card in the appropriate section of the record.

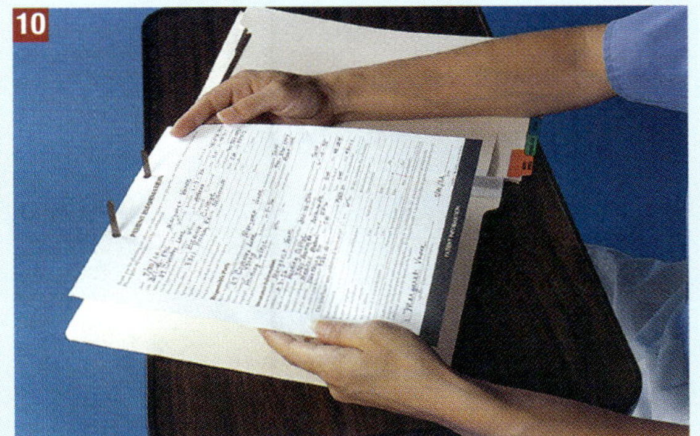
Place the patient registration form in the front of the medical record.

11. **Procedural Step.** Label preprinted forms to be placed in the record with required information such as the patient's name and date. These forms typically include the medical history form, the physical examination form, progress note sheets, and a medication record form. If the forms are not prepunched, the medical assistant must use a two-hole punch to insert two holes into the top or side of the form.
12. **Procedural Step.** Insert each form under its proper chart divider.
13. **Procedural Step.** Check the medical record to ensure that it has been prepared properly.

PROCEDURE 43.3 Filing Patient Records: Alphabetic

Outcomes

1. File paper-based patient records correctly using an alphabetic filing system
2. Maintain organization by filing

Equipment/Supplies:

- Patient records with patient names
- Alphabetic sorter
- File cabinet or shelves
- Outguides
- Index cards

1. **Procedural Step.** Gather the records that are ready to be filed and remove any elastic bands or paper clips.
   Principle. Paper clips, elastic bands, and so on prevent the record from sliding easily into and out of the file.
2. **Procedural Step.** Check the records to be sure that no loose sheets of paper are present. If loose sheets are found, insert them in the record.
3. **Procedural Step.** Sort the records alphabetically by last name, using the alphabetic sorter if available.

Continued

PROCEDURE 43.3 Filing Patient Records: Alphabetic—cont'd

4. **Procedural Step.** Find the correct location in the file for the first record, pull the outguide halfway out, slide the record in front of the outguide in the correct location in the file, and finish removing the outguide. If your office does not use outguides, use your hand to make a space between the record before and the record after the one you are filing.

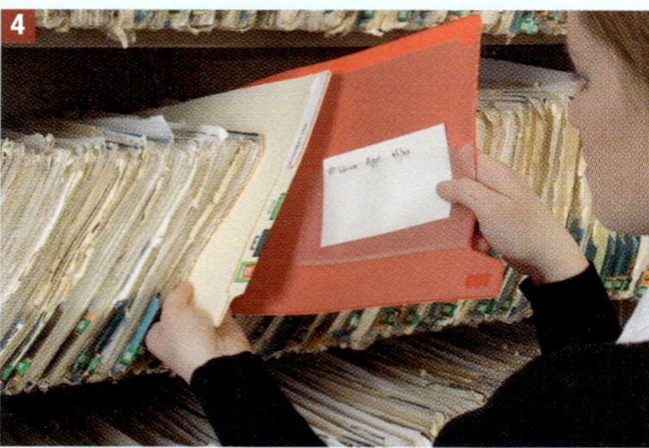

Slide the record in front of the outguide.

5. **Procedural Step.** If there is an index card in the outguide showing who had the record from the outguide, remove it. Place the outguide with other unused outguides. Some offices keep index cards for the providers in separate boxes so that new cards do not need to be written; some offices cross out the name and reuse the index cards; some offices use slips of paper that are discarded after each use.
6. **Procedural Step.** File each record in the same way until all records have been filed.

PROCEDURE 43.4 Filing Patient Records: Numeric

Outcomes

1. File paper-based patient records correctly using a terminal digit filing system
2. Maintain organization by filing

Equipment/Supplies:

- Patient records with terminal digit labels
- File cabinet or shelves
- Numeric sorter
- Outguides
- Index cards

1. **Procedural Step.** Gather the records that are ready to be filed and remove any elastic bands or paper clips.
   Principle. Paper clips, elastic bands, and so on prevent the record from sliding easily into and out of the file.
2. **Procedural Step.** Check the records to be sure that no loose sheets of paper are present. If loose sheets are found, insert them in the record.
3. **Procedural Step.** Sort the records according to the terminal digit indexing units, using the sorter if available.
4. **Procedural Step.** Find the correct location in the file for the first record, based on the final group of numbers. Refine your search based on the middle group of numbers and then the first group of numbers. At the correct location for the record, pull the outguide halfway out, slide the record in front of the outguide, and finish removing the outguide. If your office does not use outguides, use your hand to make a space between the record before and the record after the one you are filing.
5. **Procedural Step.** If there is an index card in the outguide showing who had the record from the outguide, remove it. Place the outguide with other unused outguides. Some offices keep index cards for the providers in separate boxes so that new cards do not need to be written; some offices cross out the name and reuse the index cards; some offices use slips of paper that are discarded after each use.
6. **Procedural Step.** File each record in the same way until all records have been filed.

PROCEDURE 43.5 Filing Reports

Outcomes

1. File reports, correspondence, and other material in a paper-based patient record
2. Organize a patient's paper-based medical record

Equipment/Supplies:

- Medical records
- Assorted reports
- Letters or other material to be filed
- Hole punch
- Tape
- Stapler
- Sorter

1. **Procedural Step.** Assemble materials to be filed and necessary supplies to assist in the filing process.
2. **Procedural Step.** Remove extraneous materials, such as paper clips or pins; mend any tears with tape; and staple related pages together. Punch holes if necessary.
   Principle. Preparation before filing allows all materials in the record to be maintained in good condition.
3. **Procedural Step.** Verify that each report is ready to be filed. In most offices the provider initials reports after they have seen them. If the initials are missing, the report should go back to them.
   Principle. The provider must see each report that comes to the medical office. A procedure verifying that the provider has seen the report before filing prevents reports from being accidentally overlooked.
4. **Procedural Step.** Sort the reports using the sorter alphabetically or numerically, depending on the filing system. Sort by letters, numbers, or number groups first, then sort within each letter or number group.
   Principle. Even in a small office, large numbers of reports need to be filed in patient records if a paper-based record system is used. It is more efficient to file in order, especially when patients have more than one report to be filed.
5. **Procedural Step.** Gather all reports for a particular patient, find the correct record, and insert the report(s) into the record in the correct location. In any section, reports are filed chronologically with the most recent reports at the front of the section. When several reports are shingled on a page, the oldest report goes at the bottom with newer reports progressing up the page and in front of the older reports. You may need to place a divider in the record if you are filing the first report in a given section.
   Principle. The record usually contains several sections in a specific order. Reports need to be in the correct section to be easily located.

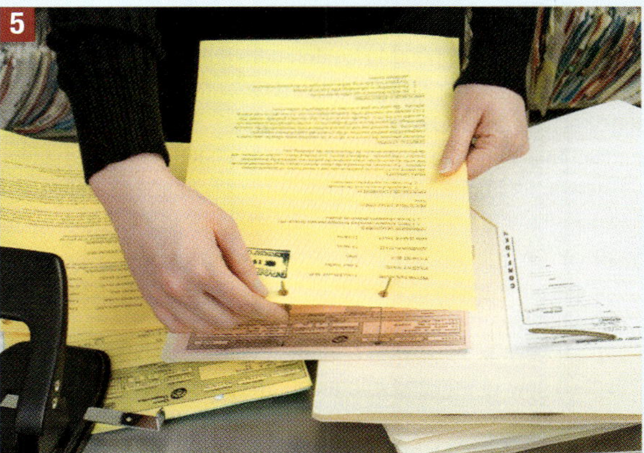

Insert the report(s) into the medical record.

6. **Procedural Step.** Put the record back together if necessary, and file with other medical records.
   Principle. It is easier to file reports in the wrong record when several records are out.
7. **Procedural Step.** If the record is not in the file, place the report back in the sorter or in the pocket of the outguide.
   Principle. It is more efficient to file reports in records you can find easily than to hunt for records just to file reports.

44 Written Communications and Mail

Check out the Evolve site at http://evolve.elsevier.com/Bonewit/today to access additional interactive activities and exercises to help you study and prepare for success.

LEARNING OUTCOMES	PROCEDURES
Business Letters	
1. Define the parts of a business letter.	
2. Identify different formats for preparing business letters.	
3. Explain how to format and compose a business letter.	Composing a business letter.
Responding to Written Communication	
4. Identify how to respond to written communication from businesses and patients.	
5. Identify postal addressing standards for envelopes and mailing labels.	
Memoranda and Other Documents	
6. Describe the process of creating memoranda.	
7. Discuss the importance of using correct grammar, spelling, and punctuation in written communication.	
8. Explain how to prepare and proofread documents.	
E-mail or Other Electronic Transmission	
9. Compare the use and style of business letters and electronic communication, such as e-mail or secure messaging within the EHR.	
10. Explain how to use e-mail and attachments for business communication.	
11. Explain how to transmit information using a fax machine.	
U.S. Mail	
12. Identify the function of the U.S. Postal Service (USPS).	
13. State the purpose of the ZIP and ZIP+4 systems.	
14. Describe the use of the following USPS mail classifications: Priority Mail Express, First-Class Mail, Priority Mail, USPS Retail Ground, and Media Mail.	
15. Correlate available insurance and delivery confirmation services with their appropriate use in the medical office.	
Processing Incoming Mail	
16. List and describe the steps for processing incoming mail.	Processing incoming mail.
Preparing Envelopes for Mailing	
17. Describe how to prepare labels and envelopes for mailing.	Preparing envelopes for mailing.
18. Compare and contrast postage meters and online postage services.	

CHAPTER OUTLINE

INTRODUCTION TO WRITTEN COMMUNICATION
Business Letters
Equipment and Supplies
Parts of a Business Letter
Heading
Inside Address
Salutation or Greeting
Body of the Letter
Complimentary Closing
Signature, Printed Signature, and Title
End Notations
FORMAT OF BUSINESS LETTERS
Setting Up a Letter
Letter Styles
Composing a Business Letter
Responding to Written Communication
POSTAL ADDRESSING STANDARDS
Letters and Large Envelopes

KEY TERMS

annotate (ANN-oh-tate)
barcode clear zone
complimentary closing
e-mail
fax
full block style
grammar
left justified
letterhead
memo (memorandum)
metered mail
modified block style
postage meter
postal bar code
proofread
right justified
salutation
semiblock style
simplified letter style
template
ZIP+4 code

INTRODUCTION TO WRITTEN COMMUNICATION

Until 20 years ago, almost all written communication between the medical office and other parties was managed by letters or forms and mailed through the U.S. Postal Service. Today, it is also common to transmit data electronically or by fax, and these data can be viewed and/or printed in paper form. Regardless of how the written material is transmitted, however, written communication must still adhere to professional standards. The medical assistant is often responsible for preparing and mailing letters, memoranda, reports, and other types of written communication. In addition, it is common to be responsible for e-mails and other electronic transmissions. To do this professionally requires thorough knowledge of grammar, spelling, format, and the technology that supports modern methods of producing written documents. In addition, the medical assistant must be familiar with the implications of Health Insurance Portability and Accountability Act (HIPAA) regulations regulating access to patient health information. These regulations are covered in detail in Chapter 3. The procedure for obtaining consent to release information from the medical record is discussed in Chapter 38.

BUSINESS LETTERS

Letters leaving the medical office—whether sent to a referring provider, a patient, an attorney, another business, or an insurance company—require proper formatting. Some letters may be dictated by the provider and prepared by the medical assistant. The medical assistant may also compose and send letters independently. The medical office may also use form letters and/or templates for routine matters. A **template** is a standard form to which additional data can be added as needed.

EQUIPMENT AND SUPPLIES

Business letters are usually created using a computer and printer. A word processing program is used to create the letter so that formatting can easily be adjusted and any necessary corrections can be made.

The medical office orders stationery and envelopes preprinted with the practice name, address, telephone number, and business logo. Individual provider names may be included if the office is small. A sheet of this type of stationery is called **letterhead.** Blank sheets of the paper of exactly the same type and weight must be purchased for letters that are longer than one page. Photocopies of letters printed on letterhead are often retained for office records in addition to the computer file used to create the letter.

PARTS OF A BUSINESS LETTER

Heading

The heading includes the return address and the date line. The return address is composed of the name and address of the business sending the letter. If office letterhead is used, no return address needs to be added. The date line is the date the letter is mailed in month, day, year order. The month is written out in full on the date line. It is usually entered on the second or third line below the return address. On letterhead stationery, it is placed a few spaces below the bottom of the letterhead.

Inside Address

The inside address includes the name and address of the party to whom the letter is being sent. It is placed above the salutation, usually with one space between the inside address and that salutation. Beginning with the inside address, information is single spaced with one or two blank lines between the separate parts of the letter. The inside address should be located in a position such that the body of the letter is centered top to bottom on the page. If the body of the letter is small, there should be more blank lines between the date line and the beginning of the inside address. If the letter is long enough to require two pages, the inside address begins on the second or third line below the date line.

Salutation or Greeting

The **salutation** (the greeting that is at the beginning of a letter) is found below the inside address separated by one or two blank lines. A business letter is formal, so the recipient's title (e.g., Mr., Mrs., Ms., Miss, Dr.) and last name should be used. The salutation is punctuated with a colon after the recipient's last name. Initials indicating credentials (such as MD or RN) are not used after names in the salutation. Correct examples include the following:

Dear Ms. Wilson:
Dear Dr. Taylor:
Dear Mr. Porto:

If the recipient's name is not known, it is permissible to use "Dear Sir," "Dear Madam," "Dear Sir or Madam," or "To Whom It May Concern." At least one line is left blank after the salutation.

Body of the Letter

The body of the letter contains the content, which should be presented clearly and concisely. A subject line may be used to begin this section. Within a paragraph the letter is single spaced, but one or two blank lines should separate each new paragraph.

Complimentary Closing

The **complimentary closing** (or *complimentary close*) is a term for the words used as a polite ending to a letter just before the writer's signature. It is a sign of respect and can be adjusted depending on how well the letter's author and the party being addressed know each other. "Sincerely" is the standard closing. A more formal closing is "Yours truly" or "Very truly yours." It is followed by a comma and separated from the body of the letter by one or two blank lines.

Signature, Printed Signature, and Title

The signature is the actual written signature of the individual sending the letter. It is added after the letter has been printed. If the letter is being sent electronically the signature can be added to the letter before it is sent. The signature line contains the printed signature of the individual sending the letter, with credentials (e.g., MD). It is entered four to five lines below the complimentary closing to leave room for the written signature. A business title (e.g., Office Manager) is capitalized if used and is entered on the line below the printed signature.

The medical assistant uses their own name and signature for a letter to a supplier or a letter to a patient responding to a billing question. Any letter dictated or composed by a provider will be signed by the provider.

End Notations

Various pieces of information may be given in notations at the bottom of the letter, usually beginning one or two lines below the typed signature. The order of the end notations may vary according to the preference of the office. A reference notation notes the initials of the person who composed the letter (in uppercase) followed by the initials of the person who typed or keyed the letter (in lowercase). The two sets of initials are separated by a colon or a slash. If the letter contains enclosures, such as a log of visits and/or billing records, this is noted in the enclosure notation, on the second line below the title. *Enclosure* or *Enc.* may be used for one enclosure. *Enclosures* followed by the number in parentheses is used for more than one enclosure. This alerts the recipient to make sure that everything the sender intended to include actually accompanies the letter. A copy notation (distribution notation) identifies the recipient(s). The letters "cc" are used, followed by a colon and the name(s) of those who are receiving copies. If a copy is sent to an individual without the knowledge of the recipient or the original letter it is called a *blind copy* (bcc). For a printed letter, the blind copy notation must be added after the original is printed. In an e-mail, the notation *Bcc* can be chosen, and a copy will be sent to the identified recipient or recipients, but there will be no notation of these copies on the original e-mail.

Fig. 44.1 shows a business letter with the parts of the letter identified.

FORMAT OF BUSINESS LETTERS

SETTING UP A LETTER

When preparing letters using a word processing program, the first step is to set the margins. The top margin of the letter should be large enough to accommodate the letterhead (usually 2 to 2½ inches). The side margins may be 1 to 2 inches. Wider margins are used for a short letter. The body of the letter is single spaced.

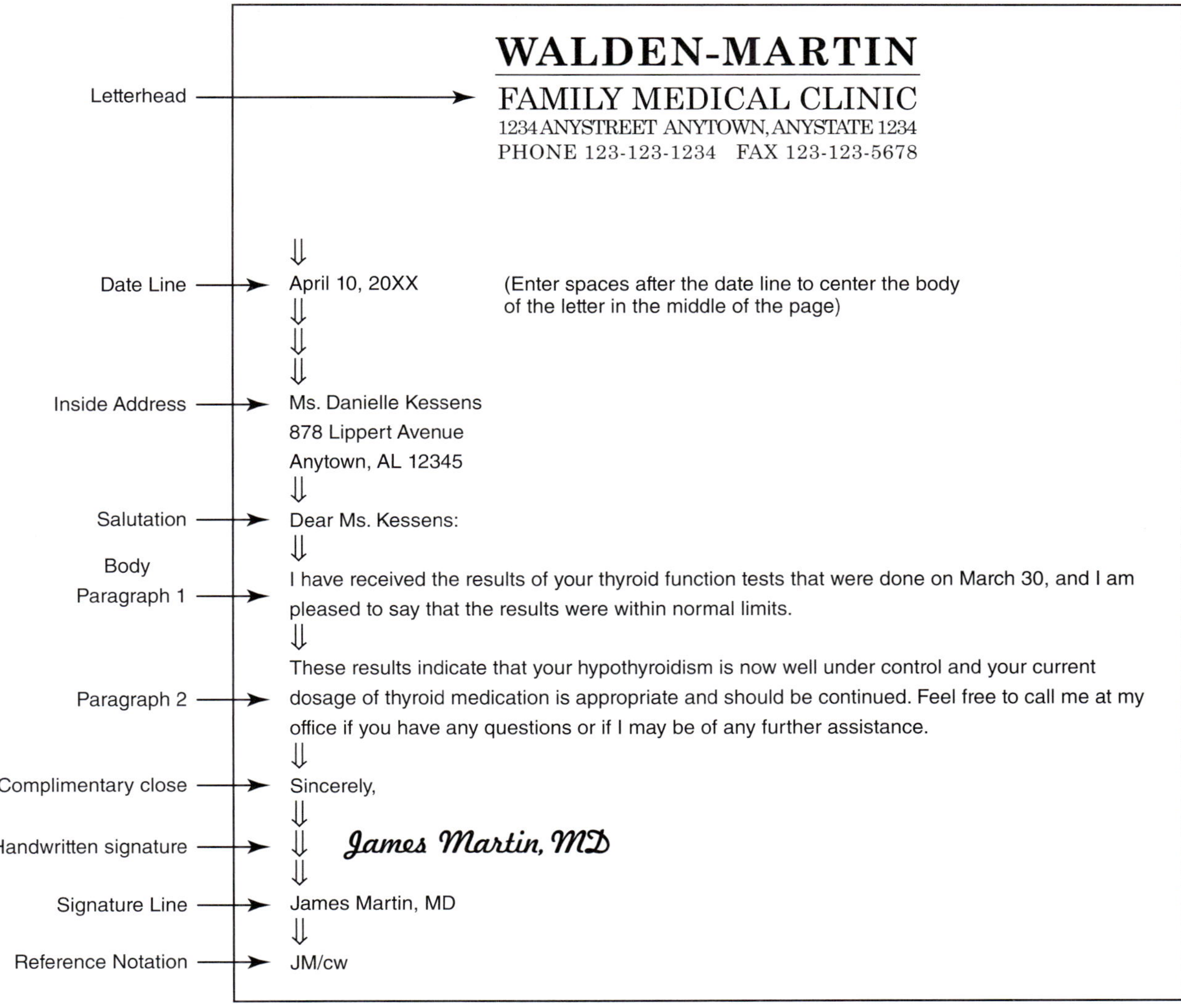
WALDEN-MARTIN
FAMILY MEDICAL CLINIC
1234 ANYSTREET ANYTOWN, ANYSTATE 1234
PHONE 123-123-1234 FAX 123-123-5678

April 10, 20XX

Ms. Danielle Kessens
878 Lippert Avenue
Anytown, AL 12345

Dear Ms. Kessens:

I have received the results of your thyroid function tests that were done on March 30, and I am pleased to say that the results were within normal limits.

These results indicate that your hypothyroidism is now well under control and your current dosage of thyroid medication is appropriate and should be continued. Feel free to call me at my office if you have any questions or if I may be of any further assistance.

Sincerely,

James Martin, MD

James Martin, MD

JM/cw

Fig. 44.1 Sample business letter with the parts of the letter identified.

In writing a business letter, a standard font should be used, such as Times New Roman 12 point. The entire letter should be created in the same font. The word processing program may include a letter wizard, which formats the letter automatically. It is also possible to use or create a letter template so that all letters from the office have the same format.

If the letter has two pages, a header should be placed at the left top margin of the second page with the name of the recipient, the page number, and the date.

LETTER STYLES

- **Full block style:** The letterhead may be centered, but all other lines are **left justified,** which means that they start at the left margin of the page. This allows rapid entry of information and easy formatting. One or two blank lines should be left between paragraphs (Fig. 44.2).
- **Modified block style:** All lines in the inside address, salutation, and body of the letter and reference lines are left justified, and there are one or two blank lines between paragraphs. However, the date line, complimentary closing, and signature lines begin in the center of the letter (they are not centered on the page) or are sometimes **right justified** (aligned with the right margin) (Fig. 44.3).
- **Semiblock style** (also called *modified block with indented paragraphs*): All lines in the inside address, salutation, and body of the letter and reference lines are left justified. Paragraphs are indented five to eight spaces, and there are double spaces between paragraphs. The date line, complimentary closing, and signature lines begin in the center of the letter or are sometimes right justified. Semiblock style is the same as modified block style, except that the first sentence of each new paragraph is indented (Fig. 44.4).

[Letterhead]

July 21, 20XX

Edith Fowler
222 Signal Hill Drive
Western Ridge, OH 44770

Dear Ms. Fowler:

After reviewing the consultation report from Morgan Nephrology Associates, we would like you to schedule a follow-up renal ultrasound in two months. Our office would be glad to schedule this test for you, or you can schedule it yourself. Please call our office at (216) 444-1100 if you need assistance with this matter.

Sincerely yours,

Richard Warner, MD

RW/mt

Fig. 44.2 Sample letter—full block style.

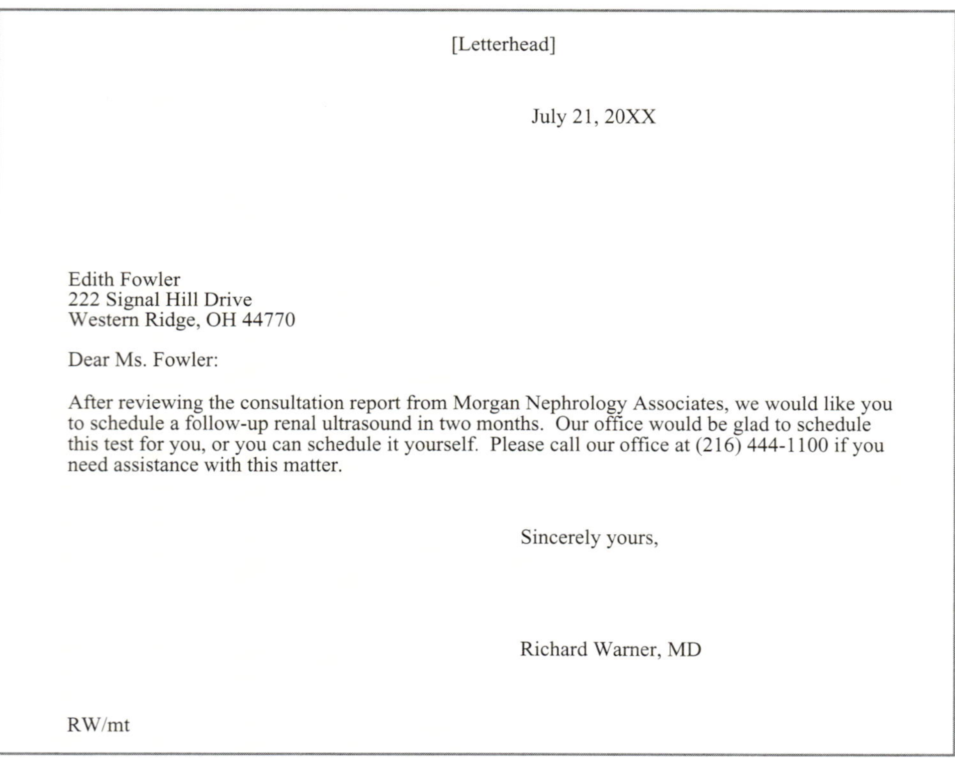

[Letterhead]

July 21, 20XX

Edith Fowler
222 Signal Hill Drive
Western Ridge, OH 44770

Dear Ms. Fowler:

After reviewing the consultation report from Morgan Nephrology Associates, we would like you to schedule a follow-up renal ultrasound in two months. Our office would be glad to schedule this test for you, or you can schedule it yourself. Please call our office at (216) 444-1100 if you need assistance with this matter.

Sincerely yours,

Richard Warner, MD

RW/mt

Fig. 44.3 Sample letter—modified block style.

- **Simplified letter style:** This style resembles a memorandum. Instead of a salutation, a subject line typed all in capital letters is placed three lines below the inside address, and the complimentary closing and signature lines are replaced by an all–capital-letter signature five lines below the letter's body. All letter formats are left justified (Fig. 44.5).

COMPOSING A BUSINESS LETTER

A medical assistant may be asked to create a form letter to send to patients or compose a business letter to order supplies, request information, or handle a problem. In addition to using a professional tone, it is important to use correct grammar and spelling to convey the desired information.

[Letterhead]

July 21, 20XX

Edith Fowler
222 Signal Hill Drive
Western Ridge, OH 44770

Dear Ms. Fowler:

After reviewing the consultation report from Morgan Nephrology Associates, we would like you to schedule a follow-up renal ultrasound in two months. Our office would be glad to schedule this test for you, or you can schedule it yourself. Please call our office at (216) 444-1100 if you need assistance with this matter.

Sincerely yours,

Richard Warner, MD

RW/mt

Fig. 44.4 Sample letter—semiblock style (also called *modified block with indented paragraphs*).

[Letterhead]

July 21, 20XX

Edith Fowler
222 Signal Hill Drive
Western Ridge, OH 44770

FOLLOW-UP RENAL ULTRASOUND

After reviewing the consultation report from Morgan Nephrology Associates, we would like you to schedule a follow-up renal ultrasound in two months. Our office would be glad to schedule this test for you, or you can schedule it yourself. Please call our office at (216) 444-1100 if you need assistance with this matter.

RICHARD WARNER, MD

RW/mt

Fig. 44.5 Sample letter—simplified style.

Before beginning the letter, it is a good idea to jot down the important points to cover in the letter and check to make sure they are presented in a logical order. If the office sends similar letters fairly often, it is helpful to review the wording of old letters. Once the content has been established, the medical assistant should enter the letter into the word processing program using the letter style preferred by the medical office. If they are unsure about the wording of the letter, a draft letter can be printed for the office manager and/or provider to review.

The letter should be proofread for accuracy, grammar, and spelling before the final version is printed. Because letters represent the medical practice, they must be as accurate and professional as possible (Procedure 44.1).

HIGHLIGHT on Letters to Inform Patients of Test Results

Although medical offices use many different methods to inform patients of results of laboratory and diagnostic tests, notifying patients by letter is a method that preserves patient confidentiality and provides consistent and reliable information to the patient about follow-up. These letters may be sent by mail and also posted on the patient portal. Studies have shown that patients prefer to receive all results, whether or not they are normal.

Many medical practices use templates or form letters that allow the medical assistant or provider to fill in the appropriate values and add comments. The final letter may include the actual results or a general statement about the results (e.g., "All your blood test results are within normal limits."). Specific time frames for follow-up testing or instructions to make a follow-up appointment are also included.

If the practice uses an electronic health record (EHR), test results can be tracked in the system to ensure that results have been received from the laboratory or testing facility. It is also possible to track that the patient has been notified and follow-up testing has been performed. Many EHR systems will create and print a letter for the patient. The system can also post an alert when follow-up testing is overdue. If the office uses a paper-based medical record, a separate log book can be kept for laboratory and diagnostic tests to track receipt of results, review by providers, and follow-up to patients.

As a means of managing provider time efficiently while maintaining the personal touch, the medical assistant may prepare the letter, enter the information about the laboratory results, and place the letter with the test results for the provider to verify accuracy, sign the letter, and add any comments. ■

RESPONDING TO WRITTEN COMMUNICATION

On a daily basis the medical office receives letters and/or e-mails that require follow-up. Unless letters are marked "personal" or "private," the medical assistant usually screens correspondence. They may respond personally to correspondence related to supply orders, billing questions, insurance-related questions, and requests for information about the practice. If an urgent response appears necessary, the telephone can be used, but in most cases the response will be in the same format as the original communication.

Correspondence relating to patient care is referred to the provider, and the medical assistant may clip the letter to the patient's medical record if a paper-based medical record system is used in the office. If the provider dictates a reply to a letter, the medical assistant may transcribe the letter or edit and print a letter dictated using voice recognition software. Many patient portals allow a patient to communicate directly with a provider via e-mail.

POSTAL ADDRESSING STANDARDS

Specific standards must be met to prepare a piece of mail so that it can be processed by automated equipment. The medical assistant should be familiar with these standards and put them into practice to ensure the most efficient and timely delivery of outgoing mail.

LETTERS AND LARGE ENVELOPES

To be mailed as a letter, an envelope must be 3½ to 6½ to inches in height and 5 to 11½ inches in length. The two most common sizes for business envelopes are the No. 10 envelope (4⅛×9½ inches) and the smaller No. 6 ¾ envelope (3⅝×6½ inches), but other sizes may be used. Square letters and letters that are too thick to pass through automated equipment require additional postage. The address may be printed directly on an envelope or on a label that will be attached to the envelope.

A large envelope requires more postage. It may be 6⅛ to 12 inches in height and 11½ to 15 inches in length. Large manila or white envelopes may be used to send patient medical records or other documents that have too many pages to fold.

COMPLETE ADDRESS

The USPS defines a complete address as one that includes all elements necessary for delivery, including the Zone Improvement Plan (ZIP)+4 code. To be complete, the address block should include the following elements in the following order:

- Recipient line (Attn: line) (and/or)
- Organization name
- Delivery address (street address including apartment number or suite number or postal box number)
- City, state, and ZIP+4 code

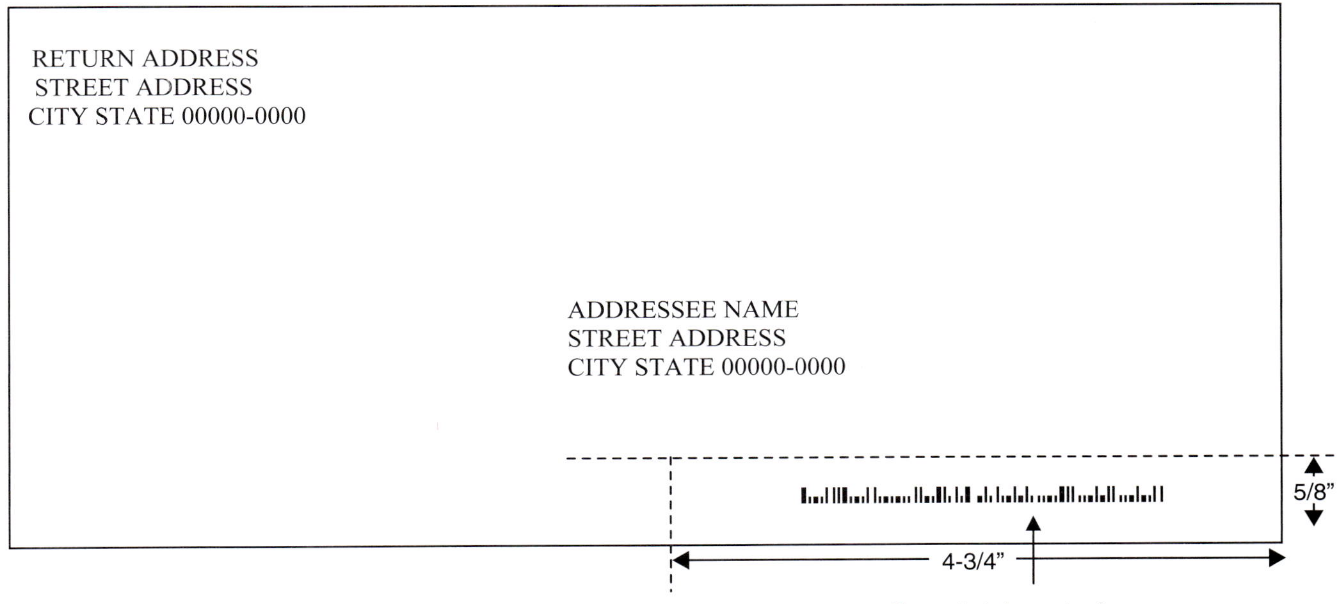

Fig. 44.6 The postal bar code is a series of long and short lines that is either printed by the sender above or below the address, or added, by the post office in the barcode clear zone at the lower right of the envelope.

The post office recommends that the address be printed legibly using upper case letters without punctuation except for the hyphen after the first five digits in the ZIP+4. Recommended abbreviations for elements of the address can be found on the USPS website.

ADDRESS FORMAT

Address format refers to how the various address elements appear on an envelope. The following standards are recommended:

1. The address should be machine printed or hand printed using plain block letters. A typeface without serifs (cross strokes at the end of the main strokes of the letter), such as Helvetica or Arial, is preferred. Script and italic styles should be avoided.
2. All lines of the address should be formatted with a uniform center margin (starting at the center of the envelope).
3. All lines of the address should be parallel to the bottom of the envelope.
4. No punctuation should be used in the address except the hyphen in the ZIP+4 code.
5. If a window envelope is used, the entire address must be visible through the window. No other print should show through the window.
6. Delivery instructions (e.g., "personal," "confidential") should be placed immediately below the return address (see next section). Special services (e.g., Registered Mail, Certified Mail, Insured Mail) should be indicated above the address and to the right of the return address, below or to the left of the area where stamps or postage will be affixed.
7. Address labels should be applied using methods and materials that prevent them from becoming damaged or removed during high-speed automated processing.
8. The address should be placed within an area that extends from ⅝ inch to 2¼ inches from the bottom edge of the envelope with a ½-inch margin on each side. This is called the *optical character recognition (OCR) read area.*
9. The **barcode clear zone** is the area on an envelope where a bar code is printed by the automated equipment. It represents an area that is ⅝ inch high × 4¾ inches long on the bottom right of an envelope. It must remain free of all printing, markings, or colored borders. Unlike supermarket bar codes, which consist of wide and narrow bars, the **postal bar code** consists of long and short bars. If the postal bar code is not included in the address, it is printed by the post office in the barcode clear zone to represent the delivery address (Fig. 44.6).

RETURN ADDRESS

The return address identifies the location to which a piece of mail should be returned if it cannot be delivered. It must be located in the upper left corner of the envelope and must not extend into the OCR read area. The return address should include the following elements:

Sender's name (optional)
Sender's delivery address
Sender's city, state, and ZIP+4 code

Letterhead envelopes or envelopes preprinted with the return address are usually used.

PREPARING MEMORANDA

A common way to communicate within the office is through the use of a **memo (memorandum),** a document

INTEROFFICE MEMORANDUM

TO:	All Staff
FROM:	Howard Lawler, MD
DATE:	6/18/XX
SUBJECT:	Introduction of new office manager

It is my pleasure to announce that effective July 1, Diane Janes, CMA (AAMA), will join our staff as office manager. Ms. Janes has had extensive experience in a variety of medical settings. Most recently she has been employed as office manager in a family care practice in Minnesota. With the relocation of her family to Wisconsin, Ms. Janes has become available to join our practice. I hope that you will join me in welcoming Ms. Janes over lunch in the office on Friday, June 28.

Fig. 44.7 A memo is used for communication within a business.

used within a company that is usually short and limited to one subject. Although a printed form can be used, it is not difficult to produce a template that can be used in a given office. The title "Memorandum" or "Interoffice Memorandum" should appear at the top of the page.

Four headings commonly appear at the top of the memo:

TO:
FROM:
DATE:
SUBJECT:

The headings may be separated from the body of the memorandum by a line that extends from 2 inches to completely across the page. The message should be informative but succinct. The body of the memo is single spaced. There is no signature at the end of the message as who it is from is indicated in the heading. A memo may be printed and circulated to all individuals included in the distribution list, or it may be sent as an e-mail attachment. If the memo is written to all staff members, a copy may be posted on a central bulletin board (Fig. 44.7).

GRAMMAR AND PUNCTUATION

It is important to respond in a timely manner to written communication using proper grammar and spelling. **Grammar** is a term for the accepted rules to create meaningful sentences in a language.

PARTS OF SPEECH

In English, words are classified as one of eight different parts of speech, a set of categories that describe how words are used. Many words can be used in more than one way.

1. *Nouns:* A noun is the name of a person, place, or thing. It can also be a word used to identify a concept or idea. *Common nouns* refer to general things or categories (e.g., *tree, house*). *Proper nouns* are names of specific individuals or places. Proper nouns are capitalized (e.g., *John Stanton, Philadelphia*).
2. *Pronouns:* A pronoun is used in place of a noun. Examples include *I, me, you, he, she, it,* and *they.* Possessive pronouns show ownership (e.g., *mine, yours, hers, its*). None of the possessive pronouns are written with an apostrophe.
3. *Verbs:* A verb shows either action or a state of being. Every sentence requires a verb in order to be complete. Verbs that show a state of being are also called *linking verbs.* Action verbs include *talk, sing, help,* and *communicate.* Verbs that show a state of being include *is, are, feel,* and *seem.*
4. *Adjectives and articles:* An adjective modifies or qualifies a noun. It is a describing word. Examples include *white, pretty, little,* and *thin.* When two or more words are used together as an adjective to modify or qualify a noun, they are often connected by a hyphen (*a 20-year-old woman*). English has three articles: *a, an,* and *the.* They may be included as adjectives or sometimes as a separate part of speech.
5. *Adverbs:* An adverb modifies a verb, adjective, or other adverb. Adverbs include words that question (*how? where?*) and words that end in *-ly* (*slowly, perfectly*).
6. *Prepositions:* A preposition shows the connection of a noun or pronoun to some other word, especially in relation to space, time, or possession. Examples include *on, in, of,* and *to.*
7. *Conjunctions:* A conjunction joins words, phrases, or clauses in a sentence. The common conjunctions include *and, but, or,* and *because.*
8. *Interjections:* An interjection is a word that expresses feelings. It is often followed by an exclamation point. Examples include *oh!, yeah!* and *ouch!* Interjections are rarely used in correspondence or reports.

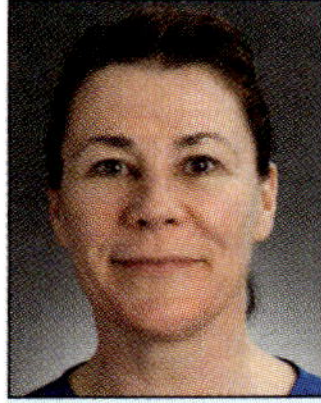

Putting It All Into Practice

My name is Christine Walters, and I am a Registered Medical Assistant. I have been working for a nephrology practice for the past 3 years. This practice was started by two doctors about 15 years ago, and their office is in a building located next to the local hospital. About a year ago a third nephrologist joined the practice, and it is surprising how much more paperwork this has created. Because the providers specialize in diseases of the kidney, our patients are usually referred by other providers. This means that our providers must communicate with the patient's primary care provider for almost every patient they see. Our providers use handheld digital recorders that are connected to our computer network. One of the providers prefers to have his reports formatted as a consultation report, which is sent with a cover letter to the referring provider. We use a template for the cover letter so that he doesn't have to dictate it each time. The other two providers usually include their findings in a letter. I am responsible for preparing these letters and reports, but it really isn't difficult because they follow a fairly regular pattern. The providers create the letters and reports using voice recognition software. I proofread and format each letter as needed, then print a final copy for mailing to the referring provider after it has been signed. It may take me up to 2 hours a day, and when the office is busy, sometimes I do get behind and I may even have to stay late to finish. I have been able to personalize the spell-checker on the computer I use, so even proofreading isn't that difficult. ■

What Would You Do? What Would You *Not* Do?

Case Study 1

The provider asks Christine to send letters to obtain brochures with information about different types of urine chemistry analyzers. He gives her the name of two manufacturers in which he is interested. The provider says, "I don't want to talk to anyone yet. I just want to see some brochures." ■

SENTENCE STRUCTURE

Sentences are composed of various combinations of independent and dependent clauses. A clause contains a subject (noun or pronoun) and a verb. If it can stand alone, it is called an *independent clause.* If it requires an additional clause in order to be meaningful, it is called a *dependent* or *subordinate clause.* Sentence classifications are as follows:

1. *Simple sentence:* A sentence composed of one independent clause. Example: *The dog was very hungry.*
2. *Compound sentence:* A sentence composed of two independent clauses connected by a conjunction. A comma separates the two clauses. Example: *The dog returned from its walk, and it drank all the water in its bowl.*
3. *Complex sentence:* A sentence composed of one independent clause and one or more dependent clauses. If the dependent clause begins the sentence, it is followed by a comma. Example: *When it returned from its walk, the dog drank all the water in its bowl.* If the dependent clause comes after the independent clause, the dependent clause is not separated by a comma. Example: *The dog drank all the water in its bowl when it returned from its walk.*

SENTENCE ERRORS

1. *Sentence fragment:* A sentence fragment is a dependent clause used to stand alone as a sentence. In this case, an additional independent clause is necessary for meaning.
   Sentence fragment: When I arrive for my appointment.
   Correct sentence: When I arrive for my appointment, I will bring my insurance card.
2. *Run-on sentence:* A run-on sentence is a sentence in which two or more independent clauses are joined without a conjunction.
   Run-on sentence: My appointment is on Thursday I will bring my insurance card.
   Correct sentence: My appointment is on Thursday, and I will bring my insurance card.
3. *Comma splice:* A comma splice is the incorrect use of a comma to separate two sentences. The sentences should be separated by using a period and beginning a new sentence or by using a semicolon. It is also permitted to separate the sentences with a comma and a conjunction.

COMMA RULES

1. Use a comma to separate the elements in a series of three or more things. The comma before the conjunction "and" is optional.
   Example: The patient complained of abdominal pain, difficulty breathing, and headache.
   Example: This 40-year-old, well-nourished, White woman was seen on 12/22/2025.
2. Use a comma before a conjunction, such as *and*, *but*, or *or*, when the conjunction connects two independent clauses. An independent clause could be used as a complete sentence.
   Example: The patient called an ambulance, and the ambulance brought her to Memorial Hospital.
   Example: We gave the patient furosemide intravenously, but after an hour her urine output was still poor.
3. Use a comma to set off introductory elements such as prepositional phrases or dependent clauses.
   Example: After the upper gastrointestinal (GI), the patient continued to experience epigastric pain.
   Example: Because we were planning surgery for next week, I did not want to prescribe any new medications.
4. Use a comma to set off information that could be omitted or placed in parentheses without changing the meaning of the sentence.
   Example: The patient, who was referred by Dr. Jenkins, is a 40-year-old woman in good health.
   Example: We will follow this patient closely in the clinic, which is open on Tuesdays and Thursdays.

5. Use a comma before quotation marks except at the end of the sentence where a period precedes the close quotation marks. Do not use a comma to introduce quoted elements introduced by the word *that.*
   Example: The patient said, "My incision burns like fire."
   Example: "My incision burns like fire," said the patient.
   Example: The patient states that her incision burns like fire.
6. Use a comma to avoid confusion.
   Example: For most the year is already finished.
   Example: For most, the year is already finished.
7. Use a comma between the city and the state, the date and the year, a name and a title, and in long numbers. No comma is necessary when only the month and year are used.
   Example: The patient was admitted to Memorial Hospital, Westford, Massachusetts in late July 20XX.
   Example: On July 5, 20XX, the patient was burned severely in a fire in Las Vegas, Nevada.
8. Use commas with terms like *not*, *however*, and *but* to express contrast.
   Example: The wound was large, but healing well.
   Example: The patient, however, had obtained antibiotics from another provider.
9. Use a comma to separate appositives, nouns of direct address, titles that follow a person's name, and introductory words from the rest of the sentence.
   Example: We will make an appointment with Dr. Cannon, a gynecologist, sometime next week.
   Example: Doctor, there is something else I wanted to ask you.
10. Separate parenthetical expressions from the rest of the sentence using commas. These expressions include the following: *I believe*, *I am sure*, *on the contrary*, *indeed*, *of course*, *nevertheless*, *in my opinion*, and *in fact.*
    Example: The report, I hope, will give you more information about multiple sclerosis.
    Example: An inadequate supply of oxygen to the myocardium, for example, is caused by narrowing of the coronary arteries.

SPELLING AND PROOFREADING

SPELLING

Although word processing programs usually provide a spell-check feature, the medical assistant must still proofread all documents for spelling. The spell-check function verifies the spelling of a given word but cannot confirm that it is the intended word or that it is used correctly in context. See Box 44.1 for a list of pairs of words that are commonly confused.

A tool to improve spelling is a personal list of words that cause difficulty. It is important to make an effort to learn these words, and remember to spell-check these words every time they are used. The medical office may purchase a medical dictionary program that can be installed on office computers for reference.

PROOFREADING

After preparing any letter or document, the medical assistant should spell-check or look up any unfamiliar words to spell them correctly. Abbreviations for medical conditions should be avoided, but abbreviations for medication times, measurements, and vital signs are usually acceptable.

It is helpful to use medical spell-check software, which is available from several companies. An ordinary spell-check program can also be personalized over time by adding medical words and abbreviations that the program does not recognize; however, additions should always be checked for correctness. After the document or letter has been keyed, the medical assistant should print a copy, **proofread** it (read it carefully and make corrections), and then correct it and print out a final copy. If there is an unintelligible word, a

BOX 44.1 Confusing Pairs of Words

Nouns and Adjectives

affect (mood) and *effect* (result)
councilor (member of a council) and *counselor* (someone who gives guidance)
ileum (last part of the small intestine) and *ilium* (a bone in the pelvis)
principal (head of a school; most important) and *principle* (basis of a system of belief)
stationary (fixed in place) and *stationery* (paper and other writing materials)

Verbs, Adjectives, and Adverbs

accept (agree or believe in) and *except* (verb: exclude; preposition or conjunction: other than)
adverse (unfavorable or bad) and *averse* (strongly disliking)
affect (to make a difference to) and *effect* (to bring about a difference)
complement (to contribute extra features) and *compliment* (to praise)
continual (happening frequently) and *continuous* (without interruption)
eminent (distinguished) and *imminent* (about to occur)
fewer (not as many) and *less* (not as much)
imply (to suggest) and *infer* (to deduce)
loose (to set free; not tight) and *lose* (to be unable to find)
precede (to go before) and *proceed* (to continue)

Pronouns

whose (shows possession) and *who's* (contraction of "who is")
your (shows possession) and *you're* (contraction of "you are")
its (shows possession) and *it's* (contraction of "it is")
their (shows possession) and *there* (shows location)

space can be left and marked in pencil for the provider to fill in before the final copy is printed.

What Would You Do? What Would You *Not* Do?

Case Study 2

Christine is proofreading a letter created by voice recognition software related to the examination of a patient with hematuria (blood in the urine). She has no difficulty proofreading the patient's history and presenting symptoms, but in the section related to diagnostic testing, there is an abbreviation that is clearly incorrect. She also does not understand the sentence in which the unknown abbreviation occurs. She proofreads the rest of the report and then returns to the section that caused difficulty. She is still unable to make any sense of the abbreviation and the rest of the sentence. ■

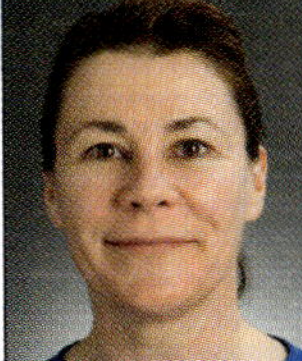

Memories *from* Practicum

Christine Walters: I did my practicum in the office of a family practitioner. I really enjoyed seeing patients of all ages because it gave me different kinds of experiences. In that office they used several different kinds of form letters. For example, their computer system kept a record of infants who were due for immunizations until the child was 2 years old. If the immunizations were more than 1 month overdue, the office sent a letter reminding the parents which immunizations were due and asking them to make an appointment. Twice while I was on my practicum, they gave me a computer printout of the children who were overdue for immunizations to prepare letters for. First, I had to check the computer system for each child to see if an appointment was scheduled in the next month. If there was an appointment, we didn't send a letter. Then I had to prepare a letter for each child still on the list. It was a form letter template, and I used the mail merge function in our word processing program to create a list of names and addresses and create the letters. When all the letters were prepared, I made copies for the medical records. I folded the letters and placed them in window envelopes so that the address was visible. I remember one patient's mother who kept apologizing for forgetting to make an appointment for her son. She said she had not been able to make the appointment when the child was in the office because she wasn't sure of her schedule, and then she just forgot about it. She thanked us for sending the reminder because she didn't want her son to get behind on his immunizations. ■

ELECTRONIC DATA TRANSMISSION

E-MAIL

E-mail (electronic mail) has become an accepted means of communication throughout the business world. **E-mail** is the exchange of information from one computer to another. Medical assistants may use e-mail to communicate with business contacts as well as patients. It is usually faster and more efficient to send an e-mail for a short message.

An e-mail message should contain an informative subject line. Successive e-mails relating to the same subject are usually created as a reply so that the recipient can read the previous correspondence related to the subject. It is polite to acknowledge receipt of an e-mail, even if there is no reply, so the sender knows that the e-mail has been received.

The tone of an e-mail is somewhat less formal than that of a letter, but correct grammar and spelling should be used without any of the abbreviated forms or emoticons that are sometimes used in personal e-mails. Many e-mail programs have spelling tools that should be used. Humor should be avoided because the recipient does not have the nonverbal cues to know when a message is meant to be humorous. The medical assistant should also avoid sending an e-mail containing criticism or other negative content because it is easier to be more negative than intended in writing than when speaking directly to an individual.

E-mails usually use plain text. At the foot of the message, the medical assistant should include the business name, contact information, and an e-mail address and telephone number. Most e-mail programs allow the medical assistant to create an e-mail signature with the contact information to be included at the bottom of every e-mail (Procedure 44.2).

It is important to remember that e-mails are not private. Even after messages have been deleted, they can often be recovered from the computer or network used to create them. E-mail should be used only for business communications that are straightforward and not confidential. It is also always important to be sure that the e-mail is being sent to the correct recipient. It is a good policy to review the recipient name(s) before hitting the "send" button. The account should be set up so that sent messages are saved, but the medical assistant may also want to create printed copies of e-mails related to orders or billing problems.

SECURE MESSAGING WITHIN THE ELECTRONIC HEALTH RECORD

Secure messaging is a common feature within an EHR system. It is also called *clinical messaging* or *clinical e-mail.* Messages sent within the EHR are considered as secure as the EHR itself. The record of an individual patient can be attached to the message. The format and tone are the same as in an ordinary e-mail. Messages can be sent only to users of the EHR system, however.

E-MAIL ATTACHMENTS

Programs for sending e-mail allow documents, images, and other types of files to be attached and transmitted with the e-mail. Unfortunately, many computer viruses are spread through e-mail attachments, so attachments should not be opened unless they are from a trusted source and/or are expected. If an attachment does contain a virus, opening the attachment launches the virus. Any e-mail with an attachment from an unknown recipient should be deleted immediately. If a medical assistant sends a file as an attachment, the recipient may also be hesitant to open the file for the same reason.

The format of an attachment may also pose a problem. The recipient may be unable to open the attachment without the software that was used to create the file in the attachment. Document files can always be saved in text format if there is any question about compatible software. Most files can also be saved as webpages, which the recipient can view with their Web browser.

FAX TRANSMISSIONS

Fax Machine

Paper copies of documents can be sent quickly from one location to another using a fax machine. The word **fax** is a short form of *facsimile* and is a method of transmitting images over telephone lines. The original document is fed into the fax machine, which encodes the images on the paper into signals to be sent over the phone. At the other end, a second fax machine prints black dots on a piece of paper that correspond to the information received. There should be a dedicated telephone line and telephone number for the fax machine, which is shown in Fig. 44.8. The phone number for the fax machine should be listed next to each telephone so that any caller can be told how to fax information to the office.

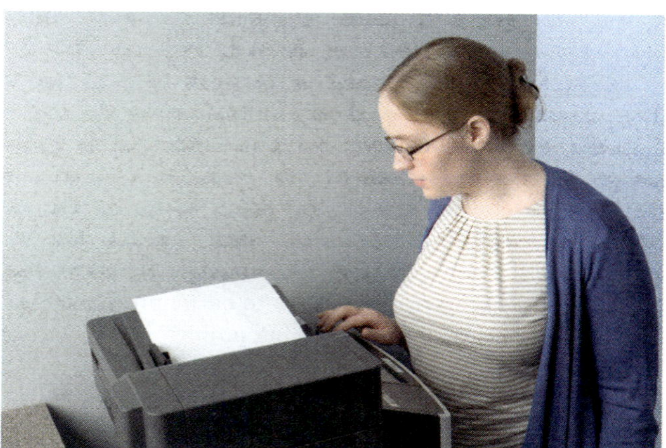

Fig. 44.8 A fax machine allows transmission of images from one location to another using a telephone line.

Sending a Fax

The fax is useful for doing business (e.g., ordering supplies) and for sending out meeting agendas or receiving résumés when hiring. To protect confidentiality, fax transmissions of patient health information should be made only when patient consent has been obtained or in an emergency situation when prompt information transfer is required. A cover sheet should be used for privacy, and the recipient should be notified by telephone when the fax is being sent so that they can remove it from the receiving fax machine promptly. The cover sheet should contain the name of the office, the name of sender, the name of the recipient, telephone numbers of both the sender and recipient, fax number of the recipient, and a confidentiality statement similar to the one in Fig. 44.9.

INTRODUCTION TO MAIL AND SHIPPING

Mail communication is an important aspect of the efficient operation of the medical office. Every day the medical assistant processes incoming mail to facilitate delivery to providers and other employees in the medical office. Preparing outgoing mail is also important.

U.S. POSTAL SYSTEM

The USPS is an independent agency with an official monopoly on the delivery of mail within the United States. It is financed primarily through the sale of postage and postage stamps. The postal service processes an average of 17.6 million pieces of mail each hour and is one of the largest employers in the United States. The USPS provides a variety of ways for mail to be transported from sender to receiver. The cost of these various services depends on the urgency with which mail must be received, as well as any special handling services provided.

CONFIDENTIALITY STATEMENT:

The documents accompanying this transmission may contain confidential information that is protected under the Privacy Act of 1974. It is being faxed to you after appropriate patient authorization or under circumstances that do not require patient authorization. This information is intended only for the use of the intended recipient(s). The authorized recipient(s) of this information is/are prohibited from disclosing this information to any other party unless permitted to do so by law or regulation.

If the reader of this message is not the intended recipient(s) or the employee or agent responsible for delivering the attached information to the intended recipient(s), please note that any dissemination, distribution, or copying of this information is strictly prohibited. **Anyone who receives this information in error should notify the sender immediately and arrange for the return or destruction of the transmitted information.**

Fig. 44.9 A medical office should include a confidentiality statement on the cover sheet for fax transmissions.

ZIP CODE SYSTEMS

In 1963 the USPS introduced the Zone Improvement Program (ZIP) code system. This system enables the postal service to process mail more accurately, quickly, and economically with automated equipment. A ZIP code consists of a five-digit code that identifies the post office to which a piece of mail is to be delivered. In 1967 it became mandatory to use the ZIP code for second- and third-class bulk mailing.

The **ZIP+4 code,** which was introduced in 1983, consists of the original five-digit code followed by a hyphen and four additional digits. These digits identify a specific geographic segment within the five-digit delivery area, such as a city block, an office building, or a group of post office boxes. The plus-four code is required for certain presorted mailings. The USPS maintains a ZIP code lookup service that makes it easy to use the internet to look up the ZIP+4 code for any address in the United States.

CLASSIFICATIONS OF DOMESTIC MAIL

Domestic mail includes mail that is collected and distributed within, among, and between the United States, its territories and possessions, the military service, and the United Nations. Classifications are based on speed of delivery, weight of individual pieces of mail, and number of pieces of mail in the mailing.

Priority Mail Express

Priority Mail Express provides overnight delivery, including on Saturday, to most U.S. locations. Sunday delivery can be provided for an extra charge. Priority Mail Express can be used for letters and packages weighing up to 70 pounds. Envelopes and packing materials are available from the post office. Medical offices may use Priority Mail Express to send laboratory specimens to an outside laboratory for testing. The postage rates for this service are considerably higher than other services, but they do include insurance against loss or damage.

First-Class Mail

First-Class Mail is used for letters or other lightweight items up to 13 ounces. The postage is based on weight, with a base rate for 1 ounce and additional postage for each additional ounce. The medical office uses this mail classification to send letters, postcards, patient statements, and sometimes insurance claim forms (if the office has permission to submit paper claims).

Sending an item First Class usually results in overnight service to local cities and second-day service nationwide. All First-Class Mail should be sealed, and it may not be opened for postal inspection without a federal search warrant.

Additional extra mailing services can be purchased for First-Class Mail, such as Certificates of Mailing, Certified Mail, Registered Mail, Collect on Delivery (COD), and Restricted Delivery. If the item that is being sent First Class is letter size, no additional designation is required on the letter. However, if the item is not letter size, it must be clearly marked "First Class."

Priority Mail

Priority Mail is used for mail weighing more than 13 ounces and up to 70 pounds that will be delivered in the same time frame as First-Class Mail. The USPS has a set rate for items up to 1 pound, and flat rate envelopes and boxes are available. For an item over 1 pound in ordinary packaging, the rate depends on both the weight of the item and the distance it must be transported. For an additional charge, Priority Mail can be combined with other services. An example of an item that might be sent from the medical office by Priority Mail is a copy of medical records.

U.S. Postal Service Retail Ground

USPS Retail Ground is used for less than urgent delivery and for oversized packages. Expected time for delivery is 2 to 8 days. The medical office rarely sends items using this service, but it may receive shipments of medical or office supplies shipped by this method.

Media Mail

Media Mail is a special classification for packages containing printed or digital educational material. It may not contain advertising, computer games, or digital drives of any kind.

What Would You Do? What Would You *Not* Do?

Case Study 3

Jerome Stone, a 68-year-old man who has had two laparoscopic surgeries in the past, calls the office and asks to have a copy of his medical record sent to his new surgeon in another state because he needs to have another surgery for the same condition. He tells Christine that the surgery is scheduled for the following week and asks if she can send the copy of the record immediately. He states that he can come into the office the following day to sign the form giving permission to release the record. He gives her the name, address, and telephone number of the new provider. ■

INSURANCE AND DELIVERY CONFIRMATION SERVICES

The USPS offers a number of extra mailing services. These services must be purchased in addition to the regular postage required to send an item. The extra services that are used most frequently in the medical office are Certified Mail and Return Receipt since these services in combination provide proof of mailing and proof of receipt of a piece of mail. A medical assistant can obtain information about other services from the USPS website. Insurance is purchased when mailing items of value. The cost of insurance is based on the declared value of the contents.

Certified Mail

Certified Mail is available for First-Class Mail and Priority Mail. It serves as legal evidence that an item was mailed by providing the sender with a mailing receipt. In addition, a record of delivery of the certified item is maintained for 2 years. A green certified mail sticker affixed to the envelope identifies the envelope as Certified Mail. The recipient must sign on delivery of a piece of Certified Mail. This service can also be combined with a Return Receipt for an additional fee (Fig. 44.10).

Return Receipt

A Return Receipt provides the sender with proof of delivery of a piece of mail and the signature of the person receiving the mail. This may be done through a postcard signed by the recipient and returned to the sender or by an e-mail with an attachment containing the recipient's signature. The sender then has a copy of the signature of the person who signed for the piece of mail. This service can be combined with other services. It is often used with Certified Mail to establish proof of mailing, as well as proof of receipt (Fig. 44.11).

PROCESSING INCOMING MAIL

Mail is delivered to the medical office in various ways. The postal carrier may deliver the mail directly to the office, or it may be placed in an outside mailbox. Some medical offices use a post office box. In this case the medical assistant must go to the post office to collect the mail each day. In a large clinic the mail may be delivered to a central mailroom, where it is sorted and distributed to each department or individual mailbox.

Once the mail is received by the medical office, it must be processed according to the preferences of individual providers. One provider may want to see all the incoming mail, whereas another provider may want the medical assistant to screen the mail and remove circulars, patient and insurance payments, and magazines for the waiting room (Procedure 44.3).

Incoming mail should be sorted in the following way. If the mail is addressed to a particular provider, it goes into that provider's mailbox or pile. Mail from another provider's office that is not addressed to a particular provider should go into the box or pile of the managing partner, medical director, or office manager.

The medical assistant handles patient and insurance payments, mail from insurance companies, and catalogs from business and medical supply companies. Table 44.1 provides a guide for sorting incoming mail.

OPENING MAIL

Once the mail has been sorted, it must be opened. The medical assistant must know which mail they are to open and which is to go unopened to the individual who must deal with it. Some providers like to open their own mail, whereas others like to have the mail opened, organized, and ready for them to read and respond to. Clearly, any mail marked "personal" or "confidential" should not be opened.

If the provider or providers prefer mail to be opened, the medical assistant should use a letter opener to open each piece carefully at the top edge. An automated letter opener facilitates this process in a larger office or clinic where there is a lot of mail. Each letter or report is stamped with the receipt date and then alphabetized by the patient's last name. The pages of each report should be stapled together,

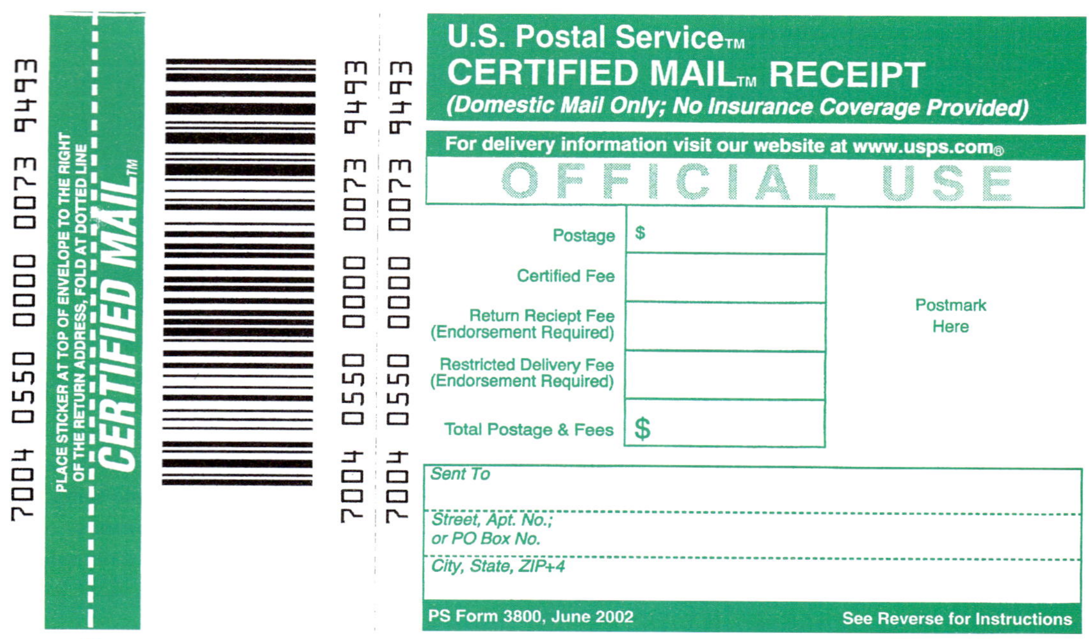

7004 0550 0000 0073 9493

PLACE STICKER AT TOP OF ENVELOPE TO THE RIGHT OF THE RETURN ADDRESS, FOLD AT DOTTED LINE

CERTIFIED MAIL™

7004 0550 0000 0073 9493

7004 0550 0000 0073 9493

U.S. Postal Service™

CERTIFIED MAIL™ RECEIPT

(Domestic Mail Only; No Insurance Coverage Provided)

For delivery information visit our website at www.usps.com®

OFFICIAL USE

Postage $

Certified Fee

Return Reciept Fee (Endorsement Required)

Restricted Delivery Fee (Endorsement Required)

Total Postage & Fees $

Postmark Here

Sent To

Street, Apt. No.; or PO Box No.

City, State, ZIP+4

PS Form 3800, June 2002 See Reverse for Instructions

Fig. 44.10 A Certified Mail Receipt form must be filled out by the sender and signed by the recipient.

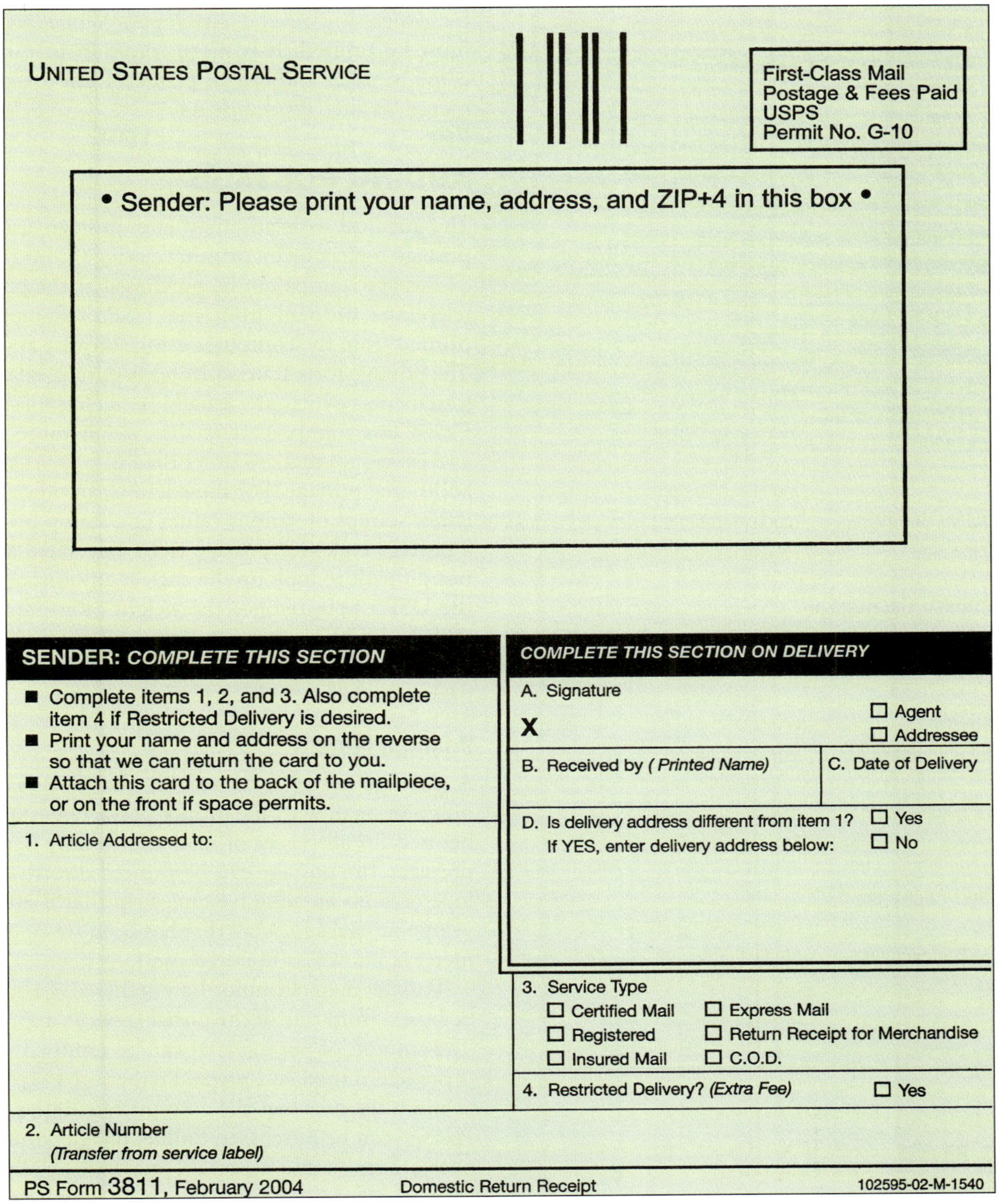

UNITED STATES POSTAL SERVICE

First-Class Mail
Postage & Fees Paid
USPS
Permit No. G-10

• Sender: Please print your name, address, and ZIP+4 in this box •

SENDER: *COMPLETE THIS SECTION*

- Complete items 1, 2, and 3. Also complete item 4 if Restricted Delivery is desired.
- Print your name and address on the reverse so that we can return the card to you.
- Attach this card to the back of the mailpiece, or on the front if space permits.

1. Article Addressed to:

2. Article Number
(Transfer from service label)

COMPLETE THIS SECTION ON DELIVERY

A. Signature
X ☐ Agent ☐ Addressee

B. Received by *(Printed Name)* C. Date of Delivery

D. Is delivery address different from item 1? ☐ Yes
If YES, enter delivery address below: ☐ No

3. Service Type
☐ Certified Mail ☐ Express Mail
☐ Registered ☐ Return Receipt for Merchandise
☐ Insured Mail ☐ C.O.D.

4. Restricted Delivery? *(Extra Fee)* ☐ Yes

PS Form 3811, February 2004 Domestic Return Receipt 102595-02-M-1540

Fig. 44.11 The sender must fill out a Return Receipt form.

if they are not already that way. A letter or report containing patient information should be attached to the patient's medical record with a paper clip if a paper-based medical record is used. Some offices use a cover sheet on the top of each report, on which the provider can check off the action they wish to occur with regard to the report (e.g., file, respond, call the patient).

Non–patient-related items are stacked together to be dealt with by the medical assistant or another member of the staff. Medical journals addressed to a particular provider can be put in their mail pile; those addressed to the practice can be put into the medical library or staff lounge. If the office is large, each staff member may have a cubicle in a central location.

Some providers may instruct the medical assistant to annotate letters. To **annotate** means to underline or highlight important words or phrases in the correspondence. This saves the provider time when reading and responding to the mail. The medical assistant may also be instructed to underline or highlight abnormal values on laboratory reports or diagnostic tests.

When a provider is on vacation, someone on the office staff is delegated to review their mail and refer any urgent mail to the provider by telephone or e-mail at the vacation location or to a covering provider. Arrange mail that is not urgent by date received for the provider to review when they return to the office.

Table 44.1 Sorting Incoming Mail

Mail Category	Recipient
First-Class Mail	
Correspondence addressed to the provider marked "Confidential" or "Personal"	Provider
Correspondence from an attorney	Provider
Laboratory reports	Provider (attach laboratory report to patient's paper-based medical record)
Patient records	Provider
Patient payments	Medical assistant
Insurance payments	Medical assistant
Bills for office supplies and equipment	Medical assistant
Bank statements	Medical assistant
Letters from insurance companies	Medical assistant
Résumés for employment	Medical assistant
Periodicals, Circulars, Catalogs	
Professional journals	Provider
Medical convention and seminar information	Provider
Pharmaceutical advertising	Provider
Advertisements for equipment and supplies	Provider or medical assistant
Magazines for the waiting room	Medical assistant
Catalogs for equipment and supplies	Medical assistant
Drug Samples and Packages	
Overnight packages	Screen appropriately
Administrative and clinical office supplies	Medical assistant
Drug samples	Medical assistant (place in drug sample storage area)

OUTGOING MAIL

The process of preparing items for mailing may include addressing envelopes, preparing mailing labels, folding letters or statements to place into envelopes, calculating and adding postage, and mailing items either in mailboxes or at the post office.

PREPARING ENVELOPES OR MAILING LABELS

Most word processing programs have a feature that creates and prints an address (and return address if desired) on various sizes of envelope. The medical assistant selects the envelope function and enters the delivery address (and return address if not preprinted on the envelope). A single envelope can then be placed in the manual feed tray for printing. Some printers have an optional envelope feed tray for processing several envelopes. When several addresses must be printed, it is more common to use labels. These come in pages and can be printed from lists using the mail merge feature (Procedure 44.4).

ADDING POSTAGE

The medical assistant may add postage using stamps or postage meters or by printing postage from the computer.

Postage stamps can be purchased at the post office or by telephone or mail from the USPS. Stamps can also be printed from the computer using software and stamp labels. The postage for a stamp printer is purchased online. Patient statements, which are usually sent First Class, require one First-Class stamp. Letters that weigh more than 1 ounce and envelopes that are larger than 6⅛ × 11½ inches require additional postage. For these letters, an office would require either stamps of various values or a stamp printer, as well as a postage scale, for postage to be calculated accurately. It is not difficult to look up the correct amount of postage using the USPS website once the weight of an item has been established. Offices that regularly send out a steady volume of mail often use a mechanical postage meter or an online postage service.

Postage Meters

A **postage meter** is a machine that automatically stamps outgoing mail with the proper postage. Postage meters may be used for all classes of mail and for any denomination of postage. The postage can be printed directly onto an envelope or onto an adhesive tape strip that is affixed to an envelope or package. Mail that has been stamped by a postage meter is known as **metered mail**.

Postage meters cannot be purchased. Instead, they must be leased from one of the postal service's approved **vendors**. The amount of postage that can be stamped with the meter is predetermined and prepaid either on a regular basis, such as monthly, or when the amount remaining is getting low. Postage can be purchased online, by telephone, or from the post office. To use a postage meter for bulk mailings, the medical office must apply for a bulk mailing permit and pay an annual fee.

Many different types of postage meters are available, ranging from simple to complex models. The simplest model has only the ability to stamp the mail. More complex models, on the other hand, have security features and may automatically weigh the mail, fold and insert letters into envelopes, seal the envelopes, and catch envelopes in a stacker tray. Complex models typically consist of two separate components: the meter that adds the postage and a base that performs the other functions. A base that is compatible with the chosen model of postage meter can be purchased outright by the medical office.

Safety Precautions

Certain safety precautions should be followed when using a postage meter:

1. Read the operating guide carefully before operating the postage meter.
2. Do not touch any moving parts of the postage meter when it is in operation.
3. Make sure to keep loose clothing, jewelry, and long hair away from all moving parts of the postage meter.
4. Do not cover the ventilation slots on the machine, to prevent overheating.
5. If a paper jam occurs, unplug the machine and make sure all machine mechanisms have come to a stop before clearing the jam.
6. Never attempt to disassemble the machine for repair. If service is required, contact the manufacturer's service representative.

Online Postage Services

The medical office may also subscribe to a service that allows the medical assistant to purchase, calculate, and print postage directly from the computer. These services usually allow the client to print stamps, print shipping labels, print postage directly on envelopes, and add special services (e.g., insurance, delivery confirmation, Return Receipt requested). The computer program can also check the accuracy of the address. Postal scales can be integrated with the computer software to calculate postage automatically. Online postage services offer increased versatility with respect to printing and personalizing labels, but if an office has a large volume of First-Class envelopes, a postage meter with envelope handling features may provide more efficient mail handling.

What Would You Do? What Would You *Not* Do? RESPONSES

Case Study 1

Page 1139

What Did Christine Do?

- ❑ Looked up the two companies mentioned by the provider using the internet to obtain the exact business names and addresses and model numbers of machines in which the provider might be interested.
- ❑ Also looked for other companies that might manufacture similar machines.
- ❑ Prepared letters to each company requesting information using the usual format for office letters.
- ❑ Used the salutation "Dear Sir or Madam."
- ❑ Proofread and signed the letters before mailing.
- ❑ Made a note to follow up after a week.

What Did Christine Not Do?

- ❑ Did not ask the provider how to find the addresses.
- ❑ Did not initiate a contact that would result in a call by a salesperson.
- ❑ Did not send the letters out with an incomplete address or with errors.

Case Study 2

Page 1141

What Did Christine Do?

- ❑ Asked another medical assistant in the office if she knew what the abbreviation should be.
- ❑ Tried to look it up in a dictionary of abbreviations to make sense of the sentence.
- ❑ If still unable to identify an appropriate abbreviation, left a blank line in the letter and indicated on a sticky note that the provider should fill in the blank.
- ❑ After the letter was reviewed by the provider, corrected the letter and printed a new copy for the provider to sign.

What Did Christine Not Do?

- ❑ Did not leave the abbreviation if it did not make sense, hoping that the provider would not notice.
- ❑ Did not mail the letter without correcting and reprinting it.
- ❑ Did not interrupt the provider to ask about the confusing abbreviation and sentence.
- ❑ Did not complain to other office staff about the voice recognition software program.

Case Study 3

Page 1143

What Did Christine Do?

- ❑ Asked Mr. Stone if he wanted her to send the form to sign for release of the medical record as an e-mail attachment.
- ❑ Informed Mr. Stone of the standard charge for copying a medical record and also whether he would be required to pay for postage.
- ❑ After receiving the consent form, took precautions to maintain privacy of Mr. Stone's record while printing a copy of it.
- ❑ Determined the best way to send the record so that it would arrive in time. Obtained authorization to send the record Priority Mail Express or Priority Mail if it was not office policy to charge the patient for postage.

What Did Christine Not Do?

- ❑ Did not tell Mr. Stone that his request could not be granted because there wasn't enough time.
- ❑ Did not send the record before receiving the signed consent form to release the record.
- ❑ Did not criticize Mr. Stone for making an unreasonable request.
- ❑ Did not fail to follow up on this request.

TERMINOLOGY REVIEW

Key Term	Definition
Annotate	To underline or highlight important words and phrases in correspondence.
Barcode clear zone	The area on the lower right-hand corner of a card or envelope that is left clear for the postal bar code to be printed.
Complimentary closing	Words used as a polite ending to a letter just before the writer's signature.
E-mail	The exchange of information from one computer to another using telecommunication.
Fax	Transmission of scanned, printed material by telephone. A short form of the word *facsimile.*
Full block style	A letter format in which all parts of the letter are left justified.
Grammar	The study of accepted rules used to create meaning in a language.
Left justified	Lines of type that begin at the left margin of a document.
Letterhead	A sheet of stationery preprinted with information about a business, including name, address, telephone number, and other information as needed.
Memo (memorandum)	A form of communication within a company that is usually short and limited to one subject.
Metered mail	Mail for which the postage has been applied using a postage meter.
Modified block style	A format for business letters in which the date line, complimentary closing, and printed signature line are on a tab at the center or right justified and all other parts of the letter are left justified.
Postage meter	A machine that automatically stamps a piece of mail with the correct postage.
Postal bar code	A series of vertical bars of two lengths, which represent the delivery address of a piece of mail.
Proofread	To identify and correct errors in a document.
Right justified	Type that is aligned with the right margin of a document.
Salutation	The greeting that begins a letter.
Semiblock style	A letter format in which the date line, complimentary closing, and printed signature line are on a tab at the center or right justified, all paragraphs are indented five to eight spaces, and the other parts of the letter are left justified.
Simplified letter style	A letter format in which all elements are left justified. The greeting is replaced by a subject line in all capital letters. The complimentary closing and typed signature are replaced by a typed signature in all capital letters.
Template	A standard form to which additional information can be added as needed.
Vendor	A company from which supplies are equipment is purchased.
ZIP+4 code	A detailed mailing code consisting of the original five-digit ZIP code followed by a hyphen and four additional digits that identifies a specific geographic segment within the delivery area.

PROCEDURE 44.1 Composing a Business Letter

Outcome Compose a professional business letter

Equipment/Supplies:

- Letterhead stationery
- Blank stationery
- Computer and printer

1. **Procedural Step.** Assemble materials, determine the address of the recipient, and decide on a format for the letter.
2. **Procedural Step.** Formulate the content for the business letter. List and organize the essential content to be sure all necessary information is included.
3. **Procedural Step.** Insert the date on the second or third line below the letterhead. For block style, the date is at the left margin. For modified block style and semiblock style, the date begins at the center of the line.
4. **Procedural Step.** Place the inside address four to 10 lines below the date at the left margin. If using a computer, adjust the number of spaces below the date line after the letter has been keyed so that the body of the letter is centered on the page.
5. **Procedural Step.** Place the salutation on the second line below the inside address, leaving a blank line between elements. The salutation should include a title and the person's last name (e.g., Dear Dr. Gordon, Dear Mrs. Wilson, Dear Rev. Meyers). It is followed by a colon.
   Principle. A business letter is more formal than personal correspondence.
6. **Procedural Step.** If desired, place a subject line on the second line below the salutation. A subject line begins

PROCEDURE 44.1 Composing a Business Letter—cont'd

with the Latin abbreviation *re* (meaning "about") followed by a colon. The abbreviation is usually capitalized (e.g., RE: Annual meeting on Thursday, June 12, 20XX).

Principle. Although optional, a subject line helps the recipient identify the subject of the letter before reading it.

7. **Procedural Step.** Begin the body of the letter on the second line below the salutation (or subject line, if used). The body of the letter is single spaced, and double spaced between paragraphs. In block and modified block letter styles, the paragraphs begin at the left margin. If semiblock style is used, indent the first line of each paragraph five to eight spaces.
8. **Procedural Step.** The final paragraph of the letter should summarize the contents and/or most important ideas.
9. **Procedural Step.** Place the complimentary closing on the second line below the final paragraph of the body of the letter. For the block letter style, the complimentary closing begins at the left margin. For the modified block letter style, it begins at a tab directly below the date line. The complimentary closing is followed by a comma.
10. **Procedural Step.** Drop down four lines and insert the first and last name of the sender followed by their credentials. Begin the typed signature directly under the complimentary closing. Place a job title, if appropriate, on the next line.

    Principle. Typing the name under the handwritten signature facilitates a response because the signature may be difficult to read.
11. **Procedural Step.** If necessary, add a reference line, enclosure notation, and/or distribution notation below the typed signature at the left margin. Double space between each notation. If you compose and key your own letter, a reference line is unnecessary. If you compose and key a letter for someone else, place your initials in lowercase letters. If you key a letter that was dictated by the person signing the letter, place their initials (uppercase) followed by your initials (lowercase) separated by a colon or slash. The enclosure notation may be written out or abbreviated "Enc." The number of enclosures is placed in parentheses if there is more than one. The distribution notation identifies individuals who receive a copy of the letter. The letters "cc" followed by a colon are used with the name of the individual receiving a copy.

    Principle. The person who receives the letter is entitled to know who prepared the letter and who received copies. If the number of enclosures is indicated, it is easier to tell if all intended material is enclosed with the letter.
12. **Procedural Step.** If the letter is longer than one page, the second page should be printed or typed on stationery of the same quality and weight as the letterhead stationery, beginning 1 inch from the top. Include the name of the recipient, the date, and the page number in the top left corner. Space the letter so that at least two lines of the body of the letter continue to the second page.
13. **Procedural Step.** Spell-check the letter and proofread it carefully. If using a computer, print the letter.

    Principle. A business letter should not contain errors. If errors are present, the credibility and professionalism of the sender may be doubted.
14. **Procedural Step.** Obtain the appropriate signature or sign the letter below the complimentary closing.
15. **Procedural Step.** Make a photocopy of the letter for your files and for any individual who will receive a copy of the letter. If the letter refers to a patient, a copy should be filed in the patient's EHR or a photocopy in a patient's paper-based medical record.

    Principle. Copies of all business letters are retained in case there are questions or further correspondence is necessary.
16. **Procedural Step.** Prepare an envelope (see Procedure 44.4) and place the letter in the designated area to be prepared for mailing. If the letter concerns a patient, a copy of the letter is filed in the patient's medical record. Other letters (e.g., letters to suppliers) are usually filed in folders by subject.

PROCEDURE 44.2 Composing a Business E-mail

Outcome Compose a professional e-mail

Equipment/Supplies:

- Computer

1. **Procedural Step.** Determine who should receive the e-mail. Add their names to the To field.
2. **Procedural Step.** Develop a concise Subject line for the e-mail.
3. **Procedural Step.** Formulate the content for the business e-mail. List and organize the essential content to be sure all necessary information is included.
4. **Procedural Step.** Place the salutation on the first line of the e-mail. When sending the e-mail to an individual the salutation should include the title and the person's last name (e.g., Dear Dr. Gordon, Dear Mrs. Wilson). When addressing a group make sure that salutation correctly addresses everyone that will be receiving it (e.g., Dear Insurance Department).
5. **Procedural Step.** Begin the body of the e-mail on the second line below the salutation. The body of the e-mail is single spaced, and double spaced between paragraphs.
6. **Procedural Step.** Place a complimentary closing on the second line below the final paragraph of the e-mail.
7. **Procedural Step.** Insert your first and last name followed by your credentials. Place a job title, if appropriate, on the next line.
8. **Procedural Step.** Proofread the e-mail. Click send.

PROCEDURE 44.3 Processing Incoming Mail

Outcome Process incoming mail

Equipment/Supplies:

- Letter opener
- Date stamp
- Paper clips
- Stapler
- Pen or highlighter
- Transparent tape

1. **Procedural Step.** Assemble supplies in a work area large enough to make several piles of mail.
2. **Procedural Step.** Stack all the envelopes so that they face in the same direction. Place any envelopes marked "personal" or "confidential" to the side.
   Principle. Letters marked "personal" or "confidential" should be opened only by the person to whom they are addressed.
3. **Procedural Step.** Tap the lower edge of the first envelope on the desk so that the contents fall to the bottom.
   Principle. Tapping the envelope prevents cutting the contents when opening the envelope.
4. **Procedural Step.** Using a letter opener, open the envelope along its top edge.
   Principle. Using a letter opener makes it easier to open the envelope neatly and preserves the return address should it be needed.
5. **Procedural Step.** Remove the contents of the envelope. Check to be sure the envelope is empty.
6. **Procedural Step.** Unfold and flatten letters. Date stamp each letter, preferably in the upper right-hand corner of the letter.
   Principle. A date stamp provides a record of when the letter was received.

PROCEDURE 44.3 Processing Incoming Mail—cont'd

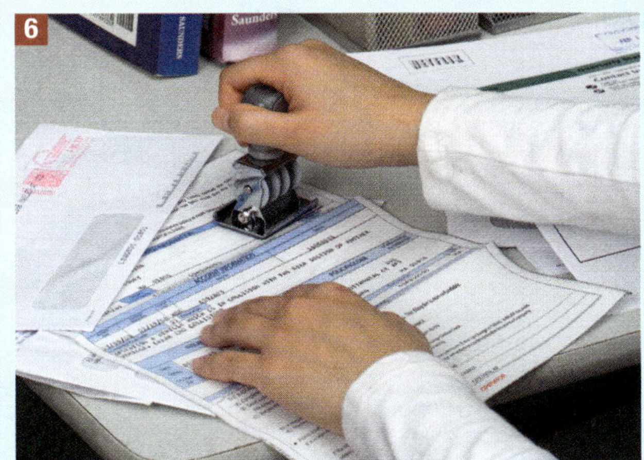

6 Date stamp each letter.

7. **Procedural Step.** Check to make sure that the letter contains an inside address. If not, staple the envelope to the letter. Discard the envelope if it is not needed, unless office policy states otherwise.
8. **Procedural Step.** Fasten enclosures to the letter with a paper clip. If a letter indicates an enclosure, but it is missing, write "No" next to the enclosure notation and circle or highlight it.
9. **Procedural Step.** Mend any torn paper with transparent tape to prevent further damage.
10. **Procedural Step.** If directed by the provider, annotate the correspondence by underlining or highlighting important words and phrases in the correspondence. Attach a sticky note indicating any action that should be taken in response to the correspondence.
    Principle. Annotating saves the provider time in reading and responding to incoming mail.
11. **Procedural Step.** Follow the same steps to open each piece of mail as described earlier, and separate the pieces of mail into categories: urgent or very important, other letters, letters or reports containing patient information or results, medical journals, and circulars or advertising.
12. **Procedural Step.** Arrange letters and reports containing patient information in alphabetic order. If the office uses paper-based medical records, find the appropriate medical record and attach each letter or report to the medical record with a paper clip.
13. **Procedural Step.** Arrange the mail for each provider with the most important mail on top and the least important on the bottom.
14. **Procedural Step.** Distribute each stack of mail to the appropriate individual.

PROCEDURE 44.4 Preparing Envelopes for Mailing

Outcome Address an envelope, and process envelopes to be mailed

Equipment/Supplies:

- Envelope
- Other items to be mailed
- Labels (optional)
- Typewriter (optional)
- Computer and printer
- Postal scale
- Postage meter (optional)
- Stamps

1. **Procedural Step.** Determine the exact address to be used to address the envelope. Addresses may be kept in a computer file or manually in an index card box or circular card file (e.g., Rolodex).
2. **Procedural Step.** Select an envelope of the appropriate size. For business letters a No. 10 envelope is most commonly used. A large manila envelope may be used for documents containing several pages.
3. **Procedural Step.** Decide on a means to address the envelope (e.g., typewriter, computer, label printer). The address may be printed directly on the envelope or on a label. Avoid addressing ordinary correspondence by hand.
   Principle. Standard business correspondence appears more professional if addressed using a typewriter or computer.
4. **Procedural Step.** Key the address near the center of the envelope in the OCR read area with the name of the recipient on the first line, the street address and apartment or suite on the second (or second and third) line, and the city, state, and nine-number ZIP code on the bottom line. Punctuation is not required

Continued

PROCEDURE 44.4

PROCEDURE 44.4 Preparing Envelopes for Mailing—cont'd

except for a hyphen after the first five numbers of the ZIP+4 code. If using an envelope without letterhead, key the return address in the upper left corner using the same guidelines.
Principle. These are guidelines recommended by the U.S. Postal Service (USPS).

5. **Procedural Step.** Add any special notations, such as "Personal" or "Confidential," below the return address and above the address at the left side of the envelope.
Principle. Nothing must be placed below the address, so the post office equipment can read the envelope correctly.
6. **Procedural Step.** Add any mailing instructions or special services (e.g., "Certified") on the right side of the envelope above the address, leaving room for a postage above.
7. **Procedural Step.** Place the item to be mailed in the envelope, folding it as needed, and seal the envelope (unless a postage meter with a sealer will be used).
8. **Procedural Step.** Weigh the piece of mail if it contains more than two sheets of paper or if an envelope larger than 6⅛×11½ inches is used.
Principle. Large envelopes, rigid envelopes, and envelopes that are not rectangular require more postage than First-Class letters weighing less than 1 ounce.
9. **Procedural Step.** Calculate and apply the correct amount of postage. One First-Class stamp or equivalent is required for First-Class letters weighing less than 1 ounce. Postage for other items may be calculated from the USPS website, using a postage meter, or using an online postage service. If a postage meter is used, all envelopes to be mailed in 1 day may be processed together.
10. **Procedural Step.** Assemble all letters and other items to be mailed.
11. **Procedural Step.** Sort envelopes according to size.
12. **Procedural Step.** Separate any items with special mailing instructions that must be taken to the post office. If necessary, add instructions to the envelopes. If the office does not have a postal scale, include any letters that may need extra postage.
13. **Procedural Step.** Place items with postage in a mailbox, or request a pickup from the postal service.
14. **Procedural Step.** Take special items to the post office. This may include items that are to be sent Return Receipt or Certified Mail, items that need to be insured, and stamped items weighing more than 13 ounces.
Principle. Items requiring delivery confirmation and Priority Mail weighing more than 13 ounces will not be accepted from a mailbox even if proper postage is attached.

Managing Practice Finances

 Check out the Evolve site at http://evolve.elsevier.com/Bonewit/today to access additional interactive activities and exercises to help you study and prepare for success.

LEARNING OBJECTIVES	PROCEDURES
1. Describe how computerized methods of maintaining patient accounts are based on former manual systems.	
2. Identify the information contained in a fee schedule and describe how it is used.	
3. Describe the information contained in a patient account ledger.	
4. List the steps to post charges, payments, and/or adjustments to the patient account.	Posting charges to the patient ledger. Posting payments and/or adjustments.
5. Describe the process to print patient ledgers, day sheets, or other reports using a practice management computer system.	
6. Differentiate between accounts receivable and accounts payable.	
7. Describe how to inform patients about financial obligations for services received.	Demonstrating professionalism and sensitivity when requesting payment for services rendered.
8. Identify various types of bank accounts.	
9. Describe precautions to take when accepting cash, checks, credit cards, or debit cards.	
10. Discuss methods to transfer funds electronically.	
11. Describe how to balance a cash drawer.	
12. Describe how a bank deposit is prepared and made.	Preparing a bank deposit.
13. Describe how entries are made in the cash disbursement journal.	
14. Describe how to maintain a petty cash fund.	

CHAPTER OUTLINE

KEY TERMS

ABA routing number
accounting
accounts payable
accounts receivable
accrual (ah-KREW-ul) basis of accounting
adjustment
assets
balance due
bookkeeping
cash basis of accounting
cashier's check
certified check
credit
day sheet
debit
disbursements
fee schedule
invoice
ledger
liabilities
Medicare advance beneficiary notice (ABN)
MICR line
payee (pay-EE)
petty cash
reconciling

INTRODUCTION TO DAILY FINANCIAL ACTIVITIES

A medical office is a business. The business of a medical office is providing medical services—one of the most important services in the entire economy. Because the medical office is a business, daily management of the medical office's finances is key to the providers' ability to provide the best services possible for patients. If the medical office's bills are not paid and fees are not collected, the medical office will cease to be a viable business and the patients will suffer.

Accounting is the term for systematic recording and reporting of financial transactions. The **cash basis of accounting**, which is usually used by medical offices, enters income when payment is received for services. This contrasts with the **accrual basis of accounting**, in which income is entered at the time of sale, even if payment has not yet been received. Companies that sell merchandise usually use the accrual basis of accounting. In both systems, expenses are entered when they are incurred, even if they have not yet been paid.

Bookkeeping refers to the process of keeping detailed records of financial transactions. Managing the daily finances is a task that often falls to a medical assistant. Professional accountants are usually responsible for general aspects of financial management, such as preparing detailed financial reports, financial planning, and preparing tax returns.

This chapter focuses on the parts of the daily financial activities involved in charging patients for the services provided each day, maintaining patient accounts and other **accounts receivable** (money owed to the medical office), and managing the **accounts payable** (money the medical office owes).

MAINTAINING PATIENT ACCOUNTS

Patient accounts make up the bulk of the medical office's income. Some income might come from rental of space—for instance, to a particular laboratory for a specimen collection station or to a social worker, psychologist, or other specialist who consults for the medical office. Other income may come from royalties—from a particular medical instrument that one or more of the providers developed, for instance, or from a book written by the professionals in the medical office. But the bulk of the medical office's income will be earned on a daily basis from the charges for services to patients.

Patient accounts may be recorded manually but most medical offices today use a computerized medical billing system, although they may maintain or print some manual records. If there is an electronic health record (EHR), the billing system (practice management system) is usually linked to all or part of it. Although a manual bookkeeping system avoids loss of data when there is a computer failure, most medical offices today use ongoing backups and therefore prefer the versatility of a computerized billing system. The trend towards large hospital-owned ambulatory care practices means that billing (including insurance billing) can be performed by the hospital billing department. Manual systems are considered outdated, although many medical office billing programs are still built on the manual model, which consisted of the following:

- A daily journal, commonly called a *day sheet*, to record all transactions that occurred on that day.
- An accounts receivable ledger for each patient, to keep a record of transactions related to that patient.
- A cumulative record of financial activity, both for the practice as a whole and for each individual provider.

When procedures are performed, charges for individual patients are entered into the medical computer billing program and automatically posted to the patient's account and the daily record of charges. In a modern practice management program that coordinates with the EHR, the provider can enter the services provided at the end of the patient visit, specify the diagnosis (and diagnosis code) that applies, and link them to the billing system. In a similar way, payments made by the patient (or an insurance company) are posted to both the patient account and the daily record of charges. The computer program can access data to generate patient bills, insurance claims, and a variety of reports, including monthly statements, activity of individual providers, and the number of specific procedures billed.

HIGHLIGHT on Bookkeeping Systems

The two most common systems for keeping records of accounts are single-entry and double-entry systems. Historically, financial transactions were recorded in a book called a *ledger* with separate pages for individual accounts. In medical offices, separate cards began to be used for individual accounts (instead of pages of a book). These cards came to be called *ledger cards*, and in medical computer billing programs, a screen showing cumulative charges and payments for a single patient is called a *patient ledger.*

The Accounting Principle

A common formulation of the accounting principle is as follows:

Assets = Liabilities + Owner's equity

where assets are property owned by the business, liabilities are debts, and owner's equity is the amount by which the owner's assets exceed liabilities.

Single-Entry Bookkeeping System

The single-entry bookkeeping system is the simplest system and is usually used in individual medical offices. It requires at least three records:

1. A chronologic journal that keeps track of all charges and patient payments, such as a daily journal.
2. A journal that keeps track of payments made by the medical office, traditionally a checkbook but now usually an electronic record of a checking account.
3. A method to keep track of individual patient accounts. These used to be recorded on pages of a book, index cards, or ledger cards, but today they are usually accounts in a computerized practice management program.

Although the single-entry system is simple, its methods for cross-checking to prevent and/or detect errors are incomplete.

Double-Entry Bookkeeping System

The double-entry system is the most complete type of bookkeeping system. It is used by manufacturing or retail businesses, hospitals, and other large health care institutions. However, it usually requires a trained bookkeeper or accountant to be used effectively.

Every transaction is posted into two different records, as a credit in one and a debit in the other. A credit is a posting that is subtracted from the balance, and a debit is a posting that is added. Records of **assets**—money and property owned by the business and money owed to the business—are balanced against records of **liabilities**—money owed to others by the business.

A charge for a service to a patient, for example, is a credit (added to the balance) in the records of assets because it increases the total assets, but it is a debit (subtracted from the balance) in the records of liabilities because it decreases the amount owed to the business.

If a double-entry bookkeeping system is used by a medical office—for example, if the medical office is owned by a hospital or other large health care institution—the medical assistant is usually responsible only for keeping the daily journal and entering charges, payments, and adjustments in the computer. The actual records of assets and liabilities are kept by an accountant. ■

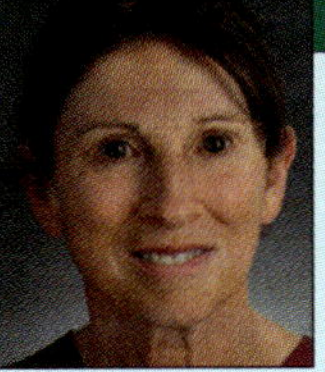

Putting It All Into Practice

My name is Maria Hernandez, and I am a Registered Medical Assistant. I work at the office of three providers who specialize in internal medicine. One of my duties is to manage patient accounts. The providers enter the service provided into the EHR at the time of the visit, and we verify the charges and enter payments and copayments. I also enter almost all of the payments we receive in the mail, including checks from patients, as well as posting insurance payments that are received by electronic transfer to individual patient accounts. I am also responsible for paying the bills for the medical office. Our patient billing is linked to our EHR, but we have another computer program to manage our accounts payable and pay bills. We also use online banking, and we have set up automatic bill payments for those bills that occur every month, including our mortgage, condominium fee, electricity, telephone, and answering service bills. We also pay many of our other bills online. The computer accounting program tracks all payments and it can print checks for new pieces of equipment or other expensive items. All of the providers are authorized to sign checks under $500.00. If we purchase an item that costs more than $500.00, a check must be signed by any two providers. When I was in school, I didn't appreciate what a big job it is to manage financial accounts. I really enjoy this part of my job now, and I have come to understand that it always saves time to work carefully and to avoid mistakes. ■

COMPUTERIZED CHARGE ENTRY

When the computerized billing system is linked to the EHR, the provider specifies the services provided and links each service to a diagnosis at the time of the visit. The front desk staff member then formalizes the charge entry by creating an electronic superbill or using a transaction entry function. Each service must be linked in the computer to a procedure code and a diagnosis code for insurance billing purposes. Coding is discussed in Chapter 46. Computerized billing programs and EHRs usually link to the ICD-10-CM so that the provider can select the correct diagnosis code for each procedure. Paper charge slips containing procedure codes and diagnosis codes (also called *superbills* or *encounter forms*) are not usually used if the practice management software is included or linked to the EHR (Fig. 45.1).

Western Medical Center
109 River Street
Western, OH 44770-0421
(490) 555-6464

Richard Warner, MDNPI # 23456781XX
Maria Gomez, MD NPI # 34567891XX
Tax ID 52-XX63777

Patient Name and Address	Birthdate	Subscriber Name	MD Name	Today's Date
DARLA SISSLE 10 MAPLE STREET WESTERN, OH 44770	2/17/1952	DARLA SISSLE	WARNER	6/26/20XX
	Account #	Insurance Company	Insurance Phone #	Time
	1015	SHHMO	(490) 565-2000	10:00 AM
Telephone No.		Insurance ID #	Group/Plan #	Sex
(490) 220-1156		21-58624	8300099	Male ☐ Female ☒

√	DESCRIPTION	CPT	FEE	√	DESCRIPTION	CPT	FEE	√	DESCRIPTION	CPT	FEE
	OFFICE VISIT				**IMMUNIZATIONS**				**PROCEDURES**		
	NEW PATIENT				Imm. admin, one	90471		√	ECG w/interpretation	93000	65--
	Straightforward/ 15–29 mins	99202			Imm. admin, each add'l	90472			Spirometry	94010	
	Low level/ 30–44 mins	99203			Influenza < 3	90657			Inhalation treatment	94640	
	Moderate level/ 45–59 mins	99204			Influenza 3 and >	90658			Remove skin tag <15	11200	
	High level/ 60–74 mins	99205			Medicare code	G0008			Cerumen removal	69210	
	ESTABLISHED PATIENT				Varicella	90716			Wart destruction < 14	17110	
	Minimal/Nurse Visit	99211			DTaP	90700			I & D abscess	10060	
	Straightforward/ 10–19 mins	99212			Td adult	90718					
	Low level/ 20–29 mins	99213			Rubella	90706					
	Moderate level/ 30–39 mins	99214			MMR	90707			**OTHER**		
	High level/ 40–54 mins	99215			Hep B Child	90744					
	WELL VISIT				Hep B Adult	90746					
	NEW PATIENT				IPV	90713					
	Infant–1 year	99381			**WELL VISIT**				**LABORATORY**		
	1 yr–4 yr	99382			ESTABLISHED PATIENT				Blood collection Vein	36415	
	5 yr – 11 yr	99383			Infant–1 year	99391			Venipuncture, Medicare	G0001	
	12 yr–17 yr	99384			1 yr–4 yr	99392			Finger stick, glucose	82948	
	18 yr –39 yr	99385			5 yr –11 yr	99393			Hemoccult, guaiac	82270	
	40 yr –64 yr	99386			12 yr–17 yr	99394			Strep, rapid	87880	
	65 yr and over	99387			18 yr –39 yr	99395			UA, dipstick (manual)	81000	
					40 yr –64 yr	99396			UA, automated	81003	
					65 yr and over	99397			Urine pregnancy	81025	

DIAGNOSTIC CODES (ICD-10-CM)			
☐ R10.9 Abdominal Pain	☐ E11.9 Diabetes II–Non Ins	☐ J02.9 Pharyngitis	☐ Z23 Immunization Encounter
☐ T78.4 Allergic Reaction	☐ K57.92 Diverticulitis	☐ M06.9 Rheumatoid Arthritis	☐ Z00.12_ Well Child Check
☐ D64.9 Anemia	☐ K57.90 Diverticulosis	☐ R06.02 Short of Breath	☐ Z00.0_ Well Adult
☐ D51.0 Anemia, Pernicious	☐ R60.9 Edema	☐ J32.9 Sinusitis	☐ ________
■ I20.9 Angina Pectoris	☐ R51 Headache	☐ L91.8 Skin Tag(s)	☐ ________
☐ I49.9 Arrhythmia, Cardiac	☐ R31.9 Hematuria	☐ J02.0 Streptococcal Sore Throat	☐ ________
☐ I70.0 Atherosclerosis, Aorta	☐ B00.9 Herpes Zoster	☐ N39.0 Urinary Tract Infection	☐ ________
☐ J45.909 Asthma	☐ I10 Hypertension		☐ ________
☐ M54.9 Back Pain	☐ E03.9 Hypothyroidism	**RETURN APPOINTMENT**	**BALANCE DUE**
☐ J20._ Bronchitis, Acute	☐ H61.2_ Impacted Cerumen	______ Days	Total Charge $ 130.00
☐ J42 Bronchitis, Chronic	☐ J11.1 Influenza	______ Weeks	Amount Paid $ 20.00
☐ R07.9 Chest Pain	☐ K58.9 Irritable Bowel Syndrome	______ Months	Previous Bal $ 35.00
☐ J44.9 COPD	☐ M19.0 Osteoarthritis	______ PRN	Adjustment $ 0.00
☐ E10.0 Diabetes I–Ins. Dep	☐ H66.9_ Otitis Media		Balance Due $ 145.00

Fig. 45.1 Completed charge slip (superbill) containing procedure and diagnosis codes (ICD-10).

FEE SCHEDULE

A **fee schedule** is a list of charges for the various procedures a provider performs. In a hospital system, it is commonly called a chargemaster. Years ago, a provider had one set of fees that they charged patients for office visits, procedures, and/or treatments. Today, however, a medical office may have to accept different amounts as payment for each service it performs, depending on which insurance provider is paying for the service. The reimbursement varies from a fixed percentage of the provider's charges to a set amount for a given service. Insurance is discussed in detail in Chapter 47.

The medical office usually has a basic fee schedule that lists the usual charges for office visits and procedures. The fee schedule is used to inform patients of charges for procedures and identifies a charge when a procedure is entered into the ledger of a patient. Sometimes medical offices offer discounts to patients who do not have insurance, patients who pay cash, and/or patients with demonstrated medical need. The decision to offer a discount should be made by the office manager, usually after discussion with the provider(s), and is often billed at the regular price with the discounted portion entered as an adjustment.

What Would You Do? What Would You *Not* Do?

Case Study 1

In the afternoon, Maria is entering charges and payments into the patient computer accounts. She notices that there are no charges for two patients on the appointment list, although she remembers that both patients arrived and were seen by one of the providers. ■

PATIENT ACCOUNT LEDGER

Each patient has their own account. It is important to verify that all the information about the account is current when the patient arrives at the office, because address information and insurance information can change between visits. A cumulative record of charges and payments is kept, usually using a computer program. It is also possible to keep account records manually. This record of charges and payments is called the patient account **ledger.** In a practice management program, the patient account ledger is linked to the patient demographic and insurance information so that periodic bills and insurance claims can be generated. Information about services provided to an individual patient and payments received for that patient show up in chronologic order on the patient ledger (Fig. 45.2). Traditionally patient ledger cards recorded a running balance, but computerized ledgers may record the balance for each line (entry) with the total patient balance at the end of the ledger.

After the provider has identified procedures done for a patient, the charges are posted to the patient ledger (Procedure 45.1).

Posting Payments to the Patient Account

Payment for services performed can be received in four ways:

1. The patient pays at the time of service, in full or in part (e.g., a copayment for managed care insurance). The office will usually accept cash and checks, and most offices also accept credit and debit cards.
2. The patient may make a payment through the mail in response to a bill.
3. The patient may make an online payment using a credit or debit card through the medical office website or the online patient portal.
4. An insurance company may make a payment either by mail or, usually, by electronic transfer.

All payments must be posted to the account of the patient for whom they are made. Some computer programs

WALDEN-MARTIN
FAMILY MEDICAL CLINIC
1234 ANYSTREET ANYTOWN, ANYSTATE 1234
PHONE 123-123-1234 FAX 123-123-5678

Ledger for Guarantor: Mora Siever

Home phone: 123-914-3584
Account #: 72534
Address: 1 Trinity Lane, Anytown, AL 12345
DOB: 01/24/19XX

Date	Patient	Service	Charges	Payment	ADJUSTMENT	Balance
12/02/20XX	Mora Siever	99396	$ 105.00	$ 20.00	$ 0.00	$ 85.00
12/02/20XX	Mora Siever	99300	$ 89.00	$ 0.00	$ 0.00	$ 89.00
10/22/20XX	Mora Siever	Ins payment	$ 0.00	$ 35.00	$ 15.00	$ −50.00
10/07/20XX	Mora Siever	99203	$ 70.00	$ 20.00	$ 0.00	$ 50.00
					Total:	$ 174.00

Fig. 45.2 Patient ledger from SimChart for the Medical Office.

have different codes for each method of payment. Cash and checks must match daily bank deposits. Payments using credit cards, online banking, or electronic transfer must later be matched to bank statements or online banking records. If checks are deposited remotely by scanning them, they must also be matched to bank statements or online banking records.

Posting Adjustments to the Patient Account

A change to the patient account that is neither a charge for services nor a payment is called an **adjustment. Credit** (negative) adjustments are subtracted from the patient balance. These are the most common type of adjustments. Examples of credit adjustments include discounts for payment at the time of service, professional courtesy discounts, and discounts given due to insurance coverage (also called *insurance write-offs*). Credit adjustments are usually discounts that are given in specific circumstances. (See Box 45.1 for common terminology used in accounting.)

Debit (positive) adjustments are added to the patient balance. Debit adjustments are discussed in more detail in Chapter 48. In most computer billing programs, the medical assistant selects a code for each charge, payment, or adjustment. The correct mathematical operation is linked to the transaction code so that the computer automatically adds charges and debit adjustments (such as a returned check) to the patient balance and subtracts payments and credit adjustments (such as an insurance write-off) (Procedure 45.2).

BOX 45.1 Common Terminology Used in Accounting

Account balance: The amount remaining in the account after all entries have been totaled.
Accounts receivable control: A summary of all unpaid accounts.
Adjustment: An entry to change an account balance that is not a charge for services or a payment, often a discount.
Credit: An entry that reduces an account balance, usually a payment.
Credit balance: The balance on an account when payments exceed charges.
Day sheet: The record of daily financial transactions.
Debit: An entry that increases an account balance, usually a charge.
Disbursements: Money paid out.
Invoice: A bill or written statement describing a purchase or service and the amount due.
Journal: The original record of financial transactions that identifies the accounts to which they belong.
Ledger: A card, book, or computer database in which financial transactions are recorded.
Payables: Amounts owed to others.
Posting: Recording financial transactions or transferring information from one record to another.
Receivables: Amounts of money owed by others.
ROA (received on account): Designation used for payments that reduce the amount owed but are not payment in full.

DAY SHEET

The **day sheet** (daily journal) keeps a running tally of the medical office's income for that day and is a record of daily transactions. Manual day sheets are rarely used, but the principle of keeping transactions from each individual day is maintained in a practice management program, and the daily journal is still called a day sheet.

For each individual patient seen, the manual day sheet records charges, payments, previous balance, adjustments, and the new balance.

Each transaction is recorded on the manual day sheet in the order in which it was recorded or entered into the computer. This includes not only patient visits but also all checks received in the mail that day. Even though the checks pay all or part of a patient balance from a previous day, they are posted to the patient account on the day they are received and deposited. At the end of the day, the day is closed (i.e., no further transactions are allowed for that day).

The use of practice management computer programs has eliminated the need for manual checking of calculations and entries that used to be done on the *proof of posting* section of a manual day sheet. Practice management programs can make all necessary calculations and use them to generate a variety of reports.

PRINTING DAY SHEETS AND OTHER REPORTS

When a computer billing program is used, the day sheet can usually be printed at the end of the day. Most computer billing programs allow the day to be closed (so that additional entries cannot be entered using that date). Usually only one day sheet can be printed for a given date. This prevents later alterations to the financial records. If an account must be corrected at a later time, any adjustments are entered on a new screen dated the day the correction is made. The original entry should never be altered after the day has been closed. Many other types of reports can be produced using billing software, including patient ledgers and various activity reports. The total of all patient accounts (plus any other outstanding income) makes up the *accounts receivable.* The computer billing program contains a report menu with standard formats, and the medical office can create custom reports depending on its needs.

OTHER FINANCIAL ACCOUNTS

In addition to taking money in, a medical office pays money out. Bills may be paid on a regular basis—for example, taking care of weekly or biweekly salaries, mortgage or rent, equipment leases, and utilities. Other payments are made in relation to specific invoices for materials or equipment.

What Would You Do? What Would You *Not* Do?

Case Study 2

After a new patient named Linda Harris has been seen, the provider asks Maria to charge the patient $15.00 less than usual for the office visit and $5.00 less than the usual charge for a flu shot because the patient was recently let go from her job. As Ms. Harris is checking out, she pays $100.00 toward the bill, which is 20% less than the usual charge for a flu shot and an office visit for a new patient. In Maria's office the usual charge for every procedure is entered for every patient. On the rare occasions when charges are reduced, any reduction is posted as a write-off. ■

Unless a bill is paid immediately when presented, it becomes part of the *accounts payable* (money owed by the business). A complete bookkeeping system notes each month any outstanding accounts payable, as well as the **disbursements** (payments) made during the month.

In addition, many offices keep a **petty cash** account, a small amount of cash available for everyday expenses. Again, petty cash must be recorded.

REQUESTING PAYMENT FOR SERVICES

Most medical offices expect patients to pay any copayment before an office visit. If a patient does not have enough cash or a checkbook with them, it is common to offer to bill the patient for a copayment of $50.00 or less if the account balance is zero. If it is known that insurance will not cover the service, such as cosmetic surgery, the patient is usually expected to pay in advance.

When discussing financial matters with patients, medical assistants are expected to display professionalism and tact. If the patient has an outstanding balance, the patient may be expected to pay it before receiving any additional services. This discussion should be held in a private area to avoid embarrassing the patient. The medical assistant should use good eye contact to convey that the request is serious and convey a sense of importance about paying the bill. At the same time, the medical assistant should be sensitive to the patient's individual circumstances. It is helpful to be able to use office policy as a justification for the need to collect payment. It may be necessary to reschedule an appointment, but if the patient has an urgent medical problem the provider or other licensed practitioner should decide how to meet the patient's needs (Procedure 45.3).

NOTIFYING PATIENTS IF INSURANCE IS NOT EXPECTED TO COVER SERVICES

Usually, insurance does not cover elective procedures such as elective cosmetic surgery. If this is the case, the medical office usually requires payment in advance of the procedure. In cases where insurance is unlikely to pay for services, the patient may be asked to sign a form agreeing to pay for the service if the claim is denied. Patients with original Medicare must be given a copy of the **Medicare Advance Beneficiary Notice (ABN)** when it is possible that Medicare might not cover the service to be provided. If Medicare never covers the service, the ABN form is not required (e.g., cosmetic surgery). This enables a patient to make a more informed decision and not be surprised by an unexpected bill (Fig. 45.3).

BANKING ACTIVITIES

If the medical office is to pay its bills, including salaries for medical assistants and other employees, it must have money in the bank. Part of the responsibility of the individual who handles the office's financial management is maintaining the medical office's bank accounts.

TYPES OF ACCOUNTS

Businesses such as medical offices will typically have one or more of the following types of bank accounts: checking, savings, or money market accounts.

Checking Account

A checking account is an account in which the money held can be withdrawn by simply writing a check against the funds available. Many banks allow businesses to earn interest on their checking accounts as long as a certain amount of money remains in the account (the minimum balance). The minimum balance can range from as little as $500 to as much as $2500. Interest is the payment the bank makes to the owner of the money on deposit for the privilege of being able to use the depositor's money to make loans to other bank customers.

If the checking account balance falls below the minimum, the account does not earn interest and there is usually a monthly service charge and a charge for each check written against the account for the entire monthly reporting period in which the balance was below the minimum. Sometimes a bank will waive the minimum balance in the medical office's checking account if the medical office agrees to keep a higher minimum balance in either a savings account or a money market account.

Savings Account

A medical office may want to keep cash that is not necessary to pay expenses in a savings account, which usually earns interest at a slightly higher rate than an interest-bearing checking account. A savings account does not have any check-writing privileges, but money can be withdrawn or transferred to the checking account if necessary.

Money Market Account

A money market account offers features of both savings and checking accounts. Money market accounts usually require a fairly high minimum balance (often $2500). However,

A. Notifier: John Doe, MD, College Clinic, 4567 Broad Avenue, Woodland Hills, XY 12345 555-486-9002

B. Patient Name: Mary Judd **C. Identification Number:** 0920XX7291

Advance Beneficiary Notice of Noncoverage (ABN)

NOTE: If Medicare doesn't pay for **D.** B12 injections below, you may have to pay.
Medicare does not pay for everything, even some care that you or your health care provider have good reason to think you need. We expect Medicare may not pay for the **D.** B12 injections below.

D.	E. Reason Medicare May Not Pay:	F. Estimated Cost
B12 injections	Medicare does not usually pay for this injection or this many injections	$35.00

WHAT YOU NEED TO DO NOW:

- Read this notice, so you can make an informed decision about your care.
- Ask us any questions that you may have after you finish reading.
- Choose an option below about whether to receive the **D.** B12 injections listed above.

Note: If you choose Option 1 or 2, we may help you to use any other insurance that you might have, but Medicare cannot require us to do this.

G. OPTIONS: Check only one box. We cannot choose a box for you.

☒ **OPTION 1.** I want the **D.** B12 injections listed above. You may ask to be paid now, but I also want Medicare billed for an official decision on payment, which is sent to me on a Medicare Summary Notice (MSN). I understand that if Medicare doesn't pay, I am responsible for payment, but **I can appeal to Medicare** by following the directions on the MSN. If Medicare does pay, you will refund any payments I made to you, less co-pays or deductibles.

☐ **OPTION 2.** I want the **D.** ____________ listed above, but do not bill Medicare. You may ask to be paid now as I am responsible for payment. **I cannot appeal if Medicare is not billed.**

☐ **OPTION 3.** I don't want the **D.** ____________ listed above. I understand with this choice I am **not** responsible for payment, and **I cannot appeal to see if Medicare would pay.**

H. Additional Information:

This notice gives our opinion, not an official Medicare decision. If you have other questions on this notice or Medicare billing, call **1-800-MEDICARE** (1-800-633-4227/**TTY:** 1-877-486-2048).
Signing below means that you have received and understand this notice. You also receive a copy.

I. Signature: Mary Judd	J. Date: March 20, 20XX

According to the Paperwork Reduction Act of 1995, no persons are required to respond to a collection of information unless it displays a valid OMB control number. The valid OMB control number for this information collection is 0938-0566. The time required to complete this information collection is estimated to average 7 minutes per response, including the time to review instructions, search existing data resources, gather the data needed, and complete and review the information collection. If you have comments concerning the accuracy of the time estimate or suggestions for improving this form, please write to: CMS, 7500 Security Boulevard, Attn: PRA Reports Clearance Officer, Baltimore, Maryland 21244-1850.

Form CMS-R-131 (03/11) Form Approved OMB No. 0938-0566

Fig. 45.3 Medicare Advance Beneficiary Notice (ABN). (From Fordney, MT: *Insurance handbook for the medical office*, ed. 14, St. Louis, 2017, Elsevier.)

they may earn interest at the money market rate—the rate at which major corporations lend to or borrow from one another for 10- to 30-day periods.

Money market accounts let the owner draw a specified number of checks per month without a processing fee. They often require checks to be for at least $500.

A medical office might want to maintain a money market account to hold money for regular but infrequent expenses, such as quarterly, semiannual, or annual payments for malpractice insurance; licenses for providers and other licensed professionals on the staff; or dues to the state, county, or local medical association or chamber of commerce.

CHECKS

Types of Checks

Checks are slips of paper used by a checking account owner to authorize payments to a third party **(payee)** for the amount of money written on the check. Paying by checks allows the medical office to maintain a permanent record of the payments it makes for goods and services.

In addition to the checks from the medical office's checkbook or money market account, the medical office may have occasion to ask its bank to prepare a cashier's check to assure the payee (person or company being paid) that funds are available. A **cashier's check** is a check drawn on the bank itself rather than on an individual account. Because the bank assumes liability for payment of the check, a cashier's check is considered more reliable than the check of an individual or business. This might be the case if the office were purchasing a large piece of equipment for which the seller is unwilling to accept a simple business check. The bank may also guarantee a personal or business check by withdrawing the funds from the checking account at the time the check is issued. This is called a **certified check.**

Check Format

At the top of each check toward the right, under the check number, is a fractional number that identifies the bank on which the check is drawn. This ABA number, which is assigned by the American Bankers Association, designates the federal reserve bank zone, the state or territory, and the unique identification number for the bank on which the check is drawn. Across the bottom of checks is a set of numbers called the **MICR line**, written in magnetic ink. When checks are processed and "cleared" for payment from the issuing bank to the account of the individual making the deposit, this set of numbers is read by a magnetic ink character recognition (MICR) system. The MICR line contains the **ABA routing number** (the unique number of the bank), the account number, and the check number. Other information that is usually printed on a check includes the name and address of the account holder and the name of the bank. The ABA routing number is also used for automatic payments, wire transfers, and direct deposit.

Business Checkbook With Stubs

One type of business checkbook that is commonly used has three checks to a page, with check stubs on the left on which to record the same information that is recorded on the check when it is written (Fig. 45.4). The checks and matching stubs are preprinted in order. In addition, the stubs have room in which to write in the amount of deposits made; the stubs therefore act as a running checkbook ledger.

Computer-Generated Checks

A number of business accounting computer programs will generate checks and immediately post the payment to the accounts payable ledger. To use these systems, the medical office will need to buy compatible blank checks for computer printing. The software can also generate the fractional bank number and MICR numbers, or they may be preprinted on the check forms.

Online Payment

Most medical offices pay bills online either as a single payment or every month. This is also popular with suppliers, who create online accounts and accept payments directly using a pay-by-computer system.

If an office handles its own payroll, it may encourage employees to use direct deposit instead of paper checks. Some medical offices may do all of their bill paying to regular suppliers, medical associations, liability insurance carriers, and other creditors online, and have their payroll checks written by an outside service provider, so checks are written only occasionally.

Preparing a Check

Checks are produced on watermarked paper to make it difficult for people to erase and then overwrite part of the check. The bank has the right to refuse to honor a check with erasures, overwrites, or other alterations. Minor corrections may be accepted if initialed by the person who signs the check. This protects the account holder from having people to whom checks are written cross out the amount and write in a larger amount. However, this also makes it important that checks be written carefully.

Most checks have at least one memo line—a line on which to write the purpose of the check. If the check is for payment of a bill or **invoice** (itemized bill), the invoice number or the account number for that particular **vendor** would go on the memo line.

If a mistake is made on a check, the medical assistant should write *void* on the check and check stub. The voided check should not be destroyed. It should be filed with bank statements and other account records so that it is available for the medical office's auditors. In some medical offices, checks exceeding a certain amount (e.g., $500, $1000) must be signed by two people; this is often a provision of that part of the medical office's general liability insurance policy that covers employee theft.

HIGHLIGHT on Check Security Features

Because of the prevalence of color copiers, many security features are built into the paper used to print checks. The paper usually has a watermark that cannot be photocopied and/or invisible florescent fibers that can be viewed under black light. The paper should have erasure protection so that the background color fades if writing or printing is altered. The paper of the check may also have a chemical stain that reacts if chemicals are used to alter information. A word such as *nonnegotiable* or *void* may appear if the check is passed through a photocopier or treated with chemicals. Various parts of the check usually have also been treated in a special way so that they will not be reproduced if the check is photocopied. The border and endorsement line usually include microprinting that will not be reproduced if the check is photocopied. ■

PRECAUTIONS FOR ACCEPTING CHECKS, CREDIT CARDS, AND/OR DEBIT CARDS

When a patient offers a check for payment at an office visit, the medical assistant should look at the check carefully to avoid accepting a phony check (see *Highlight on Check Security Features*). In addition, the medical assistant should make sure that the date and amount of the check are correct. A third-party check should never be accepted, even a payroll check. (Third-party checks are written to one party and later endorsed to pay another party.) If there is any problem with the check, it is very difficult to obtain reimbursement. Checks should be accepted for only the outstanding amount. If a patient needs cash, the medical assistant can direct them to the nearest automated teller machine (ATM). A postal money order may have only one endorsement. If the patient presents a postal money order

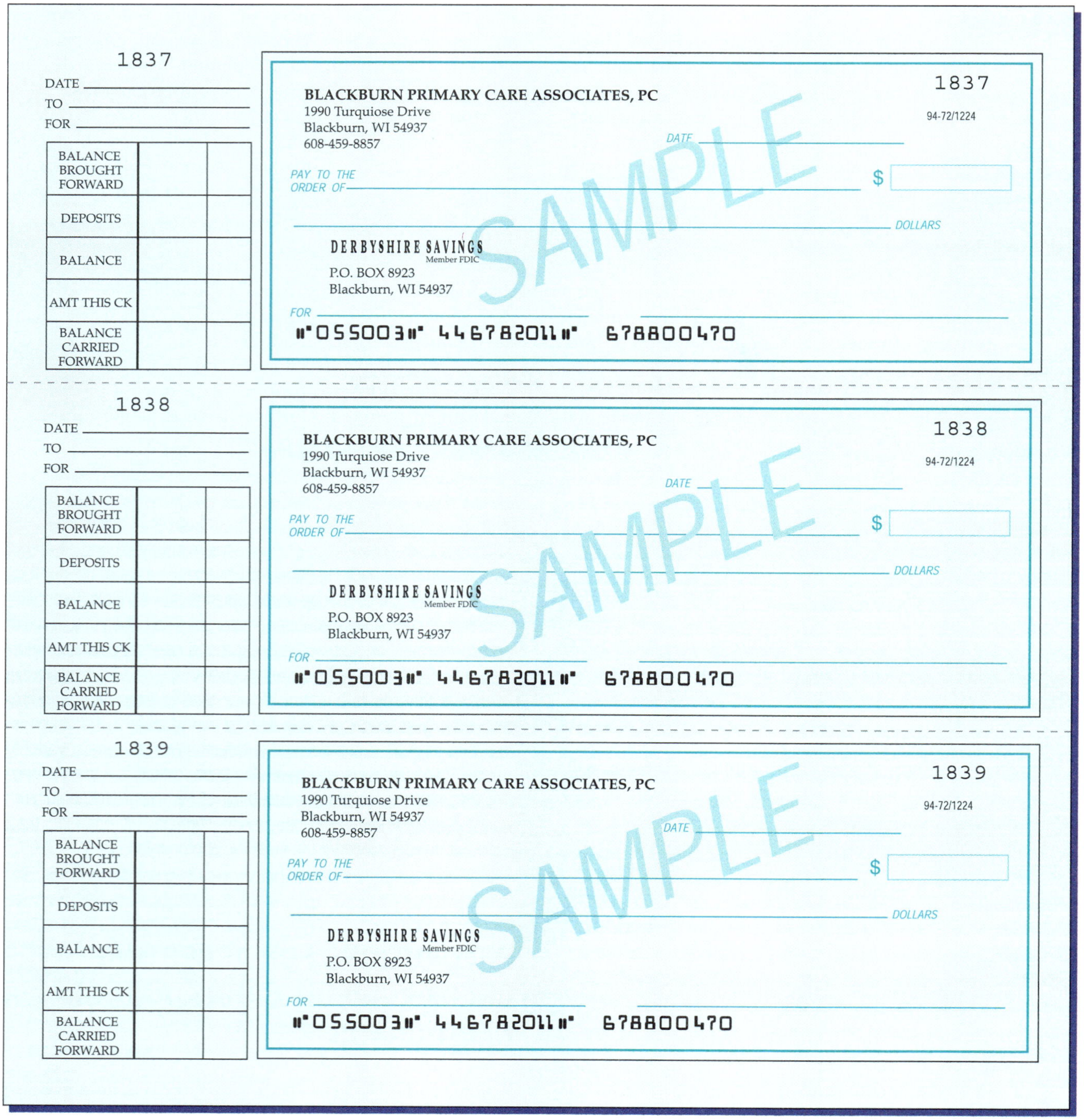

1837

DATE ______
TO ______
FOR ______

BALANCE BROUGHT FORWARD		
DEPOSITS		
BALANCE		
AMT THIS CK		
BALANCE CARRIED FORWARD		

BLACKBURN PRIMARY CARE ASSOCIATES, PC
1990 Turquiose Drive
Blackburn, WI 54937
608-459-8857

1837
94-72/1224

DATE ______

PAY TO THE ORDER OF ______ $ ______

______ DOLLARS

DERBYSHIRE SAVINGS
Member FDIC
P.O. BOX 8923
Blackburn, WI 54937

SAMPLE

FOR ______ ______

⑈055003⑈ 446782011⑈ 678800470

1838

DATE ______
TO ______
FOR ______

BALANCE BROUGHT FORWARD		
DEPOSITS		
BALANCE		
AMT THIS CK		
BALANCE CARRIED FORWARD		

BLACKBURN PRIMARY CARE ASSOCIATES, PC
1990 Turquiose Drive
Blackburn, WI 54937
608-459-8857

1838
94-72/1224

DATE ______

PAY TO THE ORDER OF ______ $ ______

______ DOLLARS

DERBYSHIRE SAVINGS
Member FDIC
P.O. BOX 8923
Blackburn, WI 54937

SAMPLE

FOR ______ ______

⑈055003⑈ 446782011⑈ 678800470

1839

DATE ______
TO ______
FOR ______

BALANCE BROUGHT FORWARD		
DEPOSITS		
BALANCE		
AMT THIS CK		
BALANCE CARRIED FORWARD		

BLACKBURN PRIMARY CARE ASSOCIATES, PC
1990 Turquiose Drive
Blackburn, WI 54937
608-459-8857

1839
94-72/1224

DATE ______

PAY TO THE ORDER OF ______ $ ______

______ DOLLARS

DERBYSHIRE SAVINGS
Member FDIC
P.O. BOX 8923
Blackburn, WI 54937

SAMPLE

FOR ______ ______

⑈055003⑈ 446782011⑈ 678800470

Fig. 45.4 A business checkbook is often arranged with three checks per page and check stubs to record transactions.

with more than one endorsement, the medical assistant should not accept It. A check with the notation *payment in full* written anywhere on the check should not be accepted unless the medical assistant is sure that the check covers the patient's entire outstanding balance. If a check is received in the mail with this notation, there are two options, and the medical assistant should follow office policy. The first option is to return the check to the patient with a letter explaining that the check cannot be accepted and requesting a new check. The other option is to write the following on the back of the check before endorsing it: "This check is deposited under protest, without prejudice, and with preservation of all rights of the payee against the drawer of this check pursuant to UCC § 1-207." The check should be endorsed under this disclaimer and can be deposited after both sides are photocopied. If the office accepts a check that claims to be "payment in full" without this disclaimer, the provider may forfeit the right to collect the rest of the **balance due**.

The number of offices accepting credit and debit cards has increased dramatically in recent years. Some offices require patients to pay with credit cards and do not keep cash in the office. (In these offices, patients without credit cards are billed.) Credit or debit card transactions should be allowed only if the actual plastic card is presented, and the patient name and signature should be verified when the card is accepted. If the patient is new, identification can be required. The office should have a policy to accept credit cards only from the individual whose name is on the card. A company should be chosen to process credit and debit transactions that has a proven track record of reliability. This company should also be using state-of-the art measures to maintain the security of customer identifying information. The processor should also provide insurance against the loss of customer data.

ELECTRONIC TRANSFER OF FUNDS

Money can be transferred from one bank account to another, either in a single financial institution or from one financial institution to another in many ways without the use of a paper check. This type of transfer includes credit and debit card payments, direct deposit payments (by which money is transferred into an account specified by the recipient), direct debit payments (by which a business debits a consumer's bank account for payment for goods and services), and online bill payment. All these services may be used by the medical office to receive payments from patients, to pay bills, and for payroll.

BANK DEPOSITS

Balancing the Cash Drawer

As a first step to preparing the bank deposit at the end of the day, the cash drawer should be balanced. Most offices maintain a cash drawer or change fund so that patients can be given change for cash payments. The money should be in a drawer with compartments for bills of different denominations. The drawer may be moved to a safe at night depending on the office. A standard sum (such as $200.00) in small bills is arranged in the drawer at the beginning of the day. At the end of the day, the money in the drawer should be counted, and the usual amount of cash on hand is returned to the drawer. Any additional cash should be removed, counted, checked against the receipts issued to patients, and added to the daily bank deposit. Usually, the person who checks patients in has the key and is responsible for maintaining the cash drawer. Note that money from the cash drawer should not be used for petty cash. The office should maintain a separate petty cash fund, which is discussed later in the chapter.

Preparing a Bank Deposit

Every time a deposit is made at the bank, it must be recorded on a deposit slip. A deposit slip is an itemized listing of the cash or checks being deposited. A deposit slip preprinted with the account number will be found in the back of the medical office's checkbook. Deposit slips (Fig. 45.5) may also be created and printed using a computer accounting program. This allows for deposits to be entered in the computer records for the office's checking account. For making a deposit, the amount of the total cash being deposited is written on the cash line, with the total of the checks on the check line. An itemized listing of the checks being deposited must be included with the deposit. The numerator of the fractional bank number (e.g., 94-72) or the check number from the top right of the check should be entered on the deposit slip in the box to the left of the amount to identify each check (Procedure 45.4).

Modern technology allows checks to be scanned and deposited into a checking account electronically. Many medical offices now use a check scanner at the registration desk. Scanning checks when they are received simplifies the process of creating a bank deposit. If the office has a safe where cash may be stored safely, deposits of cash received may be made only two or three times a week instead of daily.

What Would You Do? What Would You *Not* Do?

Case Study 3

On January 4, Leonard Simpson pays $25.00 by check as a copayment at the time of an office visit. At the end of the day when Maria is preparing the daily deposit, she notices that the date on Mr. Simpson's check is January 4 of the previous year instead of the current year. ■

Endorsing Checks

Each check being deposited must have an endorsement on its back. An endorsement authorizes a bank to cash or deposit the check. There are several types of endorsements.

Blank Endorsement

A blank endorsement is a simple signature of the party to whom the check was written. Once a check has been signed, it can be cashed by anyone holding the check.

Special Endorsement

The special endorsement begins with a statement of the party to whom the check should be paid (usually using the words *Pay to the order of...*) followed by the signature of the party to whom the check was written.

Restrictive Endorsement

The restrictive endorsement begins with instructions that specify how the check can be paid out (e.g., *for deposit only*), followed by the signature of the party to whom the check was written. The bank must follow the instructions.

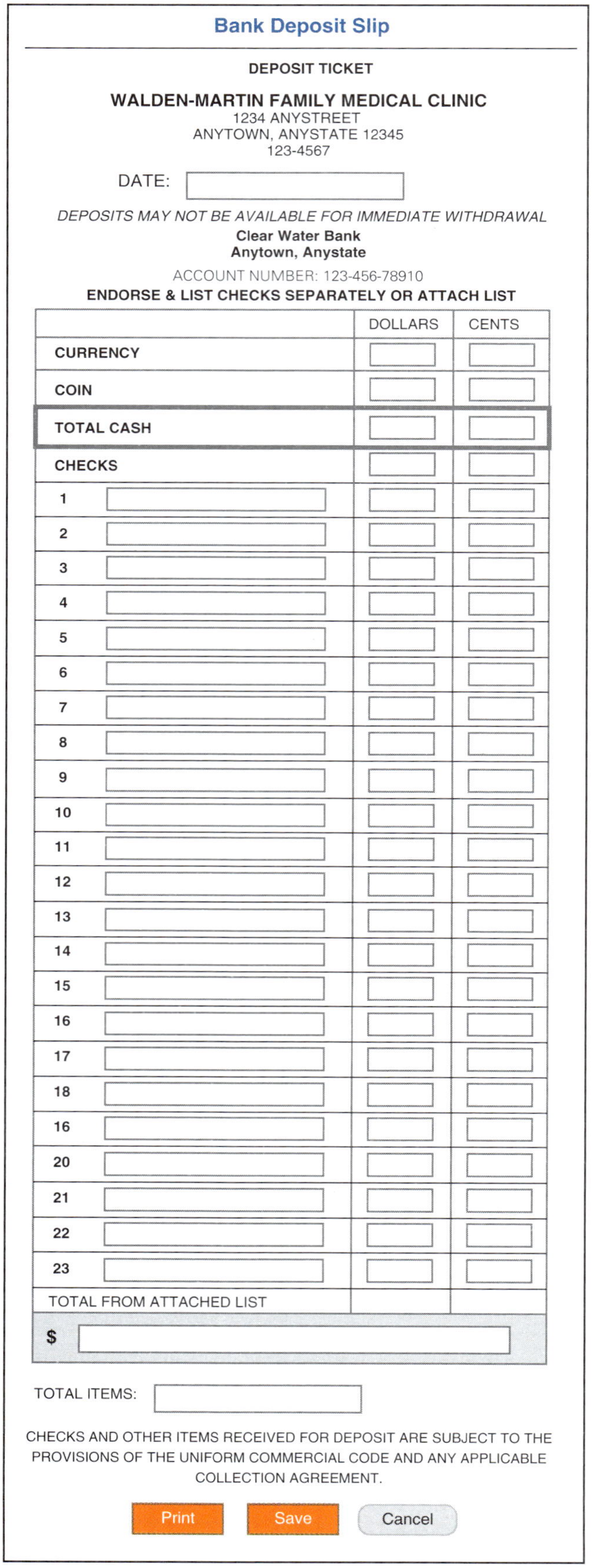

Bank Deposit Slip

DEPOSIT TICKET

WALDEN-MARTIN FAMILY MEDICAL CLINIC
1234 ANYSTREET
ANYTOWN, ANYSTATE 12345
123-4567

DATE:

DEPOSITS MAY NOT BE AVAILABLE FOR IMMEDIATE WITHDRAWAL

Clear Water Bank
Anytown, Anystate

ACCOUNT NUMBER: 123-456-78910

ENDORSE & LIST CHECKS SEPARATELY OR ATTACH LIST

	DOLLARS	CENTS
CURRENCY		
COIN		
TOTAL CASH		
CHECKS		
1		
2		
3		
4		
5		
6		
7		
8		
9		
10		
11		
12		
13		
14		
15		
16		
17		
18		
16		
20		
21		
22		
23		
TOTAL FROM ATTACHED LIST		
$		

TOTAL ITEMS:

CHECKS AND OTHER ITEMS RECEIVED FOR DEPOSIT ARE SUBJECT TO THE PROVISIONS OF THE UNIFORM COMMERCIAL CODE AND ANY APPLICABLE COLLECTION AGREEMENT.

Print Save Cancel

Fig. 45.5 Bank deposit ticket using SimChart for the Medical Office.

This type of endorsement can be entered on a check using a stamp approved by the bank that includes the words *for deposit only*, the name of the provider or medical office, and the bank account number. All checks received in the medical office should be stamped with the restrictive endorsement before deposit.

Making a Deposit

Deposits can be made in person or by using the night deposit box, usually located near the bank's front door. The night deposit box may require a key or personal identification number (PIN) code, which is supplied by the bank to customers who use it. (This prevents tampering or unauthorized use of the deposit slot.) Electronic technology now permits electronic readers to read the deposit bag's serial number, or there may be a radio frequency identification (RFID) tag in the deposit bag similar to the devices used for mass transit passes, parking passes, and inventory control. Deposits can also be made at an ATM.

RECONCILING A BANK STATEMENT

Reconciling a bank statement means making sure that the balance in the checkbook and the balance on the bank statement equal each other after adjusting for checks that were written but have not yet cleared through the bank and deposits recorded after the statement period ended.

Each month the bank will send the medical office a statement of account activity, or the medical office may access this statement online. The account balance at the end of the statement period will almost always be different from the account balance in the office's checking account ledger.

There are several reasons for this discrepancy. First, it usually takes about a week from the time the statement period ends until the office receives the statement, during which time more checks have been written. Second, checks written near the end of the statement period usually will not have cleared the account when the period ends. Third, some vendors and others do not promptly deposit or cash checks; thus, some checks will not clear the account for a month or more. Fourth, bank charges are added to the statement for such things as checks returned for insufficient funds, per-check fees, and lockbox fees. Finally, interest may accrue on the balance during the month.

For these reasons, it is important to reconcile the bank statement with the office's checkbook to verify the arithmetic used by those who have written checks. Before reconciling, enter and subtract any bank fees in the office's checking account ledger and add any interest. The amount of all outstanding checks (checks that have not cleared the bank) should be totaled and subtracted from the "new balance" shown on the bank statement. The amount of any deposits made during the month that do not appear on the statement should be added to obtain a true balance. This true balance should match the balance in the office's checking account ledger.

Petty Cash Log					
Date	Description	Add Amount	Amount	Balance	Initials
10/1/20XX	Opening balance			$ 100.00	sh
10/4/20XX	Postage due		$ 0.52	$ 99.48	sh
10/4/20XX	Cab fare for Dr. Warner		$ 12.00	$ 87.48	sh
10/15/20XX	Coffee and creamer		$ 14.72	$ 72.76	sh
10/16/20XX	Refreshments for staff meeting		$ 22.83	$ 49.93	sh
10/17/20XX	Binder clips		$ 5.52	$ 44.41	sh
10/19/20XX	Flowers for Dr. Gomez		$ 22.75	$ 21.66	sh
10/26/20XX	Blank name tags		$ 12.95	$ 8.71	sh
10/31/20XX	Check to replenish petty cash	$ 91.29		$ 100.00	sh

Fig. 45.6 Petty cash log created using Microsoft Excel.

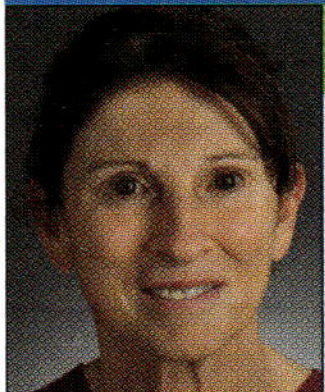

Memories *from* Practicum

Maria Hernandez: There was only one doctor in the office where I did my practicum, and in that office they used both a manual system to record patient accounts and a computer system. The office manager had been in charge for many years, and she said that she didn't trust the computer. Every morning we set up the pegboard by placing a day sheet on the bottom and receipts above. The receipts had carbon strips so that anything written would be duplicated on the layer below. As each patient checked out, we placed their ledger card between the receipt and the day sheet so that the next open line was directly above the next open line on the day sheet. The ledger cards we used were made of a special kind of carbonless paper called *NCR paper. NCR* stands for "no carbon required." When we filled in the date and charges on the receipt, it automatically was copied on the ledger card and then on the day sheet. The challenges were to be sure all three forms were lined up correctly and to be sure to apply enough pressure with the pen. The other big challenge was to add up the entries on the day sheet at the end of the day and make sure that everything balanced. The office manager said that sometimes it would take a long time to find and fix every mistake. I don't think there are very many offices left that record patient accounts this way, but I am glad I saw how it was done. It makes me appreciate how useful the computer is in managing office finances. ■

ACCOUNTS PAYABLE OR RECORD OF CASH DISBURSEMENTS

The record of cash disbursements is called the *cash disbursement journal.* The simplest form of this type of journal is a check register. In a computerized bookkeeping system, the cash disbursement journal is also automatically updated, or posted, when a check is drawn. In a single- or double-entry system, the cash disbursement journal must be separately maintained.

Each line of the cash disbursement journal has columns to record information about payments. Usually there are also columns to track expenses by categories. These features are also found in computer accounting programs.

PETTY CASH

Petty cash is the cash kept on hand to pay for small, miscellaneous items, such as tips for a delivery, postage due, reimbursement to a staff member for parking at a meeting, or even a box of Girl Scout cookies for the office break room.

A check for a predetermined amount—usually $100 to $200—is drawn to cash to establish the petty cash account. It is important to keep each office account separate. Thus, cash should never be taken from any patient payment and put into petty cash. The petty cash account should always be funded via a check drawn on the medical office's checking account.

A petty cash journal should be located near the cash box so that each disbursement can be recorded. Also, a pad of petty cash receipts should be available so that a receipt can be filled out each time a person receives money from the petty cash account. When the amount in the petty cash account falls below a predetermined amount (such as $20 or $30), or at regular intervals (daily, weekly), a new check is drawn in the amount that will return the petty cash fund to the original starting balance (Fig. 45.6).

Like any account, the petty cash account should be balanced on a regular basis. Staff members may need periodic reminders to fill out receipt forms every time they remove funds from petty cash.

What Would You Do? What Would You *Not* Do? RESPONSES

Case Study 1

Page 1157

What Did Maria Do?

- ❑ Looked at the electronic health record for both patients to determine if the provider had entered charges for services.
- ❑ If no charges were found, notified the provider that additional information was needed to bill for the patient services.
- ❑ If the provider had entered information about charges and diagnoses, followed up according to office policy so that the charges could be added to the patient accounts.

What Did Maria Not Do?

- ❑ Did not assume that there were no charges for these patients or that the information would be conveyed to the front desk eventually.
- ❑ Did not leave the day "open" because she knew that some of the charges for patient services were missing.
- ❑ Did not assume that she knew what the charges should be based on the reason for each patient's visit.

Case Study 2

Page 1159

What Did Maria Do?

- ❑ If she could not determine the reason using other means, Maria asked the provider what the reason for the discount was.
- ❑ Entered the charge for Linda Harris into the computer at the usual rate on two separate lines. In the appropriate box of each line, she entered an adjustment as directed by the provider ($15.00 for the office visit and $5.00 for the flu shot).
- ❑ Also entered the amount of the patient's payment into the patient's account.

What Did Maria Not Do?

- ❑ Did not enter the charges as the amount indicated by the provider because that was not the office policy.
- ❑ Did not enter the usual charges into the patient account without making an adjustment.

Case Study 3

Page 1163

What Did Maria Do?

- ❑ Contacted Leonard Simpson by telephone to tell him that he had used the incorrect date on his check.
- ❑ Arranged to have Mr. Simpson either send or drop off a new check. When the new check arrived, Maria returned the check with the incorrect date to Mr. Simpson.
- ❑ Maria might also have arranged for Mr. Simpson to come to the office, change the date on the check, and initial the correction.
- ❑ Waited until the new check arrived to post the payment to Mr. Simpson's account and deposit the check.
- ❑ Corrected the charge slip to remove the payment.

What Did Maria Not Do?

- ❑ Did not try to deposit the check with the incorrect date because banks will not accept checks more than 6 months after the date on the check.
- ❑ Did not alter the date and put her initials by the correction.
- ❑ Did not post the payment to Mr. Simpson's account before the new check had arrived.

TERMINOLOGY REVIEW

Key Term	Definition
ABA routing number	A nine-digit number that identifies a bank; the number is printed at the beginning of the magnetic ink character recognition (MICR) line at the bottom of a check. It also appears in fractional form at the top right of the check under the check number.
Accounting	Systematic recording and reporting of financial transactions.
Accounts payable	The outstanding bills of a business, such as a medical office.
Accounts receivable	Total amount owed to a business for goods and services.
Accrual basis of accounting	Accounting method in which income is entered at the time of sale or provision of service.
Adjustment	A change to a patient account that is neither a charge nor a payment.
Assets	In accounting, a combination of property owned and money owed to a business.
Bookkeeping	The process of keeping detailed records of financial transactions.
Cash basis of accounting	Accounting method in which income is entered when payment is received.
Cashier's check	A check drawn on a bank instead of an individual account.
Certified check	A check on an individual account that a bank assumes responsibility for, usually by withdrawing funds to cover the check from the checking account at the time the check is certified.
Credit	A posting that is subtracted from an account balance.
Day sheet	The record of daily transactions. It includes patient visits as well as all payments that were received in the mail that day.

TERMINOLOGY REVIEW—cont'd

Key Term	Definition
Debit	A posting that is added to an account balance.
Disbursements	Money paid out.
Fee schedule	List of charges (fees) for specific procedures that may be performed in a medical office.
Invoice	Itemized bill for goods or services.
Ledger	A book, card, or computer account used to record financial transactions.
Liabilities	In accounting, the amount owed by a business to creditors.
MICR line	A line of numbers containing the American Bankers Association transit routing number and the account number that appears at the bottom left of a check. These numbers are read by an MICR system.
Payee	The person to whom a check is made out.
Petty cash	A cash account kept in a business office to pay for incidentals, such as postage due and other small items.
Reconciling	Making sure that two financial records agree, such as a bank statement and bank balance.

PROCEDURE 45.1 Posting Charges

Outcome Using the information from the completed charge slip, post patient charges to a patient account

Equipment/Supplies:

- Patient charge slip
- Patient ledger or computer with SimChart for the Medical Office
- Patient day sheet (optional)
- Fee schedule
- Pen or computer

1. **Procedural Step.** If using a manual system, post the charges from a completed patient charge slip on the patient ledger and paper day sheet or SimChart day sheet (optional) using one line for all of the services provided on that date. Place the total charges for the services in the column labeled *Charges.* If using SimChart for the Medical Office, post the first service on the first line. Enter the date, patient name, Current Procedural Terminology (CPT) code, charges (from the fee schedule), payment, and adjustment. The computer will calculate the balance.
2. **Procedural Step.** If using SimChart for the Medical Office, click the *Add Row* button to post each additional charge on a new line.
3. **Procedural Step.** If using a manual system, enter the total charge in the balance column. If using SimChart for the Medical Office, click the *Save* button after all charges have been posted.
   Example:

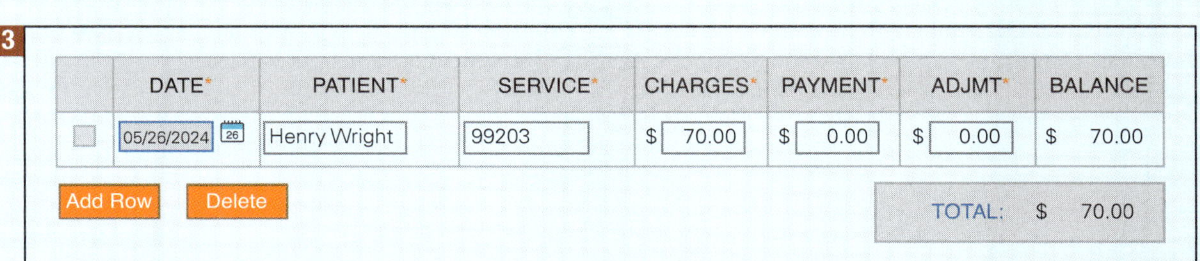

PROCEDURE 45.2 Posting Payments and/or Adjustments

Outcome Post payments and/or adjustments to a patient account

Equipment/Supplies:

- Patient ledger card or computer with SimChart for the Medical Office
- Check or cash from the patient or payment from the insurance carrier
- Calculator
- Stamp with restrictive endorsement
- Stamp pad

1. **Procedural step.** When a payment has been made, locate the patient ledger in the computer or select the patient ledger card.
   Principle. Both payments received at the patient visit and checks received in the mail must be entered to the correct patient account.
2. **Procedural step.** Compare the amount of the payment against the total amount owed.
   Principle. The total amount owed will be the balance due and charges for new services.
3. **Procedural step.** If using a manual system, post the payment from a completed patient charge slip on the patient ledger on the same line as the day's charges. If it is a check, record the number of the check. If using a computer program, post the patient payment on the same line as the charges from the day's visit.

3

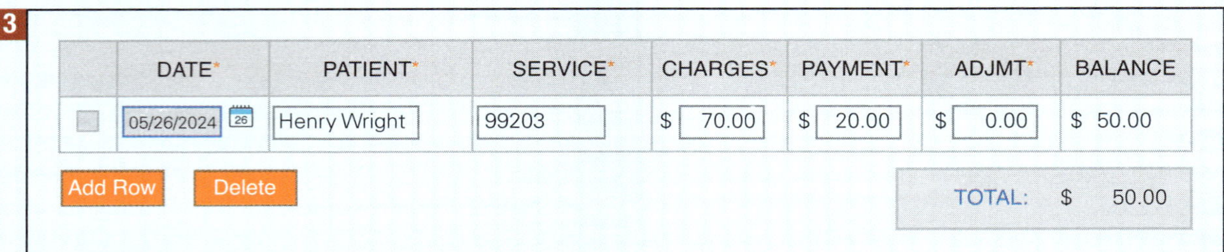

	DATE*	PATIENT*	SERVICE*	CHARGES*	PAYMENT*	ADJMT*	BALANCE
	05/26/2024	Henry Wright	99203	$ 70.00	$ 20.00	$ 0.00	$ 50.00

Charges and payments entered into the computer.

4. **Procedural step.** If posting an insurance payment or a patient check received in the mail, use a new line on a ledger card and a new line on a patient ledger in SimChart for the Medical Office.
   Principle. All payments are posted using the date of posting. In the case of insurance payments, this is not the same as the date of service.
5. **Procedural step.** If using a computer program to post an insurance payment, identify it in the service column (or use a code if the computer program requires it).
6. **Procedural step.** Determine if the amount excluded by the insurance company can be billed to the patient. If it cannot, enter the amount excluded by the insurance company as a credit adjustment in the credit column. On a ledger card, enter in the adjustment column.
   Principle. Insurance adjustments are amounts that the insurance does not allow. The insurance company provides a code to indicate them. They are credit adjustments because they are subtracted from the balance owed by the patient.
   Example. The statement from the insurance company shows that the insurance company paid $57.00 on the claim for Michael Lee. It excluded $23.00, which must be entered as a credit adjustment or write-off. The patient's copayment is $20.00.

PROCEDURE 45.2 Posting Payments and/or Adjustments—cont'd

6

UNITED WESTERN BENEFIT
1220 SIXTH STREET
WESTERN RIDGE, OH 45770

FOR SERVICES PROVIDED BY: WESTERN MEDICAL CENTER

Name of Insured: Michael Lee

Patient/ Service	Service Date(s)	Total Charge	Excluded Amounts	Patient Copayment	Plan Paid Amount
Office Visit	11/24/20XX	$ 65.00	$ 15.00 EAC	$ 20.00	$ 30.00
Cerumen Removal	11/24/20XX	$ 35.00	$ 8.00 EAC		$ 27.00
Total		**$ 100.00**	**$ 23.00**	**$ 20.00**	**$ 57.00**

EAC: This amount exceeds the allowable charge for the service. The provider is prohibited by law from billing the patient for this amount.

Insurance explanation of benefits.

7. Procedural step. Calculate the balance.
Example. The insurance payment of $57.00 has been entered as an insurance payment in the payment column, and the excluded amount has been entered in the adjustment column. The total amount subtracted from the patient's balance is $80.00.

7

DATE	PATIENT	SERVICE	CHARGES	PAYMENT	ADJMT	BALANCE
12/01/20XX	Michael Lee	Ins. pay & adjust	$ 0.00	$ 57.00	$ −23.00	$ −80.00

Insurance payment and insurance adjustment entered into the computer.

8. Procedural step. Endorse a check using a stamp containing the medical office name, the statement "For deposit only," and the number of the checking account.
Principle. This type of endorsement only allows the bank to deposit the check and prevents anyone from cashing the check or using it in any other way.

9. Procedural step. Place cash or a processed check in the designated drawer or money box for later deposit.

PROCEDURE 45.3 Demonstrating Professionalism and Sensitivity When Requesting Payment for Services Rendered

Outcome Demonstrate professionalism and sensitivity when requesting payment for services rendered

Equipment/Supplies:

- Simulated office scenario reflecting an outstanding account balance and non-urgent visit
- Patient account information reflecting past due balance

1. **Procedural Step.** Obtain office scenario from instructor and be sure that instructor is watching role play.
2. **Procedural step.** Role-play the situation with a classmate.
3. **Procedural step.** Make appropriate eye contact with the classmate who is playing the patient.
4. **Procedural step.** Establish a professional and empathetic atmosphere.
5. **Procedural step.** Using a professional manner, remind the simulated patient that office policy requires copayment at the time of the visit as well as payment of a previous balance before any new services are provided.
6. **Procedural step.** Offer suggestions for different payment options (credit card, cash, check).
7. **Procedural step.** Allow the patient an opportunity to voice any unusual circumstances that would limit the ability to pay.
8. **Procedural step.** Display sensitivity to this patient's circumstances while attempting to negotiate a reasonable resolution to this problem.
9. **Procedural step.** Decide what will be done and repeat the decision for the simulated patient.

PROCEDURE 45.4 Preparing a Bank Deposit

Outcome Prepare a bank deposit using a deposit slip and simulated checks

Equipment/Supplies:

- Account deposit slip
- Cash and checks received as payments
- Calculator or adding machine
- Bank deposit envelope or bag

1. **Procedural step.** Obtain an account deposit slip and place today's date on it. Be sure that the deposit slip contains the name of the medical office and the bank account number.
   Principle. The date, medical office name, and account number must appear on the deposit slip so that the bank can credit the deposit correctly.
2. **Procedural step.** Write the amount of currency and the amount in coins on the correct lines.
3. **Procedural step.** Stamp each check with the restrictive endorsement, and write the amount of each check on the bank deposit detail with either the numerator of the fractional American Bankers Association number or the check number.
   Principle. A reference number for each check allows the bank to verify individual items if questions arise.
4. **Procedural step.** Total all the checks and place that total on a deposit slip in the box for checks.
5. **Procedural step.** Total the cash and total amount of checks for the total amount of the bank deposit. The total amount of this deposit should be equal to the amount in the payments column on the day sheet or accounts receivable record for the given day.
6. **Procedural step.** Make a copy of the deposit slip.
   Principle. The office should keep a copy of information regarding the checks and cash included in a deposit in case there are questions at a later date.
7. **Procedural step.** Place the cash, checks, and deposit slip in a bank envelope or bank deposit bag and take or send it to the bank.
8. **Procedural step.** Record the amount of the deposit on the accounts payable record and in the check register or on the check stub nearest to the date of deposit.
   Principle. This provides information on the amount of money in the checking account against which checks can be written.
9. **Procedural step.** File the bank deposit receipt and copy of the bank deposit detail in a labeled file folder.
   Principle. All bank records must be saved for a period of time for tax and accounting purposes.

Medical Coding

 Check out the Evolve site at http://evolve.elsevier.com/Bonewit/today to access additional interactive activities and exercises to help you study and prepare for success.

LEARNING OBJECTIVES	PROCEDURES
Introduction	
1. Describe the history and rationale for using coding systems in medical care.	
Procedure Coding	
2. Describe the levels of Healthcare Common Procedure Coding System (HCPCS) codes.	
3. Describe the type of codes included in each section of the Current Procedural Terminology (CPT) manual (Level I HCPCS codes).	
4. Describe how to locate an accurate CPT code.	Performing CPT coding.
5. Identify when HCPCS Level II codes should be used.	
6. Describe how to locate an accurate HCPCS Level II code.	Performing HCPCS coding.
7. Perform procedural coding.	
Diagnostic Coding	
8. Describe the format and use of International Classification of Diseases, 10th Revision, Clinical Modification (ICD-10-CM) codes.	
9. Describe how to select an accurate code with the correct level of detail using ICD-10-CM codes.	
10. Perform diagnostic coding.	Performing ICD coding.
Improving Coding Accuracy	
11. Explain how procedure and diagnosis coding are used by third-party payors to validate medical necessity.	Demonstrating tact when discussing code selection and coding requirements with providers.
12. Give examples and explain the effects of upcoding and downcoding.	

CHAPTER OUTLINE

KEY TERMS

downcoding
established patient
inpatient
medical necessity
Medicare Severity-Diagnosis Related Groups (MS-DRGs)
modifier
NEC
new patient
NOS
outpatient
panel
relative value unit (RVU)
sequela (she-KWELL-a)
surgical package
upcoding

INTRODUCTION TO CODING

For hundreds of years, medical researchers have been interested in collecting statistics related to health and disease, including the number of individuals who contract certain diseases and the number of deaths caused by those diseases. To facilitate this undertaking, it was necessary for providers to agree on a system to classify diseases and procedures. Lists of symptoms and diseases had existed in various countries for many years, but the first comprehensive disease classification system in the United States was published in 1869 by the American Medical Association (AMA) as the American Nomenclature of Disease. (The word *nomenclature* means what things are called; in essence, this book was a dictionary of diseases.)

Turning a classification system into a coding system requires systematic replacement of names with numbers or combinations of numbers and letters. This allows information to be standardized. Numbers or combinations of numbers and letters can be easily managed and manipulated by computers.

PROCEDURE CODING

Procedure codes are a means to classify the type of care given to patients. The three main reasons for developing what have come to be called *procedure codes* are as follows:

1. To justify medical services to insurance companies by correlating procedures to diagnosis
2. To collect statistics about the outcome and effectiveness of treatments
3. To help providers and hospitals set fees based on the amount of time and skill required to provide a specific service

In 1966 the AMA published the first edition of the Current Procedural Terminology (CPT) coding system and the AMA continues to publish the most current CPT coding system. The original version focused primarily on surgical procedures and was one of many attempts to translate medical and surgical procedures into numeric codes.

LEVELS OF PROCEDURE CODES

The fourth edition of the CPT, first published in 1977, became the standard for insurance billing in the early 1980s, when it was used as the basis for a Medicare procedure coding system, the Healthcare Common Procedure Coding System (HCPCS), pronounced "hick-picks." Medicare, the government insurance program for the elderly and disabled, is administered by the Centers for Medicare and Medicaid Services (CMS). It is discussed in detail in Chapter 47. Under the Health Insurance Portability and Accountability Act (HIPAA), the commonly used code sets for procedures (HCPCS Level I codes or CPT codes and HCPCS Level II codes) must be used for electronic transactions.

Level I Codes

The first level of HCPCS codes (95%–98% of codes used for Medicare Part B) includes the current CPT codes. Level I codes are updated annually by the AMA, which publishes code books and electronic code sets.

Level II Codes

In addition, there are additional HCPCS codes for procedures, injections, and durable medical equipment covered by Medicare Part B that are not included in the CPT system. These are called Level II codes. HCPCS Level II code books are available from several publishers and can also be obtained electronically from the CMS. Each medical office must purchase updated versions of code books and/or computer files containing all codes used for insurance billing every year. In the past there were also local codes (Level III codes) used for Medicaid (the state-run insurance plan for low-income individuals), which varied from location to location. These have been phased out and are no longer in use.

CURRENT PROCEDURAL TERMINOLOGY CODES

The CPT manual contains CPT (HCPCS Level I) codes and provides both a narrative description and a five-digit code for each procedure or service a physician or other licensed provider may perform for a patient. (Hospitals use a different coding system when billing for inpatient procedures, namely the ICD-10-PCS.) There must be documentation of a diagnosis in the medical record to support the need for any procedure performed for the patient and any procedure code used in billing insurance for the patient. Diagnosis coding is discussed in the next section. In entering procedure codes on insurance claims in the outpatient setting, the five-digit CPT code is sufficient for most procedures.

RELATIVE VALUE UNITS AND DIAGNOSIS-RELATED GROUPS

Each CPT code has been assigned a **relative value unit (RVU)** that quantifies the amount of provider labor, resources, and expertise that are necessary to provide the service represented by the code. Payment by Medicare and many health maintenance organizations (HMOs) is then based on this RVU. For hospital inpatients, Medicare uses another system to determine payments based on **MS-DRGs (Medicare Severity-Diagnosis Related Groups)**. An MS-DRG is a system for grouping hospital inpatients who are expected to utilize a similar amount of hospital resources as a basis for Medicare reimbursement.

SECTIONS OF THE CURRENT PROCEDURAL TERMINOLOGY MANUAL

The CPT manual is used for most procedure coding. Its main part includes the following sections, each of which defines the procedures and services provided for specific types of medical services. The range of codes for each of the major sections, in 2024, is as follows:

Evaluation and Management	99202–99499
Anesthesia	00100–01999, 99100-99140
Surgery	10021-69990
Radiology	70010–79999
Pathology and Laboratory	80047–89398, 0001U–0419U
Medicine	90281-99199, 99500-99607, 0001A-0174A

In each annual update of the CPT, new codes may be added for new procedures, old codes may be dropped for procedures no longer in use, and modifications may be made to current procedures. A darkened circle in front of a code indicates that the code is new. A darkened triangle in front of the code indicates that the description for the code has been changed or modified (Fig. 46.1). The medical assistant must familiarize themselves with the important revisions each year when the new codes are published. In addition, codes must be updated in the office computer system (and on office forms if used) to be sure that insurance is billed correctly.

The main body of the CPT manual is organized by section, then subsection, subheading, and finally category, each providing a finer level of detail. The back of the manual contains an alphabetic index of procedures. The most common procedures performed in a given office are usually found on the charge slip and/or in the computer billing program. In the office itself, the provider identifies the procedures done during a patient visit either in the electronic health record (EHR) or on an electronic or paper charge slip. However, the patient may also be billed by the medical office for provider services in another setting—for example, when a provider examines a patient in the emergency room or a nursing home, or when they perform surgery in the hospital or an outpatient surgery setting. In most locations the office bills only for provider and office services. The patient will receive a separate bill from the hospital or surgical center. If the office bills for laboratory work done by an outside reference laboratory, this must be indicated on the insurance claim (see Chapter 47).

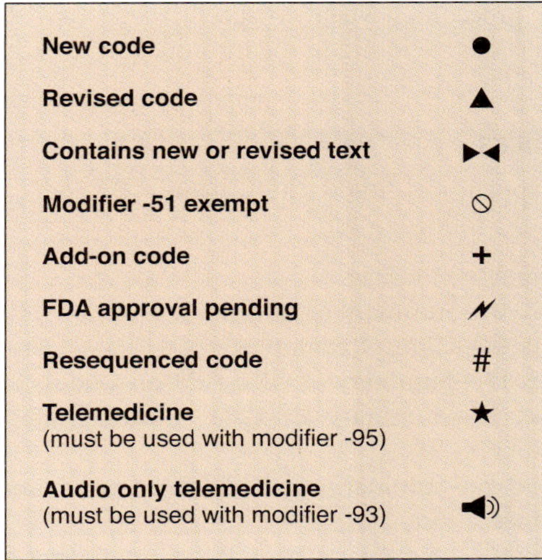

Fig. 46.1 Symbols that appear in the 2024 Current Procedural Terminology code manual.

Category II Codes

Category II codes are optional codes that may be used to track performance. They are not reported to insurance carriers. The last character of these codes is the letter *F* instead of a digit. Category II codes are found after the main sections of the CPT. In addition, they are updated twice a year, and codes that have been added since publication of the most category II codes can be found at the CPT website maintained by the AMA. Use of the code 1159F would mean that the medical record had been reviewed and a medication list was present.

Category III Codes

Category III codes are used to report services that represent emerging technology. They consist of four digits followed by the letter *T*. These codes are listed in their own section after the Category II codes with an expiration date. Category III codes are updated twice a year and, if available, must be used instead of unlisted Category I codes. (Unlisted codes are used for procedures when no specific code can be found. Unlisted codes are found in the introduction to each section of the CPT manual.)

Appendices

Several appendices follow the Category III codes as indicated in the following list:

Appendix A—Modifiers
Appendix B—Summary of Additions, Deletions, Revisions
Appendix C—Clinical Examples
Appendix D—Summary of CPT Add-on Codes
Appendix E—Summary of CPT Codes Exempt from Modifier − 51
Appendix F—Summary of CPT Codes Exempt from Modifier − 63
Appendix G—Summary of CPT Codes That Include Moderate (Conscious) Sedation
Appendix H—Alphabetical Clinical Topics Listing (aka—Alphabetical Listing)
Appendix I—Genetic Testing Code Modifiers
Appendix J—Electrodiagnostic Medicine Listing of Sensory, Motor and Mixed Nerves
Appendix K—Product Pending FDA Approval
Appendix L—Vascular Families
Appendix M—Renumbered CPT Codes-Citations Crosswalk
Appendix N—Summary of Resequenced CPT Codes
Appendix O—Multianalyte Assays with Algorithmic Analysis and Proprietary Laboratory Analyses
Appendix P—CPT Codes That May Be Used for Synchronous Real-Time Interacitve Audio-Video Services
Appendix Q—Severe Acute Respiratory Syndrome Coronavirus 2 (SARS-CoV-2) (coronavirus disease [COVID-19]) Vaccines
Appendix R—Digital Medicine—Services Taxonomy
Appendix S—Artificial Intelligence Taxonomy for Medical Services and Procedures
Appendix T—CPT Codes That May Be Used for Synchronous Real-Time Interactive Audio-Only Telemedicine Services

Appendix B is a summary of additions, deletions, and revisions from the previous year's manual. When the new manual is published, the medical assistant may not be able to find a code that has been used in the past. Appendix B provides a fast way to find out if the code has been deleted, changed, or included in another procedure.

Clinical examples of different codes are given in Appendix C. Reading these can be very helpful in learning how to decide what code to use, especially for Evaluation and Management (E/M) codes. The medical assistant should also become familiar with the other appendices to learn how to use them effectively.

MODIFIERS

A **modifier** is an addition to a procedure code that indicates unusual circumstances related to the procedure, such as a more extensive procedure or two procedures performed in the same session. All modifiers are listed in Appendix A. The modifier is added to the main code after a hyphen (Table 46.1). In addition to the two-digit modifiers, there are also two-character Level II (HCPCS/National) modifiers that can be used to specify body location. These may consist of one letter and one number (e.g., *F5—Right hand, thumb*) or two letters (e.g., *LD—Left descending coronary artery*).

Table 46.1 Selected Current Procedural Terminology Modifiers Used in the Medical Office

Modifier	Description
−22	Increased Procedural Services (not used for E/M services)
−23	Unusual Anesthesia
−26	Professional Component
−32	Mandated Services
−33	Preventative Services
−47	Anesthesia by Surgeon (not including local anesthesia)
−50	Bilateral Procedure—This code is added to the second (bilateral) procedure performed at the same operation
−57	Decision for Surgery (added to an E/M [Evaluation and Management] code when the provider makes the decision for surgery during an E/M visit)
−59	Distinct Procedural Service
−80	Assistant Surgeon
−81	Minimum Assistant Surgeon
−82	Assistant Surgeon (when qualified resident surgeon not available)
−90	Reference (Outside) Laboratory
−91	Repeat Clinical Diagnostic Laboratory Test
−92	Alternative Laboratory Platform Testing
−99	Multiple Modifiers

See the Current Procedural Terminology manual, Appendix A, for a complete list of modifiers.

LOOKING UP CURRENT PROCEDURAL TERMINOLOGY CODES IN THE INDEX

There are several steps in choosing a correct procedure code for a specific patient service. The first step in coding a procedure is to look up the procedure in the alphabetic index of a CPT manual or an online code system like TruCode in SimChart, but the code should not be recorded at this point. The medical assistant should never code directly from the index because it does not contain descriptions of the codes and may result in use of an incorrect code.

It may be necessary to look up the procedure in several ways to locate the correct code. In the index, procedures may be located by looking under the name of the procedure, the anatomic location, and sometimes the diagnosis. The terms are arranged alphabetically with the main term in boldface type and modifying terms arranged below the

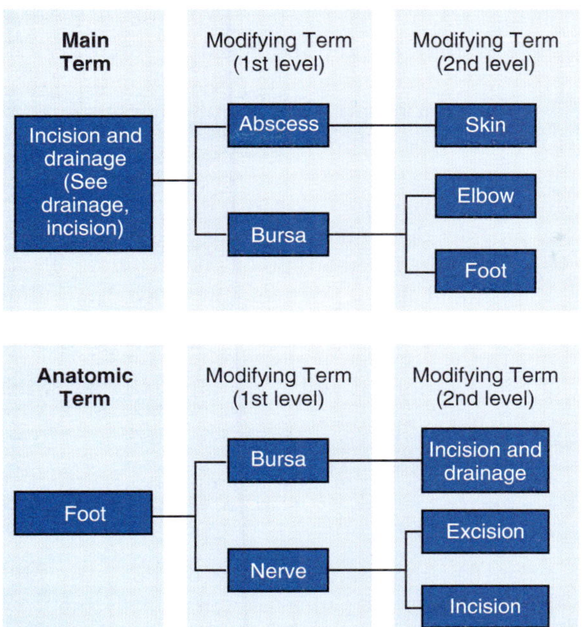

Fig. 46.2 Examples of terms in the index of the Current Procedural Terminology manual when looking up the diagnosis *Incision and drainage of a bursa of the foot.*

main term. Each level of modifying term is indented further than the level above it. For example, the main term is the main word in the procedure. The first modifying term would identify a subterm, an anatomic location, or a procedure (such as *Lesion, Nerve*, or *Repair*). When a procedure is listed in the index (as the main term or any level of modifying term), it is followed by a code or range of codes (e.g., Excision, Nerve, Foot ...... 28055). Both main terms or anatomic terms and modifying terms may point to a cross-reference using the word *See* (Fig. 46.2).

Several pieces of information may be significant when choosing the correct code for a procedure:

- Location
- Size of lesion or repair
- Method of performing the procedure, test, or surgery
- Number of minutes allotted for a treatment (e.g., acupuncture)
- Complexity of the procedure or service

SELECTING A SPECIFIC CURRENT PROCEDURAL TERMINOLOGY CODE

After identifying a code or code range from the index, the medical assistant should read all relevant codes carefully in the main text. It may also be necessary to review the guidelines at the beginning of the appropriate section of the CPT manual to obtain additional information that can be helpful in choosing a code. The medical assistant should select the code that is the best match for the medical documentation and determine if it is necessary to use a modifier or an add-on code.

There are two types of CPT codes: stand-alone codes and indented codes. The stand-alone code contains a semicolon (e.g., 93000 Electrocardiogram [ECG], routine ECG with at least 12 leads; with interpretation and report). The indented code, which follows a stand-alone code or another indented code, provides only text to replace the words after the semicolon in the stand-alone code (e.g., 93005 [indent] tracing only, without interpretation and report). In the example given, the code 93000 would be used if the ECG tracing is made and the provider interprets the tracing in the same medical office. The code 93005 (Electrocardiogram, routine ECG, with at least 12 leads; tracing only, without interpretation and report) would be used if the ECG tracing is made in one office, but insurance should not be billed for the interpretation because it will be done by another provider and billed from another office (Procedure 46.1).

Evaluation and Management

The E/M section contains codes for office visits provided by primary care practitioners and specialists. E/M codes cover the service-oriented, rather than the procedure-oriented, parts of medical care. It is important to determine where the service was provided when selecting the correct E/M code.

Although procedures are fairly easy to define—for instance, incision and drainage of a cyst—the amount of service provided by a provider during an office visit is more difficult to describe. For many of the E/M codes the history and physical examination must simply be medically appropriate and the actual code is determined by the level of medical decision-making and the amount of time spent with the patient.

The codes in the E/M section attempt to link reimbursement to the completeness of the examination and the amount of skill required to manage the patient's problems. For example, if a patient is in the office for a recheck of an ear infection, the visit would not usually take a significant amount of time. If the patient has several questions about methods other than antibiotics that could be used to treat ear infections, it will take more time for the provider to complete the examination, even though there is no additional medical problem or complication.

When determining the proper code for E/M services, the medical assistant must consider a number of factors.

1. For coding purposes, the patient is either an **established patient** (one who has been seen in the previous 3 years) or a **new patient** (one who has not had services performed by any provider in the medical office in the previous 3 years). There are separate groups of codes for each type of patient. New patients are expected to take longer to examine and are reimbursed at a higher rate. The patient is also either an **outpatient** (one who has not been admitted to a health care facility) or an **inpatient** (a patient who has been formally admitted to a health care facility). Although most services for patients who are inpatients are billed by the health care facility itself,

providers who are not employees of that facility bill for visits to the patient during a hospital admission, for inpatient consultations, for providing reports for some diagnostic tests performed at the hospital (e.g., cardiac stress tests), for critical care and intensive care services, and for care for visits to patients in nursing homes.

2. There are separate groups of codes, depending on where the service is provided and whether the provider is the patient's primary care provider or a consultant. A medical service could have been provided in the office, in a nursing home, in a hospital to a patient who has been admitted, or in a hospital emergency department. The E/M section of the CPT manual is divided into several subsections, and it is important to select a code from the correct subsection, depending on the service that the provider provided and the location where the service was provided.
3. The level of service depends primarily on two key factors:
   - The complexity of medical decision making
   - The amount of time

Medical History

The CPT manual states that there must be a medically appropriate history for each level of CPT codes. No other instructions are given. It is up to the provider to ensure that the appropriate history information is collected for the presenting problem(s).

Physical Examination

The CPT manual also states that there should be a medically appropriate physical examination done. It is up to the provider to ensure that an appropriate physical examination is done based on the problems that the patient presents with.

Medical Decision Making

Medical decision-making can be straightforward or have a low, moderate, or high level of complexity. If a patient has one problem, medical decision-making is usually straightforward. When a patient has multiple problems, especially if they are causing severe or life-threatening symptoms, the decision-making process is more complex. For example, if a new patient has poorly controlled diabetes mellitus type 1, fever, and an increased white blood count, the decision-making process for the provider would be highly complex (Fig. 46.3).

The provider determines the number and complexity of the issues presented at the time of the encounter. In addition, they should also be aware of how much data will need to be reviewed and/or analyzed for the particular patient. And finally, the provider should take into consideration the risk of complications as well as the morbitidy or mortality of the patient's condition(s).

Medical decision-making is the first key piece in determining which code is the most appropriate.

Time

The second key piece is the amount of time spent during the examination of the patient as well as analyzing the test results and diagnostic procedures that were done for the patient. Many providers are now including the amount of time spent with the patient and reviewing all of the test results in their final dicatation for the patient.

Anesthesia

Anesthesia is the administration of a drug that causes a total or partial loss of sensation. Anesthesia can be administered to provide analgesia (absence of pain) for a patient during a surgical procedure, wound closure, removal of a foreign body, childbirth, or a diagnostic test, including radiology, as well as for therapeutic radiology.

Anesthesia can be general, regional, or local. Local anesthesia by infiltration (the most common form of anesthesia used in the medical office) is included with the procedure and is not given a separate code. CPT codes for anesthesia are specified first by the anatomic region affected, then by the type of procedure. Anesthesia services are reimbursed based on a formula. Each anesthesia code is assigned a base

Type of Decision Making	Number of Diagnoses or Management Options	Amount of Complexity and/or Data to be Reviewed	Risk of Complications or Morbidity or Mortality
Straightforward	Minimal	Minimal or none	Minimal
Low complexity	Limited	Limited	Low
Moderate complexity	Multiple	Moderate	Moderate
High complexity	Extensive	Extensive	High

Fig. 46.3 In the Evaluation and Management section of the Current Procedural Terminology manual, the type of decision-making is one of the three key factors in selection of the correct level of service.

unit value (B), which can be found in the Relative Value Guide published by the American Society of Anesthesiologists. The second component of the anesthesia formula is time (T), which is measured from the time the anesthesiologist first begins to manage a patient and ends when the patient is no longer under their care. Every 15-minute period is a unit. The total anesthesia units (B + T) are multiplied by a conversion factor (CF) based on the locality of service to determine payment for anesthesia services.

The Anesthesia section has two types of modifiers: standard modifiers and physical status modifiers. Standard modifiers are those used throughout the CPT code manual; physical status modifiers indicate the patient's condition at the time anesthesia was administered. Patient condition can influence the level of complexity of administering anesthesia in the proper dose over the proper time frame. The complete descriptions of these modifiers are found in the guidelines at the beginning of the Anesthesia section of the CPT manual. Codes for moderate (conscious) sedation (medication administered intravenously over a period of time to keep a patient calm without causing loss of consciousness) are found in the Medicine section.

Surgery

The Surgery section is the largest section of the CPT manual. This section is organized by organ systems and within the systems by types of procedures.

Surgical procedures are coded as a surgical package. The term **surgical package** indicates that the code covers all routine services related to a surgery. The following areas are included in the surgical package and cannot be coded (or billed) separately:

- One E/M visit that occurs after the decision for surgery has been made, either on the day before or the day of surgery (including a history and physical examination)
- Local or topical anesthesia or a digital nerve block
- Immediate postoperative care
- Writing orders for care after surgery
- Evaluating the patient in the recovery room
- Typical follow-up postoperative care

If complications occur during the surgery or during follow-up, treatment of the complications can be coded separately.

Radiology

The Radiology section of the CPT manual includes radiology, nuclear medicine, diagnostic ultrasound, and radiation oncology. Radiology codes include both the technical component (creating the image) as well as the professional component (interpreting the image). If only one component is performed, this should be indicated by a modifier.

Most standard radiologic procedures are found in the Diagnostic Radiology subsection, including plain x-ray images, computed tomography (CT or CAT), magnetic resonance imaging (MRI), magnetic resonance angiography (MRA), and standard angiography. The codes for diagnostic radiology correspond to the anatomic site of the radiographic image, starting with the head and moving down. Some codes indicate a single view, whereas others indicate multiple views. The correct code may also indicate whether or not a contrast medium was used. In the outpatient setting, there is typically no additional charge for the provider's interpretation of the radiograph.

Pathology and Laboratory

The Pathology and Laboratory section of the CPT manual is organized by the type of tests performed, such as individual tests, panels, or assays. A **panel** is a group of laboratory tests, usually ordered together for diagnosis or screening, such as a cardiac panel (a group of tests ordered for a patient with cardiac symptoms). To use a panel code, each test in the panel must have been done. Additional or other tests are coded separately.

Different codes are used for laboratory tests performed by automated equipment and tests performed manually. When coding for a medical office, the medical assistant must be sure that patients are charged only for tests actually performed in the office (e.g., a dipstick urinalysis). If the medical assistant draws blood to be sent to an outside laboratory, the medical office charges the patient for the venipuncture (using the code 36415), but the laboratory usually bills separately for the diagnostic tests performed. The office does not charge separately for collecting urine and throat specimens if they are sent to an outside laboratory for processing.

Pathology testing, such as Papanicolaou (Pap) tests and biopsies, is usually done by a special laboratory. The medical office charges for the visit or surgery during which the specimen is collected, but the laboratory usually bills for the actual specimen testing.

Medicine

The Medicine section of the CPT manual gives the proper codes for noninvasive diagnostic and treatment services, many of which are performed in the offices of primary care providers and specialists. Invasive services, those that enter a body cavity, usually fall in the Surgery section. The Medicine section is organized according to body system.

A number of highly specialized types of testing and treatment, ranging from ECGs to ophthalmologic tests, are found in the Medicine section. In addition, the Medicine section contains the codes for immunizations and infusion therapies, including chemotherapy. Codes for procedures from this section that are performed frequently (e.g., ECGs in the office of an internist or cardiologist) are usually found in the medical billing software, although there is usually a resource where the code for a procedure that is not performed commonly in the office can be looked up.

HEALTHCARE COMMON PROCEDURE CODING SYSTEM LEVEL II CODES

HCPCS Level II codes use a five-digit alphanumeric coding system to designate specific services and equipment. Level II codes are used primarily for items and services that do

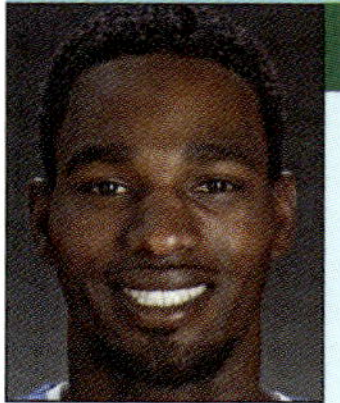

Putting It All Into Practice

My name is John Grant, and I am a Certified Medical Assistant. I work for a group of family practice providers, and we have two offices. I am responsible for entering and/or reviewing charges for every patient treated by our providers. We have found that there is more consistency if one person is responsible for this task. Our providers usually see patients in the office, but all of our providers also visit their patients if they are hospitalized, visit patients in nursing homes, and sometimes see patients in the hospital emergency department in the evenings and on weekends. Each time a patient is seen in the office, the provider enters the services and starts an electronic charge slip. I complete the charge slip, post the charge to the patient ledger, and create an insurance claim. When the providers see patients in the hospital or in nursing homes, they fill out a log sheet we developed in the office so that we can be sure that we bill patients for all services and use the correct code for each service provided. If the provider performs a procedure that is not on the electronic charge slip, I look up the correct code and enter it into the computer system. In addition, I have to be sure that the correct place of service code is entered because insurance companies will reject a claim if the place of service does not match the service provided. For example, if I use the code 99281 for an emergency department visit, I have to be sure to use the place of service code 23 (emergency department—hospital).

I also look up diagnosis codes and enter them into the computer if necessary. The most common diagnosis codes are found in our computer system, but the provider may enter a diagnosis that is not in the computer. The diagnosis has to correspond to the service, and sometimes the provider forgets to enter all of a patient's conditions with the charges. In those cases, I have to review the medical record to find the specific diagnosis that justifies a procedure. Coding is complicated, but in the long run it saves time to spend time making sure that the codes are entered correctly when the charges are entered. Otherwise, our insurance claims are rejected, and we spend a lot of time fixing mistakes and resubmitting claims. ■

What Would You Do? What Would You *Not* Do?

Case Study 1

When John is reviewing patient charges on the electronic charge slips, he finds that the primary care provider has entered the code for a straightforward medical decision-making office visit (99202) for a new patient named Peter Miller. John notices that this patient has other transactions in the computer from a previous visit about 12 months before the current visit when the patient was seen by a different provider in the practice. ■

not have Level I (CPT) codes. Examples of items with Level II codes include supplies, materials, specific medications, ambulance services, and some procedures. For example, if a patient is given a pair of metal underarm crutches after a cast has been applied, the HCPCS code E0114 would be used to bill Medicare for the crutches. Note that the code begins with a letter that corresponds to the section of the Level II code manual. All codes are in the format of one letter followed by four digits, and they are arranged alphabetically by the first character and then numerically by the subsequent digits. Like CPT codes, they also have modifiers that should be used, if necessary, to clarify an individual code.

Level II codes are updated annually by the CMS. Most commercial insurance companies also accept Level II codes for covered items or services.

LOOKING UP HEALTHCARE COMMON PROCEDURE CODING SYSTEM LEVEL II CODES

The process for locating accurate HCPCS Level II codes is almost the same as that for looking up CPT codes (Procedure 46.2). The medical assistant should first locate the item or service in the index of the HCPCS manual. The index is in the form of main term followed by subterm(s). A single code or code range may be found in the index, but the medical assistant should always find the complete description in the list of codes before making a final selection. The codes consist of one letter followed by four numbers, and they are arranged alphabetically by the initial letter and then numerically by the four digits. Codes marked ⃠ are not valid for Medicare. They are used for other insurance carriers.

Codes for medications given in the office may vary according to the dose given. These codes can be looked up in the HCPCS manual or using the TruCode tab in SimChart. Most practice management programs also have a function to look up codes as needed (Fig. 46.4).

What Would You Do? What Would You *Not* Do?

Case Study 2

While entering charges for Joan Drysdale, a 72-year-old patient with Medicare insurance, John sees that the patient was charged for an intramuscular injection (96372) of methylprednisolone in addition to the office visit (99213). No other charges are listed on the electronic charge slip. John needs to add the code for the medication itself for this patient so that Medicare can be billed. ■

DIAGNOSIS CODING

HISTORY OF DIAGNOSIS CODING

In addition to coding procedures, it is also necessary to code a patient's diagnosis or diagnoses. Diagnostic coding was originally developed to fulfill four purposes: to track disease processes, to classify the causes of death, to collect data for medical research, and to evaluate hospital service utilization.

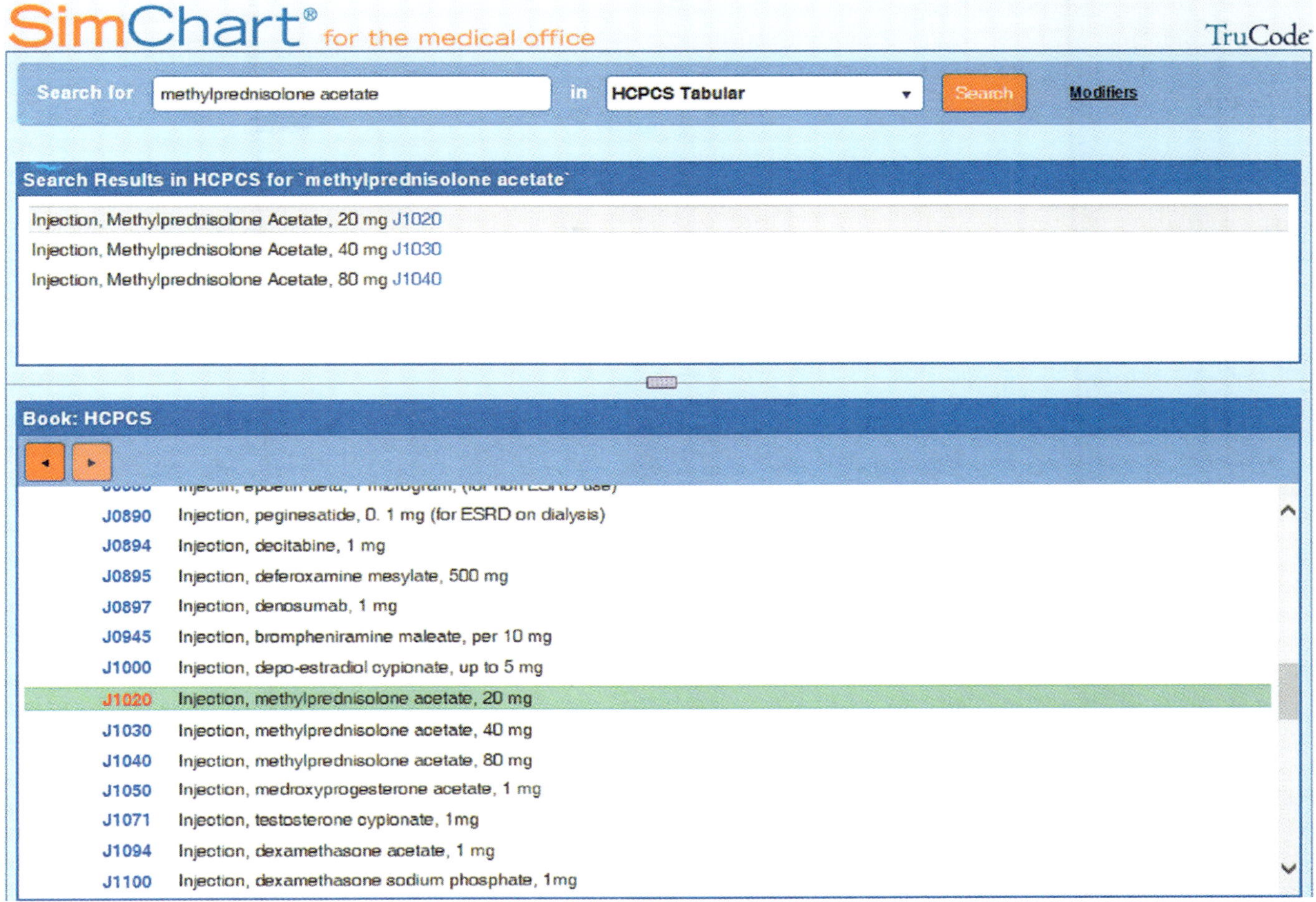

Fig. 46.4 Healthcare Common Procedure Coding System *(HCPCS)* codes can be looked up using TruCode in SimChart.

In 1948 the World Health Organization (WHO) published the first edition of the International Classification of Diseases, which assigned numbers to specific diseases. This system was developed so that more accurate statistics could be collected about how often diseases and accidents occurred and were treated. The system proved to be useful for health care review and insurance claims processing.

WHO has revised the International Classifications of Diseases (ICD) several times since 1948. For insurance coding and review of medical records, a clinical modification tool was developed to better collect and compile data about specific diseases, conditions, and medical services for healthy individuals. The acronym for this coding system was ICD-9-CM, which stands for International Classification of Diseases, 9th Revision, Clinical Modification. The ICD-9-CM became the system of choice for diagnostic coding after 1989. At that time Medicare began to require ICD-9 codes on all outpatient insurance claim forms. This soon became a requirement of all insurance companies.

The tenth edition (ICD-10) was published in 1993 by WHO. Its use in the United States was not required until October 1, 2015. Compared to the ICD-9-CM, it is important to note that there are five times more codes in the ICD-10. This allows for more precise coding of body part and patient encounter information. The ICD-9 coding system used five alphanumeric characters with a decimal point after the third character. The only character that could be a letter was the first one. Compared with the ICD-9-CM, the ICD-10-CM includes several new features:

- More extensive information related to ambulatory care and managed care encounters
- An expansion of injury codes
- New combination diagnosis and symptom codes to decrease the need for two codes
- An added sixth and seventh digit for some conditions
- Increased ability to locate and choose specific codes

In the ICD-10, for example, it is required for both diabetes mellitus and its complications to use a code that identifies the specific type or cause of the diabetes (type 1, type 2, due to drug or chemical, gestational, other, and so on). Initially coders used conversion tables, but they are primarily useful for individuals who are already very familiar with the ICD-9, and their use has diminished in the past few years.

It is necessary to use one or more diagnosis codes to have an insurance claim approved for reimbursement. If the proper ICD code(s) and coding format are not used, many insurance companies will reject a claim because the patient's diagnosis does not justify the procedures done for the patient. ICD coding is required by government-financed programs, such as Medicare and Medicaid, as well as most private insurance companies. The US Department of Health and Human Services (HHS) is responsible for mandating accepted standards of electronic transmission and required code sets as required by HIPAA.

ICD-10-CM CODES

The ICD-10-CM manual has two parts: the Index and the Tabular List. The Index is a list of diseases and conditions arranged in alphabetic order. The Tabular List is the section in which the actual codes are displayed, arranged in 22 chapters according to classification of the disease or condition or factors influencing health status or contact with health services. The ICD-9-CM had an additional volume, Volume 3, used to code inpatient hospital procedures. ICD-9-CM Volume 3 is replaced by the ICD-10-PCS (Procedure Coding System), which will not be discussed here because it is used for inpatient procedures only. CPT codes continue to be used to code outpatient procedures and provider services.

FORMAT OF ICD-10-CM CODES

The ICD-10-CM code begins with three characters followed by a decimal point. The first character is a letter, and the next two characters are usually digits. These first three characters show where the code occurs in the tabular list and stand for the basic condition. For example, Chapter 1 contains codes A00 to B99, U07.1, U09.9 which are infectious or parasitic diseases. There are 22 chapters, and most chapters contain the codes that begin with one letter of the alphabet. Chapters 3 to 14 are devoted to diseases or conditions of specific body systems. All the other chapters contain codes for types of diseases or conditions except Chapter 21, which contains codes for factors influencing health status, and Chapter 22 which contains codes for special purposes such COVID-19. The codes from Chapter 21 are usually used for individuals who seek health screening or preventative care (Table 46.2). Factors influencing health status include several reasons for an office visit besides illness, such as physical examinations, genetic carrier or genetic susceptibility, screening for various conditions, and contact with communicable diseases.

Table 46.2 Contents of the ICD-10-CM Manual

Chapter	Codes	Diseases or Conditions
1	(A00–B99, U07.1, U09.9)	Certain Infectious and Parasitic Diseases
2	(C00–D49)	Neoplasms
3	(D50–D89)	Disease of the Blood and Blood-Forming Organs and Certain Disorders Involving the Immune Mechanism
4	(E00–E89)	Endocrine, Nutritional, and Metabolic Diseases
5	(F01–F99)	Mental, Behavioral Disorders and Neurodevelopmental Disorders
6	(G00–G99)	Diseases of Nervous System
7	(H00–H59)	Diseases of Eye and Adnexa
8	(H60–H95)	Diseases of Ear and Mastoid Process
9	(I00–I99)	Diseases of Circulatory System
10	(J00–J99, U07.0)	Diseases of Respiratory System
11	(K00–K95)	Diseases of Digestive System
12	(L00–L99)	Diseases of Skin and Subcutaneous Tissue
13	(M00–M99)	Diseases of the Musculoskeletal System and Connective Tissue
14	(N00–N99)	Diseases of Genitourinary System
15	(O00–O9A)	Pregnancy, Childbirth, and the Puerperium
16	(P00–P96)	Certain Conditions Originating in the Perinatal Period
17	(Q00–Q99)	Congenital Malformations, Deformations, and Chromosomal Abnormalities
18	(R00–R99)	Symptoms, Signs, and Abnormal Clinical and Laboratory Findings, Not Elsewhere Classified
19	(S00–T88)	Injury, Poisoning, and Certain Other Consequences of External Causes
20	(V01–Y99)	External Causes of Morbidity
21	(Z00–Z99)	Factors Influencing Health Status and Contact with Health Services
22	(U00- U85)	Codes for Special Purposes

One to four characters (up to two more than for ICD-9) follow the decimal point. This allows for a total of up to seven characters in a valid code. Some three-character codes are acceptable, but ICD-10 manual indicates when additional characters are required. Characters after the decimal point make a given diagnosis more specific. The first three characters after a decimal point may be digits or letters, and the final character (if needed) is a letter. A lower-case *x* can be used as a place holder because each required digit or letter must be in the correct position (e.g., sixth character, seventh character). For example, the code for the initial encounter for a pathologic fracture in neoplastic disease in an unspecified site would be M84.50xA. The *x* is a placeholder for a sixth character that would indicate the site, which in this case is not specified. The seventh character, *A,* is required to indicate that the code refers to the initial visit.

Looking Up Diagnosis Codes in the Alphabetic Index

When coding in the outpatient setting, the medical assistant should try to find the most specific code that matches each diagnosis given by the provider. The first-listed diagnosis describes the primary reason that the patient has sought care. This may be a disease or condition, if diagnostic testing has confirmed the diagnosis. It may be one or more symptoms, if a confirmed diagnosis is pending. It may also be a reason for seeking health care when the patient is not ill (e.g., a routine physical examination). In addition, the provider may list other diagnoses if the patient has complications or coexisting conditions, especially if they are the reason for procedures or diagnostic tests.

The first step is to locate the first-listed diagnosis in the alphabetic index. As an example, assume that the provider lists the patient's first diagnosis as *Salmonella* gastroenteritis. If the medical assistant looks under *Salmonella*, they are referred to *Infection*, *Salmonella*, and the code listed is A02.9. If the medical assistant looks under *Gastroenteritis*, a subheading is found for *Salmonella* with the identical code. After locating the code in the index, the medical assistant should always follow up by reviewing the code in the tabular list to be sure that they have located the most specific code and has chosen a code with the required number of characters. It is not always possible to know from the index how many characters a specific code will require.

Codes for Individuals Who Do Not Have a Disease or Injury (Z01 to Z99)

Codes from Chapter 21 (Factors Influencing Health Status and Contact with Health Services) are used when the patient does not have a disease or injury and are referred to as *Z codes*. This code may be used as the first-listed diagnosis if the patient has sought health care to receive an immunization or for a physical examination. If the provider lists a diagnosis of family history of diabetes, the medical assistant would look up *History, family (of), diabetes mellitus* to find the code, Z83.3. Checking the tabular list would confirm that this is an acceptable first-listed or secondary diagnosis. The medical history alone justifies periodic examinations. It is important to note that even a code such as Z00.00 (*Encounter for general adult medical examination without abnormal findings*) is a diagnosis code, and it must be accompanied by a valid procedure code (CPT code) when billing the insurance company.

A Z code may also be used as a secondary code when a patient seeks care for a specific disease or condition. For example, a patient may seek care for an infection, but the care given may be influenced by the fact that the patient has a penicillin allergy that influences the care for the current condition. To code for the allergy, the medical assistant would look in the index under *History, personal allergy to, penicillin.*

External Cause Codes (V01 to Y99)

External cause codes cover external causes of injury or poisoning, such as injury resulting from collision of a motor vehicle with another motor vehicle. They facilitate the collection of statistics about causes and severity of injuries. These codes are used only in combination with other diagnosis codes to give more information about the cause of a medical problem. They are never the first-listed diagnosis. The External Cause Index is located in the Alphabetic Index after the Table of Drugs and Chemicals.

USING THE ALPHABETIC INDEX

When looking up diagnosis codes, the medical assistant must always keep in mind that insurance companies will be using the diagnosis code to pay for services. If the diagnosis codes are incorrect or incomplete, the insurance carrier may refuse to pay for the services provided.

To find the diagnosis in the index, the medical assistant may look under the main word of the patient's diagnosis. It is also possible to start from the anatomic location of the medical problem, which will be cross-referenced to the main term. The index is arranged with headings and subheadings. Each level of subheadings is also arranged alphabetically. In the examples that follow, a comma indicates that the next term is a subheading of the previous term.

During the period when the provider is still trying to determine exactly what the patient's diagnosis is, symptoms may be listed on the charge sheet. These should be coded exactly as written. If the provider writes *rule out (R/O)* with a diagnosis or condition, that condition may *not* be used for coding. Only the patient symptoms should be coded. If a patient has received ambulatory surgery, the medical assistant should look up the condition for which the surgery was done or the postoperative diagnosis, if it is different from the preoperative diagnosis.

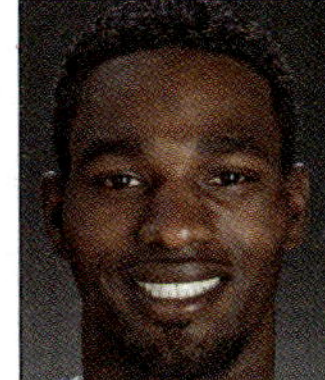

Memories *from* Practicum

John Grant: My practicum was performed in a large clinic where I spent some time in several departments. I was placed in the medical records department for 4 days, and I didn't understand why I needed to be there for such a long time. I was surprised to learn that not only was this department responsible for filing and taking care of the medical records, but also they did a considerable amount of coding. They asked me to look up diagnosis codes one day, and I spent all morning and part of the afternoon doing this. They gave me a stack of referral forms and told me to look up and write the diagnosis code on each form. If I couldn't find it or if I wasn't sure, I should put the form to one side so that someone could help me later. I was told to find the diagnosis in the index, and then look up the best code in the tabular list. I had had some practice in school, so this wasn't completely new to me. I have to admit that the pile of codes I was sure of was smaller than the pile I had questions about. I never realized that coding could be so complicated. There were some I couldn't find at all and others where I just couldn't decide what the best code was. For example, when the diagnosis was "unequal arm length due to old fracture" I found out that I should look up "Deformity, limb, unequal length, short site is ..." in the index. I also found out that I would have to look at the medical record to identify the specific bone that had been previously fractured to select a specific code. This experience showed me that coding requires real attention to detail. ■

Examples

If the progress note describes the patient's problem as "recurrent right shoulder pain, rule out bursitis," the code can be located in the index under: *Pain, shoulder* (M25.51-). The dash at the end of the code in the index indicates that at least one additional character is required (in this case to indicate if it is the right shoulder, left shoulder, or unspecified shoulder).

1. If the patient's diagnosis is "diabetic neuropathy," the medical assistant should look in the index under *Neuropathy, diabetic*. The code range is listed as E08 to E13 with .40. This means that types of diabetic neuropathy are listed under E08.40, E09.40, E10.40, E11.40, and so on. It turns out that it is necessary to correlate the underlying type of diabetes (drug induced, type 1, type 2, or other) to the neuropathy. The medical assistant should find this information in the medical record. It is also possible to locate the code by looking in the index under *Diabetes, diabetic, with, neuropathy*, although it is necessary to look under type 1 or type 2 diabetes.

USING THE TABULAR LIST

Once a code or range of codes has been identified, the medical assistant should find the correct section and determine the best code to match the information on the patient's charge slip or in the medical record. It is important to look at the additional information given relating to the diagnosis.

In the tabular list, the medical assistant should always look for the most specific code possible, remembering that the code must be supported by the information in the medical record. Parentheses are used in the index and tabular list to identify words that may be found in the diagnosis but are not required. When symbols indicate that codes require additional characters or cannot be used as a first-listed diagnosis, it is necessary to continue to look for a correct code. Codes may be identified as **NOS** (not otherwise specified) or **NEC** (not elsewhere classified) as used in the ICD-9. A code that is identified by a symbol indicating that it is used for a complication or a comorbidity (additional disease or condition) should always follow another code related to the reason the patient has sought treatment.

Instructional Notes

The word *Includes* may be used under a category and will identify additional names for conditions in the category or a description of conditions. For example, under the category code for *Mumps* (B26), the tabular list states, *Includes epidemic parotitis and infectious parotitis*. The word *Excludes* identifies specific conditions that are not included in a category and usually points to an alternative code. *Excludes 1* means that the condition is not coded here, and the patient cannot have both the excluded condition and the condition listed above it. *Excludes 2* means that the condition is not included in this code, but the patient may have two conditions, the one included in the current code, as well as the condition using the correct code for the excluded condition. For example, in the category *Allergic contact dermatitis* (L23), the patient cannot have a diagnosis of contact dermatitis that does not specify allergy (Excludes 1), and conditions such as dermatitis caused by substances taken internally are not included (Excludes 2).

More than one code may be required for a single disease or condition when a condition affects multiple body systems or is caused by or results from an underlying condition in another body system, and for late effects and complications. The instruction "Code first" instructs the coder to use another code first that will identify the cause or underlying condition. In the example of allergic contact dermatitis noted previously, an additional code that identifies the substance causing the allergic contact dermatitis should be used as the first code before the code for the dermatitis. There may also be an instruction to "Code also," which indicates that an additional code is required. In some cases, one code describes both the underlying condition and the manifestation and only one code is needed. For example, a single code is sufficient for a sore throat cause by *Streptococcus* (J02.0 *Streptococcal pharyngitis*).

Selecting the Code With the Correct Level of Detail

Codes vary in length depending on the subdivisions in the tabular list. Three-digit codes are category codes and are rarely valid codes. Codes with four digits designate a subclassification. They usually also require additional characters. Some four-digit codes are valid codes for a condition whose location, cause, or other details are unspecified. The fifth character indicates a subclassification. This may be a body part (Fig. 46.5). The sixth character often indicates a specific location or a specific type of condition. (See Table 46.3 to review an example of the meaning of characters in specific locations.)

Most codes are complete with five or six characters, but some require a seventh character (letter), usually to indicate whether it is an initial encounter, a subsequent encounter, or an encounter for a **sequela.** A sequela (pl. *sequelae*) is any condition that results from a disease, injury, or treatment for a disease or injury. The choices for the seventh character are specific for the category and will be listed in the tabular list. They apply to all subclassifications of the category. For example, in the code S32.009A (initial encounter for a unspecified fracture of an unspecified lumbar vertebra), the *A* indicates that it is the initial encounter. The letter *D* would indicate a subsequent encounter for a fracture that is healing routinely, and the letter *S* would be used for a complication (sequela) such as persistent back pain (Procedure 46.3).

IMPROVING CODING ACCURACY

MEDICAL NECESSITY

Medical necessity is a term for health care that is reasonable and necessary for a patient based on evidence-based clinical standards of care. Third-party payors make payment decisions based on medical necessity. If a covered procedure is medically necessary, a third-party payor must pay for the

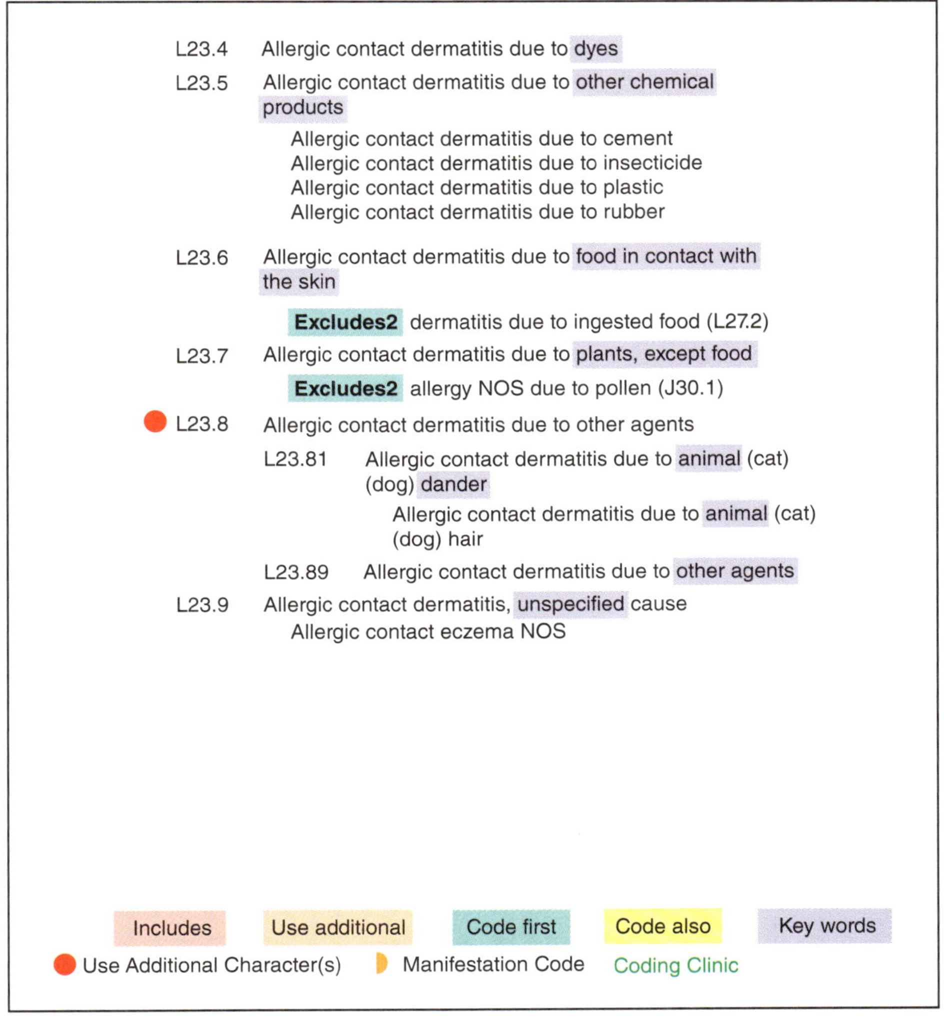
L23.4 Allergic contact dermatitis due to dyes
L23.5 Allergic contact dermatitis due to other chemical products
Allergic contact dermatitis due to cement
Allergic contact dermatitis due to insecticide
Allergic contact dermatitis due to plastic
Allergic contact dermatitis due to rubber
L23.6 Allergic contact dermatitis due to food in contact with the skin
Excludes2 dermatitis due to ingested food (L27.2)
L23.7 Allergic contact dermatitis due to plants, except food
Excludes2 allergy NOS due to pollen (J30.1)
L23.8 Allergic contact dermatitis due to other agents
L23.81 Allergic contact dermatitis due to animal (cat) (dog) dander
Allergic contact dermatitis due to animal (cat) (dog) hair
L23.89 Allergic contact dermatitis due to other agents
L23.9 Allergic contact dermatitis, unspecified cause
Allergic contact eczema NOS

Fig. 46.5 A sample from the International Classification of Diseases, 10th revision, Clinical Modification. (From Buck CJ: *2023 ICD-10-CM Physician Edition*, St. Louis, 2023, Saunders.)

Table 46.3 Specificity of ICD-10 Codes

Characters	Incomplete Code	Valid Code	Description
3	S22		Fracture of rib(s), sternum, and thoracic spine
4	S22.0		Fracture of thoracic vertebra
5	S22.01		Fracture of first thoracic vertebra
6	S22.010		Wedge compression fracture of first thoracic vertebra
7		S22.010A	Initial encounter for closed wedge compression fracture of first thoracic vertebra

procedure. Specific combinations of procedure codes and diagnosis codes may be used by third-party payors to determine medical necessity. This especially applies to Medicare, which uses National Coverage Determinations (NCDs) and Local Coverage Determinations (LCDs) to describe coverage criteria. For example, a blood test for thyroxine, thyroid-stimulating hormone (TSH), or thyroid hormone (T_3 or T_4) uptake would not be paid for by Medicare if linked to a diagnosis of precordial pain (ICD-10 code R07.2), although there is a list of more than 200 diagnosis codes that do justify such blood tests. Medicare publishes an alphabetic index of NCDs that links procedures and diagnoses on the CMS website. When coding, it is the medical assistant's obligation to verify that a procedure code is linked to the correct diagnosis code. If it is suspected that a provider has made an error when ordering a diagnostic test (e.g., ordering a chest radiograph for a patient with knee pain), the medical assistant should tactfully verify the order and point out, if necessary, that the procedure may not be reimbursed because the diagnosis does not support it (Procedure 46.4).

CODING AT THE CORRECT LEVEL OF SERVICE

When medical codes are misused in order to obtain a higher level of reimbursement than is allowed, the process is called

upcoding. Under Section 231 of the HIPAA, nearly all federal health care programs can levy fines and penalties for failure to adhere to compliance with regulations for using correct codes on claims for reimbursements. A pattern or practice of upcoding can result in large fines, and ignorance of correct procedure is not considered a defense. Medicare analyzes claims to identify atypical billing and may follow up with a more detailed analysis when a pattern has been identified for a specific provider.

Some provider offices have contracted for independent review in order to identify coding and billing errors. After such a review, it may be found that in some cases codes do not reflect a high enough level of service (**downcoding**), resulting in lower levels of reimbursement than are justified. Practitioners may avoid the higher level E/M codes out of fear of being audited. Consistently coding below the actual level of service decreases revenue, and overuse of one code level can actually trigger an audit. An independent review can also reveal cases in which the codes used on claims are higher than the level of service provided (*upcoding*). Based on an independent review, a medical office can identify problem areas and improve its coding procedures to maximize income without risking fines or other legal proceedings.

What Would You Do? What Would You *Not* Do?

Case Study 3

When entering charges for Michael Drew, a 56-year-old patient, John sees that the provider has written the diagnosis "Diabetes Type 1." Just below the code, the provider has written "with diabetic polyneuropathy." John needs to enter the charges and codes into the computer so that this patient's insurance can be billed. John's office is using ICD-10 codes. ■

What Would You Do? What Would You *Not* Do? RESPONSES

Case Study 1

Page 1178

What Did John Do?

- Double-checked the EHR to find out if the charge was entered for the correct Peter Miller and to find out if the patient had been seen before.
- Changed the CPT code to that of an established patient if it turned out that he had been seen by any practitioner in the practice within the past 3 years.
- Created a new patient ledger if it turned out from reviewing the medical record that Peter Miller was, in fact, a new patient with a different birth date and address.

What Did John Not Do?

- Did not just assume that whatever the provider entered was correct.
- Did not allow insurance to be charged for a new patient if the patient was, in fact, an established patient.
- Did not tell the provider to be more careful in the future when entering charges.

Case Study 2

Page 1178

What Did John Do?

- Looked up the Medicare code for methylprednisolone acetate in the HCPCS Level II manual, where he noted that the correct code depends on the dose given.
- Checked the medical record to identify the dose of methylprednisolone given to the patient and selected the correct HCPCS code from that information.

What Did John Not Do?

- Did not assume that all the correct codes were entered on the electronic charge slip.
- Did not guess at the dose of methylprednisolone because he knew what dose the provider usually gave.
- Did not assume that he could save time by asking the provider what dose was given.
- Did not bother the provider with the details of this coding situation.

Case Study 3

Page 1184

What Did John Do?

- Checked the ICD-10-CM manual to read all codes for diabetes mellitus and codes for diabetic polyneuropathy. He found a single code for type 1 diabetes with polyneuropathy. He used E10.42 Type 1 diabetes mellitus with polyneuropathy as the code. He selected (or entered) that code in the computer.

What Did John Not Do?

- Did not assume that two codes would be required because two codes were required when coding using the ICD-9-CM.
- Did not rely on his memory for the best code(s) for this condition.
- Did not bother the provider with the details related to this coding situation.
- Did not code from the alphabetic index of the ICD-10-CM manual.

CPT, Current Procedural Terminology; *HCPCS*, Healthcare Common Procedure Coding System.

TERMINOLOGY REVIEW

Key Term	Word Parts	Definition
Downcoding		Using procedure codes that do not reflect a high enough level of service.
Established patient		A patient who has been seen by one of the providers in the practice in the same specialty within the past 3 years.
Inpatient		A patient who has been formally admitted to a healthcare facility.
Medical necessity		Health care that is reasonable and necessary for a patient based on evidence-based clinical standards of care.
MS-DRG (Diagnosis Related Groups)		A system for grouping hospital inpatients who are expected to utilize a similar amount of hospital resources as a basis for Medicare reimbursement.
Modifier		An addition to a Current Procedural Terminology (CPT) code that indicates unusual circumstances related to the procedure, such as a more extensive procedure or two procedures performed in the same session.
NEC		A diagnosis code that is not elsewhere classified. It is used when a more specific code for the condition is not available.
New patient		For billing purposes, a patient who has not received services during the previous 3 years from a provider in a medical practice in the same specialty.
NOS		A diagnosis code that is not otherwise specified. It is used when there is not enough information given to select a more specific code.
Outpatient		A patient who has not been admitted to a healthcare facility.
Panel		A group of diagnostic tests usually ordered together for diagnosis or screening.
RVU (Relative Value Unit)		A number that quantifies the amount of provider labor, resources, and expertise necessary to provide the service represented by a CPT code.
Sequela (pl. *sequelae*)	*sequi:* follow *-a:* noun ending	Any condition that results from a disease, injury, or treatment for a disease or injury.
Surgical package		Surgical services usually covered by a single procedure code that includes a pre-operative visit, postoperative care, and local anesthesia (if applicable).
Upcoding		Using a code to obtain a higher level of reimbursement than is justified by medical procedures performed as documented in the medical record. This can result in serious fines and penalties.

PROCEDURE 46.1 Performing CPT Coding

Outcome Perform CPT coding for procedures.

Equipment/Supplies

- Patient's medical record
- Electronic charge entry with a diagnosis for which the procedure is medically necessary
- CPT manual or online resource

1. **Procedural Step.** Find the name of the procedure to look up and information about the procedure (if necessary) using the patient's electronic charge slip and/or medical record.
   Principle. The charge slip or computer charge entry identifies the procedure(s) performed, but the medical record may be necessary to identify the appropriate level of service.
2. **Procedural Step.** For Evaluation and Management (E/M) services, identify whether the patient is a new patient or an established patient.
   Principle. Different codes are used for new patients and established patients.
3. **Procedural Step.** For E/M services, identify whether the patient was seen in the medical office or at another location, such as the hospital, emergency department, or nursing home.
   Principle. Different E/M codes are used depending on the location where the patient was seen. The coding and billing for visits provided by a provider to a hospitalized patient, nursing home resident, or patient in the emergency department are often done by staff at the provider's medical office.

Continued

PROCEDURE 46.1 Performing CPT Coding—cont'd

4. **Procedural Step.** Using the index, locate the section in which the category of codes will be found. You may need to look for the name of the procedure, the diagnosis, the type of patient, the location of service, or the location of the lesion.
   Examples:
   a. To locate an initial office visit for a new patient, look in the index under New Patient, Initial Office Visit (99202–99205) or under E/M, Office and Other Outpatient (99201–99215).
   b. To locate the code for a rapid strep test, look under *Streptococcus,* Group A, Direct Optical Observation (87880).
5. **Procedural Step.** Look in the manual at the code or range of codes to read the description and determine the correct code. Do not code from the index.
   Principle. You cannot be sure that you have identified the correct code without reading the description of the code. You also may find additional information in the section to help you code properly.
6. **Procedural Step.** If the service is unusual or does not seem to fit the description of the code completely, check the list of modifiers for the section of the manual to see if a modifier is necessary.
   Example: A patient has an abscess of the left shoulder, which required incision and drainage again today:
   1: In the index, you look up Abscess, Shoulder, Incision and Drainage. It refers you to code 23030.
   2: When you look at that code, you see that it refers to a deep abscess.
   Codes[a]:

Incision	
(lines deleted)	
23020	Capsular contracture release (eg. Sever type procedure) (for incision and drainage procedures, superficial, see 10040–10060)
23030	Incision and drainage shoulder area, deep abscess or hematoma
23031	infected bursa

   3: You review the medical record and determine that the provider called the lesion a *subcutaneous abscess.*
   4: For superficial abscesses, you are referred to codes 10060, 10061. The code 10060 (incision and drainage of abscess: simple or single) appears to describe the procedure most accurately. Because the patient came for an office visit specifically for treatment of the abscess and no other E/M services were provided, you do not charge for a separate office visit.
   Codes[a]:

Incision and Drainage	
	(For excision, see 11400, et seq)
10040	Acne surgery (leg, marsupialization, opening or removal of multiple milia, comedones, cysts, pustules)
10060	Incision and drainage of abscess (eg, carbuncle, suppurative hidradenitis, cutaneous or subcutaneous abscess, cyst, furuncle, or paronychial); simple or single
10061	complicated or multiple

7. **Procedural Step.** Verify that the procedure code has a reasonable correlation with the diagnosis code(s). If there appears to be a complete lack of correlation, tactfully ask the provider which diagnosis or symptom justifies the procedure.
   Principle. Reimbursement is made by insurance companies based on the codes submitted. Procedure codes must be accurate and linked to an appropriate diagnosis.
8. **Procedural Step.** Enter the correct code(s) on the charge slip, on the encounter form, and if applicable, in the patient's record in the computer so that it can be used for insurance billing.
   Principle. Reimbursement is made by insurance companies based on the codes submitted. They must be accurate and reflect the service or procedure performed. In the example given earlier, the insurance company might refuse to pay for the service (as already provided) without a modifier to indicate that it is in fact a repeat service of a procedure performed by another provider.

Using the TruCode Encoder Software

9. **Procedural Step.** Type the main term of the procedure into the encoder Search box, and select the CPT Tabular.
10. **Procedural Step.** Scroll through the codes that appear and select the most appropriate code.
    Example: To locate the code for an initial office visit for a new patient with straightforward medical decision-making, you could enter "straightforward office visit" in the Search box. When the codes appear, you would select 99202 as the most appropriate code.

PROCEDURE 46.1 Performing CPT Coding—cont'd

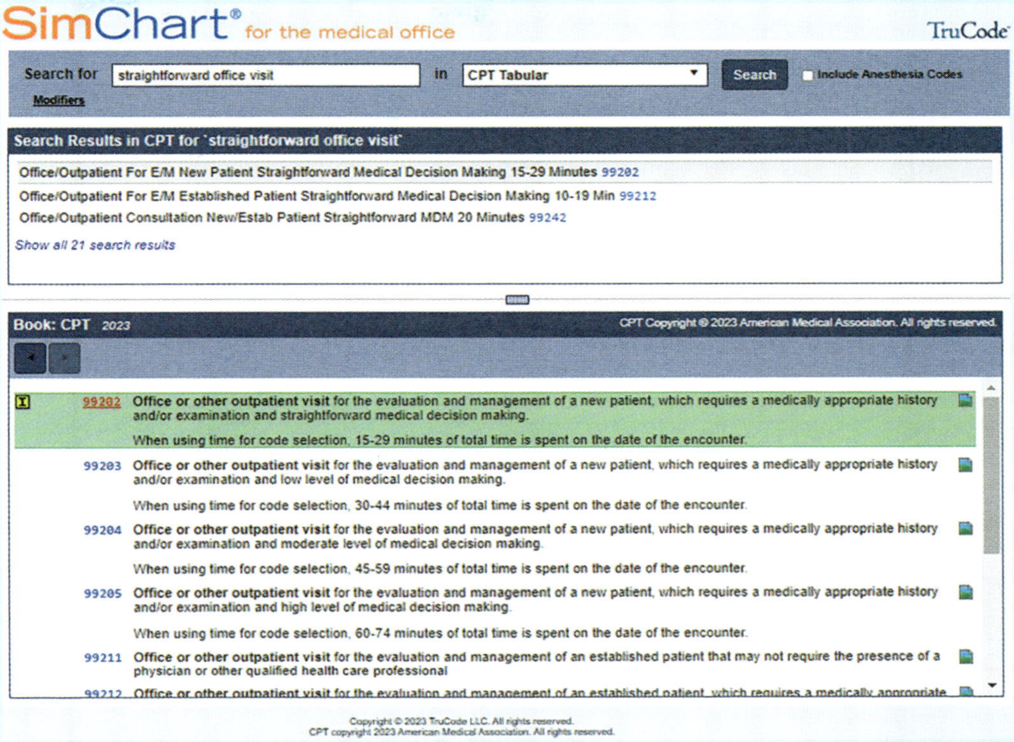

SimChart® for the medical office TruCode

Search for straightforward office visit in CPT Tabular Search Include Anesthesia Codes
Modifiers

Search Results in CPT for 'straightforward office visit'

Office/Outpatient For E/M New Patient Straightforward Medical Decision Making 15-29 Minutes 99202
Office/Outpatient For E/M Established Patient Straightforward Medical Decision Making 10-19 Min 99212
Office/Outpatient Consultation New/Estab Patient Straightforward MDM 20 Minutes 99242
Show all 21 search results

Book: CPT 2023 CPT Copyright © 2023 American Medical Association. All rights reserved.

99202 **Office or other outpatient visit** for the evaluation and management of a new patient, which requires a medically appropriate history and/or examination and straightforward medical decision making.
When using time for code selection, 15-29 minutes of total time is spent on the date of the encounter.

99203 **Office or other outpatient visit** for the evaluation and management of a new patient, which requires a medically appropriate history and/or examination and low level of medical decision making.
When using time for code selection, 30-44 minutes of total time is spent on the date of the encounter.

99204 **Office or other outpatient visit** for the evaluation and management of a new patient, which requires a medically appropriate history and/or examination and moderate level of medical decision making.
When using time for code selection, 45-59 minutes of total time is spent on the date of the encounter.

99205 **Office or other outpatient visit** for the evaluation and management of a new patient, which requires a medically appropriate history and/or examination and high level of medical decision making.
When using time for code selection, 60-74 minutes of total time is spent on the date of the encounter.

99211 **Office or other outpatient visit** for the evaluation and management of an established patient that may not require the presence of a physician or other qualified health care professional

99212 Office or other outpatient visit for the evaluation and management of an established patient, which requires a medically appropriate

PROCEDURE 46.2 Performing Healthcare Common Procedure Coding System Coding

Outcome Perform HCPCS coding for services or equipment.

Equipment/Supplies

- Patient's medical record
- Electronic charge entry
- HCPCS manual or online resource

1. **Procedural Step.** Refer to the charge entry or the patient's medical record to locate the service, supplies, or equipment requiring a HCPCS level II code.
   Principle. The charge slip usually identifies the procedure(s) performed, but the medical record may be necessary to identify more detail about the service, supplies, and so on.
2. **Procedural Step.** Using the index, locate the code or range of codes. Look up medications in the Table of Drugs.
3. **Procedural Step.** Find the code or code range by locating first the initial letter (arranged alphabetically) and then the four-digit number (arranged numerically). Read the description and determine the correct code. Do not code from the index.
   Principle. You cannot be sure that you have identified the correct code without reading the description of the code. You may also find additional information in the section to help you code properly.
4. **Procedural Step.** Check to be sure that the code is valid for the patient's insurance.
   Principle. Some HCPCS level II codes are valid for Medicaid or other insurance but not Medicare.
5. **Procedural Step.** Enter the correct code(s) on the charge slip, on the encounter form, and if applicable in the patient's record in the computer so that it can be used for insurance billing.
   Principle. Reimbursement is made by insurance companies on the basis of the codes submitted. They

Continued

PROCEDURE 46.2

PROCEDURE 46.2 Performing Healthcare Common Procedure Coding System Coding—cont'd

must be accurate and reflect the service or procedure performed.

Example:

1: To locate the code for an injection of diphenhydramine hydrochloride 25 mg, look up the drug in the index. (This medication may be given intramuscularly to treat an allergic reaction.) The code given for diphenhydramine hydrochloride is J1200.

2: Look for the code in the list of codes first under J, then under 1200. The entry J1200 states that this code covers injections up to 50 mg. It would therefore be the correct code for this example.

Using the TruCode Encoder Software

6. **Procedural Step.** Type the main term of the procedure into the encoder Search box, and select the HCPCS Tabular.
7. **Procedural Step.** Scroll through the codes that appear, and select the most appropriate code.
   See Fig. 46.4 for an example.

HCPCS, Healthcare Common Procedure Coding System.

PROCEDURE 46.3 Performing ICD Coding

Outcome Perform ICD coding for a patient's diagnosis.

Equipment/Supplies

- Patient's medical record
- Electronic charge entry
- Current ICD manual or online resource

1. **Procedural Step.** Refer to the patient's charge entry and/or medical record to identify the diagnosis. In the medical record, the provider may use the term "impression" or "diagnosis."
   Principle. The charge entry usually identifies the diagnosis, but the medical record may be necessary for additional information to select the correct code.
2. **Procedural Step.** Decide on the key word or phrase to look for the code in the alphabetic index.
3. **Procedural Step.** Locate the key word and look for the body part or other distinguishing factors. Identify the possible code(s).
4. **Procedural Step.** Locate the number(s) in the tabular list.
   Principle. You cannot be sure that you have identified the correct code without looking at the tabular list. You may also find additional information in the tabular list to help you code properly.
5. **Procedural Step.** Review the information given in the tabular list and select the most specific code that corresponds to the information on the charge slip and/or in the medical record. When there is a list of terminal characters (seventh character for ICD-10-CM), select the character that makes the code as specific as possible.
   Principle. Reimbursement may be linked to selection of the correct code.
6. **Procedural Step.** Enter the correct code(s) on the electronic charge entry so that it can be used for insurance billing.
   Principle. Reimbursement is made by insurance companies based on the codes submitted. Diagnosis codes must be accurate and justify the service provided.
7. **Procedural Step.** Verify that the diagnosis code has a reasonable correlation with the procedure code. If there appears to be a complete lack of correlation, tactfully ask the provider which diagnosis or symptom justifies the procedure.
   Principle. Reimbursement may be denied for procedures without a diagnosis that indicates medical necessity.
   Example: Patient diagnosis is "precordial chest pain, possibly angina pectoris."
   1: To locate the code in the ICD-10-CM manual, first locate *pain,* then *chest,* then *precordial* in the alphabetic index. Remember that terms in the EHR preceded by *possibly* or *rule out* should not be coded. You will find entries similar to the following:

PROCEDURE 46.3 Performing ICD Coding—cont'd

Index:[a]

PAIN

Chest (central) R07.9
- anterior wall (R07.89)
- atypical R07.89
- ischemic I20.9
- musculoskeletal R07.89
- non-cardiac R07.89
- on breathing R07.1
- pleurodynia R07.81
- precordial R07.2
- wall (anterior) R07.89

R07 Pain in throat and chest
Excludes 1 epidemic myalgia (B33.0)
Excludes 2 jaw pain R68.84
pain in breast (N64.4)

R07.0 Pain in throat
Excludes 1 chronic sore throat (J31.2)
sore throat (acute) NOS (J02.9)a
Excludes 2 dysphagia (R13.1-)
pain in neck (M54.2)

R07.1 Chest pain on breathing
Painful respiration

R07.2 Precordial pain

2: Look up the code for precordial pain (R07.2) in the tabular list to validate that it is the most specific code.

Using the TruCode Encoder Software

8. **Procedural Step.** Type the main term of the procedure into the encoder Search box, and select the Diagnosis, ICD-10-CM.
9. **Procedural Step.** Scroll through the codes that appear from the alphabetic index, and double click the most appropriate description.
10. **Procedural Step.** Review the codes in the tabular list to select the most appropriate code.
Example. Patient diagnosis is "precordial chest pain, possibly angina pectoris."

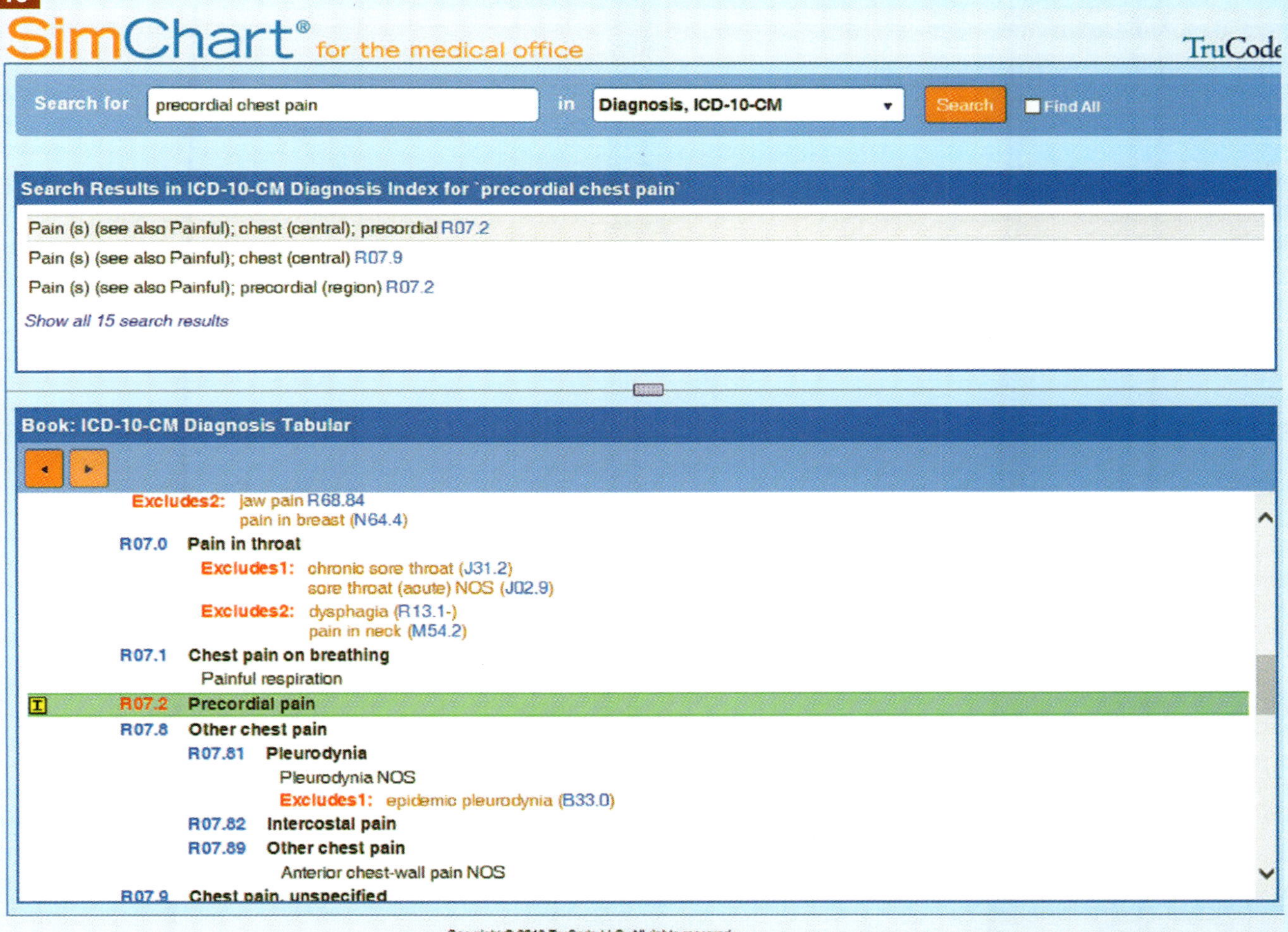

[a]Data from Buck CJ: *2023 ICD-10-CM Physician Edition*, St. Louis, 2023, Saunders.)

PROCEDURE 46.4 Demonstrating Tact When Discussing Code Selection and Coding Requirements With Providers

Outcome Demonstrate tact when discussing code selection and coding requirements with providers related to the following situation: The provider documented that a patient was given supplies for home care of a tracheostomy but did not identify which supplies in the EHR, and the patient's insurance was charged $40.00 using the CPT code 99070. The claim has been rejected because of failure to include a list of these supplies.

Equipment/Supplies

- None

1. **Procedural Step.** With the instructor observing, role play the situation described above with another student acting the part of a practice provider. Your goal is to have the provider document the supplies given to the patient in the EHR.
2. **Procedural Step.** Notify the provider tactfully that an insurance claim has been rejected because there is no list of supplies to support the CPT code 99070 for supplies given to the patient. Include the name of the patient and that the supplies in question are for home tracheostomy care.
   Principle. An insurance claim may be denied for incomplete information.
4. **Procedural Step.** Approach the provider in a respectful and professional manner.
5. **Procedural Step.** Use tact when explaining the reason for rejection of the insurance claim.
   Principle. Presenting information tactfully makes it easier to initiate a discussion about acceptable codes.
6. **Procedural Step.** Suggest that a more specific HCPCS code might be used if you knew exactly what the supplies were. This might help when resubmitting the claim.
7. **Procedural Step.** Answer any questions from the provider tactfully.
8. **Procedural Step.** Appear organized, professional, and well-groomed throughout the role play.
   Principle. Organization and good grooming reinforce professionalism.

HCPCS, Healthcare Common Procedure Coding System.

Medical Insurance

Check out the Evolve site at http://evolve.elsevier.com/Bonewit/today to access additional interactive activities and exercises to help you study and prepare for success.

LEARNING OBJECTIVES	PROCEDURES
Introduction to Insurance	
1. Trace the history of health insurance in the United States.	
2. Identify and describe three ways in which to obtain health insurance.	
3. Explain the regulations that control the amount of health insurance reimbursement for an individual claim.	
Types of Insurance	
4. Compare and contrast traditional fee-for-service health insurance plans with managed care insurance plans.	
5. Identify and define various types of managed care plans.	
6. Describe eligibility and benefits for the Medicare plan.	
7. Explain the general provisions of the Medicaid plan and the state children's insurance program.	
8. Describe government programs available to dependents of the armed services and veterans.	
9. Explain when workers' compensation covers medical care and compare it with other insurance plans.	
Insurance and Managed Care Policies and Procedures	
10. Describe how to collect information from patients for insurance billing.	
11. Describe the process for verifying eligibility and covered services.	Interpreting the information on an insurance card. Verifying insurance eligibility.
12. Correlate preauthorization and precertification requirements to the utilization review process.	Obtaining insurance preauthorization (precertification).
13. Describe the referral process for managed care.	
Insurance Claims	
14. Identify the information contained on an insurance form.	
15. Recognize potential errors in a completed insurance form.	Completing and reviewing the insurance claim form.
16. Describe the process for submission and payment of a health insurance claim following insurance guidelines.	
17. Categorize common errors that result in denied insurance claims.	
18. Demonstrate professional and tactful communication skills with third-party representatives, medical providers, and patients.	Communicating professionally and with sensitivity on matters related to managed care and/or insurance.

CHAPTER OUTLINE

KEY TERMS

assignment of benefits
beneficiary
benefit
capitation
CHAMPVA
coinsurance
coordination of benefits
copayment
deductible
eligibility
explanation of benefits (EOB)
fee-for-service insurance
formulary
group plans
guarantor
indemnity
insured
managed care
Medicaid
Medicare
Medicare Administrative Contractor (MAC)
nonparticipating provider (nonPAR)
participating provider (PAR)
preauthorization
precertification
premium
primary care provider (PCP)
primary insurance
referral
reimbursement
remittance advice (RA)
resource-based relative value scale (RBRVS)
secondary insurance
self-referral
signature on file (SOF)
third-party payor
TRICARE
usual, customary, and reasonable (UCR)
utilization review
workers' compensation

INTRODUCTION TO HEALTH INSURANCE

The growth and change in the structure of health insurance has affected American health care since the end of World War II. When industrialized countries such as Canada and many countries in Western Europe were introducing government-provided health care, the United States was turning primarily to the private market to provide insurance coverage for Americans. This created a problem, as many Americans could not afford to purchase health insurance. As health care costs continue to rise, so does the pressure to maintain high standards at a reasonable cost to both individuals and the government.

HISTORY OF HEALTH INSURANCE

Health insurance had its beginnings in accident insurance, which was first sold in the mid-1800s. In exchange for a monthly payment by a customer, the insurance carrier agreed to replace lost income resulting from an accident and later resulting from a few specific illnesses, such as smallpox, diphtheria, typhoid, and scarlet fever.

In the 1930s a group of Dallas schoolteachers made an arrangement with Baylor Hospital to have any necessary hospital care provided in exchange for monthly premiums. This arrangement was the precursor to the Blue Cross and Blue Shield programs, which were incorporated as not-for-profit companies in each state. The payments were based on the amount charged for the services provided. Other insurance companies began to offer health insurance using similar models. Labor unions began to negotiate for health insurance as an employee benefit that was not taxed as income in the same way as an increase in wages.

During World War II, Henry Kaiser created clinics in California to provide both inpatient and outpatient care for the workers in his shipyards. These clinics later opened themselves to other employers and individuals and became the Kaiser Permanente program. The employer paid a fixed amount per worker over a stated period of time for all necessary medical care. This method of payment is called **capitation**, and this type of health insurance is called a *prepaid health plan.* For many years Kaiser Permanente was the country's largest health maintenance organization (HMO). The philosophy behind the HMO movement was a belief that health care costs could be lowered if members were restricted to specific providers and facilities. Covered services also included preventive medical care in the hope of preventing conditions that would be expensive to treat. (Preventative care was not covered by traditional insurance plans.) Over time, the HMO model broadened from one in which providers were salaried employees and worked in a central facility to one in which HMOs contracted with private providers in each community.

By the 1960s, many larger and even medium-sized businesses were providing company-paid health insurance benefits as an untaxed fringe benefit instead of increasing wages or salaries. Health care costs began to increase faster than the general rate of inflation, with providers beginning to earn large incomes. But certain groups of Americans—most notably the poor, elderly, and permanently disabled—were unable to obtain medical insurance through employment.

The federal government created two programs in the Social Security Amendments of 1965 to try to close these large gaps in medical coverage. One was **Medicare**, the health insurance program for the elderly, the permanelty disabled, and those with end-stage kidney disease. Medicare is paid for with federal taxes paid by employers and workers. The second government insurance program was **Medicaid**, the health insurance program for low-income individuals and families. The Medicaid program has different names in different states, and it is administered by each state. The federal government pays for the majority of required care and a smaller percentage of optional care, such as dental care, and the states pay for the rest. Each state sets its own criteria for eligibility for the Medicaid program.

Many senators, congresspersons, and providers were against Medicare and Medicaid at the beginning, calling it "socialized medicine." But there were precedents for the government's involvement in paying for medical care. The Veterans Administration (US Department of Veterans Affairs [VA]) offered medical care for life for any man or woman who had seen active duty in the military provided that they wished to use the VA facilities. In addition, the Civilian Health and Medical Program of the Uniformed Services (CHAMPUS) program was developed to provide medical care at government expense for dependent spouses and children of active-duty military personnel. Today the former CHAMPUS program is called **TRICARE**, and has been extended with plans that cover some veterans and reservists. A companion program, the Civilian Health and Medical Program of the Department of Veterans Affairs **(CHAMPVA)**, covers dependent spouses and children of military veterans with service-connected disabilities.

In the 21st century, American society is still trying to resolve insurance issues. Low-wage workers often do not get health insurance through their employers, or they may have insurance only for themselves and not their dependents. For more than 10 years the federal government has tried to pass legislation to expand insurance coverage to all or nearly all citizens, but the costs have made it difficult to gather enough support. The federal Patient Protection and Affordable Care Act (often referred to as the Affordable Care Act, PPACA, ACA, or Obamacare), which became law in March 2010, attempts to define patients' rights and ensure that all Americans will have access to affordable, high-quality health care and preventative care. There have been changes and additions to the ACA since 2010, but it still remains the law that protects the patient's rights regarding health coverage.

OBTAINING HEALTH INSURANCE

Individuals and families have basically three ways to obtain health insurance coverage: through a group plan, by purchasing an individual policy, or through one of the government plans described earlier.

Most **group plans** are available through an employer. A group plan is one insurance policy that covers a group of people. Larger employers typically have several different plans available. The employer pays a portion of the insurance costs.

Some small business owners can purchase insurance through group plans sponsored by a trade organization. Individuals sometimes have access to group plans through professional associations or even college alumni associations. Under the Affordable Care Act, individuals and families have greater access to health insurance. The self-employed can deduct a portion of their health insurance costs from their business income, as companies do.

As part of the process of gaining the right to sell health insurance in a particular state, most insurance plans are required to offer individual policies to individuals or families who are not covered under a group plan. An open-enrollment period usually occurs at least once each year during which individuals can purchase coverage. Discussion has occurred at the federal level about allowing individuals or families who purchase their own insurance to claim a tax credit or a larger tax deduction for the cost.

Taxpayer-funded (government) health insurance is usually provided as an entitlement when other conditions are met. For instance, when an individual reaches age 65, they are entitled to Medicare benefits if they have worked for at least

10 years in Medicare-covered employment. However, the individual must still file an application because the benefits do not begin automatically. An individual must meet other criteria for other government health insurance programs.

PAYING FOR HEALTH INSURANCE AND HEALTH CARE

The amount of money paid by the consumer to purchase health insurance is called the **premium**. It can be paid monthly, quarterly, semiannually, or annually. All or part of the premium may be paid by the person enrolled in the insurance plan or by the employer. In exchange for the payment of a premium, the insurance carrier or managed care plan agrees to provide payment for specific services provided by providers, hospitals, laboratories, and other health care providers. Payment for a service covered by health insurance is called a **benefit**, and each individual covered by the health insurance plan is called a **beneficiary**, *enrollee*, or *member*. The **insured** is the individual who has the insurance, but a family plan also covers dependents of the insured, including a spouse and children.

When the premium is paid by a person's employer, even if the employee is responsible for part of the cost, that premium is often paid with pre-tax dollars. This means that the amount of the premium paid by the employer is not included in the amount of wages reported for the employee. The employee's portion may also be deducted before tax is calculated. In this case, the employee cannot use the payment for insurance as a tax deduction.

Another way to pay for health care using pre-tax dollars is a health savings account or a flexible spending account. This is a fund set up by the employer before tax is taken out of a person's earnings. The money in this fund can be used only for qualified health expenses. With a flexible spending account the funds must be used within the calendar year. Money not used is lost to the employee. With a health savings account the money is the patients and does not have to be spent during a specific timeframe.

Depending on the type of insurance policy, a patient may be responsible for paying for certain services. A **deductible** is an amount of money that must be paid for services provided to an individual or a family member in a group plan every calendar year before any insurance payments. After the deductible has been met, the patient may be required to pay a percentage of the allowed charge or a fixed fee every time service is received. If the patient is responsible for a specific percentage of the allowed charges (such as 20%), the patient portion is called **coinsurance**. An example of an insurance plan with coinsurance is Medicare Part B. A fixed dollar amount that a patient is required to pay every time they obtain medical services or fills a prescription is called a **copayment**. In some plans, the amount of the copayment is always the same, but often there are different amounts for different types of medical and/or pharmacy services.

FACTORS AFFECTING INSURANCE REIMBURSEMENT

PRIMARY, SECONDARY, AND TERTIARY INSURANCE

If a person is covered by more than one insurance policy, the insurance to which the insurance claim is sent first is called the **primary insurance**. When the patient is the insured, that insurance is the primary insurance. Insurance held by another insured (such as a spouse) that provides additional insurance coverage would be **secondary insurance**. If a third type of insurance also covers the patient, that insurance would be *tertiary insurance*. As a general rule, private insurance must be billed before government insurance, and Medicaid is always the last insurance to be billed.

COORDINATION OF BENEFITS

Some households have two working adults, both of whom are covered under separate employer health benefits. **Coordination of benefits** is a term for the rules insurance companies use to coordinate the payments for medical services so that the amount paid by all insurance carriers for any service provided is never more than 100% of the charge.

If both members of a couple have insurance with provisions for the coordination of benefits, the following rules apply:

1. If the employee who holds the policy is the patient, their insurance is the primary insurance for any services obtained. The spouse's or partner's insurance becomes the secondary insurance and can be used to pay only for any portion of the charge not covered by the primary insurance.
2. If a child is the patient, in most states the *birthday rule* applies. Under this rule, the primary insurance for the child of parents who both have a family health plan is the insurance belonging to the working adult whose birthday comes first in the year. The insurance of the adult whose birthday is later is the secondary insurance.
3. When the patient is a child of divorced parents, the rules can get somewhat complicated. If a court has decreed that one parent is the "responsible party," that parent's policy provides the primary insurance. A responsible party ruling is often made in cases of joint custody, although the responsible party can also be a noncustodial parent. If no court ruling is in place the custodial parent's policy is primary. If there is no court ruling in place, the birthday rule remains in effect.
4. Issues involving the coordination of benefits can be avoided if individuals in households with two working adults make modifications in their benefits. To reduce premium costs, some employers allow employees to take cash instead of health insurance if the family already has insurance. In cases where the company covers the complete cost for an individual but not the family, only one partner has to pay for family coverage. Of course, available

plans should be compared for cost and benefits when individuals are deciding which policy to extend to family coverage.

5. If the patient is a Medicare recipient who is also covered by an employer's policy, the employer's policy is the primary insurance and Medicare is the secondary insurance. Patients with Medicare may also have supplemental insurance to cover what would normally be a patient responsibility. These plans, which are clearly defined as Medicare supplemental insurance, are considered secondary insurance.

PARTICIPATING AND NONPARTICIPATING PROVIDERS

If the provider has a contract or agreement with a **third-party payor** (insurance carrier [company] or managed care organization), they are called a **participating provider (PAR)**. One of the requirements is often that the provider must accept the insurance carrier's determination of the allowable fee and may not bill the patient for any additional amount that the insurance carrier did not allow. The patient signs a form authorizing **assignment of benefits**. This term is used for the patient's request that the insurance carrier pay the provider directly. This authorization is usually part of the new patient information form.

A **nonparticipating provider (nonPAR)** has no contractual agreement with the third-party payor and can bill the patient for some of the difference between the insurance payment and the amount billed. A nonPAR must obtain payment from the patient (who receives *reimbursement* from the insurance carrier).

TYPES OF REIMBURSEMENT

Two basic types of insurance reimbursement exist: capitation and fee for service. (Note that the term **reimbursement** is used to designate the amount paid by insurance for health care services either to reimburse the patient or to make a direct payment to the provider of the services.)

Under capitation, the primary care provider (PCP) receives a monthly, quarterly, semiannual, or annual payment from the managed care insurance company. Specialists are usually not paid by capitation. The reimbursement per patient may vary depending on age and sex, but it does not depend on the amount of care the patient receives.

As discussed earlier, capitation moves some of the risk away from the managed care company and onto the PCP who treats the patient, and most providers prefer other payment methods. In most circumstances, there will be enough healthy patients who cost less to treat than the amount being paid by the company to make up for the few sick patients who cost more to treat.

Under **fee-for-service insurance**, the health care provider, including all providers, is reimbursed for each treatment or procedure performed. In this case the only difference between traditional fee-for-service insurance and managed care is that managed care companies often negotiate a fee schedule that is lower than traditional indemnity plans.

In many instances, however, if the provider or other medical provider agrees to accept assignment of benefits, they cannot bill the patient for any portion of the charge not paid by the insurance carrier except the deductible and copayment or coinsurance.

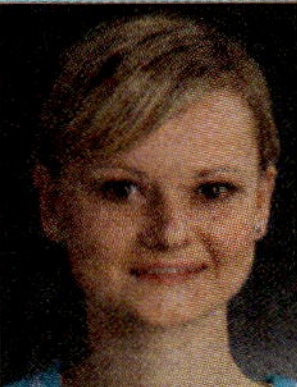

Putting It All Into Practice

My name is Sandra O'Keefe, and I am a Registered Medical Assistant. I work in the office of three dermatologists. With the advances in laser technology, there are many new procedures for removing spider veins, birthmarks, scars, hair, and tattoos. We also do Mohs micrographic surgery, a technique that removes skin cancers one layer at time with immediate tissue analysis. Using this technique, the providers can be sure that all malignant cells have been removed while taking a minimum of healthy tissue.

Billing in our office is somewhat complicated because many of the procedures are not covered by insurance. In general, insurance companies will pay for procedures that are medically necessary, such as the removal of skin cancers. They do not cover procedures that are strictly cosmetic, such as the removal of spider veins (small varicose veins on the skin). Then there are some procedures that sometimes are covered by insurance and sometimes not, such as the removal of birthmarks.

When a procedure is medically necessary, we have to obtain preauthorization from the patient's insurance carrier, and sometimes we need to provide documentation for the insurance carrier to review before they give their approval. When a procedure is not covered, we have to be sure that the patient is willing to pay for it and knows how much it will cost. We can help arrange for the patient to obtain financing to pay for the procedure over a period of time.

Our providers accept several different types of insurance, including government plans, managed care plans, and traditional insurance plans. When patients are covered by managed care plans, we have to be sure that they have the proper referrals to cover each office visit as well as the procedure. In some cases, the insurance covers a consultation visit but the proposed treatment plan is not approved; then patients must decide about paying for any recommended procedure themselves. We do our best to complete all the paperwork to obtain insurance coverage for our patients, but we are limited by the rules of each insurance carrier. ■

TYPES OF INSURANCE

Several different types of health insurance are currently available. When one is learning about insurance, it is helpful to learn the characteristics of different types of insurance, although the medical assistant may also be responsible for finding out more specific information related to individual insurance plans.

FEE-FOR-SERVICE PLANS

Traditionally, private insurance plans provided payment, either to the provider or to the patient, for each medical service provided. These traditional plans are called *fee-for-service plans* or *indemnity plans.* The term **indemnity** means an obligation to compensate an individual for loss or damage. Until the late 1980s, fee-for-service plans dominated the health care industry. They were provided through private insurance companies and also through the Blue Cross and Blue Shield plans, which were established in each state as not-for-profit, quasi-governmental agencies. Since the late 1980s, the percentage of individuals covered under traditional fee-for-service plans has steadily decreased. Fee-for-service plans usually have a deductible, and the insurance pays for a percentage of the allowed charges (commonly 80%).

The insurance carrier determines the allowed charge in two ways:

1. Through a fee schedule. A fee schedule says the insurance carrier will pay the specified percentage of a particular amount for a particular procedure. Any additional charges are the patient's responsibility.
2. Through service benefits, which define covered services but not the exact payments. Under service benefit plans, the insurance carrier will agree to pay the specified percentage of charges that are **usual, customary, and reasonable (UCR)** for the procedure and the state or region of the country in which it was performed. The usual fee is the amount that a provider usually charges or charges most often. The customary fee is the amount charged by providers in the same specialty in the same geographic area (usually the 90th percentile amount of the charges of all providers in the area). A reasonable fee meets the two criteria described earlier or is justifiable if there are special circumstances. Based on statistics kept by the insurance carrier, the fee actually charged by the provider is reviewed. The insurance carrier's payment is based on its own determination of what is UCR.

What Would You Do? What Would You *Not* Do?

Case Study 1

Diane Bennett, 35 years old, has come to the office for treatment of a lesion on her neck. She was referred from her primary care provider for up to three visits for consultation, diagnostic studies, and treatment. She is seen by one of the dermatologists in the practice, who recommends that the lesion be removed surgically, with a biopsy, in the office. During this visit Diane tells the provider that she has two other lesions she would like to have removed, one on her arm and another on her abdomen. The provider inspects the lesions and asks Sandra to contact the patient's managed care plan for authorization to treat the additional lesions. The patient says, "My provider gave me a referral to be treated by you. What's the problem? If these lesions need to be removed, I don't want any delay." ■

Under a traditional fee-for-service plan, a patient can make an appointment with any doctor, in any specialty they choose, and the insurance will pay the designated amount for the services. Some plans do have lists of approved providers for whom they pay 100% of charges; they then pay only a percentage of charges for other providers (similar to a preferred provider organization [PPO], discussed in more detail later in the chapter).

MANAGED CARE PLANS

Since the introduction of the Kaiser plan, HMOs have evolved into many forms. Both private insurance companies and government insurance plans offer HMOs as well as other types of managed care plans. The various HMO models and their descendants, collectively, are known as **managed care**. This term is used in two ways: It describes the movement to control health care costs while improving preventive care and is a general term for insurance programs reimbursing care provided in this way. Managed care plans negotiate reimbursement amounts and limit patients to those providers and facilities with whom they have contracts.

Most insurance plans today involve some form of managed care. The patient's care is managed by the insurance plan in several ways:

1. Each patient chooses one provider as a **primary care provider (PCP)**, a health care practitioner who provides most of the patient's care and also determines what other medical services the patient requires.
2. Care is usually restricted to specific providers, laboratories, and hospitals that have accepted the insurance plan's fee schedule or capitation payment plan.
3. The patient may or may not have access to providers and services outside the insurance plan. If there are tiers of providers, the patient must usually pay more for services obtained outside the plan. In addition, the patient may be subject to balance billing if they seek service from a provider who is outside the managed care plan. This means that the patient must pay the difference between the amount allowed by insurance and the amount charged for services.
4. The insurance plan may require referrals from a PCP for services including consultations with specialists, therapy such as physical therapy or speech therapy, care outside of the medical office, and some diagnostic tests. The PCP functions as a "gatekeeper" to limit and approve access to specialty services. (The process of referrals is discussed later in this chapter.)
5. The insurance plan usually requires prior notification and/or **utilization review** (reviewing proposed or current care to determine medical necessity) before authorizing referral to specialists, certain procedures, therapy, surgery, and other types of care.

Health Maintenance Organization Models

In the original HMO concept, all medical care was provided for 1 year for a fixed premium, with no deductibles or coinsurance. The patient was responsible only for a fixed amount for each visit or prescription (copayment).

HMOs have always practiced preventive medicine on the theory that much of the cost of medical care can be eliminated through routine care by PCPs. To reduce the cost of specialty care, PCPs—including providers, nurse practitioners, and physician assistants—act as gatekeepers, seeing patients first for nearly all illnesses and referring them to specialists only when necessary. The PCP is usually paid by capitation. HMOs are usually incorporated, and they are regulated state by state. They are subject to regulation requiring more comprehensive quality assurance programs than other types of insurance. Medical record audits allow the HMO to check the records of any provider's patients to make sure that the provider is not performing unnecessary procedures or ordering unnecessary tests.

Staff Model Health Maintenance Organization

The staff model HMO hires its providers directly and pays them a salary for providing health care to members. The patient can receive care only at plan facilities. This type of plan was more common when the HMO movement first began and is rare today.

Network Health Maintenance Organization

The network model HMO contracts with various group practices for services to its members. Typically, the providers also see patients who have other types of insurance. The HMO members must be referred to in-network providers if possible. Out-of-network coverage is allowed only in cases of emergency or when the need for service is urgent.

Other Managed Care Models

Health care plans that are regulated by state and federal laws as insurance plans instead of HMOs may still maintain many features of managed care. Depending on the state, there may be separate regulatory agencies.

Preferred Provider Organization

A PPO provides coverage for in-network and out-of-network services to its members, but there is a financial incentive to use in-network services. These plans usually have deductibles and coinsurance or copayments. Patients may be required to pay a copayment or percentage of in-network costs, but they must usually pay a higher percentage of out-of-network costs.

Exclusive Provider Organization

An exclusive provider organization (EPO) is similar in structure and operation to a PPO, but in order to be covered its members must receive all their health care services only within the network. Employers agree that the EPO is the only organization it will contract with for health care services to employees. If a member receives such services outside the network except for emergencies or when traveling out of the area, the cost will not be covered by insurance. In this way the EPO is similar to an HMO, but its legal structure is different. The payment method is fee-for-service.

Independent Practice Association

The providers of an independent practice association (IPA) work independently in the community but organize formally as a provider association. They are paid from funds collected from subscribers of the health plan minus administrative costs, marketing and sales costs, and other overhead costs. IPAs often have a "hold back"—a portion of the agreed-on fee that is not paid to the providers until after the end of the association's fiscal year, when the association determines if it has earned a profit or had financial losses. In this way, the association requires member providers to share some business risk.

Point-of-Service Plans

The point-of-service (POS) plan combines an in-network plan that is an HMO with an additional out-of-network plan. The POS plan functions as a combination of an HMO and a PPO. Members have a greater financial obligation when they seek out-of-network services. When they remain within the network, their only financial obligation is a copayment each time they seek service.

GOVERNMENT PLANS

Medicare

Medicare is a federally funded plan administered by the Centers for Medicare and Medicaid Services (CMS). It pays for health care services for the following individuals:

- Individuals older than age 65 who are eligible for Social Security
- Retired railroad employees and some retired federal employees
- Individuals who have been permanently disabled for 2 years
- Blind individuals
- Individuals with chronic renal disease who require dialysis or kidney transplant
- Kidney donors

The Medicare plan has several parts. Medicare Part A provides coverage for hospitalization services. Medicare Part B covers provider and other provider services. Together these two parts make up what is called the *Original Medicare Plan.* The patient's Medicare card identifies what type of coverage they have (Fig. 47.1). Until April 2019, Medicare cards were allowed to use the patient's Social Security number as an ID number, but all Medicare patients have been issued new Medicare cards with a different number. Medicare was expanded to provide more choice in the types of available plans in 1997 (also known as Part C). Several Medicare Advantage Plans, including managed care plans and fee-for-service plans, replace the Original Medicare Plan if recipients choose them. Medicare Part D was passed in 2003 and went into effect in 2006. It adds a prescription drug benefit to the Original Medicare Plan and Medicare

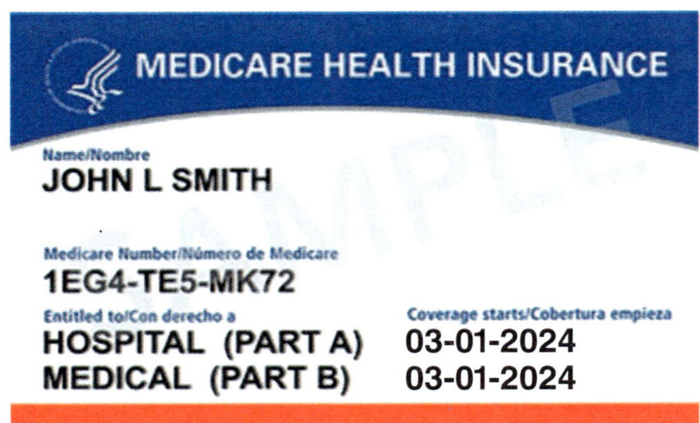

Fig. 47.1 Identification card for Medicare.

Advantage Plans that did not include this benefit. If the patient is enrolled in a Medicare Advantage plan, the provider must be a member provider of that plan for services to be covered.

Individuals aged 65 and older on Social Security, those younger than 65 years but who collect Social Security disability benefits, and those who receive railroad retirement benefits are automatically enrolled in Medicare Part A. Most people do not pay a premium for participation in Medicare Part A. There is a Part A deductible, and the amount the patient is required to pay is adjusted annually. Medicare Part A is funded through a tax paid by working individuals on all of their earned income.

Anyone eligible for Medicare Part A may also obtain Part B coverage. However, they must apply and pay a premium to obtain Medicare Part B or to enroll in one of the Medicare Advantage Plans. Former federal employees, who receive federal employee pensions rather than Social Security and who are not covered by Medicare Part A, can purchase Medicare Part B coverage.

Each Medicare claim is submitted by the medical office or other health care facility to a **Medicare Administrative Contractor (MAC)**, a multistate private health care insurer, usually for more than one state, that administers both Part A and Part B claims under a contract with CMS. The amount of payment for any service is standardized nationally.

Payment for hospitals for claims under Part A is based on Medicare Severity Diagnosis-Related Groups (MS-DRGs), a system that classifies patients according to the diagnosis, treatment, and length of hospital stay. The patient is assigned a MS-DRG based on the primary diagnosis, and the payment made by Medicare to a hospital is determined by the DRG rather than the length of time the patient remains in the hospital.

Since 1992, payments for services under Part B have been based on a **resource-based relative value scale (RBRVS)** developed by researchers at Harvard University. This system establishes *relative value units (RVUs)* for each procedure based on the amount of work involved, overhead expenses, and cost of malpractice insurance. The amount Medicare pays for each relative value unit is then adjusted annually; it is also adjusted for different geographic areas (because overhead and malpractice cost may vary). An annual fee schedule is available online for identifying the amount Medicare pays for specific procedures. A similar system is used by most commercial insurance carriers today. With the passage of the Medicare Access and CHIP Reauthorization Act (MACRA) in 2015, Medicare consolidated various incentive programs: the Physician Quality Reporting System (PQRS), and the Value-Based Payment Modifier Program (VBPM) into a single incentive program for Part B providers to reward clinicians who provide higher-value care effective January 1, 2017. Most providers participate in the Merit-Based Incentive Payment System (MIPS); it requires providers to submit reports about the care provided to Medicare patients. The payments made to providers by Medicare are increased for those providers meeting performance standards, whereas payments are reduced for those providers who do not meet performance standards.

A PAR in the Medicare program must bill for the patient, accept assignment of benefits, and accept Medicare's determination of the allowable charge for the service. Under Part B, after paying an annual deductible, the patient is responsible for 20% of the allowable charge. The amount of the deductible is adjusted yearly. If the provider, medical office, or other health care facility has any reason to believe that Medicare payment may be denied for a covered service under original Medicare Part B, the patient must be given an *Advanced Beneficiary Notice of Noncoverage (ABN)*. This form, which is discussed in Chapter 45, can be downloaded from the CMS website. The form is not required for services that Medicare never covers (e.g., cosmetic surgery).

If a provider does not participate in the Medicare program (nonPAR), usually they do not accept assignment of benefits but collect the bill from the patient up to a limiting charge (percent limit on fees above the fee-schedule amount) set by legislation.

Many patients with original Medicare purchase additional insurance (known as *Medicare supplemental* or *Medigap insurance*) that covers the annual deductible and 20% coinsurance for Part B as well as the deductible for Part A. Patients in most Medicare Advantage plans do not need supplemental insurance. Some patients may also be covered by employment plans after retirement. In this case, Medicare is the primary insurance and the Medigap or employment retiree plan is secondary. If a person continues to work after 65 years of age and obtains insurance through employment, that insurance is the primary insurance for that individual and Medicare is the secondary insurance.

Medicaid

Medicaid, formally Title XIX (Title 19) of the 1965 amendments to the Social Security laws, provides for the federal government to give each state a grant to be used toward care of low-income residents. Along with the federal government's basic funding comes an obligation for the states to provide basic health care. States may add coverage for other care to their Medicaid laws but must pay for most of those costs, with the federal government paying a portion. The name of the Medicaid program as well as procedures for gaining access to it vary from state to state.

A patient's Medicaid eligibility must be checked at every office visit. In many states patients have a Medicaid card similar to a credit card with a magnetic stripe. The medical assistant uses a machine similar to a credit card reader to verify the patient's eligibility, as discussed in Chapter 39.

Providers may agree or decline to provide services to Medicaid patients. If they agree to treat Medicaid patients, they must accept all patients with Medicaid insurance. In addition, providers must agree to accept the state's payment for services without billing patients for any difference between the state's payment and the actual charge.

Adults and children receiving basic welfare grants from a state are automatically eligible for Medicaid. Also, the children in many working households are eligible for Medicaid benefits if the parents' pay is low enough to put the family below the poverty line or if employee-provided medical insurance covers only the employed parent.

In addition to paying for medical services, Medicaid also covers the cost of long-term skilled nursing home care for low-income elderly and disabled individuals. Because nursing home care is so expensive, 20% of Medicaid beneficiaries—elderly residents of nursing homes—account for 70%–80% of the cost of the Medicaid program.

Children's Health Insurance Program

The Children's Health Insurance Program (CHIP), established in 1997, is overseen by the CMS, but it is managed by the individual states. The program has been reauthorized several times and was funded until 2027 as part of the Bipartisan Budget Act of 2018. The CHIP program is administered and partially funded on a statewide basis. Depending on the state, eligible children are enrolled in the state's Medicaid plan, a separate CHIP program, or a combination of the two. The medical assistant should familiarize themselves with the state requirements for this plan.

Insurance Plans for Dependents of Members of the Armed Services and Veterans

TRICARE is the federal insurance program that provides health benefits for the dependent spouses and children of active military personnel who are receiving care from civilian providers and health facilities. Some veterans, reservists, and retirees are also eligible. The name was changed to TRICARE when there were three types of plans, but today several plans are available.

TRICARE Prime is an HMO-type plan available to service members, reservists, dependents, and some retirees. Care is usually provided in a military treatment facility, but civilian clinics may be used in some cases.

TRICARE Select allows an individual to seek care from any provider. It is a fee-for-service insurance plan available to family members of active service personnel, veterans, and retirees.

Other TRICARE plans are limited to specific populations and/or services (such as vision or dental), and some plans specifically serve those stationed overseas and their families.

In 1973 the federal government created the Civilian Health and Medical Program of the Department of Veterans Affairs (CHAMPVA) to provide both inpatient and outpatient medical benefits for the dependent spouses and children of veterans who have sustained total, permanent, service-connected disabilities and for surviving spouses and children of veterans who have died as a result of those service-connected disabilities. The nearest VA medical center determines eligibility and issues an identification (ID) card, but CHAMPVA-covered patients are allowed to choose their own providers and other medical service providers. CHAMPVA is always secondary to Medicare.

Workers' Compensation

Workers' compensation insurance covers lost wages and the cost of medical treatment for workers injured on the job or who fall ill as a result of workplace hazards or disease. Each state has its own workers' compensation program. The cost of workers' compensation insurance is paid by employers. The premium for a given employer depends on how many previous employees have made claims under workers' compensation.

Workers are required to make a prompt claim for workers' compensation coverage after an accident or the onset of an illness. In many states the employer and the insurance company issuing the policy have the right to choose the provider who treats the patient.

If a patient visits their regular primary care provider and says the illness or injury is workplace-related, the medical assistant should check promptly with the employer to verify that the employee has made a report and that the care will be covered by the company's workers' compensation plan. It is also helpful to have the patient sign an agreement to pay for medical services if the case is declared not to be work-related, or if another condition is discovered and treated that is not work-related.

If a patient of the medical practice is seen for a workers' compensation case, separate medical and financial records should be established for that patient. Laws require that requests for medical records for compensation cases must contain only information associated with the work-related injury. If a workers' appeal board needs work-related injury records, it is important that no other medical information about the patient be released. The Health Insurance Portability and Accountability Act (HIPAA) of 1996 allows disclosure of personal health information (PHI) to workers' compensation insurers and employers without the patient's authorization.

For a workers' compensation case, the provider must supply comprehensive information, but reporting requirements vary from state to state. The individual insurance carrier or state governmental agency should be contacted to obtain instructions and proper forms. A sample form can be printed or completed online using SimChart for the Medical Office and saved to a simulated medical record for the patient.

In addition to the initial report, the provider may need to submit supplemental reports and/or a narrative letter. A completed CMS-1500 claim form is also sent to the insurance carrier for each office visit. As is the case for most government programs, the provider must accept the payment provided as payment in full. The provider submits a report and a statement monthly until care is completed.

INSURANCE AND MANAGED CARE POLICIES AND PROCEDURES

MEETING REQUIREMENTS FOR INSURANCE AND MANAGED CARE PLANS

To obtain the maximum third-party reimbursement for services provided to patients, it is very important to be familiar with the requirements of each insurance carrier and HMO providing insurance for the practice's patients. In addition, the same carrier may support more than one insurance plan. Each insurance plan works in its own way, and each has a handbook for providers. This is available in hard copy and can also usually be accessed via the internet and downloaded to the office network. The medical assistant should familiarize themselves with the various requirements of each particular insurance plan, including such things as whether a referral to a specialist must be in writing (hard copy or electronic) or can be given over the telephone. Each precertification and most referrals must be authorized by the HMO, and the authorization number should be noted on all of the certification or referral paperwork or electronic forms.

The medical assistant must also know which laboratory can do work for each plan and where patients can be referred for diagnostic follow-up. Most HMOs, for example, have contracts with a limited number of laboratories and/or medical facilities and will pay only for services provided by an approved facility.

Because many patients have prescription drug benefits, the medical assistant should also learn which pharmacies should be used for each plan and make sure that pharmacy information has been entered along with insurance plan information for each patient. The patient may have a separate pharmacy insurance card with specific information. This card should be copied for the patient's file or scanned into the office computer system.

VERIFYING ELIGIBILITY AND OBTAINING PREAUTHORIZATION (PRECERTIFICATION)

Most insurance companies have a process for reviewing services such as surgery, treatment by a specialist, physical therapy, certain diagnostic tests, and so on. The services and specific requirements vary greatly and tend to be stricter for managed care plans. The medical assistant must be able to obtain and interpret information on the patient's insurance card (Procedure 47.1). The patient's insurance card identifies telephone numbers, fax numbers, and usually a website where eligibility status can be verified (Fig. 47.2).

The first element of the process is often to verify **eligibility** status—that is, determine whether the patient has health insurance coverage and will be able to receive health insurance benefits during the proposed time period (Procedure 47.2). The second element is to verify insurance benefits—that is, determine whether the patient's insurance covers the proposed service. The insurance carrier may provide written or electronic verification, or the medical assistant may complete a form when verifying eligibility and/or benefits using the telephone.

The third element is to fulfill the insurance carrier's requirements for notifying the insurance carrier and obtaining authorization to provide the service. **Preauthorization** (or prior authorization) and **precertification** are two terms used to indicate that the patient's health insurance carrier has verified that the service is covered by the patient's insurance policy and/or that the insurance carrier has reviewed the medical necessity for a service and agreed that a procedure is medically appropriate (utilization review). Different companies may use these terms in slightly different ways. In addition, some companies require formal notification of the intent to provide or receive service, either by the provider or the patient. The requirement may be for a telephone call or submission of an electronic or written form, depending on the insurance carrier (Procedure 47.3).

Preauthorization (precertification) is usually required for certain medical procedures, therapy (e.g., physical therapy, occupational therapy, speech therapy), certain diagnostic procedures, consultations with a specialist provider, surgery, and hospitalization. Most insurance carriers prefer that requests for preauthorization (precertification) be submitted electronically using the insurance carrier's own website or an affiliate. The response is usually also provided electronically, usually with a form that can be printed and filed in a paper medical record or downloaded to an electronic health record. Paper forms can be obtained for fax or mail submission. Electronic requests can be approved more quickly.

The medical assistant should obtain the following information from the provider before initiating the request for preauthorization (precertification): a description of the service (e.g., number of visits to a specialist, type of therapy, surgery), the patient's diagnosis, any relevant information to justify the need for the service, and the proposed date of service (such as surgery or hospitalization). In addition, the medical assistant will have to provide the patient's demographic and insurance information as well as the National Provider Identifier (NPI) numbers and contact information of the primary care provider, the provider who will perform the service, and the hospital or other health care facility where the patient will receive treatment.

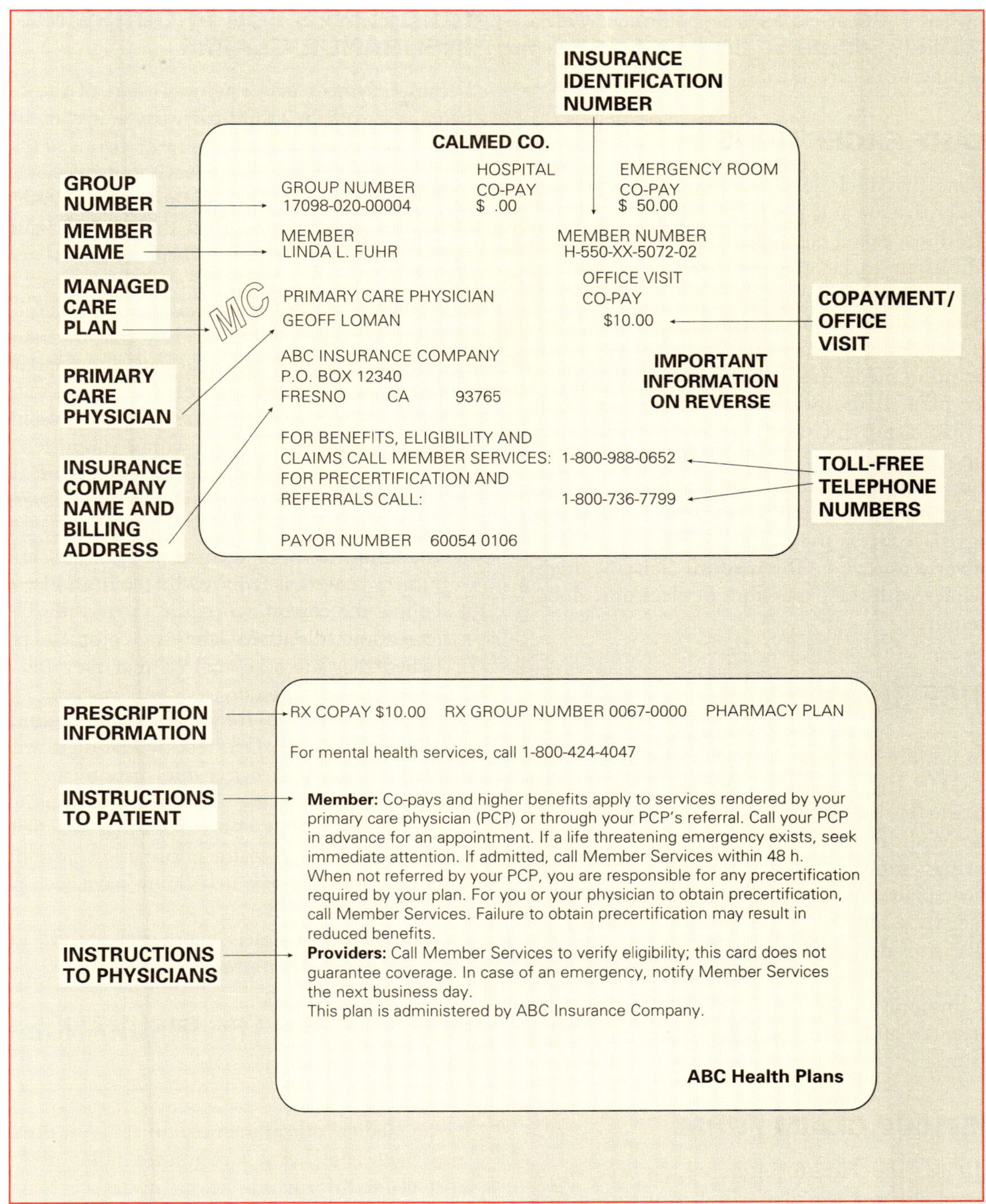

Fig. 47.2 The patient's insurance card summarizes important information about the insurance plan. (From Fordney M: *Insurance Handbook for the Medical Office*, ed 14, St. Louis, 2017, Elsevier.)

REFERRALS

A **referral** is the directing of a patient to a medical specialist by a primary care provider. (In managed care, a referral is sometimes also used as the name of an authorization for a treatment, such as a referral for physical therapy.) The PCP may be able to initiate a referral to a provider who participates in the patient's managed care plan without prior authorization, but usually a referral must be approved. This is consistent with the primary provider's role as gatekeeper, or person responsible for deciding what care is medically necessary for the patient. For many managed care plans and for patients covered by Medicaid (government insurance for low-income patients), all care other than visits to the PCP must be approved. The process is basically the same as that for obtaining prior authorization, but a different form (electronic or paper) may be required. When the patient has a traditional fee-for-service insurance plan or if the patient has Medicare, authorization to see a specialist is not required.

In this case, when a patient makes an appointment with a specialist, it is called a **self-referral**. This alerts the staff that no additional paperwork is required.

FORMULARY EXCEPTIONS

Insurance plans that include prescription drug benefits usually provide patients and providers with a list of preferred medications called a **formulary** (official list of covered medications to be used by network providers). This is an attempt to control costs by encouraging providers to prescribe generic forms of a medication. Patients may have to pay either a larger copayment or the entire cost of prescription medications that are not approved by the insurance plan. If the provider wants to prescribe a medication that is not included in the insurance plan formulary, approval can be requested from the insurance plan by using a form (electronic or paper) or by telephone. This approval will usually be granted only if formulary drugs have been tried and have failed or have caused an adverse outcome. The medical assistant might help the provider with the paperwork or electronic documentation required.

INSURANCE CLAIM FORMS

The most commonly used insurance form in the medical office is the CMS-1500. This form began as the Health Insurance Claim Form, which was approved for use by the American Medical Association in 1975. It was gradually accepted by various insurance plans for payment of claims by those plans. In 1990 this form was revised and printed in red. It became the required form for Medicare claims in 1992. It is discussed in greater detail in the next section.

Another commonly used form is the UB-04 form, which is used by hospitals and other institutions to submit paper insurance claims.

THE CMS-1500 CLAIM FORM

Since the 1950s, the Health Insurance Association of America has sought to have all medical insurance claims filed on a common form. After considerable work to develop a universal claim form, most insurance companies will accept the CMS-1500 form, either alone or as an attachment to the company's own form. This form was updated in 2005 to accept the NPI, a 10-digit identifier required for all health care providers that replaces all previous ID numbers. A claim form with minor revisions to accept the diagnosis codes of the International Classification of Diseases, 10th Revision, Clinical Modification (ICD-10-CM) was accepted in 2012 and is required for paper claim submission (Fig. 47.3). Electronic claims require the same information, and it is possible to print a completed claim form from SimChart.

GUIDELINES FOR PROCESSING INSURANCE CLAIMS

Because payment of a significant part of the bill for most patients is made by a third-party payor, it is important for the office to prepare and track insurance claims so that claims are processed in a timely manner without mistakes that would prevent or delay payment. This improves the cash flow for the office and avoids the need for the medical assistant to take extra time to correct errors. There are several general guidelines to facilitate the claim submission process.

1. Enter all patient and insurance information correctly into the computer and be sure that insurance information is updated at each visit with an updated photocopy of the patient's insurance card.
2. Be sure there is a signature on file for each patient for whom an insurance claim will be submitted.
3. Be aware of and follow requirements of all insurance companies related to verifying patient coverage, notifying before procedures, obtaining prior authorization, and using facilities such as laboratories, hospitals, and surgery centers as required by the insurance carrier.
4. Follow the correct procedure to transmit electronic information (discussed later) or complete paper claims (when they are accepted) so that they can be read by automated equipment.
5. Proofread all claims for accuracy before submitting them. Numbers that are incorrect by one digit, missing information, and/or incorrect information can result in automatic rejection of the claim. Be sure to submit any additional information with a claim that may be required.
6. Submit claims or claim information promptly and follow up to make sure that claims have been processed by the insurance carrier.
7. Follow up in a timely manner to correct and resubmit claims rejected for errors.

COMPLETING THE INSURANCE CLAIM FORM

In the medical office, the medical assistant usually prepares insurance claims using a computer billing program or submits claim information to an insurance billing clearinghouse. Since 2004, federal programs such as Medicare have required electronic claim submission unless the office has been granted a waiver that permits the submission of paper claims. Nevertheless, the medical assistant must know what information should be included so that each claim can be reviewed before submission (Procedure 47.4).

CARRIER INFORMATION

The name and address of the insurance carrier to which the claim will be sent is printed in the top section of the insurance claim form. For paper claims, this address should be entered in uppercase letters without punctuation (except for the hyphen in the ZIP+4 code).

HEALTH INSURANCE CLAIM FORM

APPROVED BY NATIONAL UNIFORM CLAIM COMMITTEE (NUCC) 02/12

PICA | PICA

CARRIER

1. MEDICARE (Medicare#) | MEDICAID (Medicaid#) | TRICARE (ID#DoD#) | CHAMPVA (Member ID#) | GROUP HEALTH PLAN (ID#) | FECA BLK LUNG (ID#) | OTHER (ID#)

1a. INSURED'S I.D. NUMBER (For Program in Item 1)

2. PATIENT'S NAME (Last Name, First Name, Middle Initial)

3. PATIENT'S BIRTH DATE MM | DD | YY SEX M F

4. INSURED'S NAME (Last Name, First Name, Middle Initial)

5. PATIENT'S ADDRESS (No., Street)

6. PATIENT RELATIONSHIP TO INSURED Self Spouse Child Other

7. INSURED'S ADDRESS (No., Street)

CITY STATE

8. RESERVED FOR NUCC USE

CITY STATE

ZIP CODE TELEPHONE (Include Area Code) ( )

ZIP CODE TELEPHONE (Include Area Code) ( )

9. OTHER INSURED'S NAME (Last Name, First Name, Middle Initial)

10. IS PATIENT'S CONDITION RELATED TO:

11. INSURED'S POLICY GROUP OR FECA NUMBER

a. OTHER INSURED'S POLICY OR GROUP NUMBER

a. EMPLOYMENT? (Current or Previous) YES NO

a. INSURED'S DATE OF BIRTH MM | DD | YY SEX M F

b. RESERVED FOR NUCC USE

b. AUTO ACCIDENT? YES NO PLACE (State)

b. OTHER CLAIM ID (Designated by NUCC)

c. RESERVED FOR NUCC USE

c. OTHER ACCIDENT? YES NO

c. INSURANCE PLAN NAME OR PROGRAM NAME

d. INSURANCE PLAN NAME OR PROGRAM NAME

10d. CLAIM CODES (Designated by NUCC)

d. IS THERE ANOTHER HEALTH BENEFIT PLAN? YES NO ***If yes***, complete items 9, 9a, and 9d.

READ BACK OF FORM BEFORE COMPLETING & SIGNING THIS FORM.

12. PATIENT'S OR AUTHORIZED PERSON'S SIGNATURE I authorize the release of any medical or other information necessary to process this claim. I also request payment of government benefits either to myself or to the party who accepts assignment below.

SIGNED ____ DATE ____

13. INSURED'S OR AUTHORIZED PERSON'S SIGNATURE I authorize payment of medical benefits to the undersigned physician or supplier for services described below.

SIGNED ____

PATIENT AND INSURED INFORMATION

14. DATE OF CURRENT ILLNESS, INJURY, or PREGNANCY(LMP) MM | DD | YY QUAL.

15. OTHER DATE QUAL. MM | DD | YY

16. DATES PATIENT UNABLE TO WORK IN CURRENT OCCUPATION FROM MM | DD | YY TO MM | DD | YY

17. NAME OF REFERRING PROVIDER OR OTHER SOURCE

17a. 17b. NPI

18. HOSPITALIZATION DATES RELATED TO CURRENT SERVICES FROM MM | DD | YY TO MM | DD | YY

19. ADDITIONAL CLAIM INFORMATION (Designated by NUCC)

20. OUTSIDE LAB? YES NO $ CHARGES

21. DIAGNOSIS OR NATURE OF ILLNESS OR INJURY Relate A-L to service line below (24E) ICD Ind.

A. B. C. D.
E. F. G. H.
I. J. K. L.

22. RESUBMISSION CODE ORIGINAL REF. NO.

23. PRIOR AUTHORIZATION NUMBER

	24. A. DATE(S) OF SERVICE From MM DD YY To MM DD YY	B. PLACE OF SERVICE	C. EMG	D. PROCEDURES, SERVICES, OR SUPPLIES (Explain Unusual Circumstances) CPT/HCPCS MODIFIER	E. DIAGNOSIS POINTER	F. $ CHARGES	G. DAYS OR UNITS	H. EPSDT Family Plan	I. ID. QUAL.	J. RENDERING PROVIDER ID. #
1									NPI	
2									NPI	
3									NPI	
4									NPI	
5									NPI	
6									NPI	

25. FEDERAL TAX I.D. NUMBER SSN EIN

26. PATIENT'S ACCOUNT NO.

27. ACCEPT ASSIGNMENT? (For govt. claims, see back) YES NO

28. TOTAL CHARGE $

29. AMOUNT PAID $

30. Rsvd for NUCC Use $

31. SIGNATURE OF PHYSICIAN OR SUPPLIER INCLUDING DEGREES OR CREDENTIALS (I certify that the statements on the reverse apply to this bill and are made a part thereof.)

SIGNED DATE

32. SERVICE FACILITY LOCATION INFORMATION

a. NPI b.

33. BILLING PROVIDER INFO & PH # ( )

a. NPI b.

PHYSICIAN OR SUPPLIER INFORMATION

NUCC Instruction Manual available at: www.nucc.org *PLEASE PRINT OR TYPE* APPROVED OMB-0938-1197 FORM 1500 (02-12)

Fig. 47.3 The CMS-1500 claim form (2/12 revision).

PATIENT AND INSURED INFORMATION

Patient Information

The patient section contains the patient's basic demographic information. This includes the patient's name, address, date of birth, and sex. It also identifies whether the provider accepts assignment of benefits, which is authorized by the patient's signature. Instead of asking patients to sign every insurance claim, the phrase **signature on file** or the abbreviation **SOF** is often used to indicate that the office maintains a copy of the patient's signature authorizing submission of the claim and assignment of benefits.

What Would You Do? What Would You *Not* Do?

Case Study 2

Daniel Litton is a 14-year-old new patient who has an appointment with one of the dermatologists in the office. He is brought to the office by his mother, who helps him fill out the new patient information form. In the section for insurance information, his mother indicates that he is covered by family insurance plans through both his father and his mother, who are married. His mother says, "I hope you will bill my insurance for him because I have better coverage for things like this." ■

Subscriber and Insurance Information

The insurance information part of the insurance claim form includes the following information about the insured (sometimes called the *subscriber* or the *guarantor*): the name of the insured, address, and relationship to the patient. It is important to be sure that the information about the **guarantor**, the individual with financial responsibility and/or insurance, has been entered into the computer (if they are not a patient). In addition, for employer-sponsored plans, the employer's name is listed. The insured has an ID number. In a family plan, other family members may use the same number as the insured, or each may be assigned a different number. For a group plan there is also a group number that is common to all members who obtain insurance from that employer or through that group.

If there is insurance in the name of a second party, this is also included on the claim form with the appropriate information about the insurance policy and ID (policy) and group numbers.

On every claim form, information must be included to identify whether the claim relates to a work injury, auto accident, or other accident. This helps the insurance carrier identify which insurance is responsible for covering the claim.

PROVIDER INFORMATION

The information about the medical services provided is entered in the lower half of the insurance claim form. In addition to information about the medical problem, the ICD-10 code for each diagnosis must be listed. Each procedure must be linked to a primary diagnosis code to justify the procedure. Below the information about the diagnosis (diagnoses), information about each procedure is given, including the date of service, place of service, procedure code, pointer to the diagnosis code, charge for the service, number of units being billed, and NPI number of the provider of each service. See Table 47.1 for a list of codes commonly used for place of service when billing from the medical office.

Table 47.1 Place-of-Service Codes Used for Billing in the Medical Office

Code	Place of Service
11	Office
12	Home
20	Urgent care facility
21	Inpatient hospital
22	On campus—outpatient hospital
23	Emergency room—hospital
24	Ambulatory surgical center
25	Birthing center
26	Military treatment facility
31	Skilled nursing facility
32	Nursing facility
33	Custodial care facility
49	Independent clinic

SUBMITTING INSURANCE CLAIMS

ELECTRONIC CLAIMS

Electronic submission speeds things up enormously. Submission is instantaneous, instead of taking a few days to move through the mail. The office may submit insurance claims directly to the insurance carrier or may submit them to a clearinghouse that processes the data and submits the claim to the appropriate carrier. The medical office may also submit information to a billing service that processes and submits claims to the various insurance companies. The procedure for submission depends on the computer software used by the office, clearinghouse, or billing service. Insurance company personnel cannot make errors inputting the information into the company's computer system because the transmission is computer to computer.

Faster delivery and faster and more accurate processing means faster reimbursement. If electronic claim submission is coupled with electronic payment from the company to the practice's operating account, the entire turnaround time from submission to money in the bank can be days instead of weeks.

All parts of the HIPAA affect insurance billing, but an important provision is the Transactions and Code Set Rule. This rule requires all health care providers to use American National Standards Institute (ANSI) technical content and format specifications for electronic transmissions. The electronic data interchange (EDI) Health Care Claim Transaction set 837P defines the format that must be used to submit health care claim billing information electronically by medical offices or to transmit this information among and within agencies involved in the reimbursement process.

PAPER CLAIMS

The CMS-1500 form is printed in red to facilitate optical scanning when paper forms are submitted. Although rarely used, paper claim forms can be purchased from medical office supply companies. For efficient processing, it is recommended to use no punctuation, to be sure that all information is within the required box, and to proofread for typographical errors that might cause the claim to be rejected. The medical assistant must be sure that the insurance carrier accepts paper claims, although most types of health insurance now require electronic claim submission.

What Would You Do? What Would You *Not* Do?

Case Study 3

Maria Santos, 33 years old, has been seen in the office for a physical examination. When she was reviewing insurance claims on the computer before submitting them, Sandra noticed that the name of the insured on the claim for Maria Santos is Jose Santos, and his date of birth is the same as her date of birth. Sandra also notices that in box 8 there is an X beside the word *Employed.* ■

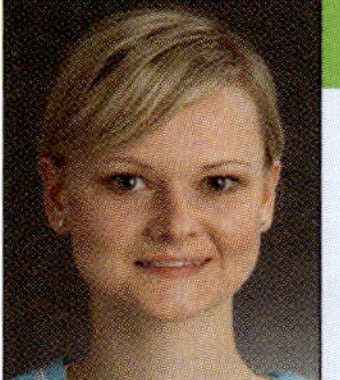

Memories *From* Practicum

Sandra O'Keefe: My practicum was done several years ago in the office of a single gynecologist in a medium-size city. Although the office had a computer billing program, we submitted most of the insurance claims on paper. After I had been at the office for several weeks, the office manager started having me fill out some insurance claim forms by hand. Then she would have me print the forms on the computer and compare my form with the computer-generated form. She said I needed to understand how to fill out the form myself, even if I didn't usually do it, so that I would know what kind of information should be in each box. At first I found it very confusing, but after a while I began to know what to look for. For example, an insurance carrier will deny a claim for a Pap test if the sex of the patient is given as male. I was always glad that I had some experience with insurance, although I don't think I realized how complex it really is until I actually began to work as a medical assistant. ■

TRACKING INSURANCE REIMBURSEMENT

Reimbursement is the payment received by the medical practice from the insurance carrier for the services performed.

USING A CLAIMS REGISTER

A record of every paper insurance claim filed should be kept using an insurance claims register. An insurance claims register can be kept manually but more commonly it is kept on a computer spreadsheet. Electronic claims have a date created within the computer system, and they can be tracked with clearinghouse claims using account aging (see Chapter 48).

If payment for a claim is delayed, the medical assistant should submit an insurance claim tracer to the insurance carrier. A form may be available on the insurance website, or there is a sample form that can be printed from SimChart for the Medical Office (see the Forms Repository).

The medical assistant should review insurance payments on a regular basis to be sure that all claims have been paid and that the insurance carrier has not denied services that should be covered or that it has paid less than it should. If a pattern of rejected claims is seen, the medical assistant should work together with other office staff to improve systems so that claims are not denied.

REMITTANCE ADVICE (EXPLANATION OF BENEFITS) FORMS

After payment has been made by the insurance carrier to the provider or if a claim is being denied, both the provider and patient receive a notification explaining payment for the claim. The provider receives a **remittance advice (RA)** or **explanation of benefits (EOB)** form. The form sent to the patient is the EOB form. The provider may elect to receive an electronic remittance advice (ERA) from Medicare or other insurance carrier. Although each insurance carrier has its own form, the type of information contained on any RA or EOB is similar, as shown in Fig. 47.4. If the insurance carrier is denying the claim, the provider will receive a RA form showing why the claim was disallowed.

Claims are usually denied for one of the following reasons: transposed names or numbers, incomplete information, incorrect or incomplete codes, or information that does not match codes or other information (Table 47.2). Claims may also be denied for late submission or late resubmission of a denied claim. (Procedure 47.5)

FOLLOW-UP AND RESUBMISSION OF CLAIMS

If a claim is denied, it should be resubmitted immediately, following any advice given by the company on the RA form. Any questions about a denial should be discussed with a provider relations representative at the company.

If claims are not being paid or denied in a timely fashion, follow-up is in order. Follow-up can be made via letter or over the telephone. The claims log can be used to find all claims to any company that are becoming delinquent and to follow up with a tracer or telephone call.

EFFECTIVE COMMUNICATION REGARDING MANAGED CARE AND/OR INSURANCE

COMMUNICATION WITH MANAGED CARE AND/OR INSURANCE PROVIDERS

When the medical assistant is communicating with managed care and/or insurance providers, it is important for them to

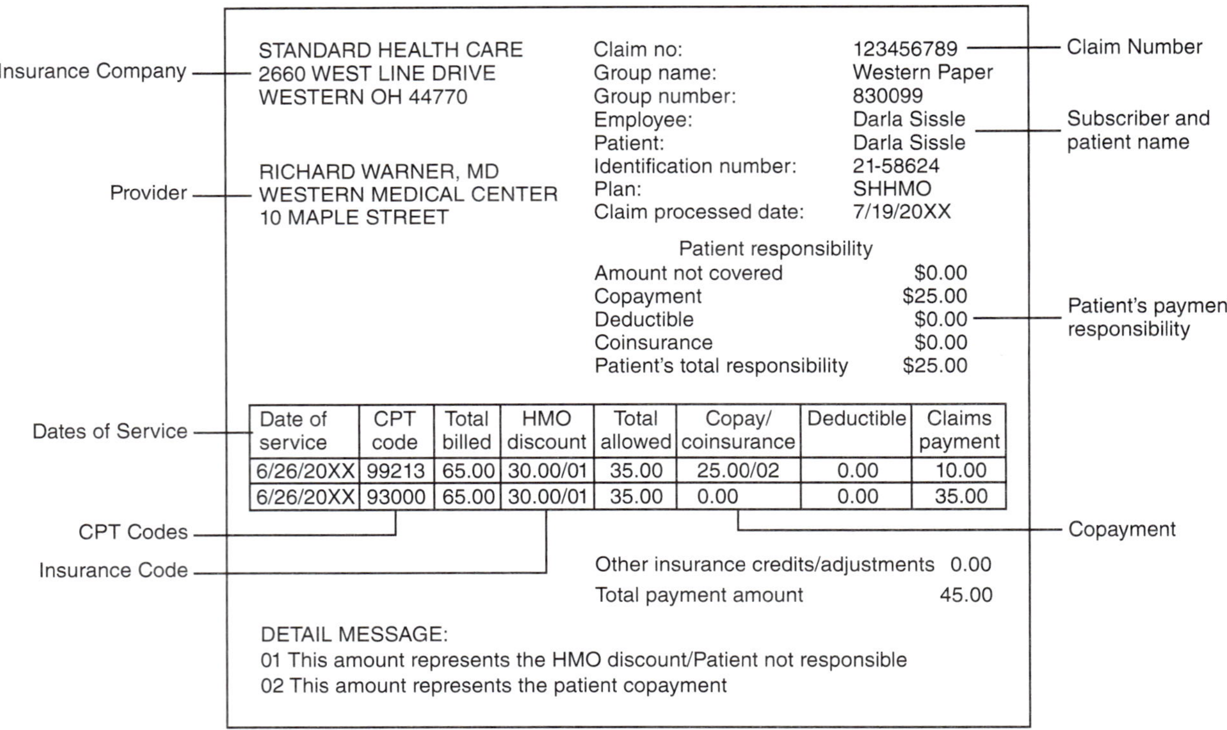
STANDARD HEALTH CARE
2660 WEST LINE DRIVE
WESTERN OH 44770

RICHARD WARNER, MD
WESTERN MEDICAL CENTER
10 MAPLE STREET

Claim no: 123456789
Group name: Western Paper
Group number: 830099
Employee: Darla Sissle
Patient: Darla Sissle
Identification number: 21-58624
Plan: SHHMO
Claim processed date: 7/19/20XX

Patient responsibility
Amount not covered $0.00
Copayment $25.00
Deductible $0.00
Coinsurance $0.00
Patient's total responsibility $25.00

Date of service	CPT code	Total billed	HMO discount	Total allowed	Copay/ coinsurance	Deductible	Claims payment
6/26/20XX	99213	65.00	30.00/01	35.00	25.00/02	0.00	10.00
6/26/20XX	93000	65.00	30.00/01	35.00	0.00	0.00	35.00

Other insurance credits/adjustments 0.00
Total payment amount 45.00

DETAIL MESSAGE:
01 This amount represents the HMO discount/Patient not responsible
02 This amount represents the patient copayment

Fig. 47.4 Sample explanation of benefits form. *CPT*, Current Procedural Terminology; *HMO*, Health Maintenance Organization.

Table 47.2 Common Errors on Insurance Claim Forms

Type of Error	Example
Transposing names or numbers	Reversing the name of the patient with the subscriber (guarantor)
	Reversing the primary insurance with the secondary insurance
	Transposing numbers in one of the identification numbers
Missing information	Missing signatures or signature stamps
	Missing or inaccurate provider National Provider Identifier number for each service, or not a provider registered with plan
	Required attachments missing (e.g., pathology report)
	Incomplete boxes
	Too little information to prove medical necessity
	No preapproval or preauthorization number
Inaccurate or incomplete codes	Inaccurate procedure or service codes (Current Procedural Terminology or Healthcare Common Procedure Coding System Level II codes)
	Missing modifier
Information does not match codes or other information	Diagnosis inconsistent with patient gender
	Diagnosis does not justify procedures performed
	Total amount of billing does not agree with services provided
	Place of service inconsistent with procedure code

be polite and tactful but also to demonstrate assertive communication techniques to maximize reimbursement. Familiarity with a specific plan's requirements and attention to detail in submitting claims help to minimize claim denials. But when a claim is denied, the medical assistant should telephone the provider and request specific information about the reason for the denial. It may be necessary to ask several questions to determine the type of documentation that will be necessary for the claim to be paid if resubmitted. If necessary, the medical assistant must ask politely for the name of an individual who can provide the requested information and should follow up with additional telephone calls.

COMMUNICATION WITH PATIENTS REGARDING MANAGED CARE AND/OR INSURANCE

The medical assistant must demonstrate different communication skills when discussing insurance benefits with patients. Although the patient has usually signed a form promising to pay for services that are not covered by insurance, the medical assistant must be willing to explain tactfully that a patient's insurance does not cover a service or that a claim has been denied and that the patient is now responsible for the bill. Patients often become upset about gaps in their insurance coverage. By imagining how they would feel in the patient's situation, the medical assistant can empathize with a patient who may be feeling angry or hostile. It is important to stay calm; express understanding for the patient's feelings; and, if necessary, suggest that the discussion be postponed to give everyone a chance to consider the situation. If a claim has been denied, the medical assistant should offer to resubmit the claim if there is any chance that additional documentation might induce the insurance provider to reverse its decision (Procedure 47.6).

What Would You Do? What Would You *Not* Do? RESPONSES

Case Study 1

Page 1196

What Did Sandra Do?

- ❑ Explained to the patient that the original referral authorized treatment of only the lesion on the patient's neck, and the insurance carrier would not pay for other treatment without authorizing it.
- ❑ Explained that Sandra would contact the insurance carrier and primary care provider and take care of any required paperwork.
- ❑ Promised to minimize delay as much as possible.
- ❑ Told the patient that she would be responsible for the cost of removal if proper authorization was not obtained from her insurance carrier.

What Did Sandra Not Do?

- ❑ Did not assume that the referral covered additional lesions not specifically mentioned on the referral form.
- ❑ Did not assure the patient that her insurance would automatically cover the cost of removing the additional lesions.
- ❑ Did not schedule the removal of the additional lesions before she received insurance authorization or the patient promised to pay for the procedure.

Case Study 2

Page 1204

What Did Sandra Do?

- ❑ Explained to Daniel's mother that there are rules governing coverage of children when both parents have insurance plans that cover their children.
- ❑ Asked Daniel's mother for her birth date and her husband's birth date.
- ❑ Explained to Daniel and his mother that usually children are covered by the insurance of the parent whose birth date comes first in the year.
- ❑ Asked Daniel's mother which insurance plan covers her children for their ordinary medical care.

What Did Sandra Not Do?

- ❑ Did not promise to send the insurance claim to the carrier the mother prefers unless it was the primary insurance carrier.
- ❑ Did not tell Daniel's mother not to worry because she would take care of it.
- ❑ Did not tell Daniel's mother that it was her responsibility to find out which insurance was the primary insurance.

Case Study 3

Page 1205

What Did Sandra Do?

- ❑ Checked the new patient information form to be sure that the insured's name and date of birth had been entered correctly, because incorrect information could lead to denial of the insurance claim.
- ❑ Checked the new patient information form to be sure that the patient had listed an employer.

What Did Sandra Not Do?

- ❑ Did not assume that it was just a coincidence that the husband and wife had the same date of birth.
- ❑ Did not assume that a few errors on the insurance claim form would not matter.
- ❑ Did not assume that the information in the computer was always correct.

TERMINOLOGY REVIEW

Key Term	Definition
Assignment of benefits	Authorization for insurance reimbursement to be made to the provider of a health service rather than the insured individual.
Beneficiary	A person who can receive benefits under an insurance plan.
Benefit	Payment for a covered service under a health insurance plan.
Capitation	A method of paying for insurance in which a fixed amount is paid to the provider per member for a specific time period regardless of the amount of care provided.
CHAMPVA	A government health insurance program that covers dependents of military veterans with service-connected disabilities.
Coinsurance	A percentage of the allowed charge for health services, which the patient is responsible for paying.
Coordination of benefits	Rules followed by insurance companies so that no claim is reimbursed at more than 100% of the charges.
Copayment	A fixed amount of money that the patient must pay for any health care service.
Deductible	An amount of money that an insured person must pay annually before health services are covered by the insurance plan.
Eligibility	Enrollment status related to a health insurance plan.
Explanation of benefits (EOB)	A statement issued by the insurance carrier explaining reimbursement for specific procedures.
Fee-for-service insurance	Insurance reimbursement that is for each treatment or procedure performed and the amount charged by the provider.
Formulary	An insurance carrier's official list of covered medications to be used by network providers.
Group plan	One insurance policy that covers a group of people.
Guarantor	A person with financial responsibility for a bill who may or may not also be a patient.
Indemnity	An obligation to provide compensation for loss or damage.
Insured	The individual who has a specific insurance plan.
Managed care	A movement in health care based on reducing health care costs while providing high-quality care. The term may be used for the techniques used to reduce costs or for the companies that pay for the care provided.
Medicaid	The government insurance program for low-income individuals and families that is funded both by the federal government and by each individual state.
Medicare	The federal health insurance program that provides insurance coverage for the elderly, permanently disabled, and individuals with end-stage renal disease.
Medicare Administrative Contractor (MAC)	A private health care insurer that administers both Medicare Part A and Medicare Part B claims, usually for more than one state, under a contract with the Centers for Medicare and Medicaid Services (CMS).
Nonparticipating provider (nonPAR)	A provider who does not have any contract with a third-party payor.
Participating provider (PAR)	A provider who has a contractual agreement with a third-party payor.
Preauthorization	Verification from a patient's insurance carrier that a procedure is covered by the patient's insurance and/or agreement, after review, that the test or procedure is medically appropriate.
Precertification	Verification from a patient's insurance carrier that a procedure is covered by the patient's insurance and/or agreement, after review, that the test or procedure is medically appropriate.
Premium	An amount of money paid in a given period to purchase health insurance.
Primary care provider (PCP)	The health care practitioner chosen by a patient to provide general medical care and also to determine and authorize additional medical services the patient may require.
Primary insurance	The insurance company that must be billed first for any individual.
Referral	The directing of a patient to a specialist provider by the primary care provider. Most managed care plans and some other insurance plans require the primary care provider to obtain prior authorization.
Reimbursement	The amount paid by insurance for health care services.
Remittance advice (RA)	A statement issued by Medicare or another third-party payor to the provider explaining reimbursement for specific procedures or denial of an insurance claim.

TERMINOLOGY REVIEW—cont'd

Key Term	Definition
Resource-based relative value scale (RBRVS)	A system to establish the Medicare fee schedule for Medicare Part B based on the service provided and the geographic location of the provider.
Secondary insurance	Insurance held by another insured (such as a spouse) that provides additional insurance coverage.
Self-referral	The process by which a patient makes an appointment with a specialist provider without requesting prior authorization from their primary care provider, usually because the patient's insurance plan does not require it.
Signature on file (SOF)	An indication on the insurance claim form that the signature of the patient is maintained by the medical office to authorize submission of insurance claims.
Third-party payor	Insurance carrier or managed care organization that pays health insurance claims.
TRICARE	A government insurance plan that provides medical care to spouses and dependents of individuals on active duty in the military. Some veterans, reservists, and retirees are also eligible. It received its name when there were three available plans.
Usual, customary, and reasonable (UCR)	A system for establishing the amount an insurance carrier will pay for a procedure. The reasonable charge is set by the insurance carrier on the basis of a provider's usual (most frequent) charge for the procedure and the customary charge of other providers in the same geographic area.
Utilization review	Reviewing proposed or current care to determine medical necessity.
Workers' compensation	An insurance program that covers lost wages and health care costs of workers injured on the job or having work-related illnesses.

PROCEDURE 47.1 Interpreting Information on an Insurance Card

Outcome Interpret information on an insurance card.

Equipment/Supplies

- Sample insurance cards (at least three)

1. **Procedural Step.** Using at least three insurance cards (see Figs. 47.1 and 47.2), make a list of information that is usually found on the front of an insurance card and information that is usually found on the back of an insurance card.
2. **Procedural Step.** Write a short paper analyzing one of the sample insurance cards, identifying and explaining how the card informs you of the insurance carrier name and contact information, the subscriber's name and identifying information, the patient's payment responsibility for various services, and the type of insurance plan.
3. **Procedural Step.** Role-play the part of a medical assistant with a classmate playing the part of the patient whose insurance card you are viewing, using the information in Fig. 47.2 from the textbook. Explain that the patient's copay is for an office visit (assuming that you work for the patient's primary care provider [PCP]). Explain how the referral process works. Tell the patient what number to call if they are admitted to a hospital because of a life-threatening emergency. Tell the patient what number to call for mental health services.
   Principle. A medical assistant obtains information about a patient's insurance plan from the insurance card and may be required to coach the patient about their insurance plan.
4. **Procedural Step.** Demonstrate sensitivity when you are communicating with the simulated patient regarding third-party requirements.
5. **Procedural Step.** Hand in your list of information on an insurance card and analysis of an insurance card to your instructor.

PROCEDURE 47.2 Verifying Insurance Eligibility and Benefits

Outcome Verify insurance or managed care eligibility; with the instructor observing directly, interact professionally with a third-party representative.

Equipment/Supplies

- Patient insurance information
- Telephone
- Computer with internet access
- Pen and paper

1. **Procedural Step.** Assemble information about the patient's insurance plan, including name of insurance or managed care company, telephone number or Web address, patient's name, patient's date of birth, subscriber's number, and group number. If possible, obtain this information from a photocopy or scan of the patient's insurance card.
   Principle: The insurance card contains all the information needed to contact a patient's insurance plan.
2. **Procedural Step.** Simulate calling the appropriate number and speaking to a representative to verify that the patient is eligible for benefits. Record the effective date and the termination date (if any).
   Principle: An individual's insurance coverage can change for many reasons. A patient must have current coverage to obtain insurance reimbursement.
3. **Procedural Step.** Ask the representative for information about the patient's deductible and copayment or coinsurance. If a service other than a routine office visit is planned, determine if it is a covered service and if precertification or preauthorization is required.
   Principle: Knowledge of deductible and copayment or coinsurance helps to determine the amount the patient should pay at the time of the visit.
4. **Procedural Step.** Ask the representative to describe the procedure for referral to specialists.
5. **Procedural Step.** Use professional communication techniques with the representative to inquire about coverage.
6. **Procedural Step.** End the call politely and professionally.
7. **Procedural Step.** Note the information according to office policy. There may be a form to fill out or a notation may be required in the patient's medical record. If the insurance carrier provides an electronic verification of eligibility, attach it to the patient's electronic medical record or print it and file it in a paper-based medical record. Include the name, title, and extension of the person contacted.

PROCEDURE 47.3 Obtaining Insurance Preauthorization (Precertification)

Outcome Obtain insurance preauthorization (precertification).

Equipment/Supplies

- Patient's medical record and insurance information
- Provider's directions about the service to be provided
- Computer or paper preauthorization (precertification) request form
- Computer with internet access
- Pen
- Telephone

1. **Procedural Step.** Assemble the following information to complete a preauthorization (precertification) request:
   - Patient's demographic information
   - Patient's insurance information
   - Information about service to be provided, including diagnosis code(s) and procedure code(s), and the patient's name, address, telephone number, and insurance information
   - Forms as needed

   It may be helpful to print and complete a Prior Authorization Request form from SimChart for the Medical Office (Forms Repository).
2. **Procedural Step.** From the patient's medical record or the provider, determine the service for which preauthorization or precertification is requested. Assemble all information needed to complete the request.
   Principle. Most requests require at a minimum the patient's name, ID number, diagnosis and diagnosis code, proposed procedure and procedure code, provider's

PROCEDURE 47.3 Obtaining Insurance Preauthorization (Precertification)—cont'd

National Provider Identifier (NPI) number, and NPI number of other provider or service provider. Assembling information ahead of time facilitates completing the request.

3. **Procedural Step.** Obtain preauthorization or precertification from the patient's insurance carrier or health maintenance organization (HMO). The preferred method is usually by completing a form on the carrier's website. Telephone, fax, or a paper form may also be used. Supply all information requested. If using the telephone, it is helpful to complete the form manually before placing the call to be sure you have all necessary information.

   Principle. The patient's medical condition must justify the service requested. Failure to obtain preauthorization or precertification required by the insurance carrier will result in denial of the patient's insurance claim.

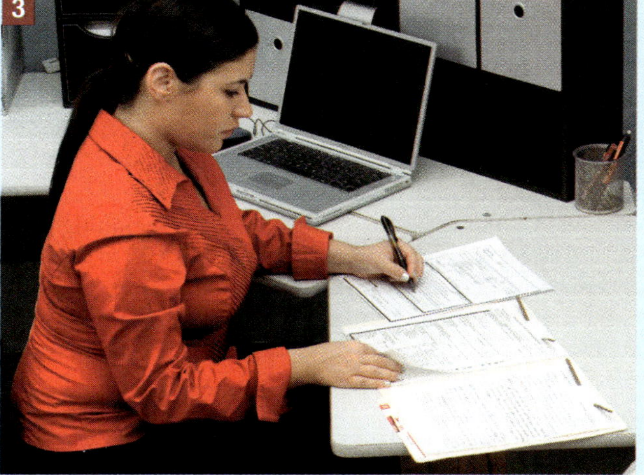

For a telephone request, it is helpful to fill out the required form before calling the insurance carrier.

4. **Procedural Step.** When the form is complete, submit the form for approval using the appropriate method.
5. **Procedural Step.** Inform the patient that they will not be able to obtain service until preauthorization or precertification is received from the insurance carrier.
6. **Procedural Step.** When approval is received, notify the patient. An electronic form should be accessible to any other health care provider using the internet. A paper copy must be sent or faxed to a specialty provider or other provider of service.
7. **Procedural Step.** Tell the patient how to make the appointment (or assist the patient in making the first appointment).
8. **Procedural Step.** File the approval form in the patient's medical record or attach an electronic form (scan a paper form) to the electronic health record.

PROCEDURE 47.4 Completing and Reviewing an Insurance Claim Form

Outcome Complete or review an insurance claim form.

Equipment/Supplies

- Patient information
- Patient account or ledger
- Copy of the patient's insurance card or computer patient information screen
- Insurance claim form
- Computer with medical billing program or SimChart for the Medical Office
- Pen
- Printer

1. **Procedural Step.** Assemble information needed to prepare an insurance claim, including a claim form, information about the patient, the patient account or ledger, and a copy of the patient's insurance card or insurance information. Review the claim form guidelines for the specific insurance carrier.
2. **Procedural Step.** Enter (or review) information as required on the paper CMS-1500 form according to the following information. If a paper claim will be submitted to be scanned by optical character recognition (OCR) or intelligent character recognition (ICR), do not use commas, dollar signs, or other punctuation unless instructed to do so.
   Principle. Most insurance companies use ICR scanning to digitize information on paper claims, and the equipment works best when the guidelines outlined earlier have been followed. It is usually no longer necessary to use only capital letters.
3. **Procedural Step.** In the carrier section, enter or validate the name and address of the insurance carrier to which the claim will be sent using the following format:
   Line 1: Name of carrier
   Line 2: First line of address
   Line 3: Second line of address (if needed)
   Line 4: City [space] State [space] ZIP
   Example—three-line address:
   Standard Health Care
   1500 Summit Avenue
   Western XY 45000
   Example—four-line address:
   Standard Health Care
   Suite 620
   1500 Summit Avenue
   Western XY 45000
4. **Procedural Step.** Complete or review the patient and insured information on the claim form.
   Box 1—The type of insurance is indicated with an X. Only one box can be marked. Insurance obtained through employment is a Group Health Plan.
   Box 1a—The ID number of the individual who is insured as shown on the insurance card.
   Box 2—The patient's last name, first name, and middle initial (separated by commas).
   Box 3—The patient's date of birth in the format MM DD YYYY and the patient's sex (M or F) marked with an X.
   Box 4—The name of the insured using the format last name, first name, middle initial (separated by commas).
   Box 5—The patient's mailing address beginning with the street. Use the two-letter state code. Do not use commas, periods, or other punctuation in the address and do not enter the hyphen in a nine-digit ZIP code. Do not use a hyphen or space as a separator in the telephone number.
   Box 6—An X in the box that defines the patient's relationship to the insured (i.e., person whose name is on the insurance policy). The choices include self, spouse, child, and other.
   Box 7—The insured's mailing address beginning with the street. Use the two-letter state code. Do not use commas, periods, or other punctuation in the address and do not enter the hyphen in a nine-digit ZIP code. Do not use a hyphen or space as a separator in the seven-digit telephone number. Complete this box if Box 4 is completed.
   Box 8—Leave this box blank.
   Box 9—If there is secondary insurance, the insured's name using the format described for Box 4.
   Box 9a—If there is secondary insurance, the subscriber's policy (ID) or group number.
   Box 9d—If there is secondary insurance, the other insured's insurance plan or program name.
   Boxes 9b and 9c have been deleted from ANSI 5010A1, the current data format for electronic claim submission, so these boxes should be left blank.
   Box 10a-c—Information related to the cause of the patient's condition(s). The correct boxes are checked (*yes* or *no*) to answer the questions. If the patient's condition was caused by an automobile accident, the state where the accident occurred is identified using the correct two-letter code.
   Box 10d—Used to report claim codes that identify additional information about the patient's condition when required by public or private payors.
   Box 11—The insured's policy group or Federal Employees' Compensation Act (FECA) number. If item

PROCEDURE 47.4 Completing and Reviewing an Insurance Claim Form—cont'd

number 4 is completed, this field should be completed. Do not enter a hyphen or space as a separator within the policy or group number.

Box 11a-d—If the patient is the insured, only box 11d must be completed. The insured's date of birth in the format MM DD YYYY and the insured's sex (M or F) marked with an X. The insured's employer and insurance plan name. An X is used in the correct box to indicate if there is additional insurance (*yes* or *no*). If *yes* is selected, Boxes 9a-d are filled out.

Box 12—If the office has on file the patient's signature on a similar permission form, the initials *SOF* or the words *Signature on File* are placed in this box. Otherwise, the patient must sign and date the form.

Box 13—If the office has on file the patient's signature on a similar permission form, the initials *SOF* or the words *Signature on File* are placed in this box. Otherwise, the patient must sign and date the form in the format MM DD YYYY.

4

1. MEDICARE (Medicare #) MEDICAID (Medicaid #) TRICARE CHAMPUS (Sponsor's SSN) CHAMPVA (Member ID#) GROUP HEALTH PLAN (SSN or ID) FECA BLK LUNG (SSN) OTHER (ID)		1a. INSURED'S I.D. NUMBER (For Program in Item 1)
2. PATIENT'S NAME (Last Name, First Name, Middle Initial)	3. PATIENT'S BIRTH DATE MM DD YY SEX M F	4. INSURED'S NAME (Last Name, First Name, Middle Initial)
5. PATIENT'S ADDRESS (No., Street)	6. PATIENT RELATIONSHIP TO INSURED Self Spouse Child Other	7. INSURED'S ADDRESS (No., Street)
CITY STATE	8. PATIENT STATUS Single Married Other	CITY STATE
ZIP CODE TELEPHONE (Include Area Code) ( )	Employed Full-Time Student Part-Time Student	ZIP CODE TELEPHONE (Include Area Code) ( )
9. OTHER INSURED'S NAME (Last Name, First Name, Middle Initial)	10. IS PATIENT'S CONDITION RELATED TO:	11. INSURED'S POLICY GROUP OR FECA NUMBER
a. OTHER INSURED'S POLICY OR GROUP NUMBER	a. EMPLOYMENT? (Current or Previous) YES NO	a. INSURED'S DATE OF BIRTH MM DD YY SEX M F
b. OTHER INSURED'S DATE OF BIRTH MM DD YY SEX M F	b. AUTO ACCIDENT? YES NO PLACE (State)	b. EMPLOYER'S NAME OR SCHOOL NAME
c. EMPLOYER'S NAME OR SCHOOL NAME	c. OTHER ACCIDENT? YES NO	c. INSURANCE PLAN NAME OR PROGRAM NAME
d. INSURANCE PLAN NAME OR PROGRAM NAME	10d. RESERVED FOR LOCAL USE	d. IS THERE ANOTHER HEALTH BENEFIT PLAN? YES NO *If yes*, return to and complete item 9 a-d.
READ BACK OF FORM BEFORE COMPLETING & SIGNING THIS FORM. 12. PATIENT'S OR AUTHORIZED PERSON'S SIGNATURE I authorize the release of any medical or other information necessary to process this claim. I also request payment of government benefits either to myself or to the party who accepts assignment below. SIGNED ___ DATE ___		13. INSURED'S OR AUTHORIZED PERSON'S SIGNATURE I authorize payment of medical benefits to the undersigned physician or supplier for services described below. SIGNED ___

PATIENT AND INSURED INFORMATION

Patient and insurance information section

5. Procedural Step. Complete the provider or supplier information.

Principle. If incomplete or incorrect information about primary and secondary insurance plans is given, the claim will be denied.

Boxes 14–16—Not usually required for Medicare, Medicaid, TRICARE, CHAMPVA, and most private insurance. If these boxes must be filled in, the dates are obtained from the patient's medical record and/or the provider. A qualifier code must be entered in box 15 using the following:

454 Initial treatment
304 Latest visit or consultation
453 Acute manifestation of a chronic condition
455 Last x-ray
471 Prescription
090 Report start (assumed care date)
091 Report end (relinquished care date)
444 First visit or consultation

Box 17—Name of the provider who ordered the service or referred the patient (first, middle initial, last) or other source followed by the credentials of the professional. If multiple providers are involved and for Medicare claims, use the following order and enter a qualifier to the left of the dotted line:

1. DN Referring provider
2. DK Ordering provider
3. DQ Supervising provider

Box 17a—Usually blank. If the provider does not have a national provider identifier (NPI) number, other identifying numbers can be used.

Box 17b—The 10-digit NPI number of the referring, ordering, or supervising provider.

Box 18—If the patient's claim is for a hospitalization, either a visit or surgery performed when the patient was hospitalized, and the dates of hospitalization. Otherwise, the box is left blank.

Continued

PROCEDURE 47.4 Completing and Reviewing an Insurance Claim Form—cont'd

Box 19—Left blank unless instructed by a specific insurance carrier to use this box for information specific to that carrier.

Box 20—*No* is usually checked. If the office paid for outside laboratory services that are not itemized on one of the lines in Box 24, *yes* is checked. If *yes* is checked, enter the charges with a space between the dollars and cents. Only one outside service can be billed per claim form.

Box 21—Enter up to 12 ICD-10-CM codes with alphanumeric characters and periods. Relate lines A to L to the lines of service in 24E by the letter of the line.

Box 22—Left blank unless the claim is a Medicaid resubmission, when the code and original reference number are entered.

Box 23—Left blank unless a referral, preauthorization, or precertification number was assigned by the insurance carrier.

6. Procedural Step. Enter information in Box 24 on lines 1–6 for each procedure that is being billed to the insurance carrier. For more than six procedures, complete an additional CMS-1500 form.

Box 24A—The date service began under the "From" section in the format MM DD YY in the unshaded area. If the service occurred on one day only, the "To" section is left blank or the "From" date may be entered again; otherwise, the date service ended.

Box 24B—The code for the place of service from Table 47.1.

Box 24C—This box is usually left blank. For some carriers, a *Y* is placed in this box if the service is an emergency service.

Box 24D—The Current Procedural Terminology (CPT) or Healthcare Common Procedure Coding System (HCPCS) Level II code and modifier(s) (if any) in the unshaded area.

Box 24E—The letter(s) (from A to L) that point to ICD-10 code(s) in Box 21 that justify the procedure. Only one letter can be used in this box for Medicare claims.

Box 24F—The charges in the unshaded area, leaving a space between the number of dollars and the number of cents instead of using a decimal point.

Box 24G—If charging for more than one of the same procedure (e.g., visits to a hospitalized patient on 3 consecutive days), the number of units of the procedure charged in the unshaded area. Otherwise, the number 1.

Box 24H—Left blank unless the patient is enrolled in the Medicaid program for Early and Periodic Screening, Diagnosis, and Treatment (EPSDT).

Box 24I—If the provider does not have an NPI number, a qualifier is entered in the shaded part of Box 24I, and the appropriate identification number is entered in the shaded part of Box 24J.

Box 24J—The 10-digit NPI number of the individual who provided service in the lower (unshaded) portion.

7. Procedural Step. Complete the remaining boxes on the CMS-1500 form.

Box 25—The tax ID number. If the Social Security number of an individual provider is used, box "SSN" is checked. If the employer ID number of a group practice is used, box "EIN" is checked.

Box 26—The patient account number. The box is left blank if there is no patient account number. Hyphens should not be used in this box.

Box 27—If the provider accepts assignment of benefits, an X is placed in the *yes* box. If assignment of benefits is not accepted, an X is placed in the *no* box.

Box 28—The total charges with a space between the number of dollars and the number of cents.

Box 29—The amount paid toward the covered charges, including any copayment. If the amount is zero, the box is left blank.

Box 30—This box should be left blank because information in it is no longer transmitted with electronic submission.

Box 31—*Signature on File* (*SOF*), or the provider's legal signature including credentials and the date.

Box 32—The name, address, city, state, and ZIP code of the facility where the services were provided, without punctuation. If services were provided at the same address as the billing address, this box as well as 32a and 32b can be left blank.

Box 32a—The 10-digit NPI number of the service facility location.

Box 32b—For purchased diagnostic services (Box 20), insert the supplier's PIN.

Box 33—The name, address, and telephone number of the provider group or supplier of services without punctuation. The telephone number is entered to the right of the title of the field without a hyphen. A hyphen is used in a nine-digit ZIP code after the fifth digit.

Box 33a—The 10-digit NPI number of the provider group or supplier of services.

Box 33b—Other ID number if the supplier of service does not have a 10-digit NPI number.

PROCEDURE 47.4 Completing and Reviewing an Insurance Claim Form—cont'd

5-7

14. DATE OF CURRENT ILLNESS, INJURY, or PREGNANCY(LMP) MM DD YY QUAL.
15. OTHER DATE QUAL. MM DD YY
16. DATES PATIENT UNABLE TO WORK IN CURRENT OCCUPATION FROM MM DD YY TO MM DD YY
17. NAME OF REFERRING PROVIDER OR OTHER SOURCE 17a. 17b. NPI
18. HOSPITALIZATION DATES RELATED TO CURRENT SERVICES FROM MM DD YY TO MM DD YY
19. ADDITIONAL CLAIM INFORMATION (Designated by NUCC)
20. OUTSIDE LAB? YES NO $ CHARGES
21. DIAGNOSIS OR NATURE OF ILLNESS OR INJURY Relate A-L to service line below (24E) ICD Ind.
A. B. C. D.
E. F. G. H.
I. J. K. L.
22. RESUBMISSION CODE ORIGINAL REF. NO.
23. PRIOR AUTHORIZATION NUMBER
24. A. DATE(S) OF SERVICE From MM DD YY To MM DD YY; B. PLACE OF SERVICE; C. EMG; D. PROCEDURES, SERVICES, OR SUPPLIES (Explain Unusual Circumstances) CPT/HCPCS MODIFIER; E. DIAGNOSIS POINTER; F. $ CHARGES; G. DAYS OR UNITS; H. EPSDT Family Plan; I. ID. QUAL.; J. RENDERING PROVIDER ID. #
1 NPI
2 NPI
3 NPI
4 NPI
5 NPI
6 NPI
PHYSICIAN OR SUPPLIER INFORMATION
25. FEDERAL TAX I.D. NUMBER SSN EIN
26. PATIENT'S ACCOUNT NO.
27. ACCEPT ASSIGNMENT? (For govt. claims, see back) YES NO
28. TOTAL CHARGE $
29. AMOUNT PAID $
30. Rsvd for NUCC Use $
31. SIGNATURE OF PHYSICIAN OR SUPPLIER INCLUDING DEGREES OR CREDENTIALS (I certify that the statements on the reverse apply to this bill and are made a part thereof.) SIGNED DATE
32. SERVICE FACILITY LOCATION INFORMATION a. NPI b.
33. BILLING PROVIDER INFO & PH # ( ) a. NPI b.

Provider and supplier section.

8. **Procedural Step.** Submit claim according to office policy. Copy a paper form before mailing and keep the copy in an insurance claims file.

Completing the Insurance Claim Form in SimChart for the Medical Office

9. **Procedural Step.** After the superbill and ledger have been created for a patient, select *Claim* from the *Info Panel* of the *Coding and Billing* screen and search for the patient.
10. **Procedural Step.** Select the correct encounter and confirm the autopopulated details on all tabs. On the *Encounter Notes* tab, select the *Yes* radio button to validate that the HIPAA form is on file for the patient, and document the day's date in the date field. Then click the *Save* button before proceeding to the *Claim Info* tab. Enter the information requested on this screen. Proceed to the *Charge Capture* screen and enter the information from the superbill as outlined earlier for Box 24.
11. **Procedural Step.** Click on the printer icon to print the claim so that you can manually double check all information before submitting the claim.
12. **Procedural Step.** When you are sure that all information is correct, click on the *Submission* tab, and then click on the "*I am ready to submit the Claim*" box. Then click the *Yes* radio button and enter the date of service in the date field. Click the *Save* button, then the *Submit Claim* button.

PROCEDURE 47.4

PROCEDURE 47.5 Assisting a Patient in Understanding an Explanation of Benefits

Outcomes

1. Explain an explanation of benefits to a patient in a reassuring and tactful manner.
2. Use critical thinking skills in the process of explaining the explanation of benefits to a patient.

Equipment/Supplies

- Explanation of benefits for the patient's visit to the provider

1. **Procedural Step.** Review the explanation of benefits prior to meeting with the patient.
2. **Procedural Step.** Clarify any questions you might have on the reasoning for the payment decision made by the insurance company before the meeting with the patient.
3. **Procedural Step.** Call the patient back to meet with you. Explain to the patient how each service was processed by the insurance company in a tactful manner.
4. **Procedural Step.** Establish a professional and empathetic atmosphere. Reassure the patient that you can work with them to resolve any issues.
5. **Procedural Step.** Using a professional manner, remind the patient of the office policies regarding payment of the balance.
6. **Procedural Step.** Decide what will be done and repeat the decision for the patient.

PROCEDURE 47.6 Communicating Professionally With Sensitivity Related to Managed Care and/or Insurance

Outcomes

1. Interact professionally with third-party representatives.
2. Display tactful behavior when communicating with medical providers regarding third-party requirements.
3. Show sensitivity when you are communicating with patients regarding third-party requirements.

Equipment/Supplies

- Pen
- Paper
- Computer with printer

1. **Procedural Step.** Review the principles of effective communication in this textbook (Chapter 4), including listening skills, measures to facilitate communication, and barriers to effective communication.
2. **Procedural Step.** Working with a group of at least two other students, assign one student to create a role-play situation for each of the following:
   a. A situation in which a medical assistant must demonstrate professional communication with a managed care provider relating to a denied insurance claim
   b. A situation in which a medical assistant must explain to a provider that a request for a diagnostic test was not approved for a patient by the patient's insurance carrier
   c. A situation in which a medical assistant must explain to a patient that the insurance carrier has denied an insurance claim and the patient will have to pay for the service

   Principle: A medical assistant must demonstrate effective communication when they are communicating with managed care and/or insurance representatives as well as with providers and patients about insurance reimbursement.
3. **Procedural Step.** Review the situations of the other students in your group to be sure that they are specific and realistic. Revise your situation as needed.
4. **Procedural Step.** Role-play each situation with your group members, demonstrating sensitivity, tact, professionalism, and/or other appropriate communication techniques.
5. **Procedural Step.** Add a short summary of the role-play experience to the situation you have created and explain how you demonstrated professional communication with a third-party representative, tact with a provider, and sensitivity to a patient in discussing a denied insurance claim.
6. **Procedural Step.** Print your paper and hand it in to your instructor.

Billing and Collections

Check out the Evolve site at http://evolve.elsevier.com/Bonewit/today to access additional interactive activities and exercises to help you study and prepare for success.

LEARNING OBJECTIVES

Billing Process

1. Describe the process of billing and collections.

Billing Problems

2. Describe problems that can occur when patients pay by check.
3. Explain how to adjust patient accounts for an overpayment and process a refund.
4. Develop a collection system.

Account Aging

5. Identify past due accounts and the actions needed.

Collection Activities

6. Describe the information to include in a collection letter.
7. Identify legal requirements that affect collections for the medical office.
8. Describe special circumstances affecting collections in the medical office.

PROCEDURES

Processing patient statements.

Posting a "non-sufficient funds" check.

Processing a credit balance and refund.

Creating and examining an accounts receivable aging record.

Writing a collection letter.

CHAPTER OUTLINE

INTRODUCTION TO BILLING
BILLING CYCLE
BILLING PROCESS
BILLING PROBLEMS
Problems With Checks
Insufficient Funds in the Office Account
Stopping Payment
Insufficient Funds in a Patient Account
Overpayments and Refunds
ACCOUNT AGING
Accounts Receivable Aging Records and Reports
Examining Accounts for Those Overdue
COLLECTION ACTIVITIES
Past Due Accounts
Collection Letters
Credit Agreements
Truth in Lending Statements
Policy for Patients With Outstanding Balances
Other Collection Techniques and Special Circumstances
Tracing "Skips"
Sending Accounts to a Collection Agency
Small Claims Court
Billing an Estate
Bankruptcy
Laws Affecting Credit and Collection Activities
Equal Credit Opportunity Act
Fair Debt Collection Practices Act
Federal Truth in Lending Act
Fair Credit Reporting Act
Bankruptcy Abuse Prevention and Consumer Protection Act of 2005

KEY TERMS

account aging
balance due
bankruptcy
claim messages
collection agency
credit balance
overdraft
patient statements
skip
Truth in Lending Statement

INTRODUCTION TO BILLING

If patients have insurance, a bill is not usually sent to the patient until after the insurance company has paid its portion of the bill. If the patient is covered by a managed care policy, the copayment is usually collected at the time of the visit, and a bill may not be necessary. Often, however, the patient has a deductible and/or coinsurance, and a bill must be sent to the patient after insurance has paid its portion of the patient charges.

If a patient visit will not be covered by insurance, most providers' offices request that payment be made at the time a medical service is provided. Medical offices usually also accept payment by credit card, which makes payment at the time of service possible and convenient for many patients. However, a number of patients still need to make arrangements to pay for their medical services over a period of time. In this case, the office must establish an account for the patient and send periodic bills. These bills are usually generated by computer software. Each bill is then placed in a window envelope and sent to the patient. Even if the patient's account is being paid by capitation, a billing record is usually kept for that patient, showing the amount of charges and payments.

The billing for provider offices that are affiliated with a hospital or large health group is usually done from a central location, and office employees are responsible only for posting charges. Patients and insurance companies make payments to the central office. Other provider offices may contract with an outside billing service. The medical assistant should understand the billing process, however, because efficient billing maximizes revenue for the medical office.

BILLING CYCLE

The bills sent to patients are called **patient statements** because they contain not only patient charges, but also payments and adjustments that affect the balance that the patient must pay. Patient statements can be sent every 2 weeks, monthly, or at any regular period, such as once every 3 months (quarterly). The time between bills is called the *billing cycle.* A bill sent out at the end of a cycle will show the balance owed at the beginning of the cycle, any payments made during the billing cycle, any new charges for new services that occurred during the billing cycle, and the **balance due** (total amount owed) at the end of the cycle.

Patient accounts are often divided into equal parts, usually alphabetically. Each week, a different section of the accounts receivable is billed. For instance, on the first week of the month, patients with a last name beginning with the letters *A* to *E* may be billed; the second week, *F* to *L*; the third week, *M* to *S*; and the fourth week, *T* to *Z*. The same cycle is followed each month. Dividing the bills in this way makes more efficient use of staff time because billing is spread out over the month instead of being performed only at the end of the month.

BILLING PROCESS

Patient statements can be produced manually using a word processing program and billing template, but in almost all medical offices that do their own billing, they are produced using the medical office practice management program or the administrative part of the electronic health record (Fig. 48.1). If an outside billing service is used, the service can either send a paper record of all of the bills sent out at the end of each cycle or transfer billing information from its computer to the office's computer, linking the information into the patient's financial record and the office's bookkeeping software.

At regular intervals, patient financial accounts should be examined, and the accounts that must be billed should be processed. Sending claims to insurance companies and billing patients are both straightforward transactions. However, the medical assistant should be aware of some special situations. A patient may have been treated for a final illness just before dying. In this case, any charges will have to be billed to the patient's estate. (Billing an estate is discussed in more detail at the end of this chapter.)

A patient may be a minor who sought treatment without their parent's knowledge. When minors are brought to a provider by a parent or guardian for treatment, the parent or guardian acknowledges that they are the responsible party for

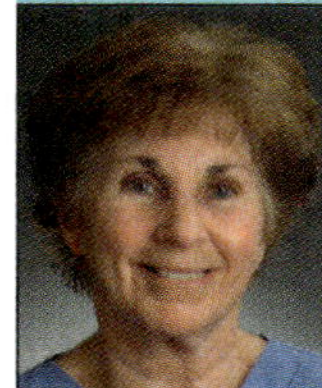

Putting It All Into Practice

My name is Christa Wilson, and I have been working in the office of three providers for the past 5 years. There are three medical assistants, and we all assist the providers during office hours, but I am responsible for most of the billing. We use cycle billing in our office. The first week of the month, we send out statements for patients whose last names begin with the letters A to F, the second week, G to L, and so on. By the end of the month, every patient with an outstanding balance has received a statement, and we begin again. I am also responsible for posting payments received in the mail. Every month, we run an aging report, and I analyze it to see which accounts are overdue. Our computer program lets us add written messages to the statements, but I add colored stickers for accounts that are older than 60 days because I think they are more likely to get the patient's attention. If there is a balance due from a patient after 90 days, I always follow up with a telephone call. When I first started making these calls, I used to get very nervous, but I have gotten accustomed to it now. I always try to stay calm and keep my cool. I have found that in most cases, there is a financial problem that makes it difficult for the individual or family to keep up with its debts. I try to work with our patients if they have an outstanding balance so that they pay something each month. Eventually, we do collect most of the money that is owed to us, and we feel that part of the reason is that we stay on top of our billing. ■

WALDEN-MARTIN
FAMILY MEDICAL CLINIC
1234 ANYSTREET ANYTOWN, ANYSTATE 1234
PHONE 123-123-1234 FAX 123-123-5678

Patient Statement

Patient Name: Sissle, Darla A
Address: 10 Maple St. Anytown AL 12345
Account #: 98866
Insurance Name: Aetna
Policy #: 12345

This statement reflects charges, payments and adjustments for Walden-Martin Family Medical Practice. Payment due upon receipt.

Date of Service	Description	Amount	Patient's Responsibility
6/26/XX	Prob Focused OV, ECG	$121.00	--
7/15/XX	INSPYMT & ADJ	$96.00	$25.00

Total Amount Due: $25.00
Please Pay in Full By: 7/26/XX

Please mail your check or money order to the above address. You can also pay by phone using your credit or debit card.

Fig. 48.1 A sample patient statement using SimChart for the Medical Office.

financial purposes. However, if a minor is treated without the parent's knowledge, the minor may want to be responsible to pay for the services in order to avoid parental questions. Minors older than 12 years may give consent for certain kinds of treatment, including treatment for sexually transmitted infections (STIs), human immunodeficiency virus (HIV) testing, and treatment for drug or alcohol abuse. Because of confidentiality, the provider may not release information to the parent or guardian about the reason for the visit.

A patient may have a credit agreement with the medical office, which allows the patient to pay bills off over time, sometimes with interest on the balance due. This is important because in such situations, although an outstanding balance may become old, it should not be considered delinquent and sent out of the office for collection (Procedure 48.1).

BILLING PROBLEMS

PROBLEMS WITH CHECKS

From time to time, the office may encounter a problem either with a check it has written or with one that has been written to the office by a patient.

Insufficient Funds in the Office Account

It is illegal to write a check for more than the amount of money in a bank account. However, this occasionally happens because of an arithmetic error in calculating the balance while writing checks or because of failure to verify the actual amount in the checking account. If the office's account accidentally becomes overdrawn, the bank may refuse to honor any check written after the account is overdrawn. In this case, the check will be returned to the person or company that deposited it, marked NSF ("non-sufficient funds" in the payer's account to cover the check). A check written on an account without adequate funds to cover it is called an **overdraft.**

It is a good practice to have overdraft protection for any office checking account. Although this protection may never be needed, it will prevent a check from bouncing or a problem with a scheduled online payment in the event that the balance in the office checking account becomes too low. In that case, funds will automatically be transferred from another office account, such as a savings account, to cover an outstanding check or make an online payment, and the bank will charge a fee for this service every time it is used.

Stopping Payment

From time to time, it may become necessary to ask the bank to stop payment on a check. A check might have been lost and a new check issued, or there may be a dispute between the medical office and a vendor about a purchase or a previous payment. Banks charge a fee for stopping payment, so this practice should be used sparingly.

Insufficient Funds in a Patient Account

The bank may not honor a check deposited by the medical office because a patient's account has insufficient funds. If a check is returned marked NSF, do not hesitate to call the patient and tell them of the problem. This may be the first of many checks that are being returned, and it is important for the person to find out why they are writing checks against insufficient funds. The bank usually charges fees both to the individual who wrote the check and to the medical office that tried to deposit the check. The amount of the NSF check must be added back to the balance owed by the patient as a positive adjustment that increases the amount owed. The fee charged by the bank is also added to the patient's balance, usually as a separate positive adjustment. As an example, assume that the patient paid a copayment of $20.00 at the time of the visit. The bank returned the check for insufficient funds and charged the medical office checking account a $15.00 fee. The medical assistant would increase the patient's account balance by $35.00 to cover both the amount of the returned check and the additional fee charged by the bank. Most offices have a sign posted in the waiting room notifying patients of the additional charge for each returned check (Procedure 48.2). When a check has been returned, the patient is often asked to make the payment using cash, a bank check, or a money order instead of another personal check. This should be done tactfully with a professional explanation of the necessity for this step.

OVERPAYMENTS AND REFUNDS

If the total of patient payments and insurance payments exceeds the allowed charge, it is called an *overpayment.* This might happen, for example, if a patient thought that they had not yet paid their annual deductible, when in fact they had. An insurance carrier might overpay if an incorrect code was used on the insurance claim. After all the payments have been posted, the balance on the account will be a negative number, or **credit balance,** indicating that the medical office owes money to the patient or the insurance carrier. Sometimes, a small credit balance is left in place when a patient has a visit scheduled in the near future because new charges will be applied. Usually, however, the medical assistant will process a refund. The amount of the refund is posted to the patient's account, bringing the account balance to zero. The medical assistant sends a letter and a check to the patient (or insurance) with a brief explanation about the overpayment (Procedure 48.3).

What Would You Do? What Would You *Not* Do?

Case Study 1

The bank returns a check from a patient for NSF. The amount on the check is $25.00, and the bank includes a notice that the medical office will be charged $15.00. Christa makes a telephone call to the patient, and she asks the patient to send the office a bank check or money order in the amount of $40.00. The patient becomes very upset. She says, "The bank will charge me the fee for the returned check, not you. All you have to do is send the check through again. There is money in the account now because I deposited my paycheck yesterday. You can't charge me a fee for this. You are just trying to make money out of this situation." ■

ACCOUNT AGING

Account aging is the process of determining how long specific account balances have been outstanding.

ACCOUNTS RECEIVABLE AGING RECORDS AND REPORTS

An accounts receivable aging record should be created to identify patient accounts that are overdue. Accounts are aged in 30-day intervals. Fig. 48.2 shows a sample accounts receivable aging record.

EXAMINING ACCOUNTS FOR THOSE OVERDUE

An account is considered overdue if it is not paid within 30 days of the date billed unless there is an outstanding credit agreement. Accounts for which all the charges are from the previous billing period are considered current (0–30 days). Overdue accounts are categorized as 30–60 days, 61–90 days, 91–120 days, and longer than 120 days.

An account with an outstanding balance after 120 days requires additional collection activity, such as sending the account out to a collection agency or writing a demand letter informing the account holder that a lawsuit will be brought if the account is not brought up to date (Procedure 48.4). Most of the time, the balance of medical office accounts is

What Would You Do? What Would You *Not* Do?

Case Study 2

A patient calls the office to say that she has received her bill, and it does not show a payment of $10.00 that she made in cash at the time of the visit. The patient is upset, and she says, "I knew I shouldn't pay cash, because now I can't prove that I made that payment. I don't see why you can't keep accurate records." Christa asks the patient if she received a receipt for the cash payment. The patient says, "How do you expect me to remember that? This happened over a month ago." ■

Enter credits in parentheses ( ) and subtract when totaling columns and P

ACCOUNTS RECEIVABLE AGING RECORD

Name	As of Date	Prepared by	Page of Page

NO.	ACCOUNT NAME	Insurance Information: Date Claim Filed	Insurance Information: Amount of Claim	Date of Last Payment	Current 1 to 30 days	31 to 60 days	61 to 90 days	91 to 120 days	121 days and over	TOTAL
	Amounts brought forward									
1	*Mary Smith*			*8/8/XX*	*120*					*120-*
2	*John Payne*			*7/6/XX*		*250-*				*250-*
3	*Jack Desmonde*			*5/25/XX*			*500*			*500-*
4	*Jill Jayne*			*4/2/XX*		*80-*		*150-*		*230-*
5										

A

Blackburn Primary Care Associates
Patient Aging

NAME	CURRENT 0 - 30	PAST 31 - 60	PAST 61 - 90	PAST 91 - 120	PAST over 120	Total Balance
Mary Smith Last Payment on 08/08/XX	$120.00					$120.00
John Payne Last Payment on 07/06/XX		$250.00				$250.00
Jack Desmonde Last Payment on 05/25/XX			$500.00			$500.00
Jill Jayne Last Payment on 04/02/XX		$80.00		$150.00		$230.00
Report Aging Totals Percent of Total Aging	$120.00 10.9%	$330.00 30.0%	$500.00 45.5%	$150.00 13.6%		$1100.00 100.0%

B

Fig. 48.2 Sample accounts receivable aging record: (A) prepared by hand; (B) prepared by computer.

small enough to permit legal action in small claims court. (Small claims court is discussed in more detail at the end of the chapter.)

COLLECTION ACTIVITIES

Many people who owe money have every intention of paying their bill but are unable to do so in the short term because of some emergency. As accounts age, it is appropriate to increase the forcefulness of any message to the patient that the account is overdue. It is important to balance a firm (or hard) approach to collections against a soft approach. When using a firm approach, it is possible that the patient will not remain with the provider. This approach is appropriate for patients who have only visited once or twice, as well as cases where it is believed that the patient could easily pay the bill but does not choose to. A softer approach is more appropriate for a patient who is experiencing financial difficulty. Patients should always be invited to call the office and make arrangements to pay over time if they have had a true emergency. Sometimes, it is medical bills themselves that are piling up, especially in the case of a patient with a chronic illness who does not have adequate insurance or has a large deductible.

Patients are also encouraged to discuss accounts for which insurance payment is expected but delayed. If an account shows an outstanding balance and insurance has not yet paid, the insurance claim should be traced to determine why payment is delayed. It may be desirable for the patient to contact the insurance company personally.

PAST DUE ACCOUNTS

Messages encouraging payment of the bill (often called **claim messages**) can be attached to bills or included in the billing envelope. Some computer programs will print a message on the bill itself.

A bill that is 60 days overdue should be accompanied by a claim message reminding the patient that the bill is overdue.

Many offices use a series of messages that become more forceful as time passes without payment.

Bills that are 90 days overdue should be followed up with a telephone call. By contacting patients directly, the medical assistant can determine why there has been no activity related to the account. The medical assistant must be careful to follow legal guidelines when discussing accounts with patients. The Fair Debt Collection Practices Act of 1966 identifies activities that are permitted and not permitted when contacting individuals who owe money. Most states also have debt collection laws with which the medical assistant should be familiar.

COLLECTION LETTERS

Bills that are aged over 120 days should be either accompanied by or followed up with a collection letter, such as the one shown in Fig. 48.3, unless arrangements have been made for the bill to be paid over time. When writing a collection letter, the medical assistant should gather information related to the account before composing the letter. The recipient should be clearly informed about what action is expected, as well as the deadline for action. The letter should not threaten legal action or transfer to a collection agency unless the office is prepared to follow through.

Each medical office has its own policy about who should sign a collection letter. In many offices, the medical assistant signs the letters. In other offices, there may be an office manager or billing specialist, or each provider may prefer to sign letters to their own patients (Procedure 48.5).

If the collection letter does not receive a response, another letter should be sent stating either that the account is now being turned over to a **collection agency** (a company that collects overdue bills for other companies) or that a lawsuit will be filed in small claims court if the account is not paid by a certain date. Some offices will continue to see patients with accounts in collection, but they usually require the patient to pay any current charges before the patient can be seen.

As in any case where it is important to have documentation that a letter was received, the letter should be sent by Certified Mail, with a Return Receipt requested. If the patient is being asked to find a new provider, the letter should allow the patient at least 2 weeks to arrange alternate care.

CREDIT AGREEMENTS

Credit agreements are documents that allow patients to set up a schedule to pay off their bills as long as they make the specified monthly payments. If a patient decides independently to pay their bill in installments (i.e., without discussing it with the medical office), no credit agreement is necessary. If the office and patient make an agreement regarding installment payments, even if no interest is charged, the agreement must be in writing. An interest charge may be added to the balance due at the end of each billing cycle when a written agreement exists.

A credit agreement with a medical office is a type of revolving credit, similar to a department store or gasoline company charge card. As long as the monthly minimum is paid, the account is considered in good standing.

Western Medical Center
107 River Street
Western, OH 44770

4/10/20XX

[Patient Address]

Dear [Patient Name],

Your account in this office is now more than 120 days overdue. We have made several previous attempts to set up a mutually agreeable payment schedule with you, but you have not followed through on your commitment. This will be your final notice. If you do not contact our office within 7 days of receipt of this letter, we will have no choice but to turn over this account to our collection agency. Please call us at (490) 220-1156 or send a check to pay the balance of your account if you wish to avoid collection activity.

Yours truly,

Richard Warner, MD

Richard Warner, MD

RW/mt

Fig. 48.3 Sample collection letter.

HIGHLIGHT on Guidelines for Telephone Collections

Things to Do

1. A creditor (person or company who is owed money) may contact the person who owes money by telephone during reasonable hours. The medical assistant should gather accurate information before placing the telephone call about an overdue account:
   a. Who owes the money?
   b. How much money is owed?
   c. How long has the money been owed?
   d. Is there any insurance claim pending?
   e. Has the insurance company processed the claim and/or made any payment?
2. A creditor may take measures to locate a person but may not divulge that they are trying to collect a bill to anyone other than the person who owes money. The medical assistant should ask to speak with the patient or the person responsible for the account when placing the call.
3. A creditor may not misrepresent themselves to trick the person who owes money into taking the call. After asking for the person responsible for the account, the medical assistant should identify themselves and the office or provider.
4. A creditor may not harass or intimidate a person who owes money. The medical assistant should speak calmly and professionally. The conversation should include a discussion of the different options for payment, including full payment, partial payment, and monthly installments. If possible, the medical assistant should obtain a verbal commitment for a date and amount of at least a first payment and/or a payment plan.
5. Although a verbal agreement is legally binding, a written agreement is easier to enforce if legal action becomes necessary. It is important to follow up any verbal agreement with a letter referring to the conversation and the agreement. If an arrangement was established for more than four monthly payments, a Truth in Lending Statement must be included, even if the patient will not pay interest.
6. Although it is not permitted to harass patients, the medical assistant may contact them again if payments are not made as agreed. Often, the knowledge that attention is being paid to the account will encourage a patient to adhere to the repayment schedule.

Things Not to Do

1. A creditor should not call too early in the day or too late at night.
2. A creditor should not divulge to employers, neighbors, or other third parties that they are trying to collect a bill from the patient.
3. A creditor should not threaten.
4. A creditor should not end the conversation on vague terms.
5. A creditor should not call repeatedly.

TRUTH IN LENDING STATEMENTS

Because a credit agreement is a type of revolving credit, it falls under federal and state government fair lending practices. Therefore, a Truth in Lending Statement must be supplied to the patient when the agreement is made. A **Truth in Lending Statement** is a written document that meets the legal requirement to disclose the terms of a loan to borrowers so that they can understand them.

This Truth in Lending Statement includes facts about such things as the maximum amount the patient may charge to the account, the interest rate, how the interest is computed (e.g., average daily balance or balance at the end of the billing period), and how the minimum monthly payment is computed (e.g., percentage of outstanding balance). Fig. 48.4 shows a sample credit agreement.

POLICY FOR PATIENTS WITH OUTSTANDING BALANCES

Most medical offices insist that a patient close out any current balance due before a credit agreement is written with that patient. If the medical office has had trouble collecting bills from a patient in the past, it may write the credit agreement for a lower maximum balance. However, the medical office cannot charge a different interest rate or compute the minimum payment in a different way for different patients depending on past payment history.

OTHER COLLECTION TECHNIQUES AND SPECIAL CIRCUMSTANCES

Tracing "Skips"

Occasionally, a bill is returned to the medical office from the post office with the notation "address unknown." This may be an innocent mistake—the result, perhaps, of an incorrect address on file or the patient's failure to notify the office after moving. On the other hand, it may be a deliberate attempt to "skip out" on the medical office's bill and the bills of other professionals and/or merchants.

A potential **skip** (account for which no billing information is available) should be followed up on immediately. The first step is to call the patient's phone number: it is very common to keep the same telephone number even if a person moves, especially if it is a mobile phone number, or a person may have had the phone company use a "new number" message to forward calls. Because caller ID is a feature on many landlines and cell phones, a telephone call from a creditor may be ignored, or the person answering the call may say that it is a wrong number.

If the patient cannot be contacted using the telephone number given at the office visit and if there is no new number listed, the next step is to call the patient's place of employment and ask to speak with the individual. The medical assistant can try to get in touch with the person by contacting professional associations, unions, or other organizations with which the person is associated.

Blackburn Primary Care Associates, PC
1990 Turquoise Drive
Blackburn, WI 54937
608-459-8857

Federal Truth in Lending Statement

Patient ____________________

Address ____________________

1. Fee for service of ____________
2. Amount down ____________
3. Amount financed ____________
4. Finance charge ____________
5. Total of payments 3 + 4 ____________
6. Number of payments ____________
7. Amount of each payment ____________

Total no. of payments _____ payable over _____ monthly installments

In the amount of $_______. The first payment is due _______.

Date ______________ Signed ____________________

Fig. 48.4 Sample credit agreement.

The medical assistant should never tell a third party that an individual owes money to the medical office and should not identify the employer; the medical assistant should say only that they wish to speak with the person. Also, it is illegal to call a third party more than once in an attempt to trace a skip unless that person asks the medical assistant to call back. For example, the medical assistant may speak with a third party where the individual with an overdue account works, and that third party might ask the medical assistant to call back at the end of the day when they are not so busy.

Another way to attempt collection is to send a letter by Registered or Certified Mail, with a Return Receipt requested, to the individual at the old address. Even if the person did not ask the post office to forward all mail, they may have asked for certain types of mail to be forwarded. In this case, the letter should be placed in a plain envelope, with just the return street address and no office name. This minimizes the chances that the individual will refuse to accept the mail.

The medical office may also use one of several internet resources to trace skips. These services usually charge a fee. The more information the office has about the individual, the more likely it is that the individual can be located.

If all of these efforts fail, the bill should be turned over to a collection agency used by the office as soon as possible. Most collection agencies handle far more "skips" than individual medical offices do and sometimes use other, more aggressive techniques. The sooner the collection agency receives the account, the better chance it has to collect the amount owed on the bill.

Sending Accounts to a Collection Agency

Collection agencies are in business specifically to collect accounts that have "aged out." This means that by the time a collection agency receives a delinquent account, the business such as a medical office has given the person who owes the money fair warning that the bill is overdue and that a professional collector is going to become involved.

Each state has specific laws under which collection agencies must work. These laws define when collection agency personnel can call, what they can say, and what other tactics they can use to collect the bill.

In general, collection agencies charge 20%–40% of the amount they collect. They are not allowed to "cut a deal" with a patient and accept less than full payment unless the medical office has agreed to the arrangement for payment.

If a patient's account is in collection, usually, the office has a policy not to see the patient unless any new charges are paid in full before the patient is seen by the provider. Other offices notify patients in writing that they will not be seen by any provider in the office until their outstanding balance has been collected.

When an account is turned over to a collection agency, the patient balance in the computer system is often adjusted to zero. The amount owed by the patient can still be seen clearly in the patient ledger, but the current balance is zero. This prevents bills to the patient from being generated, and the account no longer appears as overdue on account aging reports. The medical assistant should become familiar with the exact procedure used in their medical office. The medical office makes no further attempts at collection, and any payments received from the patient are sent directly to the collection agency. When a payment for the patient's account is received from a collection agency, it should be recorded on the daily ledger. In addition, it should be posted to the account for which it was collected. The patient's account balance, which is usually zero, is first increased (as a positive adjustment) by the amount of the payment. Then, the payment is posted as a payment, bringing the current account balance back to zero.

Small Claims Court

Small claims courts exist in each state. They are special sessions of the local district court that deal only with civil lawsuits involving small amounts of money. Most small claims lawsuits involve disputes over payments. Each state has its own rules for the maximum claim that can be brought in small claims court. This maximum amount runs from about $3500 in some states to as much as $25,000 in others.

The question for a medical office when choosing to use the court system is always whether it will sacrifice more in "good will" than it will gain in money if the collection is successful. Many offices bring suits in court only after a patient has left the medical office without paying a bill in full. Furthermore, winning a judgment in small claims court is only the first step. The office must still collect the judgment.

Small claims courts are set up to reduce the legal fees for those seeking to collect relatively small amounts of money. Because there is no lawyer, the plaintiff (an individual or business) must represent themself or itself. The office manager or medical assistant might have to assume this duty if the office uses small claims court to try to collect on patient accounts. A collection agency cannot represent the office.

The clerk of the court has all of the documents necessary to file a small claim and can usually walk a first-time claimant through the process, explaining how to fill out the forms and which documentation to submit to back up the claim. Only the defendant can appeal a small claims court judgment; for the plaintiff, a negative judgment is final.

Billing an Estate

Patients sometimes die without having paid their medical bills in full. In this instance, the office will have to collect the balance due from the estate. Estates fall into an area of the law known as *probate,* and probate law is administered by a special section of the court system in each state.

It is not appropriate to send a bill to a deceased patient's estate immediately after the death while the family is grieving; however, the bill should be sent within 30 days. The bill should be sent to "The Estate of" the patient at the patient's address rather than to a family member or other individual unless that person has made a written promise to cover the deceased's medical costs.

If the deceased patient had a will, it usually has a provision that the costs of the patient's final illness will be paid by the estate outside of the probate process. In such a case, the bill will probably be paid promptly. The will should be filed within 30 days, and the clerk of the probate court should then be able to furnish you with the name of the executor or administrator (the person responsible for handling the estate's business dealings). An itemized final bill should then be sent to this individual by Certified Mail with a Return Receipt requested.

If the patient did not have a will, the medical office's bill will be put in with other creditors' bills and paid only when payment is approved by the probate court and the administrator appointed by the court.

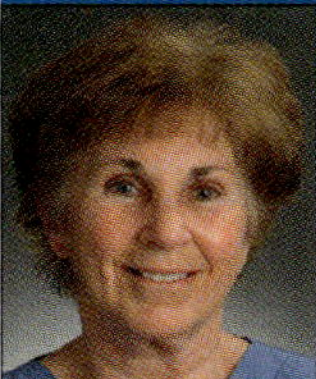

Memories *from* Practicum

Christa Wilson: During my practicum, I observed billing activities and I was allowed to assist in some ways. For example, I got a lot of practice at making sure that all statements printed correctly, checking each statement to make sure that there was an outstanding balance and that the insurance had already paid, and folding the statements to place them in window envelopes. The computer system used by the office where I did my practicum printed the statements with all activity on the account. The patient was expected to pay the balance on the bottom line of the statement. Sometimes, patients called the office because they didn't understand what amount to pay. They usually spoke to the medical assistant at the office. I noticed that she was always polite and professional when she spoke to patients. The office also taught me how to post patient payments that were sent by check. I have to say I did not realize how important good billing practices are until my practicum. I was grateful that I had experience at an office with a smooth-running system. ■

Bankruptcy

Bankruptcy laws are federal laws, meaning that they apply equally regardless of the state in which the bankrupt person lives. **Bankruptcy** is a means for an individual or business to "get out from under" a crushing load of debt, either by reorganizing the debt or by liquidating assets and dividing the funds among all of the creditors.

Individuals file for personal bankruptcy under either Chapter 7 or Chapter 13 of the bankruptcy code.

A Chapter 7 bankruptcy is a liquidation of assets. Under such a bankruptcy, only secured creditors will be paid from the proceeds from the sale of any assets. If the bankrupt patient had a credit agreement, the medical office is a secured creditor. However, if the office is merely trying to collect a bill, the office is an unsecured creditor and will not receive payment.

A Chapter 13 bankruptcy is an "Adjustment of Debts" bankruptcy. In such a bankruptcy, the debtor (patient) pays a particular amount determined by the bankruptcy court to the court-appointed trustee, who then distributes the money to creditors. The debtor, if they have a regular income, can be required to make payments from that income into the trustee account for 3 years, and the trustee makes payments to creditors under payment plans they work out.

During the period the debtor is under the jurisdiction of the bankruptcy court, no creditor may try to collect a debt outside the bankruptcy process. However, a medical office can demand payment in full for any additional service it provides to a patient from whom it is collecting old debts under a bankruptcy agreement.

What Would You Do? What Would You *Not* Do?

Case Study 3

On the day that Judith Mason is scheduled for an appointment, Christa notices that she has an outstanding balance of $58.00 from charges that were incurred 4 months ago. It is office policy that patients with a balance over 120 days are not seen until the balance has been paid. ■

LAWS AFFECTING CREDIT AND COLLECTION ACTIVITIES

Several laws affect credit and collection activities.

Equal Credit Opportunity Act

The Equal Credit Opportunity Act is a federal law that prevents discrimination on the basis of the following when offering credit:

- Sex, marital status, race, color, national origin, religion, and age
- The fact that the applicant receives public assistance income
- The fact that the applicant has exercised rights under consumer credit laws

An applicant must be informed if credit is denied and has 60 days to request, in writing, the reason for denial of credit.

Fair Debt Collection Practices Act

The Fair Debt Collection Practices Act is a federal law that requires the fair treatment of debtors and prevents unfair debt collection measures, including harassment, false statements, and threats.

- The debt collector may not make frightening, verbally abusive, or threatening calls.
- The debt collector may not call before 8 a.m. or after 9 p.m.
- The debt collector may not threaten action that cannot legally be taken or is not intended to be taken.

Federal Truth in Lending Act

Installment agreements must be in writing if more than four payments will be made (or fewer if interest is charged). The Federal Truth in Lending Act is administered by the Federal Trade Commission. It requires creditors to provide applicants with a form disclosing in a clear and obvious way all finance charges and terms.

Fair Credit Reporting Act

The Fair Credit Reporting Act requires credit bureaus to supply correct and complete information to businesses to use in evaluating a person's application for credit, insurance, or employment.

Bankruptcy Abuse Prevention and Consumer Protection Act of 2005

The Bankruptcy Abuse Prevention and Consumer Protection Act of 2005 is a revision of federal bankruptcy laws that attempts to make it more difficult for individuals to file for bankruptcy under Chapter 7, by which most of the debts are forgiven by establishing a means test to determine if individuals are able to pay some of their debts. It also makes the process of filing for bankruptcy more difficult and expensive. Debtors are still able to file for bankruptcy under Chapter 13.

What Would You Do? What Would You *Not* Do? RESPONSES

Case Study 1
Page 1220

What Did Christa Do?
- Reassured the patient that the situation is upsetting, but it can happen sometimes.
- Explained that most banks charge both the account of the individual who writes a check against an account with insufficient funds and the account where the check was deposited.
- Explained that the office has a policy of not sending a check through the bank a second time or accepting a personal check for payment after one check was returned.
- Suggested that the patient might want to consider overdraft protection.
- Explained politely that the office is only recovering its out-of-pocket expenses and was not, in fact, charging an additional fee.

What Did Christa Not Do?
- Did not get angry or raise her voice.
- Did not imply that the patient was trying to avoid payment or was a bad money manager.
- Did not make statements such as "This better not happen again!" or "How do you expect us to pay our bills if our patients' checks bounce?"

Case Study 2
Page 1220

What Did Christa Do?
- Told the patient that she would check the receipt book; then went through the duplicate receipts of the day of the patient's visit.
- If a copy of the receipt for a cash payment was found, told the patient and entered the payment into the patient's account.
- If no copy of the receipt was found, explained to the patient that it was office policy to issue a receipt for any cash payment from a book where a duplicate was made automatically.
- If no copy of the receipt was found, suggested tactfully that the patient may not remember this specific visit, and perhaps, she was unable to pay her copayment that day or forgot to pay it.
- If the patient continued to insist that she paid cash, offered to discuss the matter with the office manager or provider.

What Did Christa Not Do?
- Did not get angry at the patient or raise her voice.
- Did not say that unless the patient can show her a receipt, the office will automatically assume that she had not paid.
- Did not accuse the patient of trying to get out of paying the copayment.

Case Study 3
Page 1226

What Did Christa Do?
- Attempted to contact Ms. Mason by telephone to inform her of the office policy so that the patient would be prepared to settle her outstanding bill.
- If the patient could not be contacted before the appointment, took her to a private room when she arrived at the office to discuss her account.
- Spoke to Ms. Mason maintaining eye contact and establishing an empathetic and professional atmosphere.
- Strongly encouraged Ms. Mason to settle the account by check or credit card before being seen by the provider.
- If Ms. Mason stated that she could not pay the balance on that day, left the final decision about whether she would be seen to the provider because the patient had not been informed of the office policy before coming to the office.

What Did Christa Not Do?
- Did not take sole responsibility to tell the patient that if she did not pay, under no circumstances would she be seen by the provider.
- Did not raise her voice or get angry with Ms. Mason.
- Did not discuss Ms. Mason's financial matters where others could overhear the conversation.

TERMINOLOGY REVIEW

Key Term	Definition
Account aging	The process of finding out how long specific account balances have been outstanding.
Balance due	Total amount owed.
Bankruptcy	Legal process by which the debts of an individual or business are resolved if they cannot be paid.
Claim message	Messages encouraging payment of a bill, usually attached to or printed on the monthly statement.
Collection agency	A company that is in the business of collecting overdue accounts for other companies.
Credit balance	A negative balance on a patient account (i.e., money is owed by the medical office), usually a result of an overpayment.
Overdraft	A check (or draft) that exceeds the amount of funds in a bank account.
Patient statement	A bill sent to a patient that contains not only charges, but also payments and adjustments that affect the balance that the patient must pay.
Skip	Account for which no billing information is available.
Truth in Lending Statement	A written document that meets the legal requirement to disclose the terms of a loan in terms that the borrower can understand.

PROCEDURE 48.1 Processing Patient Statements

Outcome Prepare patient statements.

Equipment/Supplies

- Computer
- Patient accounts
- Computer program to prepare patient statements or SimChart for the Medical Office
- Window envelopes or letterhead envelopes and labels
- Word processing program
- Paper or statement forms

1. **Procedural Step.** Locate patient accounts in the computer database.
2. **Procedural Step.** Identify patient accounts with an outstanding balance for which insurance payments have been made.
   Principle. Patients are usually not billed until insurance payments have been received.
3. **Procedural Step.** Create one or more patient bills manually using a word processing program or SimChart for the Medical Office (see specific steps at the end of the procedure). If using medical billing software, compile outstanding bills using the computer program and view using *Print Preview.* Check all statements for completeness and accuracy.
   Principle. All bills must have the patient's name and address, previous activity for the account, and the amount due from the patient.
4. **Procedural Step.** Print patient statements using the office patient statement form or paper (if statement form prints with the statement). The statement form may be printed with the bills from the computer program, or statement forms may be loaded in the printer.
5. **Procedural Step.** Make sure that statements have been printed correctly.
6. **Procedural Step.** Fold statements suitable for window envelopes so that the medical office and the patient names and addresses will be visible through the windows in the envelopes. If statements are not suitable for window envelopes (such as those produced by SimChart), prepare a patient label for each statement.
7. **Procedural Step.** Insert statements in envelopes. Be sure that the names and addresses are visible if window envelopes are used. If labels are used, affix the correct mailing label to a letterhead envelope for each statement. Seal the envelopes.
8. **Procedural Step.** Place postage on envelopes and mail statements.

Preparing a Patient Statement Using SimChart for the Medical Office

9. **Procedural Step.** From the *Form Repository*, click on *Patient Statement* on the *Info Panel* at the left.
10. **Procedural Step.** Click on the *Patient Search* button at the bottom of the *Patient Statement* screen. Search for and select the correct patient.
11. **Procedural Step.** Check to be sure that the information that has populated the top part of the Patient Statement form is correct. Then, enter charges and payments that have taken place since the last statement, including the date of service, the description of the service, the amount, and the patient responsibility. All services from a single day can usually be entered on one line. The insurance payment and insurance write-off usually occur on different dates; payment is entered on a separate line (see Fig. 48.1).
12. **Procedural Step.** Click the *Save to Patient Record* button. To print the statement, find and select the patient, then open the saved statement, and click the *Print* button.

PROCEDURE 48.2 Posting a Check Returned for Non-Sufficient Funds (NSF)

Outcome Post an NSF check.

Equipment/Supplies

- Computer
- Patient accounts
- Returned check
- Patient ledger
- SimChart for the Medical Office or other practice management program
- Pen
- Calculator

1. **Procedural Step.** When the NSF check has been received, locate the patient's old balance in the computer database. In SimChart for the Medical Office, select *Ledger* on the *Info Panel* of the *Coding and Billing* tab, then select the correct patient.
2. **Procedural Step.** Add a new row, and use today's date. Enter "NSF check and fee" in the *Service* field.
3. **Procedural Step.** In SimChart for the Medical Office, enter the total of the returned check in the *Charges* field. Enter the amount charged by the bank as a positive number in the *Adjmt (Adjustment)* field.
   Principle. The amount of the returned check must be added to the patient balance because it did not clear the bank. Any fee charged by the bank is also added to the patient balance as a positive adjustment.
4. **Procedural Step.** Notify the patient by telephone or letter that the check was returned and a fee has been charged. If sending a letter, enclose a patient statement with the letter showing the total amount of the returned check, the fee, and the new balance. Demonstrate professionalism and sensitivity when discussing the returned check and informing the patient of payment conditions (such as a bank check or money order).
   Example. Darla Sissle's previous balance was $40.00. Her check for $15.00 was returned by the bank marked *NSF.* The bank also charged a fee of $15.00.

4

			Column A	Column B	Column C	Column D	Column E
DATE	PATIENT NAME	SERVICE	CHARGES	PAYMENT	ADJMT	NEW BALANCE	OLD BALANCE
6/03/XX	Darla Sissle	NSF check & fee	$ 15.00	$ 0.00	$ 15.00	$ 70.00	$ 40.00

The NSF check and bank fee are posted on the day sheet and to the patient's account.

PROCEDURE 48.2

PROCEDURE 48.3 Processing a Credit Balance and Refund

Outcome Process a credit balance and issue a refund

Equipment/Supplies

- Computer
- Patient accounts
- Payment check(s)
- SimChart for the Medical Office or other practice management program
- Pen
- Calculator

1. **Procedural Step.** When a payment has been made, locate the patient account in the computer. In SimChart for the Medical Office, select *Ledger* on the *Info Panel* of the *Coding and Billing* tab, then select the correct patient.
   Principle. Both insurance payments and patient payments must be entered in the correct patient account.
2. **Procedural Step.** Add a new row, and use today's date. Enter *Payment* and the check number (if any) in the *Service* field.
3. **Procedural Step.** Compare the amount of the payment against the total amount owed.
   Principle. The total amount owed will be the balance due and charges for new services.
4. **Procedural Step.** Even if the payment is greater than the charges, in a computer billing program, post the payment to the computer system using the correct code (i.e., patient payment, check, or insurance payment) and link to the visit for which the payment is made. In SimChart for the Medical Office, post the payment in the *Payment* field. If using a paper day sheet, post the payment in the *Payment* column.
5. **Procedural Step.** If an overpayment has occurred, note that the account balance *(Total)* is a negative number. This means that the medical office owes the patient money.
6. **Procedural Step.** Take steps to clear the balance from the system according to your office policy. If the patient has another appointment scheduled, the negative balance may be carried for a short time. In most cases, a refund should be issued promptly.
   Principle. Office policy guidelines indicate the proper management of a credit balance in a patient account.
7. **Procedural Step.** Calculate the amount to be refunded (usually the amount of the negative balance) and the recipient of the refund. If the patient overpaid because it was not known how much insurance would pay, the refund goes to the patient. If insurance overpaid (e.g., because an incorrect code was used on the claim), the refund goes to the insurance carrier.
8. **Procedural Step.** Add a new row, select the date, and enter the patient name. Enter *Refund to [recipient]* in the *Service* field. In SimChart for the Medical Office, enter the adjustment in the adjustment field with a minus number. In a practice management program, all adjustments are entered as positive numbers with the correct code, and the program performs the correct operation (addition or subtraction). Enter zeros in the other fields. The program will calculate the balance for the transaction.
9. **Procedural Step.** Verify that the *Total* (account balance) is zero.
10. **Procedural Step.** Write a check for the refund amount to the correct recipient including the date, amount in numbers, and amount in words on the line below. Leave the signature line blank.
    Principle. The medical assistant is usually not authorized to sign checks for the medical office.
11. **Procedural Step.** Record the check number, date, payee, and reason for the check on the check stub in the checkbook or in the check register.
12. **Procedural Step.** Subtract the amount of the check from the balance in the check register.
13. **Procedural Step.** Write a letter informing the recipient of the reason for the refund, and prepare an envelope.
14. **Procedural Step.** Sign the letter and your title, and leave the check, letter, and envelope in the correct place to obtain an authorized signature on the check.

PROCEDURE 48.4 Creating and Examining an Accounts Receivable Aging Record

Outcome Create and examine an accounts receivable aging record.

Equipment/Supplies

- SimChart for the Medical Office or other practice management software
- Patient accounts
- Accounts receivable aging record analysis form (optional)
- Pen

1. **Procedural Step.** In SimChart, select the *Reporting* tab under *Coding and Billing*. Under *Report*, select *Aging*. Depending on your preference, you can sort by patient or insurance to create a report for one patient or one insurance company. If you are using the reports function of a computer billing program, you can create an aging report for more than one patient and usually for all insurance companies with outstanding claims. It is also possible to create such a report manually using individual patient ledgers.
   Principle. SimChart can create an aging report for one patient. In a computerized billing system, the computer program can generate the report of all overdue accounts.
2. **Procedural Step.** Review the accounts on the report and mark the proposed action for each account according to your office policy.
   Principle. Efforts to collect outstanding accounts should become increasingly more active as the account ages. Office policy may vary with regard to specific actions.
3. **Procedural Step.** Mark all accounts that are less than 31 days old "No action needed."
   Principle. Accounts that are less than 31 days old are considered current.
4. **Procedural Step.** Mark bills with unpaid insurance claims that are older than 31 days "Follow up with insurance."
   Principle. Patients usually do not pay bills with outstanding insurance claims until they find out how much the insurance will pay. These bills, if overdue, need to be followed up with the insurance company.
5. **Procedural Step.** Mark accounts that are 31–60 days old according to office policy. For example, a note may be attached to the statement indicating "Payment is now due." It may be possible to include payment notices in the computer billing program so that they print on the statement automatically if the account is overdue.
6. **Procedural Step.** Mark accounts that are 61–90 days old according to office policy. For example, a note may be attached to the statement indicating "Payment of this bill is now overdue. Please pay the balance or contact the office."
7. **Procedural Step.** Mark accounts that are 91–120 days old according to office policy. It may be office policy to place a telephone call to the patient at this point to discuss the account. Follow up with a letter confirming any agreement made.
8. **Procedural Step.** With the instructor observing, role-play a collection telephone call with a classmate to demonstrate a professional manner for interacting with a patient who has a balance that is over 91 days old. Tell the patient a specific amount that is owed, and ask for a commitment for payment by a specific date. Remain calm, and do not threaten the patient. Inform the patient that it is office policy to turn accounts older than 120 days over to a collection agency.
   Principle: Professionalism during collection activities and sensitivity to patients help maximize collections without creating excess negativity that offends and shames patients.
9. **Procedural Step.** For accounts older than 120 days, review previous collection attempts. Unless there are known circumstances that warrant a delay in collection activity, send a collection letter stating that if payment is not received by a certain date, the account will be given to a collection agency or payment will be pursued in small claims court (depending on the procedure used by the office to collect on delinquent accounts).
   Principle. After 120 days without activity, especially if the person owing money has been contacted by telephone and letter, it is unlikely that the bill will be paid without more aggressive collection measures.
10. **Procedural Step.** Record all action taken beside each account on the report.
    Principle. This provides a written record of actions taken and results of telephone conversations.
11. **Procedural Step.** Write follow-up letters to document in writing any agreements made during telephone conversations. Attach a copy to the patient's medical record.
    Principle. A written record of verbal communications regarding bills and payments provides evidence in case further legal action is necessary.

PROCEDURE 48.5 Writing a Collection Letter

Outcome Write a collection letter.

Equipment/Supplies

- Accounts aging report
- Computer
- Patient accounts
- Letterhead stationery
- Envelope
- Printer

1. **Procedural Step.** After the accounts receivable aging record has been created, determine which accounts need a letter. In general, this will be the accounts that are 90–120 days old.
   Principle. A letter is usually sent after reminders have been sent and a telephone call has been made to collect an outstanding account balance.
2. **Procedural Step.** Review each account for the amount due, how long it has been due, any previous activity, and special situations. If the account is due from the estate of a deceased patient or insurance, or if there is a known reason why delayed payment is acceptable, do not take action on the account.
   Principle. There may be circumstances that justify the delay in payment.
3. **Procedural Step.** Otherwise, prepare a letter for each outstanding account. If using SimChart for the Medical Office, select *Collection Letter* from the *Letters* section of the *Correspondence* information panel.
4. **Procedural Step.** Identify the patient's address by selecting the correct patient in the computer billing program.
5. **Procedural Step.** Enter the information in the collection letter template including the amount of the outstanding balance, the date that the charges were incurred, the service provided, and the date by which payment is expected. The tone should be professional without threats or efforts to shame the patient.
   Principle. Although the bill is overdue, the recipient of the letter is given a reasonable amount of time to respond to this letter. Professionalism during collection activities and sensitivity to patients help maximize collections without creating excess negativity that offends and shames patients.
6. **Procedural Step.** Enter the provider name and medical assistant signature.
7. **Procedural Step.** Print the letter and save the letter to the patient record.
8. **Procedural Step.** If office policy, copy the letter and file it in a collection follow-up file.
   Principle. Future activity to collect on the account should be based on a review of your current activity.
9. **Procedural Step.** Place the letter in the envelope, address the envelope, and mail the letter.

The Medical Assistant as Office Manager

Check out the Evolve site at http://evolve.elsevier.com/Bonewit/today to access additional interactive activities and exercises to help you study and prepare for success.

LEARNING OBJECTIVES	PROCEDURES
Maintaining the Office	
1. Describe routine maintenance activities in the medical office.	
Maintaining Equipment	
2. Describe an efficient system of maintaining equipment inventory lists and operator manuals.	
3. Maintain administrative and clinical equipment.	Performing routine maintenance of equipment.
4. Describe the process of obtaining new equipment.	
Supplies	
5. Explain procedures for taking inventory.	Taking a supply or equipment inventory.
6. Describe an effective method for ordering, receiving, and storing supplies.	
Patient and Employee Safety	
7. Identify methods to maintain a safe environment and prevent injury to patients and employees.	Creating an environmental checklist and performing a safety inspection.
8. Explain how safety signs, instructions, and labels contribute to a safe office environment.	Complying with safety signs, symbols, and labels.
Employer Obligations for Payroll	
9. Explain employer obligations related to payroll.	
Creating an Environment for Teamwork	
10. Describe ways to enhance teamwork in the medical office.	
11. Describe the medical assistant's role in orienting and training new employees.	
Managing Provider and Employee Schedules	
12. Manage the provider's professional schedule.	
Locating Community Resources for Patients	
13. Locate community resources to assist patients and medical office staff.	Locating and facilitating referrals to community resources.
Risk Management	
14. List types of liability, professional (malpractice), and personal injury insurance for providers, the medical office, and medical assistants.	
15. Describe the process of compliance reporting for unsafe activities, errors in patient care, and conflicts of interest.	
16. Describe how incident reports should be used to protect the medical office.	Completing an incident report.

CHAPTER OUTLINE

General Cleaning
Cleaning Cabinets and Drawers
Miscellaneous Tasks
MAINTAINING EQUIPMENT
Inventory
Monitoring Equipment Function and Readiness for Use
Service Contracts
Service Calls
Purchases of New Equipment
SUPPLIES
Supply Inventory
Restocking
Ordering Supplies
Receiving Supplies
PATIENT AND EMPLOYEE SAFETY
Safe Work Practices
Monitoring Environmental Safety
Signs and Instructions
CREATING AN ENVIRONMENT FOR TEAMWORK
Staff Meetings
Orienting and Training Employees
Working With New Employees or Medical Assisting Students
EMPLOYER OBLIGATIONS FOR PAYROLL
Deductions
Income Taxes
Social Security and Medicare
State Taxes
Additional Obligations
Unemployment Tax
MANAGING PROVIDER AND EMPLOYEE SCHEDULES
Provider Schedules
Employee Schedules
LOCATING COMMUNITY RESOURCES FOR PATIENTS
RISK MANAGEMENT
Minimizing Risk of Injury or Illness
Liability Insurance
Compliance Reporting
Incident Reports

KEY TERMS

back order
depreciation
gross pay
inventory
invoice
minutes
net pay
per diem
purchase order (PO) number
reorder point
risk management
salary
service contract
Social Security tax
vendor
warranty
W-4 form

INTRODUCTION TO MEDICAL OFFICE MANAGEMENT

The medical assistant performs many tasks that promote the smooth running of the medical office. These tasks include maintaining the physical space, taking inventory, ordering supplies, monitoring programs such as risk management and employee safety programs, orienting new employees, and processing employee payroll. The responsibility for these management functions may be primarily that of the medical assistant in a small office or primarily that of an office manager in a larger setting. Office management always provides the basis for effective patient care, and its importance cannot be overestimated.

MAINTAINING THE OFFICE

In many medical offices, a medical assistant assumes responsibility for maintaining the physical space of the medical office and performing general maintenance. Heavy cleaning and equipment repair are usually not performed by office staff, but rather by contractors. Thus, the medical assistant may also be responsible for managing the relationship between the office and contractors, as well as medical, pharmaceutical, and office supply companies.

ADMINISTRATIVE AREA

When they are sitting at the front desk, the medical assistant must be able to effectively and efficiently answer two or three incoming calls, greet patients, and handle paperwork.

Depending on the size of the administrative area, supplies and equipment for correspondence and billing may be stored in this area, including stationery, envelopes, billing forms, and coding reference books. In addition to the telephone (discussed in detail in Chapter 41), the reception area usually contains one or more personal computers, which are linked to the office's computer network. Materials for creating new patient folders should also be at hand if a paper medical record system is used.

The administrative area must have enough room to perform the required activities without any mixing up of the patient files and other papers; it must also allow the medical assistant to maintain patient confidentiality. In addition, the administrative area should be kept clear of clutter (Fig. 49.1).

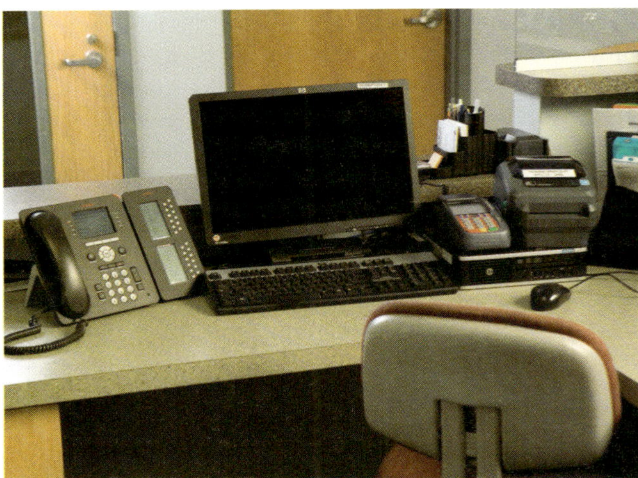

Fig. 49.1 Well-organized front office.

Again, depending on the size of the office, if business operations are performed in the office, they will take place either in the front office close to the reception area or in a separate area in the office. In the business office are the rest of the pieces of equipment necessary for administering the office, including the photocopy machine, fax machine, and postage meter or electronic mailing system. In small offices, an all-in-one printer-copier-fax machine may be used.

The medical assistant should be familiar not only with the office equipment's operation but also with the maintenance responsibilities, such as reloading paper and adding toner or printer cartridges. In addition, the medical assistant may have to follow the terms of any maintenance agreements in scheduling maintenance or repairs.

Offices should also have a paper shredder for disposing of confidential documents. Although medical records must be maintained indefinitely, old telephone logs, old payroll records, canceled checks more than 7 years old, and minutes of medical office management meetings should all be shredded rather than simply thrown away in the wastebasket or in a wastepaper recycling bin. Any documents containing patient information that have been scanned into the electronic health record (EHR) should be shredded if they are not retained. Shredded paper can still be recycled, and there is no danger that sensitive personal or business information will be seen by anyone who should not have access to it.

WAITING ROOM

The waiting room makes a first impression on a new patient. It must be neat and welcoming. The waiting room must include two to four chairs for each provider in the office at one time, a selection of current magazines, and a table or magazine stand to hold them. If the medical office sees children, some toys should be available in a separate play area. One person should be assigned to tidy up the waiting room a couple of times each day.

A waiting room should have posted signs that inform patients of office policies. The signs depend on the policies of the individual office. Common signs include the following:

- No smoking.
- Copayments are expected at the time of service (or some other phrasing regarding the expectation of payment).
- The following credit cards are accepted (followed by names of credit cards).
- No eating or drinking.
- A charge will be added for returned checks to cover any bank fees.
- Patients will be charged for canceled appointments unless at least 24 hours notice is given.

Some offices have a display rack holding health information brochures. Brochures are available from government agencies, public agencies, and many companies. With the approval of the provider(s), these brochures are often provided to help educate patients about health promotion and disease prevention.

Sometimes there is a television in the waiting room. In some medical offices, health information videos are playing. Other medical offices have a radio tuned to an easy-listening station or from an online source with quiet pop or light classical music. The medical assistant may have to turn this equipment on at the beginning of the day.

EXAMINATION AND TREATMENT ROOMS

Each examination or treatment room also needs approximately 100 sq ft of floor space to hold an examination or treatment table, cabinets and countertop, patient chair and provider stool, and a small surface for the provider to write on. The room should be laid out so that a provider and medical assistant can move freely about the room. Equipment and supplies should be within easy reach or stored in drawers or cabinets that are easy to reach.

Each examination or treatment room must have a sink as well as soap and a paper towel dispenser. Many also contain holders for containers of disinfecting wipes. Hand sanitizer may be in a wall-mounted or freestanding dispenser. The examination room must also contain a wall-mounted rigid container for the disposal of sharps, such as needles, scalpel blades, or other objects that might puncture a plastic bag. Biohazard wastebaskets with a biohazard plastic liner for materials that contain body fluids—such as blood, mucus, or pus—are located either in each examination room or in the hall. Containers for hazardous waste must be covered except when waste is being added. A foot pedal to open the cover will facilitate its use. The examination room usually contains an ordinary wastebasket for used paper towels and table paper.

For safety reasons, examination rooms should not contain syringes, needles, or medication samples. Cleaning materials and chemical solutions should never be stored under the counter in an examination room, especially if it is used for children. Having a centralized storage area will keep the examination rooms safe for all of the patients.

SECURITY SYSTEMS

A medical office maintains a number of different security systems.

First, if the office is entered from a corridor in an office building, the building owner or office condominium association will probably have an electronic security system for the building itself.

Second, regardless of whether the office is entered from a corridor or directly from the outside, the medical office should maintain an electronic security system against break-ins to the office itself.

The office's security and safety alarm system is monitored by an alarm company and may or may not also be tied to the local police and fire departments. Whether or not the system is tied in to the police and fire departments, the alarm company will call the medical office's liaison to the company whenever the alarm goes off.

This designated person is often the medical office administrator or managing partner. However, two or three people are always listed as backups in case the liaison is not available.

Third, various places within the office require another layer of security. Medication cabinets—with all medications and prescription pads inside—should be locked, and a limited number of people should have keys to the medication cabinet. The laboratory, providers' private offices, medical records cabinet or room, and business office are other areas that often have a lock and limited access.

If controlled substances are stored in the office, they should be double-locked (e.g., in a locked drawer within a locked cabinet). Two separate keys should open the two different locks.

ROUTINE MAINTENANCE

It is important to maintain the physical space of the medical office. Depending on the size of the office, many if not most routine maintenance activities are undertaken by staff. These include controlling the temperature, cleaning cabinets and drawers, changing lightbulbs, replacing batteries in battery-powered equipment, turning the security system on and off, making sure fire protection equipment is in working order, and performing some daily cleaning. In all activities, medical assistants and other staff must be sure to protect themselves and patients from hazards and injury. Good body mechanics should be used to move supplies and equipment when cleaning as well as when working with patients. The workplace should be arranged to minimize strain during all routine and maintenance activities.

TEMPERATURE AND VENTILATION

The reception area and examination rooms should be kept at a comfortable temperature. People who are ill are sensitive to cold and drafts. The reception and patient waiting areas and examination rooms should be about 70° F to 72° F. The temperature in treatment rooms, the laboratory, and providers' offices should be about 68° F to 70° F. A room used for procedures or minor surgery can be kept a little cooler because the provider and medical assistant may be wearing gowns or lab coats, gloves, and masks.

Ventilation is also important. Keeping air circulating is important both to dissipate odors and to allow germs to escape from the office atmosphere.

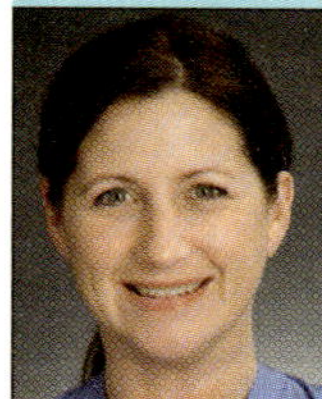

Putting It All Into Practice

My Name is Kelsey Whitman, and I am a registered medical assistant. I usually work in one of the satellite offices of a large medical group that includes primary care providers and medical specialists. The office where I usually work was formerly a house. They are planning to close it next spring, tear it down, and replace it with a modern office building. Even though there are some disadvantages to the current setting, it has a lot of charm. The waiting room and three small examination rooms are on the first floor with the providers' office, and we use the rooms upstairs for storage, a break room, and meeting rooms. I have a small office upstairs, but I never have time to sit in it. Usually, we have only one provider in the office. I work with one other medical assistant, but since I have been in the practice longer, I am responsible for making sure that everything runs smoothly. I have to go to the main office once a month for a staff meeting. The meetings are held late on Wednesday afternoons. We discuss issues affecting all work areas and have also been reviewing some of the procedures done by medical assistants to be sure that every medical assistant in every office does things the same way. The other medical assistant will be out on maternity leave in a few weeks and we have been interviewing for someone to cover for her while she is out. We will need another medical assistant when the new facility is finished and she will fill that role after covering the maternity leave. After an initial screening interview, I have been asked to talk to three applicants, to give them a tour of our office and then to offer my feedback about how they might fit into this setting. One of the applicants seemed like a real team player, and I hope they hire her. It is so important for everyone to be able to work well together. ■

GENERAL CLEANING

Larger offices may contract for cleaning services, or office cleaning may be included in the monthly rent, especially in buildings that are dedicated to medical offices. Contracted cleaning is usually done one or two times a week, so even if the major cleaning is contracted out, daily cleaning tasks must still be performed.

Daily cleaning includes tidying up all areas of the office—reception and waiting rooms, administrative space, providers' offices, examination and treatment rooms, and the laboratory.

Sinks should all be toweled dry, and rest rooms should be checked to make sure that ample toilet and facial tissue, soap, and paper towels are available. Any spills or puddles on the floor of the rest room should be mopped up, using gloves as needed.

Waste containers and recycling containers should be checked daily and emptied as needed. Biohazard sharps containers should be checked daily and replaced when they are three-quarters full. The plastic liners of biohazard waste containers should be changed as needed. Contracted cleaning services will usually not empty biohazard waste containers because they contain regulated medical waste. The medical assistant must handle biohazard waste containers carefully to prevent an exposure incident. The Occupational Safety and Health Administration (OSHA) Bloodborne Pathogens Standard outlines specific actions to take when regulated medical waste is being handled. These actions are outlined in Chapter 17.

If the office staff must do more intense cleaning, this should be done at least weekly. These tasks include mopping vinyl floors and vacuuming carpets, cleaning the glass at the reception area, polishing furniture and accessories, dusting, and thoroughly cleaning the rest rooms.

It is important to try to avoid a "medical smell" in the office. This is done by maintaining proper ventilation as well as by cleaning up spills and accidents immediately, using light or unscented air fresheners in rest rooms and examination rooms, and keeping disinfectants and cleaning materials in tightly closed containers when not in use and out of patients' reach.

CLEANING CABINETS AND DRAWERS

Storage cabinets, drawers, and bookcases are cleaned less frequently, often on a day when the provider or some of the providers in the medical office are absent so that the room is not in use. After cleaning, the medical assistant should check labels on all items before putting them back on shelves. This is a good time to check the expiration date on supplies and make a list of any items that need to be ordered or restocked from the general supply area to the cabinet. Outdated supplies must be disposed of properly. Supply cabinets should be kept tidy so items can be easily located (Fig. 49.2).

What Would You Do? What Would You *Not* Do?

Case Study 1

Jean Highsmith has brought her 1-year-old twins, Scott and Lucy, to the medical office because they have been fussy and tugging at their ears. In the waiting room, she puts the twins on the floor to play with the toys while they are waiting. When Kelsey is able to take them to an examination room, she notices that the twins, who also have runny noses, have been chewing on some of the plastic toys in the waiting room. She notices that Mrs. Highsmith has left used tissues on one of the waiting room tables. After a few minutes in the examination room, Mrs. Highsmith comes to the door holding a child under each arm and tells Kelsey that Scott has thrown up a little on the examination room table. ■

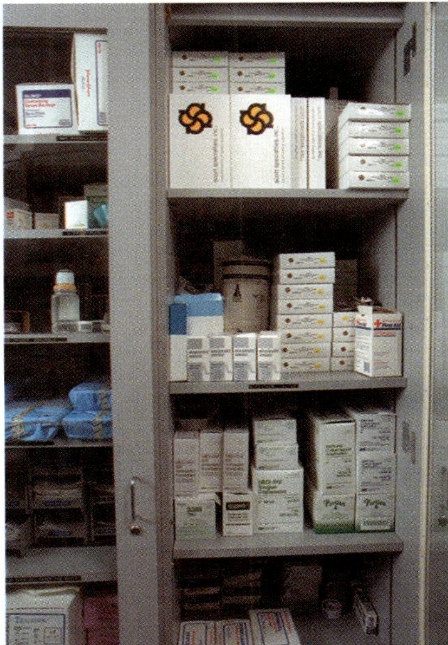

Fig. 49.2 Well-organized supply cabinet.

MISCELLANEOUS TASKS

Among the miscellaneous tasks that have to be performed daily are putting the waiting room chairs in their correct spots and replacing magazines in their racks (as well as toys if toys are available); cleaning mirrors in the rest rooms and examination rooms; and cleaning the tops, fronts, and undersides of cabinets and paper towel dispensers. Toys must be cleaned and disinfected on a regular basis because they can harbor microorganisms.

The medical assistant may be responsible for replacing light bulbs in gooseneck lamps and other special lighting. Ceiling lighting is usually a responsibility of the maintenance staff employed by the building owner. If the space is owned by the medical office, this may be a staff responsibility or may be covered by the cleaning or maintenance contract with an outside service.

MAINTAINING EQUIPMENT

Within the physical environment of the office there are many pieces of equipment both for medical purposes and for business purposes. The medical assistant who manages the office is responsible for relationship management with the individuals or companies that sell and maintain the equipment as well as with those who provide supplies for the equipment.

INVENTORY

An **inventory** is a detailed list of items in stock or in the possession of an individual or business. An equipment inventory lists each piece of equipment, the serial number, the date it was purchased, the length of the warranty, the name of the organization that services it, the manufacturer's suggested service schedule, and the date of last service. The office may also maintain a log validating maintenance and repair for larger pieces of equipment, such as computers and copiers.

An inventory is important for two reasons.

1. Tax consequences: Larger pieces of medical and office equipment are depreciated over 5 years, whereas smaller pieces of equipment and supplies can be fully deducted as an expense in the year in which they are purchased. (**Depreciation** is a name for the accounting methods used to account for the anticipated useful life of a piece of equipment and its loss of value over time.)
2. Theft or damage: In case of theft or damage, an inventory is necessary to make a complete report to the police and/or claim to the office's insurance company.

Operation manuals for the equipment can be stored centrally with the inventory list, or each manual can be stored with the piece of equipment for which it is used. Many pieces of equipment come with a plastic pouch on the side of the item or storage unit in which manuals and maintenance schedules can be kept. Often times the operation manual is offered electronically and can be accessed online. Knowing the websites to access the operation manual will be helpful. A sticker may be provided with the web address.

MONITORING EQUIPMENT FUNCTION AND READINESS FOR USE

The medical assistant should always be on the lookout for equipment problems, especially problems that could lead to a dangerous situation. All instruments should be checked when preparing them for sterilization. Before machines are used, the medical assistant should look for frayed wires, bent or damaged instruments, and machines that are not functioning properly.

Office machines should be dusted or wiped with a damp cloth regularly, following manufacturers' guidelines. Batteries, fluids, paper, toner, and other supplies should be replaced as needed. If there is a maintenance log for the piece of equipment (e.g., the autoclave log, copier log), the medical assistant should document any maintenance (Procedure 49.1).

The decision whether to repair or replace a piece of equipment will usually be made taking several factors into account:

- The age of the piece of equipment
- How expensive a new piece of equipment is
- The level of use the equipment gets
- Whether the manufacturer still produces parts for repair
- Whether any important features have been added to newer models of the equipment

If there is no service contract for the piece of equipment and the decision is made to repair it, a repair service must be located and a repair arranged. The manufacturer usually has a list of authorized repair services by region. In larger organizations, a purchase order must usually be presented in order to arrange an equipment repair.

Emergency equipment must always be ready for use. This equipment must be checked at least monthly and, in many larger facilities, more often. The contents of the emergency box or crash cart (discussed in detail in Chapter 36) should be checked for completeness by a designated person, who will initial a form to verify the presence of each item on the checklist.

Oxygen tanks are checked at the same time as emergency equipment. They should be sent to be refilled when the level falls to a predetermined point. Expiration dates of emergency medications are checked at the same time.

SERVICE CONTRACTS

Many pieces of medical office equipment are purchased with a service contract. A **service contract** is an agreement that provides for repair calls over a specific time period after the manufacturer's warranty has expired. A **warranty** is a promise by the manufacturer to repair or replace defective parts in an item during a specific time period. The service calls in a service contract may be free or require a specified charge, depending on the contract. Contracts usually call for larger pieces of equipment to be serviced at the provider's office. Smaller pieces of equipment often have a two-price contract: one price if the item is brought to a service center for repair and another if the repair is carried out on site.

SERVICE CALLS

Before calling in a service technician, the medical assistant should check the equipment thoroughly. A plug accidentally removed from a socket or a disconnected wire is often the cause of what seems like a machine breakdown.

If there is a service contract, all necessary routine maintenance should be performed in the office or an appointment should be scheduled for a technician to perform it.

The medical assistant should keep a record of all service calls, the reason the call was made, the response, whether there was a service charge, and the suggested follow-up.

PURCHASES OF NEW EQUIPMENT

Although the providers in the medical office or the clinic administrator may be responsible for purchasing equipment, the medical assistant may be asked to help look into options.

Manufacturers are glad to send information about the equipment in question. Many companies now have websites that can be browsed to see product features and costs. Some sites even have video demonstrations. A demonstration can often be arranged to take place in the office.

Some medical offices look for used equipment or furniture. Companies that sell equipment from a number of manufacturers often have used equipment in inventory. Used equipment can also be found from providers who are buying new equipment or retiring. Before purchasing a piece of used equipment, it is recommended to be sure that the manufacturer still supports the product (e.g., that replacement parts are still being produced so that the equipment can be repaired).

The medical assistant may be asked to research the "lease versus buy" decision—whether to purchase the equipment or lease it over a period of time. Most medical and office equipment can be leased. Leasing and buying each have advantages and disadvantages, mostly in terms of tax implications. The medical office lawyer should be consulted on this decision. Laboratory equipment may be provided at a reduced cost or for a low monthly rent depending on the number of tests performed, so it is important to compare options among different companies.

When new equipment is received in the office, it is a good idea to note numbers of replacement parts—such as bulbs, batteries, and cartridges—and to add them to the supply-ordering system.

SUPPLIES

A busy medical office goes through enormous quantities of supplies—both clinical and administrative—in a month. Managing the purchasing and stocking of supplies is another task that often falls to a medical assistant.

The quantity of supplies that can be ordered at one time depends on the amount of storage space in the office. A medical office can usually get a better price by ordering large amounts, but many offices are limited in the amount they can store. Sometimes it is possible to get extra storage space in the basement of the building where space is being rented.

Also, many providers receive discounts on supplies by virtue of membership in some sort of buying group or independent practice organization. Other medical offices are beginning to move toward website-based purchasing of medical supplies, which may result in significant cost savings.

It is important to develop a good system of tracking supplies, usage, and storage capacity. In this way, reordering is not done too early, when there is no room, or too late, when the medical office may actually run out of important supplies.

When a new office or office move is being planned, it is important to arrange for adequate storage space.

SUPPLY INVENTORY

A supply inventory is a listing of all the supplies regularly used in the office. This inventory can be kept in a notebook with a separate page for each supply item or it can be a set of cards—one for each. Notebook pages or cards can be grouped either by the type of supply (e.g., surgical disposable, photocopier) or by the supplier. The inventory can also be kept on the computer. A printed list of all supplies or cards for each item are used when supplies are counted, and supplies that need to be ordered are recorded on an office inventory list.

The information entered on the inventory list should contain the following:

1. The item's name
2. Any specific size used and order number if available
3. The usual supplier
4. The cost per a standard quantity (e.g., $3.50 per 100) if known
5. The type of units (e.g., each, box, package [pkg], case)
6. The quantity or number to order

The printed list of all supplies gives a **reorder point**, a number that identifies when the remaining quantity of the item is low enough that the item must be reordered. The reorder point is calculated by determining the number of items used per day or week and the number of days or weeks it takes for an order to be received. For instance, if the office uses 100 pairs of gloves per day, there are 50 pairs in each box, and it takes 5 working days to receive a new order of gloves, the reorder point would be when fewer than 15 boxes (750 gloves) are in the supply room (7.5 days' worth). The quantity to order is also noted on this list. Fig. 49.3 shows part of a sample list of bandage and dressing supplies. Lists of supplies and equipment can be maintained on one or more spreadsheets.

Most offices order supplies on a monthly basis. Some supplies are routinely reordered each ordering period, but others are ordered only on an "as-needed" basis. After the supplies in the supply closet have been counted, a supply inventory form should be completed for each supplier (Fig. 49.4).

Even if the office has been using the same supplier for a long time, it is a good practice to check other suppliers at

ITEM NAME	SUPPLIER	ITEM #	COST	REORDER AT	# TO ORDER
Bandages & Dressings					
nonsterile sponges 2" x 2"	H Medical	XY 2544	$3.50/pkg/200	5 pkg	10 pkg
nonsterile sponges 4" x 4"	H Medical	XY 7812	$8.25/pkg/200	5 pkg	10 pkg
sterile sponges 4" x 4"	H Medical	XY 5540	$22.00/box/00	2 box	5 box
non-sterile conforming bandage 2"	Winscott	49J265	$5.25/pkg/12	10 pkg	10 pkg
non-sterile conforming bandage 4"	Winscott	49J266	$8.62/pkg/12	10 pkg	10 pkg
paste bandage 4"	Winscott	57J381	$4.10 each	10	10
					10

Fig. 49.3 Sample supply inventory.

WALDEN-MARTIN
FAMILY MEDICAL CLINIC
1234 ANYSTREET ANYTOWN, ANYSTATE 1234
PHONE 123-123-1234 FAX 123-123-5678

Inventory

Submitter: K. Whitman, RMA **Date:** 9/15/20XX
PO number: S00425660

Supplier: H Medical **Phone Number:** 123-123-2046
Website: www. HMedical.com

Product	Qty	Unit	Price/unit	Cost
XY 2544 non-sterile sponges 2" x 2"	10	pkg	$3.50	$35.00
XY 7812 sterile sponges 4" x 4"	5	box	$22.00	$110.00
			Total	$145.00

Fig. 49.4 Form for inventory control.

least annually to see if a better relationship can be established. This might involve discounts for the volumes purchased, faster delivery, better prices overall, or availability of more products from another supplier than from the current supplier. If a new supplier has offered a better price, the medical assistant should always give the current supplier the opportunity to "meet or beat" the current offer. An established relationship is a known quantity in terms of delivery reliability and overall quality of the relationship. When items are ordered repeatedly from the same supplier, the medical office is usually billed instead of having to pay in advance for the supplies.

When supplies are being stored in the main supply area, supplies with the expiration date closest to the current date should be placed at the front of the area so that they are used first. New supplies are stored behind the older supplies. When the supply inventory is done, supplies may be rearranged and outdated supplies removed (Procedure 49.2).

RESTOCKING

Moving supplies from the central supply area to the place where they will be used is called *restocking*. Examination rooms should be restocked once or twice daily. General supplies in administrative areas are usually restocked weekly. The photocopy and fax machines may need more paper every day, depending on the volume of work done.

ORDERING SUPPLIES

A supply order is created by combining the list of supplies that are routinely ordered with the inventory list (or lists) that are created during a supply inventory. Most offices will try to have one or two suppliers for clinical supplies and one or two for administrative supplies. Medications may be purchased from the same company as the one used for clinical supplies or from a pharmaceutical supplier. A **purchase order (PO) number** is usually assigned by a business to authorize and keep track of each purchase request. If an order is not prepaid, a PO number is usually required before the **vendor** (a company from which supplies are purchased) will accept the order. The PO number is used as a tracking device to link an order to an invoice (itemized bill) sent separately by the vendor.

Supplies are usually ordered by telephone, by fax, or online. Even if the telephone or computer is being used, it is important to print or maintain a paper record of the transaction to reconcile against receipt of the supplies and for proper accounting. If ordering is being done by fax, it is a good idea to make a follow-up phone call to make sure the fax has come through clearly and that the order entry person at the supply house has no questions.

When the vendor cannot ship the item immediately, the item is said to be on **back order**. The order should be flagged to make sure that it will arrive when promised. A back-ordered item is usually not billed for until it is shipped.

In some states, ordering of medications, needles, and sterile solutions requires an authorization from a provider and a copy of the provider's state medical license for purchase. For purchase of controlled substances, such as narcotics, a provider authorization and a copy of the provider's federal Drug Enforcement Administration certificate are necessary.

What Would You Do? What Would You *Not* Do?

Case Study 2

Kelsey accepts a delivery of a large box of supplies from United Parcel Service (UPS) at a time when the office is especially busy. She places the box in the supply room and continues with her work. Toward the end of the day, she realizes that she has not opened the box. She goes to the supply room and opens the outer box. Inside, there are boxes and packages of dressings, bandages, tape, tissues, gauze squares, and other items. Kelsey has an appointment, and she is anxious to finish up so that she can leave the office. ■

RECEIVING SUPPLIES

Different suppliers ship in different ways, including using the US Postal Service, large national package delivery companies such as UPS or FedEx, and local courier services.

Most delivery services will ask for a signature to confirm that the delivery has been made. When supplies are received, they should immediately be brought to the storage room. At the first convenient opportunity, the packing slip should be inspected and reconciled with the order to make sure that all items have been received or that items that are to be received in a separate delivery are noted on the packing slip. If the packing slip is incorrect, the missing items should be noted and the supplier notified.

The packing slip should be clipped to the order form. When all items have been received, the order form with all the packing slips attached should be marked "all items received" and placed in the accounts payable folder. If the order was not prepaid, the **invoice** (itemized bill for items that have not been prepaid) should arrive within a few days of delivery of the final items on the order.

Once the contents of a shipping box have been placed in storage, the box should be discarded. It is not recommended to keep boxes or cartons used for shipping because they may be dirty and can harbor insects or rodents.

PATIENT AND EMPLOYEE SAFETY

In addition to maintaining the physical environment of the medical office, it is also vital for all medical facilities to maintain a safe environment both for patients and for employees. This involves several measures.

1. Manage the environment to reduce hazards.
2. Train employees in general safety and to use correct methods and processes to prevent accident or injury.
3. Maintain equipment and perform regular safety inspections.
4. Create open lines of communication so that mistakes and accidents can be reported without fear of severe consequences.
5. Analyze all incidents including "near misses" to be sure that effective systems are in place. Constant awareness of potential hazards and a culture that expects each employee to respond to potentially unsafe conditions is one of the most effective tools for preventing accident or injury.

The following are general guidelines for workplace safety as recommended by OSHA:

- Keep work areas, corridors, and hallways clear of obstacles.
- Exits should be accessible, clearly marked, and well lit. Be aware of state and/or local requirements for emergency lighting for exit signs.
- Keep floors dry, and clean up spills as soon as possible.
- Store waste in appropriate receptacles. Remove waste promptly and dispose of medical waste appropriately (see Chapter 17).
- Do not create high piles of materials that are likely to fall. Do not climb up on chairs or other unstable objects to retrieve objects stored on high shelves.
- Do not allow electrical cords to be present in areas where people walk.
- Do not leave drawers open.

SAFE WORK PRACTICES

The office should have a safety plan, and all employees in the medical office should receive training so that they can carry out their duties correctly. The prevention of the spread of infection is always important. This is discussed in detail in Chapter 17. Equipment should always be checked for frayed electrical cords and used correctly to prevent injury. Hazardous chemicals should be handled and discarded safely. Laboratory safety should be maintained following guidelines in Chapter 29. There should be a plan to respond to spills of blood, body fluids, or chemicals. Areas that are restricted for safety reasons (such as the medical laboratory) should be clearly marked. Employees should report any unsafe condition to their supervisors. Protective equipment is provided by the employer and should always be used by each employee. Chapters 36 and 37 discuss emergency and disaster response in detail.

HIGHLIGHT on Ergonomics and Worker Safety

A typical working day in a medical office puts a lot of physical stress on personnel. Bending, lifting, reaching, squatting, having a telephone stuck in the crook of the neck, and repeatedly using a typing keyboard put stress on the body. The human body was not designed by nature to perform such activities so frequently.

Common causes for disabling workplace injury include the following:

- Overexertion injuries caused by excessive lifting, carrying, or pulling an object
- Falls either on the same level or from a higher to lower level

Continued

HIGHLIGHT on Ergonomics and Worker Safety—cont'd

- Injuries caused by bending, tripping, slipping without falling, or attempting to avoid falling
- Repetitive strain injuries caused by performing a repetitive task in the same way over and over
- Being struck by or striking against an object

Ergonomics and Good Body Mechanics

The word *ergonomics* comes from the Greek root *ergon*, which means "work." Ergonomics is the study of maximizing work efficiency by adapting the work environment for optimal physical and mental function. For example, office seating should be designed to provide maximum support for the back, and computer keyboards should be positioned to reduce repetitive motion injuries to the hands, wrists, and arms. But ergonomics does not have to be "high tech"; it can be as simple as adjusting the height or angle of a computer monitor. Ergonomics can also affect selection of shelving and storage units to minimize strain when storing items or removing them from storage. In addition to adapting the environment, good body mechanics promote work efficiency and prevent injury. See the discussion in Chapter 20 of ways to use good body mechanics.

Preventing Falls

Most workplace injuries from falls occur in the service industry. Several measures can be implemented in the medical office to prevent personnel (as well as patients) from tripping and falling. Good lighting, preventing clutter in walkways, closing drawers, cleaning up spills promptly, and emphasizing safety can reduce the likelihood of falls. Medical assistants should wear sturdy shoes and avoid walking too fast, carrying items that block vision, and failing to pay attention to their surroundings. ■

MONITORING ENVIRONMENTAL SAFETY

Because constant attention is required to maintain a safe environment, it is important to create a procedure to check regularly for potential hazards. A safety checklist is a useful tool for regular safety inspections. It should include the categories to be assessed and have a space to write down any action that needs to be taken. Each part of the office should be checked for adequate lighting, clear walkways, proper storage of supplies, and removal of rubbish and biohazard waste. It is especially important to be sure that heavy boxes have not been stored in a high area where they could fall, that electrical cords are in good repair and could not cause tripping or falls, and that spills have been attended to promptly. Storage of compressed gases, medications, and chemicals should be assessed according to office policies. Emergency signs for exits should be tested, missing safety signs should be replaced, and access should be restored if safety signs are blocked (Procedure 49.3).

SIGNS AND INSTRUCTIONS

The office should post signs (or sign-sized adhesive warning labels) to instruct patients and employees as needed. As defined by OSHA, danger signs indicate that there is immediate danger and special precautions should be taken. These signs must be red on the upper panel with black lettering and a white background. They are more common in construction areas than in the medical office. Caution signs warn against potential hazards. They should be predominantly yellow with either yellow lettering on a black background or black lettering on a yellow background. Caution signs should be used if potentially hazardous procedures, such as x-ray examinations or laser treatments, are performed in the medical office (Fig. 49.5). Signs should designate areas where access is restricted. Safety instruction signs (if necessary for employees, as at an eyewash station) should have an upper panel that is green with white lettering. Labels or color coding should also be used for all biohazard boxes, biohazard waste, and flammable gases. Smoking should not be permitted in a provider's office, and signs advising patients and visitors that the office is a smoke-free environment should be clearly posted in the waiting area. Exits should be clearly marked, and an emergency evacuation map should be posted near the door to the waiting room. Exit signs should be white with red lettering not less than 6 inches high and 0.25 inch wide. Lighted exit signs should be tested by shutting off the lights in the room; bulbs should be replaced if necessary.

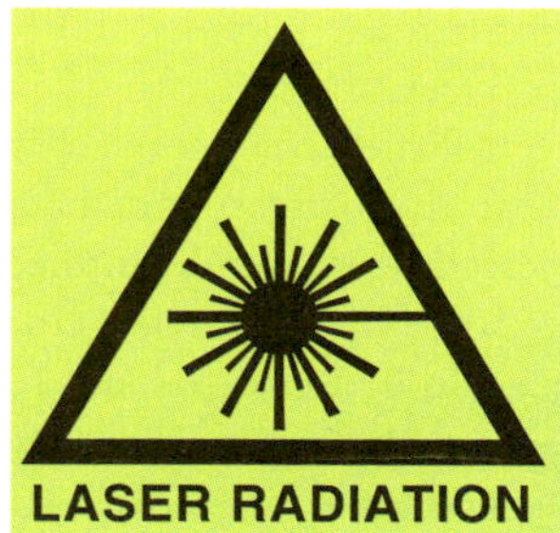

Fig. 49.5 Examples of caution signs for radiation and laser radiation.

The most commonly used safety symbol in the medical office is the biohazard symbol. This is discussed in detail in Chapter 17. If a room, refrigerator, or freezer is labeled with a biohazard warning label, only authorized personnel should be permitted to enter the room or have access to the appliance. Signs or labels with safety symbols for items that are flammable or might explode may be used, usually with explanatory text. The radiation symbol may be used on a sign with or without additional text to indicate a room with x-ray equipment or other radiation. Symbols consisting of a red circle crossed by a diagonal line indicate that an activity is prohibited. These may be used to indicate that smoking or eating is not allowed in the given area. Eyewash stations and showers may be indicated by signs or labels with a green background depicting the activity.

Labels of a bright color (orange, red, or yellow) are often placed on the front of paper medical records to identify medications to which the patient is allergic. If an EHR is used, this cannot be done, but the EHR itself monitors all new medication orders for potential allergies (Procedure 49.4).

CREATING AN ENVIRONMENT FOR TEAMWORK

Managing the medical office goes beyond the physical space, equipment, and supplies. It is also important to manage the people who work in the office. The medical assistant should help to establish an environment that supports teamwork, one in which people are willing to help one another out but are also willing to allow each individual to display their particular expertise. The medical assistant may help to set the tone for teamwork by showing respect for each employee and their skills and pitching in to help orient new employees or anyone who needs a little assistance during an especially busy time.

STAFF MEETINGS

In a busy office where each person is performing a specialized task, regular staff meetings can also promote teamwork. These meetings should occur often enough—weekly or at most monthly—that situations in need of correction can be dealt with quickly. The medical assistant may be responsible to schedule and/or lead these meetings.

The staff meeting should be used to share information or work through changes in office practice or procedures, discuss ways to improve patient satisfaction and office performance, and encourage staff to take advantage of opportunities to improve skills. Some skill improvement efforts can take place in the form of training sessions in the office on new equipment or computer systems. Others can be opportunities to attend off-site seminars and workshops.

In planning a meeting, a written agenda (list of specific items of business to be covered) assists in focusing the meeting and ensuring that all important business is considered in an organized way. One person should be assigned the task of taking **minutes** (a record of the meeting's proceedings).

Written minutes are valuable because they assist individuals who attended a meeting in following up on suggestions and decisions. The agenda should be prepared in advance, but except for a large, formal meeting, it need not be circulated until the meeting begins. Later, however, minutes should be circulated. They should be distributed as soon as possible after the meeting, although they are not usually formally approved until the beginning of the next meeting.

ORIENTING AND TRAINING EMPLOYEES

A new employee will be required to provide documentation in order to be added to the office payroll. All employees must have a Social Security number and complete an I-9 (Employment Eligibility Verification) form before they can begin working. The medical assistant may be responsible for reviewing the Social Security card and/or documents that establish identity and eligibility to work in the United States. Information about obtaining or replacing a Social Security card or changing the name on a Social Security card is available from the Social Security Administration.

Before the end of the first withholding period, a new employee must fill out a **W-4 form**, which identifies the number of exemptions claimed for proper income tax withholding. This form is updated annually, and the current version can be obtained from the Internal Revenue Service (IRS) website. An employee can submit a new form any time that their status changes—for example, if the employee gets married or has a child. If the employee elects to claim fewer exemptions than they are legally entitled to, the medical office will withhold more money from the employee's paycheck. Individuals claim fewer exemptions to be sure that adequate funds are withheld to cover their income tax liability.

A photocopy of any licenses or certificates should also be obtained from a new employee. All documents should be placed in the employee's personnel file.

WORKING WITH NEW EMPLOYEES OR MEDICAL ASSISTING STUDENTS

The medical assistant may be asked to participate in the orientation and training of a new medical assistant. This usually involves explaining provider preferences and working with the new employee to be sure that they understand how all procedures should be performed. The office may have a checklist of skills or tasks that the new employee must demonstrate before being allowed to perform them without supervision. If a new employee is not familiar with a specific piece of equipment, such as the electrocardiograph or spirometer, the medical assistant may be responsible for training the new employee in using it. A similar process is used when the office accepts medical assisting students for practicum. The medical assistant must allow a medical assisting student to observe each procedure and then perform it with supervision until the medical assistant can perform the procedure correctly without supervision (Fig. 49.6).

EMPLOYER OBLIGATIONS FOR PAYROLL

Employees must be paid regularly or the office will not be able to retain staff. The preparation of a payroll is an increasingly

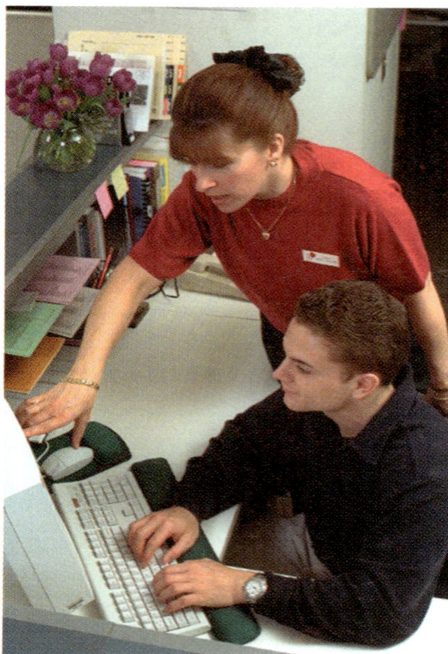

Fig. 49.6 Medical assistants may need to help medical assisting students during their practicum.

complex task. Consequently, most offices—even those that have long worked with their own payrolls—have switched to outside payroll services. Whether or not payroll is dealt with in the office, files are kept on all employees.

Payroll records for individual employees include the following:

- Name, address, Social Security number, and occupation
- The employee's withholding allowance certificate (**W-4 form**), which is used to calculate the amount withheld for federal income taxes
- Dates of employment
- Record of hours worked, wages paid, annuity, and pensions
- Record of all payroll deductions

These records must be kept for at least 4 years and be available for review by the IRS.

Employees may fill out time cards to report the hours worked, or they may clock in and out using an electronic badge reader or a computer entry. Most medical assistants are paid at an hourly rate. In this case the **gross pay,** the amount of money earned before any deductions, is calculated by multiplying the number of hours worked times the hourly rate. The **net pay** is the amount that an employee takes home after taxes are withheld. Some office employees may receive a **salary,** a fixed amount paid on a regular basis that does not depend on the number of hours worked. In this case the gross pay is the predetermined amount.

DEDUCTIONS

Income Taxes

Employers are required to withhold federal income taxes based on the amount paid to an employee and the number of withholding allowances the employee claims. The IRS publication *Employer's Tax Guide* contains detailed information including tables to determine the amount to withhold.

Social Security and Medicare

Social Security tax (called *FICA*, after the Federal Insurance Contributions Act) funds the national program of retirement benefits into which all workers pay 6.2% and employers pay 6.2% of their first $168,600 in income (for 2024). In addition, 1.45% of employee wages are withheld for Medicare taxes, and the employer must pay an additional 1.45% when the income is above a specified threshold.

State Taxes

Most states require employers to withhold state income tax based on the amount earned and the number of withholding allowances reported for the state (which may be different from the federal W-4 allowances).

ADDITIONAL OBLIGATIONS

The employer is required to deposit withheld income taxes, as well as employee and employer Social Security and Medicare taxes, following the schedule outlined in the IRS publication *Employer's Tax Guide.*

The employer is required to provide each employee with two copies of form W-2, the Wage and Tax Statement, by January 31 of each year. This form is used by the employee to complete their personal income tax forms. State income taxes are usually included on this form.

Unemployment Tax

Federal unemployment tax (FUTA) is paid by the employer on the first $7000 of income at a rate of 6% (for 2024). The money, which must be deposited quarterly, is used to pay unemployment compensation for workers who have lost their jobs. States also require employers to pay unemployment tax for their employees, and some states also require employers to withhold an unemployment tax from their employees.

MANAGING PROVIDER AND EMPLOYEE SCHEDULES

PROVIDER SCHEDULES

In addition to the medical office's appointment schedule, providers must be scheduled for other responsibilities related to patient care. In a group medical office, one provider must always be on call (i.e., available to take telephone calls from patients and make arrangements so that urgent and emergency health care needs of patients will be met). Providers in solo practice often collaborate with other providers in their community to provide this service. The medical office usually develops a standard schedule, but individual providers must be assigned to cover each on-call time period. After the schedule has been arranged, providers usually must work with one another if they want to switch or change days.

If the medical office has satellite offices, providers must be assigned times to see patients in the main office and in the other offices. If possible, coverage must be coordinated so that there is at least one provider in the satellite office every day. A master schedule is usually created, but variations occur depending on time of year and circumstances. For example, sometimes satellite offices are closed during holiday or vacation periods.

In many medical offices the providers make nursing home visits. In addition to scheduled blocks of time for these visits, there must also be a plan to provide urgent care if a nursing home resident becomes ill. Some providers always see their own patients, and in other medical offices there is one provider who is responsible for nursing home patients on a given day.

EMPLOYEE SCHEDULES

Other staff members must also be scheduled to provide coverage in both the primary office and any satellite offices. Usually employees must submit requests in writing for days off, changes to the regular schedule, and vacation. Depending on the size of the office, the medical assistant or office manager may be responsible for creating the work schedule for staff other than the providers. When one of the medical assistants or another staff member calls in sick, efforts must be made to find a replacement. The medical office often has contact with medical assistants or other employees who will work on a **per diem** basis (*per diem* is a Latin term meaning "per day" or "by the day"). Per diem employees do not have a fixed schedule. They may be given a weekly schedule depending on office needs and, in addition, they may be called in on a day when extra help is required. The office may also use an employment agency to obtain temporary employees, especially if one of the regular medical assistants is unable to work for an extended period of time.

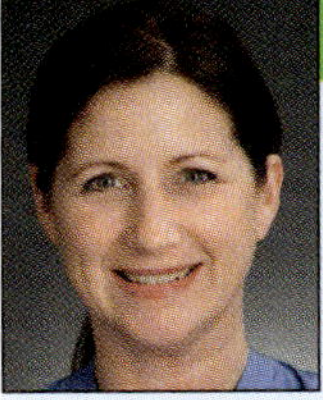

Memories *from* Practicum

Kelsey Whitman: The office where I did my practicum was in a provider office building next to the local hospital. It was a very clean, modern office, and I learned so much there. There were two providers specializing in internal medicine. At the beginning of the day, we got everything ready for the patients. We made sure that the waiting room was tidy, stocked every examination room, and turned on the online music for patients. The office closed for an hour at noon, and after the morning patients had left, we checked the waiting room, picked up the magazines, and made sure there was no trash on the tables. In the afternoon, it was my job to go through the examination rooms and make sure that all items were restocked. While I was doing my practicum, one of the providers went on vacation for a week, and we used that time to clean all the drawers and cabinets in the examination rooms. We took everything out and cleaned each area with soap and water. We found expired supplies at the backs of the cabinets, and we had to discard them. It was a lot of work, but when we were done, everything seemed much better organized. Before my practicum, I didn't realize the amount of work it is to keep everything looking neat and professional in a medical office. ■

LOCATING COMMUNITY RESOURCES FOR PATIENTS

The medical assistant can be helpful to patients by identifying community resources to meet patient health needs (Procedure 49.5). The medical office may keep a list of local organizations with telephone numbers or other contact information in the following areas:

- Support for alcoholism or addiction
- Support for caregivers of individuals with decreased mental or physical function
- Adult day care
- Visiting nurse and homemaker services
- Legal aid
- Local civic organizations including services for children, families, elders, and the homeless
- Local board of health
- Hospital-sponsored rehabilitation, weight control, and smoking cessation programs
- Immunization clinics
- Cardiopulmonary resuscitation (CPR) and first aid training

National organizations focus on many diseases. Most will provide information, and some have local chapters or can refer patients to local organizations. The medical assistant can help the patient to search the internet for these organizations. Many hospitals also have extensive programs related to specific diseases or conditions, and the medical assistant should become familiar with those in their locality, especially those sponsored by the hospital with which the medical office providers are affiliated. The hospital newsletter is a good source of information on new programs for patients.

What Would You Do? What Would You *Not* Do?

Case Study 3

Ellen Pritchard has brought her mother, Elizabeth Brown, a 76-year-old widow, to the office for a physical examination. Kelsey notices that Ellen looks upset at the checkout desk after Mrs. Brown has been seen by the provider. Kelsey asks Ellen if anything is the matter. Ellen says, "I'm worried about my mother. She has lost weight, and I don't think she is eating properly. She lives alone, and I help her as much as I can, but lately I'm not sure it's enough. I don't know what to do." ■

RISK MANAGEMENT

Risk management is the process of assessing risk and putting in place policies and procedures that minimize it. Often the focus of risk management activities is on avoiding lawsuits. Risk in a medical office comes in a number of forms.

MINIMIZING RISK OF INJURY OR ILLNESS

Physical risk involves the risk of injury or illness to employees, patients, and visitors. Business risk also exists—that is, the risk of reduced patient visits because of poor customer relations. The medical office seeks to minimize these risks and prevent lawsuits that may result from injuries related to patient care or an accident in the office.

The medical assistant or office manager is often responsible for maintaining the risk management program in close consultation with the provider or the managing partner among the providers. There may be a full-time risk manager in larger clinics or hospitals, or risk management may be a part of the duties of one of the clinic's top administrators. Policies and procedures are designed by the providers and the office's top administrator, who work closely with an attorney, an insurance professional, and a risk management professional. When a new policy is adopted, a copy is given to each employee covered by the policy. Policy and procedure manuals, once developed, should be accessible to all employees when questions arise.

LIABILITY INSURANCE

Every office should have adequate insurance protection against liability, both professional liability (commonly called *malpractice*) and liability for any accident that might occur in the office.

Professional liability insurance covers a medical professional against patient claims that diagnostic procedures, tests, or treatments either caused an injury or failed to detect an existing medical condition that should have been detected using good medical practice.

Some providers purchase insurance in their own name only and have professional staff members purchase their own professional liability policies. If this is the case, the medical assistant can purchase a professional liability policy through an organization that provides insurance to health professionals. In other cases, a medical office purchases professional liability insurance for the entire staff. If this is the case, every professional staff member should be named on the policy.

The office should also have adequate insurance to cover property damage to the office because of fire, storm, or flooding (similar to homeowner's insurance). In addition, the medical office should have adequate coverage against personal injury sustained on the office's property by a patient or employee. Many patients are ill and/or fragile, and a fall can occur at any time. The policy should cover any injury sustained on the property controlled by the medical office. If the medical office is in an office building, the public hallways are the responsibility of the landlord or medical office condominium association. If the office is in a freestanding building, the medical office is responsible for any occurrences that happen on walkways, in the parking lot, or in other outdoor areas up to the public road or sidewalk.

COMPLIANCE REPORTING

Each state board of health requires specific compliance reports for infectious diseases, other diseases, abuse, and injuries resulting from possible criminal behavior, as discussed in Chapter 3. In addition, hospitals, nursing homes, and other types of facilities must report specific serious medical incidents. Providers must also make a report to the state if a patient demonstrates failing eyesight that would interfere with the ability to maintain a driver's license. Depending on the state, reports of unsafe activities and errors in patient care (especially medication errors) must be reported, especially when they occur in relation to individuals with disabilities. Workplace disease and injury reporting is also required in most states.

The "Sunshine" provision of the Patient Protection and Affordable Care Act (PPACA) requires manufacturers of drugs, devices, and biologic and medical supplies covered by Medicare, Medicaid, or the Children's Health Insurance Program to disclose to the Centers for Medicare and Medicaid Services (CMS) any payments or other valuable transfers made to providers and teaching hospitals. It has long been felt that gifts and payments to providers by the pharmaceutical industry have created a potential conflict of interest, influencing providers to prescribe the medications of those companies who support them. Some states have placed limits on such gifts. Providers are also required to disclose any financial interest in laboratories or other health care facilities to which they refer patients.

INCIDENT REPORTS

Whenever something happens in the office for which the office could be considered liable, an incident report should be filled out. An incident can be as simple as a staff member or patient tripping over a chair, or it could be as serious as a staff member sticking themselves with a needle that has just been used to give an injection.

The incident report should be initiated by the staff member who is injured or who was closest to the patient or visitor when they were injured. A supervisor should review the report before giving it to the individual who manages the risk management program.

Incident report forms vary widely but usually ask for the following information:

- Date and time that the incident occurred
- Name and identifying information of the individual(s) involved
- Address, building, and room number where the incident occurred
- Description of how the incident occurred and exactly what occurred
- Complete description of any injury or potential injury
- Name(s) and identifying information for any witnesses
- Name and contact information for the person in the organization to whom the incident was reported
- Date of receipt and follow-up by supervisor

Incident reports should always be filled out if a patient, employee, or visitor slips or falls; if a medication error is made; if blood is drawn from the wrong patient; if the number of surgical instruments counted after a procedure does not match the number counted before the procedure; or if an employee is stuck with a needle. Any witnesses to the incident should be asked for their names, addresses, and phone numbers so that the office's insurance provider can call and investigate the incident further if necessary.

An incident report can usually be created for a patient through the EHR and filed as part of the patient's record. Paper reports are used for visitors and/or employees. A paper report should be dated and signed by the person filling it out. A provider and/or supervisor's signature also goes on the form according to the office's policy for incident reports (Procedure 49.6). If the incident relates to a reportable occurrence, the information must be forwarded to the correct government agency.

What Would You Do? What Would You *Not* Do? RESPONSES

Case Study 1

Page 1237

What Did Kelsey Do?

- ❑ Asked Mrs. Highsmith to place the used tissues in the wastebasket before taking the twins to the examination room. She then provided hand sanitizer for Mrs. Highsmith.
- ❑ Put the twins in an examination room as soon as possible.
- ❑ As soon as possible, Kelsey put on disposable gloves and removed the plastic toys that the twins had had in their mouths so that the toys could be cleaned before other children played with them.
- ❑ When told that Scott Highsmith had thrown up a little, Kelsey put on disposable gloves, used paper towels to absorb as much liquid as possible, and then promptly cleaned and disinfected the surrounding area. If she used a disposable disinfecting wipe, she let the exam table air dry.
- ❑ She reassured Mrs. Highsmith that children are ill sometimes and that cleaning up is all in a day's work.
- ❑ Kelsey noted the color and amount of vomit so that she could inform the provider.

What Did Kelsey Not Do?

- ❑ Did not ask Mrs. Highsmith to prevent the twins from playing with any toys because they had colds.
- ❑ Did not tell other mothers in the waiting room that they might not want to let their children play with the toys until they could be disinfected.
- ❑ Did not wait to perform routine cleaning until the lunch break or after office hours.
- ❑ Did not tell another staff member or Mrs. Highsmith to clean up when Scott vomited.

Case Study 2

Page 1241

What Did Kelsey Do?

- ❑ Checked the number of each type of item against the packing slip to be sure the order was complete. Made a notation if any items were missing.
- ❑ Placed all the items in their assigned storage area, either that night or the next day. Placed newer items behind older items.
- ❑ When she was placing items into storage, checked items on the shelves to be sure that none of them had expired.
- ❑ If any items were missing or back ordered, made a notation on the packing slip. Then placed the packing slip in the accounts payable folder to indicate that the order had been received.
- ❑ Removed the shipping box to the designated area for trash.

What Did Kelsey Not Do?

- ❑ After opening the large box, she did not leave the office before checking the packing slip. Another staff member might assume that the individual who opened the box had also checked the contents.
- ❑ Did not stack the items on shelves in the storage room randomly because she was in a hurry.
- ❑ Did not discard the packing slip after checking the order.
- ❑ Did not keep the shipping box. It might be dirty or harbor pests.

Case Study 3

Page 1245

What Did Kelsey Do?

- ❑ Encouraged Ellen to reach out and find out if there were services that could help her mother.
- ❑ While Mrs. Brown was present, included her in the conversation.
- ❑ If speaking to Ellen privately was an option, Kelsey offered understanding of how difficult it is to know what to do when a parent begins to be less able to function independently.
- ❑ Offered to help Ellen find resources for delivered meals or homemaking services in the community.
- ❑ Referred Ellen to local agencies that provide elder services.
- ❑ Offered to ask the provider if a referral to a visiting nurse would be appropriate.

What Did Kelsey Not Do?

- ❑ Did not exclude Mrs. Brown from the conversation or treat her like a child.
- ❑ Did not push Mrs. Brown or Ellen to accept her suggestions but rather just offered information.
- ❑ Did not promise that the provider would make specific referrals.

TERMINOLOGY REVIEW

Key Term	Definition
Back order	A term used for items ordered that cannot be shipped immediately, usually because they are out of stock.
Depreciation	Accounting methods to respond to the loss of value of a property or piece of equipment over time.
Gross pay	The total amount earned in a time period by an employee before any deductions.
Inventory	A detailed list of items in stock or in possession of an individual or business.
Invoice	An itemized bill for items whose cost has not been prepaid.
Minutes	A written record of the proceedings of a meeting.
Net pay	The actual amount of money paid directly to an employee after taxes and other deductions have been taken out.
Per diem	A term used for employees who do not have a fixed schedule but are scheduled by the day according to office needs.
Purchase order (PO) number	A number assigned by a business to authorize and keep track of a purchase request and order.
Reorder point	A number on a supply inventory that indicates when a specific item should be reordered to be sure that the supply will not run out before the new order is received.
Risk management	The process of assessing risk and putting policies and procedures in place to minimize it.
Salary	A fixed amount of money paid on a regular basis that does not depend on the number of hours worked.
Service contract	An agreement that provides for service for a piece of equipment after the warranty expires.
Social Security tax	A tax collected from employers and employees to fund the Social Security program, which provides benefits to retired workers.
Vendor	A company from whom supplies or equipment is/are purchased.
Warranty	A promise by the manufacturer to repair or replace defective parts in an item during a specific time period.
W-4 form	The form used to claim withholding allowances for federal income tax reporting.

PROCEDURE 49.1 Performing Routine Maintenance of Equipment

Outcome Perform equipment maintenance and document on equipment maintenance log.

Equipment/Supplies

- Piece of equipment to be maintained
- Cloth for dusting
- Maintenance log sheet
- Supplies necessary for the piece of equipment (e.g., paper, batteries, toner, fluids)

1. **Procedural Step.** Locate the piece of equipment to be checked.
2. **Procedural Step.** Check all electrical cords and plugs to make sure that there is no fraying or malfunction.
   Principle. Frayed electrical cords are a potential fire hazard and can cause electrical shocks.
3. **Procedural Step.** Check the piece of equipment for cracks, dents, or other damage; obvious impairment; or malfunction.
4. **Procedural Step.** Check any keyboard or keypad for cracks, faded numbers, letters, or other impairment.
5. **Procedural Step.** Dust or clean the outside or case of the piece of equipment according to the manufacturer's directions.
   Principle. Dust can interfere with the correct function of the machine.
6. **Procedural Step.** Check leads and other wires or other tubing.
7. **Procedural Step.** Check or change batteries, fluid, toner, or other essential components.

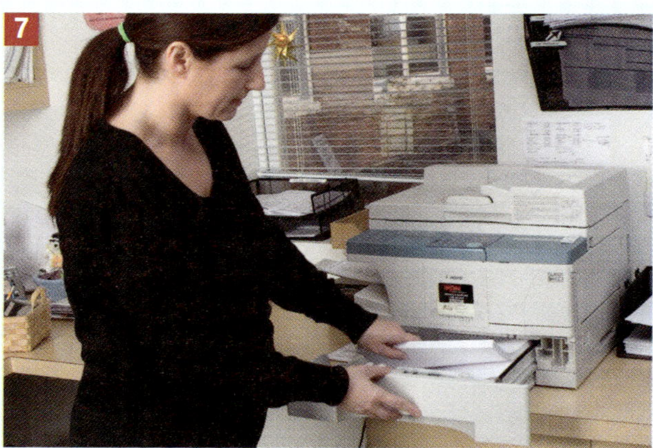

Add paper to the photocopier as needed.

PROCEDURE 49.1 Performing Routine Maintenance of Equipment—cont'd

8. **Procedural Step.** Schedule any required maintenance if appropriate.
9. **Procedural Step.** Fill out the equipment maintenance log. Example:

Equipment Description	**Bestcopy Office Photocopier**		
Serial Number	**266XXX49500**	**Model Number**	**6500AA**
Date	Action Taken/Comments	Initials	
5/26/20XX	Machine checked, glass cleaned, toner added.	KW, RMA	
5/30/20XX	Streaks on copies, service call arranged. Technician cleaned drum.	KW, RMA	
6/2/20XX	Machine checked, glass cleaned.	KW, RMA	

PROCEDURE 49.2 Taking a Supply or Equipment Inventory

Outcome Take a supply or equipment inventory.

Equipment/Supplies

- List of equipment or supplies
- Notebook or cards
- Items to inventory
- Office inventory form
- Pen

1. **Procedural Step.** Obtain a list of items in inventory from a written or computer-generated list, inventory notebook, or box of inventory cards.
   Principle. The process of taking an inventory includes validating the presence or absence of a given set of items.
2. **Procedural Step.** Check each item in the inventory record against the items present in all areas of the medical office. For equipment, validate serial numbers. For supplies, consider the supplies on hand in examination rooms and storage areas, checking expiration dates and disposing of those that are expired.
   Principle. Expired items should be thrown away and not counted as part of the inventory. The point of taking inventory is to keep track of the number of items on hand that can be used.

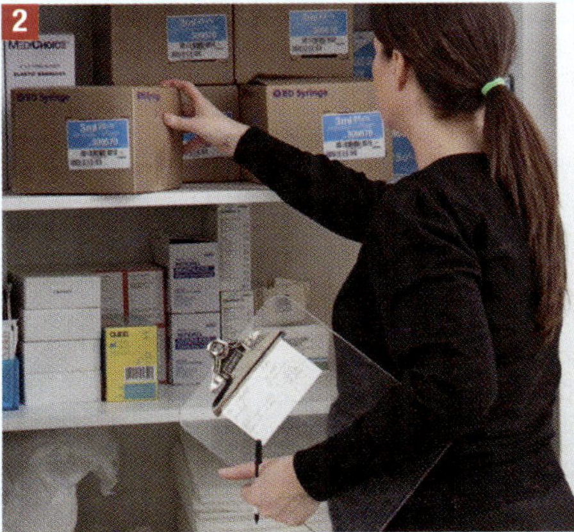

Check the quantity of supplies on hand.

3. **Procedural Step.** For an equipment inventory, make every effort to locate each piece of equipment on the list and validate that it is in working condition. Document if the item is missing or needs repair. For a supply inventory, check the quantity of supplies on hand against the quantity listed as the reorder point. If the quantity of items on hand is close to the reorder point, add the item to the office supply order list, including the name of the product (and manufacturer's or supplier's item number), the quantity to order, the type of units, and the price per unit.
   Principle. When you are preparing the supply inventory form, you must gather enough information to order a new supply of items that need to be replenished.
4. **Procedural Step.** Check that the information on the inventory card or list is correct and complete. There should be a serial number for equipment and a description of the size, color, and price as well as the name of the usual supplier.
   Principle. You will need this information when you are replacing equipment or reordering supplies.
5. **Procedural Step.** Be sure that your storage space is tidy, that items can be found when needed, and that supplies are arranged so that those with the oldest expiration dates are at the front of the storage shelf.
   Principle. Supplies are useless unless they can be found. Supplies with the oldest expiration dates should be used first.
6. **Procedural Step.** Place inventory cards, computer printout sheet, or inventory book in the proper location for follow-up, including placing orders or updating computer information and storage until needed again.

PROCEDURE 49.3 Creating an Environmental Checklist and Performing a Safety Inspection

Outcome Perform and document a safety inspection after creating an environmental checklist.

Equipment/Supplies

- Area to be inspected
- Pen and paper (or computer and word processing file) to create an environmental checklist

1. **Procedural Step.** Create a checklist of types of hazards to be inspected for, including obstructed walkways and tripping hazards; electrical hazards; improperly stored boxes; inadequate lighting; wet floors; and improperly labeled and stored biohazards, medications, and chemicals. Include a test of emergency lighting for exit signs and adequacy of safety signs.
2. **Procedural Step.** Moving from room to room in the designated area, first make a general inspection to be sure that floors are dry and all furniture and fixtures are in good repair. Then make a detailed inspection as required for each section on the checklist. Include a check for appropriate safety signs, symbols, and/or labels. If a problem is found, fix it if possible, but always note the problem on the checklist.
3. **Procedural Step.** Check for walkways that are wide enough for usual traffic without clutter. Be sure that there are no frayed carpets and no items that obstruct the walkway such as boxes, electrical cords, or debris. Be sure that there are no open drawers or cabinet doors.
4. **Procedural Step.** Check all electrical cords and plugs to ensure there is no fraying or malfunction.

   Principle. Frayed electrical cords are a potential fire hazard and can cause electrical shocks.
5. **Procedural Step.** Check all storage areas to be sure that the tops of cabinets are clear and that supplies have been stored without the potential to fall and cause injury.
6. **Procedural Step.** Assess each light to be sure that all light bulbs are in working order. Check the emergency lighting for exit signs by turning out hallway lights. Note any exceptions. Make a note if it seems that any area does not have adequate lighting.
7. **Procedural Step.** Depending on the type of area, be sure that all biohazards, chemicals, or other potentially hazardous materials are labeled correctly. Check all areas containing biohazardous materials for a biohazard sign or biohazard label. Be sure that medication cabinets are locked. Be sure that chemicals are stored in secure areas away from patients.
8. **Procedural Step.** After completing the checklist, create a written plan to respond to any problems that you could not fix during the inspection.

PROCEDURE 49.4 Complying With Safety Signs, Symbols, and Labels

Outcome Comply with safety signs, symbols, and labels.

Equipment/Supplies

- Safety signs (or pictures of safety signs)
- Biohazard trash bag in container with lid
- Paper medical record with allergy label
- Computer with printer (color if possible)

1. **Procedural Step.** Using the computer, locate and print examples of safety signs and symbols including a sign for authorized personnel only, a sign indicating radiation with a radiation symbol, and a sign for an eyewash station and/or shower. On the back of the sign, indicate where such a sign should be located in the medical office.
2. **Procedural Step.** Participate in each of the following role-play situations with a classmate as a medical assistant:
   - Instruct a patient who is preparing to enter a room with a sign for authorized personnel only.
   - Instruct a patient who asks what an eyewash station is used for.
   - Instruct a patient who is preparing to discard a tissue in a biohazard waste container.
   - Question a patient about possible pregnancy before allowing entry into a room marked with a radiation symbol.

   Principle. Medical assistants must comply with all safety signs and be sure that patients also maintain safety as instructed by safety signs.
3. **Procedural Step.** Write a short description of the role-play identifying the appropriate actions of the medical assistant.
4. **Procedural Step.** Hand in the three signs and your description of the role-play to your instructor.

PROCEDURE 49.5 Locating and Facilitating Referrals to Community Resources

Outcomes

1. Develop a current list of community resources.
2. Facilitate referrals to community resources.

Equipment/Supplies

- Local telephone book
- Office list of community resources
- Computer and printer
- Local hospital newsletter(s)
- Library access
- Local newspapers
- Pen
- Notepad

1. **Procedural Step.** Research local sources to identify community agencies with resources to assist patients. Potential sources of information include the library, local newspapers, local cable television stations, local telephone books, local hospital newsletters, and the internet.
   Principle. Familiarity with local agencies improves the medical assistant's ability to provide useful information about community resources to patients.
2. **Procedural Step.** As resources are identified, create a list including pertinent information about the resource: name, services available, address, telephone number, website address, contact name or information, and other useful information. The list may be created using pen and paper, but it should be transferred to a word processing file for ease of duplication.
3. **Procedural Step.** Include resources for organizations and support groups that can assist patients and family members of patients experiencing terminal illness.
4. **Procedural Step.** Include resources for complementary and alternative medicine practices.
5. **Procedural Step.** Once the document file has been substantially completed, group resources by subject and/or age group served. Alphabetize resources within each group.
   Principle. Arranging lists in alphabetical order facilitates finding specific information and avoids any impression of favoritism or recommending one agency more frequently than another.
6. **Procedural Step.** When the list is complete, save and print copies as needed.
7. **Procedural Step.** Ask the office providers to review and approve the list.
   Principle. Any referral made by a medical office should have the approval of the practice providers.
8. **Procedural Step.** Update the list when information changes, when a new resource is identified, and on a periodic basis to be sure information is accurate.
9. **Procedural Step.** Use the list to make appropriate recommendations to patients either in response to patient questions or when instructed to by one of the office providers.
10. **Procedural Step.** Write a two-page report identifying the specific steps a medical assistant should take to facilitate referrals for a patient who needs a handicap placard for their automobile and a patient not taking their prescribed brand name medication because the patient cannot afford it.
    Principle: A medical assistant can act as a patient navigator for patients by helping them to identify resources to obtain services such as a handicap placard, or to find out how to apply for the free drug program from the manufacturer of a brand name drug.

PROCEDURE 49.6 Completing an Incident Report

Outcome Complete an incident report.

Equipment/Supplies

- Incident report form (from SimChart for the Medical Office or OSHA Form 301)
- Index card from instructor describing an incident involving an error in patient care
- Pen
- Notes from witnesses to the incident

1. **Procedural Step.** Interview all witnesses to the incident, and make notes as needed to complete the incident report.
   Principle. The incident report is based on factual information, but individuals involved in the incident may not be available when the report is actually written.
2. **Procedural Step.** Obtain an incident report form and fill in information about the person (or persons) who are the main subject of the incident including name, date of birth, and address. If using SimChart for the Medical Office, select the Incident Report form in the Office Forms section of the Form Repository.
3. **Procedural Step.** Complete any information about health care provided, including the names and identifying information for providers or health care professionals who provided treatment.
   Principle. Risk management includes taking all possible steps to minimize an adverse result from an incident.
4. **Procedural Step.** Complete all information to describe the incident in detail including time, location (address, building, room number), what happened, and any injury or illness that resulted from the incident. Include the names and identifying information of any witnesses.
   Principle. Documentation of this information as soon as possible after the incident makes it easier to establish the facts about the incident at a later time.
5. **Procedural Step.** Depending on the form used, it may be necessary to include the name and contact information of the individual within the office to whom the incident was reported. The supervisor should add information about any follow-up that occurs at a later date. The supervisor should initiate any additional required reports to appropriate government agencies.
   Principle. Follow-up for an incident is a crucial step in effective risk management.
6. **Procedural Step.** Review the report with the subject of the incident if possible before signing the report and obtaining their signature on a paper form, also if possible. Obtain a supervisor's signature as well on a paper form.
   Principle. Signatures on an incident report indicate that parties involved have been informed of the contents of the report.
7. **Procedural Step.** If you are using SimChart for the medical office, save the report when it is complete. Create a signed paper report as well if it is office policy.

Obtaining Employment

Check out the Evolve site at http://evolve.elsevier.com/Bonewit/today to access additional interactive activities and exercises to help you study and prepare for success.

LEARNING OBJECTIVES

1. Describe the process for locating potential employers when looking for a job.
2. Discuss the steps in preparing a résumé.
3. Describe how to write a cover letter.
4. Differentiate between information placed on a résumé and information required on an employment application.
5. Explain how to provide potential employers with a résumé by mail, using a f ax, or using internet resources.
6. Prepare to answer questions commonly asked in a job interview.
7. Describe measures to prevent job burnout.
8. I dentify two professional organizations to which a medical assistant may belong.
9. Identify benefits of joining a professional organization.
10. Discuss why lifelong learning is vital for a medical assistant after graduation.

CHAPTER OUTLINE

KEY TERMS

burnout
combination résumé
continuing education unit (CEU)
cover letter
networking
résumé
reverse chronological résumé
skills based résumé

INTRODUCTION TO OBTAINING EMPLOYMENT

After graduating from a medical assisting program, most medical assistants must begin the search for their first job. Sometimes, the medical office where the graduate did a practicum asks the student to stay on as an employee. When this happens, it eases the transition from student to employed medical assistant. Because a student cannot count on this, it is important for the new graduate to see the process of learning how to seek employment as just another skill that must be mastered.

Finding a job involves more than simply answering a few online advertisements or responding to one or two help wanted notices on the school's career bulletin board. To find the right job, a medical assisting graduate needs to put time and effort into the job-hunting process.

SUCCESSFUL JOB SEARCH

Successful job hunting has two parts. The first is setting appropriate goals; the second is identifying potential employers where those goals might be met.

SETTING GOALS

Setting goals means identifying the ideal job for a medical assistant's current circumstances. The medical assistant should ask herself or himself the following questions:
- Do I want to work full-time or part-time?
- In what area of the country or region do I want to work?
- Do I want to work in a city? In the suburbs? In the country?
- What are my particular strengths and weaknesses?
- Am I interested in working in a particular medical specialty?
- Do I have a preference about the size of the organization where I would be happy?
- Do I want to specialize in either clinical or administrative duties, or, if possible, do I want to do both?

IDENTIFYING POTENTIAL EMPLOYERS

After a graduate has set goals, it is time to begin identifying potential employers. This is done by viewing online want ads and job boards to see what kinds of positions are being advertised and searching online to see what kinds of medical offices are in the community where the graduate wants to work. Larger institutions often have their own websites with employment opportunities. It is important to read carefully, because a graduate may be eligible for positions with different job titles. Many large organizations post job openings internally first. The graduate should ask family or friends who work in such institutions to keep an eye on the internal posting boards.

Larger institutions also often have personnel or human resource departments that keep files of potential employees to give to providers or department administrators who need to fill a position. When an applicant fills out an application for such a facility, the application will stay on file for a period of time—usually 6 months or 1 year. After that, a new, updated application must be submitted.

Some large institutions hire medical assistants with little experience through an affiliated temporary agency. Although the best temporary workers have significant experience, hiring new graduates as temporary employees does allow an institution to try out a new employee without a long-term commitment. If this is the case, a graduate should learn the name of the temporary agency and seek employment through it.

During the job-hunting period, it is important to set aside some time each day to look for a job. The more opportunities a graduate explores, the better the possibility of not only finding a job, but also finding the right job.

When looking for a job, it is important not to underestimate the importance of **networking**—contacting friends and acquaintances who may know of potential jobs. A personal network may include former instructors, contacts made during the medical assisting practicum, classmates, and even providers the medical assistant knows or has worked with. It is important to develop a habit of maintaining professional contacts. Staying in touch, through either occasional telephone calls, emails, or meeting for coffee or lunch, provides opportunities to gain both support and information. A contact may call in the future when there is an opening at work or when someone has asked for names of potential employees.

Potential employers may use the internet to do research about job applicants; so when the job search begins, a graduate should use a web browser and enter their own name, looking for both websites and images in order to be sure that their online image is professional. Potential employers may look at public information on Facebook, X (formerly Twitter), other social media sites, and blogs. The graduate should be sure that nothing appears that would prevent an employer from granting an interview. For example, a picture showing the graduate at a party, a comment criticizing the school the graduate attended, or even family photographs can create a negative impression. In addition, employers sometimes do credit checks, so it is recommended to review a personal credit history early in the job-hunting process and take steps to correct any errors.

TOOLS FOR A JOB SEARCH

PREPARING A RÉSUMÉ

The primary purpose of a résumé is to obtain an interview for an open position. A **résumé** is a summary of information about a person that describes education, work experience, and other information that employers may find pertinent in deciding whether or not to hire an individual.

A résumé is often important in making a first impression on a potential employer. It must be neat, professional, and informative. A paper résumé looks better if it is printed on high-quality paper. Employers, who often receive several résumés for one position, use the résumé to create a list of people with the desired training and/or experience to call in for personal interviews.

A résumé should describe a medical assistant's education, experience, and skills completely, but not in an exaggerated way. If possible, the résumé should be limited to one typewritten sheet. If the résumé is more than one page, which typically should only occur when a person has an extensive work history, the information that is especially pertinent to the job for which the medical assistant is applying should appear on the first page. If a medical assistant is applying for many different types of positions, it may be desirable to have many variations of a résumé available, each one slanted toward the requirements of certain positions.

Personal information should not be included on a résumé. Information such as marital status, children, and hobbies does not relate to a medical assistant's credentials for a position. If personal information is included, the effect is most likely to be neutral or possibly negative, providing a reason not to grant an interview. For example, the employer may be afraid that a medical assistant with two or more children may need to be absent if the children become ill.

Résumé Styles

In general, there are three styles of résumés: reverse chronological, skills based, and combination.

A **reverse chronological résumé** lists the information with the most recent items first. It contains a list of formal education, with degrees and certificates earned, followed by work experience (although work experience can come before education in this style). This is the most common type of résumé for applicants with limited work experience or those who are seeking work similar to their present work.

A **skills based résumé** categorizes experience according to skills or abilities, some of which may be a result of activities other than paid employment (e.g., volunteer work and unpaid work). A functional résumé is useful for an individual who wants to change from one type of work to a different type of work and wants to highlight how particular skills attained in one line of work can be helpful in the new position for which they are applying.

A **combination résumé** uses elements from the reverse chronological and skills based résumés. This type of résumé is often times used when an applicant has 1–3 years' experience in the field, is changing careers, or has no gaps in their work history. A combination résumé includes a short summary (no longer than two sentences), a list of the individual's skills and abilities, professional experience, and education.

Information to Include

The basic pieces of information needed for a résumé are personal demographics, objective personal statement, education, experience, skills, credentials, and references. A number of computer programs are available for preparing résumés. It used to be common practice to include an objective, but the trend is to replace this with a summary statement. If a computer program or template is used, the medical assistant should be sure to personalize the résumé. It is also helpful to use some sample résumés as guides (Figs. 50.1–50.3). Other samples may be available from the placement office of the graduate's college or medical assisting program, as well as résumé-writing books and websites.

Personal Demographics

Personal demographics include the name, address, telephone number, and email address. This information is usually placed at the top of the résumé. The email address should sound professional. If a graduate has been using an email address such as "partyanimal@server.com" or if their personal email has a link to X or Facebook, they should think about creating a new email account for the job search. The message on the cell phone and/or home phone should sound professional, without a child's voice or pet name. All identifying information should be large enough and in bold enough type to stand out.

Summary Statement

The summary statement is a branding statement that emphasizes skills and accomplishments. Because the résumé will primarily be used to decide if an interview should be scheduled, it is important to match this section to the job requirements. It is acceptable to write a new summary statement for each job application as needed.

Education

The education section includes the institutions attended and degrees or certificates received, with dates. These should be arranged in reverse chronological order (the most recent first). At least one program should be listed with a degree, certificate, or diploma and the year it was received. Usually, the high school diploma is included only if the candidate has no higher credential.

When identifying a school or program, the anticipated graduation date can be included if the résumé is prepared before the medical assistant graduates (e.g., A.S. in Medical Assisting, anticipated June 20XX). After graduation, the résumé should be revised before it is sent to other potential employers.

It is also appropriate to include the grade point average (GPA) if it is above 3.0 and any honors or awards received from the educational institution, such as Dean's List.

Previous Experience

In the section on previous experience, the following are included:

- The job title
- Years of employment
- Employer's name
- The town and state in which the work was performed

Samantha Anderson
2314 May Avenue
Western, OH 44770
Email: S.Anderson@anyserver.com
Mobile: (123) 111-1234

Certified medical assistant with proven time management and collaboration skills developed from a challenging medical assisting practicum, educational experience, and employment. Strong interpersonal skills enhanced by taking part in theatre activities to develop confidence and communication abilities. Understanding of the importance of working as part of a team and developing as a professional. Recent graduate looking for first-time employment in a medical office that provides outstanding patient care.

EDUCATION

Associate in Science, Western Community College, Western, OH **June 2025**

Major: Medical Assisting

STUDENT WORK EXPERIENCE PLACEMENT

MEDICAL ASSISTING PRACTICUM (160 HOURS) WESTERN MEDICAL ASSOCIATES **2025**

- **Patient preparation:** Prepared patients for examination, took vital signs, history and chief complaint.
- **Diagnostic testing:** Performed phlebotomy, throat cultures, rapid strep tests, ECGs, dipstick urinalysis.
- **Electronic health record:** Entered patient information and test results, took telephone messages, updated medication and allergy lists, and prepared medication refills.
- **Front office:** Answered telephones, scheduled appointments, validated insurance coverage.

OTHER EXPERIENCE

Home Health Aide, Medical Home Care, Newtown, OH **2023-2023**

- **Personal Care:** Provided personal care to English and Spanish-speaking patients in their homes.

Cashier, Western Supermarket, Western, OH **2022-2023**

CERTIFICATIONS

Certified Medical Assistant (AAMA): June 2025
BLS Healthcare Provider Level and First Aid

Fig. 50.1 Reverse chronological résumé of a recent graduate.

A new graduate may wish to present information about previous experience in two sections, titled *Related Experience* and *Other Experience.* The medical assisting practicum (practicum) can be included under the heading *Related Experience*, but if the section is titled *Work Experience*, only paid employment should be included. Most employers do not like to see gaps in a work history, which might reflect jobs that the applicant does not wish to acknowledge. If the applicant has been a homemaker, it is recommended to include the years devoted to this under *Other Experience.* Any volunteer work can also be included.

For each position or type of experience, a short summary of responsibilities should be included. If the experience was in health care or medical assisting, more details should be included than for other jobs or experience. For example, more details should be included about specific responsibilities

28 Gillian Street
Western, OH 44770
Email: saychelles@anyserver.com
Mobile: (123) 111-2345

Patricia A. Saychelles

OBJECTIVE

To obtain a challenging position as a medical assistant that will utilize my skills and training

EDUCATION

Certificate in Medical Assisting, Shamrock Institute, Western OH May 2025

Achievements

- **2018:** Attended national meeting of AAMA (American Association of Medical Assistants)
- **2017:** Recognition award for contribution to the local community and volunteering

KEY SKILLS

- Clinical skills
- Administrative skills
- Telephone skills
- Event planning
- Coordinating activities
- Laboratory tests
- Phlebotomy
- ECGs
- Electronic health record

Software Skills: Microsoft Word ~ Microsoft Excel ~ Microsoft Outlook ~ Epic ~ Edge

STUDENT WORK EXPERIENCE PLACEMENTS

Medical Assisting Practicum at Western Medical Associates 2025

COMMUNITY ACTIVITIES

- Chairperson of public library committee responsible for obtaining feedback from local community
- Volunteer for the DARE program at Western Middle School
- Secretary of the Western Women's League 2016-2017 responsible for secretarial duties, keeping the financial records and fund raising

EMPLOYMENT

Package Sorter, United Parcel Service, Western, OH **2019-2020**

Fig. 50.2 Skills based résumé of a woman who stayed home with children for several years before training as a medical assistant.

as a home health aide than as a cashier. Action verbs should be used in the description of previous experience (Fig. 50.4). Any special achievements or projects should be included (e.g., setting up an electronic tickler file in a previous job as a secretary).

When preparing the descriptions of previous experience, the medical assistant should use one of two styles consistently. Either can be written in sentence form or as a list with bullets.

Describing Responsibilities Using Verbs in the Past Tense

Example in sentence form:

Measured vital signs, prepared patients for examination, posted charges and payments, sent monthly bills, etc.

Example in bullet form:

- Measured vital signs
- Prepared patients for examination
- Posted charges and payments
- Sent monthly bills

John Davidson
16 Carriage Way
Western, OH 44770
(123) 111-3455

Energetic health professional with more than ten years of providing professional military and civilian health care, specializing in emergency treatment, supervision of personnel, physical examination, and health awareness training who seeks employment in a fast-paced urgent or emergency care setting.

- Received qualifications from the U.S. Navy as a Medical Assistant (MA), Nursing Assistant (NA), Emergency Medical Technician (EMT), Emergency Vehicle Operator (EVO) and Emergency Medical Dispatcher.
- Able to assist with and supervise personnel assisting with occupational, preventative, and emergent medical examinations, ECGs, and emergency procedures.
- Able to facilitate hospital admission and maintain paper and electronic health records.

EMPLOYMENT

United States Navy

- Hospital Corpsman First Class, Naval Air Station, Harbor Bay, OH 2014-2024
- Hospital Corpsman Second Class, Naval Air Station, Seal Beach, CA 2009-2014

OTHER CREDENTIALS

Instructor: Emergency Medical Technician (EMT-B)
Instructor: American Heart Association BLS
Advanced Life Support (ACLS) provider since 2012

EDUCATION

Attended Western Community College from 2007-2008 taking general education courses and introductory health courses.

Fig. 50.3 Combination résumé of a man who received health care training in the Armed Services.

Describing Responsibilities Using Participle Form of the Verb

Example in sentence form:

Responsible for measuring vital signs, preparing patients for examination, posting charges and payments, and sending monthly bills.

Example in bullet form:

Duties included:

- Measuring vital signs
- Preparing patients for examination
- Posting charges and payments
- Sending monthly bills

Credentials/Professional Affiliations

In the section on credentials and/or professional affiliations, the medical assistant may include certification as a certified medical assistant (CMA [AAMA]), registered medical assistant (RMA), or certified clinical medical assistant (CCMA) and any other certifications or credentials including cardiopulmonary resuscitation (CPR) and/or first aid. Membership in professional organizations, community service organizations, or disaster relief efforts may be included as well. Lists of unrelated activities, hobbies, and interests should not be included on a professional résumé.

References

Traditional résumés always included the following statement: *References will be furnished on request.* This statement is considered optional on a modern résumé because it is assumed to be the case. Actual references are not listed on the résumé because the goal is to be interviewed before the

administer	distribute	process
analyze	document	proofread
arrange	establish	propose
assist	file	purchase
authorize	instruct	reconcile
balance	list	run
calculate	log	schedule
classify	mail	send
code	measure	set up
collect	monitor	sort
compose	order	stock
contact	organize	teach
coordinate	perform	write
copy	post	
develop	prepare	

Fig. 50.4 Action verbs to use on a résumé.

potential employer checks any references. After the interview, the medical assistant provides a list of references with contact information. Before using someone's name as a reference, the medical assistant should be sure to get that person's permission. It is also polite to call individuals whose names have been used so that they can be ready to receive a phone call or written request for a reference.

For references, a medical assistant who has recently graduated should choose a balance of instructors, practicum supervisor, other job supervisors, or coworkers from volunteer activities. It is not recommended to use friends or family for references. Sometimes, the individual who will be used as a reference gives the medical assistant a letter that can be shown to a potential employer. More often, the potential employer contacts the individual given as a reference after interviewing the candidate.

Formatting the Résumé

The résumé should be formatted with at least 1-inch margins. It is important to lay out the résumé so that it looks balanced on the page with clear sections of information. After the résumé has been created, it should be proofread carefully. Spelling and grammar errors are unacceptable. A single spelling or grammar error may prevent a potential employer from offering an interview.

Often, the résumé is sent as an email attachment or is attached to an online job application. If the résumé will be sent through the mail, it should be a printed original, not a photocopy. It makes a good impression if a stationery-weight paper is used, which is slightly heavier than ordinary printer paper. Because medical assistants work in a fairly conservative segment of the job market, it is important to avoid using colored paper, unusual type fonts, or flashy formatting for the résumé.

WRITING A COVER LETTER

A **cover letter** is a letter sent with a résumé that explains briefly why the résumé is being sent. The cover letter clarifies whether the medical assistant is responding to an advertisement, has been referred by another individual, or is simply inquiring about possible job opportunities.

If sent through the mail, the cover letter should use the format for a business letter and should be printed on the same color paper as the résumé. If possible, the medical assistant should call the office to find out the name of the office manager or other individual responsible for hiring medical assistants. If sent online with a résumé, the letter should be addressed to the human resources department.

The letter should begin with the reason for writing the letter and sending the résumé. This should be followed by a brief summary of the position being sought and the candidate's qualifications for filling that position. The final paragraph should be a request for an interview.

Each cover letter should be personalized because this is the first thing the potential employer will see. Of course, it should not contain any grammar or spelling errors. The reader should be referred to the résumé for details (Fig. 50.5).

The medical assistant should keep a copy of all cover letters. The results (interview, second interview, and job offer) can be written on the copy or on a separate log that keeps track of responses to all letters sent out.

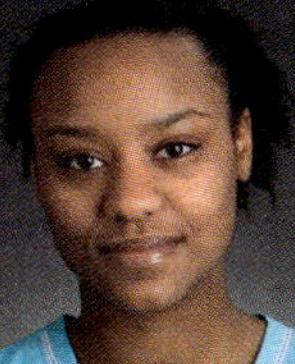

Putting It All Into Practice

My name is Deanna Taylor, and I took the CMA (AAMA) examination in June of the last year that they gave a pen-and-paper examination. During the time that I was waiting for my examination results, I went on six job interviews. I was hired in my present position 3 weeks before I found out that I passed the examination. The combination of searching for my first medical assisting job and hoping that I had passed the certification examination was very stressful. Current graduates are really lucky to take a computerized examination and get a preliminary report the same day, even if potential employers sometimes wait for the official results to hire new grads.

I was looking for a position in obstetrics and gynecology, but I sent a résumé for every medical assisting job that I saw. That turned out to be good because I had a much better idea of what different offices were like, and I became more comfortable in the interview itself. When I first walked through the door of the office that hired me, I felt comfortable. I knew that if I were a patient, I would trust the staff because they were friendly but professional. This office does specialize in obstetrics and gynecology; so I was lucky enough to find exactly the position I had hoped for.

I was interviewed by the medical office manager, a woman who works with several medical offices affiliated with a local hospital. We discussed my experience and the position. Later, she called me back for a second interview to meet with the providers and office staff. After that, she offered me the position. I was very excited, and I have to say that it has turned out very well. Even though I have been here for several years, I am always learning new things because there are so many changes. It seems that there is always a new challenge and something new to learn. ■

2314 May Avenue
Western, OH 44770
September 5, 20XX

Diane Wells, Practice Manager
Medical Practice Associates
525 Main Street
Western, OH 44770

Dear Ms. Wells:

I am sending you a copy of my résumé in response to your advertisement for a medical assistant in the Western Daily Item. As you will be able to see, I have recently completed an Associate's degree in Medical Assisting at Western Community College.

As part of our training, I was placed in an practicum for 160 hours, and I was able to practice the skills that I learned in my training program. I have also passed the national certification exam in medical assisting given by the American Association of Medical Assistants.

I look forward to hearing from you to schedule an interview. I can be reached at (490)111-1555 or at my email address S.Anderson@server.com.

Sincerely,

Susan Anderson, CMA (AAMA)

Fig. 50.5 Sample cover letter.

SENDING THE RÉSUMÉ

It is recommended to send résumés in 9- × 11-inch manila envelopes so that they do not need to be folded. If using a standard No. 10 business envelope, its color and weight should match the paper used for the résumé and cover letter if possible.

Increasingly, it is possible to respond to job openings using the internet or to fax a résumé to an office. A cover letter is still recommended.

The advantage of a faxed or emailed résumé and cover letter is that the material arrives quickly, often within minutes of making a telephone inquiry. The disadvantage is that a fax or a printout of an email does not look as crisp or professional as a mailed résumé and cover letter.

A few days after a mailed résumé should have arrived, a job applicant may call to see if the material did, indeed, arrive. At this time, it is appropriate to ask if the person doing the hiring has an idea about the time frame in which a hiring decision will be made. However, a job applicant should not call again after that, to avoid appearing too aggressive.

FILLING OUT AN EMPLOYMENT APPLICATION

Most medical facilities require a completed job application in addition to a résumé. In large facilities, it may be necessary to complete the application before an interview is scheduled. In smaller offices, the application may be filled out at the time of the interview.

It is important to keep a list of information needed to fill out the job application. This includes the name and address of previous employers, dates of employment, names and telephone numbers of supervisors, as well as the names, addresses, and telephone numbers of references. Any letters of reference should be brought to the interview so that the facility can make copies to attach them to the job application.

The medical assistant should answer all questions fully and truthfully on the application. If filling the application out by hand, the medical assistant should print legibly. All questions should be answered. It is not appropriate to refer the reader to the résumé. If a question does not apply, the medical assistant should write *N/A* or *Not Applicable.*

If the application asks for the reason for leaving a previous position, the medical assistant should avoid making any negative statements about the employer or supervisor. Common reasons for leaving are returning to school, relocation for a spouse's job, end of a temporary position, or exploration of new career options.

Some health care facilities may require applicants for medical assisting positions to take a keyboarding test or other skills test before an interview is granted.

What Would You Do? What Would You *Not* Do?

Case Study 1

Deanna is supervising a medical assisting student named Andrea in her office. Andrea had been working as a cashier at a local supermarket since graduating from high school. She had never been employed in a health care setting. When Andrea wrote her résumé, she was finished with her practicum and her graduation date was only 2 weeks away. She had many responsibilities at the practicum, but there were some skills she had learned in school, such as spirometry, that were not done where she was placed. Andrea tells Deanna, "On my résumé, I put that my practicum was work experience, because I really worked there for several weeks." ■

APPLYING FOR EMPLOYMENT USING THE INTERNET

The medical assistant may use an online employment website to create a résumé, use that résumé to apply for open positions, and also post the résumé on the web for potential employers to view it. The résumé that is created can be saved as a document file and used to post on various websites or to apply for other positions. Many employers also advertise for medical assistants and accept applications using their own websites. When looking for employment, the medical assistant should visit the websites of potential employers, review job postings in several categories, and submit an application online if a suitable position is open. By networking with other students, instructors, and friends, the medical assistant can identify online resources that others have used successfully.

GETTING THE JOB

INTERVIEW TECHNIQUES

An employment interview provides a potential employer with an opportunity to assess a candidate's interpersonal and communication skills and preparation for a position in the medical setting. The interview also provides the medical assistant with a chance to assess the potential employer. The questions asked, the flow of the discussion, and the tour of the facility help the medical assistant decide whether the position fits appropriately with their work style and personality.

For a job to be offered, the medical assistant must do well in the interview. Often, a candidate whose skills appear excellent on paper does not create a positive impression during the interview. The key for the employer is to find the person who seems to be the best fit for the position.

It is important for a medical assistant to accept any job interview offered, even if the position does not seem ideal. The more interviews a new graduate goes on, the more comfortable the job interview process becomes. It is not appropriate, however, to accept more job interviews after a position has been accepted.

Preparing for the Interview

Before the interview, the medical assistant should try to find out as much as possible about the medical office or facility. Information can be obtained by talking to someone who works there or a patient of the office, if possible. The medical assistant should ask friends and other contacts if they know anyone with information about the potential employer.

Many medical offices have a website that describes the practice. The medical assistant should enter the name of the medical office and/or providers(s) into a search engine. If the medical office has a website, it will probably include the names of the providers and other practitioners, the philosophy of the medical office, and other background information. If the office is small, it may only be possible to locate telephone and address information. This may indicate that the office is not using as much modern technology as some other offices.

When the interview is arranged, the medical assistant should find out whether one person or a committee will conduct the interview, and if one person, the name and position of the individual.

The medical assistant should ask if there are any particular things that the interviewer(s) would like to know and if any background materials should be brought to the interview.

Appearance and Behavior

As always, a professional appearance is important. A male medical assistant should wear professional clothing including dress slacks and dress shirt with a tie. A female medical assistant should wear professional clothing, such as a blouse and skirt or dress slacks. Denim skirts, denim jeans, shorts, and mid-calf pants are not appropriate for an interview. Long hair should be worn pulled back and off the collar, as it would be when working as a medical assistant. It is recommended to avoid bulky jewelry, avoid false nails and visible piercings, and present a tailored appearance (Fig. 50.6). Visible tattoos should be covered, if possible. For an interview, the medical assistant should avoid sandals or athletic shoes and never wear flip-flops. Hair, including any facial hair, should be clean and neatly trimmed.

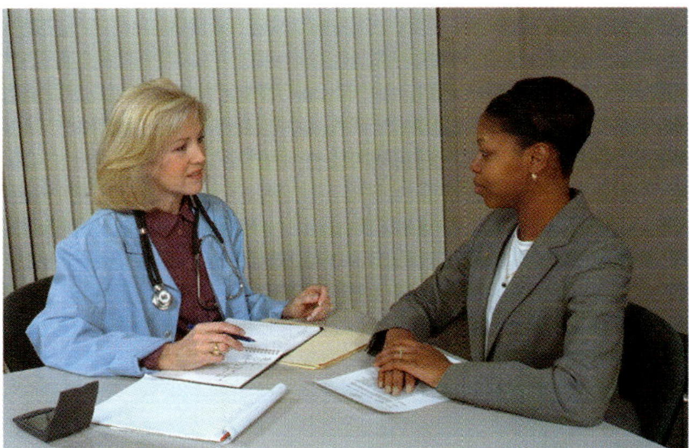

Fig. 50.6 At a job interview, the medical assistant should look and act in a professional manner.

It is important to maintain good posture and look alert during the interview. The medical assistant should sit comfortably without slouching and avoid fidgeting or displaying nervous habits. At the same time, the medical assistant presents a better impression if they are relaxed and natural instead of reserved and stiff. The interviewer is looking for an individual who interacts well with patients and can make them feel at ease. If a job applicant smiles and makes conversation easily during an interview, it is likely that they will be comfortable with patients. A job applicant should never chew gum during an interview. Before the interview, the applicant should turn off their cell phone. It is useful to have a pen and notepad handy to make notes. It is also helpful to write down questions that might be encountered in future interviews, to practice answers before the next interview.

Questions That the Interviewer Should Not Ask

Interviewers are not supposed to ask questions that do not relate to the position, including marital status, number of children, and age (unless there is a legal age requirement as part of the job). Various federal and state laws regulate these questions. The 1964 Civil Rights Act prohibits discrimination based on race, sex, color, national origin, and religion. The Age Discrimination in Employment Act prohibits questions about a person's age. The Americans with Disabilities Act of 1990 protects qualified individuals with disabilities from discrimination in employment. If the interviewer asks an illegal question, the medical assistant should try to identify or respond to the underlying concern without directly refusing to answer the question. Example:

Interviewer: "Are you a United States citizen?"

Applicant: "Are you asking whether I am authorized to work in the United States?"

What Would You Do? What Would You *Not* Do?

Case Study 2

When she was looking for a job, Deanna got lost on the way to an interview. The office was located about 30 minutes from her home. Deanna had allowed plenty of travel time, but she took the wrong turn off the highway and didn't realize it until she had gone almost 10 miles in the wrong direction. When she realized she was lost, she knew that backtracking would make her at least 15 minutes late. ■

Discussing Salary and Benefits

Specific salary is usually not discussed until a job is offered. But it is common for a salary range to be discussed. If the interviewer does not state the salary range, it is acceptable to ask about it as the interview is winding down. Asking about the salary range early in the interview may give the impression that money is the most important thing about the job. Failing to ask about a salary range may be interpreted as lack of interest.

It is also appropriate to ask a general question about benefits, such as how long an employee must work before becoming eligible for the benefits package and if health insurance is a benefit. It is customary not to ask specifically about vacation, sick days, and personal days until a job offer has been made.

When a position is offered, a discussion of salary and benefits helps the medical assistant make a decision about whether or not to accept the position. If the salary seems low or is less than that the medical assistant currently earns, it is appropriate to ask about the specific time frame when performance will be reviewed and a raise will be possible.

Often, especially in larger facilities with rigid salary structures, a position is limited to a particular salary range. It is important to be sure that the salary is adequate to meet expenses before accepting the position. Usually, an applicant can ask for 24–48 hours to consider a job offer.

Asking Questions

A good interviewer will ask a candidate at the end of the interview if they have any questions. The medical assistant may ask about who supervises the position, may ask the interviewer to clarify the job responsibilities, and/or may ask about the availability of training programs in-house or financial support for outside training or college courses. It is helpful to come to the interview with three or four written questions. If these were answered during the interview, the medical assistant can look over the list and say that it seems as though all their questions have been answered.

Determining the Timeline for Filling the Position

If the interviewer or lead interviewer on a committee does not state the employer's time frame for making a decision about filling the position, this is an important question to ask. Employers know that people must seek employment at many facilities, and most are willing to get back to applicants who have been interviewed within a few days.

FOLLOW-UP AFTER AN INTERVIEW

Although it may seem old-fashioned to write a written thank-you note after a job interview, most potential employers will be favorably impressed by this courtesy. It also provides an opportunity to include any additional information requested at the interview. See Fig. 50.7 for a sample follow-up letter.

If the interviewer has not responded by the date expected, the medical assistant may telephone to ask if the position has been filled.

LIFELONG LEARNING

The field of health care is becoming more complex all the time. It is important for every member of the health care team to improve their skills constantly and stay up to date on new techniques in their field. To provide high-quality patient care, every member of the health care team must engage in lifelong learning.

HIGHLIGHT on Responding to Questions

On the basis of previous experience at interviews and suggestions from friends about their experiences, the medical assistant should try to prepare for questions the interviewer(s) will ask. Although it may seem awkward, it is helpful to practice answering sample interview questions out loud with friends, family, or a roommate. Several common interview questions and potential answers are presented in the following discussion.

1. What can I tell you about my organization?
   It is always important to have questions prepared. The medical assistant might ask about the history of the office or clinic and/or how long it has been in its present location. They should have found out how many providers work there and what specialties are represented but could ask how many medical assistants are employed.
2. What was your favorite subject in school?
   The answer is more powerful if it demonstrates enthusiasm and has some relation to the position being applied for. Math, English, science, computer courses, and medical assisting courses are good answers. If a job applicant says that poetry was her favorite subject, the interviewer may wonder if medical assisting is the applicant's real interest.
3. Why did you choose to study medical assisting?
   People who choose this field are usually interested in health, like people, like a job where they can be active, and believe that preventive care and early diagnosis are important components of health. This question also gives the medical assistant an opportunity to demonstrate enthusiasm and caring.
4. What courses did you like least in school?
   It is better for the medical assistant to name one course and describe it as "difficult" or "challenging" (even if that does not directly respond to the question) instead of giving a long list of subjects that were boring. It is important to avoid looking like an individual who is uninterested in subjects that may relate to the job and also to avoid complaining or speaking negatively.
5. What campus activities did you participate in? What did you learn from them?
   The medical assistant can prepare by thinking of an interesting extracurricular activity they have participated in, even if there was not time to be a member of any club or organized activity in school. If the medical assistant worked for several hours while going to school, they might say so while identifying a hobby: "I worked as a cashier several hours a week to help pay for school, so I had to leave school right after class. But I'm working with a classmate to arrange for some of our graduates to get together monthly because I think that it would be too bad to lose contact with the friends I made in school."
6. Describe your responsibilities when you worked for XYZ Company.
   The medical assistant should identify their responsibilities, being sure to emphasize any special projects, promotions, or leadership roles. A medical assistant often has a part-time job while going to school, with some extra responsibility, such as opening or closing, training new employees, or rotating to different departments. If handling money was a job responsibility, it should be mentioned because it indicates reliability.
7. What types of problems have you encountered in your jobs? How did you handle them?
   The medical assistant should describe a problem that they experienced that might occur in any office setting, such as an angry or unsatisfied customer, telephones ringing off the hook, work backing up, and being overwhelmed at first. When discussing the problem, it is important to explain how the problem-solving process was applied to resolve the problem.
8. What would your instructors or previous supervisors tell me about you if I were to call them?
   The medical assistant should identify their positive attributes and practice saying them calmly, even if it seems like bragging. "They would say that I work hard," "I am organized," "I catch on quickly," "I'm good with people," and "I try hard to be accurate" are some examples. In an effective interview, the job applicant puts their best foot forward without exaggerating or distorting the truth.
9. What are some of your weaknesses or areas you need to work on?
   The medical assistant should think carefully about weaknesses that may be seen in some lights as positive, or weaknesses that everyone is subject to. Being a perfectionist, not liking to miss work for illness, and double-checking all work to be sure it is correct are examples of weaknesses that employers usually like. Being nervous in a new situation, becoming frustrated when there isn't enough time, and hating to see others sitting around when there is much work to do are traits common to many people. If a medical assistant is shy and reserved, this is a good opportunity to state that they are not always outgoing in new situations, but that it doesn't take very long to feel comfortable and open up more.
10. What are your long-term goals? or Where do you plan to be in 5 years?
    The prospective employer is trying to get a sense of how long the applicant plans to stay in the position if hired. In many areas, turnover of medical assistants is rapid, but an employer would like to be able to count on at least 2 years. If the medical assistant will be returning to school within 6 months, they should say so and identify whether part-time work would be possible at that time. ■

2314 May Avenue
Western, OH 44770
September 18, 20XX

Diane Wells, Practice Manager
Medical Practice Associates
525 Main Street
Western, OH 44770

Dear Ms. Wells:

Thank you for the opportunity to interview with you last week for the position of medical assistant. It is clear that your practice provides high quality care to patients. After meeting with you, I know that I would be glad for the opportunity to join your team.

I look forward to hearing from you about this opportunity. Please feel free to contact me at (490) 111-1555 or by email (S.Anderson@anyserver.com) if you have any questions. Thank you again for your time and consideration.

Sincerely,

Susan Anderson, CMA (AAMA)

Fig. 50.7 Sample letter after an interview.

STAYING CURRENT

Medical assistants must keep their skills current. This means keeping abreast of new techniques, as well as learning how to use the latest technology.

Administrative Skills

On the administrative side, computer software is constantly being updated. This includes operating systems and all programs used routinely in the medical office. Training to use updated versions of operating systems, word processing programs, electronic health records, or other general programs is often available online or through classes. If the office switches to an updated version of office management programs or an electronic health record, the software company often provides training for office personnel.

Another area that requires constant updating relates to changes in coding and insurance claim submission. The medical assistant should read updates and attend classes as needed to keep skills current.

Clinical Skills

On the clinical side, it is important to learn to use new diagnostic or laboratory equipment. When a new piece of equipment is purchased, training should be arranged for all staff who will use it. The medical assistant must also stay current on new medications. Pharmaceutical representatives leave informational materials for the provider, and the medical assistant should make a point of reading this information.

Preparing for Increased Responsibility

The medical assistant may be trained to assist with special procedures. The medical assistant may be sent to an outside training program at office expense, or the provider or other staff member may provide the training. It is important to pay close attention during the training and take notes to be sure that all information is retained.

The medical assistant may also be given some responsibility to supervise other staff members. Classes or workshops in supervision, appraisal, conflict management, or other subjects may be helpful to ease this transition.

AVOIDING BURNOUT

Burnout is a constant worry, especially for those in repetitive, high-stress jobs. **Burnout** is a term that has come to mean disillusionment with work and physical or emotional exhaustion. It is characterized by a loss of interest or enthusiasm and energy about work.

A person experiencing burnout may exhibit behavioral changes as well, including increased irritability, inability to empathize with patients, chronic fatigue, and poor relations with coworkers. Job burnout can be a precipitator for clinical depression and must be dealt with as a medical issue rather than a disciplinary problem.

Loss of enthusiasm at work may also result from factors outside the job. If an individual's life is out of balance, or if the individual is having problems with relationships within the family, they may not have the necessary energy to expend at work. This may appear as depression or burnout.

If a medical assistant arrives at the point where job burnout is a concern, it is important to take action. If possible, the medical assistant should reduce the hours of work, even if only for a 3- or 6-month period. Increased social activities, increased exercise, and focusing on physical and mental health can foster a more positive physical and emotional state. The medical assistant should try to find a hobby to help "decompress" from work.

Sometimes, burnout is not recognized until the problems have progressed to such a degree that professional intervention is necessary. The individual with severe burnout may need counseling, therapy, or a job change; and if the individual has developed a substance abuse problem, they may even need inpatient rehabilitation. Many large facilities have in-house employee counseling.

What Would You Do? What Would You *Not* Do?

Case Study 3

After 6 months at the obstetrics and gynecology office where she was first hired, Deanna began to wish that she had more contact with other medical assistants to discuss job-related issues. The other medical assistants in her office seemed to be busy with their families, and they didn't socialize at all after work. Deanna wished that she knew more about new trends, new medications, and new technology. She had joined the American Association of Medical Assistants (AAMA) when she graduated, but there didn't seem to be an active chapter in her area. ■

PROFESSIONAL ORGANIZATIONS AND PEER SUPPORT

The AAMA and the AMT are professional organizations for medical assistants. Even if a medical assistant has not obtained certification, they can become a member of an active chapter of one of these organizations. Through local and national meetings and workshops, medical assistants are able to enter a network of peers with whom they can share and from whom they can learn. They can also obtain insurance at reasonable cost, professional journals, and other sources of information important to the profession.

For an annual membership fee, many benefits are available, including the following:

- Peer support
- Continuing education programs
- Legislative advocacy on issues important to medical assistants
- Publications and/or newsletters with information related to the profession of medical assisting

Legislation Affecting Medical Assistants

Professional organizations can advocate for pending state and federal legislation that may affect the medical assisting profession. Changes in legislation require actions by many people. In some states, issues for medical assistants arise from actions taken by other professionals to define legally who may perform certain procedures. As a result of such actions, medical assistants may not take radiographs in most states, and they may not be permitted to administer injections or draw blood, depending on the state.

A future task for the medical assisting profession will be to organize and help draft legislation, giving medical assistants the right to perform in the workplace all skills for which they have been trained. This can best be accomplished by working with the national professional organizations and their state chapters.

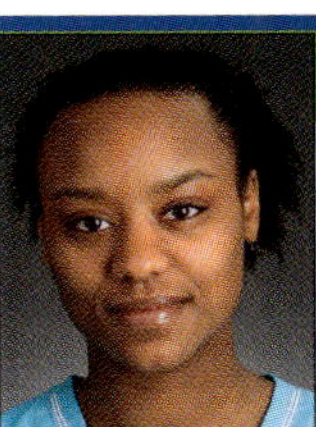

Memories *from* Practicum

Deanna Taylor: The biggest difference between a practicum and employment is that it takes more effort to stay enthusiastic about showing up every day. When I was doing my practicum, everything was new. I was always excited to go because it seemed like there was a new experience every day. Now that I have been working for several years, there are many days that seem very routine. There are new experiences, but I have to remind myself to notice them. One way that I have found to stay fresh and focused is to volunteer to be on committees to gather information or to plan the implementation of new equipment or new software. For example, I took a course and attended seminars to prepare for the transition to the ICD-10, and I worked with a committee to facilitate the changeover. I also have been taking a general business course at night for the past month. I notice things at work that I never would have before, and I am now planning to take more courses in health administration or business administration. When I was in school, all I could think of was graduating and getting a job, but now that I am a medical assistant, I realize that my career is just beginning. I realize that I am personally responsible to find a way to keep my career rewarding and satisfying. ■

CONTINUING EDUCATION UNITS

A **continuing education unit (CEU)** is a standard measure of qualified instruction as defined by a specific profession. Most health professions require a certain amount of continuing education for licensure or certification renewal. If a medical assistant has obtained national certification, it is important to validate continuing education so that the certification can be renewed. CEUs or contact hours of instruction are required for recertification as a CMA (AAMA) or RMA. The medical assistant should keep a file with the paperwork acknowledging attendance at classes or workshops, together with the CEU credits or contact hours approved for them. With the constant change in the medical field, it is not merely important but necessary to keep skills up to date, attain new skills, and obtain new information about professional practices.

Medical assisting contact hours and CEUs can be obtained from education programs that have been approved by the particular certifying agency. These education programs may be given through the state and national organization, through other educational institutions, or through home or online study programs.

PLANNING FOR JOB ADVANCEMENT OR CAREER CHANGE

One of the best ways to avoid job burnout is to chart a course of career advancement.

ADVANCING TO MANAGEMENT

If a medical assistant enjoys the administrative part of medical assisting, there are many opportunities to find a management position within the health care industry.

The larger the facility, the more the administrative and management tasks are broken into discrete parts, and the more management and administrative staff are in demand.

If a medical assistant is currently working in such a facility and would like to move up the management ladder, they should ask about the possibility of rotating through the various departments to gain experience in finance, billing, marketing, public relations, or any other department. If the medical assistant is working at a small facility or private medical office, they should take the opportunity to learn about every job within the medical office. This makes the medical assistant more versatile and more valuable as an employee. After gaining supervisory experience in a smaller facility, the medical assistant may wish to move to a larger facility.

Business courses or formal education in health administration is invaluable. A number of colleges have both bachelor's and master's degree programs in health care administration. A degree in public administration or business management would also be appropriate.

UPGRADING TECHNICAL AND CLINICAL SKILLS

To advance to a position of greater responsibility on the clinical side, it will probably be necessary to obtain more formal education. After a few years of experience, a medical assistant who wishes to remain in an outpatient setting might consider enrolling in a formal education program to become a nurse practitioner, physician's assistant, a registered nurse, a medical technologist, or an x-ray technologist.

The opportunities become broader if a medical assistant wishes to work in a hospital or rehabilitation center. The medical assistant should talk to various health professionals and explore several potential career options. Obtaining financial support for additional education may be a concern. The medical assistant must decide if financial support is available to pursue further education full time. For most candidates, it will be necessary to continue working either part time or full time at their present positions. Many employers encourage education and pay all or part of an employee's education costs.

TRANSFERRING SKILLS

Over time, the medical assistant may have built up skills that would make it possible to find a position in a field such as computers, insurance, the pharmaceutical industry, or medical equipment sales. If a medical assistant develops a strong interest in one of these areas, they should develop contacts, gather information, and develop a strategy for making a lateral career move.

This discussion would also not be complete without a word about the enormous rewards that can come from teaching—transferring knowledge and abilities to others who would like to become medical assistants.

With a medical assisting degree or certificate, a certified medical assistant may be able to get some work teaching a specific class related to medical assisting skills. A medical assistant who is interested in teaching should speak to the director of the program where they trained about teaching opportunities.

To teach full time, in addition to maintaining certification, the medical assistant should obtain a bachelor's degree and master's degree in a health care field, or in education. Depending on the financial resources available from a spouse or partner's income, family assistance, or scholarships and loans available, this may be as a part-time or full-time student.

What Would You Do? What Would You *Not* Do? RESPONSES

Case Study 1

Page 1261

What Did Deanna Do?

- ❑ Reminded Andrea that employers usually consider work experience to include only paid positions.
- ❑ Pointed out tactfully that putting the practicum in the category of work experience might indicate unreliability or lack of knowledge to a potential employer.
- ❑ Advised Andrea to include the practicum in a section on the résumé called *Related Experience.*
- ❑ Offered to look over Andrea's résumé to see if she could make other helpful suggestions.

What Did Deanna Not Do?

- ❑ Did not tell Andrea that she was being dishonest when she listed the practicum as work experience.
- ❑ Did not make a discouraging remark such as, "That won't help you get hired."

Case Study 2

Page 1262

What Did Deanna Do?

- ❑ Made sure to take with her the name and telephone number of the person with whom she was going to interview.
- ❑ When Deanna realized that she was lost, she called the individual with whom she was scheduled to interview, explained the situation, apologized, and asked if it would be better to come late or reschedule.
- ❑ At the same time, Deanna asked for directions.
- ❑ Resolved always to get very clear directions before any other interview.

What Did Deanna Not Do?

- ❑ Did not show up 15 minutes late without making every effort to contact the individual with whom she was supposed to interview.
- ❑ Did not blame any individual for giving bad directions or failing to give directions.
- ❑ Did not act like being 15 minutes late was really not important.

Case Study 3

Page 1265

What Did Deanna Do?

- ❑ Found out where there were chapters of the AAMA in her state and made a point of attending a meeting. Also, she looked into attending the national meeting of the organization.
- ❑ Asked the medical office manager if there were any continuing education programs at the local hospital that she could attend.
- ❑ Contacted graduates from her medical assisting program and arranged to get together with graduates with whom she had been friends when she was in school.
- ❑ Looked into the possibility of establishing a local chapter of the AAMA and tried to find one or two other medical assistants who might be interested in helping her.
- ❑ Looked at course offerings at the local community college to see if there were any courses or continuing education programs that she might be interested in attending.

What Did Deanna Not Do?

- ❑ Did not avoid taking responsibility for her own needs.
- ❑ Did not make excuses for putting off the process of seeking helpful contacts.
- ❑ Did not avoid reaching out to other medical assistants.

TERMINOLOGY REVIEW

Key Term	Definition
Burnout	Disillusionment with work and physical or emotional exhaustion.
Combination résumé	A résumé that uses elements from both the reverse chronological and skills based résumé. Most useful for someone with 1–3 years' experience, changing careers, or has no gaps in the work history.
Continuing education unit (CEU)	A standard measure of qualified instruction or contact hours as defined by a specific profession.
Cover letter	A letter sent with one or more documents (such as a résumé) to provide an explanation.
Networking	Contacting acquaintances and their contacts who may know of potential jobs.
Résumé	A summary of information about a person that describes education, work experience, and other information related to an individual's suitability for employment.
Reverse chronological résumé	A résumé that lists the information with the most recent items first in categories such as formal education, and work experience.
Skills based résumé	A résumé that organizes experience according to skills or abilities.

Glossary

A

ABA routing number A nine-digit number that identifies a bank; the number is printed at the beginning of the magnetic ink character recognition (MICR) line at the bottom of a check. It also appears in fractional form at the top right of the check under the check number.

Abandonment Failure to continue to provide medical care to a patient without proper notification.

Abortion The termination of the pregnancy before the fetus reaches the age of viability (20 weeks).

Abrasion A wound in which the outer layers of the skin are damaged; a scrape.

Abscess A collection of pus in a cavity surrounded by inflamed tissue.

Absorbable suture Suture material that is gradually digested and absorbed by the body.

Absorption The passage of digestive end products from the gastrointestinal tract into the blood or lymph.

Accommodation Mechanism that allows the eye to focus at various distances, primarily achieved by changing the curvature of the lens.

Account aging The process of finding out how long specific account balances have been outstanding.

Accounting Systematic recording and reporting of financial transactions.

Accounts payable The outstanding bills of a business, such as a medical office.

Accounts receivable Total amount owed to a business for goods and services.

Accreditation Credit or recognition from a regional or national organization for maintaining certain standards.

Accrual basis of accounting Accounting method in which income is entered at the time of sale or provision of service.

Acetylcholine A neurotransmitter at the neuromuscular junction.

Acetylcholinesterase An enzyme that inactivates acetylcholine.

Acronym A word formed from the first letters in a name. Written in upper case letters.

Act A bill or measure that has become law. Often refers to legislation with several parts.

Action potential A nerve impulse; a rapid change in membrane potential that involves depolarization and repolarization.

Active listening Paying close attention to a speaker without thinking of anything else.

Active transport Process that moves substances across or through a membrane and requires cellular energy.

Acute illness An illness characterized by symptoms that have a sudden and rapid onset, are usually severe and intense and subsides after a relatively short time.

Acute infection An infection that develops suddenly and lasts for a short period of time.

Added sugars Sugar and syrups that are added to food and beverages at home or during the commercial preparation of food.

Adenohypophysis Anterior portion of the pituitary gland; the gland that sits below the brain.

Adjustment A change to a patient account that is neither a charge nor a payment.

Adolescent An individual 12 to 18 years old.

Advanced Beneficiary Notice (ABN) A written notification to a patient with original Medicare that a covered service must be paid for by the patient if Medicare denies the claim as medically unnecessary.

Adventitious sounds Abnormal breath sounds.

Adverse reaction An unintended and undesirable effect produced by a drug.

Advocate A person who intercedes on another person's behalf.

Aerobe A microorganism that needs oxygen to live and grow.

Afebrile Without fever; the body temperature is normal.

Agglutination Clumping of blood cells.

Agranulocytes White blood cells that lack granules in the cytoplasm.

Allergen A substance that is capable of causing an allergic reaction.

Allergy An abnormal hypersensitivity of the body to substances that are ordinarily harmless.

Alveoli Thin-walled air sacs of the lungs in which the exchange of oxygen and carbon dioxide takes place.

Ambulation Walking or moving from one place to another.

Ambulatory Able to walk as opposed to being confined to bed or a wheelchair.

Ambulatory care Medical care that is provided on an outpatient basis. The patient is able to come to the facility providing care and return home after receiving services.

Ameboid movement Movement used by leukocytes that permits them to propel themselves from the capillaries into the tissues.

Amenorrhea The absence or cessation of the menstrual period. Amenorrhea occurs normally before puberty, during pregnancy, and after menopause.

Amphiarthrosis (*pl.*, amphiarthroses) A slightly movable joint.

Amplitude Refers to amount, extent, size, abundance, or fullness.

Ampule A small sealed glass container that holds a single dose of medication.

Anaerobe A microorganism that grows best in the absence of oxygen.

Analyte A body substance that is being identified or measured in a laboratory test.

Anaphylactic reaction A serious allergic reaction that can be life-threatening and requires immediate treatment.

Anatomic position Standard reference position for the body.

Androgens Steroid hormones that promote male characteristics.

Anemia A condition in which there is a decrease in the number of erythrocytes or amount of hemoglobin in the blood.

Anisocytosis A variation in the size of red blood cells.

Annotate To underline or highlight important words and phrases in correspondence.

Antagonist A muscle that has an action opposite to that of the prime mover.

Antecubital space The surface of the arm in front of the elbow.

Antibody A substances that is capable of combining with an antigen resulting in an antigen–antibody reaction.

Antibody-mediated immunity Immunity that is the result of B-cell action and the production of antibodies; also called humoral immunity.

Anticoagulant A substance that inhibits blood clotting.

Antigen A substances capable of stimulating the formation of antibodies.

Antioxidant A molecule that inhibits the oxidation of other molecules.

Antipyretic An agent that reduces fever.

Antiseptic An agent that inhibits the growth or kills microorganisms.

Anuria Failure of the kidneys to produce urine.

Anxiety A vague, unpleasant emotion of fear or dread often accompanied by restlessness or nervousness.

Aorta The major trunk of the arterial system of the body. The aorta arises from the upper surface of the left ventricle.

Apnea The temporary cessation of breathing.

Aponeurosis A broad flat sheet of connective tissue that connects one muscle to another.

App A specialized program, often small enough to run on a mobile device.

Appendicular skeleton Bones that are attached to the body; those of the upper and lower extremities.

Application software Software designed to accomplish a specific task (e.g., word processing); also called application program and software program.

Appointment matrix Basic pattern of available appointment times.

Appositional growth Growth resulting from material being deposited on the surface, such as the growth in diameter of long bones.

Approximation The process of bringing two parts, such as tissue, together through the use of sutures or other means.

Arbitration A formal process whereby the parties to a dispute agree to submit to the decision of a neutral party.

Arrector pili Muscle associated with hair follicles.

Articular cartilage Thin layer of hyaline cartilage that covers the ends of long bones in joints.

Articulation A joint; area of contact between two bones.

Artifact Additional electrical activity picked up by the electrocardiograph that interferes with the normal appearance of the electrocardiographic cycles.

Asepsis Free from infection. See *Medial asepsis and Surgical asepsis.*

Assets In accounting, a combination of property owned and money owed to a business.

Assignment of benefits Authorization for insurance reimbursement to be made to the provider of a health service rather than the insured individual.

Astigmatism A refractive error that causes distorted and blurred vision for both near and far objects due to a cornea that is oval shaped.

Atherosclerosis Buildup of fibrous plaques of fatty deposits and cholesterol on the inner walls of an artery that causes narrowing, obstruction, and hardening of the artery.

Atria (singular atrium) Thin-walled chambers of the heart that receive blood from veins.

Atrioventricular (AV) valve Valve between an atrium and a ventricle in the heart.

Attending provider The provider responsible for the care of a hospitalized patient.

Atypical Deviation from the normal.

Audiologist A licensed health care professional who evaluates, diagnoses, treats, and manages hearing loss and balance disorders in adults and children.

Audiometer An instrument used to measure hearing acuity.

Auscultation The process of listening to the sounds produced within the body to detect signs of disease.

Autoclave An apparatus for the sterilization of materials, using steam under pressure.

Autonomy Ability to make independent decisions without constraint or coercion by others.

Axial skeleton Bones of the head, neck, and trunk.

Axilla The area under the shoulder or armpit.

Axon The single efferent process of a neuron that carries impulses away from the cell body.

B

Bacilli (*sing.*, bacillus) Bacteria that have a rod shape.

Back order A term used for items ordered that cannot be shipped immediately, usually because they are out of stock.

Backup A duplicate copy of a program or data kept for reference in case the original is damaged, lost, or destroyed.

Bandage A strip of woven material used to wrap or cover a part of the body.

Bankruptcy Legal process by which the debts of an individual or business are resolved if they cannot be paid.

Barcode clear zone The area on the lower-right-hand corner of a card or letter that is left clear for the postal bar code to be printed.
Bariatrics The branch of medicine that deals with the treatment and control of obesity and diseases associated with obesity.
Barrier protection A physical barrier that protects against infection.
Basal ganglia Paired regions of gray matter located within the white matter of the cerebrum.
Baseline The flat horizontal line that separates the various waves of the ECG cycle.
Beneficence Acting in the best possible way; performing good deeds.
Beneficiary A person who can receive benefits under an insurance plan.
Benefit Payment for a covered service under a health insurance plan.
Bilirubin An orange-colored bile pigment that is a by-product of heme destruction from the hemoglobin molecule.
Bilirubinuria The presence of bilirubin in the urine.
Biopsy The surgical removal and examination of tissue from the living body. Biopsies are typically performed to determine whether a tumor is benign or malignant.
Bladder catheterization The passing of a sterile catheter through the urethra and into the bladder to remove urine.
Blocked Times in the appointment schedule when providers are not available to see patients.
Bloodborne disease Any disease caused by a pathogen that is carried in blood and spread through contact with blood.
Bloodborne pathogens Pathogenic microorganisms present in human blood that can cause disease in humans.
Blood chemistry testing Testing that involves the quantitative measurement of chemical substances dissolved in the plasma of the blood.
Blood pressure The pressure or force exerted by the circulating blood on the walls of the arteries.
Body language Communication that is expressed through facial expressions, body position, muscle activity, and other nonverbal means.
Body mechanics The use of the correct muscles to maintain proper balance, posture, and body alignment to accomplish a task safely and efficiently without undue strain on any muscle or joint.
Bookkeeping The process of keeping detailed records of financial transactions.
Bounding pulse A pulse with an increased volume that feels very strong and full.
Brace An orthopedic device used to support and hold a part of the body in the correct position to allow functioning of the body part while healing takes place.
Bradycardia An abnormally slow heart rate (less than 60 beats per minute).
Bradypnea An abnormal decrease in the respiratory rate of less than 12 respirations per minute.
Brain stem The portion of the brain between the diencephalon and spinal cord that contains the midbrain, pons, and medulla oblongata.
Braxton Hicks contractions Intermittent and irregular painless uterine contractions that occur throughout pregnancy. They occur more frequently toward the end of pregnancy and are sometimes mistaken for true labor pains.
Broadband A method of transmitting electronic data that handles a wide range of frequencies.
Bronchi The airways that are formed when the trachea branches.
Bronchial tree The bronchi and all their branches that function as passageways between the trachea and the alveoli.
Buffy coat A thin, light-colored layer of white blood cells and platelets that lies between a top layer of plasma and a bottom layer of red blood cells when an anticoagulant has been added to a blood specimen.
Bulbus oculi The eyeball.
Burn An injury to the tissues caused by exposure to thermal, chemical, electrical, or radioactive agents.
Burnout Disillusionment with work and physical or emotional exhaustion.

C

Calibration A mechanism to check the precision and accuracy of an automated analyzer to determine if the system is providing accurate results. Calibration is typically performed using a calibration device, often called a *standard*.
Call-in times Blocks of time when a provider accepts telephone calls from patients.
Canthus The junction of the eyelids at either corner of the eye.
Capillary action The action that causes liquid to rise along a wick, a tube, or a gauze dressing.
Capitation A method of paying for insurance in which a fixed amount is paid to the provider per member for a specific time period regardless of the amount of care provided.
Cardiac cycle One complete heartbeat.
Cash basis of accounting Accounting method in which income is entered when payment is received.
Cashier's check A check drawn on a bank instead of an individual account.
Cast A stiff cylindrical casing that is used to immobilize a body part until healing occurs.
Cell-mediated immunity Immunity that is the result of T-cell action.
Celsius scale A temperature scale on which the freezing point of water is 0° and the boiling point of water is 100°; also called the centigrade scale.
Central sulcus The groove or furrow between the frontal and parietal lobes of the cerebrum; also called the fissure of Rolando.
Cerebellum Second largest part of the human brain, located posterior to the pons and medulla oblongata and involved in the coordination of muscular movements.

Cerebrospinal fluid A fluid, similar to plasma, that fills the subarachnoid space around the brain and spinal cord and fills the ventricles of the brain.

Cerebrum The largest and uppermost part of the human brain; concerned with consciousness, learning, memory, sensations, and voluntary movements.

Certified check A check on an individual account for which a bank assumes responsibility, usually by withdrawing funds to cover the check from the checking account at the time the check is certified.

Cerumen A yellowish waxy substance secreted by glands in the ear canal which functions to lubricate and protect the ear canal. Ear wax.

Ceruminous gland A gland in the ear canal that produces cerumen or ear wax.

Cervix The lower narrow end of the uterus that opens into the vagina.

CHAMPVA A government health insurance program that covers dependents of military veterans with service-connected disabilities. The acronym stands for Civilian Health And Medical Program of the department of Veterans' Affairs.

Chemoreceptor A sensory receptor that detects the presence of chemicals; responsible for taste, smell, and monitoring of the concentration of certain chemicals in body fluids.

Chief complaint A statement of the most important symptom or symptoms for which a patient is seeking care.

Cholesterol A white waxy, fatlike substance that is essential for normal functioning of the body.

Chondrocyte Cartilage cell.

Chronic Existing over a long period of time.

Chronic illness An illness characterized by symptoms that persist for longer than six months and show little change or many worsen over time.

Chronic infection An infection that develops slowly and may worsen over an extended period of time.

Chyme The semifluid mixture of food and gastric juice that leaves the stomach through the pyloric sphincter.

Cilia Slender, hairlike projections attached to the epithelium of the respiratory tract that constantly beat in a wavelike motion to remove pathogens from the body.

Circadian rhythms Biological clock or a person's 24-hour rhythm, such as a natural sleep–wake cycle.

Civil law Law that regulates relationships and interactions between individuals and groups.

Claim message Messages encouraging payment of a bill, usually attached to or printed on the monthly statement.

CLIA-nonwaived test A complex laboratory test that does not meet the criteria for waiver and is subject to the CLIA regulations.

CLIA-waived test A laboratory test that meets the criteria for being a simple procedure that is easy to perform and has a low risk of erroneous test results.

Clinical age Method of timing a pregnancy that begins with the last menstrual period; 2 weeks more than developmental age.

Clinical diagnosis A tentative diagnosis of a patient's condition obtained through an evaluation of the health history and physical examination without the benefit of laboratory or diagnostic tests.

Clinical laboratory A facility in which tests are performed on biologic specimens to obtain information regarding the health of a patient.

Cloning Producing genetically identical cells or individuals artificially.

Closed questions Questions that anticipate a yes or no or a short answer.

Cloud computing A model where the internet is used to store and access data and programs; the servers are not physically located at the same site as the computer.

Clustering Scheduling similar types of patients or examinations on the same day or part of the day.

Coagulation The process of blood clotting.

Cocci (*sing.*, coccus) Bacteria that have a round shape.

Cochlea Spiral or snail-shaped portion of the inner ear.

Coinsurance A percentage of the allowed charge for health services that the patient is responsible for paying.

Collagenous fibers Strong, flexible connective tissue fibers that contain the protein collagen.

Collection agency A company that is in the business of collecting overdue accounts for other companies.

Colonoscope An endoscope that is specially designed for passage through the anus to permit visualization of the rectum and the entire length of the colon.

Colonoscopy The visualization of the rectum and the entire colon using a colonoscope.

Colposcope A lighted instrument with a binocular magnifying lens used to examine the vagina and cervix.

Colposcopy Examination of the vagina and cervix using a colposcope (a lighted instrument with a magnifying lens).

Combination résumé A résumé that uses elements from both the reverse-chronological and skill-based résumé. Most useful for someone with 1–3 years' experience, changing careers, or has no gaps in the work history.

Complete protein A protein that contains all of the essential amino acids needed by the body.

Complimentary closing Words used as a polite ending to a letter just before the writer's signature.

Compress A soft, moist, absorbent cloth that is folded in several layers and applied to a part of the body in the local application of heat or cold.

Computer system All of the hardware and software components making up the computer.

Conduction The transfer of energy, such as heat, from one object to another by direct contact.

Conduction myofibers Cardiac muscle cells specialized for conducting action potentials to the myocardium; part of the conduction system of the heart; also called Purkinje fibers.

Consultation report A narrative report of an opinion about a patient's condition by a practitioner other than the attending physician or primary care provider.

Contagious An infection capable of being transmitted directly or indirectly from one person to another.

Contagious disease A disease that is capable of being transmitted directly or indirectly from one person to another.

Contaminate 1. To soil, stain, or pollute; to make impure. 2. As it relates to surgical asepsis, to cause a sterile object or surface to become unsterile.

Contaminated The presence or reasonably anticipated presence of blood or OPIM on an item or surface.

Continuing Education Unit (CEU) A standard unit of measure of continuing education for professionals, defined as 1 contact hour by the American Association of Medical Assistants (AAMA) but also commonly 10 contact hours of participation.

Contractility The ability of muscle cells to shorten to produce movement.

Contrast medium A substance used to make a particular structure visible on a radiograph.

Control A solution that is used to monitor a test system to ensure reliable and accurate test results.

Controlled drug or substance A drug or substance that has restrictions placed on it by the government because of its potential for abuse and dependence.

Contusion An injury to the tissues under the skin that causes blood vessels to rupture, allowing blood to seep into the tissues; a bruise.

Convection The transfer of energy, such as heat, through air currents.

Conversion Changing from one system of measurement to another.

Coordination of benefits Rules followed by insurance companies so that no claim is reimbursed at more than 100% of the charges.

Copayment A fixed amount of money that the patient is responsible to pay at each visit.

Corpora cavernosa Two dorsal columns of erectile tissue found in the penis.

Corpus albicans Scar tissue in the ovary that forms when the corpus luteum degenerates.

Corpus luteum The yellow structure that develops from the mature follicle after ovulation.

Corpus spongiosum Ventral column of erectile tissue found in the penis.

Cover letter A letter sent with one or more documents (such as a résumé) to provide an explanation.

Crash cart A specially equipped cart for holding and transporting medications, equipment, and supplies needed for lifesaving procedures in an emergency.

Credit A posting that is subtracted from an account balance.

Credit balance A negative balance on a patient account (i.e., when money is owed by the medical office), usually the result of an overpayment.

Crepitus A grating sensation caused by fractured bone fragments rubbing against each other.

Crime An offense in violation of a law that prohibits or requires certain behavior.

Criminal law Law that regulates offenses against the public welfare.

Crisis (pertaining to fever) A sudden falling of an elevated body temperature to normal.

Crista ampullaris Receptor organ located within the ampulla of the semicircular canals of the ear, which functions in maintaining dynamic equilibrium.

Critical item An item that comes into contact with sterile tissue or the vascular system.

Critical value A laboratory test result that is dangerously abnormal and life-threatening requiring immediate attention.

Cross-contamination The process in which microorganisms are unintentionally transferred from one person, object, or place to another.

Cross-index To file under one unit and use a guide or card filed under another unit that refers to the primary filing location.

Cryosurgery The therapeutic use of freezing temperatures to destroy abnormal tissue.

Cubic centimeter The amount of space occupied by 1 milliliter (1 mL = 1 cc).

Culture The propagation of a mass of microorganisms in a laboratory culture medium.

Culture medium A mixture of nutrients on which microorganisms are grown in the laboratory.

Curative treatment A treatment that cures a disease or infection.

Cutaneous membrane A type of epithelial membrane; skin.

Cyanosis A bluish discoloration of the skin and mucous membranes.

Cytokinesis Division of the cell at the end of mitosis to form two separate daughter cells.

Cytology The science that deals with the study of cells, including their origin, structure, function, and pathology.

D

Data Raw, unorganized facts about subject matter presented to the computer for processing.

Data processing The changing of raw facts or data into usable information following a three-part sequence: input, processing, output.

Day sheet The record of daily transactions. It includes patient visits as well as all payments that were received in the mail that day.

DEA Number A registration number assigned to providers by the Drug Enforcement Administration for prescribing or dispensing controlled drugs or substances.

Debit A posting that is added to an account balance.

Decontamination The use of physical or chemical means to remove, inactivate, or destroy pathogens on a surface or item to the point where they are no longer capable of transmitting infectious particles or disease; the surface or item is rendered safe for handling, use, or disposal.

Decussation A crossing over; usually referring to motor fibers that cross over to the opposite side in the medulla oblongata.

Deductible An amount of money that an insured person must pay for medical services annually before those services are covered by an insurance plan.

Defecation The expulsion of indigestible wastes, or feces, through the anus.

Defendant The person or group against whom an action is brought in a court of law.

Deglutition The process of swallowing.

Dendrites The branching (tree-like) afferent processes of a neuron that receive impulses from other neurons and that transmit them to the cell body.

Denial Failure to acknowledge the reality of a situation.

Depreciation Accounting methods to respond to the loss of value of a property or piece of equipment over time.

Dermis Inner layer of the skin that contains the blood vessels, nerves, glands, and hair follicles.

Detergent An agent that cleanses by emulsifying dirt and oil.

Detrusor muscle The smooth muscle in the wall of the urinary bladder.

Developmental age Method of timing a pregnancy that begins with fertilization; 2 weeks less than clinical age.

Diagnosis The scientific method of determining and identifying a patient's condition.

Diagnostic procedure A procedure performed to assist in the diagnosis, management, or treatment of a patient's condition.

Diapedesis The process by which white blood cells squeeze between the cells in a vessel wall to enter the tissue spaces outside the blood vessel.

Diaphysis The long straight shaft of a long bone.

Diarthrosis (*pl.*, diarthroses) Freely movable joint characterized by a joint cavity; also called a synovial joint.

Diastole The phase in the cardiac cycle in which the heart relaxes between contractions.

Diastolic pressure The point of lesser pressure on the arterial wall, which is recorded during diastole.

Diencephalon The part of the brain between the cerebral hemispheres and the midbrain; includes the thalamus and hypothalamus.

Dietary pattern The combination of food and beverages that constitutes an individual's complete dietary intake over time.

Differential diagnosis A determination of which of two or more diseases with similar symptoms is producing a patient's symptoms.

Diffusion Movement of substances from a region of high concentration to a region of low concentration.

Digital image A picture that is stored electronically to allow viewing on a computer.

Digital subscriber line (DSL) Technology that allows digital signals to be transmitted over telephone lines at high speed even if the telephone line is also being used for voice transmission.

Dilation (of the cervix) The stretching of the external os from an opening a few millimeters wide to an opening large enough to allow the passage of an infant (approximately 10 cm).

Disaccharide A simple carbohydrate consisting of two sugar units.

Disaster A sudden event that causes damage or loss of life.

Disbursement Money paid out.

Discharge summary report A brief summary of the significant events of a patient's hospitalization.

Disinfectant An agent used to destroy pathogenic microorganisms but not their spores. Disinfectants are usually applied to inanimate objects and surfaces.

Dislocation An injury in which one end of a bone making up a joint is separated or displaced from its normal anatomic position.

Diuresis Secretion and passage of large amounts of urine.

Do-not-resuscitate (DNR) order A medical order signed by a provider that relieves health care personnel from the obligation to resuscitate a patient who stops breathing or whose heart stops.

Documenting The process of making written or electronic entries about a patient in the medical record.

Donor One who furnishes something such as blood, tissue, or organs to be used in another individual.

Dose The quantity of a drug administered at one time.

Double booking Scheduling two patients for the same appointment time.

Downcoding Using procedure codes that do not reflect a high enough level of service.

Drug A chemical used for the treatment, prevention, or diagnosis of disease.

Drug Enforcement Administration (DEA) The federal agency that enforces the Controlled Substances Act of 1970.

Ductus deferens Tubular structure that is continuous with the epididymis; it ascends through the inguinal canal and transports sperm to the ejaculatory duct.

Duty Commitment to act in a certain way.

Dysmenorrhea Pain associated with the menstrual period.

Dyspareunia Pain in the vagina or pelvis experienced by a woman during sexual intercourse.

Dysplasia The growth of abnormal cells. Dysplasia is a precancerous condition that may or may not develop into cancer.

Dyspnea Shortness of breath or difficulty breathing.

Dysrhythmia Any abnormality or irregularity in the heart's rhythm; also termed arrhythmia.

Dysuria Difficult or painful urination.

E

ECG cycle The graphic representation of a cardiac cycle.

Echocardiogram An ultrasound examination of the heart.

Ectocervix The outermost layer of the cervix that projects into the vagina.

Edema The retention of fluid in the tissues, resulting in swelling.

Effacement The thinning and shortening of the cervical canal from its normal length of 1 to 2 cm to a structure with paper-thin edges in which there is no canal at all. Effacement occurs late in pregnancy, during labor, or both. The purpose of effacement along with dilation is to permit the passage of the infant into the birth canal.

Ego defense mechanism Unconscious mental process that offers psychologic protection.
Elastic fibers Yellow connective tissue fibers that are not particularly strong but can be stretched and will return to their normal shape when released.
Elasticity The ability of tissue to return to its original shape after contraction or extension.
Electrocardiogram (ECG) The graphic representation of the electrical activity of the heart.
Electrocardiograph The instrument used to record the electrical activity of the heart.
Electrode A device placed on the skin that picks up electrical impulses given off by the heart.
Electrolyte A substance that facilitates transmission of the heart's electrical impulses.
Electronic health record (EHR) A computerized medical record of the important health information regarding a patient.
Electronic medical record (EMR) A patient health record generated by an individual health care provider or organization that is stored on a computer.
Electronic signature An electronic sound, symbol, or process added to an electronic record that indicates intent to sign.
Eligibility Enrollment status related to a health insurance plan.
E-mail The exchange of information from one computer to another using telecommunication.
Emancipated minor A person younger than the age of 18 with the rights of an adult, including the ability to consent to medical care.
Embryo The child in utero from the time of conception through the first 8 weeks of development.
Embryonic period Stage of development that lasts from the beginning of the third week until the end of the eighth week after fertilization; period during which the organ systems develop in the body.
Emergency action plan A written document that describes the actions that employees should take to ensure their safety if a fire or other emergency situation occurs.
Emergency medical services (EMS) system A network of community resources, equipment, and personnel that provides care to victims of injury or sudden illness.
Emergency preparedness The process of making plans to prevent, respond, and recover from an emergency situation.
Empathy Objective awareness and sensitivity to the feelings and emotions of others.
Empty calorie food A food that provides calories but few or no nutrients. Also known as a low-nutrient-density food.
Empirical Learned from observation or experiment.
Encryption A process by which electronic information is changed into an unreadable form that requires the original encryption software to reverse the process.
Endocardium The thin smooth inner lining of each chamber of the heart.
Endocervix The inner part of the cervix that forms a narrow canal that connects the vagina to the uterus.
Endocrine gland A gland that secretes its product directly into the blood; opposite of exocrine gland.
Endocrinology Study of the endocrine glands.
Endometrium Innermost mucous membrane layer of the uterine wall.
Endoscope An instrument that consists of a tube and an optical system used for direct visual inspection of organs or cavities.
Endosteum Membranous lining of a cavity within a bone.
Enema An injection of fluid into the rectum to aid in the elimination of feces from the colon.
Engagement The entrance of the fetal head or the presenting part into the pelvic inlet.
Enunciation The act of speaking clearly and concisely.
Epicardium The outer layer of the heart wall; the visceral pericardium.
Epidermis The outermost layer of the skin.
Epididymis A tightly coiled tubule along the posterior margin of each testicle; functions in the maturation and storage of sperm.
Epimysium Fibrous connective tissue that surrounds a whole muscle.
Epiphyseal line The remnant of the epiphyseal plate after the cartilage calcifies and growth ceases.
Epiphyseal plate The cartilaginous plate between the epiphysis and diaphysis of a bone; responsible for the lengthwise growth of a long bone.
Epiphysis The end of a long bone.
Erythema Reddening of the skin caused by the dilation of superficial blood vessels in the skin.
Erythrocyte Red blood cell. Red blood cells are responsible for transporting oxygen and carbon dioxide to the body.
Erythropoiesis The process of red blood cell formation.
Erythropoietin A hormone released by the kidneys that stimulates red blood cell production.
Essential amino acid An amino acid that is required by the body but cannot be manufactured by the body and must be obtained from food.
Established patient A patient who has been seen by one of the providers in the medical office within the past 3 years.
Estrogens Hormones that stimulate the development of female secondary sex characteristics.
Ethics The branch of knowledge that deals with standards of behavior or beliefs.
Eupnea Normal respiration. The rate is 12 to 20 respirations per minute, the rhythm is even and regular, and the depth is normal.
Evacuated blood collection tube A sterile glass or plastic blood collection tube with a color-coded closure that contains a vacuum.
Evacuation A planned systematic retreat of people to safety in an emergency situation.
Evacuation procedures Clear step-by-step procedures for the rapid, efficient, and safe removal of individuals from a building during an emergency.

Excitability The ability of muscle and nerve tissue to receive and respond to stimuli; also called irritability.
Exhalation The act of breathing out.
Exit route A continuous and unobstructed path of travel from any point within a workplace to a place of safety.
Exocrine gland A gland that secrets its product to a surface or cavity through ducts; opposite of endocrine gland.
Expected date of delivery (EDD) Projected birth date of the infant.
Explanation of benefits (EOB) A statement issued by an insurance carrier explaining reimbursement for specific procedures.
Exposure incident A specific eye, mouth, or other mucous membrane, nonintact skin, or parenteral contact with blood or OPIM that results from the performance of an employee's duties.
Expressed consent Agreement using spoken or written words.
Extensibility The ability of muscle tissue to stretch when pulled.
External os The opening of the cervical canal of the uterus into the vagina.
External respiration Exchange of gases between the lungs and the blood.
Exudate A discharge produced by the body's tissues.

F

Fahrenheit scale A temperature scale on which the freezing point of water is 32° and the boiling point of water is 212°.
False-negative result A test result denoting that a condition is absent when it is actually present.
False-positive result A test result denoting that a condition is present when it is actually absent.
Familial disease A condition that occurs in or affects members of a family more frequently than would be expected by chance.
Fasting Abstaining from food or fluids (except water) for a specified amount of time before the collection of a specimen.
Fauces Opening from the oral cavity into the oropharynx.
Fax Transmission of scanned, printed material by telephone. A short form of the word *facsimile*.
Febrile Pertaining to fever.
Fee-for-service A means of payment for health care in which the cost for each service provided is reimbursed in full or in part.
Fee-for-service insurance Insurance reimbursement that is for each treatment or procedure performed and the amount charged by the provider.
Fee schedule List of charges (fees) for specific procedures that may be performed in a medical office.
Fee splitting The practice of sharing fees with colleagues, especially for making referrals.
Felony A serious crime punishable by death or imprisonment.
Fetal heart rate The number of times per minute the fetal heart beats.
Fetal heart tones The sounds of the heartbeat of the fetus heard through the mother's abdominal wall.
Fetal period Stage of development that starts at the beginning of the ninth week after fertilization and lasts until birth.
Fetus The child in utero from the third month after conception to birth; during the first 2 months of development, it is called an *embryo*.
Fever A body temperature that is above normal; synonym for *pyrexia*.
Fibroblast An immature cell from which connective tissue can develop.
Fidelity Faithfulness.
Filing system The way in which records are arranged. Common filing systems in the medical office include alphabetic, numeric, by subject, or chronologic.
Fire extinguisher A portable device that discharges an agent designed to extinguish a fire.
Fire prevention plan A written document that identifies flammable and combustible materials stored in the workplace and ways to control workplace fire hazards.
Fire protection The implementation of safety measures to reduce the unwanted effects of fire.
Firewall A system that protects a computer network from unauthorized access by users on its own network or another network, such as the internet.
First aid The immediate care administered before complete medical care can be provided to an individual who is injured or suddenly becomes ill.
Fixed appointment scheduling An appointment scheduling method in which each patient is given a different, specific appointment time. Also called stream scheduling, time-specified scheduling, or single booking.
Flow rate The number of liters of oxygen per minute that come out of an oxygen delivery system.
Flow sheet A paper document or electronic screen that allows similar data to be recorded and viewed chronologically.
Fluoroscope An instrument used to view internal organs and structures directly in real time.
Fluoroscopy An x-ray procedure for viewing internal organs and structures directly in real time.
Forceps A two-pronged instrument used for grasping and squeezing.
Formulary An insurance carrier's official list of covered medications to be used by network providers.
Fracture Any break in a bone.
Fraud Intentional deception resulting in injury or loss.
Frenulum linguae The midline fold that connects the undersurface of the tongue with the floor of the mouth.
Frequency The condition of having to urinate often.
Full block style A letter format in which all parts of the letter are left justified.
Fundus The dome-shaped upper portion of the uterus between the fallopian tubes.
Furuncle A localized staphylococcal infection that originates deep within a hair follicle. Also known as a boil.

G

Gametes Sex cells: sperm and ova.

Gastric juice The secretions of the exocrine gastric glands.

Gastrin Hormone secreted by the endocrine glands in the stomach.

Gauge The diameter of the lumen of a needle used to administer medication.

Gene therapy Giving patients new genes or parts of genes to treat a disease or condition.

General senses Senses that are located throughout the body; somatic senses.

Genetic engineering Making, altering, or repairing genetic material.

Gestation The period of intrauterine development from conception to birth; the period of pregnancy. The average pregnancy lasts about 280 days, or 40 weeks, from the date of conception to childbirth.

Gestational age The age of the fetus between conception and birth.

Gigabyte (GB) A unit of computer storage capacity. One gigabyte is equal to a little more than 1 billion bytes or 1000 megabytes.

Gingiva Soft tissue that covers the alveolar processes of the mandible and maxillae; also called gums.

Glomerular capsule Double-layered epithelial cup that surrounds the glomerulus in a nephron; also called the Bowman capsule.

Glomerular filtration The movement of blood plasma across the filtration membrane in the renal corpuscle.

Glomerulus Cluster of capillaries in the nephron through which blood is filtered.

Glucocorticoids Hormones from the adrenal cortex that raise blood sugar levels.

Glucose The end product of carbohydrate metabolism which serves as the chief source of energy for the body.

Gluten A type of protein found in certain grains such as wheat, rye, and barley.

Glycogen The form in which glucose is stored in the body for later use.

Glycosuria The presence of glucose in the urine.

Glycosylation The process of glucose attaching to hemoglobin.

Gonadocorticoids Sex hormones secreted by the adrenal cortex.

Gonads Primary reproductive organs; organs that produce the gametes: testes in the male and ovaries in the female.

Good Samaritan Laws Provide legal immunity for individuals who administer first aid at the scene of an accident. These laws vary from state to state.

Grammar The accepted rules used to create meaning in a language.

Granulocytes Cells that develop granules in the cytoplasm; granular leukocytes.

Gross pay The total amount earned in a time period by an employee before any deductions.

Group plan One insurance policy that covers a group of people.

Guarantor A person with financial responsibility for a bill, who may or may not also be a patient.

Gustatory sense Sense of taste.

Gynecology The branch of medicine that deals with health maintenance and diseases of the female reproductive system.

H

Hand hygiene The process of cleansing or sanitizing the hands.

Hard disk drive A storage device consisting of one or more rigid, nonflexible platters coated with a magnetically sensitive material and encased in a permanently sealed, airtight container.

Hardware The physical devices making up a computer system (e.g., main computer unit, keyboard, monitor, printer).

Hazardous chemical Any chemical that is a health hazard or a physical hazard.

HAZMAT An acronym constructed from the beginnings of the two words "hazardous materials." It refers to materials that pose a danger to health or the environment and must be handled with protective equipment.

HDL (high-density lipoprotein) A lipoprotein that removes excess cholesterol from the walls of the arteries and carries it to the liver for removal by the body; known as "good" cholesterol because it is protective and beneficial to the body.

Health care proxy A legal document that names an agent to make decisions about a person's medical care if that individual becomes unable to make their wishes known.

Health coaching A process that helps patients identify their values related to health, to set health goals, and to take steps to meet their personal goals.

Health hazard The potential of a chemical to cause acute toxicity, skin corrosion or irritation, serious eye damage or irritation, respiratory or skin sensitization, germ cell mutagenicity, cancer or reproductive toxicity, or is an aspiration hazard.

Health history A collection of subjective data about a patient.

Health insurance Insurance purchased to provide protection for covered services related to health care.

Hearing range The range of sound frequencies that can be heard by a human.

Hematology The study of blood and blood-forming tissues.

Hematoma A swelling or mass of clotted blood within the tissues caused by a break in a blood vessel.

Hematopoiesis The process of blood cell formation.

Hematuria Blood present in the urine.

Hemoconcentration An increase in the concentration of the nonfilterable blood components in the blood vessels–such as red blood cells, enzymes, iron, and calcium–as a result of a decrease in the fluid content of the blood.

Hemocytoblast A stem cell in the bone marrow from which the blood cells arise.

Hemoglobin The protein- and iron-containing pigment of erythrocytes that carries oxygen to the tissues of the body.
Hemoglobin A_{1c} The compound formed when glucose attaches or glycosylates to the protein in hemoglobin.
Hemolysis The breakdown of blood cells.
Hemophilia An inherited bleeding disorder caused by a deficiency of a clotting factor needed for proper coagulation of the blood.
Hemostasis The control or stoppage of bleeding by natural or artificial means.
Hierarchy Classified according to rank or importance.
Histology Branch of microscopic anatomy that studies tissues.
Holistic Considering the whole; in medicine, considering the entire person when health care is being provided.
Home health care The provision of medical and nonmedical care in a patient's home or place of residence.
Homeostasis The state in which body systems are functioning normally and the internal environment of the body is in equilibrium, when the body is in a healthy state.
Hormone A substance secreted by an endocrine gland.
Hospice Palliative service provided for patients whose life expectancy is less than 6 months, including aiding with comfort, pain relief, and personal care. Services may be provided in the patient's home, a nursing home, or a special hospice facility.
Hospitalist A provider who cares for hospitalized patients only.
Human anatomy Study of human body shape and structure and the relationships of its parts.
Human physiology Study of the functions of humans and their separate parts.
Hydrolysis Chemical breakdown of complex molecules by the addition of water.
Hyperglycemia An abnormally high level of glucose in the blood.
Hyperopia A refractive error in which the light rays are brought to a focus behind the retina, resulting in difficulty viewing objects at a reading or working distance. Farsightedness.
Hyperpnea An abnormal increase in the rate and depth of respiration.
Hyperpyrexia An extremely high fever.
Hypertension The force of the circulating blood against the walls of the blood vessels is consistently above normal. High blood pressure.
Hyperventilation An abnormally fast and deep type of breathing, usually associated with acute anxiety conditions.
Hypochromic A red blood cell with a decreased concentration of hemoglobin.
Hypodermis Below the skin; a sheet of areolar connective tissue and adipose beneath the dermis of the skin.
Hypoglycemia An abnormally low level of glucose in the blood.
Hypopnea An abnormal decrease in the rate and depth of respiration.
Hypotension The pressure of the circulating blood against the walls of the blood vessels is below normal. Low blood pressure.
Hypothermia A life-threatening condition in which the temperature of the entire body falls to a dangerously low level or below normal body temperature.
Hypoxemia A decrease in the oxygen saturation of the blood. Hypoxemia may lead to hypoxia.
Hypoxia A reduction in the oxygen supply to the tissues of the body.

I

Ileocecal valve The valve between the small intestine and large intestine.
Immune globulin A blood product consisting of pooled human plasma containing antibodies.
Immunity The resistance of the body to pathogenic microorganisms and their toxins.
Immunization (active, artificial) The process of making an individual immune through the administration of a vaccine.
Immunoglobulins Substances produced by the body that inactivate or destroy other substances introduced into the body; antibodies.
Immunologic testing Testing that uses antigen–antibody reactions to assess the presence of a specific substance in the body or to assist in the diagnosis of an infectious disease.
Immunology The scientific study of antigen and antibody reactions.
Impacted cerumen Cerumen that is wedged firmly together in the ear so as to be immovable.
Implied consent Indication of agreement by actions instead of words.
In vivo Occurring in the living body or organism.
Incision A clean cut caused by a cutting instrument.
Incomplete protein A protein that lacks one or more of the essential amino acids needed by the body.
Incubate To provide proper conditions for growth and development. In microbiology, the act of placing a culture in a chamber (incubator) that provides optimal growth conditions for multiplication of the organisms.
Incubation period The interval of time between the invasion by a pathogenic microorganism and the appearance of the first symptoms of the disease.
Indemnity An obligation to provide compensation for loss or damage.
Indexing units Pieces of information used to identify a correct filing location.
Induration An abnormally raised, hardened area of the skin with clearly defined margins.
Infant A child from birth to 12 months of age.
Infection Invasion of the body by pathogenic microorganisms.
Infectious agent A pathogen capable of causing an infectious disease.
Infectious disease A disease caused by a pathogen that produces harmful effects in its host.

Infiltration The process by which a substance passes into and is deposited within the substance of a cell, tissue, or organ.

Inflammation A protective response of the body to trauma and the entrance of foreign matter. The purpose of inflammation is to destroy invading microorganisms and to remove damaged tissue debris from the area so that proper healing can occur.

Informed consent Agreement to a medical procedure based on understanding of the procedure and its possible consequences and effects.

Inhalation The act of breathing in.

Inhalation administration The administration of medication by way of air or another vapor being drawn into the lungs.

Initiative The ability to begin or carry through on a plan of action independently.

Inoculate To introduce microorganisms into a culture medium for growth and multiplication.

Inpatient A patient who has been admitted to a health care facility for at least one overnight stay.

Input 1. (noun) Data that have been entered into the computer. 2. (verb) The transfer of data to the computer for processing.

Input device A device for entering data into the computer (e.g., keyboard, mouse, scanner).

Inscription The part of a prescription that indicates the name of the drug and the drug dosage.

Insertion The end of a muscle that is attached to a relatively movable part; the end opposite the origin.

Inspection The process of observing a patient to detect signs of disease.

Instillation The dropping of a liquid into a body cavity.

Insufflate To blow a powder, vapor, or gas (e.g., air) into a body cavity.

Insulin A hormone secreted by the beta cells of the pancreas required for the normal use of glucose in the body.

Insured The person who is covered by a specific insurance plan.

Intercostal Between the ribs.

Internal os The internal opening of the cervical canal into the uterus.

Internal respiration Exchange of gases between the blood and tissue cells.

Internet A global system of interconnected computer networks that use the internet protocol (TCP/IP) to transmit and exchange data.

Interstitial cells Cells between the seminiferous tubules in the testes, producing testosterone; also called cells of Leydig.

Interval The length of one or more waves and a segment.

Intradermal injection Introduction of medication into the dermal layer of the skin.

Intramuscular injection The introduction of medication into the muscular layer of the body.

Inventory A detailed list of items in stock or in possession of an individual or business.

Invoice An itemized bill for goods or services.

Irrigation The washing of a body canal with a flowing solution.

Ischemia Deficiency of blood in a body part.

J

Judgmental Critical or negative; making judgments about what is good or bad based on a personal opinion.

Juxtaglomerular apparatus A complex of modified cells in the afferent arteriole and the ascending limb and distal tubule in the kidney, which helps regulate blood pressure by secreting renin. It consists of the macula densa and the juxtaglomerular cells.

K

Keratinization Process by which the cells of the epidermis become filled with keratin and move to the surface, where they are sloughed off.

Ketonuria The presence of ketone bodies in the urine.

Ketosis An accumulation of large amounts of ketone bodies in the tissues and body fluids.

Kilobyte (KB) A unit of computer storage capacity. One kilobyte is equal to 1024 bytes (characters).

Kilocalorie The amount of heat needed to raise the temperature of 1 kilogram of water by 1 degree Celsius. (Often referred to as a calorie.)

Korotkoff sounds Sounds heard during the measurement of blood pressure that are used to determine the systolic and diastolic blood pressure readings.

L

Laboratory panel A combination of laboratory tests that have been determined to be the most sensitive and specific means of identifying a disease state or evaluation a particular organ or organ system.

Laboratory test The clinical analysis and study of materials, fluids, or tissues obtained from patients to assist in the diagnosis and treatment of disease.

Laceration A wound in which the tissues are torn apart, leaving ragged and irregular edges.

Lacrimal apparatus The structures that produce and convey tears.

Lactation Milk production and ejection from the mammary glands.

Lactose A disaccharide consisting of two sugar units that is found in milk and milk products.

Laryngopharynx Portion of the pharynx that is behind the larynx and extends from the level of the hyoid bone to the lower margin of the larynx.

Larynx Passageway for air between the pharynx and trachea; commonly called the voice box.

LDL (low-density lipoprotein) A lipoprotein that picks up cholesterol from ingested fats and the liver and carries it in the blood plasma for use by the body's cells; known as "bad" cholesterol because a high level contributes to atherosclerosis.

Ledger A book, card, or computer account used to record financial transactions.

Left justified Describing lines of type that begin at the left margin of a document.

Length (recumbent) The measurement of a person from the vertex of the head to the heel of the foot in a supine position.

Letterhead A sheet of stationery preprinted with information about a business, including name, address, telephone number, and other information.

Leukocyte White blood cell. White blood cells function in defending the body against infection and foreign materials.

Leukocytosis An abnormal increase in the number of leukocytes (greater than 11,000 per cubic millimeter of blood).

Leukopenia An abnormal decrease in the number of leukocytes (less than 4500 per cubic millimeter of blood).

Liabilities Legal responsibilities. In accounting, the amount owed by a business to creditors.

License Official permission to perform an activity or practice a profession.

Licensure The process by which the state examines qualifications and gives permission to an individual or organization to engage in a profession or business.

Ligate To tie off and close a structure such as a severed blood vessel.

Lipoprotein A complex molecule consisting of protein that combines with and transports lipids (cholesterol and triglycerides) in the blood plasma.

Litigation The process of taking a lawsuit through the courts.

Living will A legal document that specifies the kind of medical treatment a patient wants or does not want if they become incapacitated.

Load The items that are being sterilized in an autoclave.

Local anesthetic A drug that produces a loss of feeling and an inability to perceive pain in only a specific part of the body.

Locum tenens A person who performs the duties of another on a temporary basis.

Long arm cast A cast that extends from the axilla to the fingers, usually with a bend at the elbow.

Long leg cast A cast that extends from the from the midthigh to the toes.

Lower esophageal sphincter Valve between the esophagus and the stomach.

Lower respiratory tract Portion of the respiratory tract that is inferior to the larynx; includes the trachea, bronchial tree, and lungs.

M

Maceration The softening and breaking down of the skin as a result of prolonged exposure to moisture.

Macrocytic An abnormally large red blood cell.

Macronutrient A nutrient required in relatively large amounts by the body. Includes carbohydrates, fat, and protein.

Macrophage Large phagocytic connective tissue cell that functions in immune responses; name given to a monocyte after it leaves the blood and enters the tissues.

Macula lutea Yellowish depression on the retina.

Malaise A vague sense of body discomfort, weakness, and fatigue that often marks the onset of a disease and continues through the course of the illness.

Malpractice Negligence by a professional.

Man-made disaster An event that causes serious damage through intentional or negligent human actions or the failure of a man-made system.

Managed care A movement in health care based on reducing health care costs while providing high-quality care. The term may be used for the techniques used to reduce costs or for the companies that pay for the care provided.

Manometer An instrument for measuring pressure.

Mast cell A connective tissue cell that produces heparin and histamine.

Mastication The process of chewing.

Mature minor An individual younger than 18 years of age with the maturity to provide informed consent for certain medical procedures.

Mechanoreceptor A sensory receptor that responds to the bending or deformation of a cell; examples include receptors for touch, pressure, hearing, and equilibrium.

Mediation Negotiation by a third party to help two parties resolve a dispute.

Medicaid The government insurance program for low-income individuals and families that is funded both by the federal government and by each individual state. The Medicaid program has a different name in each state.

Medical asepsis Practices employed to inhibit the growth and hinder the transmission of pathogenic microorganisms to prevent the spread of infection.

Medical durable power of attorney A written authorization to make health care decisions for a specified individual that is in effect if the individual becomes incapacitated.

Medical necessity Health care that is reasonable and necessary for a patient based on evidence-based clinical standards of care.

Medical practice A program that provides instructions to the computer for performing medical practice management procedures.

Medical record A written or electronic record of important information regarding a patient, including the care of that individual and the progress of the patient's condition.

Medical record format The way a medical record is organized. The two main types of medical record formats are the source-oriented record and the problem-oriented record.

Medical record management Activities related to the creation, management, use, and disposition of patients' medical records.

Medicare The federal health insurance program that provides insurance coverage for the elderly, permanently disabled, and individuals with end-stage kidney disease.

Medicare Administrative Contractor (MAC) A private health care insurer that administers both Medicare Part A and Part B claims, usually for more than one state, under a contract with the Centers for Medicare and Medicaid Services (CMS).

Megabyte (MB) A unit of computer storage capacity. One megabyte is equal to a little more than 1 million bytes or 1000 kilobytes.

Megakaryocyte A large cell that contributes to the formation of platelets.

Meiosis Type of nuclear division in which the number of chromosomes is reduced to half the number found in a body cell; this results in the formation of an egg or sperm.

Melena Darkening of the stool caused by the presence of blood in an amount of 50 mL or greater.

Melanin A dark brown or black pigment found in parts of the body, especially skin and hair.

Mature minor An individual below 18 years of age who is mature enough to provide informed consent for certain medical procedures.

Melanocyte A cell that produces the dark or black pigment melanin.

Memo (memorandum) A form of communication within a company that is usually short and limited to one subject.

Menarche First period of menstrual bleeding at puberty.

Meninges Connective tissue membranes that cover the brain and spinal cord.

Menopause The permanent cessation of menstruation, which usually occurs between the ages of 45 and 55.

Menorrhagia Excessive bleeding during a menstrual period, in the number of days or the amount of blood, or both. Also called dysfunctional uterine bleeding (DUB).

Mensuration The process of measuring a patient.

Mesentery Extensions of peritoneum associated with the intestine.

Metered mail Mail for which the postage has been applied using a postage meter.

Metrorrhagia Bleeding between menstrual periods.

Microbiology The scientific study of microorganisms and their activities.

Microcytic An abnormally small red blood cell.

Micronutrient A nutrient required in very small amounts by the body. Includes vitamins and minerals.

Microorganism A microscopic plant or animal.

Micturition Act of expelling urine from the bladder; also called voiding or urination.

MICR line A line of numbers containing the American Bankers Association (ABA) transit routing number and the account number that appears at the bottom left of a check. These numbers are read by a magnetic ink character recognition (MICR) system.

Mineral A naturally occurring inorganic substance this is essential to the proper functioning of the body.

Mineralocorticoids A group of hormones secreted by the adrenal cortex, which regulate the body's electrolyte balance.

Minutes A written record of the proceedings of a meeting.

Misdemeanor A less serious crime, punishable by a fine or imprisonment for less than 1 year.

Mitosis Process by which the nucleus of a body cell divides to form two new cells, each identical to the parent cell.

Modified block style A format for business letters in which the date line, complimentary close, and printed signature line are on a tab at the center or justified at the right and all other parts of the letter are justified at the left.

Modified wave scheduling An appointment system that has some fixed appointments and some appointment times during which patients are seen in order of arrival.

Modifier An addition to a *Current Procedural Terminology* code that indicates unusual circumstances related to the procedure, such as a more extensive procedure or two procedures performed in the same session.

Monosaccharide A simple carbohydrate consisting of one sugar unit.

Morals Beliefs about what is right and wrong.

Morphology (blood cells) The study of the size, shape, and structure of a blood cell.

Motor unit A single neuron and all the muscle fibers it stimulates.

MS-DRG (Medicare Severity-Diagnosis Related Groups) A system for grouping hospital inpatients who are expected to utilize a similar amount of hospital resources as a basis for Medicare reimbursements.

Mucous membrane Epithelial membrane that lines body cavities opening directly to the exterior; secretes mucus.

Multigravida A woman who has been pregnant more than once.

Multipara A woman who has completed two or more pregnancies to the age of fetal viability regardless of whether they ended in live infants or stillbirths.

Myelin White fatty substance that surrounds many nerve fibers.

Myocardium The middle layer of the heart wall, composed of cardiac muscle tissue.

Myometrium The thick middle layer of the uterus, composed of smooth muscle.

Myopia A refractive error in which the light rays are brought to a focus in front of the retina, resulting in difficulty viewing objects at a distance. Nearsightedness.

N

Nasopharynx Portion of the pharynx posterior to the nasal cavities, extending from the base of the skull to the uvula.

Natural disaster A catastrophic event caused by nature or the natural processes of the earth.

NEC (Not Elsewhere Classified) A diagnosis code that is used when a more specific code for the condition is not available.

Natural sugars Sugars that occur naturally in foods and beverages.

Needle biopsy A type of biopsy in which tissue from deep within the body is obtained by the insertion of a biopsy needle through the skin.

Negative feedback A mechanism of response in which a stimulus initiates reactions that reduce the stimulus.

Negligence Failure to act (or to refrain from acting) as a reasonably prudent person would in similar circumstances.
Nephron The functional unit of the kidney that filters waste substances from the blood and dilutes them with water to produce urine.
Nephron loop The hairpin loop of the renal tubule that extends into the renal pyramids.
Net pay The actual amount of money paid directly to an employee after taxes and other deductions have been taken out.
Network A group of computers that share data and resources.
Networking The process of contacting acquaintances and their contacts who may know of potential jobs.
Neurilemma The layer of cells that surrounds a nerve fiber in the peripheral nervous system and in some cases produces myelin; also called Schwann sheath.
Neuroglia Supporting cells of nervous tissue; cells in nervous tissue that do not conduct impulses; nerve glue.
Neurohypophysis Posterior portion of the pituitary gland, which lies beneath the brain and contains axons of neurons.
Neuromuscular junction The area of communication between the axon terminal of a motor neuron and the sarcolemma of a muscle fiber; also called a myoneural junction.
Neuron Nerve cell, including its processes; conducting cell of nervous tissue.
Neurotransmitter A chemical substance released at the axon terminals to stimulate a muscle fiber contraction or an impulse in another neuron.
New patient For billing purposes, a patient who has not received services during the previous 3 years from any provider in a medical office.
No-show A patient who does not keep a scheduled appointment.
Nociceptor A sensory receptor that responds to tissue damage; pain receptor.
Nocturia Excessive (voluntary) urination during the night.
Nocturnal enuresis Inability of an individual to control urination at night during sleep (bedwetting).
Nodes of Ranvier Short spaces between segments of myelin in a myelinated nerve fiber.
Nonspecific defense mechanisms Comprising the body's ability to counteract all types of harmful agents.
Nonabsorbable suture Suture material that is not absorbed by the body and either remains permanently in the body tissue and becomes encapsulated by fibrous tissue or is removed.
Noncritical item An item that comes into contact with intact skin but not with mucous membranes.
Nonessential amino acid An amino acid required by the body that can be synthesized by the body in sufficient quantities to meet its needs.
Nonintact skin Skin that has a break in its surface. It includes but is not limited to abrasions, cuts, hangnails, paper cuts, and burns.
Nonmalfeasance Ethical concept requiring that an action do no harm or do less harm than good.
Nonparticipating provider (nonPAR) A provider who does not have any contract with a third-party payor.
Nonpathogen A microorganism that is harmless and does not cause disease.
Nonverbal Communication that occurs without words, as through body posture or facial expression.
Normal flora Harmless nonpathogenic microorganisms that normally reside in many parts of the body but do not cause disease.
Normal sinus rhythm Refers to an electrocardiogram that is within normal limits.
Normochromic A red blood cell with a normal concentration of hemoglobin.
Normocytic A normal-sized red blood cell.
NOS A diagnosis code that is not otherwise specified. It is used when there is not enough information given to select a more specific code.
Nullipara A woman who has not carried a pregnancy to the point of fetal viability (20 weeks of gestation).
Nutrient A chemical substance found in food that is needed by the body for survival and well-being.
Nutrition The study of nutrients in food, including how the body uses them and their relationship to health.
Nutrition therapy The application of the science of nutrition to promote optimal heath and treat illness.

O

Obesity A medical condition in which there is an excessive accumulation of body fat to the extent that it may have an adverse effect on an individual's health and well-being.
Objective symptom A symptom that can be observed by an examiner and the patient.
Obstetrics The branch of medicine concerned with the care of the woman during pregnancy, childbirth, and the puerperium.
Occult blood Blood in such a small amount that it is not detectable by the unaided eye.
Occupational exposure Reasonably anticipated skin, eye, mucous membrane, or parenteral contact with blood or OPIM that may result from the performance of an employee's duties.
Olfaction Sense of smell.
Oliguria Decreased or scanty output of urine.
Oogenesis Process of meiosis in the female in which one ovum and three polar bodies are produced from one primary oocyte.
Oogonia Stem cells that give rise to ova or egg cells.
Open booking Patients are told to come in during a time range.
Open questions Questions that could have a variety of answers and encourage a personal response.
Operating system A type of system software that performs tasks required by the computer to function.
Ophthalmologist A physician who specializes in diagnosing and treating diseases and disorders of the eye.

Ophthalmoscope An instrument for examining the interior of the eye.

Opportunistic infection An infection resulting from a defective immune system that cannot defend the body from pathogens normally found in the environment.

Optician A technician who fits eyeglasses, contact lenses, and other vision-correcting devices.

Optimum growth temperature The temperature at which an organism grows best.

Optometrist A licensed primary health care provider who has expertise in measuring visual acuity and prescribing corrective lenses for the treatment of refractive errors.

Oral Spoken; also pertaining to the mouth.

Oral administration Administration of a medication by mouth.

Origin The end of a muscle that is attached to a relatively immovable part; the end opposite the insertion.

Oropharynx Portion of the pharynx that is posterior to the oral cavity; it extends from the uvula to the hyoid bone.

Orthopedist A physician who specializes in the diagnosis and treatment of disorders of the musculoskeletal system, which includes the bones, joints, ligaments, tendons, muscles, and nerves.

Orthopnea The condition in which breathing is easier when an individual is in a sitting or standing position.

Osmosis Diffusion of water through a selectively permeable membrane.

Osteoblast Bone-forming cell; immature bone cell.

Osteochondritis Inflammation of bone and cartilage.

Osteoclast Cell that destroys, breaks down, or resorbs bone tissue.

Osteocyte Mature bone cell.

Osteogenesis Formation of bone; also called ossification.

Osteomyelitis Inflammation of the bone or bone marrow as a result of bacterial infection.

Osteon Structural unit of bone; haversian system.

Other potentially infectious materials (OPIM) Body fluids, tissues, and organs from a human that can spread infection.

Otolaryngologist A physician who specializes in the diagnosis and treatment of disorders of the ear, nose, and throat. (Also known as an ENT physician.)

Otoliths Little stones of calcium carbonate in the macula of the inner ear.

Otologist A physician who can treat more complex ear conditions and perform more complex ear surgeries as compared with an otolaryngologist.

Otosclerosis An abnormal bone growth in the middle ear.

Otoscope An instrument used to examine the external ear canal and tympanic membrane.

Outguide A cardboard or plastic card to insert in a file when a medical record is removed.

Outpatient A patient who has not been admitted to a health care facility.

Output 1. (noun) Information that has been generated by the computer. 2. (verb) The transfer of processed data back to the user.

Output device A device that transfers processed data to the user (e.g., computer monitor, printer).

Ovarian cycle Monthly cycle of events that occur in the ovary from puberty to menopause; occurs concurrently with the uterine cycle.

Ovarian follicle An oocyte surrounded by one or more layers of cells within the ovaries.

Overdraft A check (or draft) that exceeds the funds in a bank account.

Oxygen therapy The administration of supplemental oxygen at concentrations greater than room air to treat or prevent hypoxemia.

Oxyhemoglobin Hemoglobin that has combined with oxygen.

P

Package insert (laboratory test) A printed document that provides detailed information on the use of a test and how to perform the test.

Pager An electronic device that notifies the recipient to receive a message or return a telephone call.

Palate Roof of the mouth; separates the oral cavity from the nasal cavity.

Palliative treatment Therapy that reduces the effects of a disease or condition but does not remove the disease itself.

Palpation The process of feeling with the hands to detect signs of disease.

Panel A group of diagnostic tests usually ordered together for diagnosis or screening.

Paper-based patient record (PPR) A medical record in paper form.

Paraphrasing A restatement of the words of another, often to clarify meaning.

Parenteral Brought into the body through some way other than the digestive tract; most commonly used to refer to the administration of medication by injection.

Participating provider (PAR) A provider who has a contractual agreement with a third-party payor.

Parturition Act of giving birth to an infant.

Passive transport Process that moves substances across or through a membrane and does not require cellular energy.

Pathogen A disease-producing microorganism.

Patient-centered medical home A model of primary care that emphasizes patient-centered health care based on a personal relationship between a patient, provider, and the patient's care team.

Patient incompetence Legal inability to consent to medical treatment decisions.

Patient kiosk An interactive touch screen that allows patients to check themselves in for their appointments.

Patient navigator A person whose role is to remove obstacles that patients face in accessing and receiving treatment.

Patient portal An online application that allows patients to interact with and communicate with their health care providers.

Patient self-scheduling The practice of allowing patients to have access to the computer scheduling program so that they can schedule their own appointments.
Patient statement A bill sent to a patient that contains not only charges but also payments and adjustments that affect the balance the patient must pay.
Payee The person to whom a check is made out.
Peak expiratory flow rate The maximum volume of air that can be exhaled when the patient blows into a peak flow meter as forcefully and as rapidly as possible.
Pectoral girdle Attachment for the upper extremities in the chest region; the clavicle and scapula.
Pediatrician A physician who specializes in the care and development of children and the diagnosis and treatment of children's diseases.
Pediatrics The branch of medicine that deals with the care and development of children and the diagnosis and treatment of children's diseases.
Pelvic girdle Attachment for the lower extremities; bones collectively shaped like a basin; the ilium, ischium, and pubis.
Per diem A term used for employees who do not have a fixed schedule but are scheduled by the day according to office needs.
Percent daily value (% DV) The percentage of a nutrient provided by a single serving of a food item compared with how much is required for the entire day.
Percussion The process of tapping the body to detect signs of disease.
Percussion hammer An instrument with a rubber head, used for testing reflexes.
Pericardial cavity Small space around the heart, between the parietal pericardium and visceral pericardium, that contains a small amount of serous fluid for lubrication.
Pericardium Membrane that surrounds the heart; usually referring to the pericardial sac.
Perimetrium Outermost layer of the uterus.
Perimenopause Before the onset of menopause, the phase during which the woman with regular periods changes to irregular cycles and increased periods of amenorrhea.
Perineum The external region between the vaginal orifice and the anus in a female and between the scrotum and the anus in a male.
Periosteum Tough white outer membrane that covers a bone.
Peristalsis Rhythmic contractions of the intestine that move food along the digestive tract.
Peritoneum Serous membrane associated with the abdominopelvic cavity.
Personal protective equipment (PPE) Specialized clothing or equipment worn by an employee for protection against a hazard.
Petty cash A cash account kept in a business office to pay for incidentals, such as postage due and other small items.
pH The unit that describes the acidity or alkalinity of a solution.
Phagocytosis The process whereby cells "eat"; a form of endocytosis in which solid particles are taken into the cell.
Pharmacology The study of drugs.
Pharynx Passageway for air and food; extends from the base of the skull to the larynx and esophagus; the throat.
Phlebotomist A health care professional trained in the collection of blood specimens.
Phlebotomy Incision of a vein for the removal of blood; the collection of blood.
Photoreceptor A sensory receptor that detects light; located in the retina of the eye.
Physical examination An assessment of each part of the patient's body to obtain objective data about the patient that helps the provider to determine the patient's state of health.
Physical hazard The potential of a chemical to catch fire, explode, or react with other chemicals.
Physiologic Pertaining to body processes.
Pinealocytes Secretory cells of the pineal gland that secrete melatonin.
Pinocytosis Condition of cell "drinking"; a form of endocytosis in which fluid droplets are taken into the cell.
Plaintiff The person or group that makes the complaint in a lawsuit.
Plasma The liquid part of the blood, consisting of a clear yellowish fluid that makes up approximately 55% of the total blood volume.
Pleura Serous membrane that lines the ribs (parietal layer) and surrounds the lungs (visceral layer).
Pleural cavity The small space between the parietal and visceral layers of the pleura.
Plicae circulares Circular folds in the mucosa and submucosa of the small intestine.
Poison Any substance that causes illness, injury, or death if it enters the body.
Polycythemia A disorder in which there is an increase in the number of red blood cells.
Polyp (colorectal) An abnormal noncancerous growth that protrudes from the mucous membrane of the large intestine.
Polysaccharide A complex carbohydrate made up of many sugar units strung together in a long chain.
Polyuria Increased output of urine.
Position In childbirth, the relation of the presenting part of the fetus to the maternal pelvis.
Postage meter A machine that automatically stamps pieces of mail with the correct postage.
Postal bar code A series of vertical bars of two lengths that represent the delivery address of a piece of mail. The bar code facilitates the automated sorting of mail.
Postnatal development Development that begins with birth and lasts until death.
Postoperative After a surgical operation.
Postpartum Occurring after childbirth.
Practicum A supervised work experience that is required in an educational program and is usually unpaid. Formerly called an *externship*.
Preadmission testing (PAT) A series of diagnostic tests done before surgery to establish the patient's health

status and identify any potential problems that could arise during surgery.

Preauthorization Permission from a patient's insurance company for a test, procedure, or surgery.

Precertification After review, verification from a patient's insurance carrier that a test or procedure is medically appropriate and is covered by the patient's insurance and/or agreement.

Prediabetes A condition in which glucose levels are higher than normal, but not high enough to be classified as diabetes.

Preeclampsia A major complication of pregnancy—characterized by increasing hypertension, albuminuria, and edema—the cause of which is unknown. If preeclampsia is neglected or not treated properly, it can develop into eclampsia, which can cause maternal convulsions and coma. Preeclampsia generally occurs between the 20th week of pregnancy and the end of the first week postpartum.

Preembryonic period The first 2 weeks after fertilization; the period of cleavage, implantation, and formation of primary germ layers.

Premium An amount of money paid in a given period to purchase health insurance.

Prenatal Before birth.

Prenatal development Development within the uterus.

Preoperative Before a surgical operation.

Presbycusis The gradual loss of hearing in both ears due to the normal aging process.

Presbyopia A decrease in the elasticity of the lens that occurs with aging, resulting in a decreased ability to focus on close objects.

Preschool child A child 3 to 6 years of age.

Prescription An order from a licensed provider authorizing the dispensing of a drug by a pharmacist.

Presentation Indication of the part of the fetus that is closest to the cervix and is delivered first. A cephalic presentation is a delivery in which the fetal head is presenting against the cervix. A breech presentation is a delivery in which the buttocks or feet are presented instead of the head.

Pressure point A site on the body where an artery lies close to the surface of the skin and can be compressed against an underlying bone to control bleeding.

Primary care provider (PCP) The provider chosen by a patient to provide general medical care and also to determine and authorize additional medical services the patient may require.

Primary insurance The insurance company that must be billed first for a given individual.

Prime mover The muscle that is mainly responsible for a particular body movement; also called an agonist.

Primigravida A woman who is pregnant for the first time.

Primipara A woman who has carried a pregnancy to fetal viability (20 weeks of gestation) for the first time regardless of whether the infant was stillborn or born alive.

Problem Any condition that requires further observation, diagnosis, management, or patient education.

Problem-oriented record (POR) A functional way to organize the patient information in their health record using a database, problem list, plan, and progress notes.

Processing The manipulation and reorganization of data according to the instructions in a program.

Prognosis The probable course and outcome of a patient's condition and the patient's prospects for recovery.

Program A set of instructions organized in a logical step-by-step sequence; a computer program tells the computer how to perform a specific function.

Projection Experiencing one's own emotions as those of another.

Proofread To identify and correct errors in a document.

Proprioception The sense of body position and movement; response to stimuli originating within an organism or muscle.

Proteinuria The presence of protein in the urine.

Prudent Using care or common sense.

Puerperium The period of time, usually 4 to 6 weeks after delivery, in which the uterus and body systems are returning to normal.

Pulmonary circulation The pathway that takes blood from the right side of the heart to the lungs and then returns it to the left side of the heart.

Pulse oximeter A device used to measure the oxygen saturation of arterial blood.

Pulse oximetry The use of a pulse oximeter to measure the oxygen saturation of arterial blood.

Pulse pressure The difference between the systolic and diastolic pressures.

Pulse rhythm The time interval between heartbeats.

Pulse volume The strength of the heartbeat.

Puncture A wound in the skin made by a sharp-pointed object.

Purchase order (PO) number A number assigned by a business to authorize and keep track of a purchase request and order.

Pyloric sphincter Valve between the stomach and first part of the small intestine.

Pyuria The presence of pus in the urine.

Q

Qualitative test A test that indicates whether or not a particular analyte is present in a specimen and may also provide an approximate indication of the amount of the analyte.

Quality assurance Measures to ensure that patients receive safe and appropriate services.

Quality control The application of methods to ensure that test results are reliable and accurate and that errors are detected and eliminated.

Quantitative test A test that indicates the exact amount of an analyte present in a specimen, with the results being reported in measurable units.

Quickening The first movements of the fetus in utero as felt by the mother, which usually occur between 16 and 20 weeks of gestation and are felt consistently thereafter.

R

Radiation The transfer of energy, such as heat, in the form of waves.

Radiograph The permanent image produced by x-rays acting on a radiosensitive receptor device such as a digital detector or radiographic film.

Radiography The taking of permanent images (radiographs) of internal body organs and structures by passing x-rays through the body, which then act on a radiosensitive device.

Radiologist A physician who specializes in the diagnosis and treatment of disease using radiation and other imaging techniques.

Radiology The branch of medicine that uses radiation and other imaging techniques to diagnose and treat disease.

Radiolucent Describing a structure that permits the passage of x-rays.

Radiopaque Describing a structure that obstructs the passage of x-rays.

Reagent A substance that produces a reaction with a specimen to allow the detection or measurement of an analyte.

Reciprocity Automatic issuing of a license in one state to the holder of a license in another state.

Reconciling Making sure that two financial records agree, such as a bank statement and bank balance.

Reference range A certain established and acceptable parameter or range within which the laboratory test results of a healthy individual are expected to fall. (Also known as reference value and reference interval.)

Referral The directing of a patient to a specialist provider by the primary care provider. Most managed care plans and some other insurance plans require the primary care provider to obtain prior authorization.

Reflecting In communication, expressing the meaning and emotion of another's words back to the person.

Refraction The deflection or bending of light rays by a lens.

Refractory period Time during which an excitable cell cannot respond to a stimulus that is usually adequate to initiate an action potential.

Regulated medical waste (RMW) Medical waste that may contain infectious materials posing a threat to health and safety.

Reimbursement The amount paid by insurance for health care services.

Remittance advice (RA) A statement issued by Medicare or another third-party payor to the provider explaining reimbursement for specific procedures or denial of an insurance claim.

Renal corpuscle Portion of the nephron where filtration occurs; consists of the glomerulus and glomerular capsule.

Renal cortex Outer portion of the kidney, which appears granular.

Renal erythropoietic factor A substance produced by the kidneys that activates erythropoietin to stimulate the production of red blood cells.

Renal medulla Inner portion of the kidney, consisting of the renal pyramids.

Renal pelvis Large cavity in the central region of the kidney that collects the urine as it is produced.

Renal threshold The concentration at which a substance in the blood that is not normally excreted by the kidneys begins to appear in the urine.

Renal tubule Tubular portion of the nephron that carries the filtrate away from the glomerular capsule; site where tubular reabsorption and secretion occur.

Renin An enzyme secreted by the kidneys that functions in blood pressure regulation by stimulating the formation of angiotensin.

Reorder point A number on a supply inventory that indicates when a specific item should be reordered to be sure that the supply will not run out before the new order is received.

Res ipsa loquitur A legal doctrine that assumes negligence because of the type of injury.

Reservoir host The location in which an infectious agent lives and usually grows and multiplies.

Residency A program to provide training in a medical specialty to a physician who has finished medical school.

Resident flora Harmless, nonpathogenic microorganisms that normally reside on the skin and usually do not cause disease. Also known as normal flora.

Resistance The natural ability of an organism to remain unaffected by, or to counteract, the effects of pathogens and other harmful agents in its environment.

Resource-based relative value scale (RBRVS) A system to establish the Medicare fee schedule for Medicare Part B based on the service provided and the geographic location of the provider.

Respiration Exchange of oxygen and carbon dioxide between the atmosphere and the body cells.

Respiratory membrane Any surface in the lungs where diffusion occurs; consists of the layers that the gases must pass through to get into or out of the alveoli.

Respondeat superior A legal doctrine making an employer liable for the negligent acts of employees.

Résumé A summary of information about a person that describes their education, work experience, and other information related to that person's suitability for employment.

Retention The inability to empty the bladder. The urine is being produced normally but is not being voided.

Reverse chronological order Arranging documents with the most recent document on top or in the front, which means that the oldest document is on the bottom or at the back of a section or file.

Reverse chronological résumé A résumé that lists the information with the most recent items first in categories such as formal education, and work experience.

Rhodopsin Photosensitive pigment in the rods of the retina; also called visual purple.

Right A claim that is expected to be honored.

Right justified Describing lines of type that are aligned with the right margin of a document.

Right lymphatic duct The collecting duct of the lymphatic system that collects lymph from the upper right quadrant of the body.

Risk factor A physical or behavorial condition that increases the probability that an individual will develop a particular condition.

Risk management The process of assessing risk and putting policies and procedures in place to protect a health care facility from the risk of legal action.

Router A wired or wireless device used to form or connect networks.

Rugae Longitudinal folds in the mucosa of the stomach.

RVU (Relative Value Unit) A number that quantifies the amount of provider labor, resources, and expertise necessary to provide the service represented by a CPT code.

S

Safety data sheet (SDS) A document that provides information regarding a chemical, its hazards, and measures to take to prevent injury and illness when the chemical is being handled.

Salary A fixed amount of money paid on a regular basis that does not depend on the number of hours worked.

Saltatory conduction Process in which a nerve impulse travels along a myelinated nerve fiber by jumping from one node of Ranvier to the next.

Salutation The greeting that begins a letter.

Sanitization A series of steps designed to remove debris and reduce the number of microorganisms to a safe level.

SaO_2 (saturation of arterial oxygen) Abbreviation for the percentage of hemoglobin that is saturated with oxygen in arterial blood.

Sarcolemma The covering of a muscle cell; the muscle cell membrane.

Sarcoplasm Cytoplasm of a muscle cell.

Saturated fat A type of fat that is solid at room temperature and comes primarily from animal sources.

Scalpel A surgical knife used to divide tissues.

School-age child A child 6 to 12 years of age.

Scissors A cutting instrument.

Screening test A test performed routinely on apparently healthy individuals to assist in the early detection of disease.

Sebaceous cyst A thin closed sac or capsule that contains fatty secretions from a sebaceous gland.

Sebaceous gland An oil gland of the skin that produces sebum or body oil.

Sebum Oily secretion from sebaceous glands.

Secondary insurance Insurance held by another insured (such as a spouse) that provides additional insurance coverage.

Segment The portion of the electrocardiogram between two waves.

Seizure A sudden episode of involuntary muscular contractions and relaxation, often accompanied by changes in sensation, behavior, and level of consciousness.

Self-actualization The fulfillment of each individual's potential.

Self-referral The process by which a patient makes an appointment with a specialist provider without requesting prior authorization from their primary care provider, usually because the patient's insurance plan does not require it.

Semiblock style A letter format in which the date line, complimentary close, and printed signature line are on a tab at the center or right justified, all paragraphs are indented five to eight spaces, and the other parts of the letter are left justified.

Semicritical item An item that comes into contact with nonintact skin or intact mucous membranes.

Semilunar valve Valve between a ventricle of the heart and the vessel that carries blood away from the ventricle; also pertains to the valves in veins.

Seminiferous tubules Tightly coiled structures within which sperm are produced in the testes.

Sensory adaptation Phenomenon in which some receptors respond when a stimulus is first applied but decrease their response if the stimulus is maintained; receptor sensitivity decreases with prolonged stimulation.

Sequela (*pl.*, sequelae) Any condition that results from a disease, injury, or treatment for a disease of injury.

Serous membrane Epithelial membrane that lines closed body cavities.

Serum The clear, straw-colored part of the blood (plasma) that remains after the solid elements and the clotting factor fibrinogen have been separated out of it.

Server A large computer that stores data and manages tasks for other computers on a network.

Service contract An agreement that provides for service for a piece of equipment after the warranty expires.

Sharps Objects that can penetrate the skin, such as needles and lancets.

Shock The failure of the cardiovascular system to deliver enough blood to all of the vital organs of the body.

Short arm cast A cast that extends from below the elbow to the fingers.

Short leg cast A cast that begins just below the knee and extends to the toes.

Sigmoidoscope An endoscope that is specially designed for passage through the anus to permit visualization of the rectum and sigmoid colon.

Sigmoidoscopy The visual examination of the rectum and sigmoid colon using a sigmoidoscope.

Signatura The part of a prescription that indicates the information to print on the medication label.

Signature on file (SOF) An indication on the insurance claim form that the signature of the patient is maintained by the medical office to authorize submission of insurance claims.

Simplified letter style A letter format in which all elements are left justified. The greeting is replaced by a subject line in all capital letters. The complimentary close and typed signature are replaced by a typed signature in all capital letters.

Single booking An appointment scheduling method in which each patient is given a different, specific appointment time. Also called stream scheduling or fixed appointment scheduling.

Skills based résumé A résumé that organizes experience according to skills or abilities.

Skip Account for which no billing information is available.

Smartphone A cell phone with computer capabilities.

Soak The direct immersion of a body part in water or a medicated solution.

SOAP Acronym describing a method of organizing progress notes. The SOAP note includes the following: subjective data, objective data, assessment, and plan.

Social media Applications and websites used by individuals and communities to participate in social networking.

Social Security tax (or FICA tax, according to the Federal Insurance Contributions Act) A tax collected from employers and employees to fund the Social Security program, which provides benefits to retired workers.

Software A general term for the programs or instructions that tell a computer what to do.

Solid state drive A drive that uses integrated circuits (flash memory) to store data permanently.

Somatomotor cortex The primary motor area of the brain, located in the precentral gyrus, that transmits motor impulses to the body.

Somatosensory cortex The primary sensory area of the brain; located in the postcentral gyrus; receives sensory impulses from the body.

Sonogram The image obtained with ultrasonography.

Sorter A device that facilitates putting papers or records in alphabetic or numeric order.

Special senses Senses with receptors localized in a particular area: taste, smell, vision, hearing, and equilibrium.

Specific defense mechanism Activities of the body that counteract only certain types of harmful agents.

Specific gravity The weight of a substance compared with the weight of an equal volume of a substance known as the standard. In urinalysis, the term *specific gravity* refers to the measurement of the amount of dissolved substances present in the urine compared with the same amount of distilled water.

Specimen A small sample or part taken from the body to represent the nature of the whole.

Speculum An instrument for opening a body orifice or cavity for viewing.

Spermatogenesis Process of meiosis in the male, in which four spermatids are produced from one primary spermatocyte.

Spermatogonia Stem cells that give rise to sperm cells.

Spermiogenesis Morphologic changes that transform a spermatid into a mature sperm.

Sphygmomanometer An instrument for measuring the pressure of blood within an artery.

Spirilla (*sing.*, spirillum) Bacteria that have a spiral or curved shape.

Spirometer An instrument that measures how much air is exhaled by the lungs and how fast it is exhaled.

Spirometry Measurement of an individual's breathing capacity by means of a spirometer.

Splint An orthopedic device that is rigid and removable used to support and immobilize a part of the body.

SpO_2 (saturation of peripheral oxygen) Abbreviation for the percentage of hemoglobin that is saturated with oxygen in arterial blood as measured by a pulse oximeter.

Spore A hard, thick-walled capsule formed by some bacteria that contains only the essential parts of the protoplasm of the bacterial cell.

Sprain Trauma to a joint that causes tearing of or injury to the ligaments.

Standard of care Level of appropriate care required of a health professional.

Statute of limitations A law limiting the time period for beginning a lawsuit.

Stem cells Cells that have the capacity to develop into various types of body tissue.

Sterile Free of all living microorganisms and bacterial spores.

Sterilization The process of destroying all forms of microbial life, including bacterial spores.

Stethoscope An instrument used for amplifying and hearing sounds produced by the body.

Storage capacity The maximum amount of information that a device can hold, measured in bytes.

Strain A stretching or tearing of muscles or tendons caused by trauma.

Stratum basale Bottom layer of the endometrium that is responsible for rebuilding the stratum functionale after menstruation.

Stratum corium Another name for the dermis, a layer of the skin.

Stratum corneum Outermost layer of the epidermis; consists of flattened, dead, keratinized cells.

Stratum functionale Portion of the endometrium that is sloughed off during menstruation.

Stream scheduling An appointment scheduling method in which each patient is given a different, specific appointment time. Also called fixed appointment scheduling, time-specified scheduling, or single booking.

Stress The body's response to threat or change.

Subcutaneous injection Introduction of medication beneath the skin, into the subcutaneous or fatty layer of the body.

Subcutaneous layer A sheet of areolar connective tissue and adipose tissue beneath the dermis of the skin; also called hypodermis or superficial fascia.

Subjective symptom A symptom that is felt by the patient but is not observable by an examiner.

Sublingual administration Administration of medication by placing it under the tongue, where it dissolves and is absorbed through the mucous membrane.

Subpoena A court order for a witness to appear and give testimony.

Subpoena *duces tecum* A court order to produce documents or records.

Subscription The part of the prescription that gives directions to the pharmacist and usually designates the number of doses to be dispensed.

Sudoriferous gland A gland in the skin that produces perspiration; also called sweat gland.
Summarizing Expressing the most important points of a conversation or written document.
Supernatant The clear liquid that remains at the top after a precipitate settles.
Superscription The part of a prescription consisting of the symbol Rx (from the Latin word *recipe*, meaning "take").
Suppuration The process of pus formation.
Suprapubic aspiration The passing of a sterile needle through the abdominal wall into the bladder to remove urine.
Surfactant A substance produced by certain cells in lung tissue that reduces surface tension between fluid molecules that line the respiratory membrane and helps keep the alveolus from collapsing.
Surgery The branch of medicine that deals with operative and manual procedures for correction of deformities and defects, repair of injuries, and diagnosis and treatment of certain diseases.
Surgical asepsis Practices that keep objects and areas sterile or free from microorganisms.
Surgical package Surgical services usually covered by a single procedure code that includes a preoperative visit, postoperative care, and local anesthesia (if applicable).
Surname Last name or family name of an individual; used as the first indexing unit in alphabetic filing.
Susceptibility Lack of resistance to disease.
Susceptible host One who is capable of being infected by a pathogen.
Sutures Immovable fibrous joints between the flat bones of the skull. Also, material used to approximate tissues with surgical stitches.
Swaged needle A needle with suturing material permanently attached to its end.
Sweat glands Glands in the skin that produce perspiration; also called sudoriferous glands.
Sympathy Feeling the same emotions as another.
Symptom Any change in the body or its functioning that indicates a disease might be present.
Symptomatic treatment Therapy for symptoms of a disease or condition that does not remove the disease itself.
Synapse The region of communication between two neurons.
Synarthrosis (*pl.*, synarthroses) An immovable joint.
Synergist A muscle that assists a prime mover but is not capable of producing the movement by itself, as when two or more muscles work together to produce a movement.
Synovial membrane Membrane that lines the cavities of freely movable joints.
System software A group of programs that control or maintain the operations of a computer.
Systemic circulation Pathways that transport blood from the left side of the heart to all parts of the body and return the blood to the right atrium; excludes pulmonary circulation.
Systole The phase in the cardiac cycle in which the ventricles contract, sending blood out of the heart and into the aorta and pulmonary trunk.
Systolic pressure The point of maximum pressure on the arterial walls, which is recorded during systole.

T

Tab A projection of a folder that extends beyond the top of side of the folder.
Tachycardia An abnormally fast heart rate (more than 100 beats per minute).
Tachypnea An abnormal increase in the respiratory rate of more than 20 respirations per minute.
Target tissue A tissue (cells) that responds to a particular hormone because it has receptor sites for that hormone.
Telehealth Providing healthcare via telecommunication technology.
Template A standard form to which additional information can be added as needed.
Teniae coli Bands of longitudinal muscle fibers in the large intestine.
Terabyte (TB) A unit of computer storage. One terabyte is equivalent to a little more than a trillion bytes or 1000 gigabytes.
Terminal digit filing A chronologic filing system that uses the last number or number group as the first indexing unit.
Terminal phase The last stage of illness, usually used when death is expected to occur within 6 months.
Test system A setup that includes all of the test components required to perform a laboratory test, such as testing devices, controls, and testing reagents.
Thermoreceptor A sensory receptor that detects changes in temperature.
Third-party payor Insurance carrier or managed care organization that pays health insurance claims.
Thoracic duct The primary collecting duct of the lymphatic system that collects lymph from all regions of the body except the upper right quadrant.
Thready pulse A pulse with a decreased volume that feels weak and thin.
Threshold stimulus Minimum level of stimulation that is required to start a nerve impulse or muscle contraction; also called liminal stimulus.
Thrombocyte One of the formed elements of the blood; a thrombocytes function in the blood clotting mechanism of the body; also called a platelet.
Thrombocytopenia An abnormal decrease in the number of thrombocytes (less than 150,000 platelets/cu mm of blood).
Thrombocytosis An abnormal increase in the number of thrombocytes (greater than 150
Tickler file A chronologic file containing reminders of things to be done.
Time management Skills and techniques used to manage time to accomplish tasks and meet goals.
Time-specified scheduling An appointment scheduling method in which each patient is given a different specific appointment time. Also called stream scheduling, fixed appointment scheduling, or single booking.
Tissue Group of similar cells specialized to perform a certain function.

Toddler A child 1 to 3 years old.
Topical administration Application of a drug to a particular spot, usually for a local action.
Tort An injury or wrong against a person or property that does not involve breach of contract.
Touchscreen A visual display unit that the user can touch to input data using the fingers or a stylus.
Toxemia A condition that can occur in pregnant women that includes preeclampsia and eclampsia. If preeclampsia goes undiagnosed or is not satisfactorily controlled, it can develop into eclampsia, characterized by convulsions and coma.
Toxoid A toxin (a poisonous substance produced by a bacterium) that has been treated by heat or chemicals to destroy its harmful properties. It is administered to an individual in a vaccine to prevent an infectious disease by stimulating the production of antibodies.
Trachea Passageway for air that extends inferiorly to the carina where it branches into the bronchi; commonly called the windpipe.
Transient flora Microorganisms that reside on the superficial skin layers and are picked up in the course of daily activities. They are often pathogenic but can be removed easily from the skin by sanitizing the hands.
Triage The process of separating patients by the urgency of their need for care.
TRICARE A government insurance plan that provides medical care to spouses and dependents of individuals on active duty in the military. Some veterans, reservists, and retirees are also eligible. It received its name when there were three available plans.
Triglycerides The chemical form in which most fat exists in food as well as in the body.
Trigone Triangular area in the floor of the urinary bladder formed by the openings for the urethra and the two ureters.
Trimester Three months, or one-third, of the gestational period of pregnancy.
Truth in Lending Statement A written document that meets the legal requirement to disclose the terms of a loan in terms that the borrower can understand.
Tubular reabsorption The movement of filtrate from the renal tubules back into the blood in response to the body's needs during urine formation.
Tubular secretion The movement of substances from the blood into the renal tubules in response to the body's needs during urine formation.
Tympanic membrane A thin, semitransparent membrane between the external ear canal and the middle ear that receives and transmits sound waves. Also known as the eardrum.

U

Ultrasonography The use of high-frequency sound waves to produce an image of an organ or tissue.
Unique identifier Information directly associated with an individual that reliably identifies an individual as the person for whom a service or treatment is intended.
Unsaturated fat A type of fat that is liquid at room temperature and comes primarily from plant sources.
Upcoding Using a code to obtain a higher level of reimbursement than is justified by medical procedures performed as documented in the medical record. This can result in serious fines and penalties.
Upper respiratory tract Portion of the respiratory tract that includes the nose, pharynx, and larynx.
Ureter Tubular structure that carries urine from the renal pelvis to the urinary bladder.
Urethra Passageway that conveys urine from the urinary bladder to the exterior.
Urgency The immediate need to urinate.
Urinalysis The physical, chemical, and microscopic analyses of urine.
Urinary bladder Storage reservoir for urine; located in the pelvic cavity.
Urinary incontinence The inability to retain urine in the bladder.
URL The characters and/or words used to access a specific website or file on the World Wide Web.
USB port A standard computer cable connection interface that allows several types of devices to be connected to a computer in order to transfer data across short distances.
Usual, customary, and reasonable (UCR) A system for establishing the amount an insurance carrier will pay for a procedure. The reasonable charge is set by the insurance carrier on the basis of a provider's usual (most frequent) charge for the procedure and the customary charge of other providers in the same geographic area.
Uterine cycle Monthly cycle of events that occur in the uterus from puberty to menopause; also called the menstrual cycle, which occurs concurrently with the ovarian cycle.
Uterine tubes The tubes that extend laterally from the upper portion of the uterus to the region of the ovaries; also called fallopian tubes or oviducts.
Utilization review An assessment of medical services to determine whether they were appropriate, necessary, and of high quality.

V

Vaccine A suspension of weakened microorganisms, killed microorganisms, or toxoids administered to an individual to prevent an infectious disease by stimulating the production of antibodies in that individual.
Vendor A company from which supplies or equipment is purchased.
Venipuncture Puncturing of a vein.
Venous reflux The backflow of blood (from a blood collection tube) into the patient's vein.
Venous stasis The temporary cessation or slowing of the venous blood flow.
Ventilation Movement of air into and out of the lungs; breathing.
Ventricle A pumping chamber of the heart; the right ventricle pumps blood to the lungs and the left ventricle pumps blood into the systemic circulation.
Veracity Truthfulness.
Verbal Using words to communicate.

Vertex The top of the head.
Vial A closed glass container with a rubber stopper that holds medication.
Visual acuity Acuteness or sharpness of vision. A person with normal visual acuity can see clearly and is able to distinguish fine details close up and at some distance.
Vitamin An organic compound required in small amounts by the body for normal growth and development.
VLDL (Very-low-density lipoprotein) A lipoprotein that picks up triglycerides and delivers them to the cells so that they can be used for energy by the body or stored for later use; known as "bad" cholesterol because a high level contributes to atherosclerosis.
Voicemail A method for delivery, storage, and retrieval of telephone messages that is built into the telephone system.
Void To empty the bladder.
Vulva Collective term for the external accessory structures of the female reproductive system; also called the pudendum.

W

W-4 form The form used to claim withholding allowances for federal income tax reporting.
Warranty A promise by the manufacturer to repair or replace defective parts in an item during a specific time period.
Wave scheduling A method of scheduling appointments in which several patients are given the same appointment time and are seen in the order in which they arrive.
Web browser A software program used to access the World Wide Web.
Webcam A small video camera attached to a computer that allows video to be transmitted on the internet.
Wheal A tense, pale, raised area of the skin.
Wheezing A continuous, high-pitched whistling/musical sound heard particularly during exhalation and sometimes during inhalation.
WiFi A technology for wireless local area networking and connection to the internet.
Workers' compensation An insurance program that covers lost wages and health care costs of workers injured on the job or having work-related illnesses.
World Wide Web A series of interlinked websites or files accessed via the internet.
Wound A break in the continuity of an external or internal surface caused by physical means.

Z

ZIP+4 code A more detailed mailing code consisting of the original five-digit ZIP code followed by a hyphen and four additional digits. These digits identify a specific geographic segment within the delivery area. ZIP stands for Zone Improvement Plan.
Zygote The single diploid cell that is a fertilized ovum.

Index

Note: Page numbers followed by "*f*" refer to illustrations; page numbers followed by "*t*" refer to tables; page numbers followed by "*b*" refer to boxes.

D

E

F

G

H

I

J

K

L

M

N

P

Q

R

U